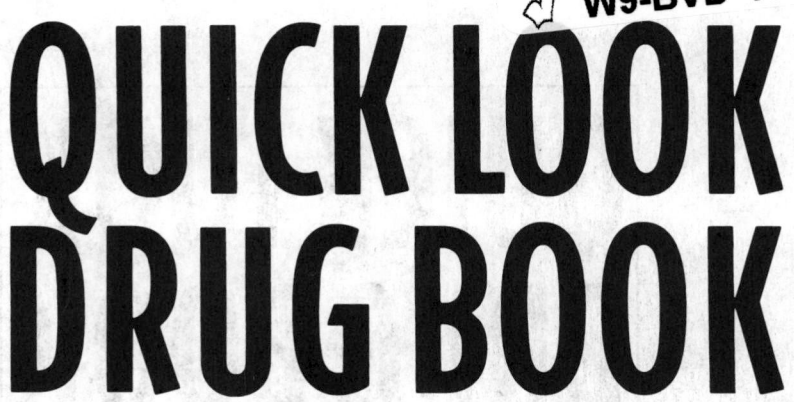

QUICK LOOK DRUG BOOK

2009

Leonard L. Lance, RPh, BSPharm
Senior Editor
Pharmacist
Lexi-Comp, Inc.
Hudson, Ohio

Charles F. Lacy, RPh, MS, PharmD, FCSHP
Editor
Vice President for Executive Affairs
Professor, Pharmacy Practice
Professor, Business Leadership
University of Southern Nevada
Las Vegas, Nevada

Morton P. Goldman, RPh, PharmD, BCPS, FCCP
Associate Editor
Director of Pharmacotherapy Services
Department of Pharmacy
Cleveland Clinic Foundation
Cleveland, Ohio

Lora L. Armstrong, RPh, PharmD, BCPS
Associate Editor
Vice President, Clinical Affairs
Pharmacy & Therapeutics Formulary Process
Clinical Program Oversight
CaremarkRx
Northbrook, Illinois

Wolters Kluwer | Lippincott Williams & Wilkins
Health

Philadelphia • Baltimore • New York • London
Buenos Aires • Hong Kong • Sydney • Tokyo

QUICK LOOK DRUG BOOK

2009

Leonard L. Lance, RPh, BSPharm
Senior Editor
Pharmacist
Lexi-Comp, Inc.
Hudson, Ohio

Charles F. Lacy, RPh, MS, PharmD, FCSHP
Editor
Vice President for Executive Affairs
Professor, Pharmacy Practice
Professor, Business Leadership
University of Southern Nevada
Las Vegas, Nevada

Morton P. Goldman, RPh, PharmD, BCPS, FCCP
Associate Editor
Director of Pharmacotherapy Services
Department of Pharmacy
Cleveland Clinic Foundation
Cleveland, Ohio

Lora L. Armstrong, RPh, PharmD, BCPS
Associate Editor
Vice President, Clinical Affairs
Pharmacy & Therapeutics Formulary Process
Clinical Program Oversight
CaremarkRx
Northbrook, Illinois

NOTICE

This data is intended to serve the user as a handy reference and not as a complete drug information resource. It does not include information on every therapeutic agent available. The publication covers over 1600 commonly used drugs and is specifically designed to present important aspects of drug data in a more concise format than is typically found in medical literature or product material supplied by manufacturers.

The nature of drug information is that it is constantly evolving because of ongoing research and clinical experience and is often subject to interpretation. While great care has been taken to ensure the accuracy of the information and recommendations presented, the reader is advised that the authors, editors, reviewers, contributors, and publishers cannot be responsible for the continued currency of the information or for any errors, omissions, or the application of this information, or for any consequences arising therefrom. Therefore, the author(s) and/or the publisher shall have no liability to any person or entity with regard to claims, loss, or damage caused, or alleged to be caused, directly or indirectly, by the use of information contained herein. Because of the dynamic nature of drug information, readers are advised that decisions regarding drug therapy must be based on the independent judgment of the clinician, changing information about a drug (eg, as reflected in the literature and manufacturer's most current product information), and changing medical practices. Therefore, this data is designed to be used in conjunction with other necessary information and is not designed to be solely relied upon by any user. The user of this data hereby and forever releases the authors and publishers of this data from any and all liability of any kind that might arise out of the use of this data. The editors are not responsible for any inaccuracy of quotation or for any false or misleading implication that may arise due to the text or formulas as used or due to the quotation of revisions no longer official.

Certain of the authors, editors, and contributors have written this book in their private capacities. No official support or endorsement by any federal or state agency or pharmaceutical company is intended or inferred.

The publishers have made every effort to trace any third party copyright holders, if any, for borrowed material. If they have inadvertently overlooked any, they will be pleased to make the necessary arrangements at the first opportunity.

Copyright © 2009 by Lexi-Comp Inc, All rights reserved.

Printed in the United States of America. No part of this publication may be reproduced, stored in a retrieval system, used as a source of information for transcription into a hospital information system or electronic health or medical record, or transmitted in any form or by any means, electronic, mechanical, photocopying, recording or otherwise, without the prior written permission of the publisher. Should you or your institution have a need for this information in a format we protect, we have solutions for you. Please contact our office at the number below.

This manual was produced using Lexi-Comp's Information Management System™ (LIMS) — a complete publishing service of Lexi-Comp Inc.

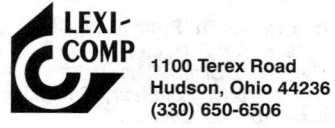

LEXI-COMP

1100 Terex Road
Hudson, Ohio 44236
(330) 650-6506

TABLE OF CONTENTS

Visit the Point http://thepoint.lww.com/QL2009 for exclusive access to:

Apothecary/Metric Conversions

Pounds/Kilograms Conversion

Temperature Conversion

Pharmaceutical Manufacturers and Distributors

Vitamin Products

Refer to the inside front cover of this book for your online access code.

ABOUT THE AUTHORS

Leonard L. Lance, RPh, BSPharm

Leonard L. (Bud) Lance has been directly involved in the pharmaceutical industry since receiving his bachelor's degree in pharmacy from Ohio Northern University in 1970. Upon graduation from ONU, Mr Lance spent four years as a navy pharmacist in various military assignments and was instrumental in the development and operation of the first whole hospital I.V. admixture program in a military (Portsmouth Naval Hospital) facility. His last 15 months in the Navy were spent on the USS Independence CV-62.

After completing his military service, he entered the retail pharmacy field and has managed both an independent and a home I.V. franchise pharmacy operation. Since the late 1970s, Mr Lance has focused much of his interest on using computers to improve pharmacy service. The independent pharmacy he worked for was one of the first retail pharmacies in the State of Ohio to computerize (1977).

His love for computers and pharmacy led him to Lexi-Comp, Inc. in 1988. He was the first pharmacist at Lexi-Comp and helped develop Lexi-Comp's first drug database in 1989 and was involved in the editing and publishing of Lexi-Comp's first *Drug Information Handbook* in 1990.

As a result of his strong publishing interest, he presently serves in the capacity of pharmacy editor and technical advisor as well as pharmacy (information) database coordinator for Lexi-Comp. Mr Lance provides technical support to Lexi-Comp's reference publications. Mr Lance also assists over 300 major hospitals in producing their own formulary (pharmacy) publications through Lexi-Comp's custom publishing service. Mr Lance is also Manager of the Dosage Forms database in the Medical Sciences Division at Lexi-Comp.

Mr Lance is past president (1984) of the Summit Pharmaceutical Association (SPA). He is a member of the Ohio Pharmacists Association (OPA), the American Pharmaceutical Association (APhA), and the American Society of Health-System Pharmacists (ASHP).

Charles F. Lacy, RPh, MS, PharmD, FCSHP

Dr Lacy is the co-founder and the current Vice President of Executive Affairs at the University of Southern Nevada. In this capacity, Dr Lacy fosters, develops, and maintains new opportunities for the university in the areas of business partnerships, foundational development, external programs development and outreach project design and coordination. Dr Lacy is Professor of Pharmacy Practice in the Nevada College of Pharmacy and Guest Professor in the MBA program and the College of Nursing.

Prior to his promotion to Executive Affairs, Dr Lacy was Vice President for Information Technologies at the University and the Facilitative Officer for Clinical Programs where he managed the clinical curriculum, clinical faculty activities, student experiential programs, pharmacy residency programs, and the college continuing education programs.

Additionally, he spent 20 years at Cedars-Sinai Medical Center, where he was the Department of Pharmacy's Clinical Coordinator. With over 20 years of clinical experience at one of the nation's largest teaching hospitals, he developed a reputation as an acknowledged expert in drug information, pharmacotherapy, and critical care drug interventions.

Dr Lacy received his doctorate from the University of Southern California School of Pharmacy. Presently, Dr Lacy holds teaching affiliations with the Nevada College of Pharmacy, the University of Southern Nevada, Showa University in Tokyo Japan, the University of Alberta at Edmonton School of Pharmacy and Health Sciences, and the Hokkaido College of Pharmacy in Sapporo Japan. He also received his master's degree from Phillips Graduate Institute in Psychology with an emphasis in Marriage and Family Therapy.

Dr Lacy is an active member of numerous professional associations including the American Society of Health-System Pharmacists (ASHP), the American College of Clinical Pharmacy (ACCP), the American Association of Colleges of Pharmacy (AACP), the American Society of Consultant Pharmacists (ASCP), the American Association of Colleges of Pharmacy (AACP), American Pharmaceutical Association (APhA), the Federation of International Pharmacy (FIP), the Japanese Pharmaceutical Association (JPA), the Nevada Pharmacy Alliance (NPA), and the California Society of Hospital Pharmacists (CSHP), through which he has chaired many committees and subcommittees. He is also an active member of the California Association of Marriage and Family Therapists (CAMFT), American Association of Marriage and Family Therapists (AAMFT), the North American Congress of Clinical Toxicology (NACCT) and the European Congress of Clinical Toxicology (ECCT).

Morton P. Goldman, RPh, PharmD, BCPS, FCCP

Dr Goldman received his bachelor's degree in pharmacy from the University of Pittsburgh, College of Pharmacy and his Doctor of Pharmacy degree from the University of Cincinnati, Division of Graduate Studies and Research. He completed his concurrent 2-year hospital pharmacy residency at the VA Medical Center in Cincinnati. Dr Goldman is presently the Director of Pharmacotherapy Services for the Department of Pharmacy at the Cleveland Clinic Foundation (CCF) after having spent over 4 years at CCF as an Infectious Disease pharmacist and 10 years as Clinical Manager/Assistant Director. He holds faculty appointments from The University of Toledo and Ohio Northern University, Colleges of Pharmacy and Case Western Reserve University, College of Medicine and is the Pharmacology Curriculum Director Coordinator for the Cleveland Clinic Lerner College of Medicine. Dr Goldman is a Board-Certified Pharmacotherapy Specialist (BCPS) with added qualifications in infectious diseases.

In his capacity as Director of Pharmacotherapy Services at CCF, Dr Goldman remains actively involved in patient care and clinical research with the Department of Infectious Disease, as well as the continuing education of the medical and pharmacy staff. He is an editor of CCF's *Guidelines for Antibiotic Use* and participates in their annual Antimicrobial Review retreat. He is a member of the Pharmacy and Therapeutics Committee and many of its subcommittees. Dr Goldman has authored numerous journal articles and lectures locally and nationally on infectious diseases topics and current drug therapies. He is currently a reviewer for the *Clinical Infectious Diseases* and the *Journal of the American Medical Association,* and coauthor of the *Infectious Diseases Handbook* and the *Drug Information Handbook for the Allied Health Professional* produced by Lexi-Comp, Inc. He also provides technical support to Lexi-Comp's Clinical Reference Library™ publications.

Dr Goldman is an active member of the Ohio College of Clinical Pharmacy, the Society of Infectious Disease Pharmacists, the American College of Clinical Pharmacy (and is a Fellow of the College), and the American Society of Health-Systems Pharmacists.

Lora L. Armstrong, RPh, PharmD, BCPS

Dr Armstrong received her bachelor's degree in pharmacy from Ferris State University and her Doctor of Pharmacy degree from Midwestern University. Dr Armstrong is a Board-Certified Pharmacotherapy Specialist (BCPS).

In her current position, Dr Armstrong serves as Vice President of Clinical Affairs with responsibility for the National Pharmacy & Therapeutics Committee process, Clinical Program Oversight process, and Pharmaceutical Pipeline Services at CVS Caremark. Prior to joining Caremark, Inc, Dr Armstrong served as the Director of Drug Information Services at the University of Chicago Hospitals. She obtained experience in a variety of clinical settings including critical care, hematology, oncology, infectious diseases, and clinical pharmacokinetics. Dr Armstrong played an active role in the education and training of medical, pharmacy, and nursing staff. She coordinated the Drug Information Center, the medical center's Adverse Drug Reaction Monitoring Program, and the continuing Education Program for pharmacists. She also maintained the hospital's strict formulary program and was the editor of the University of Chicago Hospitals' *Formulary of Accepted Drugs* and the drug information center's monthly newsletter *Topics in Drug Therapy.*

Dr Armstrong is an active member of the Academy of Managed Care Pharmacy (AMCP), the American Society of Health-Systems Pharmacists (ASHP), the American Pharmaceutical Association (APhA), the American College of Clinical Pharmacy (ACCP), and the Pharmacy & Therapeutics Society (P & T Society). Dr Armstrong wrote the chapter entitled "Drugs and Hormones Used in Endocrinology" in the 4th edition of the textbook *Endocrinology.* She is an Adjunct Clinical Instructor of Pharmacy Practice at Midwestern University. Dr Armstrong currently serves on the Drug Information Advisory Board for the American Pharmaceutical Association Scientific Review Panel for Evaluations of Drug Interactions (EDI).

EDITORIAL ADVISORY PANEL

Lawrence A. Frazee, PharmD
Pharmacotherapy Specialist in Internal Medicine
Akron General Medical Center
Akron, Ohio

Matthew A. Fuller, PharmD, BCPS, BCPP, FASHP
Clinical Pharmacy Specialist, Psychiatry
Cleveland Department of Veterans Affairs Medical
Center
Brecksville, Ohio
Associate Clinical Professor of Psychiatry
Clinical Instructor of Psychology
Case Western Reserve University
Cleveland, Ohio
Adjunct Associate Professor of Clinical Pharmacy
University of Toledo
Toledo, Ohio

Morton P. Goldman, RPh, PharmD, BCPS, FCCP
Director of Pharmacotherapy Services
The Cleveland Clinic Foundation
Cleveland, Ohio

Julie A. Golembiewski, PharmD
Clinical Associate Professor
Colleges of Pharmacy and Medicine
Clinical Pharmacist, Anesthesia/Pain
University of Illinois
Chicago, Illinois

Jeffrey P. Gonzales, PharmD, BCPS
Critical Care Clinical Pharmacy Specialist
University of Maryland Medical Center
Baltimore, Maryland

Roland Grad, MDCM, MSc, CCFP, FCFP
Department of Family Medicine
McGill University
Montreal, Quebec, Canada

Larry D. Gray, PhD, ABMM
Director of Clinical Microbiology
TriHealth
Bethesda and Good Samaritan Hospitals
Cincinnati, Ohio

Tracy Hagemann, PharmD
Associate Professor
College of Pharmacy
The University of Oklahoma
Oklahoma City, Oklahoma

Martin D. Higbee, PharmD
Associate Professor
Department of Pharmacy Practice and Science
The University of Arizona
Tucson, Arizona

Jane Hurlburt Hodding, PharmD
Director, Pharmacy
Miller Children's Hospital
Long Beach, California

Mark T. Holdsworth, PharmD, BCOP
Associate Professor of Pharmacy & Pediatrics
Pharmacy Practice Area Head
College of Pharmacy
The University of New Mexico
Albuquerque, New Mexico

Collin A. Hovinga, PharmD
Assistant Professor of Pharmacy and Pediatrics
College of Pharmacy
University of Tennessee Health Science Center
Memphis, Tennessee

Darrell T. Hulisz, PharmD
Department of Family Medicine
Case Western Reserve University
Cleveland, Ohio

Michael A. Kahn, DDS
Professor and Chairman
Department of Oral and Maxillofacial Pathology
Tufts University School of Dental Medicine
Boston, Massachusetts

Polly E. Kintzel, PharmD, BCPS, BCOP
Clinical Pharmacy Specialist-Oncology
Spectrum Health
Grand Rapids, Michigan

Daren Knoell, PharmD
Associate Professor of Pharmacy Practice and
Internal Medicine
Davis Heart and Lung Research Institute
The Ohio State University
Columbus, Ohio

Jill M. Kolesar, PharmD, FCCP, BCPS
Associate Professor
School of Pharmacy
Associate Professor
University of Wisconsin Paul P. Carbone
Comprehensive Cancer Center
University of Wisconsin
Madison, Wisconsin

Donna M. Kraus, PharmD, FAPhA
Associate Professor of Pharmacy Practice
Departments of Pharmacy Practice and Pediatrics
Pediatric Clinical Pharmacist
University of Illinois
Chicago, Illinois

Kay Kyllonen, PharmD
Clinical Specialist
The Cleveland Clinic Children's Hospital
Cleveland, Ohio

Charles Lacy, MS, PharmD, FCSHP
Vice President for Executive Affairs
Professor, Pharmacy Practice
Professor, Business Leadership
University of Southern Nevada
Las Vegas, Nevada

Brenda R. Lance, RN, MSN
Program Development Director
Northcoast HealthCare Management Company
Northcoast Infusion Network
Beachwood, Ohio

Leonard L. Lance, RPh, BSPharm
Clinical Pharmacist
Lexi-Comp, Inc
Hudson, Ohio

▶

Dominic A. Solimando, Jr, MA, FAPhA, FASHP, BCOP
Oncology Pharmacist
President, Oncology Pharmacy Services, Inc
Arlington, Virginia

Joni Lombardi Stahura, BS, PharmD, RPh
Pharmacotherapy Specialist
Lexi-Comp, Inc
Hudson, Ohio

Dan Streetman, PharmD, RPh
Pharmacotherapy Specialist
Lexi-Comp, Inc
Hudson, Ohio

Darcie-Ann Streetman, PharmD, RPh
Pharmacotherapy Specialist
Lexi-Comp, Inc
Hudson, Ohio

Carol K. Taketomo, PharmD
Pharmacy Manager
Children's Hospital Los Angeles
Los Angeles, California

Mary Temple, PharmD
Pediatric Clinical Research Specialist
Hillcrest Hospital
Mayfield Heights, Ohio

Elizabeth A. Tomsik, PharmD, BCPS
Manager
Adverse Drug Reactions Group
Lexi-Comp, Inc
Hudson, Ohio

Dana Travis, RPh
Pharmacotherapy Specialist
Lexi-Comp, Inc
Hudson, Ohio

Jennifer Trofe, PharmD
Clinical Transplant Pharmacist
Hospital of The University of Pennsylvania
Philadelphia, Pennsylvania

Beatrice B. Turkoski, RN, PhD
*Associate Professor, Graduate Faculty,
Advanced Pharmacology*
College of Nursing
Kent State University
Kent, Ohio

Amy Van Orman, PharmD
Pharmacotherapy Specialist
Lexi-Comp, Inc
Hudson, Ohio

Christine Weinstein, BS, RPh
Pharmacotherapy Specialist
Lexi-Comp, Inc
Hudson, Ohio

David M. Weinstein, PhD, RPh
Manager
Metabolism, Interactions, and Genomics Group
Lexi-Comp, Inc
Hudson, Ohio

Anne Marie Whelan, PharmD
College of Pharmacy
Dalhouise University
Halifax, Nova Scotia

Nathan Wirick, PharmD
*Infectious Disease and Antibiotic Management
Clinical Specialist*
Hillcrest Hospital
Cleveland, Ohio

Richard L. Wynn, BSPharm, PhD
Professor of Pharmacology
Baltimore College of Dental Surgery
Dental School
University of Maryland Baltimore
Baltimore, Maryland

PREFACE

Working with clinical pharmacists, hospital pharmacy and therapeutics committees, and hospital drug information centers, the editors of this handbook have directly assisted in the development and production of hospital-specific formulary documentation for several hundred major U.S. and International medical institutions. The resultant documentation provides relevant detail concerning use of medications within the hospital and other clinical settings. Current information on medications has been extracted from pertinent sources, reviewed, coalesced, and cross-referenced by the editors to create this *Quick Look Drug Book*.

Designed to meet the unique needs of medical transcription, this handbook gives the user quick access to data on 1680 medications with cross-referencing to 6228 U.S. and Canadian brand or trade names. Selection of the included medications was based on the analysis of those medications offered in a wide range of hospital formularies. The concise standardized format for data used in this handbook was developed to ensure a consistent presentation of information for all medications.

All generic drug names and synonyms appear in lower case, whereas brand or trade names appear in upper/lower case with the proper trademark information. These three items appear as individual entries in the alphabetical listing of drugs and, thus, there is no requirement for an alphabetical index of drugs names.

In this edition of the *Quick Look Drug Book*, the chemotherapy regimens and index will appear in a new section directly following the alphabetical listing of drugs. The mailing and web site addresses for pharmaceutical manufacturers and drug distributors can be accessed online using the code located on the inside front cover of this book.

The Indication/Therapeutic Category Index is an expedient mechanism for locating the medication of choice along with its classification. This index will help the user, with knowledge of the disease state, to identify medications which are most commonly used in treatment. All disease states are cross-referenced to a varying number of medications with the most frequently used medication(s) noted.

— L.L. Lance

USE OF THE HANDBOOK

The *Quick Look Drug Book* is organized into a drug information section, an appendix, and an indication/therapeutic category index.

The drug information section of the handbook, wherein all drugs are listed alphabetically, details information pertinent to each drug. Extensive cross-referencing is provided by brand name and synonyms.

Drug information is presented in a consistent format and for quick reference will provide the following:

Generic Name	U.S. Adopted Name (USAN) or International Nonproprietary Name (INN)
	If a drug product is only available in Canada, a *(Canada only)* will be attached to that product and will appear with every occurrence of that drug throughout the book
Pronunciation Guide	Subjective aid for pronouncing drug names
Sound-Alike/Look-Alike Issues	Lists drugs with similar sounding names or names that look alike
Synonyms	Official names and some slang
Tall-Man	"Tall-Man" lettering revisions recommended by the FDA
U.S./Canadian Brand Names	Common trade names used in the United States and Canada
Therapeutic Category	Lexi-Comp's own system of logical medication classification
Controlled Substance	Drug Enforcement Agency (DEA) classification for federally scheduled controlled substances
Use	Information pertaining to appropriate use of the drug
Usual Dosage	The amount of the drug to be typically given or taken during therapy
Dosage Forms	Information with regard to form, strength, and availability of the drug

Appendix

The appendix offers a compilation of tables, guidelines, and conversion information that can often be helpful when considering patient care.

Indication/Therapeutic Category Index

This index provides a listing of accepted drugs for various disease states thus focusing attention on selection of medications most frequently prescribed in relation to a clinical diagnosis. Diseases may have other nonofficial drugs for their treatment and this indication/therapeutic category index should not be used by itself to determine the appropriateness of a particular therapy. The listed indications may encompass varying degrees of severity and, since certain medications may not be appropriate for a given degree of severity, it should not be assumed that the agents listed for specific indications are interchangeable. Also included as a valuable reference is each medication's therapeutic category.

FDA NAME DIFFERENTIATION PROJECT: THE USE OF TALL-MAN LETTERS

Confusion between similar drug names is an important cause of medication errors. For years, The Institute For Safe Medication Practices (ISMP), has urged generic manufacturers to use a combination of large and small letters as well as bolding (ie, chlorpro**MAZINE** and chlorpro**PAMIDE**) to help distinguish drugs with look-alike names, especially when they share similar strengths. Recently the FDA's Division of Generic Drugs began to issue recommendation letters to manufacturers suggesting this novel way to label their products to help reduce this drug name confusion. Although this project has had marginal success, the method has successfully eliminated problems with products such as diphenhydr**AMINE** and dimenhy-**DRINATE**. Hospitals should also follow suit by making similar changes in their own labels, preprinted order forms, computer screens and printouts, and drug storage location labels.

In the *Quick Look Drug Book*, the "Tall-Man" lettering revisions for the drugs suggested by the FDA or recommended by ISMP will be listed in a field called **Tall-Man**.

The following is a list of generic product names and recommended revisions.

Drug Product	Recommended Revision
acetazolamide	aceta**ZOLAMIDE**
acetohexamide	aceto**HEXAMIDE**
alprazolam	**ALPRAZ**olam
amiloride	a**MIL**oride
amlodipine	am**LODIP**ine
azacitidine	aza**CITID**ine
azathioprine	aza**THIO**prine
bupropion	bu**PROP**ion
buspirone	bus**PIR**one
carbamazepine	car**BAM**azepine
carboplatin	**CARBO**platin
cefazolin	ce**FAZ**olin
ceftriaxone	cef**TRIAX**one
chlordiazepoxide	chlordiaze**POXIDE**
chlorpromazine	chlorpro**MAZINE**
chlorpropamide	chlorpro**PAMIDE**
cisplatin	**CIS**platin
clomiphene	clomi**PHENE**
clomipramine	clomi**PRAMINE**
clonazepam	clonaze**PAM**
clonidine	clo**NID**ine
cycloserine	cyclo**SERINE**
cyclosporine	cyclo**SPORINE**
dactinomycin	**DACTIN**omycin
daptomycin	**DAPTO**mycin
daunorubicin	**DAUNO**rubicin
dimenhydrinate	dimenhy**DRINATE**
diphenhydramine	diphenhydr**AMINE**
dobutamine	**DOBUT**amine
dopamine	**DOP**amine
doxorubicin	**DOXO**rubicin

Drug Product	Recommended Revision
duloxetine	**DUL**oxetine
ephedrine	e**PHED**rine
epinephrine	**EPINEPH**rine
fentanyl	fenta**NYL**
fluoxetine	**FLU**oxetine
glipizide	glipi**ZIDE**
glyburide	gly**BURIDE**
guaifenesin	guai**FEN**esin
guanfacine	guan**FACINE**
hydralazine	hydr**ALAZINE**
hydrocodone	**HYDRO**codone
hydromorphone	**HYDRO**morphone
hydroxyzine	hydr**OXY**zine
idarubicin	**IDA**rubicin
infliximab	in**FLIX**imab
lamivudine	lami**VUD**ine
lamotrigine	lamo**TRI**gine
lorazepam	**LOR**azepam
medroxyprogesterone	medroxy**PROGESTER**one
metformin	met**FORMIN**
methylprednisolone	methyl**PREDNIS**olone
methyltestosterone	methyl**TESTOSTER**one
metronidazole	metro**NIDAZOLE**
nicardipine	ni**CAR**dipine
nifedipine	**NIFE**dipine
nimodipine	ni**MOD**ipine
olanzapine	**OLANZ**apine
oxcarbazepine	**OX**carbazepine
oxycodone	oxy**CODONE**
paroxetine	**PAR**oxetine
pentobarbital	**PENT**obarbital
phenobarbital	**PHEN**obarbital
prednisolone	predniso**LONE**
prednisone	predni**SONE**
quetiapine	**QUE**tiapine
quinidine	qui**NID**ine
quinine	qui**NINE**
rituximab	ri**TUX**imab
sitagliptin	sita**GLIP**tin
sufentanil	**SUF**entanil
sulfadiazine	sulf**ADIAZINE**
sulfisoxazole	sulfi**SOXAZOLE**
sumatriptan	**SUMA**triptan
tiagabine	tia**GAB**ine
tizanidine	ti**ZAN**idine

Drug Product	Recommended Revision
tolazamide	**TOLAZ**amide
tolbutamide	**TOLBUT**amide
tramadol	tra**MAD**ol
trazodone	tra**ZOD**one
vinblastine	vin**BLAS**tine
vincristine	vin**CRIS**tine

Institute for Safe Medication Practices. "New Tall-Man Lettering Will Reduce Mix-Ups Due to Generic Drug Name Confusion," *ISMP Medication Safety Alert*, September 19, 2001. Available at: http://www.ismp.org.

Institute for Safe Medication Practices. "Prescription Mapping, Can Improve Efficiency While Minimizing Errors With Look-Alike Products," *ISMP Medication Safety Alert*, October 6, 1999. Available at: http://www.ismp.org.

Institute for Safe Medication Practices. "Use of Tall Man Letters Is Gaining Wide Acceptance," *ISMP Medication Safety Alert*, July 31, 2008. Available at: http://www.ismp.org.

U.S. Pharmacopeia, "USP Quality Review: Use Caution-Avoid Confusion," March 2001, No. 76. Available at: http://www.usp.org.

SAFE WRITING

Health professionals and their support personnel frequently produce handwritten copies of information they see in print; therefore, such information is subjected to even greater possibilities for error or misinterpretation on the part of others. Thus, particular care must be given to how drug names and strengths are expressed when creating written health care documents.

The following are a few examples of safe writing rules suggested by the Institute for Safe Medication Practices, Inc.*

1. There should be a space between a number and its units as it is easier to read. There should be no periods after the abbreviations mg or mL.

Correct	Incorrect
10 mg	10mg
100 mg	100mg

2. Never place a decimal and a zero after a whole number (2 mg is correct and 2.0 mg is **incorrect**). If the decimal point is not seen because it falls on a line or because individuals are working from copies where the decimal point is not seen, this causes a tenfold overdose.
3. Just the opposite is true for numbers less than one. Always place a zero before a naked decimal (0.5 mL is correct, .5 mL is **incorrect**).
4. Never abbreviate the word "unit." The handwritten U or u, looks like a 0 (zero), and may cause a tenfold overdose error to be made.
5. IU is not a safe abbreviation for international units. The handwritten IU looks like IV. Write out international units or use int. units.
6. Q.D. is not a safe abbreviation for once daily, as when the Q is followed by a sloppy dot, it looks like QID which means four times daily.
7. O.D. is not a safe abbreviation for once daily, as it is properly interpreted as meaning "right eye" and has caused liquid medications such as saturated solution of potassium iodide and Lugol's solution to be administered incorrectly. There is no safe abbreviation for once daily. It must be written out in full.
8. Do not use chemical names such as 6-mercaptopurine or 6-thioguanine, as 6-fold overdoses have been given when these were not recognized as chemical names. The proper names of these drugs are mercaptopurine or thioguanine.
9. Do not abbreviate drug names (5FC, 6MP, 5-ASA, MTX, HCTZ, CPZ, PBZ, etc) as they are misinterpreted and cause error.
10. Do not use the apothecary system or symbols.
11. Do not abbreviate microgram as µg; instead use mcg as there is less likelihood of misinterpretation.
12. When writing an outpatient prescription, write a complete prescription. A complete prescription can prevent the prescriber, the pharmacist, and/or the patient from making a mistake and can eliminate the need for further clarification. The legible prescriptions should contain:

    a. patient's full name
    b. for pediatric or geriatric patients: their age (or weight where applicable)
    c. drug name, dosage form and strength; if a drug is new or rarely prescribed, print this information
    d. number or amount to be dispensed
    e. complete instructions for the patient, including the purpose of the medication
    f. when there are recognized contraindications for a prescribed drug, indicate to the pharmacist that you are aware of this fact (ie, when prescribing a potassium salt for a patient receiving an ACE inhibitor, write "K serum leveling being monitored")

*From "Safe Writing" by Davis NM, PharmD and Cohen MR, MS, Lecturers and Consultants for Safe Medication Practices, 1143 Wright Drive, Huntington Valley, PA 19006. Phone: (215) 947-7566.

ALPHABETICAL LISTING OF DRUGS

A₁-PI *see* alpha₁-proteinase inhibitor *on page 48*
A200® Lice [US-OTC] *see* permethrin *on page 740*
A-200® Lice Treatment Kit [US-OTC] *see* pyrethrins and piperonyl butoxide *on page 806*
A-200® Maximum Strength [US-OTC] *see* pyrethrins and piperonyl butoxide *on page 806*
A and D® Original [US-OTC] *see* vitamin A and vitamin D *on page 980*

abacavir (a BAK a veer)

Synonyms abacavir sulfate; ABC
U.S./Canadian Brand Names Ziagen® [US/Can]
Therapeutic Category Antiretroviral Agent, Nucleoside Reverse Transcriptase Inhibitor (NRTI)
Use Treatment of HIV infections in combination with other antiretroviral agents
Usual Dosage Oral:
  Children: 3 months to 16 years: 8 mg/kg body weight twice daily (maximum: 300 mg twice daily) in combination with other antiretroviral agents
  Adults: 300 mg twice daily or 600 mg once daily in combination with other antiretroviral agents
Dosage Forms
  Solution, oral:
    Ziagen®: 20 mg/mL
  Tablet:
    Ziagen®: 300 mg

abacavir and lamivudine (a BAK a veer & la MI vyoo deen)

Synonyms abacavir sulfate and lamivudine; lamivudine and abacavir
U.S./Canadian Brand Names Epzicom® [US]; Kivexa™ [Can]
Therapeutic Category Antiretroviral Agent, Nucleoside Reverse Transcriptase Inhibitor (NRTI)
Use Treatment of HIV infections in combination with other antiretroviral agents
Usual Dosage Oral: Adults: HIV: One tablet (abacavir 600 mg and lamivudine 300 mg) once daily
Dosage Forms
  Tablet:
    Epzicom®: Abacavir 600 mg and lamivudine 300 mg

abacavir, lamivudine, and zidovudine

(a BAK a veer, la MI vyoo deen, & zye DOE vyoo deen)
Synonyms 3TC, abacavir, and zidovudine; azidothymidine, abacavir, and lamivudine; AZT, abacavir, and lamivudine; compound S, abacavir, and lamivudine; lamivudine, abacavir, and zidovudine; ZDV, abacavir, and lamivudine; zidovudine, abacavir, and lamivudine
U.S./Canadian Brand Names Trizivir® [US]
Therapeutic Category Antiretroviral Agent, Nucleoside Reverse Transcriptase Inhibitor (NRTI)
Use Treatment of HIV infection (either alone or in combination with other antiretroviral agents) in patients whose regimen would otherwise contain the components of Trizivir®
Usual Dosage Oral: Adolescents ≥40 kg and Adults: 1 tablet twice daily
Dosage Forms
  Tablet:
    Trizivir®: Abacavir 300 mg, lamivudine 150 mg, and zidovudine 300 mg

abacavir sulfate *see* abacavir *on page 16*
abacavir sulfate and lamivudine *see* abacavir and lamivudine *on page 16*
abarelix *(Discontinued)*

abatacept (ab a TA sept)

Sound-Alike/Look-Alike Issues
  Orencia® may be confused with Oracea™
Synonyms CTLA-4Ig
U.S./Canadian Brand Names Orencia® [US/Can]
Therapeutic Category Antirheumatic, Disease Modifying
Use

Treatment of moderately- to severely-active adult rheumatoid arthritis (RA); may be used as monotherapy or in combination with other DMARDs

Treatment of moderately- to severely-active juvenile idiopathic arthritis (JIA); may be used as monotherapy or in combination with methotrexate

Note: Abatacept should **not** be used in combination with anakinra or TNF-blocking agents

Usual Dosage I.V.:

Children 6-17 years: JIA:

<75 kg: 10 mg/kg, repeat dose at 2 and 4 weeks after initial infusion, and every 4 weeks thereafter

≥75 kg: Refer to adult dosing; maximum dose: 1000 mg

Adults: RA: Dosing is according to body weight: Repeat dose at 2 weeks and 4 weeks after initial dose, and every 4 weeks thereafter:

<60 kg: 500 mg

60-100 kg: 750 mg

>100 kg: 1000 mg

Dosage Forms

Injection, powder for reconstitution [preservative free]:

Orencia®: 250 mg

Abbokinase® *(Discontinued)* *see* urokinase *on page 965*

abbott-43818 *see* leuprolide *on page 553*

ABC *see* abacavir *on page 16*

ABCD *see* amphotericin B cholesteryl sulfate complex *on page 69*

abciximab (ab SIK si mab)

Synonyms 7E3; C7E3

U.S./Canadian Brand Names ReoPro® [US/Can]

Therapeutic Category Platelet Aggregation Inhibitor

Use Prevention of acute cardiac ischemic complications in patients at high risk for abrupt closure of the treated coronary vessel and patients at risk of restenosis; an adjunct with heparin to prevent cardiac ischemic complications in patients with unstable angina not responding to conventional therapy when a percutaneous coronary intervention (PCI) is scheduled within 24 hours

Usual Dosage

Acute coronary syndromes: PCI: I.V.: 0.25 mg/kg bolus administered 10-60 minutes before the start of intervention followed by an infusion of 0.125 mcg/kg/minute (maximum: 10 mcg/minute) for 12 hours

Patients with unstable angina not responding to conventional medical therapy and who are planning to undergo percutaneous coronary intervention within 24 hours may be treated with abciximab 0.25 mg/kg intravenous bolus followed by an 18- to 24-hour intravenous infusion of 10 mcg/minute, concluding 1 hour after the percutaneous coronary intervention.

Dosage Forms

Injection, solution:

ReoPro®: 2 mg/mL (5 mL)

Abelcet® [US/Can] *see* amphotericin B lipid complex *on page 71*

Abenol® [Can] *see* acetaminophen *on page 19*

ABI-007 *see* paclitaxel (protein bound) *on page 715*

Abilify® [US] *see* aripiprazole *on page 93*

Abilify® Discmelt™ [US] *see* aripiprazole *on page 93*

ABLC *see* amphotericin B lipid complex *on page 71*

A/B Otic [US] *see* antipyrine and benzocaine *on page 82*

Abraxane® [US] *see* paclitaxel (protein bound) *on page 715*

Abreva® [US-OTC] *see* docosanol *on page 314*

absorbable cotton *see* cellulose, oxidized regenerated *on page 193*

absorbable gelatin sponge *see* gelatin (absorbable) *on page 437*

Absorbine® Antifungal *(Discontinued)* *see* tolnaftate *on page 934*

Absorbine® Jock Itch *(Discontinued)* *see* tolnaftate *on page 934*

ABX-EGF *see* panitumumab *on page 719*

AC 2993 *see* exenatide *on page 386*

ACAM2000™ [US] *see* smallpox vaccine *on page 871*

acamprosate (a kam PROE sate)
Synonyms acamprosate calcium; calcium acetylhomotaurinate
U.S./Canadian Brand Names Campral® [US/Can]
Therapeutic Category GABA Agonist/Glutamate Antagonist
Use Maintenance of alcohol abstinence
Usual Dosage Oral: Adults: Alcohol abstinence: 666 mg 3 times/day (a lower dose may be effective in some patients)
Dosage Forms
 Tablet, enteric coated, delayed release:
  Campral®: 333 mg

acamprosate calcium *see acamprosate* *on page 18*

acarbose (AY car bose)
Sound-Alike/Look-Alike Issues
 Precose® may be confused with PreCare®
U.S./Canadian Brand Names Prandase® [Can]; Precose® [US]
Therapeutic Category Antidiabetic Agent, Oral
Use
 Monotherapy, as indicated as an adjunct to diet to lower blood glucose in patients with type 2 diabetes mellitus (noninsulin-dependent, NIDDM) whose hyperglycemia cannot be managed on diet alone
 Combination with a sulfonylurea, metformin, or insulin in patients with type 2 diabetes mellitus (noninsulin-dependent, NIDDM) when diet plus acarbose do not result in adequate glycemic control. The effect of acarbose to enhance glycemic control is additive to that of other hypoglycemic agents when used in combination.
Usual Dosage Oral:
 Adults: Dosage must be individualized on the basis of effectiveness and tolerance while not exceeding the maximum recommended dose
  Initial dose: 25 mg 3 times/day with the first bite of each main meal
  Maintenance dose: Should be adjusted at 4- to 8-week intervals based on 1-hour postprandial glucose levels and tolerance. Dosage may be increased from 25 mg 3 times/day to 50 mg 3 times/day. Some patients may benefit from increasing the dose to 100 mg 3 times/day.
  Maintenance dose ranges: 50-100 mg 3 times/day.
  Maximum dose:
   ≤60 kg: 50 mg 3 times/day
   >60 kg: 100 mg 3 times/day
 Patients receiving sulfonylureas: Acarbose given in combination with a sulfonylurea will cause a further lowering of blood glucose and may increase the hypoglycemic potential of the sulfonylurea. If hypoglycemia occurs, appropriate adjustments in the dosage of these agents should be made.
Dosage Forms
 Tablet: 25 mg, 50 mg, 100 mg
  Precose®: 25 mg, 50 mg, 100 mg

A-Caro-25 [US] *see beta-carotene* *on page 130*
Accolate® [US/Can] *see zafirlukast* *on page 989*
AccuHist® [US] *see brompheniramine and pseudoephedrine* *on page 144*
AccuHist® PDX Drops [US] *see brompheniramine, pseudoephedrine, and dextromethorphan* *on page 146*
AccuHist® Pediatric (Discontinued) *see brompheniramine and pseudoephedrine* *on page 144*
AccuNeb® [US] *see albuterol* *on page 39*
Accupril® [US/Can] *see quinapril* *on page 812*
Accuretic® [US/Can] *see quinapril and hydrochlorothiazide* *on page 813*
Accutane® [US/Can] *see isotretinoin* *on page 531*
Accuzyme® [US] *see papain and urea* *on page 721*
Accuzyme® SE [US] *see papain and urea* *on page 721*
ACE *see captopril* *on page 171*

acebutolol (a se BYOO toe lole)

Sound-Alike/Look-Alike Issues
Sectral® may be confused with Factrel®, Seconal®, Septra®

Synonyms acebutolol hydrochloride

U.S./Canadian Brand Names Apo-Acebutolol® [Can]; Gen-Acebutolol [Can]; Monitan® [Can]; Novo-Acebutolol [Can]; Nu-Acebutolol [Can]; Rhotral [Can]; Rhoxal-acebutolol [Can]; Sandoz-Acebutolol [Can]; Sectral® [US/Can]

Therapeutic Category Antiarrhythmic Agent, Class II; Beta-Adrenergic Blocker

Use Treatment of hypertension; management of ventricular arrhythmias

Usual Dosage Oral: Adults:
Hypertension: 400-800 mg/day (larger doses may be divided); maximum: 1200 mg/day; usual dose range (JNC 7): 200-800 mg/day in 2 divided doses
Ventricular arrhythmias: Initial: 400 mg/day in divided doses; maintenance: 600-1200 mg/day in divided doses

Dosage Forms
Capsule, as hydrochloride: 200 mg, 400 mg
Sectral®: 200 mg, 400 mg

acebutolol hydrochloride *see* acebutolol *on page 19*
Aceon® [US] *see* perindopril erbumine *on page 739*
Acephen® [US-OTC] *see* acetaminophen *on page 19*
Acerola [US-OTC] *see* ascorbic acid *on page 96*
Acetadote® [US] *see* acetylcysteine *on page 30*
Aceta-Gesic [US-OTC] *see* acetaminophen and phenyltoloxamine *on page 22*

acetaminophen (a seet a MIN oh fen)

Sound-Alike/Look-Alike Issues
Acephen® may be confused with AcipHex®
FeverAll® may be confused with Fiberall®
Tylenol® may be confused with atenolol, timolol, Tuinal®, Tylox®

Synonyms APAP; n-acetyl-p-aminophenol; paracetamol

U.S./Canadian Brand Names Abenol® [Can]; Acephen® [US-OTC]; Apo-Acetaminophen® [Can]; Apra Children's [US-OTC]; Aspirin Free Anacin® Maximum Strength [US-OTC]; Atasol® [Can]; Cetafen Extra® [US-OTC]; Cetafen® [US-OTC]; Comtrex® Sore Throat Maximum Strength [US-OTC]; FeverAll® [US-OTC]; Genapap™ Children [US-OTC]; Genapap™ Extra Strength [US-OTC]; Genapap™ Infant [US-OTC]; Genapap™ [US-OTC]; Genebs Extra Strength [US-OTC]; Genebs [US-OTC]; Infantaire [US-OTC]; Little Fevers™ [US-OTC]; Mapap Children's [US-OTC]; Mapap Extra Strength [US-OTC]; Mapap Infants [US-OTC]; Mapap [US-OTC]; Nortemp Children's [US-OTC]; Novo-Gesic [Can]; Pain Eze [US-OTC]; Pediatrix [Can]; Silapap® Children's [US-OTC]; Silapap® Infants [US-OTC]; Tempra® [Can]; Tycolene Maximum Strength [US-OTC]; Tycolene [US-OTC]; Tylenol® 8 Hour [US-OTC]; Tylenol® Arthritis Pain [US-OTC]; Tylenol® Children's with Flavor Creator [US-OTC]; Tylenol® Children's [US-OTC]; Tylenol® Extra Strength [US-OTC]; Tylenol® Infants [US-OTC]; Tylenol® Junior [US-OTC]; Tylenol® [US-OTC/Can]; Valorin Extra [US-OTC]; Valorin [US-OTC]

Therapeutic Category Analgesic, Nonnarcotic Antipyretic

Use Treatment of mild-to-moderate pain and fever (antipyretic/analgesic); does not have antirheumatic or antiinflammatory effects

Usual Dosage Oral, rectal:
Children <12 years: 10-15 mg/kg/dose every 4-6 hours as needed; do **not** exceed 5 doses (2.6 g) in 24 hours; alternatively, the following age-based doses may be used:
0-3 months: 40 mg
4-11 months: 80 mg
1-2 years: 120 mg
2-3 years: 160 mg
4-5 years: 240 mg
6-8 years: 320 mg
9-10 years: 400 mg
11 years: 480 mg

Note: Higher rectal doses have been studied for use in preoperative pain control in children. However, specific guidelines are not available and dosing may be product dependent. The safety and efficacy of alternating acetaminophen and ibuprofen dosing has not been established.

Adults: 325-650 mg every 4-6 hours or 1000 mg 3-4 times/day; do **not** exceed 4 g/day

Dosage Forms

Caplet: 500 mg
  Cetafen Extra® Strength [OTC], Genapap™ Extra Strength [OTC], Genebs Extra Strength [OTC], Mapap Extra Strength [OTC], Tycolene Maximum Strength [OTC], Tylenol® Extra Strength [OTC]: 500 mg

Caplet, extended release:
  Tylenol® 8 Hour [OTC], Tylenol® Arthritis Pain [OTC]: 650 mg

Capsule: 500 mg

Elixir: 160 mg/5 mL
  Apra Children's [OTC]: 160 mg/5 mL
  Mapap Children's [OTC]: 160 mg/5 mL

Gelcap: 500 mg
  Mapap Extra Strength [OTC], Tylenol® Extra Strength [OTC]: 500 mg

Geltab: 500 mg
  Tylenol® Extra Strength [OTC]: 500 mg

Liquid, oral: 500 mg/15 mL
  Comtrex® Sore Throat Maximum Strength [OTC], Tylenol® Extra Strength [OTC]: 500 mg/15 mL
  Genapap™ Children [OTC], Silapap® [OTC]: 160 mg/5 mL

Solution, oral: 160 mg/5 mL

Solution, oral [drops]: 80 mg/0.8 mL
  Genapap™ Infant [OTC], Infantaire [OTC], Silapap® Infant's [OTC]: 80 mg/0.8 mL
  Little Fevers™ [OTC]: 80 mg/1 mL

Suppository, rectal: 120 mg, 325 mg, 650 mg
  Acephen® [OTC]: 120 mg, 325 mg, 650 mg
  FeverALL® [OTC]: 80 mg, 120 mg, 325 mg, 650 mg
  Mapap [OTC]: 125 mg, 650 mg

Suspension, oral: 160 mg/5 mL
  Mapap Children's [OTC], Nortemp Children's [OTC], Tylenol® Children's [OTC], Tylenol® Children's with Flavor Creator [OTC]: 160 mg/5 mL

Suspension, oral [drops]: 80 mg/0.8 mL
  Mapap Infants [OTC], Tylenol® Infants [OTC]: 80 mg/0.8 mL

Tablet: 325 mg, 500 mg
  Aspirin Free Anacin® Extra Strength [OTC], Genapap™ Extra Strength [OTC], Genebs Extra Strength [OTC], Mapap Extra Strength [OTC], Redutemp® [OTC], Tylenol® Extra Strength [OTC], Valorin Extra [OTC]: 500 mg
  Cetafen® [OTC], Genapap™ [OTC], Genebs [OTC], Mapap [OTC], Tylenol® [OTC], Valorin [OTC]: 325 mg

Tablet, chewable: 80 mg
  Mapap Children's [OTC]: 80 mg
  Mapap Junior Strength [OTC]: 160 mg

Tablet, orally disintegrating: 80 mg, 160 mg
  Tylenol® Children's Meltaways [OTC]: 80 mg
  Tylenol® Junior Meltaways [OTC]: 160 mg

acetaminophen and butalbital *see* butalbital and acetaminophen *on page 155*

acetaminophen and chlorpheniramine *see* chlorpheniramine and acetaminophen *on page 206*

acetaminophen and codeine (a seet a MIN oh fen & KOE deen)

Sound-Alike/Look-Alike Issues
  Capital® may be confused with Capitrol®
  Tylenol® may be confused with atenolol, timolol, Tuinal®, Tylox®

Synonyms codeine and acetaminophen

U.S./Canadian Brand Names Capital® and Codeine [US]; ratio-Emtec [Can]; ratio-Lenoltec [Can]; Triatec-30 [Can]; Triatec-8 Strong [Can]; Triatec-8 [Can]; Tylenol® Elixir with Codeine [Can]; Tylenol® No. 1 Forte [Can]; Tylenol® No. 1 [Can]; Tylenol® No. 2 with Codeine [Can]; Tylenol® No. 3 with Codeine [Can]; Tylenol® No. 4 with Codeine [Can]; Tylenol® With Codeine [US]

Therapeutic Category Analgesic, Narcotic

Controlled Substance C-III; C-V

Use Relief of mild-to-moderate pain

Usual Dosage Doses should be adjusted according to severity of pain and response of the patient. Adult doses ≥60 mg codeine fail to give commensurate relief of pain but merely prolong analgesia and are associated with an appreciably increased incidence of side effects. Oral:

Children: Analgesic:
Codeine: 0.5-1 mg codeine/kg/dose every 4-6 hours
Acetaminophen: 10-15 mg/kg/dose every 4 hours up to a maximum of 2.6 g/24 hours for children <12 years; **alternatively, the following can be used:**
3-6 years: 5 mL 3-4 times/day as needed of elixir
7-12 years: 10 mL 3-4 times/day as needed of elixir
>12 years: 15 mL every 4 hours as needed of elixir

Adults:
Antitussive: Based on codeine (15-30 mg/dose) every 4-6 hours (maximum: 360 mg/24 hours based on codeine component)
Analgesic: Based on codeine (30-60 mg/dose) every 4-6 hours (maximum: 4000 mg/24 hours based on acetaminophen component)

Dosage Forms [CAN] = Canadian brand name
Caplet:
ratio-Lenoltec No. 1 [CAN], Tylenol No. 1 [CAN]: Acetaminophen 300 mg, codeine 8 mg, and caffeine 15 mg [not available in the U.S.]
Tylenol No. 1 Forte [CAN]: Acetaminophen 500 mg, codeine 8 mg, and caffeine 15 mg [not available in the U.S.]
Elixir, oral [C-V]: Acetaminophen 120 mg and codeine 12 mg per 5 mL
Tylenol Elixir with Codeine [CAN]: Acetaminophen 160 mg and codeine 8 mg per 5 mL [not available in the U.S.]
Suspension, oral [C-V]: Acetaminophen 120 mg and codeine 12 mg per 5 mL
Capital® and Codeine [C-V]: Acetaminophen 120 mg and codeine 12 mg per 5 mL
Tablet [C-III]: Acetaminophen 300 mg and codeine 15 mg; acetaminophen 300 mg and codeine 30 mg; acetaminophen 300 mg and codeine 60 mg
ratio-Emtec [CAN], Triatec-30 [CAN]: Acetaminophen 300 mg and codeine 30 mg [not available in the U.S.]
ratio-Lenoltec No. 1 [CAN]: Acetaminophen 300 mg, codeine 8 mg, and caffeine 15 mg [not available in the U.S.]
ratio-Lenoltec No. 2 [CAN], Tylenol No. 2 with Codeine [CAN]: Acetaminophen 300 mg, codeine 15 mg, and caffeine 15 mg [not available in the U.S.]
ratio-Lenoltec No. 3 [CAN], Tylenol No. 3 with Codeine [CAN]: Acetaminophen 300 mg, codeine 30 mg, and caffeine 15 mg [not available in the U.S.]
ratio-Lenoltec No. 4 [CAN], Tylenol No. 4 with Codeine [CAN]: Acetaminophen 300 mg and codeine 60 mg [not available in the U.S.]
Triatec-8 [CAN]: Acetaminophen 325 mg, codeine 8 mg, and caffeine 30 mg [not available in the U.S.]
Triatec-8 Strong [CAN]: Acetaminophen 500 mg, codeine 8 mg, and caffeine 30 mg [not available in the U.S.]
Tylenol® with Codeine No. 3: Acetaminophen 300 mg and codeine 30 mg
Tylenol® with Codeine No. 4: Acetaminophen 300 mg and codeine 60 mg

acetaminophen and diphenhydramine (a seet a MIN oh fen & dye fen HYE dra meen)

Sound-Alike/Look-Alike Issues
Excedrin® may be confused with Dexatrim®, Dexedrine®
Percogesic® may be confused with paregoric, Percodan®
Tylenol® may be confused with atenolol, timolol, Tuinal®, Tylox®

Synonyms diphenhydramine and acetaminophen

U.S./Canadian Brand Names Excedrin® P.M. [US-OTC]; Goody's PM® [US-OTC]; Legatrin PM® [US-OTC]; Percogesic® Extra Strength [US-OTC]; Tylenol® PM [US-OTC]; Tylenol® Severe Allergy [US-OTC]

Therapeutic Category Analgesic, Nonnarcotic

Use Aid in the relief of insomnia accompanied by minor pain

Usual Dosage Oral: Adults: 50 mg of diphenhydramine HCI (76 mg diphenhydramine citrate) at bedtime or as directed by physician; do not exceed recommended dosage; not for use in children <12 years of age

Dosage Forms
Caplet: Acetaminophen 500 mg and diphenhydramine 25 mg

▶

Excedrin® P.M. [OTC]: Acetaminophen 500 mg and diphenhydramine 38 mg
Legatrin PM® [OTC]: Acetaminophen 500 mg and diphenhydramine 50 mg
Percogesic® Extra Strength [OTC], Tylenol® PM [OTC]: Acetaminophen 500 mg and diphenhydramine
  25 mg
Tylenol® Severe Allergy [OTC]: Acetaminophen 500 mg and diphenhydramine 12.5 mg
Gelcap:
Tylenol® PM [OTC]: Acetaminophen 500 mg and diphenhydramine 25 mg
Geltab: Acetaminophen 500 mg and diphenhydramine 25 mg
Excedrin® P.M. [OTC]: Acetaminophen 500 mg and diphenhydramine 38 mg
Tylenol® PM [OTC]: Acetaminophen 500 mg and diphenhydramine 25 mg
Liquid:
Tylenol® PM [OTC]: Acetaminophen 500 mg and diphenhydramine 25 mg per 15 mL
Powder for oral solution:
Goody's PM® [OTC]: Acetaminophen 500 mg and diphenhydramine 38 mg
Tablet: Acetaminophen 500 mg and diphenhydramine 25 mg
Excedrin® P.M. [OTC]: Acetaminophen 500 mg and diphenhydramine 38 mg

acetaminophen and hydrocodone *see* hydrocodone and acetaminophen *on page 481*
acetaminophen and oxycodone *see* oxycodone and acetaminophen *on page 710*
acetaminophen and pentazocine *see* pentazocine and acetaminophen *on page 736*

acetaminophen and phenylephrine (a seet a MIN oh fen & fen il EF rin)
Synonyms phenylephrine hydrochloride and acetaminophen
U.S./Canadian Brand Names Alka-Seltzer Plus® Sinus Formula [US-OTC]; Contac® Cold + Flu
Maximum Strength Non-Drowsy [US-OTC]; Mapap® Sinus Congestion and Pain Daytime [US-OTC];
Sinutab® Sinus [US-OTC]; Sudafed PE® Sinus Headache [US-OTC]; Tylenol® Sinus Congestion & Pain
Daytime [US-OTC]
Therapeutic Category Analgesic, Miscellaneous; Decongestant
Use Temporary relief of sinus/nasal congestion and pressure, headache, and minor aches and pains
Usual Dosage Oral: Children ≥12 years and Adults: General dosing guidelines, refer to specific product
labeling: Sinus pain/pressure: Acetaminophen 325 mg and phenylephrine 5 mg/caplet: Take 2 caplets
every 4 hours as needed; maximum: 12 caplets/24 hours
Dosage Forms
Caplet, oral:
Contac® Cold + Flu Maximum Strength Non Drowsy [OTC]: Acetaminophen 500 mg and phenylephrine
  5 mg
Mapap® Sinus Congestion and Pain Daytime [OTC], Sinutab® Sinus [OTC], Sudafed PE® Sinus
  Headache [OTC]: Acetaminophen 325 mg and phenylephrine 5 mg
Tylenol® Sinus Congestion & Pain Daytime [OTC]: Acetaminophen 325 mg and phenylephrine 5 mg
  [Cool Burst™ flavor]
Gelcap, oral:
Tylenol® Sinus Congestion & Pain Daytime [OTC]: Acetaminophen 325 mg and phenylephrine 5 mg
Gelcap, rapid release, oral:
Tylenol® Sinus Congestion & Pain Daytime [OTC]: Acetaminophen 325 mg and phenylephrine 5 mg
Tablet for solution, oral [effervescent]:
Alka-Seltzer Plus® Sinus Formula [OTC]: Acetaminophen 250 mg and phenylephrine 5 mg

acetaminophen and phenyltoloxamine (a seet a MIN oh fen & fen il to LOKS a meen)
Sound-Alike/Look-Alike Issues
Percogesic® may be confused with paregoric, Percodan®
Synonyms phenyltoloxamine citrate and acetaminophen
U.S./Canadian Brand Names Aceta-Gesic [US-OTC]; Alpain [US]; BeFlex [US]; Dologesic® [US];
Flextra 650 [US]; Flextra-DS [US]; Genesec™ [US-OTC]; Lagesic™ [US]; Percogesic® [US-OTC];
Phenagesic [US-OTC]; Phenylgesic [US-OTC]; RhinoFlex 650 [US]; RhinoFlex™ [US]; Staflex [US]
Therapeutic Category Analgesic, Nonnarcotic
Use Relief of mild pain
Usual Dosage Oral:
Analgesic: Based on acetaminophen component:
Children: 10-15 mg/kg/dose every 4-6 hours as needed (maximum: 5 doses/24 hours)
Adults: 325-650 mg every 4-6 hours as needed (maximum: 4 g/day)

Product-specific labeling:
Flextra-650:
  Children 6 to <12 years: $^1/_2$ tablet every 6 hours (maximum: 2 tablets/day)
  Children ≥12 years and Adults: $^1/_2$-1 tablet every 6 hours (maximum: 4 tablets/day)
Flextra-DS, RhinoFlex™, RhinoFlex™-650:
  Children 6 to <12 years: $^1/_2$ tablet every 4 hours (maximum: 2.5 tablets/day)
  Children ≥12 years and Adults: $^1/_2$-1 tablet every 4 hours (maximum: 5 tablets/day)
Percogesic®:
  Children 6-12 years: 1 tablet every 4 hours (maximum: 4 tablets/24 hours)
  Adults: 1-2 tablets every 4 hours (maximum: 8 tablets/24 hours)

Dosage Forms
Caplet:
Alpain: Acetaminophen 500 mg and phenyltoloxamine citrate 60 mg
BeFlex, Staflex: Acetaminophen 500 mg and phenyltoloxamine citrate 55 mg
Dologesic®: Acetaminophen 500 mg and phenyltoloxamine citrate 30 mg
Caplet, extended release [scored]:
Lagesic™: Acetaminphen 600 mg and phenyltoloxamine citrate 66 mg
Capsule:
Dologesic®: Acetaminophen 500 mg and phenyltoloxamine citrate 30 mg
Liquid:
Dologesic®: Acetaminophen 500 mg and phenyltoloxamine citrate 30 mg per 15 mg
Tablet: Acetaminophen 325 mg and phenyltoloxamine citrate 30 mg
Aceta-Gesic [OTC], Genasec™ [OTC], Percogesic® [OTC], Phenagesic [OTC], Phenylgesic [OTC]:
  Acetaminophen 325 mg and phenyltoloxamine citrate 30 mg
Flextra-650, Vistra 650™: Acetaminophen 650 mg and phenyltoloxamine citrate 60 mg
Flextra-DS, RhinoFlex™: Acetaminophen 500 mg and phenyltoloxamine citrate 50 mg
RhinoFlex™-650: Acetaminophen 650 mg and phenyltoloxamine citrate 50 mg
Tablet, prolonged release, oral:
Zgesic: Acetaminophen 600 mg and phenyltoloxamine citrate 66 mg

acetaminophen and propoxyphene *see* propoxyphene and acetaminophen *on page 795*

acetaminophen and pseudoephedrine (a seet a MIN oh fen & soo doe e FED rin)

Sound-Alike/Look-Alike Issues
Ornex® may be confused with Orexin®, Orinase®
Sudafed® may be confused with Sufenta®
Tylenol® may be confused with atenolol, timolol, Tuinal®, Tylox®

Synonyms pseudoephedrine and acetaminophen

U.S./Canadian Brand Names Allerest® Allergy and Sinus Relief [US-OTC]; Contac® Cold and Sore Throat, Non Drowsy, Extra Strength [Can]; Dristan® N.D. [Can]; Dristan® N.D., Extra Strength [Can]; Mapap Sinus Maximum Strength [US-OTC]; Medi-Synal [US-OTC]; Oranyl Plus [US-OTC]; Ornex® Maximum Strength [US-OTC]; Ornex® [US-OTC]; Sinutab® Non Drowsy [Can]; Sudafed® Head Cold and Sinus Extra Strength [Can]; Sudafed® Multi-Symptom Sinus and Cold [US-OTC]; Tylenol® Cold Daytime, Children's [US-OTC]; Tylenol® Decongestant [Can]; Tylenol® Sinus Daytime [US-OTC]; Tylenol® Sinus [Can]

Therapeutic Category Decongestant/Analgesic

Use Relief of mild-to-moderate pain; relief of congestion

Usual Dosage Oral:
Analgesic: Based on acetaminophen component:
  Children: 10-15 mg/kg/dose every 4-6 hours as needed; do **not** exceed 5 doses in 24 hours
  Adults: 325-650 mg every 4-6 hours as needed; do **not** exceed 4 g/day
Decongestant: Based on pseudoephedrine component:
  Children:
    2-6 years: 15 mg every 4 hours; do **not** exceed 90 mg/day
    6-12 years: 30 mg every 4 hours; do **not** exceed 180 mg/day
  Children >12 years and Adults: 60 mg every 4 hours; do **not** exceed 360 mg/day

Product labeling:
Children's Tylenol® Cold Daytime: Children:
  2-5 years (24-47 lb): 1 teaspoonful every 4-6 hours (maximum: 4 doses/24 hours)
  6-11 years (48-95 lb): 2 teaspoonfuls every 4-6 hours (maximum: 4 doses/24 hours)

Sudafed® Multi-Symptom Sinus and Cold: Children ≥12 years and Adults: 2 capsules every 4-6 hours (maximum: 8 capsules/24 hours)

Tylenol® Sinus Daytime: Children ≥12 years and Adults: 2 caplets or gelcaps every 4-6 hours (maximum: 8 caplets or gelcaps/24 hours)

Dosage Forms

Caplet:

Allerest® Allergy and Sinus Relief, Ornex®: Acetaminophen 325 mg and pseudoephedrine hydrochloride 30 mg

Mapap Sinus Maximum Strength, Ornex® Maximum Strength, Tylenol® Sinus Daytime: Acetaminophen 500 mg and pseudoephedrine hydrochloride 30 mg

Capsule, liquid:

Sudafed® Multi-Symptom Sinus and Cold: Acetaminophen 325 mg and pseudoephedrine hydrochloride 30 mg

Gelcap:

Tylenol® Sinus Daytime: Acetaminophen 500 mg and pseudoephedrine hydrochloride 30 mg

Liquid:

Childrens Tylenol® Cold Daytime: Acetaminophen 160 mg and pseudoephedrine hydrochloride 15 mg per 5 mL

Tablet:

Medi-Synal: Acetaminophen 325 mg and pseudoephedrine hydrochloride 30 mg

Oranyl Plus: Acetaminophen 500 mg and pseudoephedrine hydrochloride 30 mg

acetaminophen and tramadol (a seet a MIN oh fen & TRA ma dole)

Sound-Alike/Look-Alike Issues

Ultracet™ may be confused with Ultane®, Ultram®

Synonyms APAP and tramadol; tramadol hydrochloride and acetaminophen

U.S./Canadian Brand Names Tramacet [Can]; Ultracet™ [US]

Therapeutic Category Analgesic, Miscellaneous; Analgesic, Nonnarcotic

Use Short-term (≤5 days) management of acute pain

Usual Dosage Oral: Adults: Acute pain: Two tablets every 4-6 hours as needed for pain relief (maximum: 8 tablets/day); treatment should not exceed 5 days

Dosage Forms

Tablet: Acetaminophen 325 mg and tramadol 37.5 mg

Ultracet®: Acetaminophen 325 mg and tramadol 37.5 mg

acetaminophen, aspirin, and caffeine (a seet a MIN oh fen, AS pir in, & KAF een)

Sound-Alike/Look-Alike Issues

Excedrin® may be confused with Dexatrim®, Dexedrine®

Synonyms aspirin, acetaminophen, and caffeine; aspirin, caffeine, and acetaminophen; caffeine, acetaminophen, and aspirin; caffeine, aspirin, and acetaminophen

U.S./Canadian Brand Names Excedrin® Extra Strength [US-OTC]; Excedrin® Migraine [US-OTC]; Fem-Prin® [US-OTC]; Genaced™ [US-OTC]; Goody's® Extra Strength Headache Powder [US-OTC]; Goody's® Extra Strength Pain Relief [US-OTC]; Pain-Off [US-OTC]; Vanquish® Extra Strength Pain Reliever [US-OTC]

Therapeutic Category Analgesic, Nonnarcotic

Use Relief of mild-to-moderate pain; mild-to-moderate pain associated with migraine headache

Usual Dosage Oral: Adults:

Analgesic:

Based on **acetaminophen** component:

Mild-to-moderate pain: 325-650 mg every 4-6 hours as needed; do **not** exceed 4 g/day

Mild-to-moderate pain associated with migraine headache: 500 mg/dose (in combination with 500 mg aspirin and 130 mg caffeine) every 6 hours while symptoms persist; do not use for longer than 48 hours

Based on **aspirin** component:

Mild-to-moderate pain: 325-650 mg every 4-6 hours as needed; do **not** exceed 4 g/day

Mild-to-moderate pain associated with migraine headache: 500 mg/dose (in combination with 500 mg acetaminophen and 130 mg caffeine) every 6 hours; do not use for longer than 48 hours

Product labeling:

Excedrin® Extra Strength, Excedrin® Migraine: Children >12 years and Adults: 2 doses every 6 hours (maximum: 8 doses/24 hours)

Note: When used for migraine, do not use for longer than 48 hours

Goody's® Extra Strength Headache Powder: Children >12 years and Adults: 1 powder, placed on tongue or dissolved in water, every 4-6 hours (maximum: 4 powders/24 hours)

Goody's® Extra Strength Pain Relief Tablets: Children >12 years and Adults: 2 tablets every 4-6 hours (maximum: 8 tablets/24 hours)

Vanquish® Extra Strength Pain Reliever: Children >12 years and Adults: 2 tablets every 4 hours (maximum: 12 tablets/24 hours)

Dosage Forms

Caplet: Acetaminophen 250 mg, aspirin 250 mg, and caffeine 65 mg; acetaminophen 194 mg, aspirin 227 mg, and caffeine 33 mg

Excedrin® Extra Strength [OTC], Excedrin® Migraine [OTC]: Acetaminophen 250 mg, aspirin 250 mg, and caffeine 65 mg

Vanquish® Extra Strength Pain Reliever [OTC]: Acetaminophen 194 mg, aspirin 227 mg, and caffeine 33 mg

Geltab: Acetaminophen 250 mg, aspirin 250 mg, and caffeine 65 mg

Excedrin® Extra Strength [OTC], Excedrin® Migraine [OTC]: Acetaminophen 250 mg, aspirin 250 mg, and caffeine 65 mg

Powder: Acetaminophen 260 mg, aspirin 520 mg, and caffeine 32.5 mg

Goody's® Extra Strength Headache Powder [OTC]: Acetaminophen 260 mg, aspirin 520 mg, and caffeine 32.5 mg

Tablet:

Excedrin® Extra Strength [OTC], Excedrin® Migraine [OTC], Genaced™ [OTC], Pain-Off [OTC]: Acetaminophen 250 mg, aspirin 250 mg, and caffeine 65 mg

Fem-Prin® [OTC]: Acetaminophen 194.4 mg, aspirin 226.8 mg, and caffeine 32.4 mg

Goody's® Extra Strength Pain Relief [OTC]: Acetaminophen 130 mg, aspirin 260 mg, and caffeine 16.25 mg

acetaminophen, butalbital, and caffeine *see* butalbital, acetaminophen, and caffeine *on page 155*

acetaminophen, caffeine, and dihydrocodeine
(a seet a MIN oh fen, KAF een, & dye hye droe KOE deen)

Sound-Alike/Look-Alike Issues

Panlor® DC may be confused with Pamelor®

Synonyms caffeine, dihydrocodeine, and acetaminophen; dihydrocodeine bitartrate, acetaminophen, and caffeine

U.S./Canadian Brand Names Panlor® DC [US]; Panlor® SS [US]; ZerLor™ [US]

Therapeutic Category Analgesic Combination (Opioid)

Controlled Substance C-III

Use Relief of moderate- to moderately-severe pain

Usual Dosage Oral: Adults: Relief of pain:

Panlor® DC: 2 capsules every 4 hours as needed; adjust dose based on severity of pain (maximum dose: 10 capsules/24 hours)

Panlor® SS, ZerLor™: 1 tablet every 4 hours as needed; adjust dose based on severity of pain (maximum dose: 5 tablets/24 hours)

Dosage Forms

Capsule:

Panlor® DC: Acetaminophen 356.4 mg, caffeine 30 mg, and dihydrocodeine 16 mg

Tablet:

Panlor® SS, ZerLor™: Acetaminophen 712.8 mg, caffeine 60 mg, and dihydrocodeine 32 mg

acetaminophen, caffeine, codeine, and butalbital *see* butalbital, acetaminophen, caffeine, and codeine *on page 155*

acetaminophen, chlorpheniramine, and pseudoephedrine
(a seet a MIN oh fen, klor fen IR a meen, & soo doe e FED rin)

Sound-Alike/Look-Alike Issues

Thera-Flu® may be confused with Tamiflu®, Thera-Flur-N®

Tylenol® may be confused with atenolol, timolol, Tuinal®, Tylox®

Synonyms acetaminophen, pseudoephedrine, and chlorpheniramine; chlorpheniramine, acetaminophen, and pseudoephedrine; chlorpheniramine, pseudoephedrine, and acetaminophen; pseudoephedrine, acetaminophen, and chlorpheniramine; pseudoephedrine, chlorpheniramine, and acetaminophen

▶

◀ **U.S./Canadian Brand Names** Actifed® Cold and Sinus [US-OTC]; Comtrex® Flu Therapy Nighttime [US-OTC]; Drinex [US-OTC]; Kolephrin® [US-OTC]; Sinutab® Sinus & Allergy [Can]; Sinutab® Sinus Allergy Maximum Strength [US-OTC]; Tylenol® Allergy Sinus [Can]

Therapeutic Category Antihistamine/Decongestant/Analgesic

Use Temporary relief of sinus symptoms

Usual Dosage Oral:

Analgesic: Based on **acetaminophen** component:
Children: 10-15 mg/kg/dose every 4-6 hours as needed; do **not** exceed 5 doses in 24 hours
Adults: 325-650 mg every 4-6 hours as needed; do **not** exceed 4 g/day

Antihistamine: Based on **chlorpheniramine maleate** component:
Children:
2-6 years: 1 mg every 4-6 hours (maximum: 6 mg/24 hours)
6-12 years: 2 mg every 4-6 hours (maximum: 12 mg/24 hours)
Children >12 years and Adults: 4 mg every 4-6 hours (maximum: 24 mg/24 hours)

Decongestant: Based on **pseudoephedrine** component:
Children:
2-6 years: 15 mg every 4 hours (maximum: 90 mg/24 hours)
6-12 years: 30 mg every 4 hours (maximum: 180 mg/24 hours)
Children >12 years and Adults: 60 mg every 4 hours (maximum: 360 mg/24 hours)

Product labeling:
Sinutab® Sinus Allergy Maximum Strength: Children >12 years and Adults: 2 tablets/caplets every 6 hours (maximum: 8 doses/24 hours)

Dosage Forms

Caplet: Acetaminophen 325 mg, chlorpheniramine 2 mg, and pseudoephedrine 30 mg
Actifed® Cold and Sinus [OTC], Sinutab® Sinus Allergy Maximum Strength [OTC]: Acetaminophen 500 mg, chlorpheniramine 2 mg, and pseudoephedrine 30 mg
Kolephrin® [OTC]: Acetaminophen 325 mg, chlorpheniramine 2 mg, and pseudoephedrine 30 mg

Liquid:
Comtrex® Flu Therapy Nighttime [OTC]: Acetaminophen 100 mg, chlorpheniramine 4 mg, and pseudoephedrine 60 mg per 30 mL

Tablet:
Drinex: Acetaminophen 650 mg, chlorpheniramine 4 mg, and pseudoephedrine 60 mg

acetaminophen, codeine, and doxylamine *(Canada only)*
(a seet a MIN oh fen, KOE deen, & dox IL a meen)

Synonyms codeine, doxylamine, and acetaminophen; doxylamine succinate, codeine phosphate, and acetaminophen

U.S./Canadian Brand Names Mersyndol® With Codeine [Can]

Therapeutic Category Analgesic, Opioid; Antihistamine

Controlled Substance CDSA-1

Use Relief of headache, cold symptoms, neuralgia, and muscular aches/pain

Usual Dosage Oral: Children >12 years and Adults: 1-2 tablets every 4 hours as needed; total dose should not exceed 12 tablets in a 24-hour period

Dosage Forms [CAN] = Canadian brand name

Tablet:
Mersyndol® With Codeine [CAN]: Acetaminophen 325 mg, codeine 8 mg, and doxylamine 5 mg [not available in the U.S.]

acetaminophen, dextromethorphan, and phenylephrine
(a seet a MIN oh fen, deks troe meth OR fan, & fen il EF rin)

Synonyms dextromethorphan hydrobromide, acetaminophen, and phenylephrine hydrochloride; phenylephrine, acetaminophen, and dextromethorphan; phenylephrine, dextromethorphan, and acetaminophen

U.S./Canadian Brand Names Alka-Seltzer Plus® Day Cold [US-OTC]; Mapap® Multi-Symptom Cold [US-OTC]; Tylenol® Cold Head Congestion Daytime [US-OTC]; Tylenol® Cold Multi-Symptom Daytime [US-OTC]; Vicks® DayQuil® Cold/Flu Multi-Symptom Relief [US-OTC]

Therapeutic Category Analgesic, Miscellaneous; Antitussive; Decongestant

Use Temporary relief of common cold and flu symptoms (eg, pain, fever, cough, congestion)

Usual Dosage Product labeling: Oral:

Alka-Seltzer Plus® Day Cold: Children ≥12 years and Adults: 2 capsules or 20 mL every 4 hours (maximum: 6 doses/24 hours)

Tylenol® Cold Head Congestion Daytime: Children ≥12 years and Adults: 2 caplets every 4 hours (maximum: 6 doses/24 hours)

Tylenol® Cold Multi-Symptom Daytime: Children ≥12 years and Adults: 2 caplets/gelcaps or 30 mL every 4 hours (maximum: 6 doses/24 hours)

Vicks® DayQuil® Cold/Flu Multi-Symptom Relief LiquiCaps: Children ≥12 years and Adults: 2 capsules every 4 hours (maximum: 6 doses/24 hours)

Vicks® DayQuil® Cold/Flu Multi-Symptom Relief Liquid:

Children 6-11 years: 15 mL every 4 hours, up to 5 doses/day (maximum: 75 mL/24 hours)

Children ≥12 years and Adults: 30 mL every 4 hours (maximum: 6 doses/24 hours)

Dosage Forms

Caplet:

Mapap® Multi-Symptom Cold [OTC], Tylenol® Cold Head Congestion Daytime [OTC], Tylenol® Cold Multi-Symptom Daytime [OTC]: Acetaminophen 325 mg, dextromethorphan 10 mg, and phenylephrine 5 mg

Capsule, liquid gel:

Alka-Seltzer Plus® Day Cold [OTC]: Acetaminophen 325 mg, dextromethorphan 10 mg, and phenylephrine 5 mg

Capsule, liquicap:

Vicks® DayQuil® Cold/Flu Multi-Symptom Relief [OTC]: Acetaminophen 325 mg, dextromethorphan 10 mg, and phenylephrine 5 mg

Gelcap:

Tylenol® Cold Multi-Symptom Daytime [OTC]: Acetaminophen 325 mg, dextromethorphan 10 mg, and phenylephrine 5 mg

Liquid:

Alka-Seltzer Plus® Day Cold [OTC]: Acetaminophen 162.5 mg, dextromethorphan 5 mg, and phenylephrine 2.5 mg per 5 mL

Tylenol® Cold Multi-Symptom Daytime [OTC], Vicks® DayQuil® Cold/Flu Multi-Symptom Relief [OTC]: Acetaminophen 325 mg, dextromethorphan 10 mg, and phenylephrine 5 mg per 15 mL

acetaminophen, dextromethorphan, and pseudoephedrine

(a seet a MIN oh fen, deks troe meth OR fan, & soo doe e FED rin)

Sound-Alike/Look-Alike Issues

Sudafed® may be confused with Sufenta®

Thera-Flu® may be confused with Tamiflu®, Thera-Flur-N®

Tylenol® may be confused with atenolol, timolol, Tuinal®, Tylox®

Synonyms dextromethorphan, acetaminophen, and pseudoephedrine; pseudoephedrine, acetaminophen, and dextromethorphan; pseudoephedrine, dextromethorphan, and acetaminophen

U.S./Canadian Brand Names Contac® Complete [Can]; Contac® Cough, Cold and Flu Day & Night™ [Can]; Sudafed® Cold & Cough Extra Strength [Can]; Tylenol® Cold Day Non-Drowsy [US-OTC]; Tylenol® Cold Daytime [Can]; Tylenol® Flu Non-Drowsy Maximum Strength [US-OTC]

Therapeutic Category Cold Preparation

Use Treatment of mild-to-moderate pain and fever; symptomatic relief of cough and congestion

Usual Dosage Oral:

Analgesic: Based on acetaminophen component:

Children: 10-15 mg/kg/dose every 4-6 hours as needed; do **not** exceed 5 doses/24 hours

Adults: 325-650 mg every 4-6 hours as needed; do **not** exceed 4 g/day

Cough suppressant: Based on dextromethorphan component:

Children 6-12 years: 15 mg every 6-8 hours; do **not** exceed 60 mg/24 hours

Children >12 years and Adults: 10-20 mg every 4-8 hours **or** 30 mg every 8 hours; do **not** exceed 120 mg/24 hours

Decongestant: Based on pseudoephedrine component:

Children:

2-6 years: 15 mg every 4 hours (maximum: 90 mg/24 hours)

6-12 years: 30 mg every 4 hours (maximum: 180 mg/24 hours)

Children >12 years and Adults: 60 mg every 4 hours (maximum: 360 mg/24 hours)

▶

Product labeling:
Tylenol® Cold Day Non-Drowsy:
Children 6-11 years: 1 dose every 6 hours (maximum: 4 doses/24 hours)
Children ≥12 years and Adults: 2 doses every 6 hours (maximum: 8 doses/24 hours)
Tylenol® Flu Non-Drowsy Maximum Strength: Children >12 years and Adults: 2 doses every 6 hours (maximum: 8 doses/24 hours)
Dosage Forms
Caplet:
Sudafed® Severe Cold [OTC], Tylenol® Cold Day Non-Drowsy [OTC]: Acetaminophen 325 mg, dextromethorphan 15 mg, and pseudoephedrine 30 mg
Gelcap:
Tylenol® Flu Non-Drowsy Maximum Strength [OTC]: Acetaminophen 500 mg, dextromethorphan 15 mg, and pseudoephedrine 30 mg

acetaminophen, dichloralphenazone, and isometheptene *see* acetaminophen, isometheptene, and dichloralphenazone *on page 28*

acetaminophen, isometheptene, and dichloralphenazone
(a seet a MIN oh fen, eye soe me THEP teen, & dye KLOR al FEN a zone)
Sound-Alike/Look-Alike Issues
Midrin® may be confused with Mydfrin®
Synonyms acetaminophen, dichloralphenazone, and isometheptene; dichloralphenazone, acetaminophen, and isometheptene; dichloralphenazone, isometheptene, and acetaminophen; isometheptene, acetaminophen, and dichloralphenazone; isometheptene, dichloralphenazone, and acetaminophen
U.S./Canadian Brand Names Midrin® [US]; Migratine [US]
Therapeutic Category Analgesic, Nonnarcotic
Controlled Substance C-IV
Use Relief of migraine and tension headache
Usual Dosage Oral: Adults:
Migraine headache: 2 capsules to start, followed by 1 capsule every hour until relief is obtained (maximum: 5 capsules/12 hours)
Tension headache: 1-2 capsules every 4 hours (maximum: 8 capsules/24 hours)
Dosage Forms
Capsule: Acetaminophen 325 mg, isometheptene 65 mg
Midrin®, Migratine: Acetaminophen 325 mg, isometheptene 65 mg, and dichloralphenazone 100 mg

acetaminophen, pseudoephedrine, and chlorpheniramine *see* acetaminophen, chlorpheniramine, and pseudoephedrine *on page 25*
Acetasol® HC [US] *see* acetic acid, propylene glycol diacetate, and hydrocortisone *on page 29*

acetazolamide (a set a ZOLE a mide)
Sound-Alike/Look-Alike Issues
acetaZOLAMIDE may be confused with acetoHEXAMIDE
Diamox® Sequels® may be confused with Diabinese®, Dobutrex®, Trimox®
Tall-Man acetaZOLAMIDE
U.S./Canadian Brand Names Apo-Acetazolamide® [Can]; Diamox® Sequels® [US]; Diamox® [Can]
Therapeutic Category Anticonvulsant; Carbonic Anhydrase Inhibitor
Use Treatment of glaucoma (chronic simple open-angle, secondary glaucoma, preoperatively in acute angle-closure); drug-induced edema or edema due to congestive heart failure (adjunctive therapy); centrencephalic epilepsies (immediate release dosage form); prevention or amelioration of symptoms associated with acute mountain sickness
Usual Dosage Note: I.M. administration is not recommended because of pain secondary to the alkaline pH
Children:
Glaucoma:
Oral: 8-30 mg/kg/day or 300-900 mg/m^2/day divided every 8 hours
I.V.: 20-40 mg/kg/24 hours divided every 6 hours, not to exceed 1 g/day
Edema: Oral, I.V.: 5 mg/kg or 150 mg/m^2 once every day
Epilepsy: Oral: 8-30 mg/kg/day in 1-4 divided doses, not to exceed 1 g/day; extended release capsule is not recommended for treatment of epilepsy

Adults:
Glaucoma:
Chronic simple (open-angle): Oral: 250 mg 1-4 times/day or 500 mg extended release capsule twice daily
Secondary, acute (closed-angle): I.V.: 250-500 mg, may repeat in 2-4 hours to a maximum of 1 g/day
Edema: Oral, I.V.: 250-375 mg once daily
Epilepsy: Oral: 8-30 mg/kg/day in 1-4 divided doses; **extended release capsule is not recommended for treatment of epilepsy**
Mountain sickness: Oral: 250 mg every 8-12 hours (or 500 mg extended release capsules every 12-24 hours)
Therapy should begin 24-48 hours before and continue during ascent and for at least 48 hours after arrival at the high altitude
Note: In situations of rapid ascent (such as rescue or military operations), 1000 mg/day is recommended.

Dosage Forms
Capsule, extended release:
Diamox® Sequels®: 500 mg
Injection, powder for reconstitution: 500 mg
Tablet: 125 mg, 250 mg

acetic acid (a SEE tik AS id)

Sound-Alike/Look-Alike Issues
VoSol® may be confused with Vexol®

Synonyms ethanoic acid

Therapeutic Category Antibacterial, Otic; Antibacterial, Topical

Use Irrigation of the bladder; treatment of superficial bacterial infections of the external auditory canal

Usual Dosage
Irrigation (**Note:** Dosage of an irrigating solution depends on the capacity or surface area of the structure being irrigated):
For continuous irrigation of the urinary bladder with 0.25% acetic acid irrigation, the rate of administration will approximate the rate of urine flow; usually 500-1500 mL/24 hours
For periodic irrigation of an indwelling urinary catheter to maintain patency, about 50 mL of 0.25% acetic acid irrigation is required
Otic: Insert saturated wick; keep moist 24 hours; remove wick and instill 5 drops 3-4 times/day

Dosage Forms
Solution for irrigation: 0.25% (250 mL, 500 mL, 1000 mL)
Solution, otic: 2% (15 mL)

acetic acid, hydrocortisone, and propylene glycol diacetate *see* acetic acid, propylene glycol diacetate, and hydrocortisone *on page 29*

acetic acid, propylene glycol diacetate, and hydrocortisone

(a SEE tik AS id, PRO pa leen GLY kole dye AS e tate, & hye droe KOR ti sone)

Sound-Alike/Look-Alike Issues
VoSol® may be confused with Vexol®

Synonyms acetic acid, hydrocortisone, and propylene glycol diacetate; hydrocortisone, acetic acid, and propylene glycol diacetate; propylene glycol diacetate, acetic acid, and hydrocortisone

U.S./Canadian Brand Names Acetasol® HC [US]; VoSol® HC [US]

Therapeutic Category Antibiotic/Corticosteroid, Otic

Use Treatment of superficial infections of the external auditory canal caused by organisms susceptible to the action of the antimicrobial, complicated by swelling

Usual Dosage Otic: Children ≥3 years and Adults: Instill 3-5 drops in ear(s) every 4-6 hours

Dosage Forms
Solution, otic [drops]:
Acetasol® HC, VoSol® HC: Acetic acid 2%, propylene glycol diacetate 3%, and hydrocortisone 1% (10 mL)

acetohydroxamic acid (a SEE toe hye droks am ik AS id)

Sound-Alike/Look-Alike Issues
Lithostat® may be confused with Lithobid®

▶

◀ **Synonyms** AHA

U.S./Canadian Brand Names Lithostat® [US/Can]

Therapeutic Category Urinary Tract Product

Use Adjunctive therapy in chronic urea-splitting urinary infection

Usual Dosage Oral:
  Children: Initial: 10 mg/kg/day
  Adults: 250 mg 3-4 times/day for a total daily dose of 10-15 mg/kg/day

Dosage Forms
  Tablet:
    Lithostat®: 250 mg

Acetoxyl® [Can] *see* benzoyl peroxide *on page 126*

acetoxymethylprogesterone *see* medroxyprogesterone *on page 597*

acetylcholine (a se teel KOE leen)

Sound-Alike/Look-Alike Issues
  acetylcholine may be confused with acetylcysteine

Synonyms acetylcholine chloride

U.S./Canadian Brand Names Miochol®-E [US/Can]

Therapeutic Category Cholinergic Agent

Use Produces complete miosis in cataract surgery, keratoplasty, iridectomy, and other anterior segment surgery where rapid miosis is required

Usual Dosage Intraocular: Adults: 0.5-2 mL of 1% injection (5-20 mg) instilled into anterior chamber before or after securing one or more sutures

Dosage Forms
  Powder for intraocular solution:
    Miochol®-E: 1:100 [20 mg; packaged with diluent (2 mL)]

acetylcholine chloride *see* acetylcholine *on page 30*

acetylcysteine (a se teel SIS teen)

Sound-Alike/Look-Alike Issues
  acetylcysteine may be confused with acetylcholine
  Mucomyst® may be confused with Mucinex®

Synonyms *n*-acetyl-L-cysteine; *n*-acetylcysteine; acetylcysteine sodium; mercapturic acid; NAC

U.S./Canadian Brand Names Acetadote® [US]; Acetylcysteine Solution [Can]; Mucomyst® [Can]; Parvolex® [Can]

Therapeutic Category Mucolytic Agent

Use Adjunctive mucolytic therapy in patients with abnormal or viscid mucous secretions in acute and chronic bronchopulmonary diseases; pulmonary complications of surgery and cystic fibrosis; diagnostic bronchial studies; antidote for acute acetaminophen toxicity

Usual Dosage
  Acetaminophen poisoning: Children and Adults:
    Oral: 140 mg/kg; followed by 17 doses of 70 mg/kg every 4 hours; repeat dose if emesis occurs within 1 hour of administration; therapy should continue until acetaminophen levels are undetectable and there is no evidence of hepatotoxicity.
    I.V. (Acetadote®): Loading dose: 150 mg/kg over 60 minutes; **Note:** Extended infusion time recommended by manufacturer as of February, 2006. Loading dose is followed by 2 additional infusions: Initial maintenance dose of 50 mg/kg infused over 4 hours, followed by a second maintenance dose of 100 mg/kg infused over 16 hours. To avoid fluid overload in patients <40 kg and those requiring fluid restriction, decrease volume of D_5W proportionally. Total dosage: 300 mg/kg administered over 21 hours.
    Experts suggest that the duration of acetylcysteine administration may vary depending upon serial acetaminophen levels and liver function tests obtained during treatment. In general, patients without measurable acetaminophen levels and without significant LFT elevations (>3 times the ULN) can safely stop acetylcysteine after ≤24 hours of treatment. The patients who still have detectable levels of acetaminophen, and/or LFT elevations (>1000 units/L) continue to benefit from addition acetylcysteine administration.

Adjuvant therapy in respiratory conditions: **Note:** Patients should receive an aerosolized bronchodilator 10-15 minutes prior to acetylcysteine.

Inhalation, nebulization (face mask, mouth piece, tracheostomy): Acetylcysteine 10% and 20% solution (dilute 20% solution with sodium chloride or sterile water for inhalation); 10% solution may be used undiluted

Infants: 1-2 mL of 20% solution or 2-4 mL of 10% solution until nebulized given 3-4 times/day

Children and Adults: 3-5 mL of 20% solution or 6-10 mL of 10% solution until nebulized given 3-4 times/ day; dosing range: 1-10 mL of 20% solution or 2-20 mL of 10% solution every 2-6 hours

Inhalation, nebulization (tent, croupette): Children and Adults: Dose must be individualized; may require up to 300 mL solution/treatment

Direct instillation: Adults:

Into tracheostomy: 1-2 mL of 10% to 20% solution every 1-4 hours

Through percutaneous intratracheal catheter: 1-2 mL of 20% or 2-4 mL of 10% solution every 1-4 hours via syringe attached to catheter

Diagnostic bronchogram: Nebulization or intratracheal: Adults: 1-2 mL of 20% solution or 2-4 mL of 10% solution administered 2-3 times prior to procedure

Dosage Forms
Injection, solution:
Acetadote®: 20% (30 mL) [200 mg/mL]
Solution, inhalation/oral: 10% [100 mg/mL]; 20% [200 mg/mL]

acetylcysteine sodium *see* acetylcysteine *on page 30*
Acetylcysteine Solution [Can] *see* acetylcysteine *on page 30*
acetylsalicylic acid *see* aspirin *on page 98*
Aches-N-Pain® *(Discontinued)* *see* ibuprofen *on page 495*
achromycin *see* tetracycline *on page 915*
aciclovir *see* acyclovir *on page 33*
Acid Gone [US-OTC] *see* aluminum hydroxide and magnesium carbonate *on page 53*
Acid Gone Extra Strength [US-OTC] *see* aluminum hydroxide and magnesium carbonate *on page 53*
Acid Reducer [Can] *see* ranitidine *on page 819*
Acid Reducer Maximum Strength Non Prescription [Can] *see* ranitidine *on page 819*
acidulated phosphate fluoride *see* fluoride *on page 411*
Aci-jel® *(Discontinued)* *see* acetic acid *on page 29*
Acilac [Can] *see* lactulose *on page 544*
AcipHex® [US/Can] *see* rabeprazole *on page 815*

acitretin (a si TRE tin)

Sound-Alike/Look-Alike Issues
Soriatane® may be confused with Loxitane®
U.S./Canadian Brand Names Soriatane® CK Convenience Kit™ [US]; Soriatane® [Can]
Therapeutic Category Retinoid-like Compound
Use Treatment of severe psoriasis
Usual Dosage Oral: Adults: Individualization of dosage is required to achieve maximum therapeutic response while minimizing side effects
Initial therapy: Therapy should be initiated at 25-50 mg/day, given as a single dose with the main meal
Maintenance doses of 25-50 mg/day may be given after initial response to treatment; the maintenance dose should be based on clinical efficacy and tolerability
Dosage Forms
Capsule:
Soriatane® CK Convenience Kit™: 10 mg, 25 mg

Aclaro PD™ [US] *see* hydroquinone *on page 488*
Aclasta® [Can] *see* zoledronic acid *on page 995*
Aclovate® [US] *see* alclometasone *on page 41*

acrivastine and pseudoephedrine (AK ri vas teen & soo doe e FED rin)

Synonyms pseudoephedrine hydrochloride and acrivastine
U.S./Canadian Brand Names Semprex®-D [US]

▶

◀ **Therapeutic Category** Antihistamine/Decongestant Combination

Use Temporary relief of nasal congestion, decongest sinus openings, running nose, itching of nose or throat, and itchy, watery eyes due to hay fever or other upper respiratory allergies

Usual Dosage Oral: Adults: 1 capsule 3-4 times/day

Dosage Forms
  Capsule:
    Semprex®-D: Acrivastine 8 mg and pseudoephedrine 60 mg

ACT *see* dactinomycin *on page 264*

ACT® [US-OTC] *see* fluoride *on page 411*

Act-D *see* dactinomycin *on page 264*

Actagen® Syrup *(Discontinued)* *see* triprolidine and pseudoephedrine *on page 955*

Actagen® Tablet *(Discontinued)* *see* triprolidine and pseudoephedrine *on page 955*

Act-A-Med® *(Discontinued)* *see* triprolidine and pseudoephedrine *on page 955*

ACTH *see* corticotropin *on page 249*

ActHIB® [US/Can] *see* Haemophilus B conjugate vaccine *on page 464*

Acthrel® [US] *see* corticorelin *on page 248*

Acticin® [US] *see* permethrin *on page 740*

Actidose-Aqua® [US-OTC] *see* charcoal *on page 198*

Actidose® with Sorbitol [US-OTC] *see* charcoal *on page 198*

Actifed® [Can] *see* triprolidine and pseudoephedrine *on page 955*

Actifed® Allergy Tablet (Night) *(Discontinued)* *see* diphenhydramine and pseudoephedrine *on page 306*

Actifed® Cold & Allergy [US-OTC] *[reformulation]* *see* chlorpheniramine and phenylephrine *on page 206*

Actifed® Cold and Allergy *(Discontinued)* *see* triprolidine and pseudoephedrine *on page 955*

Actifed® Cold and Sinus [US-OTC] *see* acetaminophen, chlorpheniramine, and pseudoephedrine *on page 25*

Actigall® [US] *see* ursodiol *on page 965*

Actimmune® [US/Can] *see* interferon gamma-1b *on page 518*

actinomycin *see* dactinomycin *on page 264*

actinomycin D *see* dactinomycin *on page 264*

actinomycin Cl *see* dactinomycin *on page 264*

Actiq® [US/Can] *see* fentanyl *on page 394*

Activase® [US] *see* alteplase *on page 51*

Activase® rt-PA [Can] *see* alteplase *on page 51*

activated carbon *see* charcoal *on page 198*

activated charcoal *see* charcoal *on page 198*

activated dimethicone *see* simethicone *on page 867*

activated ergosterol *see* ergocalciferol *on page 350*

activated methylpolysiloxane *see* simethicone *on page 867*

activated protein C, human, recombinant *see* drotrecogin alfa *on page 327*

Activella® [US] *see* estradiol and norethindrone *on page 362*

Actonel® [US/Can] *see* risedronate *on page 836*

Actonel® and Calcium [US] *see* risedronate and calcium *on page 837*

Actoplus Met™ [US] *see* pioglitazone and metformin *on page 755*

Actos® [US/Can] *see* pioglitazone *on page 754*

ACT® Plus [US-OTC] *see* fluoride *on page 411*

ACT® x2™ [US-OTC] *see* fluoride *on page 411*

Acular® [US/Can] *see* ketorolac *on page 538*

Acular LS™ [US/Can] *see* ketorolac *on page 538*

Acular® P.F. [US] *see* ketorolac *on page 538*

ACV *see* acyclovir *on page 33*

acycloguanosine *see* acyclovir *on page 33*

acyclovir (ay SYE kloe veer)

Sound-Alike/Look-Alike Issues
Zovirax® may be confused with Zostrix®, Zyvox®

Synonyms aciclovir; ACV; acycloguanosine

U.S./Canadian Brand Names Apo-Acyclovir® [Can]; Gen-Acyclovir [Can]; Nu-Acyclovir [Can]; ratio-Acyclovir [Can]; Zovirax® [US/Can]

Therapeutic Category Antiviral Agent

Use Treatment of genital herpes simplex virus (HSV), herpes labialis (cold sores), herpes zoster (shingles), HSV encephalitis, neonatal HSV, mucocutaneous HSV in immunocompromised patients, varicella-zoster (chickenpox)

Usual Dosage Note: Obese patients should be dosed using ideal body weight

Genital HSV:
I.V.: Children ≥12 years and Adults (immunocompetent): Initial episode, severe: 5 mg/kg every 8 hours for 5-7 days
Oral: Adults:
  Initial episode: 200 mg every 4 hours while awake (5 times/day) for 10 days (per manufacturer's labeling); 400 mg 3 times/day for 5-10 days has also been reported
  Recurrence: 200 mg every 4 hours while awake (5 times/day) for 5 days (per manufacturer's labeling; begin at earliest signs of disease); 400 mg 3 times/day for 5 days has also been reported
  Chronic suppression: 400 mg twice daily or 200 mg 3-5 times/day, for up to 12 months followed by re-evaluation (per manufacturer's labeling); 400-1200 mg/day in 2-3 divided doses has also been reported
Topical: Adults (immunocompromised): Ointment: Initial episode: 1/2" ribbon of ointment for a 4" square surface area every 3 hours (6 times/day) for 7 days

Herpes labialis (cold sores): Topical: Children ≥12 years and Adults: Cream: Apply 5 times/day for 4 days

Herpes zoster (shingles):
Oral: Adults (immunocompetent): 800 mg every 4 hours (5 times/day) for 7-10 days
I.V.:
  Children <12 years (immunocompromised): 20 mg/kg/dose every 8 hours for 7 days
  Children ≥12 years and Adults (immunocompromised): 10 mg/kg/dose or 500 mg/m^2/dose every 8 hours for 7 days

HSV encephalitis: I.V.:
  Children 3 months to 12 years: 20 mg/kg/dose every 8 hours for 10 days (per manufacturer's labeling); dosing for 14-21 days also reported
  Children ≥12 years and Adults: 10 mg/kg/dose every 8 hours for 10 days (per manufacturer's labeling); 10-15 mg/kg/dose every 8 hours for 14-21 days also reported

Mucocutaneous HSV:
I.V.:
  Children <12 years (immunocompromised): 10 mg/kg/dose every 8 hours for 7 days
  Children ≥12 years and Adults (immunocompromised): 5 mg/kg/dose every 8 hours for 7 days (per manufacturer's labeling); dosing for up to 14 days also reported
Topical: Ointment: Adults (nonlife-threatening, immunocompromised): 1/2" ribbon of ointment for a 4" square surface area every 3 hours (6 times/day) for 7 days

Neonatal HSV: I.V.: Neonate: Birth to 3 months: 10 mg/kg/dose every 8 hours for 10 days (manufacturer's labeling); 15 mg/kg/dose or 20 mg/kg/dose every 8 hours for 14-21 days has also been reported

Varicella-zoster (chickenpox): Begin treatment within the first 24 hours of rash onset:
Oral:
  Children ≥2 years and ≤40 kg (immunocompetent): 20 mg/kg/dose (up to 800 mg/dose) 4 times/day for 5 days
  Children >40 kg and Adults (immunocompetent): 800 mg/dose 4 times a day for 5 days

Dosage Forms
Capsule: 200 mg
  Zovirax®: 200 mg
Cream, topical:
  Zovirax®: 5% (2 g, 5 g)

◀ **Injection, powder for reconstitution:** 500 mg, 1000 mg
Injection, solution [preservative free]: 50 mg/mL (10 mL, 20 mL)
Ointment, topical:
Zovirax®: 5% (15 g)
Suspension, oral: 200 mg/5 mL
Zovirax®: 200 mg/5 mL
Tablet: 400 mg, 800 mg
Zovirax®: 400 mg, 800 mg

Adacel™ [US/Can] *see* diphtheria, tetanus toxoids, and acellular pertussis vaccine *on page 309*
Adagen® [US/Can] *see* pegademase (bovine) *on page 726*
Adalat® XL® [Can] *see* nifedipine *on page 672*
Adalat® CC [US] *see* nifedipine *on page 672*
Adalat® *(Discontinued) see* nifedipine *on page 672*

adalimumab (a da LIM yoo mab)

Sound-Alike/Look-Alike Issues
Humira® may be confused with Humulin®, Humalog®
Humira® Pen may be confused with HumaPen® Memoir®
Synonyms antitumor necrosis factor apha (human); D2E7; human antitumor necrosis factor alpha
U.S./Canadian Brand Names Humira® [US/Can]
Therapeutic Category Antirheumatic, Disease Modifying; Monoclonal Antibody
Use
Treatment of active rheumatoid arthritis (moderate-to-severe) and active psoriatic arthritis; may be used alone or in combination with disease-modifying antirheumatic drugs (DMARDs); treatment of ankylosing spondylitis
Treatment of moderately- to severely-active Crohn disease in patients with inadequate response to conventional treatment, or patients who have lost response to or are intolerant of infliximab
Treatment of moderate-to-severe plaque psoriasis
Treatment of moderately- to severely-active juvenile idiopathic arthritis
Usual Dosage SubQ:
Children ≥4 years: Juvenile idiopathic arthritis:
15 kg to <30 kg: 20 mg every other week
≥30 kg: 40 mg every other week
Adults:
Rheumatoid arthritis: 40 mg every other week; may be administered with other DMARDs; patients not taking methotrexate may increase dose to 40 mg every week
Ankylosing spondylitis, psoriatic arthritis: 40 mg every other week
Crohn disease: Initial: 160 mg given as 4 injections on day 1 or over 2 days, then 80 mg 2 weeks later (day 15); Maintenance: 40 mg every other week beginning day 29
Plaque psoriasis: Initial: 80 mg as a single dose; maintenance: 40 mg every other week beginning 1 week after initial dose
Dosage Forms
Injection, solution [pediatric; preservative free]:
Humira®: 20 mg/0.4 mL (0.4 mL)
Injection, solution [preservative free]:
Humira®: 40 mg/0.8 mL (0.8 mL)

adamantanamine hydrochloride *see* amantadine *on page 56*

adapalene (a DAP a leen)

U.S./Canadian Brand Names Differin® XP [Can]; Differin® [US/Can]
Therapeutic Category Acne Products
Use Treatment of acne vulgaris
Usual Dosage Topical: Children >12 years and Adults: Apply once daily at bedtime; therapeutic results should be noticed after 8-12 weeks of treatment
Dosage Forms
Cream, topical:
Differin®: 0.1% (15 g, 45 g)

Gel, topical:
Differin®: 0.1% (15 g, 45 g); 0.3% (45 g)

Addaprin [US-OTC] *see* ibuprofen *on page 495*
Adderall® [US] *see* dextroamphetamine and amphetamine *on page 283*
Adderall XR® [US/Can] *see* dextroamphetamine and amphetamine *on page 283*

adefovir (a DEF o veer)

Synonyms adefovir dipivoxil
U.S./Canadian Brand Names Hepsera™ [US/Can]
Therapeutic Category Antiretroviral Agent, Nonnucleoside Reverse Transcriptase Inhibitor (NNRTI)
Use Treatment of chronic hepatitis B with evidence of active viral replication (based on persistent elevation of ALT/AST or histologic evidence), including patients with lamivudine-resistant hepatitis B
Usual Dosage Oral: Children ≥12 years and Adults: 10 mg once daily
Dosage Forms
Tablet:
Hepsera®: 10 mg

adefovir dipivoxil *see* adefovir *on page 35*
ADEKs [US-OTC] *see* vitamins (multiple/pediatric) *on page 983*
Adenocard® [US/Can] *see* adenosine *on page 35*
Adenoscan® [US/Can] *see* adenosine *on page 35*

adenosine (a DEN oh seen)

Synonyms 9-beta-d-ribofuranosyladenine
U.S./Canadian Brand Names Adenocard® [US/Can]; Adenoscan® [US/Can]; Adenosine Injection, USP [Can]
Therapeutic Category Antiarrhythmic Agent, Class IV; Diagnostic Agent
Use
Adenocard®: Treatment of paroxysmal supraventricular tachycardia (PSVT) including that associated with accessory bypass tracts (Wolff-Parkinson-White syndrome); when clinically advisable, appropriate vagal maneuvers should be attempted prior to adenosine administration; **not effective in atrial flutter, atrial fibrillation, or ventricular tachycardia**
Adenoscan®: Pharmacologic stress agent used in myocardial perfusion thallium-201 scintigraphy
Usual Dosage
Adenocard®: **Rapid I.V. push (over 1-2 seconds) via peripheral line:**
Infants and Children:
Manufacturer's recommendation:
<50 kg: 0.05-0.1 mg/kg. If conversion of PSVT does not occur within 1-2 minutes, may increase dose by 0.05-0.1 mg/kg. May repeat until sinus rhythm is established or to a maximum single dose of 0.3 mg/kg or 12 mg. Follow each dose with normal saline flush.
≥50 kg: Refer to Adult dosing
Pediatric advanced life support (PALS): Treatment of SVT: I.V., I.O.: 0.1 mg/kg; if not effective, administer 0.2 mg/kg of PSVT; medium dose required: 0.15 mg/kg; maximum single dose: 12 mg. Follow each dose with normal saline flush.
Adults: 6 mg; if not effective within 1-2 minutes, 12 mg may be given; may repeat 12 mg bolus if needed
Maximum single dose: 12 mg
Follow each I.V. bolus of adenosine with normal saline flush
Note: Preliminary results in adults suggest adenosine may be administered via a central line at lower doses (ie, initial adult dose: 3 mg).

Adenoscan®: Stress testing: Continuous I.V. infusion via peripheral line: 140 mcg/kg/minute for 6 minutes using syringe or columetric infusion pump; total dose: 0.84 mg/kg. Thallium-201 is injected at midpoint (3 minutes) of infusion.
Dosage Forms
Injection, solution [preservative free]: 3 mg/mL (2 mL, 4 mL)
Adenocard®: 3 mg/mL (2 mL, 4 mL)
Adenoscan®: 3 mg/mL (20 mL, 30 mL)

Adenosine Injection, USP [Can] *see* adenosine *on page 35*
Adept® [US] *see* icodextrin *on page 497*

ADH *see* vasopressin *on page 972*

Adipex-P® [US] *see* phentermine *on page 744*

ADL-2698 *see* alvimopan *on page 55*

Adlone® Injection *(Discontinued)* *see* methylprednisolone *on page 623*

Adoxa® [US] *see* doxycycline *on page 323*

Adrenalin® [US/Can] *see* epinephrine *on page 344*

adrenaline *see* epinephrine *on page 344*

adrenocorticotropic hormone *see* corticotropin *on page 249*

adria *see* doxorubicin *on page 322*

Adriamycin® [US/Can] *see* doxorubicin *on page 322*

Adrucil® [US] *see* fluorouracil *on page 412*

adsorbent charcoal *see* charcoal *on page 198*

Adsorbocarpine® Ophthalmic *(Discontinued)* *see* pilocarpine *on page 753*

Adsorbonac® *(Discontinued)* *see* sodium chloride *on page 873*

Adsorbotear® Ophthalmic Solution *(Discontinued)* *see* artificial tears *on page 95*

Advagraf™ [Can] *see* tacrolimus *on page 901*

Advair® [Can] *see* fluticasone and salmeterol *on page 417*

Advair Diskus® [US/Can] *see* fluticasone and salmeterol *on page 417*

Advair® HFA [US] *see* fluticasone and salmeterol *on page 417*

Advanced Formula Oxy® Sensitive Gel *(Discontinued)* *see* benzoyl peroxide *on page 126*

Advanced NatalCare® [US] *see* vitamins (multiple/prenatal) *on page 983*

Advanced-RF NatalCare® [US] *see* vitamins (multiple/prenatal) *on page 983*

Advantage-S™ [US-OTC] *see* nonoxynol 9 *on page 677*

Advate [US] *see* antihemophilic factor (recombinant) *on page 79*

Advicor® [US/Can] *see* niacin and lovastatin *on page 669*

Advil® [US-OTC/Can] *see* ibuprofen *on page 495*

Advil® Allergy Sinus [US] *see* ibuprofen, pseudoephedrine, and chlorpheniramine *on page 497*

Advil® Children's [US-OTC] *see* ibuprofen *on page 495*

Advil® Cold and Sinus Plus [Can] *see* ibuprofen, pseudoephedrine, and chlorpheniramine *on page 497*

Advil® Cold, Children's *(Discontinued)* *see* pseudoephedrine and ibuprofen *on page 802*

Advil® Cold & Sinus [US-OTC/Can] *see* pseudoephedrine and ibuprofen *on page 802*

Advil® Infants' [US-OTC] *see* ibuprofen *on page 495*

Advil® Junior *(Discontinued)* *see* ibuprofen *on page 495*

Advil® Migraine [US-OTC] *see* ibuprofen *on page 495*

Advil® Multi-Symptom Cold [US] *see* ibuprofen, pseudoephedrine, and chlorpheniramine *on page 497*

Aerius® [Can] *see* desloratadine *on page 274*

Aeroaid® *(Discontinued)*

AeroBid® [US] *see* flunisolide *on page 408*

AeroBid®-M [US] *see* flunisolide *on page 408*

Aerodine® *(Discontinued)* *see* povidone-iodine *on page 775*

aerohist plus™ [US] *see* chlorpheniramine, phenylephrine, and methscopolamine *on page 210*

aeroKid™ [US] *see* chlorpheniramine, phenylephrine, and methscopolamine *on page 210*

Afeditab™ CR [US] *see* nifedipine *on page 672*

Afluria® [US] *see* influenza virus vaccine *on page 508*

A-Free Prenatal [US] *see* vitamins (multiple/prenatal) *on page 983*

Afrin® Children's Nose Drops *(Discontinued)* *see* oxymetazoline *on page 712*

Afrin® Extra Moisturizing [US-OTC] *see* oxymetazoline *on page 712*

Afrinol® *(Discontinued)* *see* pseudoephedrine *on page 801*

Afrin® Original [US-OTC] *see* oxymetazoline *on page 712*

Afrin® Saline Mist *(Discontinued)* *see* sodium chloride *on page 873*

Afrin® Severe Congestion [US-OTC] *see* oxymetazoline *on page 712*

Afrin® Sinus [US-OTC] *see* oxymetazoline *on page 712*

Aftate® Antifungal *(Discontinued)* see tolnaftate *on page 934*

agalsidase alfa *(Canada only)* (aye GAL si days AL fa)
Sound-Alike/Look-Alike Issues
   agalsidase alfa may be confused with agalsidase beta, alglucerase, alglucosidase alfa
Synonyms agalsidase alpha; alpha-galactosidase-A (gene-activated)
U.S./Canadian Brand Names Replagal™ [Can]
Therapeutic Category Enzyme
Use Replacement therapy for Fabry disease
Usual Dosage Note: Premedication with oral antihistamines and corticosteroids may alleviate infusion-related reactions associated with agalsidase alfa.
   I.V.: Children and Adults: Fabry disease: 0.2 mg/kg every 2 weeks
Dosage Forms [CAN] = Canadian brand name
  Injection, solution [preservative free]:
   Replagal™ [CAN]: 1 mg/1mL (3.5 mL) [not available in the U.S.]

agalsidase alpha see agalsidase alfa *(Canada only)* on page 37

agalsidase beta (aye GAL si days BAY ta)
Sound-Alike/Look-Alike Issues
   agalsidase beta may be confused with agalsidase alfa, alglucerase, alglucosidase alfa
Synonyms alpha-galactosidase-A (recombinant); r-h α-GAL
U.S./Canadian Brand Names Fabrazyme® [US/Can]
Therapeutic Category Enzyme
Use Replacement therapy for Fabry disease
Usual Dosage I.V.: Children ≥8 years and Adults: 1 mg/kg every 2 weeks
Dosage Forms
  Injection, powder for reconstitution:
   Fabrazyme®: 5 mg, 35 mg

Agenerase® [Can] *see* amprenavir *on page 74*
Agenerase® *(Discontinued)* *see* amprenavir *on page 74*
Aggrastat® [US/Can] *see* tirofiban *on page 930*
Aggrenox® [US/Can] *see* aspirin and dipyridamole *on page 100*
AGN 1135 *see* rasagiline *on page 820*
AgNO₃ *see* silver nitrate *on page 866*
Agrylin® [US/Can] *see* anagrelide *on page 75*
AHA *see* acetohydroxamic acid *on page 29*
AH-Chew® [US] *see* chlorpheniramine, phenylephrine, and methscopolamine *on page 210*
AH-Chew™ Ultra [US] *see* chlorpheniramine, phenylephrine, and methscopolamine *on page 210*
AHF (human) *see* antihemophilic factor (human) *on page 78*
AHF (human) *see* antihemophilic factor/von Willebrand factor complex (human) *on page 80*
AHF (recombinant) *see* antihemophilic factor (recombinant) *on page 79*
Ahist™ [US] *see* chlorpheniramine *on page 205*
AICC *see* antiinhibitor coagulant complex *on page 81*
Airet® *(Discontinued)* *see* albuterol *on page 39*
Airomir [Can] *see* albuterol *on page 39*
AKBeta® *(Discontinued)* *see* levobunolol *on page 555*
Ak-Chlor® Ophthalmic *(Discontinued)* *see* chloramphenicol *on page 200*
AK-Con™ [US] *see* naphazoline *on page 655*
AK-Dilate® [US] *see* phenylephrine *on page 745*
AK-Fluor® [US] *see* fluorescein *on page 410*
Ak-Homatropine® Ophthalmic *(Discontinued)* *see* homatropine *on page 475*
Akineton® *(Discontinued)*
AK-Nefrin *(Discontinued)* *see* phenylephrine *on page 745*
Akne-Mycin® [US] *see* erythromycin *on page 354*

AK-Pentolate™ [US] *see* cyclopentolate *on page 256*

AK-Poly-Bac™ [US] *see* bacitracin and polymyxin B *on page 113*

AK-Pred® [US] *see* prednisolone (ophthalmic) *on page 781*

AK-Spore® H.C. Ophthalmic *(Discontinued)* *see* bacitracin, neomycin, polymyxin B, and hydrocortisone *on page 114*

AK-Spore® H.C. Otic *(Discontinued)* *see* neomycin, polymyxin B, and hydrocortisone *on page 663*

AK-Spore® Ophthalmic Ointment *(Discontinued)* *see* bacitracin, neomycin, and polymyxin B *on page 114*

AK-Taine® *(Discontinued)* *see* proparacaine *on page 794*

AKTob® [US] *see* tobramycin *on page 931*

AK-Tracin® *(Discontinued)* *see* bacitracin *on page 113*

AK-Trol® Ophthalmic Ointment *(Discontinued)* *see* neomycin, polymyxin B, and dexamethasone *on page 662*

AK-Trol® Ophthalmic Suspension *(Discontinued)* *see* neomycin, polymyxin B, and dexamethasone *on page 662*

Akurza [US] *see* salicylic acid *on page 850*

Akwa Tears® [US-OTC] *see* artificial tears *on page 95*

Alamag [US-OTC] *see* aluminum hydroxide and magnesium hydroxide *on page 54*

Alamag Plus [US-OTC] *see* aluminum hydroxide, magnesium hydroxide, and simethicone *on page 54*

Alamast® [US/Can] *see* pemirolast *on page 730*

Alavert™ [US-OTC] *see* loratadine *on page 576*

Alavert™ Allergy and Sinus [US-OTC] *see* loratadine and pseudoephedrine *on page 576*

Alavert™ Allergy Relief 24-Hour [US-OTC] *see* loratadine *on page 576*

Alaway™ [US-OTC] *see* ketotifen *on page 538*

Alazide® *(Discontinued)* *see* hydrochlorothiazide and spironolactone *on page 480*

Albalon-A® Ophthalmic *(Discontinued)*

Albalon® *(Discontinued)* *see* naphazoline *on page 655*

albendazole (al BEN da zole)

U.S./Canadian Brand Names Albenza® [US]

Therapeutic Category Anthelmintic

Use Treatment of parenchymal neurocysticercosis caused by *Taenia solium* and cystic hydatid disease of the liver, lung, and peritoneum caused by *Echinococcus granulosus*

Usual Dosage Oral: Children and Adults:

Neurocysticercosis:

<60 kg: 15 mg/kg/day in 2 divided doses (maximum: 800 mg/day) for 8-30 days

≥60 kg: 800 mg/day in 2 divided doses for 8-30 days

Note: Give concurrent anticonvulsant and steroid therapy during first week.

Hydatid:

<60 kg: 15 mg/kg/day in 2 divided doses (maximum: 800 mg/day)

≥60 kg: 800 mg/day in 2 divided doses

Note: Administer dose for three 28-day cycles with a 14-day drug-free interval in between. The manufacturer recommends a total of 3 cycles.

Dosage Forms

Tablet:

Albenza®: 200 mg

Albenza® [US] *see* albendazole *on page 38*

Albert® Glyburide [Can] *see* glyburide *on page 448*

Albert® Pentoxifylline [Can] *see* pentoxifylline *on page 737*

Albumarc® [US] *see* albumin *on page 38*

albumin (al BYOO min)

Sound-Alike/Look-Alike Issues

Albutein® may be confused with albuterol

Buminate® may be confused with bumetanide

Synonyms albumin (human); normal human serum albumin; normal serum albumin (human); salt-poor albumin; SPA

U.S./Canadian Brand Names Albumarc® [US]; Albuminar® [US]; AlbuRx™ [US]; Albutein® [US]; Buminate® [US]; Flexbumin [US]; Plasbumin® [US]; Plasbumin®-25 [Can]; Plasbumin®-5 [Can]

Therapeutic Category Blood Product Derivative

Use Plasma volume expansion and maintenance of cardiac output in the treatment of certain types of shock or impending shock; may be useful for burn patients, ARDS, and cardiopulmonary bypass; other uses considered by some investigators (but not proven) are retroperitoneal surgery, peritonitis, and ascites; unless the condition responsible for hypoproteinemia can be corrected, albumin can provide only symptomatic relief or supportive treatment

Usual Dosage I.V.:

5% should be used in hypovolemic patients or intravascularly-depleted patients

25% should be used in patients in whom fluid and sodium intake must be minimized

Dose depends on condition of patient:

Children: Hypovolemia: 0.5-1 g/kg/dose (10-20 mL/kg/dose of albumin 5%); maximum dose: 6 g/kg/day

Adults: Usual dose: 25 g; initial dose may be repeated in 15-30 minutes if response is inadequate; no more than 250 g should be administered within 48 hours

Hypoproteinemia: 0.5-1 g/kg/dose; repeat every 1-2 days as calculated to replace ongoing losses

Hypovolemia: 5% albumin: 0.5-1 g/kg/dose; repeat as needed. **Note:** May be considered after inadequate response to crystalloid therapy and when nonprotein colloids are contraindicated. The volume administered and the speed of infusion should be adapted to individual response.

Dosage Forms

Injection, solution [preservative free; human]:

Albuminar®: 5% (50 mL, 250 mL, 500 mL) [50 mg/mL]; 25% (20 mL, 50 mL, 100 mL) [250 mg/mL]

AlbuRx™: 5% (250 mL, 500 mL) [50 mg/mL]; 25% (50 mL, 100 mL) [250 mg/mL]

Albutein®: 5% (250 mL, 500 mL) [50 mg/mL]

Buminate®: 5% (250 mL, 500 mL) [50 mg/mL]; 25% (20 mL, 50 mL, 100 mL) [250 mg/mL]

Flexbumin: 25% (50 mL, 100 mL) [250 mg/mL]

Human Albumin Grifols®: 25% (50 mL, 100 mL) [250 mg/mL]

Plasbumin®: 5% (50 mL, 250 mL) [50 mg/mL]; 25% (20 mL, 50 mL, 100 mL) [250 mg/mL]

Albuminar® [US] see albumin on page 38

albumin-bound paclitaxel see paclitaxel (protein bound) on page 715

albumin (human) see albumin on page 38

Albumisol® (Discontinued) see albumin on page 38

Albunex® (Discontinued) see albumin on page 38

AlbuRx™ [US] see albumin on page 38

Albutein® [US] see albumin on page 38

albuterol (al BYOO ter ole)

Sound-Alike/Look-Alike Issues

albuterol may be confused with Albutein®, atenolol

Proventil® may be confused with Bentyl®, Prilosec® Prinivil®

salbutamol may be confused with salmeterol

Ventolin® may be confused with phentolamine, Benylin®, Vantin®

Volmax® may be confused with Flomax®

Synonyms albuterol sulfate; salbutamol; salbutamol sulphate

U.S./Canadian Brand Names AccuNeb® [US]; Airomir [Can]; Alti-Salbutamol [Can]; Apo-Salvent® CFC Free [Can]; Apo-Salvent® Respirator Solution [Can]; Apo-Salvent® Sterules [Can]; Apo-Salvent® [Can]; Gen-Salbutamol [Can]; PMS-Salbutamol [Can]; ProAir™ HFA [US]; Proventil® HFA [US]; ratio-Inspra-Sal [Can]; ratio-Salbutamol [Can]; Rhoxal-salbutamol [Can]; Salbu-2 [Can]; Salbu-4 [Can]; Ventolin® Diskus [Can]; Ventolin® HFA [US/Can]; Ventolin® I.V. Infusion [Can]; Ventolin® [Can]; Ventrodisk [Can]; VoSpire ER® [US]

Therapeutic Category Adrenergic Agonist Agent

Use Bronchodilator in reversible airway obstruction due to asthma or COPD; prevention of exercise-induced bronchospasm

Usual Dosage

Oral:

Children: Bronchospasm:

2-6 years: 0.1-0.2 mg/kg/dose 3 times/day; maximum dose not to exceed 12 mg/day (divided doses) ▶

◄

6-12 years: 2 mg/dose 3-4 times/day; maximum dose not to exceed 24 mg/day (divided doses)
  Extended release: 4 mg every 12 hours; maximum dose not to exceed 24 mg/day (divided doses)
Children >12 years and Adults: Bronchospasm (treatment): 2-4 mg/dose 3-4 times/day; maximum dose not to exceed 32 mg/day (divided doses)
  Extended release: 8 mg every 12 hours; maximum dose not to exceed 32 mg/day (divided doses). A 4 mg dose every 12 hours may be sufficient in some patients, such as adults of low body weight.

Metered-dose inhaler (90 mcg/puff):
  Children ≤4 years *(NIH Guidelines, 2007)*:
    Quick relief: 1-2 puffs every 4-6 hours as needed
    Exacerbation of asthma (acute, severe): 4-8 puffs every 20 minutes for 3 doses, then every 1-4 hours as needed
    Exercise-induced bronchospasm (prevention): 1-2 puffs 5 minutes prior to exercise
  Children 5-11 years *(NIH Guidelines, 2007)*:
    Bronchospasm, quick relief: 2 puffs every 4-6 hours as needed
    Exacerbation of asthma (acute, severe): 4-8 puffs every 20 minutes for 3 doses, then every 1-4 hours as needed
    Exercise-induced bronchospasm (prevention): 2 puffs 5-30 minutes prior to exercise
  Children ≥12 years and Adults:
    Bronchospasm, quick relief *(NIH Guidelines, 2007)*: 2 puffs every 4-6 hours as needed
    Exacerbation of asthma (acute, severe) *(NIH Guidelines, 2007)*: 4-8 puffs every 20 minutes for up to 4 hours, then every 1-4 hours as needed
    Exercise-induced bronchospasm (prevention) *(NIH Guidelines, 2007)*: 2 puffs 5-30 minutes prior to exercise

Solution for nebulization:
  Children 2-12 years (AccuNeb®): Bronchospasm: 0.63-1.25 mg every 4-6 hours as needed
  Children ≤4 years *(NIH Guidelines, 2007)*:
    Quick relief: 0.63-2.5 mg every 4-6 hours as needed
    Exacerbation of asthma (acute, severe): 0.15 mg/kg (minimum: 2.5 mg) every 20 minutes for 3 doses, then 0.15-0.3 mg/kg (maximum: 10 mg) every 1-4 hours as needed **or** 0.5 mg/kg/hour by continuous nebulization
  Children 5-11 years *(NIH Guidelines, 2007)*:
    Quick relief: 1.25-5 mg every 4-8 hours as needed
    Exacerbation of asthma (acute, severe): 0.15 mg/kg (minimum: 2.5 mg) every 20 minutes for 3 doses, then 0.15-0.3 mg/kg (maximum: 10 mg) every 1-4 hours as needed **or** 0.5 mg/kg/hour by continuous nebulization
  Children ≥12 years and Adults:
    Bronchospasm: 2.5 mg every 4-8 hours as needed
    Quick relief *(NIH Guidelines, 2007)*: 1.25-5 mg every 4-8 hours as needed
    Exacerbation of asthma (acute, severe) *(NIH Guidelines, 2007)*: 2.5-5 mg every 20 minutes for 3 doses then 2.5-10 mg every 1-4 hours as needed, **or** 10-15 mg/hour by continuous nebulization

I.V. continuous infusion: Adults (Ventolin® I.V. solution [not available in U.S.]): Severe bronchospasm and status asthmaticus: Initial: 5 mcg/minute; may increase up to 10-20 mcg/minute at 15- to 30-minute intervals if needed

Dosage Forms [CAN] = Canadian brand name
  Aerosol, for oral inhalation
    ProAir™ HFA: 90 mcg/metered inhalation (8.5 g)
    Proventil® HFA: 90 mcg/metered inhalation (6.7 g)
    Ventolin® HFA: 90 mcg/metered inhalation (8 g, 18 g)
  Injection, solution, as sulphate:
    Ventolin® I.V. [CAN]: 1 mg/1mL (5 mL) [not available in U.S.]
  Solution for nebulization: 0.042% (3 mL); 0.083% (3 mL); 0.5% (0.5 mL, 20 mL)
    AccuNeb® [preservative free]: 0.63 mg/3 mL (3 mL) [0.021%]; 1.25 mg/3 mL (3 mL) [0.042%]
  Syrup: 2 mg/5 mL
  Tablet: 2 mg, 4 mg
  Tablet, extended release: 4 mg, 8 mg
    VoSpire ER™: 4 mg, 8 mg

albuterol and ipratropium *see* ipratropium and albuterol *on page 525*
albuterol sulfate *see* albuterol *on page 39*
Alcaine® [US/Can] *see* proparacaine *on page 794*
Alcalak [US-OTC] *see* calcium carbonate *on page 163*

alclometasone (al kloe MET a sone)
Sound-Alike/Look-Alike Issues
Aclovate® may be confused with Accolate®
Synonyms alclometasone dipropionate
U.S./Canadian Brand Names Aclovate® [US]
Therapeutic Category Corticosteroid, Topical
Use Treatment of inflammation of corticosteroid-responsive dermatosis (low to medium potency topical corticosteroid)
Usual Dosage Note: Therapy should be discontinued when control is achieved; if no improvement is seen within 2 weeks, reassessment of diagnosis may be necessary.
Topical:
Children ≥1 year: Apply thin film to affected area 2-3 times/day; do not use for >3 weeks
Adults: Apply a thin film to the affected area 2-3 times/day
Dosage Forms
Cream: 0.05% (15 g, 45 g, 60 g)
Aclovate®: 0.05% (15 g, 60 g)
Ointment: 0.05% (15 g, 45 g, 60 g)
Aclovate®: 0.05% (15 g, 45 g, 60 g)

alclometasone dipropionate *see alclometasone on page 41*
alcohol, absolute *see alcohol (ethyl) on page 41*
alcohol, dehydrated *see alcohol (ethyl) on page 41*

alcohol (ethyl) (AL koe hol, ETH il)
Sound-Alike/Look-Alike Issues
ethanol may be confused with Ethyol®, Ethamolin®
Synonyms alcohol, absolute; alcohol, dehydrated; ethanol; ethyl alcohol; EtOH
U.S./Canadian Brand Names Biobase-G™ [Can]; Biobase™ [Can]; EpiClenz™ [US-OTC]; Gel-Stat™ [US-OTC]; GelRite [US-OTC]; Isagel® [US-OTC]; Lavacol® [US-OTC]; Prevacare® [US-OTC]; Protection Plus® [US-OTC]; Purell® 2 in 1 [US-OTC]; Purell® with Aloe [US-OTC]; Purell® [US-OTC]
Therapeutic Category Intravenous Nutritional Therapy; Pharmaceutical Aid
Use Topical antiinfective; pharmaceutical aid; therapeutic neurolysis (nerve or ganglion block); replenishment of fluid and carbohydrate calories
Usual Dosage
Antiseptic: Children and Adults: Liquid denatured alcohol: Topical: Apply 1-3 times/day as needed
Therapeutic neurolysis (nerve or ganglion block): Adults: Dehydrated alcohol injection 98%: Intraneural: Dosage variable depending upon the site of injection (eg, trigeminal neuralgia: 0.05-0.5 mL as a single injection per interspace vs subarachnoid injection: 0.5-1 mL as a single injection per interspace); single doses >1.5 mL are seldom required
Replenishment of fluid and carbohydrate calories: Adults: Dehydrated alcohol infusion: Alcohol 5% and dextrose 5%: 1-2 L/day by slow infusion
Dosage Forms
Foam, topical:
Epi-Clenz™: 62% (240 mL, 480 mL)
Gel, topical:
Epi-Clenz™: 70% (45 mL, 120 mL, 480 mL)
GelRite: 67% (120 mL, 480 mL, 800 mL)
Gel-Stat™: 62% (120 mL, 480 mL)
Isagel®: 60% (59 mL, 118 mL, 621 mL, 800 mL)
Prevacare®: 60% (120 mL, 240 mL, 960 mL, 1200 mL, 1500 mL)
Protection Plus®: 62% (800 mL)
Purell®: 62% (15 mL, 30 mL, 59 mL, 120 mL, 236 mL, 250 mL, 360 mL, 500 mL, 800 mL, 1000 mL, 2000 mL)
Purell® Moisture Therapy: 62% (75 mL)
Purell® with Aloe: 62% (15 mL, 59 mL, 236 mL, 360 mL, 800 mL, 1000 mL, 2000 mL)
Injection, solution [dehydrated]: 98% (1 mL, 5 mL)
Liquid, topical [denatured]: 70% (3840 mL)
Lavacol® [OTC]: 70% (473 mL)

◄ **Lotion, topical:**
Purell® 2 in 1: 62% (60 mL, 360 mL, 1000 mL)
Towlettes, topical:
Isagel®: 60% (50s, 300s)
Purell®: 62% (35s, 175s)

Alcomicin® [Can] *see* gentamicin *on page 442*
Alconefrin® Nasal Solution *(Discontinued)* *see* phenylephrine *on page 745*
Alcortin™ [US] *see* iodoquinol and hydrocortisone *on page 520*
Aldactazide® [US] *see* hydrochlorothiazide and spironolactone *on page 480*
Aldactazide 25® [Can] *see* hydrochlorothiazide and spironolactone *on page 480*
Aldactazide 50® [Can] *see* hydrochlorothiazide and spironolactone *on page 480*
Aldactone® [US/Can] *see* spironolactone *on page 886*
Aldara® [US/Can] *see* imiquimod *on page 502*

aldesleukin (al des LOO kin)

Sound-Alike/Look-Alike Issues
aldesleukin may be confused with oprelvekin
Proleukin® may be confused with oprelvekin
Synonyms epidermal thymocyte activating factor; IL-2; interleukin-2; lymphocyte mitogenic factor; NSC-373364; T-cell growth factor; TCGF; thymocyte stimulating factor
U.S./Canadian Brand Names Proleukin® [US/Can]
Therapeutic Category Biological Response Modulator
Use Treatment of metastatic renal cell cancer, metastatic melanoma
Usual Dosage Refer to individual protocols. I.V.:
Renal cell carcinoma: 600,000 int. units/kg every 8 hours for a maximum of 14 doses; repeat after 9 days for a total of 28 doses per course. Retreat if needed 7 weeks after previous course.
Melanoma: Single-agent use: 600,000 int. units/kg every 8 hours for a maximum of 14 doses; repeat after 9 days for a total of 28 doses per course. Retreat if needed 7 weeks after previous course.
Dosage Forms
Injection, powder for reconstitution:
Proleukin®: 22 x 10^6 int. units

Aldex™ [US] *see* guaifenesin and phenylephrine *on page 456*
Aldex®D [US] *see* phenylephrine and pyrilamine *on page 747*
Aldex® DM [US] *see* phenylephrine, pyrilamine, and dextromethorphan *on page 749*
Aldomet® *(Discontinued)* *see* methyldopa *on page 620*
Aldoril® [US] *see* methyldopa and hydrochlorothiazide *on page 620*
Aldoril® D50 *(Discontinued)* *see* methyldopa and hydrochlorothiazide *on page 620*
Aldroxicon I [US-OTC] *see* aluminum hydroxide, magnesium hydroxide, and simethicone *on page 54*
Aldroxicon II [US-OTC] *see* aluminum hydroxide, magnesium hydroxide, and simethicone *on page 54*
Aldurazyme® [US/Can] *see* laronidase *on page 550*

alefacept (a LE fa sept)

Synonyms B 9273; BG 9273; human LFA-3/IgG(1) fusion protein; LFA-3/IgG(1) fusion protein, human
U.S./Canadian Brand Names Amevive® [US/Can]
Therapeutic Category Monoclonal Antibody
Use Treatment of moderate-to-severe chronic plaque psoriasis in adults who are candidates for systemic therapy or phototherapy
Usual Dosage Adults:
I.M.: 15 mg once weekly; usual duration of treatment: 12 weeks
A second course of treatment may be initiated at least 12 weeks after completion of the initial course of treatment, provided CD4+ T-lymphocyte counts are within the normal range.
Note: CD4+ T-lymphocyte counts should be monitored before initiation of treatment and every 2 weeks during therapy. Dosing should be withheld if CD4+ counts are <250 cells/μL, and dosing should be permanently discontinued if CD4+ lymphocyte counts remain at <250 cell/μL for longer than 1 month.

Dosage Forms
Injection, powder for reconstitution [I.M. administration]:
Amevive®: 15 mg

alemtuzumab (ay lem TU zoo mab)

Synonyms C1H; campath-1H; humanized IgG1 anti-CD52 monoclonal antibody; NSC-715969
U.S./Canadian Brand Names Campath® [US]; MabCampath® [Can]
Therapeutic Category Antineoplastic Agent, Monoclonal Antibody
Use Treatment of B-cell chronic lymphocytic leukemia (B-CLL)
Usual Dosage Note: Dose escalation is required; usually accomplished in 3-7 days. Do not exceed single doses >30 mg or cumulative doses >90 mg/week. Pretreatment (with acetaminophen and an oral antihistamine) is recommended prior to the first dose, with dose escalations, and as clinically indicated; I.V. hydrocortisone may be used for severe infusion-related reactions.
I.V. infusion, SubQ (unlabeled route): Adults: B-CLL:
Initial: 3 mg/day beginning on day 1; when tolerated (no grade 3 or 4 infusion reactions), increase to maintenance dose of 30 mg/dose 3 times/week on alternate days for a total duration of therapy of up to 12 weeks
Maximum dose/day: 30 mg; maximum cumulative dose/week: 90 mg
Dosage Forms
Injection, solution [preservative free]:
Campath®: 30 mg/mL (1 mL)

alendronate (a LEN droe nate)

Sound-Alike/Look-Alike Issues
Fosamax® may be confused with Flomax®
Synonyms alendronate sodium
U.S./Canadian Brand Names Apo-Alendronate® [Can]; CO Alendronate [Can]; Dom-Alendronate [Can]; Fosamax® [US/Can]; Gen-Alendronate [Can]; Novo-Alendronate [Can]; PHL-Alendronate [Can]; PHL-Alendronate-FC [Can]; PMS-Alendronate [Can]; PMS-Alendronate-FC [Can]; ratio-Alendronate [Can]; Riva-Alendronate [Can]; Sandoz Alendronate [Can]
Therapeutic Category Bisphosphonate Derivative
Use Treatment and prevention of osteoporosis in postmenopausal females; treatment of osteoporosis in males; Paget disease of the bone in patients who are symptomatic, at risk for future complications, or with alkaline phosphatase ≥2 times the upper limit of normal; treatment of glucocorticoid-induced osteoporosis in males and females with low bone mineral density who are receiving a daily dosage ≥7.5 mg of prednisone (or equivalent)
Usual Dosage Oral: Adults: **Note:** Patients treated with glucocorticoids and those with Paget disease should receive adequate amounts of calcium and vitamin D.
Osteoporosis in postmenopausal females:
Prophylaxis: 5 mg once daily **or** 35 mg once weekly
Treatment: 10 mg once daily **or** 70 mg once weekly
Osteoporosis in males: 10 mg once daily **or** 70 mg once weekly
Osteoporosis secondary to glucocorticoids in males and females: Treatment: 5 mg once daily; a dose of 10 mg once daily should be used in postmenopausal females who are not receiving estrogen.
Paget disease of bone in males and females: 40 mg once daily for 6 months
Retreatment: Relapses during the 12 months following therapy occurred in 9% of patients who responded to treatment. Specific retreatment data are not available. Following a 6-month post-treatment evaluation period, retreatment with alendronate may be considered in patients who have relapsed based on increases in serum alkaline phosphatase, which should be measured periodically. Retreatment may also be considered in those who failed to normalize their serum alkaline phosphatase.
Dosage Forms
Solution, oral:
Fosamax®: 70 mg/75 mL
Tablet: 5 mg, 10 mg, 35 mg, 40 mg, 70 mg
Fosamax®: 5 mg, 10 mg, 35 mg, 40 mg, 70 mg

alendronate and cholecalciferol (a LEN droe nate & kole e kal SI fer ole)

Synonyms alendronate sodium and cholecalciferol; cholecalciferol and alendronate; vitamin D₃ and alendronate

▶

◄ **U.S./Canadian Brand Names** Fosamax Plus D™ [US]; Fosavance [Can]

Therapeutic Category Bisphosphonate Derivative; Vitamin D Analog

Use Treatment of osteoporosis in postmenopausal females; increase bone mass in males with osteoporosis

Usual Dosage Oral: Adults: One tablet (alendronate 70 mg/cholecalciferol 2800 int. units **or** alendronate 70 mg/cholecalciferol 5600 int. units) once weekly. Appropriate dose in most osteoporotic women or men: Alendronate 70 mg/cholecalciferol 5600 int. units once weekly.

Dosage Forms

Tablet:

Fosamax Plus D™ 70/2800: Alendronate 70 mg and cholecalciferol 2800 int. units

Fosamax Plus D™ 70/5600: Alendronate 70 mg and cholecalciferol 5600 int. units

alendronate sodium *see alendronate on page 43*

alendronate sodium and cholecalciferol *see alendronate and cholecalciferol on page 43*

Alenic Alka [US-OTC] *see aluminum hydroxide and magnesium carbonate on page 53*

Alenic Alka Tablet [US-OTC] *see aluminum hydroxide and magnesium trisilicate on page 54*

Aler-Cap [US-OTC] *see diphenhydramine on page 304*

Aler-Dryl [US-OTC] *see diphenhydramine on page 304*

Aler-Tab [US-OTC] *see diphenhydramine on page 304*

Alertec® [Can] *see modafinil on page 639*

Alesse® [US/Can] *see ethinyl estradiol and levonorgestrel on page 372*

Aleve® [US-OTC] *see naproxen on page 656*

Aleve®-D Sinus & Cold [US-OTC] *see naproxen and pseudoephedrine on page 657*

Aleve® Cold & Sinus *(Discontinued)* *see naproxen and pseudoephedrine on page 657*

Aleve® Sinus & Headache [US-OTC] *see naproxen and pseudoephedrine on page 657*

Alfenta® [US/Can] *see alfentanil on page 44*

alfentanil (al FEN ta nil)

Sound-Alike/Look-Alike Issues

alfentanil may be confused with Anafranil®, fentanyl, remifentanil, sufentanil

Alfenta® may be confused with Sufenta®

Synonyms alfentanil hydrochloride

U.S./Canadian Brand Names Alfentanil Injection, USP [Can]; Alfenta® [US/Can]

Therapeutic Category Analgesic, Narcotic; General Anesthetic

Controlled Substance C-II

Use Analgesic adjunct given by continuous infusion or in incremental doses in maintenance of anesthesia with barbiturate or N_2O or a primary anesthetic agent for the induction of anesthesia in patients undergoing general surgery in which endotracheal intubation and mechanical ventilation are required

Usual Dosage Doses should be titrated to appropriate effects; wide range of doses is dependent upon desired degree of analgesia/anesthesia

Adults: Dose should be based on ideal body weight.

Dosage Forms

Injection, solution [preservative free]: 500 mcg/mL (2 mL, 5 mL)

Alfenta®: 500 mcg/mL (2 mL, 5 mL, 10 mL, 20 mL)

alfentanil hydrochloride *see alfentanil on page 44*

Alfentanil Injection, USP [Can] *see alfentanil on page 44*

Alferon® N [US/Can] *see interferon alfa-n3 on page 517*

alfuzosin (al FYOO zoe sin)

Synonyms alfuzosin hydrochloride

U.S./Canadian Brand Names Uroxatral® [US]; Xatral [Can]

Therapeutic Category Alpha-Adrenergic Blocking Agent

Use Treatment of the functional symptoms of benign prostatic hyperplasia (BPH)

Usual Dosage Oral: Adults: 10 mg once daily

Dosage Forms
Tablet, extended release:
Uroxatral®: 10 mg

alfuzosin hydrochloride *see* alfuzosin *on page 44*

alglucerase (al GLOO ser ase)

Sound-Alike/Look-Alike Issues
alglucerase may be confused with agalsidase alfa, agalsidase beta, alglucosidase alfa
Ceredase® may be confused with Cerezyme®

Synonyms glucocerebrosidase

U.S./Canadian Brand Names Ceredase® [US]

Therapeutic Category Enzyme

Use Replacement therapy for Gaucher disease (type 1)

Usual Dosage I.V.: Children and Adults: Initial: 30-60 units/kg every 2 weeks; dosing is individualized based on disease severity; average dose: 60 units/kg every 2 weeks. Range: 2.5 units/kg 3 times/week to 60 units/kg once weekly to every 4 weeks. Once patient response is well established, dose may be reduced every 3-6 months to determine maintenance therapy.

Dosage Forms
Injection, solution [preservative free]:
Ceredase®: 80 units/mL (5 mL)

alglucosidase *see* alglucosidase alfa *on page 45*

alglucosidase alfa (al gloo KOSE i dase AL fa)

Sound-Alike/Look-Alike Issues
alglucosidase alfa may be confused with agalsidase alfa, agalsidase beta, alglucerase

Synonyms alglucosidase; GAA; rhGAA

U.S./Canadian Brand Names Myozyme® [US]

Therapeutic Category Enzyme

Use Replacement therapy for Pompe disease (infantile onset)

Usual Dosage I.V.: Children 1 month to 3.5 years (at first infusion): 20 mg/kg over ~4 hours every 2 weeks

Dosage Forms
Injection, powder for reconstitution [preservative free]:
Myozyme®: 50 mg

Alimta® [US/Can] *see* pemetrexed *on page 729*

Alinia® [US] *see* nitazoxanide *on page 673*

aliskiren (a lis KYE ren)

Synonyms aliskiren hemifumarate; SPP100

U.S./Canadian Brand Names Rasilez® [Can]; Tekturna® [US]

Therapeutic Category Renin Inhibitor

Use Treatment of hypertension, alone or in combination with other antihypertensive agents

Usual Dosage Oral: Adults: Initial: 150 mg once daily; may increase to 300 mg once daily (maximum: 300 mg/day). **Note:** Prior to initiation, correct hypovolemia and/or closely monitor volume status in patients on concurrent diuretics during treatment initiation.

Dosage Forms
Tablet:
Tekturna®: 150 mg, 300 mg

aliskiren and hydrochlorothiazide (a lis KYE ren & hye droe klor oh THYE a zide)

Synonyms aliskiren hemifumarate and hydrochlorothiazide; hydrochlorothiazide and aliskiren

U.S./Canadian Brand Names Tekturna HCT® [US]

Therapeutic Category Antihypertensive Agent, Combination; Diuretic, Thiazide; Renin Inhibitor

▶

◀ **Use** Treatment of hypertension (not recommended for initial treatment)

Usual Dosage Oral: Adults: One tablet daily; dosage must be individualized (see below). May be substituted for previously titrated dosages of the individual components. Titrate at 2- to 4-week intervals as necessary.

Patients not controlled with single-agent therapy: Initiate by adding the lowest available dose of the alternative component (aliskiren 150 mg or hydrochlorothiazide 12.5 mg); titrate to effect (maximum daily aliskiren dose: 300 mg; maximum daily hydrochlorothiazide dose: 25 mg)

Dosage Forms

Tablet:

Tekturna HCT®: 150/12.5: Aliskiren 150 mg and hydrochlorothiazide 12.5 mg; 150/25: Aliskiren 150 mg and hydrochlorothiazide 25 mg; 300/12.5: Aliskiren 300 mg and hydrochlorothiazide 12.5 mg; 300/25: Aliskiren 300 mg and hydrochlorothiazide 25 mg

aliskiren hemifumarate *see* aliskiren *on page 45*

aliskiren hemifumarate and hydrochlorothiazide *see* aliskiren and hydrochlorothiazide *on page 45*

alitretinoin (a li TRET i noyn)

Sound-Alike/Look-Alike Issues

Panretin® may be confused with pancreatin

U.S./Canadian Brand Names Panretin® [US/Can]

Therapeutic Category Antineoplastic Agent, Miscellaneous; Retinoic Acid Derivative

Use Orphan drug: Topical treatment of cutaneous lesions in AIDS-related Kaposi sarcoma

Usual Dosage Topical: Apply gel twice daily to cutaneous lesions

Dosage Forms

Gel:

Panretin®: 0.1% (60 g)

Alka-Mints® [US-OTC] *see* calcium carbonate *on page 163*

Alka-Seltzer Plus® Day Cold [US-OTC] *see* acetaminophen, dextromethorphan, and phenylephrine *on page 26*

Alka-Seltzer Plus® Sinus Formula [US-OTC] *see* acetaminophen and phenylephrine *on page 22*

Alkeran® [US/Can] *see* melphalan *on page 599*

Allanderm-T™ [US] *see* trypsin, balsam peru, and castor oil *on page 958*

AllanEnzyme [US] *see* papain and urea *on page 721*

Allanfil 405 [US] *see* chlorophyllin, papain, and urea *on page 203*

Allanfil Spray [US] *see* chlorophyllin, papain, and urea *on page 203*

AllanFol RX (Discontinued) *see* folic acid, cyanocobalamin, and pyridoxine *on page 422*

AllanHist PDX [US] *see* brompheniramine, pseudoephedrine, and dextromethorphan *on page 146*

AllanTan Pediatric (Discontinued) *see* chlorpheniramine and phenylephrine *on page 206*

AllanVan-DM [US] *see* phenylephrine, pyrilamine, and dextromethorphan *on page 749*

AllanVan-S (Discontinued) *see* phenylephrine and pyrilamine *on page 747*

Allbee® C-800 [US-OTC] *see* vitamin B complex combinations *on page 981*

Allbee® C-800 + Iron [US-OTC] *see* vitamin B complex combinations *on page 981*

Allbee® with C [US-OTC] *see* vitamin B complex combinations *on page 981*

Allegra® [US/Can] *see* fexofenadine *on page 399*

Allegra® 60 mg Capsule (Discontinued) *see* fexofenadine *on page 399*

Allegra-D® [Can] *see* fexofenadine and pseudoephedrine *on page 399*

Allegra-D® 12 Hour [US] *see* fexofenadine and pseudoephedrine *on page 399*

Allegra-D® 24 Hour [US] *see* fexofenadine and pseudoephedrine *on page 399*

Allegra® ODT [US] *see* fexofenadine *on page 399*

Aller-Chlor® [US-OTC] *see* chlorpheniramine *on page 205*

Allercon® Tablet (Discontinued) *see* triprolidine and pseudoephedrine *on page 955*

Allerdryl® [Can] *see* diphenhydramine *on page 304*

AllerDur™ [US] *see* dexchlorpheniramine and pseudoephedrine *on page 280*

Allerest® 12 Hour Nasal Solution (Discontinued) *see* oxymetazoline *on page 712*

Allerest® Allergy and Sinus Relief [US-OTC] *see* acetaminophen and pseudoephedrine *on page 23*

Allerest® Eye Drops *(Discontinued)* *see* naphazoline *on page 655*

Allerest® Maximum Strength Allergy and Hay Fever [US-OTC] *see* chlorpheniramine and pseudoephedrine *on page 207*

Allerfrim® [US-OTC] *see* triprolidine and pseudoephedrine *on page 955*

Allerfrin® Syrup *(Discontinued)* *see* triprolidine and pseudoephedrine *on page 955*

Allerfrin® Tablet *(Discontinued)* *see* triprolidine and pseudoephedrine *on page 955*

Allerfrin® with Codeine *(Discontinued)* *see* triprolidine, pseudoephedrine, and codeine *(Canada only) on page 955*

Allergen® [US] *see* antipyrine and benzocaine *on page 82*

Allergy Relief [US-OTC] *see* loratadine *on page 576*

AllerMax® [US-OTC] *see* diphenhydramine *on page 304*

Allernix [Can] *see* diphenhydramine *on page 304*

AlleRx™-D [US] *see* pseudoephedrine and methscopolamine *on page 803*

AlleRx™ Dose Pack *(Discontinued)* *see* chlorpheniramine, pseudoephedrine, and methscopolamine *on page 213*

AlleRx™ Suspension [US] *see* chlorpheniramine and phenylephrine *on page 206*

Allfen-DM [US] *see* guaifenesin and dextromethorphan *on page 454*

Allfen Jr [US] *see* guaifenesin *on page 453*

Allfen *(reformulation) (Discontinued)*

Alli™ [US-OTC] *see* orlistat *on page 702*

Alloprin® [Can] *see* allopurinol *on page 47*

allopurinol (al oh PURE i nole)

Sound-Alike/Look-Alike Issues
allopurinol may be confused with Apresoline
Zyloprim® may be confused with Xylo-Pfan®, ZORprin®

Synonyms allopurinol sodium

U.S./Canadian Brand Names Alloprin® [Can]; Aloprim™ [US]; Apo-Allopurinol® [Can]; Novo-Purol [Can]; Zyloprim® [US/Can]

Therapeutic Category Xanthine Oxidase Inhibitor

Use
Oral: Prevention of attack of gouty arthritis and nephropathy; treatment of secondary hyperuricemia which may occur during treatment of tumors or leukemia; prevention of recurrent calcium oxalate calculi
I.V.: Treatment of elevated serum and urinary uric acid levels when oral therapy is not tolerated in patients with leukemia, lymphoma, and solid tumor malignancies who are receiving cancer chemotherapy

Usual Dosage
Oral: Doses >300 mg should be given in divided doses.
  Children ≤10 years: Secondary hyperuricemia associated with chemotherapy: 10 mg/kg/day in 2-3 divided doses **or** 200-300 mg/m²/day in 2-4 divided doses, maximum: 800 mg/24 hours
    Alternative (manufacturer labeling): <6 years: 150 mg/day in 3 divided doses; 6-10 years: 300 mg/day in 2-3 divided doses
  Children >10 years and Adults:
    Secondary hyperuricemia associated with chemotherapy: 600-800 mg/day in 2-3 divided doses for prevention of acute uric acid nephropathy for 2-3 days starting 1-2 days before chemotherapy
    Gout: Mild: 200-300 mg/day; Severe: 400-600 mg/day; to reduce the possibility of acute gouty attacks, initiate dose at 100 mg/day and increase weekly to recommended dosage.
    Recurrent calcium oxalate stones: 200-300 mg/day in single or divided doses
I.V.: Hyperuricemia secondary to chemotherapy: Intravenous daily dose can be given as a single infusion or in equally divided doses at 6-, 8-, or 12-hour intervals. A fluid intake sufficient to yield a daily urinary output of at least 2 L in adults and the maintenance of a neutral or, preferably, slightly alkaline urine are desirable.
  Children ≤10 years: Starting dose: 200 mg/m²/day
  Children >10 years and Adults: 200-400 mg/m²/day (maximum: 600 mg/day)

Dosage Forms
Injection, powder for reconstitution: 500 mg
  Aloprim™: 500 mg

◄ **Tablet:** 100 mg, 300 mg
Zyloprim®: 100 mg, 300 mg

allopurinol sodium *see* allopurinol *on page 47*
all-*trans*-retinoic acid *see* tretinoin (oral) *on page 946*
Almacone® [US-OTC] *see* aluminum hydroxide, magnesium hydroxide, and simethicone *on page 54*
Almacone Double Strength® [US-OTC] *see* aluminum hydroxide, magnesium hydroxide, and simethicone *on page 54*
Almora® [US-OTC] *see* magnesium gluconate *on page 585*

almotriptan (al moh TRIP tan)

Sound-Alike/Look-Alike Issues
Axert™ may be confused with Antivert®
Synonyms almotriptan malate
U.S./Canadian Brand Names Axert™ [US/Can]
Therapeutic Category Serotonin 5-HT$_{1D}$ Receptor Agonist
Use Acute treatment of migraine with or without aura
Usual Dosage Oral: Adults: Migraine: Initial: 6.25-12.5 mg in a single dose; if the headache returns, repeat the dose after 2 hours; no more than 2 doses in 24-hour period
Note: If the first dose is ineffective, diagnosis needs to be reevaluated. Safety of treating more than 4 migraines/month has not been established.
Dosage Forms
Tablet:
Axert™: 6.25 mg, 12.5 mg

almotriptan malate *see* almotriptan *on page 48*
Alocril® [US/Can] *see* nedocromil (ophthalmic) *on page 660*
Aloe Vesta® 2-n-1 Antifungal [US-OTC] *see* miconazole *on page 630*
Alomide® [US/Can] *see* lodoxamide *on page 572*
Alophen® [US-OTC] *see* bisacodyl *on page 136*
Aloprim™ [US] *see* allopurinol *on page 47*
Alor® 5/500 *(Discontinued)*
Alora® [US] *see* estradiol *on page 359*

alosetron (a LOE se tron)

Sound-Alike/Look-Alike Issues
Lotronex® may be confused with Lovenox®, Protonix®
U.S./Canadian Brand Names Lotronex® [US]
Therapeutic Category 5-HT$_3$ Receptor Antagonist
Use Treatment of women with severe diarrhea-predominant irritable bowel syndrome (IBS) who have failed to respond to conventional therapy
Usual Dosage Oral: Adults: Female: Initial: 0.5 mg twice daily for 4 weeks, with or without food; if tolerated, but response is inadequate, may be increased after 4 weeks to 1 mg twice daily. If response is inadequate after 4 weeks of 1 mg twice-daily dosing, discontinue treatment.
Note: Discontinue immediately if constipation or signs/symptoms of ischemic colitis occur. Do not reinitiate in patients who develop ischemic colitis.
Dosage Forms
Tablet:
Lotronex®: 0.5 mg, 1 mg

Aloxi® [US] *see* palonosetron *on page 716*
Alpain [US] *see* acetaminophen and phenyltoloxamine *on page 22*
alpha$_1$-antitrypsin *see* alpha$_1$-proteinase inhibitor *on page 48*
alpha$_1$-PI *see* alpha$_1$-proteinase inhibitor *on page 48*
alpha$_1$-proteinase inhibitor, human *see* alpha$_1$-proteinase inhibitor *on page 48*

alpha$_1$-proteinase inhibitor (al fa won PRO tee in ase in HI bi tor)

Synonyms A$_1$-PI; alpha$_1$-antitrypsin; alpha$_1$-PI; alpha$_1$-proteinase inhibitor, human; α$_1$-PI

U.S./Canadian Brand Names Aralast NP [US]; Aralast [US]; Prolastin® [US/Can]; Zemaira® [US]
Therapeutic Category Antitrypsin Deficiency Agent
Use Replacement therapy in congenital alpha₁-antitrypsin deficiency with clinical emphysema
Usual Dosage I.V.: Adults: 60 mg/kg once weekly
Dosage Forms
  Injection, powder for reconstitution [preservative free]:
    Aralast, Aralast NP, Prolastin®: 500 mg, 1000 mg
    Zemaira®: 1000 mg

alpha-galactosidase (AL fa ga lak TOE si days)

Synonyms *Aspergillus niger*
U.S./Canadian Brand Names beano® [US-OTC]
Therapeutic Category Enzyme
Use Prevention of flatulence and bloating attributed to a variety of grains, cereals, nuts, and vegetables containing the sugars raffinose, stachyose, and/or verbascose
Usual Dosage Oral: Children ≥12 years and Adults:
  Drops: Take 5 drops per serving of problem food; adjust according to number of problem foods per meal; usual dose/meal: 10-15 drops
  Tablet: One tablet per serving of problem food; adjust according to number of problem foods per meal; usual dose/meal: 2-3 tablets
Dosage Forms
  Liquid, oral [drops]:
    beano®: 150 galactosidase units/5 drops
  Tablet, oral:
    beano®: 150 galactosidase units/tablet

alpha-galactosidase-A (gene-activated) *see* agalsidase alfa *(Canada only) on page 37*
alpha-galactosidase-A (recombinant) *see* agalsidase beta *on page 37*
Alphagan® [Can] *see* brimonidine *on page 142*
Alphagan® (Discontinued) *see* brimonidine *on page 142*
Alphagan® P [US] *see* brimonidine *on page 142*
Alphamul® (Discontinued) *see* castor oil *on page 183*
Alphanate® [new formulation] [US] *see* antihemophilic factor/von Willebrand factor complex (human) *on page 80*
AlphaNine® SD [US] *see* factor IX *on page 388*
Alphaquin HP® [US] *see* hydroquinone *on page 488*
Alph-E [US-OTC] *see* vitamin E *on page 981*
Alph-E-Mixed [US-OTC] *see* vitamin E *on page 981*

alprazolam (al PRAY zoe lam)

Sound-Alike/Look-Alike Issues
  ALPRAZolam may be confused with alprostadil, LORazepam, triazolam
  Xanax® may be confused with Lanoxin®, Tenex®, Tylox®, Xopenex®, Zantac®, Zyrtec®
Tall-Man ALPRAZolam
U.S./Canadian Brand Names Alprazolam Intensol® [US]; Alti-Alprazolam [Can]; Apo-Alpraz® TS [Can]; Apo-Alpraz® [Can]; Gen-Alprazolam [Can]; Niravam™ [US]; Novo-Alprazol [Can]; Nu-Alprax [Can]; Xanax TS™ [Can]; Xanax XR® [US]; Xanax® [US/Can]
Therapeutic Category Benzodiazepine
Controlled Substance C-IV
Use Treatment of anxiety disorder (GAD); panic disorder, with or without agoraphobia; anxiety associated with depression
Usual Dosage Oral: **Note:** Treatment >4 months should be reevaluated to determine the patient's continued need for the drug
  Adults:
    Anxiety: Immediate release: Effective doses are 0.5-4 mg/day in divided doses; the manufacturer recommends starting at 0.25-0.5 mg 3 times/day; titrate dose upward; maximum: 4 mg/day. Patients requiring doses >4 mg/day should be increased cautiously. Periodic reassessment and consideration of dosage reduction is recommended.

▶

◀ Anxiety associated with depression: Immediate release: Average dose required: 2.5-3 mg/day in divided doses

Panic disorder:

Immediate release: Initial: 0.5 mg 3 times/day; dose may be increased every 3-4 days in increments ≤1 mg/day. Mean effective dosage: 5-6 mg/day; many patients obtain relief at 2 mg/day, as much as 10 mg/day may be required

Extended release: 0.5-1 mg once daily; may increase dose every 3-4 days in increments ≤1 mg/day (range: 3-6 mg/day)

Switching from immediate release to extended release: Patients may be switched to extended release tablets by taking the total daily dose of the immediate release tablets and giving it once daily using the extended release preparation.

Preoperative sedation: 0.5 mg in evening at bedtime and 0.5 mg 1 hour before procedure

Dose reduction: Abrupt discontinuation should be avoided. Daily dose may be decreased by 0.5 mg every 3 days, however, some patients may require a slower reduction. If withdrawal symptoms occur, resume previous dose and discontinue on a less rapid schedule.

Dosage Forms

Solution, oral [concentrate]:
Alprazolam Intensol®: 1 mg/mL
Tablet: 0.25 mg, 0.5 mg, 1 mg, 2 mg
Xanax®: 0.25 mg, 0.5 mg, 1 mg, 2 mg
Tablet, extended release: 0.5 mg, 1 mg, 2 mg, 3 mg
Xanax XR®: 0.5 mg, 1 mg, 2 mg, 3 mg
Tablet, orally disintegrating [scored]:
Niravam™: 0.25 mg, 0.5 mg, 1 mg, 2 mg

Alprazolam Intensol® [US] see alprazolam on page 49

alprozolam (al PROS ta dill)

Sound-Alike/Look-Alike Issues
alprostadil may be confused with alprazolam
Synonyms PGE$_1$; prostaglandin E$_1$
U.S./Canadian Brand Names Caverject Impulse® [US]; Caverject® [US/Can]; Edex® [US]; Muse® Pellet [Can]; Muse® [US]; Prostin VR Pediatric® [US]; Prostin® VR [Can]
Therapeutic Category Prostaglandin
Use

Prostin VR Pediatric®: Temporary maintenance of patency of ductus arteriosus in neonates with ductal-dependent congenital heart disease until surgery can be performed. These defects include cyanotic (eg, pulmonary atresia, pulmonary stenosis, tricuspid atresia, Fallot tetralogy, transposition of the great vessels) and acyanotic (eg, interruption of aortic arch, coarctation of aorta, hypoplastic left ventricle) heart disease.

Caverject®: Treatment of erectile dysfunction of vasculogenic, psychogenic, or neurogenic etiology; adjunct in the diagnosis of erectile dysfunction

Edex®, Muse®: Treatment of erectile dysfunction of vasculogenic, psychogenic, or neurogenic etiology

Usual Dosage

Patent ductus arteriosus (Prostin VR Pediatric®):

I.V. continuous infusion into a large vein, or alternatively through an umbilical artery catheter placed at the ductal opening: 0.05-0.1 mcg/kg/minute with therapeutic response, rate is reduced to lowest effective dosage; with unsatisfactory response, rate is increased gradually; maintenance: 0.01-0.4 mcg/kg/minute

PGE$_1$ is usually given at an infusion rate of 0.1 mcg/kg/minute, but it is often possible to reduce the dosage to $1/2$ or even $1/10$ without losing the therapeutic effect. The mixing schedule is as follows. Infusion rates deliver 0.1 mcg/kg/minute. **Note:** 500 mcg equals 1 ampul.

For a concentration of 2 mcg/mL, add 500 mcg to 250 mL; infuse at 0.05 mL/kg/minute (72 mL/kg/24 hours)

For a concentration of 5 mcg/mL, add 500 mcg to 100 mL; infuse at 0.02 mL/kg/minute (28.8 mL/kg/24 hours)

For a concentration of 10 mcg/mL, add 500 mcg to 50 mL; infuse at 0.01 mL/kg/minute (14.4 mL/kg/24 hours)

For a concentration of 20 mcg/mL, add 500 mcg to 25 mL; infuse at 0.005 mL/kg/minute (7.2 mL/kg/24 hours)

Therapeutic response is indicated by increased pH in those with acidosis or by an increase in oxygenation (PO$_2$) usually evident within 30 minutes

Erectile dysfunction:

Caverject®, Edex®: Intracavernous: Individualize dose by careful titration; doses >40 mcg (Edex®) or >60 mcg (Caverject®) are not recommended: Initial dose must be titrated in physicians office. Patient must stay in the physician's office until complete detumescence occurs; if there is no response, then the next higher dose may be given within 1 hour; if there is still no response, a 1-day interval before giving the next dose is recommended; increasing the dose or concentration in the treatment of impotence results in increasing pain and discomfort

Vasculogenic, psychogenic, or mixed etiology: Initiate dosage titration at 2.5 mcg, increasing by 2.5 mcg to a dose of 5 mcg and then in increments of 5-10 mcg depending on the erectile response until the dose produces an erection suitable for intercourse, not lasting >1 hour; if there is absolutely no response to initial 2.5 mcg dose, the second dose may be increased to 7.5 mcg, followed by increments of 5-10 mcg

Neurogenic etiology (eg, spinal cord injury): Initiate dosage titration at 1.25 mcg, increasing to a dose of 2.5 mcg and then 5 mcg; increase further in increments 5 mcg until the dose is reached that produces an erection suitable for intercourse, not lasting >1 hour

Maintenance: Once appropriate dose has been determined, patient may self-administer injections at a frequency of no more than 3 times/week with at least 24 hours between doses

Muse® Pellet: Intraurethral:

Initial: 125-250 mcg

Maintenance: Administer as needed to achieve an erection; duration of action is about 30-60 minutes; use only two systems per 24-hour period

Dosage Forms

Injection, powder for reconstitution:

Caverject®: 20 mcg, 40 mcg

Caverject Impulse®: 10 mcg, 20 mcg

Edex®: 10 mcg, 20 mcg, 40 mcg

Injection, solution: 500 mcg/mL (1 mL)

Prostin VR Pediatric®: 500 mcg/mL (1 mL)

Pellet, urethral:

Muse®: 250 mcg (6s), 500 mcg (6s), 1000 mcg (6s)

Alrex® [US/Can] see loteprednol on page 578

AL-Rr® Oral (Discontinued) see chlorpheniramine on page 205

Altabax™ [US] see retapamulin on page 827

Altace® [US/Can] see ramipril on page 817

Altace® HCT [Can] see ramipril and hydrochlorothiazide (Canada only) on page 818

Altace® Plus Felodipine [Can] see ramipril and felodipine (Canada only) on page 818

Altachlore [US-OTC] see sodium chloride on page 873

Altafrin [US] see phenylephrine on page 745

Altamist [US-OTC] see sodium chloride on page 873

Altarussin DM [US-OTC] see guaifenesin and dextromethorphan on page 454

Altaryl [US-OTC] see diphenhydramine on page 304

alteplase (AL te plase)

Sound-Alike/Look-Alike Issues

alteplase may be confused with Altace®

"tPA" abbreviation should not be used when writing orders for this medication; has been misread as TNKase (tenecteplase)

Synonyms alteplase, recombinant; alteplase, tissue plasminogen activator, recombinant; tPA

U.S./Canadian Brand Names Activase® rt-PA [Can]; Activase® [US]; Cathflo® Activase® [US/Can]

Therapeutic Category Fibrinolytic Agent

Use Management of acute myocardial infarction for the lysis of thrombi in coronary arteries; management of acute ischemic stroke

Acute myocardial infarction (AMI): Chest pain ≥20 minutes, ≤12-24 hours; S-T elevation ≥0.1 mV in at least two ECG leads

Acute pulmonary embolism (APE): Age ≤75 years: Documented massive pulmonary embolism by pulmonary angiography or echocardiography or high probability lung scan with clinical shock

◄ Cathflo® Activase®: Restoration of central venous catheter function

Usual Dosage

I.V.:

Coronary artery thrombi: Front loading dose (weight-based):

Patients >67 kg: Total dose: 100 mg over 1.5 hours; infuse 15 mg over 1-2 minutes. Infuse 50 mg over 30 minutes. Infuse remaining 35 mg of alteplase over the next hour. See "Note."

Patients ≤67 kg: Infuse 15 mg I.V. bolus over 1-2 minutes, then infuse 0.75 mg/kg (not to exceed 50 mg) over next 30 minutes, followed by 0.5 mg/kg over next 60 minutes (not to exceed 35 mg). See "Note."

Note: Concurrently, begin heparin 60 units/kg bolus (maximum: 4000 units) followed by continuous infusion of 12 units/kg/hour (maximum: 1000 units/hour) and adjust to aPTT target of 1.5-2 times the upper limit of control.

Acute pulmonary embolism: 100 mg over 2 hours.

Acute ischemic stroke: Doses should be given within the first 3 hours of the onset of symptoms; recommended total dose: 0.9 mg/kg (maximum dose should not exceed 90 mg) infused over 60 minutes.

Load with 0.09 mg/kg (10% of the 0.9 mg/kg dose) as an I.V. bolus over 1 minute, followed by 0.81 mg/kg (90% of the 0.9 mg/kg dose) as a continuous infusion over 60 minutes. Heparin should not be started for 24 hours or more after starting alteplase for stroke.

Intracatheter: Central venous catheter clearance: Cathflo® Activase® 1 mg/mL:

Patients <30 kg: 110% of the internal lumen volume of the catheter, not to exceed 2 mg/2 mL; retain in catheter for 0.5-2 hours; may instill a second dose if catheter remains occluded

Patients ≥30 kg: 2 mg (2 mL); retain in catheter for 0.5-2 hours; may instill a second dose if catheter remains occluded

Advisory Panel to the Society for Cardiovascular and Interventional Radiology on Thrombolytic Therapy recommendation: ≤2 mg/hour and subtherapeutic heparin (aPTT <1.5 times baseline)

Dosage Forms

Injection, powder for reconstitution, recombinant:

Activase®: 50 mg [29 million int. units]; 100 mg [58 million int. units]

Cathflo® Activase®: 2 mg

Alti-Sulfasalazine [Can] *see* sulfasalazine *on page 896*
Alti-Terazosin [Can] *see* terazosin *on page 909*
Alti-Ticlopidine [Can] *see* ticlopidine *on page 926*
Alti-Timolol [Can] *see* timolol *on page 927*
Alti-Trazodone [Can] *see* trazodone *on page 944*
Altocor™ *(Discontinued) see* lovastatin *on page 579*
Altoprev® [US] *see* lovastatin *on page 579*

altretamine (al TRET a meen)

Synonyms hexamethylmelamine; HEXM; HMM; HXM; NSC-13875
U.S./Canadian Brand Names Hexalen® [US/Can]
Therapeutic Category Antineoplastic Agent
Use Palliative treatment of persistent or recurrent ovarian cancer
Usual Dosage Refer to individual protocols. Oral: Adults: Ovarian cancer: 260 mg/m²/day in 4 divided doses for 14 or 21 days of a 28-day cycle
Dosage Forms
  Gelcap:
    Hexalen®: 50 mg

Alu-Cap® *(Discontinued) see* aluminum hydroxide *on page 53*
Aludrox® *(Discontinued) see* aluminum hydroxide and magnesium hydroxide *on page 54*

aluminum chloride hexahydrate (a LOO mi num KLOR ide heks a HYE drate)

Sound-Alike/Look-Alike Issues
  Drysol™ may be confused with Drisdol®
U.S./Canadian Brand Names Certain Dri® [US-OTC]; Drysol™ [US]; Hypercare™ [US]; Xerac AC™ [US]
Therapeutic Category Topical Skin Product
Use Astringent in the management of hyperhidrosis
Usual Dosage Topical: Adults: Apply once daily at bedtime; once excessive sweating has stopped, may decrease to once or twice weekly, or as needed. Wash treated area in the morning.
Dosage Forms
  Solution, topical:
    Certain Dri® [OTC]: 12% (36 mL)
    Drysol™, Hypercare™: 20% (35 mL, 37.5 mL, 60 mL)
    Xerac AC™: 6.25% (35 mL, 60 mL)

aluminum hydroxide (a LOO mi num hye DROKS ide)

U.S./Canadian Brand Names ALternaGel® [US-OTC]; Amphojel® [Can]; Basaljel® [Can]; Dermagran® [US-OTC]
Therapeutic Category Antacid
Use Treatment of hyperacidity; hyperphosphatemia; temporary protection of minor cuts, scrapes, and burns
Usual Dosage
  Oral:
    Hyperphosphatemia:
      Children: 50-150 mg/kg/24 hours in divided doses every 4-6 hours, titrate dosage to maintain serum phosphorus within normal range
      Adults: Initial: 300-600 mg 3 times/day with meals
    Antacid: Adults: 600-1200 mg between meals and at bedtime
  Topical: Apply to affected area as needed; reapply at least every 12 hours
Dosage Forms
  Ointment:
    Dermagran® [OTC]: 0.275% (120 g)
  Suspension, oral: 320 mg/5 mL
    ALternaGel® [OTC]: 600 mg/5 mL

aluminum hydroxide and magnesium carbonate

(a LOO mi num hye DROKS ide & mag NEE zhum KAR bun nate)
Synonyms magnesium carbonate and aluminum hydroxide

◄ **U.S./Canadian Brand Names** Acid Gone Extra Strength [US-OTC]; Acid Gone [US-OTC]; Alenic Alka [US-OTC]; Gaviscon® Extra Strength [US-OTC]; Gaviscon® Liquid [US-OTC]; Genaton™ [US-OTC]
Therapeutic Category Antacid
Use Temporary relief of symptoms associated with gastric acidity
Usual Dosage Oral: Adults:
Liquid:
Gaviscon® Regular Strength: 15-30 mL 4 times/day after meals and at bedtime
Gaviscon® Extra Strength: 15-30 mL 4 times/day after meals
Tablet (Gaviscon® Extra Strength): Chew 2-4 tablets 4 times/day
Dosage Forms
Liquid: Aluminum hydroxide 31.7 mg and magnesium carbonate 119.3 mg per 5 mL; aluminum hydroxide 84.6 mg and magnesium carbonate 79.1 mg per 5 mL
Acid Gone [OTC], Alenic Alka [OTC], Gaviscon® [OTC], Genaton™ [OTC]: Aluminum hydroxide 31.7 mg and magnesium carbonate 119.3 mg per 5 mL
Gaviscon® Extra Strength [OTC]: Aluminum hydroxide 84.6 mg and magnesium carbonate 79.1 mg per 5 mL
Tablet, chewable: Aluminum hydroxide 160 mg and magnesium carbonate 105 mg
Acid Gone Extra Strength [OTC], Gaviscon® Extra Strength [OTC]: Aluminum hydroxide 160 mg and magnesium carbonate 105 mg

aluminum hydroxide and magnesium hydroxide
(a LOO mi num hye DROKS ide & mag NEE zhum hye DROK side)
Sound-Alike/Look-Alike Issues
Maalox® may be confused with Maox®, Monodox®
Synonyms magnesium hydroxide and aluminum hydroxide
U.S./Canadian Brand Names Alamag [US-OTC]; Diovol® Ex [Can]; Diovol® [Can]; Gelusil® Extra Strength [Can]; Mylanta™ [Can]; Rulox [US-OTC]
Therapeutic Category Antacid
Use Antacid, hyperphosphatemia in renal failure
Usual Dosage Oral: 5-10 mL 4-6 times/day, between meals and at bedtime; may be used every hour for severe symptoms
Dosage Forms
Suspension: Aluminum hydroxide 225 mg and magnesium hydroxide 200 mg per 5 mL
Alamag [OTC], Rulox [OTC]: Aluminum hydroxide 225 mg and magnesium hydroxide 200 mg per 5 mL
Tablet, chewable:
Alamag [OTC]: Aluminum hydroxide 300 mg and magnesium hydroxide 150 mg

aluminum hydroxide and magnesium trisilicate
(a LOO mi num hye DROKS ide & mag NEE zhum trye SIL i kate)
Synonyms magnesium trisilicate and aluminum hydroxide
U.S./Canadian Brand Names Alenic Alka Tablet [US-OTC]; Gaviscon® Tablet [US-OTC]; Genaton Tablet [US-OTC]
Therapeutic Category Antacid
Use Temporary relief of hyperacidity
Usual Dosage Oral: Adults: Chew 2-4 tablets 4 times/day or as directed by healthcare provider
Dosage Forms
Tablet, chewable: Aluminum hydroxide 80 mg and magnesium trisilicate 20 mg
Alenic Alka [OTC], Gaviscon® [OTC], Genaton [OTC]: Aluminum hydroxide 80 mg and magnesium trisilicate 20 mg

aluminum hydroxide, magnesium hydroxide, and simethicone
(a LOO mi num hye DROKS ide, mag NEE zhum hye DROKS ide, & sye METH i kone)
Sound-Alike/Look-Alike Issues
Maalox® may be confused with Maox®, Monodox®
Mylanta® may be confused with Mynatal®
Synonyms magnesium hydroxide, aluminum hydroxide, and simethicone; simethicone, aluminum hydroxide, and magnesium hydroxide

U.S./Canadian Brand Names Alamag Plus [US-OTC]; Aldroxicon I [US-OTC]; Aldroxicon II [US-OTC]; Almacone Double Strength® [US-OTC]; Almacone® [US-OTC]; Diovol Plus® [Can]; Gelusil® [US-OTC/Can]; Maalox® Max [US-OTC]; Maalox® [US-OTC]; Mi-Acid Maximum Strength [US-OTC]; Mi-Acid [US-OTC]; Mintox Extra Strength [US-OTC]; Mintox Plus [US-OTC]; Mylanta® Double Strength [Can]; Mylanta® Extra Strength [Can]; Mylanta® Liquid [US-OTC]; Mylanta® Maximum Strength Liquid [US-OTC]; Mylanta® Regular Strength [Can]

Therapeutic Category Antacid Antiflatulent

Use Temporary relief of hyperacidity associated with gas; may also be used for indications associated with other antacids

Usual Dosage Oral: Adults: 10-20 mL or 2-4 tablets 4-6 times/day between meals and at bedtime; may be used every hour for severe symptoms

Dosage Forms

Liquid: Aluminum hydroxide 200 mg, magnesium hydroxide 200 mg, and simethicone 20 mg per 5 mL; aluminum hydroxide 400 mg, magnesium hydroxide 400 mg, and simethicone 40 mg per 5 mL

Aldroxicon I [OTC], Almacone® [OTC], Maalox® [OTC], Mi-Acid [OTC], Mylanta® [OTC]: Aluminum hydroxide 200 mg, magnesium hydroxide 200 mg, and simethicone 20 mg per 5 mL

Aldroxicon II [OTC], Almacone Double Strength [OTC], Maalox® Max® [OTC], Mi-Acid Maximum Strength [OTC], Mylanta® Maximum Strength [OTC]: Aluminum hydroxide 400 mg, magnesium hydroxide 400 mg, and simethicone 40 mg per 5 mL

Mintox Extra Strength [OTC]: Aluminum hydroxide 500 mg, magnesium hydroxide 450 mg, and simethicone 40 mg per 5 mL

Suspension:

Alamag Plus [OTC]: Aluminum hydroxide 225 mg, magnesium hydroxide 200 mg, and simethicone 25 mg per 5 mL

Tablet, chewable: Aluminum hydroxide 200 mg, magnesium hydroxide 200 mg, and simethicone 25 mg

Alamag Plus [OTC], Gelusil® [OTC], Mintox Plus [OTC]: Aluminum hydroxide 200 mg, magnesium hydroxide 200 mg, and simethicone 25 mg

Almacone® [OTC]: Aluminum hydroxide 200 mg, magnesium hydroxide 200 mg, and simethicone 20 mg

aluminum sucrose sulfate, basic *see* sucralfate *on page 890*

aluminum sulfate and calcium acetate (a LOO mi num SUL fate & KAL see um AS e tate)

Synonyms calcium acetate and aluminum sulfate

U.S./Canadian Brand Names Domeboro® [US-OTC]; Gordon Boro-Packs [US-OTC]; Pedi-Boro® [US-OTC]

Therapeutic Category Topical Skin Product

Use Astringent wet dressing for relief of inflammatory conditions of the skin; reduce weeping that may occur in dermatitis

Usual Dosage Topical: Soak affected area in the solution 2-4 times/day for 15-30 minutes or apply wet dressing soaked in the solution for more extended periods; rewet dressing with solution 2-4 times/day every 15-30 minutes

Dosage Forms

Powder, for topical solution:

Domeboro® [OTC]: Aluminum sulfate 1191 mg and calcium acetate 839 mg per packet (12s, 100s)

Gordon Boro-Packs: Aluminum sulfate 49% and calcium acetate 51% per packet (100s)

Pedi-Boro® [OTC]: Aluminum sulfate 1191 mg and calcium acetate 839 mg per packet (12s, 100s)

Alupent® [US] *see* metaproterenol *on page 609*

Alupent® Inhalation Solution *(Discontinued)* *see* metaproterenol *on page 609*

Alu-Tab® *(Discontinued)* *see* aluminum hydroxide *on page 53*

Alvesco® [US/Can] *see* ciclesonide *on page 217*

alvimopan (al vi MOE pan)

Sound-Alike/Look-Alike Issues

alvimopan may be confused with almotriptan

Synonyms ADL-2698; LY246736

U.S./Canadian Brand Names Entereg® [US]

Therapeutic Category Gastrointestinal Agent, Miscellaneous; Opioid Antagonist, Peripherally-Acting

▶

◀ **Use** Accelerate the time to upper and lower GI recovery following partial large or small bowel resection surgery with primary anastomosis

Usual Dosage Note: For hospital use only

Oral: Adults:

Initial: 12 mg administered 30 minutes to 5 hours prior to surgery

Maintenance: 12 mg twice daily beginning the day after surgery for a maximum of 7 days or until discharged from hospital (maximum total treatment doses: 15 doses)

Dosage Forms

Capsule:

Entereg®: 12 mg

amantadine (a MAN ta deen)

Sound-Alike/Look-Alike Issues

amantadine may be confused with ranitidine, rimantadine

Symmetrel® may be confused with Synthroid®

Synonyms adamantanamine hydrochloride; amantadine hydrochloride

U.S./Canadian Brand Names Endantadine® [Can]; PMS-Amantadine [Can]; Symmetrel® [US/Can]

Therapeutic Category Anti-Parkinson Agent (Dopamine Agonist); Antiviral Agent

Use Prophylaxis and treatment of influenza A viral infection (per manufacturer labeling; also refer to current ACIP guidelines for recommendations during current flu season); treatment of parkinsonism; treatment of drug-induced extrapyramidal symptoms

Note: In certain circumstances, the ACIP recommends use of amantadine in combination with oseltamivir for the treatment or prophylaxis of influenza A infection when resistance to oseltamivir is suspected.

Usual Dosage Oral:

Children:

Influenza A treatment:

1-9 years: 5 mg/kg/day in 2 divided doses (manufacturers range: 4.4-8.8 mg/kg/day); maximum dose: 150 mg/day

≥10 years and <40 kg: 5 mg/kg/day; maximum dose: 150 mg/day

≥10 years and ≥40 kg: 100 mg twice daily

Note: Initiate within 24-48 hours after onset of symptoms; discontinue as soon as possible based on clinical response (generally within 3-5 days or within 24-48 hours after symptoms disappear)

Influenza A prophylaxis: Refer to "Influenza A treatment" dosing

Note: Continue treatment throughout the peak influenza activity in the community or throughout the entire influenza season in patients who cannot be vaccinated. Development of immunity following vaccination takes ~2 weeks; amantadine therapy should be considered for high-risk patients from the time of vaccination until immunity has developed. For children <9 years receiving influenza vaccine for the first time, amantadine prophylaxis should continue for 6 weeks (4 weeks after the first dose and 2 weeks after the second dose)

Adults:

Drug-induced extrapyramidal symptoms: 100 mg twice daily; may increase to 300-400 mg/day, if needed

Influenza A viral infection: 100 mg twice daily; initiate within 24-48 hours after onset of symptoms; discontinue as soon as possible based on clinical response (generally within 3-5 days or within 24-48 hours after symptoms disappear)

Influenza A prophylaxis: 100 mg twice daily

Note: Continue treatment throughout the peak influenza activity in the community or throughout the entire influenza season in patients who cannot be vaccinated. Development of immunity following vaccination takes ~2 weeks; amantadine therapy should be considered for high-risk patients from the time of vaccination until immunity has developed

Dosage Forms

Capsule: 100 mg

Capsule, softgel: 100 mg

Solution, oral: 50 mg/5 mL

Syrup, oral: 50 mg/5 mL

Tablet: 100 mg

Symmetrel®: 100 mg

amantadine hydrochloride *see* amantadine *on page 56*

Amaphen® *(Discontinued)*

Amaryl® [US/Can] *see* glimepiride *on page 445*
Amatine® [Can] *see* midodrine *on page 633*

ambenonium (am be NOE nee um)
Synonyms ambenonium chloride
U.S./Canadian Brand Names Mytelase® [US/Can]
Therapeutic Category Cholinergic Agent
Use Treatment of myasthenia gravis
Usual Dosage Oral: Adults: 5-25 mg 3-4 times/day
Dosage Forms
  Caplet [scored]:
    Mytelase®: 10 mg

ambenonium chloride *see* ambenonium *on page 57*
Ambi 10® (Discontinued) *see* benzoyl peroxide *on page 126*
Ambien® [US] *see* zolpidem *on page 996*
Ambien CR® [US] *see* zolpidem *on page 996*
Ambifed-G [US] *see* guaifenesin and pseudoephedrine *on page 458*
Ambifed-G DM [US] *see* guaifenesin, pseudoephedrine, and dextromethorphan *on page 460*
Ambi® Skin Tone (Discontinued) *see* hydroquinone *on page 488*
AmBisome® [US/Can] *see* amphotericin B liposomal *on page 71*

ambrisentan (am bri SEN tan)
Synonyms BSF208075
U.S./Canadian Brand Names Letairis™ [US]
Therapeutic Category Endothelin Antagonist
Use Treatment of pulmonary artery hypertension (PAH) World Health Organization (WHO) Group I in patients with WHO Class II or III symptoms to improve exercise capacity and decrease the rate of clinical deterioration
Usual Dosage Oral: Adults: Initial: 5 mg once daily; if tolerated, may increase to maximum 10 mg once daily
Dosage Forms
  Tablet:
    Letairis™: 5 mg, 10 mg

amcinonide (am SIN oh nide)
U.S./Canadian Brand Names Amcort® [Can]; Cyclocort® [Can]; ratio-Amcinonide [Can]; Taro-Amcinonide [Can]
Therapeutic Category Corticosteroid, Topical
Use Relief of the inflammatory and pruritic manifestations of corticosteroid-responsive dermatoses (high potency corticosteroid)
Usual Dosage Topical: Adults: Apply in a thin film 2-3 times/day. Therapy should be discontinued when control is achieved; if no improvement is seen, reassessment of diagnosis may be necessary.
Dosage Forms
  Cream: 0.1% (15 g, 30 g, 60 g)
  Lotion: 0.1% (60 mL)
  Ointment: 0.1% (30 g, 60 g)

Amcort® [Can] *see* amcinonide *on page 57*
Amcort® Injection (Discontinued)
Amdry-C [US] *see* chlorpheniramine, pseudoephedrine, and methscopolamine *on page 213*
Amdry-D [US] *see* pseudoephedrine and methscopolamine *on page 803*
Amerge® [US/Can] *see* naratriptan *on page 657*
Americaine® Anesthetic Lubricant (Discontinued) *see* benzocaine *on page 124*
Americaine® Hemorrhoidal [US-OTC] *see* benzocaine *on page 124*
A-methapred *see* methylprednisolone *on page 623*
amethocaine hydrochloride *see* tetracaine *on page 914*

amethopterin *see* methotrexate *on page 615*
Ametop™ [Can] *see* tetracaine *on page 914*
Amevive® [US/Can] *see* alefacept *on page 42*
amfepramone *see* diethylpropion *on page 295*
AMG 073 *see* cinacalcet *on page 220*
AMG 531 *see* romiplostim *on page 843*
Amibid DM *(Discontinued)* *see* guaifenesin and dextromethorphan *on page 454*
Amibid LA *(Discontinued)* *see* guaifenesin *on page 453*
Amicar® [US] *see* aminocaproic acid *on page 60*
Amidal *(Discontinued)* *see* guaifenesin and phenylephrine *on page 456*
Amidate® [US/Can] *see* etomidate *on page 383*
Amidrine *(Discontinued)* *see* acetaminophen, isometheptene, and dichloralphenazone *on page 28*

amifostine (am i FOS teen)

Sound-Alike/Look-Alike Issues
Ethyol® may be confused with ethanol
Synonyms ethiofos; gammaphos; WR-2721; YM-08310
U.S./Canadian Brand Names Ethyol® [US/Can]
Therapeutic Category Antidote
Use Reduce the incidence of moderate to severe xerostomia in patients undergoing postoperative radiation treatment for head and neck cancer, where the radiation port includes a substantial portion of the parotid glands; reduce the cumulative renal toxicity associated with repeated administration of cisplatin
Usual Dosage Note: Antiemetic medication, including dexamethasone 20 mg I.V. and a serotonin 5-HT$_3$ receptor antagonist, is recommended prior to and in conjunction with amifostine.
Adults:
Cisplatin-induced renal toxicity, reduction: I.V.: 740-910 mg/m^2 over 15 minutes once daily 30 minutes prior to cytotoxic therapy
Note: Doses >740 mg/m^2 are associated with a higher incidence of hypotension and may require interruption of therapy or dose modification for subsequent cycles. For 910 mg/m^2 doses, the manufacturer suggests the following blood pressure-based adjustment schedule:
The infusion of amifostine should be interrupted if the systolic blood pressure decreases significantly from baseline, as defined below:
Decrease of 20 mm Hg if baseline systolic blood pressure <100
Decrease of 25 mm Hg if baseline systolic blood pressure 100-119
Decrease of 30 mm Hg if baseline systolic blood pressure 120-139
Decrease of 40 mm Hg if baseline systolic blood pressure 140-179
Decrease of 50 mm Hg if baseline systolic blood pressure ≥180
If blood pressure returns to normal within 5 minutes (assisted by fluid administration and postural management) and the patient is asymptomatic, the infusion may be restarted so that the full dose of amifostine may be administered. If the full dose of amifostine cannot be administered, the dose of amifostine for subsequent cycles should be 740 mg/m^2.
Xerostomia from head and neck cancer, reduction: I.V.: 200 mg/m^2/day over 3 minutes 15-30 minutes prior to radiation therapy
Dosage Forms
Injection, powder for reconstitution: 500 mg
Ethyol®: 500 mg

Amigesic® [Can] *see* salsalate *on page 854*
Amigesic® *(Discontinued)* *see* salsalate *on page 854*

amikacin (am i KAY sin)

Sound-Alike/Look-Alike Issues
amikacin may be confused with Amicar®, anakinra
Amikin® may be confused with Amicar®
Synonyms amikacin sulfate
U.S./Canadian Brand Names Amikacin Sulfate Injection, USP [Can]; Amikin® [Can]
Therapeutic Category Aminoglycoside (Antibiotic)

Use Treatment of serious infections (bone infections, respiratory tract infections, endocarditis, and septicemia) due to organisms resistant to gentamicin and tobramycin, including *Pseudomonas, Proteus, Serratia,* and other gram-negative bacilli; documented infection of mycobacterial organisms susceptible to amikacin

Usual Dosage Note: Individualization is critical because of the low therapeutic index

Use of ideal body weight (IBW) for determining the mg/kg/dose appears to be more accurate than dosing on the basis of total body weight (TBW)

In morbid obesity, dosage requirement may best be estimated using a dosing weight of IBW + 0.4 (TBW - IBW)

Initial and periodic peak and trough plasma drug levels should be determined, particularly in critically-ill patients with serious infections or in disease states known to significantly alter aminoglycoside pharmacokinetics (eg, cystic fibrosis, burns, or major surgery)

Usual dosage range:
Infants and Children: I.M., I.V.: 5-7.5 mg/kg/dose every 8 hours
Adults: I.M., I.V.: 5-7.5 mg/kg/dose every 8 hours
Note: Some clinicians suggest a daily dose of 15-20 mg/kg for all patients with normal renal function. This dose is at least as efficacious with similar, if not less, toxicity than conventional dosing.

Indication-specific dosing:
Adults:
Hospital-acquired pneumonia (HAP): I.V.: 20 mg/kg/day with antipseudomonal beta-lactam or carbapenem (American Thoracic Society/ATS guidelines)
Meningitis *(Pseudomonas aeruginosa):* I.V.: 5 mg/kg every 8 hours (administered with another bacteriocidal drug)
Mycobacterium fortuitum, M. chelonae, or M. abscessus: I.V.: 10-15 mg/kg daily for at least 2 weeks with high dose cefoxitin

Dosage Forms
Injection, solution: 50 mg/mL (2 mL); 250 mg/mL (2 mL, 4 mL)

amikacin sulfate *see amikacin on page 58*
Amikacin Sulfate Injection, USP [Can] *see amikacin on page 58*
Amikin® [Can] *see amikacin on page 58*

amiloride (a MIL oh ride)

Sound-Alike/Look-Alike Issues
aMILoride may be confused with amiodarone, amLODIPine, amrinone
Synonyms amiloride hydrochloride
Tall-Man aMILoride
U.S./Canadian Brand Names Apo-Amiloride® [Can]
Therapeutic Category Diuretic, Potassium Sparing
Use Counteracts potassium loss induced by other diuretics in the treatment of hypertension or edematous conditions including CHF, hepatic cirrhosis, and hypoaldosteronism; usually used in conjunction with more potent diuretics such as thiazides or loop diuretics
Usual Dosage Oral: Adults: 5-10 mg/day (up to 20 mg)
Hypertension (JNC 7): 5-10 mg/day in 1-2 divided doses
Dosage Forms
Tablet: 5 mg

amiloride and hydrochlorothiazide (a MIL oh ride & hye droe klor oh THYE a zide)

Synonyms hydrochlorothiazide and amiloride
U.S./Canadian Brand Names Apo-Amilzide® [Can]; Gen-Amilazide [Can]; Moduret [Can]; Novamilor [Can]; Nu-Amilzide [Can]
Therapeutic Category Diuretic, Combination
Use Potassium-sparing diuretic; antihypertensive
Usual Dosage Oral: Adults: Start with 1 tablet/day, then may be increased to 2 tablets/day if needed; usually given in a single dose
Dosage Forms
Tablet: 5/50: Amiloride 5 mg and hydrochlorothiazide 50 mg

amiloride hydrochloride *see amiloride on page 59*

Aminate Fe-90 [US] *see* vitamins (multiple/prenatal) *on page 983*
2-amino-6-mercaptopurine *see* thioguanine *on page 921*
2-amino-6-methoxypurine arabinoside *see* nelarabine *on page 660*
2-amino-6-trifluoromethoxy-benzothiazole *see* riluzole *on page 835*
aminobenzylpenicillin *see* ampicillin *on page 72*

aminocaproic acid (a mee noe ka PROE ik AS id)

Sound-Alike/Look-Alike Issues
Amicar® may be confused with amikacin, Amikin®, Omacor®
Synonyms EACA; epsilon aminocaproic acid
U.S./Canadian Brand Names Amicar® [US]
Therapeutic Category Hemostatic Agent
Use To enhance hemostasis when fibrinolysis contributes to bleeding (causes may include cardiac surgery, hematologic disorders, neoplastic disorders, abruption placentae, hepatic cirrhosis, and urinary fibrinolysis)
Usual Dosage Oral, I.V.: Adults: Acute bleeding syndrome: Loading dose: 4-5 g during the first hour, followed by 1 g/hour for 8 hours or until bleeding controlled (maximum daily dose: 30 g)
Dosage Forms
Injection, solution: 250 mg/mL (20 mL)
Amicar®: 250 mg/mL (20 mL)
Solution, oral: 1.25 g/5 mL (480 mL)
Syrup:
Amicar®: 1.25 g/5 mL
Tablet [scored]: 500 mg
Amicar®: 500 mg, 1000 mg

aminoglutethimide (a mee noe gloo TETH i mide)

Sound-Alike/Look-Alike Issues
Cytadren® may be confused with cytarabine
Synonyms BA-16038; elipten
U.S./Canadian Brand Names Cytadren® [US]
Therapeutic Category Antineoplastic Agent
Use Suppression of adrenal function in selected patients with Cushing syndrome
Usual Dosage Oral: Adults: **Note:** Glucocorticoid and mineralocorticoid replacement therapy may be necessary. Adrenal suppression: 250 mg every 6 hours may be increased in increments of 250 mg/day at 1- to 2-week intervals to a total of 2 g/day
Dosage Forms
Tablet [scored]:
Cytadren®: 250 mg

aminolevulinic acid (a MEE noh lev yoo lin ik AS id)

Synonyms aminolevulinic acid hydrochloride
U.S./Canadian Brand Names Levulan® Kerastick® [US]; Levulan® [Can]
Therapeutic Category Photosensitizing Agent, Topical; Porphyrin Agent, Topical
Use Treatment of minimally to moderately thick actinic keratoses (grade 1 or 2) of the face or scalp; to be used in conjunction with blue light illumination
Usual Dosage Topical: Adults: Apply to actinic keratoses (**not** perilesional skin) followed 14-18 hours later by blue light illumination. Application/treatment may be repeated at a treatment site after 8 weeks.
Dosage Forms
Powder for topical solution:
Levulan® Kerastick®: 20% (6s)

aminolevulinic acid hydrochloride *see* aminolevulinic acid *on page 60*

aminophylline (am in OFF i lin)

Sound-Alike/Look-Alike Issues
aminophylline may be confused with amitriptyline, ampicillin
Synonyms theophylline ethylenediamine

U.S./Canadian Brand Names Phyllocontin® [Can]; Phyllocontin®-350 [Can]

Therapeutic Category Theophylline Derivative

Use Bronchodilator in reversible airway obstruction due to asthma or COPD; increase diaphragmatic contractility

Usual Dosage
Treatment of acute bronchospasm: I.V.:
Loading dose (in patients not currently receiving aminophylline or theophylline): 6 mg/kg (based on aminophylline) administered I.V. over 20-30 minutes; administration rate should not exceed 25 mg/minute (aminophylline)
Approximate I.V. maintenance dosages are based upon **continuous infusions**; bolus dosing (often used in children <6 months of age) may be determined by multiplying the hourly infusion rate by 24 hours and dividing by the desired number of doses/day
6 weeks to 6 months: 0.5 mg/kg/hour
6 months to 1 year: 0.6-0.7 mg/kg/hour
1-9 years: 1 mg/kg/hour
9-16 years and smokers: 0.8 mg/kg/hour
Adults, nonsmoking: 0.5 mg/kg/hour
Older patients and patients with cor pulmonale: 0.3 mg/kg/hour
Patients with congestive heart failure: 0.1-0.2 mg/kg/hour
Dosage should be adjusted according to serum level measurements during the first 12- to 24-hour period.
Bronchodilator: Oral: Children ≥45 kg and Adults: Initial: 380 mg/day (equivalent to theophylline 300 mg/day) in divided doses every 6-8 hours; may increase dose after 3 days; maximum dose: 928 mg/day (equivalent to theophylline 800 mg/day)

Dosage Forms
Injection, solution: 25 mg/mL (10 mL, 20 mL)
Injection, solution, [preservative free]: 25 mg/mL (10 mL, 20 mL)
Tablet: 100 mg

aminosalicylate sodium *see* aminosalicylic acid *on page 61*

aminosalicylic acid (a mee noe sal i SIL ik AS id)

Synonyms 4-aminosalicylic acid; aminosalicylate sodium; para-aminosalicylate sodium; PAS; sodium PAS

U.S./Canadian Brand Names Paser® [US]

Therapeutic Category Nonsteroidal Antiinflammatory Drug (NSAID)

Use Adjunctive treatment of tuberculosis used in combination with other antitubercular agents

Usual Dosage Oral: Tuberculosis:
Children: 200-300 mg/kg/day in 3-4 equally divided doses
Adults: 150 mg/kg/day in 2-3 equally divided doses

Dosage Forms
Granules, delayed release:
Paser®: 4 g/packet

4-aminosalicylic acid *see* aminosalicylic acid *on page 61*
5-aminosalicylic acid *see* mesalamine *on page 607*
Aminoxin [US-OTC] *see* pyridoxine *on page 808*

amiodarone (a MEE oh da rone)

Sound-Alike/Look-Alike Issues
amiodarone may be confused with amiloride, amrinone
Cordarone® may be confused with Cardura®, Cordran®

Synonyms amiodarone hydrochloride

U.S./Canadian Brand Names Alti-Amiodarone [Can]; Amiodarone Hydrochloride for Injection® [Can]; Apo-Amiodarone® [Can]; Cordarone® [US/Can]; Dom-Amiodarone [Can]; Gen-Amiodarone [Can]; Novo-Amiodarone [Can]; Pacerone® [US]; PHL-Amiodarone [Can]; PMS-Amiodarone [Can]; Ratio-Amiodarone I.V. [Can]; Ratio-Amiodarone [Can]; Sandoz-Amiodarone [Can]

Therapeutic Category Antiarrhythmic Agent, Class III

◄ **Use** Management of life-threatening recurrent ventricular fibrillation (VF) or hemodynamically-unstable ventricular tachycardia (VT) refractory to other antiarrhythmic agents or in patients intolerant of other agents used for these conditions

Usual Dosage Note: Lower loading and maintenance doses are preferable in women and all patients with low body weight.

Oral: Adults: Ventricular arrhythmias: 800-1600 mg/day in 1-2 doses for 1-3 weeks, then when adequate arrhythmia control is achieved, decrease to 600-800 mg/day in 1-2 doses for 1 month; maintenance: 400 mg/day. Lower doses are recommended for supraventricular arrhythmias.

I.V.:
Children:
Pulseless VF or VT (PALS dosing): 5 mg/kg (maximum: 300 mg/dose) rapid I.V. bolus or I.O.; repeat up to a maximum daily dose of 15 mg/kg. (**Note:** Maximum recommended daily dose in adolescents is 2.2 g.)
Perfusing tachycardias (PALS dosing): Loading dose: 5 mg/kg (maximum: 300 mg/dose) I.V. over 20-60 minutes or I.O.; may repeat up to maximum dose of 15 mg/kg/day. (**Note:** Maximum recommended daily dose in adolescents is 2.2 g.)
Adults:
Breakthrough VF or VT: 150 mg supplemental doses in 100 mL D_5W over 10 minutes
Pulseless VF or VT: I.V. push: Initial: 300 mg in 20-30 mL NS or D_5W; if VF or VT recurs, supplemental dose of 150 mg followed by infusion of 1 mg/minute for 6 hours, then 0.5 mg/minute (maximum daily dose: 2.1 g)

I.V. to oral therapy conversion: Use the following as a guide:
<1-week I.V. infusion: 800-1600 mg/day
1- to 3-week I.V. infusion: 600-800 mg/day
>3-week I.V. infusion: 400 mg/day

Recommendations for conversion to intravenous amiodarone after oral administration: During long-term amiodarone therapy (ie, ≥4 months), the mean plasma-elimination half-life of the active metabolite of amiodarone is 61 days. Replacement therapy may not be necessary in such patients if oral therapy is discontinued for a period <2 weeks, since any changes in serum amiodarone concentrations during this period may **not** be clinically significant.

Dosage Forms
Injection, solution: 50 mg/mL (3 mL, 9 mL, 18 mL)
Tablet [scored]: 200 mg, 400 mg
Cordarone®: 200 mg
Pacerone®: 100 mg [not scored], 200 mg, 400 mg

amiodarone hydrochloride *see* amiodarone *on page 61*
Amiodarone Hydrochloride for Injection® [Can] *see* amiodarone *on page 61*
Ami-Tex LA *(Discontinued)* *see* guaifenesin and phenylephrine *on page 456*
Amitiza® [US] *see* lubiprostone *on page 581*
Amitone® *(Discontinued)* *see* calcium carbonate *on page 163*

amitriptyline (a mee TRIP ti leen)
Sound-Alike/Look-Alike Issues
amitriptyline may be confused with aminophylline, imipramine, nortriptyline
Elavil® may be confused with Aldoril®, Eldepryl®, enalapril, Equanil®, Mellaril®, Oruvail®, Plavix®
Synonyms amitriptyline hydrochloride
U.S./Canadian Brand Names Apo-Amitriptyline® [Can]; Levate® [Can]; Novo-Triptyn [Can]; PMS-Amitriptyline [Can]
Therapeutic Category Antidepressant, Tricyclic (Tertiary Amine)
Use Relief of symptoms of depression
Usual Dosage Oral:
Adolescents: Depressive disorders: Initial: 25-50 mg/day; may administer in divided doses; increase gradually to 100 mg/day in divided doses
Adults: Depression: 50-150 mg/day single dose at bedtime or in divided doses; dose may be gradually increased up to 300 mg/day
Dosage Forms
Tablet: 10 mg, 25 mg, 50 mg, 75 mg, 100 mg, 150 mg

amitriptyline and chlordiazepoxide (a mee TRIP ti leen & klor dye az e POKS ide)

Synonyms chlordiazepoxide and amitriptyline hydrochloride

U.S./Canadian Brand Names Limbitrol® DS [US]; Limbitrol® [US/Can]

Therapeutic Category Antidepressant, Tricyclic (Tertiary Amine)

Controlled Substance C-IV

Use Treatment of moderate-to-severe anxiety and/or agitation and depression

Usual Dosage Initial: 3-4 tablets in divided doses; this may be increased to 6 tablets/day as required; some patients respond to smaller doses and can be maintained on 2 tablets

Dosage Forms
Tablet: 12.5/5: Amitriptyline 12.5 mg and chlordiazepoxide 5 mg; 25/10: Amitriptyline 25 mg and chlordiazepoxide 10 mg
Limbitrol®: 12.5/5: Amitriptyline 12.5 mg and chlordiazepoxide 5 mg
Limbitrol® DS: 25/10: Amitriptyline 25 mg and chlordiazepoxide 10 mg

amitriptyline and perphenazine (a mee TRIP ti leen & per FEN a zeen)

Synonyms perphenazine and amitriptyline hydrochloride

U.S./Canadian Brand Names Etrafon® [Can]

Therapeutic Category Antidepressant/Phenothiazine

Use Treatment of patients with moderate-to-severe anxiety and depression

Usual Dosage Oral: 1 tablet 2-4 times/day

Dosage Forms
Tablet:
Generics:
2-10: Amitriptyline 10 mg and perphenazine 2 mg
2-25: Amitriptyline 25 mg and perphenazine 2 mg
4-10: Amitriptyline 10 mg and perphenazine 4 mg
4-25: Amitriptyline 25 mg and perphenazine 4 mg
4-50: Amitriptyline 50 mg and perphenazine 4 mg

amitriptyline hydrochloride *see* amitriptyline *on page 62*

AMJ 9701 *see* palifermin *on page 715*

AmLactin® [US-OTC] *see* lactic acid and ammonium hydroxide *on page 542*

amlexanox (am LEKS an oks)

U.S./Canadian Brand Names Aphthasol® [US]

Therapeutic Category Antiinflammatory Agent, Locally Applied

Use Treatment of aphthous ulcers (ie, canker sores)

Usual Dosage Topical: Administer (0.5 cm - 1/4") directly on ulcers 4 times/day following oral hygiene, after meals, and at bedtime

Dosage Forms
Paste, oral:
Aphthasol®: 5% (3 g)

amlodipine (am LOE di peen)

Sound-Alike/Look-Alike Issues
amLODIPine may be confused with aMILoride
Norvasc® may be confused with Navane®, Norvir®, Vascor®

Synonyms amlodipine besylate

Tall-Man amLODIPine

U.S./Canadian Brand Names Norvasc® [US/Can]

Therapeutic Category Calcium Channel Blocker

Use Treatment of hypertension; treatment of symptomatic chronic stable angina, vasospastic (Prinzmetal) angina (confirmed or suspected); prevention of hospitalization due to angina with documented CAD (limited to patients without heart failure or ejection fraction <40%)

Usual Dosage Oral:
Children 6-17 years: Hypertension: 2.5-5 mg once daily

◀ Adults:
Hypertension: Initial dose: 5 mg once daily; maximum dose: 10 mg once daily. In general, titrate in 2.5 mg increments over 7-14 days. Usual dosage range (JNC 7): 2.5-10 mg once daily.
Angina: Usual dose: 5-10 mg

Dosage Forms
Tablet: 2.5 mg, 5 mg, 10 mg
Norvasc®: 2.5 mg, 5 mg, 10 mg

amlodipine and atorvastatin (am LOW di peen & a TORE va sta tin)

Synonyms atorvastatin calcium and amlodipine besylate

U.S./Canadian Brand Names Caduet® [US/Can]

Therapeutic Category Antilipemic Agent, HMG-CoA Reductase Inhibitor; Calcium Channel Blocker

Use For use when treatment with both amlodipine and atorvastatin is appropriate:

Amlodipine: Treatment of hypertension; treatment of symptomatic chronic stable angina, vasospastic (Prinzmetal) angina (confirmed or suspected); prevention of hospitalization due to angina with documented CAD (limited to patients without heart failure or ejection fraction <40%)

Atorvastatin: Treatment of dyslipidemias or primary prevention of cardiovascular disease (atherosclerotic) as detailed here:

Primary prevention of cardiovascular disease (high-risk for CVD): To reduce the risk of MI or stroke in patients without evidence of heart disease who have multiple CVD risk factors or type 2 diabetes. Treatment reduces the risk for angina or revascularization procedures in patients with multiple risk factors.

Treatment of dyslipidemias: To reduce elevations in total cholesterol, LDL-C, apolipoprotein B, and triglycerides in patients with elevations of one or more components, and/or to increase HDL-C as present in heterozygous hypercholesterolemia (Fredrickson type IIa hyperlipidemias); treatment of primary dysbetalipoproteinemia (Fredrickson type III), elevated serum TG levels (Fredrickson type IV), and homozygous familial hypercholesterolemia

Treatment of heterozygous familial hypercholesterolemia (HeFH) in adolescent patients (10-17 years of age, females >1 year postmenarche) having LDL-C ≥190 mg/dL or LDL-C ≥160 mg/dL with positive family history of premature cardiovascular disease (CVD) or with two or more CVD risk factors.

Usual Dosage Oral:

Amlodipine:
Children >10 years: Hypertension: 2.5-5 mg once daily. **Note:** Use in ages >10 years because of atorvastatin content.

Adults:
Hypertension: Initial dose: 5 mg once daily; maximum dose: 10 mg once daily; in general, titrate in 2.5 mg increments over 7-14 days. Usual dosage range (JNC 7): 2.5-10 mg once daily
Angina: Usual dose: 5-10 mg; most patients require 10 mg for adequate effect

Atorvastatin:
Children 10-17 years (females >1 year postmenarche): HeFH: 10 mg once daily (maximum: 20 mg/day)
Adults:
Hyperlipidemias: Initial: 10-20 mg once daily; patients requiring >45% reduction in LDL-C may be started at 40 mg once daily; range: 10-80 mg once daily
Primary prevention of CVD: 10 mg once daily

Dosage Forms
Tablet:
Caduet®:
2.5/10: Amlodipine 2.5 mg and atorvastatin 10 mg
2.5/20: Amlodipine 2.5 mg and atorvastatin 20 mg
2.5/40: Amlodipine 2.5 mg and atorvastatin 40 mg
5/10: Amlodipine 5 mg and atorvastatin 10 mg
5/20: Amlodipine 5 mg and atorvastatin 20 mg
5/40: Amlodipine 5 mg and atorvastatin 40 mg
5/80: Amlodipine 5 mg and atorvastatin 80 mg
10/10: Amlodipine 10 mg and atorvastatin 10 mg
10/20: Amlodipine 10 mg and atorvastatin 20 mg
10/40: Amlodipine 10 mg and atorvastatin 40 mg
10/80: Amlodipine 10 mg and atorvastatin 80 mg

amlodipine and benazepril (am LOE di peen & ben AY ze pril)

Synonyms benazepril hydrochloride and amlodipine besylate

U.S./Canadian Brand Names Lotrel® [US]

Therapeutic Category Antihypertensive Agent, Combination

Use Treatment of hypertension

Usual Dosage Oral: Adults: 2.5-10 mg (amlodipine) and 10-40 mg (benazepril) once daily; maximum: Amlodipine: 10 mg/day; benazepril: 40 mg/day

Dosage Forms

Capsule:
2.5/10: Amlodipine 2.5 mg and benazepril 10 mg
5/10: Amlodipine 5 mg and benazepril 10 mg
5/20: Amlodipine 5 mg and benazepril 20 mg
10/20: Amlodipine 10 mg and benazepril 20 mg
Lotrel®:
2.5/10: Amlodipine 2.5 and benazepril 10 mg
5/10: Amlodipine 5 mg and benazepril 10 mg
5/20: Amlodipine 5 mg and benazepril 20 mg
5/40: Amlodipine 5 mg and benazepril 40 mg
10/20: Amlodipine 10 mg and benazepril 20 mg
10/40: Amlodipine 10 mg and benazepril 40 mg

amlodipine and olmesartan (am LOE di peen & olme SAR tan)

Synonyms amlodipine besylate and olmesartan medoxomil; olmesartan and amlodipine

U.S./Canadian Brand Names Azor™ [US]

Therapeutic Category Angiotensin II Receptor Blocker Combination; Antihypertensive Agent, Combination; Calcium Channel Blocker

Use Treatment of hypertension

Usual Dosage Oral: Dose is individualized; combination product may be substituted for individual components in patients currently maintained on both agents separately or in patients not adequately controlled with monotherapy (using one of the agents or an agent within same antihypertensive class). Adults: Hypertension: Amlodipine 5-10 mg and olmesartan 20 mg once daily; dose may be titrated after 3-4 weeks of therapy. Maximum recommended doses: Amlodipine 10 mg/day; olmesartan 40 mg/day.

Dosage Forms

Tablet:
Azor™:
5/20: Amlodipine besylate 5 mg and olmesartan medoxomil 20 mg
5/40: Amlodipine besylate 5 mg and olmesartan medoxomil 40 mg
10/20: Amlodipine besylate 10 mg and olmesartan medoxomil 20 mg
10/40: Amlodipine besylate 10 mg and olmesartan medoxomil 40 mg

amlodipine and valsartan (am LOE di peen & val SAR tan)

Synonyms amlodipine besylate and valsartan; valsartan and amlodipine

U.S./Canadian Brand Names Exforge® [US]

Therapeutic Category Angiotensin II Receptor Blocker Combination; Antihypertensive Agent, Combination; Calcium Channel Blocker

Use Treatment of hypertension

Usual Dosage Oral: Dose is individualized; combination product may be substituted for individual components in patients currently maintained on both agents separately or in patients not adequately controlled with monotherapy (using one of the agents or an agent within same antihypertensive class). Adults: Hypertension: Amlodipine 5-10 mg and valsartan 160-320 mg once daily; dose may be titrated after 3-4 weeks of therapy. Maximum recommended doses: Amlodipine 10 mg/day; valsartan 320 mg/day.

Dosage Forms

Tablet:
Exforge®:
5/160: Amlodipine 5 mg and valsartan 160 mg
5/320 mg: Amlodipine 5 mg and valsartan 320 mg
10/160: Amlodipine 10 mg and valsartan 160 mg
10/320: Amlodipine 10 mg and valsartan 320 mg

amlodipine besylate *see* amlodipine *on page 63*
amlodipine besylate and olmesartan medoxomil *see* amlodipine and olmesartan *on page 65*
amlodipine besylate and valsartan *see* amlodipine and valsartan *on page 65*
Ammens® Medicated Deodorant [US-OTC] *see* zinc oxide *on page 993*
ammonapse *see* sodium phenylbutyrate *on page 877*

ammonia spirit (aromatic) (a MOE nee ah SPEAR it, air oh MAT ik)
Synonyms smelling salts
Therapeutic Category Respiratory Stimulant
Use Respiratory and circulatory stimulant; treatment of fainting
Usual Dosage Used as "smelling salts" to treat or prevent fainting
Dosage Forms
  Solution, for inhalation: 1.7% to 2.1% (0.33 mL, 60 mL)

ammonium chloride (a MOE nee um KLOR ide)
Therapeutic Category Electrolyte Supplement, Oral
Use Treatment of hypochloremic states or metabolic alkalosis
Usual Dosage Metabolic alkalosis: The following equations represent different methods of correction utilizing either the serum HCO_3^-, the serum chloride, or the base excess
  Dosing of mEq NH_4Cl via the chloride-deficit method (hypochloremia):
    Dose of mEq NH_4Cl = [0.2 L/kg x body weight (kg)] x [103 - observed serum chloride]; administer 50% of dose over 12 hours, then reevaluate
    Note: 0.2 L/kg is the estimated chloride volume of distribution and 103 is the average normal serum chloride concentration (mEq/L)
  Dosing of mEq NH_4Cl via the bicarbonate-excess method (refractory hypochloremic metabolic alkalosis):
    Dose of NH_4Cl = [0.5 L/kg x body weight (kg)] x (observed serum HCO_3^- - 24); administer 50% of dose over 12 hours, then reevaluate
    Note: 0.5 L/kg is the estimated bicarbonate volume of distribution and 24 is the average normal serum bicarbonate concentration (mEq/L)
  These equations will yield different requirements of ammonium chloride
Dosage Forms
  Injection, solution: Ammonium 5 mEq/mL and chloride 5 mEq/mL (20 mL)

ammonium lactate *see* lactic acid and ammonium hydroxide *on page 542*
Ammonul® [US] *see* sodium phenylacetate and sodium benzoate *on page 877*
AMN107 *see* nilotinib *on page 672*
Amnesteem™ [US] *see* isotretinoin *on page 531*

amobarbital (am oh BAR bi tal)
Synonyms amobarbital sodium; amylobarbitone
U.S./Canadian Brand Names Amytal® [US/Can]
Therapeutic Category Barbiturate
Controlled Substance C-II
Use Hypnotic in short-term treatment of insomnia; reduce anxiety and provide sedation preoperatively
Usual Dosage I.M., I.V.:
  Children 6-12 years: Sedative: Manufacturer's dosing range: 65-500 mg
  Adults:
    Hypnotic: 65-200 mg at bedtime (maximum single dose: 1000 mg)
    Sedative: 30-50 mg 2-3 times/day (maximum single dose: 1000 mg)
Dosage Forms
  Injection, powder for reconstitution:
    Amytal®: 500 mg

amobarbital sodium *see* amobarbital *on page 66*
Amoclan [US] *see* amoxicillin and clavulanate potassium *on page 68*
AMO Vitrax® (Discontinued) *see* hyaluronate and derivatives *on page 476*

amoxapine (a MOKS a peen)

Sound-Alike/Look-Alike Issues
amoxapine may be confused with amoxicillin, Amoxil®
Asendin may be confused with aspirin

Therapeutic Category Antidepressant, Tricyclic (Secondary Amine)

Use Treatment of depression, psychotic depression, depression accompanied by anxiety or agitation

Usual Dosage Oral:
Adolescents: Initial: 25-50 mg/day; increase gradually to 100 mg/day; may administer as divided doses or as a single dose at bedtime
Adults: Initial: 25 mg 2-3 times/day, if tolerated, dosage may be increased to 100 mg 2-3 times/day; may be given in a single bedtime dose when dosage <300 mg/day
Maximum daily dose:
Inpatient: 600 mg
Outpatient: 400 mg

Dosage Forms
Tablet: 25 mg, 50 mg, 100 mg, 150 mg

amoxicillin (a moks i SIL in)

Sound-Alike/Look-Alike Issues
amoxicillin may be confused with amoxapine, Amoxil®, Atarax®
Amoxil® may be confused with amoxapine, amoxicillin

Synonyms *p*-hydroxyampicillin; amoxicillin trihydrate; amoxycillin

U.S./Canadian Brand Names Amoxil® [US]; Apo-Amoxi® [Can]; Gen-Amoxicillin [Can]; Lin-Amox [Can]; Novamoxin® [Can]; Nu-Amoxi [Can]; PHL-Amoxicillin [Can]; PMS-Amoxicillin [Can]

Therapeutic Category Penicillin

Use Treatment of otitis media, sinusitis, and infections caused by susceptible organisms involving the respiratory tract, skin, and urinary tract; prophylaxis of infective endocarditis in patients undergoing surgical or dental procedures; as part of a multidrug regimen for *H. pylori* eradication

Usual Dosage
Usual dosage range:
Children ≤3 months: Oral: 20-30 mg/kg/day divided every 12 hours
Children >3 months and <40 kg: Oral: 20-50 mg/kg/day in divided doses every 8-12 hours
Adults: Oral: 250-500 mg every 8 hours or 500-875 mg twice daily
Indication-specific dosing:
Children >3 months and <40 kg: Oral:
Acute otitis media: 80-90 mg/kg/day divided every 12 hours
Anthrax exposure (CDC guidelines): Note: Postexposure prophylaxis only with documented susceptible organisms: 80 mg/kg/day in divided doses every 8 hours (maximum: 500 mg/dose)
Community-acquired pneumonia:
4 months to <5 years: 80-100 mg/kg/day divided every 8 hours
5-15 years: 100 mg/kg/day divided every 8 hours; **Note:** Treatment with a macrolide or doxycycline (if age >8 years) is preferred due to higher prevalence of atypical pathogens in this age group
Ear, nose, throat, genitourinary tract, or skin/skin structure infections:
Mild to moderate: 25 mg/kg/day in divided doses every 12 hours **or** 20 mg/kg/day in divided doses every 8 hours
Severe: 45 mg/kg/day in divided doses every 12 hours **or** 40 mg/kg/day in divided doses every 8 hours
Lower respiratory tract infections: 45 mg/kg/day in divided doses every 12 hours **or** 40 mg/kg/day in divided doses every 8 hours
Lyme disease: 25-50 mg/kg/day divided every 8 hours (maximum: 500 mg)
Prophylaxis against infective endocarditis: 50 mg/kg 1 hour before procedure. **Note:** American Heart Association (AHA) guidelines now recommend prophylaxis only in patients undergoing invasive procedures and in whom underlying cardiac conditions may predispose to a higher risk of adverse outcomes should infection occur. As of April 2007, routine prophylaxis for GI/GU procedures is no longer recommended by the AHA.
Adults: Oral:
Anthrax exposure (CDC guidelines): Note: Postexposure prophylaxis in pregnant or nursing women only with documented susceptible organisms: 500 mg every 8 hours
Ear, nose, throat, genitourinary tract, or skin/skin structure infections:
Mild to moderate: 500 mg every 12 hours **or** 250 mg every 8 hours
Severe: 875 mg every 12 hours **or** 500 mg every 8 hours

◀

    Helicobacter pylori eradication: 1000 mg twice daily; requires combination therapy with at least one other antibiotic and an acid-suppressing agent (proton pump inhibitor or H$_2$ blocker)

    Lower respiratory tract infections: 875 mg every 12 hours **or** 500 mg every 8 hours

    Lyme disease: 500 mg every 6-8 hours (depending on size of patient) for 21-30 days

    Prophylaxis against infective endocarditis: 2 g 30-60 minutes before procedure. **Note:** American Heart Association (AHA) guidelines now recommend prophylaxis only in patients undergoing invasive procedures and in whom underlying cardiac conditions may predispose to a higher risk of adverse outcomes should infection occur. As of April 2007, routine prophylaxis for GI/GU procedures is no longer recommended by the AHA.

    Prophylaxis in total joint replacement patients undergoing dental procedures which produce bacteremia: 2 g 1 hour prior to procedure

Dosage Forms

    Capsule: 250 mg, 500 mg

    Amoxil®: 500 mg

    Powder for oral suspension: 125 mg/5 mL, 200 mg/5 mL, 250 mg/5 mL, 400 mg/5 mL

    Amoxil®: 250 mg/5 mL, 400 mg/5 mL

    Powder for oral suspension [drops]:

    Amoxil®: 50 mg/mL

    Tablet: 500 mg, 875 mg

    Tablet, chewable: 125 mg, 200 mg, 250 mg, 400 mg

amoxicillin and clavulanate potassium

(a moks i SIL in & klav yoo LAN ate poe TASS ee um)

Sound-Alike/Look-Alike Issues

    Augmentin® may be confused with Azulfidine®

Synonyms amoxicillin and clavulanic acid; clavulanic acid and amoxicillin

U.S./Canadian Brand Names Alti-Amoxi-Clav [Can]; Amoclan [US]; Apo-Amoxi-Clav® [Can]; Augmentin ES-600® [US]; Augmentin XR® [US]; Augmentin® [US/Can]; Clavulin® [Can]; Novo-Clavamoxin [Can]; ratio-Aclavulanate [Can]

Therapeutic Category Penicillin

Use Treatment of otitis media, sinusitis, and infections caused by susceptible organisms involving the lower respiratory tract, skin and skin structure, and urinary tract; spectrum same as amoxicillin with additional coverage of beta-lactamase producing *B. catarrhalis*, *H. influenzae*, *N. gonorrhoeae*, and *S. aureus* (not MRSA). The expanded coverage of this combination makes it a useful alternative when amoxicillin resistance is present and patients cannot tolerate alternative treatments.

Usual Dosage Note: Dose is based on the amoxicillin component

    Usual dosage range:

    Infants <3 months: Oral: 30 mg/kg/day divided every 12 hours using the 125 mg/5 mL suspension

    Children ≥3 months and <40 kg: Oral: 20-90 mg/kg/day divided every 8-12 hours

    Children >40 kg and Adults: Oral: 250-500 mg every 8 hours or 875 mg every 12 hours

    Indication-specific dosing:

    Children ≥3 months and <40 kg: Oral:

      Lower respiratory tract infections, severe infections, sinusitis: 45 mg/kg/day divided every 12 hours **or** 40 mg/kg/day divided every 8 hours

      Mild-to-moderate infections: 25 mg/kg/day divided every 12 hours or 20 mg/kg/day divided every 8 hours

      Otitis media (Augmentin® ES-600): 90 mg/kg/day divided every 12 hours for 10 days in children with severe illness and when coverage for β-lactamase-positive *H. influenzae* and *M. catarrhalis* is needed.

    Children ≥16 years and Adults: Oral:

      Acute bacterial sinusitis: Extended release tablet: Two 1000 mg tablets every 12 hours for 10 days

      Bite wounds (animal/human): 875 mg every 12 hours **or** 500 mg every 8 hours

      Chronic obstructive pulmonary disease: 875 mg every 12 hours **or** 500 mg every 8 hours

      Diabetic foot: Extended release tablet: Two 1000 mg tablets every 12 hours for 7-14 days

      Diverticulitis, perirectal abscess: Extended release tablet: Two 1000 mg tablets every 12 hours for 7-10 days

      Erysipelas: 875 mg every 12 hours **or** 500 mg every 8 hours

      Febrile neutropenia: 875 mg every 12 hours

      Pneumonia:

      Aspiration: 875 mg every 12 hours

Community-acquired: Extended release tablet: Two 1000 mg tablets every 12 hours for 7-10 days
Pyelonephritis (acute, uncomplicated): 875 mg every 12 hours **or** 500 mg every 8 hours
Skin abscess: 875 mg every 12 hours

Dosage Forms
Powder for oral suspension: 200: Amoxicillin 200 mg and clavulanate potassium 28.5 mg per 5 mL; 400: Amoxicillin 400 mg and clavulanate potassium 57 mg per 5 mL; 600: Amoxicillin 600 mg and clavulanate potassium 42.9 mg per 5 mL
Amoclan:
200: Amoxicillin 200 mg and clavulanate potassium 28.5 mg per 5 mL
400: Amoxicillin 400 mg and clavulanate potassium 57 mg per 5 mL
Augmentin®:
125: Amoxicillin 125 mg and clavulanate potassium 31.25 mg per 5 mL
250: Amoxicillin 250 mg and clavulanate potassium 62.5 mg per 5 mL
400: Amoxicillin 400 mg and clavulanate potassium 57 mg per 5 mL
Augmentin ES-600®: Amoxicillin 600 mg and clavulanate potassium 42.9 mg per 5 mL
Tablet: 500: Amoxicillin 500 mg and clavulanate potassium 125 mg; 875: Amoxicillin 875 mg and clavulanate potassium 125 mg
Augmentin®:
250: Amoxicillin 250 mg and clavulanate potassium 125 mg
500: Amoxicillin 500 mg and clavulanate potassium 125 mg
875: Amoxicillin 875 mg and clavulanate potassium 125 mg
Tablet, chewable: 200: Amoxicillin 200 mg and clavulanate potassium 28.5 mg; 400: Amoxicillin 400 mg and clavulanate potassium 57 mg
Augmentin®:
250: Amoxicillin 250 mg and clavulanate potassium 62.5 mg
Tablet, extended release:
Augmentin XR®: Amoxicillin 1000 mg and clavulanate acid 62.5 mg

amoxicillin and clavulanic acid *see* amoxicillin and clavulanate potassium *on page 68*
amoxicillin, lansoprazole, and clarithromycin *see* lansoprazole, amoxicillin, and clarithromycin *on page 549*
amoxicillin trihydrate *see* amoxicillin *on page 67*
Amoxil® [US] *see* amoxicillin *on page 67*
amoxycillin *see* amoxicillin *on page 67*
Amphadase™ [US] *see* hyaluronidase *on page 477*
amphetamine and dextroamphetamine *see* dextroamphetamine and amphetamine *on page 283*
Amphocin® *(Discontinued)* *see* amphotericin B (conventional) *on page 70*
Amphojel® [Can] *see* aluminum hydroxide *on page 53*
Amphojel® *(Discontinued)* *see* aluminum hydroxide *on page 53*
Amphotec® [US/Can] *see* amphotericin B cholesteryl sulfate complex *on page 69*
Amphotec® [Can] *see* amphotericin B lipid complex *on page 71*

amphotericin B cholesteryl sulfate complex
(am foe TER i sin bee kole LES te ril SUL fate KOM plecks)
Synonyms ABCD; amphotericin B colloidal dispersion
U.S./Canadian Brand Names Amphotec® [US/Can]
Therapeutic Category Antifungal Agent
Use Treatment of invasive aspergillosis in patients who have failed amphotericin B deoxycholate treatment, or who have renal impairment or experience unacceptable toxicity which precludes treatment with amphotericin B deoxycholate in effective doses.
Usual Dosage I.V.: Children and Adults:
Premedication: For patients who experience chills, fever, hypotension, nausea, or other nonanaphylactic infusion-related immediate reactions, premedicate with the following drugs, 30-60 minutes prior to drug administration: a nonsteroidal (eg, ibuprofen, choline magnesium trisalicylate) with or without diphenhydramine; **or** acetaminophen with diphenhydramine; **or** hydrocortisone 50-100 mg. If the patient experiences rigors during the infusion, meperidine may be administered.
Range: 3-4 mg/kg/day (infusion of 1 mg/kg/hour); maximum: 7.5 mg/kg/day
Dosage Forms
Injection, powder for reconstitution:
Amphotec®: 50 mg, 100 mg

amphotericin B colloidal dispersion *see* amphotericin B cholesteryl sulfate complex *on page 69*

amphotericin B (conventional) (am foe TER i sin bee con VEN sha nal)

Synonyms amphotericin B desoxycholate

U.S./Canadian Brand Names Fungizone® [Can]

Therapeutic Category Antifungal Agent

Use Treatment of severe systemic and central nervous system infections caused by susceptible fungi such as *Candida* species, *Histoplasma capsulatum*, *Cryptococcus neoformans*, *Aspergillus* species, *Blastomyces dermatitidis*, *Torulopsis glabrata*, and *Coccidioides immitis*; fungal peritonitis; irrigant for bladder fungal infections; used in fungal infection in patients with bone marrow transplantation, amebic meningoencephalitis, ocular aspergillosis (intraocular injection), candidal cystitis (bladder irrigation), chemoprophylaxis (low-dose I.V.), immunocompromised patients at risk of aspergillosis (intranasal/nebulized), refractory meningitis (intrathecal), coccidioidal arthritis (intraarticular/I.M.).

Low-dose amphotericin B has been administered after bone marrow transplantation to reduce the risk of invasive fungal disease.

Usual Dosage

Premedication: For patients who experience infusion-related immediate reactions, premedicate with the following drugs 30-60 minutes prior to drug administration: NSAID (with or without diphenhydramine) **or** acetaminophen with diphenhydramine **or** hydrocortisone 50-100 mg. If the patient experiences rigors during the infusion, meperidine may be administered.

Usual dosage ranges:

Infants and Children:

Test dose: I.V.: 0.1 mg/kg/dose to a maximum of 1 mg; infuse over 30-60 minutes. Many clinicians believe a test dose is unnecessary.

Maintenance dose: 0.25-1 mg/kg/day given once daily; infuse over 2-6 hours. Once therapy has been established, amphotericin B can be administered on an every-other-day basis at 1-1.5 mg/kg/dose; cumulative dose: 1.5-2 g over 6-10 weeks.

Duration of therapy: Varies with nature of infection, usual duration is 4-12 weeks or cumulative dose of 1-4 g

Adults:

Test dose: 1 mg infused over 20-30 minutes. Many clinicians believe a test dose is unnecessary.

Maintenance dose: Usual: 0.05-1.5 mg/kg/day; 1-1.5 mg/kg over 4-6 hours every other day may be given once therapy is established; aspergillosis, rhinocerebral mucormycosis, often require 1-1.5 mg/kg/day; do not exceed 1.5 mg/kg/day

Indication-specific dosing:

Children: **Meningitis, coccidioidal or cryptococcal:** I.T.: 25-100 mcg every 48-72 hours; increase to 500 mcg as tolerated

Adults:

Aspergillosis, disseminated: I.V.: 0.6-0.7 mg/kg/day for 3-6 months

Bone marrow transplantation (prophylaxis): I.V.: Low-dose amphotericin B 0.1-0.25 mg/kg/day has been administered after bone marrow transplantation to reduce the risk of invasive fungal disease.

Candidemia (neutropenic or nonneutropenic): I.V.: 0.6-1 mg/kg/day until 14 days after last positive blood culture and resolution of signs and symptoms

Candidiasis, chronic, disseminated: I.V.: 0.6-0.7 mg/kg/day for 3-6 months and resolution of radiologic lesions

Cystitis: Candidal: Bladder irrigation: Irrigate with 50 mcg/mL solution instilled periodically or continuously for 5-10 days or until cultures are clear

Dematiaceous fungi: I.V.: 0.7 mg/kg/day in combination with an azole

Endocarditis: I.V.: 0.6-1 mg/kg/day (with or without flucytosine) for 1 week, then 0.8 mg/kg/day every other day for 6-8 weeks postoperatively

Endophthalmitis, fungal: I.V.: 0.7-1 mg/kg/day (with or without flucytosine) for at least 4 weeks

Esophagitis: I.V.: 0.3-0.7 mg/kg/day for 14-21 after clinical improvement

Histoplasmosis: Chronic, severe pulmonary or disseminated: I.V.: 0.5-1 mg/kg/day for 7 days, then 0.8 mg/kg every other day (or 3 times/week) until total dose of 10-15 mg/kg; may continue itraconazole as suppressive therapy (lifelong for immunocompromised patients)

Meningitis:

Candidal: I.V.: 0.7-1 mg/kg/day (with or without flucytosine) for at least 4 weeks

Cryptococcal or Coccidioides: I.T.: Initial: 25-300 mcg every 48-72 hours; increase to 500 mcg to 1 mg as tolerated; maximum total dose: 15 mg has been suggested

Histoplasma: I.V.: 0.5-1 mg/kg/day for 7 days, then 0.8 mg/kg every other day (or 3 times/week) for 3 months total duration; follow with fluconazole suppressive therapy for up to 12 months

Meningoencephalitis, cryptococcal: I.V.:
HIV positive: 0.7-1 mg/kg/day (plus flucytosine 100 mg/kg/day) for 2 weeks, then change to oral fluconazole for at least 10 weeks; alternatively, amphotericin and flucytosine may be continued uninterrupted for 6-10 weeks
HIV negative: 0.5-0.7 mg/kg/day (plus flucytosine) for 2 weeks

Osteomyelitis: Candidal: I.V.: 0.5-1 mg/kg/day for 6-10 weeks

Penicillium marneffei: I.V.: 0.6 mg/kg/day for 2 weeks

Pneumonia: Cryptococcal (mild to moderate): I.V.:
HIV positive: 0.5-1 mg/kg/day
HIV negative: 0.5-0.7 mg/kg/day (plus flucytosine) for 2 weeks

Sporotrichosis: Pulmonary, meningeal, osteoarticular, or disseminated: I.V.: Total dose of 1-2 g, then change to oral itraconazole or fluconazole for suppressive therapy

Dosage Forms
Injection, powder for reconstitution: 50 mg

amphotericin B desoxycholate *see* amphotericin B (conventional) *on page 70*

amphotericin B lipid complex (am foe TER i sin bee LIP id KOM pleks)

Synonyms ABLC

U.S./Canadian Brand Names Abelcet® [US/Can]; Amphotec® [Can]

Therapeutic Category Antifungal Agent

Use Treatment of aspergillosis or any type of progressive fungal infection in patients who are refractory to or intolerant of conventional amphotericin B therapy

Usual Dosage I.V.: Children and Adults:
Premedication: For patients who experience infusion-related immediate reactions, premedicate with the following drugs, 30-60 minutes prior to drug administration: a nonsteroidal antiinflammatory agent ± diphenhydramine **or** acetaminophen with diphenhydramine **or** hydrocortisone 50-100 mg. If the patient experiences rigors during the infusion, meperidine may be administered.
Range: 2.5-5 mg/kg/day as a single infusion

Dosage Forms
Injection, suspension [preservative free]:
Abelcet®: 5 mg/mL (20 mL)

amphotericin B liposomal (am foe TER i sin bee lye po SO mal)

Synonyms L-AmB

U.S./Canadian Brand Names AmBisome® [US/Can]

Therapeutic Category Antifungal Agent, Systemic

Use Empirical therapy for presumed fungal infection in febrile, neutropenic patients; treatment of patients with *Aspergillus* species, *Candida* species, and/or *Cryptococcus* species infections refractory to amphotericin B desoxycholate, or in patients where renal impairment or unacceptable toxicity precludes the use of amphotericin B desoxycholate; treatment of cryptococcal meningitis in HIV-infected patients; treatment of visceral leishmaniasis

Usual Dosage
Usual dosage range:
Children ≥1 month: I.V.: 3-5 mg/kg/day
Adults: I.V.: 2-6 mg/kg/day; **Note:** Higher doses (15 mg/kg/day) have been used clinically.
Note: Premedication: For patients who experience nonanaphylactic infusion-related immediate reactions, premedicate with the following drugs 30-60 minutes prior to drug administration: A nonsteroidal antiinflammatory agent ± diphenhydramine; **or** acetaminophen with diphenhydramine; **or** hydrocortisone 50-100 mg. If the patient experiences rigors during the infusion, meperidine may be administered.

Indication-specific dosing:
Children ≥1 month: I.V.:
Candidal infection:
Endocarditis: 3-6 mg/kg/day with flucytosine 25-37.5 mg/kg 4 times daily
Meningitis: 5 mg/kg/day with flucytosine 100 mg/kg/day
Cryptococcal meningitis (HIV-positive): 6 mg/kg/day

Note: IDSA guidelines (April, 2000) report doses of 3-6 mg/kg/day, noting that 4 mg/kg/day was effective in a small, open-label trial. The manufacturer's labeled dose of 6 mg/kg/day was approved in June, 2000.

Empiric therapy: 3 mg/kg/day

Systemic fungal infections *(Aspergillus, Candida, Cryptococcus)*: 3-5 mg/kg/day

Visceral leishmaniasis:

Immunocompetent: 3 mg/kg/day on days 1-5, and 3 mg/kg/day on days 14 and 21; a repeat course may be given in patients who do not achieve parasitic clearance

Note: Alternate regimen of 10 mg/kg/day for 2 days has been reportedly effective.

Immunocompromised: 4 mg/kg/day on days 1-5, and 4 mg/kg/day on days 10, 17, 24, 31, and 38

Adults: I.V.:

Candidal infection:

Endocarditis: 3-6 mg/kg/day with flucytosine 25-37.5 mg/kg 4 times daily

Meningitis: 5 mg/kg/day with flucytosine 100 mg/kg/day

Cryptococcal meningitis (HIV-positive): 6 mg/kg/day

Note: IDSA guidelines (April, 2000) report doses of 3-6 mg/kg/day, noting that 4 mg/kg/day was effective in a small, open-label trial. The manufacturer's labeled dose of 6 mg/kg/day was approved in June, 2000.

Empiric therapy: 3 mg/kg/day

Fungal sinusitis: 5-7.5 mg/kg/day

Note: Use azole antifungal if causative organism is *Pseudallescheria boydii* (*Scedosporium* sp).

Systemic fungal infections *(Aspergillus, Candida, Cryptococcus)*: 3-5 mg/kg/day

Visceral leishmaniasis:

Immunocompetent: 3 mg/kg/day on days 1-5, and 3 mg/kg/day on days 14 and 21; a repeat course may be given in patients who do not achieve parasitic clearance

Note: Alternate regimen of 2 mg/kg/day for 5 days has been reportedly effective.

Immunocompromised: 4 mg/kg/day on days 1-5, and 4 mg/kg/day on days 10, 17, 24, 31, and 38

Dosage Forms

Injection, powder for reconstitution:

AmBisome®: 50 mg

ampicillin (am pi SIL in)

Sound-Alike/Look-Alike Issues

ampicillin may be confused with aminophylline

Synonyms aminobenzylpenicillin; ampicillin sodium; ampicillin trihydrate

U.S./Canadian Brand Names Apo-Ampi® [Can]; Novo-Ampicillin [Can]; Nu-Ampi [Can]

Therapeutic Category Penicillin

Use Treatment of susceptible bacterial infections (nonbeta-lactamase-producing organisms); treatment or prophylaxis of infective endocarditis; susceptible bacterial infections caused by streptococci, pneumococci, nonpenicillinase-producing staphylococci, *Listeria*, meningococci; some strains of *H. influenzae*, *Salmonella*, *Shigella*, *E. coli*, *Enterobacter*, and *Klebsiella*

Usual Dosage

Usual dosage range:

Infants and Children:

Oral: 50-100 mg/kg/day in doses divided every 6 hours (maximum: 2-4 g/day)

I.M., I.V.: 100-400 mg/kg/day in divided doses every 6 hours (maximum: 12 g/day)

Adults: Oral, I.M., I.V.: 250-500 mg every 6 hours

Indication-specific dosing:

Infants and Children:

Prophylaxis against Infective endocarditis:

Dental, oral, or respiratory tract procedures: I.M., I.V.: 50 mg/kg within 30-60 minutes prior to procedure in patients not allergic to penicillin and unable to take oral amoxicillin. Intramuscular injections should be avoided in patients who are receiving anticoagulant therapy. In these circumstances, orally administered regimens should be given whenever possible. Intravenously administered antibiotics should be used for patients who are unable to tolerate or absorb oral medications.

Note: American Heart Association (AHA) guidelines now recommend prophylaxis only in patients undergoing invasive procedures and in whom underlying cardiac conditions may predispose to a higher risk of adverse outcomes should infection occur.

Genitourinary and gastrointestinal tract procedures: I.M., I.V.:

High-risk patients: 50 mg/kg (maximum: 2 g) within 30 minutes prior to procedure, followed by ampicillin 25 mg/kg (or amoxicillin 25 mg/kg orally) 6 hours later; must be used in combination with gentamicin. **Note:** As of April 2007, routine prophylaxis for GI/GU procedures is no longer recommended by the AHA.

Moderate-risk patients: 50 mg/kg within 30 minutes prior to procedure

Mild-to-moderate infections:

Oral: 50-100 mg/kg/day in doses divided every 6 hours (maximum: 2-4 g/day)

I.M., I.V.: 100-150 mg/kg/day in divided doses every 6 hours (maximum: 2-4 g/day)

Severe infections, meningitis: I.M., I.V.: 200-400 mg/kg/day in divided doses every 6 hours (maximum: 6-12 g/day)

Adults:

Actinomycosis: I.V.: 50 mg/kg/day for 4-6 weeks then oral amoxicillin

Cholangitis (acute): I.V.: 2 g every 4 hours with gentamicin

Diverticulitis: I.M., I.V.: 2 g every 6 hours with metronidazole

Endocarditis:

Infective: I.V.: 12 g/day via continuous infusion or divided every 4 hours

Prophylaxis: Dental, oral, or respiratory tract: I.M., I.V.: 2 g within 30-60 minutes prior to procedure in patients not allergic to penicillin and unable to take oral amoxicillin. Intramuscular injections should be avoided in patients who are receiving anticoagulant therapy. In these circumstances, orally administered regimens should be given whenever possible. Intravenously administered antibiotics should be used for patients who are unable to tolerate or absorb oral medications.

Note: American Heart Association (AHA) guidelines now recommend prophylaxis only in patients undergoing invasive procedures and in whom underlying cardiac conditions may predispose to a higher risk of adverse outcomes should infection occur.

Prophylaxis in total joint replacement patient: I.M., I.V.: 2 g 1 hour prior to the procedure

Genitourinary and gastrointestinal tract procedures:

High-risk patients: I.M., I.V.: 2 g within 30 minutes prior to procedure, followed by ampicillin 1 g (or amoxicillin 1g orally) 6 hours later; must be used in combination with gentamicin. **Note:** As of April 2007, routine prophylaxis for GI/GU procedures is no longer recommended by the AHA.

Moderate-risk patients: I.M., I.V.: 2 g within 30 minutes prior to procedure

Group B strep prophylaxis (intrapartum): I.V.: 2 g initial dose, then 1 g every 4 hours until delivery

Listeria **infections:** I.V.: 200 mg/kg/day divided every 6 hours

Sepsis/meningitis: I.M., I.V.: 150-250 mg/kg/day divided every 3-4 hours (range: 6-12 g/day)

Urinary tract infections (enterococcus suspected): I.V.: 1-2 g every 6 hours with gentamicin

Dosage Forms

Capsule: 250 mg, 500 mg

Injection, powder for reconstitution: 125 mg, 250 mg, 500 mg, 1 g, 2 g, 10 g

Powder for oral suspension: 125 mg/5 mL, 250 mg/5 mL

ampicillin and sulbactam (am pi SIL in & SUL bak tam)

Synonyms sulbactam and ampicillin

U.S./Canadian Brand Names Unasyn® [US/Can]

Therapeutic Category Penicillin

Use Treatment of susceptible bacterial infections involved with skin and skin structure, intraabdominal infections, gynecological infections; spectrum is that of ampicillin plus organisms producing beta-lactamases such as *S. aureus, H. influenzae, E. coli, Klebsiella, Acinetobacter, Enterobacter,* and anaerobes

Usual Dosage Note: Unasyn® (ampicillin/sulbactam) is a combination product. Dosage recommendations for Unasyn® are based on the ampicillin component.

Usual dosage range:

Children ≥1 year: I.V.: 100-400 mg ampicillin/kg/day divided every 6 hours (maximum: 8 g ampicillin/day, 12 g Unasyn®). **Note:** The American Academy of Pediatrics recommends a dose of up to 300 mg/kg/day for severe infection in infants >1 month of age.

Adults: I.M., I.V.: 1-2 g ampicillin (1.5-3 g Unasyn®) every 6 hours (maximum: 8 g ampicillin/day, 12 g Unasyn®)

Indication-specific dosing:

Children:

Epiglottitis: I.V.: 100-200 mg ampicillin/kg/day divided in 4 doses

Mild-to-moderate infections: I.M., I.V.: 100-200 mg ampicillin/kg/day (150-300 mg Unasyn®) divided every 6 hours (maximum: 8 g ampicillin/day, 12 g Unasyn®)

▶

◀

Peritonsillar and retropharyngeal abscess: I.V.: 50 mg ampicillin/kg/dose every 6 hours
Severe infections: I.M., I.V.: 200-400 mg ampicillin/kg/day divided every 6 hours (maximum: 8 g ampicillin/day, 12 g Unasyn®)
  Adults: Doses expressed as ampicillin/sulbactam combination:
  Amnionitis, cholangitis, diverticulitis, endometritis, endophthalmitis, epididymitis/orchitis, liver abscess, osteomyelitis (diabetic foot), peritonitis: I.V.: 3 g every 6 hours
  Endocarditis: I.V.: 3 g every 6 hours with gentamicin or vancomycin for 4-6 weeks
  Orbital cellulitis: I.V.: 1.5 g every 6 hours
  Parapharyngeal space infections: I.V.: 3 g every 6 hours
  ***Pasteurella multocida* (human, canine/feline bites):** I.V.: 1.5-3 g every 6 hours
  Pelvic inflammatory disease: I.V.: 3 g every 6 hours with doxycycline
  Peritonitis (CAPD): Intraperitoneal:
    Anuric, intermittent: 3 g every 12 hours
    Anuric, continuous: Loading dose: 1.5 g; maintenance dose: 150 mg
  Pneumonia:
    Aspiration, community-acquired: I.V.: 1.5-3 g every 6 hours
    Hospital-acquired: I.V.: 3 g every 6 hours
  Urinary tract infections, pyelonephritis: I.V.: 3 g every 6 hours for 14 days
Dosage Forms
  Injection, powder for reconstitution: 1.5 g [ampicillin 1 g and sulbactam 0.5 g]; 3 g [ampicillin 2 g and sulbactam 1 g]; 15 g [ampicillin 10 g and sulbactam 5 g]
  Unasyn®: 1.5 g [ampicillin 1 g and sulbactam 0.5 g]; 3 g [ampicillin 2 g and sulbactam 1 g]; 15 g [ampicillin 10 g and sulbactam 5 g]; 15 g [ampicillin 10 g and sulbactam 5 g

ampicillin sodium *see* ampicillin *on page 72*
ampicillin trihydrate *see* ampicillin *on page 72*

amprenavir (am PREN a veer)

U.S./Canadian Brand Names Agenerase® [Can]
Therapeutic Category Protease Inhibitor
Use Treatment of HIV infections in combination with at least two other antiretroviral agents; oral solution should only be used when capsules or other protease inhibitors are not therapeutic options
Usual Dosage Oral: **Note:** Capsule and oral solution are **not** interchangeable on a mg-per-mg basis.
  Capsule:
    Children 4-12 years **or** 13-16 years (<50 kg): 20 mg/kg twice daily or 15 mg/kg 3 times daily; maximum: 2400 mg/day
    Children >13 years (≥50 kg) and Adults: 1200 mg twice daily
    Note: Dosage adjustments for amprenavir when administered in combination therapy:
      Efavirenz: Adjustments necessary for both agents:
        Amprenavir 1200 mg 3 times/day (single protease inhibitor) **or**
        Amprenavir 1200 mg twice daily plus ritonavir 200 mg twice daily
      Ritonavir: Adjustments necessary for both agents:
        Amprenavir 1200 mg plus ritonavir 200 mg once daily **or**
        Amprenavir 600 mg plus ritonavir 100 mg twice daily
      Note: Oral solution of ritonavir and amprenavir should not be coadministered.
  Solution:
    Children 4-12 years **or** 13-16 years (<50 kg): 22.5 mg/kg twice daily or 17 mg/kg 3 times daily; maximum: 2800 mg/day
    Children >13 years (≥50 kg) and Adults: 1400 mg twice daily

AMPT *see* metyrosine *on page 629*
amrinone lactate *see* inamrinone *on page 505*
Amrix® [US] *see* cyclobenzaprine *on page 255*
Amvisc® *(Discontinued)* *see* hyaluronate and derivatives *on page 476*
Amvisc® Plus *(Discontinued)* *see* hyaluronate and derivatives *on page 476*

amyl nitrite (AM il NYE trite)

Synonyms isoamyl nitrite
Therapeutic Category Vasodilator
Use Coronary vasodilator in angina pectoris; adjunct in treatment of cyanide poisoning; produce changes in the intensity of heart murmurs

Usual Dosage Nasal inhalation:
Cyanide poisoning: Children and Adults: Inhale the vapor from a 0.3 mL crushed ampul every minute for 15-30 seconds until I.V. sodium nitrite infusion is available
Angina: Adults: 1-6 inhalations from 1 crushed ampul; may repeat in 3-5 minutes

Dosage Forms
Vapor for inhalation [crushable covered glass capsules]: Amyl nitrite USP (0.3 mL)

amyl nitrite, sodium thiosulfate, and sodium nitrite *see* sodium nitrite, sodium thiosulfate, and amyl nitrite *on page 876*
amylobarbitone *see* amobarbital *on page 66*
Amytal® [US/Can] *see* amobarbital *on page 66*
AN100226 *see* natalizumab *on page 658*
Anabolin® (Discontinued) *see* nandrolone *on page 655*
Anacin® PM Aspirin Free (Discontinued) *see* acetaminophen and diphenhydramine *on page 21*
Anadrol®-50 [US] *see* oxymetholone *on page 712*
Anafranil® [US/Can] *see* clomipramine *on page 235*

anagrelide (an AG gre lide)

Synonyms anagrelide hydrochloride; BL4162A; NSC-724577
U.S./Canadian Brand Names Agrylin® [US/Can]; Dom-Anagrelide [Can]; Gen-Anagrelide [Can]; PHL-Anagrelide [Can]; PMS-Anagrelide [Can]; Sandoz-Anagrelide [Can]
Therapeutic Category Platelet Reducing Agent
Use Treatment of thrombocythemia associated with myeloproliferative disorders
Usual Dosage Note: Maintain for ≥1 week, then adjust to the lowest effective dose to reduce and maintain platelet count <600,000/µL ideally to the normal range; the dose must not be increased by >0.5 mg/day in any 1 week; maximum dose: 10 mg/day or 2.5 mg/dose

Oral: Thrombocythemia:
Children: Initial: 0.5 mg/day (range: 0.5 mg 1-4 times/day)
Adults: 0.5 mg 4 times/day or 1 mg twice daily (most patients will experience adequate response at dose ranges of 1.5-3 mg/day)

Dosage Forms
Capsule: 0.5 mg, 1 mg
Agrylin®: 0.5 mg

anagrelide hydrochloride *see* anagrelide *on page 75*

anakinra (an a KIN ra)

Sound-Alike/Look-Alike Issues
anakinra may be confused with amikacin
Synonyms IL-1Ra; interleukin-1 receptor antagonist
U.S./Canadian Brand Names Kineret® [US/Can]
Therapeutic Category Antirheumatic, Disease Modifying
Use Treatment of moderately- to severely-active rheumatoid arthritis in adult patients who have failed one or more disease-modifying antirheumatic drugs (DMARDs); may be used alone or in combination with DMARDs (other than tumor necrosis factor-blocking agents)
Usual Dosage SubQ: Adults: Rheumatoid arthritis: 100 mg once daily (administer at approximately the same time each day)

Dosage Forms
Injection, solution [preservative free]:
Kineret®: 100 mg/0.67 mL (1 mL)

Ana-Kit® [US] *see* epinephrine and chlorpheniramine *on page 345*
Analpram-HC® [US] *see* pramoxine and hydrocortisone *on page 778*
AnaMantle® HC [US] *see* lidocaine and hydrocortisone *on page 564*
AnaMantle HC® Forte [US] *see* lidocaine and hydrocortisone *on page 564*
Anamine® Syrup (Discontinued) *see* chlorpheniramine and pseudoephedrine *on page 207*
Anandron® [Can] *see* nilutamide *on page 672*
Anaplex® DM [US] *see* brompheniramine, pseudoephedrine, and dextromethorphan *on page 146*

Anaplex® DMX [US] *see* brompheniramine, pseudoephedrine, and dextromethorphan *on page 146*
Anaplex® Liquid *(Discontinued)* *see* chlorpheniramine and pseudoephedrine *on page 207*
Anaprox® [US/Can] *see* naproxen *on page 656*
Anaprox® DS [US/Can] *see* naproxen *on page 656*
Anaspaz® [US] *see* hyoscyamine *on page 492*

anastrozole (an AS troe zole)
Sound-Alike/Look-Alike Issues
Anastrozole may be confused with letrozole
Synonyms ICI-D1033; NSC-719344; ZD1033
U.S./Canadian Brand Names Arimidex® [US/Can]
Therapeutic Category Antineoplastic Agent
Use Treatment of locally-advanced or metastatic breast cancer (ER-positive or hormone receptor unknown) in postmenopausal women; treatment of advanced breast cancer in postmenopausal women with disease progression following tamoxifen therapy; adjuvant treatment of early ER-positive breast cancer in postmenopausal women
Usual Dosage Oral (refer to individual protocols): Adults: Breast cancer: 1 mg once daily
Dosage Forms
Tablet:
Arimidex®: 1 mg

Anatrast [US] *see* barium *on page 116*
Anbesol® [US-OTC] *see* benzocaine *on page 124*
Anbesol® Baby [US-OTC/Can] *see* benzocaine *on page 124*
Anbesol® Cold Sore Therapy [US-OTC] *see* benzocaine *on page 124*
Anbesol® Jr. [US-OTC] *see* benzocaine *on page 124*
Anbesol® Maximum Strength [US-OTC] *see* benzocaine *on page 124*
Ancobon® [US/Can] *see* flucytosine *on page 406*
Andehist DM NR [US] *see* brompheniramine, pseudoephedrine, and dextromethorphan *on page 146*
Andehist DM NR Drops *(Discontinued)*
Andehist NR Drops *(Discontinued)*
Andehist NR Syrup [US] *see* brompheniramine and pseudoephedrine *on page 144*
Andriol® [Can] *see* testosterone *on page 912*
Androcur® [Can] *see* cyproterone *(Canada only) on page 259*
Androcur® Depot [Can] *see* cyproterone *(Canada only) on page 259*
Androderm® [US/Can] *see* testosterone *on page 912*
AndroGel® [US/Can] *see* testosterone *on page 912*
Android® [US] *see* methyltestosterone *on page 624*
Andro-L.A.® Injection *(Discontinued)* *see* testosterone *on page 912*
Androlone®-D *(Discontinued)* *see* nandrolone *on page 655*
Androlone® *(Discontinued)* *see* nandrolone *on page 655*
Andropository [Can] *see* testosterone *on page 912*
Andropository® Injection *(Discontinued)* *see* testosterone *on page 912*
Androvite® [US-OTC] *see* vitamins (multiple/oral) *on page 983*
Androxy™ [US] *see* fluoxymesterone *on page 414*
Anectine® [US] *see* succinylcholine *on page 890*
Anestacon® [US] *see* lidocaine *on page 561*
Anestafoam™ [US-OTC] *see* lidocaine *on page 561*
aneurine hydrochloride *see* thiamine *on page 920*
Anexate® [Can] *see* flumazenil *on page 407*
Anexsia® [US] *see* hydrocodone and acetaminophen *on page 481*
Anextuss [US] *see* guaifenesin, dextromethorphan, and phenylephrine *on page 459*
Angeliq® [US/Can] *see* drospirenone and estradiol *on page 327*
Angiofluor™ [US] *see* fluorescein *on page 410*

Angiofluor™ Lite [US] *see* fluorescein *on page 410*
Angiomax® [US/Can] *see* bivalirudin *on page 138*
anhydrous glucose *see* dextrose *on page 286*

anidulafungin (ay nid yoo la FUN jin)

Synonyms LY303366
U.S./Canadian Brand Names Eraxis™ [US/Can]
Therapeutic Category Antifungal Agent, Parenteral; Echinocandin
Use Treatment of candidemia and other forms of *Candida* infections (including those of intraabdominal, peritoneal, and esophageal locus)
Usual Dosage I.V.: Adults:
Candidemia, intraabdominal or peritoneal candidiasis: 200 mg loading dose on day 1, followed by 100 mg daily for at least 14 days after last positive culture
Esophageal candidiasis: 100 mg loading dose on day 1, followed by 50 mg daily for at least 14 days and for at least 7 days after symptom resolution
Dosage Forms
Injection, powder for reconstitution [preservative free]:
Eraxis™: 50 mg, 100 mg

Anodynos-DHC® *(Discontinued)* *see* hydrocodone and acetaminophen *on page 481*
Anolor 300 [US] *see* butalbital, acetaminophen, and caffeine *on page 155*
Anoquan® *(Discontinued)*
Ansaid® [Can] *see* flurbiprofen *on page 416*
Ansaid® *(Discontinued)* *see* flurbiprofen *on page 416*
ansamycin *see* rifabutin *on page 833*
Antabuse® [US] *see* disulfiram *on page 312*
Antara™ [US] *see* fenofibrate *on page 393*
Antazoline-V® Ophthalmic *(Discontinued)*
Anthra-Derm® *(Discontinued)* *see* anthralin *on page 77*
Anthraforte® [Can] *see* anthralin *on page 77*

anthralin (AN thra lin)

Synonyms dithranol
U.S./Canadian Brand Names Anthraforte® [Can]; Anthranol® [Can]; Anthrascalp® [Can]; Dritho-Scalp® [US]; Micanol® [Can]; Psoriatec™ [US]
Therapeutic Category Keratolytic Agent
Use Treatment of psoriasis (quiescent or chronic psoriasis)
Usual Dosage Topical: Adults: Generally, apply once a day or as directed. The irritant potential of anthralin is directly related to the strength being used and each patient's individual tolerance. Always commence treatment using a short, daily contact time (5-10 minutes) for at least 1 week using the lowest strength possible. Contact time may be gradually increased (to 20-30 minutes) as tolerated.
Skin application: Apply sparingly only to psoriatic lesions and rub gently and carefully into the skin until absorbed. Avoid applying an excessive quantity which may cause unnecessary soiling and staining of the clothing or bed linen.
Scalp application: Comb hair to remove scalar debris, wet hair and, after suitably parting, rub cream well into the lesions, taking care to prevent the cream from spreading onto the forehead.
Remove by washing or showering; optimal period of contact will vary according to the strength used and the patient's response to treatment. Continue treatment until the skin is entirely clear (ie, when there is nothing to feel with the fingers and the texture is normal).
Dosage Forms
Cream:
Dritho-Scalp®: 0.5% (50 g)
Psoriatec™: 1% (50 g)

Anthranol® [Can] *see* anthralin *on page 77*
Anthrascalp® [Can] *see* anthralin *on page 77*

anthrax vaccine, adsorbed (AN thraks vak SEEN ad SORBED)

Synonyms AVA

U.S./Canadian Brand Names BioThrax™ [US]

Therapeutic Category Vaccine

Use Immunization against *Bacillus anthracis*. Recommended for individuals who may come in contact with animal products which come from anthrax endemic areas and may be contaminated with *Bacillus anthracis* spores; recommended for high-risk persons such as veterinarians and other handling potentially infected animals. Routine immunization for the general population is not recommended.

The Department of Defense is implementing an anthrax vaccination program against the biological warfare agent anthrax, which will be administered to all active duty and reserve personnel.

Usual Dosage SubQ: Children ≥18 years and Adults:

Primary immunization: Three injections of 0.5 mL each given 2 weeks apart, followed by three additional injections given at 6-, 12-, and 18 months; it is not necessary to restart the series if a dose is not given on time; resume as soon as practical

Subsequent booster injections: 0.5 mL at 1-year intervals are recommended for immunity to be maintained

Dosage Forms

Injection, suspension:

BioThrax™: *Bacillus anthracis* (5 mL)

anti-4 alpha integrin *see* natalizumab *on page 658*

131 I anti-B1 antibody *see* tositumomab and iodine I 131 tositumomab *on page 937*

131 I-anti-B1 monoclonal antibody *see* tositumomab and iodine I 131 tositumomab *on page 937*

Antiben® (Discontinued) *see* antipyrine and benzocaine *on page 82*

anti-CD11a *see* efalizumab *on page 335*

anti-CD20 monoclonal antibody *see* rituximab *on page 839*

anti-CD20-murine monoclonal antibody I-131 *see* tositumomab and iodine I 131 tositumomab *on page 937*

antidigoxin fab fragments, ovine *see* digoxin immune Fab *on page 297*

antidiuretic hormone *see* vasopressin *on page 972*

antihemophilic factor (human) (an tee hee moe FIL ik FAK tor HYU man)

Synonyms AHF (human); factor VIII (human)

U.S./Canadian Brand Names Hemofil M [US/Can]; Koāte®-DVI [US]; Monarc-M™ [US]; Monoclate-P® [US]

Therapeutic Category Blood Product Derivative

Use Prevention and treatment of hemorrhagic episodes in patients with hemophilia A (classic hemophilia); perioperative management of hemophilia A; can be of significant therapeutic value in patients with acquired factor VIII inhibitors not exceeding 10 Bethesda units/mL

Usual Dosage I.V.: Children and Adults: Individualize dosage based on coagulation studies performed prior to treatment and at regular intervals during treatment. In general, administration of factor VIII 1 int. unit/kg will increase circulating factor VIII levels by ~2 int. units/dL. (General guidelines presented; consult individual product labeling for specific dosing recommendations.)

Dosage based on desired factor VIII increase (%):

To calculate dosage needed based on desired factor VIII increase (%):

Body weight (kg) x 0.5 int. units/kg x desired factor VIII increase (%) = int. units factor VIII required

For example:

50 kg x 0.5 int. units/kg x 30 (% increase) = 750 int. units factor VIII

Dosage based on expected factor VIII increase (%):

It is also possible to calculate the **expected** % factor VIII increase:

(# int. units administered x 2%/int. units/kg) divided by body weight (kg) = expected % factor VIII increase

For example:

(1400 int. units x 2%/int. units/kg) divided by 70 kg = 40%

General guidelines:

Minor hemorrhage: 10-20 int. units/kg as a single dose to achieve FVIII plasma level ~20% to 40% of normal. Mild superficial or early hemorrhages may respond to a single dose; may repeat dose every 12-24 hours for 1-3 days until bleeding is resolved or healing achieved.

Moderate hemorrhage/minor surgery: 15-25 int. units/kg to achieve FVIII plasma level 30% to 50% of normal. If needed, may continue with a maintenance dose of 10-15 int. units/kg every 8-12 hours.

Major to life-threatening hemorrhage: Initial dose 40-50 int. units/kg, followed by a maintenance dose of 20-25 int. units/kg every 8-12 hours until threat is resolved, to achieve FVIII plasma level 80% to 100% of normal.

Major surgery: 50 int. units/kg given preoperatively to raise factor VIII level to 100% before surgery begins. May repeat as necessary after 6-12 hours initially and for a total of 10-14 days until healing is complete. Intensity of therapy may depend on type of surgery and postoperative regimen.

Bleeding prophylaxis: May be administered on a regular basis for bleeding prophylaxis. Doses of 24-40 int. units/kg 3 times/week have been reported in patients with severe hemophilia to prevent joint bleeding.

If bleeding is not controlled with adequate dose, test for presence of inhibitor. It may not be possible or practical to control bleeding if inhibitor titers are >10 Bethesda units/mL.

Dosage Forms

Injection, powder for reconstitution:

Hemofil M: Vial labeled with international units

Koāte®-DVI: ~250 int. units, ~500 int. units, ~1000 int. units

Monarc-M™: Vial labeled with international units

Monoclate-P®: ~250 int. units, ~500 int. units, ~1000 int. units, ~1500 int. units

antihemophilic factor (recombinant) (an tee hee moe FIL ik FAK tor ree KOM be nant)

Synonyms AHF (recombinant); factor VIII (recombinant); rAHF

U.S./Canadian Brand Names Advate [US]; Helixate® FS [US/Can]; Kogenate® FS [US/Can]; Kogenate® [Can]; Recombinate [US/Can]; ReFacto® [US/Can]

Therapeutic Category Blood Product Derivative

Use Prevention and treatment of hemorrhagic episodes in patients with hemophilia A (classic hemophilia or congenital factor VIII deficiency); perioperative management of hemophilia A; can be of significant therapeutic value in patients with acquired factor VIII inhibitors ≤10 Bethesda units/mL

Usual Dosage Children and Adults: I.V.: Individualize dosage based on coagulation studies performed prior to treatment and at regular intervals during treatment. In general, administration of factor VIII 1 int. unit/kg will increase circulating factor VIII levels by ~2 int. units/dL. (General guidelines presented; consult individual product labeling for specific dosing recommendations.)

Dosage based on desired factor VIII increase (%):

To calculate dosage needed based on desired factor VIII increase (%):

[Body weight (kg) x desired factor VIII increase (%)] divided by 2%/int. units/kg = int. units factor VIII required

For example:

50 kg x 30 (% increase) divided by 2%/int. units/kg = 750 int. units factor VIII

Dosage based on expected factor VIII increase (%):

It is also possible to calculate the **expected** % factor VIII increase:

(# int. units administered x 2%/int. units/kg) divided by body weight (kg) = expected % factor VIII increase

For example:

(1400 int. units x 2%/int. units/kg) divided by 70 kg = 40%

General guidelines:

Minor hemorrhage: 10-20 int. units/kg as a single dose to achieve FVIII plasma level ~20% to 40% of normal. Mild superficial or early hemorrhages may respond to a single dose; may repeat dose every 12-24 hours for 1-3 days until bleeding is resolved or healing achieved.

Moderate hemorrhage/minor surgery: 15-30 int. units/kg to achieve FVIII plasma level 30% to 60% of normal. May repeat 1 dose at 12-24 hours if needed. Some products suggest continuing for ≥3 days until pain and disability are resolved

Major to life-threatening hemorrhage: Initial dose 40-50 int. units/kg followed by a maintenance dose of 20-25 int. units/kg every 8-24 hours until threat is resolved, to achieve FVIII plasma level 60% to 100% of normal.

Major surgery: 50 int. units/kg given preoperatively to raise factor VIII level to 100% before surgery begins. May repeat as necessary after 6-12 hours initially and for a total of 10-14 days until healing is complete. Intensity of therapy may depend on type of surgery and postoperative regimen.

Bleeding prophylaxis: May be administered on a regular basis for bleeding prophylaxis. Doses of 24-40 int. units/kg 3 times/week have been reported in patients with severe hemophilia to prevent joint bleeding.

◀ If bleeding is not controlled with adequate dose, test for presence of inhibitor. It may not be possible or practical to control bleeding if inhibitor titers >10 Bethesda units/mL.

Dosage Forms

Injection, powder for reconstitution, recombinant [preservative free]:

Advate: 250 int. units, 500 int. units, 1000 int. units, 1500 int. units, 3000 int. units

Helixate® FS, Kogenate® FS, Recombinate: 250 int. units, 500 int. units, 1000 int. units

ReFacto®: 250 int. units, 500 units, 1000 int. units, 2000 int. units

Xyntha™: 250 int. units, 500 units, 1000 int. units, 2000 int. units

antihemophilic factor/von Willebrand factor complex (human)

(an tee hee moe FIL ik FAK tor von WILL le brand FAK tor KOM plex HYU man)

Synonyms AHF (human); factor VIII (human); FVIII/vWF; vWF:RCof

U.S./Canadian Brand Names Alphanate® *[new formulation]* [US]; Humate-P® [US/Can]

Therapeutic Category Antihemophilic Agent; Blood Product Derivative

Use

Prevention and treatment of hemorrhagic episodes in patients with hemophilia A (classical hemophilia) (Alphanate®, Humate-P®) or acquired factor VIII deficiency (Alphanate®)

Prophylaxis with surgical and/or invasive procedures in patients with von Willebrand disease (vWD) when desmopressin is either ineffective or contraindicated (Alphanate®)

Treatment of spontaneous or trauma-induced bleeding, as well as prevention of excessive bleeding during and after surgery, in patients with vWD (mild, moderate, or severe) where use of desmopressin is known or suspected to be inadequate (Humate-P®)

Usual Dosage

Hemophilia A: General guidelines (consult specific product labeling): Children and Adults: I.V.:

Individualize dosage based on coagulation studies performed prior to treatment and at regular intervals during treatment; in general, administration of factor VIII 1 int. unit/kg will increase circulating factor VIII levels by ~2 int. units/dL.

Minor hemorrhage: Loading dose: FVIII:C 15 int. units/kg to achieve FVIII:C plasma level ~30% of normal. If second infusion is needed, half the loading dose may be given once or twice daily for 1-2 days.

Moderate hemorrhage: Loading dose: FVIII:C 25 int. units/kg to achieve FVIII:C plasma level ~50% of normal; Maintenance: FVIII:C 15 int. units/kg every 8-12 hours for 1-2 days in order to maintain FVIII:C plasma levels at 30% of normal. Repeat the same dose once or twice daily for up to 7 days or until adequate wound healing.

Life-threatening hemorrhage/major surgery: Loading dose: FVIII:C 40-50 int. units/kg; Maintenance: FVIII:C 20-25 int. units/kg every 8 hours to maintain FVIII:C plasma levels at 80% to 100% of normal for 7 days. Continue same dose once or twice daily for another 7 days in order to maintain FVIII:C levels at 30% to 50% of normal.

von Willebrand disease (vWD): Treatment (Humate-P®): Children and Adults: I.V.: Individualize dosage based on coagulation studies performed prior to treatment and at regular intervals during treatment; in general, administration of factor VIII 1 int. unit/kg would be expected to raise circulating vWF:RCof ~5 int. units/dL

Type 1, mild (if desmopressin is not appropriate): Major hemorrhage:

Loading dose: vWF:RCof 40-60 int. units/kg

Maintenance dose: vWF:RCof 40-50 int. units/kg every 8-12 hours for 3 days, keeping vWF:RCof nadir >50%; follow with 40-50 int. units/kg daily for up to 7 days

Type 1, moderate or severe:

Minor hemorrhage: vWF:RCof 40-50 int. units/kg for 1-2 doses

Major hemorrhage:

Loading dose: vWF:RCof 50-75 int. units/kg

Maintenance dose: vWF:RCof 40-60 int. units/kg every 8-12 hours for 3 days to keep the vWF:RCof nadir >50%, then 40-60 int. units/kg daily for a total of up to 7 days

Types 2 and 3:

Minor hemorrhage: vWF:RCof 40-50 int. units/kg for 1-2 doses

Major hemorrhage:

Loading dose: vWF:RCof 60-80 int. units/kg

Maintenance dose: vWF:RCof 40-60 int. units/kg every 8-12 hours for 3 days, keeping the vWF:RCof nadir >50%; follow with 40-60 int. units/kg daily for a total of up to 7 days

von Willebrand disease (vWD): Surgery/procedure prophylaxis (except patients with type 3 undergoing major surgery) (Alphanate®):
Children: I.V.:
Preoperative dose: vWF:RCof 75 int. units/kg 1 hour prior to surgery
Maintenance dose: vWF:RCof 50-75 int. units/kg every 8-12 hours as clinically needed. May reduce dose after third postoperative day; continue treatment until healing is complete.
Adults: I.V.:
Preoperative dose: vWF:RCof 60 int. units/kg 1 hour prior to surgery
Maintenance dose: vWF:RCof 40-60 int. units/kg every 8-12 hours as clinically needed. May reduce dose after third postoperative day; continue treatment until healing is complete. For minor procedures, maintain vWF of 40% to 50% during postoperative days 1-3; for major procedures maintain vWF of 40% to 50% for ≥3-7 days.
von Willebrand disease (vWD): Surgery/procedure prevention of bleeding (Humate-P®): Children and Adults: I.V.:
Emergency surgery: Administer vWF:RCof 50-60 int units/kg; monitor trough coagulation factor levels for subsequent doses
Surgical management (nonemergency):
Loading dose calculation based on baseline target vWF:RCo: (Target peak vWF:RCof - Baseline vWF: RCof) x weight (in kg) / IVR = int. units vWF:RCof required. Administer loading dose 1-2 hours prior to surgery. **Note:** If IVR not available, assume 2 int. units/dL per int. units/kg of vWF:RCof product administered.
Target concentrations for vWF:RCof following loading dose:
Major surgery: 100 int. units/dL
Minor surgery: 50-60 int. units/dL
Maintenance dose: Initial: 1/2 loading dose followed by dosing determined by target tough concentrations, generally every 8-12 hours. Patients with shorter half-lives may require dosing every 6 hours.
Target maintenance trough vWF:RCof concentrations:
Major surgery: >50 int. units/dL for up to 3 days, followed by >30 int. units/dL for a minimum total treatment of 72 hours
Minor surgery: ≥30 int. units/dL for a minimum duration of 48 hours
Oral surgery: ≥30 int. units/dL for a minimum duration of 8-12 hours

Dosage Forms
Injection, powder for reconstitution [human derived]:
Alphanate®:
250 int. units [Factor VIII and vWF:RCof ratio varies by lot]
500 int. units [Factor VIII and vWF:RCof ratio varies by lot]
1000 int. units [Factor VIII and vWF:RCof ratio varies by lot]
1500 int. units [Factor VIII and vWF:RCof ratio varies by lot]
Humate-P®:
FVIII 250 int. units and vWF:RCof 600 int. units
FVIII 500 int. units and vWF:RCof 1200 int. units
FVIII 1000 int. units and vWF:RCof 2400 int. units

Antihist-1® *(Discontinued)* see clemastine *on page 228*

antiinhibitor coagulant complex (an tee in HI bi tor coe AG yoo lant KOM pleks)

Synonyms AICC; coagulant complex inhibitor
U.S./Canadian Brand Names Feiba VH Immuno [Can]; Feiba VH [US]
Therapeutic Category Hemophilic Agent
Use Hemophilia A & B patients with factor VIII inhibitors who are to undergo surgery or those who are bleeding
Usual Dosage I.V.: Children and Adults:
Feiba VH: General dosing guidelines: 50-100 units/kg (maximum: 200 units/kg)
Joint hemorrhage: 50 units/kg every 12 hours; may increase to 100 units/kg; continue until signs of clinical improvement occur
Mucous membrane bleeding: 50 units/kg every 6 hours; may increase to 100 units/kg (maximum: 2 administrations/day or 200 units/kg/day)
Soft tissue hemorrhage: 100 units/kg every 12 hours (maximum: 200 units/kg/day)
Other severe hemorrhage: 100 units/kg every 12 hours; may be used every 6 hours if needed; continue until clinical improvement

▶

◀ **Dosage Forms**
Injection, powder for reconstitution:
Feiba VH: Each bottle is labeled with Immuno units of factor VIII [heparin free; contains sodium 8 mg/mL]

Antilirium® *(Discontinued)* *see* physostigmine *on page 752*
Antiminth® *(Discontinued)* *see* pyrantel pamoate *on page 806*
Antiphlogistine Rub A-535 No Odour [Can] *see* trolamine *on page 957*

antipyrine and benzocaine (an tee PYE reen & BEN zoe kane)

Synonyms benzocaine and antipyrine
U.S./Canadian Brand Names A/B Otic [US]; Allergen® [US]; Auralgan® [Can]; Aurodex [US]
Therapeutic Category Otic Agent, Analgesic; Otic Agent, Ceruminolytic
Use Temporary relief of pain and reduction of swelling associated with acute congestive and serous otitis media, swimmer's ear, otitis externa; facilitates ear wax removal
Usual Dosage Otic: Children and Adults:
Otitis media: Fill ear canal with solution; moisten cotton pledget with solution, place in external ear, repeat every 1-2 hours until pain and congestion are relieved
Ear wax removal: Instill drops 3-4 times/day for 2-3 days
Dosage Forms
Solution, otic [drops]: Antipyrine 5.4% and benzocaine 1.4% (10 mL)
A/B Otic, Allergen®, Aurodex, Auroto: Antipyrine 5.4% and benzocaine 1.4% (15 mL)

Antispas® Injection *(Discontinued)* *see* dicyclomine *on page 293*

antithrombin III (an tee THROM bin three)

Synonyms AT-III; heparin cofactor I
U.S./Canadian Brand Names Thrombate III® [US/Can]
Therapeutic Category Blood Product Derivative
Use Treatment of hereditary antithrombin III deficiency in connection with surgical procedures, obstetrical procedures, or thromboembolism
Usual Dosage Adults:
Initial dose: Dosing is individualized based on pretherapy AT-III levels. The initial dose should raise antithrombin III levels (AT-III) to 120% and may be calculated based on the following formula:

[desired AT-III level % - baseline AT-III level %] x body weight (kg)
divided by 1.4%/int. units/kg

For example, if a 70 kg adult patient had a baseline AT-III level of 57%, the initial dose would be [(120% - 57%) x 70] divided by 1.4 = 3150 int. units

Maintenance dose: Subsequent dosing should be targeted to keep levels between 80% to 120% which may be achieved by administering 60% of the initial dose every 24 hours. Adjustments may be made by adjusting dose or interval. Maintain level within normal range for 2-8 days depending on type of procedure.
Dosage Forms
Injection, powder for reconstitution [preservative free]:
Thrombate III®: 500 int. units, 1000 int. units

antithymocyte globulin (equine) (an te THY moe site GLOB yu lin, E kwine)

Sound-Alike/Look-Alike Issues
Atgam® may be confused with Ativan®
Synonyms antithymocyte immunoglobulin; ATG; horse antihuman thymocyte gamma globulin; lymphocyte immune globulin
U.S./Canadian Brand Names Atgam® [US/Can]
Therapeutic Category Immunosuppressant Agent
Use Prevention and treatment of acute renal allograft rejection; treatment of moderate to severe aplastic anemia in patients not considered suitable candidates for bone marrow transplantation
Usual Dosage An intradermal skin test is recommended prior to administration of the initial dose of ATG; use 0.1 mL of a 1:1000 dilution of ATG in normal saline. A positive skin reaction consists of a wheal ≥10 mm in diameter. If a positive skin test occurs, the first infusion should be administered in a controlled

environment with intensive life support immediately available. A systemic reaction precludes further administration of the drug. The absence of a reaction does **not** preclude the possibility of an immediate sensitivity reaction.

Premedication with diphenhydramine, hydrocortisone, and acetaminophen is recommended prior to first dose.
Children: I.V.:
  Aplastic anemia protocol: 10-20 mg/kg/day for 8-14 days; then administer every other day for 7 more doses; addition doses may be given every other day for 21 total doses in 28 days
  Renal allograft: 5-25 mg/kg/day
Adults: I.V.:
  Aplastic anemia protocol: 10-20 mg/kg/day for 8-14 days, then administer every other day for 7 more doses, for a total of 21 doses in 28 days
  Renal allograft:
    Rejection prophylaxis: 15 mg/kg/day for 14 days followed by 14 days of alternative day therapy at the same dose; the first dose should be administered within 24 hours before or after transplantation
    Rejection treatment: 10-15 mg/kg/day for 14 days, then administer every other day for 10-14 days up to 21 doses in 28 days
Dosage Forms
Injection, solution:
  Atgam®: 50 mg/mL (5 mL)

antithymocyte globulin (rabbit) (an te THY moe site GLOB yu lin RAB bit)
Synonyms rATG
U.S./Canadian Brand Names Thymoglobulin® [US]
Therapeutic Category Immunosuppressant Agent
Use Treatment of acute rejection of renal transplant; used in conjunction with concomitant immunosuppression
Usual Dosage I.V.: Children and Adults: Treatment of acute rejection: 1.5 mg/kg/day for 7-14 days
Dosage Forms
Injection, powder for reconstitution:
  Thymoglobulin®: 25 mg

antithymocyte immunoglobulin see antithymocyte globulin (equine) on page 82
antitumor necrosis factor apha (human) see adalimumab on page 34
Anti-Tuss® Expectorant *(Discontinued)* see guaifenesin on page 453
anti-VEGF monoclonal antibody see bevacizumab on page 134
antivenin (crotalidae) polyvalent see crotalidae polyvalent immune FAB (ovine) on page 253

antivenin *(Latrodectus mactans)* (an tee VEN in lak tro DUK tus MAK tans)
Synonyms *Latrodectus mactans* antivenin; black widow spider species antivenin
Therapeutic Category Antivenin
Use Treatment of patients with symptoms of black widow spider bites
Usual Dosage
Skin test: Intradermal: Children and Adults: 0.02 mL of a 1:10 dilution in NS (also use a control solution of NS); evaluate in 10 minutes. Positive reaction is urticarial wheal surrounded by zone of erythema
Conjunctival test: Ophthalmic:
  Children: Instill 1 drop of a 1:100 dilution into the conjunctival sac
  Adults: Instill 1 drop of a 1:10 dilution into the conjunctival sac
  Note: Itching of the eye and/or reddening of conjunctiva indicates a positive reaction, usually occurring within 10 minutes.
Desensitization: Children and Adults: **Note:** In separate vials or syringes, prepare 1:10 and 1:100 dilutions of antivenin in NS.
  SubQ: Inject 0.1, 0.2, and 0.5 mL of the 1:100 dilution at 15- to 30- minute intervals. Proceed with the next dose only if no reaction has occurred following the previous. Repeat procedure using the 1:10 dilution and then undiluted antivenin.
  If a reaction occurs, apply tourniquet proximal to the injection site and administer epinephrine 1:1000. Wait at least 30 minutes, then administer another antivenin injection at the last dose which did not evoke a reaction.
  If no reaction has occurred following 0.5 mL of undiluted antivenin, continue the dose at 15-minute intervals until entire dose has been administered.

◀ Treatment of symptoms due to black widow spider bite: Administer only following the skin test or conjunctival test:
Children <12 years: I.V.: 2.5 mL
Children >12 years and Adults: I.M., I.V.: 2.5 mL

Dosage Forms
Injection, powder for reconstitution:
6000 antivenin units

antivenin *(Micrurus fulvius)* (an tee VEN in mye KRU rus FUL vee us)

Synonyms *Micrurus fulvius* antivenin; North American coral snake antivenin
Therapeutic Category Antivenin
Use Neutralization of venoms of Eastern coral snake and Texas coral snake
Usual Dosage I.V.: Children and Adults: 3-5 vials by slow injection (dependent on severity of signs/symptoms; some patients may need more than 10 vials)
Note: Each vial of antivenom neutralizes ~2 mg of venom.

Antivenin Polyvalent [Equine] *(Discontinued)* *see* crotalidae polyvalent antivenin (equine) *on page 252*
Antivert® [US] *see* meclizine *on page 595*
Antizol® [US] *see* fomepizole *on page 423*
Antrizine® *(Discontinued)* *see* meclizine *on page 595*
Anturane® *(Discontinued)*
Anucort-HC® [US] *see* hydrocortisone (rectal) *on page 484*
Anu-Med [US-OTC] *see* phenylephrine *on page 745*
Anusol-HC® [US] *see* hydrocortisone (rectal) *on page 484*
Anusol® HC-1 [US-OTC] *see* hydrocortisone (rectal) *on page 484*
Anusol® Ointment [US-OTC] *see* pramoxine *on page 777*
Anuzinc [Can] *see* zinc sulfate *on page 994*
Anxanil® Oral *(Discontinued)* *see* hydroxyzine *on page 491*
Anzemet® [US/Can] *see* dolasetron *on page 316*
Apacet® *(Discontinued)* *see* acetaminophen *on page 19*
APAP *see* acetaminophen *on page 19*
APAP and tramadol *see* acetaminophen and tramadol *on page 24*
Apaphen® *(Discontinued)* *see* acetaminophen and phenyltoloxamine *on page 22*
Apatate® [US-OTC] *see* vitamin B complex combinations *on page 981*
ApexiCon™ [US] *see* diflorasone *on page 295*
ApexiCon™ E [US] *see* diflorasone *on page 295*
Aphrodyne® *(Discontinued)* *see* yohimbine *on page 988*
Aphthasol® [US] *see* amlexanox *on page 63*
Apidra® [US/Can] *see* insulin glulisine *on page 511*
A.P.L.® *(Discontinued)* *see* chorionic gonadotropin (human) *on page 216*
Aplisol® [US] *see* tuberculin tests *on page 959*
Aplitest® *(Discontinued)* *see* tuberculin tests *on page 959*
aplonidine *see* apraclonidine *on page 90*
Apo-Acebutolol® [Can] *see* acebutolol *on page 19*
Apo-Acetaminophen® [Can] *see* acetaminophen *on page 19*
Apo-Acetazolamide® [Can] *see* acetazolamide *on page 28*
Apo-Acyclovir® [Can] *see* acyclovir *on page 33*
Apo-Alendronate® [Can] *see* alendronate *on page 43*
Apo-Allopurinol® [Can] *see* allopurinol *on page 47*
Apo-Alpraz® [Can] *see* alprazolam *on page 49*
Apo-Alpraz® TS [Can] *see* alprazolam *on page 49*
Apo-Amiloride® [Can] *see* amiloride *on page 59*
Apo-Amilzide® [Can] *see* amiloride and hydrochlorothiazide *on page 59*
Apo-Amiodarone® [Can] *see* amiodarone *on page 61*
Apo-Amitriptyline® [Can] *see* amitriptyline *on page 62*

Apo-Amoxi® [Can] *see* amoxicillin *on page 67*
Apo-Amoxi-Clav® [Can] *see* amoxicillin and clavulanate potassium *on page 68*
Apo-Ampi® [Can] *see* ampicillin *on page 72*
Apo-Atenidone® [Can] *see* atenolol and chlorthalidone *on page 102*
Apo-Atenol® [Can] *see* atenolol *on page 101*
Apo-Azathioprine® [Can] *see* azathioprine *on page 109*
Apo-Azithromycin® [Can] *see* azithromycin *on page 110*
Apo-Baclofen® [Can] *see* baclofen *on page 115*
Apo-Beclomethasone® [Can] *see* beclomethasone *on page 119*
Apo-Benazepril® [Can] *see* benazepril *on page 121*
Apo-Benztropine® [Can] *see* benztropine *on page 128*
Apo-Benzydamine® [Can] *see* benzydamine *(Canada only) on page 129*
Apo-Bisacodyl® [Can] *see* bisacodyl *on page 136*
Apo-Bisoprolol® [Can] *see* bisoprolol *on page 138*
Apo-Brimonidine® [Can] *see* brimonidine *on page 142*
Apo-Bromazepam® [Can] *see* bromazepam *(Canada only) on page 142*
Apo-Bromocriptine® [Can] *see* bromocriptine *on page 143*
Apo-Buspirone® [Can] *see* buspirone *on page 153*
Apo-Butorphanol® [Can] *see* butorphanol *on page 157*
Apo-Cal® [Can] *see* calcium carbonate *on page 163*
Apo-Calcitonin® [Can] *see* calcitonin *on page 160*
Apo-Capto® [Can] *see* captopril *on page 171*
Apo-Carbamazepine® [Can] *see* carbamazepine *on page 172*
Apo-Carvedilol® [Can] *see* carvedilol *on page 181*
Apo-Cefaclor® [Can] *see* cefaclor *on page 183*
Apo-Cefadroxil® [Can] *see* cefadroxil *on page 184*
Apo-Cefoxitin® [Can] *see* cefoxitin *on page 187*
Apo-Cefprozil® [Can] *see* cefprozil *on page 188*
Apo-Cefuroxime® [Can] *see* cefuroxime *on page 192*
Apo-Cephalex® [Can] *see* cephalexin *on page 194*
Apo-Cetirizine® [Can] *see* cetirizine *on page 196*
Apo-Chlorax® [Can] *see* clidinium and chlordiazepoxide *on page 229*
Apo-Chlordiazepoxide® [Can] *see* chlordiazepoxide *on page 201*
Apo-Chlorpropamide® [Can] *see* chlorpropamide *on page 214*
Apo-Chlorthalidone® [Can] *see* chlorthalidone *on page 214*
Apo-Cilazapril® [Can] *see* cilazapril *(Canada only) on page 219*
Apo-Cilazapril/Hctz [Can] *see* cilazapril and hydrochlorothiazide *(Canada only) on page 219*
Apo-Cimetidine® [Can] *see* cimetidine *on page 219*
Apo-Ciproflox® [Can] *see* ciprofloxacin *on page 221*
Apo-Citalopram® [Can] *see* citalopram *on page 225*
Apo-Clarithromycin [Can] *see* clarithromycin *on page 227*
Apo-Clindamycin® [Can] *see* clindamycin *on page 230*
Apo-Clobazam® [Can] *see* clobazam *(Canada only) on page 232*
Apo-Clomipramine® [Can] *see* clomipramine *on page 235*
Apo-Clonazepam® [Can] *see* clonazepam *on page 235*
Apo-Clonidine® [Can] *see* clonidine *on page 236*
Apo-Clorazepate® [Can] *see* clorazepate *on page 238*
Apo-Cloxi® [Can] *see* cloxacillin *(Canada only) on page 239*
Apo-Clozapine® [Can] *see* clozapine *on page 240*
Apo-Cromolyn® [Can] *see* cromolyn sodium *on page 251*
Apo-Cyclobenzaprine® [Can] *see* cyclobenzaprine *on page 255*
Apo-Cyproterone® [Can] *see* cyproterone *(Canada only) on page 259*
Apo-Desipramine® [Can] *see* desipramine *on page 274*

Apo-Desmopressin® [Can] *see* desmopressin acetate *on page 275*
Apo-Dexamethasone® [Can] *see* dexamethasone (systemic) *on page 278*
Apo-Diazepam® [Can] *see* diazepam *on page 289*
Apo-Diclo® [Can] *see* diclofenac *on page 292*
Apo-Diclo Rapide® [Can] *see* diclofenac *on page 292*
Apo-Diclo SR® [Can] *see* diclofenac *on page 292*
Apo-Diflunisal® [Can] *see* diflunisal *on page 296*
Apo-Digoxin® [Can] *see* digoxin *on page 296*
Apo-Diltiaz® [Can] *see* diltiazem *on page 300*
Apo-Diltiaz CD® [Can] *see* diltiazem *on page 300*
Apo-Diltiaz® Injectable [Can] *see* diltiazem *on page 300*
Apo-Diltiaz SR® [Can] *see* diltiazem *on page 300*
Apo-Diltiaz TZ® [Can] *see* diltiazem *on page 300*
Apo-Dimenhydrinate® [Can] *see* dimenhydrinate *on page 301*
Apo-Dipyridamole FC® [Can] *see* dipyridamole *on page 311*
Apo-Divalproex® [Can] *see* valproic acid and derivatives *on page 967*
Apo-Docusate-Sodium® [Can] *see* docusate *on page 314*
Apo-Domperidone® [Can] *see* domperidone *(Canada only) on page 317*
Apo-Doxazosin® [Can] *see* doxazosin *on page 320*
Apo-Doxepin® [Can] *see* doxepin *on page 321*
Apo-Doxy® [Can] *see* doxycycline *on page 323*
Apo-Doxy Tabs® [Can] *see* doxycycline *on page 323*
Apo-Enalapril® [Can] *see* enalapril *on page 339*
Apo-Erythro Base® [Can] *see* erythromycin *on page 354*
Apo-Erythro E-C® [Can] *see* erythromycin *on page 354*
Apo-Erythro-ES® [Can] *see* erythromycin *on page 354*
Apo-Erythro-S® [Can] *see* erythromycin *on page 354*
Apo-Etodolac® [Can] *see* etodolac *on page 383*
Apo-Famciclovir [Can] *see* famciclovir *on page 389*
Apo-Famotidine® [Can] *see* famotidine *on page 390*
Apo-Famotidine® Injectable [Can] *see* famotidine *on page 390*
Apo-Fenofibrate® [Can] *see* fenofibrate *on page 393*
Apo-Feno-Micro® [Can] *see* fenofibrate *on page 393*
Apo-Ferrous Gluconate® [Can] *see* ferrous gluconate *on page 398*
Apo-Ferrous Sulfate® [Can] *see* ferrous sulfate *on page 398*
Apo-Flavoxate® [Can] *see* flavoxate *on page 402*
Apo-Flecainide® [Can] *see* flecainide *on page 403*
Apo-Floctafenine® [Can] *see* floctafenine *(Canada only) on page 404*
Apo-Fluconazole® [Can] *see* fluconazole *on page 405*
Apo-Flunarizine® [Can] *see* flunarizine *(Canada only) on page 408*
Apo-Flunisolide® [Can] *see* flunisolide *on page 408*
Apo-Fluoxetine® [Can] *see* fluoxetine *on page 413*
Apo-Fluphenazine® [Can] *see* fluphenazine *on page 415*
Apo-Fluphenazine Decanoate® [Can] *see* fluphenazine *on page 415*
Apo-Flurazepam® [Can] *see* flurazepam *on page 416*
Apo-Flurbiprofen® [Can] *see* flurbiprofen *on page 416*
Apo-Flutamide® [Can] *see* flutamide *on page 416*
Apo-Fluvoxamine® [Can] *see* fluvoxamine *on page 420*
Apo-Folic® [Can] *see* folic acid *on page 421*
Apo-Fosinopril® [Can] *see* fosinopril *on page 427*
Apo-Furosemide® [Can] *see* furosemide *on page 430*
Apo-Gabapentin® [Can] *see* gabapentin *on page 431*
Apo-Gain® [Can] *see* minoxidil *on page 636*

Apo-Gemfibrozil® [Can] see gemfibrozil on page 439
Apo-Gliclazide® [Can] see gliclazide (Canada only) on page 444
Apo-Glimepiride [Can] see glimepiride on page 445
Apo-Glyburide® [Can] see glyburide on page 448
Apo-Haloperidol® [Can] see haloperidol on page 465
Apo-Haloperidol LA® [Can] see haloperidol on page 465
Apo-Hydralazine® [Can] see hydralazine on page 478
Apo-Hydro® [Can] see hydrochlorothiazide on page 479
Apo-Hydroxyquine® [Can] see hydroxychloroquine on page 489
Apo-Hydroxyurea® [Can] see hydroxyurea on page 490
Apo-Hydroxyzine® [Can] see hydroxyzine on page 491
Apo-Ibuprofen® [Can] see ibuprofen on page 495
Apo-Imipramine® [Can] see imipramine on page 501
Apo-Indapamide® [Can] see indapamide on page 505
Apo-Indomethacin® [Can] see indomethacin on page 506
Apo-Ipravent® [Can] see ipratropium on page 524
Apo-ISDN® [Can] see isosorbide dinitrate on page 530
Apo-ISMN® [Can] see isosorbide mononitrate on page 531
Apo-K® [Can] see potassium chloride on page 771
Apo-Keto® [Can] see ketoprofen on page 537
Apo-Ketoconazole® [Can] see ketoconazole on page 537
Apo-Keto-E® [Can] see ketoprofen on page 537
Apo-Ketorolac® [Can] see ketorolac on page 538
Apo-Ketorolac Injectable® [Can] see ketorolac on page 538
Apo-Keto SR® [Can] see ketoprofen on page 537
Apokyn® [US] see apomorphine on page 88
Apo-Labetalol® [Can] see labetalol on page 541
Apo-Lactulose® [Can] see lactulose on page 544
Apo-Lamotrigine® [Can] see lamotrigine on page 545
Apo-Leflunomide® [Can] see leflunomide on page 551
Apo-Levetiracetam [Can] see levetiracetam on page 554
Apo-Levobunolol® [Can] see levobunolol on page 555
Apo-Levocarb® [Can] see carbidopa and levodopa on page 177
Apo-Levocarb® CR [Can] see carbidopa and levodopa on page 177
Apo-Lisinopril® [Can] see lisinopril on page 570
Apo-Lisinopril/Hctz [Can] see lisinopril and hydrochlorothiazide on page 571
Apo-Lithium® Carbonate [Can] see lithium on page 571
Apo-Lithium® Carbonate SR [Can] see lithium on page 571
Apo-Loperamide® [Can] see loperamide on page 573
Apo-Loratadine® [Can] see loratadine on page 576
Apo-Lorazepam® [Can] see lorazepam on page 577
Apo-Lovastatin® [Can] see lovastatin on page 579
Apo-Loxapine® [Can] see loxapine on page 580
Apo-Medroxy® [Can] see medroxyprogesterone on page 597
Apo-Mefenamic® [Can] see mefenamic acid on page 598
Apo-Mefloquine® [Can] see mefloquine on page 598
Apo-Megestrol® [Can] see megestrol on page 598
Apo-Meloxicam® [Can] see meloxicam on page 599
Apo-Metformin® [Can] see metformin on page 610
Apo-Methazide® [Can] see methyldopa and hydrochlorothiazide on page 620
Apo-Methazolamide® [Can] see methazolamide on page 613
Apo-Methoprazine® [Can] see methotrimeprazine (Canada only) on page 617
Apo-Methotrexate® [Can] see methotrexate on page 615

Apo-Methyldopa® **[Can]** *see* methyldopa *on page 620*
Apo-Methylphenidate® **[Can]** *see* methylphenidate *on page 622*
Apo-Methylphenidate® **SR [Can]** *see* methylphenidate *on page 622*
Apo-Metoclop® **[Can]** *see* metoclopramide *on page 625*
Apo-Metoprolol® **[Can]** *see* metoprolol *on page 626*
Apo-Metronidazole® **[Can]** *see* metronidazole *on page 627*
Apo-Midazolam® **[Can]** *see* midazolam *on page 632*
Apo-Midodrine® **[Can]** *see* midodrine *on page 633*
Apo-Minocycline® **[Can]** *see* minocycline *on page 635*
Apo-Misoprostol® **[Can]** *see* misoprostol *on page 637*
Apo-Moclobemide® **[Can]** *see* moclobemide *(Canada only) on page 639*

apomorphine (a poe MOR feen)

Synonyms apomorphine hydrochloride; apomorphine hydrochloride hemihydrate
U.S./Canadian Brand Names Apokyn® [US]
Therapeutic Category Anti-Parkinson Agent (Dopamine Agonist)
Use Treatment of hypomobility, "off" episodes with Parkinson disease
Usual Dosage SubQ: Adults: Begin antiemetic therapy 3 days prior to initiation and continue for 2 months before reassessing need.

Parkinson disease, "off" episode: Initial test dose 2 mg, **medical supervision required; see "Note."** Subsequent dosing is based on both tolerance and response to initial test dose.

If patient tolerates test dose and responds: Starting dose: 2 mg as needed; may increase dose in 1 mg increments every few days; maximum dose: 6 mg

If patient tolerates but does not respond to 2 mg test dose: Second test dose: 4 mg

If patient tolerates and responds to 4 mg test dose: Starting dose: 3 mg, as needed for "off" episodes; may increase dose in 1 mg increments every few days; maximum dose 6 mg

If patient does not tolerate 4 mg test dose: Third test dose: 3 mg

If patient tolerates 3 mg test dose: Starting dose: 2 mg as needed for "off" episodes; may increase dose in 1 mg increments to a maximum of 3 mg

If therapy is interrupted for >1 week, restart at 2 mg and gradually titrate dose.

Note: Medical supervision is required for all test doses with standing and supine blood pressure monitoring predose and 20-, 40-, and 60 minutes postdose. If subsequent test doses are required, wait >2 hours before another test dose is given; next test dose should be timed with another "off" episode. If a single dose is ineffective for a particular "off" episode, then a second dose should not be given. The average dosing frequency was 3 times/day in the development program with limited experience in dosing >5 times/day and with total daily doses >20 mg. Apomorphine is intended to treat the "off" episodes associated with levodopa therapy of Parkinson disease and has not been studied in levodopa-naive Parkinson patients.

Dosage Forms
Injection, solution:
Apokyn®: 10 mg/mL (2 mL, 3 mL)

apomorphine hydrochloride *see* apomorphine *on page 88*
apomorphine hydrochloride hemihydrate *see* apomorphine *on page 88*
Apo-Nabumetone® **[Can]** *see* nabumetone *on page 650*
Apo-Nadol® **[Can]** *see* nadolol *on page 651*
Apo-Napro-Na® **[Can]** *see* naproxen *on page 656*
Apo-Napro-Na DS® **[Can]** *see* naproxen *on page 656*
Apo-Naproxen® **[Can]** *see* naproxen *on page 656*
Apo-Naproxen EC® **[Can]** *see* naproxen *on page 656*
Apo-Naproxen SR® **[Can]** *see* naproxen *on page 656*
Apo-Nifed® **[Can]** *see* nifedipine *on page 672*
Apo-Nifed PA® **[Can]** *see* nifedipine *on page 672*
Apo-Nitrazepam® **[Can]** *see* nitrazepam *(Canada only) on page 674*
Apo-Nitrofurantoin® **[Can]** *see* nitrofurantoin *on page 675*
Apo-Nizatidine® **[Can]** *see* nizatidine *on page 677*
Apo-Norflox® **[Can]** *see* norfloxacin *on page 679*

Apo-Nortriptyline® [Can] *see* nortriptyline *on page 680*
Apo-Oflox® [Can] *see* ofloxacin *on page 693*
Apo-Ofloxacin® [Can] *see* ofloxacin *on page 693*
Apo-Omeprazole® [Can] *see* omeprazole *on page 697*
Apo-Ondansetron® [Can] *see* ondansetron *on page 698*
Apo-Orciprenaline® [Can] *see* metaproterenol *on page 609*
Apo-Oxaprozin® [Can] *see* oxaprozin *on page 706*
Apo-Oxazepam® [Can] *see* oxazepam *on page 706*
Apo-Oxybutynin® [Can] *see* oxybutynin *on page 708*
Apo-Paclitaxel® [Can] *see* paclitaxel *on page 714*
Apo-Pantoprazole [Can] *see* pantoprazole *on page 720*
Apo-Paroxetine® [Can] *see* paroxetine *on page 724*
Apo-Pentoxifylline SR® [Can] *see* pentoxifylline *on page 737*
Apo-Pen VK® [Can] *see* penicillin V potassium *on page 734*
Apo-Perindopril® [Can] *see* perindopril erbumine *on page 739*
Apo-Perphenazine® [Can] *see* perphenazine *on page 740*
Apo-Pimozide® [Can] *see* pimozide *on page 753*
Apo-Pindol® [Can] *see* pindolol *on page 754*
Apo-Pioglitazone [Can] *see* pioglitazone *on page 754*
Apo-Piroxicam® [Can] *see* piroxicam *on page 757*
Apo-Pramipexole [Can] *see* pramipexole *on page 777*
Apo-Pravastatin® [Can] *see* pravastatin *on page 779*
Apo-Prazo® [Can] *see* prazosin *on page 780*
Apo-Prednisone® [Can] *see* prednisone *on page 782*
Apo-Primidone® [Can] *see* primidone *on page 786*
Apo-Procainamide® [Can] *see* procainamide *on page 787*
Apo-Prochlorperazine® [Can] *see* prochlorperazine *on page 788*
Apo-Propafenone® [Can] *see* propafenone *on page 793*
Apo-Propranolol® [Can] *see* propranolol *on page 796*
Apo-Quinidine® [Can] *see* quinidine *on page 813*
Apo-Quinine® [Can] *see* quinine *on page 814*
Apo-Ramipril® [Can] *see* ramipril *on page 817*
Apo-Ranitidine® [Can] *see* ranitidine *on page 819*
Apo-Risperidone® [Can] *see* risperidone *on page 837*
Apo-Salvent® [Can] *see* albuterol *on page 39*
Apo-Salvent® CFC Free [Can] *see* albuterol *on page 39*
Apo-Salvent® Respirator Solution [Can] *see* albuterol *on page 39*
Apo-Salvent® Sterules [Can] *see* albuterol *on page 39*
Apo-Selegiline® [Can] *see* selegiline *on page 860*
Apo-Sertraline® [Can] *see* sertraline *on page 863*
Apo-Simvastatin® [Can] *see* simvastatin *on page 867*
Apo-Sotalol® [Can] *see* sotalol *on page 885*
Apo-Sulfatrim® [Can] *see* sulfamethoxazole and trimethoprim *on page 894*
Apo-Sulfatrim® DS [Can] *see* sulfamethoxazole and trimethoprim *on page 894*
Apo-Sulfatrim® Pediatric [Can] *see* sulfamethoxazole and trimethoprim *on page 894*
Apo-Sulin® [Can] *see* sulindac *on page 898*
Apo-Sumatriptan® [Can] *see* sumatriptan *on page 898*
Apo-Tamox® [Can] *see* tamoxifen *on page 902*
Apo-Temazepam® [Can] *see* temazepam *on page 907*
Apo-Terazosin® [Can] *see* terazosin *on page 909*
Apo-Tetra® [Can] *see* tetracycline *on page 915*
Apo-Theo LA® [Can] *see* theophylline *on page 917*
Apo-Tiaprofenic® [Can] *see* tiaprofenic acid *(Canada only) on page 925*

Apo-Ticlopidine® [Can] *see* ticlopidine *on page 926*
Apo-Timol® [Can] *see* timolol *on page 927*
Apo-Timop® [Can] *see* timolol *on page 927*
Apo-Tizanidine® [Can] *see* tizanidine *on page 931*
Apo-Tolbutamide® [Can] *see* tolbutamide *on page 933*
Apo-Topiramate [Can] *see* topiramate *on page 935*
Apo-Trazodone® [Can] *see* trazodone *on page 944*
Apo-Trazodone D® [Can] *see* trazodone *on page 944*
Apo-Triazide® [Can] *see* hydrochlorothiazide and triamterene *on page 480*
Apo-Triazo® [Can] *see* triazolam *on page 950*
Apo-Trifluoperazine® [Can] *see* trifluoperazine *on page 951*
Apo-Trihex® [Can] *see* trihexyphenidyl *on page 952*
Apo-Trimebutine® [Can] *see* trimebutine *(Canada only) on page 952*
Apo-Trimethoprim® [Can] *see* trimethoprim *on page 953*
Apo-Trimip® [Can] *see* trimipramine *on page 954*
Apo-Valproic® [Can] *see* valproic acid and derivatives *on page 967*
Apo-Verap® [Can] *see* verapamil *on page 974*
Apo-Verap® SR [Can] *see* verapamil *on page 974*
Apo-Warfarin® [Can] *see* warfarin *on page 986*
Apo-Zidovudine® [Can] *see* zidovudine *on page 991*
Apo-Zopiclone® [Can] *see* zopiclone *(Canada only) on page 997*
APPG *see* penicillin G procaine *on page 733*
Apra Children's [US-OTC] *see* acetaminophen *on page 19*

apraclonidine (a pra KLOE ni deen)

Sound-Alike/Look-Alike Issues
Iopidine® may be confused with indapamide, iodine, Lodine®
Synonyms aplonidine; apraclonidine hydrochloride; p-aminoclonidine
U.S./Canadian Brand Names Iopidine® [US/Can]
Therapeutic Category Alpha$_2$-Adrenergic Agonist Agent, Ophthalmic
Use Prevention and treatment of postsurgical intraocular pressure (IOP) elevation; short-term, adjunctive therapy in patients who require additional reduction of IOP
Usual Dosage Ophthalmic: Adults:
0.5%: Instill 1-2 drops in the affected eye(s) 3 times/day
1%: Instill 1 drop in operative eye 1 hour prior to anterior segment laser surgery, second drop in eye immediately upon completion of procedure
Dosage Forms
Solution, ophthalmic:
Iopidine®: 0.5% (5 mL, 10 mL); 1% (0.1 mL)

apraclonidine hydrochloride *see* apraclonidine *on page 90*

aprepitant (ap RE pi tant)

Sound-Alike/Look-Alike Issues
aprepitant may be confused with fosaprepitant
Emend® (aprepitant) oral capsule formulation may be confused with Emend® for injection (fosaprepitant).
Synonyms L 754030; MK 869
U.S./Canadian Brand Names Emend® [US/Can]
Therapeutic Category Antiemetic
Use Prevention of acute and delayed nausea and vomiting associated with moderately- and highly-emetogenic chemotherapy (in combination with other antiemetics); prevention of postoperative nausea and vomiting (PONV)
Usual Dosage Oral: Adults:
Prevention of chemotherapy induced nausea/vomiting: 125 mg on day 1, followed by 80 mg on days 2 and 3 in combination with other antiemetics
Prevention of PONV: 40 mg within 3 hours prior to induction

Dosage Forms
Capsule:
Emend®: 40 mg, 80 mg, 125 mg
Combination package:
Emend®:
Capsule: 80 mg (2s)
Capsule: 125 mg (1s)

aprepitant injection *see* fosaprepitant *on page 426*
Apresoline® [Can] *see* hydralazine *on page 478*
Apresoline® (Discontinued) *see* hydralazine *on page 478*
Apri® [US] *see* ethinyl estradiol and desogestrel *on page 369*
Aprodine® [US-OTC] *see* triprolidine and pseudoephedrine *on page 955*

aprotinin (a proe TYE nin)
U.S./Canadian Brand Names Trasylol® [US/Can]
Therapeutic Category Hemostatic Agent
Use Prevention of perioperative blood loss in patients who are at increased risk for blood loss and blood transfusions in association with cardiopulmonary bypass in coronary artery bypass graft surgery
Usual Dosage Adults: Test dose: **All** patients should receive a 1 mL (1.4 mg) I.V. test dose at least 10 minutes prior to the loading dose to assess the potential for allergic reactions.
Notes:
The loading dose should be given after induction of anesthesia but prior to sternotomy. In patients with previous exposure to aprotinin, administer loading dose just prior to cannulation. A constant infusion is continued until surgery is complete.
To avoid physical incompatibility with heparin when adding to pump-prime solution, each agent should be added during recirculation to assure adequate dilution.
Regimen A (standard dose):
2 million KIU (280 mg; 200 mL) loading dose I.V. over 20-30 minutes
2 million KIU (280 mg; 200 mL) into pump prime volume
500,000 KIU/hour (70 mg/hour; 50 mL/hour) I.V. during operation
Regimen B (low dose):
1 million KIU (140 mg; 100 mL) loading dose I.V. over 20-30 minutes
1 million KIU (140 mg; 100 mL) into pump prime volume
250,000 KIU/hour (35 mg/hour; 25 mL/hour) I.V. during operation
Dosage Forms
Injection, solution:
Trasylol®: 1.4 mg/mL [10,000 KIU/mL] (100 mL, 200 mL)

Aptivus® [US/Can] *see* tipranavir *on page 930*
Aquacare® [US-OTC] *see* urea *on page 963*
Aquachloral® Supprettes® (Discontinued) *see* chloral hydrate *on page 199*
Aquacort® [Can] *see* hydrocortisone (topical) *on page 485*
AquADEKs™ [US-OTC] *see* vitamins (multiple/pediatric) *on page 983*
AquaLase™ [US] *see* balanced salt solution *on page 115*
AquaMEPHYTON® [Can] *see* phytonadione *on page 752*
AquaMEPHYTON® (Discontinued) *see* phytonadione *on page 752*
Aquanil™ HC [US-OTC] *see* hydrocortisone (topical) *on page 485*
Aquaphilic® With Carbamide [US-OTC] *see* urea *on page 963*
Aquaphyllin® (Discontinued) *see* theophylline *on page 917*
AquaSite® [US-OTC] *see* artificial tears *on page 95*
Aquasol A® [US] *see* vitamin A *on page 979*
Aquasol E® [US-OTC] *see* vitamin E *on page 981*
Aquatab® C (Discontinued) *see* guaifenesin, pseudoephedrine, and dextromethorphan *on page 460*
Aquatab® D (Discontinued) *see* guaifenesin and pseudoephedrine *on page 458*
Aquatab® DM (Discontinued) *see* guaifenesin and dextromethorphan *on page 454*
AquaTar® (Discontinued) *see* coal tar *on page 240*
Aquatensen® [Can] *see* methyclothiazide *on page 619*

Aquavit-E® [US-OTC] *see* vitamin E *on page 981*

aqueous procaine penicillin G *see* penicillin G procaine *on page 733*

Aquoral™ [US] *see* saliva substitute *on page 853*

ara-C *see* cytarabine *on page 261*

arabinosylcytosine *see* cytarabine *on page 261*

Aralast [US] *see* alpha₁-proteinase inhibitor *on page 48*

Aralast NP [US] *see* alpha₁-proteinase inhibitor *on page 48*

Aralen® [US/Can] *see* chloroquine *on page 204*

Aranelle™ [US] *see* ethinyl estradiol and norethindrone *on page 376*

Aranesp® [US/Can] *see* darbepoetin alfa *on page 267*

Arava® [US/Can] *see* leflunomide *on page 551*

Arcalyst™ [US] *see* rilonacept *on page 835*

Arduan® *(Discontinued)*

Aredia® [US/Can] *see* pamidronate *on page 716*

arformoterol (ar for MOE ter ol)

Synonyms (R,R)-formoterol L-tartrate; arformoterol tartrate

U.S./Canadian Brand Names Brovana® [US]

Therapeutic Category Beta₂-Adrenergic Agonist

Use Long-term maintenance treatment of bronchoconstriction in chronic obstructive pulmonary disease (COPD), including chronic bronchitis and emphysema

Usual Dosage Nebulization: Adults: COPD: 15 mcg twice daily; maximum: 30 mcg/day

Dosage Forms

Solution for nebulization:

Brovana®: 15 mcg/2 mL (30s, 60s)

arformoterol tartrate *see* arformoterol *on page 92*

argatroban (ar GA troh ban)

Sound-Alike/Look-Alike Issues

argatroban may be confused with Aggrastat®, Organan®

Therapeutic Category Anticoagulant, Thrombin Inhibitor

Use Prophylaxis or treatment of thrombosis in patients with heparin-induced thrombocytopenia; adjunct to percutaneous coronary intervention (PCI) in patients who have or are at risk of thrombosis associated with heparin-induced thrombocytopenia

Usual Dosage I.V.: Adults:

Heparin-induced thrombocytopenia:

Initial dose: 2 mcg/kg/minute

Maintenance dose: Patient may not be at steady-state but measure aPTT after 2 hours; adjust dose until the steady-state aPTT is 1.5-3.0 times the initial baseline value, not exceeding 100 seconds; dosage should not exceed 10 mcg/kg/minute

Conversion to oral anticoagulant: Because there may be a combined effect on the INR when argatroban is combined with warfarin, loading doses of warfarin should not be used. Warfarin therapy should be started at the expected daily dose.

Patients receiving ≤2 mcg/kg/minute of argatroban: Argatroban therapy can be stopped when the combined INR on warfarin and argatroban is >4; repeat INR measurement in 4-6 hours; if INR is below therapeutic level, argatroban therapy may be restarted. Repeat procedure daily until desired INR on warfarin alone is obtained.

Patients receiving >2 mcg/kg/minute of argatroban: Reduce dose of argatroban to 2 mcg/kg/minute; measure INR for argatroban and warfarin 4-6 hours after dose reduction; argatroban therapy can be stopped when the combined INR on warfarin and argatroban is >4. Repeat INR measurement in 4-6 hours; if INR is below therapeutic level, argatroban therapy may be restarted. Repeat procedure daily until desired INR on warfarin alone is obtained.

Note: Critically-ill patients with normal hepatic function became excessively anticoagulated with FDA-approved or lower starting doses of argatroban. Doses between 0.15-1.3 mcg/kg/minute were required to maintain aPTTs in the target range. Another report of a cardiac patient with anasarca secondary to acute renal failure had a reduction in argatroban clearance similar to patients with hepatic dysfunction. Reduced clearance may have been attributed to reduced perfusion to the liver. Consider reducing starting dose to 0.5-1 mcg/kg/minute in critically-ill patients who may have impaired hepatic perfusion (eg, patients requiring vasopressors, having decreased cardiac output, having fluid overload). In a retrospective review of critical care patients, patients with three organ system failure required 0.5 mcg/kg/minute. The mean argatroban dose of ICU patients was 0.9 mcg/kg/minute.

Percutaneous coronary intervention (PCI):
Initial: Begin infusion of 25 mcg/kg/minute and administer bolus dose of 350 mcg/kg (over 3-5 minutes). ACT should be checked 5-10 minutes after bolus infusion; proceed with procedure if ACT >300 seconds. Following initial bolus:

ACT <300 seconds: Give an additional 150 mcg/kg bolus, and increase infusion rate to 30 mcg/kg/minute (recheck ACT in 5-10 minutes)

ACT >450 seconds: Decrease infusion rate to 15 mcg/kg/minute (recheck ACT in 5-10 minutes)

Once a therapeutic ACT (300-450 seconds) is achieved, infusion should be continued at this dose for the duration of the procedure.

If dissection, impending abrupt closure, thrombus formation during PCI, or inability to achieve ACT >300 seconds: An additional bolus of 150 mcg/kg, followed by an increase in infusion rate to 40 mcg/kg/minute may be administered.

Note: Post-PCI anticoagulation, if required, may be achieved by continuing infusion at a reduced dose of 2-10 mcg/kg/minute, with close monitoring of aPTT.

Dosage Forms
Injection, solution:
100 mg/mL (2.5 mL)

arginine (AR ji neen)

Synonyms arginine hydrochloride
U.S./Canadian Brand Names R-Gene® [US]
Therapeutic Category Diagnostic Agent
Use Pituitary function test (growth hormone)
Usual Dosage I.V.: Pituitary function test:
Children: 500 mg/kg/dose administered over 30 minutes
Adults: 30 g (300 mL) administered over 30 minutes
Dosage Forms
Injection, solution:
R-Gene®: 10% (300 mL) [100 mg/mL = 950 mOsm/L]

arginine hydrochloride *see* arginine *on page 93*
8-arginine vasopressin *see* vasopressin *on page 972*
Aricept® [US/Can] *see* donepezil *on page 318*
Aricept® ODT [US] *see* donepezil *on page 318*
Aricept® RDT [Can] *see* donepezil *on page 318*
Arimidex® [US/Can] *see* anastrozole *on page 76*

aripiprazole (ay ri PIP ray zole)

Sound-Alike/Look-Alike Issues
aripiprazole may be confused with rabeprazole
Synonyms BMS-337039; OPC-14597
U.S./Canadian Brand Names Abilify® Discmelt™ [US]; Abilify® [US]
Therapeutic Category Antipsychotic Agent, Quinolone
Use
Oral: Acute and maintenance treatment of schizophrenia; stabilization, maintenance, and adjunctive therapy (to lithium or valproate) of bipolar disorder (with acute manic or mixed episodes); adjunctive treatment of major depressive disorder
Injection: Agitation associated with schizophrenia or bipolar mania

Usual Dosage Note: Oral solution may be substituted for the oral tablet on a mg-per-mg basis, up to 25 mg. Patients receiving 30 mg tablets should be given 25 mg oral solution. Orally disintegrating tablets (Abilify® Discmelt™) are bioequivalent to the immediate release tablets (Abilify®).

Children ≥10 years: Oral: Bipolar I disorder (acute manic or mixed episodes): Initial: 2 mg daily for 2 days, followed by 5 mg daily for 2 days with a further increase to target dose of 10 mg daily as monotherapy or adjunctive therapy; subsequent dose increases may be made in 5 mg increments, up to a maximum of 30 mg/day

▶

◀ Adolescents ≥13 years: Oral: Schizophrenia: Initial: 2 mg daily for 2 days, followed by 5 mg daily for 2 days with a further increase to target dose of 10 mg daily; subsequent dose increases may be made in 5 mg increments up to a maximum of 30 mg/day (30 mg/day not shown to be more efficacious than 10 mg/day)

Adults:

Acute agitation (schizophrenia/bipolar mania): I.M.: 9.75 mg as a single dose (range: 5.25-15 mg); repeated doses may be given at ≥2-hour intervals to a maximum of 30 mg/day. **Note:** If ongoing therapy with aripiprazole is necessary, transition to oral therapy as soon as possible.

Bipolar disorder (acute manic or mixed episodes): Oral:

Stabilization: Initial: 15 mg once daily as monotherapy or adjunctive to lithium or valproic acid. May increase to 30 mg once daily if clinically indicated; safety of doses >30 mg/day has not been evaluated.

Maintenance: Continue stabilization dose for up to 6 weeks; efficacy of continued treatment >6 weeks has not been established

Depression (adjunctive with antidepressants): Oral: Initial: 2-5 mg/day (range: 2-15 mg/day); dose adjustments of up to 5 mg/day may be made in intervals of ≥1 week. **Note:** Dosing based on patients already receiving antidepressant therapy.

Schizophrenia: Oral: 10-15 mg once daily; may be increased to a maximum of 30 mg once daily (efficacy at dosages above 10-15 mg has not been shown to be increased). Dosage titration should not be more frequent than every 2 weeks.

Dosage Forms

Injection, solution:
Abilify®: 7.5 mg/mL (1.3 mL)

Solution, oral:
Abilify®: 1 mg/mL

Tablet:
Abilify®: 2 mg, 5 mg, 10 mg, 15 mg, 20 mg, 30 mg

Tablet, orally disintegrating:
Abilify® Discmelt™: 10 mg, 15 mg

Aristocort® A [US] *see* triamcinolone (topical) *on page 949*
Aristospan® [US/Can] *see* triamcinolone (systemic) *on page 948*
Arixtra® [US/Can] *see* fondaparinux *on page 424*
Arm-a-Med® Isoproterenol *(Discontinued)* *see* isoproterenol *on page 529*
Arm-a-Med® Metaproterenol *(Discontinued)*

armodafinil (ar moe DAF i nil)

Synonyms R-modafinil
U.S./Canadian Brand Names Nuvigil™ [US]
Therapeutic Category Stimulant
Controlled Substance C-IV

Use Improve wakefulness in patients with excessive daytime sleepiness associated with narcolepsy and shift work sleep disorder (SWSD); adjunctive therapy for obstructive sleep apnea/hypopnea syndrome (OSAHS)

Usual Dosage Oral: Adults:

Narcolepsy: 150-250 mg once daily in the morning

Obstructive sleep apnea/hypopnea syndrome (OSAHS): 150-250 mg once daily in the morning; 250 mg was not shown to have any increased benefit over 150 mg

Shift work sleep disorder (SWSD): 150 mg given once daily ~1 hour prior to work shift

Dosage Forms

Tablet:
Nuvigil™: 50 mg, 150 mg, 250 mg

Armour® Thyroid [US] *see* thyroid, desiccated *on page 924*
Aromasin® [US/Can] *see* exemestane *on page 385*
Arranon® [US] *see* nelarabine *on page 660*
Arrestin® *(Discontinued)* *see* trimethobenzamide *on page 953*

arsenic trioxide (AR se nik tri OKS id)

Synonyms As_2O_3; NSC-706363
U.S./Canadian Brand Names Trisenox® [US]

Therapeutic Category Antineoplastic Agent, Miscellaneous

Use Induction of remission and consolidation in patients with relapsed or refractory acute promyelocytic leukemia (APL) which is specifically characterized by t(15;17) translocation or PML/RAR-alpha gene expression

Usual Dosage I.V.: Children ≥5 years and Adults: APL:
Induction: 0.15 mg/kg/day; administer daily until bone marrow remission; maximum induction: 60 doses
Consolidation: 0.15 mg/kg/day starting 3-6 weeks after completion of induction therapy; maximum consolidation: 25 doses over 5 weeks

Dosage Forms
Injection, solution [preservative free]:
Trisenox®: 1 mg/mL (10 mL)

Artane® *(Discontinued)* see trihexyphenidyl *on page 952*
Artha-G® *(Discontinued)* see salsalate *on page 854*
ArthriCare® for Women Extra Moisturizing *(Discontinued)* see capsaicin *on page 171*
ArthriCare® for Women Multi-Action *(Discontinued)* see capsaicin *on page 171*
ArthriCare® for Women Silky Dry *(Discontinued)* see capsaicin *on page 171*
ArthriCare® for Women Ultra Strength *(Discontinued)* see capsaicin *on page 171*
Arthropan® *(Discontinued)*
Arthrotec® [US/Can] see diclofenac and misoprostol *on page 293*

articaine and epinephrine (AR ti kane & ep i NEF rin)

Synonyms epinephrine and articaine hydrochloride

U.S./Canadian Brand Names Astracaine® with epinephrine 1:200,000 [Can]; Astracaine® with epinephrine forte 1:100,000 [Can]; Septanest® N [Can]; Septanest® SP [Can]; Septocaine® with epinephrine 1:100,000 [US]; Septocaine® with epinephrine 1:200,000 [US]; Ultracaine® D-S Forte [Can]; Ultracaine® D-S [Can]; Zorcaine™ [US/Can]

Therapeutic Category Local Anesthetic

Use Local, infiltrative, or conductive anesthesia in both simple and complex dental and periodontal procedures

Usual Dosage Summary of recommended volumes and concentrations for various types of anesthetic procedures; dosages (administered by submucosal injection and/or nerve block) apply to normal healthy adults:

Infiltration: Injection volume of 4% solution: 0.5-2.5 mL; total dose: 20-100 mg
Nerve block: Injection volume of 4% solution: 0.5-3.4 mL; total dose: 20-136 mg
Oral surgery: Injection volume of 4% solution: 1-5.1 mL; total dose: 40-204 mg
Note: These dosages are guides only; other dosages may be used; however, do not exceed maximum recommended dose

Dosage Forms [CAN] = Canadian brand name
Injection, solution:
Septocaine® with epinephrine 1:100,000: Articaine 4% and epinephrine 1:100,000 (1.7 mL)
Septocaine® with epinephrine 1:200,000: Articaine 4% and epinephrine 1:200,000 (1.7 mL)
Ultracaine DS® [CAN]: Articaine 4% and epinephrine 1:200,000 (1.7 mL) [not available in the U.S.]
Ultracaine DS Forte® [CAN]: Articaine 4% and epinephrine 1:100,000 (1.7 mL) [not available in the U.S.]
Zorcaine™: Articaine 4% and epinephrine 1:100,000 (1.7 mL)

artificial saliva see saliva substitute *on page 853*

artificial tears (ar ti FISH il tears)

Sound-Alike/Look-Alike Issues
Isopto® Tears may be confused with Isoptin®
Murocel® may be confused with Murocoll-2®

Synonyms hydroxyethylcellulose; polyvinyl alcohol

U.S./Canadian Brand Names Akwa Tears® [US-OTC]; AquaSite® [US-OTC]; Bion® Tears [US-OTC]; HypoTears PF [US-OTC]; HypoTears [US-OTC]; Liquifilm® Tears [US-OTC]; Moisture® Eyes PM [US-OTC]; Moisture® Eyes [US-OTC]; Murine® Tears [US-OTC]; Murocel® [US-OTC]; Nature's Tears® [US-OTC]; Nu-Tears® II [US-OTC]; Nu-Tears® [US-OTC]; OcuCoat® PF [US-OTC]; OcuCoat® [US-OTC]; Puralube® Tears [US-OTC]; Refresh Plus® [US-OTC]; Refresh Tears® [US-OTC]; Refresh® [US-OTC];

◀ Soothe® [US-OTC]; Systane® Free [US-OTC]; Systane® [US-OTC]; Teardrops® [Can]; Teargen® II [US-OTC]; Teargen® [US-OTC]; Tearisol® [US-OTC]; Tears Again® [US-OTC]; Tears Naturale® Free [US-OTC]; Tears Naturale® II [US-OTC]; Tears Naturale® [US-OTC]; Tears Plus® [US-OTC]; Tears Renewed® [US-OTC]; Ultra Tears® [US-OTC]; Viva-Drops® [US-OTC]

Therapeutic Category Ophthalmic Agent, Miscellaneous

Use Ophthalmic lubricant; for relief of dry eyes and eye irritation

Usual Dosage Ophthalmic: Children and Adults: Use as needed to relieve symptoms, 1-2 drops into eye(s) 3-4 times/day

Dosage Forms

Solution, ophthalmic: 15 mL and 30 mL dropper bottles

Akwa Tears® [OTC], AquaSite® [OTC], Bion® Tears [OTC], HypoTears PF [OTC], HypoTears [OTC], Isopto® Tears [OTC], Liquifilm® Tears [OTC], Moisture® Eyes PM [OTC], Moisture® Eyes [OTC], Murine® Tears [OTC], Murocel® [OTC], Nature's Tears® [OTC], Nu-Tears® II [OTC], Nu-Tears® [OTC], OcuCoat® PF [OTC], OcuCoat® [OTC], Puralube® Tears [OTC], Refresh® [OTC], Refresh® Plus [OTC], Refresh Tears® [OTC], Teargen® [OTC], Teargen® II [OTC], Tearisol® [OTC], Tears Again® [OTC], Tears Naturale® Free [OTC], Tears Naturale® II [OTC], Tears Naturale® [OTC], Tears Plus® [OTC], Tears Renewed® [OTC], Ultra Tears® [OTC], Viva-Drops® [OTC]: 15 mL and 30 mL dropper bottles

ASA *see* aspirin *on page 98*

As₂O₃ *see* arsenic trioxide *on page 94*

5-ASA *see* mesalamine *on page 607*

Asacol® [US/Can] *see* mesalamine *on page 607*

Asacol® 800 [Can] *see* mesalamine *on page 607*

A.S.A.® *(Discontinued)* *see* aspirin *on page 98*

Asaphen [Can] *see* aspirin *on page 98*

Asaphen E.C. [Can] *see* aspirin *on page 98*

Asco-Caps [US-OTC] *see* ascorbic acid *on page 96*

Ascocid® [US-OTC] *see* ascorbic acid *on page 96*

Ascomp® with Codeine [US] *see* butalbital, aspirin, caffeine, and codeine *on page 156*

ascorbic acid (a SKOR bik AS id)

Synonyms vitamin C

U.S./Canadian Brand Names Acerola [US-OTC]; Asco-Caps [US-OTC]; Asco-Tabs [US-OTC]; Ascocid® [US-OTC]; C-Gel [US-OTC]; C-Gram [US-OTC]; C-Time [US-OTC]; Cecon® [US-OTC]; Cemill [US-OTC]; Cenolate® [US]; Chew-C [US-OTC]; Dull-C® [US-OTC]; Mild-C® [US-OTC]; One Gram C [US-OTC]; Proflavanol C™ [Can]; Revitalose C-1000® [Can]; Time-C [US-OTC]; Time-C-Bio [US-OTC]; Vicks® Vitamin C [US-OTC]; Vita-C® [US-OTC]

Therapeutic Category Vitamin, Water Soluble

Use Prevention and treatment of scurvy; acidify the urine

Usual Dosage Oral, I.M., I.V., SubQ:

Recommended daily allowance (RDA):

<6 months: 30 mg

6 months to 1 year: 35 mg

1-3 years: 15 mg; upper limit of intake should not exceed 400 mg/day

4-8 years: 25 mg; upper limit of intake should not exceed 650 mg/day

9-13 years: 45 mg; upper limit of intake should not exceed 1200 mg/day

14-18 years: Upper limit of intake should not exceed 1800 mg/day

Male: 75 mg

Female: 65 mg

Adults: Upper limit of intake should not exceed 2000 mg/day

Male: 90 mg

Female: 75 mg

Pregnant female:

≤18 years: 80 mg; upper limit of intake should not exceed 1800 mg/day

19-50 years: 85 mg; upper limit of intake should not exceed 2000 mg/day

Lactating female:

≤18 years: 15 mg; upper limit of intake should not exceed 1800 mg/day

19-50 years: 20 mg; upper limit of intake should not exceed 2000 mg/day

Adult smoker: Add an additional 35 mg/day
Children:
  Scurvy: 100-300 mg/day in divided doses for at least 2 weeks
  Urinary acidification: 500 mg every 6-8 hours
  Dietary supplement: 35-100 mg/day
Adults:
  Scurvy: 100-250 mg 1-2 times/day for at least 2 weeks
  Urinary acidification: 4-12 g/day in 3-4 divided doses
  Prevention and treatment of colds: 1-3 g/day
  Dietary supplement: 50-200 mg/day

Dosage Forms
Caplet: 1000 mg
Caplet, timed release: 500 mg, 1000 mg
Capsule:
  Mild-C® [OTC]: 500 mg
Capsule, softgel:
  C-Gel [OTC]: 1000 mg
Capsule, sustained release:
  C-Time [OTC]: 500 mg
Capsule, timed release: 500 mg
  Asco-Caps [OTC]: 500 mg, 1000 mg
  Time-C® [OTC]: 500 mg
Crystals for solution, oral: 4 g/teaspoonful
  Mild-C® [OTC]: 3600 mg/teaspoonful
  Vita-C® [OTC]: 4 g/teaspoonful
Injection, solution: 500 mg/mL (50 mL)
  Cenolate® [OTC]: 500 mg/mL (1 mL, 2 mL)
Injection, solution [preservative free]:
  Ascor L 500®: 500 mg/mL (50 mL)
  Ascor L NC®: 500 mg/mL (50 mL)
Liquid, oral: 500 mg/5 mL
Lozenge:
  Vicks® Vitamin C [OTC]: 25 mg
Powder, for solution, oral:
  Ascocid® [OTC}: 4000 mg/5 mL; 4300 mg/5 mL; 5000 mg/5 mL
  Dull-C® [OTC]: 4 g/teaspoonful
Solution, oral:
  Cecon® [OTC]: 90 mg/mL
Tablet: 100 mg, 250 mg, 500 mg, 1000 mg
  Asco-Tabs [OTC]: 1000 mg
  Ascocid® [OTC]: 500 mg
  C-Gram [OTC]: 1000 mg
  One Gram C [OTC]: 1000 mg
Tablet, chewable: 250 mg, 500 mg
  Acerola [OTC]: 500 mg
  Chew-C [OTC]: 500 mg
  Mild-C® [OCT]: 250 mg
Tablet, timed release: 500 mg, 1000 mg
  Cemill [OTC]: 500 mg, 1000 mg
  Mild-C® [OTC]: 1000 mg
  Time-C-Bio [OTC]: 500 mg

ascorbic acid and ferrous sulfate *see* ferrous sulfate and ascorbic acid *on page 399*
Ascorbicap® *(Discontinued)* *see* ascorbic acid *on page 96*
Asco-Tabs [US-OTC] *see* ascorbic acid *on page 96*
Ascriptin® [US-OTC] *see* aspirin *on page 98*
Ascriptin® Maximum Strength [US-OTC] *see* aspirin *on page 98*
Asendin® *(Discontinued)* *see* amoxapine *on page 67*
Asmalix® *(Discontinued)* *see* theophylline *on page 917*
Asmanex® Twisthaler® [US] *see* mometasone *on page 641*

asparaginase (a SPEAR a ji nase)

Sound-Alike/Look-Alike Issues
asparaginase may be confused with pegaspargase
Elspar® may be confused with Elaprase™

Synonyms *E. coli* asparaginase; *Erwinia* asparaginase; L-asparaginase; NSC-106977 (*Erwinia*); NSC-109229 (*E. coli*)

U.S./Canadian Brand Names Elspar® [US/Can]; Kidrolase® [Can]

Therapeutic Category Antineoplastic Agent

Use Treatment of acute lymphocytic leukemia (ALL)

Usual Dosage Refer to individual protocols. **Note:** Dose, frequency, number of doses, and start date may vary by protocol and treatment phase.
Children:
I.V.:
6000 units/m^2/dose 3 times/week for ~6-9 doses **or**
1000 units/kg/day for 10 days
I.M.: 6000 units/m^2/dose 3 times/week **or** 6000 units/m^2/dose every ~3 days for ~6-9 doses
Adults:
I.V.:
6000 units/m^2/dose 3 times/week for ~6-9 doses **or**
1000 units/kg/day for 10 days
Single agent therapy (rare): 200 units/kg/day for 28 days
I.M.: 6000 units/m^2/dose 3 times/week for ~6-9 doses **or** 6000 units/m^2/dose every ~3 days for ~6-9 doses

Test dose: A test dose is often recommended prior to the first dose of asparaginase, or prior to restarting therapy after a hiatus of several days. Most commonly, 0.1 mL of a 20 units/mL (2 units) asparaginase dilution is injected intradermally, and the patient observed for at least 1 hour. False-negative rates of up to 80% to test doses of 2-50 units are reported.

Some practitioners recommend an asparaginase desensitization regimen for patients who react to a test dose, or are being retreated following a break in therapy. Doses are doubled and given every 10 minutes until the total daily dose for that day has been administered. One schedule begins with a total of 1 unit given I.V. and doubles the dose every 10 minutes until the total amount given is the planned dose for that day. For example, if a patient was to receive a total dose of 4000 units, he/she would receive injections 1 through 12 during the desensitization.

Dosage Forms
Injection, powder for reconstitution:
Elspar®: 10,000 units

aspart insulin *see* insulin aspart *on page 509*
A-Spas® (Discontinued) *see* hyoscyamine *on page 492*
Aspercin [US-OTC] *see* aspirin *on page 98*
Aspercreme® [US-OTC] *see* trolamine *on page 957*
Aspergillus niger *see* alpha-galactosidase *on page 49*
Aspergum® [US-OTC] *see* aspirin *on page 98*

aspirin (AS pir in)

Sound-Alike/Look-Alike Issues
aspirin may be confused with Afrin®, Asendin®
Ascriptin® may be confused with Aricept®
Ecotrin® may be confused with Akineton®, Edecrin®, Epogen®
Halfprin® may be confused with Halfan®, Haltran®
ZORprin® may be confused with Zyloprim®

Synonyms acetylsalicylic acid; ASA

U.S./Canadian Brand Names Asaphen E.C. [Can]; Asaphen [Can]; Ascriptin® Maximum Strength [US-OTC]; Ascriptin® [US-OTC]; Aspercin [US-OTC]; Aspergum® [US-OTC]; Aspirtab [US-OTC]; Bayer® Aspirin Extra Strength [US-OTC]; Bayer® Aspirin Regimen Adult Low Dose [US-OTC]; Bayer® Aspirin Regimen Children's [US-OTC]; Bayer® Aspirin Regimen Regular Strength [US-OTC]; Bayer® Genuine Aspirin [US-OTC]; Bayer® Plus Extra Strength [US-OTC]; Bayer® with Heart Advantage [US-OTC]; Bayer® Women's Aspirin Plus Calcium [US-OTC]; Buffasal [US-OTC]; Bufferin® Extra Strength [US-OTC]; Bufferin® [US-OTC]; Buffinol [US-OTC]; Easprin® [US]; Ecotrin® Low Strength [US-OTC];

Ecotrin® Maximum Strength [US-OTC]; Ecotrin® [US-OTC]; Entrophen® [Can]; Genacote™ [US-OTC]; Halfprin® [US-OTC]; Novasen [Can]; St. Joseph® Adult Aspirin [US-OTC]; ZORprin® [US]

Therapeutic Category Analgesic, Nonnarcotic; Antiplatelet Agent; Antipyretic; Nonsteroidal Antiinflammatory Drug (NSAID)

Use Treatment of mild-to-moderate pain, inflammation, and fever; may be used as prophylaxis of myocardial infarction; prophylaxis of stroke and/or transient ischemic episodes; management of rheumatoid arthritis, rheumatic fever, osteoarthritis, and gout (high dose); adjunctive therapy in revascularization procedures (coronary artery bypass graft [CABG], percutaneous transluminal coronary angioplasty [PTCA], carotid endarterectomy), stent implantation

Usual Dosage

Children:

Analgesic and antipyretic: Oral, rectal: 10-15 mg/kg/dose every 4-6 hours, up to a total of 4 g/day

Antiinflammatory: Oral: Initial: 60-90 mg/kg/day in divided doses; usual maintenance: 80-100 mg/kg/day divided every 6-8 hours; monitor serum concentrations

Antiplatelet effects: Adequate pediatric studies have not been performed; pediatric dosage is derived from adult studies and clinical experience and is not well established; suggested doses have ranged from 3-5 mg/kg/day to 5-10 mg/kg/day given as a single daily dose. Doses are rounded to a convenient amount (eg, 1/2 of 80 mg tablet).

Mechanical prosthetic heart valves: 6-20 mg/kg/day given as a single daily dose (used in combination with an oral anticoagulant in children who have systemic embolism despite adequate oral anticoagulation therapy (INR 2.5-3.5) and used in combination with low-dose anticoagulation (INR 2-3) and dipyridamole when full-dose oral anticoagulation is contraindicated)

Blalock-Taussig shunts: 3-5 mg/kg/day given as a single daily dose

Kawasaki disease: Oral: 80-100 mg/kg/day divided every 6 hours; monitor serum concentrations; after fever resolves: 3-5 mg/kg/day once daily; in patients without coronary artery abnormalities, give lower dose for at least 6-8 weeks or until ESR and platelet count are normal; in patients with coronary artery abnormalities, low-dose aspirin should be continued indefinitely

Antirheumatic: Oral: 60-100 mg/kg/day in divided doses every 4 hours

Adults:

Analgesic and antipyretic: Oral, rectal: 325-650 mg every 4-6 hours up to 4 g/day

Antiinflammatory: Oral: Initial: 2.4-3.6 g/day in divided doses; usual maintenance: 3.6-5.4 g/day; monitor serum concentrations

Myocardial infarction prophylaxis: 75-325 mg/day; use of a lower aspirin dosage has been recommended in patients receiving ACE inhibitors

Acute myocardial infarction: 160-325 mg/day (have patient chew tablet if not taking aspirin before presentation)

CABG: 75-325 mg/day starting 6 hours following procedure; if bleeding prevents administration at 6 hours after CABG, initiate as soon as possible

PTCA: Initial: 80-325 mg/day starting 2 hours before procedure; longer pretreatment durations (up to 24 hours) should be considered if lower dosages (80-100 mg) are used

Stent implantation: Oral: 325 mg 2 hours prior to implantation and 160-325 mg daily thereafter

Carotid endarterectomy: 81-325 mg/day preoperatively and daily thereafter

Acute stroke: 160-325 mg/day, initiated within 48 hours (in patients who are not candidates for thrombolytics and are not receiving systemic anticoagulation)

Stroke prevention/TIA: 30-325 mg/day (dosages up to 1300 mg/day in 2-4 divided doses have been used in clinical trials)

Dosage Forms

Caplet: 81 mg, 325 mg, 500 mg

Bayer® Aspirin Extra Strength [OTC], Bayer® Plus Extra Strength [OTC]: 500 mg

Bayer® Aspirin Regimen Regular Strength [OTC], Bayer® Genuine Aspirin [OTC]: 325 mg

Bayer® with Heart Advantage [OTC], Bayer® Women's Aspirin Plus Calcium [OTC]: 81 mg

Caplet, buffered: 500 mg

Ascriptin® Maximum Strength [OTC]: 500 mg

Gum:

Aspergum® [OTC]: 227 mg

Suppository, rectal: 300 mg, 600 mg

Tablet: 325 mg

Aspercin [OTC], Aspirtab [OTC], Bayer® Genuine Aspirin [OTC]: 325 mg

Tablet, buffered: 325 mg

Ascriptin® [OTC], Bufferin® [OTC], Buffasal [OTC], Buffinol [OTC]: 325 mg

Bufferin® Extra Strength [OTC]: 500 mg

Tablet, chewable: 81 mg

Bayer® Aspirin Regimen Children's [OTC], St. Joseph® Adult Aspirin [OTC]: 81 mg

▶

Tablet, controlled release: 800 mg
  ZORprin®: 800 mg
Tablet, delayed release, enteric coated:
  Easprin®: 975 mg
Tablet, enteric coated: 81 mg, 325 mg, 500 mg, 650 mg
  Bayer® Aspirin Regimen Adult Low Dose [OTC], Ecotrin® Low Strength [OTC], St. Joseph Adult Aspirin
   [OTC], Sureprin 81™ [OTC]: 81 mg
  Ecotrin® [OTC], Genacote™ [OTC]: 325 mg
  Ecotrin® Maximum Strength [OTC]: 500 mg
  Halfprin® [OTC]: 81 mg, 162 mg

aspirin, acetaminophen, and caffeine *see* acetaminophen, aspirin, and caffeine *on page 24*
aspirin and carisoprodol *see* carisoprodol and aspirin *on page 180*

aspirin and dipyridamole (AS pir in & dye peer ID a mole)
Sound-Alike/Look-Alike Issues
  Aggrenox® may be confused with Aggrastat®
Synonyms aspirin and extended-release dipyridamole; dipyridamole and aspirin
U.S./Canadian Brand Names Aggrenox® [US/Can]
Therapeutic Category Antiplatelet Agent
Use Reduction in the risk of stroke in patients who have had transient ischemia of the brain or completed ischemic stroke due to thrombosis
Usual Dosage Oral: Adults: 1 capsule (dipyridamole 200 mg, aspirin 25 mg) twice daily
Dosage Forms
  Capsule:
   Aggrenox®: Aspirin 25 mg (immediate release) and dipyridamole 200 mg (extended release)

aspirin and extended-release dipyridamole *see* aspirin and dipyridamole *on page 100*
aspirin and meprobamate *see* meprobamate and aspirin *on page 606*
aspirin and oxycodone *see* oxycodone and aspirin *on page 711*
aspirin, caffeine, and acetaminophen *see* acetaminophen, aspirin, and caffeine *on page 24*
aspirin, caffeine, and butalbital *see* butalbital, aspirin, and caffeine *on page 156*
aspirin, caffeine, and propoxyphene *see* propoxyphene, aspirin, and caffeine *on page 796*
aspirin, caffeine, codeine, and butalbital *see* butalbital, aspirin, caffeine, and codeine *on page 156*
aspirin, carisoprodol, and codeine *see* carisoprodol, aspirin, and codeine *on page 180*
Aspirin Free Anacin® *(Discontinued)* *see* acetaminophen *on page 19*
Aspirin Free Anacin® Maximum Strength [US-OTC] *see* acetaminophen *on page 19*
aspirin, orphenadrine, and caffeine *see* orphenadrine, aspirin, and caffeine *on page 703*
Aspirtab [US-OTC] *see* aspirin *on page 98*
Astelin® [US/Can] *see* azelastine *on page 110*
AsthmaHaler® Mist *(Discontinued)* *see* epinephrine *on page 344*
AsthmaNefrin® *(Discontinued)* *see* epinephrine *on page 344*
Astracaine® with epinephrine 1:200,000 [Can] *see* articaine and epinephrine *on page 95*
Astracaine® with epinephrine forte 1:100,000 [Can] *see* articaine and epinephrine *on page 95*
Astramorph/PF™ [US] *see* morphine sulfate *on page 643*
AT-III *see* antithrombin III *on page 82*
Atacand® [US/Can] *see* candesartan *on page 169*
Atacand HCT® [US] *see* candesartan and hydrochlorothiazide *on page 169*
Atacand® Plus [Can] *see* candesartan and hydrochlorothiazide *on page 169*
Atapryl® *(Discontinued)*
Atarax® [Can] *see* hydroxyzine *on page 491*
Atarax® *(Discontinued)* *see* hydroxyzine *on page 491*
Atasol® [Can] *see* acetaminophen *on page 19*

atazanavir (at a za NA veer)
Synonyms atazanavir sulfate; BMS-232632
U.S./Canadian Brand Names Reyataz® [US/Can]

Therapeutic Category Antiretroviral Agent, Protease Inhibitor

Use Treatment of HIV-1 infections in combination with at least two other antiretroviral agents

Note: In patients with prior virologic failure, coadministration with ritonavir is recommended.

Usual Dosage Oral:

Children ≥6 years and Adolescents:

Antiretroviral-naive patients:

15-24 kg: Atazanavir 150 mg once daily **plus** ritonavir 80 mg once daily

25-31 kg: Atazanavir 200 mg once daily **plus** ritonavir 100 mg once daily

32-38 kg: Atazanavir 250 mg once daily **plus** ritonavir 100 mg once daily

≥39 kg: Atazanavir 300 mg once daily **plus** 100 mg ritonavir once daily. **Note:** Treatment-naive patients ≥39 kg and ≥13 years of age who are unable to tolerate ritonavir, refer to adult dosing.

or

15-19 kg: Atazanavir 8.5 mg/kg/dose once daily (rounded to available capsule strengths) **plus** ritonavir 4 mg/kg once daily

≥20 kg: Atazanavir 7 mg/kg/dose once daily (round to available capsule strengths) (maximum: 300 mg) **plus** ritonavir 4 mg/kg once daily

Antiretroviral-experienced patients: **Note:** Atazanavir without ritonavir is not recommended in antiretroviral-experienced patients with prior virologic failure:

25-31 kg: Atazanavir 200 mg once daily **plus** ritonavir 100 mg once daily

32-38 kg: Atazanavir 250 mg once daily **plus** ritonavir 100 mg once daily

≥39 kg: Atazanavir 300 mg once daily **plus** 100 mg ritonavir once daily

Adults:

Antiretroviral-naive patients: 400 mg once daily

Antiretroviral-experienced patients: Atazanavir 300 mg once daily **plus** ritonavir 100 mg once daily. **Note:** Atazanavir without ritonavir is not recommended in antiretroviral-experienced patients with prior virologic failure.

Dosage Forms

Capsule:

Reyataz®: 100 mg, 150 mg, 200 mg, 300 mg

atazanavir sulfate *see atazanavir on page 100*

atenolol (a TEN oh lole)

Sound-Alike/Look-Alike Issues

atenolol may be confused with albuterol, Altenol®, timolol, Tylenol®

Tenormin® may be confused with Imuran®, Norpramin®, thiamine, Trovan®

U.S./Canadian Brand Names Apo-Atenol® [Can]; Gen-Atenolol [Can]; Novo-Atenol [Can]; Nu-Atenol [Can]; PMS-Atenolol [Can]; RAN™-Atenolol [Can]; Rhoxal-atenolol [Can]; Riva-Atenolol [Can]; Sandoz-Atenolol [Can]; Tenolin [Can]; Tenormin® [US/Can]

Therapeutic Category Beta-Adrenergic Blocker

Use Treatment of hypertension, alone or in combination with other agents; management of angina pectoris, postmyocardial infarction patients

Usual Dosage

Oral:

Children: Hypertension: 0.5-1 mg/kg/dose given daily; range of 0.5-1.5 mg/kg/day; maximum dose: 2 mg/kg/day up to 100 mg/day

Adults:

Hypertension: 25-50 mg once daily, may increase to 100 mg/day. Doses >100 mg are unlikely to produce any further benefit.

Angina pectoris: 50 mg once daily, may increase to 100 mg/day. Some patients may require 200 mg/day.

Postmyocardial infarction: Follow I.V. dose with 100 mg/day or 50 mg twice daily for 6-9 days postmyocardial infarction.

I.V.:

Hypertension: Dosages of 1.25-5 mg every 6-12 hours have been used in short-term management of patients unable to take oral enteral beta-blockers

Postmyocardial infarction: Early treatment: 5 mg slow I.V. over 5 minutes; may repeat in 10 minutes. If both doses are tolerated, may start oral atenolol 50 mg every 12 hours or 100 mg/day for 6-9 days postmyocardial infarction.

◀ **Dosage Forms**
  Tablet: 25 mg, 50 mg, 100 mg
    Tenormin®: 25 mg, 50 mg, 100 mg

atenolol and chlorthalidone (a TEN oh lole & klor THAL i done)

Synonyms chlorthalidone and atenolol
U.S./Canadian Brand Names Apo-Atenidone® [Can]; Novo-Atenolthalidone [Can]; Tenoretic® [US/Can]
Therapeutic Category Antihypertensive Agent, Combination
Use Treatment of hypertension with a cardioselective beta-blocker and a diuretic
Usual Dosage Oral: Adults: Initial (based on atenolol component): 50 mg once daily, then individualize dose until optimal dose is achieved
Dosage Forms
  Tablet:
    50: Atenolol 50 mg and chlorthalidone 25 mg
    100: Atenolol 100 mg and chlorthalidone 25 mg
  Tenoretic®:
    50: Atenolol 50 mg and chlorthalidone 25 mg
    100: Atenolol 100 mg and chlorthalidone 25 mg

ATG *see* antithymocyte globulin (equine) *on page 82*
Atgam® [US/Can] *see* antithymocyte globulin (equine) *on page 82*
Ativan® [US/Can] *see* lorazepam *on page 577*
ATNAA [US] *see* atropine and pralidoxime *on page 106*
Atolone® Oral *(Discontinued)*

atomoxetine (AT oh mox e teen)

Synonyms atomoxetine hydrochloride; LY139603; methylphenoxy-benzene propanamine; tomoxetine
U.S./Canadian Brand Names Strattera® [US/Can]
Therapeutic Category Norepinephrine Reuptake Inhibitor, Selective
Use Treatment of attention deficit/hyperactivity disorder (ADHD)
Usual Dosage Oral: **Note:** Atomoxetine may be discontinued without the need for tapering dose.
  Children and Adolescents ≤70 kg: ADHD: Initial: 0.5 mg/kg/day, increase after minimum of 3 days to ~1.2 mg/kg/day; may administer as either a single daily dose or 2 evenly divided doses in morning and late afternoon/early evening. Maximum daily dose: 1.4 mg/kg or 100 mg, whichever is less.
  Children and Adolescents >70 kg and Adults: ADHD: Initial: 40 mg/day, increased after minimum of 3 days to ~80 mg/day; may administer as either a single daily dose or two evenly divided doses in morning and late afternoon/early evening. May increase to 100 mg in 2-4 additional weeks to achieve optimal response.
Dosage Forms
  Capsule:
    Strattera®: 10 mg, 18 mg, 25 mg, 40 mg, 60 mg, 80 mg, 100 mg

atomoxetine hydrochloride *see* atomoxetine *on page 102*

atorvastatin (a TORE va sta tin)

Sound-Alike/Look-Alike Issues
  Lipitor® may be confused with Levatol®
U.S./Canadian Brand Names Lipitor® [US/Can]
Therapeutic Category HMG-CoA Reductase Inhibitor
Use Treatment of dyslipidemias or primary prevention of cardiovascular disease (atherosclerotic) as detailed below:

  Primary prevention of cardiovascular disease (high-risk for CVD): To reduce the risk of MI or stroke in patients without evidence of heart disease who have multiple CVD risk factors or type 2 diabetes. Treatment reduces the risk for angina or revascularization procedures in patients with multiple risk factors.
  Secondary prevention of cardiovascular disease: To reduce the risk of MI, stroke, revascularization procedures, and angina in patients with evidence of heart disease. To reduce the risk of hospitalization for heart failure.

Treatment of dyslipidemias: To reduce elevations in total cholesterol, LDL-C, apolipoprotein B, and triglycerides in patients with elevations of one or more components, and/or to increase HDL-C as present in Fredrickson type IIa, IIb, III, and IV hyperlipidemias; treatment of primary dysbetalipoproteinemia, homozygous familial hypercholesterolemia

Treatment of heterozygous familial hypercholesterolemia (HeFH) in adolescent patients (10-17 years of age, females >1 year postmenarche) having LDL-C ≥190 mg/dL or LDL-C ≥160 mg/dL with positive family history of premature cardiovascular disease (CVD) or with two or more CVD risk factors.

Usual Dosage Oral: **Note:** Doses should be individualized according to the baseline LDL-cholesterol levels, the recommended goal of therapy, and patient response; adjustments should be made at intervals of 2-4 weeks

Children 10-17 years (females >1 year postmenarche): Heterozygous familial hypercholesterolemia (HeFH): 10 mg once daily (maximum: 20 mg/day)

Adults:

Hypercholesterolemia (heterozygous familial and nonfamilial) and mixed hyperlipidemia (Fredrickson types IIa and IIb): Initial: 10-20 mg once daily; patients requiring >45% reduction in LDL-C may be started at 40 mg once daily; range: 10-80 mg once daily

Homozygous familial hypercholesterolemia: 10-80 mg once daily

Dosage Forms

Tablet:

Lipitor®: 10 mg, 20 mg, 40 mg, 80 mg

atorvastatin calcium and amlodipine besylate *see* amlodipine and atorvastatin *on page 64*

atovaquone (a TOE va kwone)

U.S./Canadian Brand Names Mepron® [US/Can]

Therapeutic Category Antiprotozoal

Use Acute oral treatment of mild-to-moderate *Pneumocystis jirovecii* pneumonia (PCP) in patients who are intolerant to co-trimoxazole; prophylaxis of PCP in patients who are intolerant to co-trimoxazole

Usual Dosage Oral: Adolescents 13-16 years and Adults:

Prevention of PCP: 1500 mg once daily with food

Treatment of mild-to-moderate PCP: 750 mg twice daily with food for 21 days

Dosage Forms

Suspension, oral:

Mepron®: 750 mg/5 mL

atovaquone and proguanil (a TOE va kwone & pro GWA nil)

Synonyms proguanil and atovaquone

U.S./Canadian Brand Names Malarone® Pediatric [Can]; Malarone® [US/Can]

Therapeutic Category Antimalarial Agent

Use Prevention or treatment of acute, uncomplicated *P. falciparum* malaria

Usual Dosage Oral:

Children (dosage based on body weight):

Prevention of malaria: Start 1-2 days prior to entering a malaria-endemic area, continue throughout the stay and for 7 days after returning. Take as a single dose, once daily.

11-20 kg: Atovaquone/proguanil 62.5 mg/25 mg

21-30 kg: Atovaquone/proguanil 125 mg/50 mg

31-40 kg: Atovaquone/proguanil 187.5 mg/75 mg

>40 kg: Atovaquone/proguanil 250 mg/100 mg

Treatment of acute malaria: Take as a single dose, once daily for 3 consecutive days.

5-8 kg: Atovaquone/proguanil 125 mg/50 mg

9-10 kg: Atovaquone/proguanil 187.5 mg/75 mg

11-20 kg: Atovaquone/proguanil 250 mg/100 mg

21-30 kg: Atovaquone/proguanil 500 mg/200 mg

31-40 kg: Atovaquone/proguanil 750 mg/300 mg

>40 kg: Atovaquone/proguanil 1 g/400 mg

Adults:

Prevention of malaria: Atovaquone/proguanil 250 mg/100 mg once daily; start 1-2 days prior to entering a malaria-endemic area, continue throughout the stay and for 7 days after returning

Treatment of acute malaria: Atovaquone/proguanil 1 g/400 mg as a single dose, once daily for 3 consecutive days

◀ **Dosage Forms**
  Tablet:
    Malarone®: Atovaquone 250 mg and proguanil 100 mg
  Tablet [pediatric]:
    Malarone®: Atovaquone 62.5 mg and proguanil 25 mg

Atozine® Oral *(Discontinued)* see hydroxyzine *on page 491*
ATRA see tretinoin (oral) *on page 946*

atracurium (a tra KYOO ree um)

Synonyms atracurium besylate
U.S./Canadian Brand Names Atracurium Besylate Injection [Can]
Therapeutic Category Skeletal Muscle Relaxant
Use Adjunct to general anesthesia to facilitate endotracheal intubation and to relax skeletal muscles during surgery; to facilitate mechanical ventilation in ICU patients; does not relieve pain or produce sedation
Usual Dosage I.V. (not to be used I.M.): Dose to effect; doses must be individualized due to interpatient variability; use ideal body weight for obese patients
  Children 1 month to 2 years: Initial: 0.3-0.4 mg/kg followed by maintenance doses as needed to maintain neuromuscular blockade
  Children >2 years to Adults: 0.4-0.5 mg/kg, then 0.08-0.1 mg/kg 20-45 minutes after initial dose to maintain neuromuscular block, followed by repeat doses of 0.08-0.1 mg/kg at 15- to 25-minute intervals
  Initial dose after succinylcholine for intubation (balanced anesthesia): Adults: 0.2-0.4 mg/kg
  Pretreatment/priming: 10% of intubating dose given 3-5 minutes before initial dose

  Continuous infusion:
    Surgery: Initial: 9-10 mcg/kg/minute at initial signs of recovery from bolus dose; block usually maintained by a rate of 5-9 mcg/kg/minute under balanced anesthesia
    ICU: Block usually maintained by rate of 11-13 mcg/kg/minute (rates for pediatric patients may be higher)
Dosage Forms
  Injection: 10 mg/mL (10 mL)
  Injection [preservative free]: 10 mg/mL (5 mL)

atracurium besylate see atracurium *on page 104*
Atracurium Besylate Injection [Can] see atracurium *on page 104*
Atralin™ [US] see tretinoin (topical) *on page 946*
Atriance™ [Can] see nelarabine *on page 660*
Atripla™ [US/Can] see efavirenz, emtricitabine, and tenofovir *on page 335*
Atropair® *(Discontinued)* see atropine *on page 104*
AtroPen® [US] see atropine *on page 104*

atropine (A troe peen)

Synonyms atropine sulfate
U.S./Canadian Brand Names AtroPen® [US]; Atropine-Care® [US]; Dioptic's Atropine Solution [Can]; Isopto® Atropine [US/Can]; Sal-Tropine™ [US]
Therapeutic Category Anticholinergic Agent
Use
  Injection: Preoperative medication to inhibit salivation and secretions; treatment of symptomatic sinus bradycardia; AV block (nodal level); ventricular asystole; antidote for anticholinesterase inhibitor poisoning (carbamate insecticides, nerve agents, organophosphate insecticides)
  Ophthalmic: Produce mydriasis and cycloplegia for examination of the retina and optic disc and accurate measurement of refractive errors; uveitis
  Oral: Inhibit salivation and secretions
Usual Dosage
  Neonates, Infants, and Children: Doses <0.1 mg have been associated with paradoxical bradycardia.
    Inhibit salivation and secretions (preanesthesia): Oral, I.M., I.V., SubQ:
      <5 kg: 0.02 mg/kg/dose 30-60 minutes preop then every 4-6 hours as needed. Use of a minimum dosage of 0.1 mg in neonates <5 kg will result in dosages >0.02 mg/kg. There is no documented minimum dosage in this age group.
      >5 kg: 0.01-0.02 mg/kg/dose to a maximum 0.4 mg/dose 30-60 minutes preop; minimum dose: 0.1 mg

Alternate dosing:
3-7 kg (7-16 lb): 0.1 mg
8-11 kg (17-24 lb): 0.15 mg
11-18 kg (24-40 lb): 0.2 mg
18-29 kg (40-65 lb): 0.3 mg
>30 kg (>65 lb): 0.4 mg

Bradycardia: I.V., intratracheal: 0.02 mg/kg, minimum dose 0.1 mg, maximum single dose: 0.5 mg in children and 1 mg in adolescents; may repeat in 5-minute intervals to a maximum total dose of 1 mg in children or 2 mg in adolescents. (**Note:** For intratracheal administration, the dosage must be diluted with normal saline to a total volume of 1-5 mL). When treating bradycardia in neonates, reserve use for those patients unresponsive to improved oxygenation and epinephrine.

Infants and Children: Nerve agent toxicity management: See **Note** under adult dosing.
Prehospital ("in the field"): I.M.:
Birth to <2 years: Mild-to-moderate symptoms: 0.05 mg/kg; severe symptoms: 0.1 mg/kg
2-10 years: Mild-to-moderate symptoms: 1 mg; severe symptoms: 2 mg
>10 years: Mild-to-moderate symptoms: 2 mg; severe symptoms: 4 mg
Hospital/emergency department: I.M.:
Birth to <2 years: Mild-to-moderate symptoms: 0.05 mg/kg I.M. **or** 0.02 mg/kg I.V.; severe symptoms: 0.1 mg/kg I.M. **or** 0.02 mg/kg I.V.
2-10 years: Mild-to-moderate symptoms: 1 mg; severe symptoms: 2 mg
>10 years: Mild-to-moderate symptoms: 2 mg; severe symptoms: 4 mg

Note: Pralidoxime is a component of the management of nerve agent toxicity; consult pralidoxime for specific route and dose. For prehospital ("in the field") management, repeat atropine I.M. (children: 0.05-0.1 mg/kg) at 5-10 minute intervals until secretions have diminished and breathing is comfortable or airway resistance has returned to near normal. For hospital management, repeat atropine I.M. (infants 1 mg; all others: 2 mg) at 5-10 minute intervals until secretions have diminished and breathing is comfortable or airway resistance has returned to near normal.

Children: Organophosphate or carbamate poisoning:
I.V.: 0.03-0.05 mg/kg every 10-20 minutes until atropine effect, then every 1-4 hours for at least 24 hours
I.M. (AtroPen®): Mild symptoms: Administer dose listed below as soon as exposure is known or suspected. If severe symptoms develop after first dose, 2 additional doses should be repeated in 10 minutes; do not administer more than 3 doses. Severe symptoms: Immediately administer 3 doses as follows:
<6.8 kg (15 lb): Use of **AtroPen® formulation not recommended;** administer atropine 0.05 mg/kg
6.8-18 kg (15-40 lb): 0.5 mg/dose
18-41 kg (40-90 lb): 1 mg/dose
>41 kg (>90 lb): 2 mg/dose

Adults (doses <0.5 mg have been associated with paradoxical bradycardia):
Asystole or pulseless electrical activity:
I.V.: 1 mg; repeat in 3-5 minutes if asystole persists; total dose of 0.04 mg/kg.
Intratracheal: Administer 2-2.5 times the recommended I.V. dose; dilute in 10 mL NS or distilled water.
Note: Absorption is greater with distilled water, but causes more adverse effects on PaO_2.
Inhibit salivation and secretions (preanesthesia):
I.M., I.V., SubQ: 0.4-0.6 mg 30-60 minutes preop and repeat every 4-6 hours as needed
Oral: 0.4 mg; may repeat in 4 hours if necessary; 0.4 mg initial dose may be exceeded in certain cases and may repeat in 4 hours if necessary
Bradycardia: I.V.: 0.5-1 mg every 5 minutes, not to exceed a total of 3 mg or 0.04 mg/kg; may give intratracheally in 10 mL NS (intratracheal dose should be 2-2.5 times the I.V. dose)
Neuromuscular blockade reversal: I.V.: 25-30 mcg/kg 30-60 seconds before neostigmine or 7-10 mcg/kg 30-60 seconds before edrophonium
Organophosphate or carbamate poisoning: **Note:** The dose of atropine required varies considerably with the severity of poisoning. Total amount of atropine used in carbamate poisoning is usually less. Severely poisoned patients may exhibit significant tolerance to atropine; ≥2 times the suggested doses may be needed. Titrate to pulmonary status (decreased bronchial secretions). Once patient is stable for a period of time, the dose/dosing frequency may be decreased. If atropinization occurs after 1-2 mg of atropine then reevaluate working diagnosis.
I.V.: Initial: 1-5 mg; doses should be doubled every 5 minutes until signs of muscarinic excess abate (clearing of bronchial secretions, bronchospasm, and adequate oxygenation). Overly aggressive dosing may cause anticholinergic toxicity (eg, delirium, hyperthermia, and muscle twitching).
I.V. Infusion: 0.5-1 mg/hour or 10% to 20% of loading dose/hour

◀ I.M. (AtroPen®): Mild symptoms: Administer 2 mg as soon as exposure is known or suspected. If severe symptoms develop after first dose, 2 additional doses should be repeated in 10 minutes; do not administer more than 3 doses. Severe symptoms: Immediately administer three 2 mg doses.

Nerve agent toxicity management: I.M.: See **Note**. Prehospital ("in the field") or hospital/emergency department: Mild-to-moderate symptoms: 2-4 mg; severe symptoms: 6 mg

Note: Pralidoxime is a component of the management of nerve agent toxicity; consult Pralidoxime for specific route and dose. For prehospital ("in the field") management, repeat atropine I.M. (2 mg) at 5-10 minute intervals until secretions have diminished and breathing is comfortable or airway resistance has returned to near normal. For hospital management, repeat atropine I.M. (2 mg) at 5-10 minute intervals until secretions have diminished and breathing is comfortable or airway resistance has returned to near normal.

Mydriasis, cycloplegia (preprocedure): Ophthalmic (1% solution): Instill 1-2 drops 1 hour before procedure.

Uveitis: Ophthalmic:
1% solution: Instill 1-2 drops 4 times/day
Ointment: Apply a small amount in the conjunctival sac up to 3 times/day; compress the lacrimal sac by digital pressure for 1-3 minutes after instillation

Dosage Forms
Injection, solution: 0.05 mg/mL (5 mL); 0.1 mg/mL (5 mL, 10 mL); 0.4 mg/0.5 mL (0.5 mL); 0.4 mg/mL (0.5 mL, 1 mL, 20 mL); 1 mg/mL (1 mL)
AtroPen®: 0.25 mg/0.3 mL (0.3 mL); 0.5 mg/0.7 mL (0.7 mL); 1 mg/0.7 mL (0.7 mL); 2 mg/0.7 mL (0.7 mL) [prefilled autoinjector]
Ointment, ophthalmic: 1% (3.5 g)
Solution, ophthalmic: 1% (2 mL, 5 mL, 15 mL)
Atropine-Care®: 1% (2 mL) [contains benzalkonium chloride]
Isopto® Atropine: 1% (5 mL, 15 mL) [contains benzalkonium chloride]
Tablet:
Sal-Tropine™: 0.4 mg

atropine and difenoxin see difenoxin and atropine on page 295
atropine and diphenoxylate see diphenoxylate and atropine on page 306

atropine and pralidoxime (A troe peen & pra li DOKS eem)

Synonyms atropine and pralidoxime chloride; Mark 1™; NAAK; nerve agent antidote kit; pralidoxime and atropine

U.S./Canadian Brand Names ATNAA [US]; Duodote™ [US]

Therapeutic Category Anticholinergic Agent Antidote

Use
ATNAA: Treatment of poisoning by susceptible organophosphorous nerve agents having anticholinesterase activity for self or buddy-administration by military personnel
Duodote™: Treatment of poisoning by organophosphorous nerve agents (eg, tabun, sarin, soman) or organophosphorous insecticide for use by trained emergency medical services personnel

Usual Dosage I.M.: Adults: Organophosphorous poisoning: **Note:** If suspected, antidotal therapy should be given immediately as soon as symptoms appear (critical to administer immediately in case of soman exposure). Definitive medical care should be sought after any injection given. One injection only may be given as self-aid. If repeat injections needed, administration must be done by another trained individual. Emergency medical personnel who have self-administered a dose must determine capacity to continue to provide care.

ATNAA:
Mild symptoms (some or all mild symptoms): Self-Aid or Buddy-Aid: 1 injection (wait 10-15 minutes for effect); if patient is able to ambulate, and knows who and where they are, then no more injections are needed. If symptoms still present: Buddy-Aid: May repeat 1-2 more injections
Severe symptoms (if most or all): Buddy-Aid: If no self-aid given, 3 injections in rapid succession; if 1 self-aid injection given, 2 injections in rapid succession
Maximum cumulative dose: 3 injections
Symptoms provided by manufacturer in ATNAA product labeling to guide therapy:
Mild symptoms: Breathing difficulties, chest tightness, coughing, difficulty in seeing, drooling, headache, localized sweating and muscular twitching, miosis, nausea (with or without vomiting), runny nose, stomach cramps, tachycardia (followed by bradycardia), wheezing

Severe symptoms: Bradycardia, confused/strange behavior, convulsions, increased wheezing and breathing difficulties, involuntary urination/defecation, miosis (severe), muscular twitching/generalized weakness (severe), red/teary eyes, respiratory failure, unconsciousness, vomiting

Duodote™:
Mild symptoms (≥2 mild symptoms): 1 injection (wait 10-15 minutes for effect); if after 10-15 minutes no severe symptoms emerge, no further injections are indicated; if any severe symptoms emerge at any point following initial injection, repeat dose by giving 2 additional injections in rapid succession. Transport to medical care facility.
Severe symptoms (≥1 severe symptom): 3 injections in rapid succession. Transport to medical care facility.
Maximum cumulative dose: 3 injections unless medical care support (eg, hospital, respiratory support) is available
Symptoms provided by manufacturer in Duodote™ product labeling to guide therapy:
Mild symptoms: Airway secretions increased, blurred vision, bradycardia, breathing difficulties, chest tightness, drooling miosis, nausea, vomiting, runny nose, salivation, stomach cramps (acute onset), tachycardia, teary eyes, tremors/muscular twitching, wheezing/coughing
Severe symptoms: Breathing difficulties (severe), confused/strange behavior, convulsions, copious secretions from lung or airway, involuntary urination/defecation, muscular twitching/generalized weakness (severe)

Dosage Forms
Injection, solution:
ATNAA, Duodote™: Atropine 2.1 mg/0.7 mL and pralidoxime chloride 600 mg/2 mL [contains benzyl alcohol; prefilled auto-injector]

atropine and pralidoxime chloride *see* atropine and pralidoxime *on page 106*
Atropine-Care® [US] *see* atropine *on page 104*
atropine, hyoscyamine, scopolamine, and phenobarbital *see* hyoscyamine, atropine, scopolamine, and phenobarbital *on page 493*
atropine soluble tablet *(Discontinued)*
atropine sulfate *see* atropine *on page 104*
atropine sulfate and edrophonium chloride *see* edrophonium and atropine *on page 334*
Atropisol® *(Discontinued)* *see* atropine *on page 104*
Atrovent® [US/Can] *see* ipratropium *on page 524*
Atrovent® HFA [US/Can] *see* ipratropium *on page 524*
Attenuvax® [US] *see* measles virus vaccine (live) *on page 594*
Atuss® HD *(Discontinued)*
Atuss® HX *(Discontinued)*
Augmentin® [US/Can] *see* amoxicillin and clavulanate potassium *on page 68*
Augmentin ES-600® [US] *see* amoxicillin and clavulanate potassium *on page 68*
Augmentin XR® [US] *see* amoxicillin and clavulanate potassium *on page 68*
Auralgan® [Can] *see* antipyrine and benzocaine *on page 82*

auranofin (au RANE oh fin)

Sound-Alike/Look-Alike Issues
Ridaura® may be confused with Cardura®
U.S./Canadian Brand Names Ridaura® [US/Can]
Therapeutic Category Gold Compound
Use Management of active stage of classic or definite rheumatoid arthritis in patients who do not respond to or tolerate other agents; psoriatic arthritis; adjunctive or alternative therapy for pemphigus
Usual Dosage Oral:
Children: Initial: 0.1 mg/kg/day divided daily; usual maintenance: 0.15 mg/kg/day in 1-2 divided doses; maximum: 0.2 mg/kg/day in 1-2 divided doses
Adults: 6 mg/day in 1-2 divided doses; after 3 months may be increased to 9 mg/day in 3 divided doses; if still no response after 3 months at 9 mg/day, discontinue drug
Dosage Forms
Capsule:
Ridaura®: 3 mg

Auraphene® B [US-OTC] *see* carbamide peroxide *on page 174*

Auro® [US-OTC] *see* carbamide peroxide *on page 174*
Aurodex [US] *see* antipyrine and benzocaine *on page 82*
Autoplex® T *(Discontinued)* *see* antiinhibitor coagulant complex *on page 81*
AVA *see* anthrax vaccine, adsorbed *on page 78*
Avagard™ [US-OTC] *see* chlorhexidine gluconate *on page 201*
Avage™ [US] *see* tazarotene *on page 904*
Avalide® [US/Can] *see* irbesartan and hydrochlorothiazide *on page 526*
Avandamet® [US/Can] *see* rosiglitazone and metformin *on page 846*
Avandaryl™ [US] *see* rosiglitazone and glimepiride *on page 845*
Avandia® [US/Can] *see* rosiglitazone *on page 845*
Avapro® [US/Can] *see* irbesartan *on page 525*
Avapro® HCT *see* irbesartan and hydrochlorothiazide *on page 526*
AVAR™ *(Discontinued)* *see* sulfur and sulfacetamide *on page 897*
AVAR™-e [US] *see* sulfur and sulfacetamide *on page 897*
AVAR™-e Green *(Discontinued)* *see* sulfur and sulfacetamide *on page 897*
Avastin® [US/Can] *see* bevacizumab *on page 134*
Avaxim® [Can] *see* hepatitis A vaccine *on page 469*
Avaxim®-Pediatric [Can] *see* hepatitis A vaccine *on page 469*
Avelox® [US/Can] *see* moxifloxacin *on page 646*
Avelox® I.V. [US/Can] *see* moxifloxacin *on page 646*
Aventyl® [Can] *see* nortriptyline *on page 680*
Aventyl® HCl *(Discontinued)* *see* nortriptyline *on page 680*
Aviane™ [US/Can] *see* ethinyl estradiol and levonorgestrel *on page 372*
avian influenza virus vaccine *see* influenza virus vaccine (H5N1) *on page 509*
Avinza® [US] *see* morphine sulfate *on page 643*
Avita® [US] *see* tretinoin (topical) *on page 946*
Avitene® [US] *see* collagen hemostat *on page 245*
Avitene® Flour [US] *see* collagen hemostat *on page 245*
Avitene® Ultrafoam [US] *see* collagen hemostat *on page 245*
Avitene® UltraWrap™ [US] *see* collagen hemostat *on page 245*
Avlosulfon® *(Discontinued)* *see* dapsone *on page 267*
Avodart® [US/Can] *see* dutasteride *on page 329*
Avonex® [US/Can] *see* interferon beta-1a *on page 517*
Axert™ [US/Can] *see* almotriptan *on page 48*
Axid® [US/Can] *see* nizatidine *on page 677*
Axid® AR [US-OTC] *see* nizatidine *on page 677*
AY-25650 *see* triptorelin *on page 956*
Aygestin® [US] *see* norethindrone *on page 679*
Ayr® Allergy Sinus [US-OTC] *see* sodium chloride *on page 873*
Ayr® Baby Saline [US-OTC] *see* sodium chloride *on page 873*
Ayr® Saline [US-OTC] *see* sodium chloride *on page 873*
Ayr® Saline No-Drip [US-OTC] *see* sodium chloride *on page 873*
5-aza-2'-deoxycytidine *see* decitabine *on page 270*
5-azaC *see* decitabine *on page 270*

azacitidine (ay za SYE ti deen)

Sound-Alike/Look-Alike Issues
   azaCITIDine may be confused with azaTHIOprine
Synonyms 5-azacytidine; 5-AZC; AZA-CR; azacytidine; ladakamycin; NSC-102816
Tall-Man azaCITIDine
U.S./Canadian Brand Names Vidaza® [US]
Therapeutic Category Antineoplastic Agent, Antimetabolite (Pyrimidine)

Use Treatment of myelodysplastic syndrome (MDS)

Usual Dosage I.V., SubQ: Adults: MDS: 75 mg/m^2/day for 7 days repeated every 4 weeks. Dose may be increased to 100 mg/m^2/day if no benefit is observed after 2 cycles and no toxicity other than nausea and vomiting have occurred. Treatment is recommended for at least 4 cycles; treatment may be continued as long as patient continues to benefit.

Dosage Forms
Injection, powder for suspension:
  Vidaza®: 100 mg

AZA-CR see azacitidine on page 108
Azactam® [US/Can] see aztreonam on page 112
azacytidine see azacitidine on page 108
5-azacytidine see azacitidine on page 108
Azasan® [US] see azathioprine on page 109
Azasite™ [US] see azithromycin on page 110

azatadine (Canada only) (a ZA ta deen)
Synonyms azatadine maleate
Therapeutic Category Antihistamine
Use Treatment of perennial and seasonal allergic rhinitis and chronic urticaria
Usual Dosage Oral: Children >12 years and Adults: 1-2 mg twice daily
Dosage Forms
Tablet, as maleate: 1 mg

azatadine maleate see azatadine (Canada only) on page 109

azathioprine (ay za THYE oh preen)
Sound-Alike/Look-Alike Issues
  azaTHIOprine may be confused with azaCITIDine, azatadine, azidothymidine, Azulfidine®
  Imuran® may be confused with Elmiron®, Enduron®, Imdur®, Inderal®, Tenormin®
Synonyms azathioprine sodium
Tall-Man azaTHIOprine
U.S./Canadian Brand Names Alti-Azathioprine [Can]; Apo-Azathioprine® [Can]; Azasan® [US]; Gen-Azathioprine [Can]; Imuran® [US/Can]; Novo-Azathioprine [Can]
Therapeutic Category Immunosuppressant Agent
Use Adjunctive therapy in prevention of rejection of kidney transplants; management of active rheumatoid arthritis (RA)
Usual Dosage I.V. dose is equivalent to oral dose (dosing should be based on ideal body weight):
  Adults:
    Renal transplantation: Oral, I.V.: Initial: 3-5 mg/kg/day usually given as a single daily dose, then 1-3 mg/kg/day maintenance
    Rheumatoid arthritis: Oral:
      Initial: 1 mg/kg/day given once daily or divided twice daily for 6-8 weeks; increase by 0.5 mg/kg every 4 weeks until response or up to 2.5 mg/kg/day; an adequate trial should be a minimum of 12 weeks
      Maintenance dose: Reduce dose by 0.5 mg/kg every 4 weeks until lowest effective dose is reached; optimum duration of therapy not specified; may be discontinued abruptly
Dosage Forms
Injection, powder for reconstitution: 100 mg
Tablet [scored]: 50 mg
  Azasan®: 75 mg, 100 mg
  Imuran®: 50 mg

azathioprine sodium see azathioprine on page 109
5-AZC see azacitidine on page 108
Azdone® (Discontinued)

azelaic acid (a zeh LAY ik AS id)
U.S./Canadian Brand Names Azelex® [US]; Finacea® [US/Can]
Therapeutic Category Topical Skin Product

▶

◀ **Use** Topical treatment of inflammatory papules and pustules of mild-to-moderate rosacea; mild-to-moderate inflammatory acne vulgaris
Finacea®: Not FDA-approved for the treatment of acne

Usual Dosage Topical:
Adolescents ≥12 years and Adults: Acne vulgaris: Cream 20%: After skin is thoroughly washed and patted dry, gently but thoroughly massage a thin film of azelaic acid cream into the affected areas twice daily, in the morning and evening. The duration of use can vary and depends on the severity of the acne. In the majority of patients with inflammatory lesions, improvement of the condition occurs within 4 weeks.

Adults: Rosacea: Gel 15%: Massage gently into affected areas of the face twice daily; use beyond 12 weeks has not been studied

Dosage Forms
Cream:
Azelex®: 20% (30 g, 50 g)
Gel:
Finacea®: 15% (50 g)

azelastine (a ZEL as teen)

Sound-Alike/Look-Alike Issues
Optivar® may be confused with Optiray®, Optive™

Synonyms azelastine hydrochloride

U.S./Canadian Brand Names Astelin® [US/Can]; Optivar® [US]

Therapeutic Category Antihistamine; Antihistamine, Ophthalmic

Use
Nasal spray: Treatment of the symptoms of seasonal allergic rhinitis such as rhinorrhea, sneezing, and nasal pruritus in children ≥5 years of age and adults; treatment of the symptoms of vasomotor rhinitis in children ≥12 years of age and adults
Ophthalmic: Treatment of itching of the eye associated with seasonal allergic conjunctivitis in children ≥3 years of age and adults

Usual Dosage
Children 5-11 years: Seasonal allergic rhinitis: Intranasal: 1 spray each nostril twice daily
Children ≥3 years and Adults: Itching eyes due to seasonal allergic conjunctivitis: Ophthalmic: Instill 1 drop into affected eye(s) twice daily
Children ≥12 years and Adults:
Seasonal allergic rhinitis: Intranasal: 1-2 sprays each nostril twice daily
Vasomotor rhinitis: Intranasal: 2 sprays each nostril twice daily.

Dosage Forms
Solution, intranasal [spray]:
Astelin®: 1 mg/mL [137 mcg/spray] (30 mL)
Solution, ophthalmic:
Optivar®: 0.05% (6 mL)

azelastine hydrochloride *see* azelastine *on page 110*
Azelex® [US] *see* azelaic acid *on page 109*
azidothymidine *see* zidovudine *on page 991*
azidothymidine, abacavir, and lamivudine *see* abacavir, lamivudine, and zidovudine *on page 16*
Azilect® [US] *see* rasagiline *on page 820*

azithromycin (az ith roe MYE sin)

Sound-Alike/Look-Alike Issues
azithromycin may be confused with erythromycin
Zithromax® may be confused with Zinacef®

Synonyms azithromycin dihydrate; azithromycin hydrogen citrate; azithromycin monohydrate; Zithromax® TRI-PAK™; Zithromax® Z-PAK®

U.S./Canadian Brand Names Apo-Azithromycin® [Can]; Azasite™ [US]; CO Azithromycin [Can]; Dom-Azithromycin [Can]; GMD-Azithromycin [Can]; Novo-Azithromycin [Can]; PHL-Azithromycin [Can]; PMS-Azithromycin [Can]; ratio-Azithromycin [Can]; Sandoz-Azithromycin [Can]; Zithromax® [US/Can]; Zmax™ [US]

Therapeutic Category Macrolide (Antibiotic)

Use

Oral, I.V.: Treatment of acute otitis media due to *H. influenzae*, *M. catarrhalis*, or *S. pneumoniae*; pharyngitis/tonsillitis due to *S. pyogenes*; treatment of mild-to-moderate upper and lower respiratory tract infections, infections of the skin and skin structure, community-acquired pneumonia, pelvic inflammatory disease (PID), sexually-transmitted diseases (urethritis/cervicitis), pharyngitis/tonsillitis (alternative to first-line therapy), and genital ulcer disease (chancroid) due to susceptible strains of *C. trachomatis*, *M. catarrhalis*, *H. influenzae*, *S. aureus*, *S. pneumoniae*, *Mycoplasma pneumoniae*, and *C. psittaci*; acute bacterial exacerbations of chronic obstructive pulmonary disease (COPD) due to *H. influenzae*, *M. catarrhalis,* or *S. pneumoniae*; acute bacterial sinusitis

Ophthalmic: Bacterial conjunctivitis

Usual Dosage Note: Extended release suspension (Zmax™) is not interchangeable with immediate release formulations. Use should be limited to approved indications. All doses are expressed as immediate release azithromycin unless otherwise specified.

Usual dosage range:
Children ≥6 months: Oral: 5-12 mg/kg given once daily (maximum: 500 mg/day) **or** 30 mg/kg as a single dose (maximum: 1500 mg)
Children ≥1 year and Adults: Ophthalmic: Instill 1 drop into affected eye(s) twice daily (8-12 hours apart) for 2 days, then 1 drop once daily for 5 days
Adolescents ≥16 years and Adults:
Oral: 250-600 mg once daily **or** 1-2 g as a single dose
I.V.: 250-500 mg once daily
Indication-specific dosing:
Children: Oral:
Bacterial sinusitis: 10 mg/kg once daily for 3 days (maximum: 500 mg/day)
Community-acquired pneumonia: 10 mg/kg on day 1 (maximum: 500 mg/day) followed by 5 mg/kg/day once daily on days 2-5 (maximum: 250 mg/day)
Otitis media:
1-day regimen: 30 mg/kg as a single dose (maximum: 1500 mg)
3-day regimen: 10 mg/kg once daily for 3 days (maximum: 500 mg/day)
5-day regimen: 10 mg/kg on day 1 (maximum: 500 mg/day) followed by 5 mg/kg/day once daily on days 2-5 (maximum: 250 mg/day)
Pharyngitis, tonsillitis: Children ≥2 years: 12 mg/kg/day once daily for 5 days (maximum: 500 mg/day)
Pertussis (CDC guidelines):
Children <6 months: 10 mg/kg/day for 5 days
Children ≥6 months: 10 mg/kg on day 1 (maximum: 500 mg/day) followed by 5 mg/kg/day once daily on days 2-5 (maximum: 250 mg/day)
Children ≥1 year and Adults: Ophthalmic:
Bacterial conjunctivitis: Instill 1 drop into affected eye(s) twice daily (8-12 hours apart) for 2 days, then 1 drop once daily for 5 days
Adolescents ≥16 years and Adults:
Bacterial sinusitis: Oral: 500 mg/day for a total of 3 days
Extended release suspension (Zmax™): 2 g as a single dose
Chancroid due to *H. ducreyi*: Oral: 1 g as a single dose
Community-acquired pneumonia:
Oral (Zmax™): 2 g as a single dose
I.V.: 500 mg as a single dose for at least 2 days, follow I.V. therapy by the oral route with a single daily dose of 500 mg to complete a 7- to 10-day course of therapy.
Mild-to-moderate respiratory tract, skin, and soft tissue infections: Oral: 500 mg in a single loading dose on day 1 followed by 250 mg/day as a single dose on days 2-5
Alternative regimen: Bacterial exacerbation of COPD: 500 mg/day for a total of 3 days
Pelvic inflammatory disease (PID): I.V.: 500 mg as a single dose for 1-2 days, follow I.V. therapy by the oral route with a single daily dose of 250 mg to complete a 7-day course of therapy
Pertussis (CDC guidelines): Oral: 500 mg on day 1 followed by 250 mg/day on days 2-5 (maximum: 500 mg/day)
Urethritis/cervicitis: Oral:
Due to C. trachomatis: 1 g as a single dose
Due to N. gonorrhoeae: 2 g as a single dose

Dosage Forms

Injection, powder for reconstitution: 500 mg
Zithromax®: 500 mg

▶

◄ **Injection, powder for reconstitution, as hydrogencitrate:** 500 mg
Injection, powder for reconstitution, as monohydrate: 500 mg
Microspheres for oral suspension, extended release:
    Zmax™: 2 g
Powder for oral suspension, as monohydrate: 100 mg/5 mL (15 mL); 200 mg/5 mL (15 mL, 22.5 mL, 30 mL)
Powder for oral suspension, immediate release:
    Zithromax®: 100 mg/5 mL, 200 mg/5 mL, 1 g/packet (3s, 10s)
Solution, ophthalmic:
    AzaSite™: 1% (2.5 mL)
Tablet: 250 mg, 500 mg, 600 mg
    Zithromax®: 250 mg, 500 mg, 600 mg
    Zithromax® TRI-PAK™ [unit-dose pack]: 500 mg (3s)
    Zithromax® Z-PAK® [unit-dose pack]: 250 mg (6s)

azithromycin dihydrate *see* azithromycin *on page 110*
azithromycin hydrogen citrate *see* azithromycin *on page 110*
azithromycin monohydrate *see* azithromycin *on page 110*
Azmacort® [US] *see* triamcinolone (inhalation, oral) *on page 948*
AZO-Gesic® [US-OTC] *see* phenazopyridine *on page 741*
Azopt® [US/Can] *see* brinzolamide *on page 142*
Azor™ [US] *see* amlodipine and olmesartan *on page 65*
AZO-Standard® [US-OTC] *see* phenazopyridine *on page 741*
AZO-Standard® Maximum Strength [US-OTC] *see* phenazopyridine *on page 741*
AZT™ [Can] *see* zidovudine *on page 991*
AZT, abacavir, and lamivudine *see* abacavir, lamivudine, and zidovudine *on page 16*
azthreonam *see* aztreonam *on page 112*

aztreonam (AZ tree oh nam)
Sound-Alike/Look-Alike Issues
    aztreonam may be confused with azidothymidine
Synonyms azthreonam
U.S./Canadian Brand Names Azactam® [US/Can]
Therapeutic Category Antibiotic, Miscellaneous
Use Treatment of patients with urinary tract infections, lower respiratory tract infections, septicemia, skin/skin structure infections, intraabdominal infections, and gynecological infections caused by susceptible gram-negative bacilli
Usual Dosage
    Children >1 month:
        Mild-to-moderate infections: I.M., I.V.: 30 mg/kg every 8 hours
        Moderate-to-severe infections: I.M., I.V.: 30 mg/kg every 6-8 hours; maximum: 120 mg/kg/day (8 g/day)
        Cystic fibrosis: I.V.: 50 mg/kg/dose every 6-8 hours (ie, up to 200 mg/kg/day); maximum: 8 g/day
    Adults:
        Urinary tract infection: I.M., I.V.: 500 mg to 1 g every 8-12 hours
        Moderately-severe systemic infections: 1 g I.V. or I.M. or 2 g I.V. every 8-12 hours
        Severe systemic or life-threatening infections (especially caused by *Pseudomonas aeruginosa*): I.V.: 2 g every 6-8 hours; maximum: 8 g/day
        Meningitis (gram-negative): I.V.: 2 g every 6-8 hours
Dosage Forms
    Infusion premixed iso-osmotic solution:
        Azactam®: 1 g (50 mL); 2 g (50 mL)
    Injection, powder for reconstitution:
        Azactam®: 1 g, 2 g

Azulfidine® [US] *see* sulfasalazine *on page 896*
Azulfidine® EN-tabs® [US] *see* sulfasalazine *on page 896*
B1 *see* tositumomab and iodine I 131 tositumomab *on page 937*
B1 antibody *see* tositumomab and iodine I 131 tositumomab *on page 937*
B-D™ Glucose [US-OTC] *see* dextrose *on page 286*

B2036-PEG *see* pegvisomant *on page 729*
B 9273 *see* alefacept *on page 42*
BA-16038 *see* aminoglutethimide *on page 60*
Babee® Cof Syrup [US-OTC] *see* dextromethorphan *on page 284*
BabyBIG® [US] *see* botulism immune globulin (intravenous-human) *on page 141*
BAC *see* benzalkonium chloride *on page 123*
Bacid® [US-OTC/Can] *see* Lactobacillus *on page 543*
Baciguent® [US-OTC/Can] *see* bacitracin *on page 113*
BaciiM® [US] *see* bacitracin *on page 113*
Baciject® [Can] *see* bacitracin *on page 113*
bacillus calmette-Guérin (BCG) live *see* BCG vaccine *on page 118*

bacitracin (bas i TRAY sin)

Sound-Alike/Look-Alike Issues
bacitracin may be confused with Bactrim®, Bactroban®
U.S./Canadian Brand Names Baciguent® [US-OTC/Can]; BaciiM® [US]; Baciject® [Can]
Therapeutic Category Antibiotic, Miscellaneous; Antibiotic, Ophthalmic; Antibiotic, Topical
Use Treatment of susceptible bacterial infections mainly; has activity against gram-positive bacilli; due to toxicity risks, systemic and irrigant uses of bacitracin should be limited to situations where less toxic alternatives would not be effective
Usual Dosage Do not administer I.V.
Infants: I.M.:
≤2.5 kg: 900 units/kg/day in 2-3 divided doses
>2.5 kg: 1000 units/kg/day in 2-3 divided doses
Children: I.M.: 800-1200 units/kg/day divided every 8 hours
Adults: Oral: Antibiotic-associated colitis: 25,000 units 4 times/day for 7-10 days
Children and Adults:
Topical: Apply 1-5 times/day
Ophthalmic, ointment: Instill 1/4" to 1/2" ribbon every 3-4 hours into conjunctival sac for acute infections, or 2-3 times/day for mild-to-moderate infections for 7-10 days
Irrigation, solution: 50-100 units/mL in normal saline, lactated Ringer's, or sterile water for irrigation; soak sponges in solution for topical compresses 1-5 times/day or as needed during surgical procedures
Dosage Forms
Injection, powder for reconstitution: 50,000 units
BaciiM®: 50,000 units
Ointment, ophthalmic: 500 units/g (3.5 g)
Ointment, topical: 500 units/g (0.9 g, 15 g, 30 g, 120 g, 454 g)
Baciguent® [OTC]: 500 units/g (15 g, 30 g)

bacitracin and polymyxin B (bas i TRAY sin & pol i MIKS in bee)

Sound-Alike/Look-Alike Issues
Betadine® may be confused with Betagan®, betaine
Synonyms polymyxin B and bacitracin
U.S./Canadian Brand Names AK-Poly-Bac™ [US]; LID-Pack® [Can]; Optimyxin® [Can]; Polysporin® [US-OTC]
Therapeutic Category Antibiotic, Ophthalmic; Antibiotic, Topical
Use Treatment of superficial infections caused by susceptible organisms
Usual Dosage Children and Adults:
Ophthalmic ointment: Instill 1/2" ribbon in the affected eye(s) every 3-4 hours for acute infections or 2-3 times/day for mild-to-moderate infections for 7-10 days
Topical ointment/powder: Apply to affected area 1-4 times/day; may cover with sterile bandage if needed
Dosage Forms
Ointment, ophthalmic: Bacitracin 500 units and polymyxin B 10,000 units per g (3.5 g)
AK-Poly-Bac™: Bacitracin 500 units and polymyxin 10,000 units per g (3.5 g)
Ointment, topical: Bacitracin 500 units and polymyxin B 10 000 units per g in white petrolatum (15 g, 30 g)
Polysporin®: Bacitracin 500 units and polymyxin B 10,000 units per g (0.9 g, 15 g, 30 g)

◀ **Powder, topical:**
Polysporin®: Bacitracin 500 units and polymyxin B 10,000 units per g (10 g)

bacitracin, neomycin, and polymyxin B
(bas i TRAY sin, nee oh MYE sin, & pol i MIKS in bee)

Synonyms neomycin, bacitracin, and polymyxin B; polymyxin B, bacitracin, and neomycin; triple antibiotic

U.S./Canadian Brand Names Neosporin® Neo To Go® [US-OTC]; Neosporin® Ophthalmic Ointment [Can]; Neosporin® Topical [US-OTC]

Therapeutic Category Antibiotic, Ophthalmic; Antibiotic, Topical

Use Helps prevent infection in minor cuts, scrapes, and burns; short-term treatment of superficial external ocular infections caused by susceptible organisms

Usual Dosage Children and Adults:
Ophthalmic: Ointment: Instill ½" into the conjunctival sac every 3-4 hours for 7-10 days for acute infections
Topical: Apply 1-3 times/day to infected area; may cover with sterile bandage as needed

Dosage Forms
Ointment, ophthalmic: Bacitracin 400 units, neomycin 3.5 mg, and polymyxin B 10,000 units per g (3.5 g)
Ointment, topical: Bacitracin 400 units, neomycin 3.5 mg, and polymyxin B 5000 units per g (0.9 g, 15 g, 30 g, 454 g)
Neosporin® [OTC]: Bacitracin 400 units, neomycin 3.5 mg, and polymyxin B 5000 units per g (15 g, 30 g)
Neosporin® Neo To Go® [OTC]: Bacitracin 400 units, neomycin 3.5 mg, and polymyxin B 5000 units per g (0.9 g)

bacitracin, neomycin, polymyxin B, and hydrocortisone
(bas i TRAY sin, nee oh MYE sin, pol i MIKS in bee, & hye droe KOR ti sone)

Synonyms hydrocortisone, bacitracin, neomycin, and polymyxin B; neomycin, bacitracin, polymyxin B, and hydrocortisone; polymyxin B, bacitracin, neomycin, and hydrocortisone

U.S./Canadian Brand Names Cortisporin® Ointment [US]; Cortisporin® Topical Ointment [Can]

Therapeutic Category Antibiotic/Corticosteroid, Ophthalmic; Antibiotic/Corticosteroid, Topical

Use Prevention and treatment of susceptible inflammatory conditions where bacterial infection (or risk of infection) is present

Usual Dosage Children and Adults:
Ophthalmic: Ointment: Instill ½ inch ribbon to inside of lower lid every 3-4 hours until improvement occurs
Topical: Apply sparingly 2-4 times/day. Therapy should be discontinued when control is achieved; if no improvement is seen, reassessment of diagnosis may be necessary.

Dosage Forms
Ointment, ophthalmic: Bacitracin 400 units, neomycin sulfate 3.5 mg, polymyxin B 10,000 units, and hydrocortisone 10 mg per g (3.5 g)
Ointment, topical:
Cortisporin®: Bacitracin 400 units, neomycin 3.5 mg, polymyxin B 5000 units, and hydrocortisone 10 mg per g (15 g)

bacitracin, neomycin, polymyxin B, and pramoxine
(bas i TRAY sin, nee oh MYE sin, pol i MIKS in bee, & pra MOKS een)

Synonyms neomycin, bacitracin, polymyxin B, and pramoxine; polymyxin B, neomycin, bacitracin, and pramoxine; pramoxine, neomycin, bacitracin, and polymyxin B

U.S./Canadian Brand Names Neosporin® + Pain Relief Ointment [US-OTC]; Tri Biozene [US-OTC]

Therapeutic Category Antibiotic, Topical

Use Prevention and treatment of susceptible superficial topical infections and provide temporary relief of pain or discomfort

Usual Dosage Children ≥2 years and Adults: Apply 1-3 times/day to infected areas; cover with sterile bandage if needed

Dosage Forms
Ointment, topical: Bacitracin 500 units, neomycin 3.5 mg, polymyxin B 10,000 units, and pramoxine 10 mg (15 g, 30 g)
Neosporin® + Pain Relief Ointment [OTC]: Bacitracin 500 units, neomycin 3.5 mg, polymyxin B 10,000 units, and pramoxine 10 mg (15 g, 30 g)

Tri Biozene: Bacitracin 500 units, neomycin 3.5 mg, polymyxin B 10,000 units, and pramoxine 10 mg (15 g)

baclofen (BAK loe fen)

Sound-Alike/Look-Alike Issues
baclofen may be confused with Bactroban®
Lioresal® may be confused with lisinopril, Lotensin®

U.S./Canadian Brand Names Apo-Baclofen® [Can]; Gen-Baclofen [Can]; Lioresal® [US/Can]; Liotec [Can]; Nu-Baclo [Can]; PMS-Baclofen [Can]

Therapeutic Category Skeletal Muscle Relaxant

Use Treatment of reversible spasticity associated with multiple sclerosis or spinal cord lesions

Orphan drug: Intrathecal: Treatment of intractable spasticity caused by spinal cord injury, multiple sclerosis, and other spinal disease (spinal ischemia or tumor, transverse myelitis, cervical spondylosis, degenerative myelopathy)

Usual Dosage
Oral (avoid abrupt withdrawal of drug): Adults: 5 mg 3 times/day, may increase 5 mg/dose every 3 days to a maximum of 80 mg/day
Intrathecal: Children and Adults:
Test dose: 50-100 mcg, doses >50 mcg should be given in 25 mcg increments, separated by 24 hours. A screening dose of 25 mcg may be considered in very small patients. Patients not responding to screening dose of 100 mcg should not be considered for chronic infusion/implanted pump.
Maintenance: After positive response to test dose, a maintenance intrathecal infusion can be administered via an implanted intrathecal pump. Initial dose via pump: Infusion at a 24-hour rate dosed at twice the test dose. Avoid abrupt discontinuation.

Dosage Forms
Injection, solution, intrathecal [preservative free]:
Lioresal®: 50 mcg/mL (1 mL); 500 mcg/mL (20 mL); 2000 mcg/mL (5 mL, 20 mL)
Tablet: 10 mg, 20 mg

BactoShield® CHG [US-OTC] see chlorhexidine gluconate on page 201

BactoShield® (Discontinued) see chlorhexidine gluconate on page 201

Bactrim™ [US] see sulfamethoxazole and trimethoprim on page 894

Bactrim™ DS [US] see sulfamethoxazole and trimethoprim on page 894

Bactrim™ I.V. Infusion (Discontinued) see sulfamethoxazole and trimethoprim on page 894

Bactroban® [US/Can] see mupirocin on page 647

Bactroban® Nasal [US] see mupirocin on page 647

baking soda see sodium bicarbonate on page 872

BAL see dimercaprol on page 302

Balacet 325™ [US] see propoxyphene and acetaminophen on page 795

balanced salt solution (BAL anced salt soe LOO shun)

U.S./Canadian Brand Names AquaLase™ [US]; BSS Plus® [US/Can]; BSS® [US/Can]; Eye-Stream® [Can]

Therapeutic Category Ophthalmic Agent, Miscellaneous

Use
Irrigation solution for ophthalmic surgery:
AquaLase™, BSS®: Intraocular or extraocular irrigating solution
BSS® Plus: Intraocular irrigating solution
Irrigation solution for eyes, ears, nose, or throat

Usual Dosage Adults: Irrigation: Based on standard for each surgical procedure

Dosage Forms
Solution, irrigation [preservative free]: Sodium chloride 0.64%, potassium chloride 0.075%, calcium chloride 0.048%, magnesium chloride 0.03%, sodium acetate 0.39%, sodium citrate 0.17% (500 mL)
Solution, ophthalmic [irrigation; preservative free]: Sodium chloride 0.64%, potassium chloride 0.075%, calcium chloride 0.048%, magnesium chloride 0.03%, sodium acetate 0.39%, sodium citrate 0.17% (18 mL, 500 mL)
AquaLase™: Sodium chloride 0.64%, potassium chloride 0.075%, calcium chloride 0.048%, magnesium chloride 0.03%, sodium acetate 0.39%, sodium citrate 0.17% (90 mL)

◀ BSS®: Sodium chloride 0.64%, potassium chloride 0.075%, calcium chloride 0.048%, magnesium chloride 0.03%, sodium acetate 0.39%, sodium citrate 0.17% (15 mL, 30 mL, 250 mL, 500 mL)
BSS Plus®: Sodium chloride 0.71%, potassium chloride 0.038%, calcium chloride 0.015%, magnesium chloride 0.02%, sodium phosphate 0.042%, sodium bicarbonate 0.21%, dextrose 0.092%, glutathione 0.018% (250 mL, 500 mL)

Baldex® *(Discontinued)*
BAL in Oil® [US] *see* dimercaprol *on page 302*
Balmex® [US-OTC] *see* zinc oxide *on page 993*
Balminil Decongestant [Can] *see* pseudoephedrine *on page 801*
Balminil DM D [Can] *see* pseudoephedrine and dextromethorphan *on page 802*
Balminil DM + Decongestant + Expectorant [Can] *see* guaifenesin, pseudoephedrine, and dextromethorphan *on page 460*
Balminil DM E [Can] *see* guaifenesin and dextromethorphan *on page 454*
Balminil Expectorant [Can] *see* guaifenesin *on page 453*
Balnetar® [US-OTC/Can] *see* coal tar *on page 240*

balsalazide (bal SAL a zide)

Sound-Alike/Look-Alike Issues
Colazal® may be confused with Clozaril®
Synonyms balsalazide disodium
U.S./Canadian Brand Names Colazal® [US]
Therapeutic Category 5-Aminosalicylic Acid Derivative; Antiinflammatory Agent
Use Treatment of mild-to-moderate active ulcerative colitis
Usual Dosage Oral:
Children 5-17 years: 750 mg 3 times/day for up to 8 weeks **or** 2.25 g (three 750 mg capsules) 3 times/day for 8 weeks
Adults: 2.25 g (three 750 mg capsules) 3 times/day for 8-12 weeks
Dosage Forms
Capsule: 750 mg
Colazal®: 750 mg

balsalazide disodium *see* balsalazide *on page 116*
balsam peru, trypsin, and castor oil *see* trypsin, balsam peru, and castor oil *on page 958*
Baltussin [US] *see* dihydrocodeine, chlorpheniramine, and phenylephrine *on page 298*
Balziva™ [US] *see* ethinyl estradiol and norethindrone *on page 376*
Band-Aid® Hurt-Free™ Antiseptic Wash [US-OTC] *see* lidocaine *on page 561*
Banophen® [US-OTC] *see* diphenhydramine *on page 304*
Banophen® Anti-Itch [US-OTC] *see* diphenhydramine *on page 304*
Banophen® Decongestant Capsule *(Discontinued) see* diphenhydramine and pseudoephedrine *on page 306*
Baraclude® [US/Can] *see* entecavir *on page 342*
Barbidonna® *(Discontinued) see* hyoscyamine, atropine, scopolamine, and phenobarbital *on page 493*
Barbita® *(Discontinued) see* phenobarbital *on page 742*
Barc™ Liquid *(Discontinued)*
Baricon™ [US] *see* barium *on page 116*
Baridium® [US-OTC] *see* phenazopyridine *on page 741*

barium (BA ree um)

Synonyms barium sulfate
U.S./Canadian Brand Names Anatrast [US]; Bar-Test [US]; Baricon™ [US]; Baro-Cat® [US]; Barobag® [US]; Barosperse® [US]; CheeTah® [US]; E-Z-Cat® Dry [US]; E-Z-Cat® [US]; E-Z-Disk™ [US]; Enhancer [US]; Entero Vu™ [US]; Entrobar® [US]; EntroEase® [US]; Esopho-Cat® [US]; HD 200® Plus [US]; Intropaste [US]; Liqui-Coat HD® [US]; Liquid Barosperse® [US]; Medebar® Plus [US]; Prepcat [US]; Readi-Cat® 2 [US]; Readi-Cat® [US]; Tomocat® 1000 [US]; Tomocat® [US]; Tonojug [US]; Tonopaque [US]; Varibar® Honey [US]; Varibar® Nectar [US]; Varibar® Pudding [US]; Varibar® Thin Honey [US]; Varibar® Thin Liquid [US]; VoLumen™ [US]

Therapeutic Category Radiopaque Agents

Use Diagnostic aid for computed tomography or x-ray examinations of the GI tract

Dosage Forms

Cream, oral:
Esopho-Cat®: 3% w/w

Paste, oral:
Varibar® Pudding: 40% w/v

Powder for suspension, oral:
Baricon™, Enhancer, HD 200® Plus: 98% w/w
E-Z-Cat® Dry: 2% w/w
Tonopaque: 95% w/w
Varibar® Thin Liquid: 40% w/v

Powder for suspension, oral/rectal:
Barosperse®, Tonojug: 95% w/w

Powder for suspension, rectal:
Barobag®: 97% w/w

Suspension, oral:
Entero Vu™: 24% w/v
EntroEase®: 13% w/v
E-Z-Cat®: 4.9% w/v
Liqui-Coat HD®: 210% w/v
Readi-Cat® 2: 2.1% w/v
Varibar® Honey, Varibar® Nectar, Varibar® Thin Honey: 40% w/v
VoLumen™: 0.1% w/v

Suspension, oral/rectal:
Baro-Cat®, Prepcat: 1.5% w/v
CheeTah®: 2.2% w/w
Liquid Barosperse®: 60% w/v
Readi-Cat®: 1.3% w/v
Readi-Cat® 2: 2.1% w/v
Tomocat®, Tomocat® 1000: 5% w/v

Suspension, paste:
Anatrast: 100% w/v
Intropaste: 70% w/v

Suspension, rectal:
Entrobar®: 50% w/v
Medebar® Plus: 100% w/v

Tablet, oral, as sulfate:
Bar-Test, E-Z-Disk™: 648 mg

barium sulfate *see* barium *on page 116*

Barobag® [US] *see* barium *on page 116*

Baro-Cat® [US] *see* barium *on page 116*

Barosperse® [US] *see* barium *on page 116*

Bar-Test [US] *see* barium *on page 116*

Basaljel® [Can] *see* aluminum hydroxide *on page 53*

base ointment *see* zinc oxide *on page 993*

basiliximab (ba si LIK si mab)

U.S./Canadian Brand Names Simulect® [US/Can]

Therapeutic Category Immunosuppressant Agent

Use Prophylaxis of acute organ rejection in renal transplantation

Usual Dosage Note: Patients previously administered basiliximab should only be reexposed to a subsequent course of therapy with extreme caution.

I.V.:

Children <35 kg: Renal transplantation: 10 mg within 2 hours prior to transplant surgery, followed by a second 10 mg dose 4 days after transplantation; the second dose should be withheld if complications occur (including severe hypersensitivity reactions or graft loss)

◀ Children ≥35 kg and Adults: Renal transplantation: 20 mg within 2 hours prior to transplant surgery, followed by a second 20 mg dose 4 days after transplantation; the second dose should be withheld if complications occur (including severe hypersensitivity reactions or graft loss)

Dosage Forms

Injection, powder for reconstitution [preservative free]:
Simulect®: 10 mg, 20 mg

Bausch & Lomb® Computer Eye Drops [US-OTC] *see* glycerin *on page 449*
BAY 43-9006 *see* sorafenib *on page 884*
Bayer® Aspirin Extra Strength [US-OTC] *see* aspirin *on page 98*
Bayer® Aspirin Regimen Adult Low Dose [US-OTC] *see* aspirin *on page 98*
Bayer® Aspirin Regimen Children's [US-OTC] *see* aspirin *on page 98*
Bayer® Aspirin Regimen Regular Strength [US-OTC] *see* aspirin *on page 98*
Bayer® Genuine Aspirin [US-OTC] *see* aspirin *on page 98*
Bayer® Plus Extra Strength [US-OTC] *see* aspirin *on page 98*
Bayer® with Heart Advantage [US-OTC] *see* aspirin *on page 98*
Bayer® Women's Aspirin Plus Calcium [US-OTC] *see* aspirin *on page 98*
BayGam® [Can] *see* immune globulin (intramuscular) *on page 502*
BayGam® *(Discontinued)* *see* immune globulin (intramuscular) *on page 502*
BayHepB® *(Discontinued)* *see* hepatitis B immune globulin *on page 470*
BayRab® *(Discontinued)* *see* rabies immune globulin (human) *on page 815*
BayRho-D® Full Dose *(Discontinued)* *see* Rho(D) immune globulin *on page 829*
BayRho-D® Mini Dose *(Discontinued)* *see* Rho(D) immune globulin *on page 829*
BayTet™ *(Discontinued)* *see* tetanus immune globulin (human) *on page 913*
Baza® Antifungal [US-OTC] *see* miconazole *on page 630*
Baza® Clear [US-OTC] *see* vitamin A and vitamin D *on page 980*
β,β-dimethylcysteine *see* penicillamine *on page 730*
B-Caro-T™ [US] *see* beta-carotene *on page 130*
BCG, live *see* BCG vaccine *on page 118*

BCG vaccine (bee see jee vak SEEN)

Synonyms bacillus calmette-Guérin (BCG) live; BCG vaccine U.S.P. *(percutaneous use product)*; BCG, live

U.S./Canadian Brand Names ImmuCyst® [Can]; Oncotice™ [Can]; Pacis™ [Can]; TheraCys® [US]; TICE® BCG [US]

Therapeutic Category Biological Response Modulator

Use Immunization against tuberculosis and immunotherapy for cancer; treatment and prophylaxis of carcinoma *in situ* of the bladder; prophylaxis of primary or recurrent superficial papillary tumors following transurethral resection

Usual Dosage

Immunization against tuberculosis: Percutaneous: **Note:** Initial lesion usually appears after 10-14 days consisting of small, red papule at injection site and reaches maximum diameter of 3 mm in 4-6 weeks.
Children <1 month: 0.2-0.3 mL (half-strength dilution). Administer tuberculin test (5 TU) after 2-3 months; repeat vaccination after 1 year of age for negative tuberculin test if indications persist.
Children >1 month and Adults: 0.2-0.3 mL (full strength dilution); conduct postvaccinal tuberculin test (5 TU of PPD) in 2-3 months; if test is negative, repeat vaccination.
Immunotherapy for bladder cancer: Intravesicular Adults:
TheraCys®: One dose instilled into bladder (for 2 hours) once weekly for 6 weeks followed by one treatment at 3, 6, 12, 18, and 24 months after initial treatment
TICE® BCG: One dose instilled into the bladder (for 2 hours) once weekly for 6 weeks followed by once monthly for 6-12 months

Dosage Forms

Injection, powder for reconstitution, intravesical [preservative free]:
TheraCys®: 81 mg
TICE® BCG: 50 mg
Injection, powder for reconstitution, percutaneous [preservative free]:
BCG Vaccine U.S.P.: 50 mg

BCG vaccine U.S.P. *(percutaneous use product)* *see* BCG vaccine *on page 118*

BCI-Fluoxetine [Can] *see* fluoxetine *on page 413*
BCI-Gabapentin [Can] *see* gabapentin *on page 431*
BCI-Metformin [Can] *see* metformin *on page 610*
BCI-Ranitidine [Can] *see* ranitidine *on page 819*
BCNU *see* carmustine *on page 180*
B complex combinations *see* vitamin B complex combinations *on page 981*
beano® [US-OTC] *see* alpha-galactosidase *on page 49*
Bebulin® VH [US] *see* factor IX complex (human) *on page 389*

becaplermin (be KAP ler min)

Sound-Alike/Look-Alike Issues
Regranex® may be confused with Granulex®, Repronex®
Synonyms recombinant human platelet-derived growth factor B; rPDGF-BB
U.S./Canadian Brand Names Regranex® [US/Can]
Therapeutic Category Topical Skin Product
Use Adjunctive treatment of diabetic neuropathic ulcers occurring on the lower limbs and feet that extend into subcutaneous tissue (or beyond) and have adequate blood supply
Usual Dosage Topical: Adults: Diabetic ulcers: Apply appropriate amount of gel once daily with a cotton swab or similar tool, as a coating over the ulcer. The amount of becaplermin to be applied will vary depending on the size of the ulcer area.
Note: If the ulcer does not decrease in size by ~30% after 10 weeks of treatment or complete healing has not occurred in 20 weeks, continued treatment with becaplermin gel should be reassessed.
To calculate the length of gel applied to the ulcer, measure the greatest length of the ulcer by the greatest width of the ulcer. Tube size and unit of measure will determine the formula used in the calculation. Recalculate amount of gel needed every 1-2 weeks, depending on the rate of change in ulcer area.
Centimeters:
15 g tube: [ulcer length (cm) x width (cm)] divided by 4 = length of gel (cm)
2 g tube: [ulcer length (cm) x width (cm)] divided by 2 = length of gel (cm)
Inches:
15 g tube: [length (in) x width (in)] x 0.6 = length of gel (in)
2 g tube: [length (in) x width (in)] x 1.3 = length of gel (in)
Dosage Forms
Gel, topical:
Regranex®: 0.01% (2 g, 15 g)

beclomethasone (be kloe METH a sone)

Sound-Alike/Look-Alike Issues
Vanceril® may be confused with Vancenase®
Synonyms beclomethasone dipropionate
U.S./Canadian Brand Names Apo-Beclomethasone® [Can]; Beconase® AQ [US]; Gen-Beclo [Can]; Nu-Beclomethasone [Can]; Propaderm® [Can]; QVAR® [US/Can]; Rivanase AQ [Can]; Vanceril® AEM [Can]
Therapeutic Category Adrenal Corticosteroid
Use
Oral inhalation: Maintenance and prophylactic treatment of asthma; includes those who require corticosteroids and those who may benefit from a dose reduction/elimination of systemically-administered corticosteroids. Not for relief of acute bronchospasm.
Nasal aerosol: Symptomatic treatment of seasonal or perennial rhinitis; prevent recurrence of nasal polyps following surgery.
Usual Dosage Nasal inhalation and oral inhalation dosage forms are not to be used interchangeably
Inhalation, nasal: Rhinitis, nasal polyps (Beconase® AQ): Children ≥6 years and Adults: 1-2 inhalations each nostril twice daily; total dose 168-336 mcg/day
Inhalation, oral: Asthma (doses should be titrated to the lowest effective dose once asthma is controlled) (QVAR®):
Children 5-11 years: Initial: 40 mcg twice daily; maximum dose: 80 mcg twice daily
Children ≥12 years and Adults:
Patients previously on bronchodilators only: Initial dose 40-80 mcg twice daily; maximum dose: 320 mcg twice day

◄ Patients previously on inhaled corticosteroids: Initial dose 40-160 mcg twice daily; maximum dose: 320 mcg twice daily

NIH Asthma Guidelines (NIH, 2007): HFA formulation (eg, QVAR®): Administer in divided doses:
Children 5-11 years:
"Low" dose: 80-160 mcg/day
"Medium" dose: >160-320 mcg/day
"High" dose: >320 mcg/day
Children ≥12 years and Adults:
"Low" dose: 80-240 mcg/day
"Medium" dose: >240-480 mcg/day
"High" dose: >480 mcg/day

Dosage Forms
Aerosol for oral inhalation:
QVAR®: 40 mcg/inhalation (7.3 g); 80 mcg/inhalation (7.3 g)
Suspension, intranasal, aqueous [spray]:
Beconase® AQ: 42 mcg/inhalation (25 g)

beclomethasone dipropionate see beclomethasone on page 119
Beclovent® (Discontinued) see beclomethasone on page 119
Beconase® AQ [US] see beclomethasone on page 119
Beconase® (Discontinued) see beclomethasone on page 119
Becotin® Pulvules® (Discontinued)
Beepen-VK® (Discontinued) see penicillin V potassium on page 734
BeFlex [US] see acetaminophen and phenyltoloxamine on page 22
behenyl alcohol see docosanol on page 314
Belix® Oral (Discontinued) see diphenhydramine on page 304
belladonna alkaloids with phenobarbital see hyoscyamine, atropine, scopolamine, and phenobarbital on page 493

belladonna and opium (bel a DON a & OH pee um)
Synonyms opium and belladonna
U.S./Canadian Brand Names B&O Supprettes® [US]
Therapeutic Category Analgesic, Narcotic
Controlled Substance C-II
Use Relief of moderate-to-severe pain associated with ureteral spasms not responsive to nonopioid analgesics and to space intervals between injections of opiates
Usual Dosage Rectal: Children >12 years and Adults: 1 suppository 1-2 times/day, up to 4 doses/day
Dosage Forms
Suppository: #15 A: Belladonna extract 16.2 mg and opium 30 mg; #16 A: Belladonna extract 16.2 mg and opium 60 mg
B&O Supprettes®: #15 A: Belladonna extract 16.2 mg and opium 30 mg; #16 A: Belladonna extract 16.2 mg and opium 60 mg

belladonna, phenobarbital, and ergotamine
(bel a DON a, fee noe BAR bi tal, & er GOT a meen)
Synonyms ergotamine tartrate, belladonna, and phenobarbital; phenobarbital, belladonna, and ergotamine tartrate
U.S./Canadian Brand Names Bellergal® Spacetabs® [Can]
Therapeutic Category Ergot Derivative
Use Management and treatment of menopausal disorders, GI disorders, and recurrent throbbing headache
Usual Dosage Oral: Adults: 1 tablet each morning and evening

Bellamine S (Discontinued) see belladonna, phenobarbital, and ergotamine on page 120
Bellatal® (Discontinued) see hyoscyamine, atropine, scopolamine, and phenobarbital on page 493
Bellergal-S® (Discontinued)
Bellergal® Spacetabs® [Can] see belladonna, phenobarbital, and ergotamine on page 120
Bel-Tabs (Discontinued) see belladonna, phenobarbital, and ergotamine on page 120
Benadryl® [Can] see diphenhydramine on page 304

Benadryl-D™ Allergy and Sinus Fastmelt™ [US-OTC] *see* diphenhydramine and pseudoephedrine *on page 306*

Benadryl-D™ Children's Allergy and Sinus [US-OTC] *see* diphenhydramine and pseudoephedrine *on page 306*

Benadryl® Allergy [US-OTC] *see* diphenhydramine *on page 304*

Benadryl® Children's Allergy [US-OTC] *see* diphenhydramine *on page 304*

Benadryl® Children's Allergy and Cold Fastmelt™ [US-OTC] *see* diphenhydramine and pseudoephedrine *on page 306*

Benadryl® Children's Allergy Fastmelt® [US-OTC] *see* diphenhydramine *on page 304*

Benadryl® Children's Dye-Free Allergy [US-OTC] *see* diphenhydramine *on page 304*

Benadryl® Itch Stopping [US-OTC] *see* diphenhydramine *on page 304*

Benadryl® Itch Stopping Extra Strength [US-OTC] *see* diphenhydramine *on page 304*

Ben-Allergin-50® Injection *(Discontinued)* *see* diphenhydramine *on page 304*

Ben-Aqua® *(Discontinued)* *see* benzoyl peroxide *on page 126*

benazepril (ben AY ze pril)

Sound-Alike/Look-Alike Issues
benazepril may be confused with Benadryl®
Lotensin® may be confused with Lioresal®, lovastatin

Synonyms benazepril hydrochloride

U.S./Canadian Brand Names Apo-Benazepril® [Can]; Lotensin® [US/Can]

Therapeutic Category Angiotensin-Converting Enzyme (ACE) Inhibitor

Use Treatment of hypertension, either alone or in combination with other antihypertensive agents

Usual Dosage Oral: Hypertension:
Children ≥6 years: Initial: 0.2 mg/kg/day (up to 10 mg/day) as monotherapy; dosing range: 0.1-0.6 mg/kg/day (maximum dose: 40 mg/day)
Adults: Initial: 10 mg/day in patients not receiving a diuretic; 20-80 mg/day as a single dose or 2 divided doses; the need for twice-daily dosing should be assessed by monitoring peak (2-6 hours after dosing) and trough responses.
Note: Patients taking diuretics should have them discontinued 2-3 days prior to starting benazepril. If they cannot be discontinued, then initial dose should be 5 mg; restart after blood pressure is stabilized if needed.

Dosage Forms
Tablet: 5 mg, 10 mg, 20 mg, 40 mg
Lotensin®: 5 mg, 10 mg, 20 mg, 40 mg

benazepril and hydrochlorothiazide (ben AY ze pril & hye droe klor oh THYE a zide)

Synonyms hydrochlorothiazide and benazepril

U.S./Canadian Brand Names Lotensin® HCT [US]

Therapeutic Category Antihypertensive Agent, Combination

Use Treatment of hypertension

Usual Dosage Oral: Dose is individualized (range: benazepril: 5-20 mg; hydrochlorothiazide: 6.25-25 mg/day)

Dosage Forms
Tablet:
Generics:
5/6.25: Benazepril 5 mg and hydrochlorothiazide 6.25 mg
10/12.5: Benazepril 10 mg and hydrochlorothiazide 12.5 mg
20/12.5: Benazepril 20 mg and hydrochlorothiazide 12.5 mg
20/25: Benazepril 20 mg and hydrochlorothiazide 25 mg
Brands:
Lotensin® HCT 5/6.25: Benazepril 5 mg and hydrochlorothiazide 6.25 mg
Lotensin® HCT 10/12.5: Benazepril 10 mg and hydrochlorothiazide 12.5 mg
Lotensin® HCT 20/12.5: Benazepril 20 mg and hydrochlorothiazide 12.5 mg
Lotensin® HCT 20/25: Benazepril 20 mg and hydrochlorothiazide 25 mg

benazepril hydrochloride *see* benazepril *on page 121*

benazepril hydrochloride and amlodipine besylate *see* amlodipine and benazepril *on page 65*

bendamustine (ben da MUS teen)

Sound-Alike/Look-Alike Issues
bendamustine may be confused with carmustine
Synonyms bendamustine hydrochloride; cytostasan; SDX-105
U.S./Canadian Brand Names Treanda® [US]
Therapeutic Category Antineoplastic Agent, Alkylating Agent
Use Treatment of chronic lymphocytic leukemia (CLL)
Usual Dosage I.V.: Adults: CLL: 100 mg/m^2 on days 1 and 2 of a 28-day treatment cycle (for up to 6 cycles)
Dosage Forms
  Injection, powder for reconstitution:
    Treanda®: 100 mg

bendamustine hydrochloride *see* bendamustine *on page 122*
bendroflumethiazide and nadolol *see* nadolol and bendroflumethiazide *on page 651*
BeneFix® [US/Can] *see* factor IX *on page 388*
Beneflur® [Can] *see* fludarabine *on page 406*
Benemid® (Discontinued) *see* probenecid *on page 786*
Benicar® [US] *see* olmesartan *on page 695*
Benicar HCT® [US] *see* olmesartan and hydrochlorothiazide *on page 695*
Benoquin® [US] *see* monobenzone *on page 642*
Benoxyl® [Can] *see* benzoyl peroxide *on page 126*

benserazide and levodopa *(Canada only)* (ben SER a zide & lee voe DOE pa)

Synonyms levodopa and benserazide
U.S./Canadian Brand Names Prolopa® [Can]
Therapeutic Category Anti-Parkinson Agent (Dopamine Agonist)
Use Treatment of Parkinson disease (except drug-induced parkinsonism)
Usual Dosage Oral: Adults: **Note:** Dosage expressed as levodopa/benserazide:
  Initial: 100/25 mg 1-2 times/day, increase every 3-4 days until therapeutic effect; optimal dosage: 400/100 mg to 800/200 mg/day divided into 4-6 doses
  Note: 200/50 mg used only when maintenance therapy is reached and not to exceed levodopa 1000-1200 mg/benserazide 250-300 mg per day
  Patients previously on levodopa: Allow 12 hours or more to lapse between last dose of levodopa; start at 15% of previous levodopa dosage
  Note: Dosages should be introduced gradually, individualized, and continued for 3-6 weeks before assessing benefit. Decrease dosage in patients with dystonia.
Dosage Forms [CAN] = Canadian brand name
  Capsule:
    Prolopa® [CAN]:
      50-12.5: Levodopa 50 mg and benserazide 12.5 mg [not available in the U.S.]
      100-25: Levodopa 100 mg and benserazide 25 mg [not available in the U.S.]
      200-50: Levodopa 200 mg and benserazide 50 mg [not available in the U.S.]

Ben-Tann [US] *see* diphenhydramine *on page 304*

bentoquatam (BEN toe kwa tam)

Synonyms quaternium-18 bentonite
U.S./Canadian Brand Names IvyBlock® [US-OTC]
Therapeutic Category Protectant, Topical
Use Skin protectant for the prevention of allergic contact dermatitis to poison oak, ivy, and sumac
Usual Dosage Topical: Children >6 years and Adults: Apply to skin 15 minutes prior to potential exposure to poison ivy, poison oak, or poison sumac, and reapply every 4 hours
Dosage Forms
  Lotion:
    IvyBlock® [OTC]: 5% (120 mL)

Bentyl® [US] *see* dicyclomine *on page 293*

Bentyl® Injection *(Discontinued)* see dicyclomine *on page 293*
Bentylol® [Can] see dicyclomine *on page 293*
Benuryl™ [Can] see probenecid *on page 786*
Benylin® 3.3 mg-D-E [Can] see guaifenesin, pseudoephedrine, and codeine *on page 460*
Benylin® D for Infants [Can] see pseudoephedrine *on page 801*
Benylin® Adult *(Discontinued)* see dextromethorphan *on page 284*
Benylin® Cough Syrup *(Discontinued)* see diphenhydramine *on page 304*
Benylin® DM-D [Can] see pseudoephedrine and dextromethorphan *on page 802*
Benylin® DM-D-E [Can] see guaifenesin, pseudoephedrine, and dextromethorphan *on page 460*
Benylin® DM *(Discontinued)* see dextromethorphan *on page 284*
Benylin® DM-E [Can] see guaifenesin and dextromethorphan *on page 454*
Benylin® E Extra Strength [Can] see guaifenesin *on page 453*
Benylin® Expectorant *(Discontinued)* see guaifenesin and dextromethorphan *on page 454*
Benylin® Pediatric *(Discontinued)* see dextromethorphan *on page 284*
Benzac® AC [US/Can] see benzoyl peroxide *on page 126*
Benzac® AC Gel *(Discontinued)* see benzoyl peroxide *on page 126*
Benzac® AC Wash [US] see benzoyl peroxide *on page 126*
BenzaClin® [US/Can] see clindamycin and benzoyl peroxide *on page 231*
Benzac® W *(Discontinued)* see benzoyl peroxide *on page 126*
Benzac® W Gel [Can] see benzoyl peroxide *on page 126*
Benzac® W Wash [US/Can] see benzoyl peroxide *on page 126*
Benzagel® [US] see benzoyl peroxide *on page 126*
Benzagel® Wash *(Discontinued)* see benzoyl peroxide *on page 126*

benzalkonium chloride (benz al KOE nee um KLOR ide)

Synonyms BAC
U.S./Canadian Brand Names HandClens® [US-OTC]; Pedi-Pro® [US]; Pronto® Plus Lice Egg Remover Kit [US-OTC]; Zephiran® [US-OTC]
Therapeutic Category Antibacterial, Topical
Use Surface antiseptic and germicidal preservative
Usual Dosage Thoroughly rinse anionic detergents and soaps from the skin or other areas prior to use of solutions because they reduce the antibacterial activity of BAC. To protect metal instruments stored in BAC solution, add crushed Anti-Rust Tablets, 4 tablets/quart, to antiseptic solution. Change solution at least once weekly. Not to be used for storage of aluminum or zinc instruments, instruments with lenses fastened by cement, lacquered catheters, or some synthetic rubber goods.
Dosage Forms
  Lotion, topical [foam]:
    HandClens®: 0.13% (50 mL, 240 mL, 1800 mL)
  Lotion, topical [spray]:
    HandClens®: 0.13% (15 mL)
  Powder, topical:
    Pedi-Pro®: 1% (60 g)
  Solution, topical:
    Pronto® Plus Lice Egg Remover Kit: 0.1% (60 mL)
    Zephiran® [OTC]: 1:750 (240 mL, 3840 mL)

Benzamycin® [US] see erythromycin and benzoyl peroxide *on page 356*
Benzamycin® Pak [US] see erythromycin and benzoyl peroxide *on page 356*
Benzashave® [US] see benzoyl peroxide *on page 126*
benzathine benzylpenicillin see penicillin G benzathine *on page 731*
benzathine penicillin G see penicillin G benzathine *on page 731*
Benzedrex® [US-OTC] see propylhexedrine *on page 798*
benzene hexachloride see lindane *on page 567*
benzhexol hydrochloride see trihexyphenidyl *on page 952*
Benziq™ [US] see benzoyl peroxide *on page 126*
Benziq™ LS [US] see benzoyl peroxide *on page 126*

benzmethyzin *see* procarbazine *on page 788*

benzocaine (BEN zoe kane)

Sound-Alike/Look-Alike Issues
Orabase®-B may be confused with Orinase®

Synonyms ethyl aminobenzoate

U.S./Canadian Brand Names Americaine® Hemorrhoidal [US-OTC]; Anbesol® Baby [US-OTC/Can]; Anbesol® Cold Sore Therapy [US-OTC]; Anbesol® Jr. [US-OTC]; Anbesol® Maximum Strength [US-OTC]; Anbesol® [US-OTC]; Benzodent® [US-OTC]; Bi-Zets [US]; Boil-Ease® Pain Relieving [US]; Cepacol® Sore Throat [US-OTC]; Chiggerex® Plus [US]; Chiggerex® [US-OTC]; Chiggertox® [US-OTC]; Cylex® [US-OTC]; Dent's Extra Strength Toothache [US-OTC]; Dentapaine [US-OTC]; Dermoplast® Antibacterial [US-OTC]; Dermoplast® Pain Relieving [US-OTC]; Detane® [US-OTC]; Foille® [US-OTC]; HDA® Toothache [US-OTC]; Hurricaine® [US-OTC]; Ivy-Rid® [US-OTC]; Kank-A® Soft Brush™ [US-OTC]; Lanacane® Maximum Strength [US-OTC]; Lanacane® [US-OTC]; Little Teethers® [US-OTC]; Mycinettes® [US-OTC]; Orabase® with Benzocaine [US-OTC]; Orajel PM® Maximum Strength [US-OTC]; Orajel® Baby Daytime and Nighttime [US-OTC]; Orajel® Baby Teething Nighttime [US-OTC]; Orajel® Baby Teething [US-OTC]; Orajel® Denture Plus [US-OTC]; Orajel® Maximum Strength [US-OTC]; Orajel® Medicated Toothache [US-OTC]; Orajel® Mouth Sore [US-OTC]; Orajel® Multi-Action Cold Sore [US-OTC]; Orajel® Ultra Mouth Sore [US-OTC]; Outgro® [US-OTC]; Red Cross™ Canker Sore [US-OTC]; Rid-A-Pain Dental [US-OTC]; Sepasoothe® [US]; Skeeter Stik [US-OTC]; Sting-Kill [US-OTC]; Tanac® [US-OTC]; Thorets [US-OTC]; Trocaine® [US-OTC]; Zilactin Baby® [Can]; Zilactin Toothache and Gum Pain® [US-OTC]; Zilactin®-B [US-OTC/Can]

Therapeutic Category Local Anesthetic

Use Temporary relief of pain associated with pruritic dermatosis, pruritus, minor burns, acute congestive, bee stings, and insect bites; mouth and gum irritations (toothache, minor sore throat pain, canker sores, dentures, orthodontia, teething, mucositis, stomatitis); sunburn; hemorrhoids; anesthetic lubricant for passage of catheters and endoscopic tubes

Usual Dosage Note: These are general dosing guidelines; refer to specific product labeling for dosing instructions.
Children ≥4 months: Topical (oral): Teething pain: 7.5% to 10%: Apply to affected gum area up to 4 times daily
Children ≥2 years and Adults:
Topical:
  Bee stings, insect bites, minor burns, sunburn: 5% to 20%: Apply to affected area 3-4 times a day as needed. In cases of bee stings, remove stinger before treatment.
  Lubricant for passage of catheters and instruments: 20%: Apply evenly to exterior of instrument prior to use.
Topical (oral): Mouth and gum irritation: 10% to 20%: Apply thin layer to affected area up to 4 times daily
Children ≥5 years and Adults: Oral: Sore throat: Allow 1 lozenge (10-15 mg) to dissolve slowly in mouth; may repeat every 2 hours as needed
Children ≥12 years and Adults: Rectal: Hemorrhoids: 5% to 20%: Apply externally to affected area up to 6 times daily

Dosage Forms
Aerosol, oral spray:
Hurricaine® [OTC]: 20% (60 mL)
Aerosol, topical spray:
Dermoplast® Antibacterial [OTC]: 20% (83 mL)
Dermoplast® Pain Relieving [OTC]: 20% (60 mL, 83 mL)
Foille® [OTC]: 5% (92 g)
Ivy-Rid® [OTC]: 2% (83 mL)
Lanacane® Maximum Strength [OTC]: 20% (120 mL)
Combination package:
Orajel® Baby Daytime and Nighttime [OTC]:
  Gel, oral [Daytime Regular Formula]: 7.5% (5.3 g)
  Gel, oral [Nighttime Formula]: 10% (5.3 g)
Cream, oral:
Benzodent® [OTC]: 20% (7.5 g, 30 g)
Orajel PM® Maximum Strength[OTC]: 20% (5.3 g, 7 g)
Cream, topical:
Lanacane® [OTC]: 6% (30 g, 60 g)
Lanacane® Maximum Strength [OTC]: 20% (30 g)

Gel, oral:
Anbesol® [OTC], Zilactin®-B [OTC]: 10% (7.5 g)
Anbesol® Baby [OTC]: 7.5% (7.5 g)
Anbesol® Jr. [OTC]: 10% (7 g)
Anbesol® Maximum Strength [OTC]: 20% (7.5 g, 10 g)
Dentapaine [OTC]: 20% (11 g)
HDA® Toothache [OTC]: 6.5% (15 mL)
Hurricaine® [OTC]: 20% (5 g, 30 g)
Kank-A® Soft Brush™ [OTC]: 20% (2 mL)
Little Teethers® [OTC]: 7.5% (9.4 g)
Orabase® with Benzocaine® [OTC]: 20% (7 g)
Orajel® [OTC]: 10% (5.3 g, 7 g, 9.4 g)
Orajel® Baby Teething [OTC]: 7.5% (9.4 g, 11.9 g)
Orajel® Baby Teething Nighttime [OTC]: 10% (5.3 g)
Orajel® Denture Plus [OTC]: 15% (9 g)
Orajel® Maximum Strength [OTC]: 20% (5.3 g, 7 g, 9.4 g, 11.9 g)
Orajel® Mouth Sore [OTC]: 20% (5.3 g, 9.4 g, 11.9 g)
Orajel® Multi-Action Cold Sore [OTC]: 20% (9.4 g)
Orajel® Ultra Mouth Sore [OTC]: 15% (9.4 g)
Gel, topical:
Detane® [OTC]: 7.5% (15 g)
Liquid, oral:
Anbesol® [OTC], Tanac® [OTC]: 10%
Anbesol® Maximum Strength [OTC], Hurricaine® [OTC], Orajel® Maximum Strength [OTC]: 20%
Orajel® Baby Teething [OTC]: 7.5%
Liquid, oral [drops]:
Rid-A-Pain Dental [OTC]: 6.3%
Liquid, topical:
Chiggertox® [OTC]: 2% (30 mL)
Outgro® [OTC]: 20% (9 mL)
Skeeter Stik [OTC]: 5% (14 mL)
Lozenge: 6 mg (18s), 15 mg (10s)
Bi-Zets: 15 mg (10s)
Cepacol® Sore Throat [OTC]: 15 mg (16s, 18s)
Cylex® [OTC], Mycinettes® [OTC]: 15 mg (12s)
Sepasoothe®: 10 mg (6s, 24s, 100s, 250s, 500s)
Thorets [OTC]: 18 mg (300s)
Trocaine® [OTC]: 10 mg (50s, 300s)
Ointment, oral:
Anbesol® Cold Sore Therapy [OTC]: 20% (7.1 g)
Red Cross™ Canker Sore [OTC]: 20% (7.5 g)
Ointment, rectal:
Americaine® Hemorrhoidal [OTC]: 20% (30 g)
Ointment, topical:
Boil-Ease® Pain Relieving: 20% (30 g)
Chiggerex® Plus: 6% (50 g)
Foille® [OTC]: 5% (3.5 g, 14 g, 28 g)
Pads, topical:
Sting-Kill [OTC]: 20% (8s)
Paste, oral:
Orabase® with Benzocaine [OTC]: 20% (6 g)
Swabs, oral:
Hurricaine® [OTC]: 20% (6s, 100s)
Orajel® Baby Teething [OTC]: 7.5% (12s)
Orajel® Medicated Mouth Sore [OTC], Orajel® Medicated Toothache [OTC]: 20% (8s, 12s)
Zilactin® Toothache and Gum Pain [OTC]: 20% (8s)
Swabs, topical:
Boil-Ease® Pain Relieving: 20% (12s)
Sting-Kill [OTC]: 20% (5s)
Wax, oral:
Dent's Extra Strength Toothache Gum [OTC]: 20% (1 g)

benzocaine and antipyrine *see* antipyrine and benzocaine *on page 82*

benzocaine, butamben, and tetracaine (BEN zoe kane, byoo TAM ben, & TET ra kane)

Synonyms benzocaine, butamben, and tetracaine hydrochloride; benzocaine, butyl aminobenzoate, and tetracaine; butamben, tetracaine, and benzocaine; tetracaine, benzocaine, and butamben

U.S./Canadian Brand Names Cetacaine® [US]; Exactacain™ [US]

Therapeutic Category Local Anesthetic

Use Topical anesthetic to control pain in surgical or endoscopic procedures; anesthetic for accessible mucous membranes except for the eyes

Usual Dosage Topical anesthetic: **Note:** Decrease dose in the acutely-ill patient:
Adults:
Cetacaine®:
Aerosol: Apply for ≤1 second; use of sprays >2 seconds is contraindicated
Gel: Apply ~1/2 inch (13 mm) x 3/16 inch (5 mm); application of >1 inch (26 cm) x 3/16 inch (5 mm) is contraindicated
Liquid: Apply 6-7 drops (0.2 mL); application of >12-14 drops (0.4 mL) is contraindicated
Exactacain™: 3 metered sprays (use of >6 metered sprays is contraindicated)

Dosage Forms
Aerosol, topical [spray]:
Cetacaine®: Benzocaine 14%, butamben 2%, and tetracaine 2% (56 g)
Exactacain™: Benzocaine 14%, butamben 2%, and tetracaine 2% (60 g)
Gel, topical:
Cetacaine®: Benzocaine 14%, butamben 2%, and tetracaine 2% (29 g)
Liquid, topical:
Cetacaine®: Benzocaine 14%, butamben 2%, and tetracaine 2% (56 g)

benzocaine, butamben, and tetracaine hydrochloride *see* benzocaine, butamben, and tetracaine *on page 126*

benzocaine, butyl aminobenzoate, and tetracaine *see* benzocaine, butamben, and tetracaine *on page 126*

Benzocol® *(Discontinued)* *see* benzocaine *on page 124*

Benzodent® [US-OTC] *see* benzocaine *on page 124*

benzoin (BEN zoin)

Synonyms gum benjamin

U.S./Canadian Brand Names Benz-Protect Swabs™ [US-OTC]; Sprayzoin™ [US-OTC]

Therapeutic Category Pharmaceutical Aid Protectant, Topical

Use Protective application for irritations of the skin; sometimes used in boiling water as steam inhalants for its expectorant and soothing action

Usual Dosage Apply 1-2 times/day

Dosage Forms
Tincture: Benzoin USP [OTC] (60 mL); Benzoin Compound USP [OTC] (30 mL, 60 mL, 120 mL, 480 mL)
Tincture [swab]:
Benz-Protect Swabs™ [OTC]: Benzoin Compound USP (50s)
Tincture [spray]: Benzoin USP [OTC] (120 mL)
Sprayzoin™ [OTC]: Benzoin Compound USP (120 mL)

benzonatate (ben ZOE na tate)

U.S./Canadian Brand Names Tessalon® [US/Can]

Therapeutic Category Antitussive

Use Symptomatic relief of nonproductive cough

Usual Dosage Oral: Children >10 years and Adults: 100 mg 3 times/day or every 4 hours up to 600 mg/day

Dosage Forms
Capsule, softgel: 100 mg, 200 mg
Tessalon®: 100 mg, 200 mg

benzoyl peroxide (BEN zoe il peer OKS ide)

Sound-Alike/Look-Alike Issues
Benoxyl® may be confused with Brevoxyl®, Peroxyl®
Benzac® may be confused with Benza®

Brevoxyl® may be confused with Benoxyl®
Fostex® may be confused with pHisoHex®

U.S./Canadian Brand Names Acetoxyl® [Can]; Benoxyl® [Can]; Benzac® AC Wash [US]; Benzac® AC [US/Can]; Benzac® W Gel [Can]; Benzac® W Wash [US/Can]; Benzagel® [US]; Benzashave® [US]; Benziq™ LS [US]; Benziq™ [US]; Brevoxyl® Cleansing [US]; Brevoxyl® Wash [US]; Brevoxyl® [US]; Clearplex [US-OTC]; Clinac™ BPO [US]; Del Aqua® [US]; Desquam-X® [US/Can]; Exact® Acne Medication [US-OTC]; Fostex® 10% BPO [US-OTC]; Inova™ [US]; NeoBenz® Micro SD [US]; NeoBenz® Micro [US]; Neutrogena® Acne Mask [US-OTC]; Neutrogena® On The Spot® Acne Treatment [US-OTC]; Oxy 10® Balance Spot Treatment [US-OTC]; Oxy 10® Balanced Medicated Face Wash [US-OTC]; Oxyderm™ [Can]; Palmer's® Skin Success Acne [US-OTC]; PanOxyl® Aqua Gel [US]; PanOxyl® Bar [US-OTC]; PanOxyl® [US/Can]; PanOxyl®-AQ [US]; Seba-Gel™ [US]; Solugel® [Can]; Triaz® Cleanser [US]; Triaz® [US]; Zapzyt® [US-OTC]; Zoderm® Hydrating Wash™ [US]; Zoderm® [US]

Therapeutic Category Acne Products

Use Adjunctive treatment of mild-to-moderate acne vulgaris and acne rosacea

Usual Dosage Children and Adults:

Cleansers: Wash once or twice daily; control amount of drying or peeling by modifying dose frequency or concentration

Topical: Apply sparingly once daily; gradually increase to 2-3 times/day if needed. If excessive dryness or peeling occurs, reduce dose frequency or concentration; if excessive stinging or burning occurs, remove with mild soap and water; resume use the next day.

Dosage Forms
Cream, topical:
BenzaShave®: 5% (120 g); 10% (120 g)
Exact® Acne Medication [OTC]: 5% (18 g)
NeoBenz® Micro: 3.5% (45 g); 5.5% (45 g); 8.5% (45 g)
NeoBenz® Micro SD: 3.5% (0.5 g); 5.5% (0.5 g); 8.5% (0.5 g)
Neutrogena® Acne Mask [OTC]: 5% (60 g)
Neutrogena® On The Spot® Acne Treatment [OTC]: 2.5% (22.5 g)
Zoderm®: 4.5% (125 mL); 6.5% (125 mL); 8.5% (125 mL)
Emulsion, topical [cleanser]:
Zoderm®: 4.5% (400 mL); 6.5% (400 mL); 8.5% (400 mL)
Gel, topical: 2.5% (60 g); 5% (45 g, 60 g, 90 g); 10% (45 g, 60 g, 90 g)
Benzac® AC [water based]: 5% (60 g); 10% (60 g)
Benzagel®: 5% (45 g); 10% (45 g)
Benziq™: 5.25% (50 g)
Benziq™ LS: 2.75% (50 g)
Brevoxyl®: 4% (43 g, 90 g); 8% (43 g, 90 g)
Clearplex [OTC]: 5% (45 g); 10% (45 g)
Clinac™ BPO: 7% (45 g)
Desquam-X®: 10% (42.5 g, 90 g)
Fostex® 10% BPO [OTC]: 10% (45 g)
Oxy 10® Balance Spot Treatment [OTC]: 5% (30 g); 10% (30 g)
PanOxyl® [alcohol based]: 5% (57 g, 113 g); 10% (57 g, 113 g)
PanOxyl® AQ [water based]: 2.5% (57 g, 113 g); 5% (57 g, 113 g); 10% (57 g, 113 g)
PanOxyl® Aqua Gel [water based]: 10% (42.5 g)
Seba-Gel™: 5% (90 g); 10% (90 g)
Triaz® Cleanser: 3% (170 g, 340 g); 6% (170 g, 340 g); 10% (170 g, 340 g)
Zapzyt® [OTC]: 10% (30 g)
Zoderm®: 4.5% (125 mL); 6.5% (125 mL); 8.5% (125 mL)
Liquid, topical: 2.5% (240 mL); 5% (120 mL, 150 mL, 240 mL); 10% (150 mL, 240 mL)
Benzac® AC Wash [water based]: 5% (240 mL); 10% (240 mL)
Benzac® W Wash [water based]: 5% (240 mL)
Benziq™ [wash]: 5.25% (175 g)
Del-Aqua®: 5% (45 mL); 10% (45 mL)
Desquam-X®: 5% (150 mL)
Oxy-10® Balance Medicated Face Wash [OTC]: 10% (240 mL)
Lotion, topical: 5% (30 mL); 5% (227 g); 10% (30 mL); 10% (227 g)
Brevoxyl® Cleansing: 4% (297 g); 8% (297 g)
Brevoxyl® Wash: 4% (170 g); 8% (170 g)
Fostex® 10% BPO [OTC]: 10% (150 mL)
Palmer's® Skin Success Acne [OTC]: 10% (30 mL)

▶

◀ **Liquid, topical** [wash]:
Zoderm® Hydrating Wash™: 5.75% (473 mL)
Pad, topical:
breze™: 4.75% (30s); 7.75% (30s)
Inova™: 4% (30s); 8% (30s)
Triaz®: 3% (30s, 60s); 6% (30s, 60s); 9% (30s)
Zoderm®: 4.5% (30s); 6.5% (30s); 8.5% (30s)
Soap, topical [bar]:
Fostex® 10% BPO [OTC]: 10% (113 g)
PanOxyl® Bar [OTC]: 5% (113 g); 10% (113 g)

benzoyl peroxide and clindamycin see clindamycin and benzoyl peroxide on page 231
benzoyl peroxide and erythromycin see erythromycin and benzoyl peroxide on page 356

benzoyl peroxide and hydrocortisone (BEN zoe il peer OKS ide & hye droe KOR ti sone)
Synonyms hydrocortisone and benzoyl peroxide
U.S./Canadian Brand Names Vanoxide-HC® [US/Can]
Therapeutic Category Acne Products
Use Treatment of acne vulgaris and oily skin
Usual Dosage Topical: Adolescents and Adults: Shake well; apply thin film 1-3 times/day, gently massage into skin
Dosage Forms
Lotion:
Vanoxide-HC®: Benzoyl peroxide 5% and hydrocortisone 0.5% (25 mL)

benzphetamine (benz FET a meen)
Synonyms benzphetamine hydrochloride
U.S./Canadian Brand Names Didrex® [US/Can]
Therapeutic Category Anorexiant
Controlled Substance C-III
Use Short-term (few weeks) adjunct in exogenous obesity
Usual Dosage Oral: Children ≥12 years and Adults: Dose should be individualized based on patient response: Initial: 25-50 mg once daily; titrate to 25-50 mg 1-3 times/day; once-daily dosing should be administered midmorning or midafternoon; maximum dose: 50 mg 3 times/day
Dosage Forms
Tablet: 50 mg
Didrex®: 50 mg

benzphetamine hydrochloride see benzphetamine on page 128
Benz-Protect Swabs™ [US-OTC] see benzoin on page 126

benztropine (BENZ troe peen)
Sound-Alike/Look-Alike Issues
benztropine may be confused with bromocriptine
Synonyms benztropine mesylate
U.S./Canadian Brand Names Apo-Benztropine® [Can]; Cogentin® [US]
Therapeutic Category Anti-Parkinson Agent; Anticholinergic Agent
Use Adjunctive treatment of Parkinson disease; treatment of drug-induced extrapyramidal symptoms (except tardive dyskinesia)
Usual Dosage Use in children ≤3 years of age should be reserved for life-threatening emergencies
Drug-induced extrapyramidal symptom: Oral, I.M., I.V.:
Children >3 years: 0.02-0.05 mg/kg/dose 1-2 times/day
Adults: 1-4 mg/dose 1-2 times/day
Acute dystonia: Adults: I.M., I.V.: 1-2 mg
Parkinsonism: Adults: Oral: 0.5-6 mg/day in 1-2 divided doses; if one dose is greater, administer at bedtime; titrate dose in 0.5 mg increments at 5- to 6-day intervals
Dosage Forms
Injection, solution:
Cogentin®: 1 mg/mL (2 mL)
Tablet: 0.5 mg, 1 mg, 2 mg

benztropine mesylate *see* benztropine *on page 128*

benzydamine *(Canada only)* (ben ZID a meen)

Synonyms benzydamine hydrochloride

U.S./Canadian Brand Names Apo-Benzydamine® [Can]; Dom-Benzydamine [Can]; Novo-Benzydamine [Can]; PMS-Benzydamine [Can]; ratio-Benzydamine [Can]; Sun-Benz® [Can]; Tantum® [Can]

Therapeutic Category Analgesic, Topical

Use Symptomatic treatment of pain associated with acute pharyngitis; treatment of pain associated with radiation-induced oropharyngeal mucositis

Usual Dosage Oral rinse: Adults:

Acute pharyngitis: Gargle with 15 mL of undiluted solution every 1½-3 hours until symptoms resolve. Patient should expel solution from mouth following use; solution should not be swallowed.

Mucositis: 15 mL of undiluted solution as a gargle or rinse 3-4 times/day; contact should be maintained for at least 30 seconds, followed by expulsion from the mouth. Clinical studies maintained contact for ~2 minutes, up to 8 times/day. Patient should not swallow the liquid. Begin treatment 1 day prior to initiation of radiation therapy and continue daily during treatment. Continue oral rinse treatments after the completion of radiation therapy until desired result/healing is achieved.

Dosage Forms [CAN] = Canadian brand name

Oral rinse: 0.15% (100 mL, 250 mL) [not available in the U.S.]

Apo-Benzydamine® [CAN], Dom-Benzydamine [CAN], Novo-Benzydamine [CAN], PMS-Benzydamine [CAN], ratio-Benzydamine [CAN], Sun-Benz® [CAN], Tantum® [CAN]: 0.15% (100 mL, 250 mL) [not available in the U.S.]

benzydamine hydrochloride *see* benzydamine *(Canada only) on page 129*

benzylpenicillin benzathine *see* penicillin G benzathine *on page 731*

benzylpenicillin potassium *see* penicillin G (parenteral/aqueous) *on page 732*

benzylpenicillin sodium *see* penicillin G (parenteral/aqueous) *on page 732*

benzylpenicilloyl-polylysine (BEN zil pen i SIL oyl pol i LIE seen)

Synonyms penicilloyl-polylysine; PPL

Therapeutic Category Diagnostic Agent

Use Adjunct in assessing the risk of administering penicillin (penicillin or benzylpenicillin) in adults with a history of clinical penicillin hypersensitivity

Usual Dosage PPL is administered by a scratch technique or by intradermal injection. For initial testing, PPL should always be applied via the scratch technique. **Do not administer intradermally to patients who have positive reactions to a scratch test.** PPL test alone does not identify those patients who react to a minor antigenic determinant and does not appear to predict reliably the occurrence of late reactions.

Scratch test: Use scratch technique with a 20-gauge needle to make 3-5 mm nonbleeding scratch on epidermis, apply a small drop of solution to scratch, rub in gently with applicator or toothpick. A positive reaction consists of a pale wheal surrounding the scratch site which develops within 10 minutes and ranges from 5-15 mm or more in diameter.

Intradermal test: Use intradermal test with a tuberculin syringe with a 26- to 30-gauge short bevel needle; a dose of 0.01-0.02 mL is injected intradermally. A control of 0.9% sodium chloride should be injected at least 1.5" from the PPL test site. Most skin responses to the intradermal test will develop within 5-15 minutes.

Interpretation:

(-) Negative: No reaction

(±) Ambiguous: Wheal only slightly larger than original bleb with or without erythematous flare and larger than control site

(+) Positive: Itching and marked increase in size of original bleb

Control site should be reactionless

beractant (ber AKT ant)

Sound-Alike/Look-Alike Issues

Survanta® may be confused with Sufenta®

Synonyms bovine lung surfactant; natural lung surfactant

U.S./Canadian Brand Names Survanta® [US/Can]

▶

◀ **Therapeutic Category** Lung Surfactant

Use Prevention and treatment of respiratory distress syndrome (RDS) in premature infants
Prophylactic therapy: Body weight <1250 g in infants at risk for developing, or with evidence of, surfactant deficiency (administer within 15 minutes of birth)
Rescue therapy: Treatment of infants with RDS confirmed by x-ray and requiring mechanical ventilation (administer as soon as possible - within 8 hours of age)

Usual Dosage
Prophylactic treatment: Administer 100 mg phospholipids (4 mL/kg) intratracheal as soon as possible; as many as 4 doses may be administered during the first 48 hours of life, no more frequently than 6 hours apart. The need for additional doses is determined by evidence of continuing respiratory distress; if the infant is still intubated and requiring at least 30% inspired oxygen to maintain a PaO_2 ≤80 torr.
Rescue treatment: Administer 100 mg phospholipids (4 mL/kg) as soon as the diagnosis of RDS is made; may repeat if needed, no more frequently than every 6 hours to a maximum of 4 doses

Dosage Forms
Suspension, intratracheal [preservative free; bovine derived]:
Survanta®: 25 mg/mL

Berocca® *(Discontinued)*
Berocca® Plus *(Discontinued)*
Berotec® [Can] *see* fenoterol *(Canada only) on page 394*
Berubigen® *(Discontinued) see* cyanocobalamin *on page 254*
Betacaine® [Can] *see* lidocaine *on page 561*

beta-carotene (BAY ta KARE oh teen)
U.S./Canadian Brand Names A-Caro-25 [US]; B-Caro-T™ [US]; Lumitene™ [US]
Therapeutic Category Vitamin, Fat Soluble
Usual Dosage Oral:
Children <14 years: 30-150 mg/day
Adults: 30-300 mg/day
Dosage Forms
Capsule, softgel: 10,000 int. units (6 mg); 25,000 int. units (15 mg)
A-Caro-25: 25,000 int. units (15 mg)
B-Caro-T™: 25,000 int. units (15 mg)
Capsule:
Lumitene™: 50,000 int. units (30 mg)
Tablet: 10,000 int. units

Betachron® *(Discontinued) see* propranolol *on page 796*
Betaderm [Can] *see* betamethasone (topical) *on page 132*
Betadine® [US-OTC/Can] *see* povidone-iodine *on page 775*
Betadine® First Aid Antibiotics + Moisturizer *(Discontinued) see* bacitracin and polymyxin B *on page 113*
Betadine® Ophthalmic [US] *see* povidone-iodine *on page 775*
9-beta-d-ribofuranosyladenine *see* adenosine *on page 35*
Betagan® [US/Can] *see* levobunolol *on page 555*
Beta-HC® [US] *see* hydrocortisone (topical) *on page 485*

betahistine *(Canada only)* (bay ta HISS teen)
Synonyms betahistine dihydrochloride
U.S./Canadian Brand Names Serc® [Can]
Therapeutic Category Antihistamine
Use Treatment of Ménière disease (to decrease episodes of vertigo)
Usual Dosage Oral: Adults: 8-16 mg 3 times/day; administration with meals is recommended
Dosage Forms [CAN] = Canadian brand name
Tablet:
Serc® [CAN]: 16 mg, 24 mg [not available in the U.S.]

betahistine dihydrochloride *see* betahistine *(Canada only) on page 130*

betaine (BAY ta een)

Sound-Alike/Look-Alike Issues
betaine may be confused with Betadine®
Cystadane® may be confused with cysteamine, cysteine
Synonyms betaine anhydrous
U.S./Canadian Brand Names Cystadane® [US/Can]
Therapeutic Category Homocystinuria Agent
Use Treatment of homocystinuria (eg, deficiencies or defects in cystathionine beta-synthase [CBS], 5,10-methylene tetrahydrofolate reductase [MTHFR], and cobalamin cofactor metabolism [CBL])
Usual Dosage Oral:
Children <3 years: Initial dose: 100 mg/kg/day given once daily or in 2 divided doses; increase weekly by 50 mg/kg increments, as needed
Children ≥3 years and Adults: Usual dose: 6 g/day administered in divided doses of 3 g twice daily; dosages of up to 20 g/day have been necessary to control homocysteine levels in some patients
Note: Dosage in all patients can be gradually increased until plasma total homocysteine is undetectable or present only in small amounts. One study in six patients with CBS deficiency, ranging from 6-17 years of age, showed minimal benefit from exceeding a twice daily dosing schedule and a 150 mg/kg/day dosage.
Dosage Forms
Powder for oral solution, anhydrous:
Cystadane®: 1 g/scoop

betaine anhydrous see betaine on page 131
Betaject™ [Can] see betamethasone (systemic) on page 132
Betalin® S (Discontinued) see thiamine on page 920
Betaloc® [Can] see metoprolol on page 626
Betaloc® Durules® [Can] see metoprolol on page 626
BetaMed [US-OTC] see pyrithione zinc on page 810

betamethasone and clotrimazole (bay ta METH a sone & kloe TRIM a zole)

Sound-Alike/Look-Alike Issues
clotrimazole may be confused with co-trimoxazole
Lotrisone® may be confused with Lotrimin®
Synonyms clotrimazole and betamethasone
U.S./Canadian Brand Names Lotriderm® [Can]; Lotrisone® [US]
Therapeutic Category Antifungal/Corticosteroid
Use Topical treatment of various dermal fungal infections (including tinea pedis, cruris, and corpora in patients ≥17 years of age)
Usual Dosage Topical: Children ≥17 years and Adults:
Allergic or inflammatory diseases: Apply to affected area twice daily, morning and evening
Tinea corporis, tinea cruris: Massage into affected area twice daily, morning and evening; do not use for longer than 2 weeks; reevaluate after 1 week if no clinical improvement; do not exceed 45 g cream/week or 45 mL lotion/week
Tinea pedis: Massage into affected area twice daily, morning and evening; do not use for longer than 4 weeks; reevaluate after 2 weeks if no clinical improvement; do not exceed 45 g cream/week or 45 mL lotion/week
Dosage Forms
Cream: Betamethasone 0.05% and clotrimazole 1% (15 g, 45 g)
Lotrisone®: Betamethasone 0.05% and clotrimazole 1% (15 g, 45 g)
Lotion: Betamethasone 0.05% and clotrimazole 1% (30 mL)
Lotrisone®: Betamethasone 0.05% and clotrimazole 1% (30 mL)

betamethasone dipropionate see betamethasone (topical) on page 132
betamethasone dipropionate and calcipotriene hydrate see calcipotriene and betamethasone on page 159
betamethasone dipropionate, augmented see betamethasone (topical) on page 132
betamethasone sodium phosphate see betamethasone (systemic) on page 132

betamethasone (systemic) (bay ta METH a sone sis TEM ik)

Synonyms betamethasone sodium phosphate

U.S./Canadian Brand Names Betaject™ [Can]; Celestone® Soluspan® [US/Can]; Celestone® [US]

Therapeutic Category Adrenal Corticosteroid

Use Antiinflammatory; immunosuppressant agent; corticosteroid replacement

Usual Dosage Base dosage on severity of disease and patient response
Children: Use lowest dose listed as initial dose for adrenocortical insufficiency (physiologic replacement)
  I.M.: 0.0175-0.125 mg base/kg/day divided every 6-12 hours **or** 0.5-7.5 mg base/m^2/day divided every 6-12 hours
  Oral: 0.0175-0.25 mg/kg/day divided every 6-8 hours **or** 0.5-7.5 mg/m^2/day divided every 6-8 hours
Adolescents and Adults:
  Oral: 2.4-4.8 mg/day in 2-4 doses; range: 0.6-7.2 mg/day
  I.M.: Betamethasone sodium phosphate and betamethasone acetate: 0.6-9 mg/day (generally, 1/3 to 1/2 of oral dose) divided every 12-24 hours
Adults:
  Intrabursal, intraarticular, intradermal: 0.25-2 mL
  Intralesional: Rheumatoid arthritis/osteoarthritis:
    Very large joints: 1-2 mL
    Large joints: 1 mL
    Medium joints: 0.5-1 mL
    Small joints: 0.25-0.5 mL

Dosage Forms
  Injection, suspension:
    Celestone® Soluspan®: Betamethasone sodium phosphate 3 mg and betamethasone acetate 3 mg per 1 mL (5 mL) [6 mg/mL]
  Solution:
    Celestone®: 0.6 mg/5 mL

betamethasone (topical) (bay ta METH a sone TOP i kal)

Sound-Alike/Look-Alike Issues
  Luxiq® may be confused with Lasix®

Synonyms betamethasone dipropionate; betamethasone dipropionate, augmented; betamethasone valerate; flubenisolone

U.S./Canadian Brand Names Beta-Val® [US]; Betaderm [Can]; Betnesol® [Can]; Betnovate® [Can]; Diprolene® AF [US]; Diprolene® Glycol [Can]; Diprolene® [US]; Diprosone® [Can]; Ectosone [Can]; Luxiq® [US]; Maxivate® [US]; Prevex® B [Can]; Taro-Sone® [Can]; Topilene® [Can]; Topisone® [Can]; Valisone® Scalp Lotion [Can]

Therapeutic Category Corticosteroid, Topical

Use Inflammatory dermatoses such as seborrheic or atopic dermatitis, neurodermatitis, anogenital pruritus, psoriasis, inflammatory phase of xerosis

Usual Dosage Topical:
  ≥13 years: Use minimal amount for shortest period of time to avoid HPA axis suppression
    Gel, augmented formulation: Apply once or twice daily; rub in gently. **Note:** Do not exceed 2 weeks of treatment or 50 g/week.
    Lotion: Apply a few drops twice daily.
      Augmented formulation: Apply a few drops once or twice daily; rub in gently. **Note:** Do not exceed 2 weeks of treatment or 50 mL/week.
    Cream/ointment: Apply one or twice daily.
      Augmented formulation: Apply once or twice daily. **Note:** Do not exceed 2 weeks of treatment or 45 g/week.
  Adults:
    Foam: Apply to the scalp twice daily, once in the morning and once at night
    Gel, augmented formulation: Apply once or twice daily; rub in gently. **Note:** Do not exceed 2 weeks of treatment or 50 g/week.
    Lotion: Apply a few drops twice daily
      Augmented formulation: Apply a few drops once or twice daily; runb in gently. **Note:** Do not exceed 2 weeks of treatment or 50 mL/week.
    Cream/ointment: Apply once or twice daily
      Augmented formulation: Apply once or twice daily. **Note:** Do not exceed 2 weeks of treatment or 45 g/week.

Dosage Forms
  Aerosol, topical [foam]:
    Luxiq®: 0.12% (50 g, 100 g, 150 g)
  Cream, topical: 0.05% (15 g, 45 g; 50 g [augmented])
    Beta-Val®: 0.1% (15 g, 45 g)
    Diprolene® AF: 0.05% (15 g, 50 g)
  Gel, topical: 0.05% (15 g, 50 g)
  Lotion, topical: 0.05% (30 mL, 60 mL); 0.1% (60 mL)
    Beta-Val®: 0.1% (60 mL)
    Diprolene®: 0.05% (30 mL, 60 mL)
  Ointment, topical: 0.05% (15 g, 45 g), 0.1% (15 g, 45 g)
    Diprolene®: 0.05% (15 g, 50 g)

betamethasone valerate *see* betamethasone (topical) *on page 132*
Betapace® [US] *see* sotalol *on page 885*
Betapace AF® [US/Can] *see* sotalol *on page 885*
Beta Sal® [US-OTC] *see* salicylic acid *on page 850*
Betasept® [US-OTC] *see* chlorhexidine gluconate *on page 201*
Betaseron® [US/Can] *see* interferon beta-1b *on page 518*
Betatar® Gel [US-OTC] *see* coal tar *on page 240*
Beta-Val® [US] *see* betamethasone (topical) *on page 132*
Betaxin® [Can] *see* thiamine *on page 920*

betaxolol (be TAKS oh lol)
Sound-Alike/Look-Alike Issues
  betaxolol may be confused with bethanechol, labetalol
  Betoptic® S may be confused with Betagan®
Synonyms betaxolol hydrochloride
U.S./Canadian Brand Names Betoptic® S [US/Can]; Kerlone® [US]; Sandoz-Betaxolol [Can]
Therapeutic Category Beta-Adrenergic Blocker
Use Treatment of chronic open-angle glaucoma or ocular hypertension; management of hypertension
Usual Dosage
  Children and Adults: Ophthalmic suspension (Betoptic® S): Instill 1 drop into affected eye(s) twice daily.
  Adults:
    Ophthalmic solution: Instill 1-2 drops into affected eye(s) twice daily.
    Oral: 5-10 mg/day; may increase dose to 20 mg/day after 7-14 days if desired response is not achieved.
Dosage Forms
  Solution, ophthalmic: 0.5% (5 mL, 10 mL, 15 mL)
  Suspension, ophthalmic:
    Betoptic® S: 0.25% (10 mL, 15 mL)
  Tablet: 10 mg, 20 mg
    Kerlone®: 10 mg, 20 mg

betaxolol hydrochloride *see* betaxolol *on page 133*

bethanechol (be THAN e kole)
Sound-Alike/Look-Alike Issues
  bethanechol may be confused with betaxolol
Synonyms bethanechol chloride
U.S./Canadian Brand Names Duvoid® [Can]; PMS-Bethanechol [Can]; Urecholine® [US]
Therapeutic Category Cholinergic Agent
Use Treatment of acute postoperative and postpartum nonobstructive (functional) urinary retention; treatment of neurogenic atony of the urinary bladder with retention
Usual Dosage Oral: Adults: Urinary retention, neurogenic bladder: Initial: 10-50 mg 3-4 times/day (some patients may require dosages of 50-100 mg 4 times/day). To determine effective dose, may initiate at a dose of 5-10 mg, with additional doses of 5-10 mg hourly until an effective cumulative dose is reached. Cholinergic effects at higher oral dosages may be cumulative.
Dosage Forms [CAN] = Canadian brand name
  Tablet: 5 mg, 10 mg, 25 mg, 50 mg

Duvoid® [CAN]: 10 mg, 25 mg, 50 mg [not available in U.S.]
Urecholine®: 5 mg, 10 mg, 25 mg, 50 mg

bethanechol chloride *see* bethanechol *on page 133*
Betimol® [US] *see* timolol *on page 927*
Betnesol® [Can] *see* betamethasone (topical) *on page 132*
Betnovate® [Can] *see* betamethasone (topical) *on page 132*
Betoptic® S [US/Can] *see* betaxolol *on page 133*

bevacizumab (be vuh SIZ uh mab)
Sound-Alike/Look-Alike Issues
bevacizumab may be confused with cetuximab
Synonyms anti-VEGF monoclonal antibody; NSC-704865; rhuMAb-VEGF
U.S./Canadian Brand Names Avastin® [US/Can]
Therapeutic Category Antineoplastic Agent, Monoclonal Antibody; Vaccine, Recombinant
Use Treatment of metastatic colorectal cancer; treatment of nonsquamous, nonsmall cell lung cancer; treatment of breast cancer (metastatic, HER-2 negative)
Usual Dosage I.V.: Adults: Details concerning dosing in combination regimens should also be consulted.
Breast cancer: 10 mg/kg every 2 weeks (in combination with paclitaxel)
Colorectal cancer: 5 or 10 mg/kg every 2 weeks (in combination with fluorouracil-based chemotherapy)
Lung cancer, nonsquamous cell nonsmall cell: 15 mg/kg every 3 weeks (in combination with carboplatin and paclitaxel)
Dosage Forms
Injection, solution [preservative free]:
Avastin®: 25 mg/mL (4 mL, 16 mL)

bexarotene (beks AIR oh teen)
U.S./Canadian Brand Names Targretin® [US/Can]
Therapeutic Category Retinoic Acid Derivative; Vitamin A Derivative; Vitamin, Fat Soluble
Use
Oral: Treatment of cutaneous manifestations of cutaneous T-cell lymphoma in patients who are refractory to at least one prior systemic therapy
Topical: Treatment of cutaneous lesions in patients with refractory cutaneous T-cell lymphoma (stage 1A and 1B) or who have not tolerated other therapies
Usual Dosage Adults:
Oral: 300-400 mg/m^2/day taken as a single daily dose.
Topical: Apply once every other day for first week, then increase on a weekly basis to once daily, 2 times/day, 3 times/day, and finally 4 times/day, according to tolerance
Dosage Forms
Capsule:
Targretin®: 75 mg
Gel:
Targretin®: 1% (60 g)

Bextra® *(Discontinued)*
Bexxar® [US] *see* tositumomab and iodine I 131 tositumomab *on page 937*

bezafibrate *(Canada only)* (be za FYE brate)
U.S./Canadian Brand Names Bezalip® [Can]; PMS-Bezafibrate [Can]
Therapeutic Category Antihyperlipidemic Agent, Miscellaneous
Use Adjunct to diet and other therapeutic measures for treatment of type IIa and IIb mixed hyperlipidemia, to regulate lipid and apoprotein levels (reduce serum TG, LDL-cholesterol, and apolipoprotein B, increase HDL-cholesterol and apolipoprotein A); treatment of adult patients with high to very high triglyceride levels (Fredrickson classification type IV and V hyperlipidemias) who are at high risk of sequelae and complications from their dyslipidemia
Usual Dosage Oral: Adults:
Immediate release: 200 mg 2-3 times/day; may reduce to 200 mg twice daily in patients with good response
Sustained release: 400 mg once daily

Dosage Forms [CAN] = Canadian brand name
   Tablet, immediate release: 200 mg [not available in the U.S.]
      PMA-Bezafibrate [CAN]: 200 mg [not available in the U.S.]
   Tablet, sustained release:
      Bezalip® [CAN]: 400 mg [not available in the U.S.]

Bezalip® [Can] *see* bezafibrate *(Canada only) on page 134*
BG 9273 *see* alefacept *on page 42*
Biavax® II *(Discontinued)*
Biaxin® [US/Can] *see* clarithromycin *on page 227*
Biaxin® XL [US/Can] *see* clarithromycin *on page 227*

bicalutamide (bye ka LOO ta mide)

Synonyms CDX; ICI-176334; NC-722665
U.S./Canadian Brand Names Casodex® [US/Can]; CO Bicalutamide [Can]; Gen-Bicalutamide [Can]; Novo-Bicalutamide [Can]; PHL-Bicalutamide [Can]; PMS-Bicalutamide [Can]; ratio-Bicalutamide [Can]; Sandoz-Bicalutamide [Can]
Therapeutic Category Androgen
Use In combination therapy with LHRH agonist analogues in treatment of metastatic prostate cancer
Usual Dosage Oral: Adults: Metastatic prostate cancer: 50 mg once daily (in combination with an LHRH analogue)
Dosage Forms
   Tablet:
      Casodex®: 50 mg

Bicillin® L-A [US/Can] *see* penicillin G benzathine *on page 731*
Bicillin® C-R [US] *see* penicillin G benzathine and penicillin G procaine *on page 731*
Bicillin® C-R 900/300 [US] *see* penicillin G benzathine and penicillin G procaine *on page 731*
BiCNU® [US/Can] *see* carmustine *on page 180*
Bidhist [US] *see* brompheniramine *on page 144*
BiDil® [US] *see* isosorbide dinitrate and hydralazine *on page 530*
BIG-IV *see* botulism immune globulin (intravenous-human) *on page 141*
Biltricide® [US/Can] *see* praziquantel *on page 779*

bimatoprost (bi MAT oh prost)

U.S./Canadian Brand Names Lumigan® [US/Can]
Therapeutic Category Ophthalmic Agent, Miscellaneous
Use Reduction of intraocular pressure (IOP) in patients with open-angle glaucoma or ocular hypertension
Usual Dosage Ophthalmic: Adults: Open-angle glaucoma or ocular hypertension: Instill 1 drop into affected eye(s) once daily in the evening; do not exceed once-daily dosing (may decrease IOP-lowering effect). If used with other topical ophthalmic agents, separate administration by at least 5 minutes.
Dosage Forms
   Solution, ophthalmic:
      Lumigan®: 0.03% (2.5 mL, 5 mL, 7.5 mL)

Biobase™ [Can] *see* alcohol (ethyl) *on page 41*
Biobase-G™ [Can] *see* alcohol (ethyl) *on page 41*
Bio-Carbamazepine [Can] *see* carbamazepine *on page 172*
Bioclate® *(Discontinued)* *see* antihemophilic factor (recombinant) *on page 79*
Biodine® *(Discontinued)* *see* povidone-iodine *on page 775*
Biolon™ *(Discontinued)* *see* hyaluronate and derivatives *on page 476*
Bionect® [US] *see* hyaluronate and derivatives *on page 476*
Bioniche Promethazine [Can] *see* promethazine *on page 791*
Bion® Tears [US-OTC] *see* artificial tears *on page 95*
Bio-Oxazepam [Can] *see* oxazepam *on page 706*
Biopatch® *(Discontinued)* *see* chlorhexidine gluconate *on page 201*
BioQuin® Durules™ [Can] *see* quinidine *on page 813*

Bio-Statin® [US] see nystatin *on page 690*

BioThrax™ [US] see anthrax vaccine, adsorbed *on page 78*

Biozyme-C® (Discontinued) see collagenase *on page 245*

biperiden (Discontinued)

Biphentin® [Can] see methylphenidate *on page 622*

bird flu vaccine see influenza virus vaccine (H5N1) *on page 509*

Bisac-Evac™ [US-OTC] see bisacodyl *on page 136*

bisacodyl (bis a KOE dil)

Sound-Alike/Look-Alike Issues
Doxidan® may be confused with doxepin

U.S./Canadian Brand Names Alophen® [US-OTC]; Apo-Bisacodyl® [Can]; Bisac-Evac™ [US-OTC]; Bisolax™ [US-OTC]; Carter's Little Pills® [Can]; Correctol® Tablets [US-OTC]; Dacodyl™ [US-OTC]; Doxidan® [US-OTC]; Dulcolax® [US-OTC/Can]; ex-lax® Ultra [US-OTC]; Fematrol [US-OTC]; Femilax™ [US-OTC]; Fleet® Bisacodyl [US-OTC]; Fleet® Stimulant Laxative [US-OTC]; Gentlax® [Can]; Veracolate [US-OTC]

Therapeutic Category Laxative

Use Treatment of constipation; colonic evacuation prior to procedures or examination

Usual Dosage
Children:
Oral: >6 years: 5-10 mg (0.3 mg/kg) at bedtime or before breakfast
Rectal suppository:
<2 years: 5 mg as a single dose
>2 years: 10 mg
Adults:
Oral: 5-15 mg as single dose (up to 30 mg when complete evacuation of bowel is required)
Rectal suppository: 10 mg as single dose

Dosage Forms
Solution, rectal [enema]:
Fleet® Bisacodyl [OTC]: 10 mg/30 mL (37 mL)
Suppository, rectal: 10 mg
Bisac-Evac™ [OTC], Biscolax™ [OTC], Dulcolax® [OTC]: 10 mg
Tablet [enteric coated]: 5 mg
Alophen® [OTC], Bisac-Evac™ [OTC], Correctol® [OTC], Dacodyl™ [OTC], Dulcolax® [OTC], ex-lax® Ultra [OTC], Fematrol [OTC], Femilax™ [OTC], Veracolate [OTC]: 5 mg
Tablet, delayed release: 5 mg
Doxidan® [OTC], Fleet® Stimulant Laxative [OTC]: 5 mg

Bisacodyl Uniserts® (Discontinued) see bisacodyl *on page 136*

bis-chloronitrosourea see carmustine *on page 180*

Bismatrol [US-OTC] see bismuth *on page 136*

Bismatrol Maximum Strength [US-OTC] see bismuth *on page 136*

bismuth (BIZ muth)

Sound-Alike/Look-Alike Issues
Kaopectate® may be confused with Kayexalate®

Synonyms bismuth subsalicylate; pink bismuth

U.S./Canadian Brand Names Bismatrol Maximum Strength [US-OTC]; Bismatrol [US-OTC]; Diotame® [US-OTC]; Kao-Tin [US-OTC]; Kaopectate® Extra Strength [US-OTC]; Kaopectate® [US-OTC]; Kapectolin [US-OTC]; Maalox® Total Stomach Relief® [US-OTC]; Peptic Relief [US-OTC]; Pepto Relief [US-OTC]; Pepto-Bismol® Maximum Strength [US-OTC]; Pepto-Bismol® [US-OTC]

Therapeutic Category Antidiarrheal

Use Subsalicylate formulation: Symptomatic treatment of mild, nonspecific diarrhea; control of traveler's diarrhea (enterotoxigenic *Escherichia coli*); as part of a multidrug regimen for *H. pylori* eradication to reduce the risk of duodenal ulcer recurrence

Usual Dosage Oral:
Treatment of nonspecific diarrhea, control/relieve traveler's diarrhea: Subsalicylate (doses based on 262 mg/15 mL liquid or 262 mg tablets):
Children: Up to 8 doses/24 hours:
  3-6 years: $1/3$ tablet or 5 mL every 30 minutes to 1 hour as needed
  6-9 years: $2/3$ tablet or 10 mL every 30 minutes to 1 hour as needed
  9-12 years: 1 tablet or 15 mL every 30 minutes to 1 hour as needed
  Children >12 years and Adults: 2 tablets or 30 mL every 30 minutes to 1 hour as needed up to 8 doses/ 24 hours
Helicobacter pylori eradication: Subsalicylate: Adults: 524 mg 4 times/day with meals and at bedtime; requires combination therapy

Dosage Forms
Caplet:
Kaopectate® [OTC]: 262 mg
Pepto-Bismol® [OTC]: 262 mg
Liquid: 262 mg/15 mL
Bismatrol [OTC], Diotame® [OTC], Kaopectate® [OTC], Kao-Tin [OTC], Peptic Relief [OTC], Pepto-Bismol® [OTC]: 262 mg/15 mL
Bismatrol Maximum Strength [OTC], Kaopectate® Extra Strength [OTC], Maalox® Total Stomach Relief® [OTC], Pepto-Bismol® Maximum Strength [OTC]: 525 mg/15 mL
Suspension: 262 mg/15 mL
Kapectolin [OTC]: 262 mg/15 mL
Tablet, chewable: 262 mg
Bismatrol [OTC], Diotame® [OTC], Peptic Relief [OTC], Pepto Relief [OTC], Pepto-Bismol® [OTC]: 262 mg

bismuth, metronidazole, and tetracycline
(BIZ muth, me troe NI da zole, & tet ra SYE kleen)
Synonyms bismuth subcitrate potassium, tetracycline, and metronidazole; bismuth subsalicylate, tetracycline, and metronidazole; metronidazole, bismuth subcitrate potassium, and tetracycline; metronidazole, bismuth subsalicylate, and tetracycline; tetracycline, metronidazole, and bismuth subcitrate potassium; tetracycline, metronidazole, and bismuth subsalicylate
U.S./Canadian Brand Names Helidac® [US]; Pylera™ [US]
Therapeutic Category Antidiarrheal
Use As part of a multidrug regimen for *H. pylori* eradication to reduce the risk of duodenal ulcer recurrence in combination with an H_2 agonist (Helidac®) or omeprazole (Pylera™)
Usual Dosage Oral: Adults:
Helidac®: Two bismuth subsalicylate 262.4 mg tablets, 1 metronidazole 250 mg tablet, and 1 tetracycline 500 mg capsule 4 times/day at meals and bedtime, plus an H_2 antagonist (at the appropriate dose) for 14 days; follow with 8 oz of water; the H_2 antagonist should be continued for a total of 28 days
Pylera™: Three capsules 4 times/day after meals and at bedtime, plus omeprazole 20 mg twice daily for 10 days; follow each dose with 8 oz of water (each capsule contains bismuth subcitrate potassium 140 mg, metronidazole 125 mg, and tetracycline 125 mg)
Dosage Forms
Capsule:
Pylera™: Bismuth subcitrate potassium 140 mg, metronidazole 125 mg, and tetracycline hydrochloride 125 mg
Combination package:
Helidac® [each package contains 14 blister cards (2-week supply); each card contains the following]:
Capsule: Tetracycline: 500 mg (4)
Tablet, chewable: Bismuth subsalicylate]: 262.4 mg (8)
Tablet: Metronidazole: 250 mg (4)

bismuth subcitrate potassium, tetracycline, and metronidazole *see* bismuth, metronidazole, and tetracycline *on page 137*
bismuth subsalicylate *see* bismuth *on page 136*
bismuth subsalicylate, tetracycline, and metronidazole *see* bismuth, metronidazole, and tetracycline *on page 137*
Bisolax™ [US-OTC] *see* bisacodyl *on page 136*

bisoprolol (bis OH proe lol)

Sound-Alike/Look-Alike Issues
Zebeta® may be confused with DiaBeta®, Zetia®
Synonyms bisoprolol fumarate
U.S./Canadian Brand Names Apo-Bisoprolol® [Can]; Monocor® [Can]; Novo-Bisoprolol [Can]; PMS-Bisoprolol [Can]; Sandoz-Bisoprolol [Can]; Zebeta® [US/Can]
Therapeutic Category Beta-Adrenergic Blocker
Use Treatment of hypertension, alone or in combination with other agents
Usual Dosage Oral: Adults: 2.5-5 mg once daily, may be increased to 10 mg, and then up to 20 mg once daily, if necessary
Hypertension (JNC 7): 2.5-10 mg once daily
Dosage Forms
  Tablet: 5 mg, 10 mg
  Zebeta®: 5 mg, 10 mg

bisoprolol and hydrochlorothiazide (bis OH proe lol & hye droe klor oh THYE a zide)

Sound-Alike/Look-Alike Issues
Ziac® may be confused with Tiazac®, Zerit®
Synonyms hydrochlorothiazide and bisoprolol
U.S./Canadian Brand Names Ziac® [US/Can]
Therapeutic Category Antihypertensive Agent, Combination
Use Treatment of hypertension
Usual Dosage Oral: Hypertension: Adults: Dose is individualized, given once daily
Dosage Forms
  Tablet: 2.5/6.25: Bisoprolol 2.5 mg and hydrochlorothiazide 6.25 mg; 5/6.25: Bisoprolol 5 mg and hydrochlorothiazide 6.25 mg; 10/6.25: Bisoprolol 10 mg and hydrochlorothiazide 6.25 mg
  Ziac®: 2.5/6.25: Bisoprolol 2.5 mg and hydrochlorothiazide 6.25 mg; 5/6.25: Bisoprolol 5 mg and hydrochlorothiazide 6.25 mg; 10/6.25: Bisoprolol 10 mg and hydrochlorothiazide 6.25 mg

bisoprolol fumarate see bisoprolol on page 138
bistropamide see tropicamide on page 957

bivalirudin (bye VAL i roo din)

Synonyms hirulog
U.S./Canadian Brand Names Angiomax® [US/Can]
Therapeutic Category Anticoagulant (Other)
Use Anticoagulant used in conjunction with aspirin for patients with unstable angina undergoing percutaneous transluminal coronary angioplasty (PTCA) or percutaneous coronary intervention (PCI) with provisional glycoprotein IIb/IIIa inhibitor; anticoagulant used in patients undergoing PCI with (or at risk of) heparin-induced thrombocytopenia (HIT) / thrombosis syndrome (HITTS)
Usual Dosage I.V.: Adults: Anticoagulant in patients undergoing PTCA/PCI or PCI with HITS/HITTS (treatment should be started just prior to procedure): Initial: Bolus: 0.75 mg/kg, followed by continuous infusion: 1.75 mg/kg/hour for the duration of procedure and up to 4 hours post-procedure if needed; determine ACT 5 minutes after bolus dose; may administer additional bolus of 0.3 mg/kg if necessary.
A glycoprotein IIb/IIIa inhibitor may be administered concomitantly during the procedure.
If needed, infusion may be continued beyond initial 4 hours at 0.2 mg/kg/hour for up to 20 hours.
Dosage Forms
  Injection, powder for reconstitution:
  Angiomax®: 250 mg

Bi-Zets [US] see benzocaine on page 124
BL4162A see anagrelide on page 75
Black-Draught Tablets [US-OTC] see senna on page 861
black widow spider species antivenin see antivenin (Latrodectus mactans) on page 83
BlemErase® Lotion (Discontinued) see benzoyl peroxide on page 126
Blenoxane® [US/Can] see bleomycin on page 139
bleo see bleomycin on page 139

bleomycin (blee oh MYE sin)

Sound-Alike/Look-Alike Issues
bleomycin may be confused with Cleocin®
Synonyms bleo; bleomycin sulfate; BLM; NSC-125066
U.S./Canadian Brand Names Blenoxane® [US/Can]; Bleomycin Injection, USP [Can]
Therapeutic Category Antineoplastic Agent
Use Treatment of squamous cell carcinomas, melanomas, sarcomas, testicular carcinoma, Hodgkin lymphoma, and non-Hodgkin lymphoma; sclerosing agent for malignant pleural effusion
Usual Dosage Maximum cumulative lifetime dose: 400 units; refer to individual protocols; 1 unit = 1 mg
May be administered I.M., I.V., SubQ, or intracavitary
Children and Adults:
Test dose for lymphoma patients: I.M., I.V., SubQ: Because of the possibility of an anaphylactoid reaction, administer 1-2 units of bleomycin before the first 1-2 doses; monitor vital signs every 15 minutes; wait a minimum of 1 hour before administering remainder of dose; if no acute reaction occurs, then the regular dosage schedule may be followed. **Note:** Test doses may produce false-negative results.
Single-agent therapy:
I.M./I.V./SubQ: Squamous cell carcinoma, lymphoma, testicular carcinoma: 0.25-0.5 units/kg (10-20 units/m^2) 1-2 times/week
CIV: 15 units/m^2 over 24 hours daily for 4 days
Pleural sclerosing: Intrapleural: 60 units as a single instillation (some recommend limiting the dose in the elderly to 40 units/m^2; usual maximum: 60 units). Dose may be repeated at intervals of several days if fluid continues to accumulate (mix in 50-100 mL of NS); may add lidocaine 100-200 mg to reduce local discomfort.
Dosage Forms
Injection, powder for reconstitution: 15 units, 30 units

Bleomycin Injection, USP [Can] *see* bleomycin *on page 139*
bleomycin sulfate *see* bleomycin *on page 139*
Bleph®-10 [US] *see* sulfacetamide *on page 892*
Blephamide® [US/Can] *see* sulfacetamide and prednisolone *on page 893*
Blis-To-Sol® [US-OTC] *see* tolnaftate *on page 934*
BLM *see* bleomycin *on page 139*
BMS-232632 *see* atazanavir *on page 100*
BMS-247550 *see* ixabepilone *on page 534*
BMS-337039 *see* aripiprazole *on page 93*
BMS-354825 *see* dasatinib *on page 268*
Boil-Ease® Pain Relieving [US] *see* benzocaine *on page 124*
Bonamine™ [Can] *see* meclizine *on page 595*
Bondronat® [Can] *see* ibandronate *on page 494*
Bonefos® [Can] *see* clodronate *(Canada only) on page 234*
Bonine® [US-OTC/Can] *see* meclizine *on page 595*
Boniva® [US] *see* ibandronate *on page 494*
Bontril® [Can] *see* phendimetrazine *on page 742*
Bontril PDM® [US] *see* phendimetrazine *on page 742*
Bontril® Slow-Release [US] *see* phendimetrazine *on page 742*
Boostrix® [US] *see* diphtheria, tetanus toxoids, and acellular pertussis vaccine *on page 309*

bortezomib (bore TEZ oh mib)

Synonyms LDP-341; MLN341; NSC-681239; PS-341
U.S./Canadian Brand Names Velcade® [US/Can]
Therapeutic Category Proteasome Inhibitor
Use Treatment of multiple myeloma; treatment of relapsed or refractory mantle cell lymphoma
Usual Dosage I.V.: Adults: Multiple myeloma, mantle cell lymphoma: 1.3 mg/m^2 twice weekly for 2 weeks on days 1, 4, 8, and 11 of a 21-day treatment cycle. Consecutive doses should be separated by at least 72 hours. Therapy extending beyond 8 cycles may be given once weekly for 4 weeks (days 1, 8, 15, and 22), followed by a 13-day rest (days 23 through 35).

◀ **Dosage Forms**
Injection, powder for reconstitution [preservative free]:
Velcade®: 3.5 mg

bosentan (boe SEN tan)

Sound-Alike/Look-Alike Issues
Tracleer® may be confused with TriCor©

U.S./Canadian Brand Names Tracleer® [US/Can]

Therapeutic Category Endothelin Antagonist

Use Treatment of pulmonary artery hypertension (PAH) (WHO Group I) in patients with World Health Organization (WHO) Class III or IV symptoms to improve exercise capacity and decrease the rate of clinical deterioration

Usual Dosage Oral: Adolescents >12 years and ≥40 kg and Adults: Initial: 62.5 mg twice daily for 4 weeks; increase to maintenance dose of 125 mg twice daily; adults <40 kg should be maintained at 62.5 mg twice daily. Doses >125 mg twice daily do not appear to confer additional clinical benefit but may increase risk of liver toxicity.

Note: When discontinuing treatment, consider a reduction in dosage to 62.5 mg twice daily for 3-7 days (to avoid clinical deterioration).

Dosage Forms
Tablet:
Tracleer®: 62.5 mg, 125 mg

B&O Supprettes® [US] see belladonna and opium on page 120
Botox® [US/Can] see botulinum toxin type A on page 140
Botox® Cosmetic [US/Can] see botulinum toxin type A on page 140

botulinum toxin type A (BOT yoo lin num TOKS in type aye)

Synonyms BTX-A

U.S./Canadian Brand Names Botox® Cosmetic [US/Can]; Botox® [US/Can]

Therapeutic Category Ophthalmic Agent, Toxin

Use Treatment of strabismus and blepharospasm associated with dystonia (including benign essential blepharospasm or VII nerve disorders) in patients ≥12 years of age; cervical dystonia (spasmodic torticollis) in patients ≥16 years of age; temporary improvement in the appearance of lines/wrinkles of the face (moderate-to-severe glabellar lines associated with corrugator and/or procerus muscle activity) in adult patients ≤65 years of age; treatment of severe primary axillary hyperhidrosis in adults not adequately controlled with topical treatments

Canadian labeling: Additional use (not in U.S. labeling): Focal spasticity, including treatment of stroke related upper limb spasticity; dynamic equines foot deformity in pediatric cerebral palsy patients

Usual Dosage

Cervical dystonia: Children ≥16 years and Adults: I.M.: For dosing guidance, the mean dose is 236 units (25th to 75th percentile range 198-300 units) divided among the affected muscles in patients previously treated with botulinum toxin. Initial dose in previously untreated patients should be lower. Sequential dosing should be based on the patient's head and neck position, localization of pain, muscle hypertrophy, patient response, and previous adverse reactions. The total dose injected into the sternocleidomastoid muscles should be ≤100 units to decrease the occurrence of dysphagia.

Blepharospasm: Children ≥12 years and Adults: I.M.: Initial dose: 1.25-2.5 units injected into the medial and lateral pretarsal orbicularis oculi of the upper and lower lid; dose may be increased up to twice the previous dose if the response from the initial dose lasted ≤2 months; maximum dose per site: 5 units; cumulative dose in a 30-day period: ≤200 units. Tolerance may occur if treatments are given more often than every 3 months, but the effect is not usually permanent.

Strabismus: Children ≥12 years and Adults: I.M.:
Initial dose:
Vertical muscles and for horizontal strabismus <20 prism diopters: 1.25-2.5 units in any one muscle
Horizontal strabismus of 20-50 prism diopters: 2.5-5 units in any one muscle
Persistent VI nerve palsy >1 month: 1.5-2.5 units in the medial rectus muscle
Reexamine patients 7-14 days after each injection to assess the effect of that dose. Subsequent doses for patients experiencing incomplete paralysis of the target may be increased up to twice the previous administered dose. The maximum recommended dose as a single injection for any one muscle is 25 units. Do not administer subsequent injections until the effects of the previous dose are gone.

Primary axillary hyperhidrosis: Adults ≥18 years: Intradermal: 50 units/axilla. Injection area should be defined by standard staining techniques. Injections should be evenly distributed into multiple sites (10-15), administered in 0.1-0.2 mL aliquots, ~1-2 cm apart.

Reduction of glabellar lines: Adults ≤65 years: I.M.: An effective dose is determined by gross observation of the patient's ability to activate the superficial muscles injected. The location, size and use of muscles may vary markedly among individuals. Inject 0.1 mL dose into each of five sites, two in each corrugator muscle and one in the procerus muscle (total dose 0.5 mL).

Dosage Forms

Injection, powder for reconstitution [preservative free]:
Botox®, Botox® Cosmetic: *Clostridium botulinum* toxin type A 100 units

botulinum toxin type B (BOT yoo lin num TOKS in type bee)

U.S./Canadian Brand Names Myobloc® [US]

Therapeutic Category Neuromuscular Blocker Agent, Toxin

Use Treatment of cervical dystonia (spasmodic torticollis)

Usual Dosage I.M.: Adults: Cervical dystonia: Initial: 2500-5000 units divided among the affected muscles in patients **previously treated** with botulinum toxin; initial dose in **previously untreated** patients should be lower. Subsequent dosing should be optimized according to patient's response.

Dosage Forms

Injection, solution [preservative free]:
Myobloc®: 5000 units/mL (0.5 mL, 1 mL, 2 mL)

botulism immune globulin (intravenous-human)

(BOT yoo lism i MYUN GLOB you lin, in tra VEE nus, YU man)

Sound-Alike/Look-Alike Issues

BabyBIG® may be confused with HBIG

Synonyms BIG-IV

U.S./Canadian Brand Names BabyBIG® [US]

Therapeutic Category Immune Globulin

Use Treatment of infant botulism caused by toxin type A or B

Usual Dosage I.V.: Children <1 year: Infant botulism: 1 mL/kg (50 mg/kg) as a single dose; infuse at 0.5 mL/kg/hour (25 mg/kg/hour) for the first 15 minutes; if well tolerated, may increase to 1 mL/kg/hour (50 mg/kg/hour)

Dosage Forms

Injection, powder for reconstitution [preservative free]:
BabyBIG® [OTC]: ~100 mg

Boudreaux's® Butt Paste [US-OTC] *see* zinc oxide *on page 993*

bovine lung surfactant *see* beractant *on page 129*

Bravelle® [US/Can] *see* urofollitropin *on page 964*

Breathe Free® [US-OTC] *see* sodium chloride *on page 873*

Breezee® Mist Antifungal *(Discontinued)* *see* miconazole *on page 630*

Breonesin® *(Discontinued)* *see* guaifenesin *on page 453*

Brethaire® *(Discontinued)* *see* terbutaline *on page 910*

Brevibloc® [US/Can] *see* esmolol *on page 357*

Brevicon® [US] *see* ethinyl estradiol and norethindrone *on page 376*

Brevicon® 0.5/35 [Can] *see* ethinyl estradiol and norethindrone *on page 376*

Brevicon® 1/35 [Can] *see* ethinyl estradiol and norethindrone *on page 376*

Brevital® [Can] *see* methohexital *on page 615*

Brevital® Sodium [US] *see* methohexital *on page 615*

Brevoxyl® [US] *see* benzoyl peroxide *on page 126*

Brevoxyl® Cleansing [US] *see* benzoyl peroxide *on page 126*

Brevoxyl® Wash [US] *see* benzoyl peroxide *on page 126*

Bricanyl® [Can] *see* terbutaline *on page 910*

Bricanyl® *(Discontinued)* *see* terbutaline *on page 910*

brimonidine (bri MOE ni deen)
Sound-Alike/Look-Alike Issues
  brimonidine may be confused with bromocriptine
Synonyms brimonidine tartrate
U.S./Canadian Brand Names Alphagan® P [US]; Alphagan® [Can]; Apo-Brimonidine® [Can]; PMS-Brimonidine Tartrate [Can]; ratio-Brimonidine [Can]; Sandoz-Brimonidine [Can]
Therapeutic Category Alpha$_2$-Adrenergic Agonist Agent, Ophthalmic
Use Lowering of intraocular pressure (IOP) in patients with open-angle glaucoma or ocular hypertension
Usual Dosage Ophthalmic: Children ≥2 years of age and Adults: Glaucoma: Instill 1 drop in affected eye(s) 3 times/day (approximately every 8 hours)
Dosage Forms
  Solution, ophthalmic: 0.2% (5 mL, 10 mL, 15 mL)
    Alphagan® P: 0.1% (5 mL, 10 mL, 15 mL); 0.15% (5 mL, 10 mL, 15 mL)

brimonidine and timolol (bri MOE ni deen & TIM oh lol)
Synonyms brimonidine tartrate and timolol maleate; timolol and brimonidine
U.S./Canadian Brand Names Combigan™ [US/Can]
Therapeutic Category Alpha$_2$ Agonist, Ophthalmic; Beta Blocker, Nonselective; Ophthalmic Agent, Antiglaucoma
Use Reduction of intraocular pressure (IOP) in patients with glaucoma or ocular hypertension
Usual Dosage Ophthalmic: Children ≥2 years and Adults: Instill 1 drop into affected eye(s) twice daily
  Note: In the Canadian labeling, use in children (at any age) is not recommended.
Dosage Forms [CAN] = Canadian availability
  Solution, ophthalmic [drops]:
    Combigan™: Brimonidine 0.2% and timolol 0.5% (5 mL, 10 mL)
    Combigan® [CAN]: Brimonidine 0.2% and timolol 0.5% (2.5 mL, 5 mL, 10 mL)

brimonidine tartrate *see brimonidine on page 142*
brimonidine tartrate and timolol maleate *see brimonidine and timolol on page 142*

brinzolamide (brin ZOH la mide)
U.S./Canadian Brand Names Azopt® [US/Can]
Therapeutic Category Carbonic Anhydrase Inhibitor
Use Lowers intraocular pressure in patients with ocular hypertension or open-angle glaucoma
Usual Dosage Ophthalmic: Adults: Instill 1 drop in affected eye(s) 3 times/day
Dosage Forms
  Suspension, ophthalmic:
    Azopt®: 1% (10 mL, 15 mL)

Brioschi® [US-OTC] *see sodium bicarbonate on page 872*
British anti-lewisite *see dimercaprol on page 302*
BRL 43694 *see granisetron on page 452*
Bromaline® [US-OTC] *see brompheniramine and pseudoephedrine on page 144*
Bromaline® DM [US-OTC] *see brompheniramine, pseudoephedrine, and dextromethorphan on page 146*
Bromarest® (Discontinued) *see brompheniramine on page 144*
Bromatane DX [US] *see brompheniramine, pseudoephedrine, and dextromethorphan on page 146*
Bromaxefed RF (Discontinued) *see brompheniramine and pseudoephedrine on page 144*

bromazepam (Canada only) (broe MA ze pam)
U.S./Canadian Brand Names Apo-Bromazepam® [Can]; Gen-Bromazepam [Can]; Lectopam® [Can]; Novo-Bromazepam [Can]; Nu-Bromazepam [Can]; Pro Doc Limitee Bromazepam [Can]
Therapeutic Category Benzodiazepine; Sedative
Use Short-term, symptomatic treatment of anxiety
Usual Dosage Oral: Adults: Initial: 6-18 mg/day in equally divided doses; initial course of treatment should not last longer than 1 week; optimal dosage range: 6-30 mg/day

Dosage Forms [CAN] = Canadian brand name
  Tablet: 1.5 mg, 3 mg, 6 mg [not available in the U.S.]
    Apo-Bromazepam® [CAN], Gen-Bromazepam [CAN], Lectopam® [CAN], Novo-Bromazepam [CAN],
    Nu-Bromazepam [CAN]: 1.5 mg, 3 mg, 6 mg [not available in the U.S.]

Brombay® *(Discontinued)* *see* brompheniramine *on page 144*
Brometane DX [US] *see* brompheniramine, pseudoephedrine, and dextromethorphan *on page 146*
Bromfed® *(Discontinued)* *see* brompheniramine and pseudoephedrine *on page 144*
Bromfed-PD® *(Discontinued)* *see* brompheniramine and pseudoephedrine *on page 144*

bromfenac (BROME fen ak)

Synonyms bromfenac sodium
U.S./Canadian Brand Names Xibrom™ [US]
Therapeutic Category Analgesic, Nonnarcotic; Nonsteroidal Antiinflammatory Drug (NSAID), Ophthalmic
Use Treatment of postoperative inflammation and reduction in ocular pain following cataract removal
Usual Dosage Ophthalmic: Adults: Instill 1 drop into affected eye(s) twice daily beginning 24 hours after surgery and continuing for 2 weeks postoperatively
Dosage Forms
  Solution, ophthalmic:
    Xibrom™: 0.09% (2.5 mL, 5 mL)

bromfenac sodium *see* bromfenac *on page 143*
Bromfenex® *(Discontinued)* *see* brompheniramine and pseudoephedrine *on page 144*
Bromfenex® PD *(Discontinued)* *see* brompheniramine and pseudoephedrine *on page 144*
Bromhist DM [US] *see* brompheniramine, pseudoephedrine, and dextromethorphan *on page 146*
Bromhist-NR [US] *see* brompheniramine and pseudoephedrine *on page 144*
Bromhist PDX [US] *see* brompheniramine, pseudoephedrine, and dextromethorphan *on page 146*
Bromhist Pediatric [US] *see* brompheniramine and pseudoephedrine *on page 144*

bromocriptine (broe moe KRIP teen)

Sound-Alike/Look-Alike Issues
  bromocriptine may be confused with benztropine, brimonidine
  Parlodel® may be confused with pindolol, Provera®
Synonyms bromocriptine mesylate
U.S./Canadian Brand Names Apo-Bromocriptine® [Can]; Parlodel® SnapTabs® [US]; Parlodel® [US/Can]; PMS-Bromocriptine [Can]
Therapeutic Category Anti-Parkinson Agent (Dopamine Agonist); Ergot Alkaloid and Derivative
Use Treatment of hyperprolactinemia associated with amenorrhea with or without galactorrhea, infertility, or hypogonadism; treatment of prolactin-secreting adenomas; treatment of acromegaly; treatment of Parkinson disease
Usual Dosage Oral:
  Children: Hyperprolactinemia:
    11-15 years (based on limited information): Initial: 1.25-2.5 mg daily; dosage may be increased as tolerated to achieve a therapeutic response (range: 2.5-10 mg daily).
    ≥16 years: Refer to adult dosing
  Adults:
    Parkinsonism: 1.25 mg twice daily, increased by 2.5 mg/day in 2- to 4-week intervals (usual dose range is 30-90 mg/day in 3 divided doses; maximum: 100 mg/day), though elderly patients can usually be managed on lower doses
    Acromegaly: Initial: 1.25-2.5 mg daily increasing by 1.25-2.5 mg daily as necessary every 3-7 days; usual dose: 20-30 mg/day (maximum: 100 mg/day)
    Hyperprolactinemia: Initial: 1.25-2.5 mg/day; may be increased by 2.5 mg/day as tolerated every 2-7 days until optimal response (range: 2.5-15 mg/day)
Dosage Forms
  Capsule: 5 mg
    Parlodel®: 5 mg
  Tablet: 2.5 mg
    Parlodel® SnapTabs®: 2.5 mg

bromocriptine mesylate *see bromocriptine on page 143*

Bromphen® *(Discontinued)* *see brompheniramine on page 144*

Bromphenex DM [US] *see brompheniramine, pseudoephedrine, and dextromethorphan on page 146*

brompheniramine (brome fen IR a meen)

Synonyms brompheniramine maleate; brompheniramine tannate

U.S./Canadian Brand Names B-Vex [US]; Bidhist [US]; BroveX™ CT [US]; BroveX™ [US]; Lodrane® 12 Hour [US]; Lodrane® 24 [US]; Lodrane® XR [US]; LoHist-12 [US]; TanaCof-XR [US]

Therapeutic Category Antihistamine

Use Symptomatic relief of perennial and seasonal allergic rhinitis, vasomotor rhinitis, and other respiratory allergies

Usual Dosage Allergic rhinitis, allergic symptoms, vasomotor rhinitis: Oral:

Children:

1-2 years (B-Vex, BroveX™): 1.25 mL every 12 hours (maximum: 2.5 mL/day)

2-6 years:

B-Vex, BroveX™: 2.5 mL every 12 hours (maximum: 5 mL/day)

BroveX™ CT: 1/2 tablet every 12 hours (maximum: 1 tablet/day)

Lodrane® XR, TanaCof-XR: 1.25 mL every 12 hours (maximum: 2.5 mL/day)

6-12 years:

B-Vex, BroveX™: 5 mL every 12 hours (maximum: 10 mL/day)

BroveX™ CT: 1/2 to 1 tablet every 12 hours (maximum: 2 tablets/day)

Lodrane® 12 Hour, LoHist-12: One tablet every 12 hours (maximum: 2 tablets/day)

Lodrane® 24: One capsule once daily

Lodrane® XR, TanaCof-XR: 2.5 mL every 12 hours (maximum: 5 mL/day)

>12 years (B-Vex, BroveX™, BroveX™ CT, Lodrane® 12 Hour, Lodrane® 24, Lodrane® XR, LoHist-12, TanaCof-XR): Refer to adult dosing

Adults:

B-Vex, BroveX™: 5-10 mL every 12 hours (maximum: 20 mL/day)

BroveX™ CT: 1-2 tablets every 12 hours (maximum: 4 tablets/day)

Lodrane® 12 Hour, LoHist: 1-2 tablets every 12 hours (maximum: 4 tablets/day)

Lodrane® 24: 1-2 capsules once daily

Lodrane® XR, TanaCof-XR: 5 mL every 12 hours (maximum: 10 mL/day)

Dosage Forms

Capsule, extended release:

Lodrane® 24: 12 mg [dye free]

Suspension, as tannate:

B-Vex, BroveX™: 12 mg/5 mL

Lodrane® XR: 8 mg/5 mL

TanaCof-XR: 8 mg/5 mL

Tablet, chewable: 12 mg

BroveX™ CT: 12 mg [banana flavor]

Tablet, extended release:

Bidhist: 6 mg

Tablet, extended release [scored]:

Lodrane® 12 Hour, LoHist-12: 6 mg [dye free]

Tablet, timed release: 6 mg

brompheniramine and pseudoephedrine (brome fen IR a meen & soo doe e FED rin)

Sound-Alike/Look-Alike Issues

Bromfed® may be confused with Bromphen®

Synonyms brompheniramine maleate and pseudoephedrine hydrochloride; brompheniramine maleate and pseudoephedrine sulfate; pseudoephedrine and brompheniramine

U.S./Canadian Brand Names AccuHist® [US]; Andehist NR Syrup [US]; Bromaline® [US-OTC]; Bromhist Pediatric [US]; Bromhist-NR [US]; Brotapp [US]; Brovex SR [US]; Dimaphen [US-OTC]; Histex® SR [US]; Lodrane® 12D [US]; Lodrane® 24D [US]; Lodrane® D [US]; LoHist 12D [US]; LoHist LQ [US]; LoHist PD [US]; Respahist® [US]; Sildec Syrup [US]; Touro® Allergy [US]

Therapeutic Category Antihistamine/Decongestant Combination

Use Temporary relief of symptoms of seasonal and perennial allergic rhinitis, and vasomotor rhinitis, including nasal obstruction

Usual Dosage Oral:
Capsule, long acting:
  Based on 60 mg pseudoephedrine:
    Children 6-12 years: 1 capsule every 12 hours
    Children ≥12 years and Adults: 1-2 capsules every 12 hours
  Based on 120 mg pseudoephedrine: Children ≥12 years and Adults: 1 capsule every 12 hours
Liquid:
  Based on brompheniramine 1 mg/pseudoephedrine 15 mg per 1 mL: Children:
    1-3 months: 0.25 mL 4 times/day
    3-6 months: 0.5 mL 4 times/day
    6-12 months: 0.75 mL 4 times/day
    12-24 months: 1 mL 4 times/day
  Based on brompheniramine 1 mg/pseudoephedrine 15 mg per 5 mL: Children:
    6-11 months (6-8 kg): 2.5 mL every 6-8 hours (maximum: 4 doses/24 hours)
    12-23 months (8-10 kg): 3.75 mL every 6-8 hours (maximum: 4 doses/24 hours)
    2-6 years: 5 mL every 6-8 hours (maximum: 4 doses/24 hours)
    6-12 years: 10 mL every 6-8 hours (maximum: 4 doses/24 hours)
    >12 years and Adults: 20 mL every 4 hours (maximum: 4 doses/24 hours)
  Based on brompheniramine 4 mg/pseudoephedrine 30 mg:
    Children 2-6 years: 2.5 mL 3 times/day
    Children >6 years and Adults: 5 mL 3 times/day
  Brompheniramine 4 mg/pseudoephedrine 45 mg per 5 mL:
    Children 2-6 years: 2.5 mL 4 times/day
    Children >6 years and Adults: 5 mL 4 times/day
Tablet, extended release: Based on pseudoephedrine 45 mg:
  Children 6-12 years: 1 tablet every 12 hours
  Children ≥12 years and Adults: 1-2 tablets every 12 hours

Dosage Forms
Caplet, extended release:
  Histex® SR: Brompheniramine 10 mg and pseudoephedrine 120 mg
Capsule, extended release:
  Lodrane® 24D: Brompheniramine 12 mg and pseudoephedrine 90 mg
Capsule, sustained release:
  Brovex SR: Brompheniramine 9 mg and pseudoephedrine 90 mg
  Respahist®: Brompheniramine 6 mg and pseudoephedrine 60 mg
Elixir:
  Dimaphen: Brompheniramine 1 mg and pseudoephedrine 15 mg per 5 mL
Liquid: Brompheniramine 4 mg and pseudoephedrine 60 mg per 5 mL (480 mL)
  Brotapp: Brompheniramine 1 mg and pseudoephedrine 15 mg per 5 mL
  LoHist LQ: Brompheniramine 4 mg and pseudoephedrine 60 mg per 5 mL
Liquid, oral [drops]:
  AccuHist®, Bromhist NR, LoHist LQ: Brompheniramine 1 mg and pseudoephedrine 12.5 mg per 1 mL
  Bromhist Pediatric: Brompheniramine 1 mg and pseudoephedrine 15 mg per 1 mL
Solution:
  Bromaline® [OTC]: Brompheniramine 1 mg and pseudoephedrine 15 mg per 5 mL
Suspension:
  Lodrane® D: Brompheniramine 8 mg and pseudoephedrine 90 mg per 5 mL
Syrup:
  Andehist NR, Sildec: Brompheniramine 4 mg and pseudoephedrine 45 mg per 5 mL
Tablet, extended release:
  Lodrane® 12D, LoHist 12D: Brompheniramine 6 mg and pseudoephedrine 45 mg
Tablet, prolonged release:
  Touro® Allergy: Brompheniramine 6 mg and pseudoephedrine 45 mg
Tablet, sustained release: Brompheniramine 6 mg and pseudoephedrine 45 mg

brompheniramine maleate *see brompheniramine on page 144*

brompheniramine maleate and pseudoephedrine hydrochloride *see brompheniramine and pseudoephedrine on page 144*

brompheniramine maleate and pseudoephedrine sulfate *see brompheniramine and pseudoephedrine on page 144*

brompheniramine, pseudoephedrine, and dextromethorphan
(brome fen IR a meen, soo doe e FED rin, & deks troe meth OR fan)

Synonyms dextromethorphan hydrobromide, brompheniramine maleate, and pseudoephedrine hydrochloride; pseudoephedrine tannate, dextromethorphan tannate, and brompheniramine tannate

U.S./Canadian Brand Names AccuHist® PDX Drops [US]; AllanHist PDX [US]; Anaplex® DM [US]; Anaplex® DMX [US]; Andehist DM NR [US]; Bromaline® DM [US-OTC]; Bromatane DX [US]; Brometane DX [US]; Bromhist DM [US]; Bromhist PDX [US]; Bromphenex DM [US]; Bromplex DX [US]; Brotapp-DM [US]; Carbofed DM [US]; EndaCof-DM [US]; EndaCof-PD [US]; Histacol™ BD [US]; Myphetane DX [US]; PediaHist DM [US]

Therapeutic Category Antihistamine; Cough Preparation; Decongestant

Use Relief of cough and upper respiratory symptoms (including nasal congestion) associated with allergy or the common cold

Usual Dosage
Children:
1-3 months (AccuHist® PDX, EndaCof-PD): 0.25 mL 4 times/day
3-6 months (AccuHist® PDX, EndaCof-PD): 0.5 mL 4 times/day
6-12 months (AccuHist® PDX, EndaCof-PD): 0.75 mL 4 times/day
12-24 months (AccuHist® PDX, EndaCof-PD): 1 mL 4 times/day
2-6 years:
Anaplex® DM, EndaCof-DM: 1.25 mL every 4-6 hours (maximum: 4 doses/24 hours)
Anaplex® DMX: 1.25 mL every 12 hours (maximum: 2.5 mL/24 hours)
6-12 years:
Anaplex® DM, EndaCof-DM: 2.5 mL every 4-6 hours (maximum: 4 doses/24 hours)
Anaplex® DMX: 2.5 mL every 12 hours (maximum: 5 mL/24 hours)
Bromaline® DM: 10 mL every 4-6 hours (maximum: 4 doses/24 hours)
Children ≥12 years and Adults:
Anaplex® DM: 5 mL every 4-6 hours (maximum: 4 doses/24 hours)
Anaplex® DMX: 5 mL every 12 hours (maximum: 10 mL/24 hours)
Bromaline® DM: 20 mL every 4-6 hours (maximum: 4 doses/24 hours)

Dosage Forms
Elixir:
Bromaline® DM [OTC]: Brompheniramine 1 mg, pseudoephedrine 15 mg, and dextromethorphan 5 mg per 5 mL
Liquid:
Bromplex DM: Brompheniramine 4 mg, pseudoephedrine 60 mg, and dextromethorphan 30 mg per 5 mL
Brotapp-DM: Brompheniramine 1 mg, pseudoephedrine 15 mg, and dextromethorphan 5 mg per 5 mL
Solution, oral [drops]:
AccuHist® PDX, AllanHist PDX, Bromhist PDX, EndaCof-PD, Histacol™ BD: Brompheniramine 1 mg, pseudoephedrine 12.5 mg, and dextromethorphan 3 mg per 1 mL
Bromhist DM, PediaHist DM: Brompheniramine 1 mg, pseudoephedrine 15 mg, and dextromethorphan 4 mg per 1 mL
Suspension: Brompheniramine 8 mg, pseudoephedrine 90 mg, and dextromethorphan 60 mg per 5 mL
Anaplex® DMX: Brompheniramine 8 mg, pseudoephedrine 90 mg, and dextromethorphan 60 mg per 5 mL
Syrup:
Anaplex® DM, Bromphenex DM, EndaCof-DM: Brompheniramine 4 mg, pseudoephedrine 60 mg, and dextromethorphan 30 mg per 5 mL
Andehist DM NR, Carbofed DM, Sildec-DM: Brompheniramine 4 mg, pseudoephedrine 45 mg, and dextromethorphan 15 mg per 5 mL
Bromatane DX, Myphetane DX: Brompheniramine 2 mg, pseudoephedrine 30 mg, and dextromethorphan 10 mg per 5 mL

brompheniramine tannate *see brompheniramine on page 144*

Brompheril® (Discontinued) *see dexbrompheniramine and pseudoephedrine on page 279*

Bromplex DX [US] *see brompheniramine, pseudoephedrine, and dextromethorphan on page 146*

Bronchial® (Discontinued) *see theophylline and guaifenesin on page 919*

Bronchial Mist® (Discontinued) *see epinephrine on page 344*

Broncho Saline® (Discontinued) *see sodium chloride on page 873*

Bronitin® Mist (Discontinued) *see epinephrine on page 344*

Brontex® [US] *see* guaifenesin and codeine *on page 454*
Brotane® (Discontinued) *see* brompheniramine *on page 144*
Brotapp [US] *see* brompheniramine and pseudoephedrine *on page 144*
Brotapp-DM [US] *see* brompheniramine, pseudoephedrine, and dextromethorphan *on page 146*
Brovana® [US] *see* arformoterol *on page 92*
BroveX™ [US] *see* brompheniramine *on page 144*
BroveX™ CT [US] *see* brompheniramine *on page 144*
Brovex SR [US] *see* brompheniramine and pseudoephedrine *on page 144*
BSF208075 *see* ambrisentan *on page 57*
BSS® [US/Can] *see* balanced salt solution *on page 115*
BSS Plus® [US/Can] *see* balanced salt solution *on page 115*
B-Tuss™ [US] *see* phenylephrine, hydrocodone, and chlorpheniramine *on page 748*
BTX-A *see* botulinum toxin type A *on page 140*
B-type natriuretic peptide (human) *see* nesiritide *on page 665*
Bubbli-Pred™ [US] *see* prednisolone (systemic) *on page 781*
Budeprion XL® [US] *see* bupropion *on page 152*
Budeprion™ SR [US] *see* bupropion *on page 152*

budesonide (byoo DES oh nide)

U.S./Canadian Brand Names Entocort® EC [US]; Entocort® [Can]; Gen-Budesonide AQ [Can]; Pulmicort Flexhaler™ [US]; Pulmicort Respules® [US]; Pulmicort® [Can]; Rhinocort® Aqua® [US/Can]; Rhinocort® Turbuhaler® [Can]
Therapeutic Category Adrenal Corticosteroid
Use
Intranasal: Management of symptoms of seasonal or perennial rhinitis
Nebulization: Maintenance and prophylactic treatment of asthma
Oral capsule: Treatment of active Crohn disease (mild-to-moderate) involving the ileum and/or ascending colon; maintenance of remission (for up to 3 months) of Crohn disease (mild-to-moderate) involving the ileum and/or ascending colon
Oral inhalation: Maintenance and prophylactic treatment of asthma; includes patients who require oral corticosteroids and those who may benefit from systemic dose reduction/elimination
Usual Dosage
Nasal inhalation: (Rhinocort® Aqua®): Rhinitis: Children ≥6 years and Adults: 64 mcg/day as a single 32 mcg spray in each nostril. Some patients who do not achieve adequate control may benefit from increased dosage. A reduced dosage may be effective after initial control is achieved.
Maximum dose: Children <12 years: 128 mcg/day; Adults: 256 mcg/day

Nebulization: Children 12 months to 8 years: Asthma: Pulmicort Respules®: Titrate to lowest effective dose once patient is stable; start at 0.25 mg/day or use as follows:
Previous therapy of bronchodilators alone: 0.5 mg/day administered as a single dose or divided twice daily (maximum daily dose: 0.5 mg)
Previous therapy of inhaled corticosteroids: 0.5 mg/day administered as a single dose or divided twice daily (maximum daily dose: 1 mg)
Previous therapy of oral corticosteroids: 1 mg/day administered as a single dose or divided twice daily (maximum daily dose: 1 mg)
NIH Asthma Guidelines (NIH, 2007):
Children 0-4 years:
"Low" dose: 0.25-0.5 mg/day
"Medium" dose: >0.5-1 mg/day
"High" dose: >1 mg/day
Children 5-11 years:
"Low" dose: 0.5 mg/day
"Medium" dose: 1 mg/day
"High" dose: 2 mg/day

Oral inhalation: Asthma:
Children ≥6 years:
Pulmicort Flexhaler™: Initial: 180 mcg twice daily (some patients may be initiated at 360 mcg twice daily); maximum 360 mcg twice daily

◄ *NIH Asthma Guidelines (NIH, 2007)* (administer in divided doses twice daily):
Children 5-11 years:
"Low" dose: 180-400 mcg/day
"Medium" dose: >400-800 mcg/day
"High" dose: >800 mcg/day
Children ≥12 years: Refer to adult dosing.
Adults:
Pulmicort Flexhaler™: Initial: 360 mcg twice daily (selected patients may be initiated at 180 mcg twice daily); maximum 720 mcg twice daily
NIH Asthma Guidelines (NIH, 2007) (administer in divided doses twice daily):
"Low" dose: 180-600 mcg/day
"Medium" dose: >600-1200 mcg/day
"High" dose: >1200 mcg/day

Oral: Crohn disease (active): Adults: 9 mg once daily in the morning for up to 8 weeks; recurring episodes may be treated with a repeat 8-week course of treatment
Note: Patients receiving CYP3A4 inhibitors should be monitored closely for signs and symptoms of hypercorticism; dosage reduction may be required. If switching from oral prednisolone, prednisolone dosage should be tapered while budesonide (Entocort™ EC) treatment is initiated.
Maintenance of remission: Following treatment of active disease (control of symptoms with CDAI <150), treatment may be continued at a dosage of 6 mg once daily for up to 3 months. If symptom control is maintained for 3 months, tapering of the dosage to complete cessation is recommended. Continued dosing beyond 3 months has not been demonstrated to result in substantial benefit.

Dosage Forms [CAN] = Canadian brand name
Capsule, enteric coated:
Entocort® EC: 3 mg
Powder for nasal inhalation:
Rhinocort® Turbuhaler® [CAN]: 100 mcg/inhalation [not available in the U.S.]
Powder for oral inhalation:
Pulmicort Flexhaler™: 90 mcg/inhalation (165 mg)
Pulmicort Flexhaler™: 180 mcg/inhalation (225 mg)
Pulmicort Turbuhaler® [CAN]: 100 mcg/inhalation, 200 mcg/inhalation, 400 mcg/inhalation [not available in the U.S.]
Suspension, intranasal [spray]:
Rhinocort® Aqua®: 32 mcg/inhalation (8.6 g)
Rhinocort® Aqua® [CAN]: 64 mcg/inhalation [not available in the U.S.]
Suspension for nebulization:
Pulmicort Respules®: 0.25 mg/2 mL, 0.5 mg/2 mL, 1 mg/2 mL

budesonide and eformoterol *see* budesonide and formoterol *on page 148*

budesonide and formoterol (byoo DES oh nide & for MOH te rol)

Synonyms budesonide and eformoterol; eformoterol and budesonide; formoterol fumarate dehydrate and budesonide
U.S./Canadian Brand Names Symbicort® [US/Can]
Therapeutic Category Beta₂-Adrenergic Agonist Agent; Corticosteroid, Inhalant (Oral)
Use Treatment of asthma in patients ≥12 years of age where combination therapy is indicated
Usual Dosage Oral inhalation:
Children 5-11 years (NIH Guidelines): Symbicort® 80/4.5: 2 inhalations twice daily. Do not exceed 4 inhalations per day.
Children ≥12 years and Adults: Symbicort® 80/4.5, Symbicort® 160/4.5: 2 inhalations twice daily. Patients currently receiving a low-to-medium dose inhaled corticosteroid may be started on the lower strength combination; those receiving a medium-to-high dose inhaled corticosteroid may be started on the higher strength combination. Consider the higher dose combination for patients not adequately controlled on the lower combination following 1-2 weeks of therapy. Do not use more than 2 inhalations twice daily of either strength.
Dosage Forms [CAN] = Canadian product
Aerosol for oral inhalation:
Symbicort® 80/4.5: Budesonide 80 mcg and formoterol fumarate dihydrate 4.5 mcg per actuation (6.9 g) [60 metered inhalations]; budesonide 80 mcg and formoterol fumarate dihydrate 4.5 mcg per actuation (10.2 g) [120 metered inhalations]

Symbicort® 160/4.5: Budesonide 160 mcg and formoterol fumarate dihydrate 4.5 mcg per actuation (6 g) [60 metered inhalations]; budesonide 160 mcg and formoterol fumarate dihydrate 4.5 mcg per actuation (10.2 g) [120 metered inhalations]

Powder for oral inhalation:

Symbicort® 100 Turbuhaler® [CAN]: Budesonide 100 mcg and formoterol dihydrate 6 mcg per inhalation (available in 60 or 120 metered doses) [delivers ~80 mcg budesonide and 4.5 mcg formoterol per inhalation; contains lactose] [not available in the U.S]

Symbicort® 200 Turbuhaler® [CAN]: Budesonide 200 mcg and formoterol dihydrate 6 mcg per inhalation (available in 60 or 120 metered doses) [delivers ~160 mcg budesonide and 4.5 mcg formoterol per inhalation; contains lactose] [not available in the U.S]

Buffasal [US-OTC] see aspirin on page 98
Bufferin® [US-OTC] see aspirin on page 98
Bufferin® Extra Strength [US-OTC] see aspirin on page 98
Buffinol [US-OTC] see aspirin on page 98
Bulk-K [US-OTC] see psyllium on page 804

bumetanide (byoo MET a nide)

Sound-Alike/Look-Alike Issues
bumetanide may be confused with Buminate®
Bumex® may be confused with Brevibloc®, Buprenex®, Permax®

U.S./Canadian Brand Names Bumex® [US/Can]; Burinex® [Can]

Therapeutic Category Diuretic, Loop

Use Management of edema secondary to congestive heart failure or hepatic or renal disease including nephrotic syndrome; may be used alone or in combination with antihypertensives in the treatment of hypertension; can be used in furosemide-allergic patients

Usual Dosage

Oral, I.M., I.V.:

Neonates: 0.01-0.05 mg/kg/dose every 24-48 hours

Infants and Children: 0.015-0.1 mg/kg/dose every 6-24 hours (maximum dose: 10 mg/day)

Adults:

Edema:

Oral: 0.5-2 mg/dose (maximum dose: 10 mg/day) 1-2 times/day

I.M., I.V.: 0.5-1 mg/dose; may repeat in 2-3 hours for up to 2 doses if needed (maximum dose: 10 mg/day)

Continuous I.V. infusion: Initial: 1 mg I.V. load then 0.5-2 mg/hour (ACC/AHA 2005 practice guidelines for chronic heart failure)

Hypertension: Oral: 0.5 mg daily (maximum dose: 5 mg/day); usual dosage range (JNC 7): 0.5-2 mg/day in 2 divided doses

Dosage Forms

Injection, solution: 0.25 mg/mL (2 mL, 4 mL, 10 mL)

Tablet: 0.5 mg, 1 mg, 2 mg

Bumex®: 1 mg

Bumex® [US/Can] see bumetanide on page 149
Bumex® Injection (Discontinued) see bumetanide on page 149
Buminate® [US] see albumin on page 38
Bupap [US] see butalbital and acetaminophen on page 155
Buphenyl® [US] see sodium phenylbutyrate on page 877

bupivacaine (byoo PIV a kane)

Sound-Alike/Look-Alike Issues
bupivacaine may be confused with mepivacaine, ropivacaine
Marcaine® may be confused with Narcan®

Synonyms bupivacaine hydrochloride

U.S./Canadian Brand Names Marcaine® Spinal [US]; Marcaine® [US/Can]; Sensorcaine® [US/Can]; Sensorcaine®-MPF Spinal [US]; Sensorcaine®-MPF [US]

Therapeutic Category Local Anesthetic

Use Local anesthetic (injectable) for peripheral nerve block, infiltration, sympathetic block, caudal or epidural block, retrobulbar block

▶

◀ **Usual Dosage** Dose varies with procedure, depth of anesthesia, vascularity of tissues, duration of anesthesia, and condition of patient. Do not use solutions containing preservatives for caudal or epidural block.

Children >12 years and Adults:

Local anesthesia: Infiltration: 0.25% infiltrated locally; maximum: 175 mg

Caudal block (preservative free): 15-30 mL of 0.25% or 0.5%

Epidural block (other than caudal block; preservative free): Administer in 3-5 mL increments, allowing sufficient time to detect toxic manifestations of inadvertent I.V. or I.T. administration: 10-20 mL of 0.25% or 0.5%

Surgical procedures requiring a high degree of muscle relaxation and prolonged effects **only**: 10-20 mL of 0.75% (**Note:** Not to be used in obstetrical cases)

Peripheral nerve block: 5 mL of 0.25% or 0.5%; maximum: 400 mg/day

Sympathetic nerve block: 20-50 mL of 0.25%

Retrobulbar anesthesia: 2-4 mL of 0.75%

Adults: Spinal anesthesia: Preservative free solution of 0.75% bupivacaine in 8.25% dextrose:

Lower extremity and perineal procedures: 1 mL

Lower abdominal procedures: 1.6 mL

Normal vaginal delivery: 0.8 mL (higher doses may be required in some patients)

Cesarean section: 1-1.4 mL

Dosage Forms

Injection, solution [preservative free]: 0.25% (10 mL, 20 mL, 30 mL, 50 mL); 0.5% (10 mL, 20 mL, 30 mL); 0.75% (10 mL, 20 mL, 30 mL)

Marcaine® [OTC]: 0.25% (10 mL, 30 mL); 0.5% (10 mL, 30 mL); 0.75% (10 mL, 30 mL)

Sensorcaine®-MPF [OTC]: 0.25% (10 mL, 30 mL); 0.5% (10 mL, 30 mL); 0.75% (10 mL, 30 mL)

Injection, solution [preservative free]: 0.75% (2 mL)

Marcaine® Spinal [OTC]: 0.75% (2 mL)

Sensorcaine®-MPF Spinal [OTC]: 0.75% (2 mL)

Injection, solution:

Marcaine® [OTC], Sensorcaine® [OTC]: 0.25% (50 mL); 0.5% (50 mL)

bupivacaine and epinephrine (byoo PIV a kane & ep i NEF rin)

Synonyms epinephrine bitartrate and bupivacaine hydrochloride

U.S./Canadian Brand Names Marcaine® with Epinephrine [US]; Sensorcaine® with Epinephrine [US/Can]; Sensorcaine®-MPF with Epinephrine [US]; Vivacaine™ [US]

Therapeutic Category Local Anesthetic

Use Local anesthetic (injectable) for peripheral nerve block, infiltration, sympathetic block, caudal or epidural block, retrobulbar block

Usual Dosage Dose varies with procedure, depth of anesthesia, vascularity of tissues, duration of anesthesia, and condition of patient. Do not use solutions containing preservatives for caudal or epidural block.

Children >12 years and Adults:

Caudal block (preservative free): 15-30 mL of 0.25% or 0.5%

Epidural block (other than caudal block, preservative free): 10-20 mL of 0.25% or 0.5%. Administer in 3-5 mL increments, allowing sufficient time to detect toxic manifestations of inadvertent I.V. or I.T. administration.

Surgical procedures requiring a high degree of muscle relaxation and prolonged effects only: 10-20 mL of 0.75% (**Note:** Not to be used in obstetrical cases)

Local anesthesia: Infiltration: 0.25% infiltrated locally (maximum: 175 mg of bupivacaine)

Peripheral nerve block: 5 mL of 0.25 or 0.5% (maximum: 400 mg/day of bupivacaine)

Retrobulbar anesthesia: 2-4 mL of 0.75%

Sympathetic nerve block: 20-50 mL of 0.25%

Infiltration and nerve block in maxillary and mandibular area: 9 mg (1.8 mL) of bupivacaine as a 0.5% solution with epinephrine 1:200,000 per injection site. A second dose may be administered if necessary to produce adequate anesthesia after allowing up to 10 minutes for onset. Up to a maximum of 90 mg of bupivacaine hydrochloride per dental appointment. The effective anesthetic dose varies with procedure, intensity of anesthesia needed, duration of anesthesia required, and physical condition of the patient; always use the lowest effective dose along with careful aspiration.

Dosage Forms

Injection, solution [preservative free]: Bupivacaine 0.25% and epinephrine 1:200,000 (10 mL, 30 mL); bupivacaine 0.5% and epinephrine 1:200,000 (1.8 mL, 10 mL, 30 mL)

Marcaine® with Epinephrine: Bupivacaine 0.25% and epinephrine 1:200,000 (10 mL, 30 mL); bupivacaine 0.5% and epinephrine 1:200,000 (1.8 mL, 3 mL, 10 mL, 30 mL); bupivacaine 0.75% and epinephrine 1:200,000 (30 mL)

Sensorcaine® MPF with Epinephrine: Bupivacaine 0.25% and epinephrine 1:200,000 (10 mL, 30 mL); bupivacaine 0.5% and epinephrine 1:200,000 (10 mL, 30 mL)

Vivacaine™: Bupivacaine hydrochloride 0.5% and epinephrine bitartrate 1:200,000

Injection, solution: Bupivacaine 0.25% and epinephrine 1:200,000 (50 mL); bupivacaine 0.5% and epinephrine 1:200,000 (50 mL)

Marcaine® with Epinephrine: Bupivacaine 0.25% and epinephrine 1:200,000 (50 mL); bupivacaine 0.5% and epinephrine 1:200,000 (50 mL)

Sensorcaine® with Epinephrine: Bupivacaine 0.25% and epinephrine 1:200,000 (50 mL); bupivacaine 0.5% and epinephrine 1:200,000 (50 mL)

bupivacaine and lidocaine see lidocaine and bupivacaine on page 563
bupivacaine hydrochloride see bupivacaine on page 149
Buprenex® [US/Can] see buprenorphine on page 151

buprenorphine (byoo pre NOR feen)

Sound-Alike/Look-Alike Issues
Buprenex® may be confused with Brevibloc®, Bumex®
Synonyms buprenorphine hydrochloride
U.S./Canadian Brand Names Buprenex® [US/Can]; Subutex® [US/Can]
Therapeutic Category Analgesic, Narcotic
Controlled Substance Injection: C-V/C-III; Tablet: C-III
Use
Injection: Management of moderate to severe pain
Tablet: Treatment of opioid dependence
Usual Dosage Long-term use is not recommended
Note: These are guidelines and do not represent the maximum doses that may be required in all patients. Doses should be titrated to pain relief/prevention. In high-risk patients (eg, elderly, debilitated, presence of respiratory disease) and/or concurrent CNS depressant use, reduce dose by one-half. Buprenorphine has an analgesic ceiling.

Acute pain (moderate to severe):
Children 2-12 years: I.M., slow I.V.: 2-6 mcg/kg every 4-6 hours
Children ≥13 years and Adults:
I.M.: Initial: Opiate-naive: 0.3 mg every 6-8 hours as needed; initial dose (up to 0.3 mg) may be repeated once in 30-60 minutes after the initial dose if needed; usual dosage range: 0.15-0.6 mg every 4-8 hours as needed
Slow I.V.: Initial: Opiate-naive: 0.3 mg every 6-8 hours as needed; initial dose (up to 0.3 mg) may be repeated once in 30-60 minutes after the initial dose if needed
Sublingual: Children ≥16 years and Adults: Opioid dependence:
Induction: Range: 12-16 mg/day (doses during an induction study used 8 mg on day 1, followed by 16 mg on day 2; induction continued over 3-4 days). Treatment should begin at least 4 hours after last use of heroin or short-acting opioid, preferably when first signs of withdrawal appear. Titrating dose to clinical effectiveness should be done as rapidly as possible to prevent undue withdrawal symptoms and patient drop-out during the induction period.
Maintenance: Target dose: 16 mg/day; range: 4-24 mg/day; patients should be switched to the buprenorphine/naloxone combination product for maintenance and unsupervised therapy
Dosage Forms
Injection, solution: 0.3 mg/mL (1 mL)
Buprenex®: 0.3 mg/mL (1 mL)
Tablet, sublingual:
Subutex®: 2 mg, 8 mg

buprenorphine and naloxone (byoo pre NOR feen & nal OKS one)

Synonyms buprenorphine hydrochloride and naloxone hydrochloride dihydrate; naloxone and buprenorphine; naloxone hydrochloride dihydrate and buprenorphine hydrochloride
U.S./Canadian Brand Names Suboxone® [US]
Therapeutic Category Analgesic, Narcotic

◀ **Controlled Substance** C-III

Use Treatment of opioid dependence

Usual Dosage Sublingual: Children ≥16 years and Adults: Opioid dependence: **Note:** This combination product is not recommended for use during the induction period; initial treatment should begin using buprenorphine oral tablets. Patients should be switched to the combination product for maintenance and unsupervised therapy.

Maintenance: Target dose (based on buprenorphine content): 16 mg/day; range: 4-24 mg/day

Dosage Forms

Tablet, sublingual:

Suboxone®: Buprenorphine 2 mg and naloxone 0.5 mg; buprenorphine 8 mg and naloxone 2 mg

buprenorphine hydrochloride *see* buprenorphine *on page 151*

buprenorphine hydrochloride and naloxone hydrochloride dihydrate *see* buprenorphine and naloxone *on page 151*

Buproban™ [US] *see* bupropion *on page 152*

bupropion (byoo PROE pee on)

Sound-Alike/Look-Alike Issues

buPROPion may be confused with busPIRone

Wellbutrin SR® may be confused with Wellbutrin XL™

Wellbutrin XL™ may be confused with Wellbutrin SR®

Zyban® may be confused with Zagam®, Diovan®

Tall-Man buPROPion

U.S./Canadian Brand Names Budeprion XL® [US]; Budeprion™ SR [US]; Buproban™ [US]; Novo-Bupropion SR [Can]; Wellbutrin SR® [US]; Wellbutrin XL™ [US/Can]; Wellbutrin® [US/Can]; Zyban® [US/Can]

Therapeutic Category Antidepressant, Aminoketone

Use Treatment of major depressive disorder, including seasonal affective disorder (SAD); adjunct in smoking cessation

Usual Dosage Oral: Adults:

Depression:

Immediate release: 100 mg 3 times/day; begin at 100 mg twice daily; may increase to a maximum dose of 450 mg/day

Sustained release: Initial: 150 mg/day in the morning; may increase to 150 mg twice daily by day 4 if tolerated; target dose: 300 mg/day given as 150 mg twice daily; maximum dose: 400 mg/day given as 200 mg twice daily

Extended release: Initial: 150 mg/day in the morning; may increase as early as day 4 of dosing to 300 mg/day; maximum dose: 450 mg/day

SAD (Wellbutrin XL™): Initial: 150 mg/day in the morning; if tolerated, may increase after 1 week to 300 mg/day

Note: Prophylactic treatment should be reserved for those patients with frequent depressive episodes and/or significant impairment. Initiate treatment in the Autumn prior to symptom onset, and discontinue in early Spring with dose tapering to 150 mg/day for 2 weeks

Smoking cessation (Zyban®): Initiate with 150 mg once daily for 3 days; increase to 150 mg twice daily; treatment should continue for 7-12 weeks

Dosage Forms

Tablet: 75 mg [generic for Wellbutrin®], 100 mg [generic for Wellbutrin®]

Wellbutrin®: 75 mg, 100 mg

Tablet, extended release: 100 mg [generic for Wellbutrin® SR], 150 mg [generic for Wellbutrin® SR], 150 mg [generic for Zyban®], 200 mg [generic for Wellbutrin® SR], 300 mg [generic for Wellbutrin XL™]

Budeprion™ SR: 100 mg [generic for Wellbutrin® SR], 150 mg [generic for Wellbutrin® SR]

Budeprion XL®: 150 mg, 300 mg [generic for Wellbutrin® XL]

Buproban™: 150 mg [generic for Zyban®]

Wellbutrin XL™: 150 mg, 300 mg

Tablet, sustained release: 100 mg [generic for Wellbutrin® SR], 150 mg [generic for Wellbutrin® SR], 150 mg [generic for Zyban®], 200 mg [generic for Wellbutrin® SR]

Wellbutrin® SR: 100 mg, 150 mg, 200 mg

Zyban®: 150 mg

Burinex® [Can] *see* bumetanide *on page 149*

Burnamycin [US-OTC] *see* lidocaine *on page 561*

Burn Jel® [US-OTC] *see* lidocaine *on page 561*
Burn-O-Jel [US-OTC] *see* lidocaine *on page 561*
Buscopan® [Can] *see* scopolamine derivatives *on page 858*

buserelin acetate *(Canada only)* (BYOO se rel in AS e tate)

Sound-Alike/Look-Alike Issues
    Suprefact® may be confused with Suprane®

U.S./Canadian Brand Names Suprefact® Depot [Can]; Suprefact® [Can]

Therapeutic Category Luteinizing Hormone-Releasing Hormone Analog

Use Palliative treatment in patients with hormone-dependent advanced prostate cancer (stage D); treatment of endometriosis in women who do not require surgical intervention as first-line therapy (length of therapy is usually 6 months, but no longer than 9 months)

Usual Dosage Adults:
    Prostate cancer: **Note:** Administration of an antiandrogen agent beginning 7 days prior to initiation of buserelin therapy and continuing for ~5 weeks with buserelin therapy is recommended in patients with prostate cancer.
    SubQ:
        Suprefact®: Initial: 500 mcg every 8 hours for 7 days. Maintenance: 200 mcg once daily
        Suprefact Depot®
            2-month: 6.3 mg implant injected into lateral abdominal wall every 8 weeks
            3-month: 9.45 mg injected into lateral abdominal wall every 12 weeks
        Intranasal (Suprefact®): Maintenance: 400 mcg (200 mcg into each nostril) 3 times/day
    Endometriosis: Intranasal (Suprefact®): 400 mcg (200 mcg into each nostril) 3 times/day for 6-9 months

Dosage Forms [CAN] = Canadian brand name
Injection, solution:
    Suprefact® [CAN]: 1 mg/mL (5.5 mL, 10 mL) [not available in U.S.]
Solution, intranasal:
    Suprefact® [CAN]: 1mg/1mL (10 mL) [not available in U.S.]
Implant, subcutaneous:
    Suprefact® [CAN] Depot: 6.3 mg, 9.45 mg [not available in U.S.]

BuSpar® [US/Can] *see* buspirone *on page 153*
Buspirex [Can] *see* buspirone *on page 153*

buspirone (byoo SPYE rone)

Sound-Alike/Look-Alike Issues
    busPIRone may be confused with buPROPion

Synonyms buspirone hydrochloride

Tall-Man busPIRone

U.S./Canadian Brand Names Apo-Buspirone® [Can]; BuSpar® [US/Can]; Buspirex [Can]; Bustab® [Can]; CO Buspirone [Can]; Dom-Buspirone [Can]; Gen-Buspirone [Can]; Lin-Buspirone [Can]; Novo-Buspirone [Can]; Nu-Buspirone [Can]; PMS-Buspirone [Can]; ratio-Buspirone [Can]; Riva-Buspirone [Can]

Therapeutic Category Antianxiety Agent

Use Management of generalized anxiety disorder (GAD)

Usual Dosage Oral:
    Generalized anxiety disorder:
        Children ≥6 years and Adolescents: Initial: 5 mg daily; increase in increments of 5 mg/day at weekly intervals as needed, to a maximum dose of 60 mg/day divided into 2-3 doses
        Adults: 15 mg/day (7.5 mg twice daily); may increase in increments of 5 mg/day every 2-3 days to a maximum of 60 mg/day; target dose for most people is 20-30 mg/day (10-15 mg twice daily)

Dosage Forms
Tablet: 5 mg, 7.5 mg, 10 mg, 15 mg, 30 mg
    BuSpar®: 5 mg, 10 mg, 15 mg, 30 mg

buspirone hydrochloride *see* buspirone *on page 153*
Bustab® [Can] *see* buspirone *on page 153*

busulfan (byoo SUL fan)

Sound-Alike/Look-Alike Issues
busulfan may be confused with Butalan®
Myleran® may be confused with Leukeran®, melphalan, Mylicon®

Synonyms NSC-750

U.S./Canadian Brand Names Busulfex® [US/Can]; Myleran® [US/Can]

Therapeutic Category Antineoplastic Agent

Use

Oral: Chronic myelogenous leukemia (CML); conditioning regimens for bone marrow transplantation
I.V.: Combination therapy with cyclophosphamide as a conditioning regimen prior to allogeneic hematopoietic progenitor cell transplantation for chronic myelogenous leukemia

Usual Dosage Note: Premedicate with prophylactic anticonvulsant therapy (eg, phenytoin) prior to high-dose busulfan treatment.

Children:

CML, remission induction: Oral: 0.06-0.12 mg/kg/day **or** 1.8-4.6 mg/m^2/day; titrate dosage to maintain leukocyte count above 40,000/mm^3; reduce dosage by 50% if the leukocyte count reaches 30,000-40,000/mm^3; discontinue drug if counts fall to ≤20,000/mm^3

BMT marrow-ablative conditioning regimen:
Oral: 1 mg/kg/dose (ideal body weight) every 6 hours for 16 doses
I.V.:
≤12 kg: 1.1 mg/kg/dose (ideal body weight) every 6 hours for 16 doses
>12 kg: 0.8 mg/kg/dose (ideal body weight) every 6 hours for 16 doses
Adjust dose to desired AUC [1125 µmol(min)] using the following formula:
Adjusted dose (mg) = Actual dose (mg) x [target AUC µmol(min) / actual AUC µmol(min)]

Adults:

CML, remission induction: Oral: 60 mcg/kg/day or 1.8 mg/m^2/day; usual range: 4-8 mg/day (may be as high as 12 mg/day); Maintenance doses: 1-4 mg/day to 2 mg/week to maintain WBC 10,000-20,000 cells/mm^3

BMT marrow-ablative conditioning regimen:
Oral: 1 mg/kg/dose (ideal body weight) every 6 hours for 16 doses
I.V.: 0.8 mg/kg (ideal body weight or actual body weight, whichever is lower); for obese or severely-obese patients adjusted ideal body weight is recommended) every 6 hours for 4 days (a total of 16 doses)

Dosage Forms

Injection, solution:
Busulfex®: 6 mg/mL (10 mL)
Tablet:
Myleran®: 2 mg

Busulfex® [US/Can] *see busulfan* *on page 154*

butabarbital (byoo ta BAR bi tal)

Sound-Alike/Look-Alike Issues
butabarbital may be confused with butalbital

U.S./Canadian Brand Names Butisol Sodium® [US]

Therapeutic Category Barbiturate

Controlled Substance C-III

Use Sedative; hypnotic

Usual Dosage Oral:

Children: Preoperative sedation: 2-6 mg/kg/dose (maximum: 100 mg)
Adults:
Sedative: 15-30 mg 3-4 times/day
Hypnotic: 50-100 mg at bedtime. When used for insomnia, treatment should be limited since barbiturates lose effectiveness for sleep induction and maintenance after 2 weeks.
Preop: 50-100 mg 1-1^1/$_2$ hours before surgery

Dosage Forms

Elixir:
Butisol Sodium®: 30 mg/5 mL
Tablet:
Butisol Sodium®: 30 mg, 50 mg

Butalan® *(Discontinued)*

butalbital, acetaminophen, and caffeine
(byoo TAL bi tal, a seet a MIN oh fen, & KAF een)

Sound-Alike/Look-Alike Issues
Fioricet® may be confused with Fiorinal®, Lorcet®
Repan® may be confused with Riopan®

Synonyms acetaminophen, butalbital, and caffeine

U.S./Canadian Brand Names Anolor 300 [US]; Dolgic® LQ [US]; Dolgic® Plus [US]; Esgic-Plus™ [US]; Esgic® [US]; Fioricet® [US]; Medigesic® [US]; Repan® [US]; Zebutal™ [US]

Therapeutic Category Barbiturate/Analgesic

Use Relief of the symptomatic complex of tension or muscle contraction headache

Usual Dosage Oral: Adults: 1-2 tablets or capsules (or 15-30 mL solution) every 4 hours; not to exceed 6 tablets or capsules (or 180 mL solution) daily

Dosage Forms
Capsule:
Anolor 300, Esgic®, Medigesic®: Butalbital 50 mg, acetaminophen 325 mg, and caffeine 40 mg
Dolgic® Plus: Butalbital 50 mg, acetaminophen 750 mg, and caffeine 40 mg
Esgic-Plus™, Zebutal™: Butalbital 50 mg, acetaminophen 500 mg, and caffeine 40 mg
Solution:
Dolgic® LQ: Butalbital 50 mg, acetaminophen 325 mg, and caffeine 40 mg per 15 mL
Tablet: Butalbital 50 mg, acetaminophen 325 mg, and caffeine 40 mg; butalbital 50 mg, acetaminophen 500 mg, and caffeine 40 mg
Esgic®, Fioricet®, Repan®: Butalbital 50 mg, acetaminophen 325 mg, and caffeine 40 mg
Esgic-Plus™: Butalbital 50 mg, acetaminophen 500 mg, and caffeine 40 mg

butalbital, acetaminophen, caffeine, and codeine
(byoo TAL bi tal, a seet a MIN oh fen, KAF een, & KOE deen)

Sound-Alike/Look-Alike Issues
Fioricet® may be confused with Fiorinal®, Florinef®, Lorcet®, Percocet®
Phrenilin® may be confused with Phenergan®, Trinalin®

Synonyms acetaminophen, caffeine, codeine, and butalbital; caffeine, acetaminophen, butalbital, and codeine; codeine, acetaminophen, butalbital, and caffeine

U.S./Canadian Brand Names Fioricet® with Codeine [US]; Phrenilin® with Caffeine and Codeine [US]

Therapeutic Category Analgesic Combination (Opioid); Barbiturate

Controlled Substance C-III

Use Relief of symptoms of complex tension (muscle contraction) headache

Usual Dosage Oral: Adults: 1-2 capsules every 4 hours. Total daily dosage should not exceed 6 capsules.

Dosage Forms
Capsule: Butalbital 50 mg, acetaminophen 325 mg, caffeine 40 mg, and codeine 30 mg
Fioricet® with Codeine: Butalbital 50 mg, acetaminophen 325 mg, caffeine 40 mg, and codeine 30 mg
Phrenilin® with Caffeine and Codeine: Butalbital 50 mg, acetaminophen 325 mg, caffeine 40 mg, and codeine 30 mg

butalbital and acetaminophen (byoo TAL bi tal & a seet a MIN oh fen)

Synonyms acetaminophen and butalbital

U.S./Canadian Brand Names Bupap [US]; Cephadyn [US]; Phrenilin® Forte [US]; Phrenilin® [US]; Promacet [US]; Sedapap® [US]

Therapeutic Category Analgesic, Miscellaneous; Barbiturate

Use Relief of the symptomatic complex of tension or muscle contraction headache

Usual Dosage Oral: Adults: One tablet/capsule every 4 hours as needed (maximum dose: 6 tablets/day)
Phrenilin®: 1-2 tablets every 4 hours as needed (maximum 6 tablets in 24 hours)

Dosage Forms
Tablet:
Phrenilin®: Butalbital 50 mg and acetaminophen 325 mg
Bupap, Cephadyn, Promacet, Sedapap®: Butalbital 50 mg and acetaminophen 650 mg
Capsule:
Phrenilin® Forte: Butalbital 50 mg and acetaminophen 650 mg

butalbital, aspirin, and caffeine (byoo TAL bi tal, AS pir in, & KAF een)

Sound-Alike/Look-Alike Issues
Fiorinal® may be confused with Fioricet®, Florical®, Florinef®

Synonyms aspirin, caffeine, and butalbital; butalbital compound

U.S./Canadian Brand Names Fiorinal® [US/Can]

Therapeutic Category Barbiturate/Analgesic

Controlled Substance C-III

Use Relief of the symptomatic complex of tension or muscle contraction headache

Usual Dosage Oral: Adults: 1-2 tablets or capsules every 4 hours; not to exceed 6 tablets/day

Dosage Forms
Capsule: Butalbital 50 mg, aspirin 325 mg, and caffeine 40 mg
Fiorinal®: Butalbital 50 mg, aspirin 325 mg, and caffeine 40 mg
Tablet: Butalbital 50 mg, aspirin 325 mg, and caffeine 40 mg

butalbital, aspirin, caffeine, and codeine
(byoo TAL bi tal, AS pir in, KAF een, & KOE deen)

Sound-Alike/Look-Alike Issues
Fiorinal® may be confused with Fioricet®, Florical®, Florinef®

Synonyms aspirin, caffeine, codeine, and butalbital; butalbital compound and codeine; codeine and butalbital compound; codeine, butalbital, aspirin, and caffeine

U.S./Canadian Brand Names Ascomp® with Codeine [US]; Fiorinal® With Codeine [US]; Fiorinal®-C 1/2 [Can]; Fiorinal®-C 1/4 [Can]; Tecnal C 1/2 [Can]; Tecnal C 1/4 [Can]

Therapeutic Category Analgesic, Narcotic; Barbiturate

Controlled Substance C-III

Use Relief of symptoms of complex tension (muscle contraction) headache

Usual Dosage Oral: Adults: 1-2 capsules every 4 hours as needed (maximum: 6 capsules/day)

Dosage Forms
Capsule: Butalbital 50 mg, aspirin 325 mg, caffeine 40 mg, and codeine 30 mg
Ascomp® with Codeine, Fiorinal® with Codeine: Butalbital 50 mg, aspirin 325 mg, caffeine 40 mg, and codeine 30 mg

butalbital compound see butalbital, aspirin, and caffeine on page 156
butalbital compound and codeine see butalbital, aspirin, caffeine, and codeine on page 156
butamben, tetracaine, and benzocaine see benzocaine, butamben, and tetracaine on page 126

butenafine (byoo TEN a feen)

Sound-Alike/Look-Alike Issues
Lotrimin® may be confused with Lotrisone®, Otrivin®

Synonyms butenafine hydrochloride

U.S./Canadian Brand Names Lotrimin® Ultra™ [US-OTC]; Mentax® [US]

Therapeutic Category Antifungal Agent

Use Topical treatment of tinea pedis (athlete's foot), tinea cruris (jock itch), tinea corporis (ringworm), and tinea versicolor

Usual Dosage Topical: Children >12 years and Adults:
Tinea corporis, tinea cruris (Lotrimin® Ultra™): Apply once daily for 2 weeks to affected area and surrounding skin
Tinea versicolor (Mentax®): Apply once daily for 2 weeks to affected area and surrounding skin
Tinea pedis (Lotrimin® Ultra™): Apply to affected skin between and around the toes, twice daily for 1 week, or once daily for 4 weeks

Dosage Forms
Cream:
Lotrimin® Ultra™ [OTC]: 1% (12 g, 24 g)
Mentax®: 1% (15 g, 30 g)

butenafine hydrochloride see butenafine on page 156
Buticaps® *(Discontinued)*
Butisol Sodium® [US] see butabarbital on page 154

butoconazole (byoo toe KOE na zole)

Synonyms butoconazole nitrate
U.S./Canadian Brand Names Femstat® One [Can]; Gynazole-1® [US/Can]
Therapeutic Category Antifungal Agent
Use Local treatment of vulvovaginal candidiasis
Usual Dosage Adults: Female: Gynazole-1®: Insert 1 applicatorful (~5 g) intravaginally as a single dose; treatment may need to be extended for up to 6 days in pregnant women (use in pregnancy during 2nd or 3rd trimester only)
Dosage Forms
  Cream, vaginal:
    Gynazole-1®: 2% (5 g)

butoconazole nitrate *see butoconazole on page 157*

butorphanol (byoo TOR fa nole)

Sound-Alike/Look-Alike Issues
  Stadol® may be confused with Haldol®, sotalol
Synonyms butorphanol tartrate
U.S./Canadian Brand Names Apo-Butorphanol® [Can]; PMS-Butorphanol [Can]
Therapeutic Category Analgesic, Narcotic
Controlled Substance C-IV
Use
  Parenteral: Management of moderate-to-severe pain; preoperative medication; supplement to balanced anesthesia; management of pain during labor
  Nasal spray: Management of moderate-to-severe pain, including migraine headache pain
Usual Dosage Note: These are guidelines and do not represent the maximum doses that may be required in all patients. Doses should be titrated to pain relief/prevention. Butorphanol has an analgesic ceiling.
Adults:
  Parenteral:
    Acute pain (moderate-to-severe):
      I.M.: Initial: 2 mg, may repeat every 3-4 hours as needed; usual range: 1-4 mg every 3-4 hours as needed
      I.V.: Initial: 1 mg, may repeat every 3-4 hours as needed; usual range: 0.5-2 mg every 3-4 hours as needed
    Preoperative medication: I.M.: 2 mg 60-90 minutes before surgery
    Supplement to balanced anesthesia: I.V.: 2 mg shortly before induction and/or an incremental dose of 0.5-1 mg (up to 0.06 mg/kg), depending on previously administered sedative, analgesic, and hypnotic medications
    Pain during labor (fetus >37 weeks gestation and no signs of fetal distress):
      I.M., I.V.: 1-2 mg; may repeat in 4 hours
      Note: Alternative analgesia should be used for pain associated with delivery or if delivery is anticipated within 4 hours.
  Nasal spray:
    Moderate-to-severe pain (including migraine headache pain): Initial: 1 spray (~1 mg per spray) in 1 nostril; if adequate pain relief is not achieved within 60-90 minutes, an additional 1 spray in 1 nostril may be given; may repeat initial dose sequence in 3-4 hours after the last dose as needed
    Alternatively, an initial dose of 2 mg (1 spray in each nostril) may be used in patients who will be able to remain recumbent (in the event drowsiness or dizziness occurs); additional 2 mg doses should not be given for 3-4 hours
    Note: In some clinical trials, an initial dose of 2 mg (as 2 doses 1 hour apart or 2 mg initially - 1 spray in each nostril) has been used, followed by 1 mg in 1 hour; side effects were greater at these dosages
Dosage Forms
  Injection, solution [preservative free]: 1 mg/mL (1 mL); 2 mg/mL (1 mL, 2 mL)
  Injection, solution [with preservative]: 2 mg/mL (10 mL)
  Solution, intranasal [spray]: 10 mg/mL (2.5 mL)

butorphanol tartrate *see butorphanol on page 157*
B-Vex [US] *see brompheniramine on page 144*
B vitamin combinations *see vitamin B complex combinations on page 981*
BW-430C *see lamotrigine on page 545*

BW524W91 *see* emtricitabine *on page 338*

Byclomine® Injection *(Discontinued)* *see* dicyclomine *on page 293*

Bydramine® Cough Syrup *(Discontinued)* *see* diphenhydramine *on page 304*

Byetta® [US] *see* exenatide *on page 386*

Bystolic™ [US] *see* nebivolol *on page 659*

C1H *see* alemtuzumab *on page 43*

C2B8 monoclonal antibody *see* rituximab *on page 839*

C7E3 *see* abciximab *on page 17*

C8-CCK *see* sincalide *on page 868*

311C90 *see* zolmitriptan *on page 995*

C225 *see* cetuximab *on page 197*

cabergoline (ca BER goe leen)

U.S./Canadian Brand Names CO Cabergoline [Can]; Dostinex® [Can]

Therapeutic Category Ergot-like Derivative

Use Treatment of hyperprolactinemic disorders, either idiopathic or due to pituitary adenomas

Usual Dosage Oral: Initial dose: 0.25 mg twice weekly; the dose may be increased by 0.25 mg twice weekly up to a maximum of 1 mg twice weekly according to the patient's serum prolactin level. Dosage increases should not occur more rapidly than every 4 weeks. Once a normal serum prolactin level is maintained for 6 months, the dose may be discontinued and prolactin levels monitored to determine if cabergoline is still required. The durability of efficacy beyond 24 months of therapy has not been established.

Dosage Forms
Tablet: 0.5 mg

Ca-DTPA *see* diethylene triamine penta-acetic acid *on page 294*

Caduet® [US/Can] *see* amlodipine and atorvastatin *on page 64*

CaEDTA *see* edetate CALCIUM disodium *on page 332*

Caelyx® [Can] *see* doxorubicin (liposomal) *on page 323*

Cafatine-PB® *(Discontinued)* *see* ergotamine *on page 352*

Cafcit® [US] *see* caffeine *on page 158*

Cafergor® [Can] *see* ergotamine and caffeine *on page 352*

Cafergot® [US] *see* ergotamine and caffeine *on page 352*

Cafetrate® *(Discontinued)* *see* ergotamine *on page 352*

caffeine (KAF een)

Synonyms caffeine and sodium benzoate; caffeine citrate; sodium benzoate and caffeine

U.S./Canadian Brand Names Cafcit® [US]; Enerjets [US-OTC]; No Doz® Maximum Strength [US-OTC]; Vivarin® [US-OTC]

Therapeutic Category Stimulant

Use
Caffeine citrate: Treatment of idiopathic apnea of prematurity
Caffeine and sodium benzoate: Treatment of acute respiratory depression (not a preferred agent)
Caffeine [OTC labeling]: Restore mental alertness or wakefulness when experiencing fatigue

Usual Dosage Note: Caffeine citrate should not be interchanged with the caffeine sodium benzoate formulation.

Caffeine citrate: Neonates: Apnea of prematurity: Oral, I.V.:
Loading dose: 10-20 mg/kg as caffeine citrate (5-10 mg/kg as caffeine base). If theophylline has been administered to the patient within the previous 3 days, a full or modified loading dose (50% to 75% of a loading dose) may be given.
Maintenance dose: 5 mg/kg/day as caffeine citrate (2.5 mg/kg/day as caffeine base) once daily starting 24 hours after the loading dose. Maintenance dose is adjusted based on patient's response and serum caffeine concentrations.

Caffeine and sodium benzoate:
Children: Stimulant: I.M., I.V., SubQ: 8 mg/kg every 4 hours as needed
Children ≥12 years and Adults: OTC labeling (stimulant): Oral: 100-200 mg every 3-4 hours as needed

Adults: Respiratory depression: I.M., I.V.: 250 mg as a single dose; may repeat as needed. Maximum single dose should be limited to 500 mg; maximum amount in any 24-hour period should generally be limited to 2500 mg.

Dosage Forms
Caplet:
NoDoz® Maximum Strength [OTC], Vivarin® [OTC]: 200 mg
Injection, solution [preservative free]: 20 mg/mL (3 mL)
Cafcit®: 20 mg/mL (3 mL)
Lozenge:
Enerjets® [OTC]: 75 mg
Solution, oral [preservative free]: 20 mg/mL (3 mL)
Cafcit®: 20 mg/mL
Tablet: 200 mg
Vivarin® [OTC]: 200 mg

caffeine, acetaminophen, and aspirin *see* acetaminophen, aspirin, and caffeine *on page 24*
caffeine, acetaminophen, butalbital, and codeine *see* butalbital, acetaminophen, caffeine, and codeine *on page 155*
caffeine and ergotamine *see* ergotamine and caffeine *on page 352*
caffeine and sodium benzoate *see* caffeine *on page 158*
caffeine, aspirin, and acetaminophen *see* acetaminophen, aspirin, and caffeine *on page 24*
caffeine citrate *see* caffeine *on page 158*
caffeine, dihydrocodeine, and acetaminophen *see* acetaminophen, caffeine, and dihydrocodeine *on page 25*
caffeine, orphenadrine, and aspirin *see* orphenadrine, aspirin, and caffeine *on page 703*
caffeine, propoxyphene, and aspirin *see* propoxyphene, aspirin, and caffeine *on page 796*
Cal-C-Caps [US-OTC] *see* calcium citrate *on page 165*
Caladryl® Clear [US-OTC] *see* pramoxine *on page 777*
CalaMycin® Cool and Clear [US-OTC] *see* pramoxine *on page 777*
Calan® [US/Can] *see* verapamil *on page 974*
Calan® SR [US] *see* verapamil *on page 974*
Calcarb 600 [US-OTC] *see* calcium carbonate *on page 163*
Cal-Cee [US-OTC] *see* calcium citrate *on page 165*
Calci-Chew® [US-OTC] *see* calcium carbonate *on page 163*
Calciday-667® *(Discontinued)* *see* calcium carbonate *on page 163*
Calciferol™ Injection *(Discontinued)* *see* ergocalciferol *on page 350*
Calcijex® [US/Can] *see* calcitriol *on page 160*
Calcimar® [Can] *see* calcitonin *on page 160*
Calcimar® *(Discontinued)* *see* calcitonin *on page 160*
Calci-Mix® [US-OTC] *see* calcium carbonate *on page 163*
Calcionate [US-OTC] *see* calcium glubionate *on page 165*

calcipotriene (kal si POE try een)
U.S./Canadian Brand Names Dovonex® [US/Can]
Therapeutic Category Antipsoriatic Agent
Use Treatment of plaque psoriasis; chronic, moderate-to-severe psoriasis of the scalp
Usual Dosage Topical: Adults:
Cream: Apply a thin film to the affected skin twice daily and rub in gently and completely, for up to 8 weeks
Solution: Apply to the affected scalp twice daily and rub in gently and completely, for up to 8 weeks
Dosage Forms
Cream:
Dovonex® [OTC]: 0.005% (60 g, 120 g)
Solution, topical: 0.005% (60 mL)
Dovonex® [OTC]: 0.005% (60 mL)

calcipotriene and betamethasone (kal si POE try een & bay ta METH a sone)
Synonyms betamethasone dipropionate and calcipotriene hydrate; calcitriol and betamethasone dipropionate

◀ **U.S./Canadian Brand Names** Dovobet® [Can]; Taclonex Scalp® [US]; Taclonex® [US]

Therapeutic Category Corticosteroid, Topical; Vitamin D Analog

Use Treatment of psoriasis vulgaris

Usual Dosage Topical: Adults: Psoriasis vulgaris:
Cream/ointment: Apply to affected area once daily for up to 4 weeks (maximum recommended dose: 100 g/week). Application to >30% of body surface area is not recommended.
Suspension: Apply to affected area of the scalp once daily for 2 weeks or until clear; may continue for up to 8 weeks (maximum recommended dose: 100 g/week)

Dosage Forms [CAN] = Canadian brand name
Cream, topical:
Dovobet® [CAN]: Calcipotriol 50 mcg and betamethasone 0.5 mg per gram (3 g, 30 g, 60 g, 100 g, 120 g) [not available in the U.S.]
Ointment, topical:
Taclonex®: Calcipotriene 0.005% and betamethasone 0.064% (60 g, 100 g)
Suspension, topical:
Taclonex Scalp®: Calcipotriene 0.005% and betamethasone 0.064% (15 g, 30 g, 60 g, 2 x 60 g)

calcipotriol and betamethasone dipropionate see calcipotriene and betamethasone on page 159

Calcite-500 [Can] see calcium carbonate on page 163

calcitonin (kal si TOE nin)

Sound-Alike/Look-Alike Issues
calcitonin may be confused with calcitriol
Miacalcin® may be confused with Micatin®

Synonyms calcitonin (salmon)

U.S./Canadian Brand Names Apo-Calcitonin® [Can]; Calcimar® [Can]; Caltine® [Can]; Fortical® [US]; Miacalcin® NS [Can]; Miacalcin® [US]

Therapeutic Category Polypeptide Hormone

Use Calcitonin (salmon): Treatment of Paget disease of bone (osteitis deformans); adjunctive therapy for hypercalcemia; treatment of osteoporosis in women >5 years postmenopause

Usual Dosage Adults:
Paget disease (Miacalcin®): Initial: I.M., SubQ: 100 units/day; maintenance: 50 units/day or 50-100 units every 1-3 days
Hypercalcemia (Miacalcin®): Initial: I.M., SubQ: 4 units/kg every 12 hours; may increase up to 8 units/kg every 12 hours to a maximum of every 6 hours
Postmenopausal osteoporosis:
I.M., SubQ: Miacalcin®: 100 units/every other day
Intranasal: Fortical®, Miacalcin®: 200 units (1 spray) in one nostril daily

Dosage Forms
Injection, solution [calcitonin-salmon]:
Miacalcin®: 200 int. units/mL (2 mL)
Solution, intranasal [spray, calcitonin-salmon]:
Fortical®: 200 int. units/0.09 mL (3.7 mL)
Miacalcin®: 200 int. units/0.09 mL (3.7 mL)

calcitonin (salmon) see calcitonin on page 160

Cal-Citrate-225 [US] see calcium citrate on page 165

Cal-Citrate® 250 (Discontinued) see calcium citrate on page 165

calcitriol (kal si TRYE ole)

Sound-Alike/Look-Alike Issues
calcitriol may be confused with calcifediol, Calciferol®, calcitonin

Synonyms 1,25 dihydroxycholecalciferol

U.S./Canadian Brand Names Calcijex® [US/Can]; Rocaltrol® [US/Can]

Therapeutic Category Vitamin D Analog

Use Management of hypocalcemia in patients on chronic renal dialysis; management of secondary hyperparathyroidism in patients with chronic kidney disease (CKD); management of hypocalcemia in hypoparathyroidism and pseudohypoparathyroidism

Usual Dosage

Hypocalcemia in patients on chronic renal dialysis (manufacturer labeling): *Adults:*
Oral: 0.25 mcg/day or every other day (may require 0.5-1 mcg/day); increases should be made at 4- to 8-week intervals
I.V.: Initial: 1-2 mcg 3 times/week (0.02 mcg/kg) approximately every other day. Adjust dose at 2-4 week intervals; dosing range: 0.5-4 mcg 3 times/week

Hypocalcemia in hypoparathyroidism/pseudohypoparathyroidism (manufacturers labeling): Oral (evaluate dosage at 2- to 4-week intervals):
Children 1-5 years: 0.25-0.75 mcg once daily
Children ≥6 years and Adults: Initial: 0.25 mcg/day, range: 0.5-2 mcg once daily

Secondary hyperparathyroidism associated with moderate-to-severe CKD in patients not on dialysis (manufacturer labeling): Oral:
Children <3 years: Initial dose: 0.01-0.015 mcg/kg/day
Children ≥3 years and Adults: 0.25 mcg/day; may increase to 0.5 mcg/day

K/DOQI guidelines for vitamin D therapy in CKD:
Children:
CKD stage 2, 3: Oral:
<10 kg: 0.05 mcg every other day
10-20 kg: 0.1-0.15 mcg/day
>20 kg: 0.25 mcg/day
Note: Treatment should only be started with serum 25(OH) D >30 ng/mL, serum iPTH >70 pg/mL, serum calcium <10 mg/dL and serum phosphorus less than or equal to the age appropriate level.
CKD stage 4: Oral:
<10 kg: 0.05 mcg every other day
10-20 kg: 0.1-0.15 mcg/day
>20 kg: 0.25 mcg/day
Note: Treatment should only be started with serum 25(OH) D >30 ng/mL, serum iPTH >110 pg/mL, serum calcium <10 mg/dL and serum phosphorus less than or equal to the age appropriate level.
CKD stage 5: Oral, I.V.: **Note:** The following initial doses are based on plasma PTH and serum calcium levels for patients with serum phosphorus <5.5 mg/dL in adolescents or <6.5 in infants and children, and Ca-P product <55 in adolescents or <65 in infants and children <12 years. Adjust dose based on serum phosphate, calcium and PTH levels. Administer dose with each dialysis session (3 times/week). Intermittent I.V./oral administration is more effective than daily oral dosing.
Plasma PTH 300-500 pg/mL and serum Ca <10 mg/dL: 0.0075 mcg/kg (maximum: 0.25 mcg/day)
Plasma PTH >500-1000 pg/mL and serum Ca <10 mg/dL: 0.015 mcg/kg (maximum: 0.5 mcg/day)
Plasma PTH >1000 pg/mL and serum Ca <10.5 mg/dL: 0.025 mcg/kg (maximum: 1 mcg/day)
Adults:
CKD stage 3: Oral: 0.25 mcg/day. Treatment should only be started with serum 25(OH) D >30 ng/mL, serum iPTH >70 pg/mL, serum calcium <9.5 mg/dL and serum phosphorus <4.6 mg/dL
CKD stage 4: Oral: 0.25 mcg/day. Treatment should only be started with serum 25(OH) D >30 ng/mL, serum iPTH >110 pg/mL, serum calcium <9.5 mg/dL and serum phosphorus <4.6 mg/dL
CKD stage 5:
Peritoneal dialysis: Oral: Initial: 0.5-1 mcg 2-3 times/week or 0.25 mcg/day
Hemodialysis: **Note:** The following initial doses are based on plasma PTH and serum calcium levels for patients with serum phosphorus <5.5 mg/dL and Ca-P product <55. Adjust dose based on serum phosphate, calcium, and PTH levels. Intermittent I.V. administration may be more effective than daily oral dosing.
Plasma PTH 300-600 pg/mL and serum Ca <9.5 mg/dL: Oral, I.V.: 0.5-1.5 mcg
Plasma PTH 600-1000 pg/mL and serum Ca <9.5 mg/dL:
Oral: 1-4 mcg
I.V : 1-3 mcg
Plasma PTH >1000 pg/mL and serum Ca <10 mg/dL:
Oral: 3-7 mcg
I.V.: 3-5 mcg

Dosage Forms

Capsule: 0.25 mcg, 0.5 mcg
Rocaltrol®: 0.25 mcg, 0.5 mcg
Injection, solution: 1 mcg/mL (1 mL)
Calcijex®: 1 mcg/mL (1 mL)
Solution, oral: 1 mcg/mL
Rocaltrol®: 1 mcg/mL

calcium acetate (KAL see um AS e tate)

Sound-Alike/Look-Alike Issues
   PhosLo® may be confused with Phos-Flur®, ProSom™

U.S./Canadian Brand Names PhosLo® [US/Can]

Therapeutic Category Electrolyte Supplement, Oral

Use Control of hyperphosphatemia in end-stage renal failure; does not promote aluminum absorption

Usual Dosage
  Dietary Reference Intake:
   0-6 months: 210 mg/day
   7-12 months: 270 mg/day
   1-3 years: 500 mg/day
   4-8 years: 800 mg/day
   Adults, Male/Female:
    9-18 years: 1300 mg/day
    19-50 years: 1000 mg/day
    ≥51 years: 1200 mg/day
   Female: Pregnancy/Lactating: Same as for Adults, Male/Female
  Oral: Adults, on dialysis: Initial: 1334 mg with each meal, can be increased gradually to bring the serum phosphate value to <6 mg/dL as long as hypercalcemia does not develop (usual dose: 2001-2868 mg calcium acetate with each meal); do not give additional calcium supplements

Dosage Forms
  Gelcap:
   PhosLo®: 667 mg [169 mg]

calcium acetate and aluminum sulfate see aluminum sulfate and calcium acetate on page 55

calcium acetylhomotaurinate see acamprosate on page 18

calcium and risedronate see risedronate and calcium on page 837

calcium and vitamin D (KAL see um & VYE ta min dee)

Synonyms vitamin D and calcium carbonate

U.S./Canadian Brand Names Cal-CYUM [US-OTC]; Caltrate® 600+ Soy™ [US-OTC]; Caltrate® 600+D [US-OTC]; Caltrate® ColonHealth™ [US-OTC]; Chew-Cal [US-OTC]; Liqua-Cal [US-OTC]; Os-Cal® 500 +D [US-OTC]; Oysco 500+D [US-OTC]; Oysco D [US-OTC]; Oyst-Cal-D 500 [US-OTC]; Oyst-Cal-D [US-OTC]

Therapeutic Category Calcium Salt; Electrolyte Supplement, Oral; Vitamin, Fat Soluble

Use Dietary supplement, antacid

Usual Dosage Oral: Adults: Refer to individual monographs for dietary reference intake.

Dosage Forms
  Capsule, softgel: Calcium 500 mg and vitamin D 500 int. units; calcium 600 mg and vitamin D 100 int. units; calcium 600 mg and vitamin D 200 int. units
   Liqua-Cal: Calcium 600 mg and vitamin D 200 int. units
  Tablet: Calcium 250 mg and vitamin D 125 int. units; calcium 500 mg and vitamin D 125 int. units; calcium 500 mg and vitamin D 200 int. units; calcium 600 mg and vitamin D 125 int. units; calcium 600 mg and vitamin D 200 int. units
   Caltrate® 600+D: Calcium 600 mg and vitamin D 200 int. units
   Caltrate® 600+ Soy™: Calcium 600 mg and vitamin D 200 int. units
   Caltrate® ColonHealth™: Calcium 600 mg and vitamin D 200 int. units
   Oysco D: Calcium 250 mg and vitamin D 125 int. units
   Oysco 500+D: Calcium 500 mg and vitamin D 200 int. units
   Oyst-Cal-D: Calcium 250 mg and vitamin D 125 int. units
   Oyst-Cal-D 500: Calcium 500 mg and vitamin D 200 int. units
  Tablet, chewable: Calcium 500 mg and vitamin D 100 int. units; calcium 600 mg and vitamin D 400 int. units
   Os-Cal® 500+D: Calcium 500 mg and vitamin D 400 int. units
  Wafer, chewable:
   Cal-CYUM: Calcium 519 mg and vitamin D 150 int. units (50s)
   Chew-Cal: Calcium 333 mg and vitamin D 40 int. units (100s, 250s)

calcium carbonate (KAL see um KAR bun ate)

Sound-Alike/Look-Alike Issues
Florical® may be confused with Fiorinal®
Mylanta® may be confused with Mynatal®
Nephro-Calci® may be confused with Nephrocaps®
Os-Cal® may be confused with Asacol®

U.S./Canadian Brand Names Alcalak [US-OTC]; Alka-Mints® [US-OTC]; Apo-Cal® [Can]; Cal-Gest [US-OTC]; Cal-Mint [US-OTC]; Calcarb 600 [US-OTC]; Calci-Chew® [US-OTC]; Calci-Mix® [US-OTC]; Calcite-500 [Can]; Caltrate® 600 [US-OTC]; Caltrate® Select [Can]; Caltrate® [Can]; Children's Pepto [US-OTC]; Chooz® [US-OTC]; Florical® [US-OTC]; Maalox® Regular Chewable [US-OTC]; Mylanta® Children's [US-OTC]; Nephro-Calci® [US-OTC]; Nutralox® [US-OTC]; Os-Cal® [Can]; Oysco 500 [US-OTC]; Oyst-Cal 500 [US-OTC]; Rolaids® Softchews [US-OTC]; Titralac™ [US-OTC]; Tums® E-X [US-OTC]; Tums® Extra Strength Sugar Free [US-OTC]; Tums® Smoothies™ [US-OTC]; Tums® Ultra [US-OTC]; Tums® [US-OTC]

Therapeutic Category Antacid; Electrolyte Supplement, Oral

Use As an antacid; treatment and prevention of calcium deficiency or hyperphosphatemia (eg, osteoporosis, osteomalacia, mild/moderate renal insufficiency, hypoparathyroidism, postmenopausal osteoporosis, rickets); has been used to bind phosphate

Usual Dosage Oral (dosage is in terms of elemental calcium):
Dietary Reference Intake:
0-6 months: 210 mg/day
7-12 months: 270 mg/day
1-3 years: 500 mg/day
4-8 years: 800 mg/day
Adults, Male/Female:
9-18 years: 1300 mg/day
19-50 years: 1000 mg/day
≥51 years: 1200 mg/day
Female: Pregnancy/Lactating: Same as for Adults, Male/Female
Hypocalcemia (dose depends on clinical condition and serum calcium level): Dose expressed in mg of **elemental calcium**
Neonates: 50-150 mg/kg/day in 4-6 divided doses; not to exceed 1 g/day
Children: 45-65 mg/kg/day in 4 divided doses
Adults: 1-2 g or more/day in 3-4 divided doses
Antacid:
Children 2-5 years (24-47 lb): Elemental calcium 161 mg as needed; maximum 483 mg per 24 hours
Children 6-11 years (48-95 lb): Elemental calcium 322 mg as needed; maximum: 966 mg per 24 hours
Adults: Dosage based on acid-neutralizing capacity of specific product; generally, 1-2 tablets or 5-10 mL every 2 hours; maximum: 7000 mg calcium carbonate per 24 hours; specific product labeling should be consulted
Dietary supplementation: Adults: 500 mg to 2 g divided 2-4 times/day
Osteoporosis: Adults >51 years: 1200 mg/day

Dosage Forms
Capsule: 364 mg, 1250 mg
Calci-Mix® [OTC]: 1250 mg
Florical® [OTC]: 364 mg
Gum, chewing: 250 mg (30s)
Chooz® [OTC]: 500 mg
Powder: 4000 mg/teaspoonful
Suspension, oral: 1250 mg/5 mL
Tablet: 1250 mg, 1500 mg
Calcarb 600 [OTC], Caltrate® 600 [OTC], Nephro-Calci® [OTC]: 1500 mg
Florical® [OTC]: 364 mg
Oysco 500 [OTC], Oyst-Cal 500 [OTC]: 1250 mg
Tablet, chewable: 500 mg, 650 mg, 750 mg
Alcalak [OTC], Nutralox® [OTC], Titralac™ [OTC]: 420 mg
Alka-Mints® [OTC]: 850 mg
Cal-Gest [OTC], Tums® [OTC]: 500 mg
Calci-Chew® [OTC]: 1250 mg
Cal-Mint [OTC]: 650 mg
Children's Pepto [OTC], Mylanta® Children's [OTC]: 400 mg

◀ Maalox® Regular [OTC]: 600 mg
Tums® E-X [OTC], Tums® Extra Strength Sugar Free [OTC], Tums® Smoothies™ [OTC]: 750 mg
Tums® Ultra® [OTC]: 1000 mg
Tablet, softchew: 1177 mg
Rolaids® [OTC]: 1177 mg

calcium carbonate and etidronate disodium *see* etidronate and calcium *on page 382*

calcium carbonate and magnesium hydroxide
(KAL see um KAR bun ate & mag NEE zhum hye DROKS ide)
Sound-Alike/Look-Alike Issues
Mylanta® may be confused with Mynatal®
Synonyms magnesium hydroxide and calcium carbonate
U.S./Canadian Brand Names Mi-Acid™ Double Strength [US-OTC]; Mylanta® Gelcaps® [US-OTC]; Mylanta® Supreme [US-OTC]; Mylanta® Ultra [US-OTC]; Rolaids® Extra Strength [US-OTC]; Rolaids® [US-OTC]
Therapeutic Category Antacid
Use Hyperacidity
Usual Dosage Oral: Adults: 2-4 tablets between meals, at bedtime, or as directed by healthcare provider
Dosage Forms
Gelcap:
Mylanta® Gelcaps® [OTC]: Calcium carbonate 550 mg and magnesium hydroxide 125 mg
Liquid:
Mylanta® Supreme [OTC]: Calcium carbonate 400 mg and magnesium hydroxide 135 mg per 5 mL
Tablet, chewable: Calcium carbonate 550 mg and magnesium hydroxide 110 mg; calcium carbonate 675 mg and magnesium hydroxide 135 mg; calcium carbonate 700 mg and magnesium hydroxide 300 mg
Mi-Acid™ Double Strength [OTC], Mylanta® Ultra [OTC]: Calcium carbonate 700 mg and magnesium hydroxide 300 mg
Rolaids® [OTC]: Calcium carbonate 550 mg and magnesium hydroxide 110 mg
Rolaids® Extra Strength [OTC]: Calcium carbonate 675 mg and magnesium hydroxide 135 mg

calcium carbonate and simethicone (KAL see um KAR bun ate & sye METH i kone)
Synonyms simethicone and calcium carbonate
U.S./Canadian Brand Names Gas Ban™ [US-OTC]; Titralac® Plus [US-OTC]
Therapeutic Category Antacid; Antiflatulent
Use Relief of acid indigestion, heartburn
Usual Dosage Oral (OTC labeling): Adults: Two tablets every 2-3 hours as needed (maximum: 19 tablets/ 24 hours)
Dosage Forms
Tablet, chewable:
Gas Ban™ [OTC]: Calcium carbonate 300 mg and simethicone 40 mg
Titralac® Plus [OTC]: Calcium carbonate 420 mg and simethicone 21 mg

calcium carbonate, magnesium hydroxide, and famotidine *see* famotidine, calcium carbonate, and magnesium hydroxide *on page 390*

calcium chloride (KAL see um KLOR ide)
Therapeutic Category Electrolyte Supplement, Oral
Use Treatment of acute symptomatic hypocalcemia; cardiac disturbances of hyperkalemia or hypocalcemia; emergent treatment of hypocalcemic tetany; treatment of severe hypermagnesemia
Usual Dosage Note: One gram of calcium chloride is equal to 270 mg of elemental calcium.
Dosages are expressed in terms of the calcium chloride salt based on a solution concentration of 100 mg/mL (10%) containing 1.4 mEq (27.3 mg)/mL elemental calcium.

Acute, symptomatic ionized hypocalcemia, hyperkalemia, or magnesium toxicity: **Note:** Routine use in cardiac arrest is not recommended due to the lack of improved survival [PALS, ACLS 2005 Guidelines]: I.V.:
Neonates: 20 mg/kg; may repeat as necessary
Infants and Children: 20 mg/kg; may repeat as necessary [PALS 2005 Guidelines]
Adults: 500-1000 mg, may repeat as necessary [ACLS 2005 Guidelines]

Hypocalcemia secondary to citrated blood transfusion: I.V.: **Note:** Routine administration of calcium, in the absence of signs/symptoms of hypocalcemia, is generally not recommended. A number of recommendations have been published seeking to address potential hypocalcemia during massive transfusion of citrated blood; however, many practitioners recommend replacement only as guided by clinical evidence of hypocalcemia and/or serial monitoring of ionized calcium. In adults, clinically-significant hypocalcemia usually dose not occur until >5 units of packed red blood cells have been administered.
Neonates, Infants, and Children: Give 32 mg (0.45 mEq elemental calcium) for each 100 mL citrated blood infused
Adults: 200-500 mg per 500 mL of citrated blood (infused into another vein)

Hypocalcemic tetany: I.V.:
Neonates: 40-60 mg/kg/dose repeated every 6-8 hours
Infants and Children: 10 mg/kg over 5-10 minutes; may repeat after 6-8 hours or follow with an infusion with a maximum dose of 200 mg/kg/day; alternatively, higher doses of 35-50 mg/kg/dose repeated every 6-8 hours have been used
Adults: 1000 mg over 10-30 minutes; may repeat after 6 hours
Dosage Forms
Injection, solution [preservative free]: 10% (10 mL)
Injection, solution: [with preservative]: 10% (10 mL)

calcium citrate (KAL see um SIT rate)
Sound-Alike/Look-Alike Issues
Citracal® may be confused with Citrucel®
U.S./Canadian Brand Names Cal-C-Caps [US-OTC]; Cal-Cee [US-OTC]; Cal-Citrate-225 [US]; Citracal® Kosher [US-OTC]; Osteocit® [Can]
Therapeutic Category Electrolyte Supplement, Oral
Use Antacid; treatment and prevention of calcium deficiency or hyperphosphatemia (eg, osteoporosis, osteomalacia, mild/moderate renal insufficiency, hypoparathyroidism, postmenopausal osteoporosis, rickets)
Usual Dosage Oral: Dosage is in terms of elemental calcium
Dietary Reference Intake:
0-6 months: 210 mg/day
7-12 months: 270 mg/day
1-3 years: 500 mg/day
4-8 years: 800 mg/day
Adults, Male/Female:
9-18 years: 1300 mg/day
19-50 years: 1000 mg/day
≥51 years: 1200 mg/day
Female: Pregnancy/Lactating: Same as for Adults, Male/Female
Dietary supplement: Usual dose: 500 mg to 2 g 2-4 times/day
Dosage Forms
Capsule:
Cal-C-Caps [OTC]: Elemental calcium 180 mg
Cal-Citrate-225: Elemental calcium 225 mg
Granules: Elemental calcium 760 mg/teaspoonful
Tablet: Elemental calcium 200 mg, 250 mg
Cal-Cee [OTC]: Elemental calcium 250 mg
Citracal® Kosher [OTC]: Elemental calcium 200 mg

calcium disodium edetate see edetate CALCIUM disodium on page 332
Calcium Disodium Versenate® [US] see edetate CALCIUM disodium on page 332

calcium glubionate (KAL see um gloo BYE oh nate)
Sound-Alike/Look-Alike Issues
calcium glubionate may be confused with calcium gluconate
U.S./Canadian Brand Names Calcionate [US-OTC]
Therapeutic Category Electrolyte Supplement, Oral

◄ **Use** Dietary supplement

Usual Dosage Dosage is in terms of **elemental** calcium
Dietary Reference Intake:
0-6 months: 210 mg/day
7-12 months: 270 mg/day
1-3 years: 500 mg/day
4-8 years: 800 mg/day
Adults, Male/Female:
9-18 years: 1300 mg/day
19-50 years: 1000 mg/day
≥51 years: 1200 mg/day
Female: Pregnancy/Lactating: Same as for Adults, Male/Female
Dietary supplement: Oral:
Infants <12 months: 1 teaspoonful 5 times a day; may mix with juice or formula
Children <4 years: 2 teaspoonsful 3 times a day
Children ≥4 years and Adults: 1 tablespoonful 3 times a day
Pregnant or lactating women: 1 tablespoonful 4 times a day

Dosage Forms
Syrup:
Calcionate: 1.8 g/5 mL

calcium gluconate (KAL see um GLOO koe nate)

Sound-Alike/Look-Alike Issues
calcium gluconate may be confused with calcium glubionate

U.S./Canadian Brand Names Cal-G [US-OTC]; Cal-GLU™ [US]

Therapeutic Category Electrolyte Supplement, Oral

Use Treatment and prevention of hypocalcemia; treatment of tetany, cardiac disturbances of hyperkalemia, cardiac resuscitation when epinephrine fails to improve myocardial contractions, hypocalcemia; calcium supplementation; hydrofluoric acid (HF) burns

Usual Dosage
Adequate Intake (as elemental calcium):
0-6 months: 210 mg/day
7-12 months: 270 mg/day
1-3 years: 500 mg/day
4-8 years: 800 mg/day
9-18 years: 1300 mg/day
Adults, Male/Female:
19-50 years: 1000 mg/day
≥51 years: 1200 mg/day
Female: Pregnancy/Lactating: Same as for Adults, Male/Female

Dosage note: Calcium chloride has 3 times more elemental calcium than calcium gluconate. Calcium chloride is 27% elemental calcium; calcium gluconate is 9% elemental calcium. One gram of calcium chloride is equal to 270 mg of elemental calcium; 1 gram of calcium gluconate is equal to 90 mg of elemental calcium. The following dosages are expressed in terms of the calcium gluconate salt based on a solution concentration of 100 mg/mL (10%) containing 0.465 mEq (9.3 mg)/mL elemental calcium:

Hypocalcemia: I.V.:
Neonates: 200-800 mg/kg/day as a continuous infusion or in 4 divided doses (maximum: 1 g/dose)
Infants and Children: 200-500 mg/kg/day as a continuous infusion or in 4 divided doses (maximum: 2-3 g/dose)
Adults: 2-15 g/24 hours as a continuous infusion or in divided doses

Hypocalcemia: Oral:
Children: 200-500 mg/kg/day divided every 6 hours
Adults: 500 mg to 2 g 2-4 times/day

Hypocalcemia secondary to citrated blood infusion: I.V.: **Note:** Routine administration of calcium, in the absence of signs/symptoms of hypocalcemia, is generally not recommended. A number of recommendations have been published seeking to address potential hypocalcemia during massive transfusion of citrated blood; however, many practitioners recommend replacement only as guided by clinical evidence of hypocalcemia and/or serial monitoring of ionized calcium.
Neonates, Infants, and Children: Give 98 mg (0.45 mEq **elemental** calcium) for each 100 mL citrated blood infused

Adults: 500 mg to 1 g per 500 mL of citrated blood (infused into another vein). Single doses up to 2 g have also been recommended.

Hypocalcemic tetany: I.V.:
  Neonates, Infants, and Children: 100-200 mg/kg/dose over 5-10 minutes; may repeat every 6-8 hours **or** follow with an infusion of 500 mg/kg/day
  Adults: 1-3 g may be administered until therapeutic response occurs
Magnesium intoxication, cardiac arrest in the presence of hyperkalemia or hypocalcemia: I.V.:
  Infants and Children: 60-100 mg/kg/dose (maximum: 3 g/dose)
  Adults: 500-800 mg/dose (maximum: 3 g/dose)
Maintenance electrolyte requirements for total parenteral nutrition: I.V.: Daily requirements: Adults: 1.7-3.4 g/1000 kcal/24 hours

Dosage Forms
  Capsule, oral:
    Cal-G: 700 mg
  Capsule, oral [preservative free]:
    Cal-GLU™: 515 mg
  Injection, solution [preservative free]: 10% (10 mL, 50 mL, 100 mL, 200 mL) [100 mg/mL]
  Powder: 347 mg/tablespoonful
  Tablet: 500 mg, 650 mg, 975 mg

calcium lactate (KAL see um LAK tate)

Therapeutic Category Electrolyte Supplement, Oral
Use Adjunct in prevention of postmenopausal osteoporosis; treatment and prevention of calcium depletion
Usual Dosage Oral (in terms of calcium lactate):
  Dietary Reference Intake (in terms of elemental calcium):
    0-6 months: 210 mg/day
    7-12 months: 270 mg/day
    1-3 years: 500 mg/day
    4-8 years: 800 mg/day
    9-18 years: 1300 mg/day
    Adults, Male/Female:
      19-50 years: 1000 mg/day
      ≥51 years: 1200 mg/day
    Female: Pregnancy/Lactating: Same as Adults, Male/Female
Dosage Forms
  Tablet: 650 mg

calcium leucovorin *see* leucovorin calcium *on page 552*
calcium levoleucovorin *see* LEVOleucovorin *on page 558*
calcium pantothenate *see* pantothenic acid *on page 721*

calcium phosphate (tribasic) (KAL see um FOS fate tri BAY sik)

Synonyms tricalcium phosphate
U.S./Canadian Brand Names Posture® [US-OTC]
Therapeutic Category Electrolyte Supplement, Oral
Use Dietary supplement
Usual Dosage Oral:
  Adequate Intake (as elemental calcium):
    0-6 months: 210 mg/day
    7-12 months: 270 mg/day
    1-3 years: 500 mg/day
    4-8 years: 800 mg/day
    9-18 years: 1300 mg/day
    Adults, Male/Female:
      19-50 years: 1000 mg/day
      ≥51 years: 1200 mg/day
    Female: Pregnancy/Lactating: Same as for Adults, Male/Female
  Dietary supplement: Adults: 2 tablets daily

▶

◄ **Dosage Forms**
Caplet:
Posture® [OTC]: Calcium 600 mg and phosphorus 280 mg

Cal-CYUM [US-OTC] *see* calcium and vitamin D *on page 162*
Caldecort® [US-OTC] *see* hydrocortisone (topical) *on page 485*

calfactant (kaf AKT ant)

U.S./Canadian Brand Names Infasurf® [US]
Therapeutic Category Lung Surfactant
Use Prevention of respiratory distress syndrome (RDS) in premature infants at high risk for RDS and for the treatment ("rescue") of premature infants who develop RDS

Prophylaxis: Therapy at birth with calfactant is indicated for premature infants <29 weeks of gestational age at significant risk for RDS. Should be administered as soon as possible, preferably within 30 minutes after birth.
Treatment: For infants ≤72 hours of age with RDS (confirmed by clinical and radiologic findings) and requiring endotracheal intubation.

Usual Dosage Intratracheal administration **only**: Each dose is 3 mL/kg body weight at birth; should be administered every 12 hours for a total of up to 3 doses
Dosage Forms
Suspension, intratracheal [preservative free]:
Infasurf®: 35 mg/mL

Cal-G [US-OTC] *see* calcium gluconate *on page 166*
Cal-Gest [US-OTC] *see* calcium carbonate *on page 163*
Cal-GLU™ [US] *see* calcium gluconate *on page 166*
Callergy Clear [US-OTC] *see* pramoxine *on page 777*
Calm-X® Oral *(Discontinued)* *see* dimenhydrinate *on page 301*
Cal-Mint [US-OTC] *see* calcium carbonate *on page 163*
Calmylin with Codeine [Can] *see* guaifenesin, pseudoephedrine, and codeine *on page 460*
Cal-Nate™ [US] *see* vitamins (multiple/prenatal) *on page 983*
CaloMist™ [US] *see* cyanocobalamin *on page 254*
Calphron® *(Discontinued)* *see* calcium acetate *on page 162*
Cal-Plus® *(Discontinued)* *see* calcium carbonate *on page 163*
Caltine® [Can] *see* calcitonin *on page 160*
Caltrate® [Can] *see* calcium carbonate *on page 163*
Caltrate® 600 [US-OTC] *see* calcium carbonate *on page 163*
Caltrate® 600+D [US-OTC] *see* calcium and vitamin D *on page 162*
Caltrate® 600+ Soy™ [US-OTC] *see* calcium and vitamin D *on page 162*
Caltrate® ColonHealth™ [US-OTC] *see* calcium and vitamin D *on page 162*
Caltrate® Jr. *(Discontinued)* *see* calcium carbonate *on page 163*
Caltrate® Select [Can] *see* calcium carbonate *on page 163*
Camila™ [US] *see* norethindrone *on page 679*
Campath® [US] *see* alemtuzumab *on page 43*
campath-1H *see* alemtuzumab *on page 43*
Campho-Phenique® [US-OTC] *see* camphor and phenol *on page 168*

camphor and phenol (KAM for & FEE nole)

Synonyms phenol and camphor
U.S./Canadian Brand Names Campho-Phenique® [US-OTC]
Therapeutic Category Topical Skin Product
Use Relief of pain and itching associated with minor burns, sunburn, minor cuts, insect bites, minor skin irritation; temporary relief of pain from cold sores
Usual Dosage Topical: Adults: Relief of pain/itching: Apply 1-3 times/day
Dosage Forms
Gel, topical:
Campho-Phenique® [OTC]: Camphor 10.8% and phenol 4.7% (7 g, 14 g)

Liquid, topical: Camphor 10.8% and phenol 4.7% (45 mL)
Campho-Phenique® [OTC]: Camphor 10.8% and phenol 4.7% (22.5 mL, 45 mL)

Campral® [US/Can] *see* acamprosate *on page 18*
Camptosar® [US/Can] *see* irinotecan *on page 526*
camptothecin-11 *see* irinotecan *on page 526*
Canasa® [US] *see* mesalamine *on page 607*
Cancidas® [US/Can] *see* caspofungin *on page 182*

candesartan (kan de SAR tan)

Synonyms candesartan cilexetil
U.S./Canadian Brand Names Atacand® [US/Can]
Therapeutic Category Angiotensin II Receptor Antagonist
Use Alone or in combination with other antihypertensive agents in treating essential hypertension; treatment of heart failure (NYHA class II-IV)
Usual Dosage Oral: Adults:
Hypertension: Usual dose is 4-32 mg once daily; dosage must be individualized. Blood pressure response is dose-related over the range of 2-32 mg. The usual recommended starting dose of 16 mg once daily when it is used as monotherapy in patients who are not volume depleted. It can be administered once or twice daily with total daily doses ranging from 8-32 mg. Larger doses do not appear to have a greater effect and there is relatively little experience with such doses.
Congestive heart failure: Initial: 4 mg once daily; double the dose at 2-week intervals, as tolerated; target dose: 32 mg
Note: In selected cases, concurrent therapy with an ACE inhibitor may provide additional benefit.
Dosage Forms
Tablet:
Atacand®: 4 mg, 8 mg, 16 mg, 32 mg

candesartan and hydrochlorothiazide (kan de SAR tan & hye droe klor oh THYE a zide)

Synonyms candesartan cilexetil and hydrochlorothiazide
U.S./Canadian Brand Names Atacand HCT® [US]; Atacand® Plus [Can]
Therapeutic Category Antihypertensive Agent, Combination
Use Treatment of hypertension; combination product should not be used for initial therapy
Usual Dosage Oral: Adults: Replacement therapy: Combination product can be substituted for individual agents; maximum therapeutic effect would be expected within 4 weeks

Usual dosage range:
Candesartan: 16-32 mg/day, given once daily or twice daily in divided doses
Hydrochlorothiazide: 12.5-25 mg once daily
Dosage Forms
Tablet:
Atacand HCT®: 16/12.5: Candesartan 16 mg and hydrochlorothiazide 12.5 mg; 32/12.5: Candesartan 32 mg and hydrochlorothiazide 12.5 mg; 32/25: Candesartan 32 mg and hydrochlorothiazide 25 mg

candesartan cilexetil *see* candesartan *on page 169*
candesartan cilexetil and hydrochlorothiazide *see* candesartan and hydrochlorothiazide *on page 169*

Candida albicans (Monilia) (KAN dee da AL bi kans mo NIL ya)

Synonyms *Monilia* skin test
U.S./Canadian Brand Names Candin® [US]
Therapeutic Category Diagnostic Agent
Use Screen for detection of nonresponsiveness to antigens in immunocompromised individuals
Usual Dosage Intradermal: 0.1 mL, examine reaction site in 24-48 hours; induration of ≥5 mm in diameter is a positive reaction
Dosage Forms
Injection, solution:
Candin®: 0.1 mL/dose (1 mL)

Candin® [US] *see* Candida albicans (Monilia) *on page 169*

Candistatin® [Can] *see* nystatin *on page 690*
Canesten® Topical [Can] *see* clotrimazole *on page 238*
Canesten® Vaginal [Can] *see* clotrimazole *on page 238*
Cankaid® [US-OTC] *see* carbamide peroxide *on page 174*
cannabidiol and tetrahydrocannabinol *see* tetrahydrocannabinol and cannabidiol *(Canada only)* *on page 915*
Canthacur® [Can] *see* cantharidin *(Canada only) on page 170*

cantharidin *(Canada only)* (kan THAR e din)
U.S./Canadian Brand Names Canthacur® [Can]; Cantharone® [Can]
Therapeutic Category Keratolytic Agent
Use Removal of ordinary and periungual warts
Usual Dosage Apply directly to lesion, cover with nonporous tape, remove tape in 24 hours, reapply if necessary

Cantharone® [Can] *see* cantharidin *(Canada only) on page 170*
Cantil® [Can] *see* mepenzolate *on page 603*
Cantil® *(Discontinued)* *see* mepenzolate *on page 603*
Capastat® Sulfate [US] *see* capreomycin *on page 170*

capecitabine (ka pe SITE a been)
Sound-Alike/Look-Alike Issues
  Xeloda® may be confused with Xenical®
Synonyms NSC-712807
U.S./Canadian Brand Names Xeloda® [US/Can]
Therapeutic Category Antineoplastic Agent, Antimetabolite
Use Treatment of metastatic colorectal cancer; adjuvant therapy of Dukes C colon cancer; treatment of metastatic breast cancer
Usual Dosage Oral:
  Adults: **Note:** Capecitabine toxicities, particularly hand-foot syndrome, may be higher in North American populations (for the treatment of colorectal cancer); therapy initiation at doses of 1000 mg/m^2 twice daily (for 2 weeks every 21 days) may be considered
  Metastatic breast cancer, metastatic colorectal cancer: 1250 mg/m^2 twice daily (morning and evening) for 2 weeks, every 21 days
  Adjuvant therapy of Dukes C colon cancer: Recommended for a total of 24 weeks (8 cycles of 2 weeks of drug administration and 1 week rest period.
Dosage Forms
  Tablet:
  Xeloda®: 150 mg, 500 mg

Capex® [US/Can] *see* fluocinolone *on page 409*
Caphosol® [US] *see* saliva substitute *on page 853*
Capital® and Codeine [US] *see* acetaminophen and codeine *on page 20*
Capitrol® *(Discontinued)*
Capoten® [US/Can] *see* captopril *on page 171*
Capozide® [US/Can] *see* captopril and hydrochlorothiazide *on page 172*

capreomycin (kap ree oh MYE sin)
Sound-Alike/Look-Alike Issues
  Capastat® may be confused with Cepastat®
Synonyms capreomycin sulfate
U.S./Canadian Brand Names Capastat® Sulfate [US]
Therapeutic Category Antibiotic, Miscellaneous
Use Treatment of tuberculosis in conjunction with at least one other antituberculosis agent
Usual Dosage I.M., I.V.: Adults: 1 g/day (maximum: 20 mg/kg/day) for 60-120 days, followed by 1 g 2-3 times/week **or** 15 mg/kg/day (maximum: 1 g/dose) for 2-4 months, followed by 15 mg/kg (maximum: 1 g/dose) 2-3 times/week

Dosage Forms
Injection, powder for reconstitution:
Capastat® Sulfate: 1 g

capreomycin sulfate *see* capreomycin *on page 170*
Capsagel® [US-OTC] *see* capsaicin *on page 171*

capsaicin (kap SAY sin)

Sound-Alike/Look-Alike Issues
Zostrix® may be confused with Zestril®, Zovirax®

U.S./Canadian Brand Names Capsagel® [US-OTC]; Capzasin-HP® [US-OTC]; Capzasin-P® [US-OTC]; Zostrix® [US-OTC/Can]; Zostrix®-HP [US-OTC/Can]

Therapeutic Category Analgesic, Topical

Use Topical treatment of pain associated with postherpetic neuralgia, rheumatoid arthritis, osteoarthritis, diabetic neuropathy; postsurgical pain

Usual Dosage Topical: Children ≥2 years and Adults: Apply to affected area at least 3-4 times/day; application frequency less than 3-4 times/day prevents the total depletion, inhibition of synthesis, and transport of substance P resulting in decreased clinical efficacy and increased local discomfort

Dosage Forms
Cream, topical: 0.025% (60 g); 0.075% (60 g)
Capzasin-P® [OTC]: 0.025% (45 g)
Capzasin-HP® [OTC]: 0.075% (45 g)
Zostrix® [OTC]: 0.025% (60 g)
Zostrix®-HP [OTC]: 0.075% (60 g)
Zostrix® Neuropathy [OTC]: 0.25% (60 g)
Gel, topical:
Capsagel® [OTC]: 0.025% (60 g); 0.05% (60 g); 0.075% (30 g)

captopril (KAP toe pril)

Sound-Alike/Look-Alike Issues
captopril may be confused with Capitrol®, carvedilol

Synonyms ACE

U.S./Canadian Brand Names Alti-Captopril [Can]; Apo-Capto® [Can]; Capoten® [US/Can]; Gen-Captopril [Can]; Novo-Captopril [Can]; Nu-Capto [Can]; PMS-Captopril [Can]

Therapeutic Category Angiotensin-Converting Enzyme (ACE) Inhibitor

Use Management of hypertension; treatment of heart failure, left ventricular dysfunction after myocardial infarction, diabetic nephropathy

Usual Dosage Note: Titrate dose according to patient's response; use lowest effective dose. Oral:
Infants: Initial: 0.15-0.3 mg/kg/dose; titrate dose upward to maximum of 6 mg/kg/day in 1-4 divided doses; usual required dose: 2.5-6 mg/kg/day
Children: Initial: 0.5 mg/kg/dose; titrate upward to maximum of 6 mg/kg/day in 2-4 divided doses
Older Children: Initial: 6.25-12.5 mg/dose every 12-24 hours; titrate upward to maximum of 6 mg/kg/day
Adolescents: Initial: 12.5-25 mg/dose given every 8-12 hours; increase by 25 mg/dose to maximum of 450 mg/day
Adults:
Acute hypertension (urgency/emergency): 12.5-25 mg, may repeat as needed (may be given sublingually, but no therapeutic advantage demonstrated)
Hypertension:
Initial dose: 12.5-25 mg 2-3 times/day; may increase by 12.5-25 mg/dose at 1- to 2-week intervals up to 50 mg 3 times/day; maximum dose: 150 mg 3 times/day; add diuretic before further dosage increases
Usual dose range (JNC 7): 25-100 mg/day in 2 divided doses
Congestive heart failure:
Initial dose: 6.25-12.5 mg 3 times/day in conjunction with cardiac glycoside and diuretic therapy; initial dose depends upon patient's fluid/electrolyte status
Target dose: 50 mg 3 times/day
LVD after MI: Initial dose: 6.25 mg followed by 12.5 mg 3 times/day; then increase to 25 mg 3 times/day during next several days and then over next several weeks to target dose of 50 mg 3 times/day
Diabetic nephropathy: 25 mg 3 times/day; other antihypertensives often given concurrently

◀ **Dosage Forms**
   Tablet: 12.5 mg, 25 mg, 50 mg, 100 mg
   Capoten®: 12.5 mg, 25 mg, 50 mg, 100 mg

captopril and hydrochlorothiazide (KAP toe pril & hye droe klor oh THYE a zide)

Synonyms hydrochlorothiazide and captopril

U.S./Canadian Brand Names Capozide® [US/Can]

Therapeutic Category Antihypertensive Agent, Combination

Use Management of hypertension

Usual Dosage Oral: Adults: Hypertension, CHF: May be substituted for previously titrated dosages of the individual components; alternatively, may initiate as follows:
   Initial: Single tablet (captopril 25 mg/hydrochlorothiazide 15 mg) taken once daily; daily dose of captopril should not exceed 150 mg; daily dose of hydrochlorothiazide should not exceed 50 mg

Dosage Forms
   Tablet:
   Generics:
      25/15: Captopril 25 mg and hydrochlorothiazide 15 mg
      25/25: Captopril 25 mg and hydrochlorothiazide 25 mg
      50/15: Captopril 50 mg and hydrochlorothiazide 15 mg
      50/25: Captopril 50 mg and hydrochlorothiazide 25 mg
   Brands:
   Capozide®:
      25/15: Captopril 25 mg and hydrochlorothiazide 15 mg
      25/25: Captopril 25 mg and hydrochlorothiazide 25 mg
      50/15: Captopril 50 mg and hydrochlorothiazide 15 mg
      50/25: Captopril 50 mg and hydrochlorothiazide 25 mg

Capzasin-HP® [US-OTC] *see* capsaicin *on page 171*

Capzasin-P® [US-OTC] *see* capsaicin *on page 171*

Carac® [US] *see* fluorouracil *on page 412*

Carafate® [US] *see* sucralfate *on page 890*

Carapres® [Can] *see* clonidine *on page 236*

carbachol (KAR ba kole)

Sound-Alike/Look-Alike Issues
   Isopto® Carbachol may be confused with Isopto® Carpine

Synonyms carbacholine; carbamylcholine chloride

U.S./Canadian Brand Names Isopto® Carbachol [US/Can]; Miostat® [US/Can]

Therapeutic Category Cholinergic Agent

Use Lowers intraocular pressure in the treatment of glaucoma; cause miosis during surgery

Usual Dosage Adults:
   Ophthalmic: Instill 1-2 drops up to 3 times/day
   Intraocular: 0.5 mL instilled into anterior chamber before or after securing sutures

Dosage Forms
   Solution, intraocular:
   Miostat® [OTC]: 0.01% (1.5 mL)
   Solution, ophthalmic:
   Isopto® Carbachol [OTC]: 1.5% (15 mL); 3% (15 mL)

carbacholine *see* carbachol *on page 172*

carbamazepine (kar ba MAZ e peen)

Sound-Alike/Look-Alike Issues
   carBAMazepine may be confused with OXcarbazepine
   Carbatrol® may be confused with Cartrol®
   Epitol® may be confused with Epinal®
   Tegretol®, Tegretol®-XR may be confused with Mebaral®, Tegrin®, Toprol-XL®, Toradol®, Trental®

Synonyms CBZ; SPD417

Tall-Man carBAMazepine

U.S./Canadian Brand Names Apo-Carbamazepine® [Can]; Bio-Carbamazepine [Can]; Carbamazepine [Can]; Carbatrol® [US]; Dom-Carbamazepine [Can]; Epitol® [US]; Equetro® [US]; Gen-Carbamazepine CR [Can]; Mapezine® [Can]; Novo-Carbamaz [Can]; Nu-Carbamazepine [Can]; PHL-Carbamazepine [Can]; PMS-Carbamazepine [Can]; Sandoz-Carbamazepine [Can]; Taro-Carbamazepine Chewable [Can]; Tegretol® [US/Can]; Tegretol®-XR [US]

Therapeutic Category Anticonvulsant

Use

Carbatrol®, Tegretol®, Tegretol®-XR: Partial seizures with complex symptomatology (psychomotor, temporal lobe), generalized tonic-clonic seizures (grand mal), mixed seizure patterns, trigeminal neuralgia

Equetro®: Acute manic and mixed episodes associated with bipolar 1 disorder

Usual Dosage Dosage must be adjusted according to patient's response and serum concentrations. Administer tablets (chewable or conventional) in 2-3 divided doses daily and suspension in 4 divided doses daily. Oral:

Epilepsy:

Children:

<6 years: Initial: 10-20 mg/kg/day divided twice or 3 times daily as tablets or 4 times/day as suspension; increase dose every week until optimal response and therapeutic levels are achieved

Maintenance dose: Divide into 3-4 doses daily (tablets or suspension); maximum recommended dose: 35 mg/kg/day

6-12 years: Initial: 200 mg/day in 2 divided doses (tablets or extended release tablets) or 4 divided doses (oral suspension); increase by up to 100 mg/day at weekly intervals using a twice daily regimen of extended release tablets or 3-4 times daily regimen of other formulations until optimal response and therapeutic levels are achieved

Maintenance: Usual: 400-800 mg/day; maximum recommended dose: 1000 mg/day

Note: Children <12 years who receive ≥400 mg/day of carbamazepine may be converted to extended release capsules (Carbatrol®) using the same total daily dosage divided twice daily

Children >12 years and Adults: Initial: 400 mg/day in 2 divided doses (tablets or extended release tablets) or 4 divided doses (oral suspension); increase by up to 200 mg/day at weekly intervals using a twice daily regimen of extended release tablets or capsules, or a 3-4 times/day regimen of other formulations until optimal response and therapeutic levels are achieved; usual dose: 800-1200 mg/day

Maximum recommended doses:

Children 12-15 years: 1000 mg/day

Children >15 years: 1200 mg/day

Adults: 1600 mg/day; however, some patients have required up to 1.6-2.4 g/day

Trigeminal or glossopharyngeal neuralgia: Adults: Initial: 200 mg/day in 2 divided doses (tablets, extended release tablets, or extended release capsules) or 4 divided doses (oral suspension) with food, gradually increasing in increments of 200 mg/day as needed

Maintenance: Usual: 400-800 mg daily in 2 divided doses (tablets, extended release tablets, or extended release capsules) or 4 divided doses (oral suspension); maximum dose: 1200 mg/day

Bipolar disorder: Adults: Initial: 400 mg/day in 2 divided doses (tablets, extended release tablets, or extended release capsules) or 4 divided doses (oral suspension), may adjust by 200 mg/day increments; maximum dose: 1600 mg/day.

Note: Equetro® is the only formulation specifically approved by the FDA for the management of bipolar disorder.

Dosage Forms

Capsule, extended release:

Carbatrol®, Equetro®: 100 mg, 200 mg, 300 mg

Suspension, oral: 100 mg/5 mL

Tegretol®: 100 mg/5 mL

Tablet: 200 mg

Epitol®, Tegretol®: 200 mg

Tablet, chewable: 100 mg

Tegretol®: 100 mg

Tablet, extended release:

Tegretol®-XR: 100 mg, 200 mg, 400 mg

Carbamazepine [Can] see carbamazepine on page 172

carbamide see urea on page 963

carbamide peroxide (KAR ba mide per OKS ide)

Synonyms urea peroxide

U.S./Canadian Brand Names Auraphene® B [US-OTC]; Auro® [US-OTC]; Cankaid® [US-OTC]; Debrox® [US-OTC]; E•R•O [US-OTC]; Gly-Oxide® [US-OTC]; Murine® Ear Wax Removal System [US-OTC]; Orajel® Perioseptic® Spot Treatment [US-OTC]; Otix® [US-OTC]

Therapeutic Category Antiinfective Agent, Oral; Otic Agent, Ceruminolytic

Use Relief of minor inflammation of gums, oral mucosal surfaces, and lips including canker sores and dental irritation; emulsify and disperse ear wax

Usual Dosage Children and Adults:

Oral: Inflammation/dental irritation: Solution (should not be used for >7 days): Oral preparation should not be used in children <2 years of age; apply several drops undiluted on affected area 4 times/day after meals and at bedtime; expectorate after 2-3 minutes **or** place 10 drops onto tongue, mix with saliva, swish for several minutes, expectorate

Otic:

Children <12 years: Tilt head sideways and individualize the dose according to patient size; 3 drops (range: 1-5 drops) twice daily for up to 4 days, tip of applicator should not enter ear canal; keep drops in ear for several minutes by keeping head tilted and placing cotton in ear

Children ≥12 years and Adults: Tilt head sideways and instill 5-10 drops twice daily up to 4 days, tip of applicator should not enter ear canal; keep drops in ear for several minutes by keeping head tilted and placing cotton in ear

Dosage Forms

Liquid, oral: 10% (60 mL)
Cankaid®: 10% (22 mL)
Gly-Oxide®: 10% (15 mL, 60 mL)
Solution, otic [drops]: 6.5% (15 mL)
Auraphene® B [OTC]: 6.5% (15 mL)
Auro® [OTC]: 6.5% (22.2 mL)
Debrox® [OTC]: 6.5% (15 mL, 30 mL)
E•R•O [OTC], Murine® Ear Wax Removal System [OTC], Otix® [OTC]: 6.5% (15 mL)

carbamylcholine chloride see carbachol on page 172
Carbaphen 12® [US] see carbetapentane, phenylephrine, and chlorpheniramine on page 176
Carbaphen 12 Ped® [US] see carbetapentane, phenylephrine, and chlorpheniramine on page 176
Carbastat® (Discontinued) see carbachol on page 172
Carbatrol® [US] see carbamazepine on page 172
Carbaxefed DM RF (Discontinued)
Carbaxefed RF (Discontinued)

carbenicillin (kar ben i SIL in)

Synonyms carbenicillin indanyl sodium; carindacillin

Therapeutic Category Penicillin

Use Treatment of serious urinary tract infections and prostatitis caused by susceptible gram-negative aerobic bacilli

Usual Dosage

Usual dosage range:
Children: Oral: 30-50 mg/kg/day divided every 6 hours (maximum dose: 2-3 g/day)
Adults: Oral: 1-2 tablets every 6 hours
Indication-specific dosing:
Adults: Oral:
Prostatitis: 2 tablets every 6 hours
Urinary tract infections: 1-2 tablets every 6 hours

carbenicillin indanyl sodium see carbenicillin on page 174

carbetapentane and chlorpheniramine (kar bay ta PEN tane & klor fen IR a meen)

Synonyms carbetapentane tannate and chlorpheniramine tannate; chlorpheniramine and carbetapentane

U.S./Canadian Brand Names C-Tanna 12 [US]; Tannate 12 S [US]; Tannic-12 S [US]; Tussi-12 S™ [US]; Tussi-12® [US]; Tussizone-12 RF™ [US]; Tustan 12S™ [US]

Therapeutic Category Antihistamine/Antitussive

Use Symptomatic relief of cough associated with upper respiratory tract conditions, such as the common cold, bronchitis, bronchial asthma

Usual Dosage Oral:

Children: Based on carbetapentane 30 mg and chlorpheniramine 4 mg per 5 mL suspension:

2-6 years: 2.5-5 mL every 12 hours

>6 years: 5-10 mL every 12 hours

Adults: Based on carbetapentane 60 mg and chlorpheniramine 5 mg per tablet: 1-2 tablets every 12 hours

Dosage Forms

Suspension:

C-Tanna 12, Tannate 12 S, Tannic-12 S, Tussi-12 S™, Tustan 12S™: Carbetapentane 30 mg and chlorpheniramine 4 mg per 5 mL

Tablet:

Tussi-12®, Tussizone-12 RF™: Carbetapentane 60 mg and chlorpheniramine 5 mg

carbetapentane and phenylephrine (kar bay ta PEN tane & fen il EF rin)

Synonyms phenylephrine tannate and carbetapentane tannate

U.S./Canadian Brand Names L-All 12 [US]

Therapeutic Category Antitussive; Antitussive/Decongestant; Sympathomimetic

Use Symptomatic relief of upper respiratory tract conditions such as the common cold, bronchial asthma, and bronchitis (acute and chronic)

Usual Dosage Oral:

Children:

2-6 years: 2.5 mL every 12 hours, not to exceed 5 mL/24 hours

6-12 years: 5 mL every 12 hours, not to exceed 10 mL/24 hours

Children >12 years and Adults: 5-10 mL every 12 hours, not to exceed 20 mL/24 hours

carbetapentane and pseudoephedrine (kar bay ta PEN tane & soo doe e FED rin)

Synonyms carbetapentane tannate and pseudoephedrine tannate; pseudoephedrine and carbetapentane

U.S./Canadian Brand Names Pseudacarb™ [US]; Respi-Tann™ [US]

Therapeutic Category Antitussive/Decongestant

Use Relief of cough and congestion due to the common cold, influenza, sinusitis, or bronchitis

Usual Dosage Relief of cough and congestion: Oral:

Children:

2-6 years: 1/2 tablet or 2.5 mL suspension every 12 hours (maximum: 4 doses/24 hours)

6-12 years: 1 tablet or 5 mL suspension every 12 hours (maximum: 4 doses/24 hours)

Children >12 years and Adults: 2 tablets or 10 mL suspension every 12 hours (maximum: 4 doses/24 hours)

Dosage Forms

Suspension: Carbetapentane 25 mg and pseudoephedrine 75 mg per 5 mL

Respi-Tann™: Carbetapentane 25 mg and pseudoephedrine 75 mg per 5 mL

Tablet, chewable:

Pseudacarb™, Respi-Tann™: Carbetapentane 25 mg and pseudoephedrine 75 mg

carbetapentane, ephedrine, phenylephrine, and chlorpheniramine *see* chlorpheniramine, ephedrine, phenylephrine, and carbetapentane *on page 208*

carbetapentane, guaifenesin, and phenylephrine

(kar bay ta PEN tane, gwye FEN e sin, & fen il EF rin)

Synonyms guaifenesin, carbetapentane citrate, and phenylephrine hydrochloride; phenylephrine hydrochloride, carbetapentane citrate, and guaifenesin

U.S./Canadian Brand Names Carbetaplex [US]; Extendryl® GCP [US]; Gentex LQ [US]; Levall™ [US]; Phencarb GG [US]

Therapeutic Category Antitussive; Expectorant; Expectorant/Decongestant/Antitussive; Sympathomimetic

Use Relief of nonproductive cough accompanying respiratory tract congestion associated with the common cold, influenza, sinusitis, and bronchitis

Usual Dosage Oral:

Children 2-6 years:

Gentex LQ: 2.5 mL every 4-6 hours

Levall™: 1.25 mL every 4-6 hours; maximum dose of phenylephrine: 15 mg/24 hours

▶

Children 6-12 years:
Gentex LQ: 5 mL every 4-6 hours
Levall™: 2.5 mL every 4-6 hours; maximum dose of phenylephrine: 30 mg/24 hours
Children ≥12 years and Adults:
Gentex LQ: 5-10 mL every 4-6 hours
Levall™: 5 mL every 4-6 hours; maximum dose of phenylephrine: 60 mg/24 hours

Dosage Forms
Liquid:
Carbetaplex: Carbetapentane 20 mg, guaifenesin 100 mg, and phenylephrine 15 mg per 5 mL
Gentex LQ: Carbetapentane 20 mg, guaifenesin 100 mg, and phenylephrine 10 mg per 5 mL
Levall™: Carbetapentane 15 mg, guaifenesin 100 mg, and phenylephrine 5 mg per 5 mL
Phencarb GG: Carbetapentane 20 mg, guaifenesin 100 mg, and phenylephrine 10 mg per 5 mL
Solution, oral:
Extendryl® GCP: Carbetapentane 15 mg, guaifenesin 100 mg, and phenylephrine 5 mg per 5 mL

carbetapentane, phenylephrine, and chlorpheniramine
(kar bay ta PEN tane, fen il EF rin, & klor fen IR a meen)

Synonyms chlorpheniramine, carbetapentane, and phenylephrine; phenylephrine, chlorpheniramine, and carbetapentane

U.S./Canadian Brand Names Carbaphen 12 Ped® [US]; Carbaphen 12® [US]

Therapeutic Category Antihistamine/Decongestant/Antitussive; Antitussive; Sympathomimetic

Use Symptomatic relief of cough, nasal congestion, and discharge associated with the common cold, bronchial asthma, acute and chronic bronchitis, and other respiratory tract conditions

Usual Dosage Oral: Relief of cough, congestion:
Children 2-6 years: Carbaphen 12 Ped®: 1-2 mL every 12 hours
Children 6-12 years: Carbaphen 12 Ped®: 2-4 mL every 12 hours
Children >12 years and Adults: Carbaphen 12®: 5-10 mL every 12 hours

Dosage Forms
Suspension:
Carbaphen 12®: Carbetapentane 60 mg, phenylephrine 20 mg, and chlorpheniramine 8 mg per 5 mL
Carbaphen 12 Ped®: Carbetapentane 15 mg, phenylephrine 2.5 mg, and chlorpheniramine 2 mg per 1 mL

carbetapentane, phenylephrine, and pyrilamine
(kar bay ta PEN tane, fen il EF rin, & peer Il a meen)

Synonyms phenylephrine tannate, carbetapentane tannate, and pyrilamine tannate; pyrilamine, phenyl-ephrine, and carbetapentane

U.S./Canadian Brand Names C-Tanna 12D [US]; Tussi-12® D [US]; Tussi-12® DS [US]

Therapeutic Category Antihistamine; Antihistamine/Decongestant/Antitussive; Antitussive; Decongestant

Use Symptomatic relief of cough associated with respiratory tract conditions such as the common cold, bronchial asthma, acute and chronic bronchitis

Usual Dosage Oral: Relief of cough:
Children:
2-6 years (Tussi-12® DS): 2.5-5 mL every 12 hours
6-11 years:
Tussi-12® D: 1/2 to 1 tablet every 12 hours
Tussi-12® DS: 5-10 mL every 12 hours
Children ≥12 years and Adults (Tussi-12® D): 1-2 tablets every 12 hours

Dosage Forms
Suspension:
C-Tanna 12D: Carbetapentane 30 mg, pyrilamine 30 mg, and phenylephrine 5 mg per 5 mL
Tussi-12® DS: Carbetapentane 30 mg, pyrilamine 30 mg, and phenylephrine 5 mg per 5 mL
Tablet:
C-Tanna 12D, Tussi-12® D: Carbetapentane 60 mg, pyrilamine 40 mg, and phenylephrine 10 mg

carbetapentane tannate and chlorpheniramine tannate *see* carbetapentane and chlorphenir-amine *on page 174*

carbetapentane tannate and pseudoephedrine tannate *see* carbetapentane and pseudoephe-drine *on page 175*

Carbetaplex [US] *see* carbetapentane, guaifenesin, and phenylephrine *on page 175*

carbetocin *(Canada only)* (kar BE toe sin)
U.S./Canadian Brand Names Duratocin™ [Can]
Therapeutic Category Uteronic Agent
Use For the prevention of uterine atony and postpartum hemorrhage following elective cesarean section under epidural or spinal anesthesia.
Usual Dosage A single I.V. dose of 100 mcg (1 mL) is administered by bolus injection, over 1 minute, only when delivery of the infant has been completed by cesarean section under epidural anesthetic. Carbetocin can be administered either before or after delivery of the placenta.
Dosage Forms
Injection: 1 mcg/mL (1 mL)

carbidopa (kar bi DOE pa)
U.S./Canadian Brand Names Lodosyn® [US]
Therapeutic Category Anti-Parkinson Agent (Dopamine Agonist)
Use Given with levodopa in the treatment of parkinsonism to enable a lower dosage of levodopa to be used and a more rapid response to be obtained and to decrease side effects; for details of administration and dosage, see Levodopa; has no effect without levodopa
Usual Dosage Oral: Adults: 70-100 mg/day; maximum daily dose: 200 mg
Dosage Forms
Tablet:
Lodosyn®: 25 mg

carbidopa and levodopa (kar bi DOE pa & lee voe DOE pa)
Synonyms levodopa and carbidopa
U.S./Canadian Brand Names Apo-Levocarb® CR [Can]; Apo-Levocarb® [Can]; Endo®-Levodopa/Carbidopa [Can]; Novo-Levocarbidopa [Can]; Nu-Levocarb [Can]; Parcopa™ [US]; Sinemet® CR [US/Can]; Sinemet® [US/Can]
Therapeutic Category Anti-Parkinson Agent (Dopamine Agonist)
Use Idiopathic Parkinson disease; postencephalitic parkinsonism; symptomatic parkinsonism
Usual Dosage Oral: Adults: Parkinson disease:
Immediate release tablet:
Initial: Carbidopa 25 mg/levodopa 100 mg 3 times/day
Dosage adjustment: Alternate tablet strengths may be substituted according to individual carbidopa/levodopa requirements. Increase by 1 tablet every other day as necessary, except when using the carbidopa 25 mg/levodopa 250 mg tablets where increases should be made using 1/2-1 tablet every 1-2 days. Use of more than 1 dosage strength or dosing 4 times/day may be required (maximum: 8 tablets of any strength/day or 200 mg of carbidopa and 2000 mg of levodopa)
Sustained release tablet:
Initial: Carbidopa 50 mg/levodopa 200 mg 2 times/day, at intervals not <6 hours
Dosage adjustment: May adjust every 3 days; intervals should be between 4-8 hours during the waking day (maximum: 8 tablets/day)
Dosage Forms
Tablet immediate release: 10/100: Carbidopa 10 mg and levodopa 100 mg; 25/100: Carbidopa 25 mg and levodopa 100 mg; 25/250: Carbidopa 25 mg and levodopa 250 mg
Sinemet®: 10/100: Carbidopa 10 mg and levodopa 100 mg; 25/100: Carbidopa 25 mg and levodopa 100 mg; 25/250: Carbidopa 25 mg and levodopa 250 mg
Tablet, immediate release, orally disintegrating:
Parcopa™: 10/100: Carbidopa 10 mg and levodopa 100 mg; 25/100: Carbidopa 25 mg and levodopa 100 mg; 25/250: Carbidopa 25 mg and levodopa 250 mg
Tablet, sustained release: Carbidopa 25 mg and levodopa 100 mg; carbidopa 50 mg and levodopa 200 mg
Sinemet® CR: Carbidopa 25 mg and levodopa 100 mg; carbidopa 50 mg and levodopa 200 mg

carbidopa, levodopa, and entacapone *see* levodopa, carbidopa, and entacapone *on page 556*
Carbihist *(Discontinued)* *see* carbinoxamine *on page 177*

carbinoxamine (kar bi NOKS a meen)
Synonyms carbinoxamine maleate
U.S./Canadian Brand Names Palgic® [US]

◀ **Therapeutic Category** Antihistamine

Use Seasonal and perennial allergic rhinitis; vasomotor rhinitis; urticaria; decrease severity of other allergic reactions

Usual Dosage Oral (Palgic®):
Children:
>3-6 years: 2-5 mg 3-4 times/day
>6 years: 4-6 mg 3-4 times/day
Adults: 4-8 mg 3-4 times/day

Dosage Forms
Solution:
Palgic®: 4 mg/5 mL
Tablet [scored]:
Palgic®: 4 mg

carbinoxamine and pseudoephedrine *(Discontinued)*

carbinoxamine maleate *see* carbinoxamine *on page 177*

Carbinoxamine PD *(Discontinued)* *see* carbinoxamine *on page 177*

carbinoxamine, pseudoephedrine, and dextromethorphan *(Discontinued)*

carbinoxamine, pseudoephedrine, and hydrocodone *see* hydrocodone, carbinoxamine, and pseudoephedrine *on page 483*

Carbiset® Tablet *(Discontinued)*

Carbiset-TR® Tablet *(Discontinued)*

Carbocaine® [US/Can] *see* mepivacaine *on page 604*

Carbocaine® 2% with Neo-Cobefrin® [US] *see* mepivacaine and levonordefrin *on page 605*

Carbodec® Syrup *(Discontinued)*

Carbodec® Tablet *(Discontinued)*

Carbodec® TR Tablet *(Discontinued)*

Carbofed DM [US] *see* brompheniramine, pseudoephedrine, and dextromethorphan *on page 146*

carbolic acid *see* phenol *on page 743*

Carbolith™ [Can] *see* lithium *on page 571*

carboplatin (KAR boe pla tin)

Sound-Alike/Look-Alike Issues
CARBOplatin may be confused with CISplatin, oxaliplatin
Paraplatin® may be confused with Platinol®

Synonyms CBDCA; NSC-241240

Tall-Man CARBOplatin

U.S./Canadian Brand Names Paraplatin-AQ [Can]

Therapeutic Category Antineoplastic Agent

Use Treatment of ovarian cancer

Usual Dosage Refer to individual protocols: **Note:** Doses for adults are usually determined by the AUC using the Calvert formula.

IVPB, I.V. infusion: Adults:
Ovarian cancer: 300-360 mg/m^2 every 4 weeks
In adults, dosing is commonly calculated using the Calvert formula:
Total dose (mg) = Target AUC x (GFR+ 25)
Usual target AUCs:
Previously untreated patients: 6-8
Previously treated patients: 4-6

Dosage Forms
Injection, powder for reconstitution: 50 mg, 150 mg, 450 mg
Injection, solution: 10 mg/mL (5 mL, 15 mL, 45 mL, 60 mL)

carboprost *see* carboprost tromethamine *on page 178*

carboprost tromethamine (KAR boe prost tro METH a meen)

Synonyms carboprost; prostaglandin F$_2$

U.S./Canadian Brand Names Hemabate® [US/Can]

Therapeutic Category Prostaglandin

Use Termination of pregnancy; treatment of refractory postpartum uterine bleeding

Usual Dosage I.M.: Adults:

Abortion: Initial: 250 mcg, then 250 mcg at 1.5- to 3.5-hour intervals, depending on uterine response; a 500 mcg dose may be given if uterine response is not adequate after several 250 mcg doses; do not exceed 12 mg total dose or continuous administration for >2 days

Refractory postpartum uterine bleeding: Initial: 250 mcg; if needed, may repeat at 15- to 90-minute intervals; maximum total dose: 2 mg (8 doses)

Dosage Forms

Injection, solution:

Hemabate®: Carboprost 250 mcg and tromethamine 83 mcg per mL (1 mL)

carbose D *see* carboxymethylcellulose *on page 179*

Carboxine *(Discontinued)* *see* carbinoxamine *on page 177*

Carboxine-PSE *(Discontinued)*

carboxymethylcellulose (kar boks ee meth il SEL yoo lose)

Sound-Alike/Look-Alike Issues

Optive™ may be confused with Optivar®

Synonyms carbose D; carboxymethylcellulose sodium

U.S./Canadian Brand Names Celluvisc™ [Can]; Optive™ [US-OTC]; Refresh Liquigel® [US-OTC]; Refresh Plus® [US-OTC/Can]; Refresh Tears® [US-OTC/Can]; Tears Again® Gel Drops™ [US-OTC]; Tears Again® Night and Day™ [US-OTC]; Theratears® [US]

Therapeutic Category Ophthalmic Agent, Miscellaneous

Use Artificial tear substitute

Usual Dosage Ophthalmic: Adults: Instill 1-2 drops into eye(s) 3-4 times/day

Dosage Forms

Gel, ophthalmic:

Tears Again® Night and Day™ [OTC]: 1.5% (3.5 g)

Solution ophthalmic [drops]:

Optive™ [OTC]: 0.5% (15 mL, 30 mL)

Refresh Liquigel® [OTC]: 1% (15 mL)

Refresh Tears® [OTC]: 0.5% (15 mL)

Tears Again® Gel Drops™ [OTC]: 0.7% (15 mL)

Theratears®: 0.25% (15 mL)

Solution ophthalmic [drops; preservative free]:

Refresh Plus®: 0.5% (0.4 mL)

Theratears®: 0.25% (0.6 mL)

carboxymethylcellulose sodium *see* carboxymethylcellulose *on page 179*

Cardene® [US] *see* nicardipine *on page 670*

Cardene® I.V. [US] *see* nicardipine *on page 670*

Cardene® SR [US] *see* nicardipine *on page 670*

Cardio-Green® *(Discontinued)* *see* indocyanine green *on page 506*

Cardioquin® *(Discontinued)* *see* quinidine *on page 813*

Cardizem® [US/Can] *see* diltiazem *on page 300*

Cardizem® CD [US/Can] *see* diltiazem *on page 300*

Cardizem® Injection *(Discontinued)* *see* diltiazem *on page 300*

Cardizem® LA [US] *see* diltiazem *on page 300*

Cardizem® SR [Can] *see* diltiazem *on page 300*

Cardizem® SR *(Discontinued)* *see* diltiazem *on page 300*

Cardura® [US] *see* doxazosin *on page 320*

Cardura-1™ [Can] *see* doxazosin *on page 320*

Cardura-2™ [Can] *see* doxazosin *on page 320*

Cardura-4™ [Can] *see* doxazosin *on page 320*

Cardura® XL [US] *see* doxazosin *on page 320*

CareNatal™ DHA [US] *see* vitamins (multiple/prenatal) *on page 983*

Carimune™ *(Discontinued)* *see* immune globulin (intravenous) *on page 503*

Carimune® NF [US] *see immune globulin (intravenous) on page 503*
carindacillin *see carbenicillin on page 174*
carisoprodate *see carisoprodol on page 180*

carisoprodol (kar eye soe PROE dole)
Synonyms carisoprodate; isobamate
U.S./Canadian Brand Names Soma® [US/Can]
Therapeutic Category Skeletal Muscle Relaxant
Use Short-term (2-3 weeks) relief of skeletal muscle pain
Usual Dosage Note: Carisoprodol should only be used for short periods (2-3 weeks) due to lack of evidence of effectiveness with prolonged use.
Oral: Children ≥16 years and Adults: 250-350 mg 3 times/day and at bedtime
Dosage Forms
 Tablet: 350 mg
  Soma®: 250 mg, 350 mg

carisoprodol and aspirin (kar eye soe PROE dole & AS pir in)
Synonyms aspirin and carisoprodol
U.S./Canadian Brand Names Soma® Compound [US]
Therapeutic Category Skeletal Muscle Relaxant
Use Skeletal muscle relaxant
Usual Dosage Oral: Adults: 1-2 tablets 4 times/day
Dosage Forms
 Tablet: Carisoprodol 200 mg and aspirin 325 mg
  Soma® Compound: Carisoprodol 200 mg and aspirin 325 mg

carisoprodol, aspirin, and codeine (kar eye soe PROE dole, AS pir in, and KOE deen)
Synonyms aspirin, carisoprodol, and codeine; codeine, aspirin, and carisoprodol
Therapeutic Category Skeletal Muscle Relaxant
Controlled Substance C-III
Use Skeletal muscle relaxant
Usual Dosage Oral: Adults: 1 or 2 tablets 4 times/day
Dosage Forms
 Tablet: Carisoprodol 200 mg, aspirin 325 mg, and codeine 16 mg

Carmol® 10 [US-OTC] *see urea on page 963*
Carmol® 20 [US-OTC] *see urea on page 963*
Carmol® 40 [US] *see urea on page 963*
Carmol® Deep Cleaning [US] *see urea on page 963*
Carmol-HC® [US] *see urea and hydrocortisone on page 964*
Carmol® Scalp Treatment [US] *see sulfacetamide on page 892*

carmustine (kar MUS teen)
Sound-Alike/Look-Alike Issues
 carmustine may be confused with bendamustine, lomustine
Synonyms BCNU; bis-chloronitrosourea; carmustinum; NSC-409962; WR-139021
U.S./Canadian Brand Names BiCNU® [US/Can]; Gliadel Wafer® [Can]; Gliadel® [US]
Therapeutic Category Antineoplastic Agent
Use
 Injection: Treatment of brain tumors (glioblastoma, brainstem glioma, medulloblastoma, astrocytoma, ependymoma, and metastatic brain tumors), multiple myeloma, Hodgkin disease (relapsed or refractory), non-Hodgkin lymphomas (relapsed or refractory),
 Wafer (implant): Adjunct to surgery in patients with recurrent glioblastoma multiforme; adjunct to surgery and radiation in patients with high-grade malignant glioma
Usual Dosage I.V. (refer to individual protocols): Adults:
 Usual dosage (per manufacturer labeling): 150-200 mg/m^2 every 6 weeks **or** 75-100 mg/m^2/day for 2 days every 6 weeks

Primary brain cancer:
150-200 mg/m^2 every 6-8 weeks as a single dose **or**
75-120 mg/m^2 days 1 and 2 every 6-8 weeks **or**
20-65 mg/m^2 every 4-6 weeks **or**
0.5-1 mg/kg every 4-6 weeks **or**
40-80 mg/m^2/day for 3 days every 6-8 weeks
Autologous BMT: ALL OF THE FOLLOWING DOSES ARE FATAL WITHOUT BMT
Combination therapy: Up to 300-900 mg/m^2
Single-agent therapy: Up to 1200 mg/m^2 (fatal necrosis is associated with doses >2 g/m^2)
Implantation (wafer): Recurrent glioblastoma multiforme, malignant glioma: Up to 8 wafers may be placed in the resection cavity (total dose 62.6 mg); should the size and shape not accommodate 8 wafers, the maximum number of wafers allowed should be placed

Dosage Forms
Implant:
Gliadel®: 7.7 mg (8s)
Injection, powder for reconstitution:
BiCNU®: 100 mg

carmustinum *see carmustine on page 180*
Carnation Instant Breakfast® [US-OTC] *see nutritional formula, enteral/oral on page 689*
Carnitor® [US/Can] *see levocarnitine on page 555*
Carnitor® SF [US] *see levocarnitine on page 555*
Carrington Antifungal [US-OTC] *see miconazole on page 630*

carteolol (KAR tee oh lole)
Sound-Alike/Look-Alike Issues
carteolol may be confused with carvedilol
Synonyms carteolol hydrochloride
U.S./Canadian Brand Names Ocupress® Ophthalmic [Can]
Therapeutic Category Beta-Adrenergic Blocker
Use Treatment of chronic open-angle glaucoma and intraocular hypertension
Usual Dosage Ophthalmic: Adults: Instill 1 drop in affected eye(s) twice daily.
Dosage Forms
Solution, ophthalmic, as hydrochloride: 1% (5 mL, 10 mL, 15 mL)

carteolol hydrochloride *see carteolol on page 181*
Carter's Little Pills® [Can] *see bisacodyl on page 136*
Carter's Little Pills® (Discontinued) *see bisacodyl on page 136*
Cartia XT™ [US] *see diltiazem on page 300*

carvedilol (KAR ve dil ole)
Sound-Alike/Look-Alike Issues
carvedilol may be confused with captopril, carteolol
U.S./Canadian Brand Names Apo-Carvedilol® [Can]; Coreg CR™ [US]; Coreg® [US/Can]; Novo-Carvedilol [Can]; PMS-Carvedilol [Can]; RAN™-Carvedilol [Can]; ratio-Carvedilol [Can]
Therapeutic Category Beta-Adrenergic Blocker
Use Mild-to-severe heart failure of ischemic or cardiomyopathic origin (usually in addition to standard therapy); left ventricular dysfunction following myocardial infarction (MI) (clinically stable with LVEF ≤40%); management of hypertension
Usual Dosage Oral: Adults: Reduce dosage if heart rate drops to <55 beats/minute.
Hypertension:
Immediate release: 6.25 mg twice daily; if tolerated, dose should be maintained for 1-2 weeks, then increased to 12.5 mg twice daily. Dosage may be increased to a maximum of 25 mg twice daily after 1-2 weeks; maximum dose: 50 mg/day.
Extended release: Initial: 20 mg once daily, if tolerated, dose should be maintained for 1-2 weeks then increased to 40 mg once daily if necessary; maximum dose: 80 mg once daily
Congestive heart failure:
Immediate release: 3.125 mg twice daily for 2 weeks; if this dose is tolerated, may increase to 6.25 mg twice daily. Double the dose every 2 weeks to the highest dose tolerated by patient. (Prior to initiating therapy, other heart failure medications should be stabilized and fluid retention minimized.) ▶

◀ Maximum recommended dose:
Mild-to-moderate heart failure:
<85 kg: 25 mg twice daily
>85 kg: 50 mg twice daily
Severe heart failure: 25 mg twice daily
Extended release: Initial: 10 mg once daily for 2 weeks; if the dose is tolerated, increase dose to 20 mg, 40 mg, and 80 mg over successive intervals of at least 2 weeks. Maintain on lower dose if higher dose is not tolerated.
Left ventricular dysfunction following MI: **Note**: Should be initiated only after patient is hemodynamically stable and fluid retention has been minimized.
Immediate release: Initial 3.125-6.25 mg twice daily; increase dosage incrementally (ie, from 6.25-12.5 mg twice daily) at intervals of 3-10 days, based on tolerance, to a target dose of 25 mg twice daily.
Extended release: Initial: 20 mg once daily; increase dosage incrementally at intervals of 3-10 days. Target dose: 80 mg once daily.

Conversion from immediate release to extended release (Coreg CR™):
Current dose immediate release tablets 3.125 mg twice daily: Convert to extended release capsules 10 mg once daily
Current dose immediate release tablets 6.25 mg twice daily: Convert to extended release capsules 20 mg once daily
Current dose immediate release tablets 12.5 mg twice daily: Convert to extended release capsules 40 mg once daily
Current dose immediate release tablets 25 mg twice daily: Convert to extended release capsules 80 mg once daily

Dosage Forms
Capsule, extended release:
Coreg CR®: 10 mg, 20 mg, 40 mg, 80 mg
Tablet: 3.125 mg, 6.25 mg, 12.5 mg, 25 mg
Coreg®: 3.125 mg, 6.25 mg, 12.5 mg, 25 mg

Casodex® [US/Can] *see* bicalutamide *on page 135*

caspofungin (kas poe FUN jin)

Synonyms caspofungin acetate
U.S./Canadian Brand Names Cancidas® [US/Can]
Therapeutic Category Antifungal Agent, Systemic
Use Treatment of invasive *Aspergillus* infections in patients who are refractory or intolerant of other therapy; treatment of candidemia and other *Candida* infections (intraabdominal abscesses, esophageal, peritonitis, pleural space); empirical treatment for presumed fungal infections in febrile neutropenic patient
Usual Dosage I.V.: Adults: **Note:** Duration of caspofungin treatment should be determined by patient status and clinical response. Empiric therapy should be given until neutropenia resolves. In patients with positive cultures, treatment should continue until 14 days after last positive culture. In neutropenic patients, treatment should be given at least 7 days after both signs and symptoms of infection **and** neutropenia resolve.
Aspergillosis, invasive: Initial dose: 70 mg on day 1; subsequent dosing: 50 mg/day. **Note:** Duration of therapy should be a minimum of 6-12 weeks or throughout period of immunosuppression.
Candidiasis: Initial dose: 70 mg on day 1; subsequent dosing: 50 mg/day
Esophageal: 50 mg/day; **Note:** The majority of patients studied for this indication also had oropharyngeal involvement.
Empiric therapy: Initial dose: 70 mg on day 1; subsequent dosing: 50 mg/day; may increase up to 70 mg/day if tolerated, but clinical response is inadequate
Concomitant use of an enzyme inducer:
Patients receiving rifampin: 70 mg caspofungin daily
Patients receiving carbamazepine, dexamethasone, efavirenz, nevirapine, **or** phenytoin (and possibly other enzyme inducers) may require an increased daily dose of caspofungin (70 mg/day).
Dosage Forms
Injection, powder for reconstitution:
Cancidas®: 50 mg, 70 mg

caspofungin acetate *see* caspofungin *on page 182*

Castellani Paint Modified [US-OTC] *see* phenol *on page 743*

castor oil (KAS tor oyl)
Synonyms oleum ricini
Therapeutic Category Laxative
Use Preparation for rectal or bowel examination or surgery; rarely used to relieve constipation; also applied to skin as emollient and protectant
Usual Dosage Oral: Oil:
  Children 2-11 years: 5-15 mL as a single dose
  Children ≥12 years and Adults: 15-60 mL as a single dose
Dosage Forms
  Oil, oral: 100%

castor oil, trypsin, and balsam peru *see* trypsin, balsam peru, and castor oil *on page 958*
Cataflam® [US/Can] *see* diclofenac *on page 292*
Catapres® [US] *see* clonidine *on page 236*
Catapres-TTS® [US] *see* clonidine *on page 236*
catechins *see* sinecatechins *on page 868*
Cathflo® Activase® [US/Can] *see* alteplase *on page 51*
Caverject® [US/Can] *see* alprostadil *on page 50*
Caverject Impulse® [US] *see* alprostadil *on page 50*
CaviRinse™ [US] *see* fluoride *on page 411*
CB-1348 *see* chlorambucil *on page 200*
CBDCA *see* carboplatin *on page 178*
CBZ *see* carbamazepine *on page 172*
CC-5013 *see* lenalidomide *on page 551*
CCI-779 *see* temsirolimus *on page 908*
CCNU *see* lomustine *on page 573*
C-Crystals® *(Discontinued)* *see* ascorbic acid *on page 96*
2-CdA *see* cladribine *on page 226*
CDDP *see* cisplatin *on page 224*
CDP870 *see* certolizumab pegol *on page 195*
CDX *see* bicalutamide *on page 135*
Cebid® *(Discontinued)* *see* ascorbic acid *on page 96*
Ceclor® [Can] *see* cefaclor *on page 183*
Ceclor® *(Discontinued)* *see* cefaclor *on page 183*
Cecon® [US-OTC] *see* ascorbic acid *on page 96*
Cedax® [US] *see* ceftibuten *on page 190*
Cedocard®-SR [Can] *see* isosorbide dinitrate *on page 530*
CEE *see* estrogens (conjugated/equine) *on page 364*
CeeNU® [US/Can] *see* lomustine *on page 573*
Ceepryn® *(Discontinued)* *see* cetylpyridinium *on page 197*

cefaclor (SEF a klor)
Sound-Alike/Look-Alike Issues
  cefaclor may be confused with cephalexin
U.S./Canadian Brand Names Apo-Cefaclor® [Can]; Ceclor® [Can]; Novo-Cefaclor [Can]; Nu-Cefaclor [Can]; PMS-Cefaclor [Can]; Raniclor™ [US]
Therapeutic Category Cephalosporin (Second Generation)
Use Treatment of susceptible bacterial infections including otitis media, lower respiratory tract infections, acute exacerbations of chronic bronchitis, pharyngitis and tonsillitis, urinary tract infections, skin and skin structure infections
Usual Dosage
  Usual dosage range:
    Children >1 month: Oral: 20-40 mg/kg/day divided every 8-12 hours (maximum dose: 1 g/day)
    Adults: Oral: 250-500 mg every 8 hours

◀ **Indication-specific dosing:**
  Children: Oral:
    Otitis media: 40 mg/kg/day divided every 12 hours
    Pharyngitis: 20 mg/kg/day divided every 12 hours
Dosage Forms
  Capsule: 250 mg, 500 mg
  Powder for oral suspension: 125 mg/5 mL, 250 mg/5 mL, 375 mg/5 mL
  Tablet, chewable:
    Raniclor™: 250 mg, 375 mg
  Tablet, extended release: 500 mg

cefadroxil (sef a DROKS il)

Synonyms cefadroxil monohydrate
U.S./Canadian Brand Names Apo-Cefadroxil® [Can]; Duricef® [Can]; Novo-Cefadroxil [Can]
Therapeutic Category Cephalosporin (First Generation)
Use Treatment of susceptible bacterial infections, including those caused by group A beta-hemolytic *Streptococcus*
Usual Dosage
  Usual dosage range: Oral:
    Children: 30 mg/kg/day divided twice daily up to a maximum of 2 g/day
    Adults: 1-2 g/day in 2 divided doses
  Indication-specific dosing: Orofacial infections: Adults: 250-500 mg every 8 hours
Dosage Forms Note: Strength is expressed as base
  Capsule: 500 mg
  Powder for oral suspension: 250 mg/5 mL, 500 mg/5 mL
  Tablet: 1 g

cefadroxil monohydrate *see* cefadroxil *on page 184*
Cefanex® *(Discontinued) see* cephalexin *on page 194*

cefazolin (sef A zoe lin)

Sound-Alike/Look-Alike Issues
  ceFAZolin may be confused with cefprozil, cefTRIAXone, cephalexin, cephalothin
  Kefzol® may be confused with Cefzil®
Synonyms cefazolin sodium
Tall-Man ceFAZolin
Therapeutic Category Cephalosporin (First Generation)
Use Treatment of respiratory tract, skin and skin structure, genital, urinary tract, biliary tract, bone and joint infections, and septicemia due to susceptible gram-positive cocci (except enterococcus); some gram-negative bacilli including *E. coli*, *Proteus*, and *Klebsiella* may be susceptible; perioperative prophylaxis
Usual Dosage
  Usual dosage range: I.M., I.V.:
    Children >1 month: 25-100 mg/kg/day divided every 6-8 hours; maximum: 6 g/day
    Adults: 250 mg to 2 g every 6-12 (usually 8) hours, depending on severity of infection; maximum dose: 12 g/day
  Indication-specific dosing: Adults: I.M., I.V.:
    Prophylaxis in total joint replacement patient: 1 g 1 hour prior to the procedure
    Mild-to-moderate infections: 500 mg to 1 g every 6-8 hours
    Mild infection with gram-positive cocci: 250-500 mg every 8 hours
    Perioperative prophylaxis: 1 g given 30 minutes prior to surgery (repeat with 500 mg to 1 g during prolonged surgery); followed by 500 mg to 1 g every 6-9 hours for 24 hours postop
    Pneumococcal pneumonia: 500 mg every 12 hours
    Severe infection: 1-2 g every 6 hours
    UTI (uncomplicated): 1 g every 12 hours
Dosage Forms
  Infusion [iso-osmotic dextrose solution]: 1 g (50 mL)
  Injection, powder for reconstitution: 500 mg, 1 g, 10 g, 20 g

cefazolin sodium *see* cefazolin *on page 184*

cefdinir (SEF di ner)

Synonyms CFDN

U.S./Canadian Brand Names Omnicef® [US/Can]

Therapeutic Category Cephalosporin (Third Generation)

Use Treatment of community-acquired pneumonia, acute exacerbations of chronic bronchitis, acute bacterial otitis media, acute maxillary sinusitis, pharyngitis/tonsillitis, and uncomplicated skin and skin structure infections.

Usual Dosage

Usual dosage range:

Children 6 months to 12 years: Oral: 7 mg/kg/dose twice daily or 14 mg/kg/dose once daily (maximum: 600 mg/day)

Adolescents and Adults: Oral: 300 mg twice daily or 600 mg once daily

Indication-specific dosing:

Children 6 months to 12 years: Oral:

Acute bacterial otitis media, pharyngitis/tonsillitis: 7 mg/kg/dose twice daily for 5-10 days **or** 14 mg/kg/dose once daily for 10 days (maximum: 600 mg/day)

Acute maxillary sinusitis: 7 mg/kg/dose twice daily **or** 14 mg/kg/dose once daily for 10 days (maximum: 600 mg/day)

Uncomplicated skin and skin structure infections: 7 mg/kg/dose twice daily for 10 days (maximum: 600 mg/day)

Adolescents and Adults:

Acute exacerbations of chronic bronchitis, pharyngitis/tonsillitis: 300 mg twice daily for 5-10 days **or** 600 mg once daily for 10 days

Acute maxillary sinusitis: 300 mg twice daily **or** 600 mg once daily for 10 days

Community-acquired pneumonia, uncomplicated skin and skin structure infections: 300 mg twice daily for 10 days

Dosage Forms

Capsule: 300 mg

Omnicef®: 300 mg

Powder for oral suspension: 125 mg/5 mL; 250 mg/5 mL

Omnicef®: 125 mg/5 mL (60 mL, 100 mL), 250 mg/5 mL (60 mL, 100 mL)

cefditoren (sef de TOR en)

Synonyms cefditoren pivoxil

U.S./Canadian Brand Names Spectracef® [US]

Therapeutic Category Antibiotic, Cephalosporin

Use Treatment of acute bacterial exacerbation of chronic bronchitis or community-acquired pneumonia (due to susceptible organisms including *Haemophilus influenzae, Haemophilus parainfluenzae, Streptococcus pneumoniae*-penicillin susceptible only, *Moraxella catarrhalis*); pharyngitis or tonsillitis (*Streptococcus pyogenes*); and uncomplicated skin and skin-structure infections (*Staphylococcus aureus* - not MRSA, *Streptococcus pyogenes*)

Usual Dosage

Usual dosage range:

Children ≥12 years and Adults: Oral: 200-400 mg twice daily

Indication-specific dosing:

Children ≥12 years and Adults: Oral:

Acute bacterial exacerbation of chronic bronchitis: 400 mg twice daily for 10 days

Community-acquired pneumonia: 400 mg twice daily for 14 days

Pharyngitis, tonsillitis, uncomplicated skin and skin structure infections: 200 mg twice daily for 10 days

Dosage Forms

Tablet:

Spectracef®: 200 mg

cefditoren pivoxil *see* cefditoren *on page 185*

cefepime (SEF e pim)

Synonyms cefepime hydrochloride

U.S./Canadian Brand Names Maxipime® [US/Can]

Therapeutic Category Cephalosporin (Fourth Generation)

▶

Use Treatment of uncomplicated and complicated urinary tract infections, including pyelonephritis caused by typical urinary tract pathogens; monotherapy for febrile neutropenia; uncomplicated skin and skin structure infections caused by *Streptococcus pyogenes*; moderate-to-severe pneumonia caused by pneumococcus, *Pseudomonas aeruginosa*, and other gram-negative organisms; complicated intra-abdominal infections (in combination with metronidazole). Also active against methicillin-susceptible staphylococci, *Enterobacter* sp, and many other gram-negative bacilli.

Children 2 months to 16 years: Empiric therapy of febrile neutropenia patients, uncomplicated skin/soft tissue infections, pneumonia, and uncomplicated/complicated urinary tract infections.

Usual Dosage
Usual dosage range:
  Children: I.M., I.V.: 50 mg/kg every 8-12 hours (maximum not to exceed adult dosing)
  Adults: I.V.: 1-2 g every 8-12 hours; I.M.: 500-1000 mg every 12 hours
Indication-specific dosing:
  Children ≥2 months to 16 years (<40 kg):
    Febrile neutropenia: I.V.: 50 mg/kg every 8 hours for 7 days or until neutropenia resolves
    Skin and skin structure infections (uncomplicated) and pneumonia: I.V.: 50 mg/kg every 12 hours for 10 days
    Urinary tract infections, complicated and uncomplicated: I.M., I.V.: 50 mg/kg every 12 hours for 7-10 days; **Note:** I.M. may be considered for mild-to-moderate infection only
  Adults:
    Febrile neutropenia, monotherapy: I.V.: 2 g every 8 hours for 7 days or until the neutropenia resolves
    Intraabdominal infections, complicated: I.V.: 2 g every 12 hours for 7-10 days with metronidazole
    Pneumonia: I.V.:
      Nosocomial (HAP/VAP): 1-2 g every 8-12 hours; **Note:** Duration of therapy may vary considerably (7-21 days); usually longer courses are required if *Pseudomonas*. In absence of *Pseudomonas*, and if appropriate empiric treatment used and patient responsive, it may be clinically appropriate to reduce duration of therapy to 7-10 days (American Thoracic Society Guidelines, 2005).
      Community-acquired (including pseudomonal): 1-2 g every 12 hours for 10 days
    Skin and skin structure, uncomplicated: I.V.: 2 g every 12 hours for 10 days
    Urinary tract infections, complicated and uncomplicated:
      Mild-to-moderate: I.M., I.V.: 500-1000 mg every 12 hours for 7-10 days
      Severe: I.V.: 2 g every 12 hours for 10 days
Dosage Forms
  Injection, powder for reconstitution: 500 mg, 1 g, 2 g
    Maxipime®: 500 mg, 1 g, 2 g

cefepime hydrochloride *see cefepime on page 185*
Cefizox® [US/Can] *see ceftizoxime on page 190*
Cefotan® *(Discontinued)*

cefotaxime (sef oh TAKS eem)

Sound-Alike/Look-Alike Issues
  cefotaxime may be confused with cefoxitin, ceftizoxime, cefuroxime
Synonyms cefotaxime sodium
U.S./Canadian Brand Names Claforan® [US/Can]
Therapeutic Category Cephalosporin (Third Generation)
Use Treatment of susceptible infection in respiratory tract, skin and skin structure, bone and joint, urinary tract, gynecologic as well as septicemia, and documented or suspected meningitis. Active against most gram-negative bacilli (not *Pseudomonas*) and gram-positive cocci (not enterococcus). Active against many penicillin-resistant pneumococci.
Usual Dosage
Usual dosage range:
  Infants and Children 1 month to 12 years <50 kg: I.M., I.V.: 50-200 mg/kg/day in divided doses every 6-8 hours
  Children >12 years and Adults: I.M., I.V.: 1-2 g every 4-12 hours
Indication-specific dosing:
  Infants and Children 1 month to 12 years:
    Epiglottitis: I.M., I.V.: 150-200 mg/kg/day in 4 divided doses with clindamycin for 7-10 days
    Meningitis: I.M., I.V.: 200 mg/kg/day in divided doses every 6 hours
    Pneumonia: I.V.: 200 mg/kg/day divided every 8 hours

Sepsis: I.V.: 150 mg/kg/day divided every 8 hours
Typhoid fever: I.M., I.V.: 150-200 mg/kg/day in 3-4 divided doses (maximum: 12 g/day); fluoroquinolone resistant: 80 mg/kg/day in 3-4 divided doses (maximum: 12 g/day)
Children >12 years and Adults:
Arthritis (septic): I.V.: 1 g every 8 hours
Brain abscess, meningitis: I.V.: 2 g every 4-6 hours
Caesarean section: I.M., I.V.: 1 g as soon as the umbilical cord is clamped, then 1 g at 6- and 12-hour intervals
Epiglottitis: I.V.: 2 g every 4-8 hours
Gonorrhea: I.M.: 1 g as a single dose
Disseminated: I.V.: 1 g every 8 hours
Life-threatening infections: I.V.: 2 g every 4 hours
Liver abscess: I.V.: 1-2 g every 6 hours
Lyme disease:
Cardiac manifestations: I.V.: 2 g every 4 hours
CNS manifestations: I.V.: 2 g every 8 hours for 14-28 days
Moderate-to-severe infections: I.M., I.V.: 1-2 g every 8 hours
Orbital cellulitis: I.V.: 2 g every 4 hours
Peritonitis (spontaneous): I.V.: 2 g every 8 hours, unless life-threatening then 2 g every 4 hours
Septicemia: I.V.: 2 g every 6-8 hours
Skin and soft tissue:
Mixed, necrotizing: I.V.: 2 g every 6 hours, with metronidazole or clindamycin
Bite wounds (animal): I.V.: 2 g every 6 hours
Surgical prophylaxis: I.M., I.V.: 1 g 30-90 minutes before surgery
Uncomplicated infections: I.M., I.V.: 1 g every 12 hours
Dosage Forms
Infusion, as sodium [premixed iso-osmotic solution]:
Claforan®: 1 g (50 mL); 2 g (50 mL)
Injection, powder for reconstitution: 500 mg, 1 g, 2 g, 10 g, 20 g
Claforan®: 500 mg, 1 g, 2 g, 10 g

cefotaxime sodium *see* cefotaxime *on page 186*

cefoxitin (se FOKS i tin)

Sound-Alike/Look-Alike Issues
cefoxitin may be confused with cefotaxime, cefotetan, Cytoxan®
Mefoxin® may be confused with Lanoxin®
Synonyms cefoxitin sodium
U.S./Canadian Brand Names Apo-Cefoxitin® [Can]
Therapeutic Category Cephalosporin (Second Generation)
Use Less active against staphylococci and streptococci than first generation cephalosporins, but active against anaerobes including *Bacteroides fragilis*; active against gram-negative enteric bacilli including *E. coli*, *Klebsiella*, and *Proteus*; used predominantly for respiratory tract, skin and skin structure, bone and joint, urinary tract and gynecologic as well as septicemia; surgical prophylaxis; intraabdominal infections and other mixed infections; indicated for bacterial *Eikenella corrodens* infections
Usual Dosage
Usual dosage range:
Infants >3 months and Children: I.M., I.V.: 80-160 mg/kg/day in divided doses every 4-6 hours (maximum dose: 12 g/day)
Adults: I.M., I.V.: 1-2 g every 6-8 hours (maximum dose: 12 g/day)
Note: I.M. injection is painful.
Indication-specific dosing:
Infants >3 months and Children:
Mild-to-moderate infection: I.M., I.V.: 80-100 mg/kg/day in divided doses every 4-6 hours
Perioperative prophylaxis: I.V.: 30-40 mg/kg 30-60 minutes prior to surgery followed by 30-40 mg/kg/dose every 6 hours for no more than 24 hours after surgery depending on the procedure
Severe infection: I.M., I.V.: 100-160 mg/kg/day in divided doses every 4-6 hours
Adolescents and Adults:
Perioperative prophylaxis: I.M., I.V.: 1-2 g 30-60 minutes prior to surgery followed by 1-2 g every 6-8 hours for no more than 24 hours after surgery depending on the procedure

◀ Adults:
  Amnionitis, endomyometritis: I.M., I.V.: 2 g every 6-8 hours
  Aspiration pneumonia, empyema, orbital cellulitis, parapharyngeal space, human bites: I.M., I.V.: 2 g every 8 hours
  Liver abscess: I.V.: 1 g every 4 hours
  Mycobacterium species, not MTB or MAI: I.V.: 12 g/day with amikacin
  Pelvic inflammatory disease:
    Inpatients: I.V.: 2 g every 6 hours **plus** doxycycline 100 mg I.V. or 100 mg orally every 12 hours until improved, followed by doxycycline 100 mg orally twice daily to complete 14 days
    Outpatients: I.M.: 2 g **plus** probenecid 1 g orally as a single dose, followed by doxycycline 100 mg orally twice daily for 14 days
Dosage Forms
  Injection, powder for reconstitution: 1 g, 2 g, 10 g
  Powder for prescription compounding: 100 g

cefoxitin sodium *see* cefoxitin *on page 187*

cefpodoxime (sef pode OKS eem)
Sound-Alike/Look-Alike Issues
  Vantin® may be confused with Ventolin®
Synonyms cefpodoxime proxetil
U.S./Canadian Brand Names Vantin® [US/Can]
Therapeutic Category Cephalosporin (Second Generation)
Use Treatment of susceptible acute, community-acquired pneumonia caused by *S. pneumoniae* or nonbeta-lactamase producing *H. influenzae*; acute uncomplicated gonorrhea caused by *N. gonorrhoeae*; uncomplicated skin and skin structure infections caused by *S. aureus* or *S. pyogenes*; acute otitis media caused by *S. pneumoniae, H. influenzae,* or *M. catarrhalis*; pharyngitis or tonsillitis; and uncomplicated urinary tract infections caused by *E. coli, Klebsiella,* and *Proteus*
Usual Dosage
  Usual dosage range:
    Children 2 months to 12 years: Oral: 10 mg/kg/day divided every 12 hours (maximum dose: 400 mg/day)
    Children ≥12 years and Adults: Oral: 100-400 mg every 12 hours
  Indication-specific dosing:
    Children 2 months to 12 years: Oral:
      Acute maxillary sinusitis: 10 mg/kg/day divided every 12 hours for 10 days (maximum: 200 mg/dose)
      Acute otitis media: 10 mg/kg/day divided every 12 hours (400 mg/day) for 5 days (maximum: 200 mg/dose)
      Pharyngitis/tonsillitis: 10 mg/kg/day in 2 divided doses for 5-10 days (maximum: 100 mg/dose)
    Children ≥12 years and Adults: Oral:
      Acute community-acquired pneumonia and bacterial exacerbations of chronic bronchitis: 200 mg every 12 hours for 14 days and 10 days, respectively
      Acute maxillary sinusitis: 200 mg every 12 hours for 10 days
      Pharyngitis/tonsillitis: 100 mg every 12 hours for 5-10 days
      Skin and skin structure: 400 mg every 12 hours for 7-14 days
      Uncomplicated gonorrhea (male and female) and rectal gonococcal infections (female): 200 mg as a single dose
      Uncomplicated urinary tract infection: 100 mg every 12 hours for 7 days
Dosage Forms
  Granules for oral suspension: 50 mg/5 mL (50 mL, 75 mL, 100 mL); 100 mg/5 mL (50 mL, 75 mL, 100 mL)
  Tablet: 100 mg, 200 mg
    Vantin®: 100 mg, 200 mg

cefpodoxime proxetil *see* cefpodoxime *on page 188*

cefprozil (sef PROE zil)
Sound-Alike/Look-Alike Issues
  cefprozil may be confused with cefazolin, cefuroxime
  Cefzil® may be confused with Cefol®, Ceftin®, Kefzol®

U.S./Canadian Brand Names Apo-Cefprozil® [Can]; Cefzil® [Can]; Ran-Cefprozil [Can]; Sandoz-Cefprozil [Can]

Therapeutic Category Cephalosporin (Second Generation)

Use Treatment of otitis media and infections involving the respiratory tract and skin and skin structure; active against methicillin-sensitive staphylococci, many streptococci, and various gram-negative bacilli including *E. coli*, some *Klebsiella*, *P. mirabilis*, *H. influenzae*, and *Moraxella*.

Usual Dosage

Usual dosage range:
Infants and Children >6 months to 12 years: Oral: 7.5-15 mg/kg/day divided every 12 hours
Children >12 years and Adults: Oral: 250-500 mg every 12 hours or 500 mg every 24 hours

Indication-specific dosing:
Infants and Children >6 months to 12 years: Oral: **Otitis media:** 15 mg/kg every 12 hours for 10 days
Children 2-12 years: Oral:
Pharyngitis/tonsillitis: 7.5-15 mg/kg/day divided every 12 hours for 10 days (administer for >10 days if due to *S. pyogenes*); maximum: 1 g/day
Uncomplicated skin and skin structure infections: 20 mg/kg every 24 hours for 10 days; maximum: 1 g/day
Children >12 years and Adults: Oral:
Pharyngitis/tonsillitis: 500 mg every 24 hours for 10 days
Secondary bacterial infection of acute bronchitis or acute bacterial exacerbation of chronic bronchitis: 500 mg every 12 hours for 10 days
Uncomplicated skin and skin structure infections: 250 mg every 12 hours or 500 mg every 12-24 hours for 10 days

Dosage Forms
Powder for oral suspension: 125 mg/5 mL, 250 mg/5 mL
Tablet: 250 mg, 500 mg

ceftazidime (SEF tay zi deem)

Sound-Alike/Look-Alike Issues
ceftazidime may be confused with ceftizoxime
Ceptaz® may be confused with Septra®
Tazicef® may be confused with Tazidime®

U.S./Canadian Brand Names Fortaz® [US/Can]; Tazicef® [US]

Therapeutic Category Cephalosporin (Third Generation)

Use Treatment of documented susceptible *Pseudomonas aeruginosa* infection and infections due to other susceptible aerobic gram-negative organisms; empiric therapy of a febrile, granulocytopenic patient

Usual Dosage

Usual dosage range:
Infants and Children 1 month to 12 years: I.V.: 30-50 mg/kg/dose every 8 hours (maximum dose: 6 g/day)
Adults: I.M., I.V.: 500 mg to 2 g every 8-12 hours

Indication-specific dosing:
Bacterial arthritis (gram-negative bacilli): I.V.: 1-2 g every 8 hours
Cystic fibrosis: I.V.: 30-50 mg/kg every 8 hours (maximum: 6 g/day)
Melioidosis: I.V.: 40 mg/kg every 8 hours for 10 days, followed by oral therapy with doxycycline or TMP/SMX
Otitis externa: I.V.: 2 g every 8 hours
Peritonitis (CAPD):
Anuric, intermittent: 1000-1500 mg/day
Anuric, continuous (per liter exchange): Loading dose: 250 mg; maintenance dose: 125 mg
Severe infections, including meningitis, complicated pneumonia, endophthalmitis, CNS infection, osteomyelitis, intraabdominal and gynecological, skin and soft tissue: I.V.: 2 g every 8 hours

Dosage Forms
Infusion [premixed iso-osmotic solution, frozen]:
Fortaz®: 1 g (50 mL); 2 g (50 mL)
Injection, powder for reconstitution: 1 g, 2 g, 6 g
Fortaz®: 500 mg, 1 g, 2 g, 6 g
Tazicef®: 1 g, 2 g, 6 g

ceftibuten (sef TYE byoo ten)

U.S./Canadian Brand Names Cedax® [US]

Therapeutic Category Cephalosporin (Third Generation)

Use Oral cephalosporin for treatment of bronchitis, otitis media, and pharyngitis/tonsillitis due to *H. influenzae* and *M. catarrhalis*, both beta-lactamase-producing and nonproducing strains, as well as *S. pneumoniae* (weak) and *S. pyogenes*

Usual Dosage
Usual dosage range:
Children <12 years: Oral: 9 mg/kg/day for 10 days (maximum dose: 400 mg/day)
Children ≥12 years and Adults: Oral: 400 mg once daily for 10 days (maximum dose: 400 mg/day)

Dosage Forms
Capsule:
Cedax®: 400 mg
Powder for oral suspension:
Cedax®: 90 mg/5 mL

Ceftin® [US/Can] *see* cefuroxime *on page 192*

Ceftin® Tablet 125 mg (Discontinued) *see* cefuroxime *on page 192*

ceftizoxime (sef ti ZOKS eem)

Sound-Alike/Look-Alike Issues
ceftizoxime may be confused with cefotaxime, ceftazidime, cefuroxime

Synonyms ceftizoxime sodium

U.S./Canadian Brand Names Cefizox® [US/Can]

Therapeutic Category Cephalosporin (Third Generation)

Use Treatment of susceptible bacterial infections, mainly respiratory tract, skin and skin structure, bone and joint, urinary tract and gynecologic, as well as septicemia; active against many gram-negative bacilli (not *Pseudomonas*), some gram-positive cocci (not *Enterococcus*), and some anaerobes

Usual Dosage
Usual dosage range:
Children ≥6 months: I.M., I.V.: 150-200 mg/kg/day divided every 6-8 hours (maximum: 12 g/24 hours)
Adults: I.M., I.V.: 1-4 g every 8-12 hours
Indication-specific dosing:
Adults:
Gonococcal:
Disseminated infection: I.M., I.V.: 1 g every 8 hours
Uncomplicated: I.M.: 1 g as single dose
Life-threatening infections: I.V.: 2 g every 4 hours or 4 g every 8 hours

Dosage Forms
Infusion [premixed iso-osmotic solution]:
Cefizox®: 1 g (50 mL); 2 g (50 mL)

ceftizoxime sodium *see* ceftizoxime *on page 190*

ceftriaxone (sef trye AKS one)

Sound-Alike/Look-Alike Issues
cefTRIAXone may be confused with ceFAZolin
Rocephin® may be confused with Roferon®

Synonyms ceftriaxone sodium

Tall-Man cefTRIAXone

U.S./Canadian Brand Names Rocephin® [US/Can]

Therapeutic Category Cephalosporin (Third Generation)

Use Treatment of lower respiratory tract infections, acute bacterial otitis media, skin and skin structure infections, bone and joint infections, intraabdominal and urinary tract infections, pelvic inflammatory disease (PID), uncomplicated gonorrhea, bacterial septicemia, and meningitis; used in surgical prophylaxis

Usual Dosage
Usual dosage range:
Infants and Children: I.M., I.V.: 50-100 mg/kg/day in 1-2 divided doses (maximum: 4 g/day)
Adults: I.M., I.V.: 1-2 g every 12-24 hours
Indication-specific dosing:
Infants and Children:
Epiglottitis: I.M., I.V.: 50-100 mg/kg once daily for 7-10 days with clindamycin
Mild-to-moderate infections: I.M., I.V.: 50-75 mg/kg/day in 1-2 divided doses every 12-24 hours (maximum: 2 g/day); continue until at least 2 days after signs and symptoms of infection have resolved
Meningitis:
Gonococcal, complicated:
<45 kg: I.V.: 50 mg/kg/day given every 12 hours (maximum: 2 g/day); usual duration of treatment is 10-14 days
>45 kg: I.V.: 1-2 g every 12 hours; usual duration of treatment is 10-14 days
Uncomplicated: I.M., I.V.: Loading dose of 100 mg/kg (maximum: 4 g), followed by 100 mg/kg/day divided every 12-24 hours (maximum: 4 g/day); usual duration of treatment is 7-14 days
Otitis media: *Acute:* I.M.: 50 mg/kg in a single dose (maximum: 1 g)
Pneumonia: I.V.: 50-75 mg/kg once daily
Prophylaxis against infective endocarditis: I.M., I.V.: 50 mg/kg 30-60 minutes before procedure; maximum dose: 1 g. Intramuscular injections should be avoided in patients who are receiving anticoagulant therapy. In these circumstances, orally administered regimens should be given whenever possible. Intravenously administered antibiotics should be used for patients who are unable to tolerate or absorb oral medications.
Note: American Heart Association (AHA) guidelines now recommend prophylaxis only in patients undergoing invasive procedures and in whom underlying cardiac conditions may predispose to a higher risk of adverse outcomes should infection occur. As of April 2007, routine prophylaxis for GI/GU procedures is no longer recommended by the AHA.
Serious infections: I.V.: 80-100 mg/kg/day in 1-2 divided doses (maximum: 4 g/day)
Typhoid fever: I.V.: 100 mg/kg once daily (maximum 4 g)
Adults:
Arthritis (septic): I.V.: 1-2 g once daily
Brain abscess and necrotizing fasciitis: I.V.: 2 g every 12 hours
Cavernous sinus thrombosis: I.V.: 1 g every 12 hours with vancomycin or linezolid
Endocarditis, native valve: I.M., I.V.: 2 g once daily for 2-4 weeks
Lyme disease: I.V.: 2 g once daily for 14-28 days
Mastoiditis (hospitalized): I.V.: 2 g once daily; >60 years old: 1 g once daily
Meningitis: I.V.: 2 g every 12 hours for 7-14 days (longer courses may be necessary for selected organisms)
Pelvic inflammatory disease: I.M.: 250 mg in a single dose
Pneumonia, community-acquired: I.V.: 1 g once daily, usually in combination with a macrolide; consider 2 g/day for patients at risk for more severe infection and/or resistant organisms (ICU status, age >65 years, disseminated infection)
Prophylaxis against infective endocarditis: I.M., I.V.: 1 g 30-60 minutes before procedure. Intramuscular injections should be avoided in patients who are receiving anticoagulant therapy. In these circumstances, orally administered regimens should be given whenever possible. Intravenously administered antibiotics should be used for patients who are unable to tolerate or absorb oral medications.
Note: American Heart Association (AHA) guidelines now recommend prophylaxis only in patients undergoing invasive procedures and in whom underlying cardiac conditions may predispose to a higher risk of adverse outcomes should infection occur. As of April 2007, routine prophylaxis for GI/GU procedures is no longer recommended by the AHA.
Septic/toxic shock: I.V.: 2 g once daily; with clindamycin for toxic shock
Surgical prophylaxis: I.V.: 1 g 30 minutes to 2 hours before surgery
Syphilis: I.M., I.V.: 1 g once daily for 8-10 days
Typhoid fever: I.V.: 2-3 g once daily for 7-14 days

Dosage Forms
Infusion [premixed in dextrose]: 1 g (50 mL); 2 g (50 mL)
Injection, powder for reconstitution: 250 mg, 500 mg, 1 g, 2 g, 10 g
Rocephin®: 500 mg, 1 g

ceftriaxone sodium *see ceftriaxone on page 190*

cefuroxime (se fyoor OKS eem)
Sound-Alike/Look-Alike Issues
cefuroxime may be confused with cefotaxime, cefprozil, ceftizoxime, deferoxamine
Ceftin® may be confused with Cefzil®, Cipro®
Zinacef® may be confused with Zithromax®

Synonyms cefuroxime axetil; cefuroxime sodium

U.S./Canadian Brand Names Apo-Cefuroxime® [Can]; Ceftin® [US/Can]; Cefuroxime For Injection [Can]; ratio-Cefuroxime [Can]; Zinacef® [US/Can]

Therapeutic Category Cephalosporin (Second Generation)

Use Treatment of infections caused by staphylococci, group B streptococci, *H. influenzae* (type A and B), *E. coli*, *Enterobacter*, *Salmonella*, and *Klebsiella*; treatment of susceptible infections of the upper and lower respiratory tract, otitis media, urinary tract, uncomplicated skin and soft tissue, bone and joint, sepsis, uncomplicated gonorrhea, and early Lyme disease; preoperative prophylaxis of susceptible infections

Usual Dosage Note: Cefuroxime axetil film-coated tablets and oral suspension are not bioequivalent and are not substitutable on a mg-per-mg basis

Usual dosage range:
Children 3 months to 12 years:
Oral: 20-30 mg/kg/day in 2 divided doses
I.M., I.V.: 75-150 mg/kg/day divided every 8 hours (maximum dose: 6 g/day)
Children ≥13 years and Adults:
Oral: 250-500 mg twice daily
I.M., I.V.: 750 mg to 1.5 g every 6-8 hours or 100-150 mg/kg/day in divided doses every 6-8 hours (maximum: 6 g/day)

Indication-specific dosing:
Children ≥3 months to 12 years:
Acute bacterial maxillary sinusitis, acute otitis media, and impetigo:
Oral: Suspension: 30 mg/kg/day in 2 divided doses for 10 days (maximum dose: 1 g/day); tablet: 250 mg twice daily for 10 days
I.M., I.V.: 75-150 mg/kg/day divided every 8 hours (maximum dose: 6 g/day)
Epiglottitis: Oral: 150 mg/kg/day in 3 divided doses for 7-10 days
Pharyngitis/tonsillitis:
Oral: Suspension: 20 mg/kg/day (maximum: 500 mg/day) in 2 divided doses for 10 days; tablet: 125 mg every 12 hours for 10 days
I.M., I.V.: 75-150 mg/kg day divided every 8 hours (maximum: 6 g/day)
Children ≥13 years and Adults (all oral doses listed are for tablet formulation):
Bronchitis (acute and exacerbations of chronic bronchitis):
Oral: 250-500 mg every 12 hours for 10 days
I.V.: 500-750 mg every 8 hours (complete therapy with oral dosing)
Cellulitis, orbital: I.V.: 1.5 g every 8 hours
Gonorrhea:
Disseminated: I.M., I.V.: 750 mg every 8 hours
Uncomplicated:
Oral: 1 g as a single dose
I.M.: 1.5 g as single dose (administer in 2 different sites with probenecid)
Lyme disease (early): Oral: 500 mg twice daily for 20 days
Pharyngitis/tonsillitis and sinusitis: Oral: 250 mg twice daily for 10 days
Pneumonia (uncomplicated): I.V.: 750 mg every 8 hours
Severe or complicated infections: I.M., I.V.: 1.5 g every 8 hours (up to 1.5 g every 6 hours in life-threatening infections)
Skin/skin structure infection (uncomplicated):
Oral: 250-500 mg every 12 hours for 10 days
I.M., I.V.: 750 mg every 8 hours
Surgical prophylaxis:
I.V.: 1.5 g 30 minutes to 1 hour prior to procedure (if procedure is prolonged can give 750 mg every 8 hours I.M.)
Open heart: I.V.: 1.5 g every 12 hours to a total of 6 g
Urinary tract infection (uncomplicated):
Oral: 125-250 mg every 12 hours for 7-10 days
I.M., I.V.: 750 mg every 8 hours

Dosage Forms Note: Strength expressed as base
  Infusion [premixed]: 750 mg (50 mL); 1.5 g (50 mL)
    Zinacef®: 750 mg (50 mL); 1.5 g (50 mL)
  Injection, powder for reconstitution: 750 mg, 1.5 g, 7.5 g, 75 g, 225 g
    Zinacef®: 750 mg, 1.5 g, 7.5 g
  Powder for suspension, oral: 125 mg/5 mL, 250 mg/5 mL
    Ceftin®: 125 mg/5 mL, 250 mg/5 mL
  Tablet: 250 mg, 500 mg
    Ceftin®: 250 mg, 500 mg

cefuroxime axetil *see* cefuroxime *on page 192*
Cefuroxime For Injection [Can] *see* cefuroxime *on page 192*
cefuroxime sodium *see* cefuroxime *on page 192*
Cefzil® [Can] *see* cefprozil *on page 188*
Celebrex® [US/Can] *see* celecoxib *on page 193*

celecoxib (se le KOKS ib)
Sound-Alike/Look-Alike Issues
  Celebrex® may be confused with Celexa®, cerebra, Cerebyx®
U.S./Canadian Brand Names Celebrex® [US/Can]; GD-Celecoxib [Can]
Therapeutic Category Nonsteroidal Antiinflammatory Drug (NSAID), COX-2 Selective
Use Relief of the signs and symptoms of osteoarthritis, ankylosing spondylitis, juvenile rheumatoid arthritis (JRA), and rheumatoid arthritis; management of acute pain; treatment of primary dysmenorrhea; to reduce the number of intestinal polyps in familial adenomatous polyposis (FAP)

  Canadian note: Celecoxib is only indicated for relief of symptoms of rheumatoid arthritis, osteoarthritis, and relief of acute pain in adults
Usual Dosage Note: Use the lowest effective dose for the shortest duration of time, consistent with individual patient goals. Oral:
  Children ≥2 years: JRA
    ≥10 kg to ≤25 kg: 50 mg twice daily
    >25 kg: 100 mg twice daily
  Adults:
    Acute pain or primary dysmenorrhea: Initial dose: 400 mg, followed by an additional 200 mg if needed on day 1; maintenance dose: 200 mg twice daily as needed
    Ankylosing spondylitis: 200 mg/day as a single dose or in divided doses twice daily; if no effect after 6 weeks, may increase to 400 mg/day. If no response following 6 weeks of treatment with 400 mg/day, consider discontinuation and alternative treatment.
    Familial adenomatous polyposis: 400 mg twice daily
    Osteoarthritis: 200 mg/day as a single dose or in divided dose twice daily
    Rheumatoid arthritis: 100-200 mg twice daily
Dosage Forms
  Capsule:
    Celebrex®: 50 mg, 100 mg, 200 mg, 400 mg

Celestone® [US] *see* betamethasone (systemic) *on page 132*
Celestone® Soluspan® [US/Can] *see* betamethasone (systemic) *on page 132*
Celexa® [US/Can] *see* citalopram *on page 225*
CellCept® [US/Can] *see* mycophenolate *on page 649*
Cellugel® [US] *see* hydroxypropyl methylcellulose *on page 490*

cellulose, oxidized regenerated (SEL yoo lose, OKS i dyzed re JEN er aye ted)
Sound-Alike/Look-Alike Issues
  Surgicel® may be confused with Serentil®
Synonyms absorbable cotton; oxidized regenerated cellulose
U.S./Canadian Brand Names Surgicel® Fibrillar [US]; Surgicel® NuKnit [US]; Surgicel® [US]
Therapeutic Category Hemostatic Agent
Use Hemostatic; temporary packing for the control of capillary, venous, or small arterial hemorrhage
Usual Dosage Minimal amounts of the fabric strip are laid on the bleeding site or held firmly against the tissues until hemostasis occurs; remove excess material

Dosage Forms
 Fabric, fibrous:
  Surgicel® Fibrillar:
   1" x 2" (10s)
   2" x 4" (10s)
   4" x 4" (10s)
 Fabric, knitted:
  Surgicel® NuKnit:
   1" x 1" (24s)
   1" x 3¹/₂" (10s)
   3" x 4" (24s)
   6" x 9" (10s)
 Fabric, sheer weave:
  Surgicel®:
   ¹/₂" x 2" (24s)
   2" x 3" (24s)
   2" x 14" (24s)
   4" x 8" (24s)

Celluvisc™ [Can] *see* carboxymethylcellulose *on page 179*
Celontin® [US/Can] *see* methsuximide *on page 619*
Celsentri™ [Can] *see* maraviroc *on page 591*
Cemill [US-OTC] *see* ascorbic acid *on page 96*
Cena-K® *(Discontinued)* *see* potassium chloride *on page 771*
Cenestin® [US/Can] *see* estrogens (conjugated A/synthetic) *on page 363*
Cenolate® [US] *see* ascorbic acid *on page 96*
Centamin [US-OTC] *see* vitamins (multiple/oral) *on page 983*
Centany™ *(Discontinued)* *see* mupirocin *on page 647*
Centrum® [US-OTC] *see* vitamins (multiple/oral) *on page 983*
Centrum Kids® Complete [US-OTC] *see* vitamins (multiple/pediatric) *on page 983*
Centrum Kids® Dora the Explorer™ Complete [US-OTC] *see* vitamins (multiple/pediatric) *on page 983*
Centrum Kids® Rugrats® Complete [US-OTC] *see* vitamins (multiple/pediatric) *on page 983*
Centrum Kids® SpongeBob™ SquarePants Complete [US-OTC] *see* vitamins (multiple/pediatric) *on page 983*
Centrum® Performance™ [US-OTC] *see* vitamins (multiple/oral) *on page 983*
Centrum® Silver® [US-OTC] *see* vitamins (multiple/oral) *on page 983*
Cēpacol® Antibacterial Mouthwash Gold [US-OTC] *see* cetylpyridinium *on page 197*
Cēpacol® Dual Action Maximum Strength [US-OTC] *see* dyclonine *on page 330*
Cēpacol® Sore Throat [US-OTC] *see* benzocaine *on page 124*
Cēpastat® [US-OTC] *see* phenol *on page 743*
Cēpastat® Extra Strength [US-OTC] *see* phenol *on page 743*
Cephadyn [US] *see* butalbital and acetaminophen *on page 155*

cephalexin (sef a LEKS in)

Sound-Alike/Look-Alike Issues
 cephalexin may be confused with cefaclor, cefazolin, cephalothin, ciprofloxacin
Synonyms cephalexin monohydrate
U.S./Canadian Brand Names Apo-Cephalex® [Can]; Keflex® [US]; Keftab® [Can]; Novo-Lexin [Can]; Nu-Cephalex [Can]
Therapeutic Category Cephalosporin (First Generation)
Use Treatment of susceptible bacterial infections including respiratory tract infections, otitis media, skin and skin structure infections, bone infections, and genitourinary tract infections, including acute prostatitis; alternative therapy for acute infective endocarditis prophylaxis
Usual Dosage
 Usual dosage range:
  Children >1 year: Oral: 25-100 mg/kg/day every 6-8 hours (maximum: 4 g/day)
  Adults: Oral: 250-1000 mg every 6 hours; maximum: 4 g/day
 Indication-specific dosing:
  Children >1 year: Oral:
   Furunculosis: 25-50 mg/kg/day in 4 divided doses
   Impetigo: 25 mg/kg/day in 4 divided doses

Otitis media: 75-100 mg/kg/day in 4 divided doses

Prophylaxis against infective endocarditis (dental, oral, or respiratory tract procedures): 50 mg/kg 30-60 minutes prior to procedure (maximum: 2 g). **Note:** American Heart Association (AHA) guidelines now recommend prophylaxis only in patients undergoing invasive procedures and in whom underlying cardiac conditions may predispose to a higher risk of adverse outcomes should infection occur.

Severe infections: 50-100 mg/kg/day in divided doses every 6-8 hours

Skin abscess: 50 mg/kg/day in 4 divided doses (maximum: 4 g)

Streptococcal pharyngitis, skin and skin structure infections: 25-50 mg/kg/day divided every 12 hours

Children >15 years and Adults: Oral:

Cellulitis and mastitis: 500 mg every 6 hours

Furunculosis/skin abscess: 250 mg 4 times/day

Prophylaxis against infective endocarditis (dental, oral, or respiratory tract procedures): 2 g 30-60 minutes prior to procedure. **Note:** American Heart Association (AHA) guidelines now recommend prophylaxis only in patients undergoing invasive procedures and in whom underlying cardiac conditions may predispose to a higher risk of adverse outcomes should infection occur.

Prophylaxis in total joint replacement patients undergoing dental procedures which produce bacteremia: 2 g 1 hour prior to procedure

Streptococcal pharyngitis, skin and skin structure infections: 500 mg every 12 hours

Uncomplicated cystitis: 500 mg every 12 hours for 7-14 days

Dosage Forms

Capsule: 250 mg, 500 mg

Keflex®: 250 mg, 500 mg, 750 mg

Powder for oral suspension: 125 mg/5 mL, 250 mg/5 mL

Keflex®: 125 mg/5 mL, 250 mg/5 mL

Tablet: 250 mg, 500 mg

cephalexin monohydrate *see* cephalexin *on page 194*

cephalothin *(Discontinued)*

Cephulac® *(Discontinued) see* lactulose *on page 544*

Ceprotin [US] *see* protein C concentrate (human) *on page 799*

Ceptaz® *(Discontinued) see* ceftazidime *on page 189*

Cerebyx® [US/Can] *see* fosphenytoin *on page 428*

Ceredase® [US] *see* alglucerase *on page 45*

Cerezyme® [US/Can] *see* imiglucerase *on page 500*

Ceron [US] *see* chlorpheniramine and phenylephrine *on page 206*

Ceron-DM [US] *see* chlorpheniramine, phenylephrine, and dextromethorphan *on page 209*

Cerovel™ [US] *see* urea *on page 963*

Certain Dri® [US-OTC] *see* aluminum chloride hexahydrate *on page 53*

certolizumab pegol (cer to LIZ u mab PEG ol)

Synonyms CDP870

U.S./Canadian Brand Names Cimzia® [US]

Therapeutic Category Gastrointestinal Agent, Miscellaneous; Tumor Necrosis Factor (TNF) Blocking Agent

Use Treatment of moderately- to severely-active Crohn disease in patients who have inadequate response to conventional therapy

Usual Dosage Note: Each 400 mg dose should be administered as 2 injections of 200 mg each

SubQ: Adults: Crohn disease: Initial: 400 mg, repeat dose 2 and 4 weeks after initial dose; Maintenance: 400 mg every 4 weeks

Dosage Forms

Injection, powder for reconstitution:

Cimzia®: 200 mg [contains sterile water for reconstitution, syringes, and needles]

Certuss-D® [US] *see* guaifenesin, dextromethorphan, and phenylephrine *on page 459*

Cerubidine® [US/Can] *see* daunorubicin hydrochloride *on page 269*

Cerumenex® *(Discontinued)*

Cervidil® [US/Can] *see* dinoprostone *on page 303*

C.E.S.® [Can] *see* estrogens (conjugated/equine) *on page 364*

Cesia™ [US] *see* ethinyl estradiol and desogestrel *on page 369*

Cetacaine® [US] *see* benzocaine, butamben, and tetracaine *on page 126*

Cetacort® [US] *see* hydrocortisone (topical) *on page 485*

Cetafen® [US-OTC] *see* acetaminophen *on page 19*

Cetafen Extra® [US-OTC] *see* acetaminophen *on page 19*

Cetamide™ [Can] *see* sulfacetamide *on page 892*

Cetapred® Ophthalmic *(Discontinued)* *see* sulfacetamide and prednisolone *on page 893*

cetirizine (se TI ra zeen)

Sound-Alike/Look-Alike Issues
 Zyrtec® may be confused with Serax®, Xanax®, Zantac®, Zyprexa®

Synonyms cetirizine hydrochloride; P-071; UCB-P071

U.S./Canadian Brand Names Apo-Cetirizine® [Can]; Reactine™ [Can]; Zyrtec® Allergy [US-OTC]; Zyrtec® [US-OTC]; Zyrtec®, Children's Allergy [US-OTC]; Zyrtec®, Children's Hives Relief [US-OTC]

Therapeutic Category Antihistamine

Use Perennial and seasonal allergic rhinitis and other allergic symptoms including urticaria; chronic idiopathic urticaria

Usual Dosage Oral:
 Children:
  6-12 months: Chronic urticaria, perennial allergic rhinitis: 2.5 mg once daily
  12 months to <2 years: Chronic urticaria, perennial allergic rhinitis: 2.5 mg once daily; may increase to 2.5 mg every 12 hours if needed
  2-5 years: Chronic urticaria, perennial or seasonal allergic rhinitis: Initial: 2.5 mg once daily; may be increased to 2.5 mg every 12 hours **or** 5 mg once daily
  Children ≥6 years and Adults: Chronic urticaria, perennial or seasonal allergic rhinitis: 5-10 mg once daily, depending upon symptom severity

Dosage Forms
 Syrup: 5 mg/5 mL (120 mL, 473 mL)
  Zyrtec® [OTC]: 5 mg/5 mL
  Zyrtec® [OTC], Children's Allergy [OTC], Zyrtec® [OTC], Children's Hives Relief [OTC]: 5 mg/5 mL
 Tablet, as hydrochloride: 5 mg, 10 mg
  Zyrtec® Allergy [OTC]: 10 mg
 Tablet, chewable, as hydrochloride:
  Zyrtec® [OTC], Children's Allergy [OTC]: 5 mg, 10 mg

cetirizine and pseudoephedrine (se TI ra zeen & soo doe e FED rin)

Sound-Alike/Look-Alike Issues
 Zyrtec® may be confused with Serax®, Xanax®, Zantac®, Zyprexa®

Synonyms cetirizine hydrochloride and pseudoephedrine hydrochloride; pseudoephedrine hydrochloride and cetirizine hydrochloride

U.S./Canadian Brand Names Reactine® Allergy and Sinus [Can]; Zytrec-D® Allergy & Congestion [US-OTC]

Therapeutic Category Antihistamine/Decongestant Combination

Use Treatment of symptoms of seasonal or perennial allergic rhinitis

Usual Dosage Oral: Children ≥12 years and Adults: Seasonal/perennial allergic rhinitis: 1 tablet twice daily

Dosage Forms
 Tablet, extended release: Cetirizine hydrochloride 5 mg and pseudoephedrine hydrochloride 120 mg
  Zytrec-D® Allergy & Congestion: Cetirizine 5 mg and pseudoephedrine 120 mg

cetirizine hydrochloride *see* cetirizine *on page 196*

cetirizine hydrochloride and pseudoephedrine hydrochloride *see* cetirizine and pseudoephedrine *on page 196*

cetrorelix (set roe REL iks)

Synonyms cetrorelix acetate

U.S./Canadian Brand Names Cetrotide® [US/Can]

Therapeutic Category Antigonadotropic Agent

Use Inhibits premature luteinizing hormone (LH) surges in women undergoing controlled ovarian stimulation

Usual Dosage SubQ: Adults: Female: Used in conjunction with controlled ovarian stimulation therapy using gonadotropins (FSH, HMG):

Single-dose regimen: 3 mg given when serum estradiol levels show appropriate stimulation response, usually stimulation day 7 (range days 5-9). If hCG is not administered within 4 days, continue cetrorelix at 0.25 mg/day until hCG is administered.

Multiple-dose regimen: 0.25 mg morning or evening of stimulation day 5, or morning of stimulation day 6; continue until hCG is administered.

Dosage Forms
Injection, powder for reconstitution:
Cetrotide®: 0.25 mg, 3 mg

cetrorelix acetate *see* cetrorelix *on page 196*
Cetrotide® [US/Can] *see* cetrorelix *on page 196*

cetuximab (se TUK see mab)

Sound-Alike/Look-Alike Issues
cetuximab may be confused with bevacizumab
Synonyms C225; IMC-C225; NSC-714692
U.S./Canadian Brand Names Erbitux® [US/Can]
Therapeutic Category Antineoplastic Agent, Monoclonal Antibody; Epidermal Growth Factor Receptor (EGFR) Inhibitor
Use Treatment of metastatic colorectal cancer; treatment of squamous cell cancer of the head and neck
Usual Dosage I.V.: Adults: **Note:** Premedicate with an antihistamine (eg, diphenhydramine) I.V. 30-60 minutes prior to the first dose; premedication for subsequent doses is based on clinical judgement.
Colorectal cancer:
Initial loading dose: 400 mg/m^2 infused over 120 minutes
Maintenance dose: 250 mg/m^2 infused over 60 minutes weekly
Head and neck cancer:
Initial loading dose: 400 mg/m^2 infused over 120 minutes
Maintenance dose: 250 mg/m^2 infused over 60 minutes weekly
Note: If given in combination with radiation therapy, administer loading dose 1 week prior to initiation of radiation course. Weekly maintenance dose should be completed 1 hour prior to radiation for the duration of radiation therapy (6-7 weeks).

Dosage Forms
Injection, solution [preservative free]:
Erbitux®: 2 mg/mL (50 mL, 100 mL)

cetylpyridinium (SEE til peer i DI nee um)

Synonyms cetylpyridinium chloride; CPC
U.S./Canadian Brand Names Cepacol® Antibacterial Mouthwash Gold [US-OTC]; DiabetAid Gingivitis Mouth Rinse [US-OTC]
Therapeutic Category Local Anesthetic
Use Antiseptic to aid in the prevention and reduction of plaque and gingivitis, and to freshen breath
Usual Dosage Oral (OTC labeling): Children ≥6 years and Adults: Rinse or gargle to freshen mouth; may be used before or after brushing
Dosage Forms
Liquid, oral [mouthwash/gargle]:
Cepacol® Antibacterial Mouthwash Gold [OTC]: 0.05%
DiabetAid Gingivitis Mouth Rinse [OTC]: 0.1%

cetylpyridinium chloride *see* cetylpyridinium *on page 197*
Cevalin® (Discontinued) *see* ascorbic acid *on page 96*

cevimeline (se vi ME leen)

Sound-Alike/Look-Alike Issues
Evoxac® may be confused with Eurax®
Synonyms cevimeline hydrochloride

▶

◀ **U.S./Canadian Brand Names** Evoxac® [US/Can]
Therapeutic Category Cholinergic Agent
Use Treatment of symptoms of dry mouth in patients with Sjögren syndrome
Usual Dosage Oral: Adults: 30 mg 3 times/day
Dosage Forms
Capsule:
Evoxac®: 30 mg

cevimeline hydrochloride *see* cevimeline *on page 197*
CFDN *see* cefdinir *on page 185*
CG *see* chorionic gonadotropin (human) *on page 216*
C-Gel [US-OTC] *see* ascorbic acid *on page 96*
CGP-42446 *see* zoledronic acid *on page 995*
CGP-57148B *see* imatinib *on page 499*
C-Gram [US-OTC] *see* ascorbic acid *on page 96*
CGS-20267 *see* letrozole *on page 552*
Champix® [Can] *see* varenicline *on page 971*
Chantix® [US] *see* varenicline *on page 971*
Charcadole® [Can] *see* charcoal *on page 198*
Charcadole®, Aqueous [Can] *see* charcoal *on page 198*
Charcadole® TFS [Can] *see* charcoal *on page 198*
Char-Caps [US-OTC] *see* charcoal *on page 198*
CharcoAid® *(Discontinued)* *see* charcoal *on page 198*
CharcoAid® G [US-OTC] *see* charcoal *on page 198*

charcoal (CHAR kole)
Sound-Alike/Look-Alike Issues
Actidose® may be confused with Actos®
Synonyms activated carbon; activated charcoal; adsorbent charcoal; liquid antidote; medicinal carbon; medicinal charcoal
U.S./Canadian Brand Names Actidose-Aqua® [US-OTC]; Actidose® with Sorbitol [US-OTC]; Char-Caps [US-OTC]; Charcadole® TFS [Can]; Charcadole® [Can]; Charcadole®, Aqueous [Can]; CharcoAid® G [US-OTC]; Charcoal Plus® DS [US-OTC]; Charcocaps® [US-OTC]; EZ-Char™ [US-OTC]; Kerr Insta-Char® [US-OTC]; Requa® Activated Charcoal [US-OTC]
Therapeutic Category Antidote
Use Emergency treatment in poisoning by drugs and chemicals; aids the elimination of certain drugs and improves decontamination of excessive ingestions of sustained-release products or in the presence of bezoars; repetitive doses have proven useful to enhance the elimination of certain drugs (eg, carbamazepine, dapsone, phenobarbital, quinine, or theophylline); repetitive doses for gastric dialysis in uremia to adsorb various waste products; dietary supplement (digestive aid)
Usual Dosage Oral:
Acute poisoning: **Note:** ~10 g of activated charcoal for each 1 g of toxin is considered adequate; this may require multiple doses. If sorbitol is also used, sorbitol dose should not exceed 1.5 g/kg. When using multiple doses of charcoal, sorbitol should be given with every other dose (not to exceed 2 doses/day). Children:
<1 year: 0.5-1 g/kg (10-25 g) as a single dose; if multiple doses are needed, give as 0.25 g/kg/hour or equivalent (eg, 0.5 g/kg every 2 hours)
1-12 years: 0.5-1 g/kg (25-50 g) as a single dose; if multiple doses are needed, give as 0.25 g/kg/hour or equivalent (eg, 0.5 g/kg every 2 hours)
Children >12 years and Adults: 25-100 g as a single dose; if multiple doses are needed, additional doses may be given as 12.5 g/hour or equivalent (eg, 25 g every 2 hours)
Dietary supplement: Adults: 500-520 mg after meals; may repeat in 2 hours if needed (maximum: 10 g/day)
Dosage Forms
Capsule:
Char-Caps [OTC], CharcoCaps® [OTC]: 260 mg
Pellets, for suspension:
EZ-Char™ [OTC]: 25 g

Powder for suspension: 30 g, 240 g
  CharcoAid® G [OTC]: 15 g
Suspension:
  Actidose-Aqua® [OTC]: 15 g, 25 g, 50 g
  Kerr Insta-Char® [OTC]: 25 g, 50 g
Suspension [with sorbitol]:
  Actidose® with Sorbitol [OTC], Kerr Insta-Char® [OTC]: 25 g, 50 g
Tablet:
  Requa® Activated Charcoal: 250 mg
Tablet, enteric coated:
  Charcoal Plus® DS [OTC]: 250 mg

Charcoal Plus® DS [US-OTC] *see* charcoal *on page 198*
Charcocaps® [US-OTC] *see* charcoal *on page 198*
Chealamide® *(Discontinued)* *see* edetate disodium *on page 333*
CheeTah® [US] *see* barium *on page 116*
Chemet® [US/Can] *see* succimer *on page 889*
Cheracol® [US] *see* guaifenesin and codeine *on page 454*
Cheracol® [US-OTC] *see* phenol *on page 743*
Cheracol® D [US-OTC] *see* guaifenesin and dextromethorphan *on page 454*
Cheracol® Plus [US-OTC] *see* guaifenesin and dextromethorphan *on page 454*
Chew-C [US-OTC] *see* ascorbic acid *on page 96*
Chew-Cal [US-OTC] *see* calcium and vitamin D *on page 162*
CHG *see* chlorhexidine gluconate *on page 201*
Chibroxin® *(Discontinued)* *see* norfloxacin *on page 679*
chickenpox vaccine *see* varicella virus vaccine *on page 971*
Chiggerex® [US-OTC] *see* benzocaine *on page 124*
Chiggerex® Plus [US] *see* benzocaine *on page 124*
Chiggertox® [US-OTC] *see* benzocaine *on page 124*
Children's Advil® Cold [Can] *see* pseudoephedrine and ibuprofen *on page 802*
Children's Dimetapp® Elixir Cold & Allergy *(Discontinued)* *see* brompheniramine and pseudoephedrine *on page 144*
Children's Hold® *(Discontinued)* *see* dextromethorphan *on page 284*
Children's Kaopectate® *(Discontinued)*
Children's Motion Sickness Liquid [Can] *see* dimenhydrinate *on page 301*
Children's Pepto [US-OTC] *see* calcium carbonate *on page 163*
children's vitamins *see* vitamins (multiple/pediatric) *on page 983*
ChiRhoStim® [US] *see* secretin *on page 860*
Chirocaine® *(Discontinued)*
Chlo-Amine® Oral *(Discontinued)* *see* chlorpheniramine *on page 205*
Chlorafed® Liquid *(Discontinued)* *see* chlorpheniramine and pseudoephedrine *on page 207*
chloral *see* chloral hydrate *on page 199*

chloral hydrate (KLOR al HYE drate)

Synonyms chloral; hydrated chloral; trichloroacetaldehyde monohydrate
U.S./Canadian Brand Names PMS-Chloral Hydrate [Can]; Somnote® [US]
Therapeutic Category Hypnotic, Nonbarbiturate
Controlled Substance C-IV
Use Short-term sedative and hypnotic (<2 weeks); sedative/hypnotic for diagnostic procedures; sedative prior to EEG evaluations
Usual Dosage
  Children:
    Sedation or anxiety: Oral, rectal: 5-15 mg/kg/dose every 8 hours (maximum: 500 mg/dose)
    Prior to EEG: Oral, rectal: 20-25 mg/kg/dose, 30-60 minutes prior to EEG; may repeat in 30 minutes to maximum of 100 mg/kg or 2 g total
    Hypnotic: Oral, rectal: 20-40 mg/kg/dose up to a maximum of 50 mg/kg/24 hours or 1 g/dose or 2 g/24 hours

▶

◀ Conscious sedation: Oral: 50-75 mg/kg/dose 30-60 minutes prior to procedure; may repeat 30 minutes after initial dose if needed, to a total maximum dose of 120 mg/kg or 1 g total
Adults: Oral, rectal:
Sedation, anxiety: 250 mg 3 times/day
Hypnotic: 500-1000 mg at bedtime or 30 minutes prior to procedure, not to exceed 2 g/24 hours
Discontinuation: Withdraw gradually over 2 weeks if patient has been maintained on high doses for prolonged period of time. Do not stop drug abruptly; sudden withdrawal may result in delirium.
Dosage Forms
Capsule:
Somnote®: 500 mg
Suppository, rectal: 500 mg
Syrup: 500 mg/5 mL

chlorambucil (klor AM byoo sil)
Sound-Alike/Look-Alike Issues
chlorambucil may be confused with Chloromycetin®
Leukeran® may be confused with Alkeran®, leucovorin, Leukine®, Myleran®
Synonyms CB-1348; chlorambucilum; chloraminophene; chlorbutinum; NSC-3088; WR-139013
U.S./Canadian Brand Names Leukeran® [US/Can]
Therapeutic Category Antineoplastic Agent
Use Management of chronic lymphocytic leukemia (CLL), Hodgkin lymphoma, non-Hodgkin lymphoma (NHL)
Usual Dosage Oral (refer to individual protocols): Adults:
CLL, NHL: 0.1 mg/kg/day for 3-6 weeks **or** 0.4 mg/kg (increased by 0.1 mg/kg/dose until response/toxicity observed) biweekly **or** 0.4 mg/kg (increased by 0.1 mg/kg/dose until response/toxicity observed) monthly **or** 0.03-0.1 mg/kg/day continuously
Hodgkin lymphoma: 0.2 mg/kg/day for 3-6 weeks **or** 0.4 mg/kg (increased by 0.1 mg/kg/dose until response/toxicity observed) biweekly **or** 0.4 mg/kg (increased by 0.1 mg/kg/dose until response/toxicity observed) monthly **or** 0.03-0.1 mg/kg/day continuously
Dosage Forms
Tablet:
Leukeran®: 2 mg

chlorambucilum *see chlorambucil on page 200*
chloraminophene *see chlorambucil on page 200*

chloramphenicol (klor am FEN i kole)
Sound-Alike/Look-Alike Issues
Chloromycetin® may be confused with chlorambucil, Chlor-Trimeton®
U.S./Canadian Brand Names Chloromycetin® Succinate [Can]; Chloromycetin® [Can]; Diochloram® [Can]; Pentamycetin® [Can]
Therapeutic Category Antibiotic, Miscellaneous; Antibiotic, Ophthalmic; Antibiotic, Otic
Use Treatment of serious infections due to organisms resistant to other less toxic antibiotics or when its penetrability into the site of infection is clinically superior to other antibiotics to which the organism is sensitive; useful in infections caused by *Bacteroides*, *H. influenzae*, *Neisseria meningitidis*, *Salmonella*, and *Rickettsia*; active against many vancomycin-resistant enterococci
Usual Dosage
Meningitis: I.V.: Infants >30 days and Children: 50-100 mg/kg/day divided every 6 hours
Other infections: I.V.:
Infants >30 days and Children: 50-75 mg/kg/day divided every 6 hours; maximum daily dose: 4 g/day
Adults: 50-100 mg/kg/day in divided doses every 6 hours; maximum daily dose: 4 g/day
Dosage Forms
Injection, powder for reconstitution: 1 g

ChloraPrep® [US-OTC] *see chlorhexidine gluconate on page 201*
ChloraPrep® Frepp® [US-OTC] *see chlorhexidine gluconate on page 201*
ChloraPrep® Sepp® [US-OTC] *see chlorhexidine gluconate on page 201*
Chlorascrub™ [US-OTC] *see chlorhexidine gluconate on page 201*
Chlorascrub™ Maxi [US-OTC] *see chlorhexidine gluconate on page 201*
Chloraseptic® Gargle [US-OTC] *see phenol on page 743*

Chloraseptic® Mouth Pain [US-OTC] *see phenol on page 743*
Chloraseptic® Pocket Pump [US-OTC] *see phenol on page 743*
Chloraseptic® Spray [US-OTC] *see phenol on page 743*
Chloraseptic® Spray for Kids [US-OTC] *see phenol on page 743*
Chlorate® Oral *(Discontinued)* *see chlorpheniramine on page 205*
chlorbutinum *see chlorambucil on page 200*
Chlordex GP [US] *see dextromethorphan, chlorpheniramine, phenylephrine, and guaifenesin on page 285*

chlordiazepoxide (klor dye az e POKS ide)

Sound-Alike/Look-Alike Issues
chlordiazePOXIDE may be confused with chlorproMAZINE
Librium® may be confused with Librax®
Synonyms methaminodiazepoxide hydrochloride
Tall-Man chlordiazePOXIDE
U.S./Canadian Brand Names Apo-Chlordiazepoxide® [Can]; Librium® [US]
Therapeutic Category Benzodiazepine
Controlled Substance C-IV
Use Management of anxiety disorder or for the short-term relief of symptoms of anxiety; withdrawal symptoms of acute alcoholism; preoperative apprehension and anxiety
Usual Dosage
Children >6 years: Anxiety: Oral, I.M.: 0.5 mg/kg/24 hours divided every 6-8 hours
Adults:
Anxiety:
Oral: 15-100 mg divided 3-4 times/day
I.M., I.V.: Initial: 50-100 mg followed by 25-50 mg 3-4 times/day as needed
Preoperative anxiety: I.M.: 50-100 mg prior to surgery
Ethanol withdrawal symptoms: Oral, I.V.: 50-100 mg to start, dose may be repeated in 2-4 hours as necessary to a maximum of 300 mg/24 hours
Note: Up to 300 mg may be given I.M. or I.V. during a 6-hour period, but not more than this in any 24-hour period.
Dosage Forms
Capsule: 5 mg, 10 mg, 25 mg
Librium®: 5 mg, 10 mg, 25 mg
Injection, powder for reconstitution:
Librium®: 100 mg

chlordiazepoxide and amitriptyline hydrochloride *see amitriptyline and chlordiazepoxide on page 63*
chlordiazepoxide and clidinium *see clidinium and chlordiazepoxide on page 229*
chlorethazine *see mechlorethamine on page 595*
chlorethazine mustard *see mechlorethamine on page 595*
Chlorex-A [US] *see chlorpheniramine, phenylephrine, and phenyltoloxamine on page 211*

chlorhexidine gluconate (klor HEKS i deen GLOO koe nate)

Sound-Alike/Look-Alike Issues
Peridex® may be confused with Precedex™
Synonyms CHG
U.S./Canadian Brand Names Avagard™ [US-OTC]; BactoShield® CHG [US-OTC]; Betasept® [US-OTC]; ChloraPrep® Frepp® [US-OTC]; ChloraPrep® Sepp® [US-OTC]; ChloraPrep® [US-OTC]; Chlorascrub™ Maxi [US-OTC]; Chlorascrub™ [US-OTC]; Dyna-Hex® [US-OTC]; Hibiclens® [US-OTC]; Hibidil® 1:2000 [Can]; Hibistat® [US-OTC]; Operand® Chlorhexidine Gluconate [US-OTC]; ORO-Clense [Can]; Peridex® Oral Rinse [Can]; Peridex® [US]; PerioChip® [US]; PerioGard® [US]
Therapeutic Category Antibiotic, Oral Rinse; Antibiotic, Topical
Use Skin cleanser for surgical scrub, cleanser for skin wounds, preoperative skin preparation, germicidal hand rinse, and as antibacterial dental rinse. Chlorhexidine is active against gram-positive and gram-negative organisms, facultative anaerobes, aerobes, and yeast.
Orphan drug: Peridex®: Oral mucositis with cytoreductive therapy when used for patients undergoing bone marrow transplant

◀ **Usual Dosage** Adults:

Oral rinse (Peridex®, PerioGard®):

Floss and brush teeth, completely rinse toothpaste from mouth and swish 15 mL (one capful) undiluted oral rinse around in mouth for 30 seconds, then expectorate. Caution patient not to swallow the medicine and instruct not to eat for 2-3 hours after treatment. (Cap on bottle measures 15 mL.)

Treatment of gingivitis: Oral prophylaxis: Swish for 30 seconds with 15 mL chlorhexidine, then expectorate; repeat twice daily (morning and evening). Patient should have a reevaluation followed by a dental prophylaxis every 6 months.

Periodontal chip: One chip is inserted into a periodontal pocket with a probing pocket depth ≥5 mm. Up to 8 chips may be inserted in a single visit. Treatment is recommended every 3 months in pockets with a remaining depth ≥5 mm. If dislodgment occurs 7 days or more after placement, the subject is considered to have had the full course of treatment. If dislodgment occurs within 48 hours, a new chip should be inserted. The chip biodegrades completely and does not need to be removed. Patients should avoid dental floss at the site of PerioChip® insertion for 10 days after placement because flossing might dislodge the chip.

Insertion of periodontal chip: Pocket should be isolated and surrounding area dried prior to chip insertion. The chip should be grasped using forceps with the rounded edges away from the forceps. The chip should be inserted into the periodontal pocket to its maximum depth. It may be maneuvered into position using the tips of the forceps or a flat instrument.

Cleanser:

Surgical scrub: Scrub 3 minutes and rinse thoroughly, wash for an additional 3 minutes

Hand sanitizer (Avagard™): Dispense 1 pumpful in palm of one hand; dip fingertips of opposite hand into solution and work it under nails. Spread remainder evenly over hand and just above elbow, covering all surfaces. Repeat on other hand. Dispense another pumpful in each hand and reapply to each hand up to the wrist. Allow to dry before gloving.

Hand wash: Wash for 15 seconds and rinse

Hand rinse: Rub 15 seconds and rinse

Dosage Forms

Chip, for periodontal pocket insertion:

PerioChip®: 2.5 mg

Liquid, topical [surgical scrub]:

BactoShield® CHG [OTC]: 2% (120 mL, 480 mL, 750 mL, 960 mL, 3840 mL); 4% (120 mL, 480 mL, 960 mL, 3840 mL)

Betasept® [OTC]: 4% 120 mL, 240 mL, 480 mL, 960 mL, 3840 mL)

ChloraPrep® [OTC]: 2% (0.67 mL, 1.5 mL, 3 mL, 10.5 mL, 26 mL)

Dyna-Hex® [OTC]: 2% (120 mL, 480 mL, 960 mL, 3840 mL); 4% (120 mL, 480 mL, 960 mL, 3840 mL)

Hibiclens® [OTC]: 4% (15 mL, 120 mL, 240 mL, 480 mL, 960 mL, 3840 mL)

Operand® Chlorhexidine Gluconate [OTC]: 2% (120 mL); 4% (120 mL, 240 mL, 480 mL, 960 mL, 3840 mL)

Liquid, oral [rinse]: 0.12%

Peridex®, PerioGard®: 0.12%

Lotion, topical [surgical scrub]:

Avagard™ [OTC]: 1% (500 mL)

Sponge/Brush, topical:

BactoShield® CHG [OTC]: 4%

Sponge, topical [surgical scrub]:

ChloraPrep® [OTC] 3 mL: 2% (25s)

ChloraPrep® [OTC] 10.5 mL: 2% (25s)

ChloraPrep® [OTC] 26 mL: 2% (25s)

ChloraPrep® Frepp® [OTC] 1.5 mL: 2% (20s)

ChloraPrep® Sepp® [OTC] 0.67 mL: 2% (200s)

Swab, topical [prep pad]:

Chlorascrub™ [OTC]: 3.15% (100s)

Swabstick, topical [surgical scrub]:

ChloraPrep® [OTC] 1.75 mL: 2% (48s)

ChloraPrep® [OTC] 5.25 mL: 2% (40s)

Chlorascrub™ [OTC] 1.6 mL: 3.15% (50s)

Chlorascrub™ Maxi [OTC] 5.1 mL: 3.15% (30s)

Wipe, topical [towlette]:

Hibistat® [OTC]: 0.5% (50s)

chlormeprazine *see prochlorperazine on page 788*

Chlor-Mes [US] *see chlorpheniramine, phenylephrine, and methscopolamine on page 210*

Chlor-Mes-D [US] *see chlorpheniramine, phenylephrine, and methscopolamine on page 210*

2-chlorodeoxyadenosine *see cladribine on page 226*

chloroethane *see ethyl chloride on page 381*

Chloromag® [US] *see magnesium chloride on page 583*

Chloromycetin® [Can] *see chloramphenicol on page 200*

Chloromycetin® Succinate [Can] *see chloramphenicol on page 200*

chlorophyll (KLOR oh fil)

Synonyms chlorophyllin

U.S./Canadian Brand Names Nullo® [US-OTC]

Therapeutic Category Gastrointestinal Agent, Miscellaneous

Use Control fecal odors in colostomy or ileostomy

Usual Dosage
Oral: Children >12 years and Adults: 100-200 mg/day in divided doses; may increase to 300 mg/day if odor is not controlled (maximum: 300 mg/day)
Ostomy: Tablet: May also place 1-2 tablets in empty pouch each time it is reused or changed.

Dosage Forms
Caplet:
Nullo® [OTC]: Chlorophyllin copper complex 100 mg

chlorophyllin *see chlorophyll on page 203*

chlorophyllin copper complex sodium, papain, and urea *see chlorophyllin, papain, and urea on page 203*

chlorophyllin, papain, and urea (KLOR oh fil in, pa PAY in, & yoor EE a)

Sound-Alike/Look-Alike Issues
Ziox™ may be confused with Zyvox®

Synonyms chlorophyllin copper complex sodium, papain, and urea; papain, urea, and chlorophyllin; urea, chlorophyllin, and papain

U.S./Canadian Brand Names Allanfil 405 [US]; Allanfil Spray [US]; Panafil® SE [US]; Panafil® [US]; Papfyll™ [US]; Ziox 405™ [US]; Ziox™ [US]

Therapeutic Category Enzyme, Topical Debridement

Use Treatment of acute and chronic lesions, such as venous, diabetic, and decubitus ulcers, burns, postoperative wounds, pilonidal cyst wounds, carbuncles, and miscellaneous traumatic or infected wounds

Usual Dosage Topical: Adults: Apply with each dressing change; daily or twice daily dressing changes are preferred, but may be every 2-3 days. Cover with dressing following application.
Ointment: Apply 1/8" thickness over the wound with clean applicator.
Spray: Completely cover the wound site so that the wound is not visible.

Dosage Forms
Aerosol, topical [foam]:
Papfyll™: Chlorophyllin copper complex sodium 0.5%, papain ≥520,000 USP units/g, and urea 10% (45 g)
Emulsion [spray]:
Panafil® SE: Chlorophyllin copper complex sodium 0.5%, papain ≥521,700 USP units/g, and urea 10% (34 mL)
Ointment:
Allanfil 405, Panafil®: Chlorophyllin copper complex sodium 0.5%, papain ≥521,700 USP units/g, and urea 10% (6 g, 30 g)
Ziox™: Chlorophyllin copper complex sodium 0.5%, papain ≥521,700 USP units/g, and urea 10% (30 g)
Ziox 405™: Chlorophyllin copper complex sodium 0.5%, papain ≥521,700 USP units/g, and urea 10% (3.5 g, 30 g)
Solution [spray]:
Allanfil: Chlorophyllin copper complex sodium 0.5%, papain ≥521,700 USP units/g, and urea 10% (33 mL)

chloroprocaine (klor oh PROE kane)

Sound-Alike/Look-Alike Issues
Nesacaine® may be confused with Neptazane®
Synonyms chloroprocaine hydrochloride
U.S./Canadian Brand Names Nesacaine® [US]; Nesacaine®-CE [Can]; Nesacaine®-MPF [US]
Therapeutic Category Local Anesthetic
Use Infiltration anesthesia and peripheral and epidural anesthesia
Usual Dosage Dosage varies with anesthetic procedure, the area to be anesthetized, the vascularity of the tissues, depth of anesthesia required, degree of muscle relaxation required, and duration of anesthesia; range.
  Children >3 years (normally developed): Maximum dose (without epinephrine): 11 mg/kg; for infiltration, concentrations of 0.5% to 1% are recommended; for nerve block, concentrations of 1% to 1.5% are recommended
  Adults:
    Maximum single dose (without epinephrine): 11 mg/kg; maximum dose: 800 mg
    Maximum single dose (with epinephrine): 14 mg/kg; maximum dose: 1000 mg
    Infiltration and peripheral nerve block:
      Mandibular: 2%: 2-3 mL; total dose 40-60 mg
      Infraorbital: 2%: 0.5-1 mL; total dose 10-20 mg
      Brachial plexus: 2%; 30-40 mL; total dose 600-800 mg
      Digital (without epinephrine): 1%; 3-4 mL; total dose: 30-40 mg
      Pudendal: 2%; 10 mL each side; total dose: 400 mg
      Paracervical: 1%; 3 mL per each of four sites
    Caudal block: Preservative-free: 2% or 3%: 15-25 mL; may repeat at 40-60 minute intervals
    Lumbar epidural block: Preservative-free: 2% or 3%: 2-2.5 mL per segment; usual total volume: 15-25 mL; may repeat with doses that are 2-6 mL less than initial dose every 40-50 minutes.
Dosage Forms
  Injection, solution: 1% (30 mL); 2% (30 mL)
    Nesacaine®: 1% (30 mL); 2% (30 mL)
  Injection, solution [preservative free]: 2% (20 mL); 3% (20 mL)
    Nesacaine®-MPF: 2% (20 mL); 3% (20 mL)

chloroprocaine hydrochloride see chloroprocaine on page 204
Chloroptic® Ophthalmic Solution (Discontinued) see chloramphenicol on page 200
Chloroptic® SOP (Discontinued) see chloramphenicol on page 200

chloroquine (KLOR oh kwin)

Synonyms chloroquine phosphate
U.S./Canadian Brand Names Aralen® [US/Can]; Novo-Chloroquine [Can]
Therapeutic Category Aminoquinoline (Antimalarial)
Use Suppression or chemoprophylaxis of malaria; treatment of uncomplicated or mild-to-moderate malaria; extraintestinal amebiasis
Usual Dosage Oral:
  Suppression or prophylaxis of malaria:
    Children: Administer 5 mg base/kg/week on the same day each week (not to exceed 300 mg base/dose); begin 1-2 weeks prior to exposure; continue for 4-6 weeks after leaving endemic area; if suppressive therapy is not begun prior to exposure, double the initial loading dose to 10 mg base/kg and administer in 2 divided doses 6 hours apart, followed by the usual dosage regimen
    Adults: 500 mg/week (300 mg base) on the same day each week; begin 1-2 weeks prior to exposure; continue for 4-6 weeks after leaving endemic area; if suppressive therapy is not begun prior to exposure, double the initial loading dose to 1 g (600 mg base) and administer in 2 divided doses 6 hours apart, followed by the usual dosage regimen
  Acute attack:
    Children: 10 mg/kg (base) on day 1, followed by 5 mg/kg (base) 6 hours later and 5 mg/kg (base) on days 2 and 3
    Adults: 1 g (600 mg base) on day 1, followed by 500 mg (300 mg base) 6 hours later, followed by 500 mg (300 mg base) on days 2 and 3
  Extraintestinal amebiasis:
    Children: 10 mg/kg (base) once daily for 2-3 weeks (up to 300 mg base/day)
    Adults: 1 g/day (600 mg base) for 2 days followed by 500 mg/day (300 mg base) for at least 2-3 weeks

Dosage Forms
Tablet: 250 mg, 500 mg
Aralen®: 500 mg

chloroquine phosphate *see* chloroquine *on page 204*

chlorothiazide (klor oh THYE a zide)

U.S./Canadian Brand Names Diuril® [US/Can]; Sodium Diuril® [US]
Therapeutic Category Diuretic, Thiazide
Use Management of mild-to-moderate hypertension; adjunctive treatment of edema
Usual Dosage Note: The manufacturer states that I.V. and oral dosing are equivalent. Some clinicians may use lower I.V. doses; however, because of chlorothiazide's poor oral absorption. I.V. dosing in infants and children has not been well established.
Infants >6 months and Children: Oral: 10-20 mg/kg/day in 1-2 divided doses (maximum dose: 375 mg/day in children <2 years or 1 g/day in children 2-12 years)
Adults:
Hypertension: Oral: 500-2000 mg/day divided in 1-2 doses (manufacturer labeling); doses of 125-500 mg/day have also been recommended (JNC 7)
Edema: Oral, I.V.: 500-1000 mg once or twice daily; intermittent treatment (eg, therapy on alternative days) may be appropriate for some patients
ACC/AHA 2005 Heart Failure guidelines:
Oral: 250-500 mg once or twice daily (maximum daily dose: 1000 mg)
I.V.: 500-1000 mg once daily plus a loop diuretic
Dosage Forms
Injection, powder for reconstitution:
Sodium Diuril®: 500 mg
Suspension, oral:
Diuril®: 250 mg/5 mL
Tablet: 250 mg, 500 mg

Chlorphed® *(Discontinued)* *see* brompheniramine *on page 144*
Chlorphed®-LA Nasal Solution *(Discontinued)* *see* oxymetazoline *on page 712*
Chlorphen [US-OTC] *see* chlorpheniramine *on page 205*

chlorpheniramine (klor fen IR a meen)

Sound-Alike/Look-Alike Issues
Chlor-Trimeton® may be confused with Chloromycetin®
Synonyms chlorpheniramine maleate; CTM
U.S./Canadian Brand Names Ahist™ [US]; Aller-Chlor® [US-OTC]; Chlor-Trimeton® [US-OTC]; Chlor-Tripolon® [Can]; Chlorphen [US-OTC]; CPM-12 [US]; Diabetic Tussin® Allergy Relief [US-OTC]; Novo-Pheniram [Can]; PediaTan™ [US]; QDALL® AR [US]; Teldrin® HBP [US-OTC]
Therapeutic Category Antihistamine
Use Perennial and seasonal allergic rhinitis and other allergic symptoms including urticaria
Usual Dosage Oral:
Children: 0.35 mg/kg/day in divided doses every 4-6 hours
2-6 years: 1 mg every 4-6 hours, not to exceed 6 mg in 24 hours
6-12 years: 2 mg every 4-6 hours, not to exceed 12 mg/day or sustained release 8 mg at bedtime
Children >12 years and Adults: 4 mg every 4-6 hours, not to exceed 24 mg/day or sustained release 8-12 mg every 8-12 hours, not to exceed 24 mg/day
Dosage Forms
Capsule, extended release:
CPM-12: Chlorpheniramine 12 mg
Capsule, variable release:
QDALL® AR: Chlorpheniramine 12 mg [immediate release and sustained release]
Suspension:
PediaTan™: 8 mg/5 mL
Syrup:
Aller-Chlor® [OTC], Diabetic Tussin® Allergy Relief [OTC]: 2 mg/5 mL
Tablet: 4 mg
Aller-Chlor® [OTC], Chlor-Trimeton® [OTC], Chlorphen [OTC], Teldrin® HBP [OTC]: 4 mg

▶

Tablet, extended release:
Chlor-Trimeton® [OTC]: 12 mg
Tablet, long acting [scored]:
Ahist™: 12 mg

chlorpheniramine, acetaminophen, and pseudoephedrine *see* acetaminophen, chlorpheniramine, and pseudoephedrine *on page 25*

chlorpheniramine and acetaminophen (klor fen IR a meen & a seet a MIN oh fen)

Synonyms acetaminophen and chlorpheniramine

U.S./Canadian Brand Names Coricidin HBP® Cold and Flu [US-OTC]

Therapeutic Category Antihistamine/Analgesic

Use Symptomatic relief of congestion, headache, aches and pains of colds and flu

Usual Dosage Oral: Adults: 2 tablets every 4 hours

Dosage Forms
Tablet:
Coricidin HBP® Cold and Flu [OTC]: Chlorpheniramine 2 mg and acetaminophen 325 mg

chlorpheniramine and carbetapentane *see* carbetapentane and chlorpheniramine *on page 174*

chlorpheniramine and phenylephrine (klor fen IR a meen & fen il EF rin)

Sound-Alike/Look-Alike Issues
Rynatan® may be confused with Rynatuss®

Synonyms chlorpheniramine maleate and phenylephrine hydrochloride; chlorpheniramine tannate and phenylephrine tannate; phenylephrine and chlorpheniramine

U.S./Canadian Brand Names Actifed® Cold & Allergy [US-OTC] *[reformulation]*; AlleRx™ Suspension [US]; C-Phen [US]; Ceron [US]; Dallergy Drops [US]; Dallergy®-JR [US]; Dec-Chlorphen [US]; Ed A-Hist™ [US]; Ed ChlorPed D [US]; NoHist [US]; P-Tann D [US]; PD-Hist-D [US]; PediaTan™ D [US]; Phenabid® [US]; R-Tanna Pediatric [US]; R-Tanna [US]; Rescon-Jr® [US]; Rinate™ Pediatric [US]; Rondec® [US]; Rynatan® Pediatric [US]; Rynatan® [US]; Sildec PE [US]; Sudafed PE® Sinus & Allergy [US-OTC]; Tannate Pediatric [US]; Triaminic® Cold and Allergy [US-OTC]

Therapeutic Category Antihistamine/Decongestant Combination

Use Temporary relief of upper respiratory conditions such as nasal congestion, runny nose, and sneezing due to the common cold, hay fever, or allergic or vasomotor rhinitis

Usual Dosage Oral: Antihistamine/decongestant:
Children:
6-12 months: Rondec® drops: 0.75 mL 4 times/day
1-2 years: Rondec® drops: 1 mL 4 times/day
2-6 years:
AlleRx™: 1.25 -2.5 mL every 12 hours
Dallergy®-JR suspension: 2.5 mL every 12 hours
Rondec® syrup: 1.25 mL every 4-6 hours; maximum 7.5 mL/24 hours
Rynatan® suspension: 2.5 -5 mL every 12 hours
6-12 years:
AlleRx™: 2.5- 5 mL every 12 hours
Dallergy®-JR: One capsule every 12 hours; maximum 2 capsules/24 hours
Dallergy®-JR suspension: 5 mL every 12 hours
Ed A-Hist™: One-half caplet every 12 hours
Rondec® syrup: 2.5 mL every 4-6 hours; maximum 15 mL/24 hours
Rynatan® suspension: 5-10 mL every 12 hours
≥12 years: Refer to adult dosing.
Adults:
AlleRx™: 15 mL every 12 hours
Dallergy®-JR: Two capsules every 12 hours; maximum 4 capsules/24 hours
Dallergy®-JR suspension: 10 mL every 12 hours
Ed A-Hist™: One caplet every 12 hours
R-Tanna: 1-2 tablets every 12 hours
Rondec® syrup: 5 mL every 4-6 hours; maximum 30 mL/24 hours
Rynatan® tablet: 1-2 tablets every 12 hours

Dosage Forms

Caplet, prolonged release:
Ed A-Hist™, NoHist: Chlorpheniramine 8 mg and phenylephrine 20 mg

Capsule, extended release:
Dallergy®-JR: Chlorpheniramine 4 mg and phenylephrine 20 mg

Liquid:
Ed A-Hist™: Chlorpheniramine 4 mg and phenylephrine 10 mg per 5 mL
Triaminic® Cold and Allergy [OTC]: Chlorpheniramine 1 mg and phenylephrine 2.5 mg per 5 mL

Liquid, oral [drops]:
Dallergy: Chlorpheniramine 1 mg and phenylephrine 2 mg per 1 mL

Solution, oral [drops]:
Ceron, C-Phen, Dec-Chlorphen, PD-Hist-D, Sildec PE: Chlorpheniramine 1 mg and phenylephrine 3.5 mg per 1 mL

Suspension, oral: Chlorpheniramine 4 mg and phenylephrine 20 mg per 5 mL
AlleRx™: Chlorpheniramine 3 mg and phenylephrine 7.5 per 5 mL
Dallergy®-JR : Chlorpheniramine 4 mg and phenylephrine 20 mg per 5 mL
P-Tann D, PediaTan™ D: Chlorpheniramine 8 mg and phenylephrine 10 mg per 5 mL
R-Tanna Pediatric, Rinate™ Pediatric, Rynatan® Pediatric, Tannate Pediatric: Chlorpheniramine 4.5 mg and phenylephrine 5 mg per 5 mL

Suspension, oral [drops]:
Ed ChlorPed D: Chlorpheniramine 2 mg and phenylephrine 6 mg per 1 mL

Syrup:
Ceron, C-Phen, Dec-Chlorphen, PD-Hist-D, Rondec®, Sildec PE: Chlorpheniramine 4 mg and phenylephrine 12.5 mg per 5 mL

Tablet:
Actifed® Cold & Allergy [OTC], Sudafed PE® Sinus & Allergy [OTC]: Chlorpheniramine 4 mg and phenylephrine 10 mg
R-Tanna, Rynatan®: Chlorpheniramine 9 mg and phenylephrine 25 mg

Tablet, chewable:
Rynatan®: Chlorpheniramine 4.5 mg and phenylephrine 5 mg

Tablet, sustained release:
Rescon-Jr: Chlorpheniramine 4 mg and phenylephrine 20 mg

Tablet, timed release:
Phenabid®: Chlorpheniramine 8 mg and phenylephrine 20 mg

chlorpheniramine and pseudoephedrine (klor fen IR a meen & soo doe e FED rin)

Sound-Alike/Look-Alike Issues
Allerest® may be confused with Sinarest®
Chlor-Trimeton® may be confused with Chloromycetin®
Sudafed® may be confused with Sufenta®

Synonyms chlorpheniramine maleate and pseudoephedrine hydrochloride; chlorpheniramine tannate and pseudoephedrine tannate; pseudoephedrine and chlorpheniramine

U.S./Canadian Brand Names Allerest® Maximum Strength Allergy and Hay Fever [US-OTC]; Deconamine® SR [US]; Dicel™ [US]; Duratuss® DA [US]; Histex™ [US]; LoHist-D [US]; Suclor™ [US]; Sudafed® Sinus & Allergy [US-OTC]; SudaHist® [US]; Sudal® 12 [US]; Triaminic® Cold & Allergy [Can]

Therapeutic Category Antihistamine/Decongestant Combination

Use Relief of nasal congestion associated with the common cold, hay fever, and other allergies, sinusitis, eustachian tube blockage, and vasomotor and allergic rhinitis

Usual Dosage General dosing guidelines; consult specific product labeling. Rhinitis/decongestant: Oral:
Children:
2-6 years:
Chlorpheniramine maleate 1 mg and pseudoephedrine hydrochloride 15 mg every 4-6 hours
Chlorpheniramine tannate 4.5 mg and pseudoephedrine tannate 75 mg: 2.5-5 mL every 12 hours (maximum: 10 mL/24 hours)
6-12 years: Chlorpheniramine maleate 2 mg and pseudoephedrine hydrochloride 30 mg every 4-6 hours (immediate release products)
Children ≥12 years and Adults:
Chlorpheniramine maleate 4 mg and pseudoephedrine hydrochloride 60 mg every 4-6 hours (immediate release products)

◀ Chlorpheniramine tannate 4.5 mg and pseudoephedrine tannate 75 mg: 10-20 mL every 12 hours (maximum: 40 mL/24 hours)

Deconamine® SR: Chlorpheniramine maleate 8 mg and pseudoephedrine hydrochloride 120 mg every 12 hours

Dosage Forms

Capsule, extended release: Chlorpheniramine 8 mg and pseudoephedrine 120 mg; chlorpheniramine 12 mg and pseudoephedrine 100 mg

Duratuss® DA: Chlorpheniramine 12 mg and pseudoephedrine 100 mg

Suclor™: Chlorpheniramine 8 mg and pseudoephedrine 120 mg

Capsule, sustained release: Chlorpheniramine 8 mg and pseudoephedrine 120 mg

Deconamine® SR: Chlorpheniramine 8 mg and pseudoephedrine 120 mg

Liquid:

Histex™, LoHist-D: Chlorpheniramine 2 mg and pseudoephedrine 30 mg per 5 mL

Suspension:

Dicel™: Chlorpheniramine tannate 5 mg and pseudoephedrine tannate 75 mg per 5 mL

Syrup: Chlorpheniramine 2 mg and pseudoephedrine 30 mg per 5 mL

Tablet: Chlorpheniramine 4 mg and pseudoephedrine 60 mg

Allerest® Maximum Strength Allergy and Hay Fever [OTC]: Chlorpheniramine 2 mg and pseudoephedrine 30 mg

Sudafed® Sinus & Allergy [OTC]: Chlorpheniramine 4 mg and pseudoephedrine 60 mg

Tablet, chewable:

Sudal® 12: Chlorpheniramine 4 mg and pseudoephedrine 30 mg

Tablet, sustained release:

SudaHist: Chlorpheniramine 12 mg and pseudoephedrine 120 mg

chlorpheniramine, carbetapentane, and phenylephrine *see* carbetapentane, phenylephrine, and chlorpheniramine *on page 176*

chlorpheniramine, dextromethorphan, phenylephrine, and guaifenesin *see* dextromethorphan, chlorpheniramine, phenylephrine, and guaifenesin *on page 285*

chlorpheniramine, ephedrine, phenylephrine, and carbetapentane
(klor fen IR a meen, e FED rin, fen il EF rin, & kar bay ta PEN tane)

Sound-Alike/Look-Alike Issues

Rynatuss® may be confused with Rynatan®

Synonyms carbetapentane, ephedrine, phenylephrine, and chlorpheniramine; ephedrine, chlorpheniramine, phenylephrine, and carbetapentane; phenylephrine, ephedrine, chlorpheniramine, and carbetapentane

U.S./Canadian Brand Names Quad Tann® Pediatric [US]; Quad Tann® [US]; Rynatuss® [US]; Tetra Tannate Pediatric [US]

Therapeutic Category Antihistamine/Decongestant/Antitussive

Use Symptomatic relief of cough with a decongestant and an antihistamine

Usual Dosage Oral:

Children:

<2 years: Titrate dose individually

2-6 years: 2.5-5 mL every 12 hours

>6 years: 5-10 mL every 12 hours

Adults: 1-2 tablets every 12 hours

Dosage Forms

Suspension:

Quad Tann® Pediatric, Tetra Tannate Pediatric: Chlorpheniramine 4 mg, ephedrine 5 mg, phenylephrine 5 mg, and carbetapentane 30 mg per 5 mL

Tablet:

Rynatuss®: Chlorpheniramine 5 mg, ephedrine 10 mg, phenylephrine 10 mg, and carbetapentane 50 mg

Tablet, long acting:

Quad Tann®: Chlorpheniramine 5 mg, ephedrine 10 mg, phenylephrine 10 mg, and carbetapentane 60 mg

chlorpheniramine maleate *see* chlorpheniramine *on page 205*

chlorpheniramine maleate and hydrocodone bitartrate *see* hydrocodone and chlorpheniramine *on page 482*

chlorpheniramine maleate and phenylephrine hydrochloride *see* chlorpheniramine and phenylephrine *on page 206*

chlorpheniramine maleate and pseudoephedrine hydrochloride *see* chlorpheniramine and pseudoephedrine *on page 207*

chlorpheniramine maleate, dihydrocodeine bitartrate, and phenylephrine hydrochloride *see* dihydrocodeine, chlorpheniramine, and phenylephrine *on page 298*

chlorpheniramine maleate, ibuprofen, and pseudoephedrine *see* ibuprofen, pseudoephedrine, and chlorpheniramine *on page 497*

chlorpheniramine maleate, phenylephrine hydrochloride, and guaifenesin *see* chlorpheniramine, phenylephrine, and guaifenesin *on page 210*

chlorpheniramine maleate, pseudoephedrine hydrochloride, and dextromethorphan hydrobromide *see* chlorpheniramine, pseudoephedrine, and dextromethorphan *on page 212*

chlorpheniramine, phenylephrine, and dextromethorphan
(klor fen IR a meen, fen il EF rin, & deks troe meth OR fan)

Synonyms dextromethorphan, chlorpheniramine, and phenylephrine; phenylephrine, chlorpheniramine, and dextromethorphan

U.S./Canadian Brand Names C-Phen DM [US]; Ceron-DM [US]; Corfen DM [US]; De-Chlor DM [US]; De-Chlor DR [US]; Dex PC [US]; Ed A-Hist DM [US]; Father John's® Plus [US-OTC]; Mintuss DR [US]; Neo DM [US]; Norel DM™ [US]; PD-Cof [US]; PE-Hist DM [US]; Phenabid DM® [US]; Poly Tussin DM [US]; Robitussin® Cough and Allergy [US-OTC]; Robitussin® Cough and Cold Nighttime [US-OTC]; Robitussin® Pediatric Cough and Cold Nighttime [US-OTC]; Rondec®-DM [US]; Sildec PE-DM [US]; Statuss™ DM [US]; Trital DM [US]; Tussplex™ DM [US]

Therapeutic Category Antihistamine/Decongestant/Antitussive

Use Temporary relief of cough and upper respiratory symptoms associated with allergies or the common cold

Usual Dosage Oral: Relief of cough and cold symptoms:
Children:
6-12 months (Rondec®-DM drops): 0.75 mL 4 times/day
1-2 years (Rondec®-DM drops): 1 mL 4 times/day
2-6 years (Rondec®-DM syrup): 1.25 mL every 4-6 hours (maximum: 7.5 mL/24 hours)
6-12 years (Rondec®-DM syrup): 2.5 mL every 4-6 hours (maximum: 15 mL/24 hours)
Children ≥12 years and Adults (Rondec®-DM syrup): 5 mL every 4-6 hours (maximum: 30 mL/24 hours)

Dosage Forms
Liquid:
Corfen DM, Norel DM™, Trital DM: Chlorpheniramine 4 mg, phenylephrine 10 mg, and dextromethorphan 15 mg per 5 mL
De-Chlor DM: Chlorpheniramine 2 mg, phenylephrine 10 mg, and dextromethorphan 15 mg per 5 mL
De-Chlor DR: Chlorpheniramine 2 mg, phenylephrine 6 mg, and dextromethorphan 15 mg per 5 mL
Father John's® Plus [OTC]: Chlorpheniramine 2 mg, phenylephrine 5 mg, and dextromethorphan 5 mg per 15 mL
Liquid, oral [drops]:
C-Phen DM, PD-Cof, Rondec® DM, Sildec PE-DM: Chlorpheniramine 1 mg, phenylephrine 3.5 mg, and dextromethorphan 3 mg per 1 mL
Neo DM: Chlorpheniramine 0.75 mg, phenylephrine 1.75 mg, and dextromethorphan 2.75 mg per 1 mL
Syrup:
Ceron-DM, C-Phen DM, PD-Cof, Rondec®-DM, Sildec PE-DM: Chlorpheniramine 4 mg, phenylephrine 12.5 mg, and dextromethorphan 15 mg per 5 mL
Dex PC, Mintuss DR: Chlorpheniramine 2 mg, phenylephrine 6 mg, and dextromethorphan 15 mg per 5 mL
Ed A-Hist DM: Chlorpheniramine 4 mg, phenylephrine 10 mg, and dextromethorphan 15 mg per 5 mL
PE-Hist DM, Poly Tussin DM, Tussplex™ DM: Chlorpheniramine 2 mg, phenylephrine 5 mg, and dextromethorphan 15 mg per 5 mL
Robitussin® Cough and Allergy: Chlorpheniramine 2 mg, phenylephrine 5 mg, and dextromethorphan 10 mg per 5 mL
Robitussin® Cough and Cold Nighttime, Robitussin® Pediatric Cough and Cold Nighttime: Chlorpheniramine 1 mg, phenylephrine 2.5 mg, and dextromethorphan 5 mg per 5 mL
Statuss™: DM: Chlorpheniramine 2 mg, phenylephrine 10 mg, and dextromethorphan 15 mg per 5 mL
Tablet, timed release:
Phenabid DM®: Chlorpheniramine 8 mg, phenylephrine 20 mg, and dextromethorphan 30 mg

chlorpheniramine, phenylephrine, and guaifenesin
(klor fen IR a meen, fen il EF rin, & gwye FEN e sin)

Synonyms chlorpheniramine maleate, phenylephrine hydrochloride, and guaifenesin; chlorpheniramine tannate, phenylephrine tannate, and guaifenesin; guaifenesin, phenylephrine, and chlorpheniramine; phenylephrine, chlorpheniramine, and guaifenesin

U.S./Canadian Brand Names P Chlor GG [US]

Therapeutic Category Cough and Cold Combination

Use Symptomatic relief of upper respiratory symptoms associated with infections such as the common cold or allergies

Usual Dosage General dosing guidelines; consult specific product labeling. Oral: Antihistamine/decongestant/expectorant:

Children <3 months: 2-3 drops per month of age every 4-6 hours as needed; not to exceed 4 doses/24 hours

Children 3-6 months: 0.3-0.6 mL every 4-6 hours as needed; not to exceed 4 doses/24 hours

Children 6 months to 1 year: 0.6-1 mL every 4-6 hours as needed; not to exceed 4 doses/24 hours

Children 1-2 years: 1-2 mL every 4-6 hours as needed; not to exceed 4 doses/24 hours

Dosage Forms

Liquid:

P Chlor GG [drops]: Chlorpheniramine 1 mg, phenylephrine 2 mg, and guaifenesin 20 mg per 1 mL

chlorpheniramine, phenylephrine, and hydrocodone *see* phenylephrine, hydrocodone, and chlorpheniramine *on page 748*

chlorpheniramine, phenylephrine, and methscopolamine
(klor fen IR a meen, fen il EF rin, & meth skoe POL a meen)

Synonyms methscopolamine nitrate, chlorpheniramine maleate, and phenylephrine hydrochloride; phenylephrine tannate, chlorpheniramine tannate, and methscopolamine nitrate

U.S./Canadian Brand Names aerohist plus™ [US]; aeroKid™ [US]; AH-Chew® [US]; AH-Chew™ Ultra [US]; Chlor-Mes [US]; Chlor-Mes-D [US]; Dallergy® [US]; Dehistine [US]; Duradyl® [US]; Durahist™ PE [US]; Extendryl® JR [US]; Extendryl® SR [US]; Extendryl® [US]; Histatab PH [US]; OMNIhist® II L.A. [US]; PCM [US]; Phenylephrine CM [US]; Ralix [US]; Rescon® MX [US]; Rescon® [US]; Triall™ [US]

Therapeutic Category Antihistamine/Decongestant/Anticholinergic

Use Treatment of upper respiratory symptoms such as respiratory congestion, allergic rhinitis, vasomotor rhinitis, sinusitis, and allergic skin reactions of urticaria and angioedema

Usual Dosage

Children 6-11 years: Relief of respiratory symptoms: Oral:

aeroKid™: 2.5-5 mL every 4 hours

AH-Chew® suspension: 2.5-5 mL every 12 hours

Dallergy®, Durahist™ PE, OMNIhist® II L.A., Rescon® MX: One-half caplet/tablet every 12 hours

Duradryl® syrup, Extendryl® syrup: 2.5-5 mL, may repeat up to every 4 hours depending on age and body weight

Extendryl® chewable tablet: One tablet every 4 hours; do not exceed 4 doses in 24 hours

Extendryl® JR: One tablet every 12 hours

Children ≥12 years and Adults: Relief of respiratory symptoms: Oral: **Note:** If disturbances in urination occur in patients without renal impairment, medication should be discontinued for 1-2 days and should then be restarted at a lower dose

aeroKid™: 5-10 mL every 3-4 hours

AH-Chew® suspension: 5-10 mL every 12 hours

Dallergy®, Durahist™ PE, Extendryl® SR, OMNIhist® II L.A., Rescon® MX: One capsule/tablet every 12 hours

Duradryl® syrup, Extendryl® syrup: 5-10 mL every 3-4 hours (4 times/day)

Extendryl®: 1-2 chewable tablets every 4 hours

Dosage Forms

Caplet, extended release:

aerohist plus™ [OTC]: Chlorpheniramine 8 mg, phenylephrine 20 mg, and methscopolamine 2.5 mg

Chlor-Mes, Dallergy® [OTC]: Chlorpheniramine 12 mg, phenylephrine 20 mg, and methscopolamine 2.5 mg

Liquid:

Chlor-Mes-D [OTC]: Chlorpheniramine 2 mg, phenylephrine 10 mg, and methscopolamine 0.625 mg per 5 mL

Suspension:
AH-Chew® [OTC]: Chlorpheniramine, phenylephrine, and methscopalamine 1.5 mg per 5 mL
Syrup:
aeroKid™ [OTC]: Chlorpheniramine 4 mg, phenylephrine 1 mg, and methscopolamine 1.25 mg per 5 mL
Dallergy [OTC]: Chlorpheniramine 2 mg, phenylephrine 8 mg, and methscopolamine 0.75 mg per 5 mL
Dehistine [OTC], Duradryl® [OTC]: Chlorpheniramine 2 mg, phenylephrine 10 mg, and methscopolamine 1.25 mg per 5 mL
Extendryl® [OTC]: Dexchlorpheniramine 1 mg, phenylephrine 10 mg, and methscopolamine 1.25 mg per 5 mL
Triall™ (OTC: Chlorpheniramine 2 mg, phenylephrine 8 mg, and methscopolamine 0.75 mg per 5 mL
Tablet [scored]:
Dallergy® [OTC]: Chlorpheniramine 4 mg, phenylephrine 10 mg, and methscopolamine 1.25 mg
Tablet, chewable:
AH-Chew™ Ultra: Chlorpheniramine 2 mg, phenylephrine 10 mg, and methscopolamine 1.5 mg
Extendryl [OTC], PCM [OTC]: Chlorpheniramine 2 mg, phenylephrine 10 mg, and methscopolamine 1.25 mg
Tablet, extended release: Chlorpheniramine 8 mg, phenylephrine 20 mg, and methscopolamine 1.25 mg
Durahist™ PE [OTC]: Chlorpheniramine 8 mg, phenylephrine 20 mg, and methscopolamine 1.25 mg [scored]
Extendryl SR [OTC]: Chlorpheniramine 8 mg, phenylephrine 20 mg, and methscopolamine 2.5 mg
Extendryl® JR [OTC]: Chlorpheniramine 4 mg, phenylephrine 10 mg, and methscopolamine 1.25 mg
Tablet, long acting [scored]:
OMNIhist® II L.A. [OTC]: Chlorpheniramine 8 mg, phenylephrine 25 mg, and methscopolamine 2.5 mg
Rescon® MX [OTC]: Chlorpheniramine 8 mg, phenylephrine 40 mg, and methscopolamine 2.5 mg
Tablet, sustained release:
Histatab PH: Chlorpheniramine 8 mg, phenylephrine 20 mg, and methscopolamine 1.25 mg
Ralix [OTC]: Chlorpheniramine 8 mg, phenylephrine 40 mg, and methscopolamine 2 mg
Tablet, timed release:
Phenylephrine CM [OTC]: Chlorpheniramine 8 mg, phenylephrine 40 mg, and methscopolamine 2.5 mg
Tablet, variable release:
Rescon® [OTC]: Chlorpheniramine 12 mg and phenylephrine 40 mg [sustained release] and methscopolamine 2 mg [immediate release] [MaxRelent release]

chlorpheniramine, phenylephrine, and phenyltoloxamine
(klor fen IR a meen, fen il EF rin, & fen il tole LOKS a meen)
Synonyms phenylephrine, chlorpheniramine, and phenyltoloxamine; phenyltoloxamine, chlorpheniramine, and phenylephrine
U.S./Canadian Brand Names Chlorex-A [US]; Nalex®-A [US]; NoHist-A [US]; Rhinacon A [US]
Therapeutic Category Antihistamine/Decongestant Combination
Use Symptomatic relief of rhinitis and nasal congestion due to colds or allergy
Usual Dosage Oral:
Children:
2-6 years: Nalex®-A liquid: 1.25-2.5 mL every 4-6 hours
6-12 years:
Nalex®-A liquid: 5 mL every 4-6 hours
Nalex®-A tablet: 1/2 tablet 2-3 times/day
Children >12 years and Adults:
Nalex®-A liquid: 10 mL every 4-6 hours
Nalex®-A tablet: 1 tablet 2-3 times/day
Dosage Forms
Liquid: Chlorpheniramine 2.5 mg, phenylephrine 5 mg, and phenyltoloxamine 7.5 mg per 5 mL
Nalex®-A, NoHist-A, Rhinacon A: Chlorpheniramine 2.5 mg, phenylephrine 5 mg, and phenyltoloxamine 7.5 mg per 5 mL
Tablet, extended release:
Rhinacon A: Chlorpheniramine 4 mg, phenylephrine 20 mg, and phenyltoloxamine 40 mg
Tablet, prolonged release:
Nalex®-A: Chlorpheniramine 4 mg, phenylephrine 20 mg, and phenyltoloxamine 40 mg
Tablet, sustained release:
Chlorex-A: Chlorpheniramine 4 mg, phenylephrine 20 mg, and phenyltoloxamine 40 mg

chlorpheniramine, phenylephrine, codeine, and potassium iodide
(klor fen IR a meen, fen il EF rin, KOE deen, & poe TASS ee um EYE oh dide)

Synonyms codeine, chlorpheniramine, phenylephrine, and potassium iodide; phenylephrine, chlorpheniramine, codeine, and potassium iodide; potassium iodide, chlorpheniramine, phenylephrine, and codeine

Therapeutic Category Antihistamine/Decongestant/Antitussive

Controlled Substance C-V

Use Symptomatic relief of rhinitis, nasal congestion and cough due to colds or allergy

Usual Dosage Children 6 months to 12 years: 1.25-10 mL every 4-6 hours

chlorpheniramine, pseudoephedrine, and acetaminophen *see* acetaminophen, chlorpheniramine, and pseudoephedrine *on page 25*

chlorpheniramine, pseudoephedrine, and codeine
(klor fen IR a meen, soo doe e FED rin, & KOE deen)

Synonyms codeine, chlorpheniramine, and pseudoephedrine; pseudoephedrine, chlorpheniramine, and codeine

Therapeutic Category Antihistamine/Decongestant/Antitussive

Controlled Substance C-V

Use Temporary relief of cough associated with minor throat or bronchial irritation or nasal congestion due to common cold, allergic rhinitis, or sinusitis

Usual Dosage Oral:
Children:
25-50 lb: 1.25-2.5 mL every 4-6 hours, up to 4 doses in 24-hour period
50-90 lb: 2.5-5 mL every 4-6 hours, up to 4 doses in 24-hour period
Adults: 10 mL every 4-6 hours, up to 4 doses in 24-hour period

chlorpheniramine, pseudoephedrine, and dextromethorphan
(klor fen IR a meen, soo doe e FED rin, & deks troe meth OR fan)

Synonyms chlorpheniramine maleate, pseudoephedrine hydrochloride, and dextromethorphan hydrobromide; chlorpheniramine tannate, pseudoephedrine tannate, and dextromethorphan tannate; dexchlorpheniramine tannate, pseudoephedrine tannate, and dextromethorphan tannate; dextromethorphan, chlorpheniramine, and pseudoephedrine; pseudoephedrine, chlorpheniramine, and dextromethorphan

U.S./Canadian Brand Names Dicel™ DM [US]; DuraTan™ Forte [US]; Kidkare Children's Cough and Cold [US-OTC]; Pedia Relief™ [US-OTC]; Rescon DM [US-OTC]; Tanafed DMX™ [US]; Tannate PD-DM [US]

Therapeutic Category Antihistamine/Decongestant/Antitussive

Use Temporarily relieves nasal congestion, runny nose, cough, and sneezing due to the common cold, hay fever, or allergic rhinitis

Usual Dosage General dosing guidelines; consult specific product labeling. Relief of cold symptoms: Oral:
Children:
2-6 years:
Dexchlorpheniramine tannate 2.5 mg, pseudoephedrine tannate 75 mg, and dextromethorphan tannate 25 mg (Tanafed DMX™): 2.5-5 mL every 12 hours (maximum: 10 mL/24 hours)
Dexchlorpheniramine tannate 3.5 mg, pseudoephedrine tannate 45 mg, and dextromethorphan tannate 30 mg (DuraTan™ Forte): 1.25-2.5 mL every 12 hours (maximum: 5 mL/24 hours)
6-12 years:
Chlorpheniramine maleate 1 mg, pseudoephedrine 15 mg, and dextromethorphan hydrobromide 7.5 mg per 5 mL: 10 mL every 6 hours
Chlorpheniramine maleate 1 mg, pseudoephedrine 15 mg, and dextromethorphan hydrobromide 5 mg per tablet or 5 mL: 2 tablets or 10 mL every 4-6 hours (maximum: 4 doses/24 hours)
Chlorpheniramine maleate 2 mg, pseudoephedrine 30 mg, and dextromethorphan hydrobromide 10 mg per tablet or 5 mL (Rescon DM): 5 mL every 4-6 hours (maximum: 4 doses/24 hours)
Dexchlorpheniramine tannate 2.5 mg, pseudoephedrine tannate 75 mg, and dextromethorphan tannate 25 mg (Tanafed DMX™): 5-10 mL every 12 hours (maximum: 20 mL/24 hours)
Dexchlorpheniramine tannate 3.5 mg, pseudoephedrine tannate 45 mg, and dextromethorphan tannate 30 mg (DuraTan™ Forte): 2.5-5 mL every 12 hours (maximum: 10 mL/24 hours)
>12 years: Refer to adult dosing

Adults:
Chlorpheniramine maleate 1 mg, pseudoephedrine 15 mg, and dextromethorphan hydrobromide 7.5 mg per 5 mL: 20 mL every 6 hours
Chlorpheniramine maleate 2 mg, pseudoephedrine 30 mg, and dextromethorphan hydrobromide 10 mg per tablet or 5 mL (Rescon DM): 10 mL every 4-6 hours (maximum: 4 doses/24 hours)
Dexchlorpheniramine tannate 2.5 mg, pseudoephedrine tannate 75 mg, and dextromethorphan tannate 25 mg (Tanafed DMX™): 10-20 mL every 12 hours (maximum: 40 mL/24 hours)
Dexchlorpheniramine tannate 3.5 mg, pseudoephedrine tannate 45 mg, and dextromethorphan tannate 30 mg (DuraTan™ Forte): 5-15 mL every 12 hours (maximum: 30 mL/24 hours)

Dosage Forms
Liquid: Chlorpheniramine 1 mg, pseudoephedrine 15 mg, and dextromethorphan 5 mg per 5 mL
Kidkare Children's Cough and Cold [OTC], Pedia Relief™ [OTC]: Chlorpheniramine 1 mg, pseudoephedrine 15 mg, and dextromethorphan 5 mg per 5 mL
Rescon DM [OTC]: Chlorpheniramine 2 mg, pseudoephedrine 30 mg, and dextromethorphan 10 mg per 5 mL
Suspension:
Dicel™ DM: Chlorpheniramine 5 mg, pseudoephedrine 75 mg, and dextromethorphan 25 mg per 5 mL
DuraTan™ Forte: Dexchlorpheniramine tannate 3.5 mg, pseudoephedrine tannate 45 mg, and dextromethorphan tannate 30 mg per 5 mL
Tanafed DMX™: Dexchlorpheniramine 2.5 mg, pseudoephedrine 75 mg, and dextromethorphan 25 mg
Tannate PD-DM: Dexchlorpheniramine 3 mg, pseudoephedrine 50 mg, and dextromethorphan 27.5 mg per 5 mL

chlorpheniramine, pseudoephedrine, and dihydrocodeine see pseudoephedrine, dihydrocodeine, and chlorpheniramine on page 803

chlorpheniramine, pseudoephedrine, and methscopolamine
(klor fen IR a meen, soo doe e FED rin, & meth skoe POL a meen)
Synonyms methscopolamine, chlorpheniramine, and pseudoephedrine; methscopolamine, pseudoephedrine, and chlorpheniramine; pseudoephedrine hydrochloride, methscopolamine nitrate, and chlorpheniramine maleate; pseudoephedrine, methscopolamine, and chlorpheniramine
U.S./Canadian Brand Names Amdry-C [US]; Coldamine [US]; Durahist™ [US]
Therapeutic Category Antihistamine/Decongestant/Anticholinergic
Use Relief of symptoms of allergic rhinitis, vasomotor rhinitis, sinusitis, and the common cold
Usual Dosage Oral:
Children 6-11 years (Durahist™): One-half tablet every 12 hours (maximum dose: 1 tablet/24 hours)
Children ≥12 years and Adults (Durahist™): One tablet every 12 hours (maximum dose: 2 tablets/24 hours).
Dosage Forms
Tablet, extended release:
Coldamine: Chlorpheniramine 8 mg, pseudoephedrine 90 mg, and methscopolamine 2.5 mg
Tablet, sustained release: Chlorpheniramine maleate 8 mg, pseudoephedrine hydrochloride 60 mg, and methscopolamine nitrate 1.25 mg; chlorpheniramine maleate 8 mg, pseudoephedrine hydrochloride 90 mg, and methscopolamine nitrate 2.5 mg
Amdry-C: Chlorpheniramine 8 mg, pseudoephedrine 120 mg, and methscopolamine 2.5 mg [scored]
Durahist™: Chlorpheniramine 8 mg, pseudoephedrine 60 mg, and methscopolamine 1.25 mg [scored]

chlorpheniramine tannate and phenylephrine tannate see chlorpheniramine and phenylephrine on page 206
chlorpheniramine tannate and pseudoephedrine tannate see chlorpheniramine and pseudoephedrine on page 207
chlorpheniramine tannate, phenylephrine tannate, and guaifenesin see chlorpheniramine, phenylephrine, and guaifenesin on page 210
chlorpheniramine tannate, pseudoephedrine tannate, and dextromethorphan tannate see chlorpheniramine, pseudoephedrine, and dextromethorphan on page 212
Chlor-Pro® Injection *(Discontinued)* see chlorpheniramine on page 205

chlorpromazine (klor PROE ma zeen)
Sound-Alike/Look-Alike Issues
chlorproMAZINE may be confused with chlordiazePOXIDE, chlorproPAMIDE, clomiPRAMINE, prochlorperazine, promethazine

◀   Thorazine® may be confused with thiamine, thioridazine

Synonyms chlorpromazine hydrochloride; CPZ

Tall-Man chlorproMAZINE

U.S./Canadian Brand Names Largactil® [Can]; Novo-Chlorpromazine [Can]

Therapeutic Category Phenothiazine Derivative

Use Control of mania; treatment of schizophrenia; control of nausea and vomiting; relief of restlessness and apprehension before surgery; acute intermittent porphyria; adjunct in the treatment of tetanus; intractable hiccups; combativeness and/or explosive hyperexcitable behavior in children 1-12 years of age and in short-term treatment of hyperactive children

Usual Dosage

Children ≥6 months:

Schizophrenia/psychoses:

Oral: 0.5-1 mg/kg/dose every 4-6 hours; older children may require 200 mg/day or higher

I.M., I.V.: 0.5-1 mg/kg/dose every 6-8 hours

<5 years (22.7 kg): Maximum: 40 mg/day

5-12 years (22.7-45.5 kg): Maximum: 75 mg/day

Nausea and vomiting:

Oral: 0.5-1 mg/kg/dose every 4-6 hours as needed

I.M., I.V.: 0.5-1 mg/kg/dose every 6-8 hours

<5 years (22.7 kg): Maximum: 40 mg/day

5-12 years (22.7-45.5 kg): Maximum: 75 mg/day

Adults:

Schizophrenia/psychoses:

Oral: Range: 30-2000 mg/day in 1-4 divided doses, initiate at lower doses and titrate as needed; usual dose: 400-600 mg/day; some patients may require 1-2 g/day

I.M., I.V.: Initial: 25 mg, may repeat (25-50 mg) in 1-4 hours, gradually increase to a maximum of 400 mg/dose every 4-6 hours until patient is controlled; usual dose: 300-800 mg/day

Intractable hiccups: Oral, I.M.: 25-50 mg 3-4 times/day

Nausea and vomiting:

Oral: 10-25 mg every 4-6 hours

I.M., I.V.: 25-50 mg every 4-6 hours

Dosage Forms

Injection, solution: 25 mg/mL (1 mL, 2 mL)

Tablet: 10 mg, 25 mg, 50 mg, 100 mg, 200 mg

chlorpromazine hydrochloride *see* chlorpromazine *on page 213*

chlorpropamide (klor PROE pa mide)

Sound-Alike/Look-Alike Issues

chlorproPAMIDE may be confused with chlorproMAZINE

Diabinese® may be confused with DiaBeta®, Dialume®, Diamox®

Tall-Man chlorproPAMIDE

U.S./Canadian Brand Names Apo-Chlorpropamide® [Can]; Diabinese® [US]; Novo-Propamide [Can]

Therapeutic Category Antidiabetic Agent, Oral

Use Management of blood sugar in type 2 diabetes mellitus (noninsulin-dependent, NIDDM)

Usual Dosage Oral: The dosage of chlorpropamide is variable and should be individualized based upon the patient's response

Initial dose: Adults: 250 mg/day in mild-to-moderate diabetes in middle-aged, stable diabetic

Subsequent dosages may be increased or decreased by 50-125 mg/day at 3- to 5-day intervals

Maintenance dose: 100-250 mg/day; severe diabetics may require 500 mg/day; avoid doses >750 mg/day

Dosage Forms

Tablet: 100 mg, 250 mg

chlorthalidone (klor THAL i done)

U.S./Canadian Brand Names Apo-Chlorthalidone® [Can]; Thalitone® [US]

Therapeutic Category Diuretic, Miscellaneous

Use Management of mild-to-moderate hypertension when used alone or in combination with other agents; treatment of edema associated with congestive heart failure or nephrotic syndrome. Recent studies have found chlorthalidone effective in the treatment of isolated systolic hypertension in the elderly.

Usual Dosage Oral: Adults:
  Hypertension: 25-100 mg/day or 100 mg 3 times/week; usual dosage range (JNC 7): 12.5-25 mg/day
  Edema: Initial: 50-100 mg/day or 100 mg on alternate days; maximum dose: 200 mg/day
  Heart failure-associated edema: 12.5-25 mg once daily; maximum daily dose: 100 mg (ACC/AHA 2005 Heart Failure Guidelines)
Dosage Forms
  Tablet: 25 mg, 50 mg, 100 mg
    Thalitone®: 15 mg

chlorthalidone and atenolol *see* atenolol and chlorthalidone *on page 102*
chlorthalidone and clonidine *see* clonidine and chlorthalidone *on page 237*
Chlor-Trimeton® [US-OTC] *see* chlorpheniramine *on page 205*
Chlor-Trimeton® Allergy D (Discontinued) *see* chlorpheniramine and pseudoephedrine *on page 207*
Chlor-Trimeton® Syrup (Discontinued) *see* chlorpheniramine *on page 205*
Chlor-Tripolon® [Can] *see* chlorpheniramine *on page 205*
Chlor-Tripolon ND® [Can] *see* loratadine and pseudoephedrine *on page 576*

chlorzoxazone (klor ZOKS a zone)

Sound-Alike/Look-Alike Issues
  Parafon Forte® may be confused with Fam-Pren Forte
U.S./Canadian Brand Names Parafon Forte® DSC [US]; Parafon Forte® [Can]; Strifon Forte® [Can]
Therapeutic Category Skeletal Muscle Relaxant
Use Symptomatic treatment of muscle spasm and pain associated with acute musculoskeletal conditions
Usual Dosage Oral:
  Children: 20 mg/kg/day or 600 mg/m^2/day in 3-4 divided doses
  Adults: 250-500 mg 3-4 times/day up to 750 mg 3-4 times/day
Dosage Forms
  Caplet: 500 mg
    Parafon Forte® DSC: 500 mg
  Tablet: 250 mg, 500 mg

cholecalciferol (kole e kal SI fer ole)

Synonyms D$_3$
U.S./Canadian Brand Names D-3 [US-OTC]; D-Vi-Sol® [Can]; D3-50™ [US-OTC]; D3-5™ [US-OTC]; Delta-D® [US-OTC]; Maximum D3® [US]; Vitamin D3 [US-OTC]
Therapeutic Category Vitamin D Analog
Use Dietary supplement, treatment of vitamin D deficiency, or prophylaxis of deficiency
Usual Dosage Oral: Adults: 400-1000 units/day
Dosage Forms
  Capsule, oral:
    D-3 [OTC]: 1000 int. units
    D3-5™ [OTC]: 5000 int. units
    D3-50™ [OTC]: 50,000 int. units
    Maximum D3®: 10,000 int. units
  Tablet:
    Delta-D® [OTC]: 400 int. units

cholecalciferol and alendronate *see* alendronate and cholecalciferol *on page 43*
cholera and traveler's diarrhea vaccine *see* traveler's diarrhea and cholera vaccine *(Canada only) on page 944*

cholestyramine resin (koe LES teer a meen REZ in)

U.S./Canadian Brand Names Novo-Cholamine Light [Can]; Novo-Cholamine [Can]; PMS-Cholestyramine [Can]; Prevalite® [US]; Questran® Light Sugar Free [Can]; Questran® Light [US]; Questran® [US/Can]
Therapeutic Category Bile Acid Sequestrant

▶

◀ **Use** Adjunct in the management of primary hypercholesterolemia; pruritus associated with elevated levels of bile acids; diarrhea associated with excess fecal bile acids; binding toxicologic agents; pseudomembraneous colitis

Usual Dosage Oral (dosages are expressed in terms of anhydrous resin):
Children: 240 mg/kg/day in 3 divided doses; need to titrate dose depending on indication
Adults: 4 g 1-2 times/day to a maximum of 24 g/day and 6 doses/day

Dosage Forms
Powder for oral suspension: Cholestyramine resin 4 g/5 g packet (60s); cholestyramine resin 4 g/5 g of powder (210 g); cholestyramine resin 4 g/5.7 g packet (60s); cholestyramine resin 4 g/5.7 g of powder (240 g can); cholestyramine resin 4 g/9 g packet (60s); cholestyramine resin 4 g of resin/9 g of powder (378 g)
Prevalite®: Cholestyramine resin 4 g/5.5 g packet (42s, 60s); cholestyramine resin 4 g/5.5 g of powder
Questran®: Cholestyramine resin 4 g/9 g packet (60s); cholestyramine resin 4 g/9 g of powder
Questran® Light: Cholestyramine resin 4 g/5 g packet (60s); cholestyramine resin 4 g/5 g of powder

choline magnesium trisalicylate (KOE leen mag NEE zhum trye sa LIS i late)

Synonyms tricosal
Therapeutic Category Analgesic, Nonnarcotic; Nonsteroidal Antiinflammatory Drug (NSAID)
Use Management of osteoarthritis, rheumatoid arthritis, and other arthritis; acute painful shoulder
Usual Dosage Oral (based on total salicylate content):
Children <37 kg: 50 mg/kg/day given in 2 divided doses; 2250 mg/day for heavier children
Adults: 500 mg to 1.5 g 2-3 times/day **or** 3 g at bedtime; usual maintenance dose: 1-4.5 g/day
Dosage Forms
Liquid: 500 mg/5 mL
Tablet: 500 mg, 750 mg, 1000 mg

Cholografin® Meglumine [US] see iodipamide meglumine on page 519
chondroitin sulfate and sodium hyaluronate see sodium chondroitin sulfate and sodium hyaluronate on page 875
Chooz® [US-OTC] see calcium carbonate on page 163
choriogonadotropin alfa see chorionic gonadotropin (recombinant) on page 217

chorionic gonadotropin (human) (kor ee ON ik goe NAD oh troe pin, HYU man)

Synonyms CG; hCG
U.S./Canadian Brand Names Humegon® [Can]; Novarel® [US]; Pregnyl® [US/Can]; Profasi® HP [Can]
Therapeutic Category Gonadotropin
Use Induces ovulation and pregnancy in anovulatory, infertile females; treatment of hypogonadotropic hypogonadism, prepubertal cryptorchidism; spermatogenesis induction with follitropin alfa
Usual Dosage I.M.:
Children: Various regimens:
Prepubertal cryptorchidism:
4000 units 3 times/week for 3 weeks **or**
5000 units every second day for 4 injections **or**
500 units 3 times/week for 4-6 weeks **or**
15 injections of 500-1000 units given over 6 weeks

Hypogonadotropic hypogonadism: Males:
500-1000 units 3 times/week for 3 weeks, followed by the same dose twice weekly for 3 weeks **or**
4000 units 3 times/week for 6-9 months, then reduce dosage to 2000 units 3 times/week for additional 3 months

Adults:
Induction of ovulation: Females: 5000-10,000 units one day following last dose of menotropins
Spermatogenesis induction associated with hypogonadotropic hypogonadism: Males: Treatment regimens vary (range: 1000-2000 units 2-3 times a week). Administer hCG until serum testosterone levels are normal (may require 2-3 months of therapy), then may add follitropin alfa or menopausal gonadotropin if needed to induce spermatogenesis; continue hCG at the dose required to maintain testosterone levels.

Dosage Forms
Injection, powder for reconstitution: 10,000 units
Novarel®, Pregnyl®: 10,000 units

chorionic gonadotropin (recombinant)
(kor ee ON ik goe NAD oh troe pin ree KOM be nant)

Synonyms choriogonadotropin alfa; r-hCG

U.S./Canadian Brand Names Ovidrel® [US/Can]

Therapeutic Category Gonadotropin; Ovulation Stimulator

Use As part of an assisted reproductive technology (ART) program, induces ovulation in infertile females who have been pretreated with follicle-stimulating hormones (FSH); induces ovulation and pregnancy in infertile females when the cause of infertility is functional

Usual Dosage SubQ: Adults: Female: Assisted reproductive technologies (ART) and ovulation induction: 250 mcg given 1 day following the last dose of follicle-stimulating agent. Use only after adequate follicular development has been determined. Hold treatment when there is an excessive ovarian response.

Dosage Forms

Injection, solution:
  Ovidrel®: 257.5 mcg/0.515 mL (0.515 mL)

Choron® *(Discontinued)* *see* chorionic gonadotropin (human) *on page 216*

chromium *see* trace metals *on page 940*

Chronovera® [Can] *see* verapamil *on page 974*

Chronulac® *(Discontinued)* *see* lactulose *on page 544*

CI-1008 *see* pregabalin *on page 783*

Cialis® [US/Can] *see* tadalafil *on page 902*

Cibacalcin® *(Discontinued)* *see* calcitonin *on page 160*

ciclesonide (sye KLES oh nide)

U.S./Canadian Brand Names Alvesco® [US/Can]; Omnaris™ [US/Can]

Therapeutic Category Corticosteroid, Inhalant (Oral); Corticosteroid, Nasal

Use
Intranasal: Management of seasonal and perennial allergic rhinitis
Oral inhalation: Prophylactic management of bronchial asthma

Usual Dosage
Intranasal (Omnaris™):
  Seasonal allergic rhinitis:
    U.S. labeling: Children ≥6 years and Adults: 2 sprays (50 mcg/spray) per nostril once daily; maximum: 200 mcg/day
    Canadian labeling: Children ≥12 years and Adults: 2 sprays (50 mcg/spray) per nostril once daily; maximum: 200 mcg/day
  Perennial allergic rhinitis: Children ≥12 years and Adults: 2 sprays (50 mcg/spray) per nostril once daily; maximum: 200 mcg/day
Oral inhalation (Alvesco®):
  Asthma: **Note:** Titrate to the lowest effective dose once asthma stability is achieved:
    U.S. labeling: Children ≥12 years and Adults:
      Prior therapy with bronchodilators alone: Initial: 80 mcg twice daily (maximum dose: 320 mcg/day)
      Prior therapy with inhaled corticosteroids: Initial: 80 mcg twice daily (maximum dose: 640 mcg/day)
      Prior therapy with oral corticosteroids: Initial: 320 mcg twice daily (maximum dose: 640 mcg/day)
    Canadian labeling: Children ≥12 years and Adults: Initial: 400 mcg once daily; maintenance: 100-800 mcg/day (1-2 puffs once or twice daily)

Conversion from oral to inhaled steroid: Initiation of oral inhalation therapy should begin in patients who have previously been stabilized on oral corticosteroids (OCS). A gradual dose reduction of OCS should begin ~7-10 days after starting inhaled therapy. U.S. labeling recommends reducing prednisone dose no more rapidly than ≤2.5 mg/day on a weekly basis. The Canadian labeling recommends decreasing the daily dose of prednisone by 1 mg (or equivalent of other OCS) every 7 days in closely monitored patients, and every 10 days in patients whom close monitoring is not possible. In the presence of withdrawal symptoms, resume previous OCS dose for 1 week before attempting further dose reductions.

Dosage Forms [CAN] = Canadian brand name

Aerosol for oral inhalation:
  Alvesco® [U.S.]: 80 mcg/inhalation (6.1 g) [60 metered doses]; 160 mcg/inhalation (6.1 g) [60 metered doses]; 160 mcg/inhalation (9.6 g) [120 metered doses]

◀ Alvesco® [CAN]: 50 mcg/inhalation [30-, 60-, and 120 metered doses] [not available in the U.S.]; 100 mcg/inhalation [30-, 60-, and 120 metered doses] [not available in the U.S.]; 200 mcg/inhalation [30-, 60-, and 120 metered doses] [not available in the U.S.]

Suspension, intranasal [spray]:
Omnaris™: 50 mcg/inhalation (12.5 g)

ciclopirox (sye kloe PEER oks)

Sound-Alike/Look-Alike Issues
Loprox® may be confused with Lonox®

Synonyms ciclopirox olamine

U.S./Canadian Brand Names Loprox® [US/Can]; Penlac® [US/Can]; Stieprox® [Can]

Therapeutic Category Antifungal Agent

Use
Cream/suspension: Treatment of tinea pedis (athlete's foot), tinea cruris (jock itch), tinea corporis (ringworm), cutaneous candidiasis, and tinea versicolor (pityriasis)
Gel: Treatment of tinea pedis (athlete's foot), tinea corporis (ringworm); seborrheic dermatitis of the scalp
Lacquer (solution): Topical treatment of mild-to-moderate onychomycosis of the fingernails and toenails due to *Trichophyton rubrum* (not involving the lunula) and the immediately-adjacent skin
Shampoo: Treatment of seborrheic dermatitis of the scalp

Usual Dosage Topical:
Children >10 years and Adults: Tinea pedis, tinea cruris, tinea corporis, cutaneous candidiasis, and tinea versicolor: Cream/suspension: Apply twice daily, gently massage into affected areas; if no improvement after 4 weeks of treatment, reevaluate the diagnosis.
Children ≥12 years and Adults: Onychomycosis of the fingernails and toenails: Lacquer (solution): Apply to adjacent skin and affected nails daily (as a part of a comprehensive management program for onychomycosis). Remove with alcohol every 7 days.
Children >16 years and Adults:
Tinea pedis, tinea corporis: Gel: Apply twice daily, gently massage into affected areas and surrounding skin; if no improvement after 4 weeks of treatment, reevaluate diagnosis
Seborrheic dermatitis of the scalp:
Gel: Apply twice daily, gently massage into affected areas and surrounding skin; if no improvement after 4 weeks of treatment, reevaluate diagnosis.
Shampoo: Apply ~5 mL (1 teaspoonful) to wet hair; lather, and leave in place ~3 minutes; rinse. May use up to 10 mL for longer hair. Repeat twice weekly for 4 weeks; allow a minimum of 3 days between applications.

Dosage Forms
Cream, topical: 0.77% (15 g, 30 g, 90 g)
Loprox®: 0.77% (15 g, 30 g, 90 g)
Gel, topical: 0.77% (30 g, 45 g, 100 g)
Loprox®: 0.77% (30 g, 45 g, 100 g)
Shampoo, topical:
Loprox®: 1% (120 mL)
Solution, topical [nail lacquer]: 8% (6.6 mL)
Penlac®: 8% (6.6 mL)
Suspension, topical: 0.77% (30 mL, 60 mL)
Loprox®: 0.77% (30 mL, 60 mL)

ciclopirox olamine *see ciclopirox on page 218*
cidecin *see daptomycin on page 267*

cidofovir (si DOF o veer)

U.S./Canadian Brand Names Vistide® [US]

Therapeutic Category Antiviral Agent

Use Treatment of cytomegalovirus (CMV) retinitis in patients with acquired immunodeficiency syndrome (AIDS). **Note:** Should be administered with probenecid.

Usual Dosage Adults:
Induction: 5 mg/kg I.V. over 1 hour once weekly for 2 consecutive weeks
Maintenance: 5 mg/kg over 1 hour once every other week
Note: Administer with probenecid 2 g orally 3 hours prior to each cidofovir dose and 1 g at 2 hours and 8 hours after completion of the infusion (total: 4 g)

Hydrate with 1 L of 0.9% NS I.V. prior to cidofovir infusion; a second liter may be administered over a 1- to 3-hour period immediately following infusion, if tolerated

Dosage Forms
Injection, solution [preservative free]:
Vistide®: 75 mg/mL (5 mL)

cilazapril and hydrochlorothiazide *(Canada only)*
(sye LAY za pril & hye droe klor oh THYE a zide)

Synonyms cilazapril monohydrate and hydrochlorothiazide; hydrochlorothiazide and cilazapril

U.S./Canadian Brand Names Apo-Cilazapril/Hctz [Can]; Inhibace® Plus [Can]

Therapeutic Category Angiotensin-Converting Enzyme (ACE) Inhibitor

Use Treatment of mild-to-moderate hypertension in patients who have been stabilized on the individual agents given in the same proportions; not indicated for initial treatment of hypertension

Usual Dosage Note: Initiate therapy with combination product only after successful titration of individual agents to adequate blood pressure response.
Oral: Adults: One tablet administered once daily; dose is individualized (range: Cilazapril: 2.5-10 mg; hydrochlorothiazide: 6.25-25 mg/day)

Dosage Forms [CAN] = Canadian brand name
Tablet: 5/12.5: Cilazapril 5 mg and hydrochlorothiazide 12.5 mg [not available in the U.S.]
Inhibace® Plus 5/12.5 [CAN]: Cilazapril 5 mg and hydrochlorothiazide 12.5 mg [not available in the U.S.; contains lactose]

cilazapril *(Canada only)* (sye LAY za pril)

Synonyms cilazapril monohydrate

U.S./Canadian Brand Names Apo-Cilazapril® [Can]; CO Cilazapril [Can]; Gen-Cilazapril [Can]; Inhibace® [Can]; Novo-Cilazapril [Can]; PMS-Cilazapril [Can]

Therapeutic Category Angiotensin-Converting Enzyme (ACE) Inhibitor

Use Management of hypertension; treatment of heart failure

Usual Dosage Oral:
Hypertension: 2.5-5 mg once daily (maximum dose: 10 mg/day)
Congestive heart failure: Initial: 0.5 mg once daily; if tolerated, after 5 days increase to 1 mg/day (lowest maintenance dose); may increase to maximum of 2.5 mg once daily

Dosage Forms [CAN] = Canadian brand name
Tablet:
Inhibace® [CAN], Novo-Cilazapril [CAN]: 1 mg, 2.5 mg, 5 mg [not available in the U.S.]

cilazapril monohydrate *see* cilazapril *(Canada only) on page 219*
cilazapril monohydrate and hydrochlorothiazide *see* cilazapril and hydrochlorothiazide *(Canada only) on page 219*

cilostazol (sil OH sta zol)

Sound-Alike/Look-Alike Issues
Pletal® may be confused with Plendil®

Synonyms OPC-13013

U.S./Canadian Brand Names Pletal® [US/Can]

Therapeutic Category Platelet Aggregation Inhibitor

Use Symptomatic management of peripheral vascular disease, primarily intermittent claudication

Usual Dosage Oral: Adults: 100 mg twice daily

Dosage Forms
Tablet: 50 mg, 100 mg
Pletal®: 50 mg, 100 mg

Ciloxan® [US/Can] *see* ciprofloxacin *on page 221*

cimetidine (sye MET i deen)

Sound-Alike/Look-Alike Issues
cimetidine may be confused with simethicone

U.S./Canadian Brand Names Apo-Cimetidine® [Can]; Gen-Cimetidine [Can]; Novo-Cimetidine [Can]; Nu-Cimet [Can]; PMS-Cimetidine [Can]; Tagamet® HB 200 [US-OTC]; Tagamet® HB [Can]

▶

◀ **Therapeutic Category** Histamine H_2 Antagonist

Use Short-term treatment of active duodenal ulcers and benign gastric ulcers; long-term prophylaxis of duodenal ulcer; gastric hypersecretory states; gastroesophageal reflux; prevention of upper GI bleeding in critically-ill patients; labeled for OTC use for prevention or relief of heartburn, acid indigestion, or sour stomach

Usual Dosage

Children: Oral, I.M., I.V.: 20-40 mg/kg/day in divided doses every 6 hours

Children ≥12 years and Adults: Oral: Heartburn, acid indigestion, sour stomach (OTC labeling): 200 mg up to twice daily; may take 30 minutes prior to eating foods or beverages expected to cause heartburn or indigestion

Adults:

Short-term treatment of active ulcers:

Oral: 300 mg 4 times/day or 800 mg at bedtime or 400 mg twice daily for up to 8 weeks

Note: Higher doses of 1600 mg at bedtime for 4 weeks may be beneficial for a subpopulation of patients with larger duodenal ulcers (>1 cm defined endoscopically) who are also heavy smokers (≥1 pack/day).

I.M., I.V.: 300 mg every 6 hours or 37.5 mg/hour by continuous infusion; I.V. dosage should be adjusted to maintain an intragastric pH ≥5

Prevention of upper GI bleed in critically-ill patients: 50 mg/hour by continuous infusion; I.V. dosage should be adjusted to maintain an intragastric pH ≥5

Note: Reduce dose by 50% if Cl_{cr} <30 mL/minute; treatment >7 days has not been evaluated.

Duodenal ulcer prophylaxis: Oral: 400 mg at bedtime

Gastric hypersecretory conditions: Oral, I.M., I.V.: 300-600 mg every 6 hours; dosage not to exceed 2.4 g/day

Gastroesophageal reflux disease: Oral: 400 mg 4 times/day or 800 mg twice daily for 12 weeks

Dosage Forms

Note: Strength is expressed as base

Infusion [premixed in NS]: 300 mg (50 mL)

Injection, solution: 150 mg/mL (2 mL, 8 mL)

Solution, oral: 300 mg/5 mL

Tablet: 200 mg [OTC], 300 mg, 400 mg, 800 mg

Tagamet® HB 200 [OTC]: 200 mg

Cimzia® [US] *see certolizumab pegol on page 195*

cinacalcet (sin a KAL cet)

Synonyms AMG 073; cinacalcet hydrochloride

U.S./Canadian Brand Names Sensipar® [US/Can]

Therapeutic Category Calcimimetic

Use Treatment of secondary hyperparathyroidism in patients with chronic kidney disease (CKD) on dialysis; treatment of hypercalcemia in patients with parathyroid carcinoma

Note: In Canada, cinacalcet is approved only for the treatment of secondary hyperparathyroidism in patients with chronic kidney disease (CKD) on dialysis

Usual Dosage Oral: Adults: **Do not titrate dose more frequently than every 2-4 weeks.**

Secondary hyperparathyroidism: Initial: 30 mg once daily (maximum daily dose: 180 mg); increase dose incrementally (60 mg, 90 mg, 120 mg, 180 mg once daily) as necessary to maintain iPTH level between 150-300 pg/mL.

Parathyroid carcinoma: Initial: 30 mg twice daily (maximum daily dose: 360 mg daily as 90 mg 4 times/day); increase dose incrementally (60 mg twice daily, 90 mg twice daily, 90 mg 3-4 times/day) as necessary to normalize serum calcium levels.

Dosage Forms

Tablet:

Sensipar®: 30 mg, 60 mg, 90 mg

cinacalcet hydrochloride *see cinacalcet on page 220*

Cipralex® [Can] *see escitalopram on page 356*

Cipro® [US/Can] *see ciprofloxacin on page 221*

Cipro® XL [Can] *see ciprofloxacin on page 221*

Ciprodex® [US/Can] *see ciprofloxacin and dexamethasone on page 223*

ciprofloxacin (sip roe FLOKS a sin)

Sound-Alike/Look-Alike Issues
ciprofloxacin may be confused with cephalexin
Ciloxan® may be confused with cinoxacin, Cytoxan®
Cipro® may be confused with Ceftin®

Synonyms ciprofloxacin hydrochloride

U.S./Canadian Brand Names Apo-Ciproflox® [Can]; Ciloxan® [US/Can]; Cipro® XL [Can]; Cipro® XR [US]; Cipro® [US/Can]; CO Ciprofloxacin [Can]; Dom-Ciprofloxacin [Can]; Gen-Ciprofloxacin [Can]; Novo-Ciprofloxacin [Can]; PHL-Ciprofloxacin [Can]; PMS-Ciprofloxacin [Can]; Proquin® XR [US]; RAN™-Ciprofloxacin [Can]; ratio-Ciprofloxacin [Can]; Riva-Ciprofloxacin [Can]; Sandoz-Ciprofloxacin [Can]; Taro-Ciprofloxacin [Can]

Therapeutic Category Antibiotic, Ophthalmic; Quinolone

Use

Children: Complicated urinary tract infections and pyelonephritis due to *E. coli*. **Note:** Although effective, ciprofloxacin is not the drug of first choice in children.

Children and Adults: To reduce incidence or progression of disease following exposure to aerolized *Bacillus anthracis*. Ophthalmologically, for superficial ocular infections (corneal ulcers, conjunctivitis) due to susceptible strains

Adults: Treatment of the following infections when caused by susceptible bacteria: Urinary tract infections; acute uncomplicated cystitis in females; chronic bacterial prostatitis; lower respiratory tract infections (including acute exacerbations of chronic bronchitis); acute sinusitis; skin and skin structure infections; bone and joint infections; complicated intraabdominal infections (in combination with metronidazole); infectious diarrhea; typhoid fever due to *Salmonella typhi* (eradication of chronic typhoid carrier state has not been proven); uncomplicated cervical and urethral gonorrhea (due to *N. gonorrhoeae*); nosocomial pneumonia; empirical therapy for febrile neutropenic patients (in combination with piperacillin)

Note: As of April 2007, the CDC no longer recommends the use of fluoroquinolones for the treatment of gonococcal disease.

Usual Dosage Note: Extended release tablets and immediate release formulations are not interchangeable. Unless otherwise specified, oral dosing reflects the use of immediate release formulations.

Usual dosage ranges:
Children:
Oral: 20-30 mg/kg/day in 2 divided doses; maximum dose: 1.5 g/day
I.V.: 20-30 mg/kg/day divided every 12 hours; maximum dose: 800 mg/day
Adults:
Oral: 250-750 mg every 12 hours
I.V.: 200-400 mg every 12 hours

Indication-specific dosing:
Children:
Anthrax:
Inhalational (postexposure prophylaxis):
Oral: 15 mg/kg/dose every 12 hours for 60 days; maximum: 500 mg/dose
I.V.: 10 mg/kg/dose every 12 hours for 60 days; do **not** exceed 400 mg/dose (800 mg/day)
Cutaneous (treatment, CDC guidelines): Oral: 10-15 mg/kg every 12 hours for 60 days (maximum: 1 g/day); amoxicillin 80 mg/kg/day divided every 8 hours is an option for completion of treatment after clinical improvement. **Note:** In the presence of systemic involvement, extensive edema, lesions on head/neck, refer to I.V. dosing for treatment of inhalational/gastrointestinal/oropharyngeal anthrax.
Inhalational/gastrointestinal/oropharyngeal (treatment, CDC guidelines): I.V.: Initial: 10-15 mg/kg every 12 hours for 60 days (maximum: 500 mg/dose); switch to oral therapy when clinically appropriate; refer to adult dosing for notes on combined therapy and duration

Bacterial conjunctivitis: See adult dosing

Corneal ulcer: See adult dosing

Urinary tract infection (complicated) or pyelonephritis:
Oral: 20-30 mg/kg/day in 2 divided doses (every 12 hours) for 10-21 days; maximum: 1.5 g/day
I.V.: 6-10 mg/kg every 8 hours for 10-21 days (maximum: 400 mg/dose)
Adults:
Anthrax:
Inhalational (postexposure prophylaxis):
Oral: 500 mg every 12 hours for 60 days
I.V.: 400 mg every 12 hours for 60 days

▶

Cutaneous (treatment, CDC guidelines): Oral: Immediate release formulation: 500 mg every 12 hours for 60 days. **Note:** In the presence of systemic involvement, extensive edema, lesions on head/neck, refer to I.V. dosing for treatment of inhalational/gastrointestinal/oropharyngeal anthrax

Inhalational/gastrointestinal/oropharyngeal (treatment, CDC guidelines): I.V.: 400 mg every 12 hours. **Note:** Initial treatment should include two or more agents predicted to be effective (per CDC recommendations). Continue combined therapy for 60 days.

Bacterial conjunctivitis:
Ophthalmic solution: Instill 1-2 drops in eye(s) every 2 hours while awake for 2 days and 1-2 drops every 4 hours while awake for the next 5 days
Ophthalmic ointment: Apply a ½" ribbon into the conjunctival sac 3 times/day for the first 2 days, followed by a ½" ribbon applied twice daily for the next 5 days

Bone/joint infections:
Oral: 500-750 mg twice daily for 4-6 weeks
I.V.: Mild-to-moderate: 400 mg every 12 hours for 4-6 weeks; Severe/complicated: 400 mg every 8 hours for 4-6 weeks

Chancroid (CDC guidelines): Oral: 500 mg twice daily for 3 days

Corneal ulcer: Ophthalmic solution: Instill 2 drops into affected eye every 15 minutes for the first 6 hours, then 2 drops into the affected eye every 30 minutes for the remainder of the first day. On day 2, instill 2 drops into the affected eye hourly. On days 3-14, instill 2 drops into affected eye every 4 hours. Treatment may continue after day 14 if reepithelialization has not occurred.

Febrile neutropenia*: I.V.: 400 mg every 8 hours for 7-14 days

Gonococcal infections:
Urethral/cervical gonococcal infections: Oral: 250-500 mg as a single dose (CDC recommends concomitant doxycycline or azithromycin due to possible coinfection with *Chlamydia*; **Note:** As of April 2007, the CDC no longer recommends the use of fluoroquinolones for the treatment of uncomplicated gonococcal disease.

Disseminated gonococcal infection (CDC guidelines): Oral: 500 mg twice daily to complete 7 days of therapy (initial treatment with ceftriaxone 1 g I.M./I.V. daily for 24-48 hours after improvement begins); **Note:** As of April 2007, the CDC no longer recommends the use of fluoroquinolones for the treatment of more serious gonococcal disease, unless no other options exist and susceptibility can be confirmed via culture.

Infectious diarrhea: Oral:
Salmonella: 500 mg twice daily for 5-7 days
Shigella: 500 mg twice daily for 3 days
Traveler's diarrhea: Mild: 750 mg for one dose; Severe: 500 mg twice daily for 3 days
Vibrio cholerae: 1 g for one dose

Intraabdominal*:
Oral: 500 mg every 12 hours for 7-14 days
I.V.: 400 mg every 12 hours for 7-14 days

Lower respiratory tract, skin/skin structure infections:
Oral: 500-750 mg twice daily for 7-14 days
I.V.: Mild-to-moderate: 400 mg every 12 hours for 7-14 days; Severe/complicated: 400 mg every 8 hours for 7-14 days

Nosocomial pneumonia: I.V.: 400 mg every 8 hours for 10-14 days

Prostatitis (chronic, bacterial): Oral: 500 mg every 12 hours for 28 days

Sinusitis (acute): Oral: 500 mg every 12 hours for 10 days

Typhoid fever: Oral: 500 mg every 12 hours for 10 days

Urinary tract infection:
Acute uncomplicated, cystitis:
Oral:
Immediate release formulation: 250 mg every 12 hours for 3 days
Extended release formulation (Cipro® XR, Proquin® XR): 500 mg every 24 hours for 3 days
I.V.: 200 mg every 12 hours for 7-14 days
Complicated (including pyelonephritis):
Oral:
Immediate release formulation: 500 mg every 12 hours for 7-14 days
Extended release formulation (Cipro® XR): 1000 mg every 24 hours for 7-14 days
I.V.: 400 mg every 12 hours for 7-14 days
*Combination therapy generally recommended.

Dosage Forms
Infusion [premixed in D_5W]: 200 mg (100 mL); 400 mg (200 mL)
Cipro®: 200 mg (100 mL); 400 mg (200 mL)

Injection, solution [concentrate]: 10 mg/mL (20 mL, 40 mL, 120 mL)
Cipro®: 10 mg/mL (20 mL, 40 mL)
Microcapsules for suspension, oral:
Cipro®: 250 mg/5 mL, 500 mg/5 mL
Ointment, ophthalmic:
Ciloxan®: 3.33 mg/g (3.5 g) [0.3% base]
Solution, ophthalmic: 3.5 mg/mL (2.5 mL, 5mL, 10 mL) [0.3% base]
Ciloxan®: 3.5 mg/mL (5 mL) [0.3% base]
Tablet: 100 mg, 250 mg, 500 mg, 750 mg
Cipro®: 250 mg, 500 mg, 750 mg
Tablet, extended release: 500 mg, 1000 mg
Cipro® XR: 500 mg, 1000 mg
Tablet, extended release:
Proquin® XR: 500 mg
Tablet, extended release [dose pack]:
Proquin® XR: 500 mg (3s)

ciprofloxacin and dexamethasone (sip roe FLOKS a sin & deks a METH a sone)

Synonyms ciprofloxacin hydrochloride and dexamethasone; dexamethasone and ciprofloxacin

U.S./Canadian Brand Names Ciprodex® [US/Can]

Therapeutic Category Antibiotic/Corticosteroid, Otic

Use Treatment of acute otitis media in pediatric patients with tympanostomy tubes or acute otitis externa in children and adults

Usual Dosage Otic:
Children: Acute otitis media in patients with tympanostomy tubes or acute otitis externa: Instill 4 drops into affected ear(s) twice daily for 7 days
Adults: Acute otitis externa: Instill 4 drops into affected ear(s) twice daily for 7 days

Dosage Forms
Suspension, otic:
Ciprodex®: Ciprofloxacin 0.3% and dexamethasone 0.1% (7.5 mL)

ciprofloxacin and hydrocortisone (sip roe FLOKS a sin & hye droe KOR ti sone)

Synonyms ciprofloxacin hydrochloride and hydrocortisone; hydrocortisone and ciprofloxacin

U.S./Canadian Brand Names Cipro® HC [US/Can]

Therapeutic Category Antibiotic/Corticosteroid, Otic

Use Treatment of acute otitis externa, sometimes known as "swimmer's ear"

Usual Dosage Otic: Children >1 year of age and Adults: The recommended dosage for all patients is three drops of the suspension in the affected ear twice daily for 7 days; twice-daily dosing schedule is more convenient for patients than that of existing treatments with hydrocortisone, which are typically administered three or four times a day; a twice-daily dosage schedule may be especially helpful for parents and caregivers of young children

Dosage Forms
Suspension, otic:
Cipro® HC: Ciprofloxacin 0.2% and hydrocortisone 1% (10 mL)

ciprofloxacin hydrochloride *see* ciprofloxacin *on page 221*
ciprofloxacin hydrochloride and dexamethasone *see* ciprofloxacin and dexamethasone *on page 223*
ciprofloxacin hydrochloride and hydrocortisone *see* ciprofloxacin and hydrocortisone *on page 223*
Cipro® HC [US/Can] *see* ciprofloxacin and hydrocortisone *on page 223*
Cipro® XR [US] *see* ciprofloxacin *on page 221*

cisapride (SIS a pride)

Sound-Alike/Look-Alike Issues
Propulsid® may be confused with propranolol

U.S./Canadian Brand Names Propulsid® [US]

Therapeutic Category Gastrointestinal Agent, Prokinetic

▶

◀ **Use** Treatment of nocturnal symptoms of gastroesophageal reflux disease (GERD); has demonstrated effectiveness for gastroparesis, refractory constipation, and nonulcer dyspepsia

Usual Dosage Oral:

Children: 0.15-0.3 mg/kg/dose 3-4 times/day; maximum: 10 mg/dose

Adults: Initial: 10 mg 4 times/day at least 15 minutes before meals and at bedtime; in some patients the dosage will need to be increased to 20 mg to obtain a satisfactory result

cisatracurium (sis a tra KYOO ree um)

Sound-Alike/Look-Alike Issues

Nimbex® may be confused with Revex®

Synonyms cisatracurium besylate

U.S./Canadian Brand Names Nimbex® [US/Can]

Therapeutic Category Skeletal Muscle Relaxant

Use Adjunct to general anesthesia to facilitate endotracheal intubation and to relax skeletal muscles during surgery; to facilitate mechanical ventilation in ICU patients; does not relieve pain or produce sedation

Usual Dosage I.V. (not to be used I.M.):

Operating room administration:

Infants 1-23 months: 0.15 mg/kg over 5-10 seconds during either halothane or opioid anesthesia

Children 2-12 years: Intubating doses: 0.1-0.15 mg/kg over 5-15 seconds during either halothane or opioid anesthesia. (**Note:** When given during stable opioid/nitrous oxide/oxygen anesthesia, 0.1 mg/kg produces maximum neuromuscular block in an average of 2.8 minutes and clinically effective block for 28 minutes.)

Adults: Intubating doses: 0.15-0.2 mg/kg as component of propofol/nitrous oxide/oxygen induction-intubation technique. (**Note:** May produce generally good or excellent conditions for tracheal intubation in 1.5-2 minutes with clinically effective duration of action during propofol anesthesia of 55-61 minutes.); initial dose after succinylcholine for intubation: 0.1 mg/kg; maintenance dose: 0.03 mg/kg 40-60 minutes after initial dose, then at ~20-minute intervals based on clinical criteria

Children ≥2 years and Adults: Continuous infusion: After an initial bolus, a diluted solution can be given by continuous infusion for maintenance of neuromuscular blockade during extended surgery; adjust the rate of administration according to the patient's response as determined by peripheral nerve stimulation. An initial infusion rate of 3 mcg/kg/minute may be required to rapidly counteract the spontaneous recovery of neuromuscular function; thereafter, a rate of 1-2 mcg/kg/minute should be adequate to maintain continuous neuromuscular block in the 89% to 99% range in most pediatric and adult patients. Consider reduction of the infusion rate by 30% to 40% when administering during stable isoflurane, enflurane, sevoflurane, or desflurane anesthesia. Spontaneous recovery from neuro-muscular blockade following discontinuation of infusion of cisatracurium may be expected to proceed at a rate comparable to that following single bolus administration.

Intensive care unit administration: Follow the principles for infusion in the operating room. At initial signs of recovery from bolus dose, begin the infusion at a dose of 3 mcg/kg/minute and adjust rates accordingly; dosage ranges of 0.5-10 mcg/kg/minute have been reported. If patient is allowed to recover from neuromuscular blockade, readministration of a bolus dose may be necessary to quickly reestablish neuromuscular block prior to reinstituting the infusion.

Dosage Forms

Injection, solution:

Nimbex®: 2 mg/mL (5 mL, 10 mL); 10 mg/mL (20 mL)

cisatracurium besylate see cisatracurium on page 224

cisplatin (SIS pla tin)

Sound-Alike/Look-Alike Issues

CISplatin may be confused with CARBOplatin

Synonyms CDDP

Tall-Man CISplatin

Therapeutic Category Antineoplastic Agent

Use Treatment of bladder, testicular, and ovarian cancer

Usual Dosage Refer to individual protocols. **VERIFY ANY CISPLATIN DOSE EXCEEDING 100 mg/m^2 PER COURSE.**

Adults:

Advanced bladder cancer: 50-70 mg/m^2 every 3-4 weeks

Malignant pleural mesothelioma in combination with pemetrexed: 75 mg/m^2 on day 1 of each 21-day cycle; see pemetrexed monograph for additional details

Metastatic ovarian cancer: 75-100 mg/m^2 every 3-4 weeks

Intraperitoneal: Cisplatin has been administered intraperitoneal with systemic sodium thiosulfate for ovarian cancer; doses up to 90-270 mg/m^2 have been administered and retained for 4 hours before draining

Testicular cancer: 10-20 mg/m^2/day for 5 days repeated every 3-4 weeks

Dosage Forms

Injection, solution [preservative free]: 1 mg/mL (50 mL, 100 mL, 200 mL)

13-*cis*-retinoic acid see isotretinoin *on page 531*

citalopram (sye TAL oh pram)

Sound-Alike/Look-Alike Issues

Celexa® may be confused with Celebrex®, Cerebra®, Cerebyx®, Ranexa™, Zyprexa®

Synonyms citalopram hydrobromide; nitalapram

U.S./Canadian Brand Names Apo-Citalopram® [Can]; Celexa® [US/Can]; CO Citalopram [Can]; Dom-Citalopram [Can]; Gen-Citalopram [Can]; Mint-Citalopram [Can]; Novo-Citalopram [Can]; PHL-Citalopram [Can]; PMS-Citalopram [Can]; RAN™-Citalopram [Can]; ratio-Citalopram [Can]; Riva-Citalopram [Can]; Sandoz-Citalopram [Can]

Therapeutic Category Antidepressant

Use Treatment of depression

Usual Dosage Oral: Adults: Depression: Initial: 20 mg/day, generally with an increase to 40 mg/day; doses of more than 40 mg are not usually necessary. Should a dose increase be necessary, it should occur in 20 mg increments at intervals of no less than 1 week. Maximum dose: 60 mg/day

Dosage Forms

Solution, oral: 10 mg/5 mL

Celexa®: 10 mg/5 mL

Tablet: 10 mg, 20 mg, 40 mg

Celexa®: 10 mg, 20 mg, 40 mg

citalopram hydrobromide see citalopram *on page 225*

Citanest® Plain [Can] see prilocaine *on page 785*

Citanest® Plain Dental [US] see prilocaine *on page 785*

Citracal® Kosher [US-OTC] see calcium citrate *on page 165*

Citracal® Prenatal 90+ DHA *(Discontinued)* see vitamins (multiple/prenatal) *on page 983*

Citracal® Prenatal + DHA *(Discontinued)* see vitamins (multiple/prenatal) *on page 983*

CitraNatal™ 90 DHA [US] see vitamins (multiple/prenatal) *on page 983*

CitraNatal™ DHA [US] see vitamins (multiple/prenatal) *on page 983*

CitraNatal™ Rx [US] see vitamins (multiple/prenatal) *on page 983*

citrate of magnesia see magnesium citrate *on page 584*

citric acid and D-gluconic acid irrigant see citric acid, magnesium carbonate, and glucono-delta-lactone *on page 225*

citric acid and potassium citrate see potassium citrate and citric acid *on page 772*

citric acid bladder mixture see citric acid, magnesium carbonate, and glucono-delta-lactone *on page 225*

citric acid, magnesium carbonate, and glucono-delta-lactone

(SI trik AS id, mag NEE see um KAR bo nate, and GLOO kon o DEL ta LAK tone)

Sound-Alike/Look-Alike Issues

Renacidin® may be confused with Remicade®

Synonyms citric acid and D-gluconic acid irrigant; citric acid bladder mixture; citric acid, magnesium hydroxycarbonate, D-gluconic acid, magnesium acid citrate, and calcium carbonate; hemiacidrin

U.S./Canadian Brand Names Renacidin® [US]

Therapeutic Category Irrigating Solution

Use Prevention of formation of calcifications of indwelling urinary tract catheters; treatment of renal and bladder calculi of the apatite or struvite type

▶

◀ **Usual Dosage** Adults:
Dissolution or prevention of calcifications: Irrigation (indwelling urethral catheters): 30-60 mL 2-3 times/
day by means of a rubber syringe
Renal calculi: Irrigation: Infuse NS at 60 mL/hour and increase until pain, elevated pressure, or maximum
flow rate of 120 mL/hour is reached. Begin flow of solution at maximum rate achieved with NS.
Bladder calculi: 30 mL instilled through urinary catheter; clamp for 30-60 minutes, then release and drain;
repeat 4-6 times/day
Dosage Forms
Solution, irrigation:
Renacidin®: Citric acid 6.602 g, magnesium carbonate 3.177 g, glucono-delta-lactone 0.198 g per 100
mL (500 mL)

**citric acid, magnesium hydroxycarbonate, D-gluconic acid, magnesium acid citrate, and
calcium carbonate** see citric acid, magnesium carbonate, and glucono-delta-lactone on page 225

citric acid, sodium citrate, and potassium citrate
(SIT rik AS id, SOW dee um SIT rate, & poe TASS ee um SIT rate)
Synonyms potassium citrate, citric acid, and sodium citrate; sodium citrate, citric acid, and potassium
citrate
U.S./Canadian Brand Names Cytra-3 [US]; Polycitra® [US]; Polycitra®-LC [US]; Tricitrates [US]
Therapeutic Category Alkalinizing Agent
Use Conditions where long-term maintenance of an alkaline urine is desirable as in control and dissolution
of uric acid and cystine calculi of the urinary tract
Usual Dosage Oral:
Children: 5-15 mL diluted in water after meals and at bedtime
Adults: 15-30 mL diluted in water after meals and at bedtime
Dosage Forms
Solution, oral:
Cytra-3, Polycitra®-LC, Tricitrates: Citric acid 334 mg, sodium citrate 500 mg, and potassium citrate
550 mg per 5 mL
Syrup, oral:
Polycitra®: Citric acid 334 mg, sodium citrate 500 mg, and potassium citrate 550 mg per 5 mL

Citroma® [US-OTC] see magnesium citrate on page 584
Citro-Mag® [Can] see magnesium citrate on page 584
Citrotein® [US-OTC] see nutritional formula, enteral/oral on page 689
citrovorum factor see leucovorin calcium on page 552
Citrucel® [US-OTC] see methylcellulose on page 619
Citrucel® Fiber Shake [US-OTC] see methylcellulose on page 619
Citrucel® Fiber Smoothie [US-OTC] see methylcellulose on page 619
CL-118,532 see triptorelin on page 956
Cl-719 see gemfibrozil on page 439
CL-825 see pentostatin on page 737
CL-184116 see porfimer on page 769
CL-232315 see mitoxantrone on page 638

cladribine (KLA dri been)
Sound-Alike/Look-Alike Issues
cladribine may be confused with clofarabine
Leustatin® may be confused with lovastatin
Synonyms 2-CdA; 2-chlorodeoxyadenosine; NSC-105014
U.S./Canadian Brand Names Leustatin® [US/Can]
Therapeutic Category Antineoplastic Agent
Use Treatment of hairy cell leukemia
Usual Dosage I.V. (refer to individual protocols): Adults: Hairy cell leukemia: Continuous infusion:
0.09 mg/kg/day days 1-7; may be repeated every 28-35 days
Dosage Forms
Injection, solution [preservative free]: 1 mg/mL (10 mL)
Leustatin®: 1 mg/mL (10 mL)

Claforan® [US/Can] *see* cefotaxime *on page 186*
Claravis™ [US] *see* isotretinoin *on page 531*
Clarifoam™ EF [US] *see* sulfur and sulfacetamide *on page 897*
Clarinex® [US] *see* desloratadine *on page 274*
Clarinex-D® 12 Hour [US] *see* desloratadine and pseudoephedrine *on page 275*
Clarinex-D® 24 Hour [US] *see* desloratadine and pseudoephedrine *on page 275*
Claripel™ [US] *see* hydroquinone *on page 488*

clarithromycin (kla RITH roe mye sin)

Sound-Alike/Look-Alike Issues
clarithromycin may be confused with erythromycin

U.S./Canadian Brand Names Apo-Clarithromycin [Can]; Biaxin® XL [US/Can]; Biaxin® [US/Can]; Gen-Clarithromycin [Can]; PMS-Clarithromycin [Can]; ratio-Clarithromycin [Can]

Therapeutic Category Macrolide (Antibiotic)

Use
Children:
Acute otitis media (*H. influenzae, M. catarrhalis,* or *S. pneumoniae*)
Community-acquired pneumonia due to susceptible *Mycoplasma pneumoniae, S. pneumoniae,* or *Chlamydia pneumoniae* (TWAR)
Pharyngitis/tonsillitis due to susceptible *S. pyogenes,* acute maxillary sinusitis due to susceptible *H. influenzae, S. pneumoniae,* or *Moraxella catarrhalis,* uncomplicated skin/skin structure infections due to susceptible *S. aureus, S. pyogenes,* and mycobacterial infections
Prevention of disseminated mycobacterial infections due to MAC disease in patients with advanced HIV infection
Adults:
Pharyngitis/tonsillitis due to susceptible *S. pyogenes*
Acute maxillary sinusitis and acute exacerbation of chronic bronchitis due to susceptible *H. influenzae, H. parainfluenzae, M. catarrhalis,* or *S. pneumoniae*
Community-acquired pneumonia due to susceptible *H. influenzae, H. parainfluenzae, Mycoplasma pneumoniae, S. pneumoniae,* or *Chlamydia pneumoniae* (TWAR), *Moraxella catarrhalis*
Uncomplicated skin/skin structure infections due to susceptible *S. aureus, S. pyogenes*
Disseminated mycobacterial infections due to *M. avium* or *M. intracellulare*
Prevention of disseminated mycobacterial infections due to *M. avium* complex (MAC) disease (eg, patients with advanced HIV infection)
Duodenal ulcer disease due to *H. pylori* in regimens with other drugs including amoxicillin and lansoprazole or omeprazole, ranitidine bismuth citrate, bismuth subsalicylate, tetracycline, and/or an H_2 antagonist

Usual Dosage
Usual dosage range:
Children ≥6 months: Oral: 7.5 mg/kg every 12 hours (maximum: 500 mg/dose)
Adults: Oral: 250-500 mg every 12 hours **or** 1000 mg (two 500 mg extended release tablets) once daily for 7-14 days
Indication-specific dosing:
Children: Oral:
Community-acquired pneumonia, sinusitis, bronchitis, skin infections: 15 mg/kg/day divided every 12 hours for 10 days
Mycobacterial infection (prevention and treatment): 7.5 mg/kg (up to 500 mg) twice daily. **Note:** Safety of clarithromycin for MAC not studied in children <20 months.
Adults: Oral:
Acute exacerbation of chronic bronchitis:
M. catarrhalis and *S. pneumoniae*: 250 mg every 12 hours for 7-14 days **or** 1000 mg (two 500 mg extended release tablets) once daily for 7 days
H. influenzae: 500 mg every 12 hours for 7-14 days or 1000 mg (two 500 mg extended release tablets) once daily for 7 days
H. parainfluenzae: 500 mg every 12 hours for 7 days or 1000 mg (two 500 mg extended release tablets) once daily for 7 days
Acute maxillary sinusitis: 500 mg every 12 hours **or** 1000 mg (two 500 mg extended release tablets) once daily for 14 days
Mycobacterial infection (prevention and treatment): 500 mg twice daily (use with other antimycobacterial drugs, eg, ethambutol or rifampin)

◀ **Peptic ulcer disease:** Eradication of *Helicobacter pylori*: Dual or triple combination regimens with bismuth subsalicylate, amoxicillin, an H_2-receptor antagonist, or proton-pump inhibitor: 500 mg every 8-12 hours for 10-14 days

Pharyngitis, tonsillitis: 250 mg every 12 hours for 10 days

Pneumonia:

C. pneumoniae, M. pneumoniae, and *S. pneumoniae*: 250 mg every 12 hours for 7-14 days **or** 1000 mg (two 500 mg extended release tablets) once daily for 7 days

H. influenzae: 250 mg every 12 hours for 7 days **or** 1000 mg (two 500 mg extended release tablets) once daily for 7 days

Skin and skin structure infection, uncomplicated: 250 mg every 12 hours for 7-14 days

Dosage Forms

Granules for oral suspension: 125 mg/5 mL (50 mL, 100 mL); 250 mg/5 mL (50 mL, 100 mL)

Biaxin®: 125 mg/5 mL, 250 mg/5 mL

Tablet: 250 mg, 500 mg

Biaxin®: 250 mg, 500 mg

Tablet, extended release: 500 mg

Biaxin® XL: 500 mg

clarithromycin, lansoprazole, and amoxicillin *see* lansoprazole, amoxicillin, and clarithromycin *on page 549*

Claritin® [Can] *see* loratadine *on page 576*

Claritin® 24 Hour Allergy [US-OTC] *see* loratadine *on page 576*

Claritin-D® 12 Hour Allergy & Congestion [US-OTC] *see* loratadine and pseudoephedrine *on page 576*

Claritin-D® 24 Hour Allergy & Congestion [US-OTC] *see* loratadine and pseudoephedrine *on page 576*

Claritin® Allergic Decongestant [Can] *see* oxymetazoline *on page 712*

Claritin® Children's [US-OTC] *see* loratadine *on page 576*

Claritin® Children's Allergy [US-OTC] *see* loratadine *on page 576*

Claritin® (Discontinued) *see* loratadine *on page 576*

Claritin® Extra [Can] *see* loratadine and pseudoephedrine *on page 576*

Claritin® Hives Relief [US-OTC] *see* loratadine *on page 576*

Claritin® Kids [Can] *see* loratadine *on page 576*

Claritin® Liberator [Can] *see* loratadine and pseudoephedrine *on page 576*

Claritin® Reditabs [OTC] (Discontinued) *see* loratadine *on page 576*

Clarus™ [Can] *see* isotretinoin *on page 531*

Clasteon® [Can] *see* clodronate *(Canada only) on page 234*

clavulanic acid and amoxicillin *see* amoxicillin and clavulanate potassium *on page 68*

Clavulin® [Can] *see* amoxicillin and clavulanate potassium *on page 68*

Clear Away® Disc (Discontinued) *see* salicylic acid *on page 850*

Clear By Design® Gel (Discontinued) *see* benzoyl peroxide *on page 126*

Clear eyes® for Dry Eyes and ACR Relief [US-OTC] *see* naphazoline *on page 655*

Clear eyes® for Dry Eyes and Redness Relief [US-OTC] *see* naphazoline *on page 655*

Clear eyes® Redness Relief [US-OTC] *see* naphazoline *on page 655*

Clear eyes® Seasonal Relief [US-OTC] *see* naphazoline *on page 655*

Clearplex [US-OTC] *see* benzoyl peroxide *on page 126*

Clearsil® Maximum Strength (Discontinued) *see* benzoyl peroxide *on page 126*

Clear Tussin® 30 (Discontinued) *see* guaifenesin and dextromethorphan *on page 454*

clemastine (KLEM as teen)

Synonyms clemastine fumarate

U.S./Canadian Brand Names Dayhist® Allergy [US-OTC]; Tavist® Allergy [US-OTC]

Therapeutic Category Antihistamine

Use Perennial and seasonal allergic rhinitis and other allergic symptoms including urticaria

Usual Dosage Oral:

Infants and Children <6 years: 0.05 mg/kg/day as **clemastine base** or 0.335-0.67 mg/day clemastine fumarate (0.25-0.5 mg base/day) divided into 2 or 3 doses; maximum daily dosage: 1.34 mg (1 mg base)

Children 6-12 years: 0.67-1.34 mg clemastine fumarate (0.5-1 mg base) twice daily; do not exceed 4.02 mg/day (3 mg/day base)

Children ≥12 years and Adults:

1.34 mg clemastine fumarate (1 mg base) twice daily to 2.68 mg (2 mg base) 3 times/day; do not exceed 8.04 mg/day (6 mg base)

OTC labeling: 1.34 mg clemastine fumarate (1 mg base) twice daily; do not exceed 2 mg base/24 hours

Dosage Forms

Syrup: 0.67 mg/5 mL [0.5 mg base/5 mL; prescription formulation]

Tablet: 1.34 mg [1 mg base; OTC], 2.68 mg [2 mg base; prescription formulation]

Dayhist® Allergy [OTC], Tavist® Allergy [OTC]: 1.34 mg [1 mg base]

clemastine fumarate *see* clemastine *on page 228*

Clenia™ [US] *see* sulfur and sulfacetamide *on page 897*

Cleocin® [US] *see* clindamycin *on page 230*

Cleocin HCl® [US] *see* clindamycin *on page 230*

Cleocin Pediatric® [US] *see* clindamycin *on page 230*

Cleocin Phosphate® [US] *see* clindamycin *on page 230*

Cleocin T® [US] *see* clindamycin *on page 230*

Cleocin® Vaginal Ovule [US] *see* clindamycin *on page 230*

clevidipine (klev ID i peen)

Sound-Alike/Look-Alike Issues

clevidipine may be confused with cladribine, clofarabine, clomiPRAMINE

Cleviprex™ may be confused with Claravis™

Synonyms clevidipine butyrate

U.S./Canadian Brand Names Cleviprex™ [US]

Therapeutic Category Calcium Channel Blocker

Use Management of hypertension when oral treatment is not feasible or not desirable

Usual Dosage I.V.: Adults: Initial: 1-2 mg/hour

Titration: Initial: dose may be doubled at 90-second intervals toward blood pressure goal. As blood pressure approaches goal, dose may be increased by less than double every 5-10 minutes. **Note:** For every 1-2 mg/hour increase in dose, an approximate reduction of 2-4 mm Hg in systolic blood pressure may occur.

Usual maintenance: 4-6 mg/hour; maximum: 21 mg/hour (1000 mL within a 24-hour period). There is limited short-term experience with doses up to 32 mg/hour. Data is limited beyond 72 hours.

Dosage Forms

Injection, emulsion:

Cleviprex™: 0.5 mg/mL (50 mL, 100 mL)

clevidipine butyrate *see* clevidipine *on page 229*

Cleviprex™ [US] *see* clevidipine *on page 229*

clidinium and chlordiazepoxide (kli DI nee um & klor dye az e POKS ide)

Sound-Alike/Look-Alike Issues

Librax® may be confused with Librium®

Synonyms chlordiazepoxide and clidinium

U.S./Canadian Brand Names Apo-Chlorax® [Can]; Librax® *[original formulation]* [US/Can]

Therapeutic Category Anticholinergic Agent

Use Adjunct treatment of peptic ulcer; treatment of irritable bowel syndrome

Usual Dosage Oral: 1-2 capsules 3-4 times/day, before meals or food and at bedtime

Dosage Forms

Capsule: Clidinium 2.5 mg and chlordiazepoxide 5 mg

Librax® [original formulation]: Clidinium 2.5 mg and chlordiazepoxide 5 mg

Climara® [US/Can] *see* estradiol *on page 359*
ClimaraPro® [US] *see* estradiol and levonorgestrel *on page 361*
Clinac™ BPO [US] *see* benzoyl peroxide *on page 126*
Clindagel® [US] *see* clindamycin *on page 230*
ClindaMax® [US] *see* clindamycin *on page 230*

clindamycin (klin da MYE sin)

Sound-Alike/Look-Alike Issues
Cleocin® may be confused with bleomycin, Clinoril®, Lincocin®

Synonyms clindamycin hydrochloride; clindamycin palmitate; clindamycin phosphate

U.S./Canadian Brand Names Alti-Clindamycin [Can]; Apo-Clindamycin® [Can]; Cleocin HCl® [US]; Cleocin Pediatric® [US]; Cleocin Phosphate® [US]; Cleocin T® [US]; Cleocin® Vaginal Ovule [US]; Cleocin® [US]; Clindagel® [US]; ClindaMax® [US]; Clindamycin Injection, USP [Can]; ClindaReach™ [US]; Clindesse™ [US]; Clindoxyl® [Can]; Dalacin® C [Can]; Dalacin® T [Can]; Dalacin® Vaginal [Can]; Evoclin® [US]; Gen-Clindamycin [Can]; Novo-Clindamycin [Can]; PMS-Clindamycin [Can]; ratio-Clindamycin [Can]; Riva-Clindamycin [Can]; Taro-Clindamycin [Can]

Therapeutic Category Acne Products; Antibiotic, Miscellaneous

Use Treatment of susceptible bacterial infections, mainly those caused by anaerobes, streptococci, pneumococci, and staphylococci; bacterial vaginosis (vaginal cream, vaginal suppository); pelvic inflammatory disease (I.V.); topically in treatment of severe acne; vaginally for *Gardnerella vaginalis*

Usual Dosage
Usual dosage ranges:
Infants and Children:
Oral: 8-20 mg/kg/day as hydrochloride; 8-25 mg/kg/day as palmitate in 3-4 divided doses (minimum dose of palmitate: 37.5 mg 3 times/day)
I.M., I.V.:
<1 month: 15-20 mg/kg/day
>1 month: 20-40 mg/kg/day in 3-4 divided doses
Adults:
Oral: 150-450 mg/dose every 6-8 hours; maximum dose: 1.8 g/day
I.M., I.V.: 1.2-1.8 g/day in 2-4 divided doses; maximum dose: 4.8 g/day
Indication-specific dosing:
Children:
Anthrax: I.V.: 7.5 mg/kg every 6 hours
Babesiosis: Oral: 20-40 mg/kg/day divided every 8 hours for 7 days plus quinine
Orofacial infections:
Oral: 10-20 mg/kg in 3-4 equally divided doses
I.V.: 15-25 mg/kg in 3-4 equally divided doses
Children ≥12 years and Adults:
Acne vulgaris: Topical:
Gel, pledget, lotion, solution: Apply a thin film twice daily
Foam (Evoclin®): Apply once daily
Adults:
Amnionitis: I.V.: 450-900 mg every 8 hours
Anthrax: I.V.: 900 mg every 8 hours with ciprofloxacin or doxycycline
Babesiosis:
Oral: 600 mg 3 times/day for 7 days with quinine
I.V.: 1.2 g twice daily
Bacterial vaginosis: Intravaginal:
Suppositories: Insert one ovule (100 mg clindamycin) daily into vagina at bedtime for 3 days
Cream:
Cleocin®: One full applicator inserted intravaginally once daily before bedtime for 3 or 7 consecutive days in nonpregnant patients or for 7 consecutive days in pregnant patients
Clindesse™: One full applicator inserted intravaginally as a single dose at anytime during the day in nonpregnant patients
Bite wounds (canine): Oral: 300 mg 4 times/day with a fluoroquinolone
Gangrenous pyomyositis: I.V.: 900 mg every 8 hours with penicillin G
Group B streptococcus (neonatal prophylaxis): I.V.: 900 mg every 8 hours until delivery
Orofacial/parapharyngeal space infections:
Oral: 150-450 mg every 6 hours for 7 days, maximum 1.8 g/day
I.V.: 600-900 mg every 8 hours

Pelvic inflammatory disease: I.V.: 900 mg every 8 hours with gentamicin 2 mg/kg, then 1.5 mg/kg every 8 hours; continue after discharge with doxycycline 100 mg twice daily to complete 14 days of total therapy

Prophylaxis in total joint replacement patients undergoing dental procedures which produce bacteremia:
Oral: 600 mg 1 hour prior to procedure
I.V.: 600 mg 1 hour prior to procedure (for patients unable to take oral medication)

Toxic shock syndrome: I.V.: 900 mg every 8 hours with penicillin G or ceftriaxone

Dosage Forms
Capsule: 75 mg, 150 mg, 300 mg
Cleocin HCl®: 75 mg, 150 mg, 300 mg
Cream, vaginal:
Cleocin®: 2% (40 g)
ClindaMax®: 2% (40 g)
Clindesse™: 2% (5 g)
Foam, topical:
Evoclin®: 1% (50 g, 100 g)
Gel, topical: 1% (30 g, 60 g)
Cleocin T®: 1% (30 g, 60 g)
Clindagel®: 1% (40 mL, 75 mL)
ClindaMax®: 1% (30 g, 60 g)
Granules for oral solution:
Cleocin Pediatric®: 75 mg/5 mL
Infusion [premixed in D_5W]:
Cleocin Phosphate®: 300 mg (50 mL); 600 mg (50 mL); 900 mg (50 mg/mL]
Injection, solution: 150 mg/mL (2 mL, 4 mL, 6 mL, 60 mL)
Cleocin Phosphate®: 150 mg/mL (2 mL, 4 mL, 6 mL, 60 mL)
Lotion: 1% (60 mL)
Cleocin T®, ClindaMax®: 1% (60 mL)
Pledgets, topical: 1% (60s, 69s)
Cleocin T®: 1% (60s)
ClindaReach™: 1% (120s)
Solution, topical: 1% (30 mL, 60 mL)
Cleocin T®: 1% (30 mL, 60 mL)
Suppository, vaginal:
Cleocin® Vaginal Ovule: 100 mg (3s)

clindamycin and benzoyl peroxide (klin da MYE sin & BEN zoe il peer OKS ide)

Synonyms benzoyl peroxide and clindamycin; clindamycin phosphate and benzoyl peroxide
U.S./Canadian Brand Names BenzaClin® [US/Can]; Duac® CS [US]
Therapeutic Category Topical Skin Product; Topical Skin Product, Acne
Use Topical treatment of acne vulgaris
Usual Dosage Topical: Children ≥12 years and Adults: Apply to affected areas after skin has been cleansed and dried
BenzaClin®: Acne: Apply twice daily (morning and evening)
Duac® CS: Inflammatory acne: Apply once daily in the evening
Dosage Forms
Gel, topical:
BenzaClin®: Clindamycin 1% and benzoyl peroxide 5% (25 g, 50 g)
Duac® CS: Clindamycin 1% and benzoyl peroxide 5% (45 g)

clindamycin and tretinoin (klin da MYE sin & TRET i noyn)

Synonyms clindamycin phosphate and tretinoin; tretinoin and clindamycin
U.S./Canadian Brand Names Ziana™ [US]
Therapeutic Category Acne Products; Retinoic Acid Derivative; Topical Skin Product; Topical Skin Product, Acne
Use Treatment of acne vulgaris
Usual Dosage Topical: Children ≥12 years and Adults: Apply pea-size amount to entire face once daily at bedtime

▶

◀ **Dosage Forms**
 Gel, topical:
 Ziana™: Clindamycin phosphate 1.2% and tretinoin 0.025% (30 g, 60 g)

clindamycin hydrochloride see clindamycin on page 230
Clindamycin Injection, USP [Can] see clindamycin on page 230
clindamycin palmitate see clindamycin on page 230
clindamycin phosphate see clindamycin on page 230
clindamycin phosphate and benzoyl peroxide see clindamycin and benzoyl peroxide on page 231
clindamycin phosphate and tretinoin see clindamycin and tretinoin on page 231
ClindaReach™ [US] see clindamycin on page 230
Clindesse™ [US] see clindamycin on page 230
Clindets® (Discontinued) see clindamycin on page 230
Clindex® (Discontinued) see clidinium and chlordiazepoxide on page 229
Clindoxyl® [Can] see clindamycin on page 230
Clinoril® [US] see sulindac on page 898

clioquinol and flumethasone (Canada only) (klye ok KWIN ole & floo METH a sone)

Synonyms flumethasone and clioquinol; iodochlorhydroxyquin and flumethasone
U.S./Canadian Brand Names Locacorten® Vioform® [Can]
Therapeutic Category Antibiotic, Topical; Corticosteroid, Topical
Use Treatment of corticosteroid-responsive dermatoses complicated by infection with bacterial and/or fungal agents
Usual Dosage Children >2 years and Adults:
 Otic solution (drops): Instill 2-3 drops into affected ear(s) 2 times/day; generally limit duration to 10 days
 Topical: Apply in a thin layer to affected area 2-3 times/day; generally limit duration to 7 days
Dosage Forms [CAN] = Canadian brand name
 Cream, topical:
 Locacorten® Vioform® [CAN]: Clioquinol 3% and flumethasone 0.02% (15 g, 50 g) [not available in the U.S.]
 Solution, otic:
 Locacorten® Vioform® [CAN]: Clioquinol 1% and flumethasone 0.02% (10 mL) [not available in the U.S.]

Clobazam-10 [Can] see clobazam (Canada only) on page 232

clobazam (Canada only) (KLOE ba zam)

U.S./Canadian Brand Names Alti-Clobazam [Can]; Apo-Clobazam® [Can]; Clobazam-10 [Can]; Dom-Clobazam [Can]; Frisium® [Can]; Novo-Clobazam [Can]; PMS-Clobazam [Can]; ratio-Clobazam [Can]
Therapeutic Category Anticonvulsant; Antidepressant
Use Adjunctive treatment of epilepsy
Usual Dosage Oral:
 Children:
 <2 years: Initial 0.5-1 mg/kg/day
 2-16 years: Initial: 5 mg/day; may be increased (no more frequently than every 5 days) to a maximum of 40 mg/day
 Adults: Initial: 5-15 mg/day; dosage may be gradually adjusted (based on tolerance and seizure control) to a maximum of 80 mg/day
Note: Daily doses of up to 30 mg may be taken as a single dose at bedtime; higher doses should be divided.
Dosage Forms [CAN] = Canadian brand name
 Tablet: 10 mg [not available in the U.S.]
 Alti-Clobazam [CAN], Apo-Clobazam® [CAN], Clobazam-10 [CAN], Dom-Clobazam [CAN], Frisium® [CAN], Novo-Clobazam [CAN], PMS-Clobazam [CAN], ration-Clobazam [CAN]: 10 mg [not available in the U.S.]

clobetasol (kloe BAY ta sol)

Synonyms clobetasol propionate

U.S./Canadian Brand Names Clobex® [US/Can]; Cormax® [US]; Dermovate® [Can]; Gen-Clobetasol [Can]; Novo-Clobetasol [Can]; Olux-E™ [US]; Olux® [US]; Taro-Clobetasol [Can]; Temovate E® [US]; Temovate® [US]

Therapeutic Category Corticosteroid, Topical

Use Short-term relief of inflammation of moderate-to-severe corticosteroid-responsive dermatoses (very high potency topical corticosteroid)

Usual Dosage Topical: Discontinue when control achieved; if improvement not seen within 2 weeks, reassessment of diagnosis may be necessary.

Children ≥12 years and Adults:

Steroid-responsive dermatoses:

Cream, emollient cream, gel, ointment: Apply twice daily for up to 2 weeks (maximum dose: 50 g/week)

Foam (Olux-E™): Apply to affected area twice daily for up to 2 weeks (maximum dose: 50 g/week); do not apply to face or intertriginous areas

Steroid-responsive dermatoses: Foam (Olux®), solution: Apply to affected scalp twice daily for up to 2 weeks (maximum dose: 50 g/week or 50 mL/week)

Mild-to-moderate plaque-type psoriasis of nonscalp areas: Foam (Olux®): Apply to affected area twice daily for up to 2 weeks (maximum dose: 50 g/week); do not apply to face or intertriginous areas

Children ≥16 years and Adults: Moderate-to-severe plaque-type psoriasis: Emollient cream, lotion: Apply twice daily for up to 2 weeks, has been used for up to 4 weeks when application is <10% of body surface area; use with caution (maximum dose: 50 g/week)

Children ≥18 years and Adults:

Moderate-to-severe plaque-type psoriasis: Spray: Apply by spraying directly onto affected area twice daily; should be gently rubbed into skin. Should be used for not longer than 4 weeks; treatment beyond 2 weeks should be limited to localized lesions which have not improved sufficiently. Total dose should not exceed 50 g/week or 59 mL/week.

Scalp psoriasis: Shampoo: Apply thin film to dry scalp once daily; leave in place for 15 minutes, then add water, lather; rinse thoroughly

Steroid-responsive dermatoses: Lotion: Apply twice daily for up to 2 weeks (maximum dose: 50 g/week)

Dosage Forms

Aerosol, topical [foam]: 0.05% (50 g, 100 g)

Olux®, Olux-E™: 0.05% (50 g, 100 g)

Cream: 0.05% (15 g, 30 g, 45 g, 60 g)

Cormax®: 0.05% (15 g, 30 g, 45 g)

Temovate®: 0.05% (30 g, 60 g)

Cream [in emollient base]: 0.05% (15 g, 30 g, 60 g)

Temovate E®: 0.05% (60 g)

Gel: 0.05% (15 g, 30 g, 60 g)

Temovate®: 0.05% (60 g)

Lotion:

Clobex®: 0.05% (30 mL, 59 mL, 118 mL)

Ointment: 0.05% (15 g, 30 g, 45 g, 60 g)

Cormax®: 0.05% (15 g, 45 g)

Temovate®: 0.05% (15 g, 30 g)

Shampoo:

Clobex®: 0.05% (120 mL)

Solution, topical [for scalp application]: 0.05% (25 mL, 50 mL)

Cormax®: 0.05% (25 mL, 50 mL)

Temovate®: 0.05% (50 mL) [contains isopropyl alcohol 40%]

Solution, topical [spray]:

Clobex®: 0.05% (60 mL, 125 mL)

clobetasol propionate see clobetasol on page 232
Clobevate® (Discontinued) see clobetasol on page 232
Clobex® [US/Can] see clobetasol on page 232

clocortolone (kloe KOR toe lone)

Sound-Alike/Look-Alike Issues

Cloderm® may be confused with Clocort®

Synonyms clocortolone pivalate

U.S./Canadian Brand Names Cloderm® [US/Can]

Therapeutic Category Corticosteroid, Topical

◄ **Use** Inflammation of corticosteroid-responsive dermatoses (intermediate-potency topical corticosteroid)

Usual Dosage Adults: Apply sparingly and gently; rub into affected area from 1-4 times/day. Therapy should be discontinued when control is achieved; if no improvement is seen, reassessment of diagnosis may be necessary.

Dosage Forms

Cream:
Cloderm®: 0.1% (30 g, 45 g, 90 g)

clocortolone pivalate see clocortolone on page 233
Cloderm® [US/Can] see clocortolone on page 233

clodronate *(Canada only)* (KLOE droh nate)

Synonyms clodronate disodium

U.S./Canadian Brand Names Bonefos® [Can]; Clasteon® [Can]

Therapeutic Category Bisphosphonate Derivative

Use Management of hypercalcemia of malignancy; management of osteolysis due to bone metastases of malignancy

Usual Dosage Adults:
Clasteon®: Hypercalcemia of malignancy/osteolytic bone metastases:
I.V.:
Single infusion: 1500 mg as a single dose
Multiple infusions: 300 mg/day; should not be prolonged beyond 10 days
Oral: Recommended daily maintenance dose following I.V. therapy: Range: 1600 mg (4 capsules) to 2400 mg (6 capsules) given in a single or 2 divided doses; maximum recommended daily dose: 3200 mg (8 capsules). Should be taken at least 1 hour before or after food since food may decrease clodronate absorption.
Bonefos®:
Hypercalcemia of malignancy:
I.V.: Multiple infusions: 300 mg/day; should not be prolonged beyond 7 days
Oral: Recommended daily maintenance dose following I.V. therapy: Range: 1600 mg (4 capsules) to 2400 mg (6 capsules) given in single or 2 divided doses; maximum recommended daily dose: 3200 mg (8 capsules). Should be taken at least 2 hours before or after food since food may decrease clodronate absorption.
Osteolytic bone metastases:
I.V.: Multiple infusions: 300 mg/day; should not be prolonged beyond 7 days
Oral: Initial: 1600 mg/day; may be increased to a maximum of 3200 mg/day

Dosage Forms [CAN] = Canadian brand name

Injection:
Bonefos® [CAN]: 60 mg/mL (5 mL) [not available in the U.S.]
Clasteon® [CAN]: 30 mg/mL (10 mL) [not available in the U.S.]

Capsule:
Bonefos® [CAN], Clasteon® [CAN]: 400 mg [not available in the U.S.]

clodronate disodium see clodronate *(Canada only)* on page 234

clofarabine (klo FARE a been)

Synonyms Clofarex; NSC606869

U.S./Canadian Brand Names Clolar™ [US]

Therapeutic Category Antineoplastic Agent, Antimetabolite (Purine Antagonist)

Use Treatment of relapsed or refractory acute lymphoblastic leukemia

Usual Dosage I.V.: Children and Adults 1-21 years: ALL: 52 mg/m^2/day days 1 through 5; repeat every 2-6 weeks

Dosage Forms

Injection, solution [preservative free]:
Clolar™: 1 mg/mL (20 mL)

Clofarex see clofarabine on page 234
Clolar™ [US] see clofarabine on page 234
Clomid® [US/Can] see clomiphene on page 235

clomiphene (KLOE mi feen)

Sound-Alike/Look-Alike Issues
clomiPHENE may be confused with clomiPRAMINE, clonidine
Clomid® may be confused with clonidine
Serophene® may be confused with Sarafem®

Synonyms clomiphene citrate

Tall-Man clomiPHENE

U.S./Canadian Brand Names Clomid® [US/Can]; Milophene® [Can]; Serophene® [US/Can]

Therapeutic Category Ovulation Stimulator

Use Treatment of ovulatory failure in patients desiring pregnancy

Usual Dosage Oral: Adults: Ovulation induction: Females:
Initial course: 50 mg once daily for 5 days. Begin on or about the fifth day of cycle if progestin-induced bleeding is scheduled or spontaneous uterine bleeding occurs prior to therapy.
Dose adjustment: Subsequent doses may be increased to 100 mg once daily for 5 days only if ovulation does not occur at the initial dose. A low dose or duration of course is recommended in patients where unusual sensitivity to pituitary gonadotropin is suspected (eg, PCOS).
Repeat courses: If needed, the 5-day cycle may be repeated as early as 30 days after the previous one. Exclude the presence of pregnancy.
Maximum dose: 100 mg once daily for 5 days for 6 cycles. Discontinue if ovulation does not occur after 3 courses of treatment; or if 3 ovulatory responses occur but pregnancy is not achieved. Reevaluate if menses does not occur following ovulatory response. Doses larger than 150 mg have been reported, however, pregnancy rates are low.

Dosage Forms
Tablet [scored]: 50 mg
Clomid®, Serophene®: 50 mg

clomiphene citrate *see* clomiphene *on page 235*

clomipramine (kloe MI pra meen)

Sound-Alike/Look-Alike Issues
clomiPRAMINE may be confused with chlorproMAZINE, clomiPHENE, desipramine, Norpramin®
Anafranil® may be confused with alfentanil, enalapril, nafarelin

Synonyms clomipramine hydrochloride

Tall-Man clomiPRAMINE

U.S./Canadian Brand Names Anafranil® [US/Can]; Apo-Clomipramine® [Can]; CO Clomipramine [Can]; Gen-Clomipramine [Can]

Therapeutic Category Antidepressant, Tricyclic (Tertiary Amine)

Use Treatment of obsessive-compulsive disorder (OCD)

Usual Dosage Oral: OCD:
Children: ≥10 years:
Initial: 25 mg/day; may gradually increase as tolerated over the first 2 weeks to 3 mg/kg/day or 100 mg/day (whichever is less) in divided doses
Maintenance: May further increase to recommended maximum of 3 mg/kg/day or 200 mg/day (whichever is less); may give as a single daily dose at bedtime once tolerated
Adults:
Initial: 25 mg/day; may gradually increase as tolerated over the first 2 weeks to 100 mg/day in divided doses
Maintenance: May further increase to recommended maximum of 250 mg/day; may give as a single daily dose at bedtime once tolerated

Dosage Forms
Capsule: 25 mg, 50 mg, 75 mg
Anafranil®: 25 mg, 50 mg, 75 mg

clomipramine hydrochloride *see* clomipramine *on page 235*
Clonapam [Can] *see* clonazepam *on page 235*

clonazepam (kloe NA ze pam)

Sound-Alike/Look-Alike Issues
clonazePAM may be confused with clofazimine, cloNIDine, clorazepate, clozapine, LORazepam

▶

◄ Klonopin® may be confused with clofazimine, clonNIDine, clorazepate, clozapine, LORazepam

Tall-Man clonazePAM

U.S./Canadian Brand Names Alti-Clonazepam [Can]; Apo-Clonazepam® [Can]; Clonapam [Can]; CO Clonazepam [Can]; Gen-Clonazepam [Can]; Klonopin® Wafers [US]; Klonopin® [US/Can]; Novo-Clonazepam [Can]; Nu-Clonazepam [Can]; PMS-Clonazepam [Can]; Rho®-Clonazepam [Can]; Rivotril® [Can]; Sandoz-Clonazepam [Can]

Therapeutic Category Benzodiazepine

Controlled Substance C-IV

Use Alone or as an adjunct in the treatment of petit mal variant (Lennox-Gastaut), akinetic, and myoclonic seizures; petit mal (absence) seizures unresponsive to succimides; panic disorder with or without agoraphobia

Usual Dosage Oral:

Children <10 years or 30 kg: Seizure disorders:

Initial daily dose: 0.01-0.03 mg/kg/day (maximum: 0.05 mg/kg/day) given in 2-3 divided doses; increase by no more than 0.5 mg every third day until seizures are controlled or adverse effects seen

Usual maintenance dose: 0.1-0.2 mg/kg/day divided 3 times/day, not to exceed 0.2 mg/kg/day

Adults:

Burning mouth syndrome (dental use): 0.25-3 mg/day in 2 divided doses, in morning and evening

Seizure disorders:

Initial daily dose not to exceed 1.5 mg given in 3 divided doses; may increase by 0.5-1 mg every third day until seizures are controlled or adverse effects seen (maximum: 20 mg/day)

Usual maintenance dose: 0.05-0.2 mg/kg; do not exceed 20 mg/day

Panic disorder: 0.25 mg twice daily; increase in increments of 0.125-0.25 mg twice daily every 3 days; target dose: 1 mg/day (maximum: 4 mg/day)

Discontinuation of treatment: To discontinue, treatment should be withdrawn gradually. Decrease dose by 0.125 mg twice daily every 3 days until medication is completely withdrawn.

Dosage Forms

Tablet: 0.5 mg, 1 mg, 2 mg

Klonopin®: 0.5 mg, 1 mg, 2 mg

Tablet, orally disintegrating: 0.125 mg, 0.25 mg, 0.5 mg, 1 mg, 2 mg

Klonopin®: 0.125 mg, 0.25 mg, 0.5 mg, 1 mg, 2 mg

clonidine (KLON i deen)

Sound-Alike/Look-Alike Issues

cloNIDine may be confused with Clomid®, clomiPHENE, clonazePAM, clozapine, Klonopin®, quiNIDine

Catapres® may be confused with Cataflam®, Cetapred®, Combipres®

Synonyms clonidine hydrochloride

Tall-Man cloNIDine

U.S./Canadian Brand Names Apo-Clonidine® [Can]; Carapres® [Can]; Catapres-TTS® [US]; Catapres® [US]; Dixarit® [Can]; Duraclon® [US]; Novo-Clonidine [Can]; Nu-Clonidine [Can]

Therapeutic Category Alpha-Adrenergic Agonist

Use Management of mild-to-moderate hypertension; either used alone or in combination with other antihypertensives

Orphan drug: Duraclon®: For continuous epidural administration as adjunctive therapy with intraspinal opiates for treatment of cancer pain in patients tolerant to or unresponsive to intraspinal opiates

Usual Dosage

Children:

Oral:

Hypertension: Children ≥12 years: Initial: 0.2 mg/day in 2 divided doses; increase gradually at 5- to 7-day intervals; maximum: 2.4 mg/day

Clonidine tolerance test (test of growth hormone release from pituitary): 0.15 mg/m^2 or 4 mcg/kg as single dose

Epidural infusion: Pain management: Reserved for patients with severe intractable pain, unresponsive to other analgesics or epidural or spinal opiates: Initial: 0.5 mcg/kg/hour; adjust with caution, based on clinical effect

Adults:

Oral:

Acute hypertension (urgency): Initial 0.1-0.2 mg; may be followed by additional doses of 0.1 mg every hour, if necessary, to a maximum total dose of 0.6 mg

Hypertension: Initial dose: 0.1 mg twice daily (maximum recommended dose: 2.4 mg/day); usual dose range (JNC 7): 0.1-0.8 mg/day in 2 divided doses

Nicotine withdrawal symptoms: 0.1 mg twice daily to maximum of 0.4 mg/day for 3-4 weeks

Transdermal: Hypertension: Apply once every 7 days; for initial therapy start with 0.1 mg and increase by 0.1 mg at 1- to 2-week intervals (dosages >0.6 mg do not improve efficacy); usual dose range (JNC 7): 0.1-0.3 mg once weekly

Note: If transitioning from oral to transdermal therapy, overlap oral regimen for 1-2 days; transdermal route takes 2-3 days to achieve therapeutic effects.

Conversion from oral to transdermal:

Day 1: Place Catapres-TTS® 1; administer 100% of oral dose.

Day 2: Administer 50% of oral dose.

Day 3: Administer 25% of oral dose.

Day 4: Patch remains, no further oral supplement necessary.

Epidural infusion: Pain management: Starting dose: 30 mcg/hour; titrate as required for relief of pain or presence of side effects; minimal experience with doses >40 mcg/hour; should be considered an adjunct to intraspinal opiate therapy

Dosage Forms

Injection, solution [epidural; preservative free]:

Duraclon®: 100 mcg/mL (10 mL); 500 mcg/mL (10 mL)

Tablet: 0.1 mg, 0.2 mg, 0.3 mg

Catapres®: 0.1 mg, 0.2 mg, 0.3 mg

Transdermal system, topical [once-weekly patch]:

Catapres-TTS®-1: 0.1 mg/24 hours (4s)

Catapres-TTS®-2: 0.2 mg/24 hours (4s)

Catapres-TTS®-3: 0.3 mg/24 hours (4s)

clonidine and chlorthalidone (KLON i deen & klor THAL i done)

Sound-Alike/Look-Alike Issues

Combipres® may be confused with Catapres®

Synonyms chlorthalidone and clonidine

U.S./Canadian Brand Names Clorpres® [US]

Therapeutic Category Antihypertensive Agent, Combination

Use Management of mild-to-moderate hypertension

Usual Dosage Oral: 1 tablet 1-2 times/day; maximum: 0.6 mg clonidine and 30 mg chlorthalidone

Dosage Forms

Tablet:

Clorpres®: 0.1: Clonidine 0.1 mg and chlorthalidone 15 mg; 0.2: Clonidine 0.2 mg and chlorthalidone 15 mg; 0.3: Clonidine 0.3 mg and chlorthalidone 15 mg

clonidine hydrochloride *see* clonidine *on page 236*

clopidogrel (kloh PID oh grel)

Sound-Alike/Look-Alike Issues

Plavix® may be confused with Elavil®, Paxil®

Synonyms clopidogrel bisulfate

U.S./Canadian Brand Names Plavix® [US/Can]

Therapeutic Category Antiplatelet Agent

Use Reduces rate of atherothrombotic events (myocardial infarction, stroke, vascular deaths) in patients with recent MI or stroke, or established peripheral arterial disease; reduces rate of atherothrombotic events in patients with unstable angina or non-ST-segment elevation acute coronary syndromes (unstable angina and non-ST-segment elevation MI) managed medically or through percutaneous coronary intervention (PCI) (with or without stent) or CABG; reduces rate of death and atherothrombotic events in patients with ST-segment elevation MI (STEMI) managed medically

Usual Dosage Oral: Adults:

Recent MI, recent stroke, or established arterial disease: 75 mg once daily

Acute coronary syndrome:

Unstable angina, non-ST-segment elevation myocardial infarction (UA/NSTEMI): Initial: 300 mg loading dose, followed by 75 mg once daily (in combination with aspirin 75-325 mg once daily). **Note:** A loading dose of 600 mg has been used in some investigations; limited research exists comparing the two doses.

◄   ST-segment elevation myocardial infarction (STEMI): 75 mg once daily (in combination with aspirin 75-162 mg/day). CLARITY used a 300 mg loading dose of clopidogrel (with thrombolysis). The duration of therapy was <28 days (usually until hospital discharge).

Note: Drug-eluting stents: Duration of clopidogrel (in combination with aspirin): Ideally 12 months following drug-eluting stent placement in patients not at high risk for bleeding; at a minimum, 1, 3, and 6 months for bare metal, sirolimus, and paclitaxel stents, respectively, for uninterrupted therapy. Interruption of therapy may result in stent thrombosis with subsequent fatal and nonfatal myocardial infarction.

Dosage Forms
Tablet:
Plavix®: 75 mg, 300 mg

clopidogrel bisulfate *see* clopidogrel *on page 237*
Clopixol® [Can] *see* zuclopenthixol *(Canada only) on page 997*
Clopixol-Acuphase® [Can] *see* zuclopenthixol *(Canada only) on page 997*
Clopixol® Depot [Can] *see* zuclopenthixol *(Canada only) on page 997*

clorazepate (klor AZ e pate)

Sound-Alike/Look-Alike Issues
clorazepate may be confused with clofibrate, clonazepam
Synonyms clorazepate dipotassium
U.S./Canadian Brand Names Apo-Clorazepate® [Can]; Novo-Clopate [Can]; Tranxene® SD™ [US]; Tranxene® SD™-Half Strength [US]; Tranxene® T-Tab® [US]
Therapeutic Category Anticonvulsant; Benzodiazepine
Controlled Substance C-IV
Use Treatment of generalized anxiety disorder; management of ethanol withdrawal; adjunct anticonvulsant in management of partial seizures
Usual Dosage Oral:
Children 9-12 years: Anticonvulsant: Initial: 3.75-7.5 mg/dose twice daily; increase dose by 3.75 mg at weekly intervals, not to exceed 60 mg/day in 2-3 divided doses
Children >12 years and Adults: Anticonvulsant: Initial: Up to 7.5 mg/dose 2-3 times/day; increase dose by 7.5 mg at weekly intervals, not to exceed 90 mg/day
Adults:
Anxiety:
Regular release tablets (Tranxene® T-Tab®): 7.5-15 mg 2-4 times/day
Sustained release (Tranxene® SD™): 11.25 or 22.5 mg once daily at bedtime
Ethanol withdrawal: Initial: 30 mg, then 15 mg 2-4 times/day on first day; maximum daily dose: 90 mg; gradually decrease dose over subsequent days
Dosage Forms
Tablet: 3.75 mg, 7.5 mg, 15 mg
Tranxene® SD™: 22.5 mg
Tranxene® SD™-Half Strength: 11.25 mg
Tranxene® T-Tab®: 3.75 mg, 7.5 mg, 15 mg

clorazepate dipotassium *see* clorazepate *on page 238*
Clorpactin® WCS-90 [US-OTC] *see* oxychlorosene *on page 709*
Clorpres® [US] *see* clonidine and chlorthalidone *on page 237*
Clotrimaderm [Can] *see* clotrimazole *on page 238*

clotrimazole (kloe TRIM a zole)

Sound-Alike/Look-Alike Issues
clotrimazole may be confused with co-trimoxazole
Lotrimin® may be confused with Lotrisone®, Otrivin®
Mycelex® may be confused with Myoflex®
U.S./Canadian Brand Names Canesten® Topical [Can]; Canesten® Vaginal [Can]; Clotrimaderm [Can]; Cruex® Cream [US-OTC]; Gyne-Lotrimin® 3 [US-OTC]; Gyne-Lotrimin® 7 [US-OTC]; Lotrimin® AF Athlete's Foot Cream [US-OTC]; Lotrimin® AF for Her [US-OTC]; Lotrimin® AF Jock Itch Cream [US-OTC]; Mycelex® [US]; Trivagizole-3® [Can]
Therapeutic Category Antifungal Agent

Use Treatment of susceptible fungal infections, including oropharyngeal candidiasis, dermatophytoses, superficial mycoses, and cutaneous candidiasis, as well as vulvovaginal candidiasis; limited data suggest that clotrimazole troches may be effective for prophylaxis against oropharyngeal candidiasis in neutropenic patients

Usual Dosage
Children >3 years and Adults:
Oral:
Prophylaxis: 10 mg troche dissolved 3 times/day for the duration of chemotherapy or until steroids are reduced to maintenance levels
Treatment: 10 mg troche dissolved slowly 5 times/day for 14 consecutive days
Topical (cream, solution): Apply twice daily; if no improvement occurs after 4 weeks of therapy, reevaluate diagnosis
Children >12 years and Adults:
Vaginal:
Cream:
1%: Insert 1 applicatorful vaginal cream daily (preferably at bedtime) for 7 consecutive days
2%: Insert 1 applicatorful vaginal cream daily (preferably at bedtime) for 3 consecutive days
Tablet: Insert 100 mg/day for 7 days or 500 mg single dose
Topical (cream, solution): Apply to affected area twice daily (morning and evening) for 7 consecutive days

Dosage Forms
Cream, topical: 1% (15 g, 30 g, 45 g)
Cruex® [OTC]: 1% (15 g)
Lotrimin® AF Athlete's Foot [OTC]: 1% (12 g)
Lotrimin® AF Jock Itch [OTC]: 1% (12 g)
Lotrimin® AF for Her: 1% (24 g)
Cream, topical/vaginal: 1% (45 g)
Gyne-Lotrimin® 7 [OTC]: 1% (45 g)
Cream, vaginal: 2% (21 g)
Gyne-Lotrimin® 3 [OTC]: 2% (21 g)
Solution, topical: 1% (10 mL, 30 mL)
Troche, oral: 10 mg
Mycelex®: 10 mg

clotrimazole and betamethasone *see* betamethasone and clotrimazole *on page 131*
Cloxacillin [Can] *see* cloxacillin *(Canada only) on page 239*

cloxacillin *(Canada only)* (kloks a SIL in)

Synonyms cloxacillin sodium

U.S./Canadian Brand Names Apo-Cloxi® [Can]; Cloxacillin [Can]; Novo-Cloxin [Can]; Nu-Cloxi [Can]

Therapeutic Category Penicillin

Use Treatment of susceptible bacterial infections, including beta-hemolytic streptococci, pneumococci, and penicillinase-producing staphylococci causing respiratory tract, skin and skin structure, bone and joint, urinary tract infections

Usual Dosage Note: Dose and duration of therapy can vary depending on infecting organism, severity of infection, and clinical response of patient. Treat beta-hemolytic streptococcal infections at least 10 days to prevent the occurrence of rheumatic fever or acute glomerulonephritis. Treat severe staphylococcal infections for at least 14 days; endocarditis and osteomyelitis require an extended duration of therapy
Usual dosage range:
Oral:
Children ≤20 kg: 25-50 mg/kg/day in divided doses every 6 hours
Children >20 kg and Adults: 250-500 mg every 6 hours (manufacturer recommended maximum adult dose: 6 g/day)
I.M., I.V.:
Children ≤20 kg: 25-50 mg/kg/day in divided doses every 6 hours; up to 200 mg/kg/day has been used in some studies for severe infections
Children >20 kg and Adults: 250-500 mg every 6 hours (manufacturer recommended maximum adult dose: 6 g/day)

Dosage Forms
Capsule: 250 mg, 500 mg [not available in the U.S.]
Injection, powder for reconstitution: 50 mg, 500 mg, 1000 mg, 2000 mg [not available in the U.S.]
Powder for suspension, oral: 125 mg/5 mL [not available in the U.S.]

cloxacillin sodium *see* cloxacillin *(Canada only) on page 239*

Cloxapen® *(Discontinued) see* cloxacillin *(Canada only) on page 239*

clozapine (KLOE za peen)

Sound-Alike/Look-Alike Issues
clozapine may be confused with clofazimine, clonidine, Klonopin®
Clozaril® may be confused with Clinoril®, Colazal®

U.S./Canadian Brand Names Apo-Clozapine® [Can]; Clozaril® [US/Can]; FazaClo® [US]; Gen-Clozapine [Can]

Therapeutic Category Antipsychotic Agent, Dibenzodiazepine

Use Treatment-refractory schizophrenia; to reduce risk of recurrent suicidal behavior in schizophrenia or schizoaffective disorder

Usual Dosage Oral: Adults:
Schizophrenia: Initial: 12.5 mg once or twice daily; increased, as tolerated, in increments of 25-50 mg/day to a target dose of 300-450 mg/day after 2-4 weeks, may require doses as high as 600-900 mg/day

Reduce risk of suicidal behavior: Initial: 12.5 mg once or twice daily; increased, as tolerated, in increments of 25-50 mg/day to a target dose of 300-450 mg/day after 2-4 weeks; median dose is ~300 mg/day (range: 12.5-900 mg)

Termination of therapy: If dosing is interrupted for ≥48 hours, therapy must be reinitiated at 12.5-25 mg/day; may be increased more rapidly than with initial titration, unless cardiopulmonary arrest occurred during initial titration.

In the event of planned termination of clozapine, gradual reduction in dose over a 1- to 2-week period is recommended. If conditions warrant abrupt discontinuation (leukopenia), monitor patient for psychosis and cholinergic rebound (headache, nausea, vomiting, diarrhea).

Patients discontinued on clozapine therapy due to WBC <2000/mm^3 or ANC <1000/mm^3 should not be restarted on clozapine.

Dosage Forms
Tablet: 25 mg, 50 mg, 100 mg, 200 mg
Clozaril®: 25 mg [scored], 100 mg [scored]
Tablet, orally disintegrating:
FazaClo®: 12.5 mg, 25 mg, 100 mg

Clozaril® [US/Can] *see* clozapine *on page 240*

Clysodrast® *(Discontinued) see* bisacodyl *on page 136*

CMA-676 *see* gemtuzumab ozogamicin *on page 439*

CMV-IGIV *see* cytomegalovirus immune globulin (intravenous-human) *on page 262*

CNJ-016™ [US] *see* vaccinia immune globulin (intravenous) *on page 966*

CoActifed® [Can] *see* triprolidine, pseudoephedrine, and codeine *(Canada only) on page 955*

coagulant complex inhibitor *see* antiinhibitor coagulant complex *on page 81*

coagulation factor VIIa *see* factor VIIa (recombinant) *on page 387*

CO Alendronate [Can] *see* alendronate *on page 43*

coal tar (KOLE tar)

Synonyms crude coal tar; LCD; pix carbonis

U.S./Canadian Brand Names Balnetar® [US-OTC/Can]; Betatar® Gel [US-OTC]; Cutar® [US-OTC]; Denorex® Original Therapeutic Strength [US-OTC]; DHS™ Tar [US-OTC]; DHS™ Targel [US-OTC]; Doak® Tar [US-OTC]; Estar® [Can]; Exorex® [US]; Fototar® [US-OTC]; MG 217® Medicated Tar [US-OTC]; MG 217® [US-OTC]; Neutrogena® T/Gel Extra Strength [US-OTC]; Neutrogena® T/Gel Stubborn Itch Control [US-OTC]; Neutrogena® T/Gel [US-OTC]; Oxipor® VHC [US-OTC]; Reme-T™ [US-OTC]; Targel® [Can]; Tera-Gel™ [US-OTC]; Zetar® [US-OTC]

Therapeutic Category Antipsoriatic Agent; Antiseborrheic Agent, Topical

Use Topically for controlling dandruff, seborrheic dermatitis, or psoriasis

Usual Dosage Topical:
Bath: Add appropriate amount to bath water; for adults usually 60-90 mL of a 5% to 20% solution or 15-25 mL of 30% lotion; soak 5-20 minutes, then pat dry; use once daily to 3 days

Shampoo: Rub shampoo onto wet hair and scalp, rinse thoroughly; repeat; leave on 5 minutes; rinse thoroughly; apply twice weekly for the first 2 weeks then once weekly or more often if needed

Soap: Use on affected areas in place of regular soap. Work into a lather using warm water; massage into skin; rinse.

Skin: Apply to the affected area 1-4 times/day; decrease frequency to 2-3 times/week once condition has been controlled

Scalp psoriasis: Tar oil bath or coal tar solution may be painted sparingly to the lesions 3-12 hours before each shampoo

Psoriasis of the body, arms, legs: Apply at bedtime; if thick scales are present, use product with salicylic acid and apply several times during the day

Dosage Forms
Cream:
  Fototar®: Coal tar 2% (85 g, 454 g)
Emulsion, topical:
  Cutar® [OTC]: Coal tar solution 7.5% (180 mL, 3840 mL)
  Exorex®: Coal tar 1% (240 mL)
Gel, shampoo:
  DHS™ Targel [OTC]: Coal tar solution 2.9% (240 mL)
Liquid:
  Doak® Tar Distillate: Coal tar 40% (60 mL)
Lotion, topical:
  Doak® Tar [OTC]: Coal tar distillate 5% (240 mL)
  Exorex®: Coal tar 1% (240 mL)
  MG 217® [OTC]: Coal tar solution 5% (120 mL)
  Oxipor® VHC [OTC]: Coal tar solution 25% (60 mL, 120 mL)
Oil, topical:
  Balnetar®: Coal tar 2.5% (225 mL) [for use in bath]
  Doak® Tar [OTC]: Coal tar distillate 2% (240 mL)
Ointment, topical:
  MG 217® [OTC]: Coal tar solution 10% (107 g, 430 g)
Shampoo, topical:
  Betatar Gel® [OTC]: Coal tar solution 5% (240 mL)
  Denorex® Original Therapeutic Strength [OTC]: Coal tar solution 12.5% (120 mL, 240 mL, 360 mL)
  DHS™ Tar [OTC]: Coal tar solution 2.9% (120 mL, 240 mL, 480 mL)
  Doak® Tar [OTC]: Coal tar distillate 3% (240 mL)
  MG 217® Medicated Tar [OTC]: Coal tar solution 15% (120 mL, 240 mL)
  Neutrogena® T/Gel [OTC]: Coal tar 0.5% (132 mL, 480 mL)
  Neutrogena® T/Gel Extra Strength [OTC]: Coal tar extract 4% (132 mL)
  Neutrogena® T/Gel Stubborn Itch Control [OTC]: Coal tar extract 2% (132 mL)
  Reme-T™ [OTC]: Coal tar 5% (236 mL)
  Tera-Gel™ [OTC]: Solubilized coal tar 0.5% (120 mL, 240 mL)
  Zetar® [OTC]: Coal tar 1% (180 mL)

coal tar and salicylic acid (KOLE tar & sal i SIL ik AS id)

Synonyms salicylic acid and coal tar

U.S./Canadian Brand Names Sebcur/T® [Can]; Tarsum® [US-OTC]; X-Seb T® Pearl [US-OTC]; X-Seb T® Plus [US-OTC]

Therapeutic Category Antipsoriatic Agent; Antiseborrheic Agent, Topical

Use Seborrheal dermatitis, dandruff, psoriasis

Usual Dosage Psoriasis: Scalp:
  Gel: Apply directly to plaques; may leave in place for up to 1 hour. Apply water and work into a lather; rinse.
  Shampoo: Apply to wet hair; massage into scalp; rinse.

Dosage Forms
  Gel [shampoo]: Coal tar solution 10% [equivalent to coal tar 2%] and salicylic acid (120 mL, 240 mL)
    Tarsum® [OTC]: Coal tar solution 10% [equivalent to coal tar 2%] and salicylic acid (120 mL, 240 mL)
  Shampoo, topical: Coal tar solution 10% [equivalent to coal tar 2%] and salicylic acid (120 mL, 240 mL)
    X-Seb T® Pearl [OTC], X-Seb T® Plus [OTC]: Coal tar solution 10% [equivalent to coal tar 2%] and salicylic acid (120 mL, 240 mL)

CO Azithromycin [Can] *see azithromycin on page 110*
Cobex® (Discontinued) *see cyanocobalamin on page 254*
CO Bicalutamide [Can] *see bicalutamide on page 135*

CO Buspirone [Can] *see* buspirone *on page 153*
CO Cabergoline [Can] *see* cabergoline *on page 158*

cocaine (koe KANE)

Synonyms cocaine hydrochloride
Therapeutic Category Local Anesthetic
Controlled Substance C-II
Use Topical anesthesia for mucous membranes
Usual Dosage Topical application (ear, nose, throat, bronchoscopy): Dosage depends on the area to be anesthetized, tissue vascularity, technique of anesthesia, and individual patient tolerance; the lowest dose necessary to produce adequate anesthesia should be used; concentrations of 1% to 10% are used (not to exceed 1 mg/kg). Use reduced dosages for children, elderly, or debilitated patients.
Dosage Forms
  Powder, for prescription compounding: 1 g, 5 g, 25 g
  Solution, topical: 4% (4 mL, 10 mL)

cocaine hydrochloride *see* cocaine *on page 242*
CO Cilazapril [Can] *see* cilazapril *(Canada only) on page 219*
CO Ciprofloxacin [Can] *see* ciprofloxacin *on page 221*
CO Citalopram [Can] *see* citalopram *on page 225*
CO Clomipramine [Can] *see* clomipramine *on page 235*
CO Clonazepam [Can] *see* clonazepam *on page 235*
Codal-DM [US-OTC] *see* phenylephrine, pyrilamine, and dextromethorphan *on page 749*
Codamine® *(Discontinued)*
Codamine® Pediatric *(Discontinued)*
Codehist® DH *(Discontinued)* *see* chlorpheniramine, pseudoephedrine, and codeine *on page 212*

codeine (KOE deen)

Sound-Alike/Look-Alike Issues
  codeine may be confused with Cardene®, Cophene®, Cordran®, iodine, Lodine®
Synonyms codeine phosphate; codeine sulfate; methylmorphine
U.S./Canadian Brand Names Codeine Contin® [Can]
Therapeutic Category Analgesic, Narcotic; Antitussive
Controlled Substance C-II
Use Treatment of mild-to-moderate pain; antitussive in lower doses; dextromethorphan has equivalent antitussive activity but has much lower toxicity in accidental overdose
Usual Dosage Note: These are guidelines and do not represent the maximum doses that may be required in all patients. Doses should be titrated to pain relief/prevention. Doses >1.5 mg/kg body weight are not recommended.
Analgesic:
  Children: Oral, I.M., SubQ: 0.5-1 mg/kg/dose every 4-6 hours as needed; maximum: 60 mg/dose
  Adults:
    Oral: 30 mg every 4-6 hours as needed; patients with prior opiate exposure may require higher initial doses. Usual range: 15-120 mg every 4-6 hours as needed
    Oral, controlled release formulation (Codeine Contin®, not available in U.S.): 50-300 mg every 12 hours. **Note:** A patient's codeine requirement should be established using prompt release formulations; conversion to long-acting products may be considered when chronic, continuous treatment is required. Higher dosages should be reserved for use only in opioid-tolerant patients.
    I.M., SubQ: 30 mg every 4-6 hours as needed; patients with prior opiate exposure may require higher initial doses. Usual range: 15-120 mg every 4-6 hours as needed; more frequent dosing may be needed
Antitussive: Oral (for nonproductive cough):
  Children: 1-1.5 mg/kg/day in divided doses every 4-6 hours as needed: Alternative dose according to age:
    2-6 years: 2.5-5 mg every 4-6 hours as needed; maximum: 30 mg/day
    6-12 years: 5-10 mg every 4-6 hours as needed; maximum: 60 mg/day
  Adults: 10-20 mg/dose every 4-6 hours as needed; maximum: 120 mg/day

Dosage Forms [CAN] = Canadian brand name
Injection: 15 mg/mL (2 mL); 30 mg/mL (2 mL)
Powder, for prescription compounding: 10 g, 25 g
Tablet: 15 mg, 30 mg, 60 mg
Tablet, controlled release: 50 mg, 100 mg, 150 mg, 200 mg
  Codeine Contin® [CAN]: 50 mg, 100 mg, 150 mg, 200 mg [not available in the U.S.]

codeine, acetaminophen, butalbital, and caffeine *see* butalbital, acetaminophen, caffeine, and codeine *on page 155*

codeine and acetaminophen *see* acetaminophen and codeine *on page 20*

codeine and butalbital compound *see* butalbital, aspirin, caffeine, and codeine *on page 156*

codeine and guaifenesin *see* guaifenesin and codeine *on page 454*

codeine and promethazine *see* promethazine and codeine *on page 791*

codeine, aspirin, and carisoprodol *see* carisoprodol, aspirin, and codeine *on page 180*

codeine, butalbital, aspirin, and caffeine *see* butalbital, aspirin, caffeine, and codeine *on page 156*

codeine, chlorpheniramine, and pseudoephedrine *see* chlorpheniramine, pseudoephedrine, and codeine *on page 212*

codeine, chlorpheniramine, phenylephrine, and potassium iodide *see* chlorpheniramine, phenylephrine, codeine, and potassium iodide *on page 212*

Codeine Contin® [Can] *see* codeine *on page 242*

codeine, doxylamine, and acetaminophen *see* acetaminophen, codeine, and doxylamine *(Canada only) on page 26*

codeine, guaifenesin, and pseudoephedrine *see* guaifenesin, pseudoephedrine, and codeine *on page 460*

codeine phosphate *see* codeine *on page 242*

codeine, promethazine, and phenylephrine *see* promethazine, phenylephrine, and codeine *on page 792*

codeine, pseudoephedrine, and triprolidine *see* triprolidine, pseudoephedrine, and codeine *(Canada only) on page 955*

codeine sulfate *see* codeine *on page 242*

codeine, triprolidine, and pseudoephedrine *see* triprolidine, pseudoephedrine, and codeine *(Canada only) on page 955*

Codiclear® DH *(Discontinued)*

codimal® DM [US-OTC] *see* phenylephrine, pyrilamine, and dextromethorphan *on page 749*

Codituss DM [US-OTC] *see* phenylephrine, pyrilamine, and dextromethorphan *on page 749*

cod liver oil *see* vitamin A and vitamin D *on page 980*

CO Enalapril [Can] *see* enalapril *on page 339*

Co-Fluconazole [Can] *see* fluconazole *on page 405*

CO Fluoxetine [Can] *see* fluoxetine *on page 413*

Cogentin® [US] *see* benztropine *on page 128*

Co-Gesic® [US] *see* hydrocodone and acetaminophen *on page 481*

CO Glimepiride [Can] *see* glimepiride *on page 445*

Cognex® [US] *see* tacrine *on page 901*

CO Ipra-Sal [Can] *see* ipratropium and albuterol *on page 525*

Colace® [US-OTC/Can] *see* docusate *on page 314*

Colace® Adult/Children Suppositories [US-OTC] *see* glycerin *on page 449*

Colace® Infant/Children Suppositories [US-OTC] *see* glycerin *on page 449*

Colax-C® [Can] *see* docusate *on page 314*

Colazal® [US] *see* balsalazide *on page 116*

ColBenemid® *(Discontinued) see* colchicine and probenecid *on page 244*

colchicine (KOL chi seen)

Sound-Alike/Look-Alike Issues
  colchicine may be confused with Cortrosyn®
Therapeutic Category Antigout Agent

▶

◄ **Use** Treatment of acute gouty arthritis attacks and prevention of recurrences of such attacks

Usual Dosage
Gouty arthritis: Adults:
Prophylaxis of acute attacks: Oral: 0.6 mg twice daily; initial and/or subsequent dosage may be decreased (ie, 0.6 mg once daily) in patients at risk of toxicity or in those who are intolerant (including weakness, loose stools, or diarrhea); range: 0.6 mg every other day to 0.6 mg 3 times/day
Acute attacks:
Oral: Initial: 0.6-1.2 mg, followed by 0.6 every 1-2 hours; some clinicians recommend a maximum of 3 doses; more aggressive approaches have recommended a maximum dose of up to 6 mg. Wait at least 3 days before initiating another course of therapy
I.V.: Initial: 1-2 mg, then 0.5 mg every 6 hours until response, not to exceed total dose of 4 mg. If pain recurs, it may be necessary to administer additional daily doses. The amount of colchicine administered intravenously in an acute treatment period (generally ~1 week) should not exceed a total dose of 4 mg. Do not administer more colchicine by any route for at least 7 days after a full course of I.V. therapy.
Note: Many experts would avoid use because of potential for serious, life-threatening complications. Should not be administered to patients with renal insufficiency, hepatobiliary obstruction, patients >70 years of age, or recent oral colchicine use. Should be reserved for hospitalized patients who are under the care of a physician experienced in the use of intravenous colchicine.
Surgery: Gouty arthritis, prophylaxis of recurrent attacks: Adults: Oral: 0.6 mg/day or every other day; patients who are to undergo surgical procedures may receive 0.6 mg 3 times/day for 3 days before and 3 days after surgery

Dosage Forms
Injection, solution: 0.5 mg/mL (2 mL)
Tablet: 0.6 mg

colchicine and probenecid (KOL chi seen & proe BEN e sid)

Synonyms probenecid and colchicine
Therapeutic Category Antigout Agent
Use Treatment of chronic gouty arthritis when complicated by frequent, recurrent acute attacks of gout
Usual Dosage Oral: Adults: 1 tablet daily for 1 week, then 1 tablet twice daily thereafter
Dosage Forms
Tablet: Colchicine 0.5 mg and probenecid 0.5 g

Coldamine [US] *see* chlorpheniramine, pseudoephedrine, and methscopolamine *on page 213*
Coldcough [US] *see* pseudoephedrine, dihydrocodeine, and chlorpheniramine *on page 803*
Coldcough HC *(Discontinued)*
Coldcough PD [US] *see* dihydrocodeine, chlorpheniramine, and phenylephrine *on page 298*
Coldlac-LA® *(Discontinued)*
Coldloc® *(Discontinued)*
Coldmist DM *(Discontinued) see* guaifenesin, pseudoephedrine, and dextromethorphan *on page 460*
Coldtuss DR *(Discontinued) see* chlorpheniramine, phenylephrine, and dextromethorphan *on page 209*

colesevelam (koh le SEV a lam)

U.S./Canadian Brand Names WelChol® [US/Can]
Therapeutic Category Antihyperlipidemic Agent, Miscellaneous; Bile Acid Sequestrant
Use Management of elevated LDL in primary hypercholesterolemia (Fredrickson type IIa) when used alone or in combination with an HMG-CoA reductase inhibitor; improve control of type 2 diabetes mellitus (noninsulin dependent, NIDDM) in conjunction with insulin or oral antidiabetic agents
Usual Dosage Oral: Adults: 3 tablets twice daily with meals or 6 tablets once daily with a meal
Dosage Forms
Tablet:
WelChol®: 625 mg

Colestid® [US/Can] *see* colestipol *on page 244*

colestipol (koe LES ti pole)

Synonyms colestipol hydrochloride
U.S./Canadian Brand Names Colestid® [US/Can]

Therapeutic Category Antihyperlipidemic Agent, Miscellaneous

Use Adjunct in management of primary hypercholesterolemia; regression of arteriolosclerosis; relief of pruritus associated with elevated levels of bile acids; possibly used to decrease plasma half-life of digoxin in toxicity

Usual Dosage Oral: Adults:

Granules: 5-30 g/day given once or in divided doses 2-4 times/day; initial dose: 5 g 1-2 times/day; increase by 5 g at 1- to 2-month intervals

Tablets: 2-16 g/day; initial dose: 2 g 1-2 times/day; increase by 2 g at 1- to 2-month intervals

Dosage Forms

Granules for suspension, oral: 5 g/packet (30s, 90s); 5 g/scoopful (500 g)

Colestid®: 5 g/packet (30s, 90s); 5 g/teaspoon (300 g, 500 g)

Colestid®, flavored: 5 g/packet (60s)

Colestid®, flavored: 5 g/scoopful (450 g)

Tablet: 1 g

Tablet, oral [micronized]:

Colestid®: 1 g

colestipol hydrochloride *see* colestipol *on page 244*
CO Levetiracetam [Can] *see* levetiracetam *on page 554*
CO Lisinopril [Can] *see* lisinopril *on page 570*

colistimethate (koe lis ti METH ate)

Synonyms colistimethate sodium; colistin methanesulfonate; colistin sulfomethate; pentasodium colistin methanesulfonate

U.S./Canadian Brand Names Coly-Mycin® M [US/Can]

Therapeutic Category Antibiotic, Miscellaneous

Use Treatment of infections due to sensitive strains of certain gram-negative bacilli which are resistant to other antibacterials or in patients allergic to other antibacterials

Usual Dosage Note: Doses should be based on ideal body weight in obese patients; dosage expressed in terms of colistin.

I.M., I.V.: Children and Adults: Susceptible infections: 2.5-5 mg/kg/day in 2-4 divided doses

Dosage Forms

Injection, powder for reconstitution, as colistin base: 150 mg

Coly-Mycin® M: 150 mg

colistimethate sodium *see* colistimethate *on page 245*
colistin methanesulfonate *see* colistimethate *on page 245*
colistin, neomycin, hydrocortisone, and thonzonium *see* neomycin, colistin, hydrocortisone, and thonzonium *on page 662*
colistin sulfomethate *see* colistimethate *on page 245*
collagen *see* collagen hemostat *on page 245*
collagen absorbable hemostat *see* collagen hemostat *on page 245*

collagenase (KOL la je nase)

U.S./Canadian Brand Names Santyl® [US]

Therapeutic Category Enzyme

Use Promotes debridement of necrotic tissue in dermal ulcers and severe burns

Orphan drug: Injection: Treatment of Peyronie disease; treatment of Dupuytren disease

Usual Dosage Topical: Apply once daily (or more frequently if the dressing becomes soiled)

Dosage Forms

Ointment:

Santyl®: 250 units/g (15 g, 30 g)

collagen hemostat (KOL la jen HEE moe stat)

Sound-Alike/Look-Alike Issues

Avitene® may be confused with Ativan®

Synonyms collagen; collagen absorbable hemostat; MCH; microfibrillar collagen hemostat

◀ **U.S./Canadian Brand Names** Avitene® Flour [US]; Avitene® Ultrafoam [US]; Avitene® UltraWrap™ [US]; Avitene® [US]; EndoAvitene® [US]; Helistat® [US]; Helitene® [US]; Instat™ MCH [US]; Instat™ [US]; SyringeAvitene™ [US]

Therapeutic Category Hemostatic Agent

Use Adjunct to hemostasis when control of bleeding by ligature is ineffective or impractical

Usual Dosage Apply dry directly to source of bleeding; remove excess material after ~10-15 minutes

Dosage Forms

Pad:
Instat™: 1 inch x 2 inch (24s); 3 inch x 4 inch (24s)

Powder:
Avitene® Flour [microfibrillar product]: 0.5 g, 1 g, 5 g
Helitene®: 0.5 g, 1 g
Instat™ MCH [microfibrillar product]: 0.5 g, 1 g
SyringeAvitene™ [microfibrillar product, prefilled syringe]: 1 g

Sheet:
Avitene® [microfibrillar product, nonwoven web]: 35 mm x 35 mm (1s); 70 mm x 35 mm (6s, 12s); 70 mm x 70 mm (6s, 12s)
EndoAvitene® [microfibrillar product, preloaded applicator]: 5 mm diameter (6s); 10 mm diameter (6s)

Sponge:
Avitene® Ultrafoam [microfibrillar product]: 2 cm x 6.25 cm x 7 mm (12s); 8 cm x 6.25 cm x 1 cm (6s); 8 cm x 12.5 cm x 1 cm (6s); 8 cm x 12.5 cm x 3 mm (6s)
Avitene® UltraWrap™ [microfibrillar product]: 8 cm x 12.5 cm (6s)
Helistat®: 0.5 inch x 1 inch x 7 mm (18s); 3 inch x 4 inch x 5 inch (10s)

Colocort® [US] *see* hydrocortisone (rectal) *on page 484*

CO Lovastatin [Can] *see* lovastatin *on page 579*

Coly-Mycin® M [US/Can] *see* colistimethate *on page 245*

Coly-Mycin® S [US] *see* neomycin, colistin, hydrocortisone, and thonzonium *on page 662*

Colyte® [US/Can] *see* polyethylene glycol-electrolyte solution *on page 766*

Combantrin™ [Can] *see* pyrantel pamoate *on page 806*

ComBgen™ [US] *see* folic acid, cyanocobalamin, and pyridoxine *on page 422*

Combigan™ [US/Can] *see* brimonidine and timolol *on page 142*

CombiPatch® [US] *see* estradiol and norethindrone *on page 362*

Combipres® (Discontinued) *see* clonidine and chlorthalidone *on page 237*

Combivent® [US/Can] *see* ipratropium and albuterol *on page 525*

Combivir® [US/Can] *see* zidovudine and lamivudine *on page 992*

Combunox™ [US] *see* oxycodone and ibuprofen *on page 711*

CO Meloxicam [Can] *see* meloxicam *on page 599*

Comfort® Ophthalmic (Discontinued) *see* naphazoline *on page 655*

Comfort® Tears Solution (Discontinued) *see* artificial tears *on page 95*

Comhist® (Discontinued) *see* chlorpheniramine, phenylephrine, and phenyltoloxamine *on page 211*

CO Mirtazapine [Can] *see* mirtazapine *on page 637*

Commit® [US-OTC] *see* nicotine *on page 670*

Compazine® [Can] *see* prochlorperazine *on page 788*

Compazine® (Discontinued) *see* prochlorperazine *on page 788*

Compound 347™ [US] *see* enflurane *on page 340*

compound E *see* cortisone acetate *on page 249*

compound F *see* hydrocortisone (systemic) *on page 484*

compound S *see* zidovudine *on page 991*

compound S, abacavir, and lamivudine *see* abacavir, lamivudine, and zidovudine *on page 16*

Compound W® [US-OTC] *see* salicylic acid *on page 850*

Compound W® One-Step Wart Remover [US-OTC] *see* salicylic acid *on page 850*

Compound W® One-Step Wart Remover for Feet [US-OTC] *see* salicylic acid *on page 850*

Compound W® One-Step Wart Remover for Kids [US-OTC] *see* salicylic acid *on page 850*

Compoz® Nighttime Sleep Aid [US-OTC] *see* diphenhydramine *on page 304*

Compro™ [US] *see* prochlorperazine *on page 788*

Comtan® [US/Can] *see* entacapone *on page 342*

Comtrex® Flu Therapy Nighttime [US-OTC] *see* acetaminophen, chlorpheniramine, and pseudoephedrine *on page 25*

Comtrex® Maximum Strength Sinus and Nasal Decongestant *(Discontinued)* *see* acetaminophen, chlorpheniramine, and pseudoephedrine *on page 25*

Comtrex® Non-Drowsy Cold and Cough Relief *(Discontinued)* *see* acetaminophen, dextromethorphan, and pseudoephedrine *on page 27*

Comtrex® Sore Throat Maximum Strength [US-OTC] *see* acetaminophen *on page 19*

Comvax® [US] *see Haemophilus* B conjugate and hepatitis B vaccine *on page 463*

Conceptrol® [US-OTC] *see* nonoxynol 9 *on page 677*

Concerta® [US/Can] *see* methylphenidate *on page 622*

Condyline™ [Can] *see* podofilox *on page 763*

Condylox® [US] *see* podofilox *on page 763*

Conex® *(Discontinued)*

Congess® Jr *(Discontinued)* *see* guaifenesin and pseudoephedrine *on page 458*

Congess® Sr *(Discontinued)* *see* guaifenesin and pseudoephedrine *on page 458*

Congestac® [US-OTC] *see* guaifenesin and pseudoephedrine *on page 458*

conivaptan (koe NYE vap tan)

Synonyms conivaptan hydrochloride; YM087

U.S./Canadian Brand Names Vaprisol® [US]

Therapeutic Category Vasopressin Antagonist

Use Treatment of euvolemic and hypervolemic hyponatremia in hospitalized patients

Usual Dosage I.V.: Adults:
Loading dose: 20 mg infused over 30 minutes, followed by continuous infusion of 20 mg over 24 hours
Maintenance: 20 mg/day as continuous infusion over 24 hours; may titrate to maximum of 40 mg/day if serum sodium not rising sufficiently; total duration of therapy not to exceed 4 days

Dosage Forms
Injection, solution:
Vaprisol®: 5 mg/mL (4 mL)

conivaptan hydrochloride *see* conivaptan *on page 247*

conjugated estrogen and methyltestosterone *see* estrogens (esterified) and methyltestosterone *on page 366*

CO Norfloxacin [Can] *see* norfloxacin *on page 679*

Conray® [US] *see* iothalamate meglumine *on page 522*

Conray® 30 [US] *see* iothalamate meglumine *on page 522*

Conray® 43 [US] *see* iothalamate meglumine *on page 522*

Conray® 400 [US] *see* iothalamate sodium *on page 523*

Constulose [US] *see* lactulose *on page 544*

Contac® Cold 12 Hour Relief Non Drowsy [Can] *see* pseudoephedrine *on page 801*

Contac® Cold 12 Hour Relief Non Drowsy *(Discontinued)* *see* pseudoephedrine *on page 801*

Contac® Cold and Sore Throat, Non Drowsy, Extra Strength [Can] *see* acetaminophen and pseudoephedrine *on page 23*

Contac® Cold-Chest Congestion, Non Drowsy, Regular Strength [Can] *see* guaifenesin and pseudoephedrine *on page 458*

Contac® Cold *(Discontinued)* *see* pseudoephedrine *on page 801*

Contac® Cold + Flu Maximum Strength Non-Drowsy [US-OTC] *see* acetaminophen and phenylephrine *on page 22*

Contac® Complete [Can] *see* acetaminophen, dextromethorphan, and pseudoephedrine *on page 27*

Contac® Cough, Cold and Flu Day & Night™ [Can] *see* acetaminophen, dextromethorphan, and pseudoephedrine *on page 27*

Contac® Cough Formula Liquid *(Discontinued)* *see* guaifenesin and dextromethorphan *on page 454*

continuous renal replacement therapy *see* electrolyte solution, renal replacement *on page 336*

ControlRx® [US] *see* fluoride *on page 411*

Contuss® *(Discontinued)*

Contuss® XT *(Discontinued)*

CO Paroxetine [Can] *see* paroxetine *on page 724*

Copaxone® [US/Can] *see* glatiramer acetate *on page 444*

COPD [US] *see* dyphylline and guaifenesin *on page 330*

Copegus® [US] *see* ribavirin *on page 831*

Cophene-B® *(Discontinued) see* brompheniramine *on page 144*

Cophene XP® *(Discontinued)*

CO Pioglitazone [Can] *see* pioglitazone *on page 754*

copolymer-1 *see* glatiramer acetate *on page 444*

copper *see* trace metals *on page 940*

CO Pravastatin [Can] *see* pravastatin *on page 779*

Co-Pyronil® 2 Pulvules® *(Discontinued) see* chlorpheniramine and pseudoephedrine *on page 207*

CO Ramipril [Can] *see* ramipril *on page 817*

CO Ranitidine [Can] *see* ranitidine *on page 819*

Cordarone® [US/Can] *see* amiodarone *on page 61*

Cordran® [US/Can] *see* flurandrenolide *on page 415*

Cordran® SP [US] *see* flurandrenolide *on page 415*

Cordron-D NR *(Discontinued)*

Cordron-DM NR *(Discontinued)*

Cordron-HC *(Discontinued)*

Cordron-HC NR *(Discontinued)*

Coreg® [US/Can] *see* carvedilol *on page 181*

Coreg CR™ [US] *see* carvedilol *on page 181*

Corfen DM [US] *see* chlorpheniramine, phenylephrine, and dextromethorphan *on page 209*

Corgard® [US/Can] *see* nadolol *on page 651*

Coricidin HBP® Chest Congestion and Cough [US-OTC] *see* guaifenesin and dextromethorphan *on page 454*

Coricidin HBP® Cold and Flu [US-OTC] *see* chlorpheniramine and acetaminophen *on page 206*

CO Risperidone [Can] *see* risperidone *on page 837*

Corlopam® [US/Can] *see* fenoldopam *on page 393*

Cormax® [US] *see* clobetasol *on page 232*

Coronex® [Can] *see* isosorbide dinitrate *on page 530*

Correctol® [US-OTC] *see* docusate *on page 314*

Correctol® Tablets [US-OTC] *see* bisacodyl *on page 136*

Cortaid® Intensive Therapy [US-OTC] *see* hydrocortisone (topical) *on page 485*

Cortaid® Maximum Strength [US-OTC] *see* hydrocortisone (topical) *on page 485*

Cortaid® Sensitive Skin [US-OTC] *see* hydrocortisone (topical) *on page 485*

Cortamed® [Can] *see* hydrocortisone (topical) *on page 485*

Cortatrigen® Otic *(Discontinued) see* neomycin, polymyxin B, and hydrocortisone *on page 663*

Cortef® [US/Can] *see* hydrocortisone (systemic) *on page 484*

Cortenema® [Can] *see* hydrocortisone (rectal) *on page 484*

Corticool® [US-OTC] *see* hydrocortisone (topical) *on page 485*

corticorelin (kor ti koe REL in)

Sound-Alike/Look-Alike Issues
corticorelin may be confused with corticotropin
Acthrel® may be confused with Acthar®

Synonyms corticorelin ovine triflutate; human corticotrophin-releasing hormone, analogue; ovine corticotrophin-releasing hormone

U.S./Canadian Brand Names Acthrel® [US]

Therapeutic Category Diagnostic Agent, ACTH-Dependent Hypercortisolism

Use Diagnostic test used in adrenocorticotropic hormone (ACTH)-dependent Cushing syndrome to differentiate between pituitary and ectopic production of ACTH

Usual Dosage I.V.: Adults: Testing pituitary corticotrophin function: 1 mcg/kg; dosages >100 mcg have been associated with an increase in adverse effects

Note: Venous blood samples should be drawn 15 minutes before and immediately prior to corticorelin administration to determine baseline ACTH and cortisol. At 15-, 30-, and 60 minutes after administration, venous blood samples should be drawn again to determine response. **Basal and peak responses differ depending on AM or PM administration; therefore, any repeat evaluations are recommended to be done at the same time of day as initial testing.**

Dosage Forms
Injection, powder for reconstitution:
Acthrel®: 100 mcg

corticorelin ovine triflutate *see corticorelin on page 248*

corticotropin (kor ti koe TROE pin)

Sound-Alike/Look-Alike Issues
corticotropin may be confused with corticorelin

Synonyms ACTH; adrenocorticotropic hormone; corticotropin, repository

U.S./Canadian Brand Names H.P. Acthar® Gel [US]

Therapeutic Category Adrenal Corticosteroid

Use Acute exacerbations of multiple sclerosis; diagnostic aid in adrenocortical insufficiency, severe muscle weakness in myasthenia gravis

Cosyntropin is preferred over corticotropin for diagnostic test of adrenocortical insufficiency (cosyntropin is less allergenic and test is shorter in duration)

Usual Dosage
Children:
Antiinflammatory/immunosuppressant: I.M.: 0.8 units/kg/day or 25 units/m^2/day divided every 12-24 hours
Infantile spasms: Various regimens have been used. Some neurologists recommend low-dose ACTH (5-40 units/day) for short periods (1-6 weeks), while others recommend larger doses of ACTH (40-160 units/day) for long periods of treatment (3-12 months). Well designed comparative dosing studies are needed. Example of low dose regimen:
Initial: I.M.: 20 units/day for 2 weeks, if patient responds, taper and discontinue; if patient does not respond, increase dose to 30 units/day for 4 weeks then taper and discontinue
I.M. usual dose: 20-40 units/day or 5-8 units/kg/day in 1-2 divided doses; range: 5-160 units/day
Oral prednisone (2 mg/kg/day) was as effective as I.M. ACTH gel (20 units/day) in controlling infantile spasms
Adults: Acute exacerbation of multiple sclerosis: I.M.: 80-120 units/day for 2-3 weeks
Repository injection: I.M., SubQ: 40-80 units every 24-72 hours
Dosage Forms
Injection, gelatin:
H.P. Acthar® Gel: 80 units/mL (5 mL)

corticotropin, repository *see corticotropin on page 249*
Cortifoam® [US/Can] *see hydrocortisone (rectal) on page 484*
Cortimyxin® [Can] *see neomycin, polymyxin B, and hydrocortisone on page 663*
cortisol *see hydrocortisone (systemic) on page 484*

cortisone acetate (KOR ti sone AS e tate)

Sound-Alike/Look-Alike Issues
cortisone may be confused with Cortizone®

Synonyms compound E

Therapeutic Category Adrenal Corticosteroid

Use Management of adrenocortical insufficiency

Usual Dosage If possible, administer glucocorticoids before 9 AM to minimize adrenocortical suppression; dosing depends upon the condition being treated and the response of the patient; **Note:** Supplemental doses may be warranted during times of stress in the course of withdrawing therapy
Children:
Antiinflammatory or immunosuppressive: Oral: 2.5-10 mg/kg/day or 20-300 mg/m^2/day in divided doses every 6-8 hours

◄ Physiologic replacement: Oral: 0.5-0.75 mg/kg/day **or** 20-25 mg/m²/day in divided doses every 8 hours
Adults:
  Antiinflammatory or immunosuppressive: Oral: 25-300 mg/day in divided doses every 12-24 hours
  Physiologic replacement: Oral: 25-35 mg/day
Dosage Forms
  Tablet: 25 mg

Cortisporin® Cream [US] *see* neomycin, polymyxin B, and hydrocortisone *on page 663*
Cortisporin® Ointment [US] *see* bacitracin, neomycin, polymyxin B, and hydrocortisone *on page 114*
Cortisporin® Ophthalmic *(Discontinued)* *see* neomycin, polymyxin B, and hydrocortisone *on page 663*
Cortisporin® Otic [US/Can] *see* neomycin, polymyxin B, and hydrocortisone *on page 663*
Cortisporin®-TC [US] *see* neomycin, colistin, hydrocortisone, and thonzonium *on page 662*
Cortisporin® Topical Cream *(Discontinued)* *see* neomycin, polymyxin B, and hydrocortisone *on page 663*
Cortisporin® Topical Ointment [Can] *see* bacitracin, neomycin, polymyxin B, and hydrocortisone *on page 114*
Cortizone®-10 Maximum Strength [US-OTC] *see* hydrocortisone (topical) *on page 485*
Cortizone®-10 Plus Maximum Strength [US-OTC] *see* hydrocortisone (topical) *on page 485*
Cortizone®-10 Quick Shot [US-OTC] *see* hydrocortisone (topical) *on page 485*
Cortone® *(Discontinued)*
Cortrosyn® [US/Can] *see* cosyntropin *on page 250*
Corvert® [US] *see* ibutilide *on page 497*
Corzide® [US] *see* nadolol and bendroflumethiazide *on page 651*
CO Sertraline [Can] *see* sertraline *on page 863*
CO Simvastatin [Can] *see* simvastatin *on page 867*
Cosmegen® [US/Can] *see* dactinomycin *on page 264*
Cosopt® [US/Can] *see* dorzolamide and timolol *on page 319*
CO Sotalol [Can] *see* sotalol *on page 885*
CO Sumatriptan [Can] *see* sumatriptan *on page 898*

cosyntropin (koe sin TROE pin)
Sound-Alike/Look-Alike Issues
  Cortrosyn® may be confused with colchicine, Cotazym®
Synonyms synacthen; tetracosactide
U.S./Canadian Brand Names Cortrosyn® [US/Can]
Therapeutic Category Diagnostic Agent
Use Diagnostic test to differentiate primary adrenal from secondary (pituitary) adrenocortical insufficiency
Usual Dosage Adrenocortical insufficiency: I.M., I.V. (over 2 minutes): Peak plasma cortisol concentrations usually occur 45-60 minutes after cosyntropin administration
  Children <2 years: 0.125 mg
  Children >2 years and Adults: 0.25-0.75 mg
  When greater cortisol stimulation is needed, an I.V. infusion may be used:
    Children >2 years and Adults: 0.25 mg administered at 0.04 mg/hour over 6 hours
Dosage Forms
  Injection, powder for reconstitution:
    Cortrosyn®: 0.25 mg

Cotazym® [Can] *see* pancrelipase *on page 718*
Cotazym® *(Discontinued)* *see* pancrelipase *on page 718*
Cotazym-S® *(Discontinued)* *see* pancrelipase *on page 718*
CO Temazepam [Can] *see* temazepam *on page 907*
Co-Topiramate [Can] *see* topiramate *on page 935*
co-trimoxazole *see* sulfamethoxazole and trimethoprim *on page 894*
Coughcold HCM *(Discontinued)*
Coughtuss [US] *see* phenylephrine, hydrocodone, and chlorpheniramine *on page 748*
Coumadin® [US/Can] *see* warfarin *on page 986*

Covan® [Can] see triprolidine, pseudoephedrine, and codeine *(Canada only) on page 955*

Covaryx™ [US] see estrogens (esterified) and methyltestosterone *on page 366*

Covaryx™ HS [US] see estrogens (esterified) and methyltestosterone *on page 366*

Co-Venlafaxine XR [Can] see venlafaxine *on page 973*

Covera® [Can] see verapamil *on page 974*

Covera-HS® [US/Can] see verapamil *on page 974*

Coversyl® [Can] see perindopril erbumine *on page 739*

Coversyl® Plus [Can] see perindopril erbumine and indapamide *(Canada only) on page 739*

co-vidarabine see pentostatin *on page 737*

coviracil see emtricitabine *on page 338*

Cozaar® [US/Can] see losartan *on page 577*

CO Zopiclone [Can] see zopiclone *(Canada only) on page 997*

CP358774 see erlotinib *on page 353*

CPC see cetylpyridinium *on page 197*

C-Phen [US] see chlorpheniramine and phenylephrine *on page 206*

C-Phen DM [US] see chlorpheniramine, phenylephrine, and dextromethorphan *on page 209*

CPM see cyclophosphamide *on page 256*

CPM-12 [US] see chlorpheniramine *on page 205*

CPT-11 see irinotecan *on page 526*

CPZ see chlorpromazine *on page 213*

Crantex HC *(Discontinued)*

Crantex LA [US] see guaifenesin and phenylephrine *on page 456*

Creomulsion® Cough [US-OTC] see dextromethorphan *on page 284*

Creomulsion® for Children [US-OTC] see dextromethorphan *on page 284*

Creon® [US/Can] see pancrelipase *on page 718*

Creo-Terpin® [US-OTC] see dextromethorphan *on page 284*

Crestor® [US/Can] see rosuvastatin *on page 846*

Cresylate® [US] see m-cresyl acetate *on page 592*

Crinone® [US/Can] see progesterone *on page 790*

Critic-Aid® Clear AF [US-OTC] see miconazole *on page 630*

Critic-Aid Skin Care® [US-OTC] see zinc oxide *on page 993*

Criticare HN® [US-OTC] see nutritional formula, enteral/oral *on page 689*

Crixivan® [US/Can] see indinavir *on page 505*

CroFab™ [US] see crotalidae polyvalent immune FAB (ovine) *on page 253*

Crolom® [US] see cromolyn sodium *on page 251*

cromoglycic acid see cromolyn sodium *on page 251*

cromolyn sodium (KROE moe lin SOW dee um)

Sound-Alike/Look-Alike Issues
Intal® may be confused with Endal®
NasalCrom® may be confused with Nasacort®, Nasalide®

Synonyms cromoglycic acid; disodium cromoglycate; DSCG

U.S./Canadian Brand Names Apo-Cromolyn® [Can]; Crolom® [US]; Gastrocrom® [US]; Intal® [US/Can]; Nalcrom® [Can]; NasalCrom® [US-OTC]; Nu-Cromolyn [Can]; Opticrom® [Can]

Therapeutic Category Mast Cell Stabilizer

Use
Inhalation: May be used as an adjunct in the prophylaxis of allergic disorders, including asthma; prevention of exercise-induced bronchospasm
Nasal: Prevention and treatment of seasonal and perennial allergic rhinitis
Oral: Systemic mastocytosis
Ophthalmic: Treatment of vernal keratoconjunctivitis, vernal conjunctivitis, and vernal keratitis

◀ **Usual Dosage**
Oral:
Systemic mastocytosis:
Children 2-12 years: 100 mg 4 times/day; not to exceed 40 mg/kg/day; given 1/2 hour prior to meals and at bedtime
Children >12 years and Adults: 200 mg 4 times/day; given 1/2 hour prior to meals and at bedtime; if control of symptoms is not seen within 2-3 weeks, dose may be increased to a maximum 40 mg/kg/day

Inhalation:
For chronic control of asthma, taper frequency to the lowest effective dose (ie, 4 times/day to 3 times/day to twice daily); **Note:** Not effective for immediate relief of symptoms in acute asthmatic attacks; must be used at regular intervals for 2-4 weeks to be effective.
Nebulization solution: Children >2 years and Adults: Initial: 20 mg 4 times/day; usual dose: 20 mg 3-4 times/day
Metered spray:
Children 5-12 years: Initial: 2 inhalations 4 times/day; usual dose: 1-2 inhalations 3-4 times/day
Children ≥12 years and Adults: Initial: 2 inhalations 4 times/day; usual dose: 2-4 inhalations 3-4 times/day
Prevention of allergen- or exercise-induced bronchospasm: Administer 10-15 minutes prior to exercise or allergen exposure but no longer than 1 hour before:
Nebulization solution: Children >2 years and Adults: Single dose of 20 mg
Metered spray: Children >5 years and Adults: Single dose of 2 inhalations
Ophthalmic: Children >4 years and Adults: 1-2 drops in each eye 4-6 times/day
Nasal: Allergic rhinitis (treatment and prophylaxis): Children ≥2 years and Adults: 1 spray into each nostril 3-4 times/day; may be increased to 6 times/day (symptomatic relief may require 2-4 weeks)

Dosage Forms
Aerosol, for oral inhalation:
Intal®: 800 mcg/inhalation (8.1 g, 14.2 g)
Solution for nebulization: 20 mg/2 mL (60s, 120s)
Intal®: 20 mg/2 mL (60s, 120s)
Solution, intranasal [spray]:
NasalCrom® [OTC]: 40 mg/mL (13 mL, 26 mL)
Solution, ophthalmic: 4% (10 mL)
Crolom®: 4% (10 mL)
Solution, oral [concentrate]:
Gastrocrom®: 100 mg/5 mL

Crosseal™ *(Discontinued)* *see* fibrin sealant kit *on page 400*
crotalidae antivenin *see* crotalidae polyvalent antivenin (equine) *on page 252*

crotalidae polyvalent antivenin (equine)
(kroe TAL ih die pol i VAY lent an tee VEN in (EE kwine))

Synonyms crotalidae antivenin; crotaline antivenin, polyvalent; North, Central, and South American antisnake-bite serum; pit viper antivenin; snake (pit vipers) antivenin

Therapeutic Category Antivenin

Use Neutralization of venoms of North, Central, and South American crotalids: Rattlesnakes (*Crotalus*, *Sistrurus*); copperhead and cottonmouth moccasins (*Agkistrodon*), including *A. halys* of Korea and Japan; the Fer-de-lance and other species of *Bothrops*; tropical rattler (*Crotalus durissus*), cantil (*A. bilineatus*); bushmaster (*Lachesis mutus*) of South and Central America

Usual Dosage I.M., I.V.: Children and Adults: Crotalid envenomation: **Note:** Clinical trials included patients as young as 11 years of age. Specific pediatric studies have not been conducted. Because the absolute venom dose is expected to be the same in adults and children, adult dosing should be used. Products contain thimerosal, which in high doses has been associated with neurological and renal toxicity. Very young children are most susceptible.
Initial sensitivity test: 0.02-0.03 mL of a 1:10 dilution of normal horse serum or antivenin given intracutaneously; also give a control test using normal saline in the opposite extremity. A positive reaction occurs within 5-30 minutes. A negative reaction does not rule out the possibility of an immediate or delayed reaction with treatment.
Minimal envenomation: 20-40 mL (2-4 vials)
Moderate envenomation: 50-90 mL (5-9 vials)
Severe envenomation: ≥100-150 mL (10-15 vials)

Note: Variability in the required dose has been reported (5-43 vials administered). The entire initial dose of antivenin should be administered as soon as possible to be most effective (within 4 hours after the bite). I.V. is the preferred route of administration. When administered I.V., infuse the initial 5-10 mL over 3-5 minutes while carefully observing the patient for signs and symptoms of sensitivity reactions. If no reaction occurs, continue infusion at a safe I.V. fluid delivery rate. Additional doses of antivenin are based on clinical response to the initial dose. If swelling continues to progress, symptoms increase in severity, hypotension occurs, or decrease in hematocrit appears, an additional 10-50 mL (1-5 vials) should be administered.

crotalidae polyvalent immune FAB (ovine)
(kroe TAL ih die pol i VAY lent i MYUN fab (oh vine))

Synonyms antivenin (crotalidae) polyvalent; crotaline antivenin, polyvalent; fabAV; North American antisnake-bite serum; snake antivenin

U.S./Canadian Brand Names CroFab™ [US]

Therapeutic Category Antivenin

Use Neutralization of venoms of North American crotalids: Rattlesnakes (*Crotalus*, *Sistrurus*); copperhead and cottonmouth moccasins (*Agkistrodon*)

Usual Dosage I.V.: Children and Adults: **Note:** Clinical trials included patients as young as 11 years of age. Specific pediatric studies have not been conducted. Because the absolute venom dose is expected to be the same in adults and children, adult dosing should be used. Products contain thimerosal, which in high doses has been associated with neurological and renal toxicity. Very young children are most susceptible.

Crotalid envenomation: Minimal or moderate:
Initial dose: 4-6 vials, dependent upon patient response. Treatment should begin within 6 hours of snakebite; monitor for 1 hour following infusion. Repeat with an additional 4-6 vials if control is not achieved with initial dose. Continue to treat with 4- to 6-vial doses until complete arrest of local manifestations, coagulation tests, and systemic signs are normal.

Maintenance dose: Once control is achieved, administer 2 vials every 6 hours for up to 18 hours. Optimal dosing past 18 hours has not been established; however, treatment may be continued if deemed necessary based on the patient's condition.

Dosage Forms
Injection, powder for reconstitution:
CroFab™: Derived from *Crotalus adamanteus*, *C. atrox*, *C. scutulatus*, and *Agkistrodon piscivorus* snake venoms

crotaline antivenin, polyvalent see crotalidae polyvalent antivenin (equine) on page 252
crotaline antivenin, polyvalent see crotalidae polyvalent immune FAB (ovine) on page 253

crotamiton (kroe TAM i tonn)

Sound-Alike/Look-Alike Issues
Eurax® may be confused with Efudex®, Eulexin®, Evoxac™, Serax®, Urex®

U.S./Canadian Brand Names Eurax® [US]

Therapeutic Category Scabicides/Pediculicides

Use Treatment of scabies (*Sarcoptes scabiei*) and symptomatic treatment of pruritus

Usual Dosage Topical:
Scabicide: Children and Adults: Wash thoroughly and scrub away loose scales, then towel dry; apply a thin layer and massage drug onto skin of the entire body from the neck to the toes (with special attention to skin folds, creases, and interdigital spaces). Repeat application in 24 hours. Take a cleansing bath 48 hours after the final application. Treatment may be repeated after 7-10 days if live mites are still present.
Pruritus: Massage into affected areas until medication is completely absorbed; repeat as necessary

Dosage Forms
Cream:
Eurax®: 10% (60 g)
Lotion:
Eurax®: 10% (60 mL, 480 mL)

CRRT see electrolyte solution, renal replacement on page 336
crude coal tar see coal tar on page 240
Cruex® Cream [US-OTC] see clotrimazole on page 238
Cryselle™ [US] see ethinyl estradiol and norgestrel on page 380

crystalline penicillin *see* penicillin G (parenteral/aqueous) *on page 732*

Crystamine® *(Discontinued)* *see* cyanocobalamin *on page 254*

Crysti 1000® *(Discontinued)* *see* cyanocobalamin *on page 254*

CsA *see* cyclosporine *on page 257*

C-Tanna 12 [US] *see* carbetapentane and chlorpheniramine *on page 174*

C-Tanna 12D [US] *see* carbetapentane, phenylephrine, and pyrilamine *on page 176*

C-Time [US-OTC] *see* ascorbic acid *on page 96*

CTLA-4Ig *see* abatacept *on page 16*

CTM *see* chlorpheniramine *on page 205*

CTX *see* cyclophosphamide *on page 256*

Cubicin® [US/Can] *see* daptomycin *on page 267*

Culturelle® [US-OTC] *see* Lactobacillus *on page 543*

Cuprimine® [US/Can] *see* penicillamine *on page 730*

Curasore [US-OTC] *see* pramoxine *on page 777*

Curosurf® [US/Can] *see* poractant alfa *on page 768*

Cutar® [US-OTC] *see* coal tar *on page 240*

Cutivate® [US/Can] *see* fluticasone (topical) *on page 419*

CVT-3146 *see* regadenoson *on page 823*

CyA *see* cyclosporine *on page 257*

cyanide antidote kit *see* sodium nitrite, sodium thiosulfate, and amyl nitrite *on page 876*

Cyanide Antidote Package [US] *see* sodium nitrite, sodium thiosulfate, and amyl nitrite *on page 876*

cyanocobalamin (sye an oh koe BAL a min)

Synonyms vitamin B_{12}

U.S./Canadian Brand Names CaloMist™ [US]; Nascobal® [US]; Twelve Resin-K [US]

Therapeutic Category Vitamin, Water Soluble

Use Treatment of pernicious anemia; vitamin B_{12} deficiency due to dietary deficiencies or malabsorption diseases, inadequate secretion of intrinsic factor, and inadequate utilization of B_{12} (eg, during neoplastic treatment); increased B_{12} requirements due to pregnancy, thyrotoxicosis, hemorrhage, malignancy, liver or kidney disease

CaloMist™: Maintenance of vitamin B_{12} concentrations after initial correction in patients with B_{12} deficiency without CNS involvement

Usual Dosage

Adequate intake:

Children:

0-6 months: 0.4 mcg/day

7-12 months: 0.5 mcg/day

Recommended intake:

Children:

1-3 years: 0.9 mcg/day

4-8 years: 1.2 mcg/day

9-13 years: 1.8 mcg/day

Children >14 years and Adults: 2.4 mcg/day

Pregnancy: 2.6 mcg/day

Lactation: 2.8 mcg/day

Vitamin B_{12} deficiency:

I.M., deep SubQ:

Children (dosage not well established): 0.2 mcg/kg for 2 days, followed by 1000 mcg/day for 2-7 days, followed by 100 mcg/week for one month; for malabsorptive causes of B_{12} deficiency, monthly maintenance doses of 100 mcg have been recommended **or** as an alternative 100 mcg/day for 10-15 days, then once or twice weekly for several months

Adults: Initial: 30 mcg/day for 5-10 days; maintenance: 100-200 mcg/month

Intranasal: Adults:

Nascobal®: 500 mcg in one nostril once weekly

CaloMist™: Maintenance therapy (following correction of vitamin B_{12} deficiency): 25 mcg in each nostril daily (50 mcg/day). If inadequate response, 25 mcg in each nostril twice daily (100 mcg/day).

Oral: Adults: 250 mcg/day

Pernicious anemia: I.M., deep SubQ (administer concomitantly with folic acid if needed, 1 mg/day for 1 month):
  Children: 30-50 mcg/day for 2 or more weeks (to a total dose of 1000-5000 mcg), then follow with 100 mcg/month as maintenance dosage
  Adults: 100 mcg/day for 6-7 days; if improvement, administer same dose on alternate days for 7 doses, then every 3-4 days for 2-3 weeks; once hematologic values have returned to normal, maintenance dosage: 100 mcg/month. **Note:** Alternative dosing of 1000 mcg/day for 5 days (followed by 500-1000 mcg/month) has been used.
  Hematologic remission (without evidence of nervous system involvement): Adults:
  Intranasal (Nascobal®): 500 mcg in one nostril once weekly
  Oral: 1000-2000 mcg/day
  I.M., SubQ: 100-1000 mcg/month
Schilling test: Adults: I.M.: 1000 mcg
Dosage Forms
  Injection, solution: 1000 mcg/mL (1 mL, 10 mL, 30 mL)
  Lozenge: 50 mcg, 100 mcg, 250 mcg, 500 mcg
  Lozenge, sublingual: 500 mcg
  Solution, intranasal [spray]:
    CaloMist™: 25 mcg/0.1 mL actuation (18 mL)
    Nascobal®: 500 mcg/0.1 mL actuation (2.3 mL)
  Tablet: 50 mcg, 100 mcg, 250 mcg, 500 mcg, 1000 mcg
    Twelve Resin-K: 1000 mcg
  Tablet, timed release: 1000 mcg, 1500 mcg
  Tablet, sublingual: 1000 mcg, 2500 mcg, 5000 mcg

cyanocobalamin, folic acid, and pyridoxine see folic acid, cyanocobalamin, and pyridoxine on page 422

Cyanoject® (Discontinued) see cyanocobalamin on page 254

Cyclen® [Can] see ethinyl estradiol and norgestimate on page 378

Cyclessa® [US/Can] see ethinyl estradiol and desogestrel on page 369

cyclobenzaprine (sye kloe BEN za preen)

Sound-Alike/Look-Alike Issues
  cyclobenzaprine may be confused with cycloSERINE, cyproheptadine
  Flexeril® may be confused with Floxin®
Synonyms cyclobenzaprine hydrochloride
U.S./Canadian Brand Names Amrix® [US]; Apo-Cyclobenzaprine® [Can]; Fexmid™ [US]; Flexeril® [US/Can]; Flexitec [Can]; Gen-Cyclobenzaprine [Can]; Novo-Cycloprine [Can]; Nu-Cyclobenzaprine [Can]
Therapeutic Category Skeletal Muscle Relaxant
Use Treatment of muscle spasm associated with acute painful musculoskeletal conditions
Usual Dosage Oral: **Note:** Do not use longer than 2-3 weeks
  Capsule, extended release: Adults: Usual: 15 mg once daily; some patients may require up to 30 mg once daily
  Tablet, immediate release: Children ≥15 years and Adults: Initial: 5 mg 3 times/day; may increase to 7.5-10 mg 3 times/day if needed
Dosage Forms
  Capsule, extended release:
    Amrix®: 15 mg, 30 mg
  Tablet: 5 mg, 10 mg
    Fexmid™: 7.5 mg
    Flexeril®: 5 mg, 10 mg

cyclobenzaprine hydrochloride see cyclobenzaprine on page 255

Cyclocort® [Can] see amcinonide on page 57

Cyclocort® (Discontinued) see amcinonide on page 57

Cyclogyl® [US/Can] see cyclopentolate on page 256

Cyclomen® [Can] see danazol on page 266

Cyclomydril® [US] see cyclopentolate and phenylephrine on page 256

cyclopentolate (sye kloe PEN toe late)

Synonyms cyclopentolate hydrochloride

U.S./Canadian Brand Names AK-Pentolate™ [US]; Cyclogyl® [US/Can]; Cylate™ [US]; Diopentolate® [Can]

Therapeutic Category Anticholinergic Agent

Use Diagnostic procedures requiring mydriasis and cycloplegia

Usual Dosage Ophthalmic:

Neonates and Infants: **Note:** Cyclopentolate and phenylephrine combination formulation is the preferred agent for use in neonates and infants due to lower cyclopentolate concentration and reduced risk for systemic reactions

Children: Instill 1 drop of 0.5%, 1%, or 2% in eye followed by 1 drop of 0.5% or 1% in 5 minutes, if necessary

Adults: Instill 1 drop of 1% followed by another drop in 5 minutes; 2% solution in heavily pigmented iris

Dosage Forms

Solution, ophthalmic: 1% (2 mL, 15 mL)

AK-Pentolate™, Cylate™: 1% (2 mL, 15 mL)

Cyclogyl®: 0.5% (15 mL); 1% (2 mL, 5 mL, 15 mL); 2% (2 mL, 5 mL, 15 mL)

cyclopentolate and phenylephrine (sye kloe PEN toe late & fen il EF rin)

Synonyms phenylephrine and cyclopentolate

U.S./Canadian Brand Names Cyclomydril® [US]

Therapeutic Category Anticholinergic/Adrenergic Agonist

Use Induce mydriasis greater than that produced with cyclopentolate HCl alone

Usual Dosage Ophthalmic: Neonates, Infants, Children, and Adults: Instill 1 drop into the eye every 5-10 minutes, for up to 3 doses, approximately 40-50 minutes before the examination

Dosage Forms

Solution, ophthalmic:

Cyclomydril®: Cyclopentolate 0.2% and phenylephrine 1% (2 mL, 5 mL)

cyclopentolate hydrochloride see cyclopentolate on page 256

cyclophosphamide (sye kloe FOS fa mide)

Sound-Alike/Look-Alike Issues

cyclophosphamide may be confused with cycloSPORINE, ifosfamide

Cytoxan® may be confused with cefoxitin, Centoxin®, Ciloxan®, cytarabine, CytoGam®, Cytosar®, Cytosar-U®, Cytotec®

Synonyms CPM; CTX; CYT; NSC-26271

U.S./Canadian Brand Names Cytoxan® [US/Can]; Procytox® [Can]

Therapeutic Category Antineoplastic Agent

Use

Oncologic: Treatment of Hodgkin and non-Hodgkin lymphoma, Burkitt lymphoma, chronic lymphocytic leukemia (CLL), chronic myelocytic leukemia (CML), acute myelocytic leukemia (AML), acute lymphocytic leukemia (ALL), mycosis fungoides, multiple myeloma, neuroblastoma, retinoblastoma, rhabdomyosarcoma, Ewing sarcoma; breast, testicular, endometrial, ovarian, and lung cancers, and in conditioning regimens for bone marrow transplantation

Nononcologic: Prophylaxis of rejection for kidney, heart, liver, and bone marrow transplants, severe rheumatoid disorders, nephrotic syndrome, Wegener granulomatosis, idiopathic pulmonary hemosideroses, myasthenia gravis, multiple sclerosis, systemic lupus erythematosus, lupus nephritis, autoimmune hemolytic anemia, idiopathic thrombocytic purpura (ITP), macroglobulinemia, and antibody-induced pure red cell aplasia

Usual Dosage Refer to individual protocols

Children:

SLE: I.V.: 500-750 mg/m^2 every month; maximum dose: 1 g/m^2

JRA/vasculitis: I.V.: 10 mg/kg every 2 weeks

Children and Adults:

Oral: 50-100 mg/m^2/day as continuous therapy or 400-1000 mg/m^2 in divided doses over 4-5 days as intermittent therapy

I.V.:
Single doses: 400-1800 mg/m^2 (30-50 mg/kg) per treatment course (1-5 days) which can be repeated at 2-4 week intervals
Continuous daily doses: 60-120 mg/m^2 (1-2.5 mg/kg) per day
Autologous BMT: IVPB: 50 mg/kg/dose x 4 days or 60 mg/kg/dose for 2 days; total dose is usually divided over 2-4 days
Nephrotic syndrome: Oral: 2-3 mg/kg/day every day for up to 12 weeks when corticosteroids are unsuccessful
Dosage Forms
 Injection, powder for reconstitution: 500 mg, 1 g, 2 g
 Tablet: 25 mg, 50 mg

cycloserine (sye kloe SER een)

Sound-Alike/Look-Alike Issues
 cycloSERINE may be confused with cyclobenzaprine, cycloSPORINE
Tall-Man cycloSERINE
U.S./Canadian Brand Names Seromycin® [US]
Therapeutic Category Antibiotic, Miscellaneous
Use Adjunctive treatment in pulmonary or extrapulmonary tuberculosis
Usual Dosage Some neurotoxic effects may be relieved or prevented by concomitant administration of pyridoxine

Tuberculosis: Oral:
 Children: 10-20 mg/kg/day in 2 divided doses up to 1000 mg/day for 18-24 months
 Adults: Initial: 250 mg every 12 hours for 14 days, then administer 500 mg to 1 g/day in 2 divided doses for 18-24 months (maximum daily dose: 1 g)
Dosage Forms
 Capsule:
 Seromycin®: 250 mg

cyclosporin A see cyclosporine on page 257

cyclosporine (SYE kloe spor een)

Sound-Alike/Look-Alike Issues
 cycloSPORINE may be confused with cyclophosphamide, Cyklokapron®, cycloSERINE
 cycloSPORINE modified (Neoral®, Gengraf®) may be confused with cycloSPORINE non-modified (Sandimmne®)
 Gengraf® may be confused with Prograf®
 Neoral® may be confused with Neurontin®, Nizoral®
 Sandimmune® may be confused with Sandostatin®
Synonyms CsA; CyA; cyclosporin A
Tall-Man cycloSPORINE
U.S./Canadian Brand Names Gengraf® [US]; Neoral® [US/Can]; Restasis® [US]; Rhoxal-cyclosporine [Can]; Sandimmune® I.V. [Can]; Sandimmune® [US]; Sandoz-Cyclosporine [Can]
Therapeutic Category Immunosuppressant Agent
Use Prophylaxis of organ rejection in kidney, liver, and heart transplants, has been used with azathioprine and/or corticosteroids; severe, active rheumatoid arthritis (RA) not responsive to methotrexate alone; severe, recalcitrant plaque psoriasis in nonimmunocompromised adults unresponsive to or unable to tolerate other systemic therapy

Ophthalmic emulsion (Restasis®): Increase tear production when suppressed tear production is presumed to be due to keratoconjunctivitis sicca-associated ocular inflammation (in patients not already using topical antiinflammatory drugs or punctal plugs)
Usual Dosage Neoral®/Genraf® and Sandimmune® are not bioequivalent and cannot be used interchangeably.
Children: Transplant: Refer to adult dosing; children may require, and are able to tolerate, larger doses than adults.
Adults:
Newly-transplanted patients: Adjunct therapy with corticosteroids is recommended. Initial dose should be given 4-12 hours prior to transplant or may be given postoperatively; adjust initial dose to achieve desired plasma concentration

◀ Oral: Dose is dependent upon type of transplant and formulation:

Cyclosporine (modified):

Renal: 9 ± 3 mg/kg/day, divided twice daily

Liver: 8 ± 4 mg/kg/day, divided twice daily

Heart: 7 ± 3 mg/kg/day, divided twice daily

Cyclosporine (nonmodified): Initial dose: 15 mg/kg/day as a single dose (range 14-18 mg/kg); lower doses of 10-14 mg/kg/day have been used for renal transplants. Continue initial dose daily for 1-2 weeks; taper by 5% per week to a maintenance dose of 5-10 mg/kg/day; some renal transplant patients may be dosed as low as 3 mg/kg/day

Note: When using the nonmodified formulation, cyclosporine levels may increase in liver transplant patients when the T-tube is closed; dose may need decreased

I.V.: Cyclosporine (nonmodified): Manufacturer's labeling: Initial dose: 5-6 mg/kg/day as a single dose (1/3 the oral dose), infused over 2-6 hours; use should be limited to patients unable to take capsules or oral solution; patients should be switched to an oral dosage form as soon as possible

Note: Many transplant centers administer cyclosporine as "divided dose" infusions (in 2-3 doses/day) or as a continuous (24-hour) infusion; dosages range from 3-7.5 mg/kg/day. Specific institutional protocols should be consulted.

Conversion to cyclosporine (modified) from cyclosporine (nonmodified): Start with daily dose previously used and adjust to obtain preconversion cyclosporine trough concentration. Plasma concentrations should be monitored every 4-7 days and dose adjusted as necessary, until desired trough level is obtained. When transferring patients with previously poor absorption of cyclosporine (nonmodified), monitor trough levels at least twice weekly (especially if initial dose exceeds 10 mg/kg/day); high plasma levels are likely to occur.

Rheumatoid arthritis: Oral: Cyclosporine (modified): Initial dose: 2.5 mg/kg/day, divided twice daily; salicylates, NSAIDs, and oral glucocorticoids may be continued; dose may be increased by 0.5-0.75 mg/kg/day if insufficient response is seen after 8 weeks of treatment; additional dosage increases may be made again at 12 weeks (maximum dose: 4 mg/kg/day). Discontinue if no benefit is seen by 16 weeks of therapy.

Note: Increase the frequency of blood pressure monitoring after each alteration in dosage of cyclosporine. Cyclosporine dosage should be decreased by 25% to 50% in patients with no history of hypertension who develop sustained hypertension during therapy and, if hypertension persists, treatment with cyclosporine should be discontinued.

Psoriasis: Oral: Cyclosporine (modified): Initial dose: 2.5 mg/kg/day, divided twice daily; dose may be increased by 0.5 mg/kg/day if insufficient response is seen after 4 weeks of treatment. Additional dosage increases may be made every 2 weeks if needed (maximum dose: 4 mg/kg/day). Discontinue if no benefit is seen by 6 weeks of therapy. Once patients are adequately controlled, the dose should be decreased to the lowest effective dose. Doses lower than 2.5 mg/kg/day may be effective. Treatment longer than 1 year is not recommended.

Note: Increase the frequency of blood pressure monitoring after each alteration in dosage of cyclosporine. Cyclosporine dosage should be decreased by 25% to 50% in patients with no history of hypertension who develop sustained hypertension during therapy and, if hypertension persists, treatment with cyclosporine should be discontinued.

Keratoconjunctivitis sicca: Ophthalmic (Restasis®): Children ≥16 years and Adults: Instill 1 drop in each eye every 12 hours

Dosage Forms

Capsule [modified]:

Gengraf®: 25 mg, 100 mg

Capsule [non-modified]: 25 mg, 100 mg

Capsule, soft gel [modified]: 25 mg, 50 mg, 100 mg

Neoral®: 25 mg, 100 mg

Capsule, soft gel [non-modified]:

Sandimmune®: 25 mg, 100 mg

Emulsion, ophthalmic [preservative free]:

Restasis®: 0.05% (0.4 mL)

Injection, solution [non-modified]: 50 mg/mL (5 mL)

Sandimmune®: 50 mg/mL (5 mL)

Solution, oral [modified]: 100 mg/mL

Gengraf®, Neoral®: 100 mg/mL

Solution, oral [non-modified]: 100 mg/mL

Sandimmune®: 100 mg/mL

Cycofed® Pediatric *(Discontinued)* see guaifenesin, pseudoephedrine, and codeine *on page 460*
Cyestra-35 [Can] see cyproterone and ethinyl estradiol *(Canada only) on page 259*
Cyklokapron® [US/Can] see tranexamic acid *on page 942*
Cylate™ [US] see cyclopentolate *on page 256*
Cylex® [US-OTC] see benzocaine *on page 124*
Cymbalta® [US/Can] see duloxetine *on page 328*
Cyomin® *(Discontinued)* see cyanocobalamin *on page 254*

cyproheptadine (si proe HEP ta deen)

Sound-Alike/Look-Alike Issues
cyproheptadine may be confused with cyclobenzaprine
Periactin may be confused with Perative®, Percodan®, Persantine®
Synonyms cyproheptadine hydrochloride
Therapeutic Category Antihistamine
Use Perennial and seasonal allergic rhinitis and other allergic symptoms including urticaria
Usual Dosage Oral:
Children:
Allergic conditions: 0.25 mg/kg/day or 8 mg/m^2/day in 2-3 divided doses **or**
2-6 years: 2 mg every 8-12 hours (not to exceed 12 mg/day)
7-14 years: 4 mg every 8-12 hours (not to exceed 16 mg/day)
Migraine headaches: 4 mg 2-3 times/day
Children ≥12 years and Adults: Spasticity associated with spinal cord damage: 4 mg at bedtime; increase by a 4 mg dose every 3-4 days; average daily dose: 16 mg in divided doses; not to exceed 36 mg/day
Children >13 years and Adults: Appetite stimulation (anorexia nervosa): 2 mg 4 times/day; may be increased gradually over a 3-week period to 8 mg 4 times/day
Adults:
Allergic conditions: 4-20 mg/day divided every 8 hours (not to exceed 0.5 mg/kg/day)
Cluster headaches: 4 mg 4 times/day
Migraine headaches: 4-8 mg 3 times/day
Dosage Forms
Syrup: 2 mg/5 mL
Tablet: 4 mg

cyproheptadine hydrochloride see cyproheptadine *on page 259*
cyproterone acetate see cyproterone *(Canada only) on page 259*

cyproterone and ethinyl estradiol *(Canada only)*
(sye PROE ter one & ETH in il es tra DYE ole)
Synonyms ethinyl estradiol and cyproterone acetate
U.S./Canadian Brand Names Cyestra-35 [Can]; Diane-35® [Can]
Therapeutic Category Acne Products; Estrogen and Androgen Combination
Use Treatment of females with severe acne, unresponsive to other therapies, with associated symptoms of androgenization (including mild hirsutism or seborrhea). **Should not be used solely for contraception;** however, will provide reliable contraception if taken as recommended for approved indications.
Usual Dosage Oral: Adults: Female: Acne: One tablet daily for 21 days, followed by 7 days off; first cycle should begin on the first day of menstrual flow. Discontinue therapy 3-4 cycles after symptoms have resolved.
Dosage Forms CAN = [Canadian brand name]
Tablet:
Diane-35 [CAN]: Cyproterone 2 mg and ethinyl estradiol 0.35 mg (21s) [not available in the U.S.]

cyproterone *(Canada only)* (sye PROE ter one)
Synonyms cyproterone acetate
U.S./Canadian Brand Names Androcur® Depot [Can]; Androcur® [Can]; Apo-Cyproterone® [Can]; Gen-Cyproterone [Can]; Novo-Cyproterone [Can]
Therapeutic Category Antiandrogen; Progestin

◀ **Use** Palliative treatment of advanced prostate carcinoma

Usual Dosage Adults: Males: Prostatic carcinoma (palliative treatment):

Oral: 200-300 mg/day in 2-3 divided doses; following orchiectomy, reduce dose to 100-200 mg/day; should be taken with meals

I.M. (depot): 300 mg (3 mL) once weekly; reduce dose in orchiectomized patients to 300 mg every 2 weeks

Dosage Forms [CAN] = Canadian brand name:

Injection, solution: 100 mg/mL (3 mL) [not available in the U.S.]

Androcur® Depot [CAN]: 100 mg/mL (3 mL) [not available in the U.S.]

Tablet: 50 mg [not available in the U.S.]

Androcur® [CAN], Apo-Cyproterone® [CAN], Gen-Cyproterone [CAN]: 50 mg [not available in the U.S.]

Cystadane® [US/Can] *see* betaine *on page 131*

Cystagon® [US] *see* cysteamine *on page 260*

cysteamine (sis TEE a meen)

Synonyms cysteamine bitartrate

U.S./Canadian Brand Names Cystagon® [US]

Therapeutic Category Urinary Tract Product

Use Treatment of nephropathic cystinosis

Usual Dosage Oral: Initiate therapy with 1/4 to 1/6 of maintenance dose; titrate slowly upward over 4-6 weeks. **Note:** Dosage may be increased if cystine levels are <1 nmol/1/2 cystine/mg protein, although intolerance and incidence of adverse events may be increased.

Children <12 years: Maintenance: 1.3 g/m^2/day or 60 mg/kg/day divided into 4 doses (maximum dose: 1.95 g/m^2/day or 90 mg/kg/day)

Children >12 years and Adults (>110 lb): 2 g/day in 4 divided doses; maximum dose: 1.95 g/m^2/day or 90 mg/kg/day

Dosage Forms

Capsule:

Cystagon®: 50 mg, 150 mg

cysteamine bitartrate *see* cysteamine *on page 260*

cysteine (SIS te een)

Synonyms cysteine hydrochloride

U.S./Canadian Brand Names Cysteine-500 [US]

Therapeutic Category Nutritional Supplement

Use Supplement to crystalline amino acid solutions, in particular the specialized pediatric formulas (eg, Aminosyn® PF, TrophAmine®) to meet the intravenous amino acid nutritional requirements of infants receiving parenteral nutrition (PN)

Usual Dosage I.V.: Neonates and Infants: Added as a fixed ratio to crystalline amino acid solution: 40 mg cysteine per g of amino acids; dosage will vary with the daily amino acid dosage (eg, 0.5-2.5 g/kg/day amino acids would result in 20-100 mg/kg/day cysteine); individual doses of cysteine of 0.8-1 mmol/kg/day have also been added directly to the daily PN solution; the duration of treatment relates to the need for PN; patients on chronic PN therapy have received cysteine until 6 months of age and in some cases until 2 years of age

Dosage Forms

Capsule:

Cysteine-500: 500 mg

Injection, solution: 50 mg/mL (10 mL, 50 mL)

Cysteine-500 [US] *see* cysteine *on page 260*

cysteine hydrochloride *see* cysteine *on page 260*

Cystistat® [Can] *see* hyaluronate and derivatives *on page 476*

Cysto-Conray® II [US] *see* iothalamate meglumine *on page 522*

Cystografin® [US] *see* diatrizoate meglumine *on page 288*

Cystografin® Dilute [US] *see* diatrizoate meglumine *on page 288*

Cystospaz® [US/Can] *see* hyoscyamine *on page 492*

Cystospaz-M® *(Discontinued)* *see* hyoscyamine *on page 492*

CYT *see* cyclophosphamide *on page 256*
Cytadren® [US] *see* aminoglutethimide *on page 60*

cytarabine (sye TARE a been)

Sound-Alike/Look-Alike Issues
cytarabine may be confused with Cytadren®, Cytosar®, Cytoxan®, vidarabine
cytarabine (conventional) may be confused with cytarabine liposomal
Cytosar-U may be confused with cytarabine, Cytovene®, Cytoxan®, Neosar®

Synonyms ara-C; arabinosylcytosine; cytarabine (conventional); cytarabine hydrochloride; Cytosar-U; cytosine arabinosine hydrochloride; NSC-63878

U.S./Canadian Brand Names Cytosar® [Can]

Therapeutic Category Antineoplastic Agent

Use Treatment of acute myeloid leukemia (AML), acute lymphocytic leukemia (ALL), chronic myelocytic leukemia (CML; blast phase), and lymphomas; prophylaxis and treatment of meningeal leukemia

Usual Dosage Refer to individual protocols. Children and Adults:
Remission induction:
I.V.: 75-200 mg/m^2/day for 5-10 days; a second course, beginning 2-4 weeks after the initial therapy, may be required in some patients.
or 100 mg/m^2 for 7 days
or 100 mg/m^2/dose every 12 hours for 7 days
I.T.: Usual dose 30 mg/m^2 every 4 days; range: 5-75 mg/m^2 every 2-7 days until CNS findings normalize; or age-based dosing (frequency of administration usually defined by protocol):
<1 year of age: 15-20 mg per dose
1-2 years of age: 16-30 mg per dose
2-3 years of age: 20-50 mg per dose
>3 years of age: 24-75 mg per dose
Remission maintenance:
I.V.: 70-200 mg/m^2/day for 2-5 days at monthly intervals
I.M., SubQ: 1-1.5 mg/kg single dose for maintenance at 1- to 4-week intervals

Dosage Forms
Injection, powder for reconstitution: 100 mg, 500 mg, 1 g, 2 g
Injection, solution: 20 mg/mL (5 mL, 25 mL, 50 mL); 100 mg/mL (20 mL)

cytarabine (conventional) *see* cytarabine *on page 261*
cytarabine hydrochloride *see* cytarabine *on page 261*

cytarabine (liposomal) (sye TARE a been lip po SOE mal)

Sound-Alike/Look-Alike Issues
cytarabine may be confused with Cytadren®, Cytosar®, Cytoxan®, vidarabine
cytarabine (liposomal) may be confused with conventional cytarabine
DepoCyt® may be confused with Depoject®

U.S./Canadian Brand Names DepoCyt® [US/Can]

Therapeutic Category Antineoplastic Agent, Antimetabolite (Purine)

Use Treatment of lymphomatous meningitis

Usual Dosage Note: Patients should be started on dexamethasone 4 mg twice daily (oral or I.V.) for 5 days, beginning on the day of cytarabine liposomal injection.

Intrathecal: Adults:
Induction: 50 mg every 14 days for a total of 2 doses (weeks 1 and 3)
Consolidation: 50 mg every 14 days for 3 doses (weeks 5, 7, and 9), followed by an additional dose at week 13
Maintenance: 50 mg every 28 days for 4 doses (weeks 17, 21, 25, and 29)

Dosage reduction for toxicity: If drug-related neurotoxicity develops, reduce dose to 25 mg. If toxicity persists, discontinue treatment.

Dosage Forms
Injection, suspension, intrathecal [preservative free]:
Depocyt®: 10 mg/mL (5 mL)

CytoGam® [US/Can] *see* cytomegalovirus immune globulin (intravenous-human) *on page 262*

cytomegalovirus immune globulin (intravenous-human)
(sye toe meg a low VYE rus i MYUN GLOB yoo lin in tra VEE nus HYU man)

Sound-Alike/Look-Alike Issues
  CytoGam® may be confused with Cytoxan®, Gamimune® N

Synonyms CMV-IGIV

U.S./Canadian Brand Names CytoGam® [US/Can]

Therapeutic Category Immune Globulin

Use Prophylaxis of cytomegalovirus (CMV) disease associated with kidney, lung, liver, pancreas, and heart transplants; concomitant use with ganciclovir should be considered in organ transplants (other than kidney) from CMV seropositive donors to CMV seronegative recipients

Usual Dosage I.V.: Adults:
  Kidney transplant:
    Initial dose (within 72 hours of transplant): 150 mg/kg/dose
    2-, 4-, 6-, and 8 weeks after transplant: 100 mg/kg/dose
    12 and 16 weeks after transplant: 50 mg/kg/dose
  Liver, lung, pancreas, or heart transplant:
    Initial dose (within 72 hours of transplant): 150 mg/kg/dose
    2-, 4-, 6-, and 8 weeks after transplant: 150 mg/kg/dose
    12 and 16 weeks after transplant: 100 mg/kg/dose

Dosage Forms
  Injection, solution [preservative free]:
    CytoGam®: 50 mg ± 10 mg/mL (50 mL)

Cytomel® [US/Can] *see* liothyronine *on page 568*

Cytosar® [Can] *see* cytarabine *on page 261*

Cytosar-U *see* cytarabine *on page 261*

cytosine arabinosine hydrochloride *see* cytarabine *on page 261*

cytostasan *see* bendamustine *on page 122*

Cytotec® [US] *see* misoprostol *on page 637*

Cytovene® [US/Can] *see* ganciclovir *on page 435*

Cytoxan® [US/Can] *see* cyclophosphamide *on page 256*

Cytra-3 [US] *see* citric acid, sodium citrate, and potassium citrate *on page 226*

Cytra-K [US] *see* potassium citrate and citric acid *on page 772*

Cytuss HC [US] *see* phenylephrine, hydrocodone, and chlorpheniramine *on page 748*

D2E7 *see* adalimumab *on page 34*

D-3 [US-OTC] *see* cholecalciferol *on page 215*

D_3 *see* cholecalciferol *on page 215*

D3-5™ [US-OTC] *see* cholecalciferol *on page 215*

D3-50™ [US-OTC] *see* cholecalciferol *on page 215*

D-3-mercaptovaline *see* penicillamine *on page 730*

d4T *see* stavudine *on page 887*

D_5W *see* dextrose *on page 286*

$D_{10}W$ *see* dextrose *on page 286*

$D_{25}W$ *see* dextrose *on page 286*

$D_{30}W$ *see* dextrose *on page 286*

$D_{40}W$ *see* dextrose *on page 286*

$D_{50}W$ *see* dextrose *on page 286*

$D_{60}W$ *see* dextrose *on page 286*

$D_{70}W$ *see* dextrose *on page 286*

$DAB_{389}IL-2$ *see* denileukin diftitox *on page 272*

dabigatran etexilate *(Canada only)* (da BIG a tran ett EX ill ate)
Synonyms dabigatran etexilate mesilate
U.S./Canadian Brand Names Pradax™ [Can]

Therapeutic Category Anticoagulant, Thrombin Inhibitor

Use Postoperative thromboprophylaxis in patients who have undergone total hip or knee replacement procedures

Usual Dosage Oral: **Note:** Therapy should not be initiated until hemostasis has been established. When transitioning from intravenous anticoagulation therapy, initiate oral dabigatran therapy no sooner than time of next regularly scheduled dose of I.V. anticoagulant. When transitioning from dabigatran to I.V. anticoagulation therapy, allow 24 hours after the last dabigatran dose before initiating I.V. anticoagulation therapy.

Adults: Postoperative thromboprophylaxis:

Knee replacement: Initial: 110 mg given 1-4 hours after completion of surgery and establishment of hemostasis **OR** 220 mg as one dose in postoperative patients in whom therapy is not initiated on day of surgery regardless of reason; maintenance: 220 mg once daily (total duration of therapy: 10 days)

Hip replacement: Initial: 110 mg given 1-4 hours after completion of surgery and establishment of hemostasis **OR** 220 mg as one dose in postoperative patients in whom therapy is not initiated on day of surgery regardless of reason; maintenance: 220 mg once daily (total duration of therapy: 28-35 days)

Dosage Forms [CAN] = Canadian brand name

Capsule:

Pradax™ [CAN]: 75 mg, 110 mg [not available in the U.S.]

dabigatran etexilate mesilate *see* dabigatran etexilate *(Canada only) on page 262*

dacarbazine (da KAR ba zeen)

Sound-Alike/Look-Alike Issues

dacarbazine may be confused with Dicarbosil®, procarbazine

Synonyms DIC; dimethyl triazeno imidazole carboxamide; DTIC; imidazole carboxamide; imidazole carboxamide dimethyltriazene; WR-139007

U.S./Canadian Brand Names DTIC® [Can]

Therapeutic Category Antineoplastic Agent

Use Treatment of malignant melanoma, Hodgkin disease, soft-tissue sarcomas, fibrosarcomas, rhabdomyosarcoma, islet cell carcinoma, medullary carcinoma of the thyroid, and neuroblastoma

Usual Dosage Refer to individual protocols. Some dosage regimens include:

Intraarterial: 50-400 mg/m^2 for 5-10 days

I.V.:

Hodgkin disease, ABVD: 375 mg/m^2 days 1 and 15 every 4 weeks **or** 100 mg/m^2/day for 5 days

Metastatic melanoma (alone or in combination with other agents): 150-250 mg/m^2 days 1-5 every 3-4 weeks

Metastatic melanoma: 850 mg/m^2 every 3 weeks

High dose: Bone marrow/blood cell transplantation: I.V.: 1-3 g/m^2; maximum dose as a single agent: 3.38 g/m^2; generally combined with other high-dose chemotherapeutic drugs

Dosage Forms

Injection, powder for reconstitution: 100 mg, 200 mg

Dacex-DM [US] *see* guaifenesin, dextromethorphan, and phenylephrine *on page 459*

daclizumab (dac KLYE zue mab)

U.S./Canadian Brand Names Zenapax® [US/Can]

Therapeutic Category Immunosuppressant Agent

Use Part of an immunosuppressive regimen (including cyclosporine and corticosteroids) for the prophylaxis of acute organ rejection in patients receiving renal transplant

Usual Dosage Daclizumab is used adjunctively with other immunosuppressants (eg, cyclosporine, corticosteroids, mycophenolate mofetil, and azathioprine): I.V.:

Children: Use same weight-based dose as adults

Adults: Immunoprophylaxis against acute renal allograft rejection: 1 mg/kg infused over 15 minutes within 24 hours before transplantation (day 0), then every 14 days for 4 additional doses

Dosage Forms

Injection, solution [concentrate; preservative free]:

Zenapax®: 5 mg/mL (5 mL)

Dacodyl™ [US-OTC] *see* bisacodyl *on page 136*

Dacogen™ [US] *see* decitabine *on page 270*
DACT *see* dactinomycin *on page 264*

dactinomycin (dak ti noe MYE sin)

Sound-Alike/Look-Alike Issues
DACTINomycin may be confused with DAPTOmycin, DAUNOrubicin
actinomycin may be confused with achromycin
Synonyms ACT; Act-D; actinomycin; actinomycin Cl; actinomycin D; DACT; NSC-3053
Tall-Man DACTINomycin
U.S./Canadian Brand Names Cosmegen® [US/Can]
Therapeutic Category Antineoplastic Agent
Use Treatment of testicular tumors, melanoma, gestational trophoblastic neoplasm, Wilms tumor, neuroblastoma, retinoblastoma, rhabdomyosarcoma, uterine sarcomas, Ewing sarcoma, Kaposi sarcoma, sarcoma botryoides, and soft tissue sarcoma
Usual Dosage Refer to individual protocols:
Note: Medication orders for dactinomycin are commonly written in MICROgrams (eg, 150 mcg) although many regimens list the dose in MILLIgrams (eg, mg/kg or mg/m^2). One-time doses for >1000 mcg, or multiple-day doses for >500 mcg/day are not common. The dose intensity per 2-week cycle for adults and children should not exceed 15 mcg/kg/day for 5 days or 400-600 mcg/m^2/day for 5 days. Some practitioners recommend calculation of the dosage for obese or edematous adult patients on the basis of body surface area in an effort to relate dosage to lean body mass.
Children >6 months: I.V.: Usual dose: 15 mcg/kg/day **or** 400-600 mcg/m^2/day for 5 days every 3-6 weeks
Wilms tumor, rhabdomyosarcoma, Ewing sarcoma: 15 mcg/kg/day for 5 days (in various combination regimens and schedules)
Adults: I.V.:
Usual doses:
2.5 mg/m^2 in divided doses over 1 week, repeated every 2 weeks **or**
0.75-2 mg/m^2 every 1-4 weeks **or**
400-600 mcg/m^2/day for 5 days, repeated every 3-6 weeks
Testicular cancer: 1000 mcg/m^2 on day 1 (as part of a combination chemotherapy regimen)
Gestational trophoblastic neoplasm: 12 mcg/kg/day for 5 days **or** 500 mcg days 1 and 2 (as part of a combination chemotherapy regimen)
Wilms tumor, Ewing sarcoma: 15 mcg/kg/day for 5 days (in various combination regimens and schedules)
Dosage Forms
Injection, powder for reconstitution:
Cosmegen®: 0.5 mg

Daily Prenatal [US] *see* vitamins (multiple/prenatal) *on page 983*
Dairyaid® [Can] *see* lactase *on page 542*
Dakin's Solution [US] *see* sodium hypochlorite solution *on page 876*
Dakrina® Ophthalmic Solution *(Discontinued)* *see* artificial tears *on page 95*
Dalacin® C [Can] *see* clindamycin *on page 230*
Dalacin® T [Can] *see* clindamycin *on page 230*
Dalacin® Vaginal [Can] *see* clindamycin *on page 230*
Dallergy® [US] *see* chlorpheniramine, phenylephrine, and methscopolamine *on page 210*
Dallergy-D® Syrup *(Discontinued)* *see* chlorpheniramine and phenylephrine *on page 206*
Dallergy Drops [US] *see* chlorpheniramine and phenylephrine *on page 206*
Dallergy®-JR [US] *see* chlorpheniramine and phenylephrine *on page 206*
Dalmane® [US/Can] *see* flurazepam *on page 416*
d-Alpha-Gems™ [US-OTC] *see* vitamin E *on page 981*
***d*-alpha tocopherol** *see* vitamin E *on page 981*

dalteparin (dal TE pa rin)

Synonyms dalteparin sodium; NSC-714371
U.S./Canadian Brand Names Fragmin® [US/Can]
Therapeutic Category Anticoagulant (Other)

Use Prevention of deep vein thrombosis which may lead to pulmonary embolism, in patients requiring abdominal surgery who are at risk for thromboembolism complications (eg, patients >40 years of age, obesity, patients with malignancy, history of deep vein thrombosis or pulmonary embolism, and surgical procedures requiring general anesthesia and lasting >30 minutes); prevention of DVT in patients undergoing hip-replacement surgery; patients immobile during an acute illness; acute treatment of unstable angina or non-Q-wave myocardial infarction; prevention of ischemic complications in patients on concurrent aspirin therapy; in patients with cancer, extended treatment (6 months) of acute symptomatic venous thromboembolism (DVT and/or PE) to reduce the recurrence of venous thromboembolism

Usual Dosage SubQ: Adults:

Abdominal surgery:

Low-to-moderate DVT risk: 2500 int. units 1-2 hours prior to surgery, then once daily for 5-10 days postoperatively

High DVT risk: 5000 int. units the evening prior to surgery and then once daily for 5-10 days postoperatively. Alternatively in patients with malignancy: 2500 int. units 1-2 hours prior to surgery, 2500 int. units 12 hours later, then 5000 int. units once daily for 5-10 days postoperatively.

Patients undergoing total hip surgery: **Note:** Three treatment options are currently available. Dose is given for 5-10 days, although up to 14 days of treatment have been tolerated in clinical trials:

Postoperative start:

Initial: 2500 int. units 4-8 hours* after surgery

Maintenance: 5000 int. units once daily; start at least 6 hours after postsurgical dose

Preoperative (starting day of surgery):

Initial: 2500 int. units within 2 hours before surgery

Adjustment: 2500 int. units 4-8 hours* after surgery

Maintenance: 5000 int. units once daily; start at least 6 hours after postsurgical dose

Preoperative (starting evening prior to surgery):

Initial: 5000 int. units 10-14 hours before surgery

Adjustment: 5000 int. units 4-8 hours* after surgery

Maintenance: 5000 int. units once daily, allowing 24 hours between doses.

*Dose may be delayed if hemostasis is not yet achieved.

Unstable angina or non-Q-wave myocardial infarction: 120 int. units/kg body weight (maximum dose: 10,000 int. units) every 12 hours for 5-8 days with concurrent aspirin therapy. Discontinue dalteparin once patient is clinically stable.

Venous thromboembolism: Cancer patients:

Initial (month 1): 200 int. units/kg (maximum dose: 18,000 int. units) once daily for 30 days

Maintenance (months 2-6): ~150 int. units/kg (maximum dose: 18,000 int. units) once daily. If platelet count between 50,000-100,000/mm^3, reduce dose by 2,500 int. units until platelet count recovers to ≥100,000/mm^3. If platelet count <50,000/mm^3, discontinue dalteparin until platelet count recover to >50,000/mm^3.

Immobility during acute illness: 5000 int. units once daily

Dosage Forms

Injection, solution:

Fragmin®: Antifactor Xa 10,000 int. units per 1 mL (9.5 mL); antifactor Xa 25,000 units per 1 mL (3.8 mL)

Injection, solution [preservative free]:

Fragmin®: Antifactor Xa 2500 int. units per 0.2 mL (0.2 mL); antifactor Xa 5000 int. units per 0.2 mL (0.2 mL); antifactor Xa 7500 int. units per 0.3 mL (0.3 mL); antifactor Xa 10,000 int. units per 1 mL (1 mL); antifactor Xa 12,500 int. units per 0.5 mL (0.5 mL); antifactor Xa 15,000 int. units per 0.6 mL (0.6 mL); antifactor Xa 18,000 int. units per 0.72 mL (0.72 mL)

dalteparin sodium *see dalteparin on page 264*

Damason-P® *(Discontinued)*

danaparoid *(Canada only)* (da NAP a roid)

Sound-Alike/Look-Alike Issues

Orgaran® may be confused with argatroban

Synonyms danaparoid sodium

U.S./Canadian Brand Names Orgaran® [Can]

Therapeutic Category Anticoagulant (Other)

Use Prevention of postoperative deep vein thrombosis following elective hip replacement surgery

Usual Dosage SubQ: Adults: Prevention of DVT following hip replacement: 750 anti-Xa units twice daily; beginning 1-4 hours before surgery and then not sooner than 2 hours after surgery and every 12 hours until the risk of DVT has diminished. The average duration of therapy is 7-10 days.

◄ **Dosage Forms** [CAN] = Canadian brand name
Injection, solution:
Orgaran® [CAN]: 750 anti-Xa units/0.6 mL (0.6 mL) [not available in the U.S.]

danaparoid sodium *see* danaparoid *(Canada only) on page 265*

danazol (DA na zole)
Sound-Alike/Look-Alike Issues
danazol may be confused with Dantrium®
Danocrine® may be confused with Dacriose®
U.S./Canadian Brand Names Cyclomen® [Can]; Danocrine® [Can]
Therapeutic Category Androgen
Use Treatment of endometriosis, fibrocystic breast disease, and hereditary angioedema
Usual Dosage Oral: Adults:
Females: Endometriosis: Initial: 200-400 mg/day in 2 divided doses for mild disease; individualize dosage. Usual maintenance dose: 800 mg/day in 2 divided doses to achieve amenorrhea and rapid response to painful symptoms. Continue therapy uninterrupted for 3-6 months (up to 9 months).
Females: Fibrocystic breast disease: Range: 100-400 mg/day in 2 divided doses
Males/Females: Hereditary angioedema: Initial: 200 mg 2-3 times/day; after favorable response, decrease the dosage by 50% or less at intervals of 1-3 months or longer if the frequency of attacks dictates. If an attack occurs, increase the dosage by up to 200 mg/day.
Dosage Forms
Capsule: 50 mg, 100 mg, 200 mg

Dandrex [US-OTC] *see* selenium sulfide *on page 861*
Danocrine® [Can] *see* danazol *on page 266*
Danocrine® *(Discontinued)* *see* danazol *on page 266*
Dantrium® [US/Can] *see* dantrolene *on page 266*

dantrolene (DAN troe leen)
Sound-Alike/Look-Alike Issues
Dantrium® may be confused with danazol, Daraprim®
Synonyms dantrolene sodium
U.S./Canadian Brand Names Dantrium® [US/Can]
Therapeutic Category Skeletal Muscle Relaxant
Use Treatment of spasticity associated with spinal cord injury, stroke, cerebral palsy, or multiple sclerosis; treatment of malignant hyperthermia
Usual Dosage
Spasticity: Oral:
Children: Initial: 0.5 mg/kg/dose twice daily, increase frequency to 3-4 times/day at 4- to 7-day intervals, then increase dose by 0.5 mg/kg to a maximum of 3 mg/kg/dose 2-4 times/day up to 400 mg/day
Adults: 25 mg/day to start, increase frequency to 2-4 times/day, then increase dose by 25 mg every 4-7 days to a maximum of 100 mg 2-4 times/day or 400 mg/day

Malignant hyperthermia: Children and Adults:
Preoperative prophylaxis:
Oral: 4-8 mg/kg/day in 4 divided doses, begin 1-2 days prior to surgery with last dose 3-4 hours prior to surgery
I.V.: 2.5 mg/kg ~1¼ hours prior to anesthesia and infused over 1 hour with additional doses as needed and individualized
Crisis: I.V.: 2.5 mg/kg; may repeat dose up to cumulative dose of 10 mg/kg; if physiologic and metabolic abnormalities reappear, repeat regimen
Postcrisis follow-up: Oral: 4-8 mg/kg/day in 4 divided doses for 1-3 days; I.V. dantrolene may be used when oral therapy is not practical; individualize dosage beginning with 1 mg/kg or more as the clinical situation dictates
Dosage Forms
Capsule: 25 mg, 50 mg, 100 mg
Dantrium®: 25 mg, 50 mg, 100 mg
Injection, powder for reconstitution:
Dantrium®: 20 mg

dantrolene sodium *see* dantrolene *on page 266*
dapcin *see* daptomycin *on page 267*
dapiprazole *(Discontinued)*

dapsone (DAP sone)

Sound-Alike/Look-Alike Issues
dapsone may be confused with Diprosone®
Synonyms diaminodiphenylsulfone
Therapeutic Category Sulfone
Use Treatment of leprosy and dermatitis herpetiformis (infections caused by *Mycobacterium leprae*)
Usual Dosage Oral:
Leprosy:
Children: 1-2 mg/kg/24 hours, up to a maximum of 100 mg/day
Adults: 50-100 mg/day for 3-10 years
Dermatitis herpetiformis: Adults: Start at 50 mg/day, increase to 300 mg/day, or higher to achieve full control, reduce dosage to minimum level as soon as possible
Dosage Forms
Tablet: 25 mg, 100 mg

Daptacel® [US] *see* diphtheria, tetanus toxoids, and acellular pertussis vaccine *on page 309*

daptomycin (DAP toe mye sin)

Sound-Alike/Look-Alike Issues
DAPTOmycin may be confused with DACTINomycin
Cubicin® may be confused with Cleocin®
Synonyms cidecin; dapcin; LY146032
Tall-Man DAPTOmycin
U.S./Canadian Brand Names Cubicin® [US/Can]
Therapeutic Category Antibiotic, Cyclic Lipopeptide
Use Treatment of complicated skin and skin structure infections caused by susceptible aerobic gram-positive organisms; *Staphylococcus aureus* bacteremia, including right-sided infective endocarditis caused by MSSA or MRSA
Usual Dosage I.V.: Adults:
Skin and soft tissue: 4 mg/kg once daily for 7-14 days
Bacteremia, right-sided endocarditis caused by MSSA or MRSA: 6 mg/kg once daily for 2-6 weeks
Dosage Forms
Injection, powder for reconstitution:
Cubicin®: 500 mg

Daranide® [US/Can] *see* dichlorphenamide *on page 291*
Daraprim® [US/Can] *see* pyrimethamine *on page 809*

darbepoetin alfa (dar be POE e tin AL fa)

Sound-Alike/Look-Alike Issues
darbepoetin alfa may be confused with epoetin alfa, epoetin beta
Synonyms erythropoiesis-stimulating agent (ESA); erythropoiesis-stimulating protein; NSC-729969
U.S./Canadian Brand Names Aranesp® [US/Can]
Therapeutic Category Colony-Stimulating Factor; Growth Factor; Recombinant Human Erythropoietin
Use Treatment of anemia (elevate/maintain red blood cell level and decrease the need for transfusions) associated with chronic renal failure (including patients on dialysis and not on dialysis); treatment of anemia due to concurrent chemotherapy in patients with metastatic cancer (nonmyeloid malignancies)
Note: Darbepoetin is **not** indicated for use in cancer patients under the following conditions:
  • receiving hormonal therapy, therapeutic biologic products, or radiation therapy unless also receiving concurrent myelosuppressive chemotherapy
  • receiving myelosuppressive therapy when the expected outcome is curative
Usual Dosage Anemia associated with CRF: Individualize dosing to achieve and maintain hemoglobin levels between 10-12 g/dL. Hemoglobin levels should not exceed 12 g/dL. **Note:** I.V. route is preferred in hemodialysis patients.

◀ **Dosage Forms**
Injection, solution [preservative free]:
Aranesp®: 25 mcg/0.42 mL (0.42 mL); 40 mcg/ 0.4 mL (0.4 mL); 60 mcg/0.3 mL (0.3 mL); 100 mcg/0.5 mL (0.5 mL); 150 mcg/0.3 mL (0.3 mL); 200 mcg/0.4 mL (0.4 mL); 300 mcg/0.6 mL (0.6 mL); 500 mcg/ mL (1 mL) [contains polysorbate 80; prefilled syringe; needle cover contains latex]
Aranesp®: 25 mcg/mL (1 mL); 40 mcg/mL (1 mL); 60 mcg/mL (1 mL); 100 mcg/mL (1 mL); 150 mcg/0.75 mL (0.75 mL); 200 mcg/mL (1 mL); 300 mcg/mL (1 mL) [contains polysorbate 80; single-dose vial]

darifenacin (dar i FEN a sin)

Synonyms darifenacin hydrobromide; UK-88,525
U.S./Canadian Brand Names Enablex® [US/Can]
Therapeutic Category Anticholinergic Agent
Use Management of symptoms of bladder overactivity (urge incontinence, urgency, and frequency)
Usual Dosage Oral: Adults: Initial: 7.5 mg once daily. If response is not adequate after a minimum of 2 weeks, dosage may be increased to 15 mg once daily.
Dosage Forms
Tablet, extended release:
Enablex®: 7.5 mg, 15 mg

darifenacin hydrobromide *see darifenacin on page 268*

darunavir (dar OO na veer)

Synonyms darunavir ethanolate; TMC-114
U.S./Canadian Brand Names Prezista™ [US]
Therapeutic Category Antiretroviral Agent, Protease Inhibitor
Use Treatment of HIV-1 infections in combination with ritonavir and other antiretroviral agents; limited to highly treatment-experienced or multiprotease inhibitor-resistant patients
Usual Dosage Oral: Adults: 600 mg twice daily with meals
Note: Coadministration with ritonavir (100 mg twice daily) is required.
Dosage Forms
Tablet:
Prezista™: 300 mg, 600 mg

darunavir ethanolate *see darunavir on page 268*
Darvocet A500® [US] *see propoxyphene and acetaminophen on page 795*
Darvocet-N® 50 [US/Can] *see propoxyphene and acetaminophen on page 795*
Darvocet-N® 100 [US/Can] *see propoxyphene and acetaminophen on page 795*
Darvon® [US] *see propoxyphene on page 795*
Darvon® Compound (Discontinued) *see propoxyphene, aspirin, and caffeine on page 796*
Darvon-N® [US/Can] *see propoxyphene on page 795*

dasatinib (da SA ti nib)

Synonyms BMS-354825; NSC-732517
U.S./Canadian Brand Names Sprycel® [US/Can]
Therapeutic Category Antineoplastic Agent, Tyrosine Kinase Inhibitor
Use Treatment of chronic myelogenous leukemia (CML) in chronic, accelerated or blast (myeloid or lymphoid) phase resistant or intolerant to prior therapy (including imatinib); treatment of Philadelphia chromosome-positive (Ph+) acute lymphoblastic leukemia (ALL) resistant or intolerant to prior therapy
Usual Dosage Oral: Adults:
CML:
Chronic phase: 100 mg once daily. In clinical studies, a dose escalation to 140 mg once daily was allowed in patients not achieving cytogenetic response at recommended initial dosage.
Canadian labeling: 70 mg twice daily (dose escalation to 90 mg twice daily was allowed).
Accelerated or blast phase: 70 mg twice daily. In clinical studies, a dose escalation to 100 mg twice daily was allowed in patients not achieving cytogenetic response at recommended initial dosage.
Ph+ ALL: 70 mg twice daily. In clinical studies, a dose escalation to 100 mg twice daily was allowed in patients not achieving cytogenetic response at recommended initial dosage.

Dosage Forms
Tablet, oral:
Sprycel®: 20 mg, 50 mg, 70 mg, 100 mg

daunomycin *see* daunorubicin hydrochloride *on page 269*

daunorubicin citrate (liposomal) (daw noe ROO bi sin SI trate lip po SOE mal)
Sound-Alike/Look-Alike Issues
DAUNOrubicin liposomal may be confused with dactinomycin, DOXOrubicin, DOXOrubicin liposomal, epirubicin, idarubicin
Liposomal formulation (DaunoXome®) may be confused with the conventional formulation (Cerubidine®, Rubex®)
Synonyms DAUNOrubicin liposomal; liposomal DAUNOrubicin; NSC-697732
Tall-Man DAUNOrubicin citrate (liposomal)
U.S./Canadian Brand Names DaunoXome® [US]
Therapeutic Category Antineoplastic Agent
Use First-line treatment of advanced HIV-associated Kaposi sarcoma (KS)
Usual Dosage I.V. (refer to individual protocols): Adults: HIV-associated KS: 40 mg/m^2 every 2 weeks
Dosage Forms
Injection, solution [preservative free]:
DaunoXome®: 2 mg/mL (25 mL)

daunorubicin hydrochloride (daw noe ROO bi sin hye droe KLOR ide)
Sound-Alike/Look-Alike Issues
DAUNOrubicin may be confused with dactinomycin, DOXOrubicin, DOXOrubicin liposomal, epirubicin, idarubicin
Conventional formulation (Cerubidine®, DAUNOrubicin hydrochloride) may be confused with the liposomal formulation (DaunoXome®)
Synonyms daunomycin; NSC-82151; rubidomycin hydrochloride
Tall-Man DAUNOrubicin hydrochloride
U.S./Canadian Brand Names Cerubidine® [US/Can]
Therapeutic Category Antineoplastic Agent
Use Treatment of acute lymphocytic (ALL) and nonlymphocytic (ANLL) leukemias
Usual Dosage I.V. (refer to individual protocols):
Children: **Note:** Cumulative dose should not exceed 300 mg/m^2 in children >2 years or 10 mg/kg in children <2 years of age; maximum cumulative doses for younger children are unknown.
Children <2 years or BSA <0.5 m^2: ALL combination therapy: 1 mg/kg/dose per protocol, with frequency dependent on regimen employed
Children ≥2 years and BSA ≥0.5 m^2:
ALL combination therapy: Remission induction: 25 mg/m^2 on day 1 every week for up to 4-6 cycles
AML combination therapy: Induction: I.V. continuous infusion: 30-60 mg/m^2/day on days 1-3 of cycle
Adults: **Note:** Cumulative dose should not exceed 550 mg/m^2 in adults without risk factors for cardiotoxicity and should not exceed 400 mg/m^2 in adults receiving chest irradiation.
Range: 30-60 mg/m^2/day for 3 days, repeat dose in 3-4 weeks
ALL combination therapy: 45 mg/m^2/day for 3 days
AML combination therapy:
Adults <60 years: Induction: 45 mg/m^2/day for 3 days of the first course of induction therapy; subsequent courses: 45 mg/m^2/day for 2 days
Adults ≥60 years: Induction: 30 mg/m^2/day for 3 days of the first course of induction therapy; subsequent courses: 30 mg/m^2/day for 2 days
Dosage Forms
Injection, powder for reconstitution: 20 mg
Cerubidine®: 20 mg
Injection, solution: 5 mg/mL (4 mL, 10 mL)

DAUNOrubicin liposomal *see* daunorubicin citrate (liposomal) *on page 269*
DaunoXome® [US] *see* daunorubicin citrate (liposomal) *on page 269*
1-Day™ [US-OTC] *see* tioconazole *on page 929*
Dayhist® Allergy [US-OTC] *see* clemastine *on page 228*

Daypro® [US/Can] *see* oxaprozin *on page 706*
Dayto Himbin® *(Discontinued) see* yohimbine *on page 988*
Daytrana™ [US] *see* methylphenidate *on page 622*
DC 240® Softgel® *(Discontinued) see* docusate *on page 314*
dCF *see* pentostatin *on page 737*
DDAVP® [US/Can] *see* desmopressin acetate *on page 275*
ddI *see* didanosine *on page 294*
1-deamino-8-D-arginine vasopressin *see* desmopressin acetate *on page 275*
Debrox® [US-OTC] *see* carbamide peroxide *on page 174*
Decadron® [US] *see* dexamethasone (systemic) *on page 278*
Decadron® Phosphate *(Discontinued) see* dexamethasone (systemic) *on page 278*
Deca-Durabolin® [Can] *see* nandrolone *on page 655*
Deca-Durabolin® *(Discontinued) see* nandrolone *on page 655*
Decahist-DM *(Discontinued)*
Decavac™ [US] *see* diphtheria and tetanus toxoid *on page 306*
Dec-Chlorphen [US] *see* chlorpheniramine and phenylephrine *on page 206*
Dec-Chlorphen DM *(Discontinued) see* chlorpheniramine, phenylephrine, and dextromethorphan *on page 209*
De-Chlor DM [US] *see* chlorpheniramine, phenylephrine, and dextromethorphan *on page 209*
De-Chlor DR [US] *see* chlorpheniramine, phenylephrine, and dextromethorphan *on page 209*
De-Chlor G *(Discontinued)*
De-Chlor HC [US] *see* phenylephrine, hydrocodone, and chlorpheniramine *on page 748*

decitabine (de SYE ta been)

Synonyms 5-aza-2'-deoxycytidine; 5-azaC; NSC-127716
U.S./Canadian Brand Names Dacogen™ [US]
Therapeutic Category Antineoplastic Agent, Antimetabolite (Pyrimidine)
Use Treatment of myelodysplastic syndrome (MDS)
Usual Dosage I.V.: Adults: MDS: 15 mg/m^2 over 3 hours every 8 hours (45 mg/m^2/day) for 3 days (135 mg/m^2/cycle) every 6 weeks. Treatment is recommended for at least 4 cycles and may continue until the patient no longer continues to benefit.
Dosage Forms
Injection, powder for reconstitution:
Dacogen™: 50 mg

Declomycin® [US/Can] *see* demeclocycline *on page 272*
Deconamine® SR [US] *see* chlorpheniramine and pseudoephedrine *on page 207*
Deconsal® II [US] *see* guaifenesin and phenylephrine *on page 456*
Deconsal® CT [US] *see* phenylephrine and pyrilamine *on page 747*
Deep Sea [US-OTC] *see* sodium chloride *on page 873*
Defen-LA® *(Discontinued) see* guaifenesin and pseudoephedrine *on page 458*

deferasirox (de FER a sir ox)

Sound-Alike/Look-Alike Issues
deferasirox may be confused with deferoxamine
Synonyms ICL670
U.S./Canadian Brand Names Exjade® [US/Can]
Therapeutic Category Antidote; Chelating Agent
Use Treatment of chronic iron overload due to blood transfusions (transfusional hemosiderosis)
Usual Dosage Oral: Children ≥2 years and Adults:
Initial: 20 mg/kg daily (calculate dose to nearest whole tablet)
Maintenance: Adjust dose every 3-6 months based on serum ferritin levels; increase by 5-10 mg/kg/day (calculate dose to nearest whole tablet); titrate. Maximum dose: 30 mg/kg/day; consider interrupting therapy for serum ferritin <500 mcg/L. **Note:** Consider dose reduction or interruption for hearing loss or visual disturbances.

Dosage Forms
  Tablet, for oral suspension:
  Exjade®: 125 mg, 250 mg, 500 mg

deferoxamine (de fer OKS a meen)

Sound-Alike/Look-Alike Issues
  deferoxamine may be confused with cefuroxime, deferasirox
  Desferal® may be confused with desflurane, Dexferrum®, Disophrol®
Synonyms deferoxamine mesylate; desferrioxamine; NSC-644468
U.S./Canadian Brand Names Desferal® [US/Can]; PMS-Deferoxamine [Can]
Therapeutic Category Antidote
Use Acute iron intoxication or when clinical signs of significant iron toxicity exist; chronic iron overload secondary to multiple transfusions
Usual Dosage
  Acute iron toxicity: **Note:** I.V. route is used when severe toxicity is evidenced by systemic symptoms (coma, shock, metabolic acidosis, or severe gastrointestinal bleeding) or potentially severe intoxications (serum iron level >500 mcg/dL). When severe symptoms are not present, the I.M. route may be preferred (per manufacturer); however, the use of deferoxamine in situations where the serum iron concentration is <500 mcg/dL or when severe toxicity is not evident is a subject of some clinical debate.
  Children ≥3 years:
    I.M.: 90 mg/kg/dose every 8 hours (maximum: 6 g/24 hours)
    I.V.: 15 mg/kg/hour (maximum: 6 g/24 hours)
  Adults: I.M., I.V.: Initial: 1000 mg, may be followed by 500 mg every 4 hours for up to 2 doses; subsequent doses of 500 mg have been administered every 4-12 hours
    Maximum recommended dose: 6 g/day (per manufacturer, however, higher doses have been administered)
  Chronic iron overload:
  Children ≥3 years:
    I.V.: 15 mg/kg/hour (maximum: 12 g/24 hours)
    SubQ: 20-40 mg/kg/day over 8-12 hours (maximum: 1000-2000 mg/day)
  Adults:
    I.M., I.V.: 500-1000 mg/day I.M.; in addition, 2000 mg should be given I.V. with each unit of blood transfused (administer separately from blood); maximum: 1 g/day in absence of transfusions; 6 g/day if patient received transfusions
    SubQ: 1-2 g every day or 20-40 mg/kg/day over 8-24 hours
Dosage Forms
  Injection, powder for reconstitution: 500 mg, 2 g
    Desferal®: 500 mg, 2 g

deferoxamine mesylate see deferoxamine on page 271
Deficol® (Discontinued) see bisacodyl on page 136
Definity® [US/Can] see perflutren lipid microspheres on page 738
Degest® 2 Ophthalmic (Discontinued) see naphazoline on page 655
Dehistine [US] see chlorpheniramine, phenylephrine, and methscopolamine on page 210
Dehydral® [Can] see methenamine on page 614
dehydrobenzperidol see droperidol on page 326
Del Aqua® [US] see benzoyl peroxide on page 126
Delatest® Injection (Discontinued) see testosterone on page 912
Delatestryl® [US/Can] see testosterone on page 912

delavirdine (de la VIR deen)

Synonyms U-90152S
U.S./Canadian Brand Names Rescriptor® [US/Can]
Therapeutic Category Antiviral Agent
Use Treatment of HIV-1 infection in combination with at least two additional antiretroviral agents
Usual Dosage Oral: Adolescents ≥16 years and Adults: 400 mg 3 times/day
Dosage Forms
  Tablet:
    Rescriptor®: 100 mg, 200 mg

Delestrogen® [US] *see* estradiol *on page 359*
Delfen® [US-OTC] *see* nonoxynol 9 *on page 677*
Delsym® [US-OTC] *see* dextromethorphan *on page 284*
delta-9-tetrahydro-cannabinol *see* dronabinol *on page 326*
delta-9-tetrahydrocannabinol and cannabinol *see* tetrahydrocannabinol and cannabidiol *(Canada only) on page 915*
delta-9 THC *see* dronabinol *on page 326*
Delta-D® [US-OTC] *see* cholecalciferol *on page 215*
deltacortisone *see* prednisone *on page 782*
deltadehydrocortisone *see* prednisone *on page 782*
deltahydrocortisone *see* prednisolone (systemic) *on page 781*
Del-Vi-A® *(Discontinued)* *see* vitamin A *on page 979*
Demadex® [US] *see* torsemide *on page 937*

demeclocycline (dem e kloe SYE kleen)

Synonyms demeclocycline hydrochloride; demethylchlortetracycline
U.S./Canadian Brand Names Declomycin® [US/Can]
Therapeutic Category Tetracycline Derivative
Use Treatment of susceptible bacterial infections (acne, gonorrhea, pertussis, and urinary tract infections) caused by both gram-negative and gram-positive organisms
Usual Dosage Oral:
  Children ≥8 years: 8-12 mg/kg/day divided every 6-12 hours
  Adults: 150 mg 4 times/day or 300 mg twice daily
Dosage Forms
  Tablet: 150 mg, 300 mg
    Declomycin®: 150 mg, 300 mg

demeclocycline hydrochloride *see* demeclocycline *on page 272*
Demerol® [US/Can] *see* meperidine *on page 603*
4-demethoxydaunorubicin *see* idarubicin *on page 498*
demethylchlortetracycline *see* demeclocycline *on page 272*
Demser® [US/Can] *see* metyrosine *on page 629*
Demulen® 30 [Can] *see* ethinyl estradiol and ethynodiol diacetate *on page 371*
Demulen® *(Discontinued)* *see* ethinyl estradiol and ethynodiol diacetate *on page 371*
Denavir® [US] *see* penciclovir *on page 730*

denileukin diftitox (de ni LOO kin DIF ti toks)

Synonyms DAB$_{389}$IL-2; NSC-714744
U.S./Canadian Brand Names ONTAK® [US]
Therapeutic Category Antineoplastic Agent, Miscellaneous
Use Treatment of persistent or recurrent cutaneous T-cell lymphoma (CTCL) whose malignant cells express the CD25 component of the IL-2 receptor
Usual Dosage I.V.: Adults: 9 or 18 mcg/kg/day days 1 through 5 every 21 days
Dosage Forms
  Injection, solution [frozen]:
    ONTAK®: 150 mcg/mL (2 mL)

Denorex® Daily Protection [US-OTC] *see* pyrithione zinc *on page 810*
Denorex® Original Therapeutic Strength [US-OTC] *see* coal tar *on page 240*
Denta 5000 Plus [US] *see* fluoride *on page 411*
DentaGel [US] *see* fluoride *on page 411*
Dentapaine [US-OTC] *see* benzocaine *on page 124*
Dent's Ear Wax *(Discontinued)* *see* carbamide peroxide *on page 174*
Dent's Extra Strength Toothache [US-OTC] *see* benzocaine *on page 124*
2'-deoxycoformycin *see* pentostatin *on page 737*
deoxycoformycin *see* pentostatin *on page 737*
Depacon® [US] *see* valproic acid and derivatives *on page 967*

Depade® [US] *see* naltrexone *on page 654*
Depakene® [US/Can] *see* valproic acid and derivatives *on page 967*
Depakote® [US] *see* valproic acid and derivatives *on page 967*
Depakote® ER [US] *see* valproic acid and derivatives *on page 967*
Depakote® Sprinkle [US] *see* valproic acid and derivatives *on page 967*
depAndro® Injection *(Discontinued)* *see* testosterone *on page 912*
Depen® [US/Can] *see* penicillamine *on page 730*
depGynogen® Injection *(Discontinued)* *see* estradiol *on page 359*
Deplin™ [US] *see* methylfolate *on page 621*
depMedalone® Injection *(Discontinued)* *see* methylprednisolone *on page 623*
DepoCyt® [US/Can] *see* cytarabine (liposomal) *on page 261*
DepoDur® [US] *see* morphine sulfate *on page 643*
Depo®-Estradiol [US/Can] *see* estradiol *on page 359*
Depoject® Injection *(Discontinued)* *see* methylprednisolone *on page 623*
Depo-Medrol® [US/Can] *see* methylprednisolone *on page 623*
Deponit® Patch *(Discontinued)* *see* nitroglycerin *on page 675*
Depo-Prevera® [Can] *see* medroxyprogesterone *on page 597*
Depo-Provera® [US/Can] *see* medroxyprogesterone *on page 597*
Depo-Provera® Contraceptive [US] *see* medroxyprogesterone *on page 597*
depo-subQ provera 104™ [US] *see* medroxyprogesterone *on page 597*
Depotest® 100 [Can] *see* testosterone *on page 912*
Depotest® Injection *(Discontinued)* *see* testosterone *on page 912*
Depo®-Testosterone [US] *see* testosterone *on page 912*
deprenyl *see* selegiline *on page 860*

dequalinium *(Canada only)* (de kwal LI ne um)

Therapeutic Category Antibacterial, Topical; Antifungal Agent, Topical
Use Treatment of mouth and throat infections
Usual Dosage Adults:
Lozenge: One lozenge sucked slowly every 2-3 hours
Oral paint: Apply freely to infected area, every 2-3 hours, or as directed by physician
Dosage Forms
Lozenge, as chloride: 0.25 mg (20s)
Oral paint, as chloride: 0.5% (25 mL)

Dermaflex® Gel *(Discontinued)* *see* lidocaine *on page 561*
DermaFungal [US-OTC] *see* miconazole *on page 630*
Dermagran® [US-OTC] *see* aluminum hydroxide *on page 53*
Dermagran® AF [US-OTC] *see* miconazole *on page 630*
Dermamycin® [US-OTC] *see* diphenhydramine *on page 304*
Dermarest Dricort® [US-OTC] *see* hydrocortisone (topical) *on page 485*
Dermarest® Psoriasis Medicated Moisturizer [US-OTC] *see* salicylic acid *on page 850*
Dermarest® Psoriasis Medicated Scalp Treatment [US-OTC] *see* salicylic acid *on page 850*
Dermarest® Psoriasis Medicated Shampoo/Conditioner [US-OTC] *see* salicylic acid *on page 850*
Dermarest® Psoriasis Medicated Skin Treatment [US-OTC] *see* salicylic acid *on page 850*
Dermarest® Psoriasis Overnight Treatment [US-OTC] *see* salicylic acid *on page 850*
Dermarest® Skin Correction Cream Plus [US-OTC] *see* hydroquinone *on page 488*
Derma-Smoothe/FS® [US/Can] *see* fluocinolone *on page 409*
Dermatop® [US/Can] *see* prednicarbate *on page 780*
Dermatophytin-O *(Discontinued)*
Dermazene® [US] *see* iodoquinol and hydrocortisone *on page 520*
DermaZinc™ [US-OTC] *see* pyrithione zinc *on page 810*
Dermazole [Can] *see* miconazole *on page 630*
Dermoplast® Antibacterial [US-OTC] *see* benzocaine *on page 124*

Dermoplast® Pain Relieving [US-OTC] *see* benzocaine *on page 124*
DermOtic® [US] *see* fluocinolone *on page 409*
Dermovate® [Can] *see* clobetasol *on page 232*
Dermtex® HC [US-OTC] *see* hydrocortisone (topical) *on page 485*
Desferal® [US/Can] *see* deferoxamine *on page 271*
desferrioxamine *see* deferoxamine *on page 271*

desflurane (DES flure ane)
Sound-Alike/Look-Alike Issues
desflurane may be confused with Desferal®
U.S./Canadian Brand Names Suprane® [US/Can]
Therapeutic Category General Anesthetic
Use Induction and maintenance of general anesthesia (adults); maintenance of anesthesia (intubated children)
Usual Dosage
Note: Concurrent use with benzodiazepines, nitrous oxide, or opioids decreases the desflurane dose.
Children (intubated): Maintenance: Surgical levels of anesthesia range between 5.2% to 10%
Adults: The minimum alveolar concentration (MAC), the concentration at which 50% of patients do not respond to surgical incision, ranges from 6.0% (45 years of age) to 7.3% (25 years of age). The concentration at which amnesia and loss of awareness occur (MAC - awake) is 2.4%. Surgical levels of anesthesia are achieved with concentrations between 2.5% to 8.5%.
Note: Because of the higher vapor pressure of desflurane, its vaporizer is heated in order to deliver a constant concentration
Dosage Forms
Liquid, for inhalation:
Suprane®: 100% (240 mL)

desiccated thyroid *see* thyroid, desiccated *on page 924*

desipramine (des IP ra meen)
Sound-Alike/Look-Alike Issues
desipramine may be confused with clomiPRAMINE, deserpidine, diphenhydrAMINE, disopyramide, imipramine, nortriptyline
Norpramin® may be confused with clomiPRAMINE, imipramine, Norpace®, nortriptyline, Tenormin®
Synonyms desipramine hydrochloride; desmethylimipramine hydrochloride
U.S./Canadian Brand Names Alti-Desipramine [Can]; Apo-Desipramine® [Can]; Norpramin® [US/Can]; Nu-Desipramine [Can]; PMS-Desipramine [Can]
Therapeutic Category Antidepressant, Tricyclic (Secondary Amine)
Use Treatment of depression
Usual Dosage Oral (dose is generally administered at bedtime): Depression:
Adolescents: Initial: 25-50 mg/day; gradually increase to 100 mg/day in single or divided doses (maximum: 150 mg/day)
Adults: Initial: 75 mg/day in divided doses; increase gradually to 150-200 mg/day in divided or single dose (maximum: 300 mg/day)
Dosage Forms
Tablet: 10 mg, 25 mg, 50 mg, 75 mg, 100 mg, 150 mg
Norpramin®: 10 mg, 25 mg, 50 mg, 75 mg, 100 mg, 150 mg

desipramine hydrochloride *see* desipramine *on page 274*
Desitin® [US-OTC] *see* zinc oxide *on page 993*
Desitin® Creamy [US-OTC] *see* zinc oxide *on page 993*

desloratadine (des lor AT a deen)
U.S./Canadian Brand Names Aerius® [Can]; Clarinex® [US]
Therapeutic Category Antihistamine, Nonsedating
Use Relief of nasal and non-nasal symptoms of seasonal allergic rhinitis (SAR) and perennial allergic rhinitis (PAR); treatment of chronic idiopathic urticaria (CIU)

Usual Dosage Oral:
Children:
  6-11 months: 1 mg once daily
  12 months to 5 years: 1.25 mg once daily
  6-11 years: 2.5 mg once daily
  Children ≥12 years and Adults: 5 mg once daily
Dosage Forms
  Syrup:
  Clarinex®: 0.5 mg/mL
  Tablet:
  Clarinex®: 5 mg
  Tablet, orally disintegrating:
  Clarinex® RediTabs®: 2.5 mg, 5 mg

desloratadine and pseudoephedrine (des lor AT a deen & soo doe e FED rin)

Synonyms pseudoephedrine and desloratadine

U.S./Canadian Brand Names Clarinex-D® 12 Hour [US]; Clarinex-D® 24 Hour [US]

Therapeutic Category Antihistamine/Decongestant Combination, Nonsedating

Use Relief of symptoms of seasonal allergic rhinitis, in children ≥12 years of age and adults

Usual Dosage Oral: Children ≥12 years and Adults:
Clarinex-D® 12 Hour: One tablet twice daily
Clarinex-D® 24 Hour: One tablet daily

Dosage Forms
  Tablet, variable release:
  Clarinex-D® 12 Hour: Desloratadine 2.5 mg [immediate release] and pseudoephedrine 120 mg [extended release]
  Clarinex-D® 24 Hour: Desloratadine 5 mg [immediate release] and pseudoephedrine 240 mg [extended release]

desmethylimipramine hydrochloride *see* desipramine *on page 274*

desmopressin acetate (des moe PRES in AS e tate)

Synonyms 1-deamino-8-D-arginine vasopressin

U.S./Canadian Brand Names Apo-Desmopressin® [Can]; DDAVP® [US/Can]; Minirin® [Can]; Nove-Desmopressin [Can]; Octostim® [Can]; PMS-Desmopressin [Can]; Stimate® [US]

Therapeutic Category Vasopressin Analog, Synthetic

Use
Injection: Treatment of diabetes insipidus; maintenance of hemostasis and control of bleeding in hemophilia A with factor VIII coagulant activity levels >5% and mild-to-moderate classic von Willebrand disease (type 1) with factor VIII coagulant activity levels >5%
Nasal solutions (DDAVP® Nasal Spray and DDAVP® Rhinal Tube): Treatment of central diabetes insipidus
Nasal spray (Stimate®): Maintenance of hemostasis and control of bleeding in hemophilia A with factor VIII coagulant activity levels >5% and mild to moderate classic von Willebrand's disease (type 1) with factor VIII coagulant activity levels >5%
Tablet: Treatment of central diabetes insipidus, temporary polyuria and polydipsia following pituitary surgery or head trauma, primary nocturnal enuresis

Usual Dosage
Children:
Diabetes insipidus:
  Intranasal (using 100 mcg/mL nasal solution): 3 months to 12 years: Initial: 5 mcg/day (0.05 mL/day) divided 1-2 times/day; range: 5-30 mcg/day (0.05-0.3 mL/day) divided 1-2 times/day; adjust morning and evening doses separately for an adequate diurnal rhythm of water turnover. **Note:** The nasal spray pump can only deliver doses of 10 mcg (0.1 mL) or multiples of 10 mcg (0.1 mL); if doses other than this are needed, the rhinal tube delivery system is preferred. Fluid restriction should be observed.
  Oral: ≥4 years: Initial: 0.05 mg twice daily; total daily dose should be increased or decreased as needed to obtain adequate antidiuresis (range: 0.1-1.2 mg divided 2-3 times/day). Fluid restriction should be observed.

◀ Hemophilia A and von Willebrand disease (type 1):
I.V.: ≥3 months: 0.3 mcg/kg by slow infusion; may repeat dose if needed; if used preoperatively, administer 30 minutes before procedure
Intranasal (using high concentration spray [1.5 mg/mL]): ≥11 months: Refer to adult dosing.
Nocturnal enuresis: Oral: ≥6 years: 0.2 mg at bedtime; dose may be titrated up to 0.6 mg to achieve desired response. Fluid intake should be limited 1 hour prior to dose until the next morning, or at least 8 hours after administration.
Children ≥12 years and Adults:
Diabetes insipidus:
I.V., SubQ: 2-4 mcg/day (0.5-1 mL) in 2 divided doses or ¹/₁₀ of the maintenance intranasal dose. Fluid restriction should be observed.
Intranasal (using 100 mcg/mL nasal solution): 10-40 mcg/day (0.1-0.4 mL) divided 1-3 times/day; adjust morning and evening doses separately for an adequate diurnal rhythm of water turnover. **Note:** The nasal spray pump can only deliver doses of 10 mcg (0.1 mL) or multiples of 10 mcg (0.1 mL); if doses other than this are needed, the rhinal tube delivery system is preferred. Fluid restriction should be observed.
Oral: Initial: 0.05 mg twice daily; total daily dose should be increased or decreased as needed to obtain adequate antidiuresis (range: 0.1-1.2 mg divided 2-3 times/day). Fluid restriction should be observed.
Hemophilia A and mild-to-moderate von Willebrand disease (type 1):
I.V.: 0.3 mcg/kg by slow infusion; if used preoperatively, administer 30 minutes before procedure
Intranasal (using high concentration spray [1.5 mg/mL]): <50 kg: 150 mcg (1 spray); >50 kg: 300 mcg (1 spray each nostril); repeat use is determined by the patient's clinical condition and laboratory work; if using preoperatively, administer 2 hours before surgery

Dosage Forms [CAN] = Canadian product
Injection, solution: 4 mcg/mL (1 mL, 10 mL)
DDAVP®: 4 mcg/mL (1 mL, 10 mL)
Solution, intranasal: 100 mcg/mL (2.5 mL)
DDAVP®: 100 mcg/mL (2.5 mL)
Solution, intranasal [spray]: 100 mcg/mL (5 mL)
DDAVP®: 100 mcg/mL (5 mL)
Stimate®: 1.5 mg/mL (2.5 mL)
Tablet, oral: 0.1 mg, 0.2 mg
DDAVP®: 0.1 mg, 0.2 mg
Tablet, sublingual:
DDAVP® Melt (CAN) [not available in U.S.]: 60 mcg, 120 mcg, 240 mcg

Desocort® [Can] see desonide on page 276
Desogen® [US] see ethinyl estradiol and desogestrel on page 369
desogestrel and ethinyl estradiol see ethinyl estradiol and desogestrel on page 369
Desonate™ [US] see desonide on page 276

desonide (DES oh nide)

U.S./Canadian Brand Names Desocort® [Can]; Desonate™ [US]; DesOwen® [US]; LoKara™ [US]; PMS-Desonide [Can]; Verdeso™ [US]
Therapeutic Category Corticosteroid, Topical
Use Adjunctive therapy for inflammation in acute and chronic corticosteroid responsive dermatosis (low potency corticosteroid); mild-to-moderate atopic dermatitis
Usual Dosage Topical:
Corticosteroid responsive dermatoses: Children and Adults: Therapy should be discontinued when control is achieved. If no improvement is seen within 2 weeks, reassessment of diagnosis may be necessary.
Cream, ointment: Apply 2-4 times/day sparingly
Lotion: Apply 2-3 times/day sparingly
Atopic dermatitis: Children ≥3 months and Adults: Aerosol, gel: Apply 2 times/day sparingly. Therapy should be discontinued when control is achieved. If no improvement is seen within 4 weeks, reassessment of diagnosis may be necessary.
Dosage Forms
Aerosol, topical [foam]:
Verdeso®: 0.05% (50 g, 100 g)
Cream, topical: 0.05% (15 g, 60 g)
DesOwen®: 0.05% (60 g)

Gel, topical [aqueous]:
  Desonate™: 0.05% (60 g)
Lotion, topical: 0.05% (60 mL, 120 mL)
  LoKara™: 0.05% (60 mL, 120 mL)
Ointment, topical: 0.05% (15 g, 60 g)
  DesOwen®: 0.05% (60 g)

DesOwen® [US] *see desonide on page 276*

desoximetasone (des oks i MET a sone)

Sound-Alike/Look-Alike Issues
  desoximetasone may be confused with dexamethasone
  Topicort® may be confused with Topic®
U.S./Canadian Brand Names Taro-Desoximetasone [Can]; Topicort® [US/Can]; Topicort®-LP [US]
Therapeutic Category Corticosteroid, Topical
Use Relieves inflammation and pruritic symptoms of corticosteroid-responsive dermatosis (intermediate-to high-potency topical corticosteroid)
Usual Dosage Desoximetasone is a potent fluorinated topical corticosteroid. Therapy should be discontinued when control is achieved; if no improvement is seen, reassessment of diagnosis may be necessary.

Cream, gel: Children and Adults: Apply a thin film to affected area twice daily
Ointment: Children ≥10 years and Adults: Apply a thin film to affected area twice daily
Dosage Forms
Cream, topical: 0.25% (15 g, 60 g); 0.05% (15 g, 60 g)
  Topicort®: 0.25% (15 g, 60 g)
  Topicort®-LP: 0.05% (15 g, 60 g)
Gel, topical: 0.05% (15 g, 60 g)
  Topicort®: 0.05% (15 g, 60 g)
Ointment, topical: 0.25% (15 g, 60 g)
  Topicort®: 0.25% (15 g, 60 g)

desoxyephedrine hydrochloride *see methamphetamine on page 613*
Desoxyn® [US/Can] *see methamphetamine on page 613*
desoxyphenobarbital *see primidone on page 786*
Desquam-X® [US/Can] *see benzoyl peroxide on page 126*
Desquam-X® Wash (Discontinued) *see benzoyl peroxide on page 126*
Desquam-E™ (Discontinued) *see benzoyl peroxide on page 126*

desvenlafaxine (des ven la FAX een)

Synonyms O-desmethylvenlafaxine; ODV
U.S./Canadian Brand Names Pristiq™ [US]
Therapeutic Category Antidepressant, Serotonin/Norepinephrine Reuptake Inhibitor
Use Treatment of major depressive disorder
Usual Dosage Oral: Adults: Depression: 50 mg once daily; up to 400 mg once daily have been studied; however, the manufacturer states there is no evidence that higher doses confer any additional benefit. A flat dose response curve for efficacy between 50-400 mg/day has been noted as well as an increase in adverse events.
Note: Gradually taper dose (by increasing dosing interval) if discontinuing.
Dosage Forms
Tablet, extended release:
  Pristiq™: 50 mg, 100 mg

Desyrel® [Can] *see trazodone on page 944*
Desyrel® (Discontinued) *see trazodone on page 944*
Detane® [US-OTC] *see benzocaine on page 124*
detemir insulin *see insulin detemir on page 510*
Detrol® [US/Can] *see tolterodine on page 935*
Detrol® LA [US/Can] *see tolterodine on page 935*
Detuss (Discontinued)

Detussin® Expectorant *(Discontinued)*

Dex4® Glucose [US-OTC] *see* dextrose *on page 286*

Dexacidin® *(Discontinued) see* neomycin, polymyxin B, and dexamethasone *on page 662*

Dexacine™ *(Discontinued) see* neomycin, polymyxin B, and dexamethasone *on page 662*

dexamethasone and ciprofloxacin *see* ciprofloxacin and dexamethasone *on page 223*

dexamethasone and tobramycin *see* tobramycin and dexamethasone *on page 932*

Dexamethasone Intensol® [US] *see* dexamethasone (systemic) *on page 278*

dexamethasone, neomycin, and polymyxin B *see* neomycin, polymyxin B, and dexamethasone *on page 662*

dexamethasone (ophthalmic) (deks a METH a sone op THAL mik)

Sound-Alike/Look-Alike Issues
  dexamethasone may be confused with desoximetasone
  Maxidex® may be confused with Maxzide®

Synonyms dexamethasone sodium phosphate

U.S./Canadian Brand Names Maxidex® [US/Can]

Therapeutic Category Adrenal Corticosteroid

Use Inflammatory or allergic conjunctivitis

Usual Dosage Ophthalmic: Adults:
  Ointment: Apply thin coating into conjunctival sac 3-4 times/day; gradually taper dose to discontinue
  Suspension: Instill 2 drops into conjunctival sac every hour during the day and every other hour during the night; gradually reduce dose to every 3-4 hours, then to 3-4 times/day

Dosage Forms
  Solution, ophthalmic: 0.1% (5 mL)
  Suspension, ophthalmic:
  Maxidex®: 0.1% (5 mL)

dexamethasone sodium phosphate *see* dexamethasone (ophthalmic) *on page 278*

dexamethasone sodium phosphate *see* dexamethasone (systemic) *on page 278*

dexamethasone (systemic) (deks a METH a sone sis TEM ik)

Sound-Alike/Look-Alike Issues
  dexamethasone may be confused with desoximetasone
  Decadron® may be confused with Percodan®

Synonyms dexamethasone sodium phosphate

U.S./Canadian Brand Names Apo-Dexamethasone® [Can]; Decadron® [US]; Dexamethasone Intensol® [US]; Dexasone® [Can]; DexPak® TaperPak® [US]; Diodex® [Can]; PMS-Dexamethasone [Can]

Therapeutic Category Adrenal Corticosteroid

Use Systemically and locally for chronic swelling; allergic, hematologic, neoplastic, and autoimmune diseases; may be used in management of cerebral edema, septic shock, as a diagnostic agent, antiemetic

Usual Dosage
  Children:
  Antiemetic (prior to chemotherapy): I.V. (should be given as sodium phosphate): 5-20 mg given 15-30 minutes before treatment
  Antiinflammatory immunosuppressant: Oral, I.M., I.V. (injections should be given as sodium phosphate): 0.08-0.3 mg/kg/day **or** 2.5-10 mg/m^2/day in divided doses every 6-12 hours
  Extubation or airway edema: Oral, I.M., I.V. (injections should be given as sodium phosphate): 0.5-2 mg/kg/day in divided doses every 6 hours beginning 24 hours prior to extubation and continuing for 4-6 doses afterwards
  Cerebral edema: I.V. (should be given as sodium phosphate): Loading dose: 1-2 mg/kg/dose as a single dose; maintenance: 1-1.5 mg/kg/day (maximum: 16 mg/day) in divided doses every 4-6 hours for 5 days then taper for 5 days, then discontinue
  Bacterial meningitis in infants and children >2 months: I.V. (should be given as sodium phosphate): 0.6 mg/kg/day in 4 divided doses every 6 hours for the first 4 days of antibiotic treatment; start dexamethasone at the time of the first dose of antibiotic
  Physiologic replacement: Oral, I.M., I.V.: 0.03-0.15 mg/kg/day **or** 0.6-0.75 mg/m^2/day in divided doses every 6-12 hours

Adults:
Antiemetic:
Prophylaxis: Oral, I.V.: 10-20 mg 15-30 minutes before treatment on each treatment day
   Continuous infusion regimen: Oral or I.V.: 10 mg every 12 hours on each treatment day
   Mildly emetogenic therapy: Oral, I.M., I.V.: 4 mg every 4-6 hours
   Delayed nausea/vomiting: Oral: 4-10 mg 1-2 times/day for 2-4 days **or**
      8 mg every 12 hours for 2 days; then
      4 mg every 12 hours for 2 days **or**
      20 mg 1 hour before chemotherapy; then
      10 mg 12 hours after chemotherapy; then
      8 mg every 12 hours for 4 doses; then
      4 mg every 12 hours for 4 doses
Antiinflammatory:
   Oral, I.M., I.V. (injections should be given as sodium phosphate): 0.75-9 mg/day in divided doses every 6-12 hours
   Intraarticular, intralesional, or soft tissue (as sodium phosphate): 0.4-6 mg/day
Chemotherapy: Oral, I.V.: 40 mg every day for 4 days, repeated every 4 weeks (VAD regimen)
Cerebral edema: I.V. 10 mg stat, 4 mg I.M./I.V. (should be given as sodium phosphate) every 6 hours until response is maximized, then switch to oral regimen, then taper off if appropriate; dosage may be reduced after 24 days and gradually discontinued over 5-7 days
Cushing syndrome, diagnostic: Oral: 1 mg at 11 PM, draw blood at 8 AM; greater accuracy for Cushing syndrome may be achieved by the following:
   Dexamethasone 0.5 mg by mouth every 6 hours for 48 hours (with 24-hour urine collection for 17-hydroxycorticosteroid excretion)
   Differentiation of Cushing syndrome due to ACTH excess from Cushing due to other causes: Oral: Dexamethasone 2 mg every 6 hours for 48 hours (with 24-hour urine collection for 17-hydroxycorticosteroid excretion)
Multiple sclerosis (acute exacerbation): 30 mg/day for 1 week, followed by 4-12 mg/day for 1 month
Physiological replacement: Oral, I.M., I.V. (should be given as sodium phosphate): 0.03-0.15 mg/kg/day **or** 0.6-0.75 mg/m^2/day in divided doses every 6-12 hours
Treatment of shock:
   Addisonian crisis/shock (ie, adrenal insufficiency/responsive to steroid therapy): I.V. (given as sodium phosphate): 4-10 mg as a single dose, which may be repeated if necessary
   Unresponsive shock (ie, unresponsive to steroid therapy): I.V. (given as sodium phosphate): 1-6 mg/kg as a single I.V. dose or up to 40 mg initially followed by repeat doses every 2-6 hours while shock persists

Dosage Forms
Elixir: 0.5 mg/5 mL
Injection, solution: 4 mg/mL (1 mL, 5 mL, 10 mL, 25 mL, 30 mL); 10 mg/mL (1 mL, 10 mL)
Injection, solution [preservative free]: 10 mg/mL (1 mL)
Solution, oral: 0.5 mg/5 mL
Solution, oral concentrate:
   Dexamethasone Intensol®: 1 mg/mL
Tablet: 0.5 mg, 0.75 mg, 1 mg, 1.5 mg, 2 mg, 4 mg, 6 mg
   DexPak® TaperPak®: 1.5 mg

Dexasone® [Can] *see* dexamethasone (systemic) *on page 278*

dexbrompheniramine and pseudoephedrine
(deks brom fen EER a meen & soo doe e FED rin)
Synonyms pseudoephedrine and dexbrompheniramine
U.S./Canadian Brand Names Drixoral® Cold & Allergy [US-OTC]; Drixoral® [Can]
Therapeutic Category Antihistamine/Decongestant Combination
Use Relief of symptoms of upper respiratory mucosal congestion in seasonal and perennial nasal allergies, acute rhinitis, rhinosinusitis, and eustachian tube blockage
Usual Dosage Oral: Children >12 years and Adults: 1 timed release tablet every 12 hours, may require 1 tablet every 8 hours
Dosage Forms
Tablet, sustained action: Dexbrompheniramine 6 mg and pseudoephedrine 120 mg
   Drixoral® Cold & Allergy [OTC]: Dexbrompheniramine 6 mg and pseudoephedrine 120 mg

Dexchlor® *(Discontinued)* see dexchlorpheniramine *on page 280*

dexchlorpheniramine (deks klor fen EER a meen)

Synonyms dexchlorpheniramine maleate

Therapeutic Category Antihistamine

Use Perennial and seasonal allergic rhinitis and other allergic symptoms including urticaria

Usual Dosage Oral:

Children:

2-5 years: 0.5 mg every 4-6 hours (do not use timed release)

6-11 years: 1 mg every 4-6 hours or 4 mg timed release at bedtime

Adults: 2 mg every 4-6 hours or 4-6 mg timed release at bedtime or every 8-10 hours

Dosage Forms

Syrup: 2 mg/5 mL

dexchlorpheniramine and pseudoephedrine

(deks klor fen EER a meen & soo doe e FED rin)

Synonyms pseudoephedrine tannate and dexchlorpheniramine tannate

U.S./Canadian Brand Names AllerDur™ [US]; SuTan [US]

Therapeutic Category Alpha/Beta Agonist; Antihistamine

Use Relief of nasal congestion associated with the common cold, hay fever, and other allergies, sinusitis, and vasomotor and allergic rhinitis

Usual Dosage Oral: Rhinitis/decongestant:

Children:

2-6 years: 2.5-5 mL every 12 hours (maximum: 10 mL/24 hours)

6-12 years: 5-7.5 mL every 12 hours (maximum: 15 mL/24 hours)

Children ≥12 years and Adults: 15 mL every 12 hours (maximum: 30 mL/24 hours)

Dosage Forms

Suspension:

AllerDur™, SuTan: Dexchlorpheniramine 3 mg and pseudoephedrine 50 mg per 5 mL

dexchlorpheniramine maleate *see dexchlorpheniramine on page 280*

dexchlorpheniramine tannate, pseudoephedrine tannate, and dextromethorphan tannate
see chlorpheniramine, pseudoephedrine, and dextromethorphan on page 212

Dexcon-DM *(Discontinued)* *see guaifenesin, dextromethorphan, and phenylephrine on page 459*

Dexcon-PE [US] *see guaifenesin, dextromethorphan, and phenylephrine on page 459*

Dexedrine® [US/Can] *see dextroamphetamine on page 283*

Dexferrum® [US] *see iron dextran complex on page 527*

DexFol™ [US] *see vitamin B complex combinations on page 981*

Dexiron™ [Can] *see iron dextran complex on page 527*

dexmedetomidine (deks MED e toe mi deen)

Sound-Alike/Look-Alike Issues

Precedex™ may be confused with Peridex®

Synonyms dexmedetomidine hydrochloride

U.S./Canadian Brand Names Precedex™ [US/Can]

Therapeutic Category Alpha-Adrenergic Agonist - Central-Acting (Alpha$_2$-Agonists); Sedative

Use Sedation of initially intubated and mechanically ventilated patients during treatment in an intensive care setting; duration of infusion should not exceed 24 hours

Usual Dosage Individualized and titrated to desired clinical effect

I.V.: Adults: Solution must be diluted prior to administration. Initial: Loading infusion of 1 mcg/kg over 10 minutes, followed by a maintenance infusion of 0.2-0.7 mcg/kg/hour; not indicated for infusions lasting >24 hours

Dosage Forms

Injection, solution [preservative free]:

Precedex™: 100 mcg/mL (2 mL)

dexmedetomidine hydrochloride *see dexmedetomidine on page 280*

dexmethylphenidate (dex meth il FEN i date)

Sound-Alike/Look-Alike Issues
dexmethylphenidate may be confused with methadone
Synonyms dexmethylphenidate hydrochloride
U.S./Canadian Brand Names Focalin® XR [US]; Focalin® [US]
Therapeutic Category Central Nervous System Stimulant, Nonamphetamine
Controlled Substance C-II
Use Treatment of attention-deficit/hyperactivity disorder (ADHD)
Usual Dosage Treatment of ADHD: Oral:
Children ≥6 years: Patients not currently taking methylphenidate:
Tablet: Initial: 2.5 mg twice daily; dosage may be adjusted in increments of 2.5-5 mg at weekly intervals (maximum dose: 20 mg/day); doses should be taken at least 4 hours apart
Capsule: Initial: 5 mg/day; dosage may be adjusted in increments of 5 mg/day at weekly intervals (maximum dose: 20 mg/day)
Adults: Patients not currently taking methylphenidate:
Tablet: Initial: 2.5 mg twice daily; dosage may be adjusted in increments of 2.5-5 mg at weekly intervals (maximum dose: 20 mg/day); doses should be taken at least 4 hours apart
Capsule: Initial: 10 mg/day; dosage may be adjusted in increments of 10 mg/day at weekly intervals (maximum dose: 20 mg/day)
Conversion to dexmethylphenidate from methylphenidate: Tablet, capsule: Initial: Half the total daily dose of racemic methylphenidate (maximum dexmethylphenidate dose: 20 mg/day)
Conversion from dexmethylphenidate immediate release to dexmethylphenidate extended release: When changing from Focalin® tablets to Focalin® XR capsules, patients may be switched to the same daily dose using Focalin® XR (maximum dose: 20 mg/day)
Dose reductions and discontinuation: Reduce dose or discontinue in patients with paradoxical aggravation of symptoms. Discontinue if no improvement is seen after one month of treatment.
Dosage Forms
Capsule, extended release:
Focalin® XR: 5 mg, 10 mg, 15 mg, 20 mg
Tablet: 2.5 mg, 5 mg, 10 mg
Focalin®: 2.5 mg, 5 mg, 10 mg

dexmethylphenidate hydrochloride *see* dexmethylphenidate *on page 281*
DexPak® TaperPak® [US] *see* dexamethasone (systemic) *on page 278*

dexpanthenol (deks PAN the nole)

Synonyms pantothenyl alcohol
Therapeutic Category Gastrointestinal Agent, Stimulant
Use Prophylactic use to minimize paralytic ileus; treatment of postoperative distention; topical to relieve itching and to aid healing of minor dermatoses
Usual Dosage I.M.: Adults:
Prevention of postoperative ileus: 250-500 mg stat, repeat in 2 hours, followed by doses every 6 hours until danger passes
Paralytic ileus: 500 mg stat, repeat in 2 hours, followed by doses every 6 hours, if needed
Dosage Forms
Injection, solution [preservative free]: 250 mg/mL (2 mL)

Dex PC [US] *see* chlorpheniramine, phenylephrine, and dextromethorphan *on page 209*

dexrazoxane (deks ray ZOKS ane)

Sound-Alike/Look-Alike Issues
Zinecard® may be confused with Gemzar®
Synonyms ICRF-187; NSC-169780
U.S./Canadian Brand Names Totect™ [US]; Zinecard® [US/Can]
Therapeutic Category Cardiovascular Agent, Other
Use
Zinecard®: Reduction of the incidence and severity of cardiomyopathy associated with doxorubicin administration in women with metastatic breast cancer who have received a cumulative doxorubicin ▶

◄   dose of 300 mg/m^2 and who would benefit from continuing therapy with doxorubicin. (It is not recommended for use with initial doxorubicin therapy.)

Totect™: Treatment of anthracycline-induced extravasation.

Usual Dosage I.V.: Adults:

Prevention of doxorubicin cardiomyopathy: A 10:1 ratio of dexrazoxane:doxorubicin (500 mg/m^2 dexrazoxane: 50 mg/m^2 doxorubicin)

Treatment of anthracycline extravasation: 1000 mg/m^2 on days 1 and 2 (maximum dose: 2000 mg), followed by 500 mg/m^2 on day 3 (maximum dose: 1000 mg); begin treatment as soon as possible, within 6 hours of extravasation

Dosage Forms

Injection, powder for reconstitution: 250 mg, 500 mg

Totect™: 500 mg

Zinecard®: 250 mg, 500 mg

dextran (DEKS tran)

Sound-Alike/Look-Alike Issues

dextran may be confused with Dexatrim®, Dexedrine®

Synonyms dextran 40; dextran 70; dextran, high molecular weight; dextran, low molecular weight

U.S./Canadian Brand Names Gentran® [US/Can]; LMD® [US]

Therapeutic Category Plasma Volume Expander

Use Blood volume expander used in treatment of shock or impending shock when blood or blood products are not available; dextran 40 is also used as a priming fluid in cardiopulmonary bypass and for prophylaxis of venous thrombosis and pulmonary embolism in surgical procedures associated with a high risk of thromboembolic complications

Usual Dosage I.V. (requires an infusion pump): Dose and infusion rate are dependent upon the patient's fluid status and must be individualized:

Volume expansion/shock:

Children (Dextran 40 or 70): Total dose should not exceed 20 mL/kg during first 24 hours

Adults:

Dextran 40: 500-1000 mL at a rate of 20-40 mL/minute (maximum: 20 mL/kg/day for first 24 hours); 10 mL/kg/day thereafter; therapy should not be continued beyond 5 days

Dextran 70: 500-1000 mL at a rate of 20-40 mL/minute (maximum: 20 mL/kg/day for first 24 hours)

Pump prime (Dextran 40): Varies with the volume of the pump oxygenator; generally, the 10% solution is added in a dose of 1-2 g/kg

Prophylaxis of venous thrombosis/pulmonary embolism (Dextran 40): Begin during surgical procedure and give 50-100 g on the day of surgery; an additional 50 g (500 mL) should be administered every 2-3 days during the period of risk (up to 2 weeks postoperatively); usual maximum infusion rate for nonemergency use: 4 mL/minute

Dosage Forms

Infusion [premixed in D$_5$W; low molecular weight]:

LMD®: 10% Dextran 40 (500 mL)

Infusion [premixed in NS; high molecular weight]:

Gentran®: 6% Dextran 70 (500 mL)

Infusion [premixed in NS; low molecular weight]:

LMD®: 10% Dextran (500 mL)

dextran 40 *see dextran on page 282*
dextran 70 *see dextran on page 282*

dextran 1 (DEKS tran won)

Sound-Alike/Look-Alike Issues

dextran may be confused with Dexatrim®, Dexedrine®

Therapeutic Category Plasma Volume Expander

Use Prophylaxis of serious anaphylactic reactions to I.V. infusion of dextran

Usual Dosage I.V. (time between dextran 1 and dextran solution should not exceed 15 minutes):

Children: 0.3 mL/kg 1-2 minutes before I.V. infusion of dextran

Adults: 20 mL 1-2 minutes before I.V. infusion of dextran

dextran, high molecular weight *see dextran on page 282*
dextran, low molecular weight *see dextran on page 282*

dextroamphetamine (deks troe am FET a meen)

Sound-Alike/Look-Alike Issues
dextroamphetamine may be confused with dexamethasone
Dexedrine® may be confused with dextran, Excedrin®

Synonyms dextroamphetamine sulfate

U.S./Canadian Brand Names Dexedrine® [US/Can]; DextroStat® [US]; Liquadd™ [US]

Therapeutic Category Amphetamine

Controlled Substance C-II

Use Narcolepsy; attention-deficit/hyperactivity disorder (ADHD)

Usual Dosage Oral:
Children:
Narcolepsy: 6-12 years: Initial: 5 mg/day; may increase at 5 mg increments in weekly intervals until side effects appear (maximum dose: 60 mg/day)
ADHD:
3-5 years: Initial: 2.5 mg/day given every morning; increase by 2.5 mg/day in weekly intervals until optimal response is obtained; usual range: 0.1-0.5 mg/kg/dose every morning with maximum of 40 mg/day
≥6 years: 5 mg once or twice daily; increase in increments of 5 mg/day at weekly intervals until optimal response is obtained; usual range: 0.1-0.5 mg/kg/dose every morning (5-20 mg/day) with maximum of 40 mg/day
Children >12 years and Adults: Narcolepsy: Initial: 10 mg/day, may increase at 10 mg increments in weekly intervals until side effects appear; maximum: 60 mg/day

Dosage Forms
Capsule, extended release: 5 mg, 10 mg, 15 mg
Capsule, sustained release:
Dexedrine® Spansule®: 5 mg, 10 mg, 15 mg
Tablet: 5 mg, 10 mg
DextroStat®: 5 mg, 10 mg
Solution, oral:
Liquadd™: 5 mg/5 mL

dextroamphetamine and amphetamine (deks troe am FET a meen & am FET a meen)

Sound-Alike/Look-Alike Issues
Adderall® may be confused with Inderal®

Synonyms amphetamine and dextroamphetamine

U.S./Canadian Brand Names Adderall XR® [US/Can]; Adderall® [US]

Therapeutic Category Amphetamine

Controlled Substance C-II

Use Attention-deficit/hyperactivity disorder (ADHD); narcolepsy

Usual Dosage Oral: **Note:** Use lowest effective individualized dose; administer first dose as soon as awake
ADHD:
Children: 3-5 years (Adderall®): Initial 2.5 mg/day given every morning; increase daily dose in 2.5 mg increments at weekly intervals until optimal response is obtained (maximum dose: 40 mg/day given in 1-3 divided doses); use intervals of 4-6 hours between additional doses
Children: ≥6 years:
Adderall®: Initial: 5 mg 1-2 times/day; increase daily dose in 5 mg increments at weekly intervals until optimal response is obtained (usual maximum dose: 40 mg/day given in 1-3 divided doses); use intervals of 4-6 hours between additional doses
Adderall XR®: 5-10 mg once daily in the morning; if needed, may increase daily dose in 5-10 mg increments at weekly intervals (maximum dose: 30 mg/day)
Adolescents 13-17 years (Adderall XR®): 10 mg once daily in the morning; may be increased to 20 mg/day after 1 week if symptoms are not controlled; higher doses (up to 60 mg)/day have been evaluated; however, there is not adequate evidence that higher doses afforded additional benefit.
Adults (Adderall XR®): Initial: 20 mg once daily in the morning; higher doses (up to 60 mg once daily) have been evaluated; however, there is not adequate evidence that higher doses afforded additional benefit

▶

◄ Narcolepsy (Adderall®):

Children: 6-12 years: Initial: 5 mg/day; increase daily dose in 5 mg at weekly intervals until optimal response is obtained (maximum dose: 60 mg/day given in 1-3 divided doses with intervals of 4-6 hours between doses)

Children >12 years and Adults: Initial: 10 mg/day; increase daily dose in 10 mg increments at weekly intervals until optimal response is obtained (maximum dose: 60 mg/day given in 1-3 divided doses with intervals of 4-6 hours between doses)

Dosage Forms

Capsule, extended release:

Adderall XR®:

5 mg [dextroamphetamine 1.25 mg, dextroamphetamine saccharate 1.25 mg, amphetamine aspartate monohydrate 1.25 mg, amphetamine sulfate 1.25 mg]

10 mg [dextroamphetamine sulfate 2.5 mg, dextroamphetamine saccharate 2.5 mg, amphetamine aspartate monohydrate 2.5 mg, amphetamine sulfate 2.5 mg]

15 mg [dextroamphetamine sulfate 3.75 mg, dextroamphetamine saccharate 3.75 mg, amphetamine aspartate monohydrate 3.75 mg, amphetamine sulfate 3.75 mg]

20 mg [dextroamphetamine sulfate 5 mg, dextroamphetamine saccharate 5 mg, amphetamine aspartate monohydrate 5 mg, amphetamine sulfate 5 mg]

25 mg [dextroamphetamine sulfate 6.25 mg, dextroamphetamine saccharate 6.25 mg, amphetamine aspartate monohydrate 6.25 mg, amphetamine sulfate 6.25 mg]

30 mg [dextroamphetamine sulfate 7.5 mg, dextroamphetamine saccharate 7.5 mg, amphetamine aspartate monohydrate 7.5 mg, amphetamine sulfate 7.5 mg]

Tablet: 5 mg, 7.5 mg, 10 mg, 12.5 mg, 15 mg, 20 mg, 30 mg

5 mg [dextroamphetamine sulfate 1.25 mg, dextroamphetamine saccharate 1.25 mg, amphetamine aspartate monohydrate 1.25 mg, amphetamine sulfate 1.25 mg]

7.5 mg [dextroamphetamine sulfate 1.875 mg, dextroamphetamine saccharate 1.875 mg, amphetamine aspartate monohydrate 1.875 mg, amphetamine sulfate 1.875 mg]

10 mg [dextroamphetamine sulfate 2.5 mg, dextroamphetamine saccharate 2.5 mg, amphetamine aspartate monohydrate 2.5 mg, amphetamine sulfate 2.5 mg]

12.5 mg [dextroamphetamine sulfate 3.125 mg, dextroamphetamine saccharate 3.125 mg, amphetamine aspartate monohydrate 3.125 mg, amphetamine sulfate 3.125 mg]

15 mg [dextroamphetamine sulfate 3.75 mg, dextroamphetamine saccharate 3.75 mg, amphetamine aspartate monohydrate 3.75 mg, amphetamine sulfate 3.75 mg]

20 mg [dextroamphetamine sulfate 5 mg, dextroamphetamine saccharate 5 mg, amphetamine aspartate monohydrate 5 mg, amphetamine sulfate 5 mg]

30 mg [dextroamphetamine sulfate 7.5 mg, dextroamphetamine saccharate 7.5 mg, amphetamine aspartate monohydrate 7.5 mg, amphetamine sulfate 7.5 mg]

Adderall®:

5 mg [dextroamphetamine sulfate 1.25 mg, dextroamphetamine saccharate 1.25 mg, amphetamine aspartate monohydrate 1.25 mg, amphetamine sulfate 1.25 mg]

7.5 mg [dextroamphetamine 1.875 mg, dextroamphetamine saccharate 1.875 mg, amphetamine aspartate monohydrate 1.875 mg, amphetamine sulfate 1.875 mg]

10 mg [dextroamphetamine sulfate 2.5 mg, dextroamphetamine saccharate 2.5 mg, amphetamine aspartate monohydrate 2.5 mg, amphetamine sulfate 2.5 mg]

12.5 mg [dextroamphetamine sulfate 3.125 mg, dextroamphetamine saccharate 3.125 mg, amphetamine aspartate monohydrate 3.125 mg, amphetamine sulfate 3.125 mg]

15 mg [dextroamphetamine sulfate 3.75 mg, dextroamphetamine saccharate 3.75 mg, amphetamine aspartate monohydrate 3.75 mg, amphetamine sulfate 3.75 mg]

20 mg [dextroamphetamine sulfate 5 mg, dextroamphetamine saccharate 5 mg, amphetamine aspartate monohydrate 5 mg, amphetamine sulfate 5 mg]

30 mg [dextroamphetamine sulfate 7.5 mg, dextroamphetamine saccharate 7.5 mg, amphetamine aspartate monohydrate 7.5 mg, amphetamine sulfate 7.5 mg]

dextroamphetamine sulfate *see* dextroamphetamine *on page 283*

dextromethorphan (deks troe meth OR fan)

Sound-Alike/Look-Alike Issues

Benylin® may be confused with Benadryl®, Ventolin®

Delsym® may be confused with Delfen®, Desyrel®

U.S./Canadian Brand Names Babee® Cof Syrup [US-OTC]; Creo-Terpin® [US-OTC]; Creomulsion® Cough [US-OTC]; Creomulsion® for Children [US-OTC]; Delsym® [US-OTC]; ElixSure® Cough [US-OTC]; Hold® DM [US-OTC]; Robitussin® CoughGels™ [US-OTC]; Robitussin® Maximum Strength

Cough [US-OTC]; Robitussin® Pediatric Cough [US-OTC]; Silphen DM® [US-OTC]; Triaminic® Thin Strips™ Long Acting Cough [US-OTC]; Vicks® 44® Cough Relief [US-OTC]

Therapeutic Category Antitussive

Use Symptomatic relief of coughs caused by minor viral upper respiratory tract infections or inhaled irritants; most effective for a chronic nonproductive cough

Usual Dosage Oral:

Children:

<2 years: Use only as directed by a physician

2-6 years (syrup): 2.5-7.5 mg every 4-8 hours; extended release is 15 mg twice daily (maximum: 30 mg/24 hours)

6-12 years: 5-10 mg every 4 hours or 15 mg every 6-8 hours; extended release is 30 mg twice daily (maximum: 60 mg/24 hours)

Children >12 years and Adults: 10-20 mg every 4 hours or 30 mg every 6-8 hours; extended release: 60 mg twice daily; maximum: 120 mg/day

Dosage Forms

Gelcap:

Robitussin® CoughGels™ [OTC]: 15 mg

Liquid, oral:

Creo-Terpin® [OTC], Vicks® 44® Cough Relief [OTC]: 10 mg/15 mL

Lozenge:

Hold® DM [OTC]: 5 mg (10s)

Strips, oral:

Triaminic® Thin Strips™ Long Acting Cough [OTC]: 7.5 mg

Suspension, extended release:

Delsym® [OTC]: 30 mg/5 mL (89 mL, 148 mL)

Syrup:

Babee® Cof Syrup [OTC], ElixSure® Cough [OTC], Robitussin® Pediatric Cough [OTC]: 7.5 mg/5 mL

Creomulsion® Cough [OTC]: 20 mg/15 mL

Creomulsion® for Children [OTC]: 5 mg/5 mL

Robitussin® Maximum Strength Cough [OTC]: 15 mg/5 mL

Silphen DM® [OTC]: 10 mg/5 mL

dextromethorphan, acetaminophen, and pseudoephedrine see acetaminophen, dextromethorphan, and pseudoephedrine on page 27

dextromethorphan and guaifenesin see guaifenesin and dextromethorphan on page 454

dextromethorphan and promethazine see promethazine and dextromethorphan on page 792

dextromethorphan and pseudoephedrine see pseudoephedrine and dextromethorphan on page 802

dextromethorphan, chlorpheniramine, and phenylephrine see chlorpheniramine, phenylephrine, and dextromethorphan on page 209

dextromethorphan, chlorpheniramine, and pseudoephedrine see chlorpheniramine, pseudoephedrine, and dextromethorphan on page 212

dextromethorphan, chlorpheniramine, phenylephrine, and guaifenesin
(deks troe meth OR fan, klor fen IR a meen, fen il EF rin, & gwye FEN e sin)

Synonyms chlorpheniramine, dextromethorphan, phenylephrine, and guaifenesin; guaifenesin, chlorpheniramine, phenylephrine, and dextromethorphan; phenylephrine hydrochloride, chlorpheniramine maleate, dextromethorphan hydrobromide, and guaifenesin

U.S./Canadian Brand Names Chlordex GP [US]; Donatussin [US]; Quartuss™ [US]

Therapeutic Category Antihistamine/Decongestant/Antitussive/Expectorant

Use Symptomatic relief of dry, nonproductive cough and upper respiratory symptoms associated with infections such as the common cold, bronchitis, or sinusitis

Usual Dosage General dosing guidelines; consult specific product labeling.

Antitussive/antihistamine/decongestant/expectorant: Oral (Donatussin):

Children:

2-6 years: 2.5 mL every 6 hours as needed (maximum: 10 mL/24 hours)

6-12 years: 5 mL every 6 hours as needed (maximum: 20 mL/24 hours)

Children ≥12 years and Adults: 10 mL every 6 hours as needed (maximum: 40 mL/24 hours)

▶

◀ **Dosage Forms**
Syrup:
Chlordex GP®: Dextromethorphan 7.5 mg, chlorpheniramine 2 mg, phenylephrine 10 mg, and guaifenesin 100 mg per 5 mL (480 mL)
Donatussin, Quartuss™: Dextromethorphan 15 mg, chlorpheniramine 2 mg, phenylephrine 10 mg, and guaifenesin 100 mg per 5 mL (480 mL)

dextromethorphan, guaifenesin, and pseudoephedrine *see guaifenesin, pseudoephedrine, and dextromethorphan on page 460*

dextromethorphan hydrobromide, acetaminophen, and phenylephrine hydrochloride *see acetaminophen, dextromethorphan, and phenylephrine on page 26*

dextromethorphan hydrobromide, brompheniramine maleate, and pseudoephedrine hydrochloride *see brompheniramine, pseudoephedrine, and dextromethorphan on page 146*

dextromethorphan tannate, pyrilamine tannate, and phenylephrine tannate *see phenylephrine, pyrilamine, and dextromethorphan on page 749*

dextropropoxyphene *see propoxyphene on page 795*

dextrose (DEKS trose)

Sound-Alike/Look-Alike Issues
Glutose™ may be confused with Glutofac®
Synonyms anhydrous glucose; $D_{10}W$; $D_{25}W$; $D_{30}W$; $D_{40}W$; $D_{50}W$; D_5W; $D_{60}W$; $D_{70}W$; dextrose monohydrate; glucose; glucose monohydrate; glycosum
U.S./Canadian Brand Names B-D™ Glucose [US-OTC]; Dex4® Glucose [US-OTC]; Enfamil® Glucose [US]; Glutol™ [US-OTC]; Glutose™ [US-OTC]; Insta-Glucose® [US-OTC]; Similac® Glucose [US]
Therapeutic Category Antidote, Hypoglycemia; Intravenous Nutritional Therapy
Use
Oral: Treatment of hypoglycemia
5% and 10% solutions: Peripheral infusion to provide calories and fluid replacement
25% (hypertonic) solution: Treatment of acute symptomatic episodes of hypoglycemia in infants and children to restore depressed blood glucose levels; adjunctive treatment of hyperkalemia when combined with insulin
50% (hypertonic) solution: Treatment of insulin-induced hypoglycemia (hyperinsulinemia or insulin shock) and adjunctive treatment of hyperkalemia in adolescents and adults
≥10% solutions: Infusion after admixture with amino acids for nutritional support
Usual Dosage
Hypoglycemia: Doses may be repeated in severe cases
I.V.:
Infants ≤6 months: 0.25-0.5 g/kg/dose (1-2 mL/kg/dose of 25% solution); maximum: 25 g/dose
Infants >6 months and Children: 0.5-1 g/kg/dose (2-4 mL/kg/dose of 25% solution); maximum: 25 g/dose
Adolescents and Adults: 10-25 g (40-100 mL of 25% solution or 20-50 mL of 50% solution)
Oral: Children >2 years and Adults: 10-20 g as single dose; repeat in 10 minutes if necessary
Treatment of Hyperkalemia: I.V. (in combination with insulin):
Infants and Children: 0.5-1 g/kg (using 25% or 50% solution) combined with regular insulin 1 unit for every 4-5 g dextrose given; infuse over 2 hours (infusions as short as 30 minutes have been recommended); repeat as needed
Adolescents and Adults: 25-50 g dextrose (250-500 mL $D_{10}W$) combined with 10 units regular insulin administered over 30-60 minutes; repeat as needed or as an alternative 25 g dextrose (50 mL $D_{50}W$) combined with 5-10 units regular insulin infused over 5 minutes; repeat as needed
Note: More rapid infusions (<30 minutes) may be associated with hyperglycemia and hyperosmolality and will exacerbate hyperkalemia; avoid use in patients who are already hyperglycemic
Dosage Forms
Gel:
Glutose™ [OTC]: 40% (15 g, 45 g)
Insta-Glucose® [OTC]: 40% (30 g)
Infusion:
Generics:
2.5% (1000 mL)
5% (25 mL, 50 mL, 100 mL, 150 mL, 250 mL, 500 mL, 1000 mL)
10% (250 mL, 500 mL, 1000 mL)
20% (500 mL, 1000 mL)

30% (500 mL, 1000 mL)
40% (500 mL, 1000 mL)
50% (500 mL, 1000 mL, 2000 mL)
60% (500 mL, 1000 mL)
70% (500 mL, 1000 mL, 2000 mL)
Injection, solution: 10% (3 mL, 5 mL); 25% (10 mL); 50% (50 mL)
Solution, oral:
  Enfamil® Glucose: 5%, 10%
  Glutol™ [OTC]: 55%
  Similac® Glucose: 5%, 10%
Tablet, chewable:
  B-D™ Glucose [OTC]: 5 g
  Dex4® Glucose [OTC]: 4 g

dextrose, levulose and phosphoric acid *see* fructose, dextrose, and phosphoric acid *on page 429*
dextrose monohydrate *see* dextrose *on page 286*
DextroStat® [US] *see* dextroamphetamine *on page 283*
Dey-Dose® Isoproterenol *(Discontinued)* *see* isoproterenol *on page 529*
Dey-Dose® Metaproterenol *(Discontinued)*
DFMO *see* eflornithine *on page 336*
DHAD *see* mitoxantrone *on page 638*
DHAQ *see* mitoxantrone *on page 638*
DHC® *(Discontinued)* *see* hydrocodone and acetaminophen *on page 481*
DHC Plus® *(Discontinued)*
DHE *see* dihydroergotamine *on page 299*
D.H.E. 45® [US] *see* dihydroergotamine *on page 299*
DHPG sodium *see* ganciclovir *on page 435*
DHS™ Sal [US-OTC] *see* salicylic acid *on page 850*
DHS™ Tar [US-OTC] *see* coal tar *on page 240*
DHS™ Targel [US-OTC] *see* coal tar *on page 240*
DHS™ Zinc [US-OTC] *see* pyrithione zinc *on page 810*
DHT™ *(Discontinued)*
DHT™ Intensol™ *(Discontinued)*
DiabetAid™ Antifungal Foot Bath [US-OTC] *see* miconazole *on page 630*
DiabetAid Gingivitis Mouth Rinse [US-OTC] *see* cetylpyridinium *on page 197*
Diabetic Tussin C® [US] *see* guaifenesin and codeine *on page 454*
Diabetic Tussin® Allergy Relief [US-OTC] *see* chlorpheniramine *on page 205*
Diabetic Tussin® DM [US-OTC] *see* guaifenesin and dextromethorphan *on page 454*
Diabetic Tussin® DM Maximum Strength [US-OTC] *see* guaifenesin and dextromethorphan *on page 454*
Diabetic Tussin® EX [US-OTC] *see* guaifenesin *on page 453*
Diabinese® [US] *see* chlorpropamide *on page 214*
Diaβeta® [US/Can] *see* glyburide *on page 448*
Dialose® Tablet *(Discontinued)* *see* docusate *on page 314*
Dialume® *(Discontinued)* *see* aluminum hydroxide *on page 53*
Diamicron® [Can] *see* gliclazide *(Canada only) on page 444*
Diamicron® MR [Can] *see* gliclazide *(Canada only) on page 444*
Diamine T.D.® *(Discontinued)* *see* brompheniramine *on page 144*
diaminocyclohexane oxalatoplatinum *see* oxaliplatin *on page 705*
diaminodiphenylsulfone *see* dapsone *on page 267*
Diamode [US-OTC] *see* loperamide *on page 573*
Diamox® [Can] *see* acetazolamide *on page 28*
Diamox® 250 mg Tablet *(Discontinued)* *see* acetazolamide *on page 28*
Diamox® Sequels® [US] *see* acetazolamide *on page 28*
Diane-35® [Can] *see* cyproterone and ethinyl estradiol *(Canada only) on page 259*
Diar-aid® *(Discontinued)* *see* loperamide *on page 573*

Diarr-Eze [Can] see loperamide on page 573
Diastat® [US/Can] see diazepam on page 289
Diastat® AcuDial™ [US] see diazepam on page 289
Diastat® Rectal Delivery System [Can] see diazepam on page 289

diatrizoate meglumine (dye a tri ZOE ate MEG loo meen)

U.S./Canadian Brand Names Cystografin® Dilute [US]; Cystografin® [US]; Reno-30® [US]; Reno-60® [US]; Reno-Dip® [US]

Therapeutic Category Iodinated Contrast Media; Radiological/Contrast Media, Ionic

Use

Solution for instillation: Retrograde cystourethrography; retrograde or ascending pyelography

Solution for injection: Arthrography, cerebral angiography, direct cholangiography, discography, drip infusion pyelography, excretory urography, peripheral arteriography, splenoportography, venography; contrast enhancement of computed tomographic head and body imaging

Usual Dosage Dosing is based upon route of administration, type of examination, age of patient, and product used. Consult specific product information for detailed dosing.

Dosage Forms

Solution, for instillation:
Cystografin®: 30% (100 mL, 300 mL)
Cystografin® Dilute: 18% (300 mL)
Reno-30®: 30% (50 mL)

Solution, injection:
Reno-60®: 60% (50 mL)
Reno-Dip®: 30% (300 mL)

diatrizoate meglumine and diatrizoate sodium
(dye a tri ZOE ate MEG loo meen & dye a tri ZOE ate SOW dee um)

Synonyms diatrizoate sodium and diatrizoate meglumine

U.S./Canadian Brand Names Gastrografin® [US]; MD-76®R [US]; MD-Gastroview® [US]; Renografin®-60 [US]

Therapeutic Category Iodinated Contrast Media; Radiological/Contrast Media, Ionic

Use

Oral/rectal: Examination of GI tract; adjunct to contrast enhancement in computed tomography of the torso

Injection: Angiocardiography, aortography, central venography, cerebral angiography, cholangiography, digital arteriography, excretory urography, nephrotomography, peripheral angiography, peripheral arteriography, renal arteriography, renal venography, splenoportography, visceral arteriography; contrast enhancement of computed tomographic imaging

Usual Dosage

Radiographic exam of GI tract segments:
Oral:
Children <5 years: 30 mL, dilute 1:1 (if <10 kg or debilitated, dilute 1:3)
Children 5-10 years: 60 mL, dilute 1:1 (if <10 kg or debilitated, dilute 1:3)
Adults: 30-90 mL
Rectal enema:
Children <5 years: Dilute 1:5 in tap water
Children >5 years: Dilute 90 mL in 500 mL tap water
Adults: Dilute 240 mL in 1000 mL tap water
Tomography: Adults: Oral: 25-77 mL in 1000 mL tap water 15-30 minutes prior to imaging

Dosage Forms

Solution, injection:
MD-76®R: Diatrizoate meglumine 660 mg and diatrizoate sodium 100 mg per 1 mL (50 mL, 100 mL, 200 mL)
Renografin®-60: Diatrizoate meglumine 520 mg and diatrizoate sodium 80 mg per 1 mL (50 mL)
Solution, oral/rectal:
Gastrografin®: Diatrizoate meglumine 660 mg and diatrizoate sodium 100 mg per 1 mL
MD-Gastroview®: Diatrizoate meglumine 660 mg and diatrizoate sodium 100 mg per 1 mL

diatrizoate meglumine and iodipamide meglumine
(dye a tri ZOE ate MEG loo meen & eye oh DI pa mide MEG loo meen)

Synonyms iodipamide meglumine and diatrizoate meglumine

U.S./Canadian Brand Names Sinografin® [US]

Therapeutic Category Iodinated Contrast Media; Radiological/Contrast Media, Ionic

Use Hysterosalpingography

Usual Dosage Intrauterine: Adults: Hysterosalpingography: Usual dose: 3-4 mL administered in fractional doses of ~1 mL; may give additional 3-4 mL to visualize tubes; total dosage range: 1.5-10 mL

Dosage Forms
Injection, solution [for intrauterine instillation]:
Sinografin®: Diatrizoate meglumine 524 mg and iodipamide meglumine 268 mg per mL (10 mL)

diatrizoate sodium (dye a tri ZOE ate SOW dee um)

U.S./Canadian Brand Names Hypaque™ Sodium [US]

Therapeutic Category Iodinated Contrast Media; Radiological/Contrast Media, Ionic

Use Radiographic examination of GI tract

Usual Dosage
Oral:
Infants and Children: 20% to 40% solution: 30-75 mL
Adults: 25% to 40% solution: 90-180 mL
Rectal: Enema:
Infants and Children: 10% to 15% solution: 100-500 mL depending on weight of patient
Adults: 15% to 25% solution: 500-1000 mL

Dosage Forms
Powder for solution, oral/rectal:
Hypaque™ Sodium: 100% (250 g)

diatrizoate sodium and diatrizoate meglumine see diatrizoate meglumine and diatrizoate sodium on page 288

Diatx®Zn [US] see vitamins (multiple/oral) on page 983

Diazemuls® [Can] see diazepam on page 289

Diazemuls® Injection (Discontinued) see diazepam on page 289

diazepam (dye AZ e pam)

Sound-Alike/Look-Alike Issues
diazepam may be confused with diazoxide, Ditropan®, lorazepam
Valium® may be confused with Valcyte™

U.S./Canadian Brand Names Apo-Diazepam® [Can]; Diastat® AcuDial™ [US]; Diastat® Rectal Delivery System [Can]; Diastat® [US/Can]; Diazemuls® [Can]; Diazepam Intensol® [US]; Novo-Dipam [Can]; Valium® [US/Can]

Therapeutic Category Benzodiazepine

Controlled Substance C-IV

Use Management of anxiety disorders, ethanol withdrawal symptoms; skeletal muscle relaxant; treatment of convulsive disorders
Rectal gel: Management of selected, refractory epilepsy patients on stable regimens of antiepileptic drugs (AEDs) requiring intermittent use of diazepam to control episodes of increased seizure activity

Usual Dosage Oral absorption is more reliable than I.M.
Children:
Conscious sedation for procedures: Oral: 0.2-0.3 mg/kg (maximum: 10 mg) 45-60 minutes prior to procedure
Sedation/muscle relaxant/anxiety:
Oral: 0.12-0.8 mg/kg/day in divided doses every 6-8 hours
I.M., I.V.: 0.04-0.3 mg/kg/dose every 2-4 hours to a maximum of 0.6 mg/kg within an 8-hour period if needed
Status epilepticus:
Infants 30 days to 5 years: I.V.: 0.05-0.3 mg/kg/dose given over 2-3 minutes, every 15-30 minutes to a maximum total dose of 5 mg; repeat in 2-4 hours as needed or 0.2-0.5 mg/dose every 2-5 minutes to a maximum total dose of 5 mg

◀ >5 years: I.V.: 0.05-0.3 mg/kg/dose given over 2-3 minutes every 15-30 minutes to a maximum total dose of 10 mg; repeat in 2-4 hours as needed **or** 1 mg/dose given over 2-3 minutes, every 2-5 minutes to a maximum total dose of 10 mg

Rectal gel: 0.5 mg/kg, then 0.25 mg/kg in 10 minutes if needed

Anticonvulsant (acute treatment): Rectal gel:

Children 2-5 years: 0.5 mg/kg

Children 6-11 years: 0.3 mg/kg

Children ≥12 years: 0.2 mg/kg

Note: Dosage should be rounded upward to the next available dose, 2.5, 5, 7.5, 10, 12.5, 15, 17.5, and 20 mg/dose; dose may be repeated in 4-12 hours if needed; do not use for more than 5 episodes per month or more than one episode every 5 days

Adolescents: Conscious sedation for procedures:

Oral: 10 mg

I.V.: 5 mg, may repeat with 1/2 dose if needed

Adults:

Anticonvulsant (acute treatment): Rectal gel: 0.2 mg/kg

Note: Dosage should be rounded upward to the next available dose, 2.5, 5, 7.5, 10, 12.5, 15, 17.5, and 20 mg/dose; dose may be repeated in 4-12 hours if needed; do not use for more than 5 episodes per month or more than one episode every 5 days.

Anxiety/sedation/skeletal muscle relaxant:

Oral: 2-10 mg 2-4 times/day

I.M., I.V.: 2-10 mg, may repeat in 3-4 hours if needed

Sedation in the ICU patient: I.V.: 0.03-0.1 mg/kg every 30 minutes to 6 hours

Status epilepticus:

I.V.: 5-10 mg every 10-20 minutes, up to 30 mg in an 8-hour period; may repeat in 2-4 hours if necessary

Rectal gel: Premonitory/out-of-hospital treatment: 10 mg once; may repeat once if necessary

Rapid tranquilization of agitated patient (administer every 30-60 minutes): Oral: 5-10 mg; average total dose for tranquilization: 20-60 mg

Dosage Forms

Gel, rectal:

Diastat®: Pediatric rectal tip [4.4 cm]: 5 mg/mL (2.5 mg, 5 mg)

Diastat® AcuDial™ delivery system:

10 mg: Pediatric/adult rectal tip [4.4 cm]: 5 mg/mL (delivers set doses of 5 mg, 7.5 mg, and 10 mg)

20 mg: Adult rectal tip [6 cm]: 5 mg/mL (delivers set doses of 10 mg, 12.5 mg, 15 mg, 17.5 mg, and 20 mg)

Injection, solution: 5 mg/mL (2 mL, 10 mL)

Solution, oral: 5 mg/5 mL

Solution, oral concentrate: 5 mg/mL

Diazepam Intensol®: 5 mg/mL

Tablet: 2 mg, 5 mg, 10 mg

Valium®: 2 mg, 5 mg, 10 mg

Diazepam Intensol® [US] *see* diazepam *on page 289*

diazoxide (dye az OKS ide)

Sound-Alike/Look-Alike Issues

diazoxide may be confused with diazepam, Dyazide®

U.S./Canadian Brand Names Proglycem® [US/Can]

Therapeutic Category Antihypertensive Agent; Antihypoglycemic Agent

Use Hypoglycemia related to islet cell adenoma, carcinoma, hyperplasia, or adenomatosis; nesidioblastosis; leucine sensitivity; extrapancreatic malignancy

Usual Dosage Oral: Hyperinsulinemic hypoglycemia:

Newborns and Infants: Initial dose: 10 mg/kg/day; dosing range: 8-15 mg/kg/day in divided doses every 8-12 hours

Children and Adults: Initial dose: 3 mg/kg/day; dosing range: 3-8 mg/kg/day in divided doses every 8-12 hours. **Note:** In certain instances, patients with refractory hypoglycemia may require higher doses.

Dosage Forms [CAN] = Canadian brand name

Capsule, oral:

Proglycem® [CAN]: 50 mg [not available in the U.S.]

Suspension, oral:
Proglycem®: 50 mg/mL

Dibent® Injection *(Discontinued)* see dicyclomine *on page 293*
Dibenzyline® [US/Can] see phenoxybenzamine *on page 744*

dibucaine (DYE byoo kane)
U.S./Canadian Brand Names Nupercainal® [US-OTC]
Therapeutic Category Local Anesthetic
Use Fast, temporary relief of pain and itching due to hemorrhoids, minor burns
Usual Dosage Topical: Children and Adults: Apply gently to the affected areas; no more than 30 g for adults or 7.5 g for children should be used in any 24-hour period
Dosage Forms
Ointment, topical: 1% (30 g)
Nupercainal® [OTC]: 1% (30 g, 60g)

DIC see dacarbazine *on page 263*
Dicarbosil® *(Discontinued)* see calcium carbonate *on page 163*
Dicel™ [US] see chlorpheniramine and pseudoephedrine *on page 207*
Dicel™ DM [US] see chlorpheniramine, pseudoephedrine, and dextromethorphan *on page 212*
Dicetel® [Can] see pinaverium *(Canada only) on page 754*
dichloralphenazone, acetaminophen, and isometheptene see acetaminophen, isometheptene, and dichloralphenazone *on page 28*
dichloralphenazone, isometheptene, and acetaminophen see acetaminophen, isometheptene, and dichloralphenazone *on page 28*

dichlorodifluoromethane and trichloromonofluoromethane
(dye klor oh dye flor oh METH ane & tri klor oh mon oh flor oh METH ane)
Synonyms trichloromonofluoromethane and dichlorodifluoromethane
U.S./Canadian Brand Names Fluori-Methane® [US]
Therapeutic Category Analgesic, Topical
Use Management of pain associated with injections
Usual Dosage Invert bottle over treatment area approximately 12" away from site of application; open dispenseal spring valve completely, allowing liquid to flow in a stream from the bottle. The rate of spraying is approximately 10 cm/second and should be continued until entire muscle has been covered.
Dosage Forms
Aerosol, topical:
Fluori-Methane®: Dichlorodifluoromethane 15% and trichloromonofluoromethane 85% (103 mL)

dichlorotetrafluoroethane and ethyl chloride see ethyl chloride and dichlorotetrafluoroethane *on page 382*

dichlorphenamide (dye klor FEN a mide)
Sound-Alike/Look-Alike Issues
Daranide® may be confused with Daraprim®
Synonyms diclofenamide
U.S./Canadian Brand Names Daranide® [US/Can]
Therapeutic Category Carbonic Anhydrase Inhibitor; Diuretic, Carbonic Anhydrase Inhibitor; Ophthalmic Agent, Antiglaucoma
Use Adjunct in treatment of open-angle glaucoma and perioperative treatment for angle-closure glaucoma
Usual Dosage Oral: Adults: 100-200 mg to start followed by 100 mg every 12 hours until desired response is obtained; maintenance dose: 25-50 mg 1-3 times/day
Dosage Forms
Tablet:
Daranide®: 50 mg

Dickinson's® Witch Hazel [US-OTC] see witch hazel *on page 987*
Diclectin® [Can] see doxylamine and pyridoxine *(Canada only) on page 325*

diclofenac (dye KLOE fen ak)

Sound-Alike/Look-Alike Issues
diclofenac may be confused with Diflucan®, Duphalac®
Cataflam® may be confused with Catapres®
Voltaren® may be confused with tramadol, Ultram®, Verelan®

Synonyms diclofenac epolamine; diclofenac potassium; diclofenac sodium

U.S./Canadian Brand Names Apo-Diclo Rapide® [Can]; Apo-Diclo SR® [Can]; Apo-Diclo® [Can]; Cataflam® [US/Can]; Dom-Diclofenac SR [Can]; Dom-Diclofenac [Can]; Flector® [US]; Novo-Difenac K [Can]; Novo-Difenac [Can]; Novo-Difenac-SR [Can]; Nu-Diclo [Can]; Nu-Diclo-SR [Can]; Pennsaid® [Can]; PMS-Diclofenac SR [Can]; PMS-Diclofenac [Can]; Riva-Diclofenac [Can]; Riva-Diclofenac-K [Can]; Sab-Diclofenac [Can]; Sandoz-Diclofenac [Can]; Solaraze® [US]; Voltaren Ophthalmic® [US]; Voltaren Ophtha® [Can]; Voltaren Rapide® [Can]; Voltaren® Gel [US]; Voltaren® [US/Can]; Voltaren®-XR [US]

Therapeutic Category Analgesic, Nonnarcotic; Nonsteroidal Antiinflammatory Drug (NSAID)

Use
Immediate release tablet: Ankylosing spondylitis; primary dysmenorrhea; acute and chronic treatment of rheumatoid arthritis, osteoarthritis
Delayed-release tablet: Acute and chronic treatment of rheumatoid arthritis, osteoarthritis, ankylosing spondylitis
Extended-release tablet: Chronic treatment of osteoarthritis, rheumatoid arthritis
Ophthalmic solution: Postoperative inflammation following cataract extraction; temporary relief of pain and photophobia in patients undergoing corneal refractive surgery
Topical gel 1%: Relief of osteoarthritis pain in joints amenable to topical therapy (eg, ankle, elbow, foot, hand, knee, wrist)
Topical gel 3%: Actinic keratosis (AK) in conjunction with sun avoidance
Topical patch: Acute pain due to minor strains, sprains, and contusions

Usual Dosage Adults:
Oral:
Analgesia/primary dysmenorrhea: Starting dose: 50 mg 3 times/day; maximum dose: 150 mg/day
Rheumatoid arthritis: 150-200 mg/day in 2-4 divided doses (100-200 mg/day of sustained release product)
Osteoarthritis: 100-150 mg/day in 2-3 divided doses (100-200 mg/day of sustained release product)
Ankylosing spondylitis: 100-125 mg/day in 4-5 divided doses
Ophthalmic:
Cataract surgery: Instill 1 drop into affected eye 4 times/day beginning 24 hours after cataract surgery and continuing for 2 weeks
Corneal refractive surgery: Instill 1-2 drops into affected eye within the hour prior to surgery, within 15 minutes following surgery, and then continue for 4 times/day, up to 3 days
Topical gel:
Actinic keratoses (Solaraze® Gel): Apply 3% gel to lesion area twice daily for 60-90 days
Osteoarthritis (Voltaren® Gel): **Note:** Maximum total body dose of 1% gel should not exceed 32 g per day
Lower extremities: Apply 4 g of 1% gel to affected area 4 times daily (maximum: 16 g per joint per day)
Upper extremities: Apply 2 g of 1% gel to affected area 4 times daily (maximum: 8 g per joint per day)
Topical patch: Acute pain (strains, sprains, contusions): Apply 1 patch twice daily to most painful area of skin

Dosage Forms
Gel:
Solaraze®: 3% (50 g, 100 g)
Voltaren® Gel: 1% (100 g)
Solution, ophthalmic [drops]: 0.1% (2.5 mL, 5 mL)
Voltaren Ophthalmic®: 0.1% (2.5 mL, 5 mL)
Tablet: 50 mg
Cataflam®: 50 mg
Tablet, delayed release, enteric coated: 50 mg, 75 mg
Voltaren®: 75 mg
Tablet, extended release: 100 mg
Voltaren®-XR: 100 mg
Transdermal system, topical:
Flector®: 1.3% (30s) [180 mg]

diclofenac and misoprostol (dye KLOE fen ak & mye soe PROST ole)

Synonyms misoprostol and diclofenac
U.S./Canadian Brand Names Arthrotec® [US/Can]
Therapeutic Category Analgesic, Nonnarcotic; Prostaglandin
Use The diclofenac component is indicated for the treatment of osteoarthritis and rheumatoid arthritis; the misoprostol component is indicated for the prophylaxis of NSAID-induced gastric and duodenal ulceration
Usual Dosage Oral: Adults:
Arthrotec® 50:
Osteoarthritis: 1 tablet 2-3 times/day
Rheumatoid arthritis: 1 tablet 3-4 times/day
For both regimens, if not tolerated by patient, the dose may be reduced to 1 tablet twice daily
Arthrotec® 75:
Patients who cannot tolerate full daily Arthrotec® 50 regimens: 1 tablet twice daily
Note: The use of these tablets may not be as effective at preventing GI ulceration
Dosage Forms
Tablet:
Arthrotec®: Diclofenac 50 mg and misoprostol 200 mcg; diclofenac 75 mg and misoprostol 200 mcg

diclofenac epolamine see diclofenac on page 292
diclofenac potassium see diclofenac on page 292
diclofenac sodium see diclofenac on page 292
diclofenamide see dichlorphenamide on page 291

dicloxacillin (dye kloks a SIL in)

Synonyms dicloxacillin sodium
U.S./Canadian Brand Names Dycill® [Can]; Pathocil® [Can]
Therapeutic Category Penicillin
Use Treatment of systemic infections such as pneumonia, skin and soft tissue infections, and osteomyelitis caused by penicillinase-producing staphylococci
Usual Dosage
Usual dosage range:
Children <40 kg: Oral: 12.5-100 mg/kg/day divided every 6 hours
Children >40 kg: Oral: 125-250 mg every 6 hours
Adults: Oral: 125-1000 mg every 6 hours
Indication-specific dosing:
Children: Oral:
Furunculosis: 25-50 mg/kg/day divided every 6 hours
Osteomyelitis: 50-100 mg/kg/day in divided doses every 6 hours
Adults: Oral:
Erysipelas, furunculosis, mastitis, otitis externa, septic bursitis, skin abscess: 500 mg every 6 hours
Impetigo: 250 mg every 6 hours
Prosthetic joint (long-term suppression therapy): 250 mg twice daily
Staphylococcus aureus,methicillin susceptible infection if no I.V. access: 500-1000 mg every 6-8 hours
Dosage Forms
Capsule: 250 mg, 500 mg

dicloxacillin sodium see dicloxacillin on page 293

dicyclomine (dye SYE kloe meen)

Sound-Alike/Look-Alike Issues
dicyclomine may be confused with diphenhydrAMINE, doxycycline, dyclonine
Bentyl® may be confused with Aventyl®, Benadryl®, Bontril®, Cantil®, Proventil®, Trental®
Synonyms dicyclomine hydrochloride; dicycloverine hydrochloride
U.S./Canadian Brand Names Bentylol® [Can]; Bentyl® [US]; Formulex® [Can]; Lomine [Can]; Riva-Dicyclomine [Can]
Therapeutic Category Anticholinergic Agent

◀ **Use** Treatment of functional bowel/irritable bowel syndrome

Usual Dosage Adults:

Oral: Initiate with 80 mg/day in 4 equally divided doses, then increase up to 160 mg/day. Duration: Safety data not available for duration >2 weeks.

I.M. **(should not be used I.V.):** 80 mg/day in 4 divided doses (20 mg/dose)

Dosage Forms

Capsule: 10 mg
Bentyl®: 10 mg
Injection, solution: 10 mg/mL (2 mL)
Bentyl®: 10 mg/mL (2 mL)
Syrup:
Bentyl®: 10 mg/5 mL
Tablet: 20 mg
Bentyl®: 20 mg

dicyclomine hydrochloride *see dicyclomine on page 293*
dicycloverine hydrochloride *see dicyclomine on page 293*
Di-Dak-Sol [US] *see sodium hypochlorite solution on page 876*

didanosine (dye DAN oh seen)

Sound-Alike/Look-Alike Issues
Videx® may be confused with Lidex®

Synonyms ddI; dideoxyinosine

U.S./Canadian Brand Names Videx® EC [US/Can]; Videx® [US/Can]

Therapeutic Category Antiviral Agent

Use Treatment of HIV infection; always to be used in combination with at least two other antiretroviral agents

Usual Dosage Treatment of HIV infection: Oral (administer on an empty stomach):

Pediatric powder for oral solution (Videx®):

Infants: 2 weeks to 8 months: 100 mg/m^2 twice daily is recommended by the manufacturer; 50 mg/m^2 may be considered in infants 2 weeks to 4 months (AIDSinfo guidelines)

Infants and Children >8 months: 120 mg/m^2 twice daily is recommended by the manufacturer. **Note:** AIDSinfo guidelines suggest a range of 90-150 mg/m^2 twice daily

Children 3-21 years (AIDSinfo guidelines): Treatment-naive: 240 mg/m^2/dose once daily (maximum: 400 mg/dose)

Adolescents and Adults: Dosing based on patient weight:

Pediatric powder for oral solution (Videx®):
<60 kg: 125 mg twice daily (preferred) or 250 mg once daily
≥60 kg: 200 mg twice daily (preferred) or 400 mg once daily

Delayed release capsule (Videx® EC):
<60 kg: 250 mg once daily
≥60 kg; 400 mg once daily

Dosage Forms

Capsule, delayed release, enteric coated pellets: 200 mg, 250 mg, 400 mg
Capsule, delayed release, enteric coated beadlets:
Videx® EC: 125 mg, 200 mg, 250 mg, 400 mg
Powder for oral solution, pediatric:
Videx®: 2 g, 4 g

dideoxyinosine *see didanosine on page 294*
Didrex® [US/Can] *see benzphetamine on page 128*
Didrocal™ [Can] *see etidronate and calcium on page 382*
Didronel® [US/Can] *see etidronate disodium on page 382*
dietary supplements *see nutritional formula, enteral/oral on page 689*

diethylene triamine penta-acetic acid
(dye ETH i leen TRYE a meen PEN ta a SEE tik AS id)

Synonyms Ca-DTPA; diethylenetriamine pentaacetic acid; DTPA; pentetate calcium trisodium; pentetate zinc trisodium; trisodium calcium diethylenetriaminepentaacetate (Ca-DTPA); zinc diethylenetriamine-pentaacetate (Zn-DTPA); Zn-DTPA

Therapeutic Category Antidote

Use Treatment of known or suspected internal contamination with plutonium, americium, or curium

Usual Dosage Internal contamination with plutonium, americium, or curium: Ca-DTPA is the preferred initial agent; sequential administration of Ca-DTPA then Zn-DTPA is recommended. I.V.:
Children <12 years:
Initial: Ca-DTPA: 14 mg/kg/day (maximum dose: 1 g/day)
Maintenance: Zn-DTPA: 14 mg/kg/day (maximum: 1 g/day); length of therapy depends on patient response and degree of contamination. **Note:** An equivalent dose of Ca-DTPA should be used for maintenance therapy only if Zn-DTPA is not available.
Children ≥12 years and Adults:
Initial: Ca-DTPA: 1 g/day
Pregnancy: Zn-DTPA 1 g/day should be used for the initial dose in pregnant women **except** in cases of high internal contamination
Maintenance: Zn-DTPA: 1 g/day; length of therapy depends on patient response and degree of contamination. **Note:** An equivalent dose of Ca-DTPA should be used for maintenance therapy only if Zn-DTPA is not available.

Dosage Forms
Injection, solution:
Ca-DTPA: 200 mg/mL (5 mL)
Zn-DTPA: 200 mg/mL (5 mL)

diethylenetriamine pentaacetic acid *see diethylene triamine penta-acetic acid on page 294*

diethylpropion (dye eth il PROE pee on)

Synonyms amfepramone; diethylpropion hydrochloride
U.S./Canadian Brand Names Tenuate® Dospan® [Can]; Tenuate® [Can]
Therapeutic Category Anorexiant
Controlled Substance C-IV
Use Short-term (few weeks) adjunct in the management of exogenous obesity
Usual Dosage Oral: Children >16 years and Adults:
Tablet: 25 mg 3 times/day before meals or food
Tablet, controlled release: 75 mg at midmorning
Dosage Forms
Tablet: 25 mg
Tablet, controlled release: 75 mg

diethylpropion hydrochloride *see diethylpropion on page 295*

difenoxin and atropine (dye fen OKS in & A troe peen)

Synonyms atropine and difenoxin
Therapeutic Category Antidiarrheal
Controlled Substance C-IV
Use Treatment of diarrhea
Usual Dosage Oral: Adults: Initial: 2 tablets (each tablet contains difenoxin hydrochloride 1 mg and atropine sulfate 0.025 mg), then 1 tablet after each loose stool; 1 tablet every 3-4 hours, up to 8 tablets in a 24-hour period; if no improvement after 48 hours, continued administration is not indicated

Differin® [US/Can] *see adapalene on page 34*
Differin® XP [Can] *see adapalene on page 34*
Difil-G [US] *see dyphylline and guaifenesin on page 330*
Difil®-G Forte [US] *see dyphylline and guaifenesin on page 330*

diflorasone (dye FLOR a sone)

Sound-Alike/Look-Alike Issues
Psorcon® may be confused with Proscar®, ProSom®, Psorion®
Synonyms diflorasone diacetate
U.S./Canadian Brand Names ApexiCon™ E [US]; ApexiCon™ [US]; Florone® [US/Can]; Psorcon® [Can]
Therapeutic Category Corticosteroid, Topical

▶

◀ **Use** Relieves inflammation and pruritic symptoms of corticosteroid-responsive dermatosis (high to very high potency topical corticosteroid)

Usual Dosage Topical: Apply ointment sparingly 1-3 times/day; apply cream sparingly 2-4 times/day. Therapy should be discontinued when control is achieved; if no improvement is seen, reassessment of diagnosis may be necessary.

Dosage Forms
Cream: 0.05% (15 g, 30 g, 60 g)
ApexiCon™ E: 0.05% (30 g, 60 g)
Ointment: 0.05% (15 g, 30 g, 60 g)
ApexiCon™: 0.05% (30 g, 60 g)

diflorasone diacetate *see* diflorasone *on page 295*
Diflucan® [US/Can] *see* fluconazole *on page 405*

diflunisal (dye FLOO ni sal)

Sound-Alike/Look-Alike Issues
Dolobid® may be confused with Slo-Bid®

Synonyms Dolobid

U.S./Canadian Brand Names Apo-Diflunisal® [Can]; Novo-Diflunisal [Can]; Nu-Diflunisal [Can]

Therapeutic Category Analgesic, Nonnarcotic; Nonsteroidal Antiinflammatory Drug (NSAID)

Use Management of inflammatory disorders usually including rheumatoid arthritis and osteoarthritis; can be used as an analgesic for treatment of mild-to-moderate pain

Usual Dosage Oral: Adults:
Mild-to-moderate pain: Initial: 500-1000 mg followed by 250-500 mg every 8-12 hours; maximum daily dose: 1.5 g
Arthritis: 500-1000 mg/day in 2 divided doses; maximum daily dose: 1.5 g

Dosage Forms
Tablet: 500 mg

Digibind® [US/Can] *see* digoxin immune Fab *on page 297*
DigiFab™ [US] *see* digoxin immune Fab *on page 297*
Digitek® [US] *see* digoxin *on page 296*

digoxin (di JOKS in)

Sound-Alike/Look-Alike Issues
digoxin may be confused with Desoxyn®, doxepin
Lanoxin® may be confused with Lasix®, Levoxyl®, Levsinex®, Lomotil®, Lonox®, Mefoxin®, Xanax®

U.S./Canadian Brand Names Apo-Digoxin® [Can]; Digitek® [US]; Digoxin CSD [Can]; Lanoxicaps® [Can]; Lanoxin® [US/Can]; Novo-Digoxin [Can]; Pediatric Digoxin CSD [Can]

Therapeutic Category Antiarrhythmic Agent, Miscellaneous; Cardiac Glycoside

Use Treatment of congestive heart failure and to slow the ventricular rate in tachyarrhythmias such as atrial fibrillation, atrial flutter, and supraventricular tachycardia (paroxysmal atrial tachycardia); cardiogenic shock

Usual Dosage When changing from oral (tablets or liquid) or I.M. to I.V. therapy, dosage should be reduced by 20% to 25%. Refer to the following:

Preterm infant[1]:
Total digitalizing dose[2]:
Oral: 20-30 mcg/kg[1]
I.V. or I.M.: 15-25 mcg/kg[1]
Daily maintenance dose[3]:
Oral: 5-7.5 mcg/kg[1]
I.V. or I.M.: 4-6 mcg/kg[1]
Full-term infant[1]:
Total digitalizing dose[2]:
Oral: 25-35 mcg/kg[1]
I.V. or I.M.: 20-30 mcg/kg[1]
Daily maintenance dose[3]:
Oral: 6-10 mcg/kg[1]
I.V. or I.M.: 5-8 mcg/kg[1]

1 month to 2 years[1]:
  Total digitalizing dose[2]:
    Oral: 35-60 mcg/kg[1]
    I.V. or I.M.: 30-50 mcg/kg[1]
  Daily maintenance dose[3]:
    Oral: 10-15 mcg/kg[1]
    I.V. or I.M.: 7.5-12 mcg/kg[1]
2-5 years[1]:
  Total digitalizing dose[2]:
    Oral: 30-40 mcg/kg[1]
    I.V. or I.M.: 25-35 mcg/kg[1]
  Daily maintenance dose[3]:
    Oral: 7.5-10 mcg/kg[1]
    I.V. or I.M.: 6-9 mcg/kg[1]
5-10 years[1]:
  Total digitalizing dose[2]:
    Oral: 20-35 mcg/kg[1]
    I.V. or I.M.: 15-30 mcg/kg[1]
  Daily maintenance dose[3]:
    Oral: 5-10 mcg/kg[1]
    I.V. or I.M.: 4-8 mcg/kg[1]
>10 years[1]:
  Total digitalizing dose[2]:
    Oral: 10-15 mcg/kg[1]
    I.V. or I.M.: 8-12 mcg/kg[1]
  Daily maintenance dose[3]:
    Oral: 2.5-5 mcg/kg[1]
    I.V. or I.M.: 2-3 mcg/kg[1]
Adults:
  Total digitalizing dose[2]:
    Oral: 0.75-1.5 mg
    I.V. or I.M.: 0.5-1 mg
  Daily maintenance dose[3]:
    Oral: 0.125-0.5 mg
    I.V. or I.M.: 0.1-0.4 mg
[1]Based on lean body weight and normal renal function for age. Decrease dose in patients with decreased renal function; digitalizing dose often not recommended in infants and children.
[2]Give one-half of the total digitalizing dose (TDD) in the initial dose, then give one-quarter of the TDD in each of two subsequent doses at 6- to 8-hour intervals. Obtain ECG 6 hours after each dose to assess potential toxicity.
[3]Divided every 12 hours in infants and children <10 years of age. Give once daily to children >10 years of age and adults.

Dosage Forms
  Injection: 250 mcg/mL (1 mL, 2 mL)
    Lanoxin®: 250 mcg/mL (2 mL)
  Injection, pediatric: 100 mcg/mL (1 mL)
  Solution, oral: 50 mcg/mL (2.5 mL, 5 mL, 60 mL)
  Tablet: 125 mcg, 250 mcg
    Digitek®, Lanoxin®: 125 mcg, 250 mcg

Digoxin CSD [Can] *see* digoxin *on page 296*

digoxin immune Fab (di JOKS in i MYUN fab)

Synonyms antidigoxin fab fragments, ovine
U.S./Canadian Brand Names Digibind® [US/Can]; DigiFab™ [US]
Therapeutic Category Antidote
Use Treatment of life-threatening or potentially life-threatening digoxin intoxication, including:
  • acute digoxin ingestion (ie, >10 mg in adults or >4 mg in children)
  • chronic ingestions leading to steady-state digoxin concentrations >6 ng/mL in adults or >4 ng/mL in children

- manifestations of digoxin toxicity due to overdose (life-threatening ventricular arrhythmias, progressive bradycardia, second- or third-degree heart block not responsive to atropine, serum potassium >5 mEq/L in adults or >6 mEq in children)

Usual Dosage Each vial of Digibind® 38 mg or DigiFab™ 40 mg will bind ~0.5 mg of digoxin or digitoxin.

Estimation of the dose is based on the body burden of digitalis. This may be calculated if the amount ingested is known or the postdistribution serum drug level is known (round dose to the nearest whole vial). Fab dose (in vials) based on number of tablets (0.25 mg) ingested.

Dosage Forms
Injection, powder for reconstitution:
  Digibind®: 38 mg
  DigiFab™: 40 mg

dihematoporphyrin ether see porfimer on page 769

Dihistine® DH *(Discontinued)* see chlorpheniramine, pseudoephedrine, and codeine on page 212

dihydrocodeine, aspirin, and caffeine (dye hye droe KOE deen, AS pir in, & KAF een)
Sound-Alike/Look-Alike Issues
  Synalgos®-DC may be confused with Synagis®
Synonyms dihydrocodeine compound
U.S./Canadian Brand Names Synalgos®-DC [US]
Therapeutic Category Analgesic, Narcotic
Controlled Substance C-III
Use Management of mild-to-moderate pain that requires relaxation
Usual Dosage Oral: Adults: 1-2 capsules every 4-6 hours as needed for pain
Dosage Forms
 Capsule:
  Synalgos®-DC: Dihydrocodeine 16 mg, aspirin 356.4 mg, and caffeine 30 mg

dihydrocodeine bitartrate, acetaminophen, and caffeine see acetaminophen, caffeine, and dihydrocodeine on page 25

dihydrocodeine bitartrate, phenylephrine hydrochloride, and chlorpheniramine maleate see phenylephrine, hydrocodone, and chlorpheniramine on page 748

dihydrocodeine bitartrate, pseudoephedrine hydrochloride, and chlorpheniramine maleate see pseudoephedrine, dihydrocodeine, and chlorpheniramine on page 803

dihydrocodeine, chlorpheniramine, and phenylephrine
(dye hye droe KOE deen, klor fen IR a meen, & fen il EF rin)
Synonyms chlorpheniramine maleate, dihydrocodeine bitartrate, and phenylephrine hydrochloride; phenylephrine, chlorpheniramine, and dihydrocodeine
U.S./Canadian Brand Names Baltussin [US]; Coldcough PD [US]; Novahistine DH [US]
Therapeutic Category Antihistamine; Antihistamine/Decongestant/Antitussive; Antitussive; Decongestant
Controlled Substance C-III/C-V
Use Symptomatic relief of cough and congestion associated with the upper respiratory tract
Usual Dosage Oral: Cough and congestion:
 Children 2-6 years (Novahistine DH): 1.25-2.5 mL every 4-6 hours as needed (maximum: 10 mL/24 hours)
 Children 6-12 years:
  Baltussin: 2.5 mL every 4-6 hours as needed
  Novahistine DH: 2.5-5 mL every 4-6 hours as needed (maximum: 20 mL/24 hours)
 Children ≥12 years and Adults:
  Baltussin: 5 mL every 4-6 hours as needed
  Novahistine DH: 5-10 mL every 4-6 hours as needed (maximum: 40 mL/24 hours)
Dosage Forms
 Liquid:
  Novahistine DH: Dihydrocodeine 7.5 mg, chlorpheniramine 2 mg and phenylephrine 5 mg per 5 mL
 Syrup:
  Baltussin: Dihydrocodeine 3 mg, chlorpheniramine 5 mg, and phenylephrine 20 mg per 5 mL
  Coldcough PD: Dihydrocodeine 3 mg, chlorpheniramine 2 mg, and phenylephrine 7.5 mg per 5 mL

dihydrocodeine compound *see dihydrocodeine, aspirin, and caffeine on page 298*

dihydrocodeine, pseudoephedrine, and guaifenesin
(dye hye droe KOE deen, soo doe e FED rin, & gwye FEN e sin)

Synonyms guaifenesin, dihydrocodeine, and pseudoephedrine; pseudoephedrine hydrochloride, guaifenesin, and dihydrocodeine bitartrate

U.S./Canadian Brand Names DiHydro-GP [US]; Pancof®-EXP [US]

Therapeutic Category Antitussive/Decongestant/Expectorant

Use Temporary relief of cough and congestion associated with upper respiratory tract infections and allergies

Usual Dosage Oral: Cough/congestion (Pancof®-EXP):

Children:

2-6 years: 1.25-2.5 mL every 4-6 hours as needed

6-12 years: 2.5-5 mL every 4-6 hours as needed

Children ≥12 years and Adults: 5-10 mL every 4-6 hours as needed

Dosage Forms

Syrup:

DiHydro-GP, Pancof®-EXP: Dihydrocodeine 7.5 mg, pseudoephedrine 15 mg, and guaifenesin 100 mg per 5 mL

DiHydro-CP [US] *see pseudoephedrine, dihydrocodeine, and chlorpheniramine on page 803*

dihydroergotamine (dye hye droe er GOT a meen)

Synonyms DHE; dihydroergotamine mesylate

U.S./Canadian Brand Names D.H.E. 45® [US]; Migranal® [US/Can]

Therapeutic Category Ergot Alkaloid and Derivative

Use Treatment of migraine headache with or without aura; injection also indicated for treatment of cluster headaches

Usual Dosage Adults:

I.M., SubQ: 1 mg at first sign of headache; repeat hourly to a maximum dose of 3 mg total; maximum dose: 6 mg/week

I.V.: 1 mg at first sign of headache; repeat hourly up to a maximum dose of 2 mg total; maximum dose: 6 mg/week

Intranasal: 1 spray (0.5 mg) of nasal spray should be administered into each nostril; if needed, repeat after 15 minutes, up to a total of 4 sprays. **Note:** Do not exceed 3 mg (6 sprays) in a 24-hour period and no more than 8 sprays in a week.

Dosage Forms

Injection, solution: 1 mg/mL (1 mL)

D.H.E. 45®: 1 mg/mL (1 mL)

Solution, intranasal spray:

Migranal®: 4 mg/mL [0.5 mg/spray] (1 mL)

dihydroergotamine mesylate *see dihydroergotamine on page 299*

dihydroergotoxine *see ergoloid mesylates on page 351*

dihydrogenated ergot alkaloids *see ergoloid mesylates on page 351*

DiHydro-GP [US] *see dihydrocodeine, pseudoephedrine, and guaifenesin on page 299*

dihydrohydroxycodeinone *see oxycodone on page 709*

dihydromorphinone *see hydromorphone on page 486*

dihydroxyanthracenedione dihydrochloride *see mitoxantrone on page 638*

1,25 dihydroxycholecalciferol *see calcitriol on page 160*

dihydroxydeoxynorvinkaleukoblastine *see vinorelbine on page 978*

dihydroxypropyl theophylline *see dyphylline on page 330*

Dihyrex® Injection *(Discontinued)* *see diphenhydramine on page 304*

diiodohydroxyquin *see iodoquinol on page 520*

Dilacor® XR [US] *see diltiazem on page 300*

Dilantin® [US/Can] *see phenytoin on page 750*

Dilatrate®-SR [US] *see isosorbide dinitrate on page 530*

Dilaudid® [US/Can] *see hydromorphone on page 486*

Dilaudid® Cough Syrup *(Discontinued)* *see* hydromorphone *on page 486*
Dilaudid-HP® [US/Can] *see* hydromorphone *on page 486*
Dilaudid-HP-Plus® [Can] *see* hydromorphone *on page 486*
Dilaudid® Sterile Powder [Can] *see* hydromorphone *on page 486*
Dilaudid-XP® [Can] *see* hydromorphone *on page 486*
Dilex-G [US] *see* dyphylline and guaifenesin *on page 330*
Dilocaine® Injection *(Discontinued)* *see* lidocaine *on page 561*
Dilomine® Injection *(Discontinued)* *see* dicyclomine *on page 293*
Dilor® [Can] *see* dyphylline *on page 330*
Dilor-G® [US] *see* dyphylline and guaifenesin *on page 330*
Dilt-CD [US] *see* diltiazem *on page 300*

diltiazem (dil TYE a zem)

Sound-Alike/Look-Alike Issues
diltiazem may be confused with Dilantin®
Cardizem® may be confused with Cardene®, Cardene SR®, Cardizem CD®, Cardizem SR®, cardiem
Cartia XT™ may be confused with Procardia XL®
Tiazac® may be confused with Tigan®, Tiazac® XC [Can], Ziac®

Synonyms diltiazem hydrochloride

U.S./Canadian Brand Names Alti-Diltiazem CD [Can]; Apo-Diltiaz CD® [Can]; Apo-Diltiaz SR® [Can]; Apo-Diltiaz TZ® [Can]; Apo-Diltiaz® Injectable [Can]; Apo-Diltiaz® [Can]; Cardizem® CD [US/Can]; Cardizem® LA [US]; Cardizem® SR [Can]; Cardizem® [US/Can]; Cartia XT™ [US]; Dilacor® XR [US]; Dilt-CD [US]; Dilt-XR [US]; Diltiazem HCl ER® [Can]; Diltiazem Hydrochloride Injection [Can]; Gen-Diltiazem CD [Can]; Gen-Diltiazem [Can]; Med-Diltiazem [Can]; Novo-Diltazem [Can]; Novo-Diltiazem-CD [Can]; Novo-Diltiazem HCl ER [Can]; Nu-Diltiaz [Can]; Nu-Diltiaz-CD [Can]; ratio-Diltiazem CD [Can]; Rhoxal-diltiazem CD [Can]; Rhoxal-diltiazem SR [Can]; Rhoxal-diltiazem T [Can]; Sandoz-Diltiazem CD [Can]; Sandoz-Diltiazem T [Can]; Syn-Diltiazem® [Can]; Taztia XT™ [US]; Tiazac® XC [Can]; Tiazac® [US/Can]

Therapeutic Category Calcium Channel Blocker

Use
Oral: Essential hypertension; chronic stable angina or angina from coronary artery spasm
Injection: Atrial fibrillation or atrial flutter; paroxysmal supraventricular tachycardia (PSVT)

Usual Dosage Adults:
Oral:
Angina:
Capsule, extended release (Cardizem® CD, Cartia XT™, Dilacor® XR, Tiazac®): Initial: 120-180 mg once daily (maximum dose: 480 mg/day)
Tablet, extended release (Cardizem® LA), Tiazac® XC [CAN; not available in U.S.]): 180 mg once daily; may increase at 7- to 14-day intervals (maximum recommended dose: 360 mg/day)
Tablet, immediate release (Cardizem®): Usual starting dose: 30 mg 4 times/day; usual range: 180-360 mg/day
Hypertension:
Capsule, extended release (Cardizem® CD, Cartia XT™, Dilacor® XR, Tiazac®): Initial: 180-240 mg once daily; dose adjustment may be made after 14 days; usual dose range (JNC 7): 180-420 mg/day; Tiazac®: usual dose range: 120-540 mg/day
Capsule, sustained release: Initial: 60-120 mg twice daily; dose adjustment may be made after 14 days; usual range: 240-360 mg/day
Tablet, extended release (Cardizem® LA, Tiazac® XC [CAN; not available in U.S.]): Initial: 180-240 mg once daily; dose adjustment may be made after 14 days; usual dose range (JNC 7): 120-540 mg/day
I.V.: Atrial fibrillation, atrial flutter, PSVT:
Initial bolus dose: 0.25 mg/kg actual body weight over 2 minutes (average adult dose: 20 mg)
Repeat bolus dose (may be administered after 15 minutes if the response is inadequate.): 0.35 mg/kg actual body weight over 2 minutes (average adult dose: 25 mg)
Continuous infusion (requires an infusion pump; infusions >24 hours or infusion rates >15 mg/hour are not recommended.): Initial infusion rate of 10 mg/hour; rate may be increased in 5 mg/hour increments up to 15 mg/hour as needed; some patients may respond to an initial rate of 5 mg/hour.
If diltiazem injection is administered by continuous infusion for >24 hours, the possibility of decreased diltiazem clearance, prolonged elimination half-life, and increased diltiazem and/or diltiazem metabolite plasma concentrations should be considered.

Conversion from I.V. diltiazem to oral diltiazem:
Oral dose (mg/day) is approximately equal to [rate (mg/hour) x 3 + 3] x 10.
3 mg/hour = 120 mg/day
5 mg/hour = 180 mg/day
7 mg/hour = 240 mg/day
11 mg/hour = 360 mg/day

Dosage Forms
Capsule, extended release [once-daily dosing]: 120 mg, 180 mg, 240 mg, 300 mg, 360 mg, 420 mg
Cardizem® CD, Taztia XT™: 120 mg, 180 mg, 240 mg, 300 mg, 360 mg
Cartia XT™: 120 mg, 180 mg, 240 mg, 300 mg
Dilacor® XR, Dilt-XR: 120 mg, 180 mg, 240 mg
Dilt-CD: 120 mg, 180 mg, 240 mg, 300 mg
Tiazac®: 120 mg, 180 mg, 240 mg, 300 mg, 360 mg, 420 mg
Capsule, extended release [twice-daily dosing]: 60 mg, 90 mg, 120 mg
Injection, solution: 5 mg/mL (5 mL, 10 mL, 25 mL)
Injection, powder for reconstitution: 100 mg
Tablet: 30 mg, 60 mg, 90 mg, 120 mg
Cardizem®: 30 mg, 60 mg, 90 mg, 120 mg
Tablet, extended release:
Cardizem® LA: 120 mg, 180 mg, 240 mg, 300 mg, 360 mg, 420 mg
Tiazac® XC [CAN; not available in U.S.]: 120 mg, 180 mg, 240 mg, 300 mg, 360 mg

Diltiazem HCl ER® [Can] *see* diltiazem *on page 300*
diltiazem hydrochloride *see* diltiazem *on page 300*
Diltiazem Hydrochloride Injection [Can] *see* diltiazem *on page 300*
Dilt-XR [US] *see* diltiazem *on page 300*
Dimaphen [US-OTC] *see* brompheniramine and pseudoephedrine *on page 144*
Dimaphen DM *(Discontinued)* *see* brompheniramine, pseudoephedrine, and dextromethorphan *on page 146*

dimenhydrinate (dye men HYE dri nate)
Sound-Alike/Look-Alike Issues
dimenhyDRINATE may be confused with diphenhydrAMINE
Tall-Man dimenhy**DRINATE**
U.S./Canadian Brand Names Apo-Dimenhydrinate® [Can]; Children's Motion Sickness Liquid [Can]; Dinate® [Can]; Dramamine® [US-OTC]; Driminate® [US-OTC]; Gravol® [Can]; Jamp® Travel Tablet [Can]; Nauseatol [Can]; Novo-Dimenate [Can]; SAB-Dimenhydrinate [Can]; TripTone® [US-OTC]
Therapeutic Category Antihistamine
Use Treatment and prevention of nausea, vertigo, and vomiting associated with motion sickness
Dosage forms available in Canada (not available in the U.S.), including parenteral formulations and suppositories, are also approved for the treatment of postoperative nausea and vomiting and treatment of radiation sickness.
Usual Dosage Oral:
Children:
2-5 years: 12.5-25 mg every 6-8 hours, maximum: 75 mg/day
6-12 years: 25-50 mg every 6-8 hours, maximum: 150 mg/day
Adults: 50-100 mg every 4-6 hours, not to exceed 400 mg/day
Gravol® L/A (not available in the U.S.): 75-150 mg every 8-12 hours, up to a maximum of five 75 mg caplets or three 100 mg caplets in 24 hours
Additional formulations/uses (approved in Canada) for parenteral/suppository formulations (not available in U.S.):
I.M., I.V., rectal: Adults:
Postoperative nausea and vomiting: 50-100 mg administered 30-60 minutes prior to radiation therapy; may be repeated as needed up to a maximum of 400 mg in 24 hours
Radiation sickness: 50-100 mg administered 30-60 minutes prior to radiation therapy. May be repeated as needed up to a maximum of 400 mg in 24 hours
Dosage Forms [CAN] = Canadian brand name
Capsule, softgel: 50 mg [not available in the U.S.]
Gravol® [CAN]: 50 mg [not available in the U.S.]
Capsule, long-acting: 75 mg, 100 mg [not available in the U.S.]
Gravol® L/A [CAN]: 75 mg, 100 mg [not available in the U.S.]

◄ **Injection, solution:** 50 mg/mL (1 mL)
Gravol® I.M. [CAN]: 50 mg/mL (1 mL, 5 mL) [not available in the U.S.]
Gravol® I.V. [CAN]: 10 mg/mL (5 mL) [not available in the U.S.]
Solution, oral: 3 mg/mL [not available in the U.S.]
Gravol® [CAN], Children's Motion Sickness [CAN]: 3 mg/mL [not available in the U.S.]
Suppository, rectal: 75 mg, 100 mg [not available in the U.S.]
Gravol® [CAN], Sab-Dimenhydrinate [CAN]: 75 mg, 100 mg [not available in the U.S.]
Tablet: 50 mg
Dinate® [CAN], Dramamine® [OTC], Jamp® Travel Tablet [CAN], Nauseatol® [CAN], TripTone®: 50 mg
Driminate®: 50 mg [scored]
Gravol® Filmkote Jr [CAN]: 25 mg [not available in the U.S.]
Gravol® Filmkote [CAN]: 50 mg [not available in the U.S.]
Tablet, chewable: 50 mg
Dramamine® [OTC]: 50 mg
Gravol® Chewable for Children [CAN]: 25 mg [not available in the U.S.]
Gravol® Chewable for Adults [CAN]: 50 mg [not available in the U.S.]

dimercaprol (dye mer KAP role)

Synonyms BAL; British anti-lewisite; dithioglycerol

U.S./Canadian Brand Names BAL in Oil® [US]

Therapeutic Category Chelating Agent

Use Antidote to gold, arsenic (except arsine), or acute mercury poisoning (except nonalkyl mercury); adjunct to edetate CALCIUM disodium in lead poisoning

Usual Dosage Note: Premedication with a histamine H_1 antagonist (eg, diphenhydramine) is recommended.

Children and Adults: Deep I.M.:
Mild arsenic or gold poisoning: 2.5 mg/kg every 6 hours for 2 days, then every 12 hours for 1 day, followed by once daily for 10 days
Severe arsenic or gold poisoning: 3 mg/kg every 4 hours for 2 days, then every 6 hours for 1 day, followed every 12 hours for 10 days
Mercury poisoning: 5 mg/kg initially, followed by 2.5 mg/kg 1-2 times/day for 10 days
Lead poisoning: **Note:** For the treatment of high blood lead levels in children, the CDC recommends chelation treatment when blood lead levels are >45 mcg/dL (CDC, 2002). Combination parenteral therapy is indicated when blood lead levels are ≥70 mcg/dL, or patients are symptomatic (AAP, 2005). In adults, available guidelines recommend chelation therapy with blood lead levels >50 mcg/dL and significant symptoms; chelation therapy may also be indicated with blood lead levels ≥100 mcg/dL and/ or symptoms.
Lead encephalopathy (in conjunction with edetate CALCIUM disodium): Dimercaprol 4 mg/kg (75 mg/ m^2) loading dose, followed by dimercaprol 4 mg/kg (75 mg/m^2) every 4 hours for 2-7 days (edetate CALCIUM disodium is **not** administered with the loading dose; begin edetate CALCIUM disodium with the second dose)
Symptomatic lead poisoning or blood lead levels ≥70 mcg/dL (in conjunction with edetate CALCIUM disodium): Dimercaprol 4 mg/kg (75 mg/m^2) loading dose, followed by dimercaprol 3 mg/kg/dose (50 mg/m^2) every 4 hours for 2-7 days (edetate CALCIUM disodium is **not** administered with the loading dose; begin edetate CALCIUM disodium with the second dose)

Dosage Forms
Injection, oil:
BAL in Oil®: 100 mg/mL (3 mL)

Dimetabs® Oral (Discontinued) see dimenhydrinate on page 301
Dimetapp® 12-Hour Non-Drowsy Extentabs® (Discontinued) see pseudoephedrine on page 801
Dimetapp® Children's ND (Discontinued) see loratadine on page 576
Dimetapp® Decongestant Infant (Discontinued) see pseudoephedrine on page 801
Dimetapp® DM Children's Cold and Cough (Discontinued) see brompheniramine, pseudoephedrine, and dextromethorphan on page 146
Dimetapp® Infant Decongestant Plus Cough (Discontinued) see pseudoephedrine and dextromethorphan on page 802
Dimetapp® ND Children's [US-OTC] see loratadine on page 576
Dimetapp® Sinus Caplets (Discontinued) see pseudoephedrine and ibuprofen on page 802

Dimetapp® Toddler's [US-OTC] *see* phenylephrine *on page 745*

dimethyl sulfoxide (dye meth il sul FOKS ide)

Synonyms DMSO

U.S./Canadian Brand Names Dimethyl Sulfoxide Irrigation, USP [Can]; Kemsol® [Can]; Rimso®-50 [US/Can]

Therapeutic Category Urinary Tract Product

Use Symptomatic relief of interstitial cystitis

Usual Dosage Adults: Bladder instillation: Instill 50 mL directly into bladder and allow to remain for 15 minutes; repeat every 2 weeks until symptoms are relieved, then increase intervals between treatments **or** 50 mL directly into bladder for 15-20 minutes every 1-2 weeks for 4-8 treatments

Dosage Forms

Solution, intravesical:

Rimso-50®: 50% [500 mg/mL] (50 mL)

Dimethyl Sulfoxide Irrigation, USP [Can] *see* dimethyl sulfoxide *on page 303*
dimethyl triazeno imidazole carboxamide *see* dacarbazine *on page 263*
Dinate® [Can] *see* dimenhydrinate *on page 301*
Dinate® Injection *(Discontinued)* *see* dimenhydrinate *on page 301*

dinoprostone (dye noe PROST one)

Sound-Alike/Look-Alike Issues

Prepidil® may be confused with Bepridil®

Synonyms PGE$_2$; prostaglandin E$_2$

U.S./Canadian Brand Names Cervidil® [US/Can]; Prepidil® [US/Can]; Prostin E$_2$® [US/Can]

Therapeutic Category Prostaglandin

Use

Gel: Promote cervical ripening in patients at or near term in whom there is a medical or obstetrical indication for the induction of labor

Suppositories: Terminate pregnancy from 12th through 20th week of gestation; evacuate uterus in cases of missed abortion or intrauterine fetal death up to 28 weeks of gestation; manage benign hydatidiform mole (nonmetastatic gestational trophoblastic disease)

Vaginal insert: Initiation and/or continuation of cervical ripening in patients at or near term in whom there is a medical or obstetrical indication for the induction of labor

Usual Dosage Females of reproductive age:

Abortifacient: Vaginal suppository: Insert 20 mg (1 suppository) high in vagina, repeat at 3- to 5-hour intervals until abortion occurs; continued administration for longer than 2 days is not advisable

Cervical ripening:

Endocervical gel: Using catheter supplied with gel, insert 0.5 mg into the cervical canal. May repeat every 6 hours if needed. Maximum cumulative dose: 1.5 mg/24 hours

Vaginal insert: Insert 10 mg transversely into the posterior fornix of the vagina (to be removed at the onset of active labor or after 12 hours)

Dosage Forms

Gel, endocervical:

Prepidil®: 0.5 mg/3 g syringe

Insert, vaginal:

Cervidil®: 10 mg

Suppository, vaginal:

Prostin E$_2$®: 20 mg

Diocaine® [Can] *see* proparacaine *on page 794*
Diocarpine [Can] *see* pilocarpine *on page 753*
Diochloram® [Can] *see* chloramphenicol *on page 200*
Diocto® [US-OTC] *see* docusate *on page 314*
Diocto C® *(Discontinued)*
Diocto-K® *(Discontinued)* *see* docusate *on page 314*
Diocto-K Plus® *(Discontinued)* *see* docusate *on page 314*
dioctyl calcium sulfosuccinate *see* docusate *on page 314*

dioctyl sodium sulfosuccinate see docusate on page 314
Diodex® [Can] see dexamethasone (systemic) on page 278
Diodoquin® [Can] see iodoquinol on page 520
Diogent® [Can] see gentamicin on page 442
Diomycin® [Can] see erythromycin on page 354
Dionephrine® [Can] see phenylephrine on page 745
Diopentolate® [Can] see cyclopentolate on page 256
Diopred® [Can] see prednisolone (systemic) on page 781
Dioptic's Atropine Solution [Can] see atropine on page 104
Dioptimyd® [Can] see sulfacetamide and prednisolone on page 893
Dioptrol® [Can] see neomycin, polymyxin B, and dexamethasone on page 662
Diosulf™ [Can] see sulfacetamide on page 892
Diotame® [US-OTC] see bismuth on page 136
Diotrope® [Can] see tropicamide on page 957
Dioval® Injection (Discontinued) see estradiol on page 359
Diovan® [US/Can] see valsartan on page 968
Diovan HCT® [US/Can] see valsartan and hydrochlorothiazide on page 969
Diovol® [Can] see aluminum hydroxide and magnesium hydroxide on page 54
Diovol® Ex [Can] see aluminum hydroxide and magnesium hydroxide on page 54
Diovol Plus® [Can] see aluminum hydroxide, magnesium hydroxide, and simethicone on page 54
Dipentum® [US/Can] see olsalazine on page 696
Diphen® [US-OTC] see diphenhydramine on page 304
Diphenacen 50® Injection (Discontinued) see diphenhydramine on page 304
Diphen® AF [US-OTC] see diphenhydramine on page 304
Diphenatol® (Discontinued) see diphenoxylate and atropine on page 306
Diphenhist [US-OTC] see diphenhydramine on page 304

diphenhydramine (dye fen HYE dra meen)

Sound-Alike/Look-Alike Issues
diphenhydrAMINE may be confused with desipramine, dicyclomine, dimenhyDRINATE
Benadryl® may be confused with benazepril, Bentyl®, Benylin®, Caladryl®

Synonyms diphenhydramine citrate; diphenhydramine hydrochloride; diphenhydramine tannate

Tall-Man diphenhydrAMINE

U.S./Canadian Brand Names Aler-Cap [US-OTC]; Aler-Dryl [US-OTC]; Aler-Tab [US-OTC]; Allerdryl® [Can]; AllerMax® [US-OTC]; Allernix [Can]; Altaryl [US-OTC]; Banophen® Anti-Itch [US-OTC]; Banophen® [US-OTC]; Ben-Tann [US]; Benadryl® Allergy [US-OTC]; Benadryl® Children's Allergy Fastmelt® [US-OTC]; Benadryl® Children's Allergy [US-OTC]; Benadryl® Children's Dye-Free Allergy [US-OTC]; Benadryl® Itch Stopping Extra Strength [US-OTC]; Benadryl® Itch Stopping [US-OTC]; Benadryl® [Can]; Compoz® Nighttime Sleep Aid [US-OTC]; Dermamycin® [US-OTC]; Diphenhist [US-OTC]; Diphen® AF [US-OTC]; Diphen® [US-OTC]; Dytan™ [US]; Genahist® [US-OTC]; Hydramine® [US-OTC]; Nytol® Extra Strength [Can]; Nytol® Quick Caps [US-OTC]; Nytol® Quick Gels [US-OTC]; Nytol® [Can]; PMS-Diphenhydramine [Can]; Siladryl® Allergy [US-OTC]; Silphen® [US-OTC]; Simply Sleep® [US-OTC/Can]; Sleep-ettes D [US-OTC]; Sleepinal® [US-OTC]; Sominex® Maximum Strength [US-OTC]; Sominex® [US-OTC]; Triaminic® Thin Strips™ Cough and Runny Nose [US-OTC]; Twilite® [US-OTC]; Unisom® Maximum Strength SleepGels® [US-OTC]

Therapeutic Category Antihistamine

Use Symptomatic relief of allergic symptoms caused by histamine release including nasal allergies and allergic dermatosis; adjunct to epinephrine in the treatment of anaphylaxis; nighttime sleep aid; prevention or treatment of motion sickness; antitussive; management of parkinsonian syndrome including drug-induced extrapyramidal symptoms; topically for relief of pain and itching associated with insect bites, minor cuts and burns, or rashes due to poison ivy, poison oak, and poison sumac

Usual Dosage Note: Dosages are expressed as the hydrochloride salt.
Children:
Allergic reactions or motion sickness: Oral, I.M., I.V.: 5 mg/kg/day or 150 mg/m^2/day in divided doses every 6-8 hours, not to exceed 300 mg/day
Alternate dosing by age: Oral:
2 to <6 years: 6.25 mg every 4-6 hours; maximum: 37.5 mg/day

6 to <12 years: 12.5-25 mg every 4-6 hours; maximum: 150 mg/day
  ≥12 years: 25-50 mg every 4-6 hours; maximum: 300 mg/day
Night-time sleep aid: Oral: Children ≥12 years: 50 mg at bedtime
Antitussive: Oral:
  2 to <6 years: 6.25 mg every 4 hours; maximum 37.5 mg/day
  6 to <12 years: 12.5 mg every 4 hours; maximum 75 mg/day
  ≥12 years: 25 mg every 4 hours; maximum 150 mg/day
Treatment of dystonic reactions: I.M., I.V.: 0.5-1 mg/kg/dose
Relief of pain and itching: Topical: Children ≥2 years: Apply 1% or 2% to affected area up to 3-4 times/
  day
Adults:
  Allergic reactions or motion sickness: Oral: 25-50 mg every 6-8 hours
  Antitussive: Oral: 25 mg every 4 hours; maximum 150 mg/24 hours
  Nighttime sleep aid: Oral: 50 mg at bedtime
  Allergic reactions or motion sickness: I.M., I.V.: 10-50 mg per dose; single doses up to 100 mg may be
    used if needed; not to exceed 400 mg/day
  Dystonic reaction: I.M., I.V.: 50 mg in a single dose; may repeat in 20-30 minutes if necessary
  Relief of pain and itching: Topical: Apply 1% or 2% to affected area up to 3-4 times/day

Dosage Forms

Caplet: 25 mg, 50 mg
  Aler-Dryl [OTC], AllerMax® [OTC], Compoz® Nighttime Sleep Aid [OTC], Sleep-ettes D [OTC],
    Sominex® Maximum Strength [OTC], Twilite® [OTC]: 50 mg
  Nytol® Quick Caps [OTC], Simply Sleep® [OTC]: 25 mg
Capsule: 25 mg, 50 mg
  Aler-Cap [OTC], Banophen® [OTC], Benadryl® Allergy [OTC], Diphen® [OTC], Diphenhist [OTC],
    Genahist® [OTC]: 25 mg
  Sleepinal® [OTC]: 50 mg
Capsule, softgel: 50 mg
  Benadryl® Dye-Free Allergy [OTC]: 25 mg
  Compoz® Nighttime Sleep Aid [OTC], Nytol® Quick Gels [OTC], Sleepinal® [OTC], Unisom® Maximum
    Strength SleepGels® [OTC]: 50 mg
Captab: 25 mg
  Diphenhist® [OTC]: 25 mg
Cream: 2% (30 g)
  Banophen® Anti-Itch [OTC], Benadryl® Itch Stopping Extra Strength [OTC], Diphenhist® [OTC]: 2% (30
    g)
  Benadryl® Itch Stopping [OTC]: 1% (30 g)
Elixir:
  Altaryl [OTC], Banophen® [OTC], Diphen AF [OTC]: 12.5 mg/5 mL
Gel, topical: 2% (120 mL, 28 g, 42 g)
  Benadryl® Itch Stopping Extra Strength [OTC]: 2% (120 mL)
Injection, solution: 50 mg/mL (1 mL, 10 mL)
Liquid, as hydrochloride:
  AllerMax® [OTC], Benadryl® Allergy [OTC], Benadryl® Children's Dye-Free Allergy [OTC], Genahist®
    [OTC], Hydramine® [OTC], Siladryl® Allergy [OTC]: 12.5 mg/5 mL
Liquid, topical [stick]:
  Benadryl® Itch Stopping Extra Strength [OTC]: 2% (14 mL)
Solution, oral:
  Diphenhis [OTC]: 12.5 mg/5mL
Solution, topical [spray]: 2% (60 mL)
  Benadryl® Itch Stopping Extra Strength [OTC], Dermamycin® [OTC]: 2% (60 mL)
Strips, oral:
  Benadryl® Allergy [OTC]: 25 mg (10s)
  Benadryl® Children's Allergy [OTC]: 12. 5 mg (10s)
  Triaminic® Thin Strips™ Cough and Runny Nose [OTC]: 12. 5 mg (16s)
Suspension:
  Ben-Tann: 25 mg/5 mL
Syrup: 12.5 mg/5 mL
  Silphen® Cough [OTC]: 12.5 mg/5 mL
Tablet: 25 mg, 50 mg
  Aler-Tab [OTC], Benadryl® Allergy [OTC], Genahist® [OTC], Sominex® [OTC]: 25 mg

▶

◀ **Tablet, chewable:**
Benadryl® Children's Allergy [OTC]: 12.5 mg
Dytan™: 25 mg
Tablet, orally disintegrating:
Benadryl® Children's Allergy Fastmelt® [OTC]: 19 mg

diphenhydramine and acetaminophen *see* acetaminophen and diphenhydramine *on page 21*

diphenhydramine and pseudoephedrine (dye fen HYE dra meen & soo doe e FED rin)

Sound-Alike/Look-Alike Issues
Benadryl® may be confused with benazepril, Bentyl®, Benylin®, Caladryl®
Synonyms pseudoephedrine and diphenhydramine
U.S./Canadian Brand Names Benadryl-D™ Allergy and Sinus Fastmelt™ [US-OTC]; Benadryl-D™ Children's Allergy and Sinus [US-OTC]; Benadryl® Children's Allergy and Cold Fastmelt™ [US-OTC]
Therapeutic Category Antihistamine/Decongestant Combination
Use Relief of symptoms of upper respiratory mucosal congestion in seasonal and perennial nasal allergies, acute rhinitis, rhinosinusitis, and eustachian tube blockage
Usual Dosage Oral: Adults: Based on **pseudoephedrine** component: 60 mg every 4-6 hours, maximum: 240 mg/day
Dosage Forms
Liquid:
Benadryl-D™ Children's Allergy and Sinus [OTC]: Diphenhydramine 12.5 mg and pseudoephedrine 30 mg per 5 mL
Tablet, quick dissolving:
Benadryl® Children's Allergy and Cold Fastmelt™ [OTC], Benadryl-D™ Allergy and Sinus Fastmelt™ [OTC]: Diphenhydramine 19 mg and pseudoephedrine 30 mg

diphenhydramine citrate *see* diphenhydramine *on page 304*
diphenhydramine hydrochloride *see* diphenhydramine *on page 304*
diphenhydramine tannate *see* diphenhydramine *on page 304*

diphenoxylate and atropine (dye fen OKS i late & A troe peen)

Sound-Alike/Look-Alike Issues
Lomotil® may be confused with Lamictal®, Lamisil®, lamotrigine, Lanoxin®, Lasix®, ludiomil
Lonox® may be confused with Lanoxin®, Loprox®
Synonyms atropine and diphenoxylate
U.S./Canadian Brand Names Lomotil® [US/Can]; Lonox® [US]
Therapeutic Category Antidiarrheal
Controlled Substance C-V
Use Treatment of diarrhea
Usual Dosage Oral:
Children 2-12 years (use with caution in young children due to variable responses): Liquid: Diphenoxylate 0.3-0.4 mg/kg/day in 4 divided doses until control achieved (maximum: 10 mg/day), then reduce dose as needed; some patients may be controlled on doses as low as 25% of the initial daily dose
Adults: Diphenoxylate 5 mg 4 times/day until control achieved (maximum: 20 mg/day), then reduce dose as needed; some patients may be controlled on doses of 5 mg/day
Dosage Forms
Solution, oral: Diphenoxylate 2.5 mg and atropine 0.025 mg per 5 mL
Lomotil®: Diphenoxylate 2.5 mg and atropine 0.025 mg per 5 mL
Tablet: Diphenoxylate 2.5 mg and atropine 0.025 mg
Lomotil®, Lonox®: Diphenoxylate 2.5 mg and atropine 0.025 mg

Diphenylan Sodium® *(Discontinued)* *see* phenytoin *on page 750*
diphenylhydantoin *see* phenytoin *on page 750*

diphtheria and tetanus toxoid (dif THEER ee a & TET a nus TOKS oyds)

Synonyms DT; Td; tetanus and diphtheria toxoid
U.S./Canadian Brand Names Decavac™ [US]; Td Adsorbed [Can]
Therapeutic Category Toxoid

Use

Diphtheria and tetanus toxoids adsorbed for pediatric use (DT): Infants and children through 6 years of age: Active immunization against diphtheria and tetanus when pertussis vaccine is contraindicated

Tetanus and diphtheria toxoids adsorbed for adult use (Td) (Decavac™): Children ≥7 years of age and Adults: Active immunization against diphtheria and tetanus; tetanus prophylaxis in wound management

The Advisory Committee on Immunization Practices (ACIP) recommends routine vaccination for the following:
- Adults and children ≥7 years should receive a booster dose of Td every 10 years; persons <65 years of age may substitute a single Td booster dose with Tdap
- Children 7-10 years, adults, and the elderly (≥65 years) who are wounded in bombings or similar mass casualty events who have penetrating injuries or nonintact skin exposure and who cannot confirm receipt of a tetanus booster within the previous 5 years, may also receive a single dose of Td; children ≥11 years may also received Td if Tdap is unavailable

Usual Dosage I.M.:

Infants and Children ≤6 years (DT): Primary immunization:

6 weeks to 1 year: Three 0.5 mL doses at least 4 weeks apart; administer a reinforcing dose 6-12 months after the third injection

1-6 years: Two 0.5 mL doses at least 4 weeks apart; reinforcing dose 6-12 months after second injection; if final dose is given after seventh birthday, use adult preparation

4-6 years (booster immunization): 0.5 mL; not necessary if the fourth dose was given after fourth birthday; routinely administer booster doses at 10-year intervals with the adult preparation

Children ≥7 years and Adults (Td):

Primary immunization: Patients previously not immunized should receive 2 primary doses of 0.5 mL each, given at an interval of 4-6 weeks; third (reinforcing) dose of 0.5 mL 6-12 months later

Booster immunization: 0.5 mL every 10 years; to be given to children 11-12 years of age if at least 5 years have elapsed since last dose of toxoid containing vaccine. Subsequent routine doses are not recommended more often than every 10 years. The ACIP prefers Tdap for use in adolescents 11-18 years; refer to diphtheria and tetanus toxoids and acellular pertussis vaccine monograph for additional information.

Tetanus prophylaxis in wound management; use of tetanus toxoid (Td) and/or tetanus immune globulin (TIG) depends upon the number of prior tetanus toxoid doses and type of wound.

Clean, minor wounds:
- Prior number of tetanus toxoid doses is unknown or <3: Td[1]
- Prior number of tetanus toxoid doses is ≥3: Td[1] only if >10 years since last dose
- If only three doses of fluid tetanus toxoid have been received, a fourth dose of toxoid, preferably an adsorbed toxoid, should be given

All other wounds:
- Prior number of tetanus toxoid doses is unknown or <3: Td[1] and TIG
- Prior number of tetanus toxoid doses is ≥3: Td[1] only if >5 years since last dose

[1]Adult tetanus and diphtheria toxoids; use pediatric preparations (DT or DTP) if the patient is <7 years old. Adapted from Report of the Committee on Infectious Diseases, American Academy of Pediatrics, Elk Grove Village, IL: American Academy of Pediatrics, 1986.

Dosage Forms

Injection, suspension [adult]: Diphtheria 2 Lf units and tetanus 5 Lf units per 0.5 mL (7.5 mL)

Decavac™: Diphtheria 2 Lf units and tetanus 5 Lf units per 0.5 mL (0.5 mL)

Injection, suspension [adult; preservative free]: Diphtheria 2 IF units and tetanus 5 Lf units per 0.5 mL (0.5 mL)

Injection, suspension [pediatric; preservative free]: Diphtheria 6.7 Lf units and tetanus 5 Lf units per 0.5 mL (0.5 mL)

diphtheria and tetanus toxoids, acellular pertussis, and poliovirus (inactivated) vaccine

(dif THEER ee a & TET a nus TOKS oyds, ay CEL yoo lar per TUS sis & POE lee oh VYE rus in ak ti VAY ted vak SEEN)

Synonyms diphtheria and tetanus toxoids and acellular pertussis adsorbed, and inactivated poliovirus vaccine combined; diphtheria, tetanus toxoids, acellular pertussis (DTaP); poliovirus, inactivated (IPV)

U.S./Canadian Brand Names Kinrix™ [US]

Therapeutic Category Vaccine, Inactivated

Use Active immunization against diphtheria, tetanus, pertussis, and poliomyelitis, used as the 5th dose in the DTaP series and the 4th dose in the IPV series

◀ **Usual Dosage** I.M.: Children 4-6 years: Immunization: 0.5 mL; **Note:** For use as the 5th dose in the DTaP series and the 4th dose in the IPV series

Dosage Forms

Injection, suspension [preservative free]:

Kinrix™: Diphtheria toxoid 25 Lf, tetanus toxoid 10 Lf, inactivated PT 25 mcg, FHA 25 mcg, pertactin 8 mcg, poliovirus type 1 40 DU, poliovirus type 2 8 DU, and poliovirus type 3 32 DU per 0.5 mL

diphtheria and tetanus toxoids, acellular pertussis, poliovirus (inactivated) and *Haemophilus* b conjugate vaccine

(dif THEER ee a & TET a nus TOKS oyds ay CEL yoo lar per TUS sis POE lee oh VYE rus in ak ti VAY ted & hem OF fi lus in floo EN za bee KON joo gate vak SEEN)

Synonyms *Haemophilus* B conjugate (Hib); *Haemophilus* B polysaccharide; diphtheria toxoid; diphtheria, tetanus toxoids, acellular pertussis (DTaP); DTaP-IPV/Hib; pertussis, acellular (adsorbed); poliovirus, inactivated (IPV); tetanus toxoid

U.S./Canadian Brand Names Pentacel® [US]

Therapeutic Category Vaccine, Inactivated

Use Active immunization against diphtheria, tetanus, pertussis, poliomyelitis, and invasive disease caused by *H. influenzae* type b in children 6 weeks through 4 years of age

Dosage Forms

Injection, suspension:

Pentacel®: Diphtheria toxoid 15 Lf, tetanus toxoid 5 Lf, acellular pertussis antigens [pertussis toxin detoxified 20 mcg, filamentous hemagglutinin 20 mcg, pertactin 3 mcg, fimbriae types 2 and 3 5 mcg], poliovirus [type 1: 40 D-antigen units, type 2: 8 D antigen units, type 3: 32 D antigen units], and *Haemophilus* b capsular polysaccharide 10 mcg [bound to tetanus toxoid 24 mcg] per 0.5 mL (0.5 mL) [contains albumin, aluminum, neomycin, polymyxin B sulfate, and polysorbate 80; supplied in two vials, one containing DTaP-IPV liquid and one containing Hib powder]

diphtheria and tetanus toxoids and acellular pertussis adsorbed, and inactivated poliovirus vaccine combined *see* diphtheria and tetanus toxoids, acellular pertussis, and poliovirus (inactivated) vaccine *on page 307*

diphtheria and tetanus toxoids and acellular pertussis adsorbed, hepatitis B (recombinant) and inactivated poliovirus vaccine combined *see* diphtheria, tetanus toxoids, acellular pertussis, hepatitis B (recombinant), and poliovirus (inactivated) vaccine *on page 308*

diphtheria antitoxin (dif THEER ee a an tee TOKS in)

Therapeutic Category Antitoxin

Use Treatment of diphtheria (neutralizes unbound toxin, available from CDC)

Usual Dosage I.M. or slow I.V. infusion: Dosage varies; range: 20,000-120,000 units

diphtheria CRM$_{197}$ protein *see* pneumococcal conjugate vaccine (7-valent) *on page 762*

diphtheria CRM$_{197}$ protein conjugate *see Haemophilus* B conjugate vaccine *on page 464*

diphtheria, tetanus toxoids, acellular pertussis (DTaP) *see* diphtheria and tetanus toxoids, acellular pertussis, and poliovirus (inactivated) vaccine *on page 307*

diphtheria, tetanus toxoids, acellular pertussis (DTaP) *see* diphtheria and tetanus toxoids, acellular pertussis, poliovirus (inactivated) and *Haemophilus* b conjugate vaccine *on page 308*

diphtheria, tetanus toxoids, acellular pertussis, hepatitis B (recombinant), and poliovirus (inactivated) vaccine

(dif THEER ee a, TET a nus TOKS oyds, ay CEL yoo lar per TUS sis, hep a TYE tis bee ree KOM be nant, & POE lee oh VYE rus, in ak ti VAY ted vak SEEN)

Synonyms diphtheria and tetanus toxoids and acellular pertussis adsorbed, hepatitis B (recombinant) and inactivated poliovirus vaccine combined

U.S./Canadian Brand Names Pediarix® [US/Can]

Therapeutic Category Vaccine

Use Combination vaccine for the active immunization against diphtheria, tetanus, pertussis, hepatitis B virus (all known subtypes), and poliomyelitis (caused by poliovirus types 1, 2, and 3)

Usual Dosage I.M.: Children 6 weeks to <7 years:

Immunization: 0.5 mL; repeat in 6-8 week intervals (preferably 8-week intervals) for a total of 3 doses. Vaccination usually begins at 2 months, but may be started as early as 6 weeks of age.

Use in children previously vaccinated with one or more component, and who are also scheduled to receive all vaccine components:

Hepatitis B vaccine: Infants born of HB$_s$Ag-negative mothers who received 1 dose of hepatitis B vaccine at birth may be given Pediarix® (safety data limited); use in infants who received more than 1 dose of hepatitis B vaccine has not been studied. Infants who received 1 or more doses of hepatitis B vaccine (recombinant) may be given Pediarix® to complete the hepatitis B series (safety and efficacy not established).

Diphtheria and tetanus toxoids, and acellular pertussis vaccine (DTaP): Infants previously vaccinated with 1 or 2 doses of Infanrix® may use Pediarix® to complete the first 3 doses of the series (safety and efficacy not established); use of Pediarix® to complete DTaP vaccination started with products other than Infanrix® is not recommended.

Inactivated polio vaccine (IPV): Infants previously vaccinated with 1 or 2 doses of IPV may use Pediarix® to complete the first 3 doses of the series (safety and efficacy not established).

Dosage Forms

Injection, suspension [preservative free]:

Pediarix®: Diphtheria toxoid 25 Lf, tetanus toxoid 10 Lf, inactivated PT 25 mcg, FHA 25 mcg, pertactin 8 mcg, HBsAg 10 mcg, poliovirus type 1 40 DU, poliovirus type 2 8 DU, and poliovirus type 3 32 DU per 0.5 mL

diphtheria, tetanus toxoids, and acellular pertussis vaccine

(dif THEER ee a, TET a nus TOKS oyds & ay CEL yoo lar per TUS sis vak SEEN)

Synonyms DTaP; dTpa; Tdap; tetanus toxoid, reduced diphtheria toxoid, and acellular pertussis, adsorbed

U.S./Canadian Brand Names Adacel™ [US/Can]; Boostrix® [US]; Daptacel® [US]; Infanrix® [US]; Tripedia® [US]

Therapeutic Category Toxoid

Use

Daptacel®, Infanrix®, Tripedia® (DTaP): Active immunization against diphtheria, tetanus, and pertussis from age 6 weeks through 6 years of age (prior to seventh birthday)

Adacel®, Boostrix® (Tdap): Active booster immunization against diphtheria, tetanus, and pertussis

The Advisory Committee on Immunization Practices (ACIP) recommends routine vaccination for the following:

Children 6 weeks to <7 years (DTaP): For primary immunization against diphtheria, tetanus and pertussis

Adolescents 11-18 years (Tdap) (Adacel®, Boostrix®):

- A single dose of Tdap as a booster dose in adolescents who have completed the recommended childhood DTaP vaccination series (preferred age of administration is 11-12 years)
- A single dose of Tdap should be given to replace a single dose of Td if the last dose of Td was ≥5 years earlier; lesser intervals may be used if the benefit outweighs the risk (not for multiple administrations; recommendations are for the replacement of a single dose of Td only)
- Persons wounded in bombings or similar mass casualty events and who cannot confirm receipt of a tetanus booster within the previous 5 years and who have penetrating injuries or nonintact skin exposure should receive a single dose of Tdap

Adults aged 19-64 (Adacel®): A single dose of Tdap should be given to replace a single dose of Td if the last dose of Td was ≥10 years earlier (not for multiple administrations; recommendations are for the replacement of a single dose of Td only). A shorter interval (<10 years but at least 2 years since last dose of Td) may be considered in the following situations:

- To protect against pertussis
- To protect against pertussis transmission to infants in adults who anticipate close contact with children <12 months of age; Tdap should be administered at least 2 weeks prior to beginning close contact
- Healthcare providers with direct patient contact
- Persons wounded in bombings or similar mass casualty events and who cannot confirm receipt of a tetanus booster within the previous 5 years and who have penetrating injuries or non-intact skin exposur, should receive a single dose of Tdap

Usual Dosage

Primary immunization: Children 6 weeks to <7 years: I.M.: **Note:** Whenever possible, the same product should be used for all doses. Interruption of recommended schedule does not require starting the series over; a delay between doses should not interfere with final immunity.

Daptacel®: 0.5 mL per dose, total of 4 doses administered as follows (data insufficient to recommend a fifth dose):

Three doses, usually given at 2-, 4-, and 6 months of age; may be given as early as 6 weeks of age and repeated every 6-8 weeks

Fourth dose: Given at ~15-20 months of age, but at least 6 months after third dose

Infanrix®, Tripedia®: 0.5 mL per dose, total of 5 doses administered as follows:

Three doses, usually given at 2-, 4-, and 6 months of age; may be given as early as 6 weeks of age and repeated every 4-8 weeks

Fourth dose: Given at ~15-20 months of age, but at least 6 months after third dose

Fifth dose: Given at 5-6 years of age, prior to starting school or kindergarten; if the fourth dose is given at ≥4 years of age, the fifth dose may be omitted

Booster immunization:

ACIP recommendations:

Adolescents 11-18 years: I.M.: 0.5 mL. A single dose of Tdap should be given instead of Td in adolescents who have completed the recommended childhood DTP/DTaP series and have not received Td or Tdap; preferred age of vaccination with Tdap is 11-12 years. Adolescents who received Td but not Tdap and who have completed the recommended childhood DTP/DTaP series are encouraged to receive Tdap; an interval of at least 5 years between Td and Tdap is recommended, but lesser intervals may be used if the benefit outweighs the risk.

Adults 19-64 years (Adacel™): I.M.: 0.5 mL. A single dose should be given instead of Td in adults if they received their last dose of Td ≥10 years previous. Shorter intervals (as short as 2 years) may used among healthcare providers, adults in contact with infants, or others in settings with increased risk for pertussis, including during pertussis outbreaks. Adacel™ should only be used to replace a single booster dose of Td.

Manufacturer's labeling:

Children 10-18 years (Boostrix®): I.M.: 0.5 mL as a single dose, administered 5 years after last dose of DTwP or DTaP vaccine.

Children ≥11 years and Adults ≤64 years (Adacel™): I.M.: 0.5 mL as a single dose, administered 5 years after last dose of DTwP or DTaP vaccine.

Wound management: Adacel™ (in patients 11-64 years of age) or Boostrix® (in patients 10-18 years of age) may be used as an alternative to Td vaccine when a tetanus toxoid-containing vaccine is needed for wound management, and in whom the pertussis component is also indicated. Td vaccine is the preferred agent in children ≥7 years and adults.

ACIP recommendations: ACIP prefers Tdap for adolescents 11-18 years requiring a tetanus toxoid product and who were vaccinated against tetanus ≥5 years earlier. Adolescents who completed the primary 3 dose series containing tetanus toxoid <5 years earlier are protected against tetanus and do not need a tetanus toxoid vaccine as part of wound management. The ACIP prefers Adacel™ for use in adults <65 years requiring a tetanus toxoid product and who were vaccinated against tetanus ≥5 years earlier if they have not previously received Tdap.

Dosage Forms

Injection, suspension:

Adacel®: Diphtheria 2 Lf units, tetanus 5 Lf units, and acellular pertussis 2.5 mcg per 0.5 mL (0.5 mL)

Boostrix®: Diphtheria 2.5 Lf units, tetanus 5 Lf units, and acellular pertussis 8 mcg per 0.5 mL (0.5 mL)

Daptacel®: Diphtheria 15 Lf units, tetanus 5 Lf units, and acellular pertussis 10 mcg per 0.5 mL (0.5 mL)

Infanrix®: Diphtheria 25 Lf units, tetanus 10 Lf units, and acellular pertussis 25 mcg per 0.5 mL (0.5 mL)

Tripedia®: Diphtheria 6.7 Lf units, tetanus 5 Lf units, and acellular pertussis 46.8 mcg per 0.5 mL (7.5 mL)

Note: Tripedia® vaccine is also used to reconstitute ActHIB® to prepare TriHIBit® vaccine (diphtheria, tetanus toxoids, and acellular pertussis and *Haemophilus influenzae* b conjugate vaccine combination)

diphtheria, tetanus toxoids, and acellular pertussis vaccine and *Haemophilus influenzae* b conjugate vaccine

(dif THEER ee a, TET a nus TOKS oyds & ay CEL yoo lar per TUS sis vak SEEN & hem OF fi lus in floo EN za bee KON joo gate vak SEEN)

Synonyms *Haemophilus influenzae* b conjugate vaccine and diphtheria, tetanus toxoids, and acellular pertussis vaccine

U.S./Canadian Brand Names TriHIBit® [US]

Therapeutic Category Toxoid; Vaccine, Inactivated Bacteria

Use Active immunization of children 15-18 months of age for prevention of diphtheria, tetanus, pertussis, and invasive disease caused by *H. influenzae* type b

Usual Dosage I.M.: Children >15 months of age: 0.5 mL (as part of a general vaccination schedule; see individual vaccines). Vaccine should be used within 30 minutes of reconstitution.

Dosage Forms
  Injection, suspension:
    TriHIBit®: 5 Lf units tetanus toxoid, 6.7 Lf units diphtheria toxoid, 46.8 mcg pertussis antigens, and 10 mcg *H. influenzae* type b purified capsular polysaccharide per 0.5 mL (0.5 mL)

diphtheria toxoid *see* diphtheria and tetanus toxoids, acellular pertussis, poliovirus (inactivated) and *Haemophilus* b conjugate vaccine *on page 308*
diphtheria toxoid conjugate *see Haemophilus* B conjugate vaccine *on page 464*
dipivalyl epinephrine *see* dipivefrin *on page 311*

dipivefrin (dye PI ve frin)
  Synonyms dipivalyl epinephrine; dipivefrin hydrochloride; DPE
  U.S./Canadian Brand Names Ophtho-Dipivefrin™ [Can]; PMS-Dipivefrin [Can]; Propine® [US/Can]
  Therapeutic Category Adrenergic Agonist Agent
  Use Reduces elevated intraocular pressure in chronic open-angle glaucoma; also used to treat ocular hypertension, low tension, and secondary glaucomas
  Usual Dosage Ophthalmic: Adults: Instill 1 drop every 12 hours into the eyes
  Dosage Forms
    Solution, ophthalmic: 0.1% (5 mL, 10 mL, 15 mL)
      Propine®: 0.1% (10 mL, 15 mL)

dipivefrin hydrochloride *see* dipivefrin *on page 311*
Diprivan® [US/Can] *see* propofol *on page 794*
Diprolene® [US] *see* betamethasone (topical) *on page 132*
Diprolene® AF [US] *see* betamethasone (topical) *on page 132*
Diprolene® Glycol [Can] *see* betamethasone (topical) *on page 132*
dipropylacetic acid *see* valproic acid and derivatives *on page 967*
Diprosone® [Can] *see* betamethasone (topical) *on page 132*

dipyridamole (dye peer ID a mole)
  Sound-Alike/Look-Alike Issues
    dipyridamole may be confused with disopyramide
    Persantine® may be confused with Periactin®, Permitil®
  U.S./Canadian Brand Names Apo-Dipyridamole FC® [Can]; Dipyridamole For Injection [Can]; Persantine® [US/Can]
  Therapeutic Category Antiplatelet Agent; Vasodilator
  Use
    Oral: Used with warfarin to decrease thrombosis in patients after artificial heart valve replacement
    I.V.: Diagnostic agent in CAD
  Usual Dosage
    Oral: Children ≥12 years and Adults: Adjunctive therapy for prophylaxis of thromboembolism with cardiac valve replacement: 75-100 mg 4 times/day
    I.V.: Adults: Evaluation of coronary artery disease: 0.14 mg/kg/minute for 4 minutes; maximum dose: 60 mg
  Dosage Forms
    Injection, solution: 5 mg/mL (2 mL, 10 mL)
    Tablet: 25 mg, 50 mg, 75 mg
      Persantine®: 25 mg, 50 mg, 75 mg

dipyridamole and aspirin *see* aspirin and dipyridamole *on page 100*
Dipyridamole For Injection [Can] *see* dipyridamole *on page 311*
Disalcid® (Discontinued) *see* salsalate *on page 854*
disalicylic acid *see* salsalate *on page 854*
DisCoVisc® [US] *see* sodium chondroitin sulfate and sodium hyaluronate *on page 875*
Disobrom® (Discontinued) *see* dexbrompheniramine and pseudoephedrine *on page 279*
disodium cromoglycate *see* cromolyn sodium *on page 251*
disodium thiosulfate pentahydrate *see* sodium thiosulfate *on page 880*
***d*-isoephedrine hydrochloride** *see* pseudoephedrine *on page 801*

Disonate® *(Discontinued)* *see docusate on page 314*

disopyramide (dye soe PEER a mide)
Sound-Alike/Look-Alike Issues
disopyramide may be confused with desipramine, dipyridamole
Norpace® may be confused with Norpramin®
Synonyms disopyramide phosphate
U.S./Canadian Brand Names Norpace® CR [US]; Norpace® [US/Can]; Rythmodan® [Can]; Rythmodan®-LA [Can]
Therapeutic Category Antiarrhythmic Agent, Class I-A
Use Suppression and prevention of unifocal and multifocal atrial and premature, ventricular premature complexes, coupled ventricular tachycardia; effective in the conversion of atrial fibrillation, atrial flutter, and paroxysmal atrial tachycardia to normal sinus rhythm and prevention of the recurrence of these arrhythmias after conversion by other methods
Usual Dosage Oral:
Children:
<1 year: 10-30 mg/kg/24 hours in 4 divided doses
1-4 years: 10-20 mg/kg/24 hours in 4 divided doses
4-12 years: 10-15 mg/kg/24 hours in 4 divided doses
12-18 years: 6-15 mg/kg/24 hours in 4 divided doses
Adults:
<50 kg: 100 mg every 6 hours or 200 mg every 12 hours (controlled release)
>50 kg: 150 mg every 6 hours or 300 mg every 12 hours (controlled release); if no response, increase to 200 mg every 6 hours. Maximum dose required for patients with severe refractory ventricular tachycardia is 400 mg every 6 hours.
Dosage Forms
Capsule: 100 mg, 150 mg
Norpace®: 100 mg, 150 mg
Capsule, controlled release: 100 mg, 150 mg
Norpace® CR: 100 mg, 150 mg

disopyramide phosphate *see disopyramide on page 312*
Disotate® *(Discontinued)* *see edetate disodium on page 333*
Di-Spaz® Injection *(Discontinued)* *see dicyclomine on page 293*
Di-Spaz® Oral *(Discontinued)* *see dicyclomine on page 293*
DisperMox™ *(Discontinued)* *see amoxicillin on page 67*

disulfiram (dye SUL fi ram)
Sound-Alike/Look-Alike Issues
disulfiram may be confused with Diflucan®
Antabuse® may be confused with Anturane®
U.S./Canadian Brand Names Antabuse® [US]
Therapeutic Category Aldehyde Dehydrogenase Inhibitor Agent
Use Management of chronic alcoholism
Usual Dosage Oral: Adults: Do not administer until the patient has abstained from ethanol for at least 12 hours

Initial: 500 mg/day as a single dose for 1-2 weeks; maximum daily dose is 500 mg
Average maintenance dose: 250 mg/day; range: 125-500 mg; duration of therapy is to continue until the patient is fully recovered socially and a basis for permanent self control has been established; maintenance therapy may be required for months or even years
Dosage Forms
Tablet:
Antabuse®: 250 mg, 500 mg

Dital® *(Discontinued)* *see phendimetrazine on page 742*
dithioglycerol *see dimercaprol on page 302*
dithranol *see anthralin on page 77*
Ditropan® [US/Can] *see oxybutynin on page 708*
Ditropan® XL [US/Can] *see oxybutynin on page 708*

Diurigen® *(Discontinued)* *see* chlorothiazide *on page 205*
Diuril® [US/Can] *see* chlorothiazide *on page 205*
divalproex sodium *see* valproic acid and derivatives *on page 967*
Divigel® [US] *see* estradiol *on page 359*
Dixarit® [Can] *see* clonidine *on page 236*
Dizac® Injectable Emulsion *(Discontinued)* *see* diazepam *on page 289*
Dizmiss® *(Discontinued)* *see* meclizine *on page 595*
5071-1DL(6) *see* megestrol *on page 598*
***dl*-alpha tocopherol** *see* vitamin E *on page 981*
4-DMDR *see* idarubicin *on page 498*
***D*-mannitol** *see* mannitol *on page 590*
D-Med® Injection *(Discontinued)* *see* methylprednisolone *on page 623*
DMSA *see* succimer *on page 889*
DMSO *see* dimethyl sulfoxide *on page 303*
Doak® Tar [US-OTC] *see* coal tar *on page 240*
Doan's® Extra Strength [US-OTC] *see* magnesium salicylate *on page 588*

dobutamine (doe BYOO ta meen)

Sound-Alike/Look-Alike Issues
DOBUTamine may be confused with DOPamine
Synonyms dobutamine hydrochloride
Tall-Man DOBUTamine
U.S./Canadian Brand Names Dobutamine Injection, USP [Can]; Dobutrex® [Can]
Therapeutic Category Adrenergic Agonist Agent
Use Short-term management of patients with cardiac decompensation
Usual Dosage Administration requires the use of an infusion pump; I.V. infusion:
Neonates: 2-15 mcg/kg/minute, titrate to desired response
Children and Adults: 2.5-20 mcg/kg/minute; maximum: 40 mcg/kg/minute, titrate to desired response.
Dosage Forms
Infusion [premixed in dextrose]: 1 mg/mL (250 mL, 500 mL); 2 mg/mL (250 mL); 4 mg/mL (250 mL)
Injection, solution: 12.5 mg/mL (20 mL, 40 mL, 100 mL)

dobutamine hydrochloride *see* dobutamine *on page 313*
Dobutamine Injection, USP [Can] *see* dobutamine *on page 313*
Dobutrex® [Can] *see* dobutamine *on page 313*

docetaxel (doe se TAKS el)

Sound-Alike/Look-Alike Issues
Taxotere® may be confused with Taxol®
Synonyms NSC-628503; RP-6976
U.S./Canadian Brand Names Taxotere® [US/Can]
Therapeutic Category Antineoplastic Agent
Use Treatment of breast cancer; locally-advanced or metastatic nonsmall cell lung cancer (NSCLC); hormone refractory, metastatic prostate cancer; advanced gastric adenocarcinoma; locally-advanced squamous cell head and neck cancer
Usual Dosage I.V. infusion: Adults: Refer to individual protocols: **Note:** Premedicate with corticosteroids, beginning the day before docetaxel administration, (administer for 1-5 days) to reduce the severity of hypersensitivity reactions and pulmonary/peripheral edema
Breast cancer:
Locally-advanced or metastatic: 60-100 mg/m^2 every 3 weeks; patients initially started at 60 mg/m^2 who do not develop toxicity may tolerate higher doses
Operable, node-positive (adjuvant treatment): 75 mg/m^2 every 3 weeks for 6 courses (in combination with doxorubicin and cyclophosphamide)
Nonsmall cell lung cancer: 75 mg/m^2 every 3 weeks (as monotherapy or in combination with cisplatin)
Prostate cancer: 75 mg/m^2 every 3 weeks (in combination with prednisone)
Gastric adenocarcinoma: 75 mg/m^2 every 3 weeks (in combination with cisplatin and fluorouracil)
Head and neck cancer: 75 mg/m^2 every 3 weeks (in combination with cisplatin and fluorouracil) for 3 or 4 cycles, followed by radiation therapy

◄ **Dosage Forms**
Injection, solution [concentrate]:
Taxotere®: 20 mg/0.5 mL (0.5 mL, 2 mL)

docosanol (doe KOE san ole)

Synonyms *n*-docosanol; behenyl alcohol

U.S./Canadian Brand Names Abreva® [US-OTC]

Therapeutic Category Antiviral Agent, Topical

Use Treatment of herpes simplex of the face or lips

Usual Dosage Topical: Children ≥12 years and Adults: Apply 5 times/day to affected area of face or lips. Start at first sign of cold sore or fever blister and continue until healed.

Dosage Forms
Cream, topical:
Abreva® [OTC]: 10% (2 g)

docusate (DOK yoo sate)

Sound-Alike/Look-Alike Issues
docusate may be confused with Doxinate®
Colace® may be confused with Calan®, Cozaar®
Surfak® may be confused with Surbex®

Synonyms dioctyl calcium sulfosuccinate; dioctyl sodium sulfosuccinate; docusate calcium; docusate potassium; docusate sodium; DOSS; DSS

U.S./Canadian Brand Names Apo-Docusate-Sodium® [Can]; Colace® [US-OTC/Can]; Colax-C® [Can]; Correctol® [US-OTC]; D-S-S® [US-OTC]; Diocto® [US-OTC]; Docu-Soft [US-OTC]; Docusoft-S™ [US-OTC]; DOK™ [US-OTC]; DOS® [US-OTC]; Dulcolax® Stool Softener [US-OTC]; Enemeez® Plus [US-OTC]; Enemeez® [US-OTC]; Fleet® Sof-Lax® [US-OTC]; Genasoft® [US-OTC]; Novo-Docusate Calcium [Can]; Novo-Docusate Sodium [Can]; Phillips'® Stool Softener Laxative [US-OTC]; PMS-Docusate Calcium [Can]; PMS-Docusate Sodium [Can]; Regulex® [Can]; Selax® [Can]; Silace [US-OTC]; Soflax™ [Can]; Surfak® [US-OTC]

Therapeutic Category Stool Softener

Use Stool softener in patients who should avoid straining during defecation and constipation associated with hard, dry stools; prophylaxis for straining (Valsalva) following myocardial infarction. A safe agent to be used in elderly; some evidence that doses <200 mg are ineffective; stool softeners are unnecessary if stool is well hydrated or "mushy" and soft; shown to be ineffective used long-term.

Usual Dosage Docusate salts are interchangeable; the amount of sodium or calcium per dosage unit is clinically insignificant

Infants and Children <3 years: Oral: 10-40 mg/day in 1-4 divided doses
Children: Oral:
3-6 years: 20-60 mg/day in 1-4 divided doses
6-12 years: 40-150 mg/day in 1-4 divided doses
Adolescents and Adults: Oral: 50-500 mg/day in 1-4 divided doses
Older Children and Adults: Rectal: Add 50-100 mg of docusate liquid to enema fluid (saline or water); administer as retention or flushing enema

Dosage Forms
Capsule, oral: 100 mg, 240 mg, 250 mg
Colace® [OTC]: 50 mg, 100 mg
Capsule, softgel, oral: 100 mg, 240 mg, 250 mg
Correctol® [OTC], Docu-Soft [OTC], Docusoft-S™ [OTC], Genasoft® [OTC], Dulcolax® Stool Softener [OTC], Fleet® Sof-Lax® [OTC], Phillips'® Stool Softener Laxative [OTC]: 100 mg
DOK™ [OTC], DOS® [OTC], D-S-S® [OTC]: 100 mg, 250 mg
Surfak® [OTC]: 240 mg
Liquid, oral: 150 mg/15 mL
Colace® [OTC], Diocto® [OTC], Silace [OTC]: 150 mg/15 mL
Solution, rectal [enema]:
Enemeez® [OTC], Enemeez® Plus [OTC]: 283 mg/5 mL
Syrup: 20 mg/5 mL, 60 mg/15 mL
Colace® [OTC], Diocto® [OTC]: 60 mg/15 mL
Silace [OTC]: 20 mg/5 mL

docusate and senna (DOK yoo sate & SEN na)

Sound-Alike/Look-Alike Issues
   Senokot® may be confused with Depakote®
Synonyms senna and docusate; senna-S
U.S./Canadian Brand Names Peri-Colace® [US-OTC]; Senokot-S® [US-OTC]; SenoSol™-SS [US-OTC]
Therapeutic Category Laxative, Stimulant; Stool Softener
Use Short-term treatment of constipation
Usual Dosage Oral: Constipation: OTC ranges:
   Children:
      2-6 years: Initial: 4.3 mg sennosides plus 25 mg docusate (1/2 tablet) once daily (maximum: 1 tablet twice daily)
      6-12 years: Initial: 8.6 sennosides plus 50 mg docusate (1 tablet) once daily (maximum: 2 tablets twice daily)
      Children ≥12 years and Adults: Initial: 2 tablets (17.2 mg sennosides plus 100 mg docusate) once daily (maximum: 4 tablets twice daily)
Dosage Forms
   Tablet: Docusate 50 mg and sennosides 8.6 mg
      Peri-Colace® [OTC], Senokot-S® [OTC], SenoSol™-SS: Docusate 50 mg and sennosides 8.6 mg

docusate calcium see docusate on page 314
docusate potassium see docusate on page 314
docusate sodium see docusate on page 314
Docu-Soft [US-OTC] see docusate on page 314
Docusoft Plus™ (Discontinued)
Docusoft-S™ [US-OTC] see docusate on page 314

dofetilide (doe FET il ide)

U.S./Canadian Brand Names Tikosyn® [US/Can]
Therapeutic Category Antiarrhythmic Agent, Class III
Use Maintenance of normal sinus rhythm in patients with chronic atrial fibrillation/atrial flutter of longer than 1-week duration who have been converted to normal sinus rhythm; conversion of atrial fibrillation and atrial flutter to normal sinus rhythm
Usual Dosage Oral: Adults: **Note:** QT or QT_c must be determined prior to first dose. If QT_c >440 msec (>500 msec in patients with ventricular conduction abnormalities), dofetilide is contraindicated.
   Initial: 500 mcg orally twice daily. Initial dosage must be adjusted in patients with estimated Cl_{cr} <60 mL/minute. Dofetilide may be initiated at lower doses than recommended based on physician discretion.
   Modification of dosage in response to initial dose: QT_c interval should be measured 2-3 hours after the initial dose. If the QT_c >15% of baseline, or if the QT_c is >500 msec (550 msec in patients with ventricular conduction abnormalities) dofetilide should be adjusted. If the starting dose is 500 mcg twice daily, then adjust to 250 mcg twice daily. If the starting dose was 250 mcg twice daily, then adjust to 125 mcg twice daily. If the starting dose was 125 mcg twice daily then adjust to 125 mcg every day.
   Continued monitoring for doses 2-5: QT_c interval must be determined 2-3 hours after each subsequent dose of dofetilide for in-hospital doses 2-5. If the measured QT_c is >500 msec (550 msec in patients with ventricular conduction abnormalities) at any time, dofetilide should be discontinued.
   Chronic therapy (following the 5th dose):
      QT or QT_c and creatinine clearance should be evaluated every 3 months. If QT_c >500 msec (>550 msec in patients with ventricular conduction abnormalities), dofetilide should be discontinued.
Dosage Forms
   Capsule:
      Tikosyn®: 125 mcg, 250 mcg, 500 mcg

Dofus [US-OTC] see Lactobacillus on page 543
DOK™ [US-OTC] see docusate on page 314
Doktors® Nasal Solution (Discontinued) see phenylephrine on page 745
Dolacet® Forte (Discontinued) see hydrocodone and acetaminophen on page 481

dolasetron (dol A se tron)

Sound-Alike/Look-Alike Issues
dolasetron may be confused with granisetron, ondansetron, palonosetron
Anzemet® may be confused with Aldomet® and Avandamet®

Synonyms dolasetron mesylate; MDL 73,147EF

U.S./Canadian Brand Names Anzemet® [US/Can]

Therapeutic Category Selective 5-HT$_3$ Receptor Antagonist

Use Prevention of nausea and vomiting associated with emetogenic cancer chemotherapy; prevention of postoperative nausea and vomiting; treatment of postoperative nausea and vomiting (injectable form only).

Note: In Canada, the use of dolasetron is contraindicated for all uses in children <18 years of age or in the treatment of postoperative nausea and vomiting in adults. These are not labeled contraindications in the U.S.

Usual Dosage Note: In Canada, the use of dolasetron is contraindicated in children <18 years of age or in the treatment of postoperative nausea and vomiting in adults. These are not labeled contraindications in the U.S.

Prevention of chemotherapy-associated nausea and vomiting (including initial and repeat courses):
Children 2-16 years:
Oral: 1.8 mg/kg within 1 hour before chemotherapy; maximum: 100 mg/dose
I.V.: 1.8 mg/kg ~30 minutes before chemotherapy; maximum: 100 mg/dose
Adults:
Oral:100 mg single dose 1 hour prior to chemotherapy
I.V.: 1.8 mg/kg or 100 mg 30 minutes prior to chemotherapy
Prevention of postoperative nausea and vomiting:
Children 2-16 years:
Oral: 1.2 mg/kg within 2 hours before surgery; maximum: 100 mg/dose
I.V.: 0.35 mg/kg (maximum: 12.5 mg) ~15 minutes before stopping anesthesia
Adults:
Oral: 100 mg within 2 hours before surgery
I.V.: 12.5 mg ~15 minutes before stopping anesthesia
Treatment of postoperative nausea and vomiting: I.V. (only):
Children: 0.35 mg/kg (maximum: 12.5 mg) as soon as needed
Adults: 12.5 mg as soon as needed

Dosage Forms
Injection, solution:
Anzemet®: 20 mg/mL (0.625 mL) [single-use Carpuject® or vial; contains mannitol 38.2 mg/mL]; 20 mg/mL (5 mL) [single-use vial; contains mannitol 38.2 mg/mL]; 20 mg/mL (25 mL) [multidose vial; contains mannitol 29 mg/mL]
Tablet:
Anzemet®: 50 mg, 100 mg

Dom-Buspirone [Can] *see* buspirone *on page 153*
Dom-Carbamazepine [Can] *see* carbamazepine *on page 172*
Dom-Ciprofloxacin [Can] *see* ciprofloxacin *on page 221*
Dom-Citalopram [Can] *see* citalopram *on page 225*
Dom-Clobazam [Can] *see* clobazam *(Canada only) on page 232*
Dom-Diclofenac [Can] *see* diclofenac *on page 292*
Dom-Diclofenac SR [Can] *see* diclofenac *on page 292*
Dom-Divalproex [Can] *see* valproic acid and derivatives *on page 967*
Dom-Domperidone [Can] *see* domperidone *(Canada only) on page 317*
Domeboro® [US-OTC] *see* aluminum sulfate and calcium acetate *on page 55*
dome paste bandage *see* zinc gelatin *on page 993*
Dom-Fenofibrate Supra [Can] *see* fenofibrate *on page 393*
Dom-Fluconazole [Can] *see* fluconazole *on page 405*
Dom-Fluoxetine [Can] *see* fluoxetine *on page 413*
Dom-Furosemide [Can] *see* furosemide *on page 430*
Dom-Loperamide [Can] *see* loperamide *on page 573*
Dom-Mefenamic Acid [Can] *see* mefenamic acid *on page 598*
Dom-Methimazole [Can] *see* methimazole *on page 614*
Dom-Metoprolol [Can] *see* metoprolol *on page 626*
Dom-Moclobemide [Can] *see* moclobemide *(Canada only) on page 639*

domperidone *(Canada only)* (dom PE ri done)

Synonyms domperidone maleate
U.S./Canadian Brand Names Apo-Domperidone® [Can]; Dom-Domperidone [Can]; Novo-Domperidone [Can]; Nu-Domperidone [Can]; PHL-Domperidone [Can]; PMS-Domperidone [Can]; RAN™-Domperidone [Can]; ratio-Domperidone [Can]
Therapeutic Category Dopamine Antagonist
Use Symptomatic management of upper GI motility disorders associated with chronic and subacute gastritis and diabetic gastroparesis; prevention of GI symptoms associated with use of dopamine-agonist anti-Parkinson agents
Usual Dosage Oral: Adults:
GI motility disorders: 10 mg 3-4 times/day, 15-30 minutes before meals; severe/resistant cases: 20 mg 3-4 times/day, 15-30 minutes before meals
Nausea/vomiting associated with dopamine-agonist anti-Parkinson agents: 20 mg 3-4 times/day
Dosage Forms [CAN] = Canadian brand name
Tablet: 10 mg [not available in the U.S.]
Alti-Domperidone [CAN], Apo-Domperidone® [CAN], Dom-Domperidone [CAN], Novo-Domperidone [CAN], Nu-Domperidone [CAN], PHL-Domperidone [CAN], PMS-Domperidone [CAN], ratio-Domperidone [CAN]: 10 mg [not available in the U.S.]

domperidone maleate *see* domperidone *(Canada only) on page 317*
Dom-Propranolol [Can] *see* propranolol *on page 796*
Dom-Ranitidine [Can] *see* ranitidine *on page 819*
Dom-Risperidone [Can] *see* risperidone *on page 837*
Dom-Sertraline [Can] *see* sertraline *on page 863*
Dom-Simvastatin [Can] *see* simvastatin *on page 867*
Dom-Sumatriptan [Can] *see* sumatriptan *on page 898*
Dom-Temazepam [Can] *see* temazepam *on page 907*
Dom-Tiaprofenic® [Can] *see* tiaprofenic acid *(Canada only) on page 925*
Dom-Topiramate [Can] *see* topiramate *on page 935*
DOM-Ursodiol C [Can] *see* ursodiol *on page 965*
Dom-Verapamil SR [Can] *see* verapamil *on page 974*
Dom-Zopiclone [Can] *see* zopiclone *(Canada only) on page 997*
Donatussin [US] *see* dextromethorphan, chlorpheniramine, phenylephrine, and guaifenesin *on page 285*
Donatussin DC *(Discontinued)*

Donatussin DM *(Discontinued)* *see* chlorpheniramine, phenylephrine, and dextromethorphan *on page 209*

Donatussin Drops [US] *see* guaifenesin and phenylephrine *on page 456*

donepezil (doh NEP e zil)

Sound-Alike/Look-Alike Issues
Aricept® may be confused with AcipHex®, Ascriptin®, and Azilect®

Synonyms E2020

U.S./Canadian Brand Names Aricept® ODT [US]; Aricept® RDT [Can]; Aricept® [US/Can]

Therapeutic Category Acetylcholinesterase Inhibitor; Cholinergic Agent

Use Treatment of mild, moderate, or severe dementia of the Alzheimer type

Usual Dosage Oral: Adults: Dementia of Alzheimer type: Initial: 5 mg/day at bedtime; may increase to 10 mg/day at bedtime after 4-6 weeks

Dosage Forms
Tablet:
Aricept®: 5 mg, 10 mg
Tablet, orally disintegrating:
Aricept® ODT: 5 mg, 10 mg

Donnamar® *(Discontinued)* *see* hyoscyamine *on page 492*

Donnapine® *(Discontinued)* *see* hyoscyamine, atropine, scopolamine, and phenobarbital *on page 493*

Donnatal® **[US]** *see* hyoscyamine, atropine, scopolamine, and phenobarbital *on page 493*

Donnatal Extentabs® **[US]** *see* hyoscyamine, atropine, scopolamine, and phenobarbital *on page 493*

dopamine (DOE pa meen)

Sound-Alike/Look-Alike Issues
DOPamine may be confused with DOBUTamine, Dopram®

Synonyms dopamine hydrochloride

Tall-Man DOPamine

Therapeutic Category Adrenergic Agonist Agent

Use Adjunct in the treatment of shock (eg, MI, open heart surgery, renal failure, cardiac decompensation) which persists after adequate fluid volume replacement

Usual Dosage I.V. infusion (administration requires the use of an infusion pump):
Neonates: 1-20 mcg/kg/minute continuous infusion, titrate to desired response.
Children: 1-20 mcg/kg/minute, maximum: 50 mcg/kg/minute continuous infusion, titrate to desired response.
Adults: 1-5 mcg/kg/minute up to 20 mcg/kg/minute, titrate to desired response (maximum: 50 mcg/kg/minute). Infusion may be increased by 1-4 mcg/kg/minute at 10- to 30-minute intervals until optimal response is obtained.
If dosages >20-30 mcg/kg/minute are needed, a more direct-acting pressor may be more beneficial (ie, epinephrine, norepinephrine).

Dosage Forms
Infusion [premixed in D_5W]: 0.8 mg/mL (250 mL, 500 mL); 1.6 mg/mL (250 mL, 500 mL); 3.2 mg/mL (250 mL)
Injection, solution: 40 mg/mL (5 mL, 10 mL); 80 mg/mL (5 mL); 160 mg/mL (5 mL)

dopamine hydrochloride *see* dopamine *on page 318*

Dopram® **[US]** *see* doxapram *on page 320*

Doral® **[US/Can]** *see* quazepam *on page 811*

Doribax™ **[US]** *see* doripenem *on page 318*

doripenem (dore i PEN em)

Synonyms S-4661

U.S./Canadian Brand Names Doribax™ [US]

Therapeutic Category Antibiotic, Carbapenem

Use Treatment of complicated intraabdominal infections and complicated urinary tract infections (including pyelonephritis) due to susceptible gram-positive, gram-negative (including *Pseudomonas aeruginosa*), and anaerobic bacteria

Usual Dosage
  Usual dosage: Adults: I.V.: 500 mg every 8 hours
  Indication-specific dosing: Adults: I.V.:
    Intraabdominal infection (complicated): 500 mg every 8 hours for 5-14 days
    Urinary tract infection (complicated) or pyelonephritis: 500 mg every 8 hours for 10-14 days
Dosage Forms
  Injection, powder for reconstitution:
    Doribax™: 500 mg

Dormarex® 2 Oral *(Discontinued)* see diphenhydramine *on page 304*

dornase alfa (DOOR nase AL fa)
Synonyms recombinant human deoxyribonuclease; rhDNase
U.S./Canadian Brand Names Pulmozyme® [US/Can]
Therapeutic Category Enzyme
Use Management of cystic fibrosis patients to reduce the frequency of respiratory infections that require parenteral antibiotics in patients with FVC ≥40% of predicted; in conjunction with standard therapies, to improve pulmonary function in patients with cystic fibrosis
Usual Dosage Inhalation:
  Children ≥3 months to Adults: 2.5 mg once daily through selected nebulizers; experience in children <5 years is limited
  Patients unable to inhale or exhale orally throughout the entire treatment period may use Pari-Baby™ nebulizer. Some patients may benefit from twice daily administration.
Dosage Forms
  Solution for nebulization [preservative free]:
    Pulmozyme®: 1 mg/mL (2.5 mL)

Doryx® [US] *see* doxycycline *on page 323*

dorzolamide (dor ZOLE a mide)
Synonyms dorzolamide hydrochloride
U.S./Canadian Brand Names Trusopt® [US/Can]
Therapeutic Category Carbonic Anhydrase Inhibitor
Use Lowers intraocular pressure in patients with ocular hypertension or open-angle glaucoma
Usual Dosage Children and Adults: Reduction of intraocular pressure: Instill 1 drop in the affected eye(s) 3 times/day
Dosage Forms
  Solution, ophthalmic:
    Trusopt®: 2% (10 mL)

dorzolamide and timolol (dor ZOLE a mide & TYE moe lole)
Synonyms timolol and dorzolamide
U.S./Canadian Brand Names Cosopt® [US/Can]; Preservative-Free Cosopt® [Can]
Therapeutic Category Beta-Adrenergic Blocker; Carbonic Anhydrase Inhibitor
Use Reduction of intraocular pressure in patients with ocular hypertension or open-angle glaucoma
Usual Dosage Ophthalmic: Children ≥2 years and Adults: Instill 1 drop in affected eye(s) twice daily
Dosage Forms
  Solution, ophthalmic:
    Cosopt®: Dorzolamide 2% and timolol 0.5% (10 mL)

dorzolamide hydrochloride *see* dorzolamide *on page 319*
DOS® [US-OTC] *see* docusate *on page 314*
DOSS *see* docusate *on page 314*
Dostinex® [Can] *see* cabergoline *on page 158*
Dostinex® *(Discontinued) see* cabergoline *on page 158*
Double Tussin DM [US-OTC] *see* guaifenesin and dextromethorphan *on page 454*
Dovobet® [Can] *see* calcipotriene and betamethasone *on page 159*
Dovonex® [US/Can] *see* calcipotriene *on page 159*

doxacurium *(Discontinued)*

doxapram (DOKS a pram)

Sound-Alike/Look-Alike Issues
doxapram may be confused with doxacurium, doxazosin, doxepin, Doxinate®, DOXOrubicin
Dopram® may be confused with DOPamine

Synonyms doxapram hydrochloride

U.S./Canadian Brand Names Dopram® [US]

Therapeutic Category Respiratory Stimulant

Use Respiratory and CNS stimulant for respiratory depression secondary to anesthesia, drug-induced CNS depression; acute hypercapnia secondary to COPD

Usual Dosage
Respiratory depression following anesthesia:
Intermittent injection: Initial: 0.5-1 mg/kg; may repeat at 5-minute intervals (only in patients who demonstrate initial response); maximum total dose: 2 mg/kg
I.V. infusion: Initial: 5 mg/minute until adequate response or adverse effects seen; decrease to 1-3 mg/minute; maximum total dose: 4 mg/kg
Drug-induced CNS depression:
Intermittent injection: Initial: Priming dose of 1-2 mg/kg, repeat after 5 minutes; may repeat at 1-2 hour intervals (until sustained consciousness); maximum: 3 g/day. May repeat in 24 hours if necessary.
I.V. infusion: Initial: Priming dose of 1-2 mg/kg, repeat after 5 minutes. If no response, wait 1-2 hours and repeat. If some stimulation is noted, initiate infusion at 1-3 mg/minute (depending on size of patient/depth of CNS depression); suspend infusion if patient begins to awaken. Infusion should not be continued for >2 hours. May reinstitute infusion as described above, including bolus, after rest interval of 30 minutes to 2 hours; maximum: 3 g/day
Acute hypercapnia secondary to COPD: I.V. infusion: Initial: Initiate infusion at 1-2 mg/minute (depending on size of patient/depth of CNS depression); may increase to maximum rate of 3 mg/minute; infusion should not be continued for >2 hours. Monitor arterial blood gases prior to initiation of infusion and at 30-minute intervals during the infusion (to identify possible development of acidosis/CO_2 retention). Additional infusions are not recommended (per manufacturer).

Dosage Forms
Injection, solution: 20 mg/mL (20 mL)
Dopram®: 20 mg/mL (20 mL)

doxapram hydrochloride *see* doxapram *on page 320*

doxazosin (doks AY zoe sin)

Sound-Alike/Look-Alike Issues
doxazosin may be confused with doxapram, doxepin, DOXOrubicin
Cardura® may be confused with Cardene®, Cordarone®, Cordran®, Coumadin®, K-Dur®, Ridaura®

Synonyms doxazosin mesylate

U.S./Canadian Brand Names Alti-Doxazosin [Can]; Apo-Doxazosin® [Can]; Cardura-1™ [Can]; Cardura-2™ [Can]; Cardura-4™ [Can]; Cardura® XL [US]; Cardura® [US]; Gen-Doxazosin [Can]; Novo-Doxazosin [Can]

Therapeutic Category Alpha-Adrenergic Blocking Agent

Use Treatment of hypertension alone or in conjunction with diuretics, ACE inhibitors, beta-blockers, or calcium antagonists; treatment of urinary outflow obstruction and/or obstructive and irritative symptoms associated with benign prostatic hyperplasia (BPH), particularly useful in patients with troublesome symptoms who are unable or unwilling to undergo invasive procedures, but who require rapid symptomatic relief; can be used in combination with finasteride

Usual Dosage Oral: Adults:
Immediate release: 1 mg once daily in morning or evening; may be increased to 2 mg once daily. Thereafter titrate upwards, if needed, over several weeks, balancing therapeutic benefit with doxazosin-induced postural hypotension.
Hypertension: Maximum dose: 16 mg/day
BPH: Goal: 4-8 mg/day; maximum dose: 8 mg/day
Extended release: BPH: 4 mg once daily with breakfast; titrate based on response and tolerability every 3-4 weeks to maximum recommended dose of 8 mg/day
Reinitiation of therapy: If therapy is discontinued for several days, restart at 4 mg dose and titrate as before.

Conversion to extended release from immediate release: Initiate with 4 mg once daily; omit final evening dose of immediate release prior to starting morning dosing with extended release product.

Dosage Forms
Tablet: 1 mg, 2 mg, 4 mg, 8 mg
Cardura®: 1 mg, 2 mg, 4 mg, 8 mg
Tablet, extended release:
Cardura® XL: 4 mg, 8 mg

doxazosin mesylate *see* doxazosin *on page 320*

doxepin (DOKS e pin)

Sound-Alike/Look-Alike Issues
doxepin may be confused with digoxin, doxapram, doxazosin, Doxidan®, doxycycline
Sinequan® may be confused with saquinavir, Serentil®, Seroquel®, Singulair®
Zonalon® may be confused with Zone-A Forte®

Synonyms doxepin hydrochloride

U.S./Canadian Brand Names Apo-Doxepin® [Can]; Novo-Doxepin [Can]; Prudoxin™ [US]; Sinequan® [Can]; Zonalon® [US/Can]

Therapeutic Category Antidepressant, Tricyclic (Tertiary Amine); Topical Skin Product

Use
Oral: Depression
Topical: Short-term (<8 days) management of moderate pruritus in adults with atopic dermatitis or lichen simplex chronicus

Usual Dosage
Oral: Topical: Burning mouth syndrome (dental use): Cream: Apply 3-4 times daily
Oral (entire daily dose may be given at bedtime):
Depression or anxiety:
Adolescents: Initial: 25-50 mg/day in single or divided doses; gradually increase to 100 mg/day
Adults: Initial: 25-150 mg/day at bedtime or in 2-3 divided doses; may gradually increase up to 300 mg/day; single dose should not exceed 150 mg; select patients may respond to 25-50 mg/day
Chronic urticaria, angioedema, nocturnal pruritus: Adults: 10-30 mg/day

Topical: Pruritus: Adults: Apply a thin film 4 times/day with at least 3- to 4-hour interval between applications; not recommended for use >8 days. **Note:** Low-dose (25-50 mg) oral administration has also been used to treat pruritus, but systemic effects are increased.

Dosage Forms
Capsule: 10 mg, 25 mg, 50 mg, 75 mg, 100 mg, 150 mg
Cream:
Prudoxin™: 5% (45 g)
Zonalon®: 5% (30 g, 45 g)
Solution, oral concentrate: 10 mg/mL

doxepin hydrochloride *see* doxepin *on page 321*

doxercalciferol (doks er kal si fe FEER ole)

Synonyms 1α-hydroxyergocalciferol

U.S./Canadian Brand Names Hectorol® [US/Can]

Therapeutic Category Vitamin D Analog

Use Treatment of secondary hyperparathyroidism in patients with chronic kidney disease

Usual Dosage
Oral:
Dialysis patients: Dose should be titrated to lower iPTH to 150-300 pg/mL; dose is adjusted at 8-week intervals (maximum dose: 20 mcg 3 times/week)
Initial dose: iPTH >400 pg/mL: 10 mcg 3 times/week at dialysis
Dose titration:
iPTH level decreased by 50% and >300 pg/mL: Dose can be increased to 12.5 mcg 3 times/week for 8 more weeks; this titration process can continue at 8-week intervals; each increase should be by 2.5 mcg/dose
iPTH level 150-300 pg/mL: Maintain current dose
iPTH level <100 pg/mL: Suspend doxercalciferol for 1 week; resume at a reduced dose; decrease each dose (not weekly dose) by at least 2.5 mcg

◄ Predialysis patients: Dose should be titrated to lower iPTH to 35-70 pg/mL with stage 3 disease or to 70-110 pg/mL with stage 4 disease: Dose may be adjusted at 2-week intervals (maximum dose: 3.5 mcg/day)

Initial dose: 1 mcg/day

Dose titration:

iPTH level >70 pg/mL with stage 3 disease or >110 pg/mL with stage 4 disease: Increase dose by 0.5 mcg every 2 weeks as necessary

iPTH level 35-70 pg/mL with stage 3 disease or 70-110 pg/mL with stage 4 disease: Maintain current dose

iPTH level is <35 pg/mL with stage 3 disease or <70 pg/mL with stage 4 disease: Suspend doxercalciferol for 1 week, then resume at a reduced dose (at least 0.5 mcg lower)

I.V.:

Dialysis patients: Dose should be titrated to lower iPTH to 150-300 pg/mL; dose is adjusted at 8-week intervals (maximum dose: 18 mcg/week)

Initial dose: iPTH level >400 pg/mL: 4 mcg 3 times/week after dialysis, administered as a bolus dose

Dose titration:

iPTH level decreased by <50% and >300 pg/mL: Dose can be increased by 1-2 mcg at 8-week intervals, as necessary

iPTH level decreased by >50% and >300 pg/mL: Maintain current dose

iPTH level 150-300 pg/mL: Maintain the current dose

iPTH level <100 pg/mL: Suspend doxercalciferol for 1 week; resume at a reduced dose (at least 1 mcg lower)

Dosage Forms

Capsule:

Hectorol®: 0.5 mcg, 2.5 mcg

Injection, solution:

Hectorol®: 2 mcg/mL (2 mL)

Doxidan® [US-OTC] *see* bisacodyl *on page 136*
Doxil® [US] *see* doxorubicin (liposomal) *on page 323*

doxorubicin (doks oh ROO bi sin)

Sound-Alike/Look-Alike Issues

DOXOrubicin may be confused with dactinomycin, DAUNOrubicin, DAUNOrubicin liposomal, doxacurium, doxapram, doxazosin, DOXOrubicin liposomal, epirubicin, idarubicin

Adriamycin PFS® may be confused with achromycin, Aredia®, Idamycin®

ADR (error-prone abbreviation)

Conventional formulation (Adriamycin PFS®, Adriamycin RDF®) may be confused with the liposomal formulation (Doxil®)

Synonyms adria; doxorubicin hydrochloride; hydroxydaunomycin hydrochloride; hydroxyldaunorubicin hydrochloride; NSC-123127

Tall-Man DOXOrubicin

U.S./Canadian Brand Names Adriamycin® [US/Can]

Therapeutic Category Antineoplastic Agent

Use Treatment of leukemias, lymphomas, multiple myeloma, osseous and nonosseous sarcomas, mesotheliomas, germ cell tumors of the ovary or testis, and carcinomas of the head and neck, thyroid, lung, breast, stomach, pancreas, liver, ovary, bladder, prostate, uterus, neuroblastoma and Wilms tumor.

Usual Dosage I.V.: Refer to individual protocols. **Note:** Lower dosage should be considered for patients with inadequate marrow reserve (due to old age, prior treatment or neoplastic marrow infiltration)

Children:

35-75 mg/m^2/dose every 21 days **or**

20-30 mg/m^2/dose once weekly **or**

60-90 mg/m^2/dose given as a continuous infusion over 96 hours every 3-4 weeks

Adults: Usual or typical dose: 60-75 mg/m^2/dose every 21 days **or**

60 mg/m^2/dose every 2 weeks (dose dense) **or**

40-60 mg/m^2/dose every 3-4 weeks **or**

20-30 mg/m^2/day for 2-3 days every 4 weeks **or**

20 mg/m^2/dose once weekly

Dosage Forms

Injection, powder for reconstitution: 10 mg, 50 mg

Adriamycin®: 10 mg, 20 mg, 50 mg

Injection, solution: 2 mg/mL (5 mL, 10 mL, 25 mL, 100 mL)
Adriamycin®: 2 mg/mL (5 mL, 10 mL, 25 mL, 100 mL)

doxorubicin hydrochloride see doxorubicin on page 322
DOXOrubicin hydrochloride (liposomal) see doxorubicin (liposomal) on page 323

doxorubicin (liposomal) (doks oh ROO bi sin lip pah SOW mal)

Sound-Alike/Look-Alike Issues
DOXOrubicin liposomal may be confused with dactinomycin, DAUNOrubicin, DAUNOrubicin liposomal, doxacurium, doxapram, doxazosin, DOXOrubicin, epirubicin, idarubicin
DOXOrubicin liposomal may be confused with DAUNOrubicin liposomal
Doxil® may be confused with Doxy®, Paxil®
Liposomal formulation (Doxil®) may be confused with the conventional formulation (Adriamycin PFS®, Adriamycin RDF®)

Synonyms DOXOrubicin hydrochloride (liposomal); liposomal DOXOrubicin; NSC-712227; pegylated liposomal DOXOrubicin

Tall-Man DOXOrubicin (liposomal)

U.S./Canadian Brand Names Caelyx® [Can]; Doxil® [US]

Therapeutic Category Antineoplastic Agent

Use Treatment of ovarian cancer, multiple myeloma, and AIDS-related Kaposi sarcoma

Usual Dosage Refer to individual protocols. **Liposomal formulations of doxorubicin should NOT be substituted for conventional doxorubicin hydrochloride on a mg-per-mg basis.**
AIDS-related Kaposi sarcoma: I.V.: 20 mg/m^2/dose once every 3 weeks
Multiple myeloma: I.V.: 30 mg/m^2/dose every 3 weeks (in combination with bortezomib)
Ovarian cancer: I.V.: 50 mg/m^2/dose every 4 weeks

Dosage Forms
Injection, solution:
Doxil®: 2 mg/mL (10 mL, 25 mL)

Doxy-100® [US] see doxycycline on page 323
Doxycin [Can] see doxycycline on page 323

doxycycline (doks i SYE kleen)

Sound-Alike/Look-Alike Issues
doxycycline may be confused with dicyclomine, doxepin, doxylamine
Doxy-100® may be confused with Doxil®
Monodox® may be confused with Maalox®
Oracea™ may be confused with Orencia®

Synonyms doxycycline calcium; doxycycline hyclate; doxycycline monohydrate

U.S./Canadian Brand Names Adoxa® [US]; Apo-Doxy Tabs® [Can]; Apo-Doxy® [Can]; Doryx® [US]; Doxy-100® [US]; Doxycin [Can]; Doxytec [Can]; Monodox® [US]; Novo-Doxylin [Can]; Nu-Doxycycline [Can]; Oracea™ [US]; Periostat® [US/Can]; Vibra-Tabs® [US/Can]; Vibramycin® [US]

Therapeutic Category Tetracycline Derivative

Use Principally in the treatment of infections caused by susceptible *Rickettsia*, *Chlamydia*, and *Mycoplasma*; alternative to mefloquine for malaria prophylaxis; treatment for syphilis, uncomplicated *Neisseria gonorrhoeae*, *Listeria*, *Actinomyces israelii*, and *Clostridium* infections in penicillin-allergic patients; used for community-acquired pneumonia and other common infections due to susceptible organisms; anthrax due to *Bacillus anthracis*, including inhalational anthrax (postexposure); treatment of infections caused by uncommon susceptible gram-negative and gram-positive organisms including *Borrelia recurrentis*, *Ureaplasma urealyticum*, *Haemophilus ducreyi*, *Yersinia pestis*, *Francisella tularensis*, *Vibrio cholerae*, *Campylobacter fetus*, *Brucella* spp, *Bartonella bacilliformis*, and *Calymmatobacterium granulomatis*, Q fever, Lyme disease; treatment of inflammatory lesions associated with rosacea; intestinal amebiasis; severe acne

Usual Dosage
Usual dosage range:
Children >8 years (<45 kg): Oral, I.V.: 2-5 mg/kg/day in 1-2 divided doses, not to exceed 200 mg/day
Children >8 years (>45 kg) and Adults: Oral, I.V.: 100-200 mg/day in 1-2 divided doses

◄ **Indication-specific dosing:**

Children:

Anthrax: Doxycycline should be used in children if antibiotic susceptibility testing, exhaustion of drug supplies, or allergic reaction preclude use of penicillin or ciprofloxacin. For treatment, the consensus recommendation does not include a loading dose for doxycycline.

Inhalational (postexposure prophylaxis) (MMWR, 2001, 50:889-893): Oral, I.V. (use oral route when possible):

≤8 years: 2.2 mg/kg every 12 hours for 60 days

>8 years and ≤45 kg: 2.2 mg/kg every 12 hours for 60 days

>8 years and >45 kg: 100 mg every 12 hours for 60 days

Cutaneous (treatment): Oral: See dosing for "Inhalational (postexposure prophylaxis)"

Note: In the presence of systemic involvement, extensive edema, and/or lesions on head/neck, doxycycline should initially be administered I.V.

Inhalational/gastrointestinal/oropharyngeal (treatment): I.V.: Refer to dosing for inhalational anthrax (postexposure prophylaxis); switch to oral therapy when clinically appropriate

Note: Initial treatment should include two or more agents predicted to be effective (per CDC recommendations). Agents suggested for use in conjunction with doxycycline or ciprofloxacin include rifampin, vancomycin, imipenem, penicillin, ampicillin, chloramphenicol, clindamycin, and clarithromycin. May switch to oral antimicrobial therapy when clinically appropriate. Continue combined therapy for 60 days

Children ≥8 years: **Malaria prophylaxis:** Oral: 2 mg/kg/day (maximum: 100 mg/day). Start 1-2 days prior to travel to endemic area; continue daily during travel and for 4 weeks after leaving endemic area

Children ≥8 years (and >45 kg) and Adults:

Chlamydial infections, uncomplicated: Oral: 100 mg twice daily for ≥7 days

Lyme disease, Q fever, or tularemia: Oral: 100 mg twice daily for 14-21 days

Rickettsial disease or ehrlichiosis: Oral, I.V.: 100 mg twice daily for 7-14 days

Adults:

Anthrax:

Inhalational (postexposure prophylaxis): Oral, I.V. (use oral route when possible): 100 mg every 12 hours for 60 days (*MMWR*, 2001, 50:889-93); **Note:** Preliminary recommendation, FDA review and update is anticipated.

Cutaneous (treatment): Oral: 100 mg every 12 hours for 60 days. **Note:** In the presence of systemic involvement, extensive edema, lesions on head/neck, refer to I.V. dosing for treatment of inhalational/gastrointestinal/oropharyngeal anthrax

Inhalational/gastrointestinal/oropharyngeal (treatment): I.V.: Initial: 100 mg every 12 hours; switch to oral therapy when clinically appropriate; some recommend initial loading dose of 200 mg, followed by 100 mg every 8-12 hours (*JAMA*, 1997, 278:399-411). **Note:** Initial treatment should include two or more agents predicted to be effective (per CDC recommendations). Agents suggested for use in conjunction with doxycycline or ciprofloxacin include rifampin, vancomycin, imipenem, penicillin, ampicillin, chloramphenicol, clindamycin, and clarithromycin. May switch to oral antimicrobial therapy when clinically appropriate. Continue combined therapy for 60 days

Brucellosis: Oral: 100 mg twice daily for 6 weeks with rifampin or streptomycin

Community-acquired pneumonia, bronchitis: Oral, I.V.: 100 mg twice daily

Endometritis, salpingitis, parametritis, or peritonitis: I.V.: 100 mg twice daily with cefoxitin 2 g every 6 hours for 4 days and for ≥48 hours after patient improves; then continue with oral therapy 100 mg twice daily to complete a 10- to 14-day course of therapy

Gonococcal infection, acute (PID) in combination with another antibiotic: I.V.: 100 mg every 12 hours until improved, followed by 100 mg orally twice daily to complete 14 days

Malaria prophylaxis: 100 mg/day. Start 1-2 days prior to travel to endemic area; continue daily during travel and for 4 weeks after leaving endemic area

Nongonococcal urethritis: Oral: 100 mg twice daily for 7 days

Periodontitis: Oral (Periostat®): 20 mg twice daily as an adjunct following scaling and root planing; may be administered for up to 9 months. Safety beyond 12 months of treatment and efficacy beyond 9 months of treatment have not been established.

Rosacea: (Oracea™): Oral: 40 mg once daily in the morning

Syphilis:

Early syphilis: Oral, I.V.: 200 mg/day in divided doses for 14 days

Late syphilis: Oral, I.V.: 200 mg/day in divided doses for 28 days

***Yersinia pestis*(plague):** Oral: 100 mg twice daily for 7 days

Vibrio cholerae: Oral: 300 mg as a single dose

Dosage Forms

Capsule: 50 mg, 100 mg

Vibramycin®: 100 mg
Monodox®: 50 mg, 75 mg, 100 mg
Capsule, variable release:
Oracea™: 40 mg [30 mg (immediate-release) and 10 mg (delayed-release)]
Injection, powder for reconstitution: 100 mg
Doxy-100®: 100 mg
Powder for oral suspension: 25 mg/5 mL (60 mL)
Vibramycin®: 25 mg/5 mL
Syrup:
Vibramycin®: 50 mg/5 mL
Tablet: 20 mg, 50 mg, 75 mg, 100 mg, 150 mg
Adoxa®: 50 mg, 75 mg, 100 mg
Adoxa® Pak™ 1/75 [unit-dose pack]: 75 mg (31s)
Adoxa® Pak™ 1/100 [unit-dose pack]: 100 mg (31s)
Adoxa® Pak™ 1/150 [unit-dose pack]: 150 mg (30s)
Adoxa® Pak™ 2/100 [unit-dose pack]: 100 mg (60s)
Periostat®: 20 mg
Vibra-Tabs®: 100 mg
Tablet, delayed-release coated pellets:
Doryx®: 75 mg, 100 mg, 150 mg

doxycycline calcium *see* doxycycline *on page 323*
doxycycline hyclate *see* doxycycline *on page 323*
doxycycline monohydrate *see* doxycycline *on page 323*

doxylamine (dox IL a meen)
Sound-Alike/Look-Alike Issues
doxylamine may be confused with doxycycline
Synonyms doxylamine succinate
U.S./Canadian Brand Names Good Sense Sleep Aid [US-OTC]; Unisom® SleepTabs® [US-OTC]
Therapeutic Category Antihistamine
Use Treatment of short-term insomnia
Usual Dosage Oral: Adults: One tablet 30 minutes before bedtime; once daily or as instructed by healthcare professional
Dosage Forms
Tablet:
Good Sense Sleep Aid [OTC], Unisom® SleepTabs® [OTC]: 25 mg

doxylamine and pyridoxine *(Canada only)* (dox IL a meen & peer i DOX een)
Sound-Alike/Look-Alike Issues
doxylamine may be confused with doxycycline
Synonyms doxylamine succinate and pyridoxine hydrochloride; pyridoxine and doxylamine
U.S./Canadian Brand Names Diclectin® [Can]
Therapeutic Category Antihistamine; Vitamin
Use Treatment of pregnancy-associated nausea and vomiting
Usual Dosage Oral: Adults: Two delayed release tablets (a total of doxylamine 20 mg and pyridoxine 20 mg) at bedtime; in severe cases or in cases with nausea/vomiting during the day, dosage may be increased by 1 tablet in the morning and/or afternoon
Dosage Forms [CAN] = Canadian brand name
Tablet, delayed release:
Diclectin® [CAN]: Doxylamine 10 mg and pyridoxine 10 mg [not available in the U.S.]

doxylamine succinate *see* doxylamine *on page 325*
doxylamine succinate and pyridoxine hydrochloride *see* doxylamine and pyridoxine *(Canada only) on page 325*
doxylamine succinate, codeine phosphate, and acetaminophen *see* acetaminophen, codeine, and doxylamine *(Canada only) on page 26*
Doxytec [Can] *see* doxycycline *on page 323*
DPA *see* valproic acid and derivatives *on page 967*
D-Pan® *(Discontinued)* *see* dexpanthenol *on page 281*

DPE *see* dipivefrin *on page 311*

D-penicillamine *see* penicillamine *on page 730*

DPH *see* phenytoin *on page 750*

D-Phen 1000 [US] *see* guaifenesin and phenylephrine *on page 456*

DPM™ [US-OTC] *see* urea *on page 963*

Dramamine® [US-OTC] *see* dimenhydrinate *on page 301*

Dramamine® Less Drowsy Formula [US-OTC] *see* meclizine *on page 595*

Dramilin® Injection *(Discontinued)* *see* dimenhydrinate *on page 301*

dried smallpox vaccine *see* smallpox vaccine *on page 871*

Driminate® [US-OTC] *see* dimenhydrinate *on page 301*

Drinex [US-OTC] *see* acetaminophen, chlorpheniramine, and pseudoephedrine *on page 25*

Drinkables® MultiVitamins [US-OTC] *see* vitamins (multiple/oral) *on page 983*

Drisdol® [US/Can] *see* ergocalciferol *on page 350*

Dristan™ 12-Hour [US-OTC] *see* oxymetazoline *on page 712*

Dristan® Long Lasting Nasal [Can] *see* oxymetazoline *on page 712*

Dristan® Long Lasting Nasal Solution *(Discontinued)* *see* oxymetazoline *on page 712*

Dristan® N.D. [Can] *see* acetaminophen and pseudoephedrine *on page 23*

Dristan® N.D., Extra Strength [Can] *see* acetaminophen and pseudoephedrine *on page 23*

Dristan® Saline Spray *(Discontinued)* *see* sodium chloride *on page 873*

Drithocreme® HP 1% *(Discontinued)* *see* anthralin *on page 77*

Dritho-Scalp® [US] *see* anthralin *on page 77*

Drixoral® [Can] *see* dexbrompheniramine and pseudoephedrine *on page 279*

Drixoral® Cold & Allergy [US-OTC] *see* dexbrompheniramine and pseudoephedrine *on page 279*

Drixoral® Cough & Congestion Liquid Caps *(Discontinued)* *see* pseudoephedrine and dextromethorphan *on page 802*

Drixoral® Cough Liquid Caps *(Discontinued)* *see* dextromethorphan *on page 284*

Drixoral® Nasal [Can] *see* oxymetazoline *on page 712*

Drixoral® ND [Can] *see* pseudoephedrine *on page 801*

Drixoral® Non-Drowsy *(Discontinued)* *see* pseudoephedrine *on page 801*

Drize®-R *(Discontinued)* *see* chlorpheniramine, phenylephrine, and methscopolamine *on page 210*

dronabinol (droe NAB i nol)

Sound-Alike/Look-Alike Issues
dronabinol may be confused with droperidol

Synonyms delta-9 THC; delta-9-tetrahydro-cannabinol; tetrahydrocannabinol; THC

U.S./Canadian Brand Names Marinol® [US/Can]

Therapeutic Category Antiemetic

Controlled Substance C-III

Use Chemotherapy-associated nausea and vomiting refractory to other antiemetic(s); AIDS-related anorexia

Usual Dosage Refer to individual protocols. Oral:
Antiemetic: Children and Adults: 5 mg/m^2 1-3 hours before chemotherapy, then 5 mg/m^2/dose every 2-4 hours after chemotherapy for a total of 4-6 doses/day; increase doses in increments of 2.5 mg/m^2 to a maximum of 15 mg/m^2/dose.
Appetite stimulant: Adults: Initial: 2.5 mg twice daily (before lunch and dinner); titrate up to a maximum of 20 mg/day.

Dosage Forms
Capsule, soft gelatin: 2.5 mg, 5 mg, 10 mg
Marinol®: 2.5 mg, 5 mg, 10 mg

droperidol (droe PER i dole)

Sound-Alike/Look-Alike Issues
droperidol may be confused with dronabinol
Inapsine® may be confused with Nebcin®

Synonyms dehydrobenzperidol

U.S./Canadian Brand Names Droperidol Injection, USP [Can]; Inapsine® [US]

Therapeutic Category Antiemetic; Antipsychotic Agent, Butyrophenone

Use Antiemetic in surgical and diagnostic procedures; preoperative medication in patients when other treatments are ineffective or inappropriate

Usual Dosage Titrate carefully to desired effect

Children 2-12 years: Nausea and vomiting: I.M., I.V.: 0.05-0.06 mg/kg (maximum initial dose: 0.1 mg/kg); additional doses may be repeated to achieve effect; administer additional doses with caution

Adults: Prevention of postoperative nausea and vomiting (PONV): I.M., I.V.: Initial: 0.625-2.5 mg; additional doses of 1.25 mg may be administered to achieve desired effect; administer additional doses with caution. Consensus guidelines recommend 0.625-1.25 mg I.V. administered after surgery

Dosage Forms

Injection, solution: 2.5 mg/mL (1 mL, 2 mL)

Inapsine®: 2.5 mg/mL (1 mL, 2 mL)

Droperidol Injection, USP [Can] *see* droperidol *on page 326*

drospirenone and estradiol (droh SPYE re none & es tra DYE ole)

Synonyms E2 and DRSP; estradiol and drospirenone

U.S./Canadian Brand Names Angeliq® [US/Can]

Therapeutic Category Estrogen and Progestin Combination

Use Treatment of moderate-to-severe vasomotor symptoms associated with menopause; treatment of vulvar and vaginal atrophy associated with menopause

Usual Dosage Oral: Adults:

Moderate-to-severe vasomotor symptoms associated with menopause: One tablet daily; reevaluate patients at 3- and 6-month intervals to determine if treatment is still necessary.

Atrophic vaginitis in females with an intact uterus: One tablet daily; reevaluate patients at 3- and 6-month intervals to determine if treatment is still necessary.

Note: The lowest dose of estrogen/progestin that will control symptoms should be used; medication should be discontinued as soon as possible.

Dosage Forms

Tablet:

Angeliq®: Drospirenone 0.5 mg and estradiol 1 mg

drospirenone and ethinyl estradiol *see* ethinyl estradiol and drospirenone *on page 370*

drotrecogin alfa (dro TRE coe jin AL fa)

Synonyms activated protein C, human, recombinant; drotrecogin alfa, activated; protein C (activated), human, recombinant

U.S./Canadian Brand Names Xigris® [US/Can]

Therapeutic Category Protein C (Activated)

Use Reduction of mortality from severe sepsis (associated with organ dysfunction) in adults at high risk of death (eg, APACHE II score ≥25)

Usual Dosage I.V.: Adults: Sepsis: 24 mcg/kg/hour for a total of 96 hours; stop infusion **immediately** if clinically-important bleeding is identified. **Note:** Use actual body weight for dosing.

Dosage Forms

Injection, powder for reconstitution [preservative free]:

Xigris®: 5 mg, 20 mg

drotrecogin alfa, activated *see* drotrecogin alfa *on page 327*

DroTuss-CP [US] *see* phenylephrine, hydrocodone, and chlorpheniramine *on page 748*

Droxia® [US] *see* hydroxyurea *on page 490*

Dry Eye® Therapy Solution *(Discontinued)* *see* artificial tears *on page 95*

Dryox® Gel *(Discontinued)* *see* benzoyl peroxide *on page 126*

Dryox® Wash *(Discontinued)* *see* benzoyl peroxide *on page 126*

Drysol™ [US] *see* aluminum chloride hexahydrate *on page 53*

Dryvax® *(Discontinued)* *see* smallpox vaccine *on page 871*

DSCG *see* cromolyn sodium *on page 251*

D-ser(but)6,Azgly10-LHRH *see* goserelin *on page 451*

D-S-S® [US-OTC] *see* docusate *on page 314*

DSS *see* docusate *on page 314*

DT *see* diphtheria and tetanus toxoid *on page 306*

D-Tann HC *(Discontinued)*

DTaP *see* diphtheria, tetanus toxoids, and acellular pertussis vaccine *on page 309*

DTaP-IPV/Hib *see* diphtheria and tetanus toxoids, acellular pertussis, poliovirus (inactivated) and *Haemophilus* b conjugate vaccine *on page 308*

DTIC® [Can] *see* dacarbazine *on page 263*

DTIC *see* dacarbazine *on page 263*

DTPA *see* diethylene triamine penta-acetic acid *on page 294*

dTpa *see* diphtheria, tetanus toxoids, and acellular pertussis vaccine *on page 309*

D-Trp(6)-LHRH *see* triptorelin *on page 956*

Duac® CS [US] *see* clindamycin and benzoyl peroxide *on page 231*

Duac® *(Discontinued)* *see* clindamycin and benzoyl peroxide *on page 231*

Duet® [US] *see* vitamins (multiple/prenatal) *on page 983*

Duetact™ [US] *see* pioglitazone and glimepiride *on page 755*

Duet™ DHA [US] *see* vitamins (multiple/prenatal) *on page 983*

Duet® DHA^ec^ [US] *see* vitamins (multiple/prenatal) *on page 983*

Dukoral™ [Can] *see* traveler's diarrhea and cholera vaccine *(Canada only) on page 944*

Dulcolax® [US-OTC/Can] *see* bisacodyl *on page 136*

Dulcolax® Stool Softener [US-OTC] *see* docusate *on page 314*

Dull-C® [US-OTC] *see* ascorbic acid *on page 96*

duloxetine (doo LOX e teen)

Sound-Alike/Look-Alike Issues
DULoxetine may be confused with FLUoxetine

Synonyms (+)-(S)-N-methyl-γ-(1-naphthyloxy)-2-thiophenepropylamine hydrochloride; duloxetine hydrochloride; LY248686

Tall-Man DULoxetine

U.S./Canadian Brand Names Cymbalta® [US/Can]

Therapeutic Category Antidepressant, Serotonin/Norepinephrine Reuptake Inhibitor

Use Acute and maintenance treatment of major depressive disorder (MDD); treatment of generalized anxiety disorder (GAD); management of pain associated with diabetic neuropathy; management of fibromyalgia

Usual Dosage Oral: Adults:
Major depressive disorder: Initial: 40-60 mg/day; dose may be divided (ie, 20 or 30 mg twice daily) or given as a single daily dose of 60 mg; maintenance: 60 mg once daily; for doses >60 mg/day, titrate dose in increments of 30 mg/day over 1 week as tolerated to a maximum dose: 120 mg/day. **Note:** Doses >60 mg/day have not been demonstrated to be more effective.

Diabetic neuropathy: 60 mg once daily; lower initial doses may be considered in patients where tolerability is a concern and/or renal impairment is present. **Note:** Doses up to 120 mg/day administered in clinical trials offered no additional benefit and were less well tolerated than dose of 60 mg/day.

Fibromyalgia: Initial: 30 mg/day for 1 week, then increase to 60 mg/day as tolerated. **Note:** Doses up to 120 mg/day administered in clinical trials offered no additional benefit and were less well tolerated than dose of 60 mg/day.

Generalized anxiety disorder: Initial: 30-60 mg/day as a single daily dose; patients initiated at 30 mg/day should be titrated to 60 mg/day after 1 week; maximum dose: 120 mg/day. **Note:** Doses >60 mg/day have not been demonstrated to be more effective than 60 mg/day.

Dosage Forms
Capsule, delayed release, enteric coated pellets:
Cymbalta®: 20 mg, 30 mg, 60 mg

duloxetine hydrochloride *see* duloxetine *on page 328*

Duocaine™ [US] *see* lidocaine and bupivacaine *on page 563*

DuoCet™ *(Discontinued)* *see* hydrocodone and acetaminophen *on page 481*

Duodote™ [US] *see* atropine and pralidoxime *on page 106*

DuoFilm® [Can] *see* salicylic acid *on page 850*

Duoforte® 27 [Can] *see* salicylic acid *on page 850*

Duomax [US] *see* guaifenesin and phenylephrine *on page 456*

DuoNeb® [US] *see* ipratropium and albuterol *on page 525*
DuoPlant® (Discontinued) *see* salicylic acid *on page 850*
Duotan PD (Discontinued) *see* dexchlorpheniramine and pseudoephedrine *on page 280*
Duo-Trach® Injection (Discontinued) *see* lidocaine *on page 561*
DuP 753 *see* losartan *on page 577*
Duphalac® (Discontinued) *see* lactulose *on page 544*
Durabolin® [Can] *see* nandrolone *on page 655*
Duraclon® [US] *see* clonidine *on page 236*
Duradrin® (Discontinued) *see* acetaminophen, isometheptene, and dichloralphenazone *on page 28*
Duradyl® [US] *see* chlorpheniramine, phenylephrine, and methscopolamine *on page 210*
Duradyne DHC® (Discontinued) *see* hydrocodone and acetaminophen *on page 481*
Duragesic® [US/Can] *see* fentanyl *on page 394*
Dura-Gest® (Discontinued)
Durahist™ [US] *see* chlorpheniramine, pseudoephedrine, and methscopolamine *on page 213*
Durahist™ PE [US] *see* chlorpheniramine, phenylephrine, and methscopolamine *on page 210*
Duralith® [Can] *see* lithium *on page 571*
Duralone® Injection (Discontinued) *see* methylprednisolone *on page 623*
Duramist® Plus [US-OTC] *see* oxymetazoline *on page 712*
Duramorph® [US] *see* morphine sulfate *on page 643*
Duraphen™ II DM [US] *see* guaifenesin, dextromethorphan, and phenylephrine *on page 459*
Duraphen™ DM (Discontinued) *see* guaifenesin, dextromethorphan, and phenylephrine *on page 459*
Duraphen™ Forte [US] *see* guaifenesin, dextromethorphan, and phenylephrine *on page 459*
DuraTan™ Forte [US] *see* chlorpheniramine, pseudoephedrine, and dextromethorphan *on page 212*
Duratest® Injection (Discontinued) *see* testosterone *on page 912*
Durathate® Injection (Discontinued) *see* testosterone *on page 912*
Duration® (Discontinued) *see* oxymetazoline *on page 712*
Duratocin™ [Can] *see* carbetocin *(Canada only) on page 177*
Duratuss® [US] *see* guaifenesin and phenylephrine *on page 456*
Duratuss® DA [US] *see* chlorpheniramine and pseudoephedrine *on page 207*
Duratuss® DM [US] *see* guaifenesin and dextromethorphan *on page 454*
Duratuss GP® [US] *see* guaifenesin and phenylephrine *on page 456*
Duratuss® HD (Discontinued)
Dura-Vent®/DA (Discontinued) *see* chlorpheniramine, phenylephrine, and methscopolamine *on page 210*
Dura-Vent® (Discontinued)
Duricef® [Can] *see* cefadroxil *on page 184*
Duricef® (Discontinued) *see* cefadroxil *on page 184*
Duricef® Oral Suspension 125 mg/5 mL (Discontinued) *see* cefadroxil *on page 184*
Durolane® [Can] *see* hyaluronate and derivatives *on page 476*
Durrax® Oral (Discontinued) *see* hydroxyzine *on page 491*

dutasteride (doo TAS teer ide)

U.S./Canadian Brand Names Avodart® [US/Can]
Therapeutic Category Antineoplastic Agent, Anthracenedione
Use Treatment of symptomatic benign prostatic hyperplasia (BPH) as monotherapy or combination therapy with tamsulosin
Usual Dosage Oral: Adults: Males: 0.5 mg once daily alone or in combination with tamsulosin
Dosage Forms
  Capsule, softgel:
    Avodart®: 0.5 mg

Duvoid® [Can] *see* bethanechol *on page 133*
Duvoid® (Discontinued) *see* bethanechol *on page 133*
D-Vi-Sol® [Can] *see* cholecalciferol *on page 215*
DW286 *see* gemifloxacin *on page 439*

Dwelle® Ophthalmic Solution *(Discontinued)* see artificial tears *on page 95*
Dyazide® [US] see hydrochlorothiazide and triamterene *on page 480*
Dycill® [Can] see dicloxacillin *on page 293*
Dycill® *(Discontinued)* see dicloxacillin *on page 293*
Dyclone® *(Discontinued)* see dyclonine *on page 330*

dyclonine (DYE kloe neen)

Sound-Alike/Look-Alike Issues
dyclonine may be confused with dicyclomine
Synonyms dyclonine hydrochloride
U.S./Canadian Brand Names Cēpacol® Dual Action Maximum Strength [US-OTC]; Sucrets® [US-OTC]
Therapeutic Category Local Anesthetic
Use Temporary relief of pain associated with oral mucosa
Usual Dosage Oral:
Lozenge: Children ≥2 years and Adults: One lozenge every 2 hours as needed (maximum: 10 lozenges/day)
Spray:
Children ≥3-12 years: 1-3 sprays, up to 4 times a day
Children ≥12 years and Adults: 1-4 sprays, up to 4 times a day
Dosage Forms
Lozenge:
Sucrets® [OTC]: 1.2 mg, 2 mg, 3 mg
Spray, oral:
Cēpacol® Dual Action Maximum Strength [OTC]: 0.1%

dyclonine hydrochloride see dyclonine *on page 330*
Dygase *(Discontinued)* see pancreatin *on page 717*
Dylix [US] see dyphylline *on page 330*
Dymenate® Injection *(Discontinued)* see dimenhydrinate *on page 301*
Dynabac® *(Discontinued)*
Dynacin® [US] see minocycline *on page 635*
DynaCirc® [Can] see isradipine *on page 532*
DynaCirc® CR [US] see isradipine *on page 532*
DynaCirc® *(Discontinued)* see isradipine *on page 532*
Dyna-Hex® [US-OTC] see chlorhexidine gluconate *on page 201*
Dynahist-ER Pediatric® *(Discontinued)* see chlorpheniramine and pseudoephedrine *on page 207*
Dynapen® *(Discontinued)* see dicloxacillin *on page 293*
Dynatuss-EX [US] see guaifenesin, dextromethorphan, and phenylephrine *on page 459*
Dynex *(Discontinued)* see guaifenesin and pseudoephedrine *on page 458*

dyphylline (DYE fi lin)

Synonyms dihydroxypropyl theophylline
U.S./Canadian Brand Names Dilor® [Can]; Dylix [US]; Lufyllin® [US/Can]
Therapeutic Category Theophylline Derivative
Use Bronchodilator in reversible airway obstruction due to asthma, chronic bronchitis, or emphysema
Usual Dosage Oral: Adults: Up to 15 mg/kg 4 times/day, individualize dosage
Dosage Forms
Elixir:
Dylix: 100 mg/15 mL
Tablet:
Lufyllin®: 200 mg, 400 mg

dyphylline and guaifenesin (DYE fi lin & gwye FEN e sin)

Synonyms guaifenesin and dyphylline
U.S./Canadian Brand Names COPD [US]; Difil-G [US]; Difil®-G Forte [US]; Dilex-G [US]; Dilor-G® [US]; Lufyllin®-GG [US]
Therapeutic Category Expectorant; Theophylline Derivative

Use Treatment of bronchial asthma and reversible bronchospasm associated with chronic bronchitis and emphysema

Usual Dosage Oral:

Children 6-12 years:

Elixir: Lufyllin®-GG: 15-30 mL 3 or 4 times/day

Syrup: Dilex-G:

18-27 kg: 1.25-1.6 mL 4 times/day

27-36 kg: 2.5-3.3 mL 4 times/day

36.5-45 kg: 3.3-3.7 mL 4 times/day

Tablet: Lufyllin®-GG: 1/2 -1 tablet 3 or 4 times/day

Children >12 years and Adults:

Elixir: Lufyllin®-GG: 30 mL 4 times/day

Syrup:

Dilex-G: 5-10 mL 4 times/day

Difil®-G Forte: 5-10 mL 3 or 4 times/day; may double or triple (in severe cases) according to patient response

Tablet: Difil-G, Dilex-G, Lufyllin®-GG: One tablet 3 or 4 times/day

Dosage Forms

Elixir: Dyphylline 100 mg and guaifenesin 100 mg per 15 mL

Lufyllin®-GG: Dyphylline 100 mg and guaifenesin 100 mg per 15 mL

Liquid: Dyphylline 100 mg and guaifenesin 100 mg per 5 mL

Difil®-G Forte: Dyphylline 100 mg and guaifenesin 100 mg per 5 mL

Syrup:

Dilex-G: Dyphylline 100 mg and guaifenesin 200 mg per 5 mL

Tablet: Dyphylline 200 mg and guaifenesin 200 mg

COPD, Lufyllin®-GG: Dyphylline 200 mg and guaifenesin 200 mg

Difil®-G: Dyphylline 200 mg and guaifenesin 300 mg

Dilex-G: Dyphylline 200 mg and guaifenesin 400 mg

Dyrenium® [US] *see* triamterene *on page 949*

Dyrexan-OD® (Discontinued) *see* phendimetrazine *on page 742*

Dytan™ [US] *see* diphenhydramine *on page 304*

E2 and DRSP *see* drospirenone and estradiol *on page 327*

7E3 *see* abciximab *on page 17*

E2020 *see* donepezil *on page 318*

EACA *see* aminocaproic acid *on page 60*

EarSol® HC [US] *see* hydrocortisone (topical) *on page 485*

Easprin® [US] *see* aspirin *on page 98*

Ebixa® [Can] *see* memantine *on page 600*

echothiophate iodide (ek oh THYE oh fate EYE oh dide)

Synonyms ecostigmine iodide

U.S./Canadian Brand Names Phospholine Iodide® [US]

Therapeutic Category Cholinesterase Inhibitor

Use Used as miotic in treatment of chronic, open-angle glaucoma; may be useful in specific cases of angle-closure glaucoma (postiridectomy or where surgery refused/contraindicated); postcataract surgery-related glaucoma; accommodative esotropia

Usual Dosage Ophthalmic:

Children: Accommodative esotropia:

Diagnosis: Instill 1 drop (0.125%) once daily into both eyes at bedtime for 2-3 weeks

Treatment: Usual dose: Instill 1 drop of 0.06% once daily or 0.125% every other day (maximum: 0.125% daily). **Note:** Use lowest concentration and frequency which gives satisfactory response; if necessary, doses >0.125% daily may be used for short periods of time.

Adults: Open-angle or secondary glaucoma:

Initial: Instill 1 drop (0.03%) twice daily into eyes with 1 dose just prior to bedtime

Maintenance: Some patients have been treated with 1 dose daily or every other day

Conversion from other ophthalmic agents: If IOP control was unsatisfactory, patients may be expected to require higher doses of echothiophate (eg, ≥0.06%); however, patients should be initially started on the 0.03% strength for a short period to better tolerance.

◄ **Dosage Forms**
  Powder for reconstitution, ophthalmic:
    Phospholine Iodide®: 6.25 mg (5 mL) [0.125%]

EC-Naprosyn® [US] *see* naproxen *on page 656*
E. coli asparaginase *see* asparaginase *on page 98*

econazole (e KONE a zole)

Synonyms econazole nitrate
Therapeutic Category Antifungal Agent
Use Topical treatment of tinea pedis (athlete's foot), tinea cruris (jock itch), tinea corporis (ringworm), tinea versicolor, and cutaneous candidiasis
Usual Dosage Topical: Children and Adults:
  Tinea pedis: Apply sufficient amount to cover affected areas once daily for 1 month
  Tinea cruris, tinea corporis, tinea versicolor: Apply sufficient amount to cover affected areas once daily for 2 weeks
  Cutaneous candidiasis: Apply sufficient quantity twice daily (morning and evening) for 2 weeks
Dosage Forms
  Cream, topical: 1% (15 g, 30 g, 85 g)

econazole nitrate *see* econazole *on page 332*
Econopred® Plus [US] *see* prednisolone (ophthalmic) *on page 781*
ecostigmine iodide *see* echothiophate iodide *on page 331*
Ecotrin® [US-OTC] *see* aspirin *on page 98*
Ecotrin® Low Strength [US-OTC] *see* aspirin *on page 98*
Ecotrin® Maximum Strength [US-OTC] *see* aspirin *on page 98*
Ectosone [Can] *see* betamethasone (topical) *on page 132*

eculizumab (e kue LIZ oo mab)

Sound-Alike/Look-Alike Issues
  eculizumab may be confused with efalizumab
U.S./Canadian Brand Names Soliris™ [US]
Therapeutic Category Monoclonal Antibody; Monoclonal Antibody, Complement Inhibitor
Use Treatment of paroxysmal nocturnal hemoglobinuria (PNH) to reduce hemolysis
Usual Dosage Note: Patients must receive meningococcal vaccine at least 2 weeks prior to treatment initiation; revaccinate according to current guidelines.
  I.V.: Adults: PNH: 600 mg once weekly (±2 days) for 4 weeks, followed by 900 mg 1 week (±2 days) later; then maintenance: 900 mg every 2 weeks (±2 days) thereafter
  Treatment should be administered at the recommended time interval, however, the administration day may be varied by ±2 days if serum LDH levels suggest increased hemolysis before the end of the dosing interval.
Dosage Forms
  Injection, solution [preservative free]:
    Soliris™: 10 mg/mL (30 mL)

Ed A-Hist™ [US] *see* chlorpheniramine and phenylephrine *on page 206*
Ed A-Hist DM [US] *see* chlorpheniramine, phenylephrine, and dextromethorphan *on page 209*
edathamil disodium *see* edetate disodium *on page 333*
Ed ChlorPed D [US] *see* chlorpheniramine and phenylephrine *on page 206*
Edecrin® [US/Can] *see* ethacrynic acid *on page 367*

edetate CALCIUM disodium (ED e tate KAL see um dye SOW dee um)

Sound-Alike/Look-Alike Issues
  edetate CALCIUM disodium may be confused with etomidate

  To avoid potentially serious errors, the abbreviation "EDTA" should **never** be used.

  edetate CALCIUM disodium (CaEDTA) may be confused with edetate disodium (Na$_2$EDTA). CDC recommends that edetate disodium should **never** be used for chelation therapy in children. Fatal hypocalcemia may result if edetate disodium is used for chelation therapy instead of edetate calcium disodium. ISMP recommends confirming the diagnosis to help distinguish between the two drugs prior to dispensing and/or administering either drug.

Synonyms CaEDTA ; calcium disodium edetate; edetate disodium CALCIUM

U.S./Canadian Brand Names Calcium Disodium Versenate® [US]

Therapeutic Category Chelating Agent

Use Treatment of symptomatic acute and chronic lead poisoning or for symptomatic patients with high blood lead levels

Usual Dosage

Treatment of lead poisoning: Children and Adults: **Note:** For the treatment of high blood lead levels in children, the CDC recommends chelation treatment when blood lead levels are >45 mcg/dL (CDC, 2002). In adults, available guidelines recommend chelation therapy with blood lead levels >50 mcg/dL and significant symptoms; chelation therapy may also be indicated with blood lead levels ≥100 mcg/dL and/or symptoms. Depending upon the blood lead level, additional courses may be necessary; repeat at least 2-4 days and preferably 2-4 weeks apart:

Asymptomatic lead poisoning with blood lead level >20 mcg/dL and <70 mcg/dL (manufacturer labeling): I.M., I.V.: 1000 mg/m^2/day (25-50 mg/kg/day) for 5 days. **Note:** The AAP recommends succimer as the drug used for initial management in asymptomatic children when blood lead levels are >45 mcg/dL and <70 mcg/dL. Edetate CALCIUM disodium can be used in children allergic to to succimer (AAP, 2005).

Symptomatic lead poisoning or blood lead levels ≥70 mcg/dL: I.M., I.V.: 1000 mg/m^2/day (25-50 mg/kg/day) for 5 days. Edetate CALCIUM disodium should be administered 4 hours after the initial dimercaprol dose. Edetate CALCIUM disodium should be used in conjunction with dimercaprol when blood lead levels are >70 mcg/dL or when symptoms of lead poisoning are present.

Lead encephalopathy: I.M., I.V.: 1500 mg/m^2/day (50-75 mg/kg/day). Edetate CALCIUM disodium should be administered 4 hours after the initial dimercaprol dose. Edetate CALCIUM disodium should be used in conjunction with dimercaprol when blood lead levels are >70 mcg/dL or when symptoms of lead poisoning are present.

Lead nephropathy: Adults: An alternative dosing regimen reflecting the reduction in renal clearance is based upon the serum creatinine. Dose of edetate CALCIUM disodium based on serum creatinine: **Note:** Repeat regimen monthly until lead levels are reduced to an acceptable level:

S_{cr} >2-3 mg/dL / Cl_{cr} 30-50 mL/minute: Reduce recommended dose by 50% and administer daily

S_{cr} >3-4 mg/dL / Cl_{cr} 20-30 mL/minute: Reduce recommended dose by 50% and administer every 48 hours

S_{cr} >4 mg/dL / Cl_{cr} <20 mL/minute: Reduce recommended dose by 50% and administer once weekly

Dosage Forms

Injection, solution:

Calcium Disodium Versenate®: 200 mg/mL (5 mL)

edetate disodium (ED e tate dye SOW dee um)

Sound-Alike/Look-Alike Issues

edetate disodium may be confused with etomidate

To avoid potentially serious errors, the abbreviation "EDTA" should **never** be used.

edetate disodium (Na$_2$EDTA) may be confused with edetate calcium disodium (CaEDTA). CDC recommends that edetate disodium should **never** be used for chelation therapy in children. Fatal hypocalcemia may result if edetate disodium is used for chelation therapy instead of edetate calcium disodium. ISMP recommends confirming the diagnosis to help distinguish between the two drugs prior to dispensing and/or administering either drug.

Synonyms edathamil disodium; Na$_2$EDTA; sodium edetate

Therapeutic Category Chelating Agent

Use Emergency treatment of hypercalcemia in adults

Usual Dosage Note: Confirm the diagnosis prior to dispensing.

I.V.: Hypercalcemia: Adults: 50 mg/kg/day over 3 or more hours to a maximum of 3 g/24 hours; a suggested regimen of 5 days followed by 2 days without drug and repeated courses up to 15 total doses

Dosage Forms

Injection, solution: 150 mg/mL (20 mL)

edetate disodium CALCIUM *see* edetate CALCIUM disodium *on page 332*

Edex® [US] *see* alprostadil *on page 50*

edrophonium and atropine (ed roe FOE nee um & A troe peen)

Synonyms atropine sulfate and edrophonium chloride; edrophonium chloride and atropine sulfate

Therapeutic Category Anticholinergic Agent; Antidote; Cholinergic Agonist

Use Reversal of nondepolarizing neuromuscular blockers; adjunct treatment of respiratory depression caused by curare overdose

Usual Dosage I.V.: Adults: Reversal of neuromuscular blockade: 0.05 mL/kg given over 45-60 seconds. The dose delivered is 0.5-1 mg/kg of edrophonium and 0.007-0.015 mg/kg of atropine. An edrophonium dose of 1 mg/kg should rarely be exceeded. **Note:** Monitor closely for bradyarrhythmias. Have atropine on hand in case needed.

edrophonium *(Canada only)* (ed roe FOE nee um)

Synonyms edrophonium chloride

U.S./Canadian Brand Names Enlon® [Can]; Tensilon® [Can]

Therapeutic Category Cholinergic Agent

Use Diagnosis of myasthenia gravis; differentiation of cholinergic crises from myasthenia crises; reversal of nondepolarizing neuromuscular blockers; adjunct treatment of respiratory depression caused by curare overdose

Usual Dosage Usually administered I.V., however, if not possible, I.M. or SubQ may be used:
Infants:
  I.M.: 0.5-1 mg
  I.V.: Initial: 0.1 mg, followed by 0.4 mg if no response; total dose = 0.5 mg
Children:
  Diagnosis: Initial: 0.04 mg/kg over 1 minute followed by 0.16 mg/kg if no response, to a maximum total dose of 5 mg for children <34 kg, or 10 mg for children >34 kg **or**
  Alternative dosing (manufacturer's recommendation):
    ≤34 kg: 1 mg; if no response after 45 seconds, repeat dosage in 1 mg increments every 30-45 seconds, up to a total of 5 mg
    >34 kg: 2 mg; if no response after 45 seconds, repeat dosage in 1 mg increments every 30-45 seconds, up to a total of 10 mg
  I.M.:
    <34 kg: 1 mg
    >34 kg: 5 mg
  Titration of oral anticholinesterase therapy: 0.04 mg/kg once given 1 hour after oral intake of the drug being used in treatment; if strength improves, an increase in neostigmine or pyridostigmine dose is indicated
Adults:
  Diagnosis:
    I.V.: 2 mg test dose administered over 15-30 seconds; 8 mg given 45 seconds later if no response is seen; test dose may be repeated after 30 minutes
    I.M.: Initial: 10 mg; if no cholinergic reaction occurs, administer 2 mg 30 minutes later to rule out false-negative reaction
  Titration of oral anticholinesterase therapy: 1-2 mg given 1 hour after oral dose of anticholinesterase; if strength improves, an increase in neostigmine or pyridostigmine dose is indicated
  Reversal of nondepolarizing neuromuscular blocking agents (neostigmine with atropine usually preferred): I.V.: 10 mg over 30-45 seconds; may repeat every 5-10 minutes up to 40 mg
  Termination of paroxysmal atrial tachycardia: I.V. rapid injection: 5-10 mg
  Differentiation of cholinergic from myasthenic crisis: I.V.: 1 mg; may repeat after 1 minute. **Note:** Intubation and controlled ventilation may be required if patient has cholinergic crisis

Dosage Forms
  Injection, solution:
    Enlon®: 10 mg/mL (15 mL)

edrophonium chloride *see* edrophonium *(Canada only) on page 334*
edrophonium chloride and atropine sulfate *see* edrophonium and atropine *on page 334*
ED-SPAZ® *(Discontinued)* *see* hyoscyamine *on page 492*
ED-TLC [US] *see* phenylephrine, hydrocodone, and chlorpheniramine *on page 748*
ED-Tuss HC [US] *see* phenylephrine, hydrocodone, and chlorpheniramine *on page 748*
E.E.M.T. D.S. [US] *see* estrogens (esterified) and methyltestosterone *on page 366*
E.E.M.T. H.S. [US] *see* estrogens (esterified) and methyltestosterone *on page 366*

E.E.S.® [US/Can] *see* erythromycin *on page 354*

efalizumab (e fa li ZOO mab)

Sound-Alike/Look-Alike Issues
efalizumab may be confused with eculizumab
Synonyms anti-CD11a; hu1124
U.S./Canadian Brand Names Raptiva® [US]
Therapeutic Category Immunosuppressant Agent; Monoclonal Antibody
Use Treatment of chronic moderate-to-severe plaque psoriasis in patients who are candidates for systemic therapy or phototherapy
Usual Dosage SubQ: Adults: Psoriasis: Initial: 0.7 mg/kg, followed by weekly dose of 1 mg/kg (maximum: 200 mg/dose)
Dosage Forms
Injection, powder for reconstitution:
Raptiva®: 150 mg

efavirenz (e FAV e renz)

U.S./Canadian Brand Names Sustiva® [US/Can]
Therapeutic Category Antiretroviral Agent, Nonnucleoside Reverse Transcriptase Inhibitor (NNRTI)
Use Treatment of HIV-1 infections in combination with at least two other antiretroviral agents
Usual Dosage Oral: Dosing at bedtime is recommended to limit central nervous system effects; should not be used as single-agent therapy

Children ≥3 years: Dosage is based on body weight
10 kg to <15 kg: 200 mg once daily
15 kg to <20 kg: 250 mg once daily
20 kg to <25 kg: 300 mg once daily
25 kg to <32.5 kg: 350 mg once daily
32.5 kg to <40 kg: 400 mg once daily
≥40 kg: 600 mg once daily
Adults: 600 mg once daily
Dosage Forms
Capsule:
Sustiva®: 50 mg, 200 mg
Tablet:
Sustiva®: 600 mg

efavirenz, emtricitabine, and tenofovir

(e FAV e renz, em trye SYE ta been, & te NOE fo veer)
Synonyms emtricitabine, efavirenz, and tenofovir; tenofovir disoproxil fumarate, efavirenz, and emtricitabine
U.S./Canadian Brand Names Atripla™ [US/Can]
Therapeutic Category Antiretroviral Agent, Nonnucleoside Reverse Transcriptase Inhibitor (NNRTI); Antiretroviral Agent, Nucleoside Reverse Transcriptase Inhibitor (NRTI); Antiretroviral Agent, Reverse Transcriptase Inhibitor (Nucleotide)
Use Treatment of HIV infection
Usual Dosage Oral: Adults: One tablet once daily to be taken on an empty stomach (at bedtime is recommended).
Dosage Forms
Tablet:
Atripla™: Efavirenz 600 mg, emtricitabine 200 mg, and tenofovir disoproxil fumarate 300 mg

Effer-K™ [US] *see* potassium bicarbonate and potassium citrate *on page 770*
Effer-Syllium® *(Discontinued)* *see* psyllium *on page 804*
Effexor® [US] *see* venlafaxine *on page 973*
Effexor XR® [US/Can] *see* venlafaxine *on page 973*
Eflone® *(Discontinued)* *see* fluorometholone *on page 412*

eflornithine (ee FLOR ni theen)

Sound-Alike/Look-Alike Issues
Vaniqa™ may be confused with Viagra®

Synonyms DFMO; eflornithine hydrochloride

U.S./Canadian Brand Names Vaniqa™ [US/Can]

Therapeutic Category Antiprotozoal; Topical Skin Product

Use Cream: Females ≥12 years: Reduce unwanted hair from face and adjacent areas under the chin

Orphan status: Injection: Treatment of meningoencephalitic stage of *Trypanosoma brucei gambiense* infection (sleeping sickness)

Usual Dosage
Children ≥12 years and Adults: Females: Topical: Apply thin layer of cream to affected areas of face and adjacent chin twice daily, at least 8 hours apart

Adults: I.V. infusion: 100 mg/kg/dose given every 6 hours (over at least 45 minutes) for 14 days

Dosage Forms
Cream, topical:
Vaniqa™: 13.9% (30 g)
Injection, solution:
Vaniqa™: 200 mg/mL (100 mL) [orphan drug status]

eflornithine hydrochloride *see eflornithine on page 336*

Efodine® (Discontinued) *see povidone-iodine on page 775*

eformoterol and budesonide *see budesonide and formoterol on page 148*

Efudex® [US/Can] *see fluorouracil on page 412*

E-Gems® [US-OTC] *see vitamin E on page 981*

E-Gems Elite® [US-OTC] *see vitamin E on page 981*

E-Gems Plus® [US-OTC] *see vitamin E on page 981*

EHDP *see etidronate disodium on page 382*

Elaprase™ [US] *see idursulfase on page 498*

Elavil® (Discontinued) *see amitriptyline on page 62*

Eldepryl® [US] *see selegiline on page 860*

Eldopaque® [US-OTC/Can] *see hydroquinone on page 488*

Eldopaque Forte® [US] *see hydroquinone on page 488*

Eldoquin® [US-OTC/Can] *see hydroquinone on page 488*

Eldoquin Forte® [US] *see hydroquinone on page 488*

electrolyte lavage solution *see polyethylene glycol-electrolyte solution on page 766*

electrolyte lavage solution *see polyethylene glycol-electrolyte solution and bisacodyl on page 766*

electrolyte solution, renal replacement
(ee LEK trow lite soe LOO shun REE nil ree PLASE ment)

Synonyms continuous renal replacement therapy; CRRT; renal replacement solution

U.S./Canadian Brand Names Normocarb HF™ [US]; PrismaSol [US]

Therapeutic Category Alkalinizing Agent; Electrolyte Supplement

Use Used as a replacement solution to replenish water, correct electrolytes, and adjust acid-base balance depleted by hemofiltration or hemodiafiltration (continuous renal replacement therapy [CRRT])

Usual Dosage Note: If using PrismaSol, ensure that compartment A and B are mixed.
Continuous renal replacement circuit: Children and Adults: Pre- or post-filter: Volume of solution administered depends upon the patient's fluid balance, target fluid balance, body weight, and amount of fluid removed during hemofiltration process.
Post-filter replacement: Volume infused/hour should not be greater than 1/3 of blood flow rate (eg, blood flow rate 100 mL/minute [6000 mL/hour], post-filter replacement rate ≤2000 mL/hour)

Dosage Forms
Injection, solution [concentrate; preservative free]:
Normocarb HF™ 25: Bicarbonate 25 mEq/L, chloride 116.5 mEq/L, magnesium 1.5 mEq/L, sodium 140 mEq/L (240 mL) [strength represents final solution after mixing; when diluted as directed, makes 3240 mL of infusate]

Normocarb HF™ 35: Bicarbonate 35 mEq/L, chloride 106.5 mEq/L, magnesium 1.5 mEq/L, sodium 140 mEq/L (240 mL) [strength represents final solution after mixing; when diluted as directed, makes 3240 mL of infusate]
Injection, solution [preservative free]:
PrismaSol BGK 0/2.5: Bicarbonate 32 mEq/L, calcium 2.5 mEq/L, chloride 109 mEq/L, dextrose 100 mg/dL, lactate 3 mEq/L, magnesium 1.5 mEq/L, sodium 140 mEq/L (5000 mL) [strength represents final solution after mixing]
PrismaSol BGK 2/0: Bicarbonate 32 mEq/L, chloride 108 mEq/L, dextrose 100 mg/dL, lactate 3 mEq/L, magnesium 1 mEq/L, potassium 2 mEq/L, sodium 140 mEq/L (5000 mL) [strength represents final solution after mixing]
PrismaSol BGK 2/3.5: Bicarbonate 32 mEq/L, calcium 3.5 mEq/L, chloride 111.5 mEq/L, dextrose 100 mg/dL, lactate 3 mEq/L, magnesium 1 mEq/L, potassium 2 mEq/L, sodium 140 mEq/L (5000 mL) [strength represents final solution after mixing]
PrismaSol BGK 4/2.5: Bicarbonate 32 mEq/L, calcium 2.5 mEq/L, chloride 113 mEq/L, dextrose 100 mg/dL, lactate 3 mEq/L, magnesium 1.5 mEq/L, potassium 4 mEq/L, sodium 140 mEq/L (5000 mL) [strength represents final solution after mixing]
PrismaSol BK 0/3.5: Bicarbonate 32 mEq/L, calcium 3.5 mEq/L, chloride 109.5 mEq/L, lactate 3 mEq/L, magnesium 1 mEq/L, sodium 140 mEq/L (5000 mL) [strength represents final solution after mixing]

Elestat™ [US] *see* epinastine *on page 344*
Elestrin™ [US] *see* estradiol *on page 359*

eletriptan (el e TRIP tan)

Synonyms eletriptan hydrobromide
U.S./Canadian Brand Names Relpax® [US/Can]
Therapeutic Category Serotonin 5-HT$_{1B, 1D}$ Receptor Agonist
Use Acute treatment of migraine, with or without aura
Usual Dosage Oral: Adults: Acute migraine: 20-40 mg; if the headache improves but returns, dose may be repeated after 2 hours have elapsed since first dose; maximum 80 mg/day.
Note: If the first dose is ineffective, diagnosis needs to be reevaluated. Safety of treating >3 headaches/month has not been established.
Dosage Forms
Tablet:
Relpax®: 20 mg, 40 mg

eletriptan hydrobromide *see* eletriptan *on page 337*
Elidel® [US/Can] *see* pimecrolimus *on page 753*
Eligard® [US/Can] *see* leuprolide *on page 553*
Elimite® [US] *see* permethrin *on page 740*
elipten *see* aminoglutethimide *on page 60*
Elitek™ [US] *see* rasburicase *on page 821*
Elixomin® (Discontinued) *see* theophylline *on page 917*
Elixophyllin® [US] *see* theophylline *on page 917*
Elixophyllin® (Discontinued) *see* theophylline *on page 917*
Elixophyllin-GG® [US] *see* theophylline and guaifenesin *on page 919*
ElixSure™ Fever/Pain (Discontinued) *see* acetaminophen *on page 19*
ElixSure® Cough [US-OTC] *see* dextromethorphan *on page 284*
Ellence® [US/Can] *see* epirubicin *on page 346*
Elmiron® [US/Can] *see* pentosan polysulfate sodium *on page 737*
Elocom® [Can] *see* mometasone *on page 641*
Elocon® [US] *see* mometasone *on page 641*
Eloxatin® [US] *see* oxaliplatin *on page 705*
Elspar® [US/Can] *see* asparaginase *on page 98*
Eltor® [Can] *see* pseudoephedrine *on page 801*
Eltroxin® [Can] *see* levothyroxine *on page 560*
Emadine® [US] *see* emedastine *on page 338*
Embeline™ (Discontinued) *see* clobetasol *on page 232*
Embeline™ E (Discontinued) *see* clobetasol *on page 232*

Emcyt® [US/Can] *see* estramustine *on page 363*
Emecheck® *(Discontinued)*

emedastine (em e DAS teen)
Synonyms emedastine difumarate
U.S./Canadian Brand Names Emadine® [US]
Therapeutic Category Antihistamine, H$_1$ Blocker, Ophthalmic
Use Treatment of allergic conjunctivitis
Usual Dosage Ophthalmic: Children ≥3 years and Adults: Instill 1 drop in affected eye up to 4 times/day
Dosage Forms
  Solution, ophthalmic:
    Emadine®: 0.05% (5 mL)

emedastine difumarate *see* emedastine *on page 338*
Emend® [US/Can] *see* aprepitant *on page 90*
Emend® for Injection [US] *see* fosaprepitant *on page 426*
Emetrol® [US-OTC] *see* fructose, dextrose, and phosphoric acid *on page 429*
Emitrip® *(Discontinued)* *see* amitriptyline *on page 62*
Emko® *(Discontinued)* *see* nonoxynol 9 *on page 677*
EMLA® [US/Can] *see* lidocaine and prilocaine *on page 565*
Emo-Cort® [Can] *see* hydrocortisone (topical) *on page 485*
Emsam® [US] *see* selegiline *on page 860*

emtricitabine (em trye SYE ta been)
Synonyms BW524W91; coviracil; FTC
U.S./Canadian Brand Names Emtriva® [US/Can]
Therapeutic Category Antiretroviral Agent, Nucleoside Reverse Transcriptase Inhibitor (NRTI)
Use Treatment of HIV infection in combination with at least two other antiretroviral agents
Usual Dosage Oral:
  Children:
    0-3 months: Solution: 3 mg/kg/day
    3 months to 17 years:
      Capsule: Children >33 kg: 200 mg once daily
      Solution: 6 mg/kg once daily; maximum: 240 mg/day
  Adults:
    Capsule: 200 mg once daily
    Solution: 240 mg once daily
Dosage Forms
  Capsule:
    Emtriva®: 200 mg
  Solution:
    Emtriva®: 10 mg/mL

emtricitabine and tenofovir (em trye SYE ta been & te NOE fo veer)
Synonyms tenofovir and emtricitabine
U.S./Canadian Brand Names Truvada® [US/Can]
Therapeutic Category Antiretroviral Agent, Nucleoside Reverse Transcriptase Inhibitor (NRTI); Antiretroviral Agent, Reverse Transcriptase Inhibitor (Nucleotide)
Use Treatment of HIV infection in combination with other antiretroviral agents
Usual Dosage Oral: Adults: One tablet (emtricitabine 200 mg and tenofovir 300 mg) once daily
Dosage Forms
  Tablet:
    Truvada®: Emtricitabine 200 mg and tenofovir 300 mg

emtricitabine, efavirenz, and tenofovir *see* efavirenz, emtricitabine, and tenofovir *on page 335*
Emtriva® [US/Can] *see* emtricitabine *on page 338*
Emulsoil® *(Discontinued)* *see* castor oil *on page 183*
E-Mycin® *(Discontinued)*

E-Mycin-E® *(Discontinued)*
ENA 713 *see* rivastigmine *on page 840*
Enablex® **[US/Can]** *see* darifenacin *on page 268*

enalapril (e NAL a pril)

Sound-Alike/Look-Alike Issues
enalapril may be confused with Anafranil®, Elavil®, Eldepryl®, nafarelin, ramipril

Synonyms enalapril maleate; enalaprilat

U.S./Canadian Brand Names Apo-Enalapril® [Can]; CO Enalapril [Can]; Gen-Enalapril [Can]; Novo-Enalapril [Can]; PMS-Enalapril [Can]; ratio-Enalapril [Can]; Riva-Enalapril [Can]; Sandoz-Enalapril [Can]; Taro-Enalapril [Can]; Vasotec® I.V. [Can]; Vasotec® [US/Can]

Therapeutic Category Angiotensin-Converting Enzyme (ACE) Inhibitor

Use Treatment of hypertension; treatment of symptomatic heart failure; treatment of asymptomatic left ventricular dysfunction

Usual Dosage Use lower listed initial dose in patients with hyponatremia, hypovolemia, severe congestive heart failure, decreased renal function, or in those receiving diuretics.

Oral: **Enalapril:** Children 1 month to 17 years: Hypertension: Initial: 0.08 mg/kg/d (up to 5 mg) in 1-2 divided doses; adjust dosage based on patient response; doses >0.58 mg/kg (40 mg) have not been evaluated in pediatric patients

Adults:
Oral: **Enalapril:**
Hypertension: 2.5-5 mg/day then increase as required, usually at 1- to 2-week intervals; usual dose range (JNC 7): 2.5-40 mg/day in 1-2 divided doses. **Note:** Initiate with 2.5 mg if patient is taking a diuretic which cannot be discontinued. May add a diuretic if blood pressure cannot be controlled with enalapril alone.

Heart failure: Initial: 2.5 mg once or twice daily (usual range: 5-40 mg/day in 2 divided doses). Titrate slowly at 1- to 2-week intervals. Target dose: 10-20 mg twice daily (ACC/AHA 2005 Heart Failure Guidelines)

Asymptomatic left ventricular dysfunction: 2.5 mg twice daily, titrated as tolerated to 20 mg/day

I.V.: **Enalaprilat:**
Hypertension: 1.25 mg/dose, given over 5 minutes every 6 hours; doses as high as 5 mg/dose every 6 hours have been tolerated for up to 36 hours. **Note:** If patients are concomitantly receiving diuretic therapy, begin with 0.625 mg I.V. over 5 minutes; if the effect is not adequate after 1 hour, repeat the dose and administer 1.25 mg at 6-hour intervals thereafter; if adequate, administer 0.625 mg I.V. every 6 hours.

Heart failure: Avoid I.V. administration in patients with unstable heart failure or those suffering acute myocardial infarction.

Conversion from I.V. to oral therapy if not concurrently on diuretics: 5 mg once daily; subsequent titration as needed; if concurrently receiving diuretics and responding to 0.625 mg I.V. every 6 hours, initiate with 2.5 mg/day.

Dosage Forms
Injection, solution: 1.25 mg/mL (1 mL, 2 mL)
Tablet: 2.5 mg, 5 mg, 10 mg, 20 mg
Vasotec®: 2.5 mg, 5 mg, 10 mg, 20 mg

enalapril and felodipine (e NAL a pril & fe LOE di peen)

Synonyms enalapril maleate and felodipine; felodipine and enalapril

U.S./Canadian Brand Names Lexxel® [Can]

Therapeutic Category Antihypertensive Agent, Combination

Use Treatment of hypertension, however, not indicated for initial treatment of hypertension; replacement therapy in patients receiving separate dosage forms (for patient convenience); when monotherapy with one component fails to achieve desired antihypertensive effect, or when dose-limiting adverse effects limit upward titration of monotherapy

Usual Dosage Oral: Adults: Enalapril 5-20 mg and felodipine 2.5-10 mg once daily

enalapril and hydrochlorothiazide (e NAL a pril & hye droe klor oh THYE a zide)

Synonyms enalapril maleate and hydrochlorothiazide; hydrochlorothiazide and enalapril

U.S./Canadian Brand Names Vaseretic® [US/Can]

Therapeutic Category Antihypertensive Agent, Combination

▶

339

◀ **Use** Treatment of hypertension

Usual Dosage Oral: Adults: Enalapril 5-10 mg and hydrochlorothiazide 12.5-25 mg once daily (maximum: 40 mg/day [enalapril]; 50 mg/day [hydrochlorothiazide])

Dosage Forms
   Tablet: 5/12.5: Enalapril 5 mg and hydrochlorothiazide 12.5 mg; 10/25: Enalapril 10 mg and hydro-chlorothiazide 25 mg
   Vaseretic®: 10/25: enalapril 10 mg and hydrochlorothiazide 25 mg

enalaprilat see enalapril on page 339
enalapril maleate see enalapril on page 339
enalapril maleate and felodipine see enalapril and felodipine on page 339
enalapril maleate and hydrochlorothiazide see enalapril and hydrochlorothiazide on page 339
Enbrel® [US/Can] see etanercept on page 367
Encare® [US-OTC] see nonoxynol 9 on page 677
Encora™ [US] see vitamins (multiple/oral) on page 983
Encort™ [US] see hydrocortisone (rectal) on page 484
EndaCof *(Discontinued)*
EndaCof-DM [US] see brompheniramine, pseudoephedrine, and dextromethorphan on page 146
EndaCof-PD [US] see brompheniramine, pseudoephedrine, and dextromethorphan on page 146
EndaCof-XP *(Discontinued)*
Endagen™-HD *(Discontinued)* see phenylephrine, hydrocodone, and chlorpheniramine on page 748
Endantadine® [Can] see amantadine on page 56
EndoAvitene® [US] see collagen hemostat on page 245
Endocet® [US/Can] see oxycodone and acetaminophen on page 710
Endocodone® *(Discontinued)* see oxycodone on page 709
Endodan® [US/Can] see oxycodone and aspirin on page 711
Endo®-Levodopa/Carbidopa [Can] see carbidopa and levodopa on page 177
Endolor® *(Discontinued)*
Endometrin® [US] see progesterone on page 790
Endrate® *(Discontinued)* see edetate disodium on page 333
Enduron® [Can] see methyclothiazide on page 619
Enduron® *(Discontinued)* see methyclothiazide on page 619
Enduronyl® Forte *(Discontinued)*
Enemeez® [US-OTC] see docusate on page 314
Enemeez® Plus [US-OTC] see docusate on page 314
Ener-B® *(Discontinued)* see cyanocobalamin on page 254
Enerjets [US-OTC] see caffeine on page 158
Enfamil® Glucose [US] see dextrose on page 286

enflurane (EN floo rane)
   Sound-Alike/Look-Alike Issues
      enflurane may be confused with isoflurane
   U.S./Canadian Brand Names Compound 347™ [US]; Ethrane® [US]
   Therapeutic Category General Anesthetic
   Use Maintenance of general anesthesia
   Usual Dosage Minimum alveolar concentration (MAC), the concentration at which 50% of patients do not respond to surgical incision, is 1.6% for enflurane. The concentration at which amnesia and loss of awareness occur (MAC - awake) is 0.4%. Surgical levels of anesthesia are achieved with concentrations between 0.5% to 3%.
   Dosage Forms
      Liquid, for inhalation:
         Compound 347™, Ethrane®: >99.9% (250 mL)

enfuvirtide (en FYOO vir tide)
   Synonyms T-20
   U.S./Canadian Brand Names Fuzeon® [US/Can]

Therapeutic Category Antiretroviral Agent, Fusion Protein Inhibitor

Use Treatment of HIV-1 infection in combination with other antiretroviral agents in treatment-experienced patients with evidence of HIV-1 replication despite ongoing antiretroviral therapy

Usual Dosage SubQ:

Children 6-16 years: 2 mg/kg twice daily (maximum dose: 90 mg twice daily)

Adolescents ≥16 years and Adults: 90 mg twice daily

Dosage Forms

Injection, powder for reconstitution [preservative free]:

Fuzeon®: 108 mg

ENG *see* etonogestrel *on page 383*

Engerix-B® [US/Can] *see* hepatitis B vaccine *on page 471*

Engerix-B® and Havrix® *see* hepatitis A inactivated and hepatitis B (recombinant) vaccine *on page 469*

enhanced-potency inactivated poliovirus vaccine *see* poliovirus vaccine (inactivated) *on page 764*

Enhancer [US] *see* barium *on page 116*

Enisyl® *(Discontinued)* *see* l-lysine *on page 572*

Enjuvia™ [US] *see* estrogens (conjugated B/synthetic) *on page 364*

Enlon® [Can] *see* edrophonium *(Canada only) on page 334*

Enlon® *(Discontinued)* *see* edrophonium *(Canada only) on page 334*

Enlon-Plus™ *(Discontinued)* *see* edrophonium and atropine *on page 334*

Enomine® *(Discontinued)*

Enovil® *(Discontinued)* *see* amitriptyline *on page 62*

enoxaparin (ee noks a PA rin)

Sound-Alike/Look-Alike Issues

Lovenox® may be confused with Lotronex®, Protonix®

Synonyms enoxaparin sodium

U.S./Canadian Brand Names Enoxaparin Injection [Can]; Lovenox® HP [Can]; Lovenox® [US/Can]

Therapeutic Category Anticoagulant (Other)

Use

Acute coronary syndromes: Unstable angina (UA), non-ST-segment elevation (NSTEMI), and ST-segment elevation myocardial infarction (STEMI)

DVT prophylaxis: Following hip or knee replacement surgery, abdominal surgery, or in medical patients with severely-restricted mobility during acute illness in patients at risk of thromboembolic complications

DVT treatment (acute): Inpatient treatment (patients with and without pulmonary embolism) and outpatient treatment (patients without pulmonary embolism)

Note: High-risk patients include those with one or more of the following risk factors: >40 years of age, obesity, general anesthesia lasting >30 minutes, malignancy, history of deep vein thrombosis or pulmonary embolism

Usual Dosage SubQ: Adults:

DVT prophylaxis:

Hip replacement surgery:

Twice-daily dosing: 30 mg twice daily, with initial dose within 12-24 hours after surgery, and every 12 hours until risk of DVT has diminished or the patient is adequately anticoagulated on warfarin.

Once-daily dosing: 40 mg once daily, with initial dose within 9-15 hours before surgery, and daily until risk of DVT has diminished or the patient is adequately anticoagulated on warfarin.

Knee replacement surgery: 30 mg twice daily, with initial dose within 12-24 hours after surgery, and every 12 hours until risk of DVT has diminished (usually 7-10 days).

Abdominal surgery: 40 mg once daily, with initial dose given 2 hours prior to surgery; continue until risk of DVT has diminished (usual 7-10 days).

Medical patients with severely-restricted mobility during acute illness: 40 mg once daily; continue until risk of DVT has diminished

DVT treatment (acute): **Note:** Start warfarin within 72 hours and continue enoxaparin until INR is between 2.0 and 3.0 (usually 7 days).

Inpatient treatment (with or without pulmonary embolism): 1 mg/kg/dose every 12 hours or 1.5 mg/kg once daily.

Outpatient treatment (without pulmonary embolism): 1 mg/kg/dose every 12 hours.

◀

ST-segment elevation myocardial infarction (STEMI):

Patients <75 years of age: Initial: 30 mg I.V. single bolus plus 1 mg/kg (maximum 100 mg for the first 2 doses only) SubQ every 12 hours. The first SubQ dose should be administered with the I.V. bolus. Maintenance: After first 2 doses, administer 1 mg/kg SubQ every 12 hours.

Patients ≥75 years of age: Initial: SubQ: 0.75 mg/kg every 12 hours (**Note:** No I.V. bolus is administered in this population); a maximum dose of 75 mg is recommended for the first 2 doses. Maintenance: After first 2 doses, administer 0.75 mg/kg SubQ every 12 hours

Additional notes on STEMI treatment: Therapy was continued for 8 days or until hospital discharge; optimal duration not defined. Unless contraindicated, all patients received aspirin (75-325 mg daily) in clinical trials. In patients with STEMI receiving thrombolytics, initiate enoxaparin dosing between 15 minutes before and 30 minutes after fibrinolytic therapy. In patients undergoing PCI, if balloon inflation occurs <8 hours after the last SubQ enoxaparin dose, no additional dosing is needed. If balloon inflation occurs ≥8 hours after last SubQ enoxaparin dose, a single I.V. dose of 0.3 mg/kg should be administered.

Unstable angina or non-ST-segment myocardial infarction (NSTEMI): 1 mg/kg every 12 hours in conjunction with oral aspirin therapy (100-325 mg once daily); continue until clinical stabilization (a minimum of at least 2 days)

Dosage Forms

Injection, solution [graduated prefilled syringe; preservative free]:

Lovenox®: 60 mg/0.6 mL (0.6 mL); 80 mg/0.8 mL (0.8 mL); 100 mg/mL (1 mL); 120 mg/0.8 mL (0.8 mL); 150 mg/mL (1 mL)

Injection, solution [multidose vial]:

Lovenox®: 100 mg/mL (3 mL)

Injection, solution [prefilled syringe; preservative free]:

Lovenox®: 30 mg/0.3 mL (0.3 mL); 40 mg/0.4 mL (0.4 mL)

Enoxaparin Injection [Can] *see* enoxaparin *on page 341*

enoxaparin sodium *see* enoxaparin *on page 341*

Enpresse™ [US] *see* ethinyl estradiol and levonorgestrel *on page 372*

Ensure® [US-OTC] *see* nutritional formula, enteral/oral *on page 689*

Ensure Plus® [US-OTC] *see* nutritional formula, enteral/oral *on page 689*

entacapone (en TA ka pone)

U.S./Canadian Brand Names Comtan® [US/Can]

Therapeutic Category Anti-Parkinson Agent; Reverse COMT Inhibitor

Use Adjunct to levodopa/carbidopa therapy in patients with idiopathic Parkinson disease who experience "wearing-off" symptoms at the end of a dosing interval

Usual Dosage Oral: Adults: 200 mg with each dose of levodopa/carbidopa, up to a maximum of 8 times/day (maximum daily dose: 1600 mg/day). To optimize therapy, the dosage of levodopa may need reduced or the dosing interval may need extended. Patients taking levodopa ≥800 mg/day or who had moderate-to-severe dyskinesias prior to therapy required an average decrease of 25% in the daily levodopa dose.

Dosage Forms

Tablet:

Comtan®: 200 mg

entacapone, carbidopa, and levodopa *see* levodopa, carbidopa, and entacapone *on page 556*

entecavir (en TE ka veer)

U.S./Canadian Brand Names Baraclude® [US/Can]

Therapeutic Category Antiretroviral Agent, Reverse Transcriptase Inhibitor (Nucleoside)

Use Treatment of chronic hepatitis B infection in adults with evidence of active viral replication and either evidence of persistent transaminase elevations or histologically-active disease

Usual Dosage Oral: Adolescents ≥16 years and Adults:

Nucleoside treatment naive: 0.5 mg daily

Lamivudine-resistant viremia (or known lamivudine-resistant mutations): 1 mg daily

Dosage Forms

Oral solution:

Baraclude®: 0.05 mg/mL

Tablet:
  Baraclude®: 0.5 mg, 1 mg

Entereg® [US] *see* alvimopan *on page 55*

enterotoxigenic *Escherichia coli* and *Vibrio cholera* vaccine *see* traveler's diarrhea and cholera vaccine *(Canada only) on page 944*

Entero Vu™ [US] *see* barium *on page 116*

Entertainer's Secret® [US-OTC] *see* saliva substitute *on page 853*

Entex® *(Discontinued)* *see* guaifenesin and phenylephrine *on page 456*

Entex® ER *(Discontinued)* *see* guaifenesin and phenylephrine *on page 456*

Entex® HC *(Discontinued)*

Entex® LA [Can] *see* guaifenesin and pseudoephedrine *on page 458*

Entex® LA *(Discontinued)* *see* guaifenesin and phenylephrine *on page 456*

Entex® PSE [US] *see* guaifenesin and pseudoephedrine *on page 458*

Entocort® [Can] *see* budesonide *on page 147*

Entocort® EC [US] *see* budesonide *on page 147*

Entrobar® [US] *see* barium *on page 116*

EntroEase® [US] *see* barium *on page 116*

Entrophen® [Can] *see* aspirin *on page 98*

Entsol® [US-OTC] *see* sodium chloride *on page 873*

Entuss-D® Liquid *(Discontinued)*

Enulose [US] *see* lactulose *on page 544*

Eperbel-S *(Discontinued)* *see* belladonna, phenobarbital, and ergotamine *on page 120*

ephedrine (e FED rin)

Sound-Alike/Look-Alike Issues
  ePHEDrine may be confused with Epifrin®, EPINEPHrine

Synonyms ephedrine sulfate

Tall-Man ePHEDrine

U.S./Canadian Brand Names Pretz-D® [US-OTC]

Therapeutic Category Adrenergic Agonist Agent

Use Treatment of bronchial asthma, nasal congestion, acute bronchospasm, idiopathic orthostatic hypotension, hypotension induced by spinal anesthesia

Usual Dosage
  Children:
    Oral, SubQ: 3 mg/kg/day or 25-100 mg/m^2/day in 4-6 divided doses every 4-6 hours
    I.M., slow I.V. push: 0.2-0.3 mg/kg/dose every 4-6 hours
  Adults:
    Oral: 25-50 mg every 3-4 hours as needed
    I.M., SubQ: 25-50 mg, parenteral adult dose should not exceed 150 mg in 24 hours
    I.M.: Hypotension induced by anesthesia: 25 mg
    I.V.: 5-25 mg/dose slow I.V. push repeated after 5-10 minutes as needed, then every 3-4 hours not to exceed 150 mg/24 hours
  Nasal spray:
    Children 6-12 years: 1-2 sprays into each nostril, not more frequently than every 4 hours
    Children ≥12 years and Adults: 2-3 sprays into each nostril, not more frequently than every 4 hours

Dosage Forms
  Capsule: 25 mg
  Injection, solution: 50 mg/mL (1 mL, 10 mL)
  Solution, intranasal spray: 0.25% (50 mL)
    Pretz-D® [OTC]: 0.25% (50 mL)

ephedrine, chlorpheniramine, phenylephrine, and carbetapentane *see* chlorpheniramine, ephedrine, phenylephrine, and carbetapentane *on page 208*

ephedrine sulfate *see* ephedrine *on page 343*

EpiClenz™ [US-OTC] *see* alcohol (ethyl) *on page 41*

epidermal thymocyte activating factor *see* aldesleukin *on page 42*

Epifoam® [US] *see* pramoxine and hydrocortisone *on page 778*

Epifrin® *(Discontinued)* see epinephrine *on page 344*

epinastine (ep i NAS teen)
Synonyms epinastine hydrochloride
U.S./Canadian Brand Names Elestat™ [US]
Therapeutic Category Antihistamine, H₁ Blocker, Ophthalmic
Use Treatment of allergic conjunctivitis
Usual Dosage Ophthalmic: Allergic conjunctivitis: Children ≥3 years and Adults: Instill 1 drop into each eye twice daily; continue throughout period of exposure, even in the absence of symptoms
Dosage Forms
Solution, ophthalmic:
Elestat™: 0.05% (5 mL)

epinastine hydrochloride see epinastine *on page 344*

epinephrine (ep i NEF rin)
Sound-Alike/Look-Alike Issues
EPINEPHrine may be confused with ePHEDrine
Epifrin® may be confused with ephedrine, EpiPen®
EpiPen® may be confused with Epifrin®
Synonyms adrenaline; epinephrine bitartrate; epinephrine hydrochloride; racepinephrine
Tall-Man EPINEPHrine
U.S./Canadian Brand Names Adrenalin® [US/Can]; EpiPen® Jr [US/Can]; EpiPen® [US/Can]; Primatene® Mist [US-OTC]; Raphon [US-OTC]; S2® [US-OTC]; Twinject™ [US/Can]
Therapeutic Category Adrenergic Agonist Agent
Use Treatment of bronchospasms, bronchial asthma, nasal congestion, viral croup, anaphylactic reactions, cardiac arrest; added to local anesthetics to decrease systemic absorption of local anesthetics and increase duration of action; decrease superficial hemorrhage
Usual Dosage
Neonates: Cardiac arrest: I.V.: 0.01-0.03 mg/kg (0.1-0.3 mL/kg of **1:10,000** solution) every 3-5 minutes as needed. Although I.V. route is preferred, may consider administration of doses up to 0.1 mg/kg through the endotracheal tube until I.V. access established; dilute intratracheal doses to 1-2 mL with normal saline.

Infants and Children:
Asystole/pulseless arrest, bradycardia, VT/VF (after failed defibrillations):
I.V., I.O.: 0.01 mg/kg (0.1 mL/kg of **1:10,000** solution) every 3-5 minutes as needed (maximum: 1 mg)
Intratracheal: 0.1 mg/kg (0.1 mL/kg of **1:1000** solution) every 3-5 minutes (maximum: 10 mg)
Continuous I.V. infusion: 0.1-1 mcg/kg/minute; doses <0.3 mcg/kg/minute generally produce β-adrenergic effects and higher doses generally produce α-adrenergic vasoconstriction; titrate dosage to desired effect
Bronchodilator: SubQ: 0.01 mg/kg (0.01 mL/kg of **1:1000**) (single doses not to exceed 0.5 mg) every 20 minutes for 3 doses
Nebulization: 1-3 inhalations up to every 3 hours using solution prepared with 10 drops of 1:100
Children <4 years: S2® (racepinephrine, OTC labeling): Croup: 0.05 mL/kg (max 0.5 mL/dose); dilute in NS 3 mL. Administer over ~15 minutes; do not administer more frequently than every 2 hours.
Inhalation: Children ≥4 years: Primatene® Mist: Refer to adult dosing.
Decongestant: Children ≥6 years: Refer to adult dosing
Hypersensitivity reaction:
SubQ, I.V.: 0.01 mg/kg every 20 minutes; larger doses or continuous infusion may be needed for some anaphylactic reactions
Self-administration following severe allergic reactions (eg, insect stings, food): **Note:** World Health Organization (WHO) and Anaphylaxis Canada recommend the availability of 1 dose for every 10-20 minutes of travel time to a medical emergency facility:
Twinject™: SubQ, I.M.:
Children 15-30 kg: 0.15 mg
Children >30 kg: 0.3 mg
EpiPen® Jr: I.M.: Children <30 kg: 0.15 mg
EpiPen®: I.M.: Children ≥30 kg: 0.3 mg

Adults:
   Asystole/pulseless arrest, bradycardia, VT/VF:
      I.V., I.O.: 1 mg every 3-5 minutes; if this approach fails, higher doses of epinephrine (up to 0.2 mg/kg) may be indicated for treatment of specific problems (eg, beta-blocker or calcium channel blocker overdose)
      Intratracheal: Administer 2-2.5 mg for VF or pulseless VT if I.V./I.O. access is delayed or cannot be established; dilute in 5-10 mL NS or distilled water. **Note:** Absorption is greater with distilled water, but causes more adverse effects on PaO_2.
   Bradycardia (symptomatic) or hypotension (not responsive to atropine or pacing): I.V. infusion: 2-10 mcg/minute; titrate to desired effect
   Bronchodilator:
      SubQ: 0.3-0.5 mg **(1:1000)** every 20 minutes for 3 doses
      Nebulization: 1-3 inhalations up to every 3 hours using solution prepared with 10 drops of the **1:100** product
         S2® (racepinephrine, OTC labeling): 0.5 mL (~10 drops). Dose may be repeated not more frequently than very 3-4 hours if needed. Solution should be diluted if using jet nebulizer.
      Inhalation: Primatene® Mist (OTC labeling): One inhalation, wait at least 1 minute; if not relieved, may use once more. Do not use again for at least 3 hours.
   Decongestant: Intranasal: Apply 1:1000 locally as drops or spray or with sterile swab
   Hypersensitivity reaction:
      SubQ, I.M.: 0.3-0.5 mg (1:1000) every 15-20 minutes if condition requires (I.M. route is preferred)
      I.V.: 0.1 mg (1:10,000) over 5 minutes. May infuse at 1-4 mcg/minute to prevent the need to repeat injections frequently.
      Self-administration following severe allergic reactions (eg, insect stings, food): **Note:** The World Health Organization (WHO) and Anaphylaxis Canada recommend the availability of one dose for every 10 to 20 minutes of travel time to a medical emergency facility. More than 2 doses should only be administered under direct medical supervision.
         Twinject™: SubQ, I.M.: 0.3 mg
         EpiPen®: I.M.: 0.3 mg

Dosage Forms
   Aerosol for oral inhalation:
      Primatene® Mist [OTC]: 0.22 mg/inhalation (15 mL, 22.5 mL)
   Injection, solution [prefilled auto injector]:
      EpiPen®: 0.3 mg/0.3 mL (2 mL) [1:1000; delivers 0.3 mg per injection; available as single unit or in double-unit pack with training unit]
      EpiPen® Jr: 0.15 mg/0.3 mL (2 mL) [1:2000 solution; delivers 0.15 mg per injection; available as single unit or in double-unit pack with training unit]
      Twinject™: 0.15 mg/0.15 mL (1.1 mL) [1:1000 solution; delivers 0.15 mg per injection; two 0.15 mg doses per injector]; 0.3 mg/0.3 mL (1.1 mL) [1:1000 solution; delivers 0.3 mg per injection; two 0.3 mg doses per injector]
   Injection, solution: 0.1 mg/mL (10 mL) [1:10,000 solution]; 1 mg/mL (1 mL) [1:1000 solution]
      Adrenalin®: 1 mg/mL (1 mL, 30 mL) [1:1000 solution]
   Solution for oral inhalation:
      Adrenalin®: 1% (7.5 mL) [10 mg/mL, 1:100 solution]
   Solution for oral inhalation [racepinephrine; preservative free]:
      S2®: 2.25% (0.5 mL, 15 mL)
   Solution, intranasal [drops, spray]:
      Adrenalin®: 1 mg/mL [1:1000 solution]
   Solution, topical [racepinephrine]:
      Raphon: 2.25% (15 mL)

epinephrine and articaine hydrochloride see articaine and epinephrine on page 95

epinephrine and chlorpheniramine (ep i NEF rin & klor fen IR a meen)

Synonyms insect sting kit
U.S./Canadian Brand Names Ana-Kit® [US]
Therapeutic Category Antidote
Use Anaphylaxis emergency treatment of insect bites or stings by the sensitive patient that may occur within minutes of insect sting or exposure to an allergic substance
Usual Dosage I.M. or SubQ: Children and Adults:
   Epinephrine:
      <2 years: 0.05-0.1 mL

345

◄
   2-6 years: 0.15 mL
   6-12 years: 0.2 mL
   >12 years : 0.3 mL
  Chlorpheniramine:
   <6 years: 1 tablet
   6-12 years: 2 tablets
   >12 years: 4 tablets

Dosage Forms
  Kit:
   Ana-Kit®: Epinephrine 1:1000 (1 mL), chlorpheniramine chewable tablet 2 mg (4), sterile alcohol pads (2), tourniquet (1)

epinephrine and lidocaine *see* lidocaine and epinephrine *on page 563*
epinephrine bitartrate *see* epinephrine *on page 344*
epinephrine bitartrate and bupivacaine hydrochloride *see* bupivacaine and epinephrine *on page 150*
epinephrine hydrochloride *see* epinephrine *on page 344*
EpiPen® [US/Can] *see* epinephrine *on page 344*
EpiPen® Jr [US/Can] *see* epinephrine *on page 344*
epipodophyllotoxin *see* etoposide *on page 384*
EpiQuin™ Micro [US] *see* hydroquinone *on page 488*

epirubicin (ep i ROO bi sin)

Sound-Alike/Look-Alike Issues
  epirubicin may be confused with DAUNOrubicin, DOXOrubicin, idarubicin
  Ellence® may be confused with Elase®

Synonyms epirubicin hydrochloride; NSC-256942; pidorubicin; pidorubicin hydrochloride

U.S./Canadian Brand Names Ellence® [US/Can]; Pharmorubicin® [Can]

Therapeutic Category Antineoplastic Agent, Anthracycline; Antineoplastic Agent, Antibiotic

Use Adjuvant therapy for primary breast cancer

Usual Dosage I.V.: Adults: 100-120 mg/m^2 once every 3-4 weeks **or** 50-60 mg/m^2 days 1 and 8 every 3-4 weeks

  Breast cancer:
   CEF-120: 60 mg/m^2 on days 1 and 8 every 28 days for 6 cycles
   FEC-100: 100 mg/m^2 on day 1 every 21 days for 6 cycles
   Note: Patients receiving 120 mg/m^2/cycle as part of combination therapy should also receive prophylactic therapy with sulfamethoxazole/trimethoprim or a fluoroquinolone.
  Dosage modifications:
   Delay day 1 dose until platelets are ≥100,000/mm^3, ANC ≥1500/mm^3, and nonhematologic toxicities have recovered to ≤grade 1
   Reduce day 1 dose in subsequent cycles to 75% of previous day 1 dose if patient experiences nadir platelet counts <50,000/mm^3, ANC <250/mm^3, neutropenic fever, or grade 3/4 nonhematologic toxicity during the previous cycle
   For divided doses (day 1 and day 8), reduce day 8 dose to 75% of day 1 dose if platelet counts are 75,000-100,000/mm^3 and ANC is 1000-1499/mm^3; omit day 8 dose if platelets are <75,000/mm^3, ANC <1000/mm^3, or grade 3/4 nonhematologic toxicity
  Dosage adjustment in bone marrow dysfunction: Heavily-treated patients, patients with preexisting bone marrow depression or neoplastic bone marrow infiltration: Lower starting doses (75-90 mg/mm^2) should be considered.

Dosage Forms
  Injection, powder for reconstitution [preservative free]: 50 mg, 200 mg
  Injection, solution [preservative free]: 2 mg/mL (5 mL, 25 mL, 75 mL, 100 mL)
   Ellence®: 2 mg/mL (25 mL, 100 mL)

epirubicin hydrochloride *see* epirubicin *on page 346*
Epitol® [US] *see* carbamazepine *on page 172*
Epival® I.V. [Can] *see* valproic acid and derivatives *on page 967*
Epivir® [US] *see* lamivudine *on page 544*
Epivir-HBV® [US] *see* lamivudine *on page 544*

eplerenone (e PLER en one)

Sound-Alike/Look-Alike Issues
Inspra™ may be confused with Spiriva®

U.S./Canadian Brand Names Inspra™ [US]

Therapeutic Category Antihypertensive Agent; Selective Aldosterone Blocker

Use Treatment of hypertension (may be used alone or in combination with other antihypertensive agents); treatment of heart failure (HF) following acute MI

Usual Dosage Oral: Adults:
Hypertension: Initial: 50 mg once daily; may increase to 50 mg twice daily if response is not adequate; may take up to 4 weeks for full therapeutic response. Doses >100 mg/day are associated with increased risk of hyperkalemia and no greater therapeutic effect.

Concurrent use with moderate CYP3A4 inhibitors: Initial: 25 mg once daily

Heart failure (post-MI): Initial: 25 mg once daily; dosage goal: Titrate to 50 mg once daily within 4 weeks, as tolerated

Dosage adjustment per serum potassium concentrations for HF (post-MI):
<5.0 mEq/L:
Increase dose from 25 mg every other day to 25 mg daily **or**
Increase dose from 25 mg daily to 50 mg daily
5.0-5.4 mEq/L: No adjustment needed
5.5-5.9 mEq/L:
Decrease dose from 50 mg daily to 25 mg daily **or**
Decrease dose from 25 mg daily to 25 mg every other day **or**
Decrease dose from 25 mg every other day to withhold medication
≥6.0 mEq/L: Withhold medication until potassium <5.5 mEq/L, then restart at 25 mg every other day

Dosage Forms
Tablet: 25 mg, 50 mg
Inspra™: 25 mg, 50 mg

EPO *see epoetin alfa* *on page 347*

epoetin alfa (e POE e tin AL fa)

Sound-Alike/Look-Alike Issues
epoetin alfa may be confused with darbepoetin alfa, epoetin beta

Synonyms rHuEPO-α; EPO; erythropoiesis-stimulating agent (ESA); erythropoietin; NSC-724223

U.S./Canadian Brand Names Epogen® [US]; Eprex® [Can]; Procrit® [US]

Therapeutic Category Colony-Stimulating Factor

Use Treatment of anemia (elevate/maintain red blood cell level and decrease the need for transfusions) associated with HIV (zidovudine) therapy, chronic renal failure (including patients on dialysis and not on dialysis); reduction of allogeneic blood transfusion for elective, noncardiac, nonvascular surgery; treatment of anemia due to concurrent chemotherapy in patients with metastatic cancer (nonmyeloid malignancies)

Note: Erythropoietin is **not** indicated for use in cancer patients under the following conditions:
• receiving hormonal therapy, therapeutic biologic products, or radiation therapy unless also receiving concurrent myelosuppressive chemotherapy
• receiving myelosuppressive therapy when the expected outcome is curative
• anemia due to other factors (eg, iron deficiency, folate deficiency or gastrointestinal bleed)

Usual Dosage Note: Hemoglobin levels should not exceed 12 g/dL and should not rise >1 g/dL per 2-week time period during therapy in any patient.

Chronic renal failure patients: Individualize dosing to achieve and maintain hemoglobin levels between 10-12 g/dL. Hemoglobin levels should not exceed 12 g/dL. **Note:** I.V. route is preferred for hemodialysis patients.

Children: I.V., SubQ: Initial dose: 50 units/kg 3 times/week
Adults: I.V., SubQ: Initial dose: 50-100 units/kg 3 times/week

Dosage adjustment in Children and Adults: SubQ, I.V.:
Decrease dose by 25%: If hemoglobin approaches 12 g/dL **or** hemoglobin increases >1 g/dL in any 2-week period. If hemoglobin continues to increase, temporarily discontinue therapy until hemoglobin begins to decrease, then resume therapy with a ~25% reduction from previous dose.
Increase dose by 25%: If hemoglobin <10 g/dL and does not increase by 1 g/dL after 4 weeks of therapy (with adequate iron stores) **or** hemoglobin decreases below 10 g/dL. Do not increase dose more frequently than at 4-week intervals.

◀ *Inadequate or lack of response:* If patient does not attain target hemoglobin range of 10-12 g/dL after appropriate dose titrations over 12 weeks:

Do not continue to increase dose and use the minimum effective dose that will maintain a hemoglobin level sufficient to avoid red blood cell transfusions **and** evaluate patient for other causes of anemia.

Monitor hemoglobin closely thereafter, and if responsiveness improves, may resume making dosage adjustments as recommended above. If responsiveness does not improve and recurrent red blood cell transfusions continue to be needed, discontinue therapy.

Maintenance dose: Individualize to target hemoglobin range of 10-12 g/dL; limit additional dosage increases to every 4 weeks (or longer)

Dialysis patients: Median dose:

Children: 167 units/kg/week (hemodialysis) **or** 76 units/kg/week (peritoneal dialysis)

Adults: 75 units/kg 3 times/week

Nondialysis patients:

Children: Dosing range: 50-250 units/kg 1-3 times/week

Adults: Median range: 75-150 units/kg/week

Zidovudine-treated, HIV-infected patients (patients with erythropoietin levels >500 mU/mL are **unlikely** to respond): Titrate dosage to use the minimum effective dose that will maintain a hemoglobin level sufficient to avoid red blood cell transfusions. Hemoglobin levels should not exceed 12 g/dL.

Children: SubQ, I.V.: Limited data available; reported dosing range: 50-400 units/kg 2-3 times/week

Adults (with serum erythropoietin levels ≤500 and zidovudine doses ≤4200 mg/week): SubQ, I.V.: 100 units/kg 3 times/week for 8 weeks

Dosage adjustment:

Increase dose by 50-100 units/kg 3 times/week: If response is not satisfactory in terms of reducing transfusion requirements **or** increasing hemoglobin after 8 weeks of therapy. Evaluate response every 4-8 weeks thereafter, and adjust the dose accordingly by 50-100 units/kg increments 3 times/week. If patients has not responded satisfactorily to a 300 units/kg/dose 3 times/week, a response to higher doses is unlikely.

Withhold dose: If hemoglobin exceeds 12 g/dL. Resume treatment with a 25% dose reduction when hemoglobin approaches a level where transfusions may be required.

Cancer patient on chemotherapy: Treatment of patients with erythropoietin levels >200 mU/mL is **not recommended.** Titrate dosage to use the minimum effective dose that will maintain a hemoglobin level sufficient to avoid red blood cell transfusions. Do not initiate therapy if hemoglobin ≥10 g/dL. Discontinue erythropoietin following completion of chemotherapy.

Children: I.V.: 600 units/kg once weekly (maximum: 40,000 units)

Dosage adjustment:

Increase dose: If response is not satisfactory after a sufficient period of evaluation (no increase in hemoglobin by ≥1 g/dL after 4 weeks of once-weekly therapy), the dose may be increased every 4 weeks (or longer) to 900 units/kg/week; maximum 60,000 units. If patient does not respond, a response to higher doses is unlikely.

Withhold dose: If hemoglobin exceeds a level needed to avoid red blood cell transfusion. Resume treatment with a 25% dose reduction when hemoglobin approaches a level where transfusions may be required.

Reduce dose by 25%: If hemoglobin increases >1 g/dL in any 2-week period **or** hemoglobin reaches a level sufficient to avoid red blood cell transfusion.

Discontinue: If after 8 weeks of therapy there is no response (ie, increased hemoglobin levels) or transfusions still required.

Adults: SubQ: Initial dose: 150 units/kg 3 times/week or 40,000 units once weekly; commonly used doses range from 10,000 units 3 times/week to 40,000-60,000 units once weekly.

Dosage adjustment:

Increase dose: If response is not satisfactory after a sufficient period of evaluation (no reduction in transfusion requirements or increase in hemoglobin after 8 weeks of 3 times/week therapy) **or** (no increase in hemoglobin by ≥1 g/dL after 4 weeks of once-weekly therapy), the dose may be increased every 4 weeks (or longer) to 300 units/kg 3 times/week, **or** when dosed weekly, increased all at once to 60,000 units weekly. If patient does not respond, a response to higher doses is unlikely.

Withhold dose: If hemoglobin exceeds a level needed to avoid red blood cell transfusion. Resume treatment with a 25% dose reduction when hemoglobin approaches a level where transfusions may be required.

Reduce dose by 25%: If hemoglobin increases >1 g/dL in any 2-week period **or** hemoglobin reaches a level sufficient to avoid red blood cell transfusion.

Discontinue: If after 8 weeks of therapy there is no response (ie, increased hemoglobin levels) or transfusions still required.

Surgery patients: Prior to initiating treatment, obtain a hemoglobin to establish that it is >10 g/dL or ≤13 g/dL: Adults: SubQ: Initial dose: 300 units/kg/day for 10 days before surgery, on the day of surgery, and for 4 days after surgery

Alternative dose: 600 units/kg in once weekly doses (21, 14, and 7 days before surgery) plus a fourth dose on the day of surgery

Dosage Forms

Injection, solution [preservative free]:

Epogen®, Procrit®: 2000 units/mL (1 mL); 3000 units/mL (1 mL); 4000 units/mL (1 mL); 10,000 units/mL (1 mL); 40,000 units/mL (1 mL)

Injection, solution [with preservative]:

Epogen®, Procrit®: 10,000 units/mL (2 mL); 20,000 units/mL (1 mL)

Epogen® [US] *see epoetin alfa on page 347*

epoprostenol (e poe PROST en ole)

Synonyms epoprostenol sodium; PGI_2; PGX; prostacyclin

U.S./Canadian Brand Names Flolan® [US/Can]

Therapeutic Category Platelet Inhibitor

Use Treatment of idiopathic pulmonary arterial hypertension (IPAH); pulmonary hypertension associated with the scleroderma spectrum of disease (SSD) in NYHA Class III and Class IV patients who do not respond adequately to conventional therapy

Usual Dosage I.V.: Adults: Initial: 1-2 ng/kg/minute, increase dose in increments of 1-2 ng/kg/minute every 15 minutes or longer until dose-limiting side effects are noted or tolerance limit to epoprostenol is observed. Significant patient variability in optimal dose exists. Maximum dose with chronic therapy has not been defined; however, doses as high as 195 ng/kg/minute have been described in children.

Note: The need for increased doses should be expected with chronic use; incremental increases occur more frequently during the first few months after the drug is initiated.

Dose adjustment:

Increase dose in 1-2 ng/kg/minute increments at intervals of at least 15 minutes if symptoms persist or recur following improvement. In clinical trials, dosing increases occurred at intervals of 24-48 hours.

Decrease dose in 2 ng/kg/minute decrements at intervals of at least 15 minutes in case of dose-limiting pharmacologic events. Avoid abrupt withdrawal or sudden large dose reductions.

Lung transplant: In patients receiving lung transplants, epoprostenol may be tapered after the initiation of cardiopulmonary bypass.

Dosage Forms

Injection, powder for reconstitution: 0.5 mg, 1.5 mg

Flolan®: 0.5 mg, 1.5 mg

epoprostenol sodium *see epoprostenol on page 349*

Eprex® [Can] *see epoetin alfa on page 347*

eprosartan (ep roe SAR tan)

U.S./Canadian Brand Names Teveten® [US/Can]

Therapeutic Category Angiotensin II Receptor Antagonist

Use Treatment of hypertension; may be used alone or in combination with other antihypertensives

Usual Dosage Oral: Adults: Dosage must be individualized; can administer once or twice daily with total daily doses of 400-800 mg. Usual starting dose is 600 mg once daily as monotherapy in patients who are euvolemic. Limited clinical experience with doses >800 mg.

Dosage Forms

Tablet:

Teveten®: 400 mg, 600 mg

eprosartan and hydrochlorothiazide (ep roe SAR tan & hye droe klor oh THYE a zide)

Synonyms eprosartan mesylate and hydrochlorothiazide; hydrochlorothiazide and eprosartan

U.S./Canadian Brand Names Teveten® HCT [US/Can]; Teveten® Plus [Can]

Therapeutic Category Angiotensin II Antagonist Combination; Antihypertensive Agent, Combination; Diuretic, Thiazide

◀ **Use** Treatment of hypertension (not indicated for initial treatment)
Usual Dosage Oral: Adults: Dose is individualized (combination substituted for individual components)
Usual recommended dose: Eprosartan 600 mg/hydrochlorothiazide 12.5 mg once daily (maximum dose: Eprosartan 600 mg/hydrochlorothiazide 25 mg once daily)

Dosage Forms
Tablet:
Teveten® HCT: 600 mg/12.5 mg: Eprosartan 600 mg and hydrochlorothiazide 12.5 mg; 600 mg/25 mg: Eprosartan 600 mg and hydrochlorothiazide 25 mg

eprosartan mesylate and hydrochlorothiazide *see* eprosartan and hydrochlorothiazide *on page 349*

epsilon aminocaproic acid *see* aminocaproic acid *on page 60*

epsom salts *see* magnesium sulfate *on page 588*

EPT *see* teniposide *on page 908*

eptacog alfa (activated) *see* factor VIIa (recombinant) *on page 387*

eptifibatide (ep TIF i ba tide)

Synonyms intrifiban

U.S./Canadian Brand Names Integrilin® [US/Can]

Therapeutic Category Antiplatelet Agent

Use Treatment of patients with acute coronary syndrome (unstable angina/non-Q wave myocardial infarction [UA/NQMI]), including patients who are to be managed medically and those undergoing percutaneous coronary intervention (PCI including angioplasty, intracoronary stenting)

Usual Dosage I.V.: Adults:
Acute coronary syndrome: Bolus of 180 mcg/kg (maximum: 22.6 mg) over 1-2 minutes, begun as soon as possible following diagnosis, followed by a continuous infusion of 2 mcg/kg/minute (maximum: 15 mg/hour) until hospital discharge or initiation of CABG surgery, up to 72 hours. Concurrent aspirin and heparin therapy (target aPTT 50-70 seconds) are recommended.
Percutaneous coronary intervention (PCI) with or without stenting: Bolus of 180 mcg/kg (maximum: 22.6 mg) administered immediately before the initiation of PCI, followed by a continuous infusion of 2 mcg/kg/minute (maximum: 15 mg/hour). A second 180 mcg/kg bolus (maximum: 22.6 mg) should be administered 10 minutes after the first bolus. Infusion should be continued until hospital discharge or for up to 18-24 hours, whichever comes first. Concurrent aspirin (160-325 mg 1-24 hours before PCI and daily thereafter) and heparin therapy (ACT 200-300 seconds during PCI) are recommended. Heparin infusion after PCI is discouraged. In patients who undergo coronary artery bypass graft surgery, discontinue infusion prior to surgery.

Dosage Forms
Injection, solution:
Integrilin®: 0.75 mg/mL (100 mL); 2 mg/mL (10 mL, 100 mL)

Epzicom® [US] *see* abacavir and lamivudine *on page 16*

Equagesic® [US] *see* meprobamate and aspirin *on page 606*

Equalactin® [US-OTC] *see* polycarbophil *on page 765*

Equalizer Gas Relief [US-OTC] *see* simethicone *on page 867*

Equanil® *(Discontinued)* *see* meprobamate *on page 605*

Equetro® [US] *see* carbamazepine *on page 172*

Equilet® *(Discontinued)* *see* calcium carbonate *on page 163*

Eraxis™ [US/Can] *see* anidulafungin *on page 77*

Erbitux® [US/Can] *see* cetuximab *on page 197*

ergocalciferol (er goe kal SIF e role)

Sound-Alike/Look-Alike Issues
Calciferol™ may be confused with calcitriol
Drisdol® may be confused with Drysol™

Synonyms activated ergosterol; viosterol; vitamin D_2

U.S./Canadian Brand Names Drisdol® [US/Can]; Ostoforte® [Can]

Therapeutic Category Vitamin D Analog

Use Treatment of refractory rickets, hypophosphatemia, hypoparathyroidism; dietary supplement

Usual Dosage Oral: **Note:** 1 mcg = 40 int. units

Adequate intake:
Infants and Children: 5 mcg/day (200 int. units/day)
Adults:
18-50 years: 5 mcg/day (200 int. units/day)
51-70 years: 10 mcg/day (400 int. units/day)

Dietary supplementation: Infants, Children, and Adults: 10 mcg/day (400 int. units/day)

Vitamin D deficiency/insufficiency in patients with CKD stages 3-4 (K/DOQI guidelines): **Note:** Dose is based on 25-hydroxyvitamin D serum level [25(OH) D]:
Children (treatment duration should be a total of 3 months):
Serum 25(OH)D <5 ng/mL:
8000 int. units/day for 4 weeks, then 4000 int. units/day for 2 months **or**
50,000 int. units/week for 4 weeks, then 50,000 int. units twice a month for 2 months
Serum 25(OH)D 5-15 ng/mL:
4000 int. units/day **or**
50,000 int. units every other week
Serum 25(OH)D 16-30 ng/mL:
2000 int. units/day **or**
50,000 int. units every 4 weeks
Adults (treatment duration should be a total of 6 months):
Serum 25(OH)D <5 ng/mL:
50,000 int. units/week for 12 weeks, then 50,000 int. units/month
Serum 25(OH)D 5-15 ng/mL:
50,000 int. units/week for 4 weeks, then 50,000 int. units/month
Serum 25(OH)D 16-30 ng/mL:
50,000 int. units/month

Hypoparathyroidism:
Children: 1.25-5 mg/day (50,000-200,000 int. units) and calcium supplements
Adults: 625 mcg to 5 mg/day (25,000-200,000 int. units) and calcium supplements

Nutritional rickets and osteomalacia:
Children and Adults (with normal absorption): 25-125 mcg/day (1000-5000 int. units)
Children with malabsorption: 250-625 mcg/day (10,000-25,000 int. units)
Adults with malabsorption: 250-7500 mcg (10,000-300,000 int. units)

Vitamin D-*dependent* rickets:
Children: 75-125 mcg/day (3000-5000 int. units); maximum: 1500 mcg/day
Adults: 250 mcg to 1.5 mg/day (10,000-60,000 int. units)

Vitamin D-*resistant* rickets: Children and Adults: 12,000-500,000 int. units/day

Familial hypophosphatemia:
Children: 40,000-80,000 int. units plus phosphate supplements; dose may be reduced once growth is complete
Adults: 10,000-60,000 int. units plus phosphate supplements

Dosage Forms
Capsule:
Drisdol®: 50,000 int. units
Liquid, oral [drops]:
Drisdol®: 8000 int. units/mL [OTC]
Tablet: 400 int. units [OTC]

ergoloid mesylates (ER goe loid MES i lates)

Synonyms dihydroergotoxine; dihydrogenated ergot alkaloids

U.S./Canadian Brand Names Hydergine® [Can]

Therapeutic Category Ergot Alkaloid and Derivative

Use Treatment of cerebrovascular insufficiency in primary progressive dementia, Alzheimer dementia, and senile onset

Usual Dosage Oral: Adults: 1 mg 3 times/day up to 4.5-12 mg/day; up to 6 months of therapy may be necessary

Dosage Forms
Tablet: 1 mg
Tablet, sublingual: 1 mg

Ergomar® [US] *see ergotamine on page 352*
ergometrine maleate *see ergonovine on page 352*

ergonovine (er goe NOE veen)

Synonyms ergometrine maleate; ergonovine maleate

U.S./Canadian Brand Names Ergotrate® [US]

Therapeutic Category Ergot Alkaloid and Derivative

Use Prevention and treatment of postpartum and postabortion hemorrhage caused by uterine atony or subinvolution

Usual Dosage Adults:

I.M., I.V. (I.V. should be reserved for emergency use only): 0.2 mg, may repeat dose in 2-4 hours if needed

Oral, SL:
Immediate post-partum: 0.2 mg (usually given I.M. or I.V)
Late post-partum: 0.2-0.4 mg every 6-12 hours until danger of uterine atony has passed (usually ~48 hours)

Dosage Forms
Injection:
Ergotrate®: 0.2 mg/mL (1 mL)
Tablet:
Ergotrate®: 0.2 mg

ergonovine maleate *see ergonovine on page 352*

ergotamine (er GOT a meen)

Synonyms ergotamine tartrate

U.S./Canadian Brand Names Ergomar® [US]

Therapeutic Category Ergot Alkaloid and Derivative

Use Abort or prevent vascular headaches, such as migraine, migraine variants, or so-called "histaminic cephalalgia"

Usual Dosage Sublingual: One tablet under tongue at first sign, then 1 tablet every 30 minutes if needed; maximum dose: 3 tablets/24 hours, 5 tablets/week

Dosage Forms
Tablet, sublingual:
Ergomar®: 2 mg

ergotamine and caffeine (er GOT a meen & KAF een)

Sound-Alike/Look-Alike Issues
Cafergot® may be confused with Carafate®

Synonyms caffeine and ergotamine; ergotamine tartrate and caffeine

U.S./Canadian Brand Names Cafergor® [Can]; Cafergot® [US]; Migergot [US]

Therapeutic Category Antimigraine Agent; Ergot Derivative; Stimulant

Use Abort or prevent vascular headaches, such as migraine, migraine variants, or so-called "histaminic cephalalgia"

Usual Dosage Adults:

Oral: Two tablets at onset of attack; then 1 tablet every 30 minutes as needed; maximum: 6 tablets per attack; do not exceed 10 tablets/week.

Rectal: One suppository rectally at first sign of an attack; follow with second dose after 1 hour, if needed; maximum: 2 per attack; do not exceed 5/week.

Dosage Forms
Suppository, rectal:
Migergot: Ergotamine tartrate 2 mg and caffeine 100 mg (12s)
Tablet: Ergotamine tartrate 1 mg and caffeine 100 mg
Cafergot®: Ergotamine tartrate 1 mg and caffeine 100 mg

ergotamine tartrate *see ergotamine on page 352*
ergotamine tartrate and caffeine *see ergotamine and caffeine on page 352*
Ergotamine Tartrate and Caffeine Cafatine® (Discontinued) *see ergotamine on page 352*

ergotamine tartrate, belladonna, and phenobarbital *see* belladonna, phenobarbital, and ergotamine *on page 120*

Ergotrate® [US] *see* ergonovine *on page 352*

erlotinib (er LOE tye nib)

Sound-Alike/Look-Alike Issues
erlotinib may be confused with gefitinib

Synonyms CP358774; erlotinib hydrochloride; NSC-718781; OSI-774; R 14-15

U.S./Canadian Brand Names Tarceva® [US/Can]

Therapeutic Category Antineoplastic, Tyrosine Kinase Inhibitor

Use Treatment of refractory locally advanced or metastatic nonsmall cell lung cancer (NSCLC); pancreatic cancer (first-line therapy in combination with gemcitabine)

Usual Dosage Oral: Adults: **Note:** Dose adjustments are likely to be needed when erlotinib is administered concomitantly with strong CYP3A4 inducers or inhibitors.
NSCLC: 150 mg/day
Pancreatic cancer: 100 mg/day in combination with gemcitabine

Dosage Forms
Tablet:
Tarceva®: 25 mg, 100 mg, 150 mg

erlotinib hydrochloride *see* erlotinib *on page 353*

Errin™ [US] *see* norethindrone *on page 679*

Ertaczo® [US] *see* sertaconazole *on page 863*

ertapenem (er ta PEN em)

Sound-Alike/Look-Alike Issues
ertapenem may be confused with imipenem, meropenem
Invanz® may be confused with Avinza™

Synonyms ertapenem sodium; L-749,345; MK0826

U.S./Canadian Brand Names Invanz® [US/Can]

Therapeutic Category Antibiotic, Carbapenem

Use Treatment of the following moderate-severe infections: Complicated intraabdominal infections, complicated skin and skin structure infections (including diabetic foot infections without osteomyelitis), complicated UTI (including pyelonephritis), acute pelvic infections (including postpartum endomyometritis, septic abortion, postsurgical gynecologic infections), and community-acquired pneumonia. Prophylaxis of surgical site infection following elective colorectal surgery. Antibacterial coverage includes aerobic gram-positive organisms, aerobic gram-negative organisms, anaerobic organisms.

Note: Methicillin-resistant *Staphylococcus*, *Enterococcus* spp, penicillin-resistant strains of *Streptococcus pneumoniae*, beta-lactamase-positive strains of *Haemophilus influenzae* are **resistant** to ertapenem, as are most *Pseudomonas aeruginosa*.

Usual Dosage Note: I.V. therapy may be administered for up to 14 days; I.M. therapy for up to 7 days

Usual dosage ranges:
Children 3 months to 12 years: I.M., I.V.: 15 mg/kg twice daily (maximum: 1 g/day)
Children ≥13 years and Adults: I.M., I.V.: 1 g/day

Indication-specific dosing:
Children 3 months to 12 years: I.M., I.V.:
Community-acquired pneumonia, complicated urinary tract infections (including pyelonephritis): 15 mg/kg twice daily (maximum: 1 g/day); duration of total antibiotic treatment: 10-14 days (**Note:** Duration includes possible switch to appropriate oral therapy after at least 3 days of parenteral treatment, once clinical improvement demonstrated.)
Intraabdominal infection: 15 mg/kg twice daily (maximum: 1 g/day) for 5-14 days
Pelvic infections (acute): 15 mg/kg twice daily (maximum: 1 g/day) for 3-10 days
Skin and skin structure infections: 15 mg/kg twice daily (maximum: 1 g/day) for 7-14 days
Children ≥13 years and Adults: I.M., I.V.:
Community-acquired pneumonia, complicated urinary tract infections (including pyelonephritis): 1 g/day; duration of total antibiotic treatment: 10-14 days (**Note:** Duration includes possible switch to appropriate oral therapy after at least 3 days of parenteral treatment, once clinical improvement demonstrated.)
Intraabdominal infection: 1 g/day for 5-14 days

◄ **Pelvic infections (acute):** 1 g/day for 3-10 days
Skin and skin structure infections (including diabetic foot infections): 1 g/day for 7-14 days
Adults: I.V.: **Prophylaxis of surgical site following colorectal surgery:** 1 g given 1 hour preoperatively

Dosage Forms
Injection, powder for reconstitution:
Invanz®: 1 g

ertapenem sodium *see ertapenem on page 353*
***Erwinia* asparaginase** *see asparaginase on page 98*
Erybid™ [Can] *see erythromycin on page 354*
Eryc® [Can] *see erythromycin on page 354*
Eryc® *(Discontinued) see erythromycin on page 354*
Eryderm® *(Discontinued) see erythromycin on page 354*
Erygel® [US] *see erythromycin on page 354*
EryPed® [US] *see erythromycin on page 354*
Ery-Tab® [US] *see erythromycin on page 354*
Erythrocin® [US] *see erythromycin on page 354*

erythromycin (er ith roe MYE sin)

Sound-Alike/Look-Alike Issues
erythromycin may be confused with azithromycin, clarithromycin, Ethmozine®
Akne-Mycin® may be confused with AK-Mycin®
E.E.S.® may be confused with DES®
Eryc® may be confused with Emcyt®, Ery-Tab®
Ery-Tab® may be confused with Eryc®
Erythrocin® may be confused with Ethmozine®

Synonyms erythromycin base; erythromycin ethylsuccinate; erythromycin lactobionate; erythromycin stearate

U.S./Canadian Brand Names Akne-Mycin® [US]; Apo-Erythro Base® [Can]; Apo-Erythro E-C® [Can]; Apo-Erythro-ES® [Can]; Apo-Erythro-S® [Can]; Diomycin® [Can]; E.E.S.® [US/Can]; Ery-Tab® [US]; Erybid™ [Can]; Eryc® [Can]; Erygel® [US]; EryPed® [US]; Erythrocin® [US]; Novo-Rythro Estolate [Can]; Novo-Rythro Ethylsuccinate [Can]; Nu-Erythromycin-S [Can]; PCE® [US/Can]; PMS-Erythromycin [Can]; Romycin® [US]; Sans Acne® [Can]

Therapeutic Category Acne Products; Antibiotic, Ophthalmic; Antibiotic, Topical; Macrolide (Antibiotic)

Use
Systemic: Treatment of susceptible bacterial infections including *S. pyogenes*, some *S. pneumoniae*, some *S. aureus*, *M. pneumoniae*, *Legionella pneumophila*, diphtheria, pertussis, *Chlamydia*, erythrasma, *N. gonorrhoeae*, *E. histolytica*, syphilis and nongonococcal urethritis, and *Campylobacter* gastroenteritis; used in conjunction with neomycin for decontaminating the bowel
Ophthalmic: Treatment of superficial eye infections involving the conjunctiva or cornea; neonatal ophthalmia
Topical: Treatment of acne vulgaris

Usual Dosage Note: Due to differences in absorption, 400 mg erythromycin ethylsuccinate produces the same serum levels as 250 mg erythromycin base or stearate.

Usual dosage range:
Neonates: Ophthalmic: Prophylaxis of neonatal gonococcal or chlamydial conjunctivitis: 0.5-1 cm ribbon of ointment should be instilled into each conjunctival sac
Infants and Children:
Oral:
Base: 30-50 mg/kg/day in 2-4 divided doses; maximum: 2 g/day
Ethylsuccinate: 30-50 mg/kg/day in 2-4 divided doses; maximum: 3.2 g/day
Stearate: 30-50 mg/kg/day in 2-4 divided doses; maximum: 2 g/day
I.V.: Lactobionate: 15-50 mg/kg/day divided every 6 hours, not to exceed 4 g/day
Children and Adults:
Ophthalmic: Instill 1/2" (1.25 cm) 2-6 times/day depending on the severity of the infection
Topical: Acne: Apply over the affected area twice daily after the skin has been thoroughly washed and patted dry

Adults:
Oral:
Base: 250-500 mg every 6-12 hours; maximum 4 g/day
Ethylsuccinate: 400-800 mg every 6-12 hours; maximum: 4 g/day
I.V.: Lactobionate: 15-20 mg/kg/day divided every 6 hours or 500 mg to 1 g every 6 hours, or given as a continuous infusion over 24 hours; maximum: 4 g/24 hours

Indication-specific dosing:
Children:
Conjunctivitis, neonatal *(C. trachomatis)*: Oral: 50 mg/kg/day (base or ethylsuccinate) in 4 divided doses for 14 days
Mild/moderate infection: Oral: 30-50 mg/kg/day in divided doses every 6-12 hours
Pertussis: Oral: 40-50 mg/kg/day in 4 divided doses for 14 days; maximum 2 g/day (not preferred agent for infants <1 month due to IHPS)
Pharyngitis, tonsillitis (streptococcal): Oral: 20 mg (base)/kg/day or 40 mg (ethylsuccinate)/kg/day in 2 divided doses for 10 days. **Note:** No longer preferred therapy due to increased organism resistance.
Pneumonia *(C. trachomatis)*: Oral: 50 mg/kg/day (base or ethylsuccinate) in 4 divided doses for 14-21 days
Preop bowel preparation: Oral: 20 mg (base)/kg at 1, 2, and 11 PM on the day before surgery combined with mechanical cleansing of the large intestine and oral neomycin
Severe infection: I.V.: 15-50 mg/kg/day; maximum: 4 g/day
Adults:
Legionnaires disease: Oral: 1.6-4 g (ethylsuccinate)/day or 1-4 g (base)/day in divided doses for 21 days. **Note:** No longer preferred therapy and only used in nonhospitalized patients.
Lymphogranuloma venereum: Oral: 500 mg (base) 4 times/day for 21 days
Nongonococcal urethritis (including coinfection with *C. trachomatis*): Oral: 500 mg (base) 4 times/day for 7 days or 800 mg (ethylsuccinate) 4 times/day for 7 days. **Note:** May use 250 mg (base) or 400 mg (ethylsuccinate) 4 times/day for 14 days if gastrointestinal intolerance.
Pelvic inflammatory disease: I.V.: 500 mg every 6 hours for 3 days, followed by 1000 mg (base)/day orally in 2-4 divided doses for 7 days. **Note:** Not recommended therapy per current treatment guidelines.
Pertussis: Oral: 500 mg (base) every 6 hours for 14 days
Syphilis, primary: Oral: 48-64 g (ethylsuccinate) or 30-40 g (base) in divided doses over 10-15 days. **Note:** Not recommended therapy per current treatment guidelines.
Dosage Forms [CAN] = Canadian brand name
Capsule, delayed release, enteric-coated pellets: 250 mg
Gel, topical: 2% (30 g, 60 g)
Granules for oral suspension:
E.E.S.®: 200 mg/5 mL
Injection, powder for reconstitution:
Erythrocin®: 500 mg, 1 g
Ointment, ophthalmic: 0.5% [5 mg/g] (1 g, 3.5 g)
Romycin®: 0.5% [5 mg/g] (3.5 g)
Ointment, topical:
Akne-Mycin®: 2% (25 g)
Powder for oral suspension:
EryPed®: 200 mg/5 mL, 400 mg/5 mL
Powder for oral suspension [drops]:
EryPed®: 100 mg/2.5 mL
Powder, for prescription compounding:
Erythro-RX: USP (50 g)
Solution, topical: 2% (60 mL)
Sans Acne® [CAN]: 2% (60 mL) [not available in the U.S.]
Suspension, oral: 200 mg/5 mL, 400 mg/5 mL
E.E.S.®: 400 mg/5 mL
Tablet: 250 mg, 400 mg, 500 mg
Erythrocin®: 250 mg, 500 mg
Tablet, delayed release, enteric coated:
Ery-Tab®: 250 mg, 333 mg, 500 mg
Tablet [polymer-coated particles]:
PCE®: 333 mg, 500 mg

erythromycin and benzoyl peroxide (er ith roe MYE sin & BEN zoe il per OKS ide)

Synonyms benzoyl peroxide and erythromycin

U.S./Canadian Brand Names Benzamycin® Pak [US]; Benzamycin® [US]

Therapeutic Category Acne Products

Use Topical control of acne vulgaris

Usual Dosage Adolescents ≥12 years and Adults: Apply twice daily, morning and evening

Dosage Forms
  Gel, topical: Erythromycin 30 mg and benzoyl peroxide 50 mg per g (23 g, 47g)
    Benzamycin®: Erythromycin 30 mg and benzoyl peroxide 50 mg per g (47 g)
    Benzamycin® Pak: Erythromycin 30 mg and benzoyl peroxide 50 mg per 0.8 g packet (60s)

erythromycin and sulfisoxazole (er ith roe MYE sin & sul fi SOKS a zole)

Sound-Alike/Look-Alike Issues
    Pediazole® may be confused with Pediapred®

Synonyms sulfisoxazole and erythromycin

U.S./Canadian Brand Names E.S.P.® [US]; Pediazole® [Can]

Therapeutic Category Macrolide (Antibiotic); Sulfonamide

Use Treatment of susceptible bacterial infections of the upper and lower respiratory tract, otitis media in children caused by susceptible strains of *Haemophilus influenzae*, and many other infections in patients allergic to penicillin

Usual Dosage Oral (dosage recommendation is based on the product's erythromycin content):
    Children ≥2 months: 50 mg/kg/day erythromycin and 150 mg/kg/day sulfisoxazole in divided doses every 6 hours; not to exceed 2 g erythromycin/day or 6 g sulfisoxazole/day for 10 days
    Adults >45 kg: 400 mg erythromycin and 1200 mg sulfisoxazole every 6 hours

Dosage Forms
  Powder for oral suspension: Erythromycin 200 mg and sulfisoxazole 600 mg per 5 mL
    E.S.P.®: Erythromycin 200 mg and sulfisoxazole 600 mg per 5 mL

erythromycin base *see erythromycin on page 354*
erythromycin ethylsuccinate *see erythromycin on page 354*
erythromycin lactobionate *see erythromycin on page 354*
erythromycin stearate *see erythromycin on page 354*
erythropoiesis-stimulating agent (ESA) *see darbepoetin alfa on page 267*
erythropoiesis-stimulating agent (ESA) *see epoetin alfa on page 347*
erythropoiesis-stimulating protein *see darbepoetin alfa on page 267*
erythropoietin *see epoetin alfa on page 347*

escitalopram (es sye TAL oh pram)

Sound-Alike/Look-Alike Issues
    Lexapro® may be confused with Loxitane®

Synonyms escitalopram oxalate; Lu-26-054; S-citalopram

U.S./Canadian Brand Names Cipralex® [Can]; Lexapro® [US]

Therapeutic Category Antidepressant, Selective Serotonin Reuptake Inhibitor

Use Treatment of major depressive disorder; generalized anxiety disorders (GAD)

Usual Dosage Oral: Adults: Depression, generalized anxiety disorder: Initial: 10 mg/day; dose may be increased to 20 mg/day after at least 1 week

Dosage Forms
  Solution, oral:
    Lexapro®: 1 mg/mL
  Tablet:
    Lexapro®: 5 mg, 10 mg, 20 mg
      Note: Cipralex® [CAN] is available only in 10 mg and 20 mg strengths.

escitalopram oxalate *see escitalopram on page 356*
Esclim® [US] *see estradiol on page 359*
Eserine® [Can] *see physostigmine on page 752*
eserine salicylate *see physostigmine on page 752*

Esgic® [US] *see* butalbital, acetaminophen, and caffeine *on page 155*
Esgic-Plus™ [US] *see* butalbital, acetaminophen, and caffeine *on page 155*
Esidrix Tablets *(Discontinued)* *see* hydrochlorothiazide *on page 479*
Eskalith CR® *(Discontinued)* *see* lithium *on page 571*
Eskalith® *(Discontinued)* *see* lithium *on page 571*

esmolol (ES moe lol)

Sound-Alike/Look-Alike Issues
esmolol may be confused with Osmitrol®
Brevibloc® may be confused with bretylium, Brevital®, Bumex®, Buprenex®

Synonyms esmolol hydrochloride

U.S./Canadian Brand Names Brevibloc® [US/Can]

Therapeutic Category Antiarrhythmic Agent, Class II; Beta-Adrenergic Blocker

Use Treatment of supraventricular tachycardia (SVT) and atrial fibrillation/flutter (control ventricular rate); treatment of tachycardia and/or hypertension (especially intraoperative or postoperative); treatment of noncompensatory sinus tachycardia

Usual Dosage I.V. infusion requires an infusion pump (must be adjusted to individual response and tolerance):
Adults:
Intraoperative tachycardia and/or hypertension (immediate control): Initial bolus: 80 mg (~1 mg/kg) over 30 seconds, followed by a 150 mcg/kg/minute infusion, if necessary. Adjust infusion rate as needed to maintain desired heart rate and/or blood pressure, up to 300 mcg/kg/minute.
For control of postoperative hypertension, as many as one-third of patients may require higher doses (250-300 mcg/kg/minute) to control blood pressure; the safety of doses >300 mcg/kg/minute has not been studied.
Supraventricular tachycardia or gradual control of postoperative tachycardia/hypertension: Loading dose: 500 mcg/kg over 1 minute; follow with a 50 mcg/kg/minute infusion for 4 minutes; response to this initial infusion rate may be a rough indication of the responsiveness of the ventricular rate.
Infusion may be continued at 50 mcg/kg/minute or, if the response is inadequate, titrated upward in 50 mcg/kg/minute increments (increased no more frequently than every 4 minutes) to a maximum of 200 mcg/kg/minute.
To achieve more rapid response, following the initial loading dose and 50 mcg/kg/minute infusion, rebolus with a second 500 mcg/kg loading dose over 1 minute, and increase the maintenance infusion to 100 mcg/kg/minute for 4 minutes. If necessary, a third (and final) 500 mcg/kg loading dose may be administered, prior to increasing to an infusion rate of 150 mcg/kg/minute. After 4 minutes of the 150 mcg/kg/minute infusion, the infusion rate may be increased to a maximum rate of 200 mcg/kg/minute (without a bolus dose).
Usual dosage range (SVT): 50-200 mcg/kg/minute with average dose of 100 mcg/kg/minute.
Guidelines for transfer to oral therapy (beta-blocker, calcium channel blocker):
Infusion should be reduced by 50% 30 minutes following the first dose of the alternative agent
Manufacturer suggests following the second dose of the alternative drug, patient's response should be monitored and if control is adequate for the first hours, esmolol may be discontinued.

Dosage Forms
Infusion [premixed in sodium chloride; preservative free]:
Brevibloc®: 2000 mg (100 mL) [20 mg/mL; double strength]; 2500 mg (250 mL) [10 mg/mL]
Injection, solution: 10 mg/mL (10 mL)
Brevibloc®:
10 mg/mL (10 mL)
20 mg/mL (5 mL, 100 mL)

esmolol hydrochloride *see* esmolol *on page 357*
E-Solve-2® Topical *(Discontinued)*

esomeprazole (es oh ME pray zol)

Sound-Alike/Look-Alike Issues
Nexium® may be confused with Nexavar®

Synonyms esomeprazole magnesium; esomeprazole sodium

U.S./Canadian Brand Names Nexium® [US/Can]

Therapeutic Category Proton Pump Inhibitor

◀ **Use**

Oral: Short-term (4-8 weeks) treatment of erosive esophagitis; maintaining symptom resolution and healing of erosive esophagitis; treatment of symptomatic gastroesophageal reflux disease (GERD); as part of a multidrug regimen for *Helicobacter pylori* eradication in patients with duodenal ulcer disease (active or history of within the past 5 years); prevention of gastric ulcers in patients at risk (age ≥60 years and/or history of gastric ulcer) associated with continuous NSAID therapy; long-term treatment of pathological hypersecretory conditions including Zollinger-Ellison syndrome

Canadian labeling: Additional use (not in U.S. labeling): Oral: Treatment of nonerosive reflux disease (NERD)

I.V.: Short-term (≤10 days) treatment of gastroesophageal reflux disease (GERD) when oral therapy is not possible or appropriate

Usual Dosage

Children 1-11 years: Oral: **Note:** Safety and efficacy of doses >1 mg/kg/day and/or therapy beyond 8 weeks have not been established.

Symptomatic GERD: 10 mg once daily for up to 8 weeks

Erosive esophagitis (healing):
<20 kg: 10 mg once daily for 8 weeks
≥20 kg: 10-20 mg once daily for 8 weeks

Nonerosive reflux disease (NERD) (Canadian labeling): 10 mg once daily for up to 8 weeks

Adolescents 12-17 years: Oral:
GERD: 20-40 mg once daily for up to 8 weeks
NERD (Canadian labeling): 20 mg once daily for 2-4 weeks; lack of symptom control after 4 weeks warrants further evaluation

Adults:
Oral:
Erosive esophagitis (healing): Initial: 20-40 mg once daily for 4-8 weeks; if incomplete healing, may continue for an additional 4-8 weeks; maintenance: 20 mg once daily (controlled studies did not extend beyond 6 months)

Symptomatic GERD: 20 mg once daily for 4 weeks; may continue an additional 4 weeks if symptoms persist

NERD (Canadian labeling): Initial: 20 mg once daily for 2-4 weeks; lack of symptom control after 4 weeks warrants further evaluation; maintenance (in patients with successful initial therapy): 20 mg once daily as needed

Helicobacter pylori eradication: 40 mg once daily for 10 days; requires combination therapy **Note:** Various regimens available.

Canadian labeling: 20 mg twice daily for 7 days; requires combination therapy

Prevention of NSAID-induced gastric ulcers: 20-40 mg once daily for up to 6 months

Treatment of NSAID-induced gastric ulcers (Canadian labeling): 20 mg once daily for 4-8 weeks.

Pathological hypersecretory conditions (Zollinger-Ellison syndrome): 40 mg twice daily; adjust regimen to individual patient needs; doses up to 240 mg/day have been administered

I.V.: GERD: 20 mg or 40 mg once daily for ≤10 days; change to oral therapy as soon as appropriate

Dosage Forms Note: Strength expressed as base. [CAN] = Canadian availability

Capsule, delayed release:
Nexium®: 20 mg, 40 mg

Granules, for oral suspension, delayed release, as magnesium:
Nexium®: 10 mg/packet (30s); 20 mg/packet (30s); 40 mg/packet (30s)
Nexium® [CAN]: 10 mg/packet (28s)

Injection, powder for reconstitution:
Nexium®: 20 mg, 40 mg

Tablet, extended release, as magnesium:
Nexium® [CAN]: 20 mg, 40 mg [not available in U.S.]

esomeprazole magnesium *see* esomeprazole *on page 357*

esomeprazole sodium *see* esomeprazole *on page 357*

Esopho-Cat® [US] *see* barium *on page 116*

Esoterica® Regular [US-OTC] *see* hydroquinone *on page 488*

E.S.P.® [US] *see* erythromycin and sulfisoxazole *on page 356*

Especol® [US-OTC] *see* fructose, dextrose, and phosphoric acid *on page 429*

Estalis® [Can] *see* estradiol and norethindrone *on page 362*

Estalis-Sequi® [Can] *see* estradiol and norethindrone *on page 362*

Estar® [Can] *see* coal tar *on page 240*

estazolam (es TA zoe lam)

Sound-Alike/Look-Alike Issues
ProSom® may be confused with PhosLo®, Proscar®, Pro-Sof® Plus, Prozac®, Psorcon®

Therapeutic Category Benzodiazepine

Controlled Substance C-IV

Use Short-term management of insomnia

Usual Dosage Oral: Adults: 1 mg at bedtime, some patients may require 2 mg; start at doses of 0.5 mg in debilitated patients

Dosage Forms
Tablet: 1 mg, 2 mg

Ester-E™ [US-OTC] *see* vitamin E *on page 981*

esterified estrogen and methyltestosterone *see* estrogens (esterified) and methyltestosterone *on page 366*

esterified estrogens *see* estrogens (esterified) *on page 365*

Estivin® II Ophthalmic *(Discontinued)* *see* naphazoline *on page 655*

Estra-L® Injection *(Discontinued)* *see* estradiol *on page 359*

Estrace® [US/Can] *see* estradiol *on page 359*

Estraderm® [US/Can] *see* estradiol *on page 359*

estradiol (es tra DYE ole)

Sound-Alike/Look-Alike Issues
Alora® may be confused with Aldara™
Elestrin™ may be confused with alosetron
Estraderm® may be confused with Testoderm®

Synonyms estradiol acetate; estradiol cypionate; estradiol hemihydrate; estradiol transdermal; estradiol valerate

U.S./Canadian Brand Names Alora® [US]; Climara® [US/Can]; Delestrogen® [US]; Depo®-Estradiol [US/Can]; Divigel® [US]; Elestrin™ [US]; Esclim® [US]; Estrace® [US/Can]; Estraderm® [US/Can]; Estradot® [Can]; Estrasorb™ [US]; Estring® [US/Can]; EstroGel® [US/Can]; Evamist™ [US]; Femring® [US]; Femtrace® [US]; Menostar® [US/Can]; Oesclim® [Can]; Sandoz-Estradiol Derm 100 [Can]; Sandoz-Estradiol Derm 50 [Can]; Sandoz-Estradiol Derm 75 [Can]; Vagifem® [US/Can]; Vivelle-Dot® [US]

Therapeutic Category Estrogen Derivative

Use Treatment of moderate-to-severe vasomotor symptoms associated with menopause; treatment of vulvar and vaginal atrophy; hypoestrogenism (due to hypogonadism, castration, or primary ovarian failure); prostatic cancer (palliation), breast cancer (palliation), osteoporosis (prophylaxis); abnormal uterine bleeding due to hormonal imbalance; postmenopausal urogenital symptoms of the lower urinary tract (urinary urgency, dysuria)

Usual Dosage All dosage needs to be adjusted based upon the patient's response
Oral:
Prostate cancer (androgen-dependent, inoperable, progressing): 10 mg 3 times/day for at least 3 months
Breast cancer (inoperable, progressing in appropriately selected patients): 10 mg 3 times/day for at least 3 months
Osteoporosis prophylaxis in postmenopausal females: 0.5 mg/day in a cyclic regimen (3 weeks on and 1 week off)
Female hypoestrogenism (due to hypogonadism, castration, or primary ovarian failure): 1-2 mg/day; titrate as necessary to control symptoms using minimal effective dose for maintenance therapy
Moderate-to-severe vasomotor symptoms associated with menopause: 1-2 mg/day, adjusted as necessary to limit symptoms; administration should be cyclic (3 weeks on, 1 week off). Patients should be reevaluated at 3- to 6-month intervals to determine if treatment is still necessary.
I.M.:
Prostate cancer: Valerate: ≥30 mg or more every 1-2 weeks
Moderate-to-severe vasomotor symptoms associated with menopause:
Cypionate: 1-5 mg every 3-4 weeks
Valerate: 10-20 mg every 4 weeks
Female hypoestrogenism (due to hypogonadism):
Cypionate: 1.5-2 mg monthly
Valerate: 10-20 mg every 4 weeks

◀ Topical:

Emulsion: Moderate-to-severe vasomotor symptoms associated with menopause: 3.84 g applied once daily in the morning

Gel:

Moderate-to-severe vasomotor symptoms associated with menopause:

Divigel®: 0.25 g/day; adjust dose based on patient response. Dosing range: 0.25-1 g/day

Elestrin™: 0.87g/day applied at the same time each day

EstroGel®: 1.25 g/day applied at the same time each day

Vulvar and vaginal atrophy:

Elestrin™: 0.87g/day applied at the same time each day

EstroGel®: 1.25 g/day applied at the same time each day

Spray: Moderate-to-severe vasomotor symptoms associated with menopause (Evamist™): Initial: One spray (1.53 mg) per day. Adjust dose based on patient response. Dosing range: 1-3 sprays per day.

Transdermal: Indicated dose may be used continuously in patients without an intact uterus. May be given continuously or cyclically (3 weeks on, 1 week off) in patients with an intact uterus **(exception - Menostar®, see specific dosing instructions).** When changing patients from oral to transdermal therapy, start transdermal patch 1 week after discontinuing oral hormone (may begin sooner if symptoms reappear within 1 week):

Once-weekly patch:

Moderate to severe vasomotor symptoms associated with menopause, vulvar and vaginal atrophy associated with menopause, female hypoestrogenism (Climara®): Apply 0.025 mg/day patch once weekly. Adjust dose as necessary to control symptoms. Patients should be reevaluated at 3- to 6-month intervals to determine if treatment is still necessary.

Osteoporosis prophylaxis in postmenopausal women:

Climara®: Apply patch once weekly; minimum effective dose 0.025 mg/day; adjust response to therapy by biochemical markers and bone mineral density

Menostar®: Apply patch once weekly. In women with a uterus, also administer a progestin for 14 days every 6-12 months

Twice-weekly patch:

Moderate-to-severe vasomotor symptoms associated with menopause, vulvar/vaginal atrophy, female hypogonadism: Titrate to lowest dose possible to control symptoms, adjusting initial dose after the first month of therapy; reevaluate therapy at 3- to 6-month intervals to taper or discontinue medication: Alora®, Esclim®, Estraderm®, Vivelle-Dot®: Apply 0.05 mg patch twice weekly

Prevention of osteoporosis in postmenopausal women:

Alora®, Vivelle-Dot®: Apply 0.025 mg patch twice weekly, increase dose as necessary

Estraderm®: Apply 0.05 mg patch twice weekly

Vaginal cream: Vulvar and vaginal atrophy: Insert 2-4 g/day intravaginally for 2 weeks, then gradually reduce to 1/2 the initial dose for 2 weeks, followed by a maintenance dose of 1 g 1-3 times/week

Vaginal ring:

Postmenopausal vaginal atrophy, urogenital symptoms: Estring®: 2 mg intravaginally; following insertion, ring should remain in place for 90 days

Moderate-to-severe vasomotor symptoms associated with menopause; vulvar/vaginal atrophy: Femring®: 0.05 mg intravaginally; following insertion, ring should remain in place for 3 months; dose may be increased to 0.1 mg if needed

Vaginal tablets: Atrophic vaginitis: Vagifem®: Initial: Insert 1 tablet once daily for 2 weeks; maintenance: Insert 1 tablet twice weekly; attempts to discontinue or taper medication should be made at 3- to 6-month intervals

Dosage Forms

Cream, vaginal:

Estrace®: 0.1 mg/g (12 g) [refill]; 0.1 mg/g (42.5 g) [packaged with applicator]

Emulsion, topical:

Estrasorb™: 2.5 mg/g (56s) [each pouch contains 4.35 mg estradiol hemihydrate; contents of two pouches delivers estradiol 0.05 mg/day]

Gel, topical:

Divigel®: 0.1% (0.25 g) [foil packet; delivers estradiol 0.25 mg/packet]; (0.5 g) [foil packet; delivers 0.5 mg estradiol/packet]; (1 g) [foil packet; delivers estradiol 1 mg/packet]

Elestrin™: 0.06% (144 g) [pump; delivers estradiol 0.52 mg/0.87 g; 100 actuations]

EstroGel®: 0.06% (50 g) [pump; delivers estradiol 0.75 mg/1.25 g; 32 actuations]

Injection, oil:

Depo®-Estradiol: 5 mg/mL (5 mL)

Injection, oil: 10 mg/mL (5 mL); 20 mg/mL (5 mL); 40 mg/mL (5 mL)

Delestrogen®: 10 mg/mL (5 mL); 20 mg/mL (5 mL); 40 mg/mL (5 mL)

Ring, vaginal:
Estring®: 2 mg (1s) [total estradiol 2 mg; releases 7.5 mcg/day over 90 days]
Femring®: 0.05 mg (1s) [total estradiol 12.4 mg; releases 0.05 mg/day over 3 months]; 0.1 mg (1s) [total estradiol 24.8 mg; releases 0.1 mg/day over 3 months]

Solution, topical [spray]:
Evamist™: 1.53 mg/spray (8.1 mL)

Tablet, oral: 0.45 mg, 0.9 mg, 1.8 mg
Femtrace®: 0.45 mg, 0.9 mg, 1.8 mg

Tablet, oral, micronized: 0.5 mg, 1 mg, 2 mg
Estrace®: 0.5 mg, 1 mg, 2 mg

Tablet, vaginal:
Vagifem®: 25 mcg

Transdermal system: 0.025 mg/24 hours (4s) [once-weekly patch]; 0.0375 mg/24 hours (4s) [once weekly patch]; 0.05 mg/24 hours (4s) [once-weekly patch]; 0.06 mg/24 hours (4s) [once weekly patch]; 0.075 mg/24 hours [once-weekly patch]; 0.1 mg/24 hours (4s) [once-weekly patch]

Brands:
Alora® [twice-weekly patch]:
  0.025 mg/24 hours (8s) [9 cm^2, total estradiol 0.77 mg]
  0.05 mg/24 hours (8s, 24s) [18 cm^2, total estradiol 1.5 mg]
  0.075 mg/24 hours (8s) [27 cm^2, total estradiol 2.3 mg]
  0.1 mg/24 hours (8s) [36 cm^2, total estradiol 3.1 mg]
Climara® [once-weekly patch]:
  0.025 mg/24 hours (4s) [6.5 cm^2, total estradiol 2.04 mg]
  0.0375 mg/24 hours (4s) [9.375 cm^2, total estradiol 2.85 mg]
  0.05 mg/24 hours (4s) [12.5 cm^2, total estradiol 3.8 mg]
  0.06 mg/24 hours (4s) [15 cm^2, total estradiol 4.55 mg]
  0.075 mg/24 hours (4s) [18.75 cm^2, total estradiol 5.7 mg]
  0.1 mg/24 hours (4s) [25 cm^2, total estradiol 7.6 mg]
Esclim® [twice-weekly patch]:
  0.025 mg/day (8s) [11 cm^2, total estradiol 5 mg]
  0.0375 mg/day (8s) [16.5 cm^2, total estradiol 7.5 mg]
  0.05 mg/day (8s) [22 cm^2, total estradiol 10 mg]
  0.075 mg/day (8s) [33 cm^2, total estradiol 15 mg]
  0.1 mg/day (8s) [44 cm^2, total estradiol 20 mg]
Estraderm® [twice-weekly patch]:
  0.05 mg/24 hours (8s) [10 cm^2, total estradiol 4 mg]
  0.1 mg/24 hours (8s) [20 cm^2, total estradiol 8 mg]
Menostar® [once-weekly patch]: 0.014 mg/24 hours (4s) [3.25 cm^2, total estradiol 1 mg]
Vivelle-Dot® [twice-weekly patch]:
  0.025 mg/day (8s) [2.5 cm^2, total estradiol 0.39 mg]
  0.0375 mg/day (8s) [3.75 cm^2, total estradiol 0.585 mg]
  0.05 mg/day (8s) [5 cm^2, total estradiol 0.78 mg]
  0.075 mg/day (8s) [7.5 cm^2, total estradiol 1.17 mg]
  0.1 mg/day (8s) [10 cm^2, total estradiol 1.56 mg]

estradiol acetate *see* estradiol *on page 359*

estradiol and drospirenone *see* drospirenone and estradiol *on page 327*

estradiol and levonorgestrel (es tra DYE ole & LEE voe nor jes trel)

Synonyms levonorgestrel and estradiol

U.S./Canadian Brand Names ClimaraPro® [US]

Therapeutic Category Estrogen and Progestin Combination

Use Women with an intact uterus: Treatment of moderate-to-severe vasomotor symptoms associated with menopause; prevention of postmenopausal osteoporosis

Usual Dosage Topical: Adult females with an intact uterus: Treatment of moderate-to-severe vasomotor symptoms associated with menopause or prevention of postmenopausal osteoporosis:
Estradiol 0.045 mg/levonorgestrel 0.015 mg: Apply one patch weekly

▶

◀ **Dosage Forms**
Transdermal system:
ClimaraPro®: Estradiol 0.045 mg/24 hours and levonorgestrel 0.015 mg/24 hours (4s) [once-weekly patch]

estradiol and NGM see estradiol and norgestimate on page 362

estradiol and norethindrone (es tra DYE ole & nor eth IN drone)

Synonyms norethindrone and estradiol
U.S./Canadian Brand Names Activella® [US]; CombiPatch® [US]; Estalis-Sequi® [Can]; Estalis® [Can]
Therapeutic Category Estrogen and Progestin Combination
Use Women with an intact uterus:
Tablet: Treatment of moderate-to-severe vasomotor symptoms associated with menopause; treatment of vulvar and vaginal atrophy; prophylaxis for postmenopausal osteoporosis
Transdermal patch: Treatment of moderate-to-severe vasomotor symptoms associated with menopause; treatment of vulvar and vaginal atrophy; treatment of hypoestrogenism due to hypogonadism, castration, or primary ovarian failure
Usual Dosage Note: Patients should be treated with the lowest effective dose and for the shortest duration, consistent with treatment goals. Adults:
Oral (Activella®): One tablet daily
Transdermal patch (CombiPatch®):
Continuous combined regimen: Apply 1 patch twice weekly
Continuous sequential regimen: Apply estradiol-only patch for first 14 days of cycle, followed by one CombiPatch® applied twice weekly for the remaining 14 days of a 28-day cycle
Transdermal patch, combination pack (product-specific dosing for Canadian formulation):
Estalis®: Continuous combined regimen: Apply a new patch twice weekly during a 28-day cycle
Estalis-Sequi®: Continuous sequential regimen: Apply estradiol-only patch for first 14 days, followed by one Estalis® patch applied twice weekly during the last 14 days of a 28-day cycle
Note: In women previously receiving oral estrogens, initiate upon reappearance of menopausal symptoms following discontinuation of oral therapy.
Dosage Forms [CAN] = Canadian brand name
Combination pack:
Estalis-Sequi® 140/50 [CAN; not available in U.S.]:
Transdermal system (Vivelle®): Estradiol 50 mcg per day (4s) [14.5 sq cm; total estradiol 4.33 mg]
Transdermal system (Estalis®): Norethindrone 140 mcg and estradiol 50 mcg per day (4s) [9 sq cm; total norethindrone 2.7 mg, total estradiol 0.62 mg; not available in the U.S.]
Estalis-Sequi® 250/50 [CAN; not available in U.S.]:
Transdermal system (Vivelle®): Estradiol 50 mcg per day (4s) [14.5 sq cm; total estradiol 4.33 mg]
Transdermal system (Estalis®): Norethindrone250 mcg and estradiol 50 mcg per day (4s) [16 sq cm; total norethindrone 4.8 mg, total estradiol 0.51 mg; not available in the U.S.]
Tablet:
Activella® 0.5/0.1: Estradiol 0.5 mg and norethindrone acetate 0.1mg (28s)
Activella® 1/0.5: Estradiol 1 mg and norethindrone acetate 0.5 mg (28s)
Transdermal system:
CombiPatch®:
0.05/0.14: Estradiol 0.05 mg and norethindrone 0.14 mg per day (8s) [9 sq cm]
0.05/0.25: Estradiol 0.05 mg and norethindrone 0.25 mg per day (8s) [16 sq cm]
Estalis® [CAN]:
140/50: Norethindrone 140 mcg and estradiol 50 mcg per day (8s) [9 sq cm; total norethindrone 2.7 mg, total estradiol 0.62 mg; not available in the U.S.]
250/50 Norethindrone 250 mcg and estradiol 50 mcg per day (8s) [16 sq cm; total norethindrone 4.8 mg, total estradiol 0.51 mg; not available in U.S.]

estradiol and norgestimate (es tra DYE ole & nor JES ti mate)

Synonyms estradiol and NGM; norgestimate and estradiol; ortho prefest
U.S./Canadian Brand Names Prefest™ [US]
Therapeutic Category Estrogen and Progestin Combination
Use Women with an intact uterus: Treatment of moderate to severe vasomotor symptoms associated with menopause; treatment of atrophic vaginitis; prevention of osteoporosis
Usual Dosage Oral: Adults: Females with an intact uterus: Treatment of menopausal symptoms, atrophic vaginitis, prevention of osteoporosis: Treatment is cyclical and consists of the following: One tablet of

estradiol 1 mg (pink tablet) once daily for 3 days, followed by 1 tablet of estradiol 1 mg and norgestimate 0.09 mg (white tablet) once daily for 3 days; repeat sequence continuously. **Note:** This dose may not be the lowest effective combination for these indications. In case of a missed tablet, restart therapy with next available tablet in sequence (taking only 1 tablet each day).

Dosage Forms
Tablet:
Prefest™: Estradiol 1 mg [15 pink tablets] and estradiol 1 mg and norgestimate 0.09 mg [15 white tablets] (supplied in blister card of 30)

estradiol cypionate *see* estradiol *on page 359*
estradiol hemihydrate *see* estradiol *on page 359*
estradiol transdermal *see* estradiol *on page 359*
estradiol valerate *see* estradiol *on page 359*
Estradot® [Can] *see* estradiol *on page 359*

estramustine (es tra MUS teen)
Sound-Alike/Look-Alike Issues
estramustine may be confused with exemestane
Emcyt® may be confused with Eryc®
Synonyms estramustine phosphate; estramustine phosphate sodium; NSC-89199
U.S./Canadian Brand Names Emcyt® [US/Can]
Therapeutic Category Antineoplastic Agent
Use Palliative treatment of prostatic carcinoma (progressive or metastatic)
Usual Dosage Oral (refer to individual protocols): Adults: Males: 14 mg/kg/day (range: 10-16 mg/kg/day) in 3 or 4 divided doses
Dosage Forms
Capsule:
Emcyt®: 140 mg

estramustine phosphate *see* estramustine *on page 363*
estramustine phosphate sodium *see* estramustine *on page 363*
Estrasorb™ [US] *see* estradiol *on page 359*
Estratab® [Can] *see* estrogens (esterified) *on page 365*
Estratab® (Discontinued) *see* estrogens (esterified) *on page 365*
Estratest® [US/Can] *see* estrogens (esterified) and methyltestosterone *on page 366*
Estratest® H.S. [US] *see* estrogens (esterified) and methyltestosterone *on page 366*
Estring® [US/Can] *see* estradiol *on page 359*
Estro-Cyp® Injection (Discontinued) *see* estradiol *on page 359*
EstroGel® [US/Can] *see* estradiol *on page 359*
estrogenic substances, conjugated *see* estrogens (conjugated/equine) *on page 364*

estrogens (conjugated A/synthetic) (ES troe jenz, KON joo gate ed, aye, sin THET ik)
Sound-Alike/Look-Alike Issues
Cenestin® may be confused with Senexon®
U.S./Canadian Brand Names Cenestin® [US/Can]
Therapeutic Category Estrogen Derivative
Use Treatment of moderate-to-severe vasomotor symptoms of menopause; treatment of vulvar and vaginal atrophy
Usual Dosage The lowest dose that will control symptoms should be used; medication should be discontinued as soon as possible. Oral: Adults:
Moderate-to-severe vasomotor symptoms: 0.45 mg/day; may be titrated up to 1.25 mg/day. Attempts to discontinue medication should be made at 3- to 6-month intervals.
Vulvar and vaginal atrophy: 0.3 mg/day
Dosage Forms
Tablet:
Cenestin®: 0.3 mg, 0.45 mg, 0.625 mg, 0.9 mg, 1.25 mg

estrogens (conjugated B/synthetic) (ES troe jenz, KON joo gate ed, bee, sin THET ik)

U.S./Canadian Brand Names Enjuvia™ [US]

Therapeutic Category Estrogen Derivative

Use Treatment of moderate-to-severe vasomotor symptoms of menopause; treatment of vulvar and vaginal atrophy associated with menopause; treatment of moderate-to-severe vaginal dryness and pain with intercourse associated with menopause

Usual Dosage The lowest dose that will control symptoms should be used; medication should be discontinued as soon as possible. Oral:

Adults:

Moderate-to-severe vasomotor symptoms associated with menopause: 0.3 mg/day; may be titrated up to 1.25 mg/day. Attempts to discontinue medication should be made at 3- to 6-month intervals.

Vaginal dryness/vulvar and vaginal atrophy associated with menopause: 0.3 mg/day. Attempts to discontinue medication should be made at 3- to 6-month intervals.

Dosage Forms

Tablet:

Enjuvia™: 0.3 mg, 0.45 mg, 0.625 mg, 0.9 mg, 1.25 mg

estrogens (conjugated/equine) (ES troe jenz KON joo gate ed, EE kwine)

Sound-Alike/Look-Alike Issues

Premarin® may be confused with Primaxin®, Provera®, Remeron®

Synonyms CEE; estrogenic substances, conjugated

U.S./Canadian Brand Names C.E.S.® [Can]; Premarin® [US/Can]

Therapeutic Category Estrogen Derivative

Use Treatment of moderate-to-severe vasomotor symptoms associated with menopause; treatment of vulvar and vaginal atrophy; hypoestrogenism (due to hypogonadism, castration, or primary ovarian failure); prostatic cancer (palliation); breast cancer (palliation); osteoporosis (prophylaxis, postmenopausal women at significant risk only); abnormal uterine bleeding

Usual Dosage Adults:

Male: Androgen-dependent prostate cancer palliation: Oral: 1.25-2.5 mg 3 times/day

Female:

Prevention of postmenopausal osteoporosis: Oral: Initial: 0.3 mg/day cyclically* or daily, depending on medical assessment of patient. Dose may be adjusted based on bone mineral density and clinical response. The lowest effective dose should be used.

Moderate-to-severe vasomotor symptoms associated with menopause: Oral: Initial: 0.3 mg/day, cyclically* or daily, depending on medical assessment of patient. The lowest dose that will control symptoms should be used. Medication should be discontinued as soon as possible.

Vulvar and vaginal atrophy:

Oral: Initial: 0.3 mg/day; the lowest dose that will control symptoms should be used. May be given cyclically* or daily, depending on medical assessment of patient. Medication should be discontinued as soon as possible.

Vaginal cream: Intravaginal: 1/2 to 2 g/day given cyclically*

Abnormal uterine bleeding:

Acute/heavy bleeding:

I.M., I.V.: 25 mg, may repeat in 6-12 hours if needed

Note: Treatment should be followed by a low-dose oral contraceptive; medroxyprogesterone acetate along with or following estrogen therapy can also be given

Female hypogonadism: Oral: 0.3-0.625 mg/day given cyclically*; dose may be titrated in 6- to 12-month intervals; progestin treatment should be added to maintain bone mineral density once skeletal maturity is achieved.

Female castration, primary ovarian failure: Oral: 1.25 mg/day given cyclically*; adjust according to severity of symptoms and patient response. For maintenance, adjust to the lowest effective dose.

*Cyclic administration: Either 3 weeks on, 1 week off **or** 25 days on, 5 days off

Male and Female: Breast cancer palliation, metastatic disease in selected patients: Oral: 10 mg 3 times/day for at least 3 months

Dosage Forms

Cream, vaginal:

Premarin®: 0.625 mg/g (42.5 g)

Injection, powder for reconstitution:

Premarin®: 25 mg

Tablet:
Premarin®: 0.3 mg, 0.45 mg, 0.625 mg, 0.9 mg, 1.25 mg

estrogens (conjugated/equine) and medroxyprogesterone
(ES troe jenz KON joo gate ed/EE kwine & me DROKS ee proe JES te rone)

Sound-Alike/Look-Alike Issues
Premphase® may be confused with Prempro™
Prempro™ may be confused with Premphase®

Synonyms medroxyprogesterone and estrogens (conjugated); MPA and estrogens (conjugated)

U.S./Canadian Brand Names Premphase® [US/Can]; Premplus® [Can]; Prempro™ [US/Can]

Therapeutic Category Estrogen and Progestin Combination

Use Women with an intact uterus: Treatment of moderate-to-severe vasomotor symptoms associated with menopause; treatment of atrophic vaginitis; osteoporosis (prophylaxis)

Usual Dosage Oral: Adults:
Treatment of moderate-to-severe vasomotor symptoms associated with menopause or treatment of atrophic vaginitis in females with an intact uterus. (The lowest dose that will control symptoms should be used; medication should be discontinued as soon as possible):
Premphase®: One maroon conjugated estrogen 0.625 mg tablet daily on days 1 through 14 and one light blue conjugated estrogen 0.625 mg/MPA 5 mg tablet daily on days 15 through 28; reevaluate patients at 3- and 6-month intervals to determine if treatment is still necessary; monitor patients for signs of endometrial cancer; rule out malignancy if unexplained vaginal bleeding occurs
Prempro™: One conjugated estrogen 0.3 mg/MPA 1.5 mg tablet daily; reevaluate at 3-and 6-month intervals to determine if therapy is still needed; dose may be increased to a maximum of one conjugated estrogen 0.625 mg/MPA 5 mg tablet daily in patients with bleeding or spotting, once malignancy has been ruled out
Osteoporosis prophylaxis in females with an intact uterus:
Premphase®: One maroon conjugated estrogen 0.625 tablet daily on days 1 through 14 and one light blue conjugated estrogen 0.625 mg/MPA 5 mg tablet daily on days 15 through 28; monitor patients for signs of endometrial cancer; rule out malignancy if unexplained vaginal bleeding occurs
Prempro™: One conjugated estrogen 0.3 mg/MPA 1.5 mg tablet daily; dose may be increased to one conjugated estrogen 0.625 mg/MPA 5 mg tablet daily; in patients with bleeding or spotting, once malignancy has been ruled out

Dosage Forms
Tablet:
Premphase® [therapy pack contains two separate tablet formulations]: Conjugated estrogens 0.625 mg [14 maroon tablets] and conjugated estrogen 0.625 mg/medroxyprogesterone 5 mg [14 light blue tablets] (28s)
Prempro™:
0.3/1.5: Conjugated estrogens 0.3 mg and medroxyprogesterone 1.5 mg (28s)
0.45/1.5: Conjugated estrogens 0.45 mg and medroxyprogesterone 1.5 mg (28s)
0.625/2.5: Conjugated estrogens 0.625 mg and medroxyprogesterone 2.5 mg (28s)
0.625/5: Conjugated estrogens 0.625 mg and medroxyprogesterone 5 mg (28s)

estrogens (esterified) (ES troe jenz, es TER i fied)

Sound-Alike/Look-Alike Issues
Estratab® may be confused with Estratest®, Estratest® H.S.

Synonyms esterified estrogens

U.S./Canadian Brand Names Estratab® [Can]; Menest® [US/Can]

Therapeutic Category Estrogen Derivative

Use Treatment of moderate to severe vasomotor symptoms associated with menopause; treatment of vulvar and vaginal atrophy; hypoestrogenism (due to hypogonadism, castration, or primary ovarian failure); prostatic cancer (palliation); breast cancer (palliation); osteoporosis (prophylaxis, in women at significant risk only)

Usual Dosage Oral: Adults:
Prostate cancer (palliation): 1.25-2.5 mg 3 times/day
Female hypogonadism: 2.5-7.5 mg of estrogen daily for 20 days followed by a 10-day rest period. Administer cyclically (3 weeks on and 1 week off). If bleeding does not occur by the end of the 10-day period, repeat the same dosing schedule; the number of courses is dependent upon the responsiveness of the endometrium. If bleeding occurs before the end of the 10-day period, begin an estrogen-progestin cyclic regimen of 2.5-7.5 mg esterified estrogens daily for 20 days. During the last 5 days of estrogen ▶

therapy, give an oral progestin. If bleeding occurs before regimen is concluded, discontinue therapy and resume on the fifth day of bleeding.

Moderate to severe vasomotor symptoms associated with menopause: 1.25 mg/day administered cyclically (3 weeks on and 1 week off). If patient has not menstruated within the last 2 months or more, cyclic administration is started arbitrary. If the patient is menstruating, cyclic administration is started on day 5 of the bleeding. For short-term use only and should be discontinued as soon as possible. Reevaluate at 3- to 6-month intervals for tapering or discontinuation of therapy.

Atopic vaginitis and kraurosis vulvae: 0.3 to ≥1.25 mg/day, depending on the tissue response of the individual patient. Administer cyclically. For short-term use only and should be discontinued as soon as possible. Reevaluate at 3- to 6-month intervals for tapering or discontinuation of therapy.

Breast cancer (palliation): 10 mg 3 times/day for at least 3 months

Osteoporosis in postmenopausal women: Initial: 0.3 mg/day and increase to a maximum daily dose of 1.25 mg/day; initiate therapy as soon as possible after menopause; cyclically or daily, depending on medical assessment of patient. Monitor patients with an intact uterus for signs of endometrial cancer; rule out malignancy if unexplained vaginal bleeding occurs

Female castration and primary ovarian failure: 1.25 mg/day, cyclically. Adjust dosage upward or downward, according to the severity of symptoms and patient response. For maintenance, adjust dosage to lowest level that will provide effective control.

Dosage Forms
Tablet:
Menest®: 0.3 mg, 0.625 mg, 1.25 mg, 2.5 mg

estrogens (esterified) and methyltestosterone
(ES troe jenz es TER i fied & meth il tes TOS te rone)
Sound-Alike/Look-Alike Issues
Estratest® may be confused with Eskalith®, Estratab®, Estratest® H.S.
Estratest® H.S. may be confused with Eskalith®, Estratab®, Estratest®

Synonyms conjugated estrogen and methyltestosterone; esterified estrogen and methyltestosterone

U.S./Canadian Brand Names Covaryx™ HS [US]; Covaryx™ [US]; E.E.M.T. D.S. [US]; E.E.M.T. H.S. [US]; Estratest® H.S. [US]; Estratest® [US/Can]

Therapeutic Category Estrogen and Androgen Combination

Use Vasomotor symptoms of menopause

Usual Dosage Oral: Adults: Females: Lowest dose that will control symptoms should be chosen, normally given 3 weeks on and 1 week off

Dosage Forms
Tablet: Esterified estrogens 1.25 mg and methyltestosterone 2.5 mg; esterified estrogen 0.625 mg and methyltestosterone 1.25 mg
Covaryx™, Covaryx™ H.S., Estratest®, E.E.M.T D.S.: Esterified estrogen 1.25 mg and methyltestosterone 2.5 mg
Estratest® H.S., E.E.M.T. H.S.: Esterified estrogen 0.625 mg and methyltestosterone 1.25 mg

estropipate (ES troe pih pate)
Synonyms piperazine estrone sulfate

U.S./Canadian Brand Names Ogen® [US/Can]; Ortho-Est® [US]

Therapeutic Category Estrogen Derivative

Use Treatment of moderate-to-severe vasomotor symptoms associated with menopause; treatment of vulvar and vaginal atrophy; hypoestrogenism (due to hypogonadism, castration, or primary ovarian failure); osteoporosis (prophylaxis, in women at significant risk only)

Usual Dosage Oral: Adults:
Moderate to severe vasomotor symptoms associated with menopause: Usual dosage range: 0.75-6 mg estropipate daily; use the lowest dose and regimen that will control symptoms, and discontinue as soon as possible. Attempt to discontinue or taper medication at 3- to 6-month intervals. If a patient with vasomotor symptoms has not menstruated within the last ≥2 months, start the cyclic administration arbitrarily. If the patient has menstruated, start cyclic administration on day 5 of bleeding.

Female hypogonadism: 1.5-9 mg estropipate daily for the first 3 weeks, followed by a rest period of 8-10 days; use the lowest dose and regimen that will control symptoms. Repeat if bleeding does not occur by the end of the rest period. The duration of therapy necessary to product the withdrawal bleeding will vary according to the responsiveness of the endometrium. If satisfactory withdrawal bleeding does not occur, give an oral progestin in addition to estrogen during the third week of the cycle.

Female castration or primary ovarian failure: 1.5-9 mg estropipate daily for the first 3 weeks of a theoretical cycle, followed by a rest period of 8-10 days; use the lowest dose and regimen that will control symptoms

Osteoporosis prophylaxis: 0.75 mg estropipate daily for 25 days of a 31-day cycle

Atrophic vaginitis or kraurosis vulvae: 0.75-6 mg estropipate daily; administer cyclically. Use the lowest dose and regimen that will control symptoms; discontinue as soon as possible.

Dosage Forms

Tablet: 0.625 mg [estropipate 0.75 mg]; 1.25 mg [estropipate 1.5 mg]; 2.5 mg [estropipate 3 mg]
Ogen®: 0.625 mg [estropipate 0.75 mg]; 1.25 mg [estropipate 1.5 mg]; 2.5 mg [estropipate 3 mg]
Ortho-Est®: 0.625 mg [estropipate 0.75 mg]; 1.25 mg [estropipate 1.5 mg]

Estrostep® 21 *(Discontinued)* *see* ethinyl estradiol and norethindrone *on page 376*

Estrostep® Fe [US] *see* ethinyl estradiol and norethindrone *on page 376*

eszopiclone (es zoe PIK lone)

Sound-Alike/Look-Alike Issues
Lunesta® may be confused with Neulasta®

U.S./Canadian Brand Names Lunesta® [US]

Therapeutic Category Hypnotic, Nonbenzodiazepine

Controlled Substance C-IV

Use Treatment of insomnia

Usual Dosage Oral: Adults: Insomnia: Initial: 2 mg immediately before bedtime (maximum dose: 3 mg)
Concurrent use with strong CYP3A4 inhibitor: 1 mg immediately before bedtime; if needed, dose may be increased to 2 mg

Dosage Forms
Tablet:
Lunesta®: 1 mg, 2 mg, 3 mg

etanercept (et a NER sept)

U.S./Canadian Brand Names Enbrel® [US/Can]

Therapeutic Category Antirheumatic, Disease Modifying

Use Treatment of moderately- to severely-active rheumatoid arthritis (RA); moderately- to severely-active polyarticular juvenile idiopathic arthritis (JIA); psoriatic arthritis; active ankylosing spondylitis (AS); moderate-to-severe chronic plaque psoriasis

Usual Dosage SubQ:
Children 2-17 years: Juvenile idiopathic arthritis:
Once-weekly dosing: 0.8 mg/kg (maximum: 50 mg/dose) once weekly
Twice-weekly dosing: 0.4 mg/kg (maximum: 25 mg/dose) twice weekly (individual doses should be separated by 72-96 hours)
Adults:
Rheumatoid arthritis, psoriatic arthritis, ankylosing spondylitis:
Once-weekly dosing: 50 mg once weekly
Twice weekly dosing: 25 mg given twice weekly (individual doses should be separated by 72-96 hours)
Plaque psoriasis:
Initial: 50 mg twice weekly, 3-4 days apart (starting doses of 25 or 50 mg once weekly have also been used successfully); maintain initial dose for 3 months
Maintenance dose: 50 mg once weekly

Dosage Forms
Injection, powder for reconstitution:
Enbrel®: 25 mg
Injection, solution [preservative free]:
Enbrel®: 50 mg/mL (0.51 mL, 0.98 mL)

ethacrynate sodium *see* ethacrynic acid *on page 367*

ethacrynic acid (eth a KRIN ik AS id)

Sound-Alike/Look-Alike Issues
Edecrin® may be confused with Eulexin®, Ecotrin®

Synonyms ethacrynate sodium

U.S./Canadian Brand Names Edecrin® [US/Can]

◀ **Therapeutic Category** Diuretic, Loop

Use Management of edema associated with congestive heart failure; hepatic cirrhosis or renal disease; short-term management of ascites due to malignancy, idiopathic edema, and lymphedema

Usual Dosage I.V. formulation should be diluted in D_5W or NS (1 mg/mL) and infused over several minutes.

Children: Oral: 1 mg/kg/dose once daily; increase at intervals of 2-3 days as needed, to a maximum of 3 mg/kg/day.

Adults:

Oral: 50-200 mg/day in 1-2 divided doses; may increase in increments of 25-50 mg at intervals of several days; doses up to 200 mg twice daily may be required with severe, refractory edema.

I.V.: 0.5-1 mg/kg/dose (maximum: 100 mg/dose); repeat doses not routinely recommended; however, if indicated, repeat doses every 8-12 hours.

Dosage Forms

Injection, powder for reconstitution:

Edecrin®: 50 mg

Tablet:

Edecrin®: 25 mg

ethambutol (e THAM byoo tole)

Sound-Alike/Look-Alike Issues

Myambutol® may be confused with Nembutal®

Synonyms ethambutol hydrochloride

U.S./Canadian Brand Names Etibi® [Can]; Myambutol® [US]

Therapeutic Category Antimycobacterial Agent

Use Treatment of tuberculosis and other mycobacterial diseases in conjunction with other antituberculosis agents

Usual Dosage

Usual dosage range: Oral:

Children: 15-20 mg/kg/day (maximum: 1 g/day) **or** 50 mg/kg/dose twice weekly (maximum: 4 g/dose)

Adults: 15-25 mg/kg daily **or** 25-30 mg/kg/dose 3 times/week (maximum: 2.5 g/dose) **or** 50 mg/kg/dose twice weekly (maximum: 4 g/dose)

Indication-specific dosing: Oral:

Disseminated *Mycobacterium avium* complex (MAC) in patients with advanced HIV infection: Adults: 15 mg/kg ethambutol in combination with azithromycin 600 mg daily

Tuberculosis, active:Note: Used as part of a multidrug regimen; treatment regimens consist of an initial 2 month phase, followed by a continuation phase of 4 or 7 additional months; frequency of dosing may differ depending on phase of therapy.

Children:

Daily therapy: 15-20 mg/kg/day (maximum: 1 g/day)

Twice weekly directly observed therapy (DOT): 50 mg/kg (maximum: 4 g/dose)

Adults (suggested doses by lean body weight):

Daily therapy: 15-25 mg/kg

40-55 kg: 800 mg

56-75 kg: 1200 mg

76-90 kg: 1600 mg (maximum dose regardless of weight)

Twice weekly directly observed therapy (DOT): 50 mg/kg

40-55 kg: 2000 mg

56-75 kg: 2800 mg

76-90 kg: 4000 mg (maximum dose regardless of weight)

Three times/week DOT: 25-30 mg/kg (maximum: 2.5 g)

40-55 kg: 1200 mg

56-75 kg: 2000 mg

76-90 kg: 2400 mg (maximum dose regardless of weight)

Dosage Forms

Tablet: 100 mg, 400 mg

Myambutol®: 100 mg, 400 mg

ethambutol hydrochloride *see* ethambutol *on page 368*

Ethamolin® [US] *see* ethanolamine oleate *on page 369*

ethanoic acid *see* acetic acid *on page 29*

ethanol *see* alcohol (ethyl) *on page 41*

ethanolamine oleate (ETH a nol a meen OH lee ate)

Sound-Alike/Look-Alike Issues
Ethamolin® may be confused with ethanol
Synonyms monoethanolamine
U.S./Canadian Brand Names Ethamolin® [US]
Therapeutic Category Sclerosing Agent
Use Orphan drug: Sclerosing agent used for bleeding esophageal varices
Usual Dosage Adults: 1.5-5 mL per varix, up to 20 mL total or 0.4 mL/kg for a 50 kg patient; doses should be decreased in patients with severe hepatic dysfunction and should receive less than recommended maximum dose
Dosage Forms
Injection, solution:
Ethamolin®: 5% [50 mg/mL] (2 mL)

EtheDent™ [US] *see* fluoride *on page 411*
Ethezyme™ 650 [US] *see* papain and urea *on page 721*
Ethezyme™ 830 (Discontinued) *see* papain and urea *on page 721*
Ethezyme™ (Discontinued) *see* papain and urea *on page 721*
ethinyl estradiol and cyproterone acetate *see* cyproterone and ethinyl estradiol *(Canada only) on page 259*

ethinyl estradiol and desogestrel (ETH in il es tra DYE ole & des oh JES trel)

Sound-Alike/Look-Alike Issues
Ortho-Cept® may be confused with Ortho-Cyclen®
Synonyms desogestrel and ethinyl estradiol
U.S./Canadian Brand Names Apri® [US]; Cesia™ [US]; Cyclessa® [US/Can]; Desogen® [US]; Kariva™ [US]; Linessa® [Can]; Marvelon® [Can]; Mircette® [US]; Ortho-Cept® [US/Can]; Reclipsen™ [US]; Solia™ [US]; Velivet™ [US]
Therapeutic Category Contraceptive, Oral
Use Prevention of pregnancy
Usual Dosage Oral: Adults: Females: Contraception:
Schedule 1 (Sunday starter): Dose begins on first Sunday after onset of menstruation; if the menstrual period starts on Sunday, take first tablet that very same day. **With a Sunday start, an additional method of contraception should be used until after the first 7 days of consecutive administration.**
For 21-tablet package: Dosage is 1 tablet daily for 21 consecutive days, followed by 7 days off of the medication; a new course begins on the 8th day after the last tablet is taken.
For 28-tablet package: Dosage is 1 tablet daily without interruption.
Schedule 2 (Day 1 starter): Dose starts on first day of menstrual cycle taking 1 tablet daily.
For 21-tablet package: Dosage is 1 tablet daily for 21 consecutive days, followed by 7 days off of the medication; a new course begins on the 8th day after the last tablet is taken.
For 28-tablet package: Dosage is 1 tablet daily without interruption.
If all doses have been taken on schedule and one menstrual period is missed, continue dosing cycle. If two consecutive menstrual periods are missed, pregnancy test is required before new dosing cycle is started.
Missed doses **monophasic formulations** (refer to package insert for complete information):
One dose missed: Take as soon as remembered or take 2 tablets next day
Two consecutive doses missed in the first 2 weeks: Take 2 tablets as soon as remembered or 2 tablets next 2 days. **An additional method of contraception should be used for 7 days after missed dose.**
Two consecutive doses missed in week 3 or three consecutive doses missed at any time:
Schedule 1 (Sunday starter): Continue to take 1 tablet daily until Sunday, then discard the rest of the pack, and a new pack is started that same day.
Schedule 2 (Day 1 starter): Current pack should be discarded, and a new pack started that same day. **An additional method of contraception should be used for 7 days after missed dose.**
Missed doses **biphasic/triphasic formulations** (refer to package insert for complete information):
One dose missed: Take as soon as remembered or take 2 tablets next day.
Two consecutive doses missed in week 1 or week 2 of the pack: Take 2 tablets as soon as remembered and 2 tablets the next day. Resume taking 1 tablet daily until the pack is empty. **An additional method of contraception should be used for 7 days after a missed dose.**

Two consecutive doses missed in week 3 of the pack; **an additional method of contraception must be used for 7 days after a missed dose**:

Schedule 1 (Sunday starter): Take 1 tablet every day until Sunday. Discard the remaining pack and start a new pack of pills on the same day.

Schedule 2 (Day 1 starter): Discard the remaining pack and start a new pack the same day.

Three or more consecutive doses missed; **an additional method of contraception must be used for 7 days after a missed dose**:

Schedule 1 (Sunday starter): Take 1 tablet every day until Sunday; on Sunday, discard the pack and start a new pack.

Schedule 2 (Day 1 starter): Discard the remaining pack and begin new pack of tablets starting on the same day.

Dosage Forms

Tablet, low-dose formulations:

Kariva™:
Day 1-21: Ethinyl estradiol 0.02 mg and desogestrel 0.15 mg [21 white tablets]
Day 22-23: 2 inactive light green tablets
Day 24-28: Ethinyl estradiol 0.01 mg [5 light blue tablets] (28s)

Mircette®:
Day 1-21: Ethinyl estradiol 0.02 mg and desogestrel 0.15 mg [21 white tablets]
Day 22-23: 2 inactive green tablets
Day 24-28: Ethinyl estradiol 0.01 mg [5 yellow tablets] (28s)

Tablet, monophasic formulations:

Apri® 28: Ethinyl estradiol 0.03 mg and desogestrel 0.15 mg (28s) [21 rose tablets and 7 white inactive tablets]

Desogen®, Reclipsen™, Solia™: Ethinyl estradiol 0.03 mg and desogestrel 0.15 mg (28s) [21 white tablets and 7 green inactive tablets]

Ortho-Cept® 28: Ethinyl estradiol 0.03 mg and desogestrel 0.15 mg (28s) [21 orange tablets and 7 green inactive tablets]

Tablet, triphasic formulations:

Cesia™, Cyclessa®:
Day 1-7: Ethinyl estradiol 0.025 mg and desogestrel 0.1 mg [7 light yellow tablets]
Day 8-14: Ethinyl estradiol 0.025 mg and desogestrel 0.125 mg [7 orange tablets]
Day 14-21: Ethinyl estradiol 0.025 mg and desogestrel 0.15 mg [7 red tablets]
Day 21-28: 7 green inactive tablets (28s)

Velivet™:
Day 1-7: Ethinyl estradiol 0.025 mg and desogestrel 0.1 mg [7 beige tablets]
Day 8-14: Ethinyl estradiol 0.025 mg and desogestrel 0.125 mg [7 orange tablets]
Day 14-21: Ethinyl estradiol 0.025 mg and desogestrel 0.15 mg [7 pink tablets]
Day 21-28: 7 white inactive tablets (28s)

ethinyl estradiol and drospirenone (ETH in il es tra DYE ole & droh SPYE re none)

Synonyms drospirenone and ethinyl estradiol

U.S./Canadian Brand Names Yasmin® [US/Can]; Yaz [US]

Therapeutic Category Contraceptive, Oral

Use Females: Prevention of pregnancy; treatment of premenstrual dysphoric disorder (PMDD); treatment of acne

Usual Dosage Oral:

Children ≥14 years and Adults: Females: Acne (Yaz): Refer to dosing for contraception

Adults: Females: Contraception (Yasmin®, Yaz), PMDD (Yaz): Dosage is 1 tablet daily for 28 consecutive days. Dose should be taken at the same time each day, either after the evening meal or at bedtime. Dosing may be started on the first day of menstrual period (Day 1 starter) or on the first Sunday after the onset of the menstrual period (Sunday starter).

Day 1 starter: Dose starts on first day of menstrual cycle taking 1 tablet daily.

Sunday starter: Dose begins on first Sunday after onset of menstruation; if the menstrual period starts on Sunday, take first tablet that very same day. **With a Sunday start, an additional method of contraception should be used until after the first 7 days of consecutive administration.**

If all doses have been taken on schedule and one menstrual period is missed, continue dosing cycle. If two consecutive menstrual periods are missed, pregnancy test is required before new dosing cycle is started.

If doses have been missed during the first 3 weeks and the menstrual period is missed, pregnancy should be ruled out prior to continuing treatment.

Missed doses (monophasic formulations) (refer to package insert for complete information):
One dose missed: Take as soon as remembered or take 2 tablets next day
Two consecutive doses missed in the first 2 weeks: Take 2 tablets as soon as remembered or 2 tablets next 2 days. **An additional method of contraception should be used for 7 days after missed dose.**
Two consecutive doses missed in week 3 or three consecutive doses missed at any time: **An additional method of contraception must be used for 7 days after a missed dose.**
Day 1 starter: Current pack should be discarded, and a new pack should be started that same day.
Sunday starter: Continue dose of 1 tablet daily until Sunday, then discard the rest of the pack, and a new pack should be started that same day.
Any number of doses missed in week 4: Continue taking one pill each day until pack is empty; no backup method of contraception is needed

Dosage Forms
Tablet:
Ocella™, Yasmin®: Ethinyl estradiol 0.03 mg and drospirenone 3 mg [21 yellow active tablets and 7 white inactive tablets] (28s)
Yaz®: Ethinyl estradiol 0.02 mg and drospirenone 3 mg [24 light pink tablets and 4 white inactive tablets] (28s)

ethinyl estradiol and ethynodiol diacetate
(ETH in il es tra DYE ole & e thye noe DYE ole dye AS e tate)
Sound-Alike/Look-Alike Issues
Demulen® may be confused with Dalmane®, Demerol®
Synonyms ethynodiol diacetate and ethinyl estradiol
U.S./Canadian Brand Names Demulen® 30 [Can]; Kelnor™ [US]; Zovia® [US]
Therapeutic Category Contraceptive, Oral
Use Prevention of pregnancy
Usual Dosage Oral: Adults: Females: Contraception:
Schedule 1 (Sunday starter): Dose begins on first Sunday after onset of menstruation; if the menstrual period starts on Sunday, take first tablet that very same day. **With a Sunday start, an additional method of contraception should be used until after the first 7 days of consecutive administration.**
For 21-tablet package: 1 tablet/day for 21 consecutive days, followed by 7 days off of the medication; a new course begins on the 8th day after the last tablet is taken.
For 28-tablet package: 1 tablet/day without interruption.
Schedule 2 (Day 1 starter): Dose starts on first day of menstrual cycle taking 1 tablet daily.
For 21-tablet package: 1 tablet/day for 21 consecutive days, followed by 7 days off of the medication; a new course begins on the 8th day after the last tablet is taken.
For 28-tablet package: 1 tablet/day without interruption.
If all doses have been taken on schedule and one menstrual period is missed, continue dosing cycle. If two consecutive menstrual periods are missed, pregnancy test is required before new dosing cycle is started.
Missed doses **monophasic formulations** (refer to package insert for complete information):
One dose missed: Take as soon as remembered or take 2 tablets next day
Two consecutive doses missed in the first 2 weeks: Take 2 tablets as soon as remembered or 2 tablets next 2 days. **An additional method of contraception should be used for 7 days after missed dose.**
Two consecutive doses missed in week 3 or three consecutive doses missed at any time: **An additional method of contraception should be used for 7 days after missed dose:**
Schedule 1 (Sunday starter): Continue dose of 1 tablet daily until Sunday, then discard the rest of the pack, and a new pack should be started that same day.
Schedule 2 (Day 1 starter): Current package should be discarded, and a new pack should be started that same day.
Dosage Forms
Tablet, monophasic formulations:
Kelnor™ 1/35: Ethinyl estradiol 0.035 mg and ethynodiol diacetate 1 mg [21 light yellow tablets and 7 white inactive tablets] (28s)
Zovia® 1/35-28: Ethinyl estradiol 0.035 mg and ethynodiol diacetate 1 mg [21 light pink tablets and 7 white inactive tablets] (28s)
Zovia® 1/50-28: Ethinyl estradiol 0.05 mg and ethynodiol diacetate 1 mg [21 pink tablets and 7 white inactive tablets] (28s)

ethinyl estradiol and etonogestrel (ETH in il es tra DYE ole & et oh noe JES trel)

Synonyms etonogestrel and ethinyl estradiol

U.S./Canadian Brand Names NuvaRing® [US/Can]

Therapeutic Category Contraceptive, Oral; Estrogen and Progestin Combination

Use Prevention of pregnancy

Usual Dosage Vaginal: Adults: Females: Contraception: One ring, inserted vaginally and left in place for 3 consecutive weeks, then removed for 1 week. A new ring is inserted 7 days after the last was removed (even if bleeding is not complete) and should be inserted at approximately the same time of day the ring was removed the previous week.

Initial treatment should begin as follows (pregnancy should always be ruled out first):

No hormonal contraceptive use in the past month: Insert ring on the first day of menstrual cycle ("Day 1"). May also insert on days 2-5 even if bleeding is not complete, however, **a spermicide or barrier method of contraception should be used for the following 7 days.***

Switching from combination oral contraceptive: Ring can be inserted on any day within 7 days after the last **active** tablet in the cycle was taken and no later than the first day a new cycle of tablets would begin. Additional forms of contraception are not needed.

Switching from progestin-only contraceptive: **A spermicide or barrier method of contraception should be used for the following 7 days with any of the following.***

If previously using a progestin-only mini-pill, insert the ring on any day of the month; do not skip days between the last pill and insertion of the ring.

If previously using an implant, insert the ring on the same day of implant removal.

If previously using a progestin-containing IUD, insert the ring on day of IUD removal.

If previously using a progestin injection, insert the ring on the day the next injection would be given.

Following complete 1st trimester abortion: Insert ring within the first 5 days of abortion. If not inserted within 5 days, follow instructions for "No hormonal contraceptive use within the past month" and instruct patient to use a nonhormonal contraceptive in the interim.

Following delivery or 2nd trimester abortion: Insert ring 4 weeks postpartum (in women who are not breast-feeding) or following 2nd trimester abortion. **A spermicide or barrier method of contraception should be used for the following 7 days.***

If the ring is accidentally removed from the vagina at anytime during the 3-week period of use, it may be rinsed with cool or lukewarm water (not hot) and reinserted as soon as possible. If the ring is not reinserted within 3 hours, contraceptive effectiveness will be decreased. **A spermicide or barrier method of contraception should be used until the ring has been in place for 7 consecutive days.***

If the ring has been removed for longer than 1 week, pregnancy must be ruled out prior to restarting therapy. **A spermicide or barrier method of contraception should be used for the following 7 days.***

If the ring has been left in place for >3 weeks, a new ring should be inserted following a 1-week (ring-free) interval. Protection continues during week 4, however, if the ring is left in place >4 weeks, pregnancy must be ruled out prior to insertion and **a spermicide or barrier method of contraception should be used for the following 7 days.***

Disconnected ring: In the event the ring disconnects at the weld joint, discard and replace with a new ring.

***Note:** Diaphragms may interfere with proper ring placement, and therefore, are not recommended for use as an additional form of contraception.

Dosage Forms

Ring, vaginal:

NuvaRing®: Ethinyl estradiol 0.015 mg/day and etonogestrel 0.12 mg/day (1s) [3-week duration]

ethinyl estradiol and levonorgestrel (ETH in il es tra DYE ole & LEE voe nor jes trel)

Sound-Alike/Look-Alike Issues

Alesse® may be confused with Aleve®

Nordette® may be confused with Nicorette®

Seasonale® may be confused with Seasonique™

Seasonique™ may be confused with Seasonale®

Tri-Levlen® may be confused with Trilafon®

Triphasil® may be confused with Tri-Norinyl®

Synonyms levonorgestrel and ethinyl estradiol

U.S./Canadian Brand Names Alesse® [US/Can]; Aviane™ [US/Can]; Enpresse™ [US]; Jolessa™ [US]; Lessina™ [US]; Levlen® [US]; Levlite™ [US]; Levora® [US]; Lutera™ [US]; Lybrel™ [US]; Min-Ovral® [Can]; Nordette® [US]; Portia™ [US]; Quasense™ [US]; Seasonale® [US/Can]; Seasonique™ [US]; Sronyx™ [US]; Triphasil® [US/Can]; Triquilar® [Can]; Trivora® [US]

Therapeutic Category Contraceptive, Oral

Use Prevention of pregnancy; postcoital contraception

Usual Dosage Oral: Adults: Females:

Contraception, 28-day cycle:

Schedule 1 (Sunday starter): Dose begins on first Sunday after onset of menstruation; if the menstrual period starts on Sunday, take first tablet that very same day. With a Sunday start, an additional method of contraception should be used until after the first 7 days of consecutive administration:

For 21-tablet package: 1 tablet/day for 21 consecutive days, followed by 7 days off of the medication; a new course begins on the 8th day after the last tablet is taken

For 28-tablet package: 1 tablet/day without interruption

Schedule 2 (Day 1 starter): Dose starts on first day of menstrual cycle taking 1 tablet/day:

For 21-tablet package: 1 tablet/day for 21 consecutive days, followed by 7 days off of the medication; a new course begins on the 8th day after the last tablet is taken

For 28-tablet package: 1 tablet/day without interruption

If all doses have been taken on schedule and one menstrual period is missed, continue dosing cycle. If two consecutive menstrual periods are missed, pregnancy test is required before new dosing cycle is started.

Missed doses **monophasic formulations** (refer to package insert for complete information):

One dose missed: Take as soon as remembered or take 2 tablets next day

Two consecutive doses missed in the first 2 weeks: Take 2 tablets as soon as remembered or 2 tablets next 2 days. An additional method of contraception should be used for 7 days after missed dose.

Two consecutive doses missed in week 3 or three consecutive doses missed at any time: An additional method of contraception must be used for 7 days after a missed dose:

Schedule 1 (Sunday starter): Continue dose of 1 tablet daily until Sunday, then discard the rest of the pack, and a new pack should be started that same day.

Schedule 2 (Day 1 starter): Current pack should be discarded, and a new pack should be started that same day.

Missed doses **biphasic/triphasic formulations** (refer to package insert for complete information):

One dose missed: Take as soon as remembered or take 2 tablets next day.

Two consecutive doses missed in week 1 or week 2 of the pack: Take 2 tablets as soon as remembered and 2 tablets the next day. Resume taking 1 tablet daily until the pack is empty. An additional method of contraception should be used for 7 days after a missed dose.

Two consecutive doses missed in week 3 of the pack: An additional method of contraception must be used for 7 days after a missed dose.

Schedule 1 (Sunday starter): Take 1 tablet every day until Sunday. Discard the remaining pack and start a new pack of pills on the same day.

Schedule 2 (Day 1 starter): Discard the remaining pack and start a new pack the same day.

Three or more consecutive doses missed: An additional method of contraception must be used for 7 days after a missed dose.

Schedule 1 (Sunday starter): Take 1 tablet every day until Sunday; on Sunday, discard the pack and start a new pack.

Schedule 2 (Day 1 starter): Discard the remaining pack and begin new pack of tablets starting on the same day.

Contraception, 91-day cycle (extended cycle regimen): Dose begins on first Sunday after onset of menstruation; if the menstrual period starts on Sunday, take first tablet that very same day. An additional method of contraception should be used until after the first 7 days of consecutive administration:

Seasonale®: One active tablet/day for 84 consecutive days, followed by 1 inactive tablet/day for 7 days; if all doses have been taken on schedule and one menstrual period is missed, pregnancy should be ruled out prior to continuing therapy.

Seasonique™: One active tablet/day for 84 consecutive days, followed by 1 low dose estrogen tablet/day for 7 days; if all doses have been taken on schedule and one menstrual period is missed, pregnancy should be ruled out prior to continuing therapy.

Missed doses:

One dose missed: Take as soon as remembered or take 2 tablets the next day

Two consecutive doses missed: Take 2 tablets as soon as remembered or 2 tablets the next 2 days. An additional nonhormonal method of contraception should be used for 7 consecutive days after the missed dose.

Three or more consecutive doses missed: Do not take the missed doses; continue taking 1 tablet/day until pack is complete. Bleeding may occur during the following week. An additional nonhormonal method of contraception should be used for 7 consecutive days after the missed dose.

Any number of pills during week 13: Throw away the missed pills and keep taking scheduled pills until the pack is finished. A backup method of contraception is not needed

Contraception, continuous use (extended cycle regimen): Lybrel™: Take one tablet daily, at the same time each day, without a tablet-free interval. Therapy should be initiated as follows:

No previous contraception: Begin on the first day of menstrual cycle. Backup contraception is not needed.

Previously taking a 21-day or 28-day combination hormonal contraceptive: Begin on day 1 of the withdrawal bleed (at the latest, 7 days after the last active tablet). Backup contraception is not needed.

Previously using a progestin-only pill: Begin the day after taking a progestin only pill. Backup contraception is needed for the first 7 days of therapy.

Previously using contraceptive implant: Begin the day of implant removal. Backup contraception is needed for the first 7 days of therapy.

Previously using contraceptive injection: Begin when the next injection is due. Backup contraception is needed for the first 7 days of therapy.

Missed doses:

One dose missed: Take as soon as remembered then take the next tablet at the regular time (2 tablets in 1 day). An additional nonhormonal method of contraception should also be used for 7 consecutive days.

Two consecutive doses missed: If remembered the day of the second missed tablet, take 2 tablets as soon as remembered, then 1 tablet the next day. If remembered the day after the second tablet is missed, take 2 tablets the day remembered, then 2 tablets the next day. An additional nonhormonal method of contraception should also be used for 7 consecutive days.

Three or more consecutive doses missed: Take 1 tablet daily and contact healthcare provider; do not take the missed pills. An additional nonhormonal method of contraception should also be used for 7 consecutive days.

Dosage Forms

Tablet, low-dose formulations:

Alesse® 28: Ethinyl estradiol 0.02 mg and levonorgestrel 0.1 mg (28s) [21 pink tablets and 7 light green inactive tablets]

Aviane™ 28: Ethinyl estradiol 0.02 mg and levonorgestrel 0.1 mg (28s) [21 orange tablets and 7 light green inactive tablets]

Lessina™ 28, Levlite™ 28: Ethinyl estradiol 0.02 mg and levonorgestrel 0.1 mg (28s) [21 pink tablets and 7 white inactive tablets]

Lutera™, Sronyx™: Ethinyl estradiol 0.02 mg and levonorgestrel 0.1 mg (28s) [21 white tablets and 7 peach inactive tablets]

Lybrel™: Ethinyl estradiol 0.02 mg and levonorgestrel 0.09 mg (28s) [28 yellow tablets]

Tablet, monophasic formulations:

Levlen® 28: Ethinyl estradiol 0.03 mg and levonorgestrel 0.15 mg (28s) [21 light orange tablets and 7 pink inactive tablets]

Levora® 28: Ethinyl estradiol 0.03 mg and levonorgestrel 0.15 mg (28s) [21 white tablets and 7 peach inactive tablets]

Nordette® 28: Ethinyl estradiol 0.03 mg and levonorgestrel 0.15 mg (28s) [21 light orange tablets and 7 pink inactive tablets]

Portia™ 28: Ethinyl estradiol 0.03 mg and levonorgestrel 0.15 mg (28s) [21 pink tablets and 7 white inactive tablets]

Tablet, monophasic formulations [extended cycle regimen]:

Jolessa™, Seasonale®: Ethinyl estradiol 0.03 mg and levonorgestrel 0.15 mg (91s) [84 pink tablets and 7 white inactive tablets]

Quasense™: Ethinyl estradiol 0.03 mg and levonorgestrel 0.15 mg] (91s) [84 white tablets and 7 peach inactive tablets

Seasonique™: Ethinyl estradiol 0.03 mg and levonorgestrel 0.15 mg (91s) [84 light blue-green tablets] and ethinyl estradiol 0.01 mg [7 yellow tablets]

Tablet, triphasic formulations:

Enpresse™:

Day 1-6: Ethinyl estradiol 0.03 mg and levonorgestrel 0.05 mg [6 pink tablets]

Day 7-11: Ethinyl estradiol 0.04 mg and levonorgestrel 0.075 mg [5 white tablets]

Day 12-21: Ethinyl estradiol 0.03 mg and levonorgestrel 0.125 mg [10 orange tablets]

Day 22-28: 7 light green inactive tablets (28s)

Triphasil® 28:

Day 1-6: Ethinyl estradiol 0.03 mg and levonorgestrel 0.05 mg [6 brown tablets]

Day 7-11: Ethinyl estradiol 0.04 mg and levonorgestrel 0.075 mg [5 white tablets]
Day 12-21: Ethinyl estradiol 0.03 mg and levonorgestrel 0.125 mg [10 light yellow tablets]
Day 22-28: 7 light green inactive tablets (28s)
Trivora® 28:
Day 1-6: Ethinyl estradiol 0.03 mg and levonorgestrel 0.05 mg [6 blue tablets]
Day 7-11: Ethinyl estradiol 0.04 mg and levonorgestrel 0.075 mg [5 white tablets]
Day 12-21: Ethinyl estradiol 0.03 mg and levonorgestrel 0.125 mg [10 pink tablets]
Day 22-28: 7 peach inactive tablets (28s)

ethinyl estradiol and NGM *see* ethinyl estradiol and norgestimate *on page 378*

ethinyl estradiol and norelgestromin (ETH in il es tra DYE ole & nor el JES troe min)

Synonyms norelgestromin and ethinyl estradiol

U.S./Canadian Brand Names Evra® [Can]; Ortho Evra® [US]

Therapeutic Category Contraceptive, Oral; Estrogen and Progestin Combination

Use Prevention of pregnancy

Usual Dosage Topical: Adults: Females:

Contraception: Apply one patch each week for 3 weeks (21 total days); followed by one week that is patch-free. Each patch should be applied on the same day each week ("patch change day") and only one patch should be worn at a time. No more than 7 days should pass during the patch-free interval.

Schedule 1 (Sunday starter): Dose begins on first Sunday after onset of menstruation; if the menstrual period starts on Sunday, apply one patch that very same day. **With a Sunday start, an additional method of contraception (nonhormonal) should be used until after the first 7 days of consecutive administration.** Each patch change will then occur on Sunday.

Schedule 2 (Day 1 starter): Dose starts on first day of menstrual cycle, applying one patch during the first 24 hours of menstrual cycle. No backup method of contraception is needed as long as the patch is applied on the first day of cycle. Each patch change will then occur on that same day of the week.

Additional dosing considerations:

No bleeding during patch-free week/missed menstrual period: If patch has been applied as directed, continue treatment on usual "patch change day". If used correctly, no bleeding during patch-free week does not necessarily indicate pregnancy. However, if no withdrawal bleeding occurs for 2 consecutive cycles, pregnancy should be ruled out. If patch has not been applied as directed, and one menstrual period is missed, pregnancy should be ruled out prior to continuing treatment.

If a patch becomes partially or completely detached for <24 hours: Try to reapply to same place, or replace with a new patch immediately. Do not reapply if patch is no longer sticky, if it is sticking to itself or another surface, or if it has material sticking to it.

If a patch becomes partially or completely detached for >24 hours (or time period is unknown): Apply a new patch and use this day of the week as the new "patch change day" from this point on. **An additional method of contraception (nonhormonal) should be used until after the first 7 days of consecutive administration.**

Switching from oral contraceptives: Apply first patch on the first day of withdrawal bleeding. If there is no bleeding within 5 days of taking the last active tablet, pregnancy must first be ruled out. If patch is applied later than the first day of bleeding, **an additional method of contraception (nonhormonal) should be used until after the first 7 days of consecutive administration**

Use after childbirth: Therapy should not be started <4 weeks after childbirth. Pregnancy should be ruled out prior to treatment if menstrual periods have not restarted. **An additional method of contraception (nonhormonal) should be used until after the first 7 days of consecutive administration.**

Use after abortion or miscarriage: Therapy may be started immediately if abortion/miscarriage occur within the first trimester. If therapy is not started within 5 days, follow instructions for first time use. If abortion/miscarriage occur during the second trimester, therapy should not be started for at least 4 weeks. Follow directions for use after childbirth.

Dosage Forms The Canadian formulation differs from the U.S. product in both composition and manufacturing process (although delivery rates appear similar). [CAN] = Canadian brand name.

Patch, transdermal:

Evra® [CAN]: Ethinyl estradiol 0.6 mg and norelgestromin 6 mg [releases ethinyl estradiol 20 mcg and norelgestromin 150 mcg per day] (1s, 3s) [not available in the U.S.]

Ortho Evra®: Ethinyl estradiol 0.75 mg and norelgestromin 6 mg [releases ethinyl estradiol 20 mcg and norelgestromin 150 mcg per day] (1s, 3s)

ethinyl estradiol and norethindrone (ETH in il es tra DYE ole & nor eth IN drone)

Sound-Alike/Look-Alike Issues
femhrt® may be confused with Femara®
Modicon® may be confused with Mylicon®
Norinyl® may be confused with Nardil®
Tri-Norinyl® may be confused with Triphasil®

Synonyms norethindrone acetate and ethinyl estradiol

U.S./Canadian Brand Names Aranelle™ [US]; Balziva™ [US]; Brevicon® 0.5/35 [Can]; Brevicon® 1/35 [Can]; Brevicon® [US]; Estrostep® Fe [US]; Femcon™ Fe [US]; femhrt® [US/Can]; Junel™ Fe [US]; Junel™ [US]; Leena™ [US]; Loestrin® 24 Fe [US]; Loestrin® Fe [US]; Loestrin® [US]; Loestrin™ 1.5/30 [Can]; Microgestin™ Fe [US]; Microgestin™ [US]; Minestrin™ 1/20 [Can]; Modicon® [US]; Necon® 0.5/35 [US]; Necon® 1/35 [US]; Necon® 10/11 [US]; Necon® 7/7/7 [US]; Norinyl® 1+35 [US]; Nortrel™ 7/7/7 [US]; Nortrel™ [US]; Ortho-Novum® [US]; Ortho® 0.5/35 [Can]; Ortho® 1/35 [Can]; Ortho® 7/7/7 [Can]; Ovcon® [US]; Select™ 1/35 [Can]; Synphasic® [Can]; Tilia™ Fe [US]; Tri-Norinyl® [US]; Zenchent™ [US]

Therapeutic Category Contraceptive, Oral

Use Prevention of pregnancy; treatment of acne; moderate-to-severe vasomotor symptoms associated with menopause; prevention of osteoporosis (in women at significant risk only)

Usual Dosage Oral:

Adolescents ≥15 years and Adults: Females: Acne: Estrostep® Fe: Refer to dosing for contraception

Adults: Females:
Moderate-to-severe vasomotor symptoms associated with menopause: Initial: femhrt® 0.5/2.5: 1 tablet daily; patient should be re-evaluated at 3- to 6-month intervals to determine if treatment is still necessary; patient should be maintained at the lowest effective dose

Prevention of osteoporosis: Initial: femhrt® 0.5/2.5: 1 tablet daily; patient should be maintained on the lowest effective dose

Contraception:
Schedule 1 (Sunday starter): Dose begins on first Sunday after onset of menstruation; if the menstrual period starts on Sunday, take first tablet that very same day. With a Sunday start, an additional method of contraception should be used until after the first 7 days of consecutive administration.
For 21-tablet package: Dosage is 1 tablet daily for 21 consecutive days, followed by 7 days off of the medication; a new course begins on the 8th day after the last tablet is taken.
For 28-tablet package: Dosage is 1 tablet daily without interruption.
Schedule 2 (Day 1 starter): Dose starts on first day of menstrual cycle taking 1 tablet daily.
For 21-tablet package: Dosage is 1 tablet daily for 21 consecutive days, followed by 7 days off the medication; a new course begins on the 8th day after the last tablet is taken.
For 28-tablet package: Dosage is 1 tablet daily without interruption.
If all doses have been taken on schedule and one menstrual period is missed, continue dosing cycle. If two consecutive menstrual periods are missed, pregnancy test is required before new dosing cycle is started.
Missed doses **monophasic formulations** (refer to package insert for complete information):
One dose missed: Take as soon as remembered or take 2 tablets next day Two consecutive doses missed in the first 2 weeks: Take 2 tablets as soon as remembered or 2 tablets next 2 days. An additional method of contraception should be used for 7 days after missed dose.
Two consecutive doses missed in week 3 or three consecutive doses missed at any time: An additional method of contraception must be used for 7 days after a missed dose.
Schedule 1 (Sunday starter): Continue dose of 1 tablet daily until Sunday, then discard the rest of the pack, and a new pack should be started that same day.
Schedule 2 (Day 1 starter): Current pack should be discarded, and a new pack should be started that same day.
Missed doses **biphasic/triphasic formulations** (refer to package insert for complete information):
One dose missed: Take as soon as remembered or take 2 tablets next day.
Two consecutive doses missed in week 1 or week 2 of the pack: Take 2 tablets as soon as remembered and 2 tablets the next day. Resume taking 1 tablet daily until the pack is empty. An additional method of contraception should be used for 7 days after a missed dose.
Two consecutive doses missed in week 3 of the pack: An additional method of contraception must be used for 7 days after a missed dose.
Schedule 1 (Sunday Starter): Take 1 tablet every day until Sunday. Discard the remaining pack and start a new pack of pills on the same day.
Schedule 2 (Day 1 starter): Discard the remaining pack and start a new pack the same day.

Three or more consecutive doses missed: An additional method of contraception must be used for 7 days after a missed dose.

Schedule 1 (Sunday Starter): Take 1 tablet every day until Sunday; on Sunday, discard the pack and start a new pack.

Schedule 2 (Day 1 Starter): Discard the remaining pack and begin new pack of tablets starting on the same day.

Dosage Forms

Tablet:

femhrt®: 1/5: Ethinyl estradiol 5 mcg and norethindrone 1 mg [white tablets]; 0.5/2.5: Ethinyl estradiol 2.5 mcg and norethindrone 0.5 mg [white tablets]

Tablet, monophasic formulations:

Balziva™: Ethinyl estradiol 0.035 mg and norethindrone 0.4 mg (28s) [21 light peach tablets and 7 white inactive tablets]

Brevicon®: Ethinyl estradiol 0.035 mg and norethindrone 0.5 mg (28s) [21 blue tablets and 7 orange inactive tablets]

Junel™ 21 1/20: Ethinyl estradiol 0.02 mg and norethindrone 1 mg (21s) [yellow tablets]

Junel™ 21 1.5/30: Ethinyl estradiol 0.03 mg and norethindrone 1.5 mg (21s) [pink tablets]

Junel™ Fe 1/20: Ethinyl estradiol 0.02 mg and norethindrone 1 mg (28s) [21 yellow tablets] and ferrous fumarate 75 mg [7 brown tablets]

Junel™ Fe 1.5/30: Ethinyl estradiol 0.03 mg and norethindrone 1.5 mg (28s) [21 pink tablets] and ferrous fumarate 75 mg [7 brown tablets]

Loestrin® 21 1/20, Microgestin™ 1/20: Ethinyl estradiol 0.02 mg and norethindrone 1 mg (21s) [white tablets]

Loestrin® 21 1.5/30, Microgestin™ 1.5/30: Ethinyl estradiol 0.03 mg and norethindrone 1.5 mg (21s) [green tablets]

Loestrin® 24 Fe: 1/20: Ethinyl estradiol 0.02 mg and norethindrone acetate 1 mg (28s) [24 white tablets] and ferrous fumarate 75 mg [4 brown tablets]

Loestrin® Fe 1/20, Microgestin™ Fe 1/20: Ethinyl estradiol 0.02 mg and norethindrone 1 mg (28s) [21 white tablets] and ferrous fumarate 75 mg [7 brown tablets]

Loestrin® Fe 1.5/30, Microgestin™ Fe 1.5/30: Ethinyl estradiol 0.03 mg and norethindrone 1.5 mg (28s) [21 green tablets] and ferrous fumarate 75 mg [7 brown tablets]

Modicon® 28: Ethinyl estradiol 0.035 mg and norethindrone 0.5 mg (28s) [21 white tablets and 7 green inactive tablets]

Necon® 0.5/35-28: Ethinyl estradiol 0.035 mg and norethindrone 0.5 mg (28s) [21 light yellow tablets and 7 white inactive tablets]

Necon® 1/35-28: Ethinyl estradiol 0.035 mg and norethindrone 1 mg (28s) [21 dark yellow tablets and 7 white inactive tablets]

Norinyl® 1+35: Ethinyl estradiol 0.035 mg and norethindrone 1 mg (28s) [21 yellow-green tablets and 7 orange inactive tablets]

Nortrel™ 0.5/35 mg:

Ethinyl estradiol 0.035 mg and norethindrone 0.5 mg (21s) [light yellow tablets]

Ethinyl estradiol 0.035 mg and norethindrone 0.5 mg (28s) [21 light yellow tablets and 7 white inactive tablets]

Nortrel™ 1/35 mg:

Ethinyl estradiol 0.035 mg and norethindrone 1 mg (21s) [yellow tablets]

Ethinyl estradiol 0.035 mg and norethindrone 1 mg (21s) [21 yellow tablets and 7 white inactive tablets]

Ortho-Novum® 1/35 28: Ethinyl estradiol 0.035 mg and norethindrone 1 mg (28s) [21 peach tablets and 7 green inactive tablets]

Ovcon® 35 21-day: Ethinyl estradiol 0.035 mg and norethindrone 0.4 mg (21s) [peach tablets]

Ovcon® 35 28-day: Ethinyl estradiol 0.035 mg and norethindrone 0.4 mg (28s) [21 peach tablets and 7 green inactive tablets]

Ovcon® 50: Ethinyl estradiol 0.05 mg and norethindrone 1 mg (28s) [21 yellow tablets and 7 green inactive tablets]

Zenchent™: Ethinyl estradiol 0.035 mg and norethindrone 0.4 mg (28s) [21 light peach tablets and 7 white inactive tablets]

Tablet, chewable, monophasic formulations:

Femcon™ Fe: Ethinyl estradiol 0.035 mg and norethindrone 0.4 mg (28s) [21 white tablets and 7 brown inactive tablets] [spearmint flavor]

Tablet, biphasic formulations:

Necon® 10/11-28:

Day 1-10: Ethinyl estradiol 0.035 mg and norethindrone 0.5 mg [10 light yellow tablets]

◀ Day 11-21: Ethinyl estradiol 0.035 mg and norethindrone 1 mg [11 dark yellow tablets]
Day 22-28: 7 white inactive tablets (28s)
Ortho-Novum® 10/11-28:
  Day 1-10: Ethinyl estradiol 0.035 mg and norethindrone 0.5 mg [10 white tablets]
  Day 11-21: Ethinyl estradiol 0.035 mg and norethindrone 1 mg [11 peach tablets]
  Day 22-28: 7 green inactive tablets (28s)

Tablet, triphasic formulations:
Aranelle™:
  Day 1-7: Ethinyl estradiol 0.035 mg and norethindrone 0.5 mg [7 light yellow tablets]
  Day 8-16: Ethinyl estradiol 0.035 mg and norethindrone 1 mg [9 white tablets]
  Day 17-21: Ethinyl estradiol 0.035 mg and norethindrone 0.5 mg [5 light yellow tablets]
  Day 22-28: 7 peach inactive tablets (28s)
Estrostep® Fe:
  Day 1-5: Ethinyl estradiol 0.02 mg and norethindrone 1 mg [5 white triangular tablets]
  Day 6-12: Ethinyl estradiol 0.03 mg and norethindrone 1 mg [7 white square tablets]
  Day 13-21: Ethinyl estradiol 0.035 mg and norethindrone 1 mg [9 white round tablets]
  Day 22-28: Ferrous fumarate 75 mg [7 brown tablets] (28s)
Leena™:
  Day 1-7: Ethinyl estradiol 0.035 mg and norethindrone 0.5 mg [7 light blue tablets]
  Day 8-16: Ethinyl estradiol 0.035 mg and norethindrone 1 mg [9 light yellow-green tablets]
  Day 17-21: Ethinyl estradiol 0.035 mg and norethindrone 0.5 mg [5 light blue tablets]
  Day 22-28: 7 orange inactive tablets (28s)
Necon® 7/7/7, Ortho-Novum® 7/7/7 28:
  Day 1-7: Ethinyl estradiol 0.035 mg and norethindrone 0.5 mg [7 white tablets]
  Day 8-14: Ethinyl estradiol 0.035 mg and norethindrone 0.75 mg [7 light peach tablets]
  Day 15-21: Ethinyl estradiol 0.035 mg and norethindrone 1 mg [7 peach tablets]
  Day 22-28: 7 green inactive tablets (28s)
Nortrel™ 7/7/7 28:
  Day 1-7: Ethinyl estradiol 0.035 mg and norethindrone 0.5 mg [7 light yellow tablets]
  Day 8-14: Ethinyl estradiol 0.035 mg and norethindrone 0.75 mg [7 blue tablets]
  Day 15-21: Ethinyl estradiol 0.035 mg and norethindrone 1 mg [7 peach tablets]
  Day 22-28: 7 white inactive tablets (28s)
Ortho-Novum® 7/7/7 28:
  Day 1-7: Ethinyl estradiol 0.035 mg and norethindrone 0.5 mg [7 white tablets]
  Day 8-14: Ethinyl estradiol 0.035 mg and norethindrone 0.75 mg [7 light peach tablets]
  Day 15-21: Ethinyl estradiol 0.035 mg and norethindrone 1 mg [7 peach tablets]
  Day 22-28: 7 green inactive tablets (28s)
Tilia™ Fe:
  Day 1-5: Ethinyl estradiol 0.02 mg and norethindrone acetate 1 mg [5 white triangular tablets]
  Day 6-12: Ethinyl estradiol 0.03 mg and norethindrone acetate 1 mg [7 white square tablets]
  Day 13-21: Ethinyl estradiol 0.035 mg and norethindrone acetate 1 mg [9 white round tablets]
  Day 22-28: Ferrous fumarate 75 mg [7 brown tablets] (28s)
Tri-Norinyl® 28:
  Day 1-7: Ethinyl estradiol 0.035 mg and norethindrone 0.5 mg [7 blue tablets]
  Day 8-16: Ethinyl estradiol 0.035 mg and norethindrone 1 mg [9 yellow-green tablets]
  Day 17-21: Ethinyl estradiol 0.035 mg and norethindrone 0.5 mg [5 blue tablets]
  Day 22-28: 7 orange inactive tablets (28s)

ethinyl estradiol and norgestimate (ETH in il es tra DYE ole & nor JES ti mate)

Sound-Alike/Look-Alike Issues
Ortho-Cyclen® may be confused with Ortho-Cept®

Synonyms ethinyl estradiol and NGM; norgestimate and ethinyl estradiol

U.S./Canadian Brand Names Cyclen® [Can]; MonoNessa™ [US]; Ortho Tri-Cyclen® Lo [US]; Ortho Tri-Cyclen® [US]; Ortho-Cyclen® [US]; Previfem™ [US]; Sprintec™ [US]; Tri-Cyclen® Lo [Can]; Tri-Cyclen® [Can]; Tri-Previfem™ [US]; Tri-Sprintec™ [US]; TriNessa™ [US]

Therapeutic Category Contraceptive, Oral

Use Prevention of pregnancy; treatment of acne

Usual Dosage Oral:
  Children ≥15 years and Adults: Females: Acne (Ortho Tri-Cyclen®): Refer to dosing for contraception

Adults: Females:
Contraception:
  Schedule 1 (Sunday starter): Dose begins on first Sunday after onset of menstruation; if the menstrual period starts on Sunday, take first tablet that very same day. **With a Sunday start, an additional method of contraception should be used until after the first 7 days of consecutive administration.**
    For 21-tablet package: Dosage is 1 tablet daily for 21 consecutive days, followed by 7 days off of the medication; a new course begins on the 8th day after the last tablet is taken.
    For 28-tablet package: Dosage is 1 tablet daily without interruption.
  Schedule 2 (Day 1 starter): Dose starts on first day of menstrual cycle taking 1 tablet daily.
    For 21-tablet package: Dosage is 1 tablet daily for 21 consecutive days, followed by 7 days off of the medication; a new course begins on the 8th day after the last tablet is taken.
    For 28-tablet package: Dosage is 1 tablet daily without interruption.
  If all doses have been taken on schedule and one menstrual period is missed, continue dosing cycle. If two consecutive menstrual periods are missed, pregnancy test is required before new dosing cycle is started.
  Missed doses **monophasic formulations** (refer to package insert for complete information):
    One dose missed: Take as soon as remembered or take 2 tablets next day
    Two consecutive doses missed in the first 2 weeks: Take 2 tablets as soon as remembered or 2 tablets next 2 days. **An additional method of contraception should be used for 7 days after missed dose.**
    Two consecutive doses missed in week 3 or three consecutive doses missed at any time: **An additional method of contraception must be used for 7 days after a missed dose:**
      Schedule 1 (Sunday starter): Continue dose of 1 tablet daily until Sunday, then discard the rest of the pack, and a new pack should be started that same day.
      Schedule 2 (Day 1 starter): Current pack should be discarded, and a new pack should be started that same day.
  Missed doses **biphasic/triphasic formulations** (refer to package insert for complete information):
    One dose missed: Take as soon as remembered or take 2 tablets next day.
    Two consecutive doses missed in week 1 or week 2 of the pack: Take 2 tablets as soon as remembered and 2 tablets the next day. Resume taking 1 tablet daily until the pack is empty. **An additional method of contraception must be used for 7 days after a missed dose.**
    Two consecutive doses missed in week 3 of the pack. **An additional method of contraception must be used for 7 days after a missed dose.**
      Schedule 1 (Sunday starter): Take 1 tablet every day until Sunday. Discard the remaining pack and start a new pack of pills on the same day.
      Schedule 2 (Day 1 starter): Discard the remaining pack and start a new pack the same day.
    Three or more consecutive doses missed. **An additional method of contraception must be used for 7 days after a missed dose.**
      Schedule 1 (Sunday starter): Take 1 tablet every day until Sunday; on Sunday, discard the pack and start a new pack.
      Schedule 2 (Day 1 starter): Discard the remaining pack and begin new pack of tablets starting on the same day.

Dosage Forms
Tablet, monophasic formulations:
MonoNessa™, Ortho-Cyclen®: Ethinyl estradiol 0.035 mg and norgestimate 0.25 mg (28s) [21 blue tablets and 7 green inactive tablets]
Previfem™: Ethinyl estradiol 0.035 mg and norgestimate 0.25 mg (28s) [21 blue tablets and 7 teal inactive tablets]
Sprintec™: Ethinyl estradiol 0.035 mg and norgestimate 0.25 mg (28s) [21 blue tablets and 7 white inactive tablets]

Tablet, triphasic formulations:
Ortho Tri-Cyclen®, TriNessa™:
  Day 1-7: Ethinyl estradiol 0.035 mg and norgestimate 0.18 mg [7 white tablets]
  Day 8-14: Ethinyl estradiol 0.035 mg and norgestimate 0.215 mg [7 light blue tablets]
  Day 15-21: Ethinyl estradiol 0.035 mg and norgestimate 0.25 mg [7 blue tablets]
  Day 22-28: 7 green inactive tablets (28s)
Tri-Previfem™:
  Day 1-7: Ethinyl estradiol 0.035 mg and norgestimate 0.18 mg [7 white tablets]
  Day 8-14: Ethinyl estradiol 0.035 mg and norgestimate 0.215 mg [7 light blue tablets]
  Day 15-21: Ethinyl estradiol 0.035 mg and norgestimate 0.25 mg [7 blue tablets]
  Day 22-28: 7 teal inactive tablets (28s)

Tri-Sprintec™:
Day 1-7: Ethinyl estradiol 0.035 mg and norgestimate 0.18 mg [7 gray tablets]
Day 8-14: Ethinyl estradiol 0.035 mg and norgestimate 0.215 mg [7 light blue tablets]
Day 15-21: Ethinyl estradiol 0.035 mg and norgestimate 0.25 mg [7 blue tablets]
Day 22-28: 7 white inactive tablets (28s)
Ortho Tri-Cyclen® Lo:
Day 1-7: Ethinyl estradiol 0.025 mg and norgestimate 0.18 mg [7 white tablets]
Day 8-14: Ethinyl estradiol 0.025 mg and norgestimate 0.215 mg [7 light blue tablets]
Day 15-21: Ethinyl estradiol 0.025 mg and norgestimate 0.25 mg [7 dark blue tablets]
Day 22-28: 7 green inactive tablets (28s)

ethinyl estradiol and norgestrel (ETH in il es tra DYE ole & nor JES trel)

Synonyms morning after pill; norgestrel and ethinyl estradiol

U.S./Canadian Brand Names Cryselle™ [US]; Lo/Ovral® [US]; Low-Ogestrel® [US]; Ogestrel® [US]; Ovral® [Can]

Therapeutic Category Contraceptive, Oral

Use Prevention of pregnancy; postcoital contraceptive or "morning after" pill

Usual Dosage Oral: Adults: Females:
Contraception:
Schedule 1 (Sunday starter): Dose begins on first Sunday after onset of menstruation; if the menstrual period starts on Sunday, take first tablet that very same day. **With a Sunday start, an additional method of contraception should be used until after the first 7 days of consecutive administration.**
For 21-tablet package: Dosage is 1 tablet daily for 21 consecutive days, followed by 7 days off of the medication; a new course begins on the 8th day after the last tablet is taken.
For 28-tablet package: Dosage is 1 tablet daily without interruption.
Schedule 2 (Day 1 starter): Dose starts on first day of menstrual cycle taking 1 tablet daily.
For 21-tablet package: Dosage is 1 tablet daily for 21 consecutive days, followed by 7 days off of the medication; a new course begins on the 8th day after the last tablet is taken.
For 28-tablet package: Dosage is 1 tablet daily without interruption.
If all doses have been taken on schedule and one menstrual period is missed, continue dosing cycle. If two consecutive menstrual periods are missed, pregnancy test is required before new dosing cycle is started.
Missed doses **monophasic formulations** (refer to package insert for complete information):
One dose missed: Take as soon as remembered or take 2 tablets next day
Two consecutive doses missed in the first 2 weeks: Take 2 tablets as soon as remembered or 2 tablets next 2 days. **An additional method of contraception should be used for 7 days after missed dose.**
Two consecutive doses missed in week 3 or three consecutive doses missed at any time:
Schedule 1 (Sunday starter): Continue to take 1 tablet daily until Sunday, then discard the rest of the pack, and a new pack is started that same day.
Schedule 2 (Day 1 starter): Current pack should be discarded, and a new pack started that same day.
An additional method of contraception should be used for 7 days after missed dose.

Postcoital contraception:
Ethinyl estradiol 0.03 mg and norgestrel 0.3 mg formulation: 4 tablets within 72 hours of unprotected intercourse and 4 tablets 12 hours after first dose
Ethinyl estradiol 0.05 mg and norgestrel 0.5 mg formulation: 2 tablets within 72 hours of unprotected intercourse and 2 tablets 12 hours after first dose

Dosage Forms

Tablet, monophasic formulations:
Cryselle™: Ethinyl estradiol 0.03 mg and norgestrel 0.3 mg [21 white tablets and 7 light green inactive tablets] (28s)
Low-Ogestrel® 28: Ethinyl estradiol 0.03 mg and norgestrel 0.3 mg [21 white tablets and 7 peach inactive tablets] (28s)
Lo/Ovral® 28: Ethinyl estradiol 0.03 mg and norgestrel 0.3 mg [21 white tablets and 7 pink inactive tablets] (28s)
Ogestrel® 28: Ethinyl estradiol 0.05 mg and norgestrel 0.5 mg [21 white tablets and 7 peach inactive tablets] (28s)

ethiofos see amifostine on page 58

ethionamide (e thye on AM ide)

U.S./Canadian Brand Names Trecator® [US/Can]
Therapeutic Category Antimycobacterial Agent

Use Treatment of tuberculosis and other mycobacterial diseases, in conjunction with other antituberculosis agents, when first-line agents have failed or resistance has been demonstrated

Usual Dosage Oral:

Children: 15-20 mg/kg/day in 2-3 divided doses, not to exceed 1 g/day

Adults: 15-20 mg/kg/day; initiate dose at 250 mg/day for 1-2 days, then increase to 250 mg twice daily for 1-2 days, with gradual increases to highest tolerated dose; average adult dose: 750 mg/day (maximum: 1 g/day in 3-4 divided doses)

Dosage Forms

Tablet:

Trecator®: 250 mg

Ethmozine® [Can] *see* moricizine *on page 643*

Ethmozine® (Discontinued) *see* moricizine *on page 643*

ethosuximide (eth oh SUKS i mide)

Sound-Alike/Look-Alike Issues

ethosuximide may be confused with methsuximide

Zarontin® may be confused with Xalatan®, Zantac®, Zaroxolyn®

U.S./Canadian Brand Names Zarontin® [US/Can]

Therapeutic Category Anticonvulsant

Use Management of absence (petit mal) seizures

Usual Dosage Oral:

Children 3-6 years: Initial: 250 mg/day; increase every 4-7 days; usual maintenance dose: 20 mg/kg/day; maximum dose: 1.5 g/day in divided doses

Children >6 years and Adults: Initial: 500 mg/day; increase by 250 mg as needed every 4-7 days, up to 1.5 g/day in divided doses; usual maintenance dose for most pediatric patients is 20 mg/kg/day.

Dosage Forms

Capsule: 250 mg

Zarontin®: 250 mg

Syrup: 250 mg/5 mL

Zarontin®: 250 mg/5 mL

ethotoin (ETH oh toyn)

Synonyms ethylphenylhydantoin

U.S./Canadian Brand Names Peganone® [US/Can]

Therapeutic Category Hydantoin

Use Generalized tonic-clonic or complex-partial seizures

Usual Dosage Oral: **Note:** Administer in 4-6 divided doses daily; titrate over several days based on patient response

Children ≥1 year: Maximum initial dose: 750 mg/day; usual maintenance dose: 0.5-1 g/day; maximum dose: 3 g/day

Adults: Initial dose: ≤1 g/day; usual maintenance dose: 2-3 g/day

Dosage Forms

Tablet:

Peganone®: 250 mg

ETH-Oxydose™ [US] *see* oxycodone *on page 709*

ethoxynaphthamido penicillin sodium *see* nafcillin *on page 652*

Ethrane® [US] *see* enflurane *on page 340*

ethyl alcohol *see* alcohol (ethyl) *on page 41*

ethyl aminobenzoate *see* benzocaine *on page 124*

ethyl chloride (ETH il KLOR ide)

Synonyms chloroethane

U.S./Canadian Brand Names Gebauer's Ethyl Chloride® [US]

Therapeutic Category Local Anesthetic

Use Local anesthetic in minor operative procedures and to relieve pain caused by insect stings and burns, and irritation caused by myofascial and visceral pain syndromes

◄ **Usual Dosage** Dosage varies with use
Dosage Forms
Aerosol:
Gebauer's Ethyl Chloride®: 100% (103 mL)

ethyl chloride and dichlorotetrafluoroethane
(ETH il KLOR ide & dye klor oh te tra floo or oh ETH ane)
Synonyms dichlorotetrafluoroethane and ethyl chloride
U.S./Canadian Brand Names Fluro-Ethyl® [US]
Therapeutic Category Local Anesthetic
Use Topical refrigerant anesthetic to control pain associated with minor surgical procedures, dermabrasion, injections, contusions, and minor strains
Usual Dosage Press gently on side of spray valve allowing the liquid to emerge as a fine mist approximately 2" to 4" from site of application
Dosage Forms
Aerosol:
Fluro-Ethyl®: Ethyl chloride 25% and dichlorotetrafluoroethane 75% (148 mL)

ethyl esters of omega-3 fatty acids *see* omega-3-acid ethyl esters *on page 697*
ethylphenylhydantoin *see* ethotoin *on page 381*
ethynodiol diacetate and ethinyl estradiol *see* ethinyl estradiol and ethynodiol diacetate *on page 371*
Ethyol® [US/Can] *see* amifostine *on page 58*
Etibi® [Can] *see* ethambutol *on page 368*

etidronate and calcium (e ti DROE nate & KAL see um)
Synonyms calcium carbonate and etidronate disodium
U.S./Canadian Brand Names Didrocal™ [Can]
Therapeutic Category Bisphosphonate Derivative; Calcium Salt
Use Treatment and prevention of postmenopausal osteoporosis; prevention of corticosteroid-induced osteoporosis
Usual Dosage Note: 90-day treatment regimen involves sequential administration of two products within the packaging; not to be taken concurrently. The first blister card contains white tablets containing etidronate disodium, while the remaining four blister cards contains blue, capsule-shaped tablets containing calcium carbonate.
Oral: Adults: Etidronate disodium 400 mg once daily for 14 days, followed by calcium carbonate 1250 mg (500 mg elemental calcium) once daily for 76 days
Dosage Forms [CAN] = Canadian brand name
Combination package [each package contains five blister cards (90-day supply)]:
Didrocal™ [CAN; not available in the U.S.]
Tablet, etidronate: 400 mg (14s) [first card (white tablets)]
Tablet, calcium: 1250 mg (76s) [remaining cards (blue tablets)]

etidronate disodium (e ti DROE nate dye SOW dee um)
Sound-Alike/Look-Alike Issues
etidronate may be confused with etidocaine, etomidate, etretinate
Synonyms EHDP; sodium etidronate
U.S./Canadian Brand Names Didronel® [US/Can]; Gen-Etidronate [Can]
Therapeutic Category Bisphosphonate Derivative
Use Symptomatic treatment of Paget disease; prevention and treatment of heterotopic ossification due to spinal cord injury or after total hip replacement
Usual Dosage Oral: Adults:
Paget disease:
Initial: 5-10 mg/kg/day (not to exceed 6 months) or 11-20 mg/kg/day (not to exceed 3 months). Doses >20 mg/kg/day are **not** recommended.
Retreatment: Initiate only after etidronate-free period ≥90 days. Monitor patients every 3-6 months. Retreatment regimens are the same as for initial treatment.

Heterotopic ossification:
Caused by spinal cord injury: 20 mg/kg/day for 2 weeks, then 10 mg/kg/day for 10 weeks; total treatment period: 12 weeks
Complicating total hip replacement: 20 mg/kg/day for 1 month preoperatively then 20 mg/kg/day for 3 months postoperatively; total treatment period is 4 months

Dosage Forms
Tablet:
Didronel®: 200 mg, 400 mg

etodolac (ee toe DOE lak)

Sound-Alike/Look-Alike Issues
Lodine® may be confused with codeine, iodine, Iopidine®, Lopid®

Synonyms etodolic acid

U.S./Canadian Brand Names Apo-Etodolac® [Can]; Utradol™ [Can]

Therapeutic Category Analgesic, Nonnarcotic; Nonsteroidal Antiinflammatory Drug (NSAID)

Use Acute and long-term use in the management of signs and symptoms of osteoarthritis; rheumatoid arthritis and juvenile rheumatoid arthritis; management of acute pain

Usual Dosage Note: For chronic conditions, response is usually observed within 2 weeks.
Adults: Oral:
Acute pain: 200-400 mg every 6-8 hours, as needed, not to exceed total daily doses of 1000 mg
Rheumatoid arthritis, osteoarthritis: 400 mg 2 times/day **or** 300 mg 2-3 times/day **or** 500 mg 2 times/day (doses >1000 mg/day have not been evaluated)

Dosage Forms
Capsule: 200 mg, 300 mg
Tablet: 400 mg, 500 mg
Tablet, extended release: 400 mg, 500 mg, 600 mg

etodolic acid *see etodolac on page 383*
EtOH *see alcohol (ethyl) on page 41*

etomidate (e TOM i date)

Sound-Alike/Look-Alike Issues
etomidate may be confused with etidronate

U.S./Canadian Brand Names Amidate® [US/Can]

Therapeutic Category General Anesthetic

Use Induction and maintenance of general anesthesia

Usual Dosage I.V.: Children >10 years and Adults: Initial: 0.2-0.6 mg/kg over 30-60 seconds for induction of anesthesia; maintenance: 5-20 mcg/kg/minute

Dosage Forms
Injection, solution: 2 mg/mL (10 mL, 20 mL)
Amidate®: 2 mg/mL (10 mL, 20 mL)

etonogestrel (e toe noe JES trel)

Synonyms 3-keto-desogestrel; ENG

U.S./Canadian Brand Names Implanon™ [US]

Therapeutic Category Contraceptive; Progestin

Use Prevention of pregnancy; for use in women who request long-acting (up to 3 years) contraception

Usual Dosage
Children: Not for use prior to menarche.
Adults: Contraception: Subdermal: Implant 1 rod in the inner side of the upper, nondominant arm. Remove no later than 3 years after the date of insertion. After ruling out pregnancy, timing of insertion is based on the patient's contraceptive history:
No hormonal contraceptives within the past month: Insert between days 1 through 5 of menstruation, even if woman is still bleeding
Switching from combination hormonal contraceptive:
Oral tablet: Insert anytime within 7 days after the last active tablet
Vaginal ring: Insert anytime during the 7-day ring-free period
Transdermal system: Insert anytime during the 7-day patch-free period

▶

◄ Switching from a progestin-only contraceptive:
Oral pill: Any day during the month; do not skip days between the last pill and implant insertion
Implant: Insert on same day as removal of implant
IUD: Insert on same day as removal of IUD
Injection: Insert on day next injection is due
First trimester abortion or miscarriage: Insert immediately. If not inserted within first 5 days follow directions for "no hormonal contraception within the past month"
Following delivery or second trimester abortion: May insert between 21 and 28 days (if not exclusively breast-feeding) or after 4 weeks (if exclusively breast-feeding). Patients should use a second form of contraception for the first 7 days if insertion occurs at >4 weeks.
Note: If following above insertion schedule, no backup contraception needed. If deviating, use back-up method for 7 days postinsertion.
Dosage Forms
Rod, subdermal:
Implanon™: 68 mg

etonogestrel and ethinyl estradiol *see* ethinyl estradiol and etonogestrel *on page 372*
Etopophos® [US] *see* etoposide phosphate *on page 384*

etoposide (e toe POE side)
Sound-Alike/Look-Alike Issues
etoposide may be confused with teniposide
VePesid® may be confused with Versed
Synonyms epipodophyllotoxin; VP-16; VP-16-213
U.S./Canadian Brand Names Toposar® [US]; VePesid® [Can]
Therapeutic Category Antineoplastic Agent
Use Treatment of refractory testicular tumors; treatment of small cell lung cancer
Usual Dosage Refer to individual protocols:
Adults:
Small cell lung cancer (in combination with other approved chemotherapeutic drugs):
Oral: Due to poor bioavailability, oral doses should be twice the I.V. dose, rounded to the nearest 50 mg given once daily
I.V.: 35 mg/m^2/day for 4 days or 50 mg/m^2/day for 5 days every 3-4 weeks
IVPB: 60-100 mg/m^2/day for 3 days (with cisplatin)
CIV: 500 mg/m^2 over 24 hours every 3 weeks
Testicular cancer (in combination with other approved chemotherapeutic drugs):
IVPB: 50-100 mg/m^2/day for 5 days repeated every 3-4 weeks
I.V.: 100 mg/m^2 every other day for 3 doses repeated every 3-4 weeks
Dosage Forms
Capsule, softgel: 50 mg
Injection, solution: 20 mg/mL (5 mL, 25 mL, 50 mL)
Toposar®: 20 mg/mL (5 mL, 25 mL, 50 mL)

etoposide phosphate (e toe POE side FOS fate)
Sound-Alike/Look-Alike Issues
etoposide may be confused with teniposide
U.S./Canadian Brand Names Etopophos® [US]
Therapeutic Category Antineoplastic Agent
Use Treatment of refractory testicular tumors; treatment of small cell lung cancer
Usual Dosage Refer to individual protocols. Adults: **Note:** Etoposide phosphate is a prodrug of etoposide, doses should be expressed as the desired **ETOPOSIDE** dose; **not** as the etoposide phosphate dose. (eg, etoposide phosphate equivalent to ____ mg etoposide).
Small cell lung cancer (in combination with other approved chemotherapeutic drugs): I.V.: Etoposide 35 mg/m^2/day for 4 days to 50 mg/m^2/day for 5 days. Courses are repeated at 3- to 4-week intervals after adequate recovery from any toxicity.
Testicular cancer (in combination with other approved chemotherapeutic agents): I.V.: Etoposide 50-100 mg/m^2/day on days 1-5 to 100 mg/m^2/day on days 1, 3, and 5. Courses are repeated at 3- to 4-week intervals after adequate recovery from any toxicity.

Dosage Forms
Injection, powder for reconstitution:
Etopophos®: 100 mg

Etrafon® [Can] *see* amitriptyline and perphenazine *on page 63*

etravirine (et ra VIR een)

Synonyms TMC125
U.S./Canadian Brand Names Intelence™ [US/Can]
Therapeutic Category Antiretroviral Agent, Nonnucleoside Reverse Transcriptase Inhibitor (NNRTI)
Use Treatment of HIV-1 infection in combination with at least two additional antiretroviral agents in treatment-experienced patients exhibiting viral replication with documented nonnucleoside reverse transcriptase inhibitor (NNRTI) resistance
Usual Dosage Oral: Adults: 200 mg twice daily after meals
Dosage Forms
Tablet:
Intelence™: 100 mg

ETS-2% Topical *(Discontinued)*
Eudal®-SR [US] *see* guaifenesin and pseudoephedrine *on page 458*
Euflex® [Can] *see* flutamide *on page 416*
Euflexxa™ [US] *see* hyaluronate and derivatives *on page 476*
Euglucon® [Can] *see* glyburide *on page 448*
Eulexin® [US/Can] *see* flutamide *on page 416*
Eurax® [US] *see* crotamiton *on page 253*
Evac-Q-Mag® *(Discontinued)* *see* magnesium citrate *on page 584*
Evac-U-Gen [US-OTC] *see* senna *on page 861*
Evalose® *(Discontinued)* *see* lactulose *on page 544*
Evamist™ [US] *see* estradiol *on page 359*
Everone® 200 [Can] *see* testosterone *on page 912*
Everone® Injection *(Discontinued)* *see* testosterone *on page 912*
Evicel™ [US] *see* fibrin sealant kit *on page 400*
Evista® [US/Can] *see* raloxifene *on page 816*
Evithrom™ [US] *see* thrombin (topical) *on page 923*
Evoclin® [US] *see* clindamycin *on page 230*
Evoxac® [US/Can] *see* cevimeline *on page 197*
Evra® [Can] *see* ethinyl estradiol and norelgestromin *on page 375*
Exactacain™ [US] *see* benzocaine, butamben, and tetracaine *on page 126*
Exact® Acne Medication [US-OTC] *see* benzoyl peroxide *on page 126*
Excedrin® Extra Strength [US-OTC] *see* acetaminophen, aspirin, and caffeine *on page 24*
Excedrin® IB *(Discontinued)* *see* ibuprofen *on page 495*
Excedrin® Migraine [US-OTC] *see* acetaminophen, aspirin, and caffeine *on page 24*
Excedrin® P.M. [US-OTC] *see* acetaminophen and diphenhydramine *on page 21*
ExeClear *(Discontinued)*
ExeCof [US] *see* guaifenesin, dextromethorphan, and phenylephrine *on page 459*
ExeCof-XP *(Discontinued)*
ExeFen [US] *see* guaifenesin and pseudoephedrine *on page 458*
ExeFen-DMX [US] *see* guaifenesin, pseudoephedrine, and dextromethorphan *on page 460*
ExeFen-PD [US] *see* guaifenesin and phenylephrine *on page 456*
Exelderm® [US/Can] *see* sulconazole *on page 892*
Exelon® [US/Can] *see* rivastigmine *on page 840*

exemestane (ex e MES tane)

Sound-Alike/Look-Alike Issues
exemestane may be confused with estramustine.
U.S./Canadian Brand Names Aromasin® [US/Can]

▶

◀ **Therapeutic Category** Antineoplastic Agent, Miscellaneous
Use Treatment of advanced breast cancer in postmenopausal women whose disease has progressed following tamoxifen therapy; adjuvant treatment of postmenopausal estrogen receptor-positive early breast cancer following 2-3 years of tamoxifen (for a total of 5 years of adjuvant therapy)
Usual Dosage Oral: Adults: 25 mg once daily
Dosage Forms
 Tablet:
  Aromasin®: 25 mg

exenatide (ex EN a tide)

Synonyms AC 2993; AC002993; exendin-4 ; LY2148568
U.S./Canadian Brand Names Byetta® [US]
Therapeutic Category Antidiabetic Agent, Incretin Mimetic
Use Management (adjunctive) of type 2 diabetes mellitus (noninsulin dependent, NIDDM) in patients receiving a sulfonylurea, thiazolidinedione, or metformin (or a combination of these agents)
Usual Dosage SubQ: Adults: Initial: 5 mcg twice daily within 60 minutes prior to a meal; after 1 month, may be increased to 10 mcg twice daily (based on response)
Dosage Forms
 Injection, solution:
  Byetta®: 250 mcg/mL (1.2 mL [5 mcg/0.02 mL; 60-dose pen]); (2.4 mL [10 mcg/0.04 mL; 60-dose pen])

exendin-4 see exenatide on page 386
ExeTuss (Discontinued) see guaifenesin and phenylephrine on page 456
ExeTuss-DM [US] see guaifenesin, dextromethorphan, and phenylephrine on page 459
ExeTuss-GP [US] see guaifenesin and phenylephrine on page 456
ExeTuss HC (Discontinued)
Exforge® [US] see amlodipine and valsartan on page 65
Exidine® Scrub (Discontinued) see chlorhexidine gluconate on page 201
Exjade® [US/Can] see deferasirox on page 270
ex-lax® [US-OTC] see senna on page 861
ex-lax® Maximum Strength [US-OTC] see senna on page 861
ex-lax® Ultra [US-OTC] see bisacodyl on page 136
Exorex® [US] see coal tar on page 240
Exsel® (Discontinued) see selenium sulfide on page 861
Extendryl® [US] see chlorpheniramine, phenylephrine, and methscopolamine on page 210
Extendryl® GCP [US] see carbetapentane, guaifenesin, and phenylephrine on page 175
Extendryl® HC (Discontinued)
Extendryl® JR [US] see chlorpheniramine, phenylephrine, and methscopolamine on page 210
Extendryl PSE [US] see pseudoephedrine and methscopolamine on page 803
Extendryl® SR [US] see chlorpheniramine, phenylephrine, and methscopolamine on page 210
Extina® [US] see ketoconazole on page 537
Extra Action Cough Syrup (Discontinued) see guaifenesin and dextromethorphan on page 454
Extraneal® [US] see icodextrin on page 497
Exubera® (Discontinued) see insulin inhalation on page 511
EYE001 see pegaptanib on page 726
Eye-Lube-A® Solution (Discontinued) see artificial tears on page 95
Eye-Sed® Ophthalmic (Discontinued) see zinc sulfate on page 994
Eye-Sine™ (Discontinued) see tetrahydrozoline on page 916
Eyestil [Can] see hyaluronate and derivatives on page 476
Eye-Stream® [Can] see balanced salt solution on page 115
E-Z-Cat® [US] see barium on page 116
E-Z-Cat® Dry [US] see barium on page 116
EZ-Char™ [US-OTC] see charcoal on page 198
E-Z-Disk™ [US] see barium on page 116

ezetimibe (ez ET i mibe)

Sound-Alike/Look-Alike Issues
Zetia® may be confused with Zebeta®, Zestril®
U.S./Canadian Brand Names Ezetrol® [Can]; Zetia® [US]
Therapeutic Category Antilipemic Agent, 2-Azetidinone
Use Use in combination with dietary therapy for the treatment of primary hypercholesterolemia (as monotherapy or in combination with HMG-CoA reductase inhibitors); homozygous sitosterolemia; homozygous familial hypercholesterolemia (in combination with atorvastatin or simvastatin); mixed hyperlipidemia (in combination with fenofibrate)
Usual Dosage Oral: Children ≥10 years and Adults: 10 mg/day
Dosage Forms
  Tablet:
    Zetia®: 10 mg

ezetimibe and simvastatin (ez ET i mibe & SIM va stat in)

Sound-Alike/Look-Alike Issues
Vytorin® may be confused with Vyvanse™
Synonyms Simvastatin and Ezetimibe
U.S./Canadian Brand Names Vytorin® [US]
Therapeutic Category Antilipemic Agent, 2-Azetidinone
Use Used in combination with dietary modification for the treatment of primary hypercholesterolemia and homozygous familial hypercholesterolemia
Usual Dosage Oral: Adults:
  Homozygous familial hypercholesterolemia: Ezetimibe 10 mg and simvastatin 40 mg once daily or ezetimibe 10 mg and simvastatin 80 mg once daily in the evening. Dosing range: Ezetimibe 10 mg and simvastatin 10-80 mg once daily.
  Hyperlipidemias: Initial: Ezetimibe 10 mg and simvastatin 20 mg once daily in the evening
    Patients who require less aggressive reduction in LDL-C: Initial: Ezetimibe 10 mg and simvastatin 10 mg once daily
    Patients who require >55% reduction in LDL-C: Initial: Ezetimibe 10 mg and simvastatin 40 mg once daily
Dosage Forms
  Tablet:
    Vytorin®:
      10/10: Ezetimibe 10 mg and simvastatin 10 mg
      10/20: Ezetimibe 10 mg and simvastatin 20 mg
      10/40: Ezetimibe 10 mg and simvastatin 40 mg
      10/80: Ezetimibe 10 mg and simvastatin 80 mg

Ezetrol® [Can] *see ezetimibe on page 387*

Ezide® (Discontinued) *see hydrochlorothiazide on page 479*

E•R•O [US-OTC] *see carbamide peroxide on page 174*

F₃T *see trifluridine on page 952*

fabAV *see crotalidae polyvalent immune FAB (ovine) on page 253*

Fabrazyme® [US/Can] *see agalsidase beta on page 37*

Factive® [US/Can] *see gemifloxacin on page 439*

factor VIIa (recombinant) (FAK ter SEV en aye ree KOM be nant)

Sound-Alike/Look-Alike Issues
NovoSeven® may be confused with Novacet®
Synonyms coagulation factor VIIa; eptacog alfa (activated); rFVIIa
U.S./Canadian Brand Names Niastase® [Can]; NovoSeven® RT [US]
Therapeutic Category Antihemophilic Agent; Blood Product Derivative

▶

Use Treatment of bleeding episodes and prevention of bleeding in surgical interventions in patients with hemophilia A or B with inhibitors to factor VIII or factor IX, acquired hemophilia, and in patients with congenital factor VII deficiency

Usual Dosage Children and Adults: I.V. administration only: Hemophilia A or B with inhibitors:

Bleeding episodes: 90 mcg/kg every 2 hours until hemostasis is achieved or until the treatment is judged ineffective. The dose and interval may be adjusted based upon the severity of bleeding and the degree of hemostasis achieved. For patients experiencing severe bleeds, dosing should be continued at 3- to 6-hour intervals after hemostasis has been achieved and the duration of dosing should be minimized.

Surgical interventions: 90 mcg/kg immediately before surgery, repeat at 2-hour intervals for the duration of surgery. Continue every 2 hours for 48 hours, then every 2-6 hours until healed for minor surgery; continue every 2 hours for 5 days, then every 4 hours until healed for major surgery.

Congenital factor VII deficiency: Bleeding episodes and surgical interventions: 15-30 mcg/kg every 4-6 hours until hemostasis. Doses as low as 10 mcg/kg have been effective.

Dosage Forms

Injection, powder for reconstitution [preservative free]:
NovoSeven® RT: 1 mg, 2 mg, 5 mg

factor VIII (human) *see* antihemophilic factor (human) *on page 78*

factor VIII (human) *see* antihemophilic factor/von Willebrand factor complex (human) *on page 80*

factor VIII (recombinant) *see* antihemophilic factor (recombinant) *on page 79*

factor IX (FAK ter nyne)

Synonyms factor IX concentrate

U.S./Canadian Brand Names AlphaNine® SD [US]; BeneFix® [US/Can]; Immunine® VH [Can]; Mononine® [US/Can]

Therapeutic Category Antihemophilic Agent

Use Control bleeding in patients with factor IX deficiency (hemophilia B or Christmas disease)

Usual Dosage Dosage is expressed in int. units of factor IX activity; dosing must be individualized based on severity of factor IX deficiency, extent and location of bleeding, and clinical status of patient. I.V.:

Formula for int. units required to raise blood level %:

AlphaNine® SD, Mononine®: Children and Adults:

Number of factor IX int. units required = body weight (in kg) x desired factor IX level increase (int. units/dL or % of normal) x 1 int. unit/kg

For example, for a 100% level a 70 kg patient who has an actual level of 20%: Number of factor IX int. units needed = 70 kg x 80% x 1 int. unit/kg = 5600 int. units

BeneFix®:

Children <15 years:

Number of factor IX int. units required = body weight (in kg) x desired factor IX level increase (int. units/dL or % of normal) x 1.4 int. units/kg

Children ≥15 years and Adults:

Number of factor IX int. units required = body weight (in kg) x desired factor IX level increase (int. units/dL or % of normal) x 1.3 int. units/kg

Guidelines: As a general rule, the level of factor IX required for treatment of different conditions is listed below:

Minor spontaneous hemorrhage, prophylaxis:

Desired levels of factor IX for hemostasis: 15% to 25%

Initial loading dose to achieve desired level: 20-30 int. units/kg

Frequency of dosing: Every 12-24 hours if necessary

Duration of treatment: 1-2 days

Moderate hemorrhage:

Desired levels of factor IX for hemostasis: 25% to 50%

Initial loading dose to achieve desired level: 25-50 int. units/kg

Frequency of dosing: Every 12-24 hours

Duration of treatment: 2-7 days

Major hemorrhage:

Desired levels of factor IX for hemostasis: >50%

Initial loading dose to achieve desired level: 30-50 int. units/kg

Frequency of dosing: Every 12-24 hours, depending on half-life and measured factor IX levels (after 3-5 days, maintain at least 20% activity)

Duration of treatment: 7-10 days, depending upon nature of insult

Surgery or major trauma:

Desired levels of factor IX for hemostasis: 50% to 100%

Initial loading dose to achieve desired level: ≤75 int. units/kg or 50-100 int. units/kg

Frequency of dosing: Every 12-24 hours or every 18-30 hours, depending on half-life and measured factor IX levels

Duration of treatment: 7-10 days, depending upon nature of insult

Dosage Forms

Injection, powder for reconstitution (exact potency labeled on each vial):
AlphaNine® SD, BeneFix®, Mononine®

factor IX complex (human) (FAK ter nyne KOM pleks HYU man)

Synonyms prothrombin complex concentrate

U.S./Canadian Brand Names Bebulin® VH [US]; Profilnine® SD [US]

Therapeutic Category Antihemophilic Agent

Use Control bleeding in patients with factor IX deficiency (hemophilia B or Christmas disease) **Note:** Factor IX concentrate containing **only** factor IX is also available and preferable for this indication.

Usual Dosage Children and Adults: Dosage is expressed in units of factor IX activity and must be individualized. I.V. only:

Formula for units required to raise blood level %:

Total blood volume (mL blood/kg) = 70 mL/kg (adults), 80 mL/kg (children)

Plasma volume = total blood volume (mL) x [1 - Hct (in decimals)]

For example, for a 70 kg adult with a Hct = 40%: Plasma volume = [70 kg x 70 mL/kg] x [1 - 0.4] = 2940 mL

To calculate number of units needed to increase level to desired range (highly individualized and dependent on patient's condition): Number of units = desired level increase [desired level - actual level] x plasma volume (in mL).

For example, for a 100% level in the above patient who has an actual level of 20%: Number of units needed = [1 (for a 100% level) - 0.2] x 2940 mL = 2352 units

As a general rule, the level of factor IX required for treatment of different conditions is listed below:

Minor Spontaneous Hemorrhage, Prophylaxis:

Desired levels of factor IX for hemostasis: 15% to 25%

Initial loading dose to achieve desired level: <20-30 units/kg

Frequency of dosing: Once; repeated in 24 hours if necessary

Duration of treatment: Once; repeated if necessary

Major Trauma or Surgery:

Desired levels of factor IX for hemostasis: 25% to 50%

Initial loading dose to achieve desired level: <75 units/kg

Frequency of dosing: Every 18-30 hours, depending on half-life and measured factor IX levels

Duration of treatment: Up to 10 days, depending upon nature of insult

Dosage Forms

Injection, powder for reconstitution [single-dose vial; exact potency labeled on each vial]:
Bebulin® VH, Profilnine® SD

factor IX concentrate *see factor IX on page 388*

Factrel® [US] *see gonadorelin on page 451*

famciclovir (fam SYE kloe veer)

Sound-Alike/Look-Alike Issues

Sound-alike/look-alike issues:
Famvir® may be confused with Femara®

U.S./Canadian Brand Names Apo-Famciclovir [Can]; Famvir® [US/Can]; PMS-Famciclovir [Can]; Sandoz-Famciclovir [Can]

Therapeutic Category Antiviral Agent

Use Treatment of acute herpes zoster (shingles); treatment and suppression of recurrent episodes of genital herpes in immunocompetent patients; treatment of herpes labialis (cold sores) in immunocompetent patients; treatment of recurrent mucocutaneous/genital herpes simplex in HIV-infected patients

Usual Dosage Oral: Adults:

Acute herpes zoster: 500 mg every 8 hours for 7 days (**Note:** Initiate therapy within 72 hours of rash onset.)

Recurrent genital herpes simplex in immunocompetent patients:

Initial: 1000 mg twice daily for 1 day (**Note:** initiate therapy within 6 hours of symptoms/lesions.)

Suppressive therapy: 250 mg twice daily for up to 1 year

Recurrent herpes labialis (cold sores): 1500 mg as a single dose; initiate therapy at first sign or symptom such as tingling, burning, or itching (initiated within 1 hour in clinical studies) ▶

Recurrent mucocutaneous/genital herpes simplex in HIV patients: 500 mg twice daily for 7 days

Dosage Forms
Tablet: 125 mg, 250 mg, 500 mg
Famvir®: 125 mg, 250 mg, 500 mg

famotidine (fa MOE ti deen)

U.S./Canadian Brand Names Apo-Famotidine® Injectable [Can]; Apo-Famotidine® [Can]; Famotidine Omega [Can]; Gen-Famotidine [Can]; Novo-Famotidine [Can]; Nu-Famotidine [Can]; Pepcid® AC Maximum Strength [US-OTC]; Pepcid® AC [US-OTC/Can]; Pepcid® I.V. [Can]; Pepcid® [US/Can]; ratio-Famotidine [Can]; Riva-Famotidine [Can]; Ulcidine [Can]

Therapeutic Category Histamine H_2 Antagonist

Use Maintenance therapy and treatment of duodenal ulcer; treatment of gastroesophageal reflux, active benign gastric ulcer, and pathological hypersecretory conditions
OTC labeling: Relief of heartburn, acid indigestion, and sour stomach

Usual Dosage
Children: Treatment duration and dose should be individualized
Peptic ulcer: 1-16 years:
Oral: 0.5 mg/kg/day at bedtime or divided twice daily (maximum dose: 40 mg/day); doses of up to 1 mg/kg/day have been used in clinical studies
I.V.: 0.25 mg/kg every 12 hours (maximum dose: 40 mg/day); doses of up to 0.5 mg/kg have been used in clinical studies
GERD: Oral:
<3 months: 0.5 mg/kg once daily
3-12 months: 0.5 mg/kg twice daily
1-16 years: 1 mg/kg/day divided twice daily (maximum dose: 40 mg twice daily); doses of up to 2 mg/kg/day have been used in clinical studies

Children ≥12 years and Adults: Heartburn, indigestion, sour stomach: OTC labeling: Oral: 10-20 mg every 12 hours; dose may be taken 15-60 minutes before eating foods known to cause heartburn

Adults:
Duodenal ulcer: Oral: Acute therapy: 40 mg/day at bedtime for 4-8 weeks; maintenance therapy: 20 mg/day at bedtime
Gastric ulcer: Oral: Acute therapy: 40 mg/day at bedtime
Hypersecretory conditions: Oral: Initial: 20 mg every 6 hours, may increase in increments up to 160 mg every 6 hours
GERD: Oral: 20 mg twice daily for 6 weeks
Esophagitis and accompanying symptoms due to GERD: Oral: 20 mg or 40 mg twice daily for up to 12 weeks
Patients unable to take oral medication: I.V.: 20 mg every 12 hours

Dosage Forms
Gelcap:
Pepcid® AC: 10 mg
Infusion [premixed in NS]:
Pepcid®: 20 mg (50 mL)
Injection, solution: 10 mg/mL (4 mL, 20 mL, 50 mL)
Pepcid®: 10 mg/mL (20 mL)
Injection, solution [preservative free]: 10 mg/mL (2 mL)
Pepcid®: 10 mg/mL (2 mL)
Powder for oral suspension:
Pepcid®: 40 mg/5 mL
Tablet: 10 mg [OTC], 20 mg, 40 mg
Pepcid®: 20 mg, 40 mg
Pepcid® AC [OTC]: 10 mg, 20 mg
Pepcid® AC Maximum Strength [OTC]: 20 mg

famotidine, calcium carbonate, and magnesium hydroxide
(fa MOE ti deen, KAL see um KAR bun ate, & mag NEE zhum hye DROKS ide)

Synonyms calcium carbonate, magnesium hydroxide, and famotidine; magnesium hydroxide, famotidine, and calcium carbonate

U.S./Canadian Brand Names Pepcid® Complete [US-OTC/Can]

Therapeutic Category Antacid; Histamine H_2 Antagonist

Use Relief of heartburn due to acid indigestion

Usual Dosage Oral: Children ≥12 years and Adults: Relief of heartburn due to acid indigestion: Pepcid® Complete: 1 tablet as needed; no more than 2 tablets in 24 hours; do **not** swallow whole, chew tablet completely before swallowing; do not use for longer than 14 days

Dosage Forms
Tablet, chewable:
Pepcid® Complete [OTC]: Famotidine 10 mg, calcium carbonate 800 mg, and magnesium hydroxide 165 mg

Famotidine Omega [Can] see famotidine on page 390

Famvir® [US/Can] see famciclovir on page 389

Fansidar® [US] see sulfadoxine and pyrimethamine on page 894

Fareston® [US/Can] see toremifene on page 937

Faslodex® [US] see fulvestrant on page 430

Fasturtec® [Can] see rasburicase on page 821

fat emulsion (fat e MUL shun)

Synonyms intravenous fat emulsion

U.S./Canadian Brand Names Intralipid® [US/Can]; Liposyn® II [US/Can]; Liposyn® III [US]

Therapeutic Category Intravenous Nutritional Therapy

Use Source of calories and essential fatty acids for patients requiring parenteral nutrition of extended duration; prevention and treatment of essential fatty acid deficiency (EFAD)

Usual Dosage I.V.: **Note:** At the onset of therapy, the patient should be observed for any immediate allergic reactions.
Nutrition:
Premature infants: Initial dose: 0.25-0.5 g/kg/day, increase by 0.25-0.5 g/kg/day to a maximum of 3 g/kg/day depending on needs/nutritional goals; limit to 1 g/kg/day if on phototherapy; should be administered over 24 hours (A.S.P.E.N. guidelines)
Infants and Children: Initial dose: 0.5-1 g/kg/day, increase by 0.5 g/kg/day to a maximum of 3 g/kg/day depending on needs/nutritional goals; may administer over 24 hours (A.S.P.E.N. guidelines)
Note: Pediatric patients: Monitor triglycerides while receiving intralipids. If serum triglyceride levels >200 mg/dL, stop infusion and restart at 0.5-1g/kg/day. Intravenous heparin (1 unit/mL of parenteral nutrition) may enhance the clearance of lipid emulsions.
Adults: Initial dose: 1 g/kg/day, increase by 0.5-1 g/kg/day to a maximum of 2.5-3 g/kg/day
Prevention of essential fatty acid deficiency (EFAD): Adults: Administer 8% to 10% of total caloric intake as fat emulsion (may be higher in stressed patients with EFAD); may be given 2-3 times weekly to meet essential fatty acid requirements

Dosage Forms
Injection, emulsion [soybean oil]:
Intralipid®: 20% [200 mg/mL] (50 mL, 100 mL, 250 mL, 500 mL, 1000 mL); 30% [300 mg/mL] (500 mL)
Liposyn® II: 10% (500 mL); 20% (500 mL)
Liposyn® III: 10% [100 mg/mL] (200 mL, 500 mL); 20% [200 mg/mL] (200 mL, 500 mL); 30% [300 mg/mL] (500 mL)

Father John's® Plus [US-OTC] see chlorpheniramine, phenylephrine, and dextromethorphan on page 209

FazaClo® [US] see clozapine on page 240

5-FC see flucytosine on page 406

FC1157a see toremifene on page 937

Fedahist® Expectorant *(Discontinued)* see guaifenesin and pseudoephedrine on page 458

Fedahist® Expectorant Pediatric *(Discontinued)* see guaifenesin and pseudoephedrine on page 458

Fedahist® Tablet *(Discontinued)* see chlorpheniramine and pseudoephedrine on page 207

Feen-A-Mint® *(Discontinued)* see bisacodyl on page 136

Feiba VH [US] see antiinhibitor coagulant complex on page 81

Feiba VH Immuno [Can] see antiinhibitor coagulant complex on page 81

felbamate (FEL ba mate)

U.S./Canadian Brand Names Felbatol® [US]
Therapeutic Category Anticonvulsant

▶

◄ **Use** Not as a first-line antiepileptic treatment; only in those patients who respond inadequately to alternative treatments and whose epilepsy is so severe that a substantial risk of aplastic anemia and/or liver failure is deemed acceptable in light of the benefits conferred by its use. Patient must be fully advised of risk and provide signed written informed consent. Felbamate can be used as either monotherapy or adjunctive therapy in the treatment of partial seizures (with and without generalization) and in adults with epilepsy. Used as adjunctive therapy in the treatment of partial and generalized seizures associated with Lennox-Gastaut syndrome in children.

Usual Dosage Anticonvulsant:

Monotherapy: Children >14 years and Adults:

Initial: 1200 mg/day in divided doses 3 or 4 times/day; titrate previously untreated patients under close clinical supervision, increasing the dosage in 600 mg increments every 2 weeks to 2400 mg/day based on clinical response and thereafter to 3600 mg/day as clinically indicated

Conversion to monotherapy: Initiate at 1200 mg/day in divided doses 3 or 4 times/day, reduce the dosage of the concomitant anticonvulsant(s) by 20% to 33% at the initiation of felbamate therapy; at week 2, increase the felbamate dosage to 2400 mg/day while reducing the dosage of the other anticonvulsant(s) up to an additional 33% of their original dosage; at week 3, increase the felbamate dosage up to 3600 mg/day and continue to reduce the dosage of the other anticonvulsant(s) as clinically indicated

Adjunctive therapy: **Note:** Dose of concomitant carbamazepine, phenobarbital, phenytoin, or valproic acid should be decreased by 20% to 33% when initiating felbamate therapy. Further dosage reductions may be necessary as dose of felbamate is increased.

Children 2-14 years with Lennox-Gastaut syndrome: Initial: 15 mg/kg/day in divided doses 3 or 4 times/day; may increase once per week by 15 mg/kg/day increments up to 45 mg/kg/day in divided doses 3 or 4 times/day.

Children >14 years and Adults: Initial: 1200 mg/day in divided doses 3 or 4 times/day; may increase once per week by 1200 mg/day increments up to 3600 mg/day in divided doses 3 or 4 times/day.

Dosage Forms

Suspension, oral:

Felbatol®: 600 mg/5 mL

Tablet:

Felbatol®: 400 mg, 600 mg

Felbatol® [US] see felbamate on page 391
Feldene® [US] see piroxicam on page 757

felodipine (fe LOE di peen)

Sound-Alike/Look-Alike Issues

Plendil® may be confused with Isordil®, pindolol, Pletal®, Prilosec®, Prinivil®

U.S./Canadian Brand Names Plendil® [US/Can]; Renedil® [Can]

Therapeutic Category Calcium Channel Blocker

Use Treatment of hypertension

Usual Dosage Oral: Adults: Hypertension: 2.5-10 mg once daily; usual initial dose: 5 mg; increase by 5 mg at 2-week intervals, as needed, to a maximum of 20 mg/day

Usual dose range (JNC 7) for hypertension: 2.5-20 mg once daily

Dosage Forms

Tablet, extended release:

Plendil®: 2.5 mg, 5 mg, 10 mg

felodipine and enalapril see enalapril and felodipine on page 339
felodipine and ramipril see ramipril and felodipine (Canada only) on page 818
Femara® [US/Can] see letrozole on page 552
Fematrol [US-OTC] see bisacodyl on page 136
Femcet® (Discontinued)
Femcon™ Fe [US] see ethinyl estradiol and norethindrone on page 376
Femguard® (Discontinued) see sulfabenzamide, sulfacetamide, and sulfathiazole on page 892
femhrt® [US/Can] see ethinyl estradiol and norethindrone on page 376
Femilax™ [US-OTC] see bisacodyl on page 136
Femiron® [US-OTC] see ferrous fumarate on page 397

Fem-Prin® [US-OTC] *see* acetaminophen, aspirin, and caffeine *on page 24*
Femring® [US] *see* estradiol *on page 359*
Femstat® One [Can] *see* butoconazole *on page 157*
Femtrace® [US] *see* estradiol *on page 359*
Fenesin DM IR [US] *see* guaifenesin and dextromethorphan *on page 454*
Fenesin IR [US] *see* guaifenesin *on page 453*
Fenesin PE IR [US] *see* guaifenesin and phenylephrine *on page 456*

fenofibrate (fen oh FYE brate)

Sound-Alike/Look-Alike Issues
TriCor® may be confused with Tracleer®
Synonyms procetofene; proctofene
U.S./Canadian Brand Names Antara™ [US]; Apo-Feno-Micro® [Can]; Apo-Fenofibrate® [Can]; Dom-Fenofibrate Supra [Can]; Fenoglide™ [US]; Gen-Fenofibrate Micro [Can]; Lipidil EZ® [Can]; Lipidil Micro® [Can]; Lipidil Supra® [Can]; Lipofen™ [US]; Lofibra® [US]; Novo-Fenofibrate [Can]; Novo-Fenofibrate-S [Can]; Nu-Fenofibrate [Can]; PHL-Fenofibrate Supra [Can]; PMS-Fenofibrate Micro [Can]; PMS-Fenofibrate Supra [Can]; ratio-Fenofibrate MC [Can]; Sandoz Fenofibrate S [Can]; TriCor® [US/Can]; Triglide™ [US]
Therapeutic Category Antihyperlipidemic Agent, Miscellaneous
Use Adjunct to dietary therapy for the treatment of adults with elevations of serum triglyceride levels (types IV and V hyperlipidemia); adjunct to dietary therapy for the reduction of low density lipoprotein cholesterol (LDL-C), total cholesterol (total-C), triglycerides, and apolipoprotein B (apo B) in adult patients with primary hypercholesterolemia or mixed dyslipidemia (Fredrickson types IIa and IIb)
Usual Dosage Oral: Adults:
Hypertriglyceridemia: Initial:
Antara™ (micronized): 43-130 mg/day; maximum dose: 130 mg/day
Fenoglide™: 40-120 mg/day; maximum dose: 120 mg/day
Lipofen™: 50-150 mg/day; maximum dose: 150 mg/day
Lofibra® (micronized): 67-200 mg/day with meals; maximum dose: 200 mg/day
Lofibra® (tablets): 54-160 mg/day; maximum dose: 160 mg/day
TriCor®: 48-145 mg/day; maximum dose: 145 mg/day
Triglide™: 50-160 mg/day; maximum dose: 160 mg/day
Hypercholesterolemia or mixed hyperlipidemia:
Antara™ (micronized): 130 mg/day
Fenoglide™: 120 mg/day
Lipofen™: 150 mg/day
Lofibra® (micronized): 200 mg/day
Lofibra® (tablets): 160 mg/day
TriCor®: 145 mg/day
Triglide™: 160 mg/day
Dosage Forms
Capsule:
Lipofen™: 50 mg, 150 mg
Capsule [micronized]: 67 mg, 134 mg, 200 mg
Antara™: 43 mg, 130 mg
Lofibra®: 67 mg, 134 mg, 200 mg
Tablet: 54 mg, 160 mg
Fenoglide™: 40 mg, 120 mg
Lofibra®: 54 mg, 160 mg
TriCor®: 48 mg, 145 mg
Triglide™: 50 mg, 160 mg

Fenoglide™ [US] *see* fenofibrate *on page 393*

fenoldopam (fe NOL doe pam)

Synonyms fenoldopam mesylate
U.S./Canadian Brand Names Corlopam® [US/Can]
Therapeutic Category Antihypertensive Agent
Use Treatment of severe hypertension (up to 48 hours in adults), including in patients with renal compromise; short-term (up to 4 hours) blood pressure reduction in pediatric patients

◄ **Usual Dosage** I.V.: Hypertension, severe:
Children: Initial: 0.2 mcg/kg/minute; may be increased to dosages of 0.3-0.5 mcg/kg/minute every 20-30 minutes (maximum dose: 0.8 mcg/kg/minute); limited to short-term (4 hours) use
Adults: Initial: 0.1-0.3 mcg/kg/minute (lower initial doses may be associated with less reflex tachycardia); may be increased in increments of 0.05-0.1 mcg/kg/minute every 15 minutes until target blood pressure is reached; the maximal infusion rate reported in clinical studies was 1.6 mcg/kg/minute

Dosage Forms
Injection, solution: 10 mg/mL (1 mL, 2 mL)
Corlopam®: 10 mg/mL (1 mL, 2 mL)

fenoldopam mesylate see fenoldopam on page 393

fenoprofen (fen oh PROE fen)

Sound-Alike/Look-Alike Issues
fenoprofen may be confused with flurbiprofen
Nalfon® may be confused with Naldecon®

Synonyms fenoprofen calcium

U.S./Canadian Brand Names Nalfon® [US/Can]

Therapeutic Category Analgesic, Nonnarcotic Nonsteroidal Antiinflammatory Drug (NSAID)

Use Symptomatic treatment of acute and chronic rheumatoid arthritis and osteoarthritis; relief of mild to moderate pain

Usual Dosage Oral: Adults:
Rheumatoid arthritis, osteoarthritis: 300-600 mg 3-4 times/day; maximum dose: 3.2 g/day
Mild-to-moderate pain: 200 mg every 4-6 hours as needed; maximum dose: 3.2 g/day

Dosage Forms
Capsule:
Nalfon®: 200 mg
Tablet: 600 mg

fenoprofen calcium see fenoprofen on page 394

fenoterol *(Canada only)* (fen oh TER ole)

Synonyms fenoterol hydrobromide

U.S./Canadian Brand Names Berotec® [Can]

Therapeutic Category Beta$_2$-Adrenergic Agonist Agent

Use Treatment and prevention of symptoms of reversible obstructive pulmonary disease (including asthma and acute bronchospasm), chronic bronchitis, emphysema

Usual Dosage Inhalation: Children ≥12 years of age and Adults:
MDI:
Acute treatment: 1 puff initially; may repeat in 5 minutes; if relief is not evident, additional doses and/or other therapy may be necessary
Intermittent/long-term treatment: 1-2 puffs 3-4 times/day (maximum of 8 puffs/24 hours)
Solution: 0.5-1 mg (up to maximum of 2.5 mg)

Dosage Forms [CAN] = Canadian brand name
Aerosol for inhalation: MDI:
Berotec® [CAN]: 100 mcg/dose [not available in the U.S.]
Solution for inhalation:
Berotec® [CAN] 0.625 mg/mL (2 mL); 0.25 mg/mL (2 mL) [not available in the U.S.]

fenoterol hydrobromide see fenoterol *(Canada only)* on page 394

fentanyl (FEN ta nil)

Sound-Alike/Look-Alike Issues
fentaNYL may be confused with alfentanil, SUFentanil

Synonyms fentanyl citrate; fentanyl hydrochloride; OTFC (oral transmucosal fentanyl citrate)

Tall-Man fentaNYL

U.S./Canadian Brand Names Actiq® [US/Can]; Duragesic® [US/Can]; Fentanyl Citrate Injection, USP [Can]; Fentora® [US]; Ionsys™ [US]; RAN™-Fentanyl Transdermal System [Can]; ratio-Fentanyl [Can]; Sublimaze® [US]

Therapeutic Category Analgesic, Narcotic; General Anesthetic

Controlled Substance C-II

Use

Injection: Sedation, relief of pain, preoperative medication, adjunct to general or regional anesthesia

Transdermal patch (eg, Duragesic®): Management of persistent moderate-to-severe chronic pain

Transmucosal lozenge (eg, Actiq®), buccal tablet (Fentora®): Management of breakthrough cancer pain in opioid-tolerant patients

Usual Dosage Note: These are guidelines and do not represent the maximum doses that may be required in all patients. Doses and dosage intervals should be titrated to pain relief/prevention. Monitor vital signs routinely. Single I.M. doses have a duration of 1-2 hours, single I.V. doses last 0.5-1 hour.

Surgery:

Children ≥2 years: Adjunct to anesthesia (induction and maintenance): Slow I.V.: 2-3 mcg/kg/dose every 1-2 hours as needed

Adults:

Premedication: I.M., slow I.V.: 50-100 mcg/dose 30-60 minutes prior to surgery

Adjunct to regional anesthesia: Slow I.V.: 25-100 mcg/dose over 1-2 minutes. **Note:** An I.V. should be in place with regional anesthesia so the I.M. route is rarely used but still maintained as an option in the package labeling.

Adjunct to general anesthesia: Slow I.V.:

Low dose: 0.5-2 mcg/kg/dose depending on the indication

Moderate dose: Initial: 2-20 mcg/kg/dose; Maintenance (bolus or infusion): 1-2 mcg/kg/hour. Discontinuing fentanyl infusion 30-60 minutes prior to the end of surgery will usually allow adequate ventilation upon emergence from anesthesia. For "fast-tracking" and early extubation following major surgery, total fentanyl doses are limited to 10-15 mcg/kg.

High-dose: 20-50 mcg/kg/dose; **Note:** Fentanyl is rarely used, but is still maintained in the package labeling.

Pain management: Adults: Iontophoretic transdermal system: 40 mcg per activation on-demand (maximum: 6 doses/hour). **Note:** Patient's pain should be controlled prior to initiating system. Instruct patient how to operate system. Only the patient should initiate system. Each system operates for 24 hours or until 80 doses have been administered, whichever comes first. Maximum duration of therapy: 72 hours.

Breakthrough cancer pain: For patients who are tolerant to and currently receiving opioid therapy for persistent cancer pain; dosing should be individually titrated to provide adequate analgesia with minimal side effects. Dose titration should be done if patient requires more than 1 dose/breakthrough pain episode for several consecutive episodes. Patients experiencing >4 breakthrough pain episodes/day should have the dose of their long-term opioid re-evaluated.

Children ≥16 years and Adults: Lozenge: Initial dose: 200 mcg; the second dose may be started 15 minutes after completion of the first dose. Consumption should be limited to ≤4 units/day. Additional requirements suggest need for improved baseline therapy.

Adults: Buccal tablet (Fentora®): Initial dose: 100 mcg; a second 100 mcg dose, if needed, may be started 30 minutes after the start of the first dose. **Note:** For patients previously using the transmucosal lozenge (Actiq®), the initial dose should be selected using the conversions listed below (maximum: 2 doses per breakthrough pain episode every 4 hours).

Dose titration, if required, should be done using multiples of the 100 mcg tablets. Patient can take two 100 mcg tablets (one on each side of mouth). If that dose is not successful, can use four 100 mcg tablets (two on each side of mouth). If titration requires >400 mcg/dose, then use 200 mcg tablets.

Conversion from lozenge to buccal tablet (Fentora®):

Lozenge dose 200-400 mcg, then buccal tablet 100 mcg

Lozenge dose 600-800 mcg, then buccal tablet 200 mcg

Lozenge dose 1200-1600 mcg, then buccal tablet 400 mcg

Note: Four 100 mcg buccal tablets deliver approximately 12% and 13% higher values of C_{max} and AUC, respectively, compared to one 400 mcg buccal tablet. To prevent confusion, patient should only have one strength available at a time. Using more than four buccal tablets at a time has not been studied.

Chronic pain management: Children ≥2 years and Adults (opioid-tolerant patients): Transdermal patch (eg, Duragesic®):

Initial: To convert patients from oral or parenteral opioids to transdermal patch, a 24-hour analgesic requirement should be calculated (based on prior opiate use). Using the tables, the appropriate initial dose can be determined. The initial fentanyl dosage may be approximated from the 24-hour morphine dosage equivalent and titrated to minimize adverse effects and provide analgesia. With the initial application, the absorption of transdermal fentanyl requires several hours to reach plateau; therefore transdermal fentanyl is inappropriate for management of acute pain. Change patch every 72 hours.

Conversion from continuous infusion of fentanyl: In patients who have adequate pain relief with a fentanyl infusion, fentanyl may be converted to transdermal dosing at a rate equivalent to the intravenous rate. A two-step taper of the infusion to be completed over 12 hours has been recommended after the patch is applied. The infusion is decreased to 50% of the original rate six hours after the application of the first patch, and subsequently discontinued twelve hours after application.

Titration: Short-acting agents may be required until analgesic efficacy is established and/or as supplements for "breakthrough" pain. The amount of supplemental doses should be closely monitored. Appropriate dosage increases may be based on daily supplemental dosage using the ratio of 45 mg/24 hours of oral morphine to a 12.5 mcg/hour increase in fentanyl dosage.

Frequency of adjustment: The dosage should not be titrated more frequently than every 3 days after the initial dose or every 6 days thereafter. Patients should wear a consistent fentanyl dosage through two applications (6 days) before dosage increase based on supplemental opiate dosages can be estimated. **Note:** Upon discontinuation, ~17 hours are required for a 50% decrease in fentanyl levels.

Frequency of application: The majority of patients may be controlled on every 72-hour administration; however, a small number of patients require every 48-hour administration.

Dosage Forms

Infusion, premixed in NS: 0.05 mg (10 mL); 1 mg (100 mL); 1.25 mg (250 mL); 2 mg (100 mL); 2.5 mg (250 mL)

Injection, solution [preservative free]: 0.05 mg/mL (2 mL, 5 mL, 10 mL, 20 mL, 50 mL)
  Sublimaze®: 0.05 mg/mL (2 mL, 5 mL, 10 mL, 20 mL)

Lozenge, oral [transmucosal]: 200 mcg, 400 mcg, 600 mcg, 800 mcg, 1200 mcg, 1600 mcg
  Actiq®: 200 mcg, 400 mcg, 600 mcg, 800 mcg, 1200 mcg, 1600 mcg

Tablet, for buccal application:
  Fentora®: 100 mcg, 200 mcg, 300 mcg, 400 mcg, 600 mcg, 800 mcg

Transdermal system, topical: 12 (5s) [delivers 12.5 mcg/hour; 3.13 cm^2]; 12 (5s) [delivers 12.5 mcg/hour; 5 cm^2]; 25 (5s) [delivers 25 mcg/hour; 10 cm^2]; 25 (5s) [delivers 25 mcg/hour; 6.25 cm^2]; 50 (5s) [delivers 50 mcg/hour; 12.5 cm^2]; 50 (5s) [delivers 50 mcg/hour; 20 cm^2]; 75 (5s) [delivers 75 mcg/hour; 18.75 cm^2]; 75 (5s) [delivers 75 mcg/hour; 30 cm^2]; 100 (5s) [delivers 100 mcg/hour; 25 cm^2]; 100 (5s) [delivers 100 mcg/hour; 40 cm^2]
  Duragesic®: 12 [delivers 12.5 mcg/hour; 5 cm^2] (5s); 25 [delivers 25 mcg/hour; 10 cm^2] (5s); 50 [delivers 50 mcg/hour; 20 cm^2] (5s); 75 [delivers 75 mcg/hour; 30 cm^2]; 100 [delivers 100 mcg/hour; 40 cm^2] (5s)

fentanyl citrate *see fentanyl on page 394*
Fentanyl Citrate Injection, USP [Can] *see fentanyl on page 394*
fentanyl hydrochloride *see fentanyl on page 394*
Fentanyl Oralet® *(Discontinued)* *see fentanyl on page 394*
Fentora® [US] *see fentanyl on page 394*
Feosol® [US-OTC] *see ferrous sulfate on page 398*
Feosol® Elixir *(Discontinued)* *see ferrous sulfate on page 398*
Feostat® *(Discontinued)* *see ferrous fumarate on page 397*
Ferancee® *(Discontinued)* *see ferrous sulfate and ascorbic acid on page 399*
Feratab® [US-OTC] *see ferrous sulfate on page 398*
Fer-Gen-Sol [US-OTC] *see ferrous sulfate on page 398*
Fergon® [US-OTC] *see ferrous gluconate on page 398*
Feridex I.V.® [US] *see ferumoxides on page 399*
Fer-In-Sol® [US-OTC/Can] *see ferrous sulfate on page 398*
Fer-In-Sol® Syrup *(Discontinued)* *see ferrous sulfate on page 398*
Fer-Iron® [US-OTC] *see ferrous sulfate on page 398*
Fermalac [Can] *see Lactobacillus on page 543*
Ferodan™ [Can] *see ferrous sulfate on page 398*
Fero-Grad 500® [US-OTC] *see ferrous sulfate and ascorbic acid on page 399*
Fero-Gradumet® *(Discontinued)* *see ferrous sulfate on page 398*
Ferospace® *(Discontinued)* *see ferrous sulfate on page 398*
Ferralet® *(Discontinued)* *see ferrous gluconate on page 398*
Ferralyn® Lanacaps® *(Discontinued)* *see ferrous sulfate on page 398*
Ferra-TD® *(Discontinued)* *see ferrous sulfate on page 398*
Ferretts [US-OTC] *see ferrous fumarate on page 397*
Ferrex 150 [US-OTC] *see polysaccharide-iron complex on page 768*

ferric (III) hexacyanoferrate (II) *see ferric hexacyanoferrate on page 397*

ferric gluconate (FER ik GLOO koe nate)

Sound-Alike/Look-Alike Issues
Ferrlecit® may be confused with Ferralet®

Synonyms sodium ferric gluconate

U.S./Canadian Brand Names Ferrlecit® [US/Can]

Therapeutic Category Iron Salt

Use Repletion of total body iron content in patients with iron-deficiency anemia who are undergoing hemodialysis in conjunction with erythropoietin therapy

Usual Dosage I.V.: Repletion of iron in hemodialysis patients:
Children ≥6 years: 1.5 mg/kg of elemental iron (maximum: 125 mg/dose) diluted in NS 25 mL, administered over 60 minutes at 8 sequential dialysis sessions
Adults: 125 mg elemental iron per 10 mL (either by I.V. infusion or slow I.V. injection). Most patients will require a cumulative dose of 1 g elemental iron over approximately 8 sequential dialysis treatments to achieve a favorable response.
Note: A test dose of 2 mL diluted in NS 50 mL administered over 60 minutes was previously recommended (not in current manufacturer labeling). Doses >125 mg are associated with increased adverse events.

Dosage Forms
Injection, solution:
Ferrlecit®: Elemental iron 12.5 mg/mL (5 mL)

ferric hexacyanoferrate (FER ik hex a SYE an oh fer ate)

Synonyms ferric (III) hexacyanoferrate (II); insoluble prussian blue; prussian blue

U.S./Canadian Brand Names Radiogardase™ [US]

Therapeutic Category Antidote

Use Treatment of known or suspected internal contamination with radioactive cesium and/or radioactive or nonradioactive thallium

Usual Dosage Oral: Internal contamination with radioactive cesium and/or radioactive or nonradioactive thallium:
Children 2-12 years: 1 g 3 times/day; treatment should begin as soon as possible following exposure, but is also effective if therapy is delayed
Children >12 years and Adults: 3 g 3 times/day; treatment should begin as soon as possible following exposure, but is also effective if therapy is delayed
Note: Cesium exposure: Once internal radioactivity is substantially decreased, dosage may be reduced to 1-2 g 3 times/day to improve gastrointestinal tolerance

Dosage Forms
Capsule:
Radiogardase®: 0.5 g

Ferrlecit® [US/Can] *see ferric gluconate on page 397*
Ferro-Sequels® [US-OTC] *see ferrous fumarate on page 397*

ferrous fumarate (FER us FYOO ma rate)

Sound-Alike/Look-Alike Issues
Feostat® may be confused with Feosol®

Synonyms iron fumarate

U.S./Canadian Brand Names Femiron® [US-OTC]; Ferretts [US-OTC]; Ferro-Sequels® [US-OTC]; Hemocyte® [US-OTC]; Ircon® [US-OTC]; Nephro-Fer® [US-OTC]; Palafer® [Can]

Therapeutic Category Electrolyte Supplement, Oral

Use Prevention and treatment of iron-deficiency anemias

Usual Dosage Oral **(dose expressed in terms of elemental iron):**
Children:
Severe iron-deficiency anemia: 4-6 mg Fe/kg/day in 3 divided doses
Mild-to-moderate iron-deficiency anemia: 3 mg Fe/kg/day in 1-2 divided doses
Prophylaxis: 1-2 mg Fe/kg/day
Adults:
Iron deficiency: 60-100 mg twice daily up to 60 mg 2 times/day

◀ Prophylaxis: 60-100 mg/day
To avoid GI upset, start with a single daily dose and increase by 1 tablet/day each week or as tolerated until desired daily dose is achieved

Dosage Forms
Tablet: 324 mg
Femiron® [OTC]: 63 mg
Ferretts [OTC]: 325 mg
Hemocyte® [OTC]: 324 mg
Ircon® [OTC]: 200 mg
Nephro-Fer® [OTC]: 350 mg
Tablet, timed release:
Ferro-Sequels® [OTC]: 150 mg

ferrous gluconate (FER us GLOO koe nate)

Synonyms iron gluconate
U.S./Canadian Brand Names Apo-Ferrous Gluconate® [Can]; Fergon® [US-OTC]; Novo-Ferrogluc [Can]
Therapeutic Category Electrolyte Supplement, Oral
Use Prevention and treatment of iron-deficiency anemias
Usual Dosage Oral **(dose expressed in terms of elemental iron):**
Children:
Severe iron-deficiency anemia: 4-6 mg Fe/kg/day in 3 divided doses
Mild-to-moderate iron-deficiency anemia: 3 mg Fe/kg/day in 1-2 divided doses
Prophylaxis: 1-2 mg Fe/kg/day
Adults:
Iron deficiency: 60 mg twice daily up to 60 mg 4 times/day
Prophylaxis: 60 mg/day
Dosage Forms
Tablet: 246 mg, 325 mg
Fergon® [OTC]: 240 mg

ferrous sulfate (FER us SUL fate)

Sound-Alike/Look-Alike Issues
Feosol® may be confused with Feostat®, Fer-In-Sol®
Fer-In-Sol® may be confused with Feosol®
Slow FE® may be confused with Slow-K®
Synonyms FeSO$_4$; iron sulfate
U.S./Canadian Brand Names Apo-Ferrous Sulfate® [Can]; Feosol® [US-OTC]; Fer-Gen-Sol [US-OTC]; Fer-In-Sol® [US-OTC/Can]; Fer-Iron® [US-OTC]; Feratab® [US-OTC]; Ferodan™ [Can]; Slow FE® [US-OTC]
Therapeutic Category Electrolyte Supplement, Oral
Use Prevention and treatment of iron-deficiency anemias
Usual Dosage Oral:
Children **(dose expressed in terms of elemental iron)**:
Severe iron-deficiency anemia: 4-6 mg Fe/kg/day in 3 divided doses
Mild-to-moderate iron-deficiency anemia: 3 mg Fe/kg/day in 1-2 divided doses
Prophylaxis: 1-2 mg Fe/kg/day up to a maximum of 15 mg/day
Adults **(dose expressed in terms of ferrous sulfate)**:
Iron deficiency: 300 mg twice daily up to 300 mg 4 times/day or 250 mg (extended release) 1-2 times/day
Prophylaxis: 300 mg/day
Dosage Forms [CAN] = Canadian brand-specific information
Elixir: 220 mg/5 mL
Liquid, oral drops: 75 mg/0.6 mL
Fer-Gen-Sol [OTC], Fer-In-Sol® [OTC], Fer-Iron® [OTC]: 75 mg/0.6 mL
Fer-In-Sol® [CAN]: 75 mg/1 mL
Tablet: 324 mg, 325 mg
Feratab® [OTC]: 300 mg
Tablet, exsiccated: 200 mg
Feosol® [OTC]: 200 mg

Tablet, exsiccated, timed release: 160 mg
Slow FE® [OTC]: 160 mg

ferrous sulfate and ascorbic acid (FER us SUL fate & a SKOR bik AS id)

Synonyms ascorbic acid and ferrous sulfate; iron sulfate and vitamin C

U.S./Canadian Brand Names Fero-Grad 500® [US-OTC]

Therapeutic Category Vitamin

Use Treatment of iron deficiency in nonpregnant adults; treatment and prevention of iron deficiency in pregnant adults

Usual Dosage Oral: Adults: 1 tablet daily

Dosage Forms
Tablet, controlled release:
Fero-Grad 500® [OTC]: Ferrous sulfate 525 mg and ascorbic acid 500 mg

Fertinorm® H.P. [Can] *see* urofollitropin *on page 964*

ferumoxides (fer yoo MOX ides)

Sound-Alike/Look-Alike Issues
Feridex I.V.® may be confused with Fertinex®

U.S./Canadian Brand Names Feridex I.V.® [US]

Therapeutic Category Radiopaque Agents

Use For I.V. administration as an adjunct to MRI (in adult patients) to enhance the T2 weighted images used in the detection and evaluation of lesions of the liver

Usual Dosage Adults: 0.56 mg of iron (0.05 mL Feridex I.V.®)/kg body weight diluted in 100 mL of 5% dextrose and infused over 30 minutes; a 5-micron filter is recommended; do not administer undiluted

Dosage Forms
Injection, solution:
Feridex I.V.®: Iron 11.2 mg/mL (5 mL)

FeSO$_4$ *see* ferrous sulfate *on page 398*
Fe-Tinic™ 150 *(Discontinued)* *see* polysaccharide-iron complex *on page 768*
FeverAll® [US-OTC] *see* acetaminophen *on page 19*
Fexmid™ [US] *see* cyclobenzaprine *on page 255*

fexofenadine (feks oh FEN a deen)

Sound-Alike/Look-Alike Issues
Allegra® may be confused with Viagra®

Synonyms fexofenadine hydrochloride

U.S./Canadian Brand Names Allegra® ODT [US]; Allegra® [US/Can]

Therapeutic Category Antihistamine

Use Relief of symptoms associated with seasonal allergic rhinitis; treatment of chronic idiopathic urticaria

Usual Dosage Oral:
Chronic idiopathic urticaria: Children 6 months to <2 years: 15 mg twice daily
Chronic idiopathic urticaria, seasonal allergic rhinitis:
Children 2-11 years: 30 mg twice daily
Children ≥12 years and Adults: 60 mg twice daily **or** 180 mg once daily

Dosage Forms
Suspension:
Allegra®: 6 mg/mL
Tablet: 30 mg, 60 mg, 180 mg
Allegra®: 60 mg, 180 mg
Tablet, orally disintegrating:
Allegra® ODT: 30 mg

fexofenadine and pseudoephedrine (feks oh FEN a deen & soo doe e FED rin)

Sound-Alike/Look-Alike Issues
Allegra-D® may be confused with Viagra®

Synonyms pseudoephedrine and fexofenadine

U.S./Canadian Brand Names Allegra-D® 12 Hour [US]; Allegra-D® 24 Hour [US]; Allegra-D® [Can] ▶

◀ **Therapeutic Category** Antihistamine/Decongestant Combination

Use Relief of symptoms associated with seasonal allergic rhinitis in adults and children ≥12 years of age

Usual Dosage Oral: Children ≥12 years and Adults:
Allegra-D® 12 Hour: One tablet twice daily
Allegra-D® 24 Hour: One tablet once daily

Dosage Forms

Tablet, extended release:
Allegra-D® 12 Hour: Fexofenadine 60 mg [immediate release] and pseudoephedrine 120 mg [extended release]
Allegra-D® 24 Hour: Fexofenadine 180 mg [immediate release] and pseudoephedrine 240 mg [extended release]

fexofenadine hydrochloride *see fexofenadine on page 399*
Fiberall® [US] *see psyllium on page 804*
FiberCon® [US-OTC] *see polycarbophil on page 765*
Fiber-Lax® [US-OTC] *see polycarbophil on page 765*
Fiber-Tabs™ [US-OTC] *see polycarbophil on page 765*
fibrin sealant (human) *see fibrin sealant kit on page 400*

fibrin sealant kit (FI brin SEEL ent kit)

Synonyms fibrin sealant (human); FS

U.S./Canadian Brand Names Evicel™ [US]; Tisseel® VH [US/Can]

Therapeutic Category Hemostatic Agent

Use

Evicel™: Adjunct to hemostasis in surgery when control of bleeding by conventional surgical techniques is ineffective or impractical

Tisseel® VH: Adjunct to hemostasis in cardiopulmonary bypass surgery and splenic injury (due to blunt or penetrating trauma to the abdomen) when the control of bleeding by conventional surgical techniques is ineffective or impractical; adjunctive sealant for closure of colostomies; hemostatic agent in heparinized patients undergoing cardiopulmonary bypass

Usual Dosage Adjunct to hemostasis: Apply topically; actual dose is based on size of surface to be covered:

Evicel™: Children and Adults: Spray or drop onto surface of bleeding tissue in short bursts (0.1-0.2 mL); if hemostatic effect is not complete, apply a second layer. To cover a layer of 1 mm thickness:
Maximum area to be sealed: 20 cm^2
Required size of Evicel™ kit: 2 mL
Maximum area to be sealed: 40 cm^2
Required size of Evicel™ kit: 4 mL
Maximum area to be sealed: 100 cm^2
Required size of Evicel™ kit: 10 mL

Tisseel® VH: Adults: Apply in thin layers to avoid excess formation of granulation tissue and slow absorption of the sealant. Following application, hold the sealed parts in the desired position for 3-5 minutes. To prevent sealant from adhering to gloves or surgical instruments, wet them with saline prior to contact.
Maximum area to be sealed: 8 cm^2
Required package size of Tisseel® VH: 2 mL
Maximum area to be sealed: 16 cm^2
Required package size of Tisseel® VH: 4 mL
Maximum area to be sealed: 40 cm^2
Required package size of Tisseel® VH: 10 mL

Dosage Forms

Topical: Kit:
Evicel™ [preservative free; each 2 mL kit contains]:
Solution, topical: Fibrinogen 55-85 mg/mL (1 mL)
Solution, topical: Thrombin 800-1200 int. units/mL and calcium chloride 5.6-6.2 mg/mL (1 mL)
Evicel™ [preservative free; each 4 mL kit contains]:
Solution, topical: Fibrinogen 55-85 mg/mL (2 mL)
Solution, topical: Thrombin 800-1200 int. units/mL and calcium chloride 5.6-6.2 mg/mL (2 mL)

Evicel™ [preservative free; each 10 mL kit contains]:
Solution, topical: Fibrinogen 55-85 mg/mL (5 mL)
Solution, topical: Thrombin 800-1200 int. units/mL and calcium chloride 5.6-6.2 mg/mL (5 mL)
Tisseel VH [each 2 mL, 4 mL, or 10 mL kit contains]:
Powder, for solution, topical: Fibrinogen 67-106 mg/mL
Powder, for solution, topical: Thrombin 400-625 int. units/mL
Solution, topical: Calcium chloride 36-44 μmol/mL
Solution, topical: Aprotinin 2250-3750 KIU/mL
Tisseel VH [each dual-chamber 2 mL, 4 mL, or 10 mL prefilled syringe contains]:
Solution, topical:
Sealer protein chamber: Fibrinogen 67-106 mg/mL and aprotinin 2250-3750 KIU/mL
Thrombin chamber: Thrombin 400-625 int. units/mL and calcium chloride 36-44 μmol/mL

Fibro-XL [US-OTC] *see psyllium on page 804*
Fibro-Lax [US-OTC] *see psyllium on page 804*

filgrastim (fil GRA stim)

Sound-Alike/Look-Alike Issues
Neupogen® may be confused with Epogen®, Neumega®, Neupro®, Nutramigen®
Synonyms G-CSF; granulocyte colony-stimulating factor; NSC-614629
U.S./Canadian Brand Names Neupogen® [US/Can]
Therapeutic Category Colony-Stimulating Factor
Use Stimulation of granulocyte production in chemotherapy-induced neutropenia (nonmyeloid malignancies, acute myeloid leukemia, and bone marrow transplantation); severe chronic neutropenia (SCN); patients undergoing peripheral blood progenitor cell (PBPC) collection
Usual Dosage Refer to individual protocols.
Dosing, even in morbidly obese patients, should be based on actual body weight. Rounding doses to the nearest vial size often enhances patient convenience and reduces costs without compromising clinical response.
Children and Adults:
Chemotherapy-induced neutropenia: SubQ, I.V.: 5 mcg/kg/day; doses may be increased by 5 mcg/kg according to the duration and severity of the neutropenia; continue for up to 14 days or until the ANC reaches 10,000/mm^3
Bone marrow transplantation: SubQ, I.V.: 10 mcg/kg/day; adjust the dose according to the duration and severity of neutropenia; recommended steps based on neutrophil response:
When ANC >1000/mm^3 for 3 consecutive days: Reduce filgrastim dose to 5 mcg/kg/day
If ANC remains >1000/mm^3 for 3 more consecutive days: Discontinue filgrastim
If ANC decreases to <1000/mm^3: Resume at 5 mcg/kg/day
If ANC decreases <1000/mm^3 during the 5 mcg/kg/day dose, increase filgrastim to 10 mcg/kg/day and follow the above steps
Peripheral blood progenitor cell (PBPC) collection: SubQ: 10 mcg/kg daily in donors, usually for 6-7 days. Begin at least 4 days before the first leukopheresis and continue until the last leukopheresis; consider dose adjustment for WBC >100,000/mm^3
Severe chronic neutropenia: SubQ:
Congenital: 6 mcg/kg twice daily; adjust the dose based on ANC and clinical response
Idiopathic/cyclic: 5 mcg/kg/day; adjust the dose based on ANC and clinical response
Dosage Forms
Injection, solution [preservative free]:
Neupogen®: 300 mcg/mL (1 mL, 1.6 mL) [vial]; 600 mcg/mL (0.5 mL, 0.8 mL) [prefilled Singleject® syringe]

Finacea® [US/Can] *see azelaic acid on page 109*

finasteride (fi NAS teer ide)

Sound-Alike/Look-Alike Issues
Proscar® may be confused with ProSom®, Prozac®, Psorcon®
U.S./Canadian Brand Names Propecia® [US/Can]; Proscar® [US/Can]
Therapeutic Category Antiandrogen
Use
Propecia®: Treatment of male pattern hair loss in **men only**. Safety and efficacy were demonstrated in men between 18-41 years of age.

◀ Proscar®: Treatment of symptomatic benign prostatic hyperplasia (BPH); can be used in combination with an alpha-blocker, doxazosin

Usual Dosage Oral: Adults: Male:

Benign prostatic hyperplasia (Proscar®): 5 mg/day as a single dose; clinical responses occur within 12 weeks to 6 months of initiation of therapy; long-term administration is recommended for maximal response

Male pattern baldness (Propecia®): 1 mg daily

Dosage Forms
Tablet: 5 mg
Propecia®: 1 mg
Proscar®: 5 mg

Fiorgen PF® *(Discontinued)*

Fioricet® [US] *see* butalbital, acetaminophen, and caffeine *on page 155*

Fioricet® with Codeine [US] *see* butalbital, acetaminophen, caffeine, and codeine *on page 155*

Fiorinal® [US/Can] *see* butalbital, aspirin, and caffeine *on page 156*

Fiorinal®-C 1/2 [Can] *see* butalbital, aspirin, caffeine, and codeine *on page 156*

Fiorinal®-C 1/4 [Can] *see* butalbital, aspirin, caffeine, and codeine *on page 156*

Fiorinal® With Codeine [US] *see* butalbital, aspirin, caffeine, and codeine *on page 156*

First™-Progesterone VGS [US] *see* progesterone *on page 790*

First® Testosterone [US] *see* testosterone *on page 912*

First® Testosterone MC [US] *see* testosterone *on page 912*

fisalamine *see* mesalamine *on page 607*

fish oil *see* omega-3-acid ethyl esters *on page 697*

FK506 *see* tacrolimus *on page 901*

Flagyl® [US/Can] *see* metronidazole *on page 627*

Flagyl ER® [US] *see* metronidazole *on page 627*

Flagystatin® [Can] *see* metronidazole and nystatin *(Canada only) on page 629*

Flamazine® [Can] *see* silver sulfadiazine *on page 866*

Flarex® [US/Can] *see* fluorometholone *on page 412*

flavan *see* flavocoxid *on page 402*

flavocoxid (fla vo KOKS id)
Synonyms flavan; flavonoid
U.S./Canadian Brand Names Limbrel™ [US]
Therapeutic Category Antiinflammatory Agent
Use Clinical dietary management of osteoarthritis, including associated inflammation
Usual Dosage Oral: 250 mg every 8-12 hours
Dosage Forms
Capsule:
Limbrel™: 250 mg, 500 mg

flavonoid *see* flavocoxid *on page 402*

Flavorcee® *(Discontinued)* *see* ascorbic acid *on page 96*

flavoxate (fla VOKS ate)
Sound-Alike/Look-Alike Issues
flavoxate may be confused with fluvoxamine
Urispas® may be confused with Urised®
Synonyms flavoxate hydrochloride
U.S./Canadian Brand Names Apo-Flavoxate® [Can]; Urispas® [US/Can]
Therapeutic Category Antispasmodic Agent, Urinary
Use Antispasmodic to provide symptomatic relief of dysuria, nocturia, suprapubic pain, urgency, and incontinence due to detrusor instability and hyperreflexia in elderly with cystitis, urethritis, urethrocystitis, urethrotrigonitis, and prostatitis

Usual Dosage Oral: Children >12 years and Adults: 100-200 mg 3-4 times/day; reduce the dose when symptoms improve

Dosage Forms
Tablet: 100 mg
Urispas®: 100 mg

flavoxate hydrochloride *see* flavoxate *on page 402*

Flebogamma® [US] *see* immune globulin (intravenous) *on page 503*

flecainide (fle KAY nide)

Sound-Alike/Look-Alike Issues
flecainide may be confused with fluconazole
Tambocor™ may be confused with tamoxifen

Synonyms flecainide acetate

U.S./Canadian Brand Names Apo-Flecainide® [Can]; Tambocor™ [US/Can]

Therapeutic Category Antiarrhythmic Agent, Class I-C

Use Prevention and suppression of documented life-threatening ventricular arrhythmias (eg, sustained ventricular tachycardia); controlling symptomatic, disabling supraventricular tachycardias in patients without structural heart disease in whom other agents fail

Usual Dosage Oral:
Children:
Initial: 3 mg/kg/day or 50-100 mg/m^2/day in 3 divided doses
Usual: 3-6 mg/kg/day or 100-150 mg/m^2/day in 3 divided doses; up to 11 mg/kg/day or 200 mg/m^2/day for uncontrolled patients with subtherapeutic levels
Adults:
Life-threatening ventricular arrhythmias:
Initial: 100 mg every 12 hours
Increase by 50-100 mg/day (given in 2 doses/day) every 4 days; maximum: 400 mg/day.
Use of higher initial doses and more rapid dosage adjustments have resulted in an increased incidence of proarrhythmic events and congestive heart failure, particularly during the first few days. Do not use a loading dose. Use very cautiously in patients with history of congestive heart failure or myocardial infarction.
Prevention of paroxysmal supraventricular arrhythmias in patients with disabling symptoms but no structural heart disease:
Initial: 50 mg every 12 hours
Increase by 50 mg twice daily at 4-day intervals; maximum: 300 mg/day.

Dosage Forms
Tablet: 50 mg, 100 mg, 150 mg
Tambocor™: 50 mg, 100 mg, 150 mg

flecainide acetate *see* flecainide *on page 403*

Flector® [US] *see* diclofenac *on page 292*

Fleet® Babylax® [US-OTC] *see* glycerin *on page 449*

Fleet® Bisacodyl [US-OTC] *see* bisacodyl *on page 136*

Fleet® Enema [US-OTC/Can] *see* sodium phosphates *on page 878*

Fleet® Enema Extra® [US-OTC] *see* sodium phosphates *on page 878*

Fleet® Enema for Children [US-OTC] *see* sodium phosphates *on page 878*

Fleet® Flavored Castor Oil *(Discontinued)* *see* castor oil *on page 183*

Fleet® Glycerin Suppositories [US-OTC] *see* glycerin *on page 449*

Fleet® Glycerin Suppositories Maximum Strength [US-OTC] *see* glycerin *on page 449*

Fleet® Laxative *(Discontinued)* *see* bisacodyl *on page 136*

Fleet® Liquid Glycerin Suppositories [US-OTC] *see* glycerin *on page 449*

Fleet® Phospho-soda® [US-OTC] *see* sodium phosphates *on page 878*

Fleet® Phospho-soda® EZ-Prep™ [US-OTC] *see* sodium phosphates *on page 878*

Fleet® Phospho-Soda® Oral Laxative [Can] *see* sodium phosphates *on page 878*

Fleet® Sof-Lax® [US-OTC] *see* docusate *on page 314*

Fleet® Stimulant Laxative [US-OTC] *see* bisacodyl *on page 136*

Fletcher's® [US-OTC] *see* senna *on page 861*

Flexaphen® *(Discontinued)* *see* chlorzoxazone *on page 215*

Flexbumin [US] *see* albumin *on page 38*

Flexeril® [US/Can] *see* cyclobenzaprine *on page 255*

Flexitec [Can] *see* cyclobenzaprine *on page 255*

Flex-Power [US-OTC] *see* trolamine *on page 957*

Flextra 650 [US] *see* acetaminophen and phenyltoloxamine *on page 22*

Flextra-DS [US] *see* acetaminophen and phenyltoloxamine *on page 22*

Flintstones® Complete [US-OTC] *see* vitamins (multiple/pediatric) *on page 983*

Flintstones™ Gummies [US-OTC] *see* vitamins (multiple/pediatric) *on page 983*

Flintstones™ Plus Immunity Support [US-OTC] *see* vitamins (multiple/pediatric) *on page 983*

Flintstones® Plus Iron [US-OTC] *see* vitamins (multiple/pediatric) *on page 983*

Flintstones™ Sour Gummies [US-OTC] *see* vitamins (multiple/pediatric) *on page 983*

floctafenina *see* floctafenine *(Canada only) on page 404*

floctafenine *(Canada only)* (flok ta FEN een)

Synonyms floctafenina; floctafeninum

U.S./Canadian Brand Names Apo-Floctafenine® [Can]

Therapeutic Category Nonsteroidal Antiinflammatory Drug (NSAID), Oral

Use Short-term management of acute, mild-to-moderate pain

Usual Dosage Oral: Adults: 200-400 mg every 6-8 hours as needed, up to a maximum of 1200 mg/day

Dosage Forms [CAN] = Canadian brand name

Tablet:

Apo-Floctafenine® [CAN]: 200 mg, 400 mg [not available in the U.S.]

floctafeninum *see* floctafenine *(Canada only) on page 404*

Flolan® [US/Can] *see* epoprostenol *on page 349*

Flomax® [US/Can] *see* tamsulosin *on page 903*

Flomax® CR [Can] *see* tamsulosin *on page 903*

Flonase® [US/Can] *see* fluticasone (nasal) *on page 418*

Flora-Q™ [US-OTC] *see* Lactobacillus *on page 543*

Florastor® [US-OTC] *see* Saccharomyces boulardii *on page 849*

Florastor® Kids [US-OTC] *see* Saccharomyces boulardii *on page 849*

Florazole® ER [Can] *see* metronidazole *on page 627*

Florical® [US-OTC] *see* calcium carbonate *on page 163*

Florinef® [Can] *see* fludrocortisone *on page 406*

Florinef® *(Discontinued)* *see* fludrocortisone *on page 406*

Florone® [US/Can] *see* diflorasone *on page 295*

Florone E® *(Discontinued)* *see* diflorasone *on page 295*

Flovent® Diskus® [Can] *see* fluticasone (oral inhalation) *on page 419*

Flovent® HFA [US/Can] *see* fluticasone (oral inhalation) *on page 419*

Floxin® [US/Can] *see* ofloxacin *on page 693*

floxuridine (floks YOOR i deen)

Sound-Alike/Look-Alike Issues

floxuridine may be confused with Fludara®, fludarabine

FUDR® may be confused with Fludara®

Synonyms 5-FUDR; fluorodeoxyuridine; NSC-27640

U.S./Canadian Brand Names FUDR® [US/Can]

Therapeutic Category Antineoplastic Agent

Use Management of hepatic metastases of colorectal and gastric cancers

Usual Dosage Refer to individual protocols.

Intraarterial:

0.1-0.6 mg/kg/day

4-20 mg/day

Dosage Forms
Injection, powder for reconstitution: 500 mg
FUDR®: 500 mg

Fluanxol® [Can] see flupenthixol (Canada only) on page 414
Fluarix® [US] see influenza virus vaccine on page 508
flubenisolone see betamethasone (topical) on page 132
Flucaine® [US] see proparacaine and fluorescein on page 794

fluconazole (floo KOE na zole)

Sound-Alike/Look-Alike Issues
fluconazole may be confused with flecainide
Diflucan® may be confused with diclofenac, Diprivan®, disulfiram
U.S./Canadian Brand Names Apo-Fluconazole® [Can]; Co-Fluconazole [Can]; Diflucan® [US/Can]; Dom-Fluconazole [Can]; Fluconazole Injection [Can]; Fluconazole Omega [Can]; Gen-Fluconazole [Can]; GMD-Fluconazole [Can]; Novo-Fluconazole [Can]; PHL-Fluconazole [Can]; PMS-Fluconazole [Can]; Riva-Fluconazole [Can]; Taro-Fluconazole [Can]; Zym-Fluconazole [Can]
Therapeutic Category Antifungal Agent
Use Treatment of candidiasis (vaginal, oropharyngeal, esophageal, urinary tract infections, peritonitis, pneumonia, and systemic infections); cryptococcal meningitis; antifungal prophylaxis in allogeneic bone marrow transplant recipients
Usual Dosage The daily dose of fluconazole is the same for oral and I.V. administration
Usual dosage ranges:
Neonates: First 2 weeks of life, especially premature neonates: Same dose as older children every 72 hours
Children: Loading dose: 6-12 mg/kg; maintenance: 3-12 mg/kg/day; duration and dosage depends on severity of infection
Adults: 200-800 mg/day; duration and dosage depends on severity of infection

Indication-specific dosing:
Children:
Candidiasis:
Oropharyngeal: Loading dose: 6 mg/kg; maintenance: 3 mg/kg/day for 2 weeks
Esophageal: Loading dose: 6 mg/kg; maintenance: 3-12 mg/kg/day for 21 days and at least 2 weeks following resolution of symptoms
Systemic infection: 6 mg/kg every 12 hours for 28 days
Meningitis, cryptococcal: Loading dose: 12 mg/kg; maintenance: 6-12 mg/kg/day for 10-12 weeks following negative CSF culture; relapse suppression (HIV-positive): 6 mg/kg/day
Adults:
Candidiasis:
Candidemia (neutropenic and nonneutropenic): 400-800 mg/day for 14 days after last positive blood culture and resolution of signs/symptoms
Chronic, disseminated: 400-800 mg/day for 3-6 months
Oropharyngeal (long-term suppression): 200 mg/day; chronic therapy is recommended in immunocompromised patients with history of oropharyngeal candidiasis (OPC)
Osteomyelitis: 400-800 mg/day for 6-12 months
Esophageal: 200 mg on day 1, then 100-200 mg/day for 2-3 weeks after clinical improvement
Prophylaxis in bone marrow transplant: 400 mg/day; begin 3 days before onset of neutropenia and continue for 7 days after neutrophils >1000 cells/mm^3
Urinary: 200 mg/day for 1-2 weeks
Vaginal: 150 mg as a single dose
Endophthalmitis: 400-800 mg/day for 6-12 weeks after surgical intervention.
Meningitis, cryptococcal: Amphotericin 0.7-1 mg/kg +/- 5-FC for 2 weeks then fluconazole 400 mg/day for at least 10 weeks (consider life-long in HIV-positive); maintenance (HIV-positive): 200-400 mg/day life-long

Dosage Forms
Infusion [premixed in sodium chloride or dextrose]: 200 mg (100 mL); 400 mg (200 mL)
Diflucan® [premixed in sodium chloride or dextrose]: 200 mg (100 mL); 400 mg (200 mL)
Powder for oral suspension: 10 mg/mL, 40 mg/mL
Diflucan®: 10 mg/mL, 40 mg/mL
Tablet: 50 mg, 100 mg, 150 mg, 200 mg
Diflucan®: 50 mg, 100 mg, 150 mg, 200 mg

Fluconazole Injection [Can] *see* fluconazole *on page 405*
Fluconazole Omega [Can] *see* fluconazole *on page 405*

flucytosine (floo SYE toe seen)

Sound-Alike/Look-Alike Issues
flucytosine may be confused with fluorouracil
Ancobon® may be confused with Oncovin®
Synonyms 5-FC; 5-fluorocytosine; 5-flurocytosine
U.S./Canadian Brand Names Ancobon® [US/Can]
Therapeutic Category Antifungal Agent
Use Adjunctive treatment of systemic fungal infections (eg, septicemia, endocarditis, UTI, meningitis, or pulmonary) caused by susceptible strains of *Candida* or *Cryptococcus*
Usual Dosage
Usual dosage ranges:
Oral: Adults: 50-150 mg/kg/day in divided doses every 6 hours

Indication-specific dosing:
Oral: Adults:
Endocarditis: 25-37.5 mg/kg every 6 hours (with amphotericin B) for at least 6 weeks after valve replacement
Meningoencephalitis, cryptococcal: Induction: 25 mg/kg/dose (with amphotericin B) every 6 hours for 2 weeks; if clinical improvement, may discontinue both amphotericin and flucytosine and follow with an extended course of fluconazole (400 mg/day); alternatively, may continue flucytosine for 6-10 weeks (with amphotericin B) without conversion to fluconazole treatment
Dosage Forms
Capsule:
Ancobon®: 250 mg, 500 mg

Fludara® [US/Can] *see* fludarabine *on page 406*

fludarabine (floo DARE a been)

Sound-Alike/Look-Alike Issues
fludarabine may be confused with floxuridine, Flumadine®
Fludara® may be confused with FUDR®
Synonyms fludarabine phosphate; NSC-312887
U.S./Canadian Brand Names Beneflur® [Can]; Fludara® [US/Can]
Therapeutic Category Antineoplastic Agent
Use
U.S. labeling: I.V.: Treatment of chronic lymphocytic leukemia (CLL) (including refractory CLL)
Canadian labeling:
I.V.: Treatment of chronic lymphocytic leukemia (CLL) (including refractory CLL); treatment of low-grade, refractory non-Hodgkin lymphoma (NHL)
Oral (formulation not available in U.S.): Treatment of CLL
Usual Dosage Adults:
I.V.: CLL: 25 mg/m^2/day for 5 days every 28 days
Oral: **Note:** Formulation available in Canada; not available in U.S.: CLL: 40 mg/m^2 once daily for 5 days every 28 days
Dosage Forms [CAN] = Canadian brand name
Injection, powder for reconstitution: 50 mg
Fludara®: 50 mg
Tablet: 10 mg [not available in the U.S.]
Fludara® [CAN]: 10 mg [not available in the U.S.]

fludarabine phosphate *see* fludarabine *on page 406*

fludrocortisone (floo droe KOR ti sone)

Sound-Alike/Look-Alike Issues
Florinef® may be confused with Fioricet®, Fiorinal®

Synonyms 9α-fluorohydrocortisone acetate; fludrocortisone acetate; fluohydrisone acetate; fluohydrocortisone acetate

U.S./Canadian Brand Names Florinef® [Can]

Therapeutic Category Adrenal Corticosteroid (Mineralocorticoid)

Use Partial replacement therapy for primary and secondary adrenocortical insufficiency in Addison disease; treatment of salt-losing adrenogenital syndrome

Usual Dosage Oral:

Infants and Children: 0.05-0.1 mg/day

Adults: 0.1-0.2 mg/day with ranges of 0.1 mg 3 times/week to 0.2 mg/day

Addison disease: Initial: 0.1 mg/day; if transient hypertension develops, reduce the dose to 0.05 mg/day. Preferred administration with cortisone (10-37.5 mg/day) or hydrocortisone (10-30 mg/day).

Salt-losing adrenogenital syndrome: 0.1-0.2 mg/day

Dosage Forms

Tablet: 0.1 mg

fludrocortisone acetate *see* fludrocortisone *on page 406*

FluLaval™ [US] *see* influenza virus vaccine *on page 508*

Flumadine® [US/Can] *see* rimantadine *on page 835*

flumazenil (FLOO may ze nil)

U.S./Canadian Brand Names Anexate® [Can]; Flumazenil Injection [Can]; Flumazenil Injection, USP [Can]; Romazicon® [US/Can]

Therapeutic Category Antidote

Use Benzodiazepine antagonist; reverses sedative effects of benzodiazepines used in conscious sedation and general anesthesia; treatment of benzodiazepine overdose

Usual Dosage I.V.:

Children: Reversal of conscious sedation and general anesthesia:

Initial dose: 0.01 mg/kg over 15 seconds (maximum: 0.2 mg)

Repeat doses (maximum: 4 doses): 0.005-0.01 mg/kg (maximum: 0.2 mg) repeated at 1-minute intervals

Maximum total cumulative dose: 1 mg or 0.05 mg/kg (whichever is lower)

Adults:

Reversal of conscious sedation and general anesthesia:

Initial dose: 0.2 mg over 15 seconds

Repeat doses (maximum: 4 doses): If desired level of consciousness is not obtained, 0.2 mg may be repeated at 1-minute intervals.

Maximum total cumulative dose: 1 mg (usual dose: 0.6-1 mg). In the event of resedation: Repeat doses may be given at 20-minute intervals with maximum of 1 mg/dose and 3 mg/hour

Suspected benzodiazepine overdose:

Initial dose: 0.2 mg over 30 seconds; if the desired level of consciousness is not obtained, 0.3 mg can be given over 30 seconds

Repeat doses: 0.5 mg over 30 seconds repeated at 1-minute intervals

Maximum total cumulative dose: 3 mg (usual dose: 1-3 mg). Patients with a partial response at 3 mg may require additional titration up to a total dose of 5 mg. If a patient has not responded 5 minutes after cumulative dose of 5 mg, the major cause of sedation is not likely due to benzodiazepines. In the event of resedation: May repeat doses at 20-minute intervals with maximum of 1 mg/dose and 3 mg/hour.

Resedation: Repeated doses may be given at 20-minute intervals as needed; repeat treatment doses of 1 mg (at a rate of 0.5 mg/minute) should be given at any time and no more than 3 mg should be given in any hour. After intoxication with high doses of benzodiazepines, the duration of a single dose of flumazenil is not expected to exceed 1 hour; if desired, the period of wakefulness may be prolonged with repeated low intravenous doses of flumazenil, or by an infusion of 0.1-0.4 mg/hour. Most patients with benzodiazepine overdose will respond to a cumulative dose of 1-3 mg and doses >3 mg do not reliably produce additional effects. Rarely, patients with a partial response at 3 mg may require additional titration up to a total dose of 5 mg. **If a patient has not responded 5 minutes after receiving a cumulative dose of 5 mg, the major cause of sedation is not likely to be due to benzodiazepines.**

Dosage Forms

Injection, solution: 0.1 mg/mL (5 mL, 10 mL)

Romazicon®: 0.1 mg/mL (5 mL, 10 mL)

Flumazenil Injection [Can] *see* flumazenil *on page 407*
Flumazenil Injection, USP [Can] *see* flumazenil *on page 407*
flumethasone and clioquinol *see* clioquinol and flumethasone *(Canada only) on page 232*
FluMist® [US] *see* influenza virus vaccine *on page 508*

flunarizine *(Canada only)* (floo NAR i zeen)

Synonyms flunarizine hydrochloride
U.S./Canadian Brand Names Apo-Flunarizine® [Can]; Novo-Flunarizine [Can]; Sibelium® [Can]
Therapeutic Category Calcium-Entry Blocker (Selective)
Use Prophylaxis of classic (with aura) or common (without aura) migraine; symptomatic treatment of vestibular vertigo (due to a diagnosed functional disorder of the vestibular system)
Usual Dosage Oral: Adults (<65 years): Usual dose: 5-10 mg/day, usually administered at bedtime
  Migraine prophylaxis: Initial dose: 10 mg at bedtime
    Maintenance dose (following initial control of symptoms): 10 mg at bedtime administered 5 consecutive days, followed by 2 consecutive medication-free days each week.
    Duration of therapy: In nonresponders, discontinue if no response occurs within 2 months. If response is noted, discontinue after 6 months; restart if patient relapses.
  Vertigo: Initial dose: 10 mg at bedtime until symptoms are controlled
    Duration of therapy:
    Chronic vertigo: Discontinue if no response within 1 month.
    Paroxysmal vertigo: Discontinue if no response is noted within 2 months.
Dosage Forms [CAN] = Canadian brand name
  Capsule:
    Apo-Flunarizine® [CAN], Novo-Flunarizine [CAN], Sibelium® [CAN]: 5 mg [not available in the U.S.]

flunarizine hydrochloride *see* flunarizine *(Canada only) on page 408*

flunisolide (floo NISS oh lide)

Sound-Alike/Look-Alike Issues
  flunisolide may be confused with Flumadine®, fluocinonide
  Nasarel® may be confused with Nizoral®
U.S./Canadian Brand Names AeroBid® [US]; AeroBid®-M [US]; Alti-Flunisolide [Can]; Apo-Flunisolide® [Can]; Nasalide® [Can]; Nasarel® [US]; PMS-Flunisolide [Can]; Rhinalar® [Can]
Therapeutic Category Adrenal Corticosteroid
Use Steroid-dependent asthma; nasal solution is used for seasonal or perennial rhinitis
Usual Dosage
  Oral inhalation: Asthma:
    AeroBid®:
      Children 6-15 years: 2 inhalations twice daily (morning and evening); up to 4 inhalations/day
      Children ≥16 years and Adults: 2 inhalations twice daily (morning and evening); up to 8 inhalations/day maximum
    NIH Asthma Guidelines (NIH, 2007) (administer in divided doses twice daily):
      Children 5-11 years:
        "Low" dose: 500-750 mcg/day
        "Medium" dose: 1000-1250 mcg/day
        "High" dose: >1250 mcg/day
      Children ≥12 years and Adults:
        "Low" dose: 500-1000 mcg/day
        "Medium" dose: >1000-2000 mcg/day
        "High" dose: >2000 mcg/day
  Intranasal: Rhinitis:
    Children 6-14 years: 1 spray each nostril 3 times daily **or** 2 sprays in each nostril twice daily; not to exceed 4 sprays/day in each nostril (200 mcg/day)
    Children ≥15 years and Adults: 2 sprays each nostril twice daily (morning and evening); may increase to 2 sprays 3 times daily; maximum dose: 8 sprays/day in each nostril (400 mcg/day)
Dosage Forms
  Aerosol for oral inhalation:
    AeroBid®, AeroBid®-M: 250 mcg/actuation (7 g)
  Solution, intranasal [spray]: 25 mcg/actuation (25 mL); 29 mcg/actuation (25 mL)
    Nasarel®: 29 mcg/actuation (25 mL)

fluocinolone (floo oh SIN oh lone)

Sound-Alike/Look-Alike Issues
fluocinolone may be confused with fluocinonide

Synonyms fluocinolone acetonide

U.S./Canadian Brand Names Capex® [US/Can]; Derma-Smoothe/FS® [US/Can]; DermOtic® [US]; Retisert® [US]; Synalar® [Can]

Therapeutic Category Corticosteroid, Topical

Use Relief of susceptible inflammatory dermatosis [low, medium corticosteroid]; dermatitis or psoriasis of the scalp; atopic dermatitis in adults and children ≥3 months of age
Ocular implant (Retisert®): Treatment of chronic, noninfectious uveitis affecting the posterior segment of the eye
Otic (DermOtic® Oil): Relief of chronic eczematous external otitis in adults and children ≥2 years of age.

Usual Dosage
Ocular implant: Chronic uveitis: Children ≥12 years and Adults: One silicone-encased tablet (0.59 mg) surgically implanted into the posterior segment of the eye is designed to initially release 0.6 mcg/day, decreasing over 30 days to a steady-state release rate of 0.3-0.4 mcg/day for 30 months. Recurrence of uveitis denotes depletion of tablet, requiring reimplantation.
Otic: Chronic eczematous external otitis: Children ≥2 years and Adults: 5 drops into the affected ear twice daily for 1-2 weeks
Topical:
Atopic dermatitis (Derma-Smoothe/FS® body oil):
Children ≥3 months: Moisten skin; apply a thin film to affected area twice daily; do not use for longer than 4 weeks
Adults: Apply a thin film to affected area 3 times/day
Corticosteroid-responsive dermatoses: Children and Adults: Cream, ointment, solution: Apply a thin layer to affected area 2-4 times/day; may use occlusive dressings to manage psoriasis or recalcitrant conditions
Inflammatory and pruritic manifestations (dental use): Adults: Apply to oral lesion 4 times/day, after meals and at bedtime
Scalp psoriasis (Derma-Smoothe/FS® scalp oil): Adults: Massage thoroughly into wet or dampened hair/scalp; cover with shower cap. Leave on overnight (or for at least 4 hours). Remove by washing hair with shampoo and rinsing thoroughly.
Seborrheic dermatitis of the scalp (Capex®): Adults: Apply no more than 1 ounce to scalp once daily; work into lather and allow to remain on scalp for ~5 minutes. Remove from hair and scalp by rinsing thoroughly with water.

Dosage Forms
Cream: 0.01% (15 g, 60 g); 0.025% (15 g, 60 g)
Implant, intravitreal:
Retisert®: 0.59 mg
Oil:
Derma-Smoothe/FS® [body oil]: 0.01% (120 mL)
Derma-Smoothe/FS® [scalp oil]: 0.01% (120 mL)
DermaOtic® [otic drops]: 0.01% (20 mL)
Ointment: 0.025% (15 g, 60 g)
Shampoo:
Capex®: 0.01% (120 mL)
Solution: 0.01% (60 mL)

fluocinolone acetonide see fluocinolone on page 409

fluocinolone, hydroquinone, and tretinoin
(floo oh SIN oh lone, HYE droe kwin one, & TRET i noyn)

Synonyms hydroquinone, fluocinolone acetonide, and tretinoin; tretinoin, fluocinolone acetonide, and hydroquinone

U.S./Canadian Brand Names Tri-Luma™ [US]

Therapeutic Category Corticosteroid, Topical; Depigmenting Agent; Retinoic Acid Derivative

Use Short-term treatment of moderate-to-severe melasma of the face

Usual Dosage Topical: Adults: Melasma: Apply a thin film once daily to hyperpigmented areas of melasma (including 1/2 inch of normal-appearing surrounding skin). Apply 30 minutes prior to bedtime; not indicated for use beyond 8 weeks. Do not use occlusive dressings.

◀ **Dosage Forms**
Cream, topical:
Tri-Luma™: Hydroquinone 4%, tretinoin 0.05%, fluocinolone 0.01% (30 g)

fluocinonide (floo oh SIN oh nide)

Sound-Alike/Look-Alike Issues
fluocinonide may be confused with flunisolide, fluocinolone
Lidex® may be confused with Lasix®, Videx®, Wydase®

U.S./Canadian Brand Names Lidemol® [Can]; Lidex® [Can]; Lyderm® [Can]; Tiamol® [Can]; Topsyn® [Can]; Vanos™ [US]

Therapeutic Category Corticosteroid, Topical

Use Antiinflammatory, antipruritic; treatment of plaque-type psoriasis (up to 10% of body surface area) [high-potency topical corticosteroid]

Usual Dosage
Children and Adults: Pruritus and inflammation: Topical (0.5% cream): Apply thin layer to affected area 2-4 times/day depending on the severity of the condition. Therapy should be discontinued when control is achieved; if no improvement is seen, reassessment of diagnosis may be necessary.
Children ≥12 years and Adults: Plaque-type psoriasis (Vanos™): Topical (0.1% cream): Apply a thin layer once or twice daily to affected areas (limited to <10% of body surface area). **Note:** Not recommended for use >2 consecutive weeks or >60 g/week total exposure. Discontinue when control is achieved.

Dosage Forms
Cream: 0.1% (30 g, 60 g)
Vanos™: 0.1% (30 g, 60 g)
Cream, anhydrous, emollient: 0.05% (15 g, 30 g, 60 g, 120 g)
Cream, aqueous, emollient: 0.05% (15 g, 30 g, 60 g)
Gel: 0.05% (15 g, 30 g, 60 g)
Ointment: 0.05% (15 g, 30 g, 60 g)
Solution: 0.05% (20 mL, 60 mL)

fluohydrisone acetate see fludrocortisone on page 406
fluohydrocortisone acetate see fludrocortisone on page 406
Fluonid® Topical (Discontinued) see fluocinolone on page 409
Fluor-I-Strip-AT® [US] see fluorescein on page 410
Fluor-I-Strip® (Discontinued) see fluorescein on page 410
Fluoracaine® (Discontinued) see proparacaine and fluorescein on page 794
Fluor-A-Day [US/Can] see fluoride on page 411
FluorCare® Neutral (Discontinued) see fluoride on page 411

fluorescein (FLURE e seen)

Synonyms fluorescein sodium; sodium fluorescein; soluble fluorescein

U.S./Canadian Brand Names AK-Fluor® [US]; Angiofluor™ Lite [US]; Angiofluor™ [US]; Fluor-I-Strip-AT® [US]; Fluorescite® [US/Can]; Fluorets® [US]; Ful-Glo® [US]

Therapeutic Category Diagnostic Agent

Use
Injection: Diagnostic aid in ophthalmic angiography and angioscopy
Topical: To stain the anterior segment of the eye for procedures (such as fitting contact lenses), disclosing corneal injury, and in applanation tonometry

Usual Dosage
Ophthalmic: Strips: Children and Adults: Moisten strip with sterile water, saline or ophthalmic fluid. Touch conjunctiva or fornix with tip of strip until adequately stained. For best results, patient should blink several times after application.
Injection:
Children: 3.5 mg/lb (7.7 mg/kg) injected rapidly into antecubital vein
Adults: 500-750 mg injected rapidly into antecubital vein
Note: Prior to use, an intradermal test dose of 0.05 mL may be used if an allergy is suspected. Evaluate 30-60 minutes following intradermal injection.
Oral: Adults: 1 g of injection solution has been administered orally in patients with inaccessible veins and when early phases of an angiogram are not needed.

Dosage Forms
  Injection, solution: 10% (5 mL); 25% (2 mL)
    AK-Fluor, Angiofluor™, Angiofluor™ Lite, Fluorescite®: 10% (5 mL); 25% (2 mL)
  Strip, ophthalmic: 1 mg
    Fluorets®: 1 mg (100)
    Ful-Glo®: 0.6 mg (300); 1 mg (300)

fluorescein and proparacaine *see* proparacaine and fluorescein *on page 794*
fluorescein sodium *see* fluorescein *on page 410*
Fluorescite® [US/Can] *see* fluorescein *on page 410*
Fluorets® [US] *see* fluorescein *on page 410*

fluoride (FLOR ide)

Sound-Alike/Look-Alike Issues
  Luride® may be confused with Lortab®
  Phos-Flur® may be confused with PhosLo®
  Thera-Flur-N® may be confused with Thera-Flu®
Synonyms acidulated phosphate fluoride; sodium fluoride; stannous fluoride
U.S./Canadian Brand Names ACT® Plus [US-OTC]; ACT® x2™ [US-OTC]; ACT® [US-OTC]; CaviRinse™ [US]; ControlRx® [US]; Denta 5000 Plus [US]; DentaGel [US]; EtheDent™ [US]; Fluor-A-Day [US/Can]; Fluorigard® [US-OTC]; Fluorinse® [US]; Flura-Drops® [US]; Gel-Kam® Rinse [US]; Gel-Kam® [US-OTC]; Just for Kids™ [US-OTC]; Lozi-Flur™ [US]; Luride® Lozi-Tab® [US]; NeutraCare® [US]; NeutraGard® Advanced [US]; NeutraGard® Plus [US]; NeutraGard® [US-OTC]; Omnii Gel™ [US-OTC]; PerioMed™ [US]; Pharmaflur® 1.1 [US]; Pharmaflur® [US]; Phos-Flur® Rinse [US-OTC]; Phos-Flur® [US]; PreviDent® 5000 Plus™ [US]; PreviDent® [US]; StanGard® Perio [US]; StanGard® [US]; Stop® [US]
Therapeutic Category Mineral, Oral
Use Prevention of dental caries
Usual Dosage Oral:
  The recommended daily dose of oral fluoride supplement (mg), based on fluoride ion content (ppm) in drinking water (2.2 mg of sodium fluoride is equivalent to 1 mg of fluoride ion): Adapted from Recommeded Dosage Schedule of The American Dental Association, The American Academy of Pediatric Dentistry, and The American Academy of Pediatrics:
  Less than 0.3 ppm:
    Birth to 6 months: 0 mg
    6 months to 3 years: 0.25 mg
    3-6 years: 0.5 mg
    6-16 years: 1 mg
  0.3-0.6 ppm:
    Birth to 3 years: 0 mg
    3-6 years: 0.25 mg
    6-16 years: 0.5 mg

  Cream: Children ≥6 years and Adults: Brush teeth with cream once daily regardless of fluoride content of drinking water
  Dental rinse or gel:
    Children 6-12 years: 5-10 mL rinse or apply to teeth and spit daily after brushing
    Adults: 10 mL rinse or apply to teeth and spit daily after brushing
    PreviDent® rinse: Children >6 years and Adults: Once weekly, rinse 10 mL vigorously around and between teeth for 1 minute, then spit; this should be done preferably at bedtime, after thoroughly brushing teeth; for maximum benefit, do not eat, drink, or rinse mouth for at least 30 minutes after treatment; do not swallow
    Fluorinse®: Children >6 years and Adults: Once weekly, vigorously swish 5-10 mL in mouth for 1 minute, then spit
  Lozenge (Lozi-Flur™): Adults: One lozenge daily regardless of fluoride content of drinking water
Dosage Forms
  Cream, oral [toothpaste]: 1.1% (51 g)
    Denta 5000 Plus, EtheDent™: 1.1% (51g)
  Gel, topical: 1.1% (56 g)
    DentaGel, EtheDent™: 1.1% (56 g)
    Gel-Kam® [OTC]: 0.4% (129 g)

▶

◀ Just for Kids™ [OTC], Omnii Gel™ [OTC], StanGard®: 0.4% (122 g)
NeutraCare®, NeutraGard® Advanced, Phos-Flur®, PreviDent®: 1.1% (60 g)
Stop®: 0.4% (120 g)
Lozenge:
Lozi-Flur™: 2.21 mg
Paste, oral [toothpaste]: 1.1% (56 g)
ControlRx®: 1.1% (56 g)
Solution, oral drops: 1.1 mg/mL
Flura-Drops®: 0.55 mg/drop
Solution, oral rinse: 0.05%, 0.2%, 0.44%, 0.5%
ACT® [OTC], ACT® Plus [OCT], Fluorigard® [OTC], NeutraGard® [OTC]: 0.05%
ACT® x2™ [OTCT]: 0.5%
CaviRinse™, Fluorinse®, NeutraGard® Plus, PreviDent®: 0.2%
Phos-Flur® [OTC]: 0.44%
Solution, oral rinse concentrate: 0.63%
Gel-Kam®, PerioMed™, StanGard® Perio: 0.63%
Tablet, chewable: 0.5 mg, 1.1 mg, 2.2 mg
EtheDent™: 0.55 mg, 1.1 mg, 2.2 mg
Fluor-A-Day: 0.56 mg, 1.1 mg, 2.21 mg
Luride® Lozi-Tab®: 0.55 mg, 1.1 mg

Fluorigard® [US-OTC] *see fluoride on page 411*

Fluori-Methane® [US] *see dichlorodifluoromethane and trichloromonofluoromethane on page 291*

Fluorinse® [US] *see fluoride on page 411*

Fluoritab® (Discontinued) *see fluoride on page 411*

5-fluorocytosine *see flucytosine on page 406*

fluorodeoxyuridine *see floxuridine on page 404*

9α-fluorohydrocortisone acetate *see fludrocortisone on page 406*

fluorometholone (flure oh METH oh lone)

U.S./Canadian Brand Names Flarex® [US/Can]; FML® Forte [US/Can]; FML® [US/Can]; PMS-Fluorometholone [Can]

Therapeutic Category Adrenal Corticosteroid

Use Treatment of steroid-responsive inflammatory conditions of the eye

Usual Dosage Ophthalmic:
Children >2 years and Adults: Reevaluate therapy if improvement is not seen within 2 days; use care not to discontinue prematurely; in chronic conditions, gradually decrease dosing frequency prior to discontinuing treatment
Ointment (FML®): Apply small amount (~1/2 inch ribbon) to conjunctival sac 1-3 times/day; may increase application to every 4 hours during the initial 24-48 hours
Suspension:
FML®: Instill 1 drop into conjunctival sac 2-4 times/day; may instill 1 drop every 4 hours during initial 24-48 hours
FML® Forte: Instill 1 drop into conjunctival sac 2-4 times/day
Adults: Suspension (Flarex®): Instill 1-2 drops into conjunctival sac 4 times/day; may increase application to 2 drops every 2 hours during initial 24-48 hours. Consult prescriber if no improvement after 14 days.

Dosage Forms
Ointment, ophthalmic:
FML®: 0.1% (3.5 g)
Suspension, ophthalmic: 0.1% (5 mL, 10 mL, 15 mL)
Flarex®: 0.1% (5 mL)
FML®: 0.1% (5 mL, 10 mL, 15 mL)
FML® Forte: 0.25% (2 mL, 5 mL, 10 mL, 15 mL)

Fluor-Op® (Discontinued) *see fluorometholone on page 412*

Fluoroplex® [US] *see fluorouracil on page 412*

fluorouracil (flure oh YOOR a sil)

Sound-Alike/Look-Alike Issues
fluorouracil may be confused with flucytosine
Efudex® may be confused with Efidac (Efidac 24®), Eurax®

Synonyms 5-fluorouracil; 5-FU; FU

U.S./Canadian Brand Names Adrucil® [US]; Carac® [US]; Efudex® [US/Can]; Fluoroplex® [US]; Fluorouracil® [US]

Therapeutic Category Antineoplastic Agent

Use Treatment of carcinomas of the breast, colon, head and neck, pancreas, rectum, or stomach; topically for the management of actinic or solar keratoses and superficial basal cell carcinomas

Usual Dosage Adults:
Refer to individual protocols:
I.V. bolus: 500-600 mg/m^2 every 3-4 weeks **or** 425 mg/m^2 on days 1-5 every 4 weeks
Continuous I.V. infusion: 1000 mg/m^2/day for 4-5 days every 3-4 weeks **or**
2300-2600 mg/m^2 on day 1 every week **or**
300-400 mg/m^2/day **or**
225 mg/m^2/day for 5-8 weeks (with radiation therapy)
Actinic keratoses: Topical:
Carac™: Apply thin film to lesions once daily for up to 4 weeks, as tolerated
Efudex®: Apply to lesions twice daily for 2-4 weeks; complete healing may not be evident for 1-2 months following treatment
Fluoroplex®: Apply to lesions twice daily for 2-6 weeks
Superficial basal cell carcinoma: Topical: Efudex® 5%: Apply to affected lesions twice daily for 3-6 weeks; treatment may be continued for up to 10-12 weeks

Dosage Forms
Cream, topical:
Carac™: 0.5% (30 g)
Efudex®: 5% (40 g)
Fluoroplex®: 1% (30 g)
Injection, solution: 50 mg/mL (10 mL, 20 mL, 50 mL, 100 mL)
Adrucil®: 50 mg/mL (10 mL, 50 mL, 100 mL)
Solution, topical: 2% (10 mL); 5% (10 mL)
Efudex®: 2% (10 mL); 5% (10 mL)
Fluorouracil®: 5% (10 mL)

Fluorouracil® [US] *see fluorouracil on page 412*

5-fluorouracil *see fluorouracil on page 412*

Fluothane® *(Discontinued)* *see halothane on page 466*

fluoxetine (floo OKS e teen)

Sound-Alike/Look-Alike Issues
FLUoxetine may be confused with DULoxetine, fluvastatin, fluvoxamine, PARoxetine
Prozac® may be confused with Prilosec®, Prograf®, Proscar®, ProSom®, ProStep®
Sarafem® may be confused with Serophene®

Synonyms fluoxetine hydrochloride

Tall-Man FLUoxetine

U.S./Canadian Brand Names Apo-Fluoxetine® [Can]; BCI-Fluoxetine [Can]; CO Fluoxetine [Can]; Dom-Fluoxetine [Can]; FXT [Can]; Gen-Fluoxetine [Can]; Novo-Fluoxetine [Can]; Nu-Fluoxetine [Can]; PHL-Fluoxetine [Can]; PMS-Fluoxetine [Can]; Prozac® Weekly™ [US]; Prozac® [US/Can]; ratio-Fluoxetine [Can]; Rhoxal-fluoxetine [Can]; Riva-Fluoxetine [Can]; Sandoz-Fluoxetine [Can]; Sarafem® [US]; Selfemra™ [US]

Therapeutic Category Antidepressant, Selective Serotonin Reuptake Inhibitor

Use Treatment of major depressive disorder (MDD); treatment of binge-eating and vomiting in patients with moderate-to-severe bulimia nervosa; obsessive-compulsive disorder (OCD); premenstrual dysphoric disorder (PMDD); panic disorder with or without agoraphobia

Usual Dosage Oral: **Note:** Upon discontinuation of fluoxetine therapy, gradually taper dose. If intolerable symptoms occur following a dose reduction, consider resuming the previously prescribed dose and/or decrease dose at a more gradual rate.
Children:
Depression: 8-18 years: 10-20 mg/day; lower-weight children can be started at 10 mg/day, may increase to 20 mg/day after 1 week if needed
Obsessive-compulsive disorder: 7-18 years: Initial: 10 mg/day; in adolescents and higher-weight children, dose may be increased to 20 mg/day after 2 weeks. Range: 10-60 mg/day.

Adults: 20 mg/day in the morning; may increase after several weeks by 20 mg/day increments; maximum: 80 mg/day; doses >20 mg may be given once daily or divided twice daily. **Note:** Lower doses of 5-10 mg/day have been used for initial treatment.
Usual dosage range:
Bulimia nervosa: 60-80 mg/day
Depression: 20-40 mg/day; patients maintained on Prozac® 20 mg/day may be changed to Prozac® Weekly™ 90 mg/week, starting dose 7 days after the last 20 mg/day dose
Obsessive-compulsive disorder: 40-80 mg/day
Panic disorder: Initial: 10 mg/day; after 1 week, increase to 20 mg/day; may increase after several weeks; doses >60 mg/day have not been evaluated
Premenstrual dysphoric disorder (Sarafem®): 20 mg/day continuously, **or** 20 mg/day starting 14 days prior to menstruation and through first full day of menses (repeat with each cycle)

Dosage Forms
Capsule: 10 mg, 20 mg, 40 mg
Prozac®: 10 mg, 20 mg, 40 mg
Selfemra™: 10 mg, 20 mg
Capsule, delayed release:
Prozac® Weekly™: 90 mg
Solution, oral: 20 mg/5 mL
Prozac®: 20 mg/5 mL
Tablet: 10 mg, 20 mg
Sarafem®: 10 mg, 20 mg

fluoxetine and olanzapine see olanzapine and fluoxetine on page 694
fluoxetine hydrochloride see fluoxetine on page 413

fluoxymesterone (floo oks i MES te rone)

U.S./Canadian Brand Names Androxy™ [US]
Therapeutic Category Androgen
Controlled Substance C-III
Use Replacement of endogenous testicular hormone; in females, palliative treatment of breast cancer
Usual Dosage Oral: Adults:
Male:
Hypogonadism: 5-20 mg/day
Delayed puberty: 2.5-20 mg/day for 4-6 months
Female: Inoperable breast carcinoma: 10-40 mg/day in divided doses for 1-3 months
Dosage Forms
Tablet: 10 mg
Androxy™: 10 mg

flupenthixol *(Canada only)* (floo pen THIKS ol)

Synonyms flupenthixol decanoate; flupenthixol dihydrochloride
U.S./Canadian Brand Names Fluanxol® [Can]
Therapeutic Category Antipsychotic Agent; Thioxanthene Derivative
Use Maintenance therapy of chronic schizophrenic patients whose main manifestations do **not** include excitement, agitation, or hyperactivity
Usual Dosage
I.M. (depot): Flupenthixol is administered by deep I.M. injection, preferably in the gluteus maximus, **NOT for I.V. use**; maintenance dosages are given at 2- to 3-week intervals
Patients not previously treated with long-acting depot neuroleptics should be given an initial test dose of 5-20 mg. An initial dose of 20 mg is usually well tolerated; however, a 5 mg test dose is recommended in elderly, frail, and cachectic patients, and in patients whose individual or family history suggests a predisposition to extrapyramidal reactions. In the subsequent 5-10 days, the therapeutic response and the appearance of extrapyramidal symptoms should be carefully monitored. Oral neuroleptic drugs may be continued, but dosage should be reduced during this overlapping period and eventually discontinued.
Oral: Initial: 1 mg 3 times/day; dose must be individualized. May be increased by 1 mg every 2-3 days based on tolerance and control of symptoms. Usual maintenance dosage: 3-6 mg/day in divided doses (doses ≥12 mg/day used in some patients).

Dosage Forms [CAN] = Canadian brand name
Injection, solution [depot]:
Fluanxol® [CAN]: 20 mg/mL (10 mL); 100 mg/mL (2 mL) [not available in the U.S.]
Tablet:
Fluanxol® [CAN]: 0.5 mg, 3 mg [not available in the U.S.]

flupenthixol decanoate see flupenthixol (Canada only) on page 414
flupenthixol dihydrochloride see flupenthixol (Canada only) on page 414

fluphenazine (floo FEN a zeen)

Sound-Alike/Look-Alike Issues
Prolixin® may be confused with Proloprim®
Synonyms fluphenazine decanoate
U.S./Canadian Brand Names Apo-Fluphenazine Decanoate® [Can]; Apo-Fluphenazine® [Can]; Modecate® Concentrate [Can]; Modecate® [Can]; PMS-Fluphenazine Decanoate [Can]
Therapeutic Category Phenothiazine Derivative
Use Management of manifestations of psychotic disorders and schizophrenia; depot formulation may offer improved outcome in individuals with psychosis who are nonadherent with oral antipsychotics
Usual Dosage Adults: Psychoses:
Oral: 0.5-10 mg/day in divided doses at 6- to 8-hour intervals; some patients may require up to 40 mg/day
I.M.: 2.5-10 mg/day in divided doses at 6- to 8-hour intervals (parenteral dose is 1/3 to 1/2 the oral dose for the hydrochloride salts)
I.M. (decanoate): 12.5-37.5 mg every 2 weeks
Conversion from hydrochloride to decanoate I.M. 0.5 mL (12.5 mg) decanoate every 3 weeks is approximately equivalent to 10 mg hydrochloride/day
Dosage Forms
Injection, oil: 25 mg/mL (5 mL)
Injection, solution: 2.5 mg/mL (10 mL)
Tablet: 1 mg, 2.5 mg, 5 mg, 10 mg

fluphenazine decanoate see fluphenazine on page 415
Flura® (Discontinued) see fluoride on page 411
Flura-Drops® [US] see fluoride on page 411

flurandrenolide (flure an DREN oh lide)

Sound-Alike/Look-Alike Issues
Cordran® may be confused with Cardura®, codeine, Cordarone®
Synonyms flurandrenolone
U.S./Canadian Brand Names Cordran® SP [US]; Cordran® [US/Can]
Therapeutic Category Corticosteroid, Topical
Use Inflammation of corticosteroid-responsive dermatoses [medium potency topical corticosteroid]
Usual Dosage Topical: Therapy should be discontinued when control is achieved; if no improvement is seen, reassessment of diagnosis may be necessary.
Children:
Cream: Apply sparingly 1-2 times/day
Tape: Apply once daily
Adults: Cream, lotion: Apply sparingly 2-3 times/day
Dosage Forms
Cream, emulsified:
Cordran® SP: 0.05% (15 g, 30 g, 60 g)
Lotion:
Cordran®: 0.05% (15 mL, 60 mL)
Tape, topical [roll]:
Cordran®: 4 mcg/cm^2 (24 inch, 80 inch)

flurandrenolone see flurandrenolide on page 415
Flurate® Ophthalmic Solution (Discontinued) see fluorescein on page 410

flurazepam (flure AZ e pam)

Sound-Alike/Look-Alike Issues
flurazepam may be confused with temazepam
Dalmane® may be confused with Demulen®, Dialume®
Synonyms flurazepam hydrochloride
U.S./Canadian Brand Names Apo-Flurazepam® [Can]; Dalmane® [US/Can]; Som Pam [Can]
Therapeutic Category Benzodiazepine
Controlled Substance C-IV
Use Short-term treatment of insomnia
Usual Dosage Oral: Insomnia:
Children: ≥15 years: 15 mg at bedtime
Adults: 15-30 mg at bedtime
Dosage Forms
Capsule: 15 mg, 30 mg
Dalmane®: 15 mg, 30 mg

flurazepam hydrochloride *see* flurazepam *on page 416*

flurbiprofen (flure BI proe fen)

Sound-Alike/Look-Alike Issues
flurbiprofen may be confused with fenoprofen
Ansaid® may be confused with Asacol®, Axid®
Ocufen® may be confused with Ocuflox®, Ocupress®
Synonyms flurbiprofen sodium
U.S./Canadian Brand Names Alti-Flurbiprofen [Can]; Ansaid® [Can]; Apo-Flurbiprofen® [Can]; Froben-SR® [Can]; Froben® [Can]; Novo-Flurprofen [Can]; Nu-Flurprofen [Can]; Ocufen® [US/Can]
Therapeutic Category Analgesic, Nonnarcotic Nonsteroidal Antiinflammatory Drug (NSAID)
Use
Oral: Treatment of rheumatoid arthritis and osteoarthritis
Ophthalmic: Inhibition of intraoperative miosis
Usual Dosage
Oral:
Rheumatoid arthritis and osteoarthritis: 200-300 mg/day in 2-, 3-, or 4 divided doses; do not administer more than 100 mg for any single dose; maximum: 300 mg/day
Dental: Management of postoperative pain: 100 mg every 12 hours
Ophthalmic: Instill 1 drop every 30 minutes, beginning 2 hours prior to surgery (total of 4 drops in each affected eye)
Dosage Forms
Solution, ophthalmic: 0.03% (2.5 mL)
Ocufen®: 0.03% (2.5 mL)
Tablet: 50 mg, 100 mg

flurbiprofen sodium *see* flurbiprofen *on page 416*
5-flurocytosine *see* flucytosine *on page 406*
Fluro-Ethyl® [US] *see* ethyl chloride and dichlorotetrafluoroethane *on page 382*
Flurosyn® Topical *(Discontinued)* *see* fluocinolone *on page 409*
FluShield® *(Discontinued)* *see* influenza virus vaccine *on page 508*

flutamide (FLOO ta mide)

Sound-Alike/Look-Alike Issues
flutamide may be confused with Flumadine®, thalidomide
Eulexin® may be confused with Edecrin®, Eurax®
Synonyms 4'-nitro-3'-trifluoromethylisobutyrantide; niftolid; NSC-147834; SCH 13521
U.S./Canadian Brand Names Apo-Flutamide® [Can]; Euflex® [Can]; Eulexin® [US/Can]; Novo-Flutamide [Can]
Therapeutic Category Antiandrogen

Use Treatment of metastatic prostatic carcinoma in combination therapy with LHRH agonist analogues

Usual Dosage Oral: Adults: Prostatic carcinoma: 250 mg 3 times/day

Dosage Forms
 Capsule: 125 mg
  Eulexin®: 125 mg

fluticasone and salmeterol (floo TIK a sone & sal ME te role)

Sound-Alike/Look-Alike Issues
 Advair may be confused with Advicor®

Synonyms fluticasone propionate and salmeterol xinafoate; salmeterol and fluticasone

U.S./Canadian Brand Names Advair Diskus® [US/Can]; Advair® HFA [US]; Advair® [Can]

Therapeutic Category Beta$_2$-Adrenergic Agonist Agent; Corticosteroid, Inhalant

Use Maintenance treatment of asthma; maintenance treatment of COPD

Usual Dosage Oral inhalation: **Note:** Do not use to transfer patients from systemic corticosteroid therapy.
 COPD: Adults:
  Advair Diskus®: Fluticasone 250 mcg/salmeterol 50 mcg twice daily, 12 hours apart. **Note:** This is the maximum dose.
  Advair Diskus® [Canadian labeling; not in approved U.S. labeling]: Fluticasone 250 mcg/salmeterol 50 mcg **or** fluticasone 500 mcg/salmeterol 50 mcg twice daily, 12 hours apart.
  Maximum dose: Fluticasone 500 mcg/salmeterol 50 mcg per inhalation (2 inhalations/day)

 Asthma:
  Children 4-11 years: Advair Diskus®: Fluticasone 100 mcg/salmeterol 50 mcg twice daily, 12 hours apart. **Note:** This is the maximum dose.
  Children ≥12 and Adults:
   Advair Diskus®: One inhalation twice daily, morning and evening, 12 hours apart
    Maximum dose: Fluticasone 500 mcg/salmeterol 50 mcg per inhalation (2 inhalations/day)
   Advair® HFA: Two inhalations twice daily, morning and evening, 12 hours apart
    Maximum dose: Fluticasone 230 mcg/salmeterol 21 mcg per inhalation (4 inhalations/day)
   Advair® 125 or Advair® 250 [Canadian labeling; not in approved U.S. labeling]: Two inhalations twice daily, morning and evening, 12 hours apart
    Maximum dose: Fluticasone 250 mcg/salmeterol 25 mcg per inhalation (4 inhalations/day)
 Note: Initial dose prescribed should be based upon previous dose of inhaled-steroid asthma therapy. Dose should be increased after 2 weeks if adequate response is not achieved. Patients should be titrated to lowest effective dose once stable. Each suggestion below specifies the product strength to use; remember to **use 1 inhalation for Diskus® and 2 inhalations for HFA.**

 Patients not currently on inhaled corticosteroids:
  Advair Diskus®: Fluticasone 100 mcg/salmeterol 50 mcg **or** fluticasone 250 mcg/salmeterol 50 mcg
  Advair® HFA: Fluticasone 45 mcg/salmeterol 21 mcg **or** fluticasone 115 mcg/salmeterol 21 mcg
 Patients currently using inhaled beclomethasone dipropionate:
  ≤160 mcg/day: Fluticasone 100 mcg/salmeterol 50 mcg **or** Advair® HFA: Fluticasone 45 mcg/salmeterol 21 mcg
  320 mcg/day: Fluticasone 250 mcg/salmeterol 50 mcg **or** Advair® HFA: Fluticasone 115 mcg/salmeterol 21 mcg
  640 mcg/day: Fluticasone 500 mcg/salmeterol 50 mcg **or** Advair® HFA: Fluticasone 230 mcg/salmeterol 21 mcg
 Patients currently using inhaled budesonide:
  ≤400 mcg/day: Fluticasone 100 mcg/salmeterol 50 mcg **or** Advair® HFA: Fluticasone 45 mcg/salmeterol 21 mcg
  800-1200 mcg/day: Fluticasone 250 mcg/salmeterol 50 mcg **or** Advair® HFA: Fluticasone 115 mcg/salmeterol 21mcg
  1600 mcg/day: Fluticasone 500 mcg/salmeterol 50 mcg **or** Advair® HFA: Fluticasone 230 mcg/salmeterol 21 mcg
 Patients currently using inhaled flunisolide CFC aerosol:
  ≤1000 mcg/day: Fluticasone 100 mcg/salmeterol 50 mcg **or** Advair® HFA: Fluticasone 45 mcg/salmeterol 21 mcg
  1250-2000 mcg/day: Fluticasone 250 mcg/salmeterol 50 mcg **or** Advair® HFA: Fluticasone 115 mcg/salmeterol 21 mcg
 Patients currently using inhaled flunisolide HFA inhalation aerosol:
  ≤320 mcg/day: Fluticasone 100 mcg/salmeterol 50 mcg **or** Advair® HFA: Fluticasone 45 mcg/salmeterol 21 mcg

◄ 640 mcg/day: Fluticasone 250 mcg/salmeterol 50 mcg **or** Advair® HFA: Fluticasone 115 mcg/salmeterol 21 mcg
Patients currently using inhaled fluticasone HFA aerosol:
≤176 mcg/day: Fluticasone 100 mcg/salmeterol 50 mcg **or** Advair® HFA: Fluticasone 45 mcg/salmeterol 21 mcg
440 mcg/day: Fluticasone 250 mcg/salmeterol 50 mcg **or** Advair® HFA: Fluticasone 115 mcg/salmeterol 21 mcg
660-880 mcg/day: Fluticasone 500 mcg/salmeterol 50 mcg **or** Advair® HFA: Fluticasone 230 mcg/salmeterol 21 mcg
Patients currently using inhaled fluticasone propionate powder:
≤200 mcg/day: Fluticasone 100 mcg/salmeterol 50 mcg **or** Advair® HFA: Fluticasone 45 mcg/salmeterol 21 mcg
500 mcg/day: Fluticasone 250 mcg/salmeterol 50 mcg **or** Advair® HFA: Fluticasone 115 mcg/salmeterol 21 mcg
1000 mcg/day: Fluticasone 500 mcg/salmeterol 50 mcg **or** Advair® HFA: Fluticasone 230 mcg/salmeterol 21 mcg
Patients currently using inhaled mometasone furoate powder:
220 mcg/day: Fluticasone 100 mcg/salmeterol 50 mcg **or** Advair® HFA: Fluticasone 45 mcg/salmeterol 21 mcg
440 mcg/day: Fluticasone 250 mcg/salmeterol 50 mcg **or** Advair® HFA: Fluticasone 115 mcg/salmeterol 21 mcg
880 mcg/day: Fluticasone 500 mcg/salmeterol 50 mcg **or** Advair® HFA: Fluticasone 230 mcg/salmeterol 21 mcg
Patients currently using inhaled triamcinolone acetonide:
≤1000 mcg/day: Fluticasone 100 mcg/salmeterol 50 mcg **or** Advair® HFA: Fluticasone 45 mcg/salmeterol 21 mcg
1100-1600 mcg/day: Fluticasone 250 mcg/salmeterol 50 mcg **or** Advair® HFA: Fluticasone 115 mcg/salmeterol 21 mcg

Dosage Forms Excipient information presented when available (limited, particularly for generics); consult specific product labeling. [DSC] = Discontinued product; [CAN] = Canadian brand name/formulation
Aerosol, for oral inhalation:
Advair® HFA:
45/21: Fluticasone propionate 45 mcg and salmeterol 21 mcg (12 g)
115/21: Fluticasone propionate 115 mcg and salmeterol 21 mcg (12 g)
230/21: Fluticasone propionate 230 mcg and salmeterol 21 mcg (12 g)
Advair® [CAN]:
125/25: Fluticasone propionate 125 mcg and salmeterol 25 mcg (12 g) [not available in the U.S.]
250/25: Fluticasone propionate 250 mcg and salmeterol 25 mcg (12 g) [not available in the U.S.]
Powder, for oral inhalation:
Advair Diskus®:
100/50: Fluticasone propionate 100 mcg and salmeterol 50 mcg (14s, 28s, 60s)
250/50: Fluticasone propionate 250 mcg and salmeterol 50 mcg (14s, 60s)
500/50: Fluticasone propionate 500 mcg and salmeterol 50 mcg (14s, 60s)

fluticasone (nasal) (floo TIK a sone NAY sal)

U.S./Canadian Brand Names Flonase® [US/Can]

Therapeutic Category Adrenal Corticosteroid

Use Intranasal: Management of seasonal and perennial allergic rhinitis and nonallergic rhinitis in patients ≥4 years of age

Usual Dosage Intranasal: Rhinitis:
Children ≥4 years and Adolescents: Initial: 1 spray (50 mcg/spray) per nostril once daily; patients not adequately responding or patients with more severe symptoms may use 2 sprays (100 mcg) per nostril. Depending on response, dosage may be reduced to 100 mcg daily. Total daily dosage should not exceed 2 sprays in each nostril (200 mcg)/day. Dosing should be at regular intervals.
Adults: Initial: 2 sprays (50 mcg/spray) per nostril once daily; may also be divided into 100 mcg twice a day. After the first few days, dosage may be reduced to 1 spray per nostril once daily for maintenance therapy. Dosing should be at regular intervals.

Dosage Forms
Suspension, intranasal, as furoate [spray]:
Veramyst™: 27.5 mcg/inhalation (10 g)
Suspension, intranasal, as propionate [spray]: 50 mcg/inhalation (16 g)
Flonase®: 50 mcg/inhalation (16 g)

fluticasone (oral inhalation) (floo TIK a sone or al in ha LAY shun)

U.S./Canadian Brand Names Flovent® Diskus® [Can]; Flovent® HFA [US/Can]

Therapeutic Category Adrenal Corticosteroid

Use Inhalation: Maintenance treatment of asthma as prophylactic therapy. It is also indicated for patients requiring oral corticosteroid therapy for asthma to assist in total discontinuation or reduction of total oral dose. NOT indicated for the relief of acute bronchospasm.

Usual Dosage Inhalation, oral: Asthma:

Flovent® HFA: Children ≥12 years: Refer to Adults dosing.

Flovent® Diskus® [Can]:

  Children 4-16 years: Usual starting dose: 50-100 mcg twice daily; may increase to 200 mcg twice daily in patients not adequately controlled; titrate to the lowest effective dose once asthma stability is achieved
  Children ≥16 years: Refer to Adults dosing.

Adults: **Note:** Titrate to the lowest effective dose once asthma stability is achieved

  Flovent® HFA: Manufacturers labeling: Dosing based on previous therapy
    Bronchodilator alone: Recommended starting dose: 88 mcg twice daily; highest recommended dose: 440 mcg twice daily
    Inhaled corticosteroids: Recommended starting dose: 88-220 mcg twice daily; highest recommended dose: 440 mcg twice daily; a higher starting dose may be considered in patients previously requiring higher doses of inhaled corticosteroids
    Oral corticosteroids: Recommended starting dose:
    Flovent® HFA: 440 mcg twice daily
    Highest recommended dose: 880 mcg twice daily; starting dose is patient dependent. In patients on chronic oral corticosteroids therapy, reduce prednisone dose no faster than 2.5-5 mg/day on a weekly basis; begin taper after 1 week of fluticasone therapy
  NIH Asthma Guidelines (administer in divided doses twice daily).
    "Low" dose: 88-264 mcg/day
    "Medium" dose: 264-660 mcg/day
    "High" dose: >660 mcg/day
  Flovent® Diskus® [CAN]:
    Mild asthma: 100-250 mcg twice daily
    Moderate asthma: 250-500 mcg twice da
    Severe asthma: 500 mcg twice daily; may increase to 1000 mcg twice daily in very severe patients requiring high doses of corticosteroids

Dosage Forms [CAN] = Canadian brand name

Aerosol for oral inhalation [CFC free]:
  Flovent® HFA: 44 mcg/inhalation (10.6 g); 110 mcg/inhalation (12 g); 220 mcg/inhalation (12 g)

Powder for oral inhalation [prefilled blister pack]:
  Flovent® Diskus® [U.S.]: 50 mcg (60s)
  Flovent® Diskus®) [CAN]: 50 mcg (28s, 60s); 100 mcg (28s, 60s); 250 mcg (28s, 60s); 500 mcg (28s, 60s) [not available in the U.S.]

fluticasone propionate and salmeterol xinafoate *see* fluticasone and salmeterol *on page 417*

fluticasone (topical) (floo TIK a sone TOP i kal)

Sound-Alike/Look-Alike Issues
  Cutivate® may be confused with Ultravate®

U.S./Canadian Brand Names Cutivate® [US/Can]

Therapeutic Category Adrenal Corticosteroid; Corticosteroid, Topical

Use Relief of inflammation and pruritus associated with corticosteroid-responsive dermatoses; atopic dermatitis

Usual Dosage Topical:

Corticosteroid-responsive dermatoses:
  Children ≥3 months: Cream: Apply sparingly to affected area twice daily. If no improvement is seen within 2 weeks, reassessment of diagnosis may be necessary
  Adults: Cream, lotion, ointment: Apply sparingly to affected area twice daily. If no improvement is seen within 2 weeks, reassessment of diagnosis may be necessary.

Atopic dermatitis:
  Children ≥3 months: Cream: Apply sparingly to affected area twice daily. If no improvement is seen within 2 weeks, reassessment of diagnosis may be necessary.

▶

◄ Children ≥1 year: Lotion: Apply sparingly to affected area twice daily
Adults: Cream, lotion: Apply sparingly to affected area once or twice daily. If no improvement is seen within 2 weeks, reassessment of diagnosis may be necessary

Dosage Forms
Cream: 0.05% (15 g, 30 g, 60 g)
Cutivate®: 0.05% (30 g, 60 g)
Lotion:
Cutivate®: 0.05% (60 mL)
Ointment: 0.005% (15 g, 30 g, 60 g)
Cutivate®: 0.005% (30 g, 60 g)

fluvastatin (FLOO va sta tin)

Sound-Alike/Look-Alike Issues
fluvastatin may be confused with fluoxetine

U.S./Canadian Brand Names Lescol® XL [US/Can]; Lescol® [US/Can]

Therapeutic Category HMG-CoA Reductase Inhibitor

Use To be used as a component of multiple risk factor intervention in patients at risk for atherosclerosis vascular disease due to hypercholesterolemia

Adjunct to dietary therapy to reduce elevated total cholesterol (total-C), LDL-C, triglyceride, and apolipoprotein B (apo-B) levels and to increase HDL-C in primary hypercholesterolemia and mixed dyslipidemia (Fredrickson types IIa and IIb); to slow the progression of coronary atherosclerosis in patients with coronary heart disease; reduce risk of coronary revascularization procedures in patients with coronary heart disease

Usual Dosage Oral:
Adolescents 10-16 years: Heterozygous familial hypercholesterolemia: Initial: 20 mg once daily; may increase every 6 weeks based on tolerability and response to a maximum recommended dose of 80 mg/day, given in 2 divided doses (immediate release capsule) or as a single daily dose (extended release tablet)
Note: Indicated only for adjunctive therapy when diet alone cannot reduce LDL-C below 190 mg/dL, or 160 mg/dL (with cardiovascular risk factors). Female patients must be 1 year postmenarche.
Adults:
Patients requiring ≥25% decrease in LDL-C: 40 mg capsule once daily in the evening, 80 mg extended release tablet once daily (anytime), or 40 mg capsule twice daily
Patients requiring <25% decrease in LDL-C: Initial: 20 mg capsule once daily in the evening; may increase based on tolerability and response to a maximum recommended dose of 80 mg/day, given in 2 divided doses (immediate release capsule) or as a single daily dose (extended release tablet)

Dosage Forms
Capsule:
Lescol®: 20 mg, 40 mg
Tablet, extended release:
Lescol® XL: 80 mg

Fluviral S/F® [Can] *see* influenza virus vaccine *on page 508*
Fluvirin® [US] *see* influenza virus vaccine *on page 508*

fluvoxamine (floo VOKS a meen)

Sound-Alike/Look-Alike Issues
fluvoxamine may be confused with flavoxate, fluoxetine
Luvox may be confused with Lasix®, Levoxyl®, Lovenox®

U.S./Canadian Brand Names Alti-Fluvoxamine [Can]; Apo-Fluvoxamine® [Can]; Luvox® CR [US]; Luvox® [Can]; Novo-Fluvoxamine [Can]; Nu-Fluvoxamine [Can]; PMS-Fluvoxamine [Can]; Rhoxal-fluvoxamine [Can]; Sandoz-Fluvoxamine [Can]

Therapeutic Category Antidepressant, Selective Serotonin Reuptake Inhibitor

Use Treatment of obsessive-compulsive disorder (OCD); treatment of social anxiety disorder

Usual Dosage Oral:
Obsessive-compulsive disorder:
Children 8-17 years: Immediate release: Initial: 25 mg once daily at bedtime; may be increased in 25 mg increments at 4- to 7-day intervals, as tolerated, to maximum therapeutic benefit; usual dose range: 50-200 mg/day. **Note:** When total daily dose exceeds 50 mg, the dose should be given in 2 divided doses with larger portion administered at bedtime.

Maximum: Children: 8-11 years: 200 mg/day, adolescents: 300 mg/day; lower doses may be effective in female versus male patients

Adults:

Immediate release: Initial: 50 mg once daily at bedtime; may be increased in 50 mg increments at 4- to 7-day intervals, as tolerated; usual dose range: 100-300 mg/day; maximum dose: 300 mg/day. **Note:** When total daily dose exceeds 100 mg, the dose should be given in 2 divided doses with larger portion administered at bedtime.

Controlled release: Initial: 100 mg once daily at bedtime; may be increased in 50 mg increments at intervals of at least 1 week; usual dosage range: 100-300 mg/day; maximum dose: 300 mg/day

Social anxiety disorder: Adults: Controlled release: Initial: 100 mg once daily at bedtime; may be increased in 50 mg increments at intervals of at least 1 week; usual dosage range: 100-300 mg/day; maximum dose: 300 mg/day

Dosage Forms

Tablet:

25 mg, 50 mg, 100 mg

Capsule, extended release:

Luvox® CR: 100 mg, 150 mg

Fluzone® [US] *see* influenza virus vaccine *on page 508*

FML® [US/Can] *see* fluorometholone *on page 412*

FML® Forte [US/Can] *see* fluorometholone *on page 412*

FML-S® *(Discontinued)*

Focalin® [US] *see* dexmethylphenidate *on page 281*

Focalin® XR [US] *see* dexmethylphenidate *on page 281*

Foille® [US-OTC] *see* benzocaine *on page 124*

folacin *see* folic acid *on page 421*

folacin, vitamin B$_{12}$, and vitamin B$_6$ *see* folic acid, cyanocobalamin, and pyridoxine *on page 422*

Folamin™ [US] *see* folic acid, cyanocobalamin, and pyridoxine *on page 422*

folate *see* folic acid *on page 421*

Folbee [US] *see* folic acid, cyanocobalamin, and pyridoxine *on page 422*

Folex® PFS™ *(Discontinued) see* methotrexate *on page 615*

Folgard® [US-OTC] *see* folic acid, cyanocobalamin, and pyridoxine *on page 422*

Folgard® RX [US] *see* folic acid, cyanocobalamin, and pyridoxine *on page 422*

Folgard RX 2.2® *(Discontinued) see* folic acid, cyanocobalamin, and pyridoxine *on page 422*

folic acid (FOE lik AS id)

Sound-Alike/Look-Alike Issues

folic acid may be confused with folinic acid

Synonyms folacin; folate; pteroylglutamic acid

U.S./Canadian Brand Names Apo-Folic® [Can]

Therapeutic Category Vitamin, Water Soluble

Use Treatment of megaloblastic and macrocytic anemias due to folate deficiency; dietary supplement to prevent neural tube defects

Usual Dosage

Oral, I.M., I.V., SubQ: Anemia:

Infants: 0.1 mg/day

Children <4 years: Up to 0.3 mg/day

Children >4 years and Adults: 0.4 mg/day

Pregnant and lactating women: 0.8 mg/day

Oral:

RDA: Expressed as dietary folate equivalents:

Children:

1-3 years: 150 mcg/day

4-8 years: 200 mcg/day

9-13 years: 300 mcg/day

Children ≥14 years and Adults: 400 mcg/day

Prevention of neural tube defects:

Females of childbearing potential: 400 mcg/day

Females at high risk or with family history of neural tube defects: 4 mg/day

Dosage Forms
Injection, solution: 5 mg/mL (10 mL)
Tablet: 0.4 mg, 0.8 mg, 1 mg

folic acid, cyanocobalamin, and pyridoxine
(FOE lik AS id, sye an oh koe BAL a min, & peer i DOKS een)

Synonyms cyanocobalamin, folic acid, and pyridoxine; folacin, vitamin B_{12}, and vitamin B_6; pyridoxine, folic acid, and cyanocobalamin

U.S./Canadian Brand Names ComBgen™ [US]; Folamin™ [US]; Folbee [US]; Folgard® RX [US]; Folgard® [US-OTC]; Foltx® [US]; Tricardio B [US]

Therapeutic Category Vitamin

Use Nutritional supplement in end-stage renal failure, dialysis, hyperhomocysteinemia, homocystinuria, malabsorption syndromes, dietary deficiencies

Usual Dosage Oral: Adults: 1 tablet daily

Dosage Forms
Tablet: Folic acid 0.8 mg, cyanocobalamin 1000 mcg, and pyridoxine 50 mg
  Folgard® RX: Folic acid 2.2 mg, cyanocobalamin 1000 mcg, and pyridoxine 25 mg
  ComBgen™: Folic acid 2.2 mg, cyanocobalamin 500 mcg, and pyridoxine 25 mg
  Folamin™, Foltx®: Folic acid 2.5 mg, cyanocobalamin 2000 mcg, and pyridoxine 25 mg
  Folbee: Folic acid 2.5 mg, cyanocobalamin 1000 mcg, and pyridoxine 25 mg
  Folgard® [OTC]: Folic acid 0.8 mg, cyanocobalamin 115 mcg, and pyridoxine 10 mg
  Tricardio B: Folic acid 0.4 mg, cyanocobalamin 250 mcg, and pyridoxine 25 mg

follicle stimulating hormone, human *see* urofollitropin *on page 964*
follicle stimulating hormone, recombinant *see* follitropin alfa *on page 422*
follicle stimulating hormone, recombinant *see* follitropin beta *on page 423*
Follistim® AQ [US] *see* follitropin beta *on page 423*
Follistim® AQ Cartridge [US] *see* follitropin beta *on page 423*

follitropin alfa (foe li TRO pin AL fa)

Synonyms follicle stimulating hormone, recombinant; FSH; rFSH-alpha; rhFSH-alpha

U.S./Canadian Brand Names Gonal-f® Pen [Can]; Gonal-f® RFF [US]; Gonal-f® [US/Can]

Therapeutic Category Ovulation Stimulator

Use
Gonal-f®: Ovulation induction in patients in whom the cause of infertility is functional and not caused by primary ovarian failure; development of multiple follicles with Assisted Reproductive Technology (ART); spermatogenesis induction
Gonal-f® RFF: Ovulation induction in patients in whom the cause of infertility is functional and not caused by primary ovarian failure; development of multiple follicles with ART

Usual Dosage Adults: **Note:** Dose should be individualized. Use the lowest dose consistent with the expectation of good results. Over the course of treatment, doses may vary depending on individual patient response.
Gonal-f®, Gonal-f® RFF: Females:
  Ovulation induction: SubQ: Initial: 75 int. units/day; incremental dose adjustments of up to 37.5 int. units may be considered after 14 days; further dose increases of the same magnitude can be made, if necessary, every 7 days (maximum dose: 300 int. units/day). If response to follitropin is appropriate, hCG is given 1 day following the last dose. Withhold hCG if serum estradiol is >2000 pg/mL, if the ovaries are abnormally enlarged, or if abdominal pain occurs. In general, therapy should not exceed 35 days.
  ART: SubQ: Initiate therapy with follitropin alfa in the early follicular phase (cycle day 2 or day 3) at a dose of 150 int. units/day, until sufficient follicular development is attained. In most cases, therapy should not exceed 10 days. In patients ≥35 years whose endogenous gonadotropin levels are suppressed, initiate follitropin alfa at a dose of 225 int. units/day. Continue treatment until adequate follicular development is indicated as determined by ultrasound in combination with measurement of serum estradiol levels. Consider adjustments to dose after 5 days based on the patient's response; adjust subsequent dosage every 3-5 days by ≤75-150 int. units additionally at each adjustment. Doses >450 int. units/day are not recommended. Once adequate follicular development is evident, administer hCG to induce final follicular maturation in preparation for oocyte. Withhold hCG if the ovaries are abnormally enlarged.

Gonal-f®: Males: Spermatogenesis induction: SubQ: Therapy should begin with hCG pretreatment until serum testosterone is in normal range, then 150 int. units 3 times/week with hCG 3 times/week; continue with lowest dose needed to induce spermatogenesis (maximum dose: 300 int. units 3 times/week); may be given for up to 18 months

Dosage Forms
Injection, powder for reconstitution [rDNA origin]:
Gonal-f®: 450 int. units
Gonal-f® RFF: 75 int. units
Injection, solution [rDNA origin]:
Gonal-f® RFF: 300 int. units/0.5 mL (0.5 mL); 450 int. units/0.75 mL (0.75 mL); 900 int. units/1.5 mL (1.5 mL)

follitropin beta (foe li TRO pin BAY ta)

Synonyms follicle stimulating hormone, recombinant; rFSH-beta; rhFSH-beta
U.S./Canadian Brand Names Follistim® AQ Cartridge [US]; Follistim® AQ [US]; Puregon® [Can]
Therapeutic Category Ovulation Stimulator
Use Ovulation induction in patients in whom the cause of infertility is functional and not caused by primary ovarian failure; development of multiple follicles with Assisted Reproductive Technology (ART)
Usual Dosage Adults: Females: **Note:** Dose should be individualized. Use the lowest dose consistent with the expectation of good results. Over the course of treatment, doses may vary depending on individual patient response.
Ovulation induction:
Follistim® AQ: I.M., SubQ: Stepwise approach: Initiate therapy with 75 int. units/day for up to 14 days. Increase by 37.5 int. units at weekly intervals until follicular growth or serum estradiol levels indicate an adequate response. The maximum (individualized) daily dose that has been safely used for ovulation induction in patients during clinical trials is 300 int. units. If response to follitropin is appropriate, hCG is given 1 day following the last dose. Withhold hCG if the ovaries are abnormally enlarged, or if abdominal pain occurs.
Follistim® AQ Cartridge: SubQ: Stepwise approach: Initiate therapy with 75 int. units/day for up to 7 days. Increase by 25 or 50 int. units at weekly intervals until follicular growth or serum estradiol levels indicate an adequate response. The maximum (individualized) daily dose that has been safely used for ovulation induction in patients during clinical trials is 175 int. units. If response to follitropin is appropriate, hCG is given 1 day following the last dose. Withhold hCG if the ovaries are abnormally enlarged, or if abdominal pain occurs.
ART:
Follistim® AQ: I.M., SubQ: A starting dose of 150-225 int. units is recommended for at least the first 4 days of treatment. The dose may be adjusted for the individual patient based upon their ovarian response. The usual maintenance dose was 75-300 int. units for 6-12 days; 375-600 int. units in patients who were poor responders. The maximum daily dose used in clinical studies is 600 int. units. When a sufficient number of follicles of adequate size are present, the final maturation of the follicles is induced by administering hCG. Oocyte retrieval is performed 34-36 hours later. Withhold hCG in cases where the ovaries are abnormally enlarged on the last day of follitropin beta therapy.
Follistim® AQ Cartridge: SubQ: A starting dose of 150-225 int. units is recommended for at least the first 5 days of treatment. The dose may be adjusted for the individual patient based upon their ovarian response. The maximum daily dose used in clinical studies is 450 int. units. When a sufficient number of follicles of adequate size are present, the final maturation of the follicles is induced by administering hCG. Oocyte retrieval is performed 34-36 hours later. Withhold hCG in cases where the ovaries are abnormally enlarged on the last day of follitropin beta therapy.

Dosage Forms
Injection, solution [rDNA origin]:
Follistim® AQ Cartridge: 175 int. units/0.21 mL (0.21 mL); 350 int. units/0.42 mL (0.42 mL); 650 int. units/0.78 mL (0.78 mL); 975 int. units/1.17 mL (1.17 mL)
Injection, solution [rDNA origin; single-dose]:
Follistim® AQ: 75 int. units/0.5 mL (0.5 mL); 150 int. units/0.5 mL (0.5 mL)

Foltx® [US] see folic acid, cyanocobalamin, and pyridoxine on page 422
Folvite® (Discontinued) see folic acid on page 421

fomepizole (foe ME pi zole)

Synonyms 4-methylpyrazole; 4-MP
U.S./Canadian Brand Names Antizol® [US]

▶

◀ **Therapeutic Category** Antidote

Use Treatment of methanol or ethylene glycol poisoning alone or in combination with hemodialysis

Usual Dosage Note: Fomepizole therapy should begin immediately upon suspicion of ethylene glycol or methanol ingestion.

Adults: Ethylene glycol and methanol toxicity: I.V.: A loading dose of 15 mg/kg should be administered, followed by doses of 10 mg/kg every 12 hours for 4 doses, then 15 mg/kg every 12 hours thereafter until ethylene glycol levels have been reduced <20 mg/dL and patient is asymptomatic with normal pH

Dosage Forms

Injection, solution [preservative free]: 1 g/mL (1.5 mL)
Antizol®: 1 g/mL (1.5 mL)

fondaparinux (fon da PARE i nuks)

Synonyms fondaparinux sodium

U.S./Canadian Brand Names Arixtra® [US/Can]

Therapeutic Category Factor Xa Inhibitor

Use Prophylaxis of deep vein thrombosis (DVT) in patients undergoing surgery for hip replacement, knee replacement, hip fracture (including extended prophylaxis following hip fracture surgery), or abdominal surgery (in patients at risk for thromboembolic complications); treatment of acute pulmonary embolism (PE); treatment of acute DVT without PE

Note: Additional Canadian approvals (not approved in U.S.): Unstable angina or non-ST segment elevation myocardial infarction (UA/NSTEMI) for the prevention of death and subsequent MI; ST segment elevation MI (STEMI) for the prevention of death and myocardial reinfarction

Usual Dosage SubQ: Adults:

DVT prophylaxis: Adults ≥50 kg: 2.5 mg once daily. **Note:** Initiate dose after hemostasis has been established, 6-8 hours postoperatively.

Usual duration: 5-9 days (up to 10 days following abdominal surgery or up to 11 days following hip replacement or knee replacement)

Extended prophylaxis is recommended following hip fracture surgery (has been tolerated for up to 32 days).

Acute DVT/PE treatment: **Note:** Concomitant treatment with warfarin sodium should be initiated as soon as possible, usually within 72 hours:

<50 kg: 5 mg once daily
50-100 kg: 7.5 mg once daily
>100 kg: 10 mg once daily

Usual duration: 5-9 days (has been administered up to 26 days)

Canadian labeling only: Adults:

UA/NSTEMI: SubQ: 2.5 mg once daily; initiate as soon as possible after diagnosis; treat for up to 8 days or until hospital discharge.

STEMI: I.V.: 2.5 mg once; subsequent doses: SubQ: 2.5 mg once daily; treat for up to 8 days or until hospital discharge

Dosage Forms

Injection, solution:

Arixtra®: 2.5 mg/0.5 mL (0.5 mL); 5 mg/0.4 mL (0.4 mL); 7.5 mg/0.6 mL (0.6 mL); 10 mg/0.8 mL (0.8 mL)

fondaparinux sodium see fondaparinux on page 424

Foradil® [Can] see formoterol on page 424

Foradil® Aerolizer® [US] see formoterol on page 424

Forane® [US/Can] see isoflurane on page 528

formoterol (for MOH te rol)

Sound-Alike/Look-Alike Issues

Foradil® may be confused with Toradol®

Synonyms formoterol fumarate; formoterol fumarate dihydrate

U.S./Canadian Brand Names Foradil® Aerolizer® [US]; Foradil® [Can]; Oxeze® Turbuhaler® [Can]; Perforomist™ [US]

Therapeutic Category Beta₂-Adrenergic Agonist Agent

Use Maintenance treatment of asthma and prevention of bronchospasm in patients ≥5 years of age with reversible obstructive airway disease, including patients with symptoms of nocturnal asthma, who require regular treatment with inhaled, short-acting beta$_2$-agonists; maintenance treatment of bronchoconstriction in patients with COPD; prevention of exercise-induced bronchospasm in patients ≥5 years of age

Note:
Oxeze® is also approved in Canada for acute relief of symptoms ("on demand" treatment) in patients ≥6 years of age.
Perforomist™ is only indicated for maintenance treatment of bronchoconstriction in patients with COPD.

Usual Dosage
Asthma maintenance treatment: Children ≥5 years and Adults: Inhalation:
Foradil®: 12 mcg capsule inhaled every 12 hours via Aerolizer™ device
Oxeze® (CAN): **Note:** Not labeled for use in the U.S.: Children ≥6 years and Adults: Inhalation: 6 mcg or 12 mcg every 12 hours. Maximum dose: Children: 24 mcg/day; Adults: 48 mcg/day
Prevention of exercise-induced bronchospasm: Children ≥5 years and Adults: Inhalation:
Foradil®:12 mcg capsule inhaled via Aerolizer™ device at least 15 minutes before exercise on an "as needed" basis; additional doses should not be used for another 12 hours. **Note:** If already using for asthma maintenance, then should not use additional doses for exercise-induced bronchospasm.
Oxeze® (CAN): **Note:** Not labeled for use in the U.S.: Children ≥6 years and Adults: Inhalation: 6 mcg or 12 mcg at least 15 minutes before exercise.
COPD maintenance treatment: Adults: Inhalation:
Foradil®: 12 mcg capsule inhaled every 12 hours via Aerolizer™ device
Perforomist™: 20 mcg unit-dose vial twice daily (maximum dose: 40 mcg/day)

Additional indication for Oxeze® (approved in Canada): Acute ("on demand") relief of bronchoconstriction: Children ≥12 years and Adults: 6 mcg or 12 mcg as a single dose (maximum dose: 72 mcg in any 24-hour period). The prolonged use of high dosages (48 mcg/day for ≥3 consecutive days) may be a sign of suboptimal control, and should prompt the re-evaluation of therapy.

Dosage Forms [CAN] = Canadian brand name
Powder for oral inhalation:
Foradil® Aerolizer®: 12 mcg/capsule (12s, 60s)
Oxeze® Turbuhaler® [CAN]: 6 mcg/inhalation, 12 mcg/inhalation [not available in the U.S.]
Solution for nebulization:
Perforomist™: 20 mcg/2 mL (2 mL)

formoterol fumarate *see formoterol on page 424*

formoterol fumarate dehydrate and budesonide *see budesonide and formoterol on page 148*

formoterol fumarate dihydrate *see formoterol on page 424*

Formula EM [US-OTC] *see fructose, dextrose, and phosphoric acid on page 429*

Formula Q® *(Discontinued) see quinine on page 814*

Formulation R™ [US-OTC] *see phenylephrine on page 745*

Formulex® [Can] *see dicyclomine on page 293*

5-formyl tetrahydrofolate *see leucovorin calcium on page 552*

Fortamet® [US] *see metformin on page 610*

Fortaz® [US/Can] *see ceftazidime on page 189*

Forteo® [US/Can] *see teriparatide on page 911*

Fortical® [US] *see calcitonin on page 160*

Fortovase® *(Discontinued) see saquinavir on page 856*

Fosamax® [US/Can] *see alendronate on page 43*

Fosamax Plus D™ [US] *see alendronate and cholecalciferol on page 43*

fosamprenavir (FOS am pren a veer)
Sound-Alike/Look-Alike Issues
Lexiva® may be confused with Levitra®
Synonyms fosamprenavir calcium; GW433908G
U.S./Canadian Brand Names Lexiva® [US]; Telzir® [Can]
Therapeutic Category Antiretroviral Agent, Protease Inhibitor

◀ **Use** Treatment of HIV infections in combination with at least two other antiretroviral agents

Usual Dosage Oral: HIV infection:

Children:

Antiretroviral therapy-naive patients:

Children 2-5 years of age: Fosamprenavir 30 mg/kg twice daily (not to exceed adult dosage of 1400 mg twice daily)

Children ≥6 years of age:

Unboosted regimen: Fosamprenavir 30 mg/kg twice daily (not to exceed adult dosage of 1400 mg twice daily)

Ritonavir-boosted regimen: Fosamprenavir 18 mg/kg twice daily plus ritonavir 3 mg/kg twice daily (not to exceed the adult dose of 700 mg plus ritonavir 100 mg twice daily)

Protease inhibitor-experienced patients: Children ≥6 years of age: Fosamprenavir 18 mg/kg plus ritonavir 3 mg/kg twice daily (not to exceed the adult dose of 700 mg plus ritonavir 100 mg twice daily)

Notes: The adult regimen of 1400 mg twice daily may be used for pediatric patients who weigh ≥47 kg. When combined with ritonavir, fosamprenavir tablets may be administered to children who weigh ≥39 kg while ritonavir capsules may be used for pediatric patients who weigh ≥33 kg.

Adults:

Antiretroviral therapy-naive patients:

Unboosted regimen: 1400 mg twice daily (without ritonavir)

Ritonavir-boosted regimens:

Once-daily regimen: Fosamprenavir 1400 mg plus ritonavir 100-200 mg once daily

Twice-daily regimen: Fosamprenavir 700 mg plus ritonavir 100 mg twice daily

Protease inhibitor-experienced patients: Fosamprenavir 700 mg plus ritonavir 100 mg twice daily.

Note: Once-daily administration is not recommended in protease inhibitor-experienced patients.

Combination therapy with efavirenz (ritonavir-boosted regimen):

Once-daily regimen: Fosamprenavir 1400 mg daily plus ritonavir 300 mg once daily

Twice-daily regimen: No dosage adjustment recommended for twice-daily regimen

Combination therapy with nevirapine (ritonavir-boosted regimen): Fosamprenavir 700 mg plus ritonavir 100 mg twice daily

Dosage Forms [CAN] = Canadian brand name

Tablet:

Lexiva®: 700 mg

Telzir® [CAN]: 700 mg [not available in the U.S.]

Suspension, oral:

Lexiva®: 50 mg/mL

Telzir® [CAN]: 50 mg/mL [not available in the U.S.]

fosamprenavir calcium *see* fosamprenavir *on page 425*

fosaprepitant (fos a PRE pi tant)

Sound-Alike/Look-Alike Issues

fosaprepitant may be confused with aprepitant, fosamprenavir

Emend® for injection (fosaprepitant) may be confused with Emend® (aprepitant) which is an oral capsule formulation.

Synonyms aprepitant injection; fosaprepitant dimeglumine; L-758,298; MK 0517

U.S./Canadian Brand Names Emend® for Injection [US]

Therapeutic Category Antiemetic; Substance P/Neurokinin 1 Receptor Antagonist

Use Prevention of acute and delayed nausea and vomiting associated with moderately- and highly-emetogenic chemotherapy (in combination with other antiemetics)

Usual Dosage I.V.: Adults: Prevention of chemotherapy-induced nausea/vomiting: 115 mg 30 minutes prior to chemotherapy on day 1 (followed by aprepitant 80 mg orally on days 2 and 3) in combination with other antiemetics

Dosage Forms

Injection, powder for reconstitution:

Emend® for Injection: 115 mg

fosaprepitant dimeglumine *see* fosaprepitant *on page 426*

Fosavance [Can] *see* alendronate and cholecalciferol *on page 43*

foscarnet (fos KAR net)

Synonyms PFA; phosphonoformate; phosphonoformic acid

U.S./Canadian Brand Names Foscavir® [US/Can]

Therapeutic Category Antiviral Agent

Use Treatment of acyclovir-resistant mucocutaneous herpes simplex virus (HSV) infections in immunocompromised persons (eg, with advanced AIDS); treatment of CMV retinitis in persons with HIV

Usual Dosage
CMV retinitis: I.V.:
Induction treatment: 60 mg/kg/dose every 8 hours **or** 90 mg/kg every 12 hours for 14-21 days
Maintenance therapy: 90-120 mg/kg/day as a single daily infusion
Herpes simplex infections (acyclovir-resistant): Induction: I.V.: 40 mg/kg/dose every 8-12 hours for 14-21 days

Dosage Forms
Injection, solution [preservative-free]: 24 mg/mL (250 mL, 500 mL)
Foscavir®: 24 mg/mL (500 mL)

Foscavir® [US/Can] see foscarnet *on page 427*

fosfomycin (fos foe MYE sin)

Sound-Alike/Look-Alike Issues
Monurol® may be confused with Monopril®

Synonyms fosfomycin tromethamine

U.S./Canadian Brand Names Monurol® [US/Can]

Therapeutic Category Antibiotic, Miscellaneous

Use Single oral dose in the treatment of uncomplicated urinary tract infections in women due to susceptible strains of *E. coli* and *Enterococcus faecalis*

Usual Dosage Oral: Adults: Females: Uncomplicated UTI: Single dose of 3 g in 3-4 oz (90-120 mL) of water

Dosage Forms
Powder for solution:
Monurol®: 3 g/sachet (3s)

fosfomycin tromethamine see fosfomycin *on page 427*

fosinopril (foe SIN oh pril)

Sound-Alike/Look-Alike Issues
fosinopril may be confused with lisinopril
Monopril® may be confused with Accupril®, minoxidil, moexipril, Monoket®, Monurol™, ramipril

Synonyms fosinopril sodium

U.S./Canadian Brand Names Apo-Fosinopril® [Can]; Gen-Fosinopril [Can]; Lin-Fosinopril [Can]; Monopril® [US/Can]; Novo-Fosinopril [Can]; PMS-Fosinopril [Can]; RAN-Fosinopril [Can]; ratio-Fosinopril [Can]; Riva-Fosinopril [Can]

Therapeutic Category Angiotensin-Converting Enzyme (ACE) Inhibitor

Use Treatment of hypertension, either alone or in combination with other antihypertensive agents; treatment of heart failure (HF)

Usual Dosage Oral:
Children ≥6 years and >50 kg: Hypertension: Initial: 5-10 mg once daily (maximum: 40 mg/day)
Adults:
Hypertension: Initial: 10 mg/day; most patients are maintained on 20-40 mg/day (maximum: 80 mg/day). May need to divide the dose into two if trough effect is inadequate; discontinue the diuretic, if possible 2-3 days before initiation of therapy; resume diuretic therapy carefully, if needed.
Heart failure: Initial: 10 mg/day (5 mg if renal dysfunction present) and increase, as needed, to a maximum of 40 mg once daily over several weeks; usual dose: 20-40 mg/day. If hypotension, orthostasis, or azotemia occur during titration, consider decreasing concomitant diuretic dose, if any.

Dosage Forms
Tablet: 10 mg, 20 mg, 40 mg
Monopril®: 10 mg, 20 mg, 40 mg

fosinopril and hydrochlorothiazide (foe SIN oh pril & hye droe klor oh THYE a zide)

Sound-Alike/Look-Alike Issues
Monopril® may be confused with Accupril®, minoxidil, moexipril, Monoket®, Monurol™, ramipril

Synonyms hydrochlorothiazide and fosinopril

U.S./Canadian Brand Names Monopril-HCT® [US/Can]

Therapeutic Category Angiotensin-Converting Enzyme (ACE) Inhibitor

Use Treatment of hypertension; not indicated for first-line treatment

Usual Dosage Note: A patient whose blood pressure is not adequately controlled with fosinopril or hydrochlorothiazide monotherapy may be switched to combination therapy; **not** for initial treatment. Oral: Adults: Hypertension: Fosinopril 10-80 mg per day, hydrochlorothiazide 12.5-50 mg per day

Dosage Forms
Tablet: 0/12.5: Fosinopril 10 mg and hydrochlorothiazide 12.5 mg; 20/12.5: Fosinopril 20 mg and hydrochlorothiazide 12.5 mg
Monopril-HCT®: 10/12.5: Fosinopril 10 mg and hydrochlorothiazide 12.5 mg; 20/12.5: Fosinopril 20 mg and hydrochlorothiazide 12.5 mg

fosinopril sodium *see fosinopril on page 427*

fosphenytoin (FOS fen i toyn)

Sound-Alike/Look-Alike Issues
Cerebyx® may be confused with Celebrex®, Celexa™, Cerezyme®

Synonyms fosphenytoin sodium

U.S./Canadian Brand Names Cerebyx® [US/Can]

Therapeutic Category Hydantoin

Use Used for the control of generalized convulsive status epilepticus and prevention and treatment of seizures occurring during neurosurgery; indicated for short-term parenteral administration when other means of phenytoin administration are unavailable, inappropriate, or deemed less advantageous (the safety and effectiveness of fosphenytoin in this use has not been systematically evaluated for more than 5 days)

Usual Dosage The dose, concentration in solutions, and infusion rates for fosphenytoin are expressed as phenytoin sodium equivalents (PE); fosphenytoin should always be prescribed and dispensed in phenytoin sodium equivalents (PE)

Adults:
Status epilepticus: I.V.: Loading dose: 15-20 mg PE/kg I.V. administered at 100-150 mg PE/minute
Nonemergent loading and maintenance dosing: I.V. or I.M.:
Loading dose: 10-20 mg PE/kg I.V. or I.M. (maximum I.V. rate: 150 mg PE/minute)
Initial daily maintenance dose: 4-6 mg PE/kg/day I.V. or I.M.
I.M. or I.V. substitution for oral phenytoin therapy: May be substituted for oral phenytoin sodium at the same total daily dose; however, Dilantin® capsules are ~90% bioavailable by the oral route; phenytoin, supplied as fosphenytoin, is 100% bioavailable by both the I.M. and I.V. routes; for this reason, plasma phenytoin concentrations may increase when I.M. or I.V. fosphenytoin is substituted for oral phenytoin sodium therapy; in clinical trials I.M. fosphenytoin was administered as a single daily dose utilizing either 1 or 2 injection sites; some patients may require more frequent dosing

Dosage Forms
Injection, solution: 75 mg/mL (2 mL, 10 mL) [equivalent to phenytoin sodium 50 mg/mL]
Cerebyx®: 75 mg/mL (2 mL, 10 mL) [equivalent to phenytoin sodium 50 mg/mL]

fosphenytoin sodium *see fosphenytoin on page 428*
Fosrenol® [US/Can] *see lanthanum on page 549*
Fostex® 10% BPO [US-OTC] *see benzoyl peroxide on page 126*
Fototar® [US-OTC] *see coal tar on page 240*
Fragmin® [US/Can] *see dalteparin on page 264*

framycetin *(Canada only)* (fra mye CEE tin)

U.S./Canadian Brand Names Sofra-Tulle® [Can]

Therapeutic Category Antibiotic, Topical

Use Treatment of infected or potentially infected burns, wounds, ulcers, and graft sites

Usual Dosage A single layer to be applied directly to the wound and covered with an appropriate dressing. If exudative, dressings should be changed at least daily. In case of leg ulcers, cut dressing accurately to size of ulcer to decrease the risk of sensitization and to avoid contact with surrounding healthy skin.

Dosage Forms

Gauze dressing: 1% (10 cm x 10 cm)

Fraxiparine™ [Can] *see* nadroparin *(Canada only) on page 651*

Fraxiparine™ Forte [Can] *see* nadroparin *(Canada only) on page 651*

Freedavite [US-OTC] *see* vitamins (multiple/oral) *on page 983*

Freezone® [US-OTC] *see* salicylic acid *on page 850*

Frisium® [Can] *see* clobazam *(Canada only) on page 232*

Froben® [Can] *see* flurbiprofen *on page 416*

Froben-SR® [Can] *see* flurbiprofen *on page 416*

Frova® [US] *see* frovatriptan *on page 429*

frovatriptan (froe va TRIP tan)

Synonyms frovatriptan succinate

U.S./Canadian Brand Names Frova® [US]

Therapeutic Category Antimigraine Agent; Serotonin $5\text{-HT}_{1B, 1D}$ Receptor Agonist

Use Acute treatment of migraine with or without aura in adults

Usual Dosage Oral: Adults: Migraine: 2.5 mg; if headache recurs, a second dose may be given if first dose provided some relief and at least 2 hours have elapsed since the first dose (maximum daily dose: 7.5 mg)

Dosage Forms

Tablet:

Frova®: 2.5 mg

frovatriptan succinate *see* frovatriptan *on page 429*

fructose, dextrose, and phosphoric acid (FRUK tose, DEKS trose, & foss FOR ik AS id)

Sound-Alike/Look-Alike Issues

Emetrol® may be confused with emetine

Synonyms dextrose, levulose and phosphoric acid; levulose, dextrose and phosphoric acid; phosphorated carbohydrate solution; phosphoric acid, levulose and dextrose

U.S./Canadian Brand Names Emetrol® [US-OTC]; Especol® [US-OTC]; Formula EM [US-OTC]; Kalmz [US-OTC]; Nausea Relief [US-OTC]; Nausetrol® [US-OTC]

Therapeutic Category Antiemetic

Use Relief of nausea associated with upset stomach that occurs with intestinal or stomach flu, and food indiscretions

Usual Dosage Oral: Nausea:

Children 2-12 years: 5-10 mL; repeat dose every 15 minutes until distress subsides; do not take for more than 1 hour (5 doses)

Children ≥12 years and Adults: 15-30 mL; repeat dose every 15 minutes until distress subsides; do not take for more than 1 hour (5 doses)

Dosage Forms

Liquid, oral: Fructose 1.87 g, dextrose 1.87 g, and phosphoric acid 21.5 mg per 5 mL

Emetrol® [OTC], Especol® [OTC], Formula EM [OTC], Kalmz [OTC], Nausea Relief [OTC], Nausetrol® [OTC]: Fructose 1.87 g, dextrose 1.87 g, and phosphoric acid 21.5 mg per 5 mL

frusemide *see* furosemide *on page 430*

FS *see* fibrin sealant kit *on page 400*

FSH *see* follitropin alfa *on page 422*

FSH *see* urofollitropin *on page 964*

FS Shampoo® Topical (Discontinued) *see* fluocinolone *on page 409*

FTC *see* emtricitabine *on page 338*

FU *see* fluorouracil *on page 412*

5-FU *see* fluorouracil *on page 412*

Fucidin® [Can] *see* fusidic acid *(Canada only) on page 431*

Fucithalmic® [Can] *see* fusidic acid *(Canada only) on page 431*
FUDR® [US/Can] *see* floxuridine *on page 404*
5-FUDR *see* floxuridine *on page 404*
Ful-Glo® [US] *see* fluorescein *on page 410*

fulvestrant (fool VES trant)
Synonyms ICI-182,780; zeneca 182,780; ZM-182,780
U.S./Canadian Brand Names Faslodex® [US]
Therapeutic Category Antineoplastic Agent, Estrogen Receptor Antagonist
Use Treatment of hormone receptor positive metastatic breast cancer in postmenopausal women with disease progression following antiestrogen therapy
Usual Dosage I.M.: Adults (postmenopausal women): 250 mg at 1-month intervals
Dosage Forms
  Injection, solution [prefilled syringe]:
    Faslodex®: 50 mg/mL (2.5 mL, 5 mL)

Fumasorb® *(Discontinued)* *see* ferrous fumarate *on page 397*
Fumerin® *(Discontinued)* *see* ferrous fumarate *on page 397*
Funduscein® Injection *(Discontinued)* *see* fluorescein *on page 410*
FungiGuard [US-OTC] *see* tolnaftate *on page 934*
Fungi-Nail® [US-OTC] *see* undecylenic acid and derivatives *on page 962*
Fungizone® [Can] *see* amphotericin B (conventional) *on page 70*
Fung-O® [US-OTC] *see* salicylic acid *on page 850*
Fungoid® Tincture [US-OTC] *see* miconazole *on page 630*
Furacin® Topical *(Discontinued)*
Furadantin® [US] *see* nitrofurantoin *on page 675*
Furalan® *(Discontinued)* *see* nitrofurantoin *on page 675*
Furan® *(Discontinued)* *see* nitrofurantoin *on page 675*
Furanite® *(Discontinued)* *see* nitrofurantoin *on page 675*
furazosin *see* prazosin *on page 780*

furosemide (fyoor OH se mide)
Sound-Alike/Look-Alike Issues
  furosemide may be confused with torsemide
  Lasix® may be confused with Esidrix®, Lanoxin®, Lidex®, Lomotil®, Luvox®, Luxiq®
Synonyms frusemide
U.S./Canadian Brand Names Apo-Furosemide® [Can]; Dom-Furosemide [Can]; Furosemide Injection, USP [Can]; Furosemide Special [Can]; Lasix® Special [Can]; Lasix® [US/Can]; Novo-Semide [Can]; Nu-Furosemide [Can]; PMS-Furosemide [Can]
Therapeutic Category Diuretic, Loop
Use Management of edema associated with congestive heart failure and hepatic or renal disease; alone or in combination with antihypertensives in treatment of hypertension
Usual Dosage
Infants and Children:
  Oral: 0.5-2 mg/kg/dose increased in increments of 1 mg/kg/dose with each succeeding dose until a satisfactory effect is achieved to a maximum of 6 mg/kg/dose no more frequently than 6 hours.
  I.M., I.V.: 1 mg/kg/dose, increasing by each succeeding dose at 1 mg/kg/dose at intervals of 6-12 hours until a satisfactory response up to 6 mg/kg/dose.
Adults:
  Oral: 20-80 mg/dose initially increased in increments of 20-40 mg/dose at intervals of 6-8 hours; usual maintenance dose interval is twice daily or every day; may be titrated up to 600 mg/day with severe edematous states.
  Hypertension (JNC 7): 20-80 mg/day in 2 divided doses
  I.M., I.V.: 20-40 mg/dose, may be repeated in 1-2 hours as needed and increased by 20 mg/dose until the desired effect has been obtained. Usual dosing interval: 6-12 hours; for acute pulmonary edema, the usual dose is 40 mg I.V. over 1-2 minutes. If not adequate, may increase dose to 80 mg. **Note:** ACC/AHA 2005 guidelines for chronic congestive heart failure recommend a maximum single dose of 160-200 mg.

Continuous I.V. infusion: Initial I.V. bolus dose 20-40 mg, followed by continuous I.V. infusion doses of 10-40 mg/hour. If urine output is <1 mL/kg/hour, double as necessary to a maximum of 80-160 mg/hour. The risk associated with higher infusion rates (80-160 mg/hour) must be weighed against alternative strategies. **Note:** ACC/AHA 2005 guidelines for chronic congestive heart failure recommend 40 mg I.V. load, then 10-40 mg/hour infusion.

Refractory heart failure: Oral, I.V.: Doses up to 8 g/day have been used.

Dosage Forms
Injection, solution: 10 mg/mL (2 mL, 4 mL, 8 mL, 10 mL)
Solution, oral: 10 mg/mL, 40 mg/5 mL
Tablet: 20 mg, 40 mg, 80 mg
    Lasix®: 20 mg
    Lasix®: 40 mg, 80 mg [scored]

Furosemide Injection, USP [Can] *see* furosemide *on page 430*
Furosemide Special [Can] *see* furosemide *on page 430*

fusidic acid *(Canada only)* (fyoo SI dik AS id)

Synonyms sodium fusidate
U.S./Canadian Brand Names Fucidin® [Can]; Fucithalmic® [Can]
Therapeutic Category Antifungal Agent, Systemic
Use

Systemic: Treatment of skin and soft tissue infections, or osteomyelitis, caused by susceptible organisms, including *Staphylococcus aureus* (penicillinase-producing or nonpenicillinase strains); may be used in the treatment of pneumonia, septicemia, endocarditis, burns, and cystic fibrosis caused by susceptible organisms when other antibiotics have failed

Topical: Treatment of primary and secondary skin infections caused by susceptible organisms

Ophthalmic: Treatment of superficial infections of the eye and conjunctiva caused by susceptible organisms

Usual Dosage
I.V.:
    Children ≤12 years: 20 mg/kg/day in 3 divided doses
    Children >12 years and Adults: 500 mg sodium fusidate 3 times/day
Ophthalmic: Children ≥2 years and Adults: Instill 1 drop in each eye every 12 hours for 7 days
Topical: Children and Adults: Apply to affected area 3-4 times/day until favorable results are achieved. If a gauze dressing is used, frequency of application may be reduced to 1-2 times/day.
Oral: Adults: 500 mg sodium fusidate 3 times/day. (**Note:** Oral dosage may be increased to 1000 mg 3 times/day in fulminating infections.)

Dosage Forms [CAN] = Canadian brand name
Cream:
    Fucidin® [CAN]: 2% (15 g, 30 g) [not available in the U.S.]
Injection, powder for reconstitution:
    Fucidin® [CAN]: 500 mg [not available in the U.S.]
Ointment, topical:
    Fucidin® [CAN]: 2% (15 g, 30 g) [not available in the U.S.]
Suspension, ophthalmic:
    Fucithalmic® [CAN]: 10 mg/g [1%] (0.2 g) [unit-dose, without preservative]; (3 g, 5 g) [multidose, contains benzalkonium chloride] [not available in the U.S.]
Tablet:
    Fucidin® [CAN]: 250 mg [not available in the U.S.]

Fuzeon® [US/Can] *see* enfuvirtide *on page 340*
FVIII/vWF *see* antihemophilic factor/von Willebrand factor complex (human) *on page 80*
FXT [Can] *see* fluoxetine *on page 413*
GAA *see* alglucosidase alfa *on page 45*

gabapentin (GA ba pen tin)

Sound-Alike/Look-Alike Issues
Neurontin® may be confused with Neoral®, Noroxin®
U.S./Canadian Brand Names Apo-Gabapentin® [Can]; BCI-Gabapentin [Can]; Gen-Gabapentin [Can]; Neurontin® [US/Can]; Novo-Gabapentin [Can]; Nu-Gabapentin [Can]; PMS-Gabapentin [Can]
Therapeutic Category Anticonvulsant

◀ **Use** Adjunct for treatment of partial seizures with and without secondary generalized seizures in patients >12 years of age with epilepsy; adjunct for treatment of partial seizures in pediatric patients 3-12 years of age; management of postherpetic neuralgia (PHN) in adults

Usual Dosage Oral:

Children: Anticonvulsant:

3-12 years: Initial: 10-15 mg/kg/day in 3 divided doses; titrate to effective dose over ~3 days; dosages of up to 50 mg/kg/day have been tolerated in clinical studies

3-4 years: Effective dose: 40 mg/kg/day in 3 divided doses

≥5-12 years: Effective dose: 25-35 mg/kg/day in 3 divided doses

See "Note" in Adults dosing.

Children >12 years and Adults:

Anticonvulsant: Initial: 300 mg 3 times/day; if necessary the dose may be increased up to 1800 mg/day. Doses of up to 2400 mg/day have been tolerated in long-term clinical studies; up to 3600 mg/day has been tolerated in short-term studies.

Note: If gabapentin is discontinued or if another anticonvulsant is added to therapy, it should be done slowly over a minimum of 1 week.

Adults: Postherpetic neuralgia or neuropathic pain: Day 1: 300 mg, Day 2: 300 mg twice daily, Day 3: 300 mg 3 times/day; dose may be titrated as needed for pain relief (range: 1800-3600 mg/day, daily doses >1800 mg do not generally show greater benefit)

Dosage Forms

Capsule: 100 mg, 300 mg, 400 mg

Neurontin®: 100 mg, 300 mg, 400 mg

Solution, oral:

Neurontin®: 250 mg/5 mL

Tablet: 100 mg, 300 mg, 400 mg, 600 mg, 800 mg

Neurontin®: 600 mg, 800 mg

Gabitril® [US/Can] see tiagabine on page 925

gadobenate dimeglumine (gad oh BEN ate dye MEG loo meen)

Synonyms gadolinum-BOPTA; Gd-BOPTA

U.S./Canadian Brand Names Multihance® Multipak™ [US]; Multihance® [US]

Therapeutic Category Diagnostic Agent; Radiological/Contrast Media, Nonionic

Use Contrast medium for magnetic resonance imaging (MRI) to visualize CNS lesions with abnormal vascularity in the brain, spine, and associated tissues

Usual Dosage I.V.: Adults: CNS lesions: 0.1 mmol/kg (0.2 mL/kg)

Dosage Forms

Injection, solution [preservative free]:

Multihance®: 529 mg/mL (5 mL, 10 mL, 15 mL, 20 mL)

Multihance® Multipack™: 529 mg/mL (50 mL, 100 mL)

gadobutrol (Canada only) (gad oh BYOO trol)

Sound-Alike/Look-Alike Issues

Gadovist® may be confused with Magnevist®, Vasovist™

Synonyms gadovist 1.0

U.S./Canadian Brand Names Gadovist® [Can]

Therapeutic Category Gadolinium-Containing Contrast Agent; Radiological/Contrast Media, Nonionic

Use Contrast medium for magnetic resonance imaging (MRI) of CNS lesions (brain, spine, and associated tissues); perfusion studies to diagnose stroke, or to detect focal cerebral ischemia or tumor perfusion; contrast-enhanced magnetic resonance angiography (CE-MRA)

Usual Dosage I.V.: Adults:

General CNS imaging: 0.1 mmol/kg (0.1 mL/kg); if needed, a second dose of 0.1-0.2 mmol/kg (0.1-0.2 mL/kg) may be repeated once within 30 minutes of the first dose

Exclusion of metastatic or recurrent tumors: 0.3 mmol/kg (0.3 mL/kg)

Perfusion studies: 0.3 mmol/kg (0.3 mL/kg)

CE-MRA:

Imaging of a single field of view (FOV):

Patient weight <75 kg: 7.5 mL

Patient weight ≥75 kg: 10 mL

Imaging >1 FOV:
  Patient weight <75 kg: 15 mL
  Patient weight ≥75 kg: 20 mL
Dosage Forms [CAN] = Canadian brand name
  Injection, solution [preservative free]:
  Gadovist® [CAN]: 604.72 mg/mL (15 mL) [not available in U.S.]

gadodiamide (gad oh DYE a mide)

Synonyms gadolinium-DTPA-BMA; Gd-DTPA-BMA

U.S./Canadian Brand Names Omniscan™ [US]

Therapeutic Category Radiological/Contrast Media, Nonionic

Use Contrast medium for magnetic resonance imaging (MRI) to visualize CNS lesions with abnormal vascularity in the brain, spine, and associated tissues, and to visualize body lesions with abnormal vascularity within the thoracic (noncardiac), abdominal, pelvic cavities, and retroperitoneal space

Usual Dosage I.V.:
Children ≥2 years:
  Body imaging:
    Kidney: 0.05 mmol/kg (0.1 mL/kg); the safety of additional doses has not been studied
    Intrathoracic (noncardiac), intraabdominal, pelvic cavities: 0.1 mmol/kg (0.2 mL/kg)
  CNS imaging: 0.1 mmol/kg (0.2 mL/kg); the safety of additional doses has not been studied
Adults:
  Body imaging:
    Kidney: 0.05 mmol/kg (0.1 mL/kg); the safety of additional doses has not been studied
    Intrathoracic (noncardiac), intraabdominal, pelvic cavities: 0.1 mmol/kg (0.2 mL/kg); the safety of additional doses has not been studied
  CNS imaging: 0.1 mmol/kg (0.2 mL/kg); if needed, a second dose of 0.2 mmol/kg (0.4 mL/kg) may be repeated once within 20 minutes of the first dose

Dosage Forms
  Injection, solution [preservative free]:
  Omniscan™: 287 mg/mL (5 mL, 10 mL, 15 mL, 20 mL, 50 mL)

gadofosveset *(Canada only)* (gad oh FOS ve set)

Sound-Alike/Look-Alike Issues
  Vasovist® may be confused with Magnevist®, Gadovist®

Synonyms gadofosveset trisodium

U.S./Canadian Brand Names Vasovist® [Can]

Therapeutic Category Gadolinium-Containing Contrast Agent; Radiological/Contrast Media, Paramagnetic Agent

Use Contrast medium used to enhance visualization of abdominal or limb vasculature in magnetic resonance angiography (MRA)

Usual Dosage I.V.: Adults: MRA: 0.03 mmol/kg (0.12 mL/kg); doses >0.03 mmol/kg are not recommended

Dosage Forms [CAN] = Canadian brand name
  Injection, solution [preservative free]:
  Vasovist® [CAN]: 0.25 mmoL/mL (10 mL, 15 mL, 20 mL) [not available in U.S.]

gadofosveset trisodium *see* gadofosveset *(Canada only) on page 433*
gadolinium-DTPA *see* gadopentetate dimeglumine *on page 433*
gadolinium-DTPA-BMA *see* gadodiamide *on page 433*
gadolinium-DTPA-BMEA *see* gadoversetamide *on page 434*
gadolinium-HP-DO3A *see* gadoteridol *on page 434*
gadolinum-BOPTA *see* gadobenate dimeglumine *on page 432*

gadopentetate dimeglumine (gad oh PEN te tate dye MEG loo meen)

Synonyms gadolinium-DTPA; Gd-DTPA

U.S./Canadian Brand Names Magnevist® [US/Can]

Therapeutic Category Radiological/Contrast Media, Paramagnetic Agent

Use Contrast medium for magnetic resonance imaging (MRI) to visualize lesions with abnormal vascularity in the brain, spine and associated tissues, head and neck, and body (excluding the heart)

◀ **Usual Dosage** I.V.: Children ≥2 years and Adults: MRI: 0.1 mmol/kg (0.2 mL/kg)
Note: Dosing for patients >130 kg (286 pounds) has not been studied.
Dosage Forms
Injection, solution [preservative free]:
   Magnevist®: Gadopentetate dimeglumine 469.01 mg/mL (5 mL, 10 mL, 15 mL, 20 mL, 50 mL, 100 mL)

gadoteridol (gad oh TER i dol)

Synonyms gadolinium-HP-DO3A; Gd-HP-DO3A
U.S./Canadian Brand Names ProHance® [US]
Therapeutic Category Radiological/Contrast Media, Nonionic
Use Contrast medium for magnetic resonance imaging (MRI) to visualize CNS lesions with abnormal vascularity in the brain, spine, and associated tissues and to visualize extracranial/extraspinal tissues in the head and neck
Usual Dosage I.V.:
   Children ≥2 years: CNS imaging: 0.1 mmol/kg (0.2 mL/kg); the safety of additional doses has not been studied
   Adults:
   CNS imaging: 0.1 mmol/kg (0.2 mL/kg); if needed, a second dose of 0.2 mmol/kg (0.4 mL/kg) may be repeated once within 30 minutes of the first dose
   Extracranial/extraspinal tissue: 0.1 mmol/kg (0.2 mL/kg)
Dosage Forms
Injection, solution [preservative free]:
   ProHance®: 279.3 mg/mL (5 mL, 10 mL, 15 mL, 17 mL, 20 mL, 50 mL) [contains calteridol calcium 0.23 mg/mL and tromethamine 1.21 mg/mL]
   ProHance® Multipack™: 279.3 mg/mL (50 mL) [contains calteridol calcium 0.23 mg/mL and tromethamine 1.21 mg/mL; pharmacy bulk package]

gadoversetamide (gad oh ver SET a mide)

Synonyms gadolinium-DTPA-BMEA; Gd-DTPA-BMEA
U.S./Canadian Brand Names OptiMARK® [US]
Therapeutic Category Radiological/Contrast Media, Nonionic
Use Contrast medium for magnetic resonance imaging (MRI) to visualize lesions with abnormal vascularity in the liver or CNS (brain, spine, and associated tissues)
Usual Dosage I.V.: Adults: CNS or liver lesions: 0.1 mmol/kg (0.2 mL/kg)
Dosage Forms
Injection, solution [preservative free]:
   OptiMARK®: 330.9 mg/mL (5 mL, 10 mL, 15 mL, 20 mL, 30 mL, 50 mL)

Gadovist® [Can] see gadobutrol (Canada only) on page 432
gadovist 1.0 see gadobutrol (Canada only) on page 432

galantamine (ga LAN ta meen)

Sound-Alike/Look-Alike Issues
   Razadyne™ may be confused with Rozerem™
   Reminyl® may be confused with Amaryl®
Synonyms galantamine hydrobromide
U.S./Canadian Brand Names Razadyne™ ER [US]; Razadyne™ [US]; Reminyl® ER [Can]; Reminyl® [Can]
Therapeutic Category Acetylcholinesterase Inhibitor (Central)
Use Treatment of mild-to-moderate dementia of Alzheimer disease
Usual Dosage Oral: Adults:
Note: Oral solution and tablet should be taken with breakfast and dinner; capsule should be taken with breakfast. If therapy is interrupted for ≥3 days, restart at the lowest dose and increase to current dose.
   Immediate release tablet or solution: Mild-to-moderate dementia of Alzheimer: Initial: 4 mg twice a day for 4 weeks; if tolerated, increase to 8 mg twice daily for ≥4 weeks; if tolerated, increase to 12 mg twice daily
   Range: 16-24 mg/day in 2 divided doses
   Extended release capsule: Initial: 8 mg once daily for 4 weeks; if tolerated, increase to 16 mg once daily for ≥4 weeks; if tolerated, increase to 24 mg once daily

Range: 16-24 mg once daily

Conversion to galantamine from other cholinesterase inhibitors: Patients experiencing poor tolerability with donepezil or rivastigmine should wait until side effects subside or allow a 7-day washout period prior to beginning galantamine. Patients not experiencing side effects with donepezil or rivastigmine may begin galantamine therapy the day immediately following discontinuation of previous therapy.

Dosage Forms

Capsule, extended release:
Razadyne™ ER: 8 mg, 16 mg, 24 mg
Solution, oral:
Razadyne™: 4 mg/mL
Tablet:
Razadyne™: 4 mg, 8 mg, 12 mg

galantamine hydrobromide *see galantamine on page 434*

galsulfase (gal SUL fase)

Synonyms recombinant N-acetylgalactosamine 4-sulfatase; rhASB

U.S./Canadian Brand Names Naglazyme™ [US]

Therapeutic Category Enzyme

Use Replacement therapy in mucopolysaccharidosis VI (MPS VI; Maroteaux-Lamy Syndrome) for improvement of walking and stair-climbing capacity

Usual Dosage Note: Premedicate with antihistamines with/without antipyretics 30-60 minutes prior to infusion. MPS VI: Children >5 years and Adults: I.V.: 1 mg/kg once weekly

Dosage Forms

Injection, solution [preservative free]:
Naglazyme™: 5 mg/5 mL (5 mL)

Gamimune® N [Can] *see immune globulin (intravenous) on page 503*

Gamimune® N Injection *(Discontinued)* *see immune globulin (intravenous) on page 503*

gamma benzene hexachloride *see lindane on page 567*

Gamma E-Gems® [US-OTC] *see vitamin E on page 981*

Gamma-E Plus [US-OTC] *see vitamin E on page 981*

Gammagard Liquid [US/Can] *see immune globulin (intravenous) on page 503*

Gammagard S/D [US/Can] *see immune globulin (intravenous) on page 503*

gamma globulin *see immune globulin (intramuscular) on page 502*

gamma hydroxybutyric acid *see sodium oxybate on page 877*

gammaphos *see amifostine on page 58*

Gammar®-P I.V. *(Discontinued)* *see immune globulin (intravenous) on page 503*

GammaSTAN™ S/D [US] *see immune globulin (intramuscular) on page 502*

Gamulin® Rh *(Discontinued)*

Gamunex® [US/Can] *see immune globulin (intravenous) on page 503*

ganciclovir (gan SYE kloe veer)

Sound-Alike/Look-Alike Issues
Cytovene® may be confused with Cytosar®, Cytosar-U®

Synonyms DHPG sodium; GCV sodium; nordeoxyguanosine

U.S./Canadian Brand Names Cytovene® [US/Can]; Vitrasert® [US/Can]

Therapeutic Category Antiviral Agent

Use
Parenteral: Treatment of CMV retinitis in immunocompromised individuals, including patients with acquired immunodeficiency syndrome; prophylaxis of CMV infection in transplant patients

Oral: Alternative to the I.V. formulation for maintenance treatment of CMV retinitis in immunocompromised patients, including patients with AIDS, in whom retinitis is stable following appropriate induction therapy and for whom the risk of more rapid progression is balanced by the benefit associated with avoiding daily I.V. infusions.

Implant: Treatment of CMV retinitis

◀ **Usual Dosage**
CMV retinitis: Slow I.V. infusion (dosing is based on total body weight):
Children >3 months and Adults:
Induction therapy: 5 mg/kg/dose every 12 hours for 14-21 days followed by maintenance therapy
Maintenance therapy: 5 mg/kg/day as a single daily dose for 7 days/week or 6 mg/kg/day for 5 days/week
CMV retinitis: Oral: 1000 mg 3 times/day with food **or** 500 mg 6 times/day with food
Prevention of CMV disease in patients with advanced HIV infection and normal renal function: Oral: 1000 mg 3 times/day with food
Prevention of CMV disease in transplant patients: Same initial and maintenance dose as CMV retinitis except duration of initial course is 7-14 days, duration of maintenance therapy is dependent on clinical condition and degree of immunosuppression
Intravitreal implant: One implant for 5- to 8-month period; following depletion of ganciclovir, as evidenced by progression of retinitis, implant may be removed and replaced

Dosage Forms
Capsule: 250 mg, 500 mg
Implant, intravitreal:
Vitrasert®: 4.5 mg [released gradually over 5-8 months]
Injection, powder for reconstitution:
Cytovene®: 500 mg

Ganidin NR [US] *see* guaifenesin *on page 453*

ganirelix (ga ni REL ix)

Synonyms ganirelix acetate
U.S./Canadian Brand Names Orgalutran® [Can]
Therapeutic Category Antigonadotropic Agent
Use Inhibits premature luteinizing hormone (LH) surges in women undergoing controlled ovarian hyperstimulation
Usual Dosage SubQ: Adults: 250 mcg/day during the mid-to-late phase after initiating follicle-stimulating hormone on day 2 or 3 of cycle. Treatment should be continued daily until the day of chorionic gonadotropin administration.
Dosage Forms
Injection, solution: 250 mcg/0.5 mL

ganirelix acetate *see* ganirelix *on page 436*
Gani-Tuss DM NR [US] *see* guaifenesin and dextromethorphan *on page 454*
Gani-Tuss® NR [US] *see* guaifenesin and codeine *on page 454*
Gantrisin® [US] *see* sulfisoxazole *on page 896*
GAR-936 *see* tigecycline *on page 927*
Garamycin® [Can] *see* gentamicin *on page 442*
Garamycin® *(Discontinued)* *see* gentamicin *on page 442*
Gardasil® [US/Can] *see* papillomavirus (Types 6, 11, 16, 18) recombinant vaccine *on page 722*
Gas-X® [US-OTC] *see* simethicone *on page 867*
Gas-X®, Children's Tongue Twisters™ [US-OTC] *see* simethicone *on page 867*
Gas-X® Extra Strength [US-OTC] *see* simethicone *on page 867*
Gas-X® Infant [US-OTC] *see* simethicone *on page 867*
Gas-X® Maximum Strength [US-OTC] *see* simethicone *on page 867*
Gas-X® Thin Strips™ [US-OTC] *see* simethicone *on page 867*
Gas Ban™ [US-OTC] *see* calcium carbonate and simethicone *on page 164*
Gas-Ban DS® *(Discontinued)* *see* aluminum hydroxide, magnesium hydroxide, and simethicone *on page 54*
Gastrocrom® [US] *see* cromolyn sodium *on page 251*
Gastrografin® [US] *see* diatrizoate meglumine and diatrizoate sodium *on page 288*
Gastrosed™ *(Discontinued)* *see* hyoscyamine *on page 492*

gatifloxacin (gat i FLOKS a sin)

U.S./Canadian Brand Names Zymar® [US/Can]
Therapeutic Category Antibiotic, Quinolone

Use Treatment of bacterial conjunctivitis

Usual Dosage Ophthalmic: Children ≥1 year and Adults: Bacterial conjunctivitis:
 Days 1 and 2: Instill 1 drop into affected eye(s) every 2 hours while awake (maximum: 8 times/day)
 Days 3-7: Instill 1 drop into affected eye(s) up to 4 times/day while awake

Dosage Forms
 Solution, ophthalmic:
  Zymar®: 0.3% (5 mL)

Gaviscon® Extra Strength [US-OTC] *see* aluminum hydroxide and magnesium carbonate *on page 53*

Gaviscon® Liquid [US-OTC] *see* aluminum hydroxide and magnesium carbonate *on page 53*

Gaviscon® Tablet [US-OTC] *see* aluminum hydroxide and magnesium trisilicate *on page 54*

G-CSF *see* filgrastim *on page 401*

G-CSF (PEG conjugate) *see* pegfilgrastim *on page 727*

GCV sodium *see* ganciclovir *on page 435*

Gd-BOPTA *see* gadobenate dimeglumine *on page 432*

GD-Celecoxib [Can] *see* celecoxib *on page 193*

Gd-DTPA *see* gadopentetate dimeglumine *on page 433*

Gd-DTPA-BMA *see* gadodiamide *on page 433*

Gd-DTPA-BMEA *see* gadoversetamide *on page 434*

Gd-HP-DO3A *see* gadoteridol *on page 434*

GD-Quinapril [Can] *see* quinapril *on page 812*

Gebauer's Ethyl Chloride® [US] *see* ethyl chloride *on page 381*

Gee Gee® (Discontinued) *see* guaifenesin *on page 453*

gefitinib (ge FI tye nib)

Sound-Alike/Look-Alike Issues
 gefitinib may be confused with erlotinib

Synonyms NSC-715055; ZD1839

U.S./Canadian Brand Names IRESSA® [US]

Therapeutic Category Antineoplastic, Tyrosine Kinase Inhibitor

Use
 U.S. labeling: Treatment of locally advanced or metastatic nonsmall cell lung cancer after failure of platinum-based and docetaxel therapies. Treatment is limited to patients who are benefiting or have benefited from treatment with gefitinib.
 Note: Due to the lack of improved survival data from clinical trials of gefitinib, and in response to positive survival data with another EGFR inhibitor, physicians are advised to use other treatment options in advanced nonsmall cell lung cancer patients following one or two prior chemotherapy regimens when they are refractory/intolerant to their most recent regimen.

 Canada labeling: Approved indication is limited to NSCLC patients with epidermal growth factor receptor (EGFR) expression status positive or unknown.

Usual Dosage Note: In response to the lack of improved survival data from the ISEL trial, AstraZeneca has temporarily suspended promotion of this drug.
 Oral: Adults: 250 mg/day; consider 500 mg/day in patients receiving effective CYP3A4 inducers (eg, rifampin, phenytoin)

Dosage Forms
 Tablet:
  IRESSA®: 250 mg

gelatin (absorbable) (JEL a tin, ab SORB a ble)

Synonyms absorbable gelatin sponge

U.S./Canadian Brand Names Gelfilm® [US]; Gelfoam® [US]

Therapeutic Category Hemostatic Agent

Use Adjunct to provide hemostasis in surgery; open prostatic surgery

Usual Dosage Hemostasis: Apply packs or sponges dry or saturated with sodium chloride. When applied dry, hold in place with moderate pressure. When applied wet, squeeze to remove air bubbles. The ▶

◄ powder is applied as a paste prepared by adding approximately 4 mL of sterile saline solution to the powder.

Dosage Forms
 Film, ophthalmic:
  Gelfilm®: 25 mm x 50 mm (6s)
 Film, topical:
  Gelfilm®: 100 mm x 125 mm (1s)
 Powder, topical:
  Gelfoam®: 1 g
 Sponge, dental:
  Gelfoam®: Size 4 (12s)
 Sponge, topical:
  Gelfoam®:
   Size 50 (4s)
   Size 100 (6s)
   Size 200 (6s)
   Size 2 cm (1s)
   Size 6 cm (6s)
   Size 12-7 mm (12s)

gelatin, pectin, and methylcellulose (JEL a tin, PEK tin, & meth il SEL yoo lose)

Synonyms methylcellulose, gelatin, and pectin; pectin, gelatin, and methylcellulose

Therapeutic Category Protectant, Topical

Use Temporary relief from minor oral irritations

Usual Dosage Press small dabs into place until the involved area is coated with a thin film; do not try to spread onto area; may be used as often as needed

Gelfilm® [US] *see* gelatin (absorbable) *on page 437*

Gelfoam® [US] *see* gelatin (absorbable) *on page 437*

Gel-Kam® [US-OTC] *see* fluoride *on page 411*

Gel-Kam® Rinse [US] *see* fluoride *on page 411*

GelRite [US-OTC] *see* alcohol (ethyl) *on page 41*

Gel-Stat™ [US-OTC] *see* alcohol (ethyl) *on page 41*

Gel-Tin® (Discontinued) *see* fluoride *on page 411*

Gelucast® [US] *see* zinc gelatin *on page 993*

Gelusil® [US-OTC/Can] *see* aluminum hydroxide, magnesium hydroxide, and simethicone *on page 54*

Gelusil® Extra Strength [Can] *see* aluminum hydroxide and magnesium hydroxide *on page 54*

gemcitabine (jem SITE a been)

Sound-Alike/Look-Alike Issues
 Gemzar® may be confused with Zinecard®

Synonyms gemcitabine hydrochloride; NSC-613327

U.S./Canadian Brand Names Gemzar® [US/Can]

Therapeutic Category Antineoplastic Agent

Use Treatment of metastatic breast cancer; locally-advanced or metastatic nonsmall cell lung cancer (NSCLC) or pancreatic cancer; advanced, relapsed ovarian cancer

Usual Dosage Refer to individual protocols. **Note**: Prolongation of the infusion time >60 minutes and administration more frequently than once weekly have been shown to increase toxicity. I.V.:
Pancreatic cancer: Initial: 1000 mg/m^2 weekly for up to 7 weeks followed by 1 week rest; then weekly for 3 weeks out of every 4 weeks.
 Dose adjustment: Patients who complete an entire cycle of therapy may have the dose in subsequent cycles increased by 25% as long as the absolute granulocyte count (AGC) nadir is >1500 x 10^6/L, platelet nadir is >100,000 x 10^6/L, and nonhematologic toxicity is less than WHO Grade 1. If the increased dose is tolerated (with the same parameters) the dose in subsequent cycles may again be increased by 20%.
Nonsmall cell lung cancer:
 1000 mg/m^2 days 1, 8, and 15; repeat cycle every 28 days
 or
 1250 mg/m^2 days 1 and 8; repeat cycle every 21 days

Breast cancer: 1250 mg/m^2 days 1 and 8; repeat cycle every 21 days
Ovarian cancer: 1000 mg/m^2 days 1 and 8; repeat cycle every 21 days

Dosage Forms
Injection, powder for reconstitution:
  Gemzar®: 200 mg, 1 g

gemcitabine hydrochloride *see gemcitabine on page 438*

gemfibrozil (jem FI broe zil)

Sound-Alike/Look-Alike Issues
  Lopid® may be confused with Levbid®, Lodine®, Lorabid®, Slo-bid™
Synonyms CI-719
U.S./Canadian Brand Names Apo-Gemfibrozil® [Can]; Gen-Gemfibrozil [Can]; GMD-Gemfibrozil [Can]; Lopid® [US/Can]; Novo-Gemfibrozil [Can]; Nu-Gemfibrozil [Can]; PMS-Gemfibrozil [Can]
Therapeutic Category Antihyperlipidemic Agent, Miscellaneous
Use Treatment of hypertriglyceridemia in types IV and V hyperlipidemia for patients who are at greater risk for pancreatitis and who have not responded to dietary intervention
Usual Dosage Oral: Adults: 1200 mg/day in 2 divided doses, 30 minutes before breakfast and dinner
Dosage Forms
Tablet, oral: 600 mg
  Lopid®: 600 mg

gemifloxacin (je mi FLOKS a sin)

Synonyms DW286; gemifloxacin mesylate; LA 20304a; SB-265805
U.S./Canadian Brand Names Factive® [US/Can]
Therapeutic Category Antibiotic, Quinolone
Use Treatment of acute exacerbation of chronic bronchitis; treatment of community-acquired pneumonia (CAP), including pneumonia caused by multidrug-resistant strains of *S. pneumoniae* (MDRSP)
Usual Dosage
Usual dosage range:
  Oral: Adults: 320 mg once daily
Indication-specific dosing:
  Oral: Adults:
    Acute exacerbations of chronic bronchitis: 320 mg once daily for 5 days
    Community-acquired pneumonia (mild to moderate): 320 mg once daily for 5 or 7 days (decision to use 5- or 7-day regimen should be guided by initial sputum culture; 7 days are recommended for MDRSP, *Klebsiella*, or *M. catarrhalis* infection)
Dosage Forms
Tablet:
  Factive®: 320 mg

gemifloxacin mesylate *see gemifloxacin on page 439*

gemtuzumab ozogamicin (gem TOO zoo mab oh zog a MY sin)

Synonyms CMA-676; NSC-720568
U.S./Canadian Brand Names Mylotarg® [US/Can]
Therapeutic Category Antineoplastic Agent, Natural Source (Plant) Derivative
Use Treatment of relapsed CD33 positive acute myeloid leukemia (AML) in patients ≥60 years of age who are not candidates for cytotoxic chemotherapy
Usual Dosage I.V.:
  Children: **Note:** Patients should receive diphenhydramine (1 mg/kg) 1 hour prior to infusion and acetaminophen 15 mg/kg 1 hour prior to infusion and every 4 hours for 2 additional doses.
  Adults: **Note:** Patients should receive diphenhydramine 50 mg orally and acetaminophen 650-1000 mg orally 1 hour prior to administration of each dose. Acetaminophen dosage should be repeated as needed every 4 hours for 2 additional doses. Pretreatment with methylprednisolone may ameliorate infusion-related symptoms.
  AML: ≥60 years: 9 mg/m^2 infused over 2 hours. A full treatment course is a total of 2 doses administered with 14 days between doses. Full hematologic recovery is not necessary for administration of the second dose. There has been only limited experience with repeat courses of gemtuzumab ozogamicin. ▶

◀ **Dosage Forms**
Injection, powder for reconstitution [preservative free]:
Mylotarg®: 5 mg

Gemzar® [US/Can] *see* gemcitabine *on page 438*

Genabid® *(Discontinued)*

Genac® [US-OTC] *see* triprolidine and pseudoephedrine *on page 955*

Gen-Acebutolol [Can] *see* acebutolol *on page 19*

Genaced™ [US-OTC] *see* acetaminophen, aspirin, and caffeine *on page 24*

Genacote™ [US-OTC] *see* aspirin *on page 98*

Gen-Acyclovir [Can] *see* acyclovir *on page 33*

Genahist® [US-OTC] *see* diphenhydramine *on page 304*

Gen-Alendronate [Can] *see* alendronate *on page 43*

Gen-Alprazolam [Can] *see* alprazolam *on page 49*

Gen-Amilazide [Can] *see* amiloride and hydrochlorothiazide *on page 59*

Genamin® Expectorant *(Discontinued)*

Gen-Amiodarone [Can] *see* amiodarone *on page 61*

Gen-Amoxicillin [Can] *see* amoxicillin *on page 67*

Gen-Anagrelide [Can] *see* anagrelide *on page 75*

Genapap™ [US-OTC] *see* acetaminophen *on page 19*

Genapap™ Children [US-OTC] *see* acetaminophen *on page 19*

Genapap™ Extra Strength [US-OTC] *see* acetaminophen *on page 19*

Genapap™ Infant [US-OTC] *see* acetaminophen *on page 19*

Genapap™ Sinus Maximum Strength *(Discontinued)* *see* acetaminophen and pseudoephedrine *on page 23*

Genaphed® [US-OTC] *see* pseudoephedrine *on page 801*

Genasal [US-OTC] *see* oxymetazoline *on page 712*

Genasoft® [US-OTC] *see* docusate *on page 314*

Genasyme® [US-OTC] *see* simethicone *on page 867*

Gen-Atenolol [Can] *see* atenolol *on page 101*

Genaton™ [US-OTC] *see* aluminum hydroxide and magnesium carbonate *on page 53*

Genaton Tablet [US-OTC] *see* aluminum hydroxide and magnesium trisilicate *on page 54*

Genatuss® *(Discontinued)* *see* guaifenesin *on page 453*

Genatuss DM® [US-OTC] *see* guaifenesin and dextromethorphan *on page 454*

Gen-Azathioprine [Can] *see* azathioprine *on page 109*

Gen-Baclofen [Can] *see* baclofen *on page 115*

Gen-Beclo [Can] *see* beclomethasone *on page 119*

Gen-Bicalutamide [Can] *see* bicalutamide *on page 135*

Gen-Bromazepam [Can] *see* bromazepam *(Canada only) on page 142*

Gen-Budesonide AQ [Can] *see* budesonide *on page 147*

Gen-Buspirone [Can] *see* buspirone *on page 153*

Gencalc® 600 *(Discontinued)* *see* calcium carbonate *on page 163*

Gen-Captopril [Can] *see* captopril *on page 171*

Gen-Carbamazepine CR [Can] *see* carbamazepine *on page 172*

Gen-Cilazapril [Can] *see* cilazapril *(Canada only) on page 219*

Gen-Cimetidine [Can] *see* cimetidine *on page 219*

Gen-Ciprofloxacin [Can] *see* ciprofloxacin *on page 221*

Gen-Citalopram [Can] *see* citalopram *on page 225*

Gen-Clarithromycin [Can] *see* clarithromycin *on page 227*

Gen-Clindamycin [Can] *see* clindamycin *on page 230*

Gen-Clobetasol [Can] *see* clobetasol *on page 232*

Gen-Clomipramine [Can] *see* clomipramine *on page 235*

Gen-Clonazepam [Can] *see* clonazepam *on page 235*

Gen-Clozapine [Can] *see* clozapine *on page 240*

Gen-Combo Sterinebs [Can] *see* ipratropium and albuterol *on page 525*
Gen-Cyclobenzaprine [Can] *see* cyclobenzaprine *on page 255*
Gen-Cyproterone [Can] *see* cyproterone *(Canada only) on page 259*
Gen-Diltiazem [Can] *see* diltiazem *on page 300*
Gen-Diltiazem CD [Can] *see* diltiazem *on page 300*
Gen-Divalproex [Can] *see* valproic acid and derivatives *on page 967*
Gen-Doxazosin [Can] *see* doxazosin *on page 320*
Genebs [US-OTC] *see* acetaminophen *on page 19*
Genebs Extra Strength [US-OTC] *see* acetaminophen *on page 19*
Gen-Enalapril [Can] *see* enalapril *on page 339*
Generlac [US] *see* lactulose *on page 544*
Genesec™ [US-OTC] *see* acetaminophen and phenyltoloxamine *on page 22*
Gen-Etidronate [Can] *see* etidronate disodium *on page 382*
Genexa™ LA *(Discontinued)* *see* guaifenesin and phenylephrine *on page 456*
Geneye [US-OTC] *see* tetrahydrozoline *on page 916*
Gen-Famotidine [Can] *see* famotidine *on page 390*
Gen-Fenofibrate Micro [Can] *see* fenofibrate *on page 393*
Genfiber™ [US-OTC] *see* psyllium *on page 804*
Gen-Fluconazole [Can] *see* fluconazole *on page 405*
Gen-Fluoxetine [Can] *see* fluoxetine *on page 413*
Gen-Fosinopril [Can] *see* fosinopril *on page 427*
Gen-Gabapentin [Can] *see* gabapentin *on page 431*
Gen-Gemfibrozil [Can] *see* gemfibrozil *on page 439*
Gen-Gliclazide [Can] *see* gliclazide *(Canada only) on page 444*
Gen-Glybe [Can] *see* glyburide *on page 448*
Gengraf® [US] *see* cyclosporine *on page 257*
Gen-Hydroxychloroquine [Can] *see* hydroxychloroquine *on page 489*
Gen-Hydroxyurea [Can] *see* hydroxyurea *on page 490*
Gen-Indapamide [Can] *see* indapamide *on page 505*
Gen-Ipratropium [Can] *see* ipratropium *on page 524*
Gen-K® *(Discontinued)* *see* potassium chloride *on page 771*
Gen-Lamotrigine [Can] *see* lamotrigine *on page 545*
Gen-Levothyroxine [Can] *see* levothyroxine *on page 560*
Gen-Lisinopril [Can] *see* lisinopril *on page 570*
Gen-Lisinopril/Hctz [Can] *see* lisinopril and hydrochlorothiazide *on page 571*
Gen-Lovastatin [Can] *see* lovastatin *on page 579*
Gen-Medroxy [Can] *see* medroxyprogesterone *on page 597*
Gen-Meloxicam [Can] *see* meloxicam *on page 599*
Gen-Metformin [Can] *see* metformin *on page 610*
Gen-Metoprolol [Can] *see* metoprolol *on page 626*
Gen-Minocycline [Can] *see* minocycline *on page 635*
Gen-Mirtazapine [Can] *see* mirtazapine *on page 637*
Gen-Nabumetone [Can] *see* nabumetone *on page 650*
Gen-Naproxen EC [Can] *see* naproxen *on page 656*
Gen-Nitro [Can] *see* nitroglycerin *on page 675*
Gen-Nizatidine [Can] *see* nizatidine *on page 677*
Gen-Nortriptyline [Can] *see* nortriptyline *on page 680*
Gen-Ondansetron [Can] *see* ondansetron *on page 698*
Genoptic® *(Discontinued)* *see* gentamicin *on page 442*
Genora® 0.5/35 *(Discontinued)* *see* ethinyl estradiol and norethindrone *on page 376*
Genora® 1/35 *(Discontinued)* *see* ethinyl estradiol and norethindrone *on page 376*
Genora® 1/50 *(Discontinued)* *see* mestranol and norethindrone *on page 608*
Genotropin® [US] *see* somatropin *on page 881*

Genotropin Miniquick® [US] *see* somatropin *on page 881*
Gen-Oxybutynin [Can] *see* oxybutynin *on page 708*
Gen-Paroxetine [Can] *see* paroxetine *on page 724*
Gen-Pindolol [Can] *see* pindolol *on page 754*
Gen-Pioglitazone [Can] *see* pioglitazone *on page 754*
Gen-Piroxicam [Can] *see* piroxicam *on page 757*
Genpril® *(Discontinued)* *see* ibuprofen *on page 495*
Gen-Ranidine [Can] *see* ranitidine *on page 819*
Gen-Risperidone [Can] *see* risperidone *on page 837*
Gen-Salbutamol [Can] *see* albuterol *on page 39*
Gen-Selegiline [Can] *see* selegiline *on page 860*
Gen-Sertraline [Can] *see* sertraline *on page 863*
Gen-Simvastatin [Can] *see* simvastatin *on page 867*
Gen-Sotalol [Can] *see* sotalol *on page 885*
Gen-Sumatriptan [Can] *see* sumatriptan *on page 898*
Gentacidin® *(Discontinued)* *see* gentamicin *on page 442*
Gentak® [US] *see* gentamicin *on page 442*

gentamicin (jen ta MYE sin)

Sound-Alike/Look-Alike Issues
gentamicin may be confused with gentian violet, kanamycin
Garamycin® may be confused with kanamycin, Terramycin®

Synonyms gentamicin sulfate

U.S./Canadian Brand Names Alcomicin® [Can]; Diogent® [Can]; Garamycin® [Can]; Gentak® [US]; Gentamicin Injection, USP [Can]; Gentasol™ [US]; SAB-Gentamicin [Can]

Therapeutic Category Aminoglycoside (Antibiotic); Antibiotic, Ophthalmic; Antibiotic, Topical

Use Treatment of susceptible bacterial infections, normally gram-negative organisms including *Pseudomonas*, *Proteus*, *Serratia*, and gram-positive *Staphylococcus*; treatment of bone infections, respiratory tract infections, skin and soft tissue infections, as well as abdominal and urinary tract infections, and septicemia; treatment of infective endocarditis; used topically to treat superficial infections of the skin or ophthalmic infections caused by susceptible bacteria

Usual Dosage Note: Dosage Individualization is **critical** because of the low therapeutic index.

Use of ideal body weight (IBW) for determining the mg/kg/dose appears to be more accurate than dosing on the basis of total body weight (TBW). In morbid obesity, dosage requirement may best be estimated using a dosing weight of IBW + 0.4 (TBW - IBW).

Initial and periodic plasma drug levels (eg, peak and trough with conventional dosing) should be determined, particularly in critically-ill patients with serious infections or in disease states known to significantly alter aminoglycoside pharmacokinetics (eg, cystic fibrosis, burns, or major surgery).

Usual dosage ranges:
Infants and Children <5 years: I.M., I.V.: 2.5 mg/kg/dose every 8 hours*
Children ≥5 years: I.M., I.V.: 2-2.5 mg/kg/dose every 8 hours*
*Note: Higher individual doses and/or more frequent intervals (eg, every 6 hours) may be required in selected clinical situations (cystic fibrosis) or serum levels document the need
Children and Adults:
Ophthalmic:
Ointment: Instill 1/2" (1.25 cm) 2-3 times/day to every 3-4 hours
Solution: Instill 1-2 drops every 2-4 hours, up to 2 drops every hour for severe infections
Topical: Apply 3-4 times/day to affected area
Adults:
I.M., I.V.:
Conventional: 1-2.5 mg/kg/dose every 8-12 hours; to ensure adequate peak concentrations early in therapy, higher initial dosage may be considered in selected patients when extracellular water is increased (edema, septic shock, postsurgical, or trauma)
Once daily: 4-7 mg/kg/dose once daily; some clinicians recommend this approach for all patients with normal renal function; this dose is at least as efficacious with similar, if not less, toxicity than conventional dosing
Intrathecal: 4-8 mg/day

Indication-specific dosing:
Neonates: I.V.:
  Meningitis:
    0-7 days of age: <2000 g: 2.5 mg/kg every 18-24 hours; >2000 g: 2.5 mg/kg every 12 hours
    8-28 days of age: <2000 g: 2.5 mg/kg every 8-12 hours; >2000 g: 2.5 mg/kg every 8 hours
Children and Adults: I.M., I.V.:
  Brucellosis: 240 mg (I.M.) daily or 5 mg/kg (I.V.) daily for 7 days; either regimen recommended in combination with doxycycline
  Cholangitis: 4-6 mg/kg once daily with ampicillin
  Diverticulitis (complicated): 1.5-2 mg/kg every 8 hours (with ampicillin and metronidazole)
  Endocarditis: Treatment: 3 mg/kg/day in 1-3 divided doses
  Meningitis:
    (Enterococcus sp or *Pseudomonas aeruginosa)*: Loading dose 2 mg/kg, then 1.7 mg/kg/dose every 8 hours (administered with another bacteriocidal drug)
    Listeria: 5-7 mg/kg/day (with penicillin) for 1 week
  Pelvic inflammatory disease: Loading dose: 2 mg/kg, then 1.5 mg/kg every 8 hours
    Alternate therapy: 4.5 mg/kg once daily
  Plague (*Yersinia pestis*): Treatment: 5 mg/kg/day, followed by postexposure prophylaxis with doxycycline
  Pneumonia, hospital- or ventilator-associated: 7 mg/kg/day (with antipseudomonal beta-lactam or carbapenem)
  Synergy (for gram-positive infections): 3 mg/kg/day in 1-3 divided doses (with ampicillin)
  Tularemia: 5 mg/kg/day divided every 8 hours for 1-2 weeks
  Urinary tract infection: 1.5 mg/kg/dose every 8 hours
Dosage Forms
  Cream, topical: 0.1% (15 g, 30 g)
  Infusion [premixed in NS]: 40 mg (50 mL); 60 mg (50 mL, 100 mL); 70 mg (50 mL); 80 mg (50 mL, 100 mL); 90 mg (100 mL); 100 mg (50 mL, 100 mL); 120 mg (100 mL)
  Injection, solution: 10 mg/mL (6 mL, 8 mL, 10 mL); 40 mg/mL (2 mL, 20 mL)
  Injection, solution [pediatric]: 10 mg/mL (2 mL)
  Injection, solution [pediatric; preservative free]: 10 mg/mL (2 mL)
  Ointment, ophthalmic: 0.3% [3 mg/g] (3.5 g)
    Gentak®: 0.3% [3 mg/g] (3.5 g)
  Ointment, topical: 0.1% (15 g, 30 g)
  Solution, ophthalmic: 0.3% (5 mL, 15 mL)
    Gentak®: 0.3% (5 mL)
    Gentasol™: 0.3% (5 mL)

gentamicin and prednisolone *see* prednisolone and gentamicin *on page 780*
Gentamicin Injection, USP [Can] *see* gentamicin *on page 442*
gentamicin sulfate *see* gentamicin *on page 442*
Gen-Tamoxifen [Can] *see* tamoxifen *on page 902*
Gen-Tamsulosin [Can] *see* tamsulosin *on page 903*
Gentasol™ [US] *see* gentamicin *on page 442*
GenTeal® [US-OTC/Can] *see* hydroxypropyl methylcellulose *on page 490*
GenTeal® Mild [US-OTC] *see* hydroxypropyl methylcellulose *on page 490*
Gen-Temazepam [Can] *see* temazepam *on page 907*
Gentex HC *(Discontinued)*
Gentex LA *(Discontinued)* *see* guaifenesin and phenylephrine *on page 456*
Gentex LQ [US] *see* carbetapentane, guaifenesin, and phenylephrine *on page 175*
Gen-Ticlopidine [Can] *see* ticlopidine *on page 926*
Gen-Timolol [Can] *see* timolol *on page 927*
Gen-Tizanidine [Can] *see* tizanidine *on page 931*
Gentlax® [Can] *see* bisacodyl *on page 136*
Gentlax® *(Discontinued)* *see* bisacodyl *on page 136*
Gen-Topiramate [Can] *see* topiramate *on page 935*
Gentran® [US/Can] *see* dextran *on page 282*
Gentrasul® *(Discontinued)* *see* gentamicin *on page 442*
Gen-Trazodone [Can] *see* trazodone *on page 944*

Gen-Triazolam [Can] *see* triazolam *on page 950*
Gentuss-HC *(Discontinued)*
Gen-Verapamil [Can] *see* verapamil *on page 974*
Gen-Verapamil SR [Can] *see* verapamil *on page 974*
Gen-Warfarin [Can] *see* warfarin *on page 986*
Gen-Zopiclone [Can] *see* zopiclone *(Canada only) on page 997*
Geocillin® *(Discontinued) see* carbenicillin *on page 174*
Geodon® [US] *see* ziprasidone *on page 994*
Geref® Diagnostic [US] *see* sermorelin acetate *on page 863*
Geref® *(Discontinued) see* sermorelin acetate *on page 863*
Geriation [US-OTC] *see* vitamins (multiple/oral) *on page 983*
Geridium® *(Discontinued) see* phenazopyridine *on page 741*
Geri-Freeda [US-OTC] *see* vitamins (multiple/oral) *on page 983*
Geri-Hydrolac™ [US-OTC] *see* lactic acid and ammonium hydroxide *on page 542*
Geri-Hydrolac™-12 [US-OTC] *see* lactic acid and ammonium hydroxide *on page 542*
Geritol Complete® [US-OTC] *see* vitamins (multiple/oral) *on page 983*
Geritol Extend® [US-OTC] *see* vitamins (multiple/oral) *on page 983*
Geritol® Tonic [US-OTC] *see* vitamins (multiple/oral) *on page 983*
German measles vaccine *see* rubella virus vaccine (live) *on page 848*
Gevrabon® [US-OTC] *see* vitamin B complex combinations *on page 981*
GF196960 *see* tadalafil *on page 902*
GG *see* guaifenesin *on page 453*
GG-Cen® *(Discontinued) see* guaifenesin *on page 453*
GHB *see* sodium oxybate *on page 877*
GI87084B *see* remifentanil *on page 824*
Gilphex TR® [US] *see* guaifenesin and phenylephrine *on page 456*
Giltuss® [US] *see* guaifenesin, dextromethorphan, and phenylephrine *on page 459*
Giltuss HC® *(Discontinued)*
Giltuss Pediatric® [US] *see* guaifenesin, dextromethorphan, and phenylephrine *on page 459*
Giltuss TR® [US] *see* guaifenesin, dextromethorphan, and phenylephrine *on page 459*
glargine insulin *see* insulin glargine *on page 510*

glatiramer acetate (gla TIR a mer AS e tate)

Sound-Alike/Look-Alike Issues
Copaxone® may be confused with Compazine®
Synonyms copolymer-1
U.S./Canadian Brand Names Copaxone® [US/Can]
Therapeutic Category Biological, Miscellaneous
Use Management of relapsing-remitting type multiple sclerosis
Usual Dosage SubQ: Adults: 20 mg daily
Dosage Forms
  Injection, solution [preservative free]:
    Copaxone®: 20 mg/mL (1 mL)

Glaucon® *(Discontinued) see* epinephrine *on page 344*
Gleevec® [US/Can] *see* imatinib *on page 499*
Gliadel® [US] *see* carmustine *on page 180*
Gliadel Wafer® [Can] *see* carmustine *on page 180*
glibenclamide *see* glyburide *on page 448*
Gliclazide-80 [Can] *see* gliclazide *(Canada only) on page 444*

gliclazide *(Canada only)* (GLYE kla zide)

U.S./Canadian Brand Names Apo-Gliclazide® [Can]; Diamicron® MR [Can]; Diamicron® [Can]; Gen-Gliclazide [Can]; Gliclazide-80 [Can]; Novo-Gliclazide [Can]; PMS-Gliclazide [Can]; Sandoz-Gliclazide [Can]

Therapeutic Category Antidiabetic Agent; Hypoglycemic Agent, Oral; Sulfonylurea Agent

Use Management of type 2 diabetes mellitus (noninsulin-dependent, NIDDM)

Usual Dosage Oral: Adults:

Immediate release tablet: Initial: 80-160 mg/day; typical dose range 80-320 mg/day; dosage of ≥160 mg should be divided into 2 equal parts for twice-daily administration; maximum dose: 320 mg/day; should be taken with meals

Sustained release tablet: 30-120 mg once daily

Note: There is no fixed dosage regimen for the management of diabetes mellitus with gliclazide or any other hypoglycemic agent. Dose must be individualized based on frequent determinations of blood glucose during dose titration and throughout maintenance.

Dosage Forms [CAN] = Canadian brand name

Tablet: 80 mg [not available in the U.S.]

Diamicron® [CAN]: 80 mg [not available in the U.S.]

Tablet, sustained release:

Diamicron® MR [CAN]: 30 mg [not available in the U.S.]

glimepiride (GLYE me pye ride)

Sound-Alike/Look-Alike Issues

glimepiride may be confused with glipiZIDE

Amaryl® may be confused with Altace®, Amerge®, Reminyl®

U.S./Canadian Brand Names Amaryl® [US/Can]; Apo-Glimepiride [Can]; CO Glimepiride [Can]; Novo-Glimepiride [Can]; PMS-Glimepiride [Can]; ratio-Glimepiride [Can]; Rhoxal-glimepiride [Can]; Sandoz-Glimepiride [Can]

Therapeutic Category Antidiabetic Agent, Oral

Use Management of type 2 diabetes mellitus (noninsulin-dependent, NIDDM) as an adjunct to diet and exercise to lower blood glucose; may be used in combination with metformin or insulin in patients whose hyperglycemia cannot be controlled by diet and exercise in conjunction with a single oral hypoglycemic agent

Usual Dosage Oral: Adults: Initial: 1-2 mg once daily, administered with breakfast or the first main meal; usual maintenance dose: 1-4 mg once daily; after a dose of 2 mg once daily, increase in increments of 2 mg at 1- to 2-week intervals based upon the patient's blood glucose response to a maximum of 8 mg once daily. If inadequate response to maximal dose, combination therapy with metformin may be considered.

Combination with insulin therapy (fasting glucose level for instituting combination therapy is in the range of >150 mg/dL in plasma or serum depending on the patient): initial recommended dose: 8 mg once daily with the first main meal

After starting with low-dose insulin, upward adjustments of insulin can be done approximately weekly as guided by frequent measurements of fasting blood glucose. Once stable, combination-therapy patients should monitor their capillary blood glucose on an ongoing basis, preferably daily.

Conversion from therapy with long half-life agents: Observe patient carefully for 1-2 weeks when converting from a longer half-life agent (eg, chlorpropamide) to glimepiride due to overlapping hypoglycemic effects.

Dosage Forms

Tablet: 1 mg, 2 mg, 4 mg

Amaryl®: 1 mg, 2 mg, 4 mg

glimepiride and pioglitazone *see* pioglitazone and glimepiride *on page 755*

glimepiride and pioglitazone hydrochloride *see* pioglitazone and glimepiride *on page 755*

glimepiride and rosiglitazone maleate *see* rosiglitazone and glimepiride *on page 845*

glipizide (GLIP i zide)

Sound-Alike/Look-Alike Issues

glipiZIDE may be confused with glimepiride, glyBURIDE

Glucotrol® may be confused with Glucophage®, Glucotrol® XL, glyBURIDE

Glucotrol® XL may be confused with Glucotrol®

Synonyms glydiazinamide

Tall-Man glipiZIDE

U.S./Canadian Brand Names Glucotrol® XL [US]; Glucotrol® [US]

Therapeutic Category Antidiabetic Agent, Oral

◀ **Use** Management of type 2 diabetes mellitus (noninsulin-dependent, NIDDM)

Usual Dosage Oral (allow several days between dose titrations): Adults: Initial: 5 mg/day; adjust dosage at 2.5-5 mg daily increments as determined by blood glucose response at intervals of several days.

   Immediate release tablet: Maximum recommended once-daily dose: 15 mg; maximum recommended total daily dose: 40 mg. Doses >15 mg/day should be administered in divided doses.

   Extended release tablet (Glucotrol® XL): Maximum recommended dose: 20 mg

   When transferring from insulin to glipizide:

   Current insulin requirement ≤20 units: Discontinue insulin and initiate glipizide at usual dose

   Current insulin requirement >20 units: Decrease insulin by 50% and initiate glipizide at usual dose; gradually decrease insulin dose based on patient response. Several days should elapse between dosage changes.

Dosage Forms

   Tablet: 5 mg, 10 mg

   Glucotrol®: 5 mg, 10 mg

   Tablet, extended release: 2.5 mg, 5 mg, 10 mg

   Glucotrol XL®: 2.5 mg, 5 mg, 10 mg

glipizide and metformin (GLIP i zide & met FOR min)

Synonyms glipizide and metformin hydrochloride; metformin and glipizide

U.S./Canadian Brand Names Metaglip™ [US]

Therapeutic Category Antidiabetic Agent (Biguanide); Antidiabetic Agent (Sulfonylurea)

Use Initial therapy for management of type 2 diabetes mellitus (noninsulin-dependent, NIDDM) when hyperglycemia cannot be managed with diet and exercise alone. Second-line therapy for management of type 2 diabetes (NIDDM) when hyperglycemia cannot be managed with a sulfonylurea or metformin along with diet and exercise.

Usual Dosage Oral: Adults:

   Type 2 diabetes, first-line therapy: Initial: Glipizide 2.5 mg/metformin 250 mg once daily with a meal. Dose adjustment: Increase dose by 1 tablet/day every 2 weeks, up to a maximum of glipizide 10 mg/metformin 1000 mg daily

   Patients with fasting plasma glucose (FPG) 280-320 mg/dL: Consider glipizide 2.5 mg/metformin 500 mg twice daily. Dose adjustment: Increase dose by 1 tablet/day every 2 weeks, up to a maximum of glipizide 10 mg/metformin 2000 mg daily in divided doses

   Type 2 diabetes, second-line therapy: Glipizide 2.5 mg/metformin 500 mg **or** glipizide 5 mg/metformin 500 mg twice daily with morning and evening meals; starting dose should not exceed current daily dose of glipizide (or sulfonylurea equivalent) or metformin. Dose adjustment: Titrate dose in increments of no more than glipizide 5 mg/metformin 500 mg, up to a maximum dose of glipizide 20 mg/metformin 2000 mg daily.

Dosage Forms

   Tablet: 2.5/250: Glipizide 2.5 mg and metformin 250 mg; 2.5/500: Glipizide 2.5 mg and metformin 500 mg; 5/500: Glipizide 5 mg and metformin 500 mg

   Metaglip™: 2.5/250: Glipizide 2.5 mg and metformin 250 mg; 2.5/500: Glipizide 2.5 mg and metformin 500 mg; 5/500: Glipizide 5 mg and metformin 500 mg

glipizide and metformin hydrochloride see glipizide and metformin on page 446

glivec see imatinib on page 499

GlucaGen® [US] see glucagon on page 446

GlucaGen® Diagnostic Kit [US] see glucagon on page 446

GlucaGen® HypoKit™ [US] see glucagon on page 446

glucagon (GLOO ka gon)

Sound-Alike/Look-Alike Issues

   glucagon may be confused with Glaucon®

Synonyms glucagon hydrochloride

U.S./Canadian Brand Names GlucaGen® Diagnostic Kit [US]; GlucaGen® HypoKit™ [US]; GlucaGen® [US]; Glucagon Emergency Kit [US]

Therapeutic Category Antihypoglycemic Agent

Use Management of hypoglycemia; diagnostic aid in radiologic examinations to temporarily inhibit GI tract movement

Usual Dosage
Hypoglycemia or insulin shock therapy: I.M., I.V., SubQ:
Children <20 kg: 0.5 mg or 20-30 mcg/kg/dose; repeated in 20 minutes as needed
Children ≥20 kg and Adults: 1 mg; may repeat in 20 minutes as needed
Note: I.V. dextrose should be administered as soon as it is available; if patient fails to respond to glucagon, I.V. dextrose must be given.
Diagnostic aid: Adults: I.M., I.V.: 0.25-2 mg 10 minutes prior to procedure
Dosage Forms
Injection, powder for reconstitution:
GlucaGen®, GlucaGen® Diagnostic Kit, GlucaGen® HypoKit™, Glucagon Emergency Kit: 1 mg

Glucagon Diagnostic Kit *(Discontinued)* *see* glucagon *on page 446*
Glucagon Emergency Kit [US] *see* glucagon *on page 446*
glucagon hydrochloride *see* glucagon *on page 446*
glucocerebrosidase *see* alglucerase *on page 45*
GlucoNorm® [Can] *see* repaglinide *on page 825*
Glucophage® [US/Can] *see* metformin *on page 610*
Glucophage® XR [US] *see* metformin *on page 610*
glucose *see* dextrose *on page 286*
glucose monohydrate *see* dextrose *on page 286*

glucose polymers (GLOO kose POL i merz)
U.S./Canadian Brand Names Moducal® [US-OTC]; Polycose® [US-OTC]
Therapeutic Category Nutritional Supplement
Use Supplies calories for those persons not able to meet the caloric requirement with usual food intake
Usual Dosage Oral: Adults: Add to foods or beverages or mix in water
Dosage Forms
Liquid:
Polycose® [OTC]: 43%
Powder:
Moducal® [OTC]: 368 g
Polycose® [OTC]: 350 g

Glucotrol® [US] *see* glipizide *on page 445*
Glucotrol® XL [US] *see* glipizide *on page 445*
Glucovance® [US] *see* glyburide and metformin *on page 448*
glulisine insulin *see* insulin glulisine *on page 511*
Glumetza™ [US/Can] *see* metformin *on page 610*

glutamic acid (gloo TAM ik AS id)
Synonyms glutamic acid hydrochloride
Therapeutic Category Gastrointestinal Agent, Miscellaneous
Use Treatment of hypochlorhydria and achlorhydria
Usual Dosage Oral: Adults: 500-1000 mg/day before meals or food
Dosage Forms
Tablet: 500 mg

glutamic acid hydrochloride *see* glutamic acid *on page 447*
Glutofac®-MX [US] *see* vitamins (multiple/oral) *on page 983*
Glutofac®-ZX [US] *see* vitamins (multiple/oral) *on page 983*
Glutol™ [US-OTC] *see* dextrose *on page 286*
Glutose™ [US-OTC] *see* dextrose *on page 286*
Glyate® *(Discontinued)* *see* guaifenesin *on page 453*
glybenclamide *see* glyburide *on page 448*
glybenzcyclamide *see* glyburide *on page 448*

glyburide (GLYE byoor ide)

Sound-Alike/Look-Alike Issues
glyBURIDE may be confused with glipiZIDE, Glucotrol®
Diaβeta® may be confused with Diabinese®, Zebeta®
Micronase® may be confused with microK®, miconazole, Micronor®, Microzide™

Synonyms glibenclamide; glybenclamide; glybenzcyclamide

Tall-Man glyBURIDE

U.S./Canadian Brand Names Albert® Glyburide [Can]; Apo-Glyburide® [Can]; Diaβeta® [US/Can]; Euglucon® [Can]; Gen-Glybe [Can]; Glynase® PresTab® [US]; Micronase® [US]; Novo-Glyburide [Can]; Nu-Glyburide [Can]; PMS-Glyburide [Can]; ratio-Glyburide [Can]; Sandoz-Glyburide [Can]

Therapeutic Category Antidiabetic Agent, Oral

Use Management of type 2 diabetes mellitus (noninsulin-dependent, NIDDM)

Usual Dosage Oral: Adults:
Diaβeta®, Micronase®:
Initial: 2.5-5 mg/day, administered with breakfast or the first main meal of the day. In patients who are more sensitive to hypoglycemic drugs, start at 1.25 mg/day.
Increase in increments of no more than 2.5 mg/day at weekly intervals based on the patient's blood glucose response
Maintenance: 1.25-20 mg/day given as single or divided doses; maximum: 20 mg/day
Micronized tablets (Glynase® PresTab®): Adults:
Initial: 1.5-3 mg/day, administered with breakfast or the first main meal of the day in patients who are more sensitive to hypoglycemic drugs, start at 0.75 mg/day. Increase in increments of no more than 1.5 mg/day in weekly intervals based on the patient's blood glucose response.
Maintenance: 0.75-12 mg/day given as a single dose or in divided doses. Some patients (especially those receiving >6 mg/day) may have a more satisfactory response with twice-daily dosing. Maximum: 12 mg/day

Dosage Forms
Tablet: 1.25 mg, 2.5 mg, 5 mg
Diaβeta®, Micronase®: 1.25 mg, 2.5 mg, 5 mg
Tablet, micronized: 1.5 mg, 3 mg, 6 mg
Glynase® PresTab®: 1.5 mg, 3 mg, 6 mg

glyburide and metformin (GLYE byoor ide & met FOR min)

Sound-Alike/Look-Alike Issues
Glucovance® may be confused with Vyvanse™

Synonyms glyburide and metformin hydrochloride; metformin and glyburide

U.S./Canadian Brand Names Glucovance® [US]

Therapeutic Category Antidiabetic Agent (Sulfonylurea); Antidiabetic Agent, Oral

Use Initial therapy for management of type 2 diabetes mellitus (noninsulin-dependent, NIDDM). Second-line therapy for management of type 2 diabetes (NIDDM) when hyperglycemia cannot be managed with a sulfonylurea or metformin; combination therapy with a thiazolidinedione may be required to achieve additional control.

Usual Dosage Note: Dose must be individualized. Dosages expressed as glyburide/metformin components.
Adults: Oral:
Initial therapy (no prior treatment with sulfonylurea or metformin): 1.25 mg/250 mg once daily with a meal; patients with Hb A$_{1c}$ >9% or fasting plasma glucose (FPG) >200 mg/dL may start with 1.25 mg/250 mg twice daily
Dosage may be increased in increments of 1.25 mg/250 mg, at intervals of not less than 2 weeks; maximum daily dose: 10 mg/2000 mg (limited experience with higher doses)
Previously treated with a sulfonylurea or metformin alone: Initial: 2.5 mg/500 mg or 5 mg/500 mg twice daily; increase in increments no greater than 5 mg/500 mg; maximum daily dose: 20 mg/2000 mg
When switching patients previously on a sulfonylurea and metformin together, do not exceed the daily dose of glyburide (or glyburide equivalent) or metformin.
Note: May combine with a thiazolidinedione in patients with an inadequate response to glyburide/metformin therapy (risk of hypoglycemia may be increased).

Dosage Forms
Tablet: Glyburide 1.25 mg and metformin 250 mg; glyburide 2.5 mg and metformin 500 mg; glyburide 5 mg and metformin 500 mg

Glucovance®: 1.25 mg/250 mg: Glyburide 1.25 mg and metformin 250 mg; 2.5 mg/500 mg: Glyburide 2.5 mg and metformin 500 mg; 5 mg/500 mg: Glyburide 5 mg and metformin 500 mg

glyburide and metformin hydrochloride *see* glyburide and metformin *on page 448*

glycerin (GLIS er in)

Synonyms glycerol

U.S./Canadian Brand Names Bausch & Lomb® Computer Eye Drops [US-OTC]; Colace® Adult/Children Suppositories [US-OTC]; Colace® Infant/Children Suppositories [US-OTC]; Fleet® Babylax® [US-OTC]; Fleet® Glycerin Suppositories Maximum Strength [US-OTC]; Fleet® Glycerin Suppositories [US-OTC]; Fleet® Liquid Glycerin Suppositories [US-OTC]; Sani-Supp® [US-OTC]

Therapeutic Category Laxative; Ophthalmic Agent, Miscellaneous

Use Constipation; reduction of intraocular pressure; reduction of corneal edema; glycerin has been administered orally to reduce intracranial pressure

Usual Dosage

Constipation: Rectal:

Children <6 years: 1 infant suppository 1-2 times/day as needed or 2-5 mL as an enema

Children >6 years and Adults: 1 adult suppository 1-2 times/day as needed or 5-15 mL as an enema

Children and Adults:

Reduction of intraocular pressure: Oral: 1-1.8 g/kg 1-1½ hours preoperatively; additional doses may be administered at 5-hour intervals

Reduction of intracranial pressure: Oral: 1.5 g/kg/day divided every 4 hours; 1 g/kg/dose every 6 hours has also been used

Reduction of corneal edema: Ophthalmic solution: Instill 1-2 drops in eye(s) prior to examination OR for lubricant effect, instill 1-2 drops in eye(s) every 3-4 hours

Dosage Forms

Solution, ophthalmic, sterile:

Bausch & Lomb® Computer Eye Drops [OTC]: 1% (15 mL)

Solution, rectal:

Fleet® Babylax® [OTC]: 2.3 g/2.3 mL (4 mL)

Fleet® Liquid Glycerin Suppositories [OTC]: 5.6 g/5.5 mL (7.5 mL)

Suppository, rectal: 82.5% (12s, 25s) [pediatric size]; 82.5% (12s, 24s, 25s, 50s, 100s) [adult size]

Colace® Adult/Children [OTC]: 2.1 g (12s, 24s, 48s, 100s)

Colace® Infant/Children [OTC]: 1.2 g (12s, 24s)

Fleet® Glycerin Suppositories [OTC]: 1 g (12s) [pediatric size]; 2g (12s, 24s, 50s) [adult size]

Fleet® Glycerin Suppositories Maximum Strength [OTC]: 3g (18s) [adult size]

Sani-Supp® [OTC]: 82.5% (10s, 25s) [pediatric size]; 82.5% (10s, 25s, 50s) [adult size]

glycerol *see* glycerin *on page 449*

glycerol guaiacolate *see* guaifenesin *on page 453*

Glycerol-T® *(Discontinued)* *see* theophylline and guaifenesin *on page 919*

glycerol triacetate *see* triacetin *on page 947*

glyceryl trinitrate *see* nitroglycerin *on page 675*

Glycofed® *(Discontinued)* *see* guaifenesin and pseudoephedrine *on page 458*

GlycoLax® [US] *see* polyethylene glycol 3350 *on page 765*

Glycon [Can] *see* metformin *on page 610*

glycopyrrolate (glye koe PYE roe late)

Synonyms glycopyrronium bromide

U.S./Canadian Brand Names Glycopyrrolate Injection, USP [Can]; Robinul® Forte [US]; Robinul® [US]

Therapeutic Category Anticholinergic Agent

Use Inhibit salivation and excessive secretions of the respiratory tract preoperatively; reversal of neuromuscular blockade; control of upper airway secretions; adjunct in treatment of peptic ulcer

Usual Dosage

Children:

Reduction of secretions (preanesthetic):

Oral: 40-100 mcg/kg/dose 3-4 times/day

I.M., I.V.: 4-10 mcg/kg/dose every 3-4 hours; maximum: 0.2 mg/dose or 0.8 mg/24 hours

Intraoperative: I.V.: 4 mcg/kg not to exceed 0.1 mg; repeat at 2- to 3-minute intervals as needed

Preoperative: I.M.:
  <2 years: 4-9 mcg/kg 30-60 minutes before procedure
  >2 years: 4 mcg/kg 30-60 minutes before procedure
Children and Adults: Reverse neuromuscular blockade: I.V.: 0.2 mg for each 1 mg of neostigmine or 5 mg of pyridostigmine administered or 5-15 mcg/kg glycopyrrolate with 25-70 mcg/kg of neostigmine or 0.1-0.3 mg/kg of pyridostigmine (agents usually administered simultaneously, but glycopyrrolate may be administered first if bradycardia is present)
Adults:
  Reduction of secretions:
    Intraoperative: I.V.: 0.1 mg repeated as needed at 2- to 3-minute intervals
    Preoperative: I.M.: 4 mcg/kg 30-60 minutes before procedure
  Peptic ulcer:
    Oral: 1-2 mg 2-3 times/day
    I.M., I.V.: 0.1-0.2 mg 3-4 times/day
Dosage Forms
  Injection, solution: 0.2 mg/mL (1 mL, 2 mL, 5 mL, 20 mL)
    Robinul®: 0.2 mg/mL (1 mL, 2 mL, 5 mL)
  Tablet:
    Robinul®: 1 mg
    Robinul® Forte: 2 mg

Glycopyrrolate Injection, USP [Can] *see* glycopyrrolate *on page 449*
glycopyrronium bromide *see* glycopyrrolate *on page 449*
glycosum *see* dextrose *on page 286*
Glycotuss® *(Discontinued)* *see* guaifenesin *on page 453*
Glycotuss-dM® *(Discontinued)* *see* guaifenesin and dextromethorphan *on page 454*
glydiazinamide *see* glipizide *on page 445*
Glynase® PresTab® [US] *see* glyburide *on page 448*
Gly-Oxide® [US-OTC] *see* carbamide peroxide *on page 174*
Glyquin® [US] *see* hydroquinone *on page 488*
Glyquin-XM™ [US/Can] *see* hydroquinone *on page 488*
Glyset® [US/Can] *see* miglitol *on page 634*
GM-CSF *see* sargramostim *on page 857*
GMD-Azithromycin [Can] *see* azithromycin *on page 110*
GMD-Fluconazole [Can] *see* fluconazole *on page 405*
GMD-Gemfibrozil [Can] *see* gemfibrozil *on page 439*
GMD-Sertraline [Can] *see* sertraline *on page 863*
G-myticin® *(Discontinued)* *see* gentamicin *on page 442*
GnRH *see* gonadorelin *on page 451*
Gold Bond® Antifungal *(Discontinued)* *see* tolnaftate *on page 934*

gold sodium thiomalate (gold SOW dee um thye oh MAL ate)
Synonyms sodium aurothiomalate
U.S./Canadian Brand Names Myochrysine® [US/Can]
Therapeutic Category Gold Compound
Use Treatment of progressive rheumatoid arthritis
Usual Dosage I.M.:
  Children: Initial: Test dose of 10 mg is recommended, followed by 1 mg/kg/week for 20 weeks; maintenance: 1 mg/kg/dose at 2- to 4-week intervals thereafter for as long as therapy is clinically beneficial and toxicity does not develop. Administration for 2-4 months is usually required before clinical improvement is observed.
  Adults: 10 mg first week; 25 mg second week; then 25-50 mg/week until 1 g cumulative dose has been given; if improvement occurs without adverse reactions, administer 25-50 mg every 2-3 weeks for 2-20 weeks, then every 3-4 weeks indefinitely
Dosage Forms
  Injection, solution:
    Myochrysine®: 50 mg/mL (1 mL, 10 mL)

GoLYTELY® [US] *see* polyethylene glycol-electrolyte solution *on page 766*

gonadorelin (goe nad oh RELL in)

Sound-Alike/Look-Alike Issues
gonadorelin may be confused with gonadotropin, guanadrel
Factrel® may be confused with Sectral®
gonadotropin may be confused with gonadorelin

Synonyms GnRH; gonadorelin acetate; gonadorelin hydrochloride; gonadotropin releasing hormone; LHRH; LRH; luteinizing hormone releasing hormone

U.S./Canadian Brand Names Factrel® [US]; Lutrepulse™ [Can]

Therapeutic Category Diagnostic Agent; Gonadotropin

Use Evaluation of functional capacity and response of gonadotrophic hormones; evaluate abnormal gonadotropin regulation as in precocious puberty and delayed puberty.
Orphan drug: Lutrepulse®: Induction of ovulation in females with hypothalamic amenorrhea

Usual Dosage
Diagnostic test: Children >12 years and Female Adults: I.V., SubQ hydrochloride salt: 100 mcg administered in women during early phase of menstrual cycle (day 1-7)
Primary hypothalamic amenorrhea: Female Adults: Acetate: I.V.: 5 mcg every 90 minutes via Lutrepulse® pump kit at treatment intervals of 21 days (pump will pulsate every 90 minutes for 7 days)

Dosage Forms
Injection, powder for reconstitution:
Factrel®: 100 mcg

gonadorelin acetate see gonadorelin on page 451
gonadorelin hydrochloride see gonadorelin on page 451
gonadotropin releasing hormone see gonadorelin on page 451
Gonak™ [US-OTC] see hydroxypropyl methylcellulose on page 490
Gonal-f® [US/Can] see follitropin alfa on page 422
Gonal-f® Pen [Can] see follitropin alfa on page 422
Gonal-f® RFF [US] see follitropin alfa on page 422
gonioscopic ophthalmic solution see hydroxypropyl methylcellulose on page 490
Goniosoft™ [US] see hydroxypropyl methylcellulose on page 490
Goniosol® (Discontinued) see hydroxypropyl methylcellulose on page 490
Good Sense Sleep Aid [US-OTC] see doxylamine on page 325
Goody's® Extra Strength Headache Powder [US-OTC] see acetaminophen, aspirin, and caffeine on page 24
Goody's® Extra Strength Pain Relief [US-OTC] see acetaminophen, aspirin, and caffeine on page 24
Goody's PM® [US-OTC] see acetaminophen and diphenhydramine on page 21
Gordofilm® [US-OTC] see salicylic acid on page 850
Gordon Boro-Packs [US-OTC] see aluminum sulfate and calcium acetate on page 55
Gormel® [US-OTC] see urea on page 963

goserelin (GOE se rel in)

Synonyms D-ser(bu^t)^6,Azgly^{10}-LHRH; goserelin acetate; ICI-118630; NSC-606864

U.S./Canadian Brand Names Zoladex® LA [Can]; Zoladex® [US/Can]

Therapeutic Category Gonadotropin-Releasing Hormone Analog

Use Palliative treatment of advanced breast cancer and carcinoma of the prostate; treatment of endometriosis, including pain relief and reduction of endometriotic lesions; endometrial thinning agent as part of treatment for dysfunctional uterine bleeding

Usual Dosage SubQ: Adults:
Prostate cancer:
Monthly implant: 3.6 mg injected into upper abdomen every 28 days
3-month implant: 10.8 mg injected into the upper abdominal wall every 12 weeks
Breast cancer, endometriosis, endometrial thinning: Monthly implant: 3.6 mg injected into upper abdomen every 28 days
Note: For breast cancer, treatment may continue indefinitely; for endometriosis, it is recommended that duration of treatment not exceed 6 months. Only 1-2 doses are recommended for endometrial thinning. ▶

◀ **Dosage Forms**
Implant, subcutaneous:
Zoladex®: 3.6 mg [1-month implant packaged with 16-gauge hypodermic needle]; 10.8 mg [3-month implant packaged with 14-gauge hypodermic needle]

goserelin acetate *see goserelin on page 451*
GP 47680 *see oxcarbazepine on page 706*
GR38032R *see ondansetron on page 698*
gramicidin, neomycin, and polymyxin B *see neomycin, polymyxin B, and gramicidin on page 663*

granisetron (gra NI se tron)

Sound-Alike/Look-Alike Issues
granisetron may be confused with dolasetron, ondansetron, palonosetron
Synonyms BRL 43694
U.S./Canadian Brand Names Granisol™ [US]; Kytril® [US/Can]
Therapeutic Category Selective 5-HT$_3$ Receptor Antagonist
Use Prophylaxis of nausea and vomiting associated with emetogenic chemotherapy and radiation therapy, (including total body irradiation and fractionated abdominal radiation); prophylaxis and treatment of postoperative nausea and vomiting (PONV)

Generally **not** recommended for treatment of existing chemotherapy-induced emesis (CIE) or for prophylaxis of nausea from agents with a low emetogenic potential.

Usual Dosage
Oral: Adults:
Prophylaxis of chemotherapy-related emesis: 2 mg once daily up to 1 hour before chemotherapy or 1 mg twice daily; the first 1 mg dose should be given up to 1 hour before chemotherapy.
Prophylaxis of radiation therapy-associated emesis: 2 mg once daily given 1 hour before radiation therapy.
I.V.:
Children ≥2 years and Adults: Prophylaxis of chemotherapy-related emesis:
Within U.S.: 10 mcg/kg/dose (maximum: 1 mg/dose) given 30 minutes prior to chemotherapy; for some drugs (eg, carboplatin, cyclophosphamide) with a later onset of emetic action, 10 mcg/kg every 12 hours may be necessary.
Outside U.S.: 40 mcg/kg/dose (or 3 mg/dose); maximum: 9 mg/24 hours
Breakthrough: Granisetron has not been shown to be effective in teminating nausea or vomiting once it occurs and should not be used for this purpose.
Adults: PONV:
Prevention: 1 mg given undiluted over 30 seconds; administer before induction of anesthesia or immediately before reversal of anesthesia
Treatment: 1 mg given undiluted over 30 seconds

Dosage Forms
Injection, solution: 1 mg/mL (1 mL, 4 mL)
Granisol™: 2 mg/10 mL (30 mL)
Kytril®: 1 mg/mL (1 mL, 4 mL)
Injection, solution [preservative free]: 0.1 mg/mL (1 mL); 1 mg/mL (1 mL)
Kytril®: 0.1 mg/mL (1 mL)
Tablet: 1 mg
Kytril®: 1 mg

Granisol™ [US] *see granisetron on page 452*
Granulex® [US] *see trypsin, balsam peru, and castor oil on page 958*
granulocyte colony-stimulating factor *see filgrastim on page 401*
granulocyte colony-stimulating factor (PEG conjugate) *see pegfilgrastim on page 727*
granulocyte-macrophage colony-stimulating factor *see sargramostim on page 857*
Gravol® [Can] *see dimenhydrinate on page 301*
green tea extract *see sinecatechins on page 868*
Grifulvin® V [US] *see griseofulvin on page 453*
Grifulvin® V Tablet 250 mg and 500 mg *(Discontinued)* *see griseofulvin on page 453*
Grisactin® Ultra *(Discontinued)* *see griseofulvin on page 453*

griseofulvin (gri see oh FUL vin)

Synonyms griseofulvin microsize; griseofulvin ultramicrosize

U.S./Canadian Brand Names Grifulvin® V [US]; Gris-PEG® [US]

Therapeutic Category Antifungal Agent

Use Treatment of susceptible tinea infections of the skin, hair, and nails

Usual Dosage Oral:
  Children >2 years:
    Microsize: 10-20 mg/kg/day in single or 2 divided doses.
    Ultramicrosize: Usual: 7.3 mg/kg/day in single dose or 2 divided doses; range: 5-15 mg/kg/day in single dose or 2 divided doses (maximum: 750 mg/day)
  Adults:
    Microsize: 500-1000 mg/day in single or divided doses
    Ultramicrosize: 375 mg/day in single or divided doses; doses up to 750 mg/day have been used for infections more difficult to eradicate such as tinea unguium and tinea pedis
  Duration of therapy depends on the site of infection:
    Tinea corporis: 2-4 weeks
    Tinea capitis: 4-6 weeks or longer (up to 8-12 weeks)
    Tinea pedis: 4-8 weeks
    Tinea unguium: 3-6 months or longer

Dosage Forms
  Suspension, oral [microsize]: 125 mg/5 mL
    Grifulvin® V: 125 mg/5 mL
  Tablet, oral [microsize]:
    Grifulvin® V: 500 mg
  Tablet, oral [ultramicrosize]:
    Gris-PEG®: 125 mg, 250 mg

griseofulvin microsize *see griseofulvin on page 453*

griseofulvin ultramicrosize *see griseofulvin on page 453*

Gris-PEG® [US] *see griseofulvin on page 453*

Guaicon DM [US-OTC] *see guaifenesin and dextromethorphan on page 454*

Guaifed® [US] *see guaifenesin and phenylephrine on page 456*

Guaifed-PD® [US] *see guaifenesin and phenylephrine on page 456*

Guaifen™ DM (Discontinued) *see guaifenesin, dextromethorphan, and phenylephrine on page 459*

guaifenesin (gwye FEN e sin)

Sound-Alike/Look-Alike Issues
  guaiFENesin may be confused with guanFACINE
  Mucinex® may be confused with Mucomyst®
  Naldecon® may be confused with Nalfon®

Synonyms GG; glycerol guaiacolate

Tall-Man guaiFENesin

U.S./Canadian Brand Names Allfen Jr [US]; Balminil Expectorant [Can]; Benylin® E Extra Strength [Can]; Diabetic Tussin® EX [US-OTC]; Fenesin IR [US]; Ganidin NR [US]; Guiatuss™ [US-OTC]; Koffex Expectorant [Can]; Mucinex® Maximum Strength [US-OTC]; Mucinex® [US-OTC]; Mucinex®, Children's Mini-Melts™ [US-OTC]; Mucinex®, Children's [US-OTC]; Mucinex®, Junior Mini-Melts™ [US-OTC]; Organidin® NR [US]; Phanasin® Diabetic Choice [US-OTC]; Phanasin® [US-OTC]; Refenesen™ 400 [US-OTC]; Refenesen™ [US-OTC]; Robitussin® [US-OTC/Can]; Scot-Tussin® Expectorant [US-OTC]; Siltussin DAS [US-OTC]; Siltussin SA [US-OTC]; Vicks® Casero™ Chest Congestion Relief [US-OTC]; XPECT™ [US-OTC]

Therapeutic Category Expectorant

Use Help loosen phlegm and thin bronchial secretions to make coughs more productive

Usual Dosage Oral:
  Children:
    6 months to 2 years: 25-50 mg every 4 hours, not to exceed 300 mg/day
    2-5 years: 50-100 mg every 4 hours, not to exceed 600 mg/day
    6-11 years: 100-200 mg every 4 hours, not to exceed 1.2 g/day
  Children >12 years and Adults: 200-400 mg every 4 hours to a maximum of 2.4 g/day
    Extended release tablet: 600-1200 mg every 12 hours, not to exceed 2.4 g/day

▶

◀ **Dosage Forms**
Caplet:
Fenesin IR, Refenesen™ 400 [OTC]: 400 mg
Granules, oral:
Mucinex® Children's Mini-Melts™ [OTC]: 50 mg/packet (12s)
Mucinex® Junior Mini-Melts™ [OTC]: 100 mg/packet (12s)
Liquid: 100 mg/5 mL
Diabetic Tussin EX® [OTC], Ganidin NR, Mucinex® Children's [OTC], Organidin® NR, Siltussin DAS [OTC]: 100 mg/5 mL
Syrup: 100 mg/5 mL
Guiatuss™ [OTC], Phanasin® [OTC], Phanasin® Diabetic Choice [OTC], Robitussin® [OTC], Scot-Tussin® Expectorant [OTC], Siltussin SA [OTC]: 100 mg/5 mL
Vicks® Casero™ [OTC]: 100 mg/6.25 mL
Tablet: 200 mg
Allfen Jr: 400 mg
Organidin® NR: 200 mg
Refenesen™ [OTC]: 200 mg
XPECT™ [OTC]: 400 mg
Tablet, extended release:
Mucinex® [OTC]: 600 mg
Mucinex® Maximum Strength [OTC]: 1200 mg

Guaifenesin AC [US] *see guaifenesin and codeine on page 454*

guaifenesin and codeine (gwye FEN e sin & KOE deen)

Synonyms codeine and guaifenesin
U.S./Canadian Brand Names Brontex® [US]; Cheracol® [US]; Diabetic Tussin C® [US]; Gani-Tuss® NR [US]; Guaifenesin AC [US]; Guaituss AC [US]; Kolephrin® #1 [US]; Mytussin® AC [US]; Robafen® AC [US]; Romilar® AC [US]; Tussi-Organidin® NR [US]; Tussi-Organidin® S-NR [US]; Tusso-C™ [US]
Therapeutic Category Antitussive/Expectorant
Controlled Substance C-V
Use Temporary control of cough due to minor throat and bronchial irritation
Usual Dosage Oral: **Note:** Also refer to specific product labeling:
Children:
2-6 years (Diabetic Tussin C® liquid, Tussi-Organidin® NR): Codeine 1 mg/kg/day in 4 divided doses
6-12 years (Diabetic Tussin C®, Kolephrin® #1, Romilar® AC, Tussi-Organidin® NR liquid): 5 mL every 4 hours; maximum 30 mL/24 hours
Children ≥12 years and Adults:
Brontex® tablets: 1 tablet every 4 hours; maximum 6 tablets/24 hours
Diabetic Tussin C®, Kolephrin® #1, Romilar® AC, Tussi-Organidin® NR liquid: 10 mL every 4 hours; maximum 60 mL/24 hours
Dosage Forms
Liquid: Guaifenesin 300 mg and codeine 10 mg per 5 mL
Brontex®: Guaifenesin 75 mg and codeine 2.5 mg per 5 mL
Diabetic Tussin C®, Tusso-C™: Guaifenesin 200 mg and codeine 10 mg per 5 mL
Gani-Tuss® NR, Guaifenesin AC, Kolephrin® #1: Guaifenesin 100 mg and codeine 10 mg per 5 mL
Tussi-Organidin® NR, Tussi-Organidin® S-NR: Guaifenesin 300 mg and codeine 10 mg per 5 mL
Syrup:
Cheracol®, Guaituss AC, Mytussin® AC, Robafen® AC, Romilar® AC: Guaifenesin 100 mg and codeine 10 mg per 5 mL
Tablet: Guaifenesin 300 mg and codeine 10 mg
Brontex®: Guaifenesin 300 mg and codeine 10 mg

guaifenesin and dextromethorphan (gwye FEN e sin & deks troe meth OR fan)

Sound-Alike/Look-Alike Issues
Benylin® may be confused with Benadryl®, Ventolin®
Synonyms dextromethorphan and guaifenesin
U.S./Canadian Brand Names Allfen-DM [US]; Altarussin DM [US-OTC]; Balminil DM E [Can]; Benylin® DM-E [Can]; Cheracol® D [US-OTC]; Cheracol® Plus [US-OTC]; Coricidin HBP® Chest Congestion and Cough [US-OTC]; Diabetic Tussin® DM Maximum Strength [US-OTC]; Diabetic Tussin® DM [US-OTC]; Double Tussin DM [US-OTC]; Duratuss® DM [US]; Fenesin DM IR [US]; Gani-Tuss DM NR [US];

Genatuss DM® [US-OTC]; Guaicon DM [US-OTC]; Guia-D [US]; Guiacon DMS [US-OTC]; Guiatuss-DM® [US-OTC]; Hydro-Tussin™ DM [US]; Koffex DM-Expectorant [Can]; Kolephrin® GG/DM [US-OTC]; Mintab DM [US]; Mucinex® Children's Cough [US-OTC]; Mucinex® DM Maximum Strength [US-OTC]; Mucinex® DM [US-OTC]; Phanatuss® DM [US-OTC]; Phlemex [US]; Refenesen™ DM [US-OTC]; Respa-DM® [US]; Robafen DM Clear [US-OTC]; Robafen DM [US-OTC]; Robitussin® Cough and Congestion [US-OTC]; Robitussin® DM [US-OTC/Can]; Robitussin® Sugar Free Cough [US-OTC]; Safe Tussin® DM [US-OTC]; Scot-Tussin® Senior [US-OTC]; Silexin [US-OTC]; Siltussin DM DAS [US-OTC]; Siltussin DM [US-OTC]; Simuc-DM [US]; Su-Tuss DM [US]; Touro® DM [US]; Tussi-Organidin® DM NR [US]; Tussi-Organidin® DM-S NR [US]; Vicks® 44E [US-OTC]; Vicks® Pediatric Formula 44E [US-OTC]; Z-Cof LA™ [US]

Therapeutic Category Antitussive/Expectorant

Use Temporary control of cough due to minor throat and bronchial irritation

Usual Dosage Oral:

Children 2-6 years:
General dosing guidelines: Guaifenesin 50-100 mg and dextromethorphan 2.5-5 mg every 4 hours (maximum dose: Guaifenesin 600 mg and dextromethorphan 30 mg per day)
Product-specific labeling:
Touro® DM: 1/2 tablet every 12 hours (maximum: 1 tablet/24 hour)
Robitussin® DM, Robitussin® Sugar Free Cough: 2.5 mL every 4 hours (maximum: 6 doses/24 hours)
Vicks® Pediatric Formula 44E: 7.5 mL every 4 hours (maximum: 6 doses/24 hours)

Children: 6-12 years:
General dosing guidelines: Guaifenesin 100-200 mg and dextromethorphan 5-10 mg every 4 hours (maximum dose: Guaifenesin 1200 mg and dextromethorphan 60 mg per day)
Product-specific labeling:
Touro® DM: 1 tablet every 12 hours (maximum: 2 tablets/24 hours)
Robitussin® DM, Robitussin® Sugar Free Cough: 5 mL every 4 hours (maximum: 6 doses/24 hours)
Vicks® 44E: 7.5 mL every 4 hours (maximum: 6 doses/24 hours)
Vicks® Pediatric Formula 44E: 15 mL every 4 hours (maximum: 6 doses/24 hours)
Z-Cof LA™: 1/2 tablet very 12 hours

Children ≥12 years and Adults:
General dosing guidelines: Guaifenesin 200-400 mg and dextromethorphan 10-20 mg every 4 hours (maximum dose: Guaifenesin 2400 mg and dextromethorphan 120 mg per day)
Product-specific labeling:
Mucinex® DM, Touro® DM: 1-2 tablets every 12 hours (maximum: 4 tablets/24 hours)
Robitussin® DM, Robitussin® Sugar Free Cough: 10 mL every 4 hours (maximum: 6 doses/24 hours)
Vicks® 44E: 15 mL every 4 hours (maximum: 6 doses/24 hours)
Vicks® Pediatric Formula 44E: 30 mL every 4 hours (maximum: 6 doses/24 hours)
Z-Cof LA™: 1 tablet every 12 hours

Dosage Forms

Caplet:
Fenesin DM IR: Guaifenesin 400 mg and dextromethorphan 15 mg
Refenesen™ DM [OTC]: Guaifenesin 400 mg and dextromethorphan 20 mg

Capsule, softgel:
Coricidin HBP® Chest Congestion and Cough [OTC]: Guaifenesin 200 mg and dextromethorphan 10 mg

Elixir:
Duratuss DM®, Simuc-DM: Guaifenesin 225 mg and dextromethorphan 25 mg per 5 mL
Su-Tuss DM: Guaifenesin 200 mg and dextromethorphan 20 mg per 5 mL
Liquid: Guaifenesin 100 mg and dextromethorphan 10 mg per 5 mL; guaifenesin 300 mg and dextromethorphan 10 mg per 5 mL
Diabetic Tussin® DM [OTC], Gani-Tuss® DM NR: Guaifenesin 100 mg and dextromethorphan 10 mg per 5 mL
Diabetic Tussin® DM Maximum Strength [OTC]: Guaifenesin 200 mg and dextromethorphan 10 mg per 5 mL
Double Tussin DM [OTC]: Guaifenesin 300 mg and dextromethorphan 200 mg per 5 mL
Hydro-Tussin™ DM: Guaifenesin 200 mg and dextromethorphan 20 mg per 5 mL
Kolephrin® GG/DM [OTC]: Guaifenesin 150 mg and dextromethorphan 10 mg per 5 mL
Mucinex® Children's Cough [OTC]: Guaifenesin 100 mg and dextromethorphan 5 mg per 5 mL
Safe Tussin® DM [OTC]: Guaifenesin 100 mg and dextromethorphan 15 mg per 5 mL
Scot-Tussin® Senior [OTC]: Guaifenesin 200 mg and dextromethorphan 15 mg per 5 mL
Tussi-Organidin® DM NR: Guaifenesin 300 mg and dextromethorphan 10 mg per 5 mL
Tussi-Organidin® DM-S NR: Guaifenesin 300 mg and dextromethorphan 10 mg per 5 mL

▶

Vicks® 44E [OTC]: Guaifenesin 200 mg and dextromethorphan hydrobromide 20 mg per 15 mL
Vicks® Pediatric Formula 44E [OTC]: Guaifenesin 100 mg and dextromethorphan hydrobromide 10 mg per 15 mL
Syrup: Guaifenesin 100 mg and dextromethorphan 10 mg per 5 mL
Altarussin DM [OTC], Cheracol® D [OTC], Cheracol® Plus [OTC], Genatuss DM® [OTC], Guiatuss® DM [OTC], Guaicon DM [OTC], Guaicon DMS [OTC], Phanatuss® DM [OTC], Robafen® DM [OTC], Robafen DM Clear [OTC], Robitussin® Cough and Congestion [OTC], Robitussin®-DM [OTC], Robitussin® Sugar Free Cough [OTC], Silexin [OTC], Siltussin DM [OTC], Siltussin DM DAS [OTC]: Guaifenesin 100 mg and dextromethorphan 10 mg per 5 mL
Mintab DM: Guaifenesin 200 mg and dextromethorphan hydrobromide 10 mg per 5 mL
Tablet: Guaifenesin 1000 mg and dextromethorphan hydrobromide 60 mg; guaifenesin 1200 mg and dextromethorphan hydrobromide 60 mg
Silexin: Guaifenesin 100 mg and dextromethorphan hydrobromide 10 mg
Tablet, extended release: 800/30: Guaifenesin 800 mg and dextromethorphan 30 mg; 1200/20: Guaifenesin 1200 mg and dextromethorphan 20 mg
Mucinex® DM [OTC], Respa-DM®: Guaifenesin 600 mg and dextromethorphan 30 mg
Mucophen® DM: Guaifenesin 1000 mg and dextromethorphan 60 mg
Mucinex® DM Maximum Strength: Guaifenesin 1200 mg and dextromethorphan 60 mg
Phlemex: Guaifenesin 1200 mg and dextromethorphan 20 mg
Touro® DM: Guaifenesin 575 mg and dextromethorphan 30 mg
Tablet, long-acting: Guaifenesin 1000 mg and dextromethorphan 60 mg
Z-Cof LA [scored]: Guaifenesin 650 mg and dextromethorphan 30 mg
Tablet, sustained release:
Allfen-DM: Guaifenesin 1000 mg and dextromethorphan 55 mg
Relacon LAX: Guaifenesin 835 mg and dextromethorphan 30 mg
Tussi-Bid®: Guaifenesin 1200 mg and dextromethorphan 60 mg
Tablet, timed release [scored]: Guaifenesin 1200 mg and dextromethorphan 60 mg
Guia-D: Guaifenesin 1000 mg and dextromethorphan 60 mg

guaifenesin and dyphylline *see* dyphylline and guaifenesin *on page 330*

guaifenesin and phenylephrine (gwye FEN e sin & fen il EF rin)

Sound-Alike/Look-Alike Issues
Entex® may be confused with Tenex®
Entex® LA brand name represents a different product in the U.S. than it does in Canada. In the U.S., Entex® LA contains guaifenesin and phenylephrine, while in Canada the product bearing this brand name contains guaifenesin and pseudoephedrine.
Synonyms guaifenesin and phenylephrine tannate; phenylephrine hydrochloride and guaifenesin
U.S./Canadian Brand Names Aldex™ [US]; Crantex LA [US]; D-Phen 1000 [US]; Deconsal® II [US]; Donatussin Drops [US]; Duomax [US]; Duratuss GP® [US]; Duratuss® [US]; ExeFen-PD [US]; ExeTuss-GP [US]; Fenesin PE IR [US]; Gilphex TR® [US]; Guaifed-PD® [US]; Guaifed® [US]; Guaiphen-D 1200 [US]; Guaiphen-D [US]; Guaiphen-PD [US]; Liquibid-D® [US]; MyDex [US]; Nasex-G [US]; Nexphen PD [US]; norel® EX [US]; Pendex [US]; Refenesen™ PE [US-OTC]; Rescon GG [US-OTC]; Sil-Tex [US]; Sina-12X [US]; SINUvent® PE [US]
Therapeutic Category Cold Preparation
Use Temporary relief of nasal congestion, sinusitis, rhinitis, and hay fever; temporary relief of cough associated with upper respiratory tract conditions, especially when associated with dry, nonproductive cough
Usual Dosage Oral:
Children 3-6 months (Donatussin): 0.3-0.6 mL; may repeat every 4-6 hours as needed; maximum 4 doses/24 hours
Children 6 months to 1 year (Donatussin): 0.6-1 mL; may repeat every 4-6 hours as needed; maximum: 4 doses/24 hours
Children 1-2 years (Donatussin): 1-2 mL; may repeat every 4-6 hours as needed; maximum: 4 doses/24 hours
Children 2-6 years:
Rescon GG, Sil-Tex: 2.5 mL every 4-6 hours; maximum: 10 mL/24 hours
Sina-12X suspension: 2.5-5 mL every 12 hours
Children 6-12 years:
Aldex™, Crantex LA, Duomax, Liquibid-D®, Sina-12X tablet: One-half tablet every 12 hours; maximum: 1 tablet/24 hours
Deconsal® II: One capsule daily

Rescon GG: 5 mL every 4-6 hours; maximum: 20 mL/24 hours
ExeFen-PD: One-half to 1 tablet every 12 hours
Guaifed-PD®: One capsule every 12 hours
SINUvent® PE: One tablet every 12 hours; maximum: 2 tablets/24 hours
Sina-12X suspension: Refer to adult dosing.
Children ≥12 years:
  Aldex™, Crantex LA, Deconsal® II, Duomax, ExeFen-PD, ExeTuss-GP, Guaifed®, Guaifed-PD®,
  Liquibid-D®, Rescon GG, Sil-Tex, Sina-12X, SINUvent® PE: Refer to adult dosing
Adults:
  Aldex™, Crantex LA, Duomax, ExeTuss-GP, Liquibid-D®: One tablet every 12 hours
  Deconsal® II: 1-2 capsules every 12 hours; maximum: 3 capsules/24 hours
  Sil-Tex: 5-10 mL every 4-6 hours; maximum: 40 mL/24 hours
  Guaifed-PD®: 1-2 capsules every 12 hours
  Guaifed®: One capsule every 12 hours; maximum: 2 capsules/24 hours
  ExeFen-PD: 1-2 tablets every 12 hours
  SINUvent® PE: Two tablets every 12 hours
  Rescon GG: 10 mL every 4-6 hours; maximum: 40 mL/24 hours
  Sina-12X suspension: 5-10 mL every 12 hours
  Sina-12X tablet: 1-2 tablets every 12 hours; maximum: 4 tablets/24 hours

Dosage Forms

Caplet:
  Fenesin PE IR, Refenesen™ PE [OTC]: Guaifenesin 400 mg and phenylephrine 10 mg
Capsule:
  Nexphen PD: Guaifenesin 200 mg and phenylephrine hydrochloride 7 mg
Capsule, variable release:
  Deconsal® II: Guaifenesin 375 mg [immediate release] and phenylephrine 20 mg [extended release]
  Guaifed®: Guaifenesin 400 mg [immediate release] and phenylephrine 15 mg [extended release]
  Guaifed-PD®: Guaifenesin 200 mg [immediate release] and phenylephrine 7.5 mg [extended release]
Liquid: Guaifenesin 100 mg and phenylephrine 7.5 mg per 5 mL
  Rescon GG [OTC]: Guaifenesin 100 mg and phenylephrine 5 mg per 5 mL
  Sil-Tex: Guaifenesin 100 mg and phenylephrine 7.5 mg per 5 mL
Liquid [drops]:
  Donatussin: Guaifenesin 20 mg and phenylephrine hydrochloride 1.5 mg
Suspension:
  Sina-12X: Guaifenesin 100 mg and phenylephrine 5 mg per 5 mL
Tablet: Guaifenesin 900 mg and phenylephrine 30 mg
  Sina-12X: Guaifenesin 200 mg and phenylephrine 25 mg
Tablet, extended release: Guaifenesin 600 mg and phenylephrine 20 mg; guaifenesin 600 mg and
  phenylephrine 40 mg; guaifenesin 1200 mg and phenylephrine 40 mg
  Aldex™: Guaifenesin 650 mg and phenylephrine 25 mg
  D-Phen: Guaifenesin 1000 mg and phenylephrine 30 mg
  ExeFen-PD: Guaifenesin 600 mg and phenylephrine 10 mg
  SINUvent® PE: Guaifenesin 600 mg and phenylephrine 15 mg
Tablet, long acting: Guaifenesin 900 mg and phenylephrine 25 mg; guaifenesin 1200 mg and
  phenylephrine hydrochloride 25 mg
Tablet, prolonged release: Guaifenesin 600 mg and phenylephrine 15 mg
Tablet, sustained release: Guaifenesin 600 mg and phenylephrine 30 mg; guaifenesin 1200 mg and
  phenylephrine 30 mg
  Crantex LA: Guaifenesin 600 mg and phenylephrine 30 mg
  Duratuss®: Guaifenesin 1200 mg and phenylephrine 25 mg
  Duratuss GP®, ExeTuss-GP: Guaifenesin 1200 mg and phenylephrine hydrochloride 25 mg
  MyDex: Guaifenesin 900 mg and phenylephrine hydrochloride 30 mg
  Nasex-G: Guaifenesin 835 mg and phenylephrine hydrochloride 25 mg
  Pendex, Prolex®-PD: Guaifenesin 600 mg and phenylephrine hydrochloride 10 mg
Tablet, timed release:
  Gilphex TR®: Guaifenesin 600 mg and phenylephrine hydrochloride 25 mg [sugar free, dye free;
  scored]
  Guaiphen-D: Guaifenesin 600 mg and phenylephrine hydrochloride 40 mg
  Guaiphen-D 1200: Guaifenesin 1200 mg and phenylephrine hydrochloride 40 mg
  Guaiphen-PD: Guaifenesin 275 mg and phenylephrine hydrochloride 25 mg

◀ **Tablet, variable release:**
Liquibid-D®: Guaifenesin 400 mg and phenylephrine 10 mg [immediate release] and guaifenesin 800 mg and phenylephrine 30 mg [sustained release]
norel® EX: Guaifenesin 400 mg [immediate release] and guaifenesin 400 mg and phenylephrine hydrochloride 40 mg [extended release]

guaifenesin and phenylephrine tannate *see* guaifenesin and phenylephrine *on page 456*
guaifenesin and potassium guaiacolsulfonate *(Discontinued)*

guaifenesin and pseudoephedrine (gwye FEN e sin & soo doe e FED rin)

Sound-Alike/Look-Alike Issues
Entex® may be confused with Tenex®
Entex® LA brand name represents a different product in the U.S. than it does in Canada. In the U.S., Entex® LA contains guaifenesin and phenylephrine, while in Canada the product bearing this brand name contains guaifenesin and pseudoephedrine.
Profen II® may be confused with Profen II DM®, Profen Forte®, Profen Forte™ DM

Synonyms pseudoephedrine and guaifenesin

U.S./Canadian Brand Names Ambifed-G [US]; Congestac® [US-OTC]; Contac® Cold-Chest Congestion, Non Drowsy, Regular Strength [Can]; Entex® LA [Can]; Entex® PSE [US]; Eudal®-SR [US]; ExeFen [US]; Guaimax-D® [US]; Levall G [US]; Maxifed-G® [US]; Maxifed® [US]; Medent LD [US]; Mucinex® D Maximum Strength [US-OTC]; Mucinex®-D [US-OTC]; Nasatab® LA [US]; Novahistex® Expectorant with Decongestant [Can]; Pseudo GG TR [US]; Pseudo Max [US]; Refenesen Plus [US-OTC]; Respa®-1st [US]; Rutuss Jr [US]; Sinutab® Non-Drying [US-OTC]; SudaTex-G [US]; Touro LA® [US]

Therapeutic Category Expectorant/Decongestant

Use Temporary relief of nasal congestion and to help loosen phlegm and thin bronchial secretions in the treatment of cough

Usual Dosage Oral:
Children 2-6 years: Maxifed-G®: One-third to 1/2 tablet every 12 hours (maximum: 1 tablet/12 hours)
Children 6-12 years:
Ambifed-G, Eudal®-SR, Guaimax-D®, Maxifed®, Nasatab® LA: One-half caplet or tablet every 12 hours (maximum: 1 tablet/24 hours)
Congestac®: One-half caplet every 4-6 hours (maximum: 2 caplets/24 hours)
Levall G: One capsule every 24 hours
Maxifed-G®: One-half to 1 tablet every 12 hours (maximum: 2 tablets/24 hours)
Children >12 years and Adults:
Ambifed-G, Entex® PSE, Eudal®- SR, Guaimax-D®, Levall G, Mucinex® D 1200/120, Nasatab® LA, Touro LA®: One tablet or capsule every 12 hours (maximum: 2 tablets or capsules in 24 hours)
Congestac®: One caplet every 4-6 hours (maximum: 4 caplets in 24 hours)
Maxifed-G®, Mucinex® D 600/60: 1-2 tablets or capsules every 12 hours (maximum: 4 tablets or capsules/24 hours)
Maxifed®: One to 11/2 tablets every 12 hours (maximum: 3 tablets/24 hours)

Dosage Forms
Caplet:
Congestac® [OTC], Refenesen Plus [OTC]: Guaifenesin 400 mg and pseudoephedrine 60 mg
Caplet, long-acting:
Touro LA®: Guaifenesin 500 mg and pseudoephedrine 120 mg
Caplet, prolonged release:
Ambifed-G: Guaifenesin 1000 mg and pseudoephedrine 60 mg
Capsule, liquicap:
Sinutab® Non-Drying [OTC]: Guaifenesin 200 mg and pseudoephedrine 30 mg
Capsule, variable release:
Entex® PSE: Guaifenesin 400 mg [immediate release] and pseudoephedrine 120 mg [extended release]
Levall G: Guaifenesin 400 mg [immediate release] and pseudoephedrine 90 mg [extended release]
Syrup: Guaifenesin 200 mg and pseudoephedrine 40 mg per 5 mL
Tablet:
ExeFen: Guaifenesin 780 mg and pseudoephedrine 80 mg
Rutuss Jr: 600/45: Guaifenesin 600 mg and pseudoephedrine 45 mg
Tablet, extended release:
Mucinex® D Maximum Strength [OTC]: Guaifenesin 1200 mg and pseudoephedrine 120 mg

Guaimax-D®: Guaifenesin 600 mg and pseudoephedrine 120 mg
Maxifed®: Guaifenesin 780 mg and pseudoephedrine 80 mg
Maxifed-G®: Guaifenesin 580 mg and pseudoephedrine 60 mg
Mucinex®-D [OTC] 600/60: Guaifenesin 600 mg and pseudoephedrine 60 mg
Pseudo Max: Guaifenesin 700 mg and pseudoephedrine 80 mg
Tablet, long acting:
Medent LD: Guaifenesin 800 mg and pseudoephedrine 60 mg
Tablet, sustained release:
Nasatab® LA: Guaifenesin 500 mg and pseudoephedrine 120 mg
Respa®-1st: Guaifenesin 600 mg and pseudoephedrine 58 mg
SudaTex-G: Guaifenesin 580 mg and pseudoephedrine 60 mg

guaifenesin and theophylline *see* theophylline and guaifenesin *on page 919*
guaifenesin, carbetapentane citrate, and phenylephrine hydrochloride *see* carbetapentane, guaifenesin, and phenylephrine *on page 175*
guaifenesin, chlorpheniramine, phenylephrine, and dextromethorphan *see* dextromethorphan, chlorpheniramine, phenylephrine, and guaifenesin *on page 285*

guaifenesin, dextromethorphan, and phenylephrine
(gwye FEN e sin, deks troe meth OR fan, & fen il EF rin)

Synonyms guaifenesin, dextromethorphan hydrobromide, and phenylephrine hydrochloride; phenylephrine hydrochloride, guaifenesin, and dextromethorphan hydrobromide

U.S./Canadian Brand Names Anextuss [US]; Certuss-D® [US]; Dacex-DM [US]; Dexcon-PE [US]; Duraphen™ Forte [US]; Duraphen™ II DM [US]; Dynatuss-EX [US]; ExeCof [US]; ExeTuss-DM [US]; Giltuss Pediatric® [US]; Giltuss TR® [US]; Giltuss® [US]; Maxiphen DM [US]; Robitussin® Cold and Cough CF [US-OTC]; Robitussin® Pediatric Cold and Cough CF [US-OTC]; SINUtuss® DM [US]; TriTuss® ER [US]; TriTuss® [US]; Tusso™-DMR [US]

Therapeutic Category Antitussive; Decongestant

Use Symptomatic relief of dry nonproductive coughs and upper respiratory symptoms associated with hay fever, colds, or the flu

Usual Dosage
Also refer to specific product labeling.
Oral:
Children 6-12 years (Certuss-D®, Duraphen™ Forte, Duraphen™ II DM, Maxiphen DM): One-half tablet every 12 hours, not to exceed 1 tablet/24 hours
Children ≥12 years and Adults:
Certuss-D®, Duraphen™ Forte, Maxiphen DM: One tablet every 12 hours, not to exceed 2 tablets/24 hours
Duraphen™ II DM: 1-1¹/₂ tablets twice daily, not to exceed 3 tablets/24 hours

Dosage Forms
Caplet:
Dexcon-PE: Guaifenesin 550 mg, dextromethorphan 25 mg, and phenylephrine 20 mg
Caplet, extended release:
TriTuss®-ER: Guaifenesin 600 mg, dextromethorphan 30 mg, and phenylephrine 10 mg
Capsule:
Tusso™-DMR: Guaifenesin 288 mg, dextromethorphan 14 mg, and phenylephrine 7 mg
Liquid:
Giltuss®: Guaifenesin 300 mg, dextromethorphan 15 mg, and phenylephrine 10 mg per 5 mL
Giltuss Pediatric®: Guaifenesin 50 mg, dextromethorphan 5 mg, and phenylephrine 2.5 mg per mL
Liquid, oral [drops]: Guaifenesin 50 mg, dextromethorphan 5 mg, and phenylephrine 2.5 mg per mL
Robitussin® Pediatric Cold and Cough CF: Guaifenesin 100 mg, dextromethorphan 5 mg, and phenylephrine 2.5 mg per 2.5 mL
Syrup: Guaifenesin 200 mg, dextromethorphan 30 mg, and phenylephrine 10 mg
Dacex-DM, TriTuss®: Guaifenesin 175 mg, dextromethorphan 25 mg, and phenylephrine 12.5 mg per 5 mL
Dynatuss-Ex: Guaifenesin 200 mg, dextromethorphan 30 mg, and phenylephrine 10 mg (473 mL)
Robitussin® Cold and Cough CF: Guaifenesin 100 mg, dextromethorphan 10 mg, and phenylephrine 5 mg per 5 mL
Tablet [scored]:
SINUtuss™ DM: Guaifenesin 600 mg, dextromethorphan hydrobromide 30 mg, and phenylephrine hydrochloride 15 mg

Tablet, extended release [scored]:
Duraphen™ II DM: Guaifenesin 800 mg, dextromethorphan 20 mg, and phenylephrine 20 mg
Duraphen™ Forte: Guaifenesin 1200 mg, dextromethorphan 30 mg, and phenylephrine 30 mg
Tablet, prolonged release [scored]:
Maxiphen DM: Guaifenesin 1000 mg, dextromethorphan 60 mg, and phenylephrine 40 mg
Tablet, sustained release: Guaifenesin 1200 mg, dextromethorphan 20 mg, and phenylephrine 40 mg
Anextuss: Guaifenesin 600 mg, dextromethorphan 60 mg, and phenylephrine 40 mg
Certuss-D® [scored]: Guaifenesin 600 mg, dextromethorphan 60 mg, and phenylephrine 40 mg
ExeCof: Guaifenesin 100 mg, dextromethorphan 60 mg, and phenylephrine 40 mg
ExeTuss-DM: Guaifenesin 600 mg, dextromethorphan 25 mg, and phenylephrine 20 mg
Tablet, timed release [scored]:
Giltuss TR®: Guaifenesin 600 mg, dextromethorphan 30 mg, and phenylephrine 20 mg

guaifenesin, dextromethorphan hydrobromide, and phenylephrine hydrochloride *see* guaifenesin, dextromethorphan, and phenylephrine *on page 459*

guaifenesin, dihydrocodeine, and pseudoephedrine *see* dihydrocodeine, pseudoephedrine, and guaifenesin *on page 299*

guaifenesin, phenylephrine, and chlorpheniramine *see* chlorpheniramine, phenylephrine, and guaifenesin *on page 210*

guaifenesin, pseudoephedrine, and codeine
(gwye FEN e sin, soo doe e FED rin, & KOE deen)
Synonyms codeine, guaifenesin, and pseudoephedrine; pseudoephedrine, guaifenesin, and codeine
U.S./Canadian Brand Names Benylin® 3.3 mg-D-E [Can]; Calmylin with Codeine [Can]; Guiatuss DAC [US]; Mytussin® DAC [US]
Therapeutic Category Antitussive/Decongestant/Expectorant
Controlled Substance C-III; C-V
Use Temporarily relieves nasal congestion and controls cough associated with upper respiratory infections and related conditions (common cold, sinusitis, bronchitis, influenza)
Usual Dosage Oral:
Children 6-12 years (Guiatuss DAC): 5 mL every 4 hours (maximum: 20 mL/24 hours)
Children >12 years and Adults (Guiatuss DAC): 10 mL every 4 hours (maximum: 40 mL/24 hours)
Dosage Forms
Syrup: Guaifenesin 100 mg, pseudoephedrine 30 mg, and codeine 10 mg per 5 mL; guaifenesin 200 mg, pseudoephedrine 60 mg, and codeine 20 mg per 5 mL
Guiatuss DAC, Mytussin® DAC: Guaifenesin 100 mg, pseudoephedrine 30 mg, and codeine 10 mg per 5 mL

guaifenesin, pseudoephedrine, and dextromethorphan
(gwye FEN e sin, soo doe e FED rin, & deks troe meth OR fan)
Sound-Alike/Look-Alike Issues
Profen II DM® may be confused with Profen II®, Profen Forte®, Profen Forte™ DM
Profen Forte™ DM may be confused with Profen II®, Profen II DM®, Profen Forte®
Synonyms dextromethorphan, guaifenesin, and pseudoephedrine; pseudoephedrine, dextromethorphan, and guaifenesin
U.S./Canadian Brand Names Ambifed-G DM [US]; Balminil DM + Decongestant + Expectorant [Can]; Benylin® DM-D-E [Can]; ExeFen-DMX [US]; Koffex DM + Decongestant + Expectorant [Can]; Maxifed DM [US]; Maxifed DMX [US]; Medent-DM [US]; Novahistex® DM Decongestant Expectorant [Can]; Novahistine® DM Decongestant Expectorant [Can]; Profen Forte™ DM [US]; Profen II DM® [US]; Pseudo Max DMX [US]; Relacon-DM NR [US]; Robitussin® Cough and Cold CF [US-OTC]; Robitussin® Cough and Cold Infant CF [US-OTC]; Robitussin® Cough and Cold [US-OTC/Can]; Ru-Tuss DM [US]; SudaTex-DM [US]; Touro® CC [US]; Touro® CC-LD [US]; Tusnel Liquid® [US]; Tusnel Pediatric® [US]; Tusnel-DM Pediatric® [US]; Z-Cof™ 12DM [US]
Therapeutic Category Cold Preparation
Use Temporarily relieves nasal congestion and controls cough due to minor throat and bronchial irritation; helps loosen phlegm and thin bronchial secretions to make coughs more productive
Usual Dosage Note: Also refer to specific product labeling.
Children 2-6 years:
Maxifed DM: 1/3 to 1/2 tablet every 12 hours, not to exceed 1 tablet/24 hours
Profen II DM® (syrup): 1.25-2.5 mL every 4 hours, not to exceed 15 mL/24 hours
Robitussin® Cough and Cold Infant CF: 2.5 mL every 4-6 hours, not to exceed 4 doses/24 hours

Touro® CC: ½ tablet every 12 hour, not to exceed 1 tablet/24 hours
Z-Cof™ 12DM: 2.5 mL 2-3 times/day, not to exceed 7.5 mL/24 hours

Children 6-12 years:
Ambifed-G DM, Profen Forte™ DM, Profen II DM®: ½ tablet every 12 hours not to exceed 1 tablet/24 hours
Maxifed DM: ½ to 1 tablet every 12 hours, not to exceed 2 tablets/24 hours
Touro® CC: 1 tablet every 12 hours, not to exceed 2 tablets/24 hours
Profen II DM® (syrup): 2.5-5 mL every 4 hours, not to exceed 30 mL/24 hours
Z-Cof™ 12DM: 5 mL 2-3 times/day, not to exceed 15 mL/24 hours

Children ≥12 years and Adults:
Ambifed-G DM, Profen Forte™ DM: 1 tablet every 12 hours not to exceed 2 tablets/24 hours
Maxifed DM, Touro® CC: 1-2 tablets every 12 hours, not to exceed 4 tablets/24 hours
Profen II DM® (tablet): 1 to 1½ tablets every 12 hours, not to exceed 3 tablets/24 hours
Profen II DM® (syrup): 5-10 mL every 4 hours, not to exceed 60 mL/24 hours
Z-Cof™ 12DM: 10 mL 2-3 times/day, not to exceed 30 mL/24 hours

Dosage Forms

Caplet, prolonged release:
Ambifed-G DM: Guaifenesin 1000 mg, pseudoephedrine 60 mg, and dextromethorphan 30 mg

Caplet, sustained release:
Touro® CC: Guaifenesin 575 mg, pseudoephedrine 60 mg, and dextromethorphan 30 mg
Touro® CC-LD: Guaifenesin 575 mg, pseudoephedrine 25 mg, and dextromethorphan 30 mg

Capsule, softgel:
Robitussin® Cough and Cold [OTC]: Guaifenesin 200 mg, pseudoephedrine 30 mg, and dextromethorphan 10 mg

Liquid: Guaifenesin 100 mg, pseudoephedrine 30 mg, and dextromethorphan 10 mg per 5 mL
Profen II DM®: Guaifenesin 200 mg, pseudoephedrine 15 mg, and dextromethorphan 10 mg per 5 mL
Relacon-DM NR, Z-Cof™ DM: Guaifenesin 200 mg, pseudoephedrine 40 mg, and dextromethorphan 15 mg
Tusnel Liquid®: Guaifenesin 200 mg, pseudoephedrine 30 mg, and dextromethorphan 15 mg per 5 mL
Tusnel Pediatric®: Guaifenesin 50 mg, pseudoephedrine 15 mg, and dextromethorphan 5 mg per 5 mL

Liquid, oral [drops]:
Robitussin® Cough and Cold Infant CF [OTC]: Guaifenesin 100 mg, pseudoephedrine 15 mg, and dextromethorphan 5 mg per 2.5 mL
Tusnel-DM Pediatric®: Guaifenesin 25 mg, pseudoephedrine 5 mg, and dextromethorphan 5 mg per 1 mL

Suspension:
Z-Cof™ 12DM: Guaifenesin 175 mg, pseudoephedrine 30 mg, and dextromethorphan 15 mg per 5 mL

Syrup: Guaifenesin 100 mg, pseudoephedrine 45 mg, and dextromethorphan 15 mg per 5 mL
Robitussin® Cough and Cold CF [OTC]: Guaifenesin 100 mg, pseudoephedrine 30 mg, and dextromethorphan 10 mg per 5 mL
Ru-Tuss DM: Guaifenesin 100 mg, pseudoephedrine 45 mg, and dextromethorphan 15 mg per 5 mL

Tablet, extended release: Guaifenesin 100 mg, pseudoephedrine hydrochloride 30 mg, and dextromethorphan hydrobromide 10 mg; guaifenesin 800 mg, pseudoephedrine 60 mg, and dextromethorphan30 mg; guaifenesin 1200 mg, pseudoephedrine 60 mg, and dextromethorphan 60 mg; guaifenesin 1200 mg, pseudoephedrine 120 mg, and dextromethorphan 60 mg; guaifenesin 800 mg, pseudoephedrine90 mg, and dextromethorphan 60 mg; guaifenesin 550 mg, pseudoephedrine 60 mg, and dextromethorphan 30 mg; guaifenesin 595 mg, pseudoephedrine 48 mg, and dextromethorphan 32 mg; guaifenesin 600 mg, pseudoephedrine 60 mg, and dextromethorphan 30 mg
Profen Forte™ DM: Guaifenesin 800 mg, pseudoephedrine 90 mg, and dextromethorphan 60 mg
Profen II DM®: Guaifenesin 800 mg, pseudoephedrine 45 mg, and dextromethorphan 30 mg

Tablet, long acting: Guaifenesin 800 mg, pseudoephedrine 60 mg, and dextromethorphan 30 mg
Medent-DM: Guaifenesin 800 mg, pseudoephedrine 60 mg, and dextromethorphan 30 mg

Tablet, sustained release:
ExeFen-DMX, Maxifed DM: Guaifenesin 780 mg, pseudoephedrine 80 mg, and dextromethorphan 40 mg
Maxifed DM, SudaTex-DM: Guaifenesin 580 mg, pseudoephedrine 60 mg, and dextromethorphan 30 mg
Pseudo Max DMX: Guaifenesin 700 mg, pseudoephedrine 80 mg, and dextromethorphan 40 mg

Guaifenex® (Discontinued)
Guaifenex® DM (Discontinued) see guaifenesin and dextromethorphan *on page 454*

Guaifenex® GP *(Discontinued)* see guaifenesin and pseudoephedrine *on page 458*
Guaifenex® PPA 75 *(Discontinued)*
Guaifenex® PSE *(Discontinued)* see guaifenesin and pseudoephedrine *on page 458*
Guaifenex™-Rx *(Discontinued)* see guaifenesin and pseudoephedrine *on page 458*
Guaifenex™-Rx DM *(Discontinued)* see guaifenesin, pseudoephedrine, and dextromethorphan *on page 460*
Guaimax-D® [US] see guaifenesin and pseudoephedrine *on page 458*
Guaipax® *(Discontinued)*
Guaiphen-D [US] see guaifenesin and phenylephrine *on page 456*
Guaiphen-D 1200 [US] see guaifenesin and phenylephrine *on page 456*
Guaiphen-PD [US] see guaifenesin and phenylephrine *on page 456*
Guaitab® *(Discontinued)* see guaifenesin and pseudoephedrine *on page 458*
Guaituss AC [US] see guaifenesin and codeine *on page 454*
Guaituss CF® *(Discontinued)*
Guaivent® *(Discontinued)* see guaifenesin and pseudoephedrine *on page 458*

guanabenz (GWAHN a benz)

Sound-Alike/Look-Alike Issues
   guanabenz may be confused with guanadrel, guanfacine
Synonyms guanabenz acetate
U.S./Canadian Brand Names Wytensin® [Can]
Therapeutic Category Alpha-Adrenergic Agonist
Use Management of hypertension
Usual Dosage Oral: Adults: Initial: 4 mg twice daily; increase in increments of 4-8 mg/day every 1-2 weeks to a maximum of 32 mg twice daily
Dosage Forms
   Tablet: 4 mg, 8 mg

guanabenz acetate see guanabenz *on page 462*

guanfacine (GWAHN fa seen)

Sound-Alike/Look-Alike Issues
   guanFACINE may be confused with guaiFENesin, guanabenz, guanidine
   Tenex® may be confused with Entex®, Ten-K®, Xanax®
Synonyms guanfacine hydrochloride
Tall-Man guanFACINE
U.S./Canadian Brand Names Tenex® [US/Can]
Therapeutic Category Alpha-Adrenergic Agonist
Use Management of hypertension
Usual Dosage Oral: Adults: Hypertension: 1 mg usually at bedtime, may increase if needed at 3- to 4-week intervals; usual dose range (JNC 7): 0.5-2 mg once daily
Dosage Forms
   Tablet: 1 mg, 2 mg
   Tenex®: 1 mg, 2 mg

guanfacine hydrochloride see guanfacine *on page 462*

guanidine (GWAHN i deen)

Sound-Alike/Look-Alike Issues
   guanidine may be confused with guanfacine, guanethidine
Synonyms guanidine hydrochloride
Therapeutic Category Cholinergic Agent
Use Reduction of the symptoms of muscle weakness associated with the myasthenic syndrome of Eaton-Lambert, not for myasthenia gravis
Usual Dosage Oral: Adults: Eaton-Lambert syndrome: Initial: 10-15 mg/kg/day in 3-4 divided doses, gradually increase to 35 mg/kg/day or up to development of side effects

Dosage Forms
  Tablet: 125 mg

guanidine hydrochloride *see* guanidine *on page 462*

Guia-D [US] *see* guaifenesin and dextromethorphan *on page 454*

Guiacon DMS [US-OTC] *see* guaifenesin and dextromethorphan *on page 454*

GuiaCough® (Discontinued) *see* guaifenesin and dextromethorphan *on page 454*

GuiaCough® Expectorant (Discontinued) *see* guaifenesin *on page 453*

Guiaplex™ HC (Discontinued)

Guiatex® (Discontinued)

Guiatuss™ [US-OTC] *see* guaifenesin *on page 453*

Guiatuss DAC [US] *see* guaifenesin, pseudoephedrine, and codeine *on page 460*

Guiatuss-DM® [US-OTC] *see* guaifenesin and dextromethorphan *on page 454*

gum benjamin *see* benzoin *on page 126*

GW506U78 *see* nelarabine *on page 660*

GW-1000-02 *see* tetrahydrocannabinol and cannabidiol *(Canada only) on page 915*

GW433908G *see* fosamprenavir *on page 425*

GW572016 *see* lapatinib *on page 550*

G-well® (Discontinued) *see* lindane *on page 567*

Gynazole-1® [US/Can] *see* butoconazole *on page 157*

Gyne-Lotrimin® 3 [US-OTC] *see* clotrimazole *on page 238*

Gyne-Lotrimin® 7 [US-OTC] *see* clotrimazole *on page 238*

Gyne-Sulf® (Discontinued) *see* sulfabenzamide, sulfacetamide, and sulfathiazole *on page 892*

Gynodiol® (Discontinued) *see* estradiol *on page 359*

Gynogen L.A.® Injection (Discontinued) *see* estradiol *on page 359*

Gynol II® [US-OTC] *see* nonoxynol 9 *on page 677*

Gynol II® Extra Strength [US-OTC] *see* nonoxynol 9 *on page 677*

Gynovite® Plus [US-OTC] *see* vitamins (multiple/oral) *on page 983*

H5N1 influenza vaccine *see* influenza virus vaccine (H5N1) *on page 509*

Habitrol® [Can] *see* nicotine *on page 670*

Haemophilus B conjugate and hepatitis B vaccine
(he MOF i lus bee KON joo gate & hep a TYE tis bee vak SEEN)

Sound-Alike/Look-Alike Issues
  Comvax® may be confused with Recombivax [Recombivax HB®]

Synonyms *Haemophilus* b (meningococcal protein conjugate) conjugate vaccine; hepatitis b vaccine (recombinant); Hib conjugate vaccine

U.S./Canadian Brand Names Comvax® [US]

Therapeutic Category Vaccine, Inactivated Virus

Use
  Immunization against invasive disease caused by *H. influenzae* type b and against infection caused by all known subtypes of hepatitis B virus in infants 6 weeks to 15 months of age born of hepatitis B surface antigen (HB$_s$Ag) negative mothers
  Infants born of HB$_s$Ag-positive mothers or mothers of unknown HB$_s$Ag status should receive hepatitis B immune globulin and hepatitis B vaccine (recombinant) at birth and should complete the hepatitis B vaccination series given according to a particular schedule

Usual Dosage I.M.: Infants: 0.5 mL at 2, 4, and 12-15 months of age (total of 3 doses)
  If the recommended schedule cannot be followed, the interval between the first two doses should be at least 6 weeks and the interval between the second and third dose should be as close as possible to 8-11 months. Minimum age for first dose is 6 weeks.
  Modified Schedule: Children who receive one dose of hepatitis B vaccine at or shortly after birth may receive Comvax® on a schedule of 2, 4, and 12-15 months of age

Dosage Forms
  Injection, suspension [preservative free]:
    Comvax®: *Haemophilus* b PRP 7.5 mcg and HB$_s$Ag 5 mcg per 0.5 mL (0.5 mL)

Haemophilus B conjugate (Hib) *see* diphtheria and tetanus toxoids, acellular pertussis, poliovirus (inactivated) and *Haemophilus* b conjugate vaccine *on page 308*

Haemophilus B conjugate vaccine (he MOF fi lus bee KON joo gate vak SEEN)

Synonyms *Haemophilus* b oligosaccharide conjugate vaccine; *Haemophilus* b polysaccharide vaccine; diphtheria CRM$_{197}$ protein conjugate; diphtheria toxoid conjugate; HbCV; HbOC; Hib conjugate vaccine; Hib polysaccharide conjugate; PRP-OMP; PRP-T

U.S./Canadian Brand Names ActHIB® [US/Can]; PedvaxHIB® [US/Can]

Therapeutic Category Vaccine, Inactivated Bacteria

Use Routine immunization of children 2 months to 5 years of age against invasive disease caused by *H. influenzae* type b

Unimmunized children ≥5 years of age with a chronic illness known to be associated with increased risk of *Haemophilus influenzae* type b disease, specifically, persons with anatomic or functional asplenia or sickle cell anemia or those who have undergone splenectomy, should receive *Haemophilus influenzae* type b (Hib) vaccine.

Haemophilus b conjugate vaccines are not indicated for prevention of bronchitis or other infections due to *H. influenzae* in adults; adults with specific dysfunction or certain complement deficiencies who are at especially high risk of *H. influenzae* type b infection (HIV-infected adults); patients with Hodgkin disease (vaccinated at least 2 weeks before the initiation of chemotherapy or 3 months after the end of chemotherapy)

Usual Dosage I.M.: Children: 0.5 mL as a single dose should be administered; do not inject I.V.

Dosage Forms
Injection, powder for reconstitution [preservative free]:
ActHIB®: *Haemophilus* b capsular polysaccharide 10 mcg and tetanus toxoid 24 mcg per dose
Injection, suspension:
PedvaxHIB®: *Haemophilus* b capsular polysaccharide 7.5 mcg and *Neisseria meningitidis* OMPC 125 mcg per 0.5 mL (0.5 mL)

Haemophilus b (meningococcal protein conjugate) conjugate vaccine *see Haemophilus* B conjugate and hepatitis B vaccine *on page 463*
Haemophilus b oligosaccharide conjugate vaccine *see Haemophilus* B conjugate vaccine *on page 464*
Haemophilus B polysaccharide *see* diphtheria and tetanus toxoids, acellular pertussis, poliovirus (inactivated) and *Haemophilus* b conjugate vaccine *on page 308*
Haemophilus b polysaccharide vaccine *see Haemophilus* B conjugate vaccine *on page 464*
Haemophilus influenzae b conjugate vaccine and diphtheria, tetanus toxoids, and acellular pertussis vaccine *see* diphtheria, tetanus toxoids, and acellular pertussis vaccine and *Haemophilus influenzae* b conjugate vaccine *on page 310*

halcinonide (hal SIN oh nide)

Sound-Alike/Look-Alike Issues
halcinonide may be confused with Halcion®
Halog® may be confused with Haldol®, Mycolog®

U.S./Canadian Brand Names Halog® [US/Can]

Therapeutic Category Corticosteroid, Topical

Use Inflammation of corticosteroid-responsive dermatoses [high potency topical corticosteroid]

Usual Dosage Topical: Children and Adults: Steroid-responsive dermatoses: Apply sparingly 1-3 times/ day, occlusive dressing may be used for severe or resistant dermatoses; a thin film is effective; do not overuse. Therapy should be discontinued when control is achieved; if no improvement is seen, reassessment of diagnosis may be necessary.

Dosage Forms
Cream:
Halog®: 0.1% (30 g, 60 g)
Ointment:
Halog®: 0.1% (30 g, 60 g)

Halcion® [US/Can] *see* triazolam *on page 950*
Haldol® [US] *see* haloperidol *on page 465*
Haldol® Decanoate [US] *see* haloperidol *on page 465*

Haley's M-O *see* magnesium hydroxide and mineral oil *on page 586*

HalfLytely® and Bisacodyl [US] *see* polyethylene glycol-electrolyte solution and bisacodyl *on page 766*

Halfprin® [US-OTC] *see* aspirin *on page 98*

halobetasol (hal oh BAY ta sol)

Sound-Alike/Look-Alike Issues
Ultravate® may be confused with Cutivate®

Synonyms halobetasol propionate

U.S./Canadian Brand Names Ultravate® [US/Can]

Therapeutic Category Corticosteroid, Topical

Use Relief of inflammatory and pruritic manifestations of corticosteroid-response dermatoses [super high potency topical corticosteroid]

Usual Dosage Topical: Children ≥12 years and Adults:
Inflammatory and pruritic manifestations (dental use): Cream: Apply sparingly to lesion twice daily. Treatment should not exceed 2 consecutive weeks and total dosage should not exceed 50 g/week. Therapy should be discontinued when control is achieved; if no improvement is seen, reassessment of diagnosis may be necessary.
Steroid-responsive dermatoses: Apply sparingly to skin twice daily, rub in gently and completely; treatment should not exceed 2 consecutive weeks and total dosage should not exceed 50 g/week. Therapy should be discontinued when control is achieved; if no improvement is seen, reassessment of diagnosis may be necessary.

Dosage Forms
Cream: 0.05% (15 g, 50 g)
Ultravate®: 0.05% (15 g, 50 g)
Ointment: 0.05% (15 g, 50 g)
Ultravate®: 0.05% (15 g, 50 g)

halobetasol propionate *see* halobetasol *on page 465*

Halog® [US/Can] *see* halcinonide *on page 464*

Halog®-E (Discontinued) *see* halcinonide *on page 464*

haloperidol (ha loe PER i dole)

Sound-Alike/Look-Alike Issues
haloperidol may be confused Halotestin®
Haldol® may be confused with Halcion®, Halenol®, Halog®, Halotestin®, Stadol®

Synonyms haloperidol decanoate; haloperidol lactate

U.S./Canadian Brand Names Apo-Haloperidol LA® [Can]; Apo-Haloperidol® [Can]; Haldol® Decanoate [US]; Haldol® [US]; Haloperidol Injection, USP [Can]; Haloperidol Long Acting [Can]; Haloperidol-LA Omega [Can]; Haloperidol-LA [Can]; Novo-Peridol [Can]; Peridol [Can]; PMS-Haloperidol LA [Can]

Therapeutic Category Antipsychotic Agent, Butyrophenone

Use Management of schizophrenia; control of tics and vocal utterances of Tourette disorder in children and adults; severe behavioral problems in children

Usual Dosage
Children: 3-12 years (15-40 kg): Oral:
Initial: 0.05 mg/kg/day or 0.25-0.5 mg/day given in 2-3 divided doses; increase by 0.25-0.5 mg every 5-7 days; maximum: 0.15 mg/kg/day
Usual maintenance:
Agitation or hyperkinesia: 0.01-0.03 mg/kg/day once daily
Nonpsychotic disorders: 0.05-0.075 mg/kg/day in 2-3 divided doses
Psychotic disorders: 0.05-0.15 mg/kg/day in 2-3 divided doses
Children 6-12 years: Sedation/psychotic disorders: I.M. (as lactate): 1-3 mg/dose every 4-8 hours to a maximum of 0.15 mg/kg/day; change over to oral therapy as soon as able
Adults: Psychosis:
Oral: 0.5-5 mg 2-3 times/day; usual maximum: 30 mg/day
I.M. (as lactate): 2-5 mg every 4-8 hours as needed
I.M. (as decanoate): Initial: 10-20 times the daily oral dose administered at 4-week intervals
Maintenance dose: 10-15 times initial oral dose; used to stabilize psychiatric symptoms

◀ **Dosage Forms**
Injection, oil: 50 mg/mL (1 mL, 5 mL); 100 mg/mL (1 mL, 5 mL)
Injection, solution: 5 mg/mL (1 mL, 10 mL)
  Haldol®: 5 mg/mL (1 mL)
Solution, oral concentrate: 2 mg/mL
Tablet: 0.5 mg, 1 mg, 2 mg, 5 mg, 10 mg, 20 mg

haloperidol decanoate see haloperidol on page 465
Haloperidol Injection, USP [Can] see haloperidol on page 465
Haloperidol-LA [Can] see haloperidol on page 465
haloperidol lactate see haloperidol on page 465
Haloperidol-LA Omega [Can] see haloperidol on page 465
Haloperidol Long Acting [Can] see haloperidol on page 465

halothane (HA loe thane)

Sound-Alike/Look-Alike Issues
  halothane may be confused with Halotestin®
Therapeutic Category General Anesthetic
Use Induction and maintenance of general anesthesia
Usual Dosage Minimum alveolar concentration (MAC), the concentration at which 50% of patients do not respond to surgical incision, is 0.74% for halothane. The concentration at which amnesia and loss of awareness occur (MAC - awake) is 0.41%. Surgical levels of anesthesia are maintained with concentrations between 0.5% to 2%; inspired concentrations of up to 3% required for induction of anesthesia.

Halotussin® (Discontinued) see guaifenesin on page 453
Halotussin® DM (Discontinued) see guaifenesin and dextromethorphan on page 454
Halotussin® PE (Discontinued) see guaifenesin and pseudoephedrine on page 458
Haltran® (Discontinued) see ibuprofen on page 495
hamamelis water see witch hazel on page 987
HandClens® [US-OTC] see benzalkonium chloride on page 123
HAVRIX® [US/Can] see hepatitis A vaccine on page 469
Havrix® and Engerix-B® see hepatitis A inactivated and hepatitis B (recombinant) vaccine on page 469
HbCV see Haemophilus B conjugate vaccine on page 464
HBIG see hepatitis B immune globulin on page 470
hBNP see nesiritide on page 665
HbOC see Haemophilus B conjugate vaccine on page 464
hCG see chorionic gonadotropin (human) on page 216
HD 200® Plus [US] see barium on page 116
HDA® Toothache [US-OTC] see benzocaine on page 124
HDCV see rabies virus vaccine on page 816
Head & Shoulders® Citrus Breeze [US-OTC] see pyrithione zinc on page 810
Head & Shoulders® Citrus Breeze 2-in-1 [US-OTC] see pyrithione zinc on page 810
Head & Shoulders® Classic Clean [US-OTC] see pyrithione zinc on page 810
Head & Shoulders® Classic Clean 2-In-1 [US-OTC] see pyrithione zinc on page 810
Head & Shoulders® Dry Scalp Care [US-OTC] see pyrithione zinc on page 810
Head & Shoulders® Dry Scalp Care 2-in-1 [US-OTC] see pyrithione zinc on page 810
Head & Shoulders® Extra Volume [US-OTC] see pyrithione zinc on page 810
Head & Shoulders® intensive solutions 2-in-1 [US-OTC] see pyrithione zinc on page 810
Head & Shoulders® intensive solutions for dry/damaged hair [US-OTC] see pyrithione zinc on page 810
Head & Shoulders® intensive solutions for fine/oily hair [US-OTC] see pyrithione zinc on page 810
Head & Shoulders® intensive solutions for normal hair [US-OTC] see pyrithione zinc on page 810
Head & Shoulders® Intensive Treatment [US-OTC] see selenium sulfide on page 861

Head & Shoulders® Ocean Lift [US-OTC] *see* pyrithione zinc *on page 810*

Head & Shoulders® Ocean Lift 2-in-1 [US-OTC] *see* pyrithione zinc *on page 810*

Head & Shoulders® Refresh [US-OTC] *see* pyrithione zinc *on page 810*

Head & Shoulders® Refresh 2-in-1 [US-OTC] *see* pyrithione zinc *on page 810*

Head & Shoulders® Restoring Shine [US-OTC] *see* pyrithione zinc *on page 810*

Head & Shoulders® Restoring Shine 2-in-1 [US-OTC] *see* pyrithione zinc *on page 810*

Head & Shoulders® Sensitive Care [US-OTC] *see* pyrithione zinc *on page 810*

Head & Shoulders® Sensitive Care 2-in-1 [US-OTC] *see* pyrithione zinc *on page 810*

Head & Shoulders® Smooth & Silky [US-OTC] *see* pyrithione zinc *on page 810*

Head & Shoulders® Smooth & Silky 2-In-1 [US-OTC] *see* pyrithione zinc *on page 810*

Healon® [US/Can] *see* hyaluronate and derivatives *on page 476*

Healon®5 [US] *see* hyaluronate and derivatives *on page 476*

Healon GV® [US/Can] *see* hyaluronate and derivatives *on page 476*

Hectorol® [US/Can] *see* doxercalciferol *on page 321*

Helidac® [US] *see* bismuth, metronidazole, and tetracycline *on page 137*

Helistat® [US] *see* collagen hemostat *on page 245*

Helitene® [US] *see* collagen hemostat *on page 245*

Helixate® FS [US/Can] *see* antihemophilic factor (recombinant) *on page 79*

Hemabate® [US/Can] *see* carboprost tromethamine *on page 178*

hematin *see* hemin *on page 467*

hemiacidrin *see* citric acid, magnesium carbonate, and glucono-delta-lactone *on page 225*

hemin (HEE min)

Synonyms hematin

U.S./Canadian Brand Names Panhematin® [US]

Therapeutic Category Blood Modifiers

Use Treatment of recurrent attacks of acute intermittent porphyria (AIP)

Usual Dosage I.V.: Children ≥16 years and Adults: 1-4 mg/kg/day administered over 10-15 minutes for 3-14 days; may be repeated no earlier than every 12 hours; not to exceed 6 mg/kg in any 24-hour period

Dosage Forms

Injection, powder for reconstitution [preservative free]:

Panhematin®: 313 mg

Hemocyte® [US-OTC] *see* ferrous fumarate *on page 397*

Hemocyte Plus® [US] *see* vitamins (multiple/oral) *on page 983*

Hemofil M [US/Can] *see* antihemophilic factor (human) *on page 78*

Hemril®-30 [US] *see* hydrocortisone (rectal) *on page 484*

HepaGam B™ [US/Can] *see* hepatitis B immune globulin *on page 470*

Hepalean® [Can] *see* heparin *on page 467*

Hepalean® Leo [Can] *see* heparin *on page 467*

Hepalean®-LOK [Can] *see* heparin *on page 467*

heparin (HEP a rin)

Sound-Alike/Look-Alike Issues

heparin may be confused with Hespan®

Synonyms heparin calcium; heparin lock flush; heparin sodium

U.S./Canadian Brand Names Hep-Lock U/P [US]; Hep-Lock® [US]; Hepalean® Leo [Can]; Hepalean® [Can]; Hepalean®-LOK [Can]; HepFlush®-10 [US]

Therapeutic Category Anticoagulant (Other)

Use Prophylaxis and treatment of thromboembolic disorders

Note: Heparin lock flush solution is intended only to maintain patency of I.V. devices and is **not** to be used for anticoagulant therapy.

Usual Dosage

Children:

Intermittent I.V.: Initial: 50-100 units/kg, then 50-100 units/kg every 4 hours

◀ I.V. infusion: Initial: 50 units/kg, then 15-25 units/kg/hour; increase dose by 2-4 units/kg/hour every 6-8 hours as required

Adults:

Prophylaxis (low-dose heparin): SubQ: 5000 units every 8-12 hours

Intermittent I.V.: Initial: 10,000 units, then 50-70 units/kg (5000-10,000 units) every 4-6 hours

I.V. infusion (weight-based dosing per institutional nomogram recommended):

Acute coronary syndromes: MI: Fibrinolytic therapy:

Full-dose alteplase, reteplase, or tenecteplase with dosing as follows: Concurrent bolus of 60 units/kg (maximum: 4000 units), then 12 units/kg/hour (maximum: 1000 units/hour) as continuous infusion. Check aPTT every 4-6 hours; adjust to target of 1.5-2 times the upper limit of control (50-70 seconds in clinical trials); usual range 10-30 units/kg/hour. Duration of heparin therapy depends on concurrent therapy and the specific patient risks for systemic or venous thromboembolism.

Streptokinase: Heparin use optional depending on concurrent therapy and specific patient risks for systemic or venous thromboembolism (anterior MI, CHF, previous embolus, atrial fibrillation, LV thrombus): If heparin is administered, start when aPTT <2 times the upper limit of control; do not use a bolus, but initiate infusion adjusted to a target aPTT of 1.5-2 times the upper limit of control (50-70 seconds in clinical trials). If heparin is not administered by infusion, 7500-12,500 units SubQ every 12 hours (when aPTT <2 times the upper limit of control) is recommended.

Percutaneous coronary intervention: Heparin bolus and infusion may be administered to an activated clotting time (ACT) of 300-350 seconds if no concurrent GPIIb/IIIa receptor antagonist is administered or 200-250 seconds if a GPIIb/IIIa receptor antagonist is administered.

Treatment of unstable angina (high-risk and some intermediate-risk patients): Initial bolus of 60-70 units/kg (maximum: 5000 units), followed by an initial infusion of 12-15 units/kg/hour (maximum: 1000 units/hour). The American College of Chest Physicians consensus conference has recommended dosage adjustments to correspond to a therapeutic range equivalent to heparin levels of 0.3-0.7 units/mL by antifactor Xa determinations.

Treatment of venous thromboembolism:

DVT/PE: I.V. push: 80 units/kg followed by continuous infusion of 18 units/kg/hour

DVT: SubQ: 17,500 units every 12 hours

Line flushing: When using daily flushes of heparin to maintain patency of single and double lumen central catheters, 10 units/mL is commonly used for younger infants (eg, <10 kg) while 100 units/mL is used for older infants, children, and adults. Capped PVC catheters and peripheral heparin locks require flushing more frequently (eg, every 6-8 hours). Volume of heparin flush is usually similar to volume of catheter (or slightly greater). Additional flushes should be given when stagnant blood is observed in catheter, after catheter is used for drug or blood administration, and after blood withdrawal from catheter.

Addition of heparin (0.5-3 unit/mL) to peripheral and central parenteral nutrition has not been shown to decrease catheter-related thrombosis. The final concentration of heparin used for TPN solutions may need to be decreased to 0.5 units/mL in small infants receiving larger amounts of volume in order to avoid approaching therapeutic amounts. Arterial lines are heparinized with a final concentration of 1 unit/mL.

Dosage Forms

Infusion [premixed in NaCl 0.45%; porcine intestinal mucosa source]: 12,500 units (250 mL); 25,000 units (250 mL, 500 mL)

Infusion [preservative free; premixed in D_5W; porcine intestinal mucosa source]: 10,000 units (100 mL); 12,500 units (250 mL); 20,000 units (500 mL); 25,000 units (250 mL, 500 mL)

Infusion [preservative free; premixed in NaCl 0.9%; porcine intestinal mucosa source]: 1000 units (500 mL); 2000 units (1000 mL)

Injection, solution [lock flush preparation; porcine intestinal mucosa source; multidose vial]: 10 units/mL (1 mL, 10 mL, 30 mL); 100 units/mL (1 mL, 5 mL, 10 mL, 30 mL)

Hep-Lock®: 10 units/mL (1 mL, 2 mL, 10 mL, 30 mL); 100 units/mL (1 mL, 2 mL, 10 mL, 30 mL)

Injection, solution [lock flush preparation; porcine intestinal mucosa source; prefilled syringe]: 10 units/mL (1 mL, 2 mL, 3 mL, 5 mL); 100 units/mL (1 mL, 2 mL, 3 mL, 5 mL)

Injection, solution [preservative free; lock flush preparation; porcine intestinal mucosa source; prefilled syringe]: 1 unit/mL (2 mL, 3 mL, 5 mL); 2 units/mL (3 mL); 10 units/mL (2.5 mL, 3 mL, 5 mL, 10 mL); 100 units/mL (3 mL, 5 mL, 10 mL)

Injection, solution [preservative free; lock flush preparation; porcine intestinal mucosa source; vial]: 10 units/mL (10 mL)

HepFlush®-10: 10 units/mL (10 mL)

Hep-Lock U/P: 10 units/mL (1 mL); 100 units/mL (1 mL)

Injection, solution [porcine intestinal mucosa source; multidose vial]: 1000 units/mL (1 mL, 10 mL, 30 mL); 5000 units/mL (1 mL, 10 mL); 10,000 units/mL (1 mL, 4 mL, 5 mL); 20,000 units/mL (1 mL)

Injection, solution [porcine intestinal mucosa source; prefilled syringe]: 5000 units/mL (1 mL)
Injection, solution [preservative free; porcine intestinal mucosa source; prefilled syringe]: 10,000 units/mL (0.5 mL)
Injection, solution [preservative free; porcine intestinal mucosa source; vial]: 1000 units/mL (2 mL); 2000 units/mL (5 mL); 2500 units/mL (10 mL)

heparin calcium *see* heparin *on page 467*
heparin cofactor I *see* antithrombin III *on page 82*
heparin lock flush *see* heparin *on page 467*
heparin sodium *see* heparin *on page 467*

hepatitis A inactivated and hepatitis B (recombinant) vaccine
(hep a TYE tis aye in ak ti VAY ted & hep a TYE tis bee ree KOM be nant vak SEEN)

Synonyms Engerix-B® and Havrix®; Havrix® and Engerix-B®; hepatitis B (recombinant) and hepatitis A inactivated vaccine

U.S./Canadian Brand Names Twinrix® [US/Can]

Therapeutic Category Vaccine

Use Active immunization against disease caused by hepatitis A virus and hepatitis B virus (all known subtypes) in populations desiring protection against or at high risk of exposure to these viruses.

Populations include travelers to areas of intermediate/high endemicity for **both** HAV and HBV; those at increased risk of HBV infection due to behavioral or occupational factors; patients with chronic liver disease; laboratory workers who handle live HAV and HBV; healthcare workers, police, and other personnel who render first-aid or medical assistance; workers who come in contact with sewage; employees of day care centers and correctional facilities; patients/staff of hemodialysis units; male homosexuals; patients frequently receiving blood products; military personnel; users of injectable illicit drugs; close household contacts of patients with hepatitis A and hepatitis B infection; residents of drug and alcohol treatment centers

Usual Dosage I.M.: Adults: Primary immunization: Three doses (1 mL each) given on a 0-, 1-, and 6-month schedule
Alternative regimen: Accelerated regimen (1 mL doses at day 0, 7, and 21-30, followed by a booster at 12 months) has demonstrated similar safety, tolerability, and immunogenicity to the standard regimen.

Dosage Forms

Injection, suspension [preservative free]:
Twinrix®: Inactivated hepatitis A virus 720 ELISA units and hepatitis B surface antigen 20 mcg per mL (1 mL)

hepatitis A vaccine (hep a TYE tis aye vak SEEN)

U.S./Canadian Brand Names Avaxim® [Can]; Avaxim®-Pediatric [Can]; HAVRIX® [US/Can]; VAQTA® [US/Can]

Therapeutic Category Vaccine, Inactivated Virus

Use
Active immunization against disease caused by hepatitis A virus (HAV) in persons ≥12 months of age. The Centers for Disease Control and Prevention (CDC)/Advisory Committee on Immunization Practices (ACIP) recommends routine vaccination for all children ≥12 months of age (CDC, 2006). In addition, the CDC/ACIP recommends vaccination in patients at high risk for HAV infection (CDC, 2006), including:
- Travelers to countries with intermediate to high endemicity of HAV (a list of countries is available at http://wwwn.cdc.gov/travel/contentdiseases.aspx)
- Men who have sex with men
- Illegal drug users
- Patients with chronic liver disease
- Patients who receive clotting-factor concentrates
- Persons who work with HAV-infected primates or with HAV in a research laboratory setting

Usual Dosage I.M.: **Note:** The manufacturer recommends that primary immunization be given at least 2 weeks prior to expected HAV exposure; however, the CDC recommends that travelers receive their first dose at least 4 weeks prior to departure for optimal protection:
HAVRIX®:
Children 12 months to 18 years: 720 ELISA units (0.5 mL) with a booster dose of 720 ELISA units to be given 6-12 months following primary immunization
Adults: 1440 ELISA units (1 mL) with a booster dose of 1440 ELISA units to be given 6-12 months following primary immunization

◀ VAQTA®:
Children 12 months to 18 years: 25 units (0.5 mL) with 25 units (0.5 mL) booster dose of 25 units to be given 6-18 months after primary immunization (6-12 months if initial dose was with HAVRIX®)
Adults: 50 units (1 mL) with 50 units (1 mL) booster dose of 50 units to be given 6-18 months after primary immunization (6-12 months if initial dose was with HAVRIX®)

Dosage Forms
Injection, suspension [adult formulation; preservative free]:
HAVRIX®: Viral antigen 1440 ELISA units/mL (1 mL)
VAQTA®: HAV antigen 50 units/mL (1 mL)
Injection, suspension [pediatric formulation; preservative free]:
HAVRIX®: Viral antigen 720 ELISA units/0.5 mL (0.5 mL)
Injection, suspension [pediatric/adolescent formulation; preservative free]:
VAQTA®: HAV antigen 25 units/0.5 mL (0.5 mL)

hepatitis B immune globulin (hep a TYE tis bee i MYUN GLOB yoo lin)

Sound-Alike/Look-Alike Issues
HBIG may be confused with BabyBIG
Synonyms HBIG
U.S./Canadian Brand Names HepaGam B™ [US/Can]; HyperHep B® [Can]; HyperHEP B™ S/D [US]; Nabi-HB® [US]
Therapeutic Category Immune Globulin
Use
Passive prophylactic immunity to hepatitis B following: Acute exposure to blood containing hepatitis B surface antigen (HB$_s$Ag); perinatal exposure of infants born to HB$_s$Ag-positive mothers; sexual exposure to HB$_s$Ag-positive persons; household exposure to persons with acute HBV infection
Prevention of hepatitis B virus recurrence after liver transplantation in HB$_s$Ag-positive transplant patients
Note: Hepatitis B immune globulin is not indicated for treatment of active hepatitis B infection and is ineffective in the treatment of chronic active hepatitis B infection.
Usual Dosage
I.M.:
Newborns: Perinatal exposure of infants born to HB$_s$Ag-positive mothers: 0.5 mL as soon after birth as possible (within 12 hours); active vaccination with hepatitis B vaccine may begin at the same time in a different site (if not contraindicated). If first dose of hepatitis B vaccine is delayed for as long as 3 months, dose may be repeated. If hepatitis B vaccine is refused, dose may be repeated at 3 and 6 months.
Infants <12 months: Household exposure prophylaxis: 0.5 mL (to be administered if mother or primary caregiver has acute HBV infection)
Children ≥12 months and Adults: Postexposure prophylaxis: 0.06 mL/kg as soon as possible after exposure (ie, within 24 hours of needlestick, ocular, or mucosal exposure or within 14 days of sexual exposure); usual dose: 3-5 mL; repeat at 28-30 days after exposure in nonresponders to hepatitis B vaccine or in patients who refuse vaccination
Note: HBIG may be administered at the same time (but at a different site) or up to 1 month preceding hepatitis B vaccination without impairing the active immune response

I.V.: Adults: Prevention of hepatitis B virus recurrence after liver transplantation (HepaGam B™): 20,000 int. units/dose according to the following schedule:
Anhepatic phase (Initial dose): One dose given with the liver transplant
Week 1 postop: One dose daily for 7 days (days 1-7)
Weeks 2-12 postop: One dose every 2 weeks starting day 14
Month 4 onward: One dose monthly starting on month 4
Dose adjustment: Adjust dose to reach anti-HBs levels of 500 int. units/L within the first week after transplantation. In patients with surgical bleeding, abdominal fluid drainage >500 mL or those undergoing plasmapheresis, administer 10,000 int. units/dose every 6 hours until target anti-HBs levels are reached.
Dosage Forms Note: Potency expressed in international units (as compared to the WHO standard) is noted by individual lot on the vial label.
Injection, solution [preservative free]:
HyperHEP B™ S/D: 15% to 18% (0.5 mL, 1 mL, 5 mL)
Nabi-HB®: 5% (1 mL, 5 mL) [>312 int. units/mL]
HepaGam B™: 5% (1 mL, 5 mL) [>312 int. units/mL]

hepatitis B inactivated virus vaccine (recombinant DNA) *see* hepatitis B vaccine *on page 471*

hepatitis B (recombinant) and hepatitis A inactivated vaccine *see* hepatitis A inactivated and hepatitis B (recombinant) vaccine *on page 469*

hepatitis B vaccine (hep a TYE tis bee vak SEEN)

Sound-Alike/Look-Alike Issues
Recombivax HB® may be confused with Comvax®

Synonyms hepatitis B inactivated virus vaccine (recombinant DNA)

U.S./Canadian Brand Names Engerix-B® [US/Can]; Recombivax HB® [US/Can]

Therapeutic Category Vaccine, Inactivated Virus

Use Immunization against infection caused by all known subtypes of hepatitis B virus (HBV), in individuals seeking protection from HBV infection and/or in the following individuals considered at high risk of potential exposure to hepatitis B virus or HB_sAg-positive materials:

Workplace Exposure:
- Healthcare workers[1] (including students, custodial staff, lab personnel, etc)
- Police and fire personnel
- Military personnel
- Morticians and embalmers
- Clients/staff of institutions for the developmentally disabled

Lifestyle Factors:
- Homosexual men
- Heterosexually-active persons with multiple partners in a 6-month period or those with recently acquired sexually-transmitted disease
- Intravenous drug users

Specific Patient Groups:
- Those on hemodialysis[2], receiving transfusions[3], or in hematology/oncology units
- Adolescents
- Infants born of HB_sAG-positive mothers
- Individuals with chronic liver disease
- Individual with HIV infection

Others:
- Prison inmates and staff of correctional facilities
- Household and sexual contacts of HBV carriers
- Residents, immigrants, adoptees, and refugees from areas with endemic HBV infection (eg, Alaskan Eskimos, Pacific Islanders, Indochinese, and Haitian descent)
- International travelers to areas of endemic HBV
- Children born after 11/21/1991

[1]The risk of hepatitis B virus (HBV) infection for healthcare workers varies both between hospitals and within hospitals. Hepatitis B vaccination is recommended for all healthcare workers with blood exposure.
[2]Hemodialysis patients often respond poorly to hepatitis B vaccination; higher vaccine doses or increased number of doses are required. A special formulation of one vaccine is now available for such persons (Recombivax HB®, 40 mcg/mL). The anti-HB_s(antibody to hepatitis B surface antigen) response of such persons should be tested after they are vaccinated, and those who have not responded should be revaccinated with 1-3 additional doses. Patients with chronic renal disease should be vaccinated as early as possible, ideally before they require hemodialysis. In addition, their anti-HB_s levels should be monitored at 6- to 12-month intervals to assess the need for revaccination.
[3]Patients with hemophilia should be immunized subcutaneously, not intramuscularly.

Usual Dosage I.M.:
Immunization regimen: Regimen consists of 3 doses (0, 1, and 6 months): First dose given on the elected date, second dose given 1 month later, third dose given 6 months after the first dose.
Note: Infants born to mothers whose HB_sAg status is unknown should follow the regimen for HB_sAg-positive mothers, omitting the dose of HBIG.
Note: Preterm infants <2000 g and born to HB_sAg-negative mothers should have the first dose delayed until 1 month after birth or hospital discharge due to decreased immune response in underweight infants.

Initial dose:
Birth (infants born of HB_s Ag-negative mothers) to 19 years:
Recombivax HB®: 0.5 mL (5 mcg/0.5 mL pediatric/adolescent formulation) **or**
Engerix-B®: 0.5 mL (10 mcg/0.5 mL formulation)

▶

20 years and older:
Recombivax HB®: 1 mL (10 mcg/mL adult formulation) **or**
Engerix-B®: 1 mL (20 mcg/mL formulation)
Dialysis or immunocompromised patients (revaccinate if anti-HB$_s$ <10 mIU/mL ≥1-2 months after third dose):
Recombivax HB®: 1 mL (40 mcg/mL dialysis formulation) **or**
Engerix-B®: 2 mL (two 1 mL doses given at different sites using the 20 mcg/mL formulation)
1-month dose:
Birth (infants born of HB$_s$Ag-negative mothers) to 19 years:
Recombivax HB®: 0.5 mL (5 mcg/0.5 mL pediatric/adolescent formulation) **or**
Engerix-B®: 0.5 mL (10 mcg/0.5 mL formulation)
20 years and older:
Recombivax HB®: 1 mL (10 mcg/mL adult formulation) **or**
Engerix-B®: 1 mL (20 mcg/mL formulation)
Dialysis or immunocompromised patients (revaccinate if anti-HB$_s$ <10 mIU/mL ≥1-2 months after third dose):
Recombivax HB®: 1 mL (40 mcg/mL dialysis formulation) **or**
Engerix-B®: 2 mL (two 1 mL doses given at different sites using the 20 mcg/mL formulation)
2-month dose:
Dialysis or immunocompromised patients (revaccinate if anti-HB$_s$ <10 mIU/mL ≥1-2 months after third dose):
Engerix-B®: 2 mL (two 1 mL doses given at different sites using the 20 mcg/mL formulation)
6-month dose (final dose in series should not be administered before age of 24 weeks):
Birth (infants born of HB$_s$Ag-negative mothers) to 19 years:
Recombivax HB®: 0.5 mL (5 mcg/0.5 mL pediatric/adolescent formulation)
Engerix-B®: 0.5 mL (10 mcg/0.5 mL formulation)
20 years and older:
Recombivax HB®: 1 mL (10 mcg/mL adult formulation) **or**
Engerix-B®: 1 mL (20 mcg/mL formulation)
Dialysis or immunocompromised patients (revaccinate if anti-HB$_s$ <10 mIU/mL ≥1-2 months after third dose):
Recombivax HB®: 1 mL (40 mcg/mL dialysis formulation) **or**
Engerix-B®: 2 mL (two 1 mL doses given at different sites using the 20 mcg/mL formulation)
Alternative dosing schedule for **Recombivax HB®:**
Children 11-15 years (10 mcg/mL adult formulation): First dose of 1 mL given on the elected date, second dose given 4-6 months later
Adults ≥20 years: Doses may be administered at 0, 1, and 4 months **or** at 0, 2, and 4 months
Alternative dosing schedules for **Engerix-B®:**
Children ≤10 years (10 mcg/0.5 mL formulation): High-risk children: 0.5 mL at 0, 1, 2, and 12 months; lower-risk children ages 5-10 who are candidates for an extended administration schedule may receive an alternative regimen of 0.5 mL at 0, 12, and 24 months. If booster dose is needed, revaccinate with 0.5 mL.
Adolescents 11-19 years (20 mcg/mL formulation): 1 mL at 0, 1, and 6 months. High-risk adolescents: 1 mL at 0, 1, 2, and 12 months; lower-risk adolescents 11-16 years who are candidates for an extended administration schedule may receive an alternative regimen of 0.5 mL (using the 10 mcg/0.5 mL) formulation at 0, 12, and 24 months. If booster dose is needed, revaccinate with 20 mcg.
Adults ≥20 years:
Doses may be administered at 0, 1, and 4 months **or** at 0, 2, and 4 months
High-risk adults (20 mcg/mL formulation): 1 mL at 0, 1, 2, and 12 months. If booster dose is needed, revaccinate with 1 mL.
Postexposure prophylaxis **Note:** High-risk individuals may include children born of hepatitis B-infected mothers, those who have been or might be exposed or those who have traveled to high-risk areas.

Postexposure prophylaxis recommended dosage for infants born to HB$_s$Ag-positive mothers (by product/age):
Engerix-B® (pediatric formulation 10 mcg/0.5 mL):
Give 0.5 mL at birth (≤12 hours); repeat 0.5 mL at 1 month and 6 months.
The first dose may be given at birth at the same time as HBIG, but give in the opposite anterolateral thigh. This may better ensure vaccine absorption.
An alternate regimen is administration of the vaccine at birth, and at 1, 2, and 12 months later.
Recombivax HB® (pediatric/adolescent formulation 5 mcg/0.5 mL):
Give 0.5 mL at birth (≤12 hours); repeat 0.5 mL at 1 month and 6 months

The first dose may be given at birth at the same time as HBIG, but give in the opposite anterolateral thigh. This may better ensure vaccine absorption.

Hepatitis B immune globulin: Give 0.5 mL at birth (or within 7 days of birth).

Dosage Forms

Injection, suspension [preservative free; recombinant DNA]:

Engerix-B®:

Hepatitis B surface antigen 20 mcg/mL (1 mL) [adult formulation]

Hepatitis B surface antigen 10 mcg/0.5 mL (0.5 mL) [pediatric/adolescent formulation]

Recombivax HB®:

Hepatitis B surface antigen 10 mcg/mL (1 mL, 3 mL) [adult formulation]

Hepatitis B surface antigen 40 mcg/mL (1 mL) [dialysis formulation]

Hepatitis B surface antigen 5 mcg/0.5 mL (0.5 mL) [pediatric/adolescent formulation]

hepatitis b vaccine (recombinant) see *Haemophilus* B conjugate and hepatitis B vaccine *on page 463*

HepFlush®-10 [US] *see* heparin *on page 467*

Hep-Lock® [US] *see* heparin *on page 467*

Hep-Lock U/P [US] *see* heparin *on page 467*

Hepsera™ [US/Can] *see* adefovir *on page 35*

Heptalac® (Discontinued) *see* lactulose *on page 544*

Heptovir® [Can] *see* lamivudine *on page 544*

Herceptin® [US/Can] *see* trastuzumab *on page 943*

HES *see* hetastarch *on page 473*

Hespan® [US] *see* hetastarch *on page 473*

hetastarch (HET a starch)

Sound-Alike/Look-Alike Issues

Hespan® may be confused with heparin

Synonyms HES; hydroxyethyl starch

U.S./Canadian Brand Names Hespan® [US]; Hextend® [US/Can]; Voluven® [Can]

Therapeutic Category Plasma Volume Expander

Use Blood volume expander used in treatment of hypovolemia; prevention of hypovolemia (Voluven®); adjunct in leukapheresis to improve harvesting and increase the yield of granulocytes by centrifugation (Hespan®)

Usual Dosage I.V. infusion (requires an infusion pump):

Plasma volume expansion: Adults: 500-1000 mL (up to 1500 mL/day) or 20 mL/kg/day (up to 1500 mL/day); larger volumes (15,000 mL/24 hours) have been used safely in small numbers of patients

Leukapheresis: 250-700 mL; **Note:** Citrate anticoagulant is added before use.

Dosage Forms

Infusion [premixed in lactated electrolyte injection]:

Hextend®: 6% (500 mL)

Infusion, solution [premixed in NaCl 0.9%]: 6% (500 mL)

Hespan®, Voluven®: 6% (500 mL)

Hexabrix™ [US] *see* ioxaglate meglumine and ioxaglate sodium *on page 523*

hexachlorocyclohexane *see* lindane *on page 567*

hexachlorophene (heks a KLOR oh feen)

Sound-Alike/Look-Alike Issues

pHisoHex® may be confused with Fostex®, pHisoDerm®

U.S./Canadian Brand Names pHisoHex® [US/Can]

Therapeutic Category Antibacterial, Topical

Use Surgical scrub and as a bacteriostatic skin cleanser; control an outbreak of gram-positive infection when other procedures have been unsuccessful

Usual Dosage Topical: Children and Adults: Apply 5 mL cleanser and water to area to be cleansed; lather and rinse thoroughly under running water

Dosage Forms

Liquid, topical:

pHisoHex®: 3% (150 mL, 500 mL, 3840 mL)

Hexalen® [US/Can] *see* altretamine *on page 53*
hexamethylenetetramine *see* methenamine *on page 614*
hexamethylmelamine *see* altretamine *on page 53*
Hexit™ [Can] *see* lindane *on page 567*
HEXM *see* altretamine *on page 53*
Hextend® [US/Can] *see* hetastarch *on page 473*

hexylresorcinol (heks il re ZOR si nole)

U.S./Canadian Brand Names S.T. 37® [US-OTC]; Sucrets® Original [US-OTC]
Therapeutic Category Local Anesthetic
Use Minor antiseptic and local anesthetic for sore throat; topical antiseptic for minor cuts or abrasions
Usual Dosage Children ≥2 years and Adults:
  Antiseptic: Topical: Solution: Apply to affected area 1-3 times/day
  Sore throat: Oral:
    Lozenge: May be used as needed, allow to dissolve slowly in mouth (maximum: 10 lozenges/day)
    Solution: Gargle or swish in mouth up to 4 times/day
Dosage Forms
  Lozenge:
    Sucrets® Original [OTC]: 2.4 mg
  Solution:
    S.T. 37® [OTC]: 0.1%

hFSH *see* urofollitropin *on page 964*
hGH *see* somatropin *on page 881*
Hib conjugate vaccine *see* Haemophilus B conjugate and hepatitis B vaccine *on page 463*
Hib conjugate vaccine *see* Haemophilus B conjugate vaccine *on page 464*
Hibiclens® [US-OTC] *see* chlorhexidine gluconate *on page 201*
Hibidil® 1:2000 [Can] *see* chlorhexidine gluconate *on page 201*
Hibistat® [US-OTC] *see* chlorhexidine gluconate *on page 201*
Hib polysaccharide conjugate *see* Haemophilus B conjugate vaccine *on page 464*
HibTITER® (Discontinued) *see* Haemophilus B conjugate vaccine *on page 464*
High Gamma Vitamin E Complete™ [US-OTC] *see* vitamin E *on page 981*
Hi-Kovite [US-OTC] *see* vitamins (multiple/oral) *on page 983*
Hiprex® [US/Can] *see* methenamine *on page 614*
hirulog *see* bivalirudin *on page 138*
Histacol™ BD [US] *see* brompheniramine, pseudoephedrine, and dextromethorphan *on page 146*
Histade™ (Discontinued) *see* chlorpheniramine and pseudoephedrine *on page 207*
Histalet® X (Discontinued) *see* guaifenesin and pseudoephedrine *on page 458*
Histantil [Can] *see* promethazine *on page 791*
Histatab PH [US] *see* chlorpheniramine, phenylephrine, and methscopolamine *on page 210*
Histatab® Plus (Discontinued) *see* chlorpheniramine and phenylephrine *on page 206*
Hista-Vent® DA (Discontinued) *see* chlorpheniramine, phenylephrine, and methscopolamine *on page 210*
Hista-Vent® PSE (Discontinued) *see* chlorpheniramine, pseudoephedrine, and methscopolamine *on page 213*
Histerone® Injection (Discontinued) *see* testosterone *on page 912*
Histex™ [US] *see* chlorpheniramine and pseudoephedrine *on page 207*
Histex™ I/E (Discontinued) *see* carbinoxamine *on page 177*
Histex® SR [US] *see* brompheniramine and pseudoephedrine *on page 144*
Histinex® D Liquid (Discontinued)
Histinex® HC [US] *see* phenylephrine, hydrocodone, and chlorpheniramine *on page 748*
Histinex® PV (Discontinued)
Histor-D® Syrup (Discontinued) *see* chlorpheniramine and phenylephrine *on page 206*
Histor-D® Timecelles® (Discontinued) *see* chlorpheniramine, phenylephrine, and methscopolamine *on page 210*
Histrodrix® (Discontinued) *see* dexbrompheniramine and pseudoephedrine *on page 279*

Histussin D® *(Discontinued)*

Histussin® HC *(Discontinued)* *see* phenylephrine, hydrocodone, and chlorpheniramine *on page 748*

Hi-Vegi-Lip [US-OTC] *see* pancreatin *on page 717*

Hivid® *(Discontinued)*

hMG *see* menotropins *on page 602*

HMM *see* altretamine *on page 53*

HMR 3647 *see* telithromycin *on page 906*

HMS Liquifilm® *(Discontinued)* *see* medrysone *on page 597*

HN₂ *see* mechlorethamine *on page 595*

Hold® DM [US-OTC] *see* dextromethorphan *on page 284*

homatropine (hoe MA troe peen)

Synonyms homatropine hydrobromide

U.S./Canadian Brand Names Isopto® Homatropine [US]

Therapeutic Category Anticholinergic Agent

Use Producing cycloplegia and mydriasis for refraction; treatment of acute inflammatory conditions of the uveal tract; optical aid in axial lens opacities

Usual Dosage Ophthalmic:

Children:

Mydriasis and cycloplegia for refraction: Instill 1 drop of 2% solution immediately before the procedure; repeat at 10-minute intervals as needed

Uveitis: Instill 1 drop of 2% solution 2-3 times/day

Adults:

Mydriasis and cycloplegia for refraction: Instill 1-2 drops of 2% solution or 1 drop of 5% solution before the procedure; repeat at 5- to 10-minute intervals as needed; maximum of 3 doses for refraction

Uveitis: Instill 1-2 drops of 2% or 5% 2-3 times/day up to every 3-4 hours as needed

Dosage Forms

Solution, ophthalmic:

Isopto® Homatropine: 2% (5 mL); 5% (5 mL, 15 mL)

homatropine and hydrocodone *see* hydrocodone and homatropine *on page 482*

homatropine hydrobromide *see* homatropine *on page 475*

horse antihuman thymocyte gamma globulin *see* antithymocyte globulin (equine) *on page 82*

H.P. Acthar® Gel [US] *see* corticotropin *on page 249*

Hp-PAC® [Can] *see* lansoprazole, amoxicillin, and clarithromycin *on page 549*

HPV Vaccine *see* papillomavirus (Types 6, 11, 16, 18) recombinant vaccine *on page 722*

HTF919 *see* tegaserod *on page 905*

hu1124 *see* efalizumab *on page 335*

Humalog® [US/Can] *see* insulin lispro *on page 511*

Humalog® Mix 25 [Can] *see* insulin lispro protamine and insulin lispro *on page 512*

Humalog® Mix 50/50™ [US] *see* insulin lispro protamine and insulin lispro *on page 512*

Humalog® Mix 50/50 Insulin *(Discontinued)*

Humalog® Mix 75/25™ [US] *see* insulin lispro protamine and insulin lispro *on page 512*

human antitumor necrosis factor alpha *see* adalimumab *on page 34*

human corticotrophin-releasing hormone, analogue *see* corticorelin *on page 248*

human diploid cell cultures rabies vaccine *see* rabies virus vaccine *on page 816*

human growth hormone *see* somatropin *on page 881*

humanized IgG1 anti-CD52 monoclonal antibody *see* alemtuzumab *on page 43*

human LFA-3/IgG(1) fusion protein *see* alefacept *on page 42*

human menopausal gonadotropin *see* menotropins *on page 602*

human papillomavirus vaccine *see* papillomavirus (Types 6, 11, 16, 18) recombinant vaccine *on page 722*

human rotavirus vaccine, attenuated (HRV) *see* rotavirus vaccine *on page 847*

human thyroid stimulating hormone *see* thyrotropin alpha *on page 924*

Humate-P® [US/Can] *see* antihemophilic factor/von Willebrand factor complex (human) *on page 80*

Humatin® [Can] *see* paromomycin *on page 723*

Humatin® *(Discontinued)* *see* paromomycin *on page 723*

Humatrope® [US/Can] *see* somatropin *on page 881*

Humegon® [Can] *see* chorionic gonadotropin (human) *on page 216*

Humegon® *(Discontinued)* *see* menotropins *on page 602*

Humibid® CS *(Discontinued)* *see* guaifenesin and dextromethorphan *on page 454*

Humibid® DM *(Discontinued)* *see* guaifenesin and dextromethorphan *on page 454*

Humibid® e *(Discontinued)* *see* guaifenesin *on page 453*

Humibid® LA *(Discontinued)* *see* guaifenesin *on page 453*

Humibid® LA *(reformulation)* *(Discontinued)*

Humibid® Pediatric *(Discontinued)* *see* guaifenesin *on page 453*

Humibid® Sprinkle *(Discontinued)* *see* guaifenesin *on page 453*

Humira® [US/Can] *see* adalimumab *on page 34*

Humist® [US-OTC] *see* sodium chloride *on page 873*

Humist® for Kids [US-OTC] *see* sodium chloride *on page 873*

Humulin® 20/80 [Can] *see* insulin NPH and insulin regular *on page 512*

Humulin® 50/50 [US] *see* insulin NPH and insulin regular *on page 512*

Humulin® L *(Discontinued)*

Humulin® 70/30 [US/Can] *see* insulin NPH and insulin regular *on page 512*

Humulin® N [US/Can] *see* insulin NPH *on page 512*

Humulin® R [US/Can] *see* insulin regular *on page 513*

Humulin® R U-500 [US] *see* insulin regular *on page 513*

Humulin® U *(Discontinued)*

Hurricaine® [US-OTC] *see* benzocaine *on page 124*

HXM *see* altretamine *on page 53*

Hyalgan® [US] *see* hyaluronate and derivatives *on page 476*

hyaluronan *see* hyaluronate and derivatives *on page 476*

hyaluronate and derivatives (hye al yoor ON ate & dah RIV ah tives)

Sound-Alike/Look-Alike Issues
Synvisc® may be confused with Synagis®

Synonyms hyaluronan; hyaluronic acid; hylan polymers; sodium hyaluronate

U.S./Canadian Brand Names Bionect® [US]; Cystistat® [Can]; Durolane® [Can]; Euflexxa™ [US]; Eyestil [Can]; Healon GV® [US/Can]; Healon® [US/Can]; Healon®5 [US]; Hyalgan® [US]; Hylaform® Plus [US]; Hylaform® [US]; Hylira™ [US]; IPM Wound Gel™ [US-OTC]; Juvederm™ 24HV [US]; Juvederm™ 30 [US]; Juvederm™ 30HV [US]; Orthovisc® [US/Can]; Perlane® [US]; Provisc® [US]; Restylane® [US]; Supartz™ [US]; Suplasyn® [Can]; Synvisc® [US]; Vitrax® [US]

Therapeutic Category Antirheumatic Miscellaneous; Ophthalmic Agent, Viscoelastic; Skin and Mucous Membrane Agent

Use
Intraarticular injection: Treatment of pain in osteoarthritis in knee in patients who have failed nonpharmacologic treatment and simple analgesics

Intradermal: Correction of moderate-to-severe facial wrinkles or folds

Ophthalmic: Surgical aid in cataract extraction, intraocular implantation, corneal transplant, glaucoma filtration, and retinal attachment surgery

Topical cream, gel, spray: Management of skin ulcers and wounds

Topical lotion: Treatment of xerosis (dry, scaly skin)

Usual Dosage Adults:

Osteoarthritis of the knee: Intraarticular:
Eulexxa™: Inject 20 mg (2 mL) once weekly for 3 weeks

Hyalgan®: Inject 20 mg (2 mL) once weekly for 5 weeks; some patients may benefit with a total of 3 injections

Orthovisc®: Inject 30 mg (2 mL) once weekly for 3-4 weeks

Supartz™: Inject 25 mg (2.5 mL) once weekly for 5 weeks

Synvisc®: Inject 16 mg (2 mL) once weekly for 3 weeks (total of 3 injections)

Facial wrinkles: Intradermal:
Note: Formulations differ in terms of recommended injection depth: Juvederm™, Hylaform®, and Restylane® are intended for mid to deep intradermal injection; Perlane® is intended for injection into the deep dermis to superficial subcutis

Hylaform®, Hylaform® Plus: Inject as required for cosmetic result; typical treatment regimen requires <2 mL; limit injection to ≤1.5 mL per injection site; maximum: 20 mL/60 kg/year

Juvederm™ (all formulations): Inject as required for cosmetic result; typical treatment regimen requires <2 mL; limit injection to 1.6 mL per injection site; maximum: 20 mL/60 kg/year

Perlane®: Inject as required into deep dermis/superficial subcutis for cosmetic result; typical treatment regimen requires 1.9-4.6 mL; maximum 6 mL per treatment

Restylane®: Inject as required for cosmetic result; typical treatment regimen requires <2 mL; limit injection to ≤1.5 mL per injection site

Ophthalmic (Healon®, Provisc®, Vitrax®): Depends upon procedure (slowly introduce a sufficient quantity into eye)

Topical:Note: Formulations are used for different indications:

Bionect® cream, gel, and spray: Apply a thin layer to clean and disinfected wound or ulcer 2-3 times/day, and cover with sterile gauze pad. If needed, cover with elastic or compressive bandage.

IPM Wound Gel™: Apply to clean dry ulcer or wound, and cover with nonstick dressing; repeat daily. Discontinue if wound size increase after 3-4 applications.

Hylira™ lotion: Apply to affected area and rub in thoroughly 2-3 times daily. Discontinue if condition worsens.

Dosage Forms
Hylan B:
Injection, gel:
Hylaform® [500 micron particle]: 5.5 mg/mL (0.75 mL)
Hylaform® Plus [700 micron particle]: 5.5 mg/mL (0.75 mL)
Hylan Polymers A and B (Hylan G-F 20):
Injection, solution, intraarticular:
Synvisc®: 8 mg/mL (2 mL)
Hyaluronate:
Cream, topical:
Bionect®: 0.2% (25 g)
Gel, topical:
Bionect®: 0.2% (30 g, 60 g)
IPM Wound Gel™ [OTC]: 2.5% (10 g)
Lotion, topical:
Hylira™ Lotion: 0.1% (340 g, 1000 g)
Injection, gel, intradermal:
Juvederm™ 24HV, Juvederm™ 30, Juvederm™ 30HV: 24 mg/mL [prefilled syringe]
Perlane®: 20 mg/mL (1mL) [prefilled syringe]
Restylane®: 20 mg/mL
Injection, solution, intraarticular:
Euflexxa™, Hyalgan®: 10 mg/mL (2 mL)
Orthovisc®: 15 mg/mL (2 mL)
Supartz™: 10 mg/mL (2.5 mL)
Synvisc®: 8 mg/mL (2 mL)
Injection, solution, intraocular:
Healon®: 10 mg/mL (0.4 mL, 0.55 mL, 0.85 mL, 2 mL)
Healon®5: 23 mg/mL
Healon GV®: 14 mg/mL (0.55 mL, 0.85 mL)
Provisc®: 10 mg/mL (0.4 mL, 0.55 mL, 0.8 mL)
Vitrax®: 30 mg/mL (0.65 mL)

hyaluronic acid *see* hyaluronate and derivatives *on page 476*

hyaluronidase (hye al yoor ON i dase)
Sound-Alike/Look-Alike Issues
Wydase® may be confused with Lidex®, Wyamine®
U.S./Canadian Brand Names Amphadase™ [US]; Hydase™ [US]; Hylenex™ [US]; Vitrase® [US]
Therapeutic Category Enzyme

▶

Use Increase the dispersion and absorption of other drugs; increase rate of absorption of parenteral fluids given by hypodermoclysis; adjunct in subcutaneous urography for improving resorption of radiopaque agents

Usual Dosage Note: A preliminary skin test for hypersensitivity can be performed. ACTH, antihistamines, corticosteroids, estrogens, and salicylates, when used in large doses, may cause tissues to be partly resistant to hyaluronidase. May require larger doses of hyaluronidase for the same effect.

Skin test: Intradermal: 0.02 mL (3 units) of a 150 units/mL solution. Positive reaction consists of a wheal with pseudopods appearing within 5 minutes and persisting for 20-30 minutes with localized itching.

Hypodermoclysis: SubQ: 15 units is added to each 100 mL of I.V. fluid to be administered; 150 units facilitates absorption of >1000 mL of solution

Premature Infants and Neonates: Volume of a single clysis should not exceed 25 mL/kg and the rate of administration should not exceed 2 mL/minute

Children <3 years: Volume of a single clysis should not exceed 200 mL

Children ≥3 years and Adults: Rate and volume of a single clysis should not exceed those used for infusion of I.V. fluids

Urography: Children and Adults: SubQ: 75 units over each scapula followed by injection of contrast medium at the same site; patient should be in the prone position.

Dosage Forms

Injection, powder for reconstitution:
Vitrase®: 6200 units

Injection, solution:
Amphadase™: 150 units/mL (1 mL)

Injection, solution [preservative free]:
Hydase™: 150 units/mL (1 mL)
Hylenex™: 150 units/mL (1 mL, 2 mL)
Vitrase®: 200 units/mL (2 mL)

hycamptamine *see* topotecan *on page 936*

Hycamtin® [US/Can] *see* topotecan *on page 936*

hycet™ [US] *see* hydrocodone and acetaminophen *on page 481*

HycoClear Tuss® *(Discontinued)*

Hycodan® *(Discontinued) see* hydrocodone and homatropine *on page 482*

Hycomine® Compound *(Discontinued)*

Hycomine® *(Discontinued)*

Hycomine® Pediatric *(Discontinued)*

Hycort™ [Can] *see* hydrocortisone (topical) *on page 485*

Hycotuss® *(Discontinued)*

Hydase™ [US] *see* hyaluronidase *on page 477*

Hydeltra T.B.A.® [Can] *see* prednisolone (systemic) *on page 781*

Hydergine® [Can] *see* ergoloid mesylates *on page 351*

Hydergine® *(Discontinued) see* ergoloid mesylates *on page 351*

Hyderm [Can] *see* hydrocortisone (topical) *on page 485*

hydralazine (hye DRAL a zeen)

Sound-Alike/Look-Alike Issues
hydrALAZINE may be confused with hydrOXYzine

Synonyms hydralazine hydrochloride

Tall-Man hydrALAZINE

U.S./Canadian Brand Names Apo-Hydralazine® [Can]; Apresoline® [Can]; Novo-Hylazin [Can]; Nu-Hydral [Can]

Therapeutic Category Vasodilator

Use Management of moderate-to-severe hypertension, congestive heart failure, hypertension secondary to preeclampsia/eclampsia; treatment of primary pulmonary hypertension

Usual Dosage
Children:
Oral: Initial: 0.75-1 mg/kg/day in 2-4 divided doses; increase over 3-4 weeks to maximum of 7.5 mg/kg/day in 2-4 divided doses; maximum daily dose: 200 mg/day
I.M., I.V.: 0.1-0.2 mg/kg/dose (not to exceed 20 mg) every 4-6 hours as needed, up to 1.7-3.5 mg/kg/day in 4-6 divided doses

Adults:
Oral:
Hypertension:
Initial dose: 10 mg 4 times/day for first 2-4 days; increase to 25 mg 4 times/day for the balance of the first week
Increase by 10-25 mg/dose gradually to 50 mg 4 times/day (maximum: 300 mg/day); usual dose range (JNC 7): 25-100 mg/day in 2 divided doses
Congestive heart failure:
Initial dose: 10-25 mg 3-4 times/day
Adjustment: Dosage must be adjusted based on individual response
Target dose: 225-300 mg/day in divided doses; use in combination with isosorbide dinitrate
I.M., I.V.:
Hypertension: Initial: 10-20 mg/dose every 4-6 hours as needed, may increase to 40 mg/dose; change to oral therapy as soon as possible.
Preeclampsia/eclampsia: 5 mg/dose then 5-10 mg every 20-30 minutes as needed.
Dosage Forms
Injection, solution: 20 mg/mL (1 mL)
Tablet: 10 mg, 25 mg, 50 mg, 100 mg

hydralazine and hydrochlorothiazide (hye DRAL a zeen & hye droe klor oh THYE a zide)
Synonyms hydrochlorothiazide and hydralazine
Therapeutic Category Antihypertensive Agent, Combination
Use Management of moderate-to-severe hypertension and treatment of congestive heart failure
Usual Dosage Oral: Adults: Hydralazine 25-100 mg/day and hydrochlorothiazide 25-50 mg/day in 2 divided doses (maximum: hydrochlorothiazide: 50 mg/day)
Dosage Forms
Capsule: 25/25: Hydralazine 25 mg and hydrochlorothiazide 25 mg; 50/50: Hydralazine 50 mg and hydrochlorothiazide 50 mg; 100/50: Hydralazine 100 mg and hydrochlorothiazide 50 mg

hydralazine and isosorbide dinitrate see isosorbide dinitrate and hydralazine on page 530
hydralazine hydrochloride see hydralazine on page 478
Hydramine® [US-OTC] see diphenhydramine on page 304
hydrated chloral see chloral hydrate on page 199
Hydrate® (Discontinued) see dimenhydrinate on page 301
Hydrea® [US/Can] see hydroxyurea on page 490
Hydrisalic™ [US-OTC] see salicylic acid on page 850
Hydro 40™ [US] see urea on page 963
Hydrocet® (Discontinued) see hydrocodone and acetaminophen on page 481

hydrochlorothiazide (hye droe klor oh THYE a zide)
Sound-Alike/Look-Alike Issues
hydrochlorothiazide may be confused with hydrocortisone, hydroflumethiazide
Esidrix may be confused with Lasix®
HCTZ is an error-prone abbreviation (mistaken as hydrocortisone)
Microzide™ may be confused with Maxzide®, Micronase®
U.S./Canadian Brand Names Apo-Hydro® [Can]; Microzide™ [US]; Novo-Hydrazide [Can]; PMS-Hydrochlorothiazide [Can]
Therapeutic Category Diuretic, Thiazide
Use Management of mild-to-moderate hypertension; treatment of edema in congestive heart failure and nephrotic syndrome
Usual Dosage Oral (effect of drug may be decreased when used every day):
Children (in pediatric patients, chlorothiazide may be preferred over hydrochlorothiazide as there are more dosage formulations [eg, suspension] available): Edema, hypertension:
<6 months: 1-3 mg/kg/day in 2 divided doses
>6 months to 2 years: 1-3 mg/kg/day in 2 divided doses; maximum: 37.5 mg/day
>2-17 years: Initial: 1 mg/kg/day; maximum: 3 mg/kg/day (50 mg/day)
Adults:
Edema: 25-100 mg/day in 1-2 doses; maximum: 200 mg/day

◄ Hypertension: 12.5-50 mg/day; minimal increase in response and more electrolyte disturbances are seen with doses >50 mg/day

Dosage Forms
Capsule: 12.5 mg
Microzide™: 12.5 mg
Tablet: 25 mg, 50 mg

hydrochlorothiazide and aliskiren *see aliskiren and hydrochlorothiazide on page 45*
hydrochlorothiazide and amiloride *see amiloride and hydrochlorothiazide on page 59*
hydrochlorothiazide and benazepril *see benazepril and hydrochlorothiazide on page 121*
hydrochlorothiazide and bisoprolol *see bisoprolol and hydrochlorothiazide on page 138*
hydrochlorothiazide and captopril *see captopril and hydrochlorothiazide on page 172*
hydrochlorothiazide and cilazapril *see cilazapril and hydrochlorothiazide (Canada only) on page 219*
hydrochlorothiazide and enalapril *see enalapril and hydrochlorothiazide on page 339*
hydrochlorothiazide and eprosartan *see eprosartan and hydrochlorothiazide on page 349*
hydrochlorothiazide and fosinopril *see fosinopril and hydrochlorothiazide on page 428*
hydrochlorothiazide and hydralazine *see hydralazine and hydrochlorothiazide on page 479*
hydrochlorothiazide and irbesartan *see irbesartan and hydrochlorothiazide on page 526*
hydrochlorothiazide and lisinopril *see lisinopril and hydrochlorothiazide on page 571*
hydrochlorothiazide and losartan *see losartan and hydrochlorothiazide on page 578*
hydrochlorothiazide and methyldopa *see methyldopa and hydrochlorothiazide on page 620*
hydrochlorothiazide and metoprolol *see metoprolol and hydrochlorothiazide on page 627*
hydrochlorothiazide and metoprolol tartrate *see metoprolol and hydrochlorothiazide on page 627*
hydrochlorothiazide and moexipril *see moexipril and hydrochlorothiazide on page 640*
hydrochlorothiazide and olmesartan medoxomil *see olmesartan and hydrochlorothiazide on page 695*
hydrochlorothiazide and propranolol *see propranolol and hydrochlorothiazide on page 797*
hydrochlorothiazide and quinapril *see quinapril and hydrochlorothiazide on page 813*
hydrochlorothiazide and ramipril *see ramipril and hydrochlorothiazide (Canada only) on page 818*

hydrochlorothiazide and spironolactone
(hye droe klor oh THYE a zide & speer on oh LAK tone)

Sound-Alike/Look-Alike Issues
Aldactazide® may be confused with Aldactone®

Synonyms spironolactone and hydrochlorothiazide

U.S./Canadian Brand Names Aldactazide 25® [Can]; Aldactazide 50® [Can]; Aldactazide® [US]; Novo-Spirozine [Can]

Therapeutic Category Antihypertensive Agent, Combination

Use Management of mild-to-moderate hypertension; treatment of edema in congestive heart failure and nephrotic syndrome, and cirrhosis of the liver accompanied by edema and/or ascites

Usual Dosage Oral:
Children: 1.5-3 mg/kg/day in 2-4 divided doses (maximum: 200 mg/day)
Adults: Hydrochlorothiazide 12.5-50 mg/day and spironolactone 12.5-50 mg/day; manufacturer labeling states hydrochlorothiazide maximum 200 mg/day, however, usual dose in JNC-7 is 12.5-50 mg/day

Dosage Forms
Tablet: Hydrochlorothiazide 25 mg and spironolactone 25 mg
Aldactazide®: 25/25: Hydrochlorothiazide 25 mg and spironolactone 25 mg; 50/50: Hydrochlorothiazide 50 mg and spironolactone 50 mg

hydrochlorothiazide and telmisartan *see telmisartan and hydrochlorothiazide on page 906*

hydrochlorothiazide and triamterene (hye droe klor oh THYE a zide & trye AM ter een)

Sound-Alike/Look-Alike Issues
Dyazide® may be confused with diazoxide, Dynacin®
Maxzide® may be confused with Maxidex®, Microzide™

Synonyms triamterene and hydrochlorothiazide

U.S./Canadian Brand Names Apo-Triazide® [Can]; Dyazide® [US]; Maxzide® [US]; Maxzide®-25 [US]; Novo-Triamzide [Can]; Nu-Triazide [Can]; Penta-Triamterene HCTZ [Can]; Riva-Zide [Can]

Therapeutic Category Antihypertensive Agent, Combination

Use Treatment of hypertension or edema (not recommended for initial treatment) when hypokalemia has developed on hydrochlorothiazide alone or when the development of hypokalemia must be avoided

Usual Dosage Oral: Adults:

Hydrochlorothiazide 25 mg and triamterene 37.5 mg: 1-2 tablets/capsules once daily
Hydrochlorothiazide 50 mg and triamterene 75 mg: 1/2-1 tablet daily

Dosage Forms

Capsule: Hydrochlorothiazide 25 mg and triamterene 37.5 mg; hydrochlorothiazide 25 mg and triamterene 50 mg

Dyazide®: Hydrochlorothiazide 25 mg and triamterene 37.5 mg

Tablet: Hydrochlorothiazide 25 mg and triamterene 37.5 mg; hydrochlorothiazide 50 mg and triamterene 75 mg

Maxzide®: Hydrochlorothiazide 50 mg and triamterene 75 mg [scored]

Maxzide®-25: Hydrochlorothiazide 25 mg and triamterene 37.5 mg [scored]

hydrochlorothiazide and valsartan *see valsartan and hydrochlorothiazide on page 969*
Hydrocil® Instant [US-OTC] *see psyllium on page 804*

hydrocodone and acetaminophen (hye droe KOE done & a seet a MIN oh fen)

Sound-Alike/Look-Alike Issues

Lorcet® may be confused with Fioricet®
Lortab® may be confused with Cortef®, Lorabid®, Luride®
Vicodin® may be confused with Hycodan®, Hycomine®, Indocin®, Uridon®
Zydone® may be confused with Vytone®

Synonyms acetaminophen and hydrocodone

U.S./Canadian Brand Names Anexsia® [US]; Co-Gesic® [US]; hycet™ [US]; Lorcet® 10/650 [US]; Lorcet® Plus [US]; Lortab® [US]; Margesic® H [US]; Maxidone™ [US]; Norco® [US]; Stagesic® [US]; Vicodin® ES [US]; Vicodin® HP [US]; Vicodin® [US]; Xodol® 10/300 [US]; Xodol® 5/300 [US]; Xodol® 7.5/300 [US]; Zydone® [US]

Therapeutic Category Analgesic, Narcotic

Controlled Substance C-III

Use Relief of moderate-to-severe pain

Usual Dosage Oral (doses should be titrated to appropriate analgesic effect): Analgesic:

Children 2-13 years or <50 kg: Hydrocodone 0.135 mg/kg/dose every 4-6 hours; do not exceed 6 doses/day or the maximum recommended dose of acetaminophen

Children and Adults ≥50 kg: Average starting dose in opioid-naive patients: Hydrocodone 5-10 mg 4 times/day; the dosage of acetaminophen should be limited to ≤4 g/day (and possibly less in patients with hepatic impairment or ethanol use).

Dosage ranges (based on specific product labeling): Hydrocodone 2.5-10 mg every 4-6 hours; maximum: 60 mg hydrocodone/day (maximum dose of hydrocodone may be limited by the acetaminophen content of specific product)

Dosage Forms

Capsule: Hydrocodone 5 mg and acetaminophen 500 mg

Margesic® H, Stagesic®: Hydrocodone 5 mg and acetaminophen 500 mg

Elixir: Hydrocodone 7.5 mg and acetaminophen 500 mg per 15 mL

Lortab®: Hydrocodone 7.5 mg and acetaminophen 500 mg per 15 mL

Solution, oral: Hydrocodone 7.5 mg and acetaminophen 325 mg per 15 mL

hycet™: Hydrocodone 7.5 mg and acetaminophen 325 mg per 15 mL

Tablet:

Generics:

Hydrocodone 2.5 mg and acetaminophen 500 mg
Hydrocodone 5 mg and acetaminophen 325 mg
Hydrocodone 5 mg and acetaminophen 500 mg
Hydrocodone 7.5 mg and acetaminophen 325 mg
Hydrocodone 7.5 mg and acetaminophen 500 mg
Hydrocodone 7.5 mg and acetaminophen 650 mg
Hydrocodone 7.5 mg and acetaminophen 750 mg
Hydrocodone 10 mg and acetaminophen 325 mg
Hydrocodone 10 mg and acetaminophen 500 mg
Hydrocodone 10 mg and acetaminophen 650 mg

◀ Hydrocodone 10 mg and acetaminophen 660 mg
Hydrocodone 10 mg and acetaminophen 750 mg
Brands:
  Anexsia®: 5/325: Hydrocodone 5 mg and acetaminophen 320 mg
  Co-Gesic® 5/500: Hydrocodone 5 mg and acetaminophen 500 mg
  Lorcet® 10/650: Hydrocodone 10 mg and acetaminophen 650 mg
  Lorcet® Plus: Hydrocodone 7.5 mg and acetaminophen 650 mg
  Lortab®: /500: Hydrocodone 5 mg and acetaminophen 500 mg; 7.5/500: Hydrocodone 7.5 mg and acetaminophen 500 mg; 10/500: Hydrocodone 10 mg and acetaminophen 500 mg
  Maxidone™: Hydrocodone 10 mg and acetaminophen 750 mg
  Norco®: Hydrocodone 5 mg and acetaminophen 325 mg; hydrocodone 7.5 mg and acetaminophen 325 mg; hydrocodone 10 mg and acetaminophen 325 mg
  Vicodin®: Hydrocodone 5 mg and acetaminophen 500 mg
  Vicodin® ES: Hydrocodone 7.5 mg and acetaminophen 750 mg
  Vicodin® HP: Hydrocodone 10 mg and acetaminophen 660 mg
  Xodol®: 10/300: Hydrocodone 10 mg and acetaminophen 300 mg; 5/300: Hydrocodone 5 mg and acetaminophen 300 mg; 7/300: Hydrocodone 7 mg and acetaminophen 300 mg
  Zydone®: Hydrocodone 5 mg and acetaminophen 400 mg; hydrocodone 7.5 mg and acetaminophen 400 mg; hydrocodone 10 mg and acetaminophen 400 mg

hydrocodone and aspirin *(Discontinued)*

hydrocodone and chlorpheniramine (hye droe KOE done & klor fen IR a meen)
Synonyms chlorpheniramine maleate and hydrocodone bitartrate; hydrocodone tannate and chlorpheniramine tannate
U.S./Canadian Brand Names Tussionex® [US]
Therapeutic Category Antihistamine/Antitussive
Controlled Substance C-III
Use Symptomatic relief of cough and upper respiratory symptoms associated with cold and allergy
Usual Dosage Oral:
  Children 6-12 years (Tussionex®): 2.5 mL every 12 hours; do not exceed 5 mL/24 hours
  Children >12 years and Adults (Tussionex®): 5 mL every 12 hours; do not exceed 10 mL/24 hours
Dosage Forms
  Capsule, extended release:
    TussiCaps™ 5 mg/4 mg: Hydrocodone bitartrate 5 mg and chlorpheniramine maleate 4 mg
    TussiCaps™ 10 mg/8 mg: Hydrocodone bitartrate 10 mg and chlorpheniramine maleate 8 mg
  Suspension, extended release:
    Tussionex®: Hydrocodone bitartrate 10 mg and chlorpheniramine maleate 8 mg per 5 mL

hydrocodone and guaifenesin *(Discontinued)*

hydrocodone and homatropine (hye droe KOE done & hoe MA troe peen)
Sound-Alike/Look-Alike Issues
  Hycodan® may be confused with Hycomine®, Vicodin®
Synonyms homatropine and hydrocodone
U.S./Canadian Brand Names Hydromet® [US]; Tussigon® [US]
Therapeutic Category Antitussive
Controlled Substance C-III
Use Symptomatic relief of cough
Usual Dosage Oral:
  Children 6-12 years: 1/2 tablet or 2.5 mL every 4-6 hours as needed (maximum: 3 tablets or 15 mL/24 hours)
  Children ≥12 years and Adults: 1 tablet or 5 mL every 4-6 hours as needed (maximum: 6 tablets/24 hours or 30 mL/24 hours)
Dosage Forms
  Syrup: Hydrocodone 5 mg and homatropine 1.5 mg per 5 mL
    Hydromet®: Hydrocodone 5 mg and homatropine 1.5 mg per 5 mL
  Tablet:
    Tussigon®: Hydrocodone 5 mg and homatropine 1.5 mg

hydrocodone and ibuprofen (hye droe KOE done & eye byoo PROE fen)
Synonyms ibuprofen and hydrocodone
U.S./Canadian Brand Names Ibudone™ [US]; Reprexain® [US]; Vicoprofen® [US/Can]
Therapeutic Category Analgesic, Narcotic
Controlled Substance C-III
Use Short-term (generally <10 days) management of moderate-to-severe acute pain; is not indicated for treatment of such conditions as osteoarthritis or rheumatoid arthritis
Usual Dosage Oral: Adults: 1 tablet every 4-6 hours as needed for pain; maximum: 5 tablets/day
Dosage Forms
    Tablet: Hydrocodone 5 mg and ibuprofen 200 mg; hydrocodone 7.5 mg and ibuprofen 200 mg
    Ibudone™: 5/200: Hydrocodone bitartrate 5 mg and ibuprofen 200 mg; 10/200: Hydrocodone bitartrate 10 mg and ibuprofen 200 mg
    Reprexain®: Hydrocodone 5 mg and ibuprofen 200 mg; hydrocodone 7.5 mg and ibuprofen 200 mg
    Vicoprofen®: Hydrocodone 7.5 mg and ibuprofen 200 mg

hydrocodone and pseudoephedrine *(Discontinued)*
hydrocodone bitartrate, carbinoxamine maleate, and pseudoephedrine hydrochloride *see* hydrocodone, carbinoxamine, and pseudoephedrine *on page 483*

hydrocodone, carbinoxamine, and pseudoephedrine
(hye droe KOE done, kar bi NOKS a meen, & soo doe e FED rin)
Synonyms carbinoxamine, pseudoephedrine, and hydrocodone; hydrocodone bitartrate, carbinoxamine maleate, and pseudoephedrine hydrochloride; pseudoephedrine, hydrocodone, and carbinoxamine
Therapeutic Category Antihistamine/Decongestant/Antitussive
Controlled Substance C-III
Use Symptomatic relief of cough, congestion, and rhinorrhea associated with the common cold, influenza, bronchitis, or sinusitis
Usual Dosage Oral: Relief of cough, congestion, and runny nose:
Children:
    2-10 years: Dosing based on hydrocodone content: 0.6 mg/kg/day given in 4 divided doses. Alternately, the following dosing may be used based on age:
    2-4 years: 1.25 mL every 4-6 hours; maximum dose: 7.5 mL/24 hours
    4-10 years: 2.5 mL every 4-6 hours; maximum dose: 15 mL/24 hours
    >10 years: Refer to Adults dosing
Adults: 5-10 mL every 4-6 hours; maximum dose: 30 mL/24 hours

hydrocodone, chlorpheniramine, phenylephrine, acetaminophen, and caffeine *(Discontinued)*
Hydrocodone PA® Syrup *(Discontinued)*
hydrocodone, phenylephrine, and chlorpheniramine *see* phenylephrine, hydrocodone, and chlorpheniramine *on page 748*
hydrocodone, phenylephrine, and diphenhydramine *(Discontinued)*
hydrocodone, phenylephrine, and guaifenesin *(Discontinued)*
hydrocodone, pseudoephedrine, and guaifenesin *(Discontinued)*
hydrocodone tannate and chlorpheniramine tannate *see* hydrocodone and chlorpheniramine *on page 482*
hydrocortisone acetate *see* hydrocortisone (rectal) *on page 484*
hydrocortisone, acetic acid, and propylene glycol diacetate *see* acetic acid, propylene glycol diacetate, and hydrocortisone *on page 29*
hydrocortisone and benzoyl peroxide *see* benzoyl peroxide and hydrocortisone *on page 128*
hydrocortisone and ciprofloxacin *see* ciprofloxacin and hydrocortisone *on page 223*
hydrocortisone and iodoquinol *see* iodoquinol and hydrocortisone *on page 520*
hydrocortisone and lidocaine *see* lidocaine and hydrocortisone *on page 564*
hydrocortisone and pramoxine *see* pramoxine and hydrocortisone *on page 778*
hydrocortisone and urea *see* urea and hydrocortisone *on page 964*
hydrocortisone, bacitracin, neomycin, and polymyxin B *see* bacitracin, neomycin, polymyxin B, and hydrocortisone *on page 114*
hydrocortisone butyrate *see* hydrocortisone (topical) *on page 485*

hydrocortisone, neomycin, and polymyxin B *see* neomycin, polymyxin B, and hydrocortisone *on page 663*

hydrocortisone, neomycin, colistin, and thonzonium *see* neomycin, colistin, hydrocortisone, and thonzonium *on page 662*

hydrocortisone probutate *see* hydrocortisone (topical) *on page 485*

hydrocortisone (rectal) (hye droe KOR ti sone REK tal)

Sound-Alike/Look-Alike Issues
hydrocortisone may be confused with hydrocodone, hydroxychloroquine, hydrochlorothiazide
Anusol-HC® may be confused with Anusol®
Anusol® may be confused with Anusol-HC®, Aplisol®, Aquasol®
Proctocort® may be confused with ProctoCream®
ProctoCream® may be confused with Proctocort®
HCT (occasional abbreviation for hydrocortisone) is an error-prone abbreviation (mistaken as hydrochlorothiazide)

Synonyms hydrocortisone acetate

U.S./Canadian Brand Names Anucort-HC® [US]; Anusol-HC® [US]; Anusol® HC-1 [US-OTC]; Colocort® [US]; Cortenema® [Can]; Cortifoam® [US/Can]; Encort™ [US]; Hemril®-30 [US]; Nupercainal® Hydrocortisone Cream [US-OTC]; Preparation H® Hydrocortisone [US-OTC]; Procto-Kit™ [US]; Procto-Pak™ [US]; Proctocort® [US]; ProctoCream® HC [US]; Proctosert [US]; Proctosol-HC® [US]; Proctozone-HC™ [US]; Tucks® Anti-Itch [US-OTC]

Therapeutic Category Adrenal Corticosteroid

Use Adjunctive treatment of ulcerative colitis; rectal itching; hemorrhoids

Usual Dosage Rectal: Adults: Ulcerative colitis: 10-100 mg 1-2 times/day for 2-3 weeks

Dosage Forms
Aerosol, rectal:
Cortifoam®: 10% (15 g)
Cream, rectal: 1% (30 g)
Cortizone®-10 [OTC]: 1% (30 g)
Nupercainal® Hydrocortisone Cream [OTC]: 1% (27 g, 30 g)
Preparation H® Hydrocortisone [OTC]: 1% (27 g)
Suppository, rectal: 25 mg (12s, 24s, 100s)
Anucort-HC®, Tucks® Anti-Itch [OTC]: 25 mg (12s, 24s, 100s)
Anusol-HC®, Proctosol-HC®: 25 mg (12s, 24s)
Encort™, Proctocort®: 30 mg (12s)
Hemril®-30, Proctosert: 30 mg (12s, 24s)
Suspension, rectal: 100 mg/60 mL (7s)
Colocort®: 100 mg/60 mL (1s, 7s)

hydrocortisone sodium succinate *see* hydrocortisone (systemic) *on page 484*

hydrocortisone (systemic) (hye droe KOR ti sone sis TEM ik)

Sound-Alike/Look-Alike Issues
hydrocortisone may be confused with hydrocodone, hydroxychloroquine, hydrochlorothiazide
Cortef® may be confused with Lortab®
HCT (occasional abbreviation for hydrocortisone) is an error-prone abbreviation (mistaken as hydrochlorothiazide)

Synonyms compound F; cortisol; hydrocortisone sodium succinate

U.S./Canadian Brand Names Cortef® [US/Can]; Solu-Cortef® [US/Can]

Therapeutic Category Adrenal Corticosteroid

Use Management of adrenocortical insufficiency

Usual Dosage Dose should be based on severity of disease and patient response
Acute adrenal insufficiency: I.M., I.V.:
Infants and young Children: Succinate: 1-2 mg/kg/dose bolus, then 25-150 mg/day in divided doses every 6-8 hours
Older Children: Succinate: 1-2 mg/kg bolus then 150-250 mg/day in divided doses every 6-8 hours
Adults: Succinate: 100 mg I.V. bolus, then 300 mg/day in divided doses every 8 hours or as a continuous infusion for 48 hours; once patient is stable change to oral, 50 mg every 8 hours for 6 doses, then taper to 30-50 mg/day in divided doses
Chronic adrenal corticoid insufficiency: Adults: Oral: 20-30 mg/day

Antiinflammatory or immunosuppressive:
Infants and Children:
Oral: 2.5-10 mg/kg/day **or** 75-300 mg/m^2/day every 6-8 hours
I.M., I.V.: Succinate: 1-5 mg/kg/day **or** 30-150 mg/m^2/day divided every 12-24 hours
Adolescents and Adults: Oral, I.M., I.V.: Succinate: 15-240 mg every 12 hours
Congenital adrenal hyperplasia: Oral: Initial: 10-20 mg/m^2/day in 3 divided doses; a variety of dosing schedules have been used. **Note:** Inconsistencies have occurred with liquid formulations; tablets may provide more reliable levels. Doses must be individualized by monitoring growth, bone age, and hormonal levels. Mineralocorticoid and sodium supplementation may be required based upon electrolyte regulation and plasma renin activity.
Physiologic replacement: Children:
Oral: 0.5-0.75 mg/kg/day **or** 20-25 mg/m^2/day every 8 hours
I.M.: Succinate: 0.25-0.35 mg/kg/day **or** 12-15 mg/m^2/day once daily
Shock: I.M., I.V.: Succinate:
Children: Initial: 50 mg/kg, then repeated in 4 hours and/or every 24 hours as needed
Adolescents and Adults: 500 mg to 2 g every 2-6 hours
Status asthmaticus: Children and Adults: I.V.: Succinate: 1-2 mg/kg/dose every 6 hours for 24 hours, then maintenance of 0.5-1 mg/kg every 6 hours
Adults:
Rheumatic diseases:
Intralesional, intraarticular, soft tissue injection: Acetate:
Large joints: 25 mg (up to 37.5 mg)
Small joints: 10-25 mg
Tendon sheaths: 5-12.5 mg
Soft tissue infiltration: 25-50 mg (up to 75 mg)
Bursae: 25-37.5 mg
Ganglia: 12.5-25 mg
Stress dosing (surgery) in patients known to be adrenally-suppressed or on chronic systemic steroids: I.V.:
Minor stress (ie, inguinal herniorrhaphy): 25 mg/day for 1 day
Moderate stress (ie, joint replacement, cholecystectomy): 50-75 mg/day (25 mg every 8-12 hours) for 1-2 days
Major stress (pancreatoduodenectomy, esophagogastrectomy, cardiac surgery): 100-150 mg/day (50 mg every 8-12 hours) for 2-3 days

Dosage Forms
Injection, powder for reconstitution:
Solu-Cortef®: 100 mg, 250 mg, 500 mg, 1 g
Tablet: 20 mg
Cortef®: 5 mg, 10 mg, 20 mg

hydrocortisone (topical) (hye droe KOR ti sone TOP i kal)

Sound-Alike/Look-Alike Issues
hydrocortisone may be confused with hydrocodone, hydroxychloroquine, hydrochlorothiazide
Cortizone® may be confused with cortisone
HCT (occasional abbreviation for hydrocortisone) is an error-prone abbreviation (mistaken as hydrochlorothiazide)
Hytone® may be confused with Vytone®

Synonyms hydrocortisone butyrate; hydrocortisone probutate; hydrocortisone valerate

U.S./Canadian Brand Names Aquacort® [Can]; Aquanil™ HC [US-OTC]; Beta-HC® [US]; Caldecort® [US-OTC]; Cetacort® [US]; Cortaid® Intensive Therapy [US-OTC]; Cortaid® Maximum Strength [US-OTC]; Cortaid® Sensitive Skin [US-OTC]; Cortamed® [Can]; Corticool® [US-OTC]; Cortizone®-10 Maximum Strength [US-OTC]; Cortizone®-10 Plus Maximum Strength [US-OTC]; Cortizone®-10 Quick Shot [US-OTC]; Dermarest Dricort® [US-OTC]; Dermtex® HC [US-OTC]; EarSol® HC [US]; Emo-Cort® [Can]; Hycort™ [Can]; Hyderm [Can]; HydroVal® [Can]; HydroZone Plus [US-OTC]; Hytone® [US]; IvySoothe® [US-OTC]; Locoid Lipocream® [US]; Locoid® [US/Can]; Nutracort® [US]; Pandel® [US]; Post Peel Healing Balm [US-OTC]; Prevex® HC [Can]; Sarna® HC [Can]; Sarnol®-HC [US-OTC]; Texacort® [US]; Westcort® [US/Can]

Therapeutic Category Corticosteroid, Topical

Use Relief of inflammation of corticosteroid-responsive dermatoses (low and medium potency topical corticosteroid)

◄ **Usual Dosage** Topical: Children >2 years and Adults: Dermatosis: Apply to affected area 2-4 times/day (Buteprate: Apply once or twice daily). Therapy should be discontinued when control is achieved; if no improvement is seen, reassessment of diagnosis may be necessary.

Dosage Forms

Cream, topical: 0.2% (15 g, 45 g, 60 g); 0.5% (9 g, 30 g, 60 g); 1% (1.5 g, 30 g, 114 g, 454 g); 2.5% (20 g, 30 g, 454 g)

Anusol-HC®: 2.5% (30 g)

Caldecort® [OTC], HydroZone Plus [OTC], IvySoothe® [OTC], Proctocort®, Procto-Pak™, Procto-Kit™: 1% (30 g)

Cortaid® Intensive Therapy [OTC]: 1% (60 g)

Cortaid® Maximum Strength [OTC]: 1% (15 g, 30 g, 40 g, 60 g)

Cortaid® Sensitive Skin [OTC]: 0.5% (15 g)

Cortizone®-10 Maximum Strength [OTC]: 1% (15 g, 30 g, 60 g)

Cortizone®-10 Plus Maximum Strength [OTC]: 1% (30 g, 60 g)

Dermarest® Dricort® [OTC]: 1% (15 g, 30 g)

Hytone®: 2.5% (30 g, 60 g)

Locoid®, Locoid Lipocream®: 0.1% (15 g, 45 g)

Pandel®: 0.1% (15 g, 45 g, 80 g)

Post Peel Healing Balm [OTC]: 1% (23 g)

ProctoCream® HC, Proctosol-HC®, Proctozone-HC™: 2.5% (30 g)

Westcort®: 0.2% (15 g, 45 g, 60 g)

Gel, topical:

Corticool®: 1% (45 g)

Lotion, topical: 1% (120 mL); 2.5% (60 mL)

Aquanil™ HC [OTC], HydroZone Plus: 1% (120 mL)

Beta-HC®, Sarnol®-HC [OTC]: 1% (60 mL)

Hytone®: 2.5% (60 mL)

Nutracort®: 1% (60 mL, 120 mL); 2.5% (60 mL, 120 mL)

Ointment, topical: 0.2% (15 g, 45 g, 60 g); 0.5% (30 g); 1% (30 g, 454 g); 2.5% (20 g, 30 g, 454 g)

Anusol® HC-1 [OTC]: 1% (21 g)

Cortaid® Maximum Strength [OTC]: 1% (15 g, 30 g)

Cortizone®-10 Maximum Strength [OTC]: 1% (30 g, 60 g)

Locoid®: 0.1% (15 g, 45 g)

Westcort®: 0.2% (15 g, 45 g, 60 g)

Solution, otic:

EarSol® HC: 1% (30 mL)

Solution, topical: 0.1% (20 mL, 60 mL); 2.5% (30 mL)

Texacort®: 2.5% (30 mL)

Locoid®: 0.1% (20 mL, 60 mL)

Solution, topical spray:

Cortaid® Intensive Therapy [OTC]: 1% (60 mL)

Cortizone®-10 Quick Shot [OTC]: 1% (44 mL)

Dermtex® HC [OTC]: 1% (52 mL)

hydrocortisone valerate see hydrocortisone (topical) on page 485

HydroDIURIL® (Discontinued) see hydrochlorothiazide on page 479

Hydro DP (Discontinued)

HydroFed (Discontinued)

Hydrogesic® (Discontinued) see hydrocodone and acetaminophen on page 481

Hydro-GP (Discontinued)

Hydromet® [US] see hydrocodone and homatropine on page 482

Hydromorph Contin® [Can] see hydromorphone on page 486

Hydromorph-IR® [Can] see hydromorphone on page 486

hydromorphone (hye droe MOR fone)

Sound-Alike/Look-Alike Issues

Dilaudid® may be confused with Demerol®, Dilantin®

HYDROmorphone may be confused with morphine; significant overdoses have occurred when hydromorphone products have been inadvertently administered instead of morphine sulfate. Commercially available prefilled syringes of both products looks similar and are often stored in close proximity to each other. **Note:** Hydromorphone 1 mg oral is approximately equal to morphine 4 mg oral; hydromorphone 1 mg I.V. is approximately equal to morphine 5 mg I.V.

Dilaudid®, Dilaudid-HP®: Extreme caution should be taken to avoid confusing the highly-concentrated (Dilaudid-HP®) injection with the less-concentrated (Dilaudid®) injectable product.

Synonyms dihydromorphinone; hydromorphone hydrochloride

Tall-Man HYDROmorphone

U.S./Canadian Brand Names Dilaudid-HP-Plus® [Can]; Dilaudid-HP® [US/Can]; Dilaudid-XP® [Can]; Dilaudid® Sterile Powder [Can]; Dilaudid® [US/Can]; Hydromorph Contin® [Can]; Hydromorph-IR® [Can]; Hydromorphone HP [Can]; Hydromorphone HP® 10 [Can]; Hydromorphone HP® 20 [Can]; Hydromorphone HP® 50 [Can]; Hydromorphone HP® Forte [Can]; Hydromorphone Hydrochloride Injection, USP [Can]; PMS-Hydromorphone [Can]

Therapeutic Category Analgesic, Narcotic

Controlled Substance C-II

Use Management of moderate-to-severe pain

Usual Dosage
Acute pain (moderate to severe): **Note:** These are guidelines and do not represent the maximum doses that may be required in all patients. Doses should be titrated to pain relief/prevention.
Children ≥6 months and <50 kg:
Oral: 0.03-0.08 mg/kg/dose every 3-4 hours as needed
I.V.: 0.015 mg/kg/dose every 3-6 hours as needed
Children >50 kg and Adults:
Oral: Initial: Opiate-naive: 2-4 mg every 3-6 hours as needed; elderly/debilitated patients may require lower doses; patients with prior opiate exposure may require higher initial doses; usual dosage range: 2-8 mg every 3-4 hours as needed
I.V.: Initial: Opiate-naive: 0.2-0.6 mg every 2-3 hours as needed; patients with prior opiate exposure may tolerate higher initial doses
Patient-controlled analgesia (PCA): (Opiate-naive: Consider lower end of dosing range)
Usual concentration: 0.2 mg/mL
Demand dose: Usual: 0.1-0.2 mg; range: 0.05-0.5 mg
Lockout interval: 5-15 minutes
4-hour limit: 4-6 mg
Epidural:
Bolus dose: 1-1.5 mg
Infusion concentration: 0.05-0.075 mg/mL
Infusion rate: 0.04-0.4 mg/hour
Demand dose: 0.15 mg
Lockout interval: 30 minutes
I.M., SubQ: **Note:** I.M. use may result in variable absorption and a lag time to peak effect.
Initial: Opiate-naive: 0.8-1 mg every 4-6 hours as needed; patients with prior opiate exposure may require higher initial doses; usual dosage range: 1-2 mg every 3-6 hours as needed
Rectal: 3 mg every 4-8 hours as needed

Chronic pain: Adults: Oral: **Note:** Patients taking opioids chronically may become tolerant and require doses higher than the usual dosage range to maintain the desired effect. Tolerance can be managed by appropriate dose titration. There is no optimal or maximal dose for hydromorphone in chronic pain. The appropriate dose is one that relieves pain throughout its dosing interval without causing unmanageable side effects.
Controlled release formulation (Hydromorph Contin®, not available in U.S.): 3-30 mg every 12 hours.
Note: A patient's hydromorphone requirement should be established using prompt release formulations; conversion to long acting products may be considered when chronic, continuous treatment is required. Higher dosages should be reserved for use only in opioid-tolerant patients.

Dosage Forms [CAN] = Canadian brand name
Capsule, controlled release:
Hydromorph Contin® [CAN]: 3 mg, 6 mg, 12 mg, 18 mg, 24 mg, 30 mg [not available in U.S.]
Injection, powder for reconstitution:
Dilaudid-HP®: 250 mg
Injection, solution: 1 mg/mL (1 mL); 2 mg/mL (1 mL, 20 mL); 4 mg/mL (1 mL)
Dilaudid®: 1 mg/mL (1 mL); 2 mg/mL (1 mL, 20 mL); 4 mg/mL (1 mL)
Injection, solution [preservative free]: 10 mg/mL (1 mL, 5 mL, 50 mL)
Dilaudid-HP®: 10 mg/mL (1 mL, 5 mL, 50 mL)

▶

◀ **Liquid, oral:**
Dilaudid®: 1 mg/mL (480 mL)
Powder, for prescription compounding: 100% (15 grain)
Suppository, rectal: 3 mg
Dilaudid®: 3 mg (6s)
Tablet: 2 mg, 4 mg, 8 mg
Dilaudid®: 2 mg, 4 mg, 8 mg

Hydromorphone HP [Can] *see* hydromorphone *on page 486*
Hydromorphone HP® 10 [Can] *see* hydromorphone *on page 486*
Hydromorphone HP® 20 [Can] *see* hydromorphone *on page 486*
Hydromorphone HP® 50 [Can] *see* hydromorphone *on page 486*
Hydromorphone HP® Forte [Can] *see* hydromorphone *on page 486*
hydromorphone hydrochloride *see* hydromorphone *on page 486*
Hydromorphone Hydrochloride Injection, USP [Can] *see* hydromorphone *on page 486*
Hydromox® *(Discontinued)*
Hydron CP [US] *see* phenylephrine, hydrocodone, and chlorpheniramine *on page 748*
Hydron PSC *(Discontinued)*
Hydro-Par® *(Discontinued) see* hydrochlorothiazide *on page 479*
Hydro-PC II [US] *see* phenylephrine, hydrocodone, and chlorpheniramine *on page 748*
Hydro PC II Plus [US] *see* phenylephrine, hydrocodone, and chlorpheniramine *on page 748*
hydroquinol *see* hydroquinone *on page 488*

hydroquinone (HYE droe kwin one)

Sound-Alike/Look-Alike Issues
Eldopaque® may be confused with Eldoquin®
Eldoquin® may be confused with Eldopaque®
Eldopaque Forte® may be confused with Eldoquin Forte®
Eldoquin Forte® may be confused with Eldopaque Forte®

Synonyms hydroquinol; quinol

U.S./Canadian Brand Names Aclaro PD™ [US]; Alphaquin HP® [US]; Claripel™ [US]; Dermarest® Skin Correction Cream Plus [US-OTC]; Eldopaque Forte® [US]; Eldopaque® [US-OTC/Can]; Eldoquin Forte® [US]; Eldoquin® [US-OTC/Can]; EpiQuin™ Micro [US]; Esoterica® Regular [US-OTC]; Glyquin-XM™ [US/Can]; Glyquin® [US]; Lustra-AF™ [US]; Lustra® [US/Can]; Melanex® [US]; Melpaque HP® [US]; Melquin HP® [US]; Melquin-3® [US]; NeoStrata® AHA [US-OTC]; NeoStrata® HQ [Can]; Nuquin HP® [US]; Palmer's® Skin Success Eventone® Fade Cream [US-OTC]; Solaquin Forte® [US/Can]; Solaquin® [US-OTC/Can]; Ultraquin™ [Can]

Therapeutic Category Topical Skin Product

Use Gradual bleaching of hyperpigmented skin conditions

Usual Dosage Topical: Children >12 years and Adults: Apply thin layer and rub in twice daily

Dosage Forms

Cream, topical: 4% (30 g)
Alphaquin HP®: 4% (30 g, 60 g)
Eldoquin® [OTC]: 2% (15 g, 30 g)
Eldoquin Forte®, EpiQuin™ Micro, Lustra®: 4% (30 g)
Esoterica® Regular [OTC]: 2% (85 g)
Melquin HP®: 4% (15 g, 30 g)
Cream, topical [with sunscreen]: 4% (30 g)
Claripel™: 4% (30 g, 45 g)
Dermarest® Skin Correcting Cream Plus [OTC]: 2% (85 g)
Eldopaque® [OTC]: 2% (15 g, 30 g)
Eldopaque Forte®, Glyquin®, Glyquin-XM™, Solaquin Forte®: 4% (30 g)
Lustra-AF™: 4% (30 g, 60 g)
Melpaque HP®: 4% (15 g, 30 g)
Nuquin HP®: 4% (15 g, 30 g, 60 g)
Palmer's® Skin Success Eventone® Fade Cream [OTC]: 2% (81 g, 132 g)
Solaquin® [OTC]: 2% (30 g)
Emulsion, topical:
Aclaro PD™: 4% (42.5 g)

Gel, topical:
  NeoStrata® AHA [OTC]: 2% (45 g)
Gel, topical [with sunscreen]: 4% (30 g)
  Nuquin HP: 4% (15 g, 30 g)
  Solaquin Forte®: 4% (30 g)
Solution, topical:
  Melanex®, Melquin-3®: 3% (30 mL)

hydroquinone, fluocinolone acetonide, and tretinoin *see* fluocinolone, hydroquinone, and tretinoin *on page 409*

Hydrotropine® *(Discontinued) see* hydrocodone and homatropine *on page 482*

Hydro-Tussin™-CBX *(Discontinued)*

Hydro-Tussin™ DHC *(Discontinued) see* pseudoephedrine, dihydrocodeine, and chlorpheniramine *on page 803*

Hydro-Tussin™ DM [US] *see* guaifenesin and dextromethorphan *on page 454*

Hydro-Tussin™ EXP *(Discontinued) see* dihydrocodeine, pseudoephedrine, and guaifenesin *on page 299*

Hydro-Tussin™ HC *(Discontinued)*

Hydro-Tussin™ HD *(Discontinued)*

Hydro-Tussin™ XP *(Discontinued)*

HydroVal® [Can] *see* hydrocortisone (topical) *on page 485*

hydroxyamphetamine and tropicamide (hye droks ee am FET a meen & troe PIK a mide)

Synonyms hydroxyamphetamine hydrobromide and tropicamide; tropicamide and hydroxyamphetamine

U.S./Canadian Brand Names Paremyd® [US]

Therapeutic Category Adrenergic Agonist Agent, Ophthalmic

Use Short-term pupil dilation for diagnostic procedures and exams

Usual Dosage Ophthalmic: Adults: Instill 1-2 drops into conjunctival sac(s)

Dosage Forms
  Solution, ophthalmic:
    Paremyd®: Hydroxyamphetamine 1% and tropicamide 0.25% (15 mL)

hydroxyamphetamine hydrobromide and tropicamide *see* hydroxyamphetamine and tropicamide *on page 489*

4-hydroxybutyrate *see* sodium oxybate *on page 877*

hydroxycarbamide *see* hydroxyurea *on page 490*

hydroxychloroquine (hye droks ee KLOR oh kwin)

Sound-Alike/Look-Alike Issues
  hydroxychloroquine may be confused with hydrocortisone
  Plaquenil® may be confused with Platinol®

Synonyms hydroxychloroquine sulfate

U.S./Canadian Brand Names Apo-Hydroxyquine® [Can]; Gen-Hydroxychloroquine [Can]; Plaquenil® [US/Can]

Therapeutic Category Aminoquinoline (Antimalarial)

Use Suppression and treatment of acute attacks of malaria; treatment of systemic lupus erythematosus (SLE) and rheumatoid arthritis

Usual Dosage Note: Hydroxychloroquine sulfate 200 mg is equivalent to 155 mg hydroxychloroquine base and 250 mg chloroquine phosphate. Second-line alternative treatment (chloroquine is preferred).
Oral:
Children:
  Chemoprophylaxis of malaria: 5 mg/kg (base) once weekly; should not exceed the recommended adult dose; begin 2 weeks before exposure; continue for 4 weeks (per CDC guidelines) after leaving endemic area; if suppressive therapy is not begun prior to the exposure, double the initial dose and give in 2 doses, 6 hours apart and continue treatment for 8 weeks
  Acute attack: 10 mg/kg (base) initially, followed by 5 mg/kg at 6, 24, and 48 hours
Adults:
  Chemoprophylaxis of malaria: 310 mg (base) weekly on same day each week; begin 2 weeks before exposure; continue for 4 weeks (per CDC guidelines) after leaving endemic area; if suppressive ▶

◀ therapy is not begun prior to the exposure, double the initial dose and give in 2 doses, 6 hours apart and continue treatment for 8 weeks

Acute attack: 620 mg (base) initially, followed by 310 mg (base) at 6, 24, and 48 hours

Rheumatoid arthritis: Initial: 310-465 mg/day (base) taken with food or milk; increase dose gradually until optimum response level is reached; usually after 4-12 weeks dose should be reduced by 1/2 to a maintenance dose of 155-310 mg/day (base)

Lupus erythematosus: 310 mg (base) every day or twice daily for several weeks-months depending on response; 155-310 mg/day (base) for prolonged maintenance therapy

Dosage Forms
Tablet: 200 mg
Plaquenil®: 200 mg

hydroxychloroquine sulfate see hydroxychloroquine on page 489
hydroxydaunomycin hydrochloride see doxorubicin on page 322
1α-hydroxyergocalciferol see doxercalciferol on page 321
hydroxyethylcellulose see artificial tears on page 95
hydroxyethyl starch see hetastarch on page 473
hydroxyldaunorubicin hydrochloride see doxorubicin on page 322

hydroxypropyl cellulose (hye droks ee PROE pil SEL yoo lose)
U.S./Canadian Brand Names Lacrisert® [US/Can]
Therapeutic Category Ophthalmic Agent, Miscellaneous
Use Dry eyes (moderate to severe)
Usual Dosage Ophthalmic: Adults: Apply once daily into the inferior cul-de-sac beneath the base of tarsus, not in apposition to the cornea nor beneath the eyelid at the level of the tarsal plate
Dosage Forms
Insert, ophthalmic [preservative free]:
Lacrisert®: 5 mg

hydroxypropyl methylcellulose (hye droks ee PROE pil meth il SEL yoo lose)
Sound-Alike/Look-Alike Issues
Isopto® Tears may be confused with Isoptin®
Synonyms gonioscopic ophthalmic solution; hypromellose
U.S./Canadian Brand Names Cellugel® [US]; GenTeal® Mild [US-OTC]; GenTeal® [US-OTC/Can]; Gonak™ [US-OTC]; Goniosoft™ [US]; Isopto® Tears [US-OTC/Can]; Tearisol® [US-OTC]; Tears Again® MC [US-OTC]
Therapeutic Category Ophthalmic Agent, Miscellaneous
Use Relief of burning and minor irritation due to dry eyes; diagnostic agent in gonioscopic examination
Usual Dosage Ophthalmic: Adults: Dry eyes: Instill 1-2 drops in affected eye(s) as needed
Dosage Forms
Gel, ophthalmic:
GenTeal® [OTC]: 0.3% (10 mL)
Solution, ophthalmic: 0.4% (15 mL)
GenTeal® [OTC]: 0.3% (15 mL, 25 mL)
GenTeal® Mild [OTC]: 0.2% (15 mL, 25 mL)
Gonak™ [OTC], Goniosoft™: 2.5% (15 mL)
Isopto® Tears [OTC], Tearisol® [OTC]: 0.5% (15 mL)
Tears Again® MC [OTC]: 0.3% (15 mL)
Solution, ophthalmic [for injection]:
Cellugel®: 2% (1 mL)

9-hydroxy-risperidone see paliperidone on page 715

hydroxyurea (hye droks ee yoor EE a)
Sound-Alike/Look-Alike Issues
hydroxyurea may be confused with hydrOXYzine
Synonyms hydroxycarbamide
U.S./Canadian Brand Names Apo-Hydroxyurea® [Can]; Droxia® [US]; Gen-Hydroxyurea [Can]; Hydrea® [US/Can]; Mylocel™ [US]

Therapeutic Category Antineoplastic Agent

Use Treatment of melanoma, refractory chronic myelocytic leukemia (CML), relapsed and refractory metastatic ovarian cancer; radiosensitizing agent in the treatment of squamous cell head and neck cancer (excluding lip cancer); adjunct in the management of sickle cell patients who have had at least three painful crises in the previous 12 months (to reduce frequency of these crises and the need for blood transfusions)

Usual Dosage Oral (refer to individual protocols): All doses should be based on ideal or actual body weight, whichever is less:

Adults: Dose should always be titrated to patient response and WBC counts; usual oral doses range from 10-30 mg/kg/day or 500-3000 mg/day; if WBC count falls to <2500 cells/mm^3, or the platelet count to <100,000/mm^3, therapy should be stopped for at least 3 days and resumed when values rise toward normal

Solid tumors:
Intermittent therapy: 80 mg/kg as a single dose every third day
Continuous therapy: 20-30 mg/kg/day given as a single dose/day
Concomitant therapy with irradiation: 80 mg/kg as a single dose every third day starting at least 7 days before initiation of irradiation
Resistant chronic myelocytic leukemia: Continuous therapy: 20-30 mg/kg once daily
Sickle cell anemia (moderate/severe disease): Initial: 15 mg/kg/day, increased by 5 mg/kg every 12 weeks if blood counts are in an acceptable range until the maximum tolerated dose of 35 mg/kg/day is achieved or the dose that does not produce toxic effects

Acceptable range:
Neutrophils ≥2500 cells/mm^3
Platelets ≥95,000/mm^3
Hemoglobin >5.3 g/dL, and
Reticulocytes ≥95,000/mm^3 if the hemoglobin concentration is <9 g/dL

Toxic range:
Neutrophils <2000 cells/mm^3
Platelets <80,000/mm^3
Hemoglobin <4.5 g/dL
Reticulocytes <80,000/mm^3 if the hemoglobin concentration is <9 g/dL

Monitor for toxicity every 2 weeks; if toxicity occurs, stop treatment until the bone marrow recovers; restart at 2.5 mg/kg/day less than the dose at which toxicity occurs; if no toxicity occurs over the next 12 weeks, then the subsequent dose should be increased by 2.5 mg/kg/day; reduced dosage of hydroxyurea alternating with erythropoietin may decrease myelotoxicity and increase levels of fetal hemoglobin in patients who have not been helped by hydroxyurea alone

Dosage Forms
Capsule: 500 mg
Droxia®: 200 mg, 300 mg, 400 mg
Hydrea®: 500 mg
Tablet:
Mylocel™: 1000 mg

hydroxyzine (hye DROKS i zeen)

Sound-Alike/Look-Alike Issues
hydrOXYzine may be confused with hydrALAZINE, hydroxyurea
Atarax® may be confused with amoxicillin, Ativan®
Vistaril® may be confused with Restoril®, Versed, Zestril®

Synonyms hydroxyzine hydrochloride; hydroxyzine pamoate

Tall-Man hydroOXYzine

U.S./Canadian Brand Names Apo-Hydroxyzine® [Can]; Atarax® [Can]; Hydroxyzine Hydrochloride Injection, USP [Can]; Novo-Hydroxyzin [Can]; PMS-Hydroxyzine [Can]; Vistaril® [US/Can]

Therapeutic Category Antiemetic; Antihistamine

Use Treatment of anxiety; preoperative sedative; antipruritic

Usual Dosage
Children:
Preoperative sedation:
Oral: 0.6 mg/kg/dose
I.M.: 0.5-1 mg/kg/dose
Pruritus, anxiety: Oral:
<6 years: 50 mg daily in divided doses
≥6 years: 50-100 mg daily in divided doses

▶

◀ Adults:
Anxiety: Oral, I.M.: 50-100 mg 4 times/day
Preoperative sedation:
Oral: 50-100 mg
I.M.: 25-100 mg
Pruritus: Oral, I.M.: 25 mg 3-4 times/day
Dosage Forms
Capsule: 25 mg, 50 mg, 100 mg
Vistaril®: 25 mg, 50 mg
Injection, solution: 25 mg/mL (1 mL); 50 mg/mL (1 mL, 2 mL, 10 mL)
Syrup: 10 mg/5 mL
Tablet: 10 mg, 25 mg, 50 mg

hydroxyzine hydrochloride *see* hydroxyzine *on page 491*
Hydroxyzine Hydrochloride Injection, USP [Can] *see* hydroxyzine *on page 491*
hydroxyzine pamoate *see* hydroxyzine *on page 491*
HydroZone Plus [US-OTC] *see* hydrocortisone (topical) *on page 485*
Hyflex-DS® *(Discontinued)* *see* acetaminophen and phenyltoloxamine *on page 22*
Hygroton® *(Discontinued)* *see* chlorthalidone *on page 214*
Hylaform® [US] *see* hyaluronate and derivatives *on page 476*
Hylaform® Plus [US] *see* hyaluronate and derivatives *on page 476*
hylan polymers *see* hyaluronate and derivatives *on page 476*
Hylenex™ [US] *see* hyaluronidase *on page 477*
Hylira™ [US] *see* hyaluronate and derivatives *on page 476*
Hylutin Injection *(Discontinued)*
hyoscine butylbromide *see* scopolamine derivatives *on page 858*
hyoscine hydrobromide *see* scopolamine derivatives *on page 858*

hyoscyamine (hye oh SYE a meen)

Sound-Alike/Look-Alike Issues
Anaspaz® may be confused with Anaprox®, Antispas®
Levbid® may be confused with Lithobid®, Lopid®, Lorabid®
Levsinex® may be confused with Lanoxin®
Synonyms *l*-hyoscyamine sulfate; hyoscyamine sulfate
U.S./Canadian Brand Names Anaspaz® [US]; Cystospaz® [US/Can]; Hyosyne [US]; Levbid® [US]; Levsin/SL® [US]; Levsinex® [US]; Levsin® [US/Can]; Symax SL [US]; Symax SR [US]
Therapeutic Category Anticholinergic Agent
Use
Oral: Adjunctive therapy for peptic ulcers, irritable bowel, neurogenic bladder/bowel; treatment of infant colic, GI tract disorders caused by spasm; to reduce rigidity, tremors, sialorrhea, and hyperhidrosis associated with parkinsonism; as a drying agent in acute rhinitis
Injection: Preoperative antimuscarinic to reduce secretions and block cardiac vagal inhibitory reflexes; to improve radiologic visibility of the kidneys; symptomatic relief of biliary and renal colic; reduce GI motility to facilitate diagnostic procedures (ie, endoscopy, hypotonic duodenography); reduce pain and hypersecretion in pancreatitis, certain cases of partial heart block associated with vagal activity; reversal of neuromuscular blockade
Usual Dosage
Oral: Children: Gastrointestinal disorders: Dose as listed, based on age and weight (kg) using 0.125 mg/mL drops; repeat dose every 4 hours as needed:
Children <2 years:
3.4 kg: 4 drops; maximum: 24 drops/24 hours
5 kg: 5 drops; maximum: 30 drops/24 hours
7 kg: 6 drops; maximum: 36 drops/24 hours
10 kg: 8 drops; maximum: 48 drops/24 hours
Oral, S.L.:
Children 2-12 years: Gastrointestinal disorders: Dose as listed, based on age and weight (kg); repeat dose every 4 hours as needed:
10 kg: 0.031-0.033 mg; maximum: 0.75 mg/24 hours

20 kg: 0.0625 mg; maximum: 0.75 mg/24 hours
40 kg: 0.0938 mg; maximum: 0.75 mg/24 hours
50 kg: 0.125 mg; maximum: 0.75 mg/24 hours
Children >12 years and Adults: Gastrointestinal disorders: 0.125-0.25 mg every 4 hours or as needed (before meals or food); maximum: 1.5 mg/24 hours
Cystospaz®: 0.15-0.3 mg up to 4 times/day
Oral (timed release): Children >12 years and Adults: Gastrointestinal disorders: 0.375-0.75 mg every 12 hours; maximum: 1.5 mg/24 hours
I.M., I.V., SubQ: Children >12 years and Adults: Gastrointestinal disorders: 0.25-0.5 mg; may repeat as needed up to 4 times/day, at 4-hour intervals
I.V.: Children >2 year and Adults: I.V.: Preanesthesia: 5 mcg/kg given 30-60 minutes prior to induction of anesthesia or at the time preoperative narcotics or sedatives are administered
I.V.: Adults: Diagnostic procedures: 0.25-0.5 mg given 5-10 minutes prior to procedure
To reduce drug-induced bradycardia during surgery: 0.125 mg; repeat as needed
To reverse neuromuscular blockade: 0.2 mg for every 1 mg neostigmine (or the physostigmine/pyridostigmine equivalent)

Dosage Forms
Capsule, timed release: 0.375 mg
Levsinex®: 0.375 mg
Elixir: 0.125 mg/5 mL
Hyosyne, Levsin®: 0.125 mg/5 mL
Injection, solution: 0.5 mg/mL (1 mL)
Levsin®: 0.5 mg/mL (1 mL)
Solution, oral [drops]: 0.125 mg/mL
Hyosyne, Levsin®: 0.125 mg/mL
Tablet: 0.125 mg
Anaspaz®, Levsin®: 0.125 mg
Tablet, extended release: 0.375 mg
Levbid®, Symax SR: 0.375 mg
Tablet, sublingual: 0.125 mg
Levsin/SL®, Symax SL: 0.125 mg

hyoscyamine, atropine, scopolamine, and phenobarbital
(hye oh SYE a meen, A troe peen, skoe POL a meen, & fee noe BAR bi tal)
Sound-Alike/Look-Alike Issues
Donnatal® may be confused with Donnagel®
Synonyms atropine, hyoscyamine, scopolamine, and phenobarbital; belladonna alkaloids with phenobarbital; phenobarbital, hyoscyamine, atropine, and scopolamine; scopolamine, hyoscyamine, atropine, and phenobarbital
U.S./Canadian Brand Names Donnatal Extentabs® [US]; Donnatal® [US]
Therapeutic Category Anticholinergic Agent
Use Adjunct in treatment of irritable bowel syndrome, acute enterocolitis, duodenal ulcer
Usual Dosage Oral:
Children: Donnatal® elixir: To be given every 4-6 hours; initial dose based on weight:
4.5 kg: 0.5 mL every 4 hours **or** 0.75 mL every 6 hours
10 kg: 1 mL every 4 hours **or** 1.5 mL every 6 hours
14 kg: 1.5 mL every 4 hours **or** 2 mL every 6 hours
23 kg: 2.5 mL every 4 hours **or** 3.8 mL every 6 hours
34 kg: 3.8 mL every 4 hours **or** 5 mL every 6 hours
≥45 kg: 5 mL every 4 hours **or** 7.5 mL every 6 hours
Adults:
Donnatal®: 1-2 tablets or 5-10 mL of elixir 3-4 times/day
Donnatal Extentabs®: 1 tablet every 12 hours; may increase to 1 tablet every 8 hours if needed
Dosage Forms
Elixir:
Donnatal®: Hyoscyamine 0.1037 mg, atropine 0.0194 mg, scopolamine 0.0065 mg, and phenobarbital 16.2 mg per 5 mL
Tablet: Hyoscyamine 0.1037 mg, atropine 0.0194 mg, scopolamine 0.0065 mg, and phenobarbital 16.2 mg
Donnatal®: Hyoscyamine 0.1037 mg, atropine 0.0194 mg, scopolamine 0.0065 mg, and phenobarbital 16.2 mg

Tablet, extended release:
Donnatal Extentabs®: Hyoscyamine 0.3111 mg, atropine 0.0582 mg, scopolamine 0.0195 mg, and phenobarbital 48.6 mg

hyoscyamine sulfate *see* hyoscyamine *on page 492*
Hyosyne [US] *see* hyoscyamine *on page 492*
Hy-Pam® Oral *(Discontinued)* *see* hydroxyzine *on page 491*
Hypaque™ Sodium [US] *see* diatrizoate sodium *on page 289*
Hyperab® *(Discontinued)* *see* rabies immune globulin (human) *on page 815*
hyperal *see* total parenteral nutrition *on page 938*
hyperalimentation *see* total parenteral nutrition *on page 938*
Hypercare™ [US] *see* aluminum chloride hexahydrate *on page 53*
HyperHep B® [Can] *see* hepatitis B immune globulin *on page 470*
HyperHEP B™ S/D [US] *see* hepatitis B immune globulin *on page 470*
HyperRAB™ S/D [US/Can] *see* rabies immune globulin (human) *on page 815*
HyperRHO™ S/D Full Dose [US] *see* Rh$_o$(D) immune globulin *on page 829*
HyperRHO™ S/D Mini Dose [US] *see* Rh$_o$(D) immune globulin *on page 829*
Hyper-Sal™ [US] *see* sodium chloride *on page 873*
Hyperstat® *(Discontinued)* *see* diazoxide *on page 290*
HyperTET™ S/D [US/Can] *see* tetanus immune globulin (human) *on page 913*
Hyphed *(Discontinued)*
Hy-Phen® *(Discontinued)* *see* hydrocodone and acetaminophen *on page 481*
HypoTears [US-OTC] *see* artificial tears *on page 95*
HypoTears PF [US-OTC] *see* artificial tears *on page 95*
HypRho®-D *(Discontinued)*
HypRho®-D Mini-Dose *(Discontinued)*
Hyprogest® 250 *(Discontinued)*
hypromellose *see* hydroxypropyl methylcellulose *on page 490*
Hytakerol® *(Discontinued)*
HyTan™ *(Discontinued)* *see* hydrocodone and chlorpheniramine *on page 482*
Hytone® [US] *see* hydrocortisone (topical) *on page 485*
Hytrin® [Can] *see* terazosin *on page 909*
Hytrin® *(Discontinued)* *see* terazosin *on page 909*
Hyzaar® [US/Can] *see* losartan and hydrochlorothiazide *on page 578*
Hyzaar® DS [Can] *see* losartan and hydrochlorothiazide *on page 578*
Hyzine® *(Discontinued)* *see* hydroxyzine *on page 491*

ibandronate (eye BAN droh nate)
Synonyms ibandronate sodium; ibandronic acid; NSC-722623
U.S./Canadian Brand Names Bondronat® [Can]; Boniva® [US]
Therapeutic Category Bisphosphonate Derivative
Use Treatment and prevention of osteoporosis in postmenopausal females
Usual Dosage
Oral:
Treatment of postmenopausal osteoporosis: 2.5 mg/day or 150 mg once a month
Prevention of postmenopausal osteoporosis: 2.5 mg/day; 150 mg once a month may be considered
I.V.: Treatment of postmenopausal osteoporosis: 3 mg every 3 months
Dosage Forms
Injection, solution:
Boniva®: 1 mg/mL (3 mL)
Tablet:
Boniva®: 2.5 mg [once-daily formulation]; 150 mg [once-monthly formulation]

ibandronate sodium *see* ibandronate *on page 494*
ibandronic acid *see* ibandronate *on page 494*
Iberet® [US-OTC] *see* vitamins (multiple/oral) *on page 983*

Iberet®-500 [US-OTC] *see* vitamins (multiple/oral) *on page 983*
ibidomide hydrochloride *see* labetalol *on page 541*

ibritumomab (ib ri TYOO mo mab)

Synonyms ibritumomab tiuxetan; IDEC-Y2B8; In-111 ibritumomab; In-111 zevalin; Y-90 ibritumomab; Y-90 zevalin

U.S./Canadian Brand Names Zevalin® [US/Can]

Therapeutic Category Antineoplastic Agent, Monoclonal Antibody; Radiopharmaceutical

Use Treatment of relapsed or refractory low-grade, follicular, or transformed B-cell non-Hodgkin lymphoma

Usual Dosage I.V.: Adults: **Note:** Premedication with acetaminophen and diphenhydramine is recommended for rituximab infusions. Ibritumomab is administered **only** as part of the Zevalin® therapeutic regimen (a combined treatment regimen with rituximab). The regimen consists of two steps:

Step 1:
Rituximab infusion: 250 mg/m^2 at an initial rate of 50 mg/hour. If hypersensitivity or infusion-related events do not occur, increase infusion in increments of 50 mg/hour every 30 minutes, to a maximum of 400 mg/hour. Infusions should be temporarily slowed or interrupted if hypersensitivity or infusion-related events occur. The infusion may be resumed at one-half the previous rate upon improvement of symptoms.

In-111 ibritumomab infusion: Within 4 hours of the completion of rituximab infusion, inject 5 mCi (1.6 mg total antibody dose) over 10 minutes.

Biodistribution of In-111 ibritumomab should be assessed by imaging at 48-72 hours postinjection. Optional additional imaging may be performed to resolve ambiguities. If biodistribution is not acceptable, the patient should not proceed to Step 2.

Step 2 (initiated 7-9 days following Step 1):
Rituximab infusion: 250 mg/m^2 at an initial rate of 100 mg/hour (50 mg/hour if infusion-related events occurred with the first infusion). If hypersensitivity or infusion-related events do not occur, increase infusion in increments of 100 mg/hour every 30 minutes, to a maximum of 400 mg/hour, as tolerated.

Y-90 ibritumomab infusion: Within 4 hours of the completion of rituximab infusion:
Platelet count ≥150,000 cells/mm^3: Inject 0.4 mCi/kg (14.8 MBq/kg actual body weight) over 10 minutes; maximum dose: 32 mCi (1184 MBq)

Platelet count between 100,000-149,000 cells/mm^3: Inject 0.3 mCi/kg (11.1 MBq/kg actual body weight) over 10 minutes; maximum dose: 32 mCi (1184 MBq)

Platelet count <100,000 cells/mm^3: Do **not** administer

Maximum dose: The prescribed, measured, and administered dose of Y-90 ibritumomab must not exceed 32 mCi (1184 MBq), regardless of the patient's body weight

Dosage Forms Each kit contains 4 vials for preparation of either In-111 or Y-90 conjugate (as indicated on container label)

Injection, solution:
Zevalin®: 1.6 mg/mL (2 mL)

ibritumomab tiuxetan *see* ibritumomab *on page 495*
Ibu® [US] *see* ibuprofen *on page 495*
Ibu-200 [US-OTC] *see* ibuprofen *on page 495*
Ibudone™ [US] *see* hydrocodone and ibuprofen *on page 483*
Ibuprin® (Discontinued) *see* ibuprofen *on page 495*

ibuprofen (eye byoo PROE fen)

Sound-Alike/Look-Alike Issues
Haltran® may be confused with Halfprin®

Synonyms p-isobutylhydratropic acid; ibuprofen lysine

U.S./Canadian Brand Names Addaprin [US-OTC]; Advil® Children's [US-OTC]; Advil® Infants' [US-OTC]; Advil® Migraine [US-OTC]; Advil® [US-OTC/Can]; Apo-Ibuprofen® [Can]; I-Prin [US-OTC]; Ibu-200 [US-OTC]; Ibu® [US]; Midol® Cramp and Body Aches [US-OTC]; Motrin® Children's [US-OTC/Can]; Motrin® IB [US-OTC/Can]; Motrin® Infants' [US-OTC]; Motrin® Junior Strength [US-OTC]; NeoProfen® [US]; Novo-Profen [Can]; Nu-Ibuprofen [Can]; Proprinal [US-OTC]; Ultraprin [US-OTC]

Therapeutic Category Analgesic, Nonnarcotic; Antipyretic; Nonsteroidal Antiinflammatory Drug (NSAID)

Use
Oral: Inflammatory diseases and rheumatoid disorders including juvenile rheumatoid arthritis, mild-to-moderate pain, fever, dysmenorrhea

◄ Injection: Ibuprofen lysine is for use in premature infants weighing between 500-1500 g and who are ≤32 weeks gestational age (GA) to induce closure of a clinically-significant patent ductus arteriosus (PDA) when usual treatments are ineffective

Usual Dosage

I.V.: Infants between 500-1500 g and ≤32 weeks GA: Patent ductus arteriosus: Initial dose: Ibuprofen 10 mg/kg, followed by two doses of 5 mg/kg at 24 and 48 hours. Dose should be based on birth weight.

Oral:
Children:
Antipyretic: 6 months to 12 years: Temperature <102.5°F (39°C): 5 mg/kg/dose; temperature >102.5°F: 10 mg/kg/dose given every 6-8 hours (maximum daily dose: 40 mg/kg/day)
Juvenile rheumatoid arthritis: 30-50 mg/kg/24 hours divided every 8 hours; start at lower end of dosing range and titrate upward (maximum: 2.4 g/day)
Analgesic: 4-10 mg/kg/dose every 6-8 hours
OTC labeling (analgesic, antipyretic):
Children 6 months to 11 years: See below; use of weight to select dose is preferred; doses may be repeated every 6-8 hours (maximum: 4 doses/day)
Children ≥12 years: 200 mg every 4-6 hours as needed (maximum: 1200 mg/24 hours)
Ibuprofen Dosing:
Weight 12-17 lbs (6-11 months of age): 50 mg
Weight 18-23 lbs (12-23 months of age): 75 mg
Weight 24-35 lbs (2-3 years of age): 100 mg
Weight 35-47 lbs (4-5 years of age): 150 mg
Weight 48-59 lbs (6-8 years of age): 200 mg
Weight 60-71 lbs (9-10 years of age): 250 mg
Weight 72-95 lbs (11 years of age): 300 mg
Adults:
Inflammatory disease: 400-800 mg/dose 3-4 times/day (maximum dose: 3.2 g/day)
Analgesia/pain/fever/dysmenorrhea: 200-400 mg/dose every 4-6 hours (maximum daily dose: 1.2 g, unless directed by physician; under physician supervision daily doses ≤2.4 g may be used)
OTC labeling (analgesic, antipyretic): 200 mg every 4-6 hours as needed (maximum: 1200 mg/24 hours)

Dosage Forms
Caplet: 200 mg [OTC]
Advil® [OTC], Ibu-200 [OTC], Motrin® IB [OTC]: 200 mg
Motrin® Junior [OTC]: 100 mg [scored]
Capsule, liquid-filled:
Advil® [OTC], Advil® Migraine [OTC]: 200 mg
Gelcap:
Advil® [OTC]: 200 mg
Injection, solution, as lysine [preservative free]:
NeoProfen®: 17.1 mg/mL (2 mL) [equivalent to ibuprofen 10 mg/mL]
Suspension, oral: 100 mg/5 mL
Advil® Children's [OTC], Motrin® Children's [OTC]: 100 mg/5 mL
Suspension, oral [concentrate, drops]: 40 mg/mL
Advil® Infants' [OTC], Motrin® Infants' [OTC]: 40 mg/mL
Tablet: 200 mg, 400 mg, 600 mg, 800 mg
Addaprin [OTC], Advil® [OTC], I-Prin [OTC], Ibu-200 [OTC], Midol® Cramp and Body Aches [OTC], Motrin® IB [OTC], Proprinal [OTC], Ultraprin [OTC]: 200 mg
Ibu®: 400 mg, 600 mg, 800 mg
Tablet, chewable:
Advil® Children's [OTC]: 50 mg
Advil® Junior [OTC], Motrin® Junior [OTC]: 100 mg

ibuprofen and hydrocodone *see* hydrocodone and ibuprofen *on page 483*

ibuprofen and oxycodone *see* oxycodone and ibuprofen *on page 711*

ibuprofen and pseudoephedrine *see* pseudoephedrine and ibuprofen *on page 802*

ibuprofen lysine *see* ibuprofen *on page 495*

ibuprofen, pseudoephedrine, and chlorpheniramine
(eye byoo PROE fen, soo doe e FED rin, & klor fen IR a meen)

Synonyms chlorpheniramine maleate, ibuprofen, and pseudoephedrine; ibuprofen, pseudoephedrine, and chlorpheniramine maleate; pseudoephedrine, chlorpheniramine, and ibuprofen

U.S./Canadian Brand Names Advil® Allergy Sinus [US]; Advil® Cold and Sinus Plus [Can]; Advil® Multi-Symptom Cold [US]

Therapeutic Category Antihistamine/Decongestant/Analgesic

Use Temporary relief of symptoms associated with the common cold, hay fever, or other respiratory allergies

Usual Dosage Oral: Children ≥12 years and Adults: One caplet every 4-6 hours while symptoms persist (maximum: 6 caplets/24 hours)

Dosage Forms
Caplet:
Advil® Allergy Sinus, Advil® Multi-Symptom Cold: Ibuprofen 200 mg, pseudoephedrine 30 mg, and chlorpheniramine 2 mg

ibuprofen, pseudoephedrine, and chlorpheniramine maleate *see* ibuprofen, pseudoephedrine, and chlorpheniramine *on page 497*

ibutilide (i BYOO ti lide)

Synonyms ibutilide fumarate

U.S./Canadian Brand Names Corvert® [US]

Therapeutic Category Antiarrhythmic Agent, Class III

Use Acute termination of atrial fibrillation or flutter of recent onset; the effectiveness of ibutilide has not been determined in patients with arrhythmias >90 days in duration

Usual Dosage I.V.: Initial: Adults:
<60 kg: 0.01 mg/kg over 10 minutes
≥60 kg: 1 mg over 10 minutes
If the arrhythmia does not terminate within 10 minutes after the end of the initial infusion, a second infusion of equal strength may be infused over a 10-minute period

Dosage Forms
Injection, solution:
Corvert®: 0.1 mg/mL (10 mL)

ibutilide fumarate *see* ibutilide *on page 497*

Icar™ Prenatal [US] *see* vitamins (multiple/prenatal) *on page 983*

IC-Green™ [US] *see* indocyanine green *on page 506*

ICI-182,780 *see* fulvestrant *on page 430*

ICI-204,219 *see* zafirlukast *on page 989*

ICI-46474 *see* tamoxifen *on page 902*

ICI-118630 *see* goserelin *on page 451*

ICI-176334 *see* bicalutamide *on page 135*

ICI-D1033 *see* anastrozole *on page 76*

ICI-D1694 *see* raltitrexed *(Canada only) on page 817*

ICL670 *see* deferasirox *on page 270*

icodextrin (eye KOE dex trin)

U.S./Canadian Brand Names Adept® [US]; Extraneal® [US]

Therapeutic Category Adhesiolytic; Peritoneal Dialysate, Osmotic

Use
Adept®: Reduction of postsurgical adhesions in gynecologic laparoscopic procedures
Extraneal®: Daily exchange for the long dwell (8- to 16-hour) during continuous ambulatory peritoneal dialysis (CAPD) or automated peritoneal dialysis (APD) for the management of end-stage renal disease (ESRD); improvement of long-dwell ultrafiltration and clearance of creatinine and urea nitrogen (compared to 4.25% dextrose) in patients with high/average or greater transport characteristics as measured by peritoneal equilibration test (PET)

◄ **Usual Dosage** Intraperitoneal: Adults:
  CAPD or APD (Extraneal®): Given as a single daily exchange in CAPD or APD; dwell time of 8-16 hours is suggested
  Laparoscopic gynecologic surgery (Adept®): Irrigate with at least 100 mL every 30 minutes during surgery; aspirate remaining fluid after surgery is completed, then instill 1 L into the cavity
Dosage Forms
  Solution, intraperitoneal:
    Adept®: 4% (1.5 L) [for laparoscopic surgery]
    Extraneal: 7.5% (1.5 L, 2 L, 2.5 L) [for peritoneal dialysis]

ICRF-187 *see* dexrazoxane *on page 281*

Idamycin® [Can] *see* idarubicin *on page 498*

Idamycin® (Discontinued) *see* idarubicin *on page 498*

Idamycin PFS® [US] *see* idarubicin *on page 498*

idarubicin (eye da ROO bi sin)

Sound-Alike/Look-Alike Issues
  IDArubicin may be confused with DOXOrubicin, DAUNOrubicin, epirubicin
  Idamycin PFS® may be confused with Adriamycin
Synonyms 4-demethoxydaunorubicin; 4-DMDR; idarubicin hydrochloride; IDR; IMI 30; NSC-256439; SC 33428
Tall-Man IDArubicin
U.S./Canadian Brand Names Idamycin PFS® [US]; Idamycin® [Can]
Therapeutic Category Antineoplastic Agent
Use Treatment of acute leukemias (AML, ANLL, ALL), accelerated phase or blast crisis of chronic myelogenous leukemia (CML), breast cancer
Usual Dosage I.V. (refer to individual protocols):
  Children:
    Leukemia: 10-12 mg/m²/day for 3 days every 3 weeks
    Solid tumors: 5 mg/m²/day for 3 days every 3 weeks
  Adults:
    Leukemia induction: 12 mg/m²/day for 3 days
    Leukemia consolidation: 10-12 mg/m²/day for 2 days
Dosage Forms
  Injection, solution [preservative free]: 1 mg/mL (5 mL, 10 mL, 20 mL)
    Idamycin PFS®: 1 mg/mL (5 mL, 10 mL, 20 mL)

idarubicin hydrochloride *see* idarubicin *on page 498*

IDEC-C2B8 *see* rituximab *on page 839*

IDEC-Y2B8 *see* ibritumomab *on page 495*

IDR *see* idarubicin *on page 498*

idursulfase (eye dur SUL fase)

Sound-Alike/Look-Alike Issues
  Elaprase™ may be confused with Elspar®
U.S./Canadian Brand Names Elaprase™ [US]
Therapeutic Category Enzyme
Use Replacement therapy in mucopolysaccharidosis II (MPS II, Hunter syndrome) for improvement of walking capacity
Usual Dosage I.V.: Children ≥5 years and Adults: MPS II: 0.5 mg/kg once weekly
Dosage Forms
  Injection, solution [preservative free]:
    Elaprase™: 2 mg/mL (5 mL)

Ifex® [US/Can] *see* ifosfamide *on page 499*

IFLrA *see* interferon alfa-2a *on page 514*

ifosfamide (eye FOSS fa mide)

Sound-Alike/Look-Alike Issues
ifosfamide may be confused with cyclophosphamide
Synonyms isophosphamide; NSC-109724; Z4942
U.S./Canadian Brand Names Ifex® [US/Can]
Therapeutic Category Antineoplastic Agent
Use Treatment of testicular cancer
Usual Dosage Refer to individual protocols. To prevent bladder toxicity, ifosfamide should be given with the urinary protector mesna and hydration of at least 2 L of oral or I.V. fluid per day.
I.V.: Adults: Testicular cancer: 1200 mg/m^2/day for 5 days every 3 weeks
Dosage Forms
Injection, powder for reconstitution: 1 g
Ifex®: 1 g, 3 g
Injection, solution:
50 mg/mL (20 mL, 60 mL)

IG *see* immune globulin (intramuscular) *on page 502*
IgG4-kappa monoclonal antibody *see* natalizumab *on page 658*
IGIM *see* immune globulin (intramuscular) *on page 502*
IL-1Ra *see* anakinra *on page 75*
IL-2 *see* aldesleukin *on page 42*
IL-11 *see* oprelvekin *on page 701*
Ilopan-Choline® Oral *(Discontinued)* *see* dexpanthenol *on page 281*
Ilopan® Injection *(Discontinued)* *see* dexpanthenol *on page 281*

iloprost (EYE loe prost)

Synonyms iloprost tromethamine; prostacyclin PGI_2
U.S./Canadian Brand Names Ventavis® [US]
Therapeutic Category Prostaglandin
Use Treatment of idiopathic pulmonary arterial hypertension in patients with NYHA Class III or IV symptoms
Usual Dosage Inhalation: Adults: Initial: 2.5 mcg/dose; if tolerated, increase to 5 mcg/dose; administer 6-9 times daily (dosing at intervals ≥2 hours while awake); maintenance dose: 2.5-5 mcg/dose; maximum daily dose: 45 mcg
Dosage Forms
Solution for oral inhalation [preservative-free]:
Ventavis®: 10 mcg/mL (1 mL, 2 mL)

iloprost tromethamine *see* iloprost *on page 499*
Ilozyme® *(Discontinued)* *see* pancrelipase *on page 718*

imatinib (eye MAT eh nib)

Synonyms CGP-57148B; glivec; imatinib mesylate; NSC-716051; STI571
U.S./Canadian Brand Names Gleevec® [US/Can]
Therapeutic Category Antineoplastic, Tyrosine Kinase Inhibitor
Use Treatment of:
Gastrointestinal stromal tumors (GIST) kit-positive (CD117) unresectable and/or (metastatic) malignant
Philadelphia chromosome-positive (Ph+) chronic myeloid leukemia (CML) in chronic phase (newly-diagnosed)
Ph+ CML in blast crisis, accelerated phase, or chronic phase after failure of interferon therapy
Ph+ acute lymphoblastic leukemia (ALL) (relapsed or refractory)
Ph+ ALL induction therapy (newly diagnosed) [**not** an approved indication in the U.S.]

Note: The following indications are **not** approved in Canada:
Aggressive systemic mastocytosis (ASM) without D816V c-Kit mutation (or c-Kit mutation status unknown)
Dermatofibrosarcoma protuberans (DFSP) (unresectable, recurrent and metastatic)
Hypereosinophilic syndrome (HES) and/or chronic eosinophilic leukemia (CEL)

▶

◀ Myelodysplastic/myeloproliferative disease (MDS/MPD) associated with platelet-derived growth factor receptor (PDGFR) gene rearrangements

Ph+ CML in chronic phase in pediatric patients recurring following stem cell transplant or who are resistant to interferon-alpha therapy

Usual Dosage Oral: **Note:** For concurrent use with a strong CYP3A4 enzyme-inducing agent (eg, rifampin, phenytoin), imatinib dosage should be increased by at least 50%.

Children ≥2 years: **Note:** May be administered once daily or in 2 divided doses.

Ph+ CML (chronic phase, recurrent or resistant): 260 mg/m^2/day

Ph+ CML (chronic phase, newly diagnosed): 340 mg/m^2/day; maximum: 600 mg /day

Adults:

Ph+ CML:

Chronic phase: 400 mg once daily; may be increased to 600 mg daily

Canadian labeling: Includes range up to 800 mg/day (400 mg twice daily)

Accelerated phase or blast crisis: 600 mg once daily; may be increased to 800 mg daily (400 mg twice daily)

Ph+ ALL (induction, newly diagnosed): *Canadian labeling* (not an approved use in the U.S.): 600 mg once daily

Ph+ ALL (relapsed or refractory): 600 mg once daily

GIST: 400-600 mg/day

Canadian labeling: Includes range up to 800 mg/ day (400 mg twice daily)

ASM with eosinophilia: Initiate at 100 mg once daily; titrate up to a maximum of 400 mg once daily (if tolerated) for insufficient response to lower dose

ASM without D816V c-Kit mutation or c-Kit mutation status unknown: 400 mg once daily

DFSP: 400 mg twice daily

HES/CEL: 400 mg once daily

HES/CEL with FIP1L1-PDGFRα fusion kinase: Initiate at 100 mg once daily; titrate up to a maximum of 400 mg once daily (if tolerated) if insufficient response to lower dose

MDS/MPD: 400 mg once daily

Dosage Forms

Tablet:

Gleevec®: 100 mg; 400 mg

imatinib mesylate *see* imatinib *on page 499*

IMC-C225 *see* cetuximab *on page 197*

Imdur® [US/Can] *see* isosorbide mononitrate *on page 531*

IMI 30 *see* idarubicin *on page 498*

IMid-3 *see* lenalidomide *on page 551*

imidazole carboxamide *see* dacarbazine *on page 263*

imidazole carboxamide dimethyltriazene *see* dacarbazine *on page 263*

imiglucerase (i mi GLOO ser ace)

Sound-Alike/Look-Alike Issues

Cerezyme® may be confused with Cerebyx®, Ceredase®

U.S./Canadian Brand Names Cerezyme® [US/Can]

Therapeutic Category Enzyme

Use Long-term enzyme replacement therapy for patients with Type 1 Gaucher disease

Usual Dosage I.V.: Children ≥2 years and Adults: Initial: 30-60 units/kg every 2 weeks; dosing is individualized based on disease severity. Dosing range: 2.5 units/kg 3 times/week up to as much as 60 units/kg administered as frequently as once a week or as infrequently as every 4 weeks. Average dose: 60 units/kg administered every 2 weeks

Dosage Forms

Injection, powder for reconstitution:

Cerezyme®: 200 units, 400 units

imipemide *see* imipenem and cilastatin *on page 500*

imipenem and cilastatin (i mi PEN em & sye la STAT in)

Sound-Alike/Look-Alike Issues

imipenem may be confused with ertapenem, meropenem

Primaxin® may be confused with Premarin®, Primacor®

Synonyms imipemide

U.S./Canadian Brand Names Primaxin® I.V. [Can]; Primaxin® [US/Can]

Therapeutic Category Carbapenem (Antibiotic)

Use Treatment of lower respiratory tract, urinary tract, intraabdominal, gynecologic, bone and joint, skin and skin structure, and polymicrobic infections as well as bacterial septicemia and endocarditis. Antibacterial activity includes resistant gram-negative bacilli (*Pseudomonas aeruginosa* and *Enterobacter* sp), gram-positive bacteria (methicillin-sensitive *Staphylococcus aureus* and *Streptococcus* sp) and anaerobes.

Usual Dosage

Usual dosage ranges: Note: Dosage based on **imipenem** content:

Neonates ≤3 months and weight ≥1500 g: Non-CNS infections: I.V.:

  <1 week: 25 mg/kg every 12 hours

  1-4 weeks: 25 mg/kg every 8 hours

  4 weeks to 3 months: 25 mg/kg every 6 hours

Children >3 months: Non-CNS infections: I.V.: 15-25 mg/kg every 6 hours; maximum dosage: Susceptible infections: 2 g/day; moderately-susceptible organisms: 4 g/day

Adults:

  I.M.: 500-750 mg every 12 hours; maximum: 1500 mg/day

  I.V.: Weight ≥70 kg: 250-1000 mg every 6-8 hours; maximum: 4 g/day

Indication-specific dosing: Note: Doses based on imipenem content. I.M. administration is not intended for severe or life-threatening infections (eg, septicemia, endocarditis, shock), UTI, bone/joint or polymicrobic infections:

Children: I.V.: **Cystic fibrosis:** Doses up to 90 mg/kg/day have been used

Adults:

Intraabdominal infections:

  I.V.: Mild infection: 250-500 mg every 6 hours; severe: 500 mg every 6 hours

  I.M.: Mild-to-moderate infection: 750 mg every 12 hours

Lower respiratory tract, skins/skin structure, gynecologic infections: I.M.: Mild/moderate: 500-750 mg every 12 hours

Mild infection: Note: Rarely a suitable option in mild infections; normally reserved for moderate-severe cases:

  I.M.: 500 mg every 12 hours

  I.V.:

    Fully-susceptible organisms: 250 mg every 6 hours

    Moderately-susceptible organisms: 500 mg every 6 hours

Moderate infection:

  I.M.: 750 mg every 12 hours

  I.V.:

    Fully-susceptible organisms: 500 mg every 6-8 hours

    Moderately-susceptible organisms: 500 mg every 6 hours or 1 g every 8 hours

Pseudomonas infections: I.V.: 500 mg every 6 hours; **Note:** Higher doses may be required based on organism sensitivity.

Severe infection: I.V.:

  Fully-susceptible organisms: 500 mg every 6 hours

  Moderately-susceptible organisms: 1 g every 6-8 hours

  Maximum daily dose should not exceed 50 mg/kg or 4 g/day, whichever is lower

Urinary tract infection: I.V.:

  Uncomplicated: 250 mg every 6 hours

  Complicated: 500 mg every 6 hours

Dosage Forms

Injection, powder for reconstitution [I.M.]:

  Primaxin®: Imipenem 500 mg and cilastatin 500 mg

Injection, powder for reconstitution [I.V.]:

  Primaxin®: Imipenem 250 mg and cilastatin 250 mg; imipenem 500 mg and cilastatin 500 mg

imipramine (im IP ra meen)

Sound-Alike/Look-Alike Issues

imipramine may be confused with amitriptyline, desipramine, Norpramin®

Synonyms imipramine hydrochloride; imipramine pamoate

U.S./Canadian Brand Names Apo-Imipramine® [Can]; Novo-Pramine [Can]; Tofranil-PM® [US]; Tofranil® [US/Can]

▶

◀ **Therapeutic Category** Antidepressant, Tricyclic (Tertiary Amine)

Use Treatment of depression; treatment of nocturnal enuresis in children

Usual Dosage Oral:

Children: Enuresis: ≥6 years: Initial: 25 mg at bedtime, if inadequate response still seen after 1 week of therapy, increase by 25 mg/day; dose should not exceed 2.5 mg/kg/day or 50 mg at bedtime if 6-12 years of age or 75 mg at bedtime if ≥12 years of age

Adolescents: Depression: Initial: 25-50 mg/day; increase gradually; maximum: 100 mg/day in single or divided doses

Adults: Depression:

Outpatients: Initial: 75 mg/day; may increase gradually to 150 mg/day. May be given in divided doses or as a single bedtime dose; maximum: 200 mg/day

Inpatients: Initial: 100-150 mg/day; may increase gradually to 200 mg/day; if no response after 2 weeks, may further increase to 250-300 mg/day. May be given in divided doses or as a single bedtime dose; maximum: 300 mg/day.

Dosage Forms

Capsule: 75 mg, 100 mg, 125 mg, 150 mg
Tofranil-PM®: 75 mg, 100 mg, 125 mg, 150 mg
Tablet: 10 mg, 25 mg, 50 mg
Tofranil®: 10 mg, 25 mg, 50 mg

imipramine hydrochloride *see* imipramine *on page 501*
imipramine pamoate *see* imipramine *on page 501*

imiquimod (i mi KWI mod)

Sound-Alike/Look-Alike Issues

Aldara® may be confused with Alora®, Lialda™

U.S./Canadian Brand Names Aldara® [US/Can]

Therapeutic Category Immune Response Modifier

Use Treatment of external genital and perianal warts/condyloma acuminata; nonhyperkeratotic, nonhypertrophic actinic keratosis on face or scalp; superficial basal cell carcinoma (sBCC) with a maximum tumor diameter of 2 cm located on the trunk, neck, or extremities (excluding hands or feet)

Usual Dosage Topical: **Note:** A rest period of several days may be taken if required by the patient's discomfort or severity of the local skin reaction. Treatment may resume once the reaction subsides.

Children ≥12 years and Adults: Perianal warts/condyloma acuminata: Apply a thin layer 3 times/week prior to bedtime and leave on skin for 6-10 hours. Remove with mild soap and water. Examples of 3 times/week application schedules are: Monday, Wednesday, Friday; or Tuesday, Thursday, Saturday. Continue imiquimod treatment until there is total clearance of the genital/perianal warts for ≤16 weeks.

Adults:

Actinic keratosis: Apply twice weekly for 16 weeks to a treatment area on face or scalp (but not both concurrently); apply prior to bedtime and leave on skin for 8 hours. Remove with mild soap and water.

Common oral warts (dental use): Apply once daily prior to bedtime

Superficial basal cell carcinoma: Apply once daily prior to bedtime, 5 days/week for 6 weeks. Treatment area should include a 1 cm margin of skin around the tumor. Leave on skin for 8 hours. Remove with mild soap and water.

Dosage Forms

Cream:
Aldara®: 5% (12s, 24s)

Imitrex® [US/Can] *see* sumatriptan *on page 898*
Imitrex® DF [Can] *see* sumatriptan *on page 898*
Imitrex® Nasal Spray [Can] *see* sumatriptan *on page 898*
ImmuCyst® [Can] *see* BCG vaccine *on page 118*

immune globulin (intramuscular) (i MYUN GLOB yoo lin, IN tra MUS kyoo ler)

Synonyms gamma globulin; IG; IGIM; immune serum globulin; ISG

U.S./Canadian Brand Names BayGam® [Can]; GammaSTAN™ S/D [US]

Therapeutic Category Immune Globulin

Use To provide passive immunity in susceptible individuals under the following circumstances:

Hepatitis A: Within 14 days of exposure and prior to manifestation of disease

Measles: For use within 6 days of exposure in an unvaccinated person, who has not previously had measles

Varicella: When Varicella Zoster Immune Globulin is not available

Rubella: Postexposure prophylaxis (within 72 hours) to reduce the risk of infection in exposed pregnant women who will not consider therapeutic abortion

Immunoglobulin deficiency: To help prevent serious infections

Usual Dosage I.M.: Children and Adults:

Hepatitis A:

Preexposure prophylaxis upon travel into endemic areas (hepatitis A vaccine preferred):

0.02 mL/kg for anticipated risk of exposure <3 months

0.06 mL/kg for anticipated risk of exposure ≥3 months

Repeat approximate dose every 5 months if exposure continues

Postexposure prophylaxis: 0.02 mL/kg given within 14 days of exposure. IG is not needed if at least 1 dose of hepatitis A vaccine was given at ≥1 month before exposure

Measles:

Prophylaxis, immunocompetent: 0.25 mL/kg/dose (maximum dose: 15 mL) given within 6 days of exposure followed by live attenuated measles vaccine in 5-6 months when indicated

Prophylaxis, immunocompromised: 0.5 mL/kg (maximum dose: 15 mL) immediately following exposure

Rubella: Prophylaxis during pregnancy: 0.55 mL/kg/dose within 72 hours of exposure

Varicella: Prophylaxis: 0.6-1.2 mL/kg (varicella zoster immune globulin preferred) within 72 hours of exposure

IgG deficiency: 0.66 mL/kg/dose every 3-4 weeks. A double dose may be given at onset of therapy; some patients may require more frequent injections.

Dosage Forms

Injection, solution [preservative free; solvent detergent-treated]:

GamaSTAN™ S/D: 15% to 18% (2 mL, 10 mL)

immune globulin (intravenous) (i MYUN GLOB yoo lin, IN tra VEE nus)

Sound-Alike/Look-Alike Issues

Gamimune® N may be confused with CytoGam®

Synonyms IVIG

U.S./Canadian Brand Names Carimune® NF [US]; Flebogamma® [US]; Gamimune® N [Can]; Gammagard Liquid [US/Can]; Gammagard S/D [US/Can]; Gamunex® [US/Can]; Octagam® [US]; Privigen™ [US]

Therapeutic Category Immune Globulin

Use

Treatment of primary immunodeficiency syndromes (congenital agammaglobulinemia, severe combined immunodeficiency syndromes [SCIDS], common variable immunodeficiency, X-linked immunodeficiency, Wiskott-Aldrich syndrome) (Carimune® NF, Flebogamma®, Gammagard Liquid, Gammagard S/D, Gamunex®, Octagam®, Privigen™)

Treatment of immune (idiopathic) thrombocytopenic purpura (ITP) (Carimune® NF, Gammagard S/D, Gamunex®, Privigen™)

Prevention of coronary artery aneurysms associated with Kawasaki disease (in combination with aspirin) (Gammagard S/D)

Prevention of bacterial infection in B-cell chronic lymphocytic leukemia (CLL) (Gammagard S/D)

Usual Dosage Approved doses and regimens may vary between brands; check manufacturer guidelines. **Note:** Some clinicians dose IVIG on ideal body weight or an adjusted ideal body weight in morbidly-obese patients.

Children: I.V.: Pediatric HIV, prevention of infection (CDC guidelines): 400 mg/kg every 2-4 weeks

Children and Adults: I.V.:

Primary immunodeficiency disorders: **Note:** Adjust dose/frequency based desired IgG levels and clinical response:

General dosing range: 200-800 mg/kg per month

Carimune® NF: 200 mg/kg every 4 weeks. May increase dose to 300 mg/kg every 4 weeks or may increase frequency based on patient response.

Flebogamma®, Gammagard Liquid, Gammagard S/D, Gamunex®, Octagam®: 300-600 mg/kg every 3-4 weeks; adjusted based on dosage and interval in conjunction with monitored serum IgG concentrations

Privigen™: 200-800 mg/kg every 3-4 weeks; adjusted based on dosage and interval in conjunction with monitored serum IgG concentrations

B-cell chronic lymphocytic leukemia (CLL) (Gammagard S/D): 400 mg/kg/dose every 3-4 weeks

Immune (idiopathic) thrombocytopenic purpura (ITP):
Carimune® NF:
Acute: 400 mg/kg/day for 2-5 days
Chronic: 400 mg/kg as needed to maintain platelet count ≥30,000/mm^3 or to control significant bleeding; may increase dose if needed (range: 800-1000 mg/kg)
Gammagard S/D: 1000 mg/kg; adjust additional doses based on patient response or platelet count. Up to 3 separate doses may be administered on alternate days if required.
Gamunex®: 1000 mg/kg/day for 1-2 days, **or** 400 mg/kg/day for 5 days
Privigen™: 1000 mg/kg/day for 2 consecutive days
Kawasaki disease: Initiate IVIG therapy within 10 days of disease onset: Must be used in combination with aspirin: 80-100 mg/kg/day in 4 divided doses for 14 days; when fever subsides, dose aspirin at 3-5 mg/kg once daily for ≥6-8 weeks
AHA guidelines: 2000 mg/kg as a single dose
Gammagard S/D: 1000 mg/kg as a single dose administered over 10 hours, **or** 400 mg/kg/day for 4 days. Begin within 7 days of onset of fever.
Hematopoietic stem cell transplantation with hypogammaglobulinemia (CDC guidelines):
Children: 400 mg/kg per month; increase dose or frequency to maintain IgG levels >400 mg/dL
Adolescents and Adults: 500 mg/kg/week

Dosage Forms
Injection, powder for reconstitution [preservative free, nanofiltered]:
Carimune® NF: 3 g, 6 g, 12 g
Injection, powder for reconstitution [preservative free, solvent detergent-treated]:
Gammagard S/D: 2.5 g, 5 g, 10 g
Injection, solution [preservative free; solvent detergent-treated]:
Gammagard Liquid: 10% (10 mL, 25 mL, 50 mL, 100 mL, 200 mL)
Injection, solution [preservative free]:
Flebogamma®: 5% (10 mL, 50 mL, 100 mL, 200 mL)
Gamunex®: 10% (10 mL, 25 mL, 50 mL, 100 mL, 200 mL)
Privigen™: 10% (50 mL, 100 mL, 200 mL)

immune globulin (subcutaneous) (i MYUN GLOB yoo lin sub kyoo TAY nee us)
Synonyms immune globulin subcutaneous (human); SCIG
U.S./Canadian Brand Names Vivaglobin® [US]
Therapeutic Category Immune Globulin
Use Treatment of primary immune deficiency (PID)
Usual Dosage Note: Consider premedicating with acetaminophen and diphenhydramine.
SubQ infusion: Children ≥2 years and Adults: 100-200 mg/kg weekly (maximum rate: 20 mL/hour; doses >15 mL should be divided between sites); adjust the dose over time to achieve desired clinical response or target IgG levels
Conversion from I.V. to SubQ: Multiply previous I.V. dose by 1.37, then divide into a weekly regimen by dividing by the previous I.V. dosing interval (eg, if the dosing interval was every 3 weeks, divide by 3); adjust the dose over time to achieve desired clinical response or target IgG levels. SubQ infusion administration should begin 1 week after the last I.V. dose.
Dosage Forms
Injection, solution [preservative free]:
Vivaglobin®: IgG 160 mg/mL (3 mL, 10 mL, 20 mL)

immune globulin subcutaneous (human) *see* immune globulin (subcutaneous) *on page 504*
immune serum globulin *see* immune globulin (intramuscular) *on page 502*
Immunine® VH [Can] *see* factor IX *on page 388*
Imodium® [Can] *see* loperamide *on page 573*
Imodium® A-D [US-OTC] *see* loperamide *on page 573*
Imodium® Advanced [US] *see* loperamide and simethicone *on page 574*
Imogam® Rabies-HT [US] *see* rabies immune globulin (human) *on page 815*
Imogam® Rabies Pasteurized [Can] *see* rabies immune globulin (human) *on page 815*
Imovane® [Can] *see* zopiclone *(Canada only) on page 997*
Imovax® Rabies [US/Can] *see* rabies virus vaccine *on page 816*
Implanon™ [US] *see* etonogestrel *on page 383*
Imuran® [US/Can] *see* azathioprine *on page 109*

In-111 ibritumomab *see* ibritumomab *on page 495*
In-111 zevalin *see* ibritumomab *on page 495*

inamrinone (eye NAM ri none)
Sound-Alike/Look-Alike Issues
amrinone may be confused with aMILoride, amiodarone
Synonyms amrinone lactate
Therapeutic Category Adrenergic Agonist Agent
Use Short-term therapy in patients with intractable heart failure
Usual Dosage Dosage is based on clinical response (**Note:** Dose should not exceed 10 mg/kg/24 hours).
Adults: 0.75 mg/kg I.V. bolus over 2-3 minutes followed by maintenance infusion of 5-10 mcg/kg/minute; I.V. bolus may need to be repeated in 30 minutes.
Dosage Forms
Injection, solution: 5 mg/mL (20 mL)

I-Naphline® Ophthalmic *(Discontinued)* *see* naphazoline *on page 655*
Inapsine® [US] *see* droperidol *on page 326*
Increlex™ [US] *see* mecasermin *on page 595*

indapamide (in DAP a mide)
Sound-Alike/Look-Alike Issues
indapamide may be confused with Iopidine®
U.S./Canadian Brand Names Apo-Indapamide® [Can]; Gen-Indapamide [Can]; Lozide® [Can]; Lozol® [Can]; Novo-Indapamide [Can]; Nu-Indapamide [Can]; PMS-Indapamide [Can]
Therapeutic Category Diuretic, Miscellaneous
Use Management of mild-to-moderate hypertension; treatment of edema in congestive heart failure and nephrotic syndrome
Usual Dosage Oral: Adults:
Edema: 2.5-5 mg/day. **Note:** There is little therapeutic benefit to increasing the dose >5 mg/day; there is, however, an increased risk of electrolyte disturbances
Hypertension: 1.25 mg in the morning, may increase to 5 mg/day by increments of 1.25-2.5 mg; consider adding another antihypertensive and decreasing the dose if response is not adequate
Dosage Forms
Tablet: 1.25 mg, 2.5 mg

indapamide and perindopril erbumine *see* perindopril erbumine and indapamide *(Canada only) on page 739*
Inderal® [US/Can] *see* propranolol *on page 796*
Inderal® LA [US/Can] *see* propranolol *on page 796*
Inderide® [US] *see* propranolol and hydrochlorothiazide *on page 797*

indinavir (in DIN a veer)
Sound-Alike/Look-Alike Issues
indinavir may be confused with Denavir™
Synonyms indinavir sulfate
U.S./Canadian Brand Names Crixivan® [US/Can]
Therapeutic Category Antiviral Agent
Use Treatment of HIV infection; should always be used as part of a multidrug regimen (at least three antiretroviral agents)
Usual Dosage Oral: Adults:
Unboosted regimen: 800 mg every 8 hours
Ritonavir-boosted regimens:
Ritonavir 100-200 mg twice daily plus indinavir 800 mg twice daily **or**
Ritonavir 400 mg twice daily plus indinavir 400 mg twice daily
Dosage adjustments for indinavir when administered in combination therapy:
Delavirdine, itraconazole, or ketoconazole: Reduce indinavir dose to 600 mg every 8 hours
Efavirenz: Increase indinavir dose to 1000 mg every 8 hours
Lopinavir and ritonavir (Kaletra™): Indinavir 600 mg twice daily
Nelfinavir: Increase indinavir dose to 1200 mg twice daily

▶

Nevirapine: Increase indinavir dose to 1000 mg every 8 hours
Rifabutin: Reduce rifabutin to ½ the standard dose plus increase indinavir to 1000 mg every 8 hours
Dosage Forms
Capsule:
Crixivan®: 100 mg, 200 mg, 333 mg, 400 mg

indinavir sulfate *see indinavir on page 505*
Indocid® P.D.A. [Can] *see indomethacin on page 506*
Indocin® [US/Can] *see indomethacin on page 506*
Indocin® I.V. [US] *see indomethacin on page 506*

indocyanine green (in doe SYE a neen green)
U.S./Canadian Brand Names IC-Green™ [US]
Therapeutic Category Diagnostic Agent
Use Determining hepatic function, cardiac output, and liver blood flow; ophthalmic angiography
Usual Dosage Adults:
Ophthalmic angiography: Use doses of up to 40 mg of dye in 2 mL of aqueous solvent, in some patients, half the volume (1 mL) has been found to produce angiograms of comparable resolution; immediately following the bolus dose of dye, a bolus of sodium chloride 0.9% 5 mL is given; this regimen will deliver a spatially limited dye bolus of optimal concentration to the choroidal vasculature following I.V. injection into the antecubital vein.
Cardiac output determination: Dye is injected as rapidly as possible through a cardiac catheter; the usual dose is 1.25 mg for infants, 2.5 mg for children, and 5 mg for adults; total dose should not exceed 2 mg/kg; the dye should be flushed from the catheter with sodium chloride 0.9% to prevent hemolysis
Dosage Forms
Injection, powder for reconstitution: 25 mg
IC-Green®: 25 mg

Indo-Lemmon [Can] *see indomethacin on page 506*
indometacin *see indomethacin on page 506*

indomethacin (in doe METH a sin)
Sound-Alike/Look-Alike Issues
Indocin® may be confused with Imodium®, Lincocin®, Minocin®, Vicodin®
Synonyms indometacin; indomethacin sodium trihydrate
U.S./Canadian Brand Names Apo-Indomethacin® [Can]; Indo-Lemmon [Can]; Indocid® P.D.A. [Can]; Indocin® I.V. [US]; Indocin® [US/Can]; Indotec [Can]; Novo-Methacin [Can]; Nu-Indo [Can]; Rhodacine® [Can]
Therapeutic Category Analgesic, Nonnarcotic Nonsteroidal Antiinflammatory Drug (NSAID)
Use Acute gouty arthritis, acute bursitis/tendonitis, moderate-to-severe osteoarthritis, rheumatoid arthritis, ankylosing spondylitis; I.V. form used as alternative to surgery for closure of patent ductus arteriosus in neonates
Usual Dosage
Patent ductus arteriosus:
Neonates: I.V.: Initial: 0.2 mg/kg, followed by 2 doses depending on postnatal age (PNA):
PNA **at time of first dose** <48 hours: 0.1 mg/kg at 12- to 24-hour intervals
PNA **at time of first dose** 2-7 days: 0.2 mg/kg at 12- to 24-hour intervals
PNA **at time of first dose** >7 days: 0.25 mg/kg at 12- to 24-hour intervals
In general, may use 12-hour dosing interval if urine output >1 mL/kg/hour after prior dose; use 24-hour dosing interval if urine output is <1 mL/kg/hour but >0.6 mL/kg/hour; doses should be withheld if patient has oliguria (urine output <0.6 mL/kg/hour) or anuria
Inflammatory/rheumatoid disorders: Oral: Use lowest effective dose.
Children ≥2 years: 1-2 mg/kg/day in 2-4 divided doses; maximum dose: 4 mg/kg/day; not to exceed 150-200 mg/day
Adults: 25-50 mg/dose 2-3 times/day; maximum dose: 200 mg/day. In patients with arthritis and persistent night pain and/or morning stiffness may give the larger portion (up to 100 mg) of the total daily dose at bedtime.
Bursitis/tendonitis: Oral: Adults: Initial dose: 75-150 mg/day in 3-4 divided doses; usual treatment is 7-14 days

Acute gouty arthritis: Oral: Adults: 50 mg 3 times daily until pain is tolerable then reduce dose; usual treatment <3-5 days

Dosage Forms
Capsule: 25 mg, 50 mg
Injection, powder for reconstitution:
Indocin® I.V.: 1 mg
Suppository, rectal: 50 mg (30s)
Suspension, oral: 25 mg/5 mL
Indocin®: 25 mg/5 mL

indomethacin sodium trihydrate *see* indomethacin *on page 506*
Indotec [Can] *see* indomethacin *on page 506*
INF-alpha 2 *see* interferon alfa-2b *on page 515*
Infanrix® [US] *see* diphtheria, tetanus toxoids, and acellular pertussis vaccine *on page 309*
Infantaire [US-OTC] *see* acetaminophen *on page 19*
Infantaire Gas Drops [US-OTC] *see* simethicone *on page 867*
Infants' Tylenol® Cold Plus Cough Concentrated Drops *(Discontinued)* *see* acetaminophen, dextromethorphan, and pseudoephedrine *on page 27*
Infasurf® [US] *see* calfactant *on page 168*
INFeD® [US] *see* iron dextran complex *on page 527*
Infergen® [US] *see* interferon alfacon-1 *on page 517*
Inflamase® Mild [Can] *see* prednisolone (ophthalmic) *on page 781*

infliximab (in FLIKS e mab)

Sound-Alike/Look-Alike Issues
inFLIXimab may be confused with riTUXimab
Remicade® may be confused with Renacidin®, Rituxan®
Synonyms infliximab, recombinant; NSC-728729
Tall-Man inFLIXimab
U.S./Canadian Brand Names Remicade® [US/Can]
Therapeutic Category Monoclonal Antibody
Use Treatment of rheumatoid arthritis (moderate-to-severe, with methotrexate); treatment of Crohn disease (moderate-to-severe with inadequate response to conventional therapy) for induction and maintenance of remission, and/or to reduce the number of draining enterocutaneous and rectovaginal fistulas, and to maintain fistula closure; treatment of psoriatic arthritis; treatment of plaque psoriasis (chronic severe); treatment of ankylosing spondylitis; treatment of and maintenance of healing of ulcerative colitis (moderately- to severely-active with inadequate response to conventional therapy)
Usual Dosage I.V.: **Note:** Premedication with antihistamines (anti-H$_1$ and/or anti-H$_2$), acetaminophen and/ or corticosteroids may be considered to prevent and/or manage infusion-related reactions:
Children: U.S. labeling ≥6 years, Canadian labeling ≥9 years: Crohn disease: 5 mg/kg at 0, 2, and 6 weeks, followed by a maintenance dose of 5 mg/kg every 8 weeks; if no response by week 14, consider discontinuing therapy
Adults:
Crohn disease: Induction regimen: 5 mg/kg at 0, 2, and 6 weeks, followed by 5 mg/kg every 8 weeks thereafter; dose may be increased to 10 mg/kg in patients who respond but then lose their response. If no response by week 14, consider discontinuing therapy.
Psoriatic arthritis (with or without methotrexate): 5 mg/kg at 0, 2, and 6 weeks, then every 8 weeks
Rheumatoid arthritis (in combination with methotrexate therapy): 3 mg/kg at 0, 2, and 6 weeks, then every 8 weeks thereafter; doses have ranged from 3-10 mg/kg intravenous infusion repeated at 4- to 8-week intervals
Ankylosing spondylitis: 5 mg/kg at 0, 2, and 6 weeks, followed by 5 mg/kg every 6 weeks thereafter
Plaque psoriasis: 5 mg/kg at 0, 2, and 6 weeks, then every 8 weeks thereafter
Ulcerative colitis: 5 mg/kg at 0, 2, and 6 weeks, followed by 5 mg/kg every 8 weeks thereafter
Dosage Forms
Injection, powder for reconstitution [preservative free]:
Remicade®: 100 mg

infliximab, recombinant *see* infliximab *on page 507*

influenza virus vaccine (in floo EN za VYE rus vak SEEN)

Sound-Alike/Look-Alike Issues

influenza virus vaccine (human strain) may be confused with the avian strain (H5N1) of influenza virus vaccine

Fluarix® may be confused with Flarex®

influenza virus vaccine may be confused with tetanus toxoid and tuberculin products. Medication errors have occurred when tuberculin skin tests (PPD) have been inadvertently administered instead of tetanus toxoid products and influenza virus vaccine. These products are refrigerated and often stored in close proximity to each other.

Synonyms influenza virus vaccine (purified surface antigen); influenza virus vaccine (split-virus); influenza virus vaccine (trivalent, live); live attenuated influenza vaccine (LAIV); trivalent inactivated influenza vaccine (TIV)

U.S./Canadian Brand Names Afluria® [US]; Fluarix® [US]; FluLaval™ [US]; FluMist® [US]; Fluviral S/F® [Can]; Fluvirin® [US]; Fluzone® [US]; Vaxigrip® [Can]

Therapeutic Category Vaccine, Inactivated Virus

Use Provide active immunity to influenza virus strains contained in the vaccine

Advisory Committee on Immunization Practices (ACIP) target groups for vaccination:
- Persons ≥50 years of age
- Residents of nursing homes and other chronic-care facilities that house persons of any age with chronic medical conditions
- Adults and children with chronic disorders of the pulmonary or cardiovascular systems, including asthma
- Adults and children who have required regular medical follow-up or hospitalization during the preceding year because of chronic metabolic diseases (including diabetes mellitus), hepatic disease, renal dysfunction, hematologic disorders, hemoglobinopathies, or immunosuppression (including immunosuppression caused by medications or HIV)
- Adults and children with conditions which may compromise respiratory function, the handling of respiratory secretions, or that can increase the risk of aspiration (eg, cognitive dysfunction, spinal; cord injuries, seizure disorders, other neuromuscular disorders)
- Children and adolescents (6 months to 18 years of age) who are receiving long-term aspirin therapy and therefore, may be at risk for developing Reye syndrome after influenza
- Women who will be pregnant during the influenza season
- Children 6-59 months of age

The ACIP also recommends vaccination for close contacts of children 0-59 months of age, healthy persons who may transmit influenza to those at risk, all healthcare workers, and all persons (including school-aged children) who want to decrease their risk of influenza infection or transmitting influenza to others.

Usual Dosage It is important to note that influenza seasons vary in their timing and duration from year to year. In general, the optimal time to receive vaccine is October-November, prior to exposure to influenza; however, vaccination should continue into December and throughout the influenza season as long as vaccine is available.

Note: Children <9 years who are not previously vaccinated or who received only 1 dose of vaccine during the previous season (if it was their first year of vaccination) should receive 2 doses, in order to achieve satisfactory antibody response per ACIP recommendations.

I.M.:
Fluzone®:
  Children 6-35 months: 0.25 mL/dose (1 or 2 doses per season; see **Note**)
  Children 3-8 years: 0.5 mL/dose (1 or 2 doses per season; see **Note**)
  Children ≥9 years and Adults: 0.5 mL/dose (1 dose per season)
Fluvirin®:
  Children 4-8 years: 0.5 mL/dose (1 or 2 doses per season; see **Note**)
  Children ≥9 years and Adults: 0.5 mL/dose (1 dose per season)
Afluria®, Fluarix®, FluLaval™: Adults: 0.5 mL/dose (1 dose per season)
Intranasal (FluMist®):
  Children 2-8 years, previously **not vaccinated** with influenza vaccine: Initial season: Two 0.2 mL doses separated by at least 4 weeks
  Children 2-8 years, previously **vaccinated** with influenza vaccine: 0.2 mL/dose (1 or 2 doses separated by at least 4 weeks; see **Note**)
  Children ≥9 years and Adults ≤49 years: 0.2 mL/dose (1 dose per season)

Dosage Forms
  Injection, suspension [purified split-virus]:
   Afluria®, FluLaval™, Fluvirin®, Fluzone®: 5 mL
  Injection, suspension [purified split-virus; preservative free]:
   Afluria®, Fluarix®, Fluvirin®: 0.5 mL
   Fluzone®: 0.25 mL, 0.5 mL
  Solution, intranasal [preservative free; trivalent; live virus; spray]:
   FluMist®: 0.2 mL

influenza virus vaccine (H5N1) (in floo EN za VYE rus vak SEEN H5N1)

Sound-Alike/Look-Alike Issues
   influenza virus vaccine (H5N1) may be confused with the nonavian strain of influenza virus vaccine
Synonyms avian influenza virus vaccine; bird flu vaccine; H5N1 influenza vaccine; influenza virus vaccine (monovalent)
Therapeutic Category Vaccine
Use Active immunization of adults at increased risk of exposure to the H5N1 viral subtype of influenza
Usual Dosage I.M.: Adults 18-64 years: 1 mL, followed by second 1 mL dose given 28 days later (acceptable range: 21-35 days)
Dosage Forms
  Injection, suspension [monovalent]: Hemagglutinin (H5N1 strain) 90 mcg/1 mL (5 mL)

influenza virus vaccine (monovalent) *see* influenza virus vaccine (H5N1) *on page 509*
influenza virus vaccine (purified surface antigen) *see* influenza virus vaccine *on page 508*
influenza virus vaccine (split-virus) *see* influenza virus vaccine *on page 508*
influenza virus vaccine (trivalent, live) *see* influenza virus vaccine *on page 508*
Infufer® [Can] *see* iron dextran complex *on page 527*
Infumorph® [US] *see* morphine sulfate *on page 643*
Infuvite® Adult [US] *see* vitamins (multiple/injectable) *on page 982*
Infuvite® Pediatric [US] *see* vitamins (multiple/injectable) *on page 982*
INH *see* isoniazid *on page 528*
inhaled insulin *see* insulin inhalation *on page 511*
Inhibace® [Can] *see* cilazapril *(Canada only) on page 219*
Inhibace® Plus [Can] *see* cilazapril and hydrochlorothiazide *(Canada only) on page 219*
Innohep® [US/Can] *see* tinzaparin *on page 929*
InnoPran XL™ [US] *see* propranolol *on page 796*
Inocor® *(Discontinued)*
INOmax® [US/Can] *see* nitric oxide *on page 674*
Inova™ [US] *see* benzoyl peroxide *on page 126*
insect sting kit *see* epinephrine and chlorpheniramine *on page 345*
insoluble prussian blue *see* ferric hexacyanoferrate *on page 397*
Inspra™ [US] *see* eplerenone *on page 347*
Insta-Glucose® [US-OTC] *see* dextrose *on page 286*
Instat™ [US] *see* collagen hemostat *on page 245*
Instat™ MCH [US] *see* collagen hemostat *on page 245*

insulin aspart (IN soo lin AS part)

Sound-Alike/Look-Alike Issues
   NovoLog® may be confused with Novolin®
   NovoLog® Mix 70/30 may be confused with NovoLog®
Synonyms aspart insulin
U.S./Canadian Brand Names NovoLog® [US]; NovoRapid® [Can]
Therapeutic Category Antidiabetic Agent, Insulin
Use Treatment of type 1 diabetes mellitus (insulin-dependent, IDDM) and type 2 diabetes mellitus (noninsulin-dependent, NIDDM) to improve glycemic control
Usual Dosage Refer to Insulin Regular on page 513. Insulin aspart is a rapid-acting insulin analog which is normally administered as a premeal component of the insulin regimen. It is normally used along with a long-acting (basal) form of insulin or continuous basal administration of insulin via a SubQ infusion pump. ▶

I.V.: Insulin aspart may be administered I.V. in selected clinical situations to control hyperglycemia. Appropriate medical supervision is required.

SubQ: When used in a meal-related treatment regimen, 50% to 70% of total daily insulin requirement may be provided by insulin aspart as divided premeal boluses and the remainder provided by an intermediate or long-acting insulin or continuous basal administration of insulin via a SubQ infusion pump. Due to rapid onset and short duration, some patients may require more basal insulin to prevent premeal hyperglycemia when using insulin aspart as opposed to regular insulin.

SubQ infusion pump: Initial programming of the pump may be based upon the total daily dose of insulin (TDD) given in the previous regimen with ~50% of the TDD given as divided premeal boluses and ~50% of TDD given as a basal infusion; adjust dose as necessary.

Dosage Forms
Injection, solution:
NovoLog®: 100 units/mL (3 mL) [FlexPen® prefilled syringe or PenFill® prefilled cartridge]; (10 mL)

insulin aspart and insulin aspart protamine see insulin aspart protamine and insulin aspart on page 510

insulin aspart protamine and insulin aspart
(IN soo lin AS part PROE ta meen & IN soo lin AS part)

Sound-Alike/Look-Alike Issues
NovoLog® Mix 70/30 may be confused with Novolin® 70/30

Synonyms insulin aspart and insulin aspart protamine

U.S./Canadian Brand Names NovoLog® Mix 70/30 [US]; NovoMix® 30 [Can]

Therapeutic Category Antidiabetic Agent, Insulin

Use Treatment of type 1 diabetes mellitus (insulin-dependent, IDDM) and type 2 diabetes mellitus (noninsulin-dependent, NIDDM) to improve glycemic control

Usual Dosage Refer to insulin regular monograph on page 513. Fixed ratio insulins (such as insulin aspart protamine and insulin aspart combination) are normally administered in 2 daily doses.

Dosage Forms
Injection, suspension:
NovoLog® Mix 70/30: Insulin aspart protamine suspension 70% [intermediate acting] and insulin aspart solution 30% [rapid acting]: 100 units/mL (3 mL) [FlexPen® prefilled syringe]; (10 mL) [vial]

insulin detemir (IN soo lin DE te mir)

Synonyms detemir insulin

U.S./Canadian Brand Names Levemir® [US/Can]

Therapeutic Category Antidiabetic Agent, Insulin

Use Treatment of type 1 diabetes mellitus (insulin-dependent, IDDM) and type 2 diabetes mellitus (noninsulin-dependent, NIDDM) to improve glycemic control

Usual Dosage Also refer to insulin regular on page 513.

Note: Duration is dose-dependent. Dosage must be carefully titrated (adjustment of dose and timing. Adjustment of concomitant antidiabetic treatment (short-acting insulins or oral antidiabetic agents) may be required. In Canada, insulin detemir is not approved for use in children.

SubQ: Children ≥6 years and Adults:
Basal insulin or basal-bolus (Type 1 or type 2 diabetes): May be substituted on a unit-per-unit basis. Adjust dose to achieve glycemic targets.
Insulin-naive patients (type 2 diabetes only): 0.1-0.2 units/kg once daily in the evening or 10 units once or twice daily. Adjust dose to achieve glycemic targets. **Note:** Canadian labeling recommends 10 units once daily (twice daily dosing is not included).

Dosage Forms
Injection, solution:
Levemir®: 100 units/mL (3 mL) [FlexPen® prefilled syringe]; (10 mL) [vial]

insulin glargine (IN soo lin GLAR jeen)

Sound-Alike/Look-Alike Issues
insulin glargine may be confused with insulin glulisine
Lantus® may be confused with Lente®

Synonyms glargine insulin

U.S./Canadian Brand Names Lantus® OptiSet® [Can]; Lantus® [US/Can]

Therapeutic Category Antidiabetic Agent, Insulin

Use Treatment of type 1 diabetes mellitus (insulin-dependent, IDDM) and type 2 diabetes mellitus (noninsulin-dependent, NIDDM) requiring basal (long-acting) insulin to improve glycemic control

Usual Dosage SubQ: Children ≥6 years and Adults:

Type 1 diabetes: As a basal component of combination insulin regimen, normally 50% to 75% of daily insulin requirement is administered as a long-acting form. More rapid acting forms are usually used in association with meals. Refer to Insulin Regular on page 513.

Type 2 diabetes:

Patient not already on insulin: 10 units once daily, adjusted according to patient response (range in clinical study: 2-100 units/day)

Patient already receiving insulin: In clinical studies, when changing to insulin glargine from once-daily NPH or Ultralente® insulin, the initial dose was not changed; when changing from twice-daily NPH to once-daily insulin glargine, the total daily dose was reduced by 20% and adjusted according to patient response

Dosage Forms

Injection, solution:

Lantus®: 100 units/mL (3 mL) [OptiClik® prefilled cartridge or SoloStar® disposable insulin device]; (10 mL) [vial]

insulin glulisine (IN soo lin gloo LIS een)

Sound-Alike/Look-Alike Issues

insulin glulisine may be confused with insulin glargine

Synonyms glulisine insulin

U.S./Canadian Brand Names Apidra® [US/Can]

Therapeutic Category Antidiabetic Agent, Insulin

Use Treatment of type 1 diabetes mellitus (insulin-dependent, IDDM) and type 2 diabetes mellitus (noninsulin-dependent, NIDDM) to improve glycemic control

Usual Dosage Refer to Insulin Regular on page 513. Insulin glulisine is a rapid-acting insulin analog which is normally administered as a premeal component of the insulin regimen. It is normally used along with a long-acting (basal) form of insulin or continuous basal administration of insulin via a SubQ infusion pump.

SubQ: When used in a meal-related treatment regimen, 50% to 70% of total daily insulin requirement may be provided by insulin glulisine (in divided doses) and the remainder provided by an intermediate- or long-acting insulin. Insulin glulisine may also be administered by external subcutaneous infusion pumps.

I.V.: Under close medical supervision, insulin glulisine may be administered by infusion.

Dosage Forms

Injection, solution:

Apidra®: 100 units/mL (3 mL [cartridge], 10 mL [vial])

insulin inhalation (IN soo lin in ha LAY shun)

Synonyms inhaled insulin

Therapeutic Category Antidiabetic Agent, Insulin

Use Treatment of type 1 diabetes mellitus (insulin-dependent, IDDM); type 2 diabetes mellitus (noninsulin-dependent, NIDDM)

Usual Dosage Inhalation: Children ≥6 years and Adults:

Initial: 0.05 mg/kg (rounded down to nearest whole milligram) 3 times/daily administered within 10 minutes of a meal

Adjustment: Dosage may be increased or decreased based on serum glucose monitoring, meal size, nutrient composition, time of day, and exercise patterns.

Note: A 1 mg blister is approximately equivalent to 3 units of regular insulin, while a 3 mg blister is approximately equivalent to 8 units of regular insulin administered subcutaneously. Patients should combine 1 mg and 3 mg blisters so that the fewest blisters are required to achieve the prescribed dose. Consecutive inhalation of three 1 mg blisters results in significantly higher insulin levels as compared to inhalation of a single 3 mg blister (do not substitute). In a patient stabilized on a dosage which uses 3 mg blisters, if 3 mg blister is temporarily unavailable, inhalation of two 1 mg blisters may be substituted.

insulin lispro (IN soo lin LYE sproe)

Sound-Alike/Look-Alike Issues

Humalog® may be confused with Humulin®, Humira®

▶

◀ **Synonyms** lispro insulin

U.S./Canadian Brand Names Humalog® [US/Can]

Therapeutic Category Antidiabetic Agent, Insulin

Use Treatment of type 1 diabetes mellitus (insulin-dependent, IDDM) and type 2 diabetes mellitus (noninsulin-dependent, NIDDM) to improve glycemic control

Usual Dosage Refer to insulin regular monograph on page 513. Insulin lispro is equipotent to insulin regular, but has a more rapid onset.

Dosage Forms

Injection, solution:

Humalog®: 100 units/mL (3 mL) [prefilled cartridge or prefilled disposable pen]; (10 mL) [vial]

insulin lispro and insulin lispro protamine *see* insulin lispro protamine and insulin lispro *on page 512*

insulin lispro protamine and insulin lispro

(IN soo lin LYE sproe PROE ta meen & IN soo lin LYE sproe)

Sound-Alike/Look-Alike Issues

Humalog® Mix 75/25™ may be confused with Humulin® 70/30.

Synonyms insulin lispro and insulin lispro protamine

U.S./Canadian Brand Names Humalog® Mix 25 [Can]; Humalog® Mix 50/50™ [US]; Humalog® Mix 75/25™ [US]

Therapeutic Category Antidiabetic Agent, Insulin

Use Treatment of type 1 diabetes mellitus (insulin-dependent, IDDM) and type 2 diabetes mellitus (noninsulin-dependent, NIDDM) to improve glycemic control

Usual Dosage Refer to insulin regular monograph on page 513. Fixed ratio insulins (such as insulin lispro protamine and insulin lispro) are normally administered in 2 daily doses.

Dosage Forms

Injection, suspension:

Humalog® Mix 50/50™: Insulin lispro protamine suspension 50% [intermediate acting] and insulin lispro solution 50% [rapid acting]: 100 units/mL (3 mL) [disposable pen]

Humalog® Mix 75/25™: Insulin lispro protamine suspension 75% [intermediate acting] and insulin lispro solution 25% [rapid acting]: 100 units/mL (3 mL) [disposable pen]; (10 mL) [vial]

insulin NPH (IN soo lin N P H)

Sound-Alike/Look-Alike Issues

Humulin® may be confused with Humalog®, Humira®

Novolin® may be confused with NovoLog®

Synonyms isophane insulin; NPH insulin

U.S./Canadian Brand Names Humulin® N [US/Can]; Novolin® ge NPH [Can]; Novolin® N [US]

Therapeutic Category Insulin, Intermediate-Acting

Use Treatment of type 1 diabetes mellitus (insulin-dependent, IDDM) and type 2 diabetes mellitus (noninsulin-dependent, NIDDM) to improve glycemic control

Usual Dosage Refer to insulin regular monograph on page 513. Insulin NPH is usually administered 1-2 times daily.

Dosage Forms [CAN] = Canadian brand name

Injection, suspension:

Humulin® N, Novolin® N: 100 units/mL (3 mL, 10 mL)

Novolin® ge NPH [CAN]: 100 units/mL (3 mL, 10 mL) [not available in the U.S.]

insulin NPH and insulin regular (IN soo lin N P H & IN soo lin REG yoo ler)

Sound-Alike/Look-Alike Issues

Humulin® 70/30 may be confused with Humalog® Mix 75/25

Novolin® 70/30 may be confused with NovoLog® Mix 70/30

Synonyms insulin regular and insulin NPH; isophane insulin and regular insulin; NPH insulin and regular insulin

U.S./Canadian Brand Names Humulin® 20/80 [Can]; Humulin® 50/50 [US]; Humulin® 70/30 [US/Can]; Novolin® 70/30 [US]; Novolin® ge 10/90 [Can]; Novolin® ge 20/80 [Can]; Novolin® ge 30/70 [Can]; Novolin® ge 40/60 [Can]; Novolin® ge 50/50 [Can]

Therapeutic Category Antidiabetic Agent, Insulin

Use Treatment of type 1 diabetes mellitus (insulin-dependent, IDDM) and type 2 diabetes mellitus (noninsulin-dependent, NIDDM) to improve glycemic control

Usual Dosage Refer to insulin regular monograph on page 513. Fixed ratio insulins are normally administered in 1-2 daily doses.

Dosage Forms
Injection, suspension:
Humulin® 50/50: Insulin NPH suspension 50% [intermediate acting] and insulin regular solution 50% [short acting]: 100 units/mL (10 mL)
Humulin® 70/30: Insulin NPH suspension 70% [intermediate acting] and insulin regular solution 30% [short acting]: 100 units/mL (3 mL, 10 mL)
Novolin® 70/30: Insulin NPH suspension 70% [intermediate acting] and insulin regular solution 30% [short acting]: 100 units/mL (3 mL, 10 mL)

Additional formulations available in Canada [not available in the U.S.]:
Injection, suspension:
Humulin® 20/80: Insulin regular solution 20% [short acting] and insulin NPH suspension 80% [intermediate acting]: 100 units/mL (3 mL)
Novolin® ge 30/70: Insulin regular solution 30% [short acting] and insulin NPH suspension 70% [intermediate acting]: 100 units/mL (3 mL)
Novolin® ge 40/60: Insulin regular solution 40% [short acting] and insulin NPH suspension 60% [intermediate acting]: 100 units/mL (3 mL)
Novolin® ge 50/50: Insulin regular solution 50% [short acting] and insulin NPH suspension 50% [intermediate acting]: 100 units/mL (3 mL)

insulin regular (IN soo lin REG yoo ler)
Sound-Alike/Look-Alike Issues
Humulin® may be confused with Humalog®, Humira®
Novolin® may be confused with NovoLog®

Synonyms regular insulin

U.S./Canadian Brand Names Humulin® R U-500 [US]; Humulin® R [US/Can]; Novolin® ge Toronto [Can]; Novolin® R [US]

Therapeutic Category Antidiabetic Agent, Insulin Antidote

Use Treatment of type 1 diabetes mellitus (insulin-dependent, IDDM); type 2 diabetes mellitus (noninsulin-dependent, NIDDM) unresponsive to treatment with diet and/or oral hypoglycemics, to improve glycemic control; adjunct to parenteral nutrition; diabetic ketoacidosis (DKA)

Usual Dosage SubQ (regular insulin may also be administered I.V.): The number and size of daily doses, time of administration, and diet and exercise require continuous medical supervision. In addition, specific formulations may require distinct administration procedures.
Type 1 Diabetes Mellitus: Children and Adults: **Note:** Multiple daily doses guided by blood glucose monitoring are the standard of diabetes care. Combinations of insulin are commonly used.
Initial dose: 0.2-0.6 units/kg/day in divided doses. Conservative initial doses of 0.2-0.4 units/kg/day are often recommended to avoid the potential for hypoglycemia.
Division of daily insulin requirement: Generally, 50% to 75% of the daily insulin dose is given as an intermediate- or long-acting form of insulin (in 1-2 daily injections). The remaining portion of the 24-hour insulin requirement is divided and administered as a rapid-acting or short-acting form of insulin. These may be given with meals (before or at the time of meals depending on the form of insulin) or at the same time as injections of intermediate forms (some premixed combinations are intended for this purpose).
Adjustment of dose: Dosage must be titrated to achieve glucose control and avoid hypoglycemia. Adjust dose to maintain premeal and bedtime glucose of 80-140 mg/dL (children <5 years: 100-200 mg/dL). Since combinations of agents are frequently used, dosage adjustment must address the individual component of the insulin regimen which most directly influences the blood glucose value in question, based on the known onset and duration of the insulin component.
Usual maintenance range: 0.5-1.2 units/kg/day in divided doses. An estimate of anticipated needs may be based on body weight and/or activity factors as follows:
Adolescents: May require ≤1.5 units/kg/day during growth spurts
Nonobese: 0.4-0.6 units/kg/day
Obese: 0.8-1.2 units/kg/day
Renal failure: Due to alterations in pharmacokinetics of insulin, may require <0.2 units/kg/day
Type 2 Diabetes Mellitus:
Augmentation therapy: Dosage must be carefully adjusted.

◀ Insulins other than glargine: Initial dosage of 0.15-0.2 units/kg/day have been recommended

Insulin glargine: Initial dose: 10 units/day

Note: Administered when residual beta-cell function is present, as a supplemental agent when oral hypoglycemics have not achieved goal glucose control. Twice daily NPH, or an evening dose of NPH, lente, or glargine insulin may be added to oral therapy with metformin or a sulfonylurea. Augmentation to control postprandial glucose may be accomplished with regular, glulisine, aspart, or lispro insulin.

Monotherapy: Initial dose: Highly variable: See Augmentation therapy dosing.

Note: An empirically-defined scheme for dosage estimation based on fasting plasma glucose and degree of obesity has been published with recommended doses ranging from 6-77 units/day. In the setting of glucose toxicity (loss of beta-cell sensitivity to glucose concentrations), insulin therapy may be used for short-term management to restore sensitivity of beta-cells; in these cases, the dose may need to be rapidly reduced/withdrawn when sensitivity is reestablished.

Diabetic ketoacidosis:

Children <20 years:

I.V.: Regular insulin infused at 0.1 units/kg/hour; continue until acidosis clears, then decrease to 0.05 units/kg/hour until SubQ replacement dosing can be initiated

SubQ, I.M.: If no I.V. infusion access, regular insulin 0.1 units/kg I.M. bolus followed by 0.1 units/kg/hour SubQ or I.M.; continue until acidosis clears, then decrease to 0.05 units/kg/hour until SubQ replacement dosing can be initiated

Adults:

I.V.: Regular insulin 0.15 units/kg initially followed by an infusion of 0.1 units/kg/hour

SubQ, I.M.: Regular insulin 0.4 units/kg given half as I.V. bolus and half as SubQ or I.M., followed by 0.1 units/kg/hour SubQ or I.M.

If serum glucose does not fall by 50-70 mg/dL in the first hour, double insulin dose hourly until glucose falls at an hourly rate of 50-70 mg/dL. Decrease dose to 0.05-0.1 units/kg/hour once serum glucose reaches 250 mg/dL.

Note: Newly-diagnosed patients with IDDM presenting in DKA and patients with blood sugars <800 mg/dL may be relatively "sensitive" to insulin and should receive loading and initial maintenance doses ~50% of those indicated.

Infusion should continue until reversal of acid-base derangement/ketonemia. Serum glucose is not a direct indicator of these abnormalities, and may decrease more rapidly than correction of the range of metabolic abnormalities.

Dosage Forms

Injection, solution:

Humulin® R: 100 units/mL (10 mL)

Novolin® R: 100 units/mL (3 mL) [InnoLet® prefilled syringe or PenFill® prefilled cartridge]; (10 mL) [vial]

Injection, solution [concentrate]:

Humulin® R U-500: 500 units/mL (20 mL vial)

insulin regular and insulin NPH *see* insulin NPH and insulin regular *on page 512*

Intal® [US/Can] *see* cromolyn sodium *on page 251*

Integrilin® [US/Can] *see* eptifibatide *on page 350*

Intelence™ [US/Can] *see* etravirine *on page 385*

Intensol® Solution (Discontinued) *see* metoclopramide *on page 625*

α-2-interferon *see* interferon alfa-2b *on page 515*

interferon alfa-2a (PEG conjugate) *see* peginterferon alfa-2a *on page 727*

interferon alfa-2b and ribavirin combination pack *see* interferon alfa-2b and ribavirin *on page 516*

interferon alfa-2b (PEG conjugate) *see* peginterferon alfa-2b *on page 728*

interferon alfa-2a (in ter FEER on AL fa too aye)

Sound-Alike/Look-Alike Issues

interferon alfa-2a may be confused with interferon alfa-2b, interferon alfa-n3, pegylated interferon alfa-2b

Roferon-A® may be confused with Rocephin®

Synonyms IFLrA; interferon alpha-2a; NSC-367982; rIFN-A

U.S./Canadian Brand Names Roferon-A® [Can]

Therapeutic Category Biological Response Modulator

Use

Patients >18 years of age: Treatment of hairy cell leukemia, chronic hepatitis C

Children and Adults: Treatment of Philadelphia chromosome-positive (Ph+) chronic myelogenous leukemia (CML) in chronic phase, within 1 year of diagnosis (limited experience in children)

Usual Dosage Refer to individual protocols

Children (limited data): Ph+ chronic myelogenous leukemia (CML): I.M.: 2.5-5 million units/m^2/day; **Note:** In juveniles, higher dosages (30 million units/m^2/day) have been associated with severe adverse events, including death

Adults:

Hairy cell leukemia: SubQ: 3 million units/day for 16-24 weeks, then 3 million units 3 times/week for up to 6-24 months

Ph+ chronic myelogenous leukemia (CML): SubQ: 9 million units/day, continue treatment until disease progression **or** 3 million units/day for 3 days, followed by 6 million units/day for 3 days, followed by 9 million units daily until disease progression

Chronic hepatitis C: SubQ: 3 million units 3 times/week for 12 months **or** 6 million units 3 times/week for 12 weeks followed by 3 million units 3 times/week for 36 weeks

interferon alfa-2b (in ter FEER on AL fa too bee)

Sound-Alike/Look-Alike Issues

interferon alfa-2b may be confused with interferon alfa-2a, interferon alfa-n3, pegylated interferon alfa-2b

Intron® A may be confused with PEG-Intron®

Synonyms INF-alpha 2; interferon alpha-2b; NSC-377523; rLFN-α2; α-2-interferon

U.S./Canadian Brand Names Intron® A [US/Can]

Therapeutic Category Biological Response Modulator

Use

Patients ≥1 year of age: Chronic hepatitis B

Patients ≥3 years of age: Chronic hepatitis C (in combination with ribavirin)

Patients ≥18 years of age: Condyloma acuminata, chronic hepatitis B, chronic hepatitis C, hairy cell leukemia, malignant melanoma, AIDS-related Kaposi sarcoma, follicular non-Hodgkin lymphoma

Usual Dosage Refer to individual protocols. **Note:** Withhold treatment for ANC <500/mm^3 or platelets <25,000/mm^3. Consider premedication with acetaminophen prior to administration to reduce the incidence of some adverse reactions. Not all dosage forms and strengths are appropriate for all indications; refer to product labeling for details.

Children 1-17 years: Chronic hepatitis B: SubQ: 3 million units/m^2 3 times/week for 1 week; then 6 million units/m^2 3 times/week; maximum: 10 million units 3 times/week; total duration of therapy 16-24 weeks

Children ≥3 years: Chronic hepatitis C: In combination with ribavirin (refer to interferon alfa-2b/ribavirin combination pack monograph)

Adults:

Hairy cell leukemia: I.M., SubQ: 2 million units/m^2 3 times/week for up to 6 months (may continue treatment with continued treatment response)

Lymphoma (follicular): SubQ: 5 million units 3 times/week for up to 18 months

Malignant melanoma: Induction: 20 million units/m^2 I.V. for 5 consecutive days per week for 4 weeks, followed by maintenance dosing of 10 million units/m^2 SubQ 3 times/week for 48 weeks

AIDS-related Kaposi sarcoma: I.M., SubQ: 30 million units/m^2 3 times/week

Chronic hepatitis B: I.M., SubQ: 5 million units/day or 10 million units 3 times/week for 16 weeks

Chronic hepatitis C: I.M., SubQ: 3 million units 3 times/week for 16 weeks. In patients with normalization of ALT at 16 weeks, continue treatment for 18-24 months; consider discontinuation if normalization does not occur at 16 weeks. **Note:** May be used in combination therapy with ribavirin in previously untreated patients or in patients who relapse following alpha interferon therapy.

Condyloma acuminata: Intralesionally: 1 million units/lesion (maximum: 5 lesions/treatment) 3 times/ week (on alternate days) for 3 weeks; may administer a second course at 12-16 weeks

Dosage Forms

Injection, powder for reconstitution [preservative free]

Intron® A: 10 million units; 18 million units; 50 million units

Injection, solution [multidose prefilled pen]:

Intron® A:

Delivers 3 million units/0.2 mL (1.5 mL)

Delivers 5 million units/0.2 mL (1.5 mL)

Delivers 10 million units/0.2 mL (1.5 mL)

Injection, solution [multidose vial]:

Intron® A: 6 million units/mL (3 mL); 10 million units/mL (2.5 mL)

interferon alfa-2b and ribavirin (in ter FEER on AL fa too bee & rye ba VYE rin)

Synonyms interferon alfa-2b and ribavirin combination pack; ribavirin and interferon alfa-2b combination pack

U.S./Canadian Brand Names Rebetron® [US]

Therapeutic Category Antiviral Agent; Biological Response Modulator

Use Combination therapy for the treatment of chronic hepatitis C in patients with compensated liver disease previously untreated with alpha interferon or who have relapsed after alpha interferon therapy

Usual Dosage

Children ≥3 years: Chronic hepatitis C: **Note:** Treatment duration may vary. Consult current guidelines and literature. Combination therapy:

Intron® A: SubQ:

25-61 kg: 3 million int. units/m^2 3 times/week

>61 kg: Refer to Adults dosing

Rebetol®: Oral: **Note:** Oral solution should be used in children 3-5 years of age, children ≤25 kg, or those unable to swallow capsules.

Capsule/solution: 15 mg/kg/day in 2 divided doses (morning and evening)

Capsule dosing recommendations:

25-36 kg: 400 mg/day (200 mg morning and evening)

37-49 kg: 600 mg/day (200 mg in the morning and two 200 mg capsules in the evening)

50-61 kg: 800 mg/day (two 200 mg capsules morning and evening)

>61 kg: Refer to Adults dosing

Adults: Chronic hepatitis C: Recommended dosage of combination therapy:

Intron® A: SubQ: 3 million int. units 3 times/week **and**

Rebetol® capsule: Oral:

≤75 kg (165 lb): 1000 mg/day (two 200 mg capsules in the morning and three 200 mg capsules in the evening)

>75 kg: 1200 mg/day (three 200 mg capsules in the morning and three 200 mg capsules in the evening)

Note: Treatment duration may vary. Consult current guidelines and literature.

Dosage Forms

Combination package:

Rebetron®:

For patients ≤75 kg [contains single-dose vials]:

Injection, solution: Interferon alfa-2b (Intron® A): 3 million int. units/0.5 mL (0.5 mL)

Capsule: Ribavirin (Rebetol®): 200 mg (70s)

For patients ≤75 kg [contains multidose vials]:

Injection, solution: Interferon alfa-2b (Intron® A): 3 million int. units/0.5 mL (3.8 mL)

Capsule: Ribavirin (Rebetol®): 200 mg (70s)

For patients ≤75 kg [contains multidose pen]:

Injection, solution: Interferon alfa-2b (Intron® A): 3 million int. units/0.2 mL (1.5 mL)

Capsule: Ribavirin (Rebetol®): 200 mg (70s)

For patients >75 kg [contains single-dose vials]:

Injection, solution: Interferon alfa-2b (Intron® A): 3 million int. units/0.5 mL (0.5 mL)

Capsule: Ribavirin (Rebetol®): 200 mg (84s)

For patients >75 kg [contains multidose vials]:

Injection, solution: Interferon alfa-2b (Intron® A): 3 million int. units/0.5 mL (3.8 mL)

Capsule: Ribavirin (Rebetol®): 200 mg (84s)

For patients >75 kg [contains multidose pen]:

Injection, solution: Interferon alfa-2b (Intron® A): 3 million int. units/0.2 mL (1.5 mL)

Capsule: Ribavirin (Rebetol®): 200 mg (84s)

For Rebetol® dose reduction [contains single-dose vials]:

Injection, solution: Interferon alfa-2b (Intron® A): 3 million int. units/0.5 mL (0.5 mL)

Capsule: Ribavirin (Rebetol®): 200 mg (42s)

For Rebetol® dose reduction [contains multidose vials]:

Injection, solution: Interferon alfa-2b (Intron® A): 3 million int. units/0.5 mL (3.8 mL)

Capsule: Ribavirin (Rebetol®): 200 mg (42s)

For Rebetol® dose reduction [contains multidose pen]:

Injection, solution: Interferon alfa-2b (Intron® A): 3 million int. units/0.2 mL (1.5 mL)

Capsule: Ribavirin (Rebetol®): 200 mg (42s)

interferon alfacon-1 (in ter FEER on AL fa con one)

Sound-Alike/Look-Alike Issues
interferon alfacon-1 may be confused with interferon alfa-2a, interferon alfa-2b, interferon alfa-n3, peginterferon alfa-2b

U.S./Canadian Brand Names Infergen® [US]

Therapeutic Category Interferon

Use Treatment of chronic hepatitis C virus (HCV) infection in patients ≥18 years of age with compensated liver disease and anti-HCV serum antibodies or HCV RNA.

Usual Dosage SubQ: Adults ≥18 years:
Chronic HCV infection: 9 mcg 3 times/week for 24 weeks; allow 48 hours between doses
Patients who have previously tolerated interferon therapy but did not respond or relapsed: 15 mcg 3 times/week for up to 48 weeks
Dose reduction for toxicity: Dose should be held in patients who experience a severe adverse reaction, and treatment should be stopped or decreased if the reaction does not become tolerable.
Doses were reduced from 9 mcg to 7.5 mcg in the pivotal study.
For patients receiving 15 mcg/dose, doses were reduced in 3 mcg decrements. Efficacy is decreased with doses <7.5 mcg

Dosage Forms
Injection, solution [preservative free]:
Infergen®: 30 mcg/mL (0.3 mL, 0.5 mL)

interferon alfa-n3 (in ter FEER on AL fa en three)

Sound-Alike/Look-Alike Issues
Alferon® may be confused with Alkeran®

U.S./Canadian Brand Names Alferon® N [US/Can]

Therapeutic Category Biological Response Modulator

Use Patients ≥18 years of age: Intralesional treatment of refractory or recurring genital or venereal warts (condylomata acuminata)

Usual Dosage Adults: Inject 250,000 units (0.05 mL) in each wart twice weekly for a maximum of 8 weeks; therapy should not be repeated for at least 3 months after the initial 8-week course of therapy

Dosage Forms
Injection, solution:
Alferon® N: 5 million int. units (1 mL)

interferon alpha-2a *see* interferon alfa-2a *on page 514*
interferon alpha-2b *see* interferon alfa-2b *on page 515*

interferon beta-1a (in ter FEER on BAY ta won aye)

Sound-Alike/Look-Alike Issues
Avonex® may be confused with Avelox®

Synonyms rIFN beta-1a

U.S./Canadian Brand Names Avonex® [US/Can]; Rebif® [US/Can]

Therapeutic Category Biological Response Modulator

Use Treatment of relapsing forms of multiple sclerosis (MS)

Usual Dosage Adults: **Note:** Analgesics and/or antipyretics may help decrease flu-like symptoms on treatment days:
I.M. (Avonex®): 30 mcg once weekly
SubQ (Rebif®): Doses should be separated by at least 48 hours:
Target dose 44 mcg 3 times/week:
Initial: 8.8 mcg (20% of final dose) 3 times/week for 2 weeks
Titration: 22 mcg (50% of final dose) 3 times/week for 2 weeks
Final dose: 44 mcg 3 times/week
Target dose 22 mcg 3 times/week:
Initial: 4.4 mcg (20% of final dose) 3 times/week for 2 weeks
Titration: 11 mcg (50% of final dose) 3 times/week for 2 weeks
Final dose: 22 mcg 3 times/week

◀ **Dosage Forms**
    Combination package [preservative free]:
      Rebif® Titration Pack:
        Injection, solution: 8.8 mcg/0.2 mL (0.2 mL) [6 prefilled syringes]
        Injection, solution: 22 mcg/0.5 mL (0.5 mL) [6 prefilled syringes]
    Injection, powder for reconstitution:
      Avonex®: 33 mcg [6.6 million units; provides 30 mcg/mL following reconstitution]
    Injection, solution:
      Avonex®: 30 mcg/0.5 mL (0.5 mL)
    Injection, solution [preservative free]:
      Rebif®: 22 mcg/0.5 mL (0.5 mL) [prefilled syringe]; 44 mcg/0.5 mL (0.5 mL) [prefilled syringe]

interferon beta-1b (in ter FEER on BAY ta won bee)

Synonyms rIFN beta-1b
U.S./Canadian Brand Names Betaseron® [US/Can]
Therapeutic Category Biological Response Modulator
Use Treatment of relapsing forms of multiple sclerosis (MS); treatment of first clinical episode with MRI features consistent with MS
Usual Dosage SubQ: **Note:** Gradual dose-titration, analgesics, and/or antipyretics may help decrease flu-like symptoms on treatment days:
    Adults: Initial: 0.0625 mg (2 million units; 0.25 mL) every other day; gradually increase dose by 0.0625 every 2 weeks
    Target dose: 0.25 mg (8 million units; 1 mL) every other day
Dosage Forms
    Injection, powder for reconstitution [preservative free]:
      Betaseron®: 0.3 mg [9.6 million units] [prefilled syringe]

interferon gamma-1b (in ter FEER on GAM ah won bee)

U.S./Canadian Brand Names Actimmune® [US/Can]
Therapeutic Category Biological Response Modulator
Use Reduce frequency and severity of serious infections associated with chronic granulomatous disease; delay time to disease progression in patients with severe, malignant osteopetrosis
Usual Dosage If severe reactions occur, reduce dose by 50% or therapy should be interrupted until adverse reaction abates.

Children: Severe, malignant osteopetrosis: SubQ:
    BSA ≤0.5 m^2: 1.5 mcg/kg/dose 3 times/week
    BSA >0.5 m^2: 50 mcg/m^2 (1 million int. units/m^2) 3 times/week
Children and Adults: Chronic granulomatous disease: SubQ:
    BSA ≤0.5 m^2: 1.5 mcg/kg/dose 3 times/week
    BSA >0.5 m^2: 50 mcg/m^2 (1 million int. units/m^2) 3 times/week

Note: Previously expressed as 1.5 million units/m^2; 50 mcg is equivalent to 1 million int. units/m^2.
Dosage Forms
    Injection, solution [preservative free]:
      Actimmune®: 100 mcg [2 million int. units] (0.5 mL)

Invirase® [US/Can] *see* saquinavir *on page 856*
Iodex [US-OTC] *see* iodine *on page 519*
Iodex-p® *(Discontinued)* *see* povidone-iodine *on page 775*

iodine (EYE oh dyne)
Sound-Alike/Look-Alike Issues
iodine may be confused with codeine, Iopidine®, Lodine®
U.S./Canadian Brand Names Iodex [US-OTC]; Iodoflex™ [US]; Iodosorb® [US]
Therapeutic Category Topical Skin Product
Use Used topically as an antiseptic in the management of minor, superficial skin wounds and has been used to disinfect the skin preoperatively
Usual Dosage
Topical:
Cleaning wet ulcers and wounds (Iodosorb®, Iodoflex™): Apply to clean wound; maximum: 50 g/application and 150 g/week. Change dressing ~3 times/week; reduce applications as exudate decreases. Do not use for >3 months; discontinue when wound is free of exudate.
Antiseptic for minor cuts, scrapes, burns: Apply small amount to affected area 1-3 times/day
Oral: RDA:
Children:
1-8 years: 90 mcg/day
9-13 years: 120 mcg/day
≥14 years: Refer to adult dosing
Adults: 150 mcg/day
Pregnancy: 220 mcg/day
Breast-feeding: 290 mcg/day
Dosage Forms
Dressing, topical [gel pad]:
Iodoflex™: 0.9% (5 g, 10 g)
Gel, topical:
Iodosorb®: 0.9% (40 g)
Ointment, topical:
Iodex [OTC]: 4.7% (30 g, 720 g)
Tincture, topical: 2% (30 mL, 480 mL); 7% (30 mL, 480 mL)

iodine *see* trace metals *on page 940*
iodine I 131 tositumomab and tositumomab *see* tositumomab and iodine I 131 tositumomab *on page 937*

iodipamide meglumine (eye oh DI pa mide MEG loo meen)
U.S./Canadian Brand Names Cholografin® Meglumine [US]
Therapeutic Category Iodinated Contrast Media; Radiological/Contrast Media, Ionic
Use Contrast medium for intravenous cholangiography and cholecystography
Usual Dosage Note: Do not repeat for 24 hours
I.V.: Cholangiography and cholecystography:
Infants and Children: 0.3-0.6 mL/kg (maximum: 20 mL)
Adults: 20 mL
Dosage Forms
Injection, solution:
Cholografin® Meglumine: 520 mg/mL (20 mL)

iodipamide meglumine and diatrizoate meglumine *see* diatrizoate meglumine and iodipamide meglumine *on page 289*

iodixanol (EYE oh dix an ole)
U.S./Canadian Brand Names Visipaque™ [US]
Therapeutic Category Iodinated Contrast Media; Radiological/Contrast Media, Nonionic
Use
Intraarterial: Digital subtraction angiography, angiocardiography, peripheral arteriography, visceral arteriography, cerebral arteriography

◄ Intravenous: Contrast enhanced computed tomography imaging, excretory urography, and peripheral venography

Usual Dosage

Children >1 year: **Note:** Maximum recommended total dose of iodine: Not been established
Intraarterial (cerebral, cardiac chambers, and related major arteries and visceral studies): Iodixanol 320 mg iodine/mL: 1-2 mL/kg; maximum dose: 4 mL/kg
I.V. (contrast-enhanced computer tomography or excretory urography): Iodixanol 270 mg iodine /mL: 1-2 mL/kg; maximum dose: 2 mL/kg

Children >12 years and Adults: **Note:** Maximum recommended total dose of iodine: 80 g
Intraarterial: Iodixanol 320 mg iodine/mL: Dose individualized based on injection site and study type; refer to product labeling
I.V.: Iodixanol 270 mg and 320 mg iodine/mL: concentration and dose vary based on study type; refer to product labeling.

Dosage Forms

Injection, solution [preservative free]:
Visipaque™ 270: 550 mg/mL (50 mL, 100 mL, 125 mL, 150 mL, 200 mL)
Visipaque™ 320: 652 mg/mL (50 mL, 100 mL, 125 mL, 150 mL, 200 mL)

iodochlorhydroxyquin and flumethasone see clioquinol and flumethasone (Canada only) on page 232

Iodoflex™ [US] see iodine on page 519

iodoquinol (eye oh doe KWIN ole)

Synonyms diiodohydroxyquin

U.S./Canadian Brand Names Diodoquin® [Can]; Yodoxin® [US]

Therapeutic Category Amebicide

Use Treatment of acute and chronic intestinal amebiasis; asymptomatic cyst passers; *Blastocystis hominis* infections; ineffective for amebic hepatitis or hepatic abscess

Usual Dosage Oral:
Children: 30-40 mg/kg/day (maximum: 650 mg/dose) in 3 divided doses for 20 days; not to exceed 1.95 g/day
Adults: 650 mg 3 times/day after meals for 20 days; not to exceed 1.95 g/day

Dosage Forms
Tablet:
Yodoxin®: 210 mg, 650 mg

iodoquinol and hydrocortisone (eye oh doe KWIN ole & hye droe KOR ti sone)

Sound-Alike/Look-Alike Issues
Vytone® may be confused with Hytone®, Zydone®

Synonyms hydrocortisone and iodoquinol

U.S./Canadian Brand Names Alcortin™ [US]; Dermazene® [US]; Vytone® [US]

Therapeutic Category Antifungal/Corticosteroid

Use Treatment of eczema (including impetiginized, nuchal, and nummular); acne urticaria; anogenital pruritus, atopic dermatitis, chronic infectious dermatitis; chronic eczematoid otitis externa; folliculitis, intertrigo; lichen simplex chronicus; moniliasis; mycotic dermatoses; neurodermatitis (localized or systemic); pyoderma, stasis dermatitis

Usual Dosage Topical: Children ≥12 years and Adults: Apply 3-4 times/day

Dosage Forms
Cream: Iodoquinol 1% and hydrocortisone 1% (30 g)
Dermazene®: Iodoquinol 1% and hydrocortisone 1% (30 g, 45 g)
Vytone®: Iodoquinol 1% and hydrocortisone 1% (30 g)
Gel:
Alcortin™: Iodoquinol 1% and hydrocortisone 2% (2 g)

Iodosorb® [US] see iodine on page 519

iohexol (eye oh HEX ole)

U.S./Canadian Brand Names Omnipaque™ [US]

Therapeutic Category Polypeptide Hormone; Radiological/Contrast Media, Nonionic

Use
Intrathecal: Myelography; contrast enhancement for computerized tomography
Intravascular: Angiocardiography, aortography, digital subtraction angiography, peripheral arteriography, excretory urography; contrast enhancement for computed tomographic imaging
Oral/body cavity: Arthrography, GI tract examination, hysterosalpingography, pancreatography, cholangiopancreatography, herniography, cystourethrography; enhanced computed tomography of the abdomen

Dosage Forms
Solution, injection [preservative free]:
Omnipaque™:
140: 302 mg/mL (50 mL)
180: 388 mg/mL (10 mL, 20 mL)
240: 518 mg/mL (10 mL, 20 mL, 100 mL, 150 mL, 200 mL)
300: 647 mg/mL (10 mL, 30 mL, 50 mL, 75 mL, 100 mL, 125 mL, 150 mL, 200 mL)
350: 755 mg/mL (50 mL, 75 mL, 100 mL, 125 mL, 150 mL, 200 mL, 250 mL)

Ionamin® [US/Can] *see* phentermine *on page 744*

Ionil® [US-OTC] *see* salicylic acid *on page 850*

Ionil Plus® [US-OTC] *see* salicylic acid *on page 850*

Ionil T® Plus (Discontinued) *see* coal tar *on page 240*

Ionsys™ [US] *see* fentanyl *on page 394*

iopamidol (eye oh PA mi dole)
U.S./Canadian Brand Names Isovue Multipack® [US]; Isovue-M® [US]; Isovue® [US]
Therapeutic Category Iodinated Contrast Media; Radiological/Contrast Media, Nonionic
Use
Intrathecal (Isovue-M®): Neuroradiology; contrast enhancement of computed tomographic cisternography and ventriculography; thoracolumbar myelography
Intravascular (Isovue®, Isovue Multipack®): Angiography, excretory urography; contrast enhancement of computed tomographic imaging; evaluation of certain malignancies; image enhancement of non-neoplastic lesions

Dosage Forms
Injection, solution:
Isovue®:
200: 41% (50 mL, 200 mL)
250: 51% (50 mL, 100 mL, 150 mL)
300: 61% (30 mL, 50 mL, 75 mL, 100 mL, 125 mL, 150 mL, 175 mL)
370: 76% (20 mL, 30 mL, 50 mL, 75 mL, 100 mL, 125 mL, 150 mL, 200 mL)
Isovue-M®:
200: 41% (10 mL, 20 mL)
300: 61% (15 mL)
Isovue Multipack® [pharmacy bulk package]:
250: 51% (200 mL)
300: 61% (200 mL, 500 mL)
370: 76% (200 mL, 500 mL)

Iopidine® [US/Can] *see* apraclonidine *on page 90*

iopromide (eye oh PROE mide)
U.S./Canadian Brand Names Ultravist® [US]
Therapeutic Category Radiological/Contrast Media, Nonionic
Use Enhance imaging in cerebral arteriography and peripheral arteriography; coronary arteriography and left ventriculography, visceral angiography and aortography; contrast-enhanced computed tomographic imaging of the head and body, excretory urography, intraarterial digital subtraction angiography, peripheral venography

Usual Dosage
Children >2 years: I.V.:
Cardiac chambers and related arteries (370 mg iodine/mL): 1-2 mL/kg; maximum dose for procedure: 4 mL/kg
Contrast-enhanced CT (300 mg iodine/mL): 1-2 mL/kg; maximum dose for procedure: 3 mL/kg

◄ Adults: **Note:** Maximum recommended total dose of iodine is 86 g. Individualize dose based upon patient's age, body weight, size of the vessel, and the rate of blood flow within the vessel.

Intravascular:

Aortography and visceral angiography (370 mg iodine/mL): Volume and rate of administration based on blood flow and specific characteristics of vessels being studied; maximum dose for procedure: 225 mL

Cerebral arteriography (300 mg iodine/mL): Maximum dose for procedure: 150 mL

Carotid artery visualization: 3-12 mL

Vertebral artery visualization: 4-12 mL

Aortic arch injection: 20-50 mL

Coronary arteriography and left ventriculography (370 mg iodine/mL): Maximum dose for procedure: 225 mL

Left coronary: 3-14 mL

Right coronary: 3-14 mL

Left ventricle: 30-60 mL

Intraarterial digital subtraction angiography (150 mg iodine/mL): Maximum dose for procedure: 250 mL

Carotid arteries: 6-10 mL

Vertebral: 4-8 mL

Aorta: 20-50 mL

Major branches of the abdominal aorta: 2-20 mL

Peripheral arteriography (300 mg iodine/mL): Maximum dose for procedure: 250 mL. **Note:** The artery needs a pulse to be injected.

Subclavian or femoral artery: 5-40 mL

Aortic bifurcation for distal runoff 25-50 mL

I.V.:

Contrast-enhanced CT (300 mg iodine/mL):

Head: 50-200 mL; maximum dose for procedure: 200 mL

Body: 50-200 mL (usual dose for infusion is 100-200 mL); **Note:** Can be given by bolus injection, by rapid infusion, or both; maximum dose for procedure: 200 mL

Excretory urography (normal renal function; 300 mg iodine/mL): 1 mL/kg; maximum dose for procedure: 100 mL

Peripheral venography (240 mg iodine/mL): Minimum amount to clearly visualize the structure under examination; maximum dose for procedure: 250 mL

Dosage Forms

Injection, solution:

Ultravist®:

Iodine 150 mg/mL (provides iopromide 311.7 mg/mL) (50 mL)

Iodine 240 mg/mL (provides iopromide 498.72 mg/mL) (50 mL, 100 mL, 200 mL)

Iodine 300 mg/mL (provides iopromide 623.4 mg/mL) (50 mL, 100 mL, 150 mL, 500 mL)

Iodine 370 mg/mL (provides iopromide 768.86 mg/mL) (50 mL, 100 mL, 150 mL, 200 mL, 500 mL)

Iosat™ [US-OTC] see potassium iodide *on page 773*

iothalamate meglumine (eye oh thal A mate MEG loo meen)

U.S./Canadian Brand Names Conray® 30 [US]; Conray® 43 [US]; Conray® [US]; Cysto-Conray® II [US]

Therapeutic Category Iodinated Contrast Media; Radiological/Contrast Media, Ionic

Use

Solution for injection: Arthrography, cerebral angiography, cranial computerized angiotomography, digital subtraction angiography, direct cholangiography, endoscopic retrograde cholangiopancreatography, excretory urography, peripheral arteriography, urography, venography; contrast enhancement of computed tomographic images

Solution for instillation: Retrograde cystography and cystourethrography

Dosage Forms

Injection, solution:

Conray®: 60% (30 mL, 50 mL, 100 mL, 150 mL)

Conray® 30: 30% (50 mL, 150 mL)

Conray® 43: 43% (50 mL, 100 mL, 200 mL, 250 mL)

Injection, solution for instillation:

Cysto-Conray® II: 17.2% (250 mL, 500 mL)

iothalamate sodium (eye oh thal A mate SOW dee um)
U.S./Canadian Brand Names Conray® 400 [US]
Therapeutic Category Iodinated Contrast Media; Radiological/Contrast Media, Ionic
Use Excretory urography, angiocardiography, aortography; contrast enhancement of computed tomographic brain images
Dosage Forms
Injection, solution:
Conray® 400: 66.8% (50 mL)

ioversol (EYE oh ver sole)
U.S./Canadian Brand Names Optiray® [US]
Therapeutic Category Iodinated Contrast Media; Radiological/Contrast Media, Nonionic
Use Arteriography, angiography, angiocardiography, ventriculography, excretory urography, and venography procedures; contrast enhanced tomographic imaging
Dosage Forms
Injection, solution [preservative free]:
Optiray®:
160: 34% (50 mL)
240: 51% (50 mL, 100 mL, 125 mL, 200 mL, 500 mL)
300: 64% (50 mL, 100 mL, 150 mL, 200 mL)
320: 68% (20 mL, 30 mL, 50 mL, 75 mL, 100 mL, 125 mL, 150 mL, 200 mL, 250 mL)
350: 74% (50 mL, 75 mL, 100 mL, 150 mL, 200 mL, 250 mL, 500 mL)

ioxaglate meglumine and ioxaglate sodium
(eye ox AG late MEG loo meen & eye ox AG late SOW dee um)
Synonyms ioxaglate sodium and ioxaglate meglumine
U.S./Canadian Brand Names Hexabrix™ [US]
Therapeutic Category Iodinated Contrast Media; Radiological/Contrast Media, Ionic
Use Angiocardiography, arteriography, aortography, arthrography, angiography, hysterosalpingography, venography, and urography procedures; contrast enhancement of computed tomographic imaging
Dosage Forms
Injection, solution:
Hexabrix™: ioxaglate meglumine 39.3% and ioxaglate sodium 19.6% (20 mL, 50 mL, 100 mL, 150 mL, 200 mL)

ioxaglate sodium and ioxaglate meglumine *see* ioxaglate meglumine and ioxaglate sodium
on page 523

ioxilan (eye OKS ee lan)
U.S./Canadian Brand Names Oxilan® 300 [Can]; Oxilan® 350 [Can]; Oxilan® [US]
Therapeutic Category Iodinated Contrast Media; Radiological/Contrast Media, Nonionic
Use
Intraarterial: Ioxilan 300 mgI/mL is indicated for cerebral arteriography. Ioxilan 350 mgI/mL is indicated for coronary arteriography and left ventriculography, visceral angiography, aortography, and peripheral arteriography
Intravenous: Both products are indicated for excretory urography and contrast-enhanced computed tomographic (CECT) imaging of the head and body
Usual Dosage Adults:
Intraarterial: Coronary arteriography and left ventriculography: For visualization of coronary arteries and left ventricle, ioxilan injection with a concentration of 350 mg iodine/mL is recommended
Usual injection volumes:
Left and right coronary: 2-10 mL (0.7-3.5 g iodine)
Left ventricle: 25-50 mL (8.75-17.5 g iodine)
Total doses should not exceed 250 mL; the injection rate of ioxilan should approximate the flow rate in the vessel injected
Cerebral arteriography: For evaluation of arterial lesions of the brain, a concentration of 300 mg iodine/mL is indicated
Recommended doses: 8-12 mL (2.4-3.6 g iodine)
Total dose should not exceed 150 mL

▶

◀ **Dosage Forms**
Injection, solution [preservative free]:
Oxilan®: 300: 62% (50 mL, 100 mL, 150 mL, 200 mL); 350: 73% (50 mL, 100 mL, 150 mL, 200 mL)

ipecac syrup (IP e kak SIR up)

Synonyms syrup of ipecac
Therapeutic Category Antidote
Use Treatment of acute oral drug overdosage and in certain poisonings
Usual Dosage Oral:
Children:
6-12 months: 5-10 mL followed by 10-20 mL/kg of water; repeat dose one time if vomiting does not occur within 20 minutes
1-12 years: 15 mL followed by 10-20 mL/kg of water; repeat dose one time if vomiting does not occur within 20 minutes
If emesis does not occur within 30 minutes after second dose, ipecac must be removed from stomach by gastric lavage
Adults: 15-30 mL followed by 200-300 mL of water; repeat dose one time if vomiting does not occur within 20 minutes
Dosage Forms
Syrup: 70 mg/mL (30 mL)

I-Pentolate® *(Discontinued)* see cyclopentolate on page 256
I-Phrine® Ophthalmic Solution *(Discontinued)* see phenylephrine on page 745
I-Picamide® *(Discontinued)* see tropicamide on page 957
Iplex™ *(Discontinued)* see mecasermin on page 595
IPM Wound Gel™ [US-OTC] see hyaluronate and derivatives on page 476
IPOL® [US/Can] see poliovirus vaccine (inactivated) on page 764

ipratropium (i pra TROE pee um)

Sound-Alike/Look-Alike Issues
Atrovent® may be confused with Alupent®
Synonyms ipratropium bromide
U.S./Canadian Brand Names Alti-Ipratropium [Can]; Apo-Ipravent® [Can]; Atrovent® HFA [US/Can]; Atrovent® [US/Can]; Gen-Ipratropium [Can]; Novo-Ipramide [Can]; Nu-Ipratropium [Can]; PMS-Ipratropium [Can]
Therapeutic Category Anticholinergic Agent
Use
Oral inhalation: Anticholinergic bronchodilator used in bronchospasm associated with COPD, bronchitis, and emphysema
Nasal spray: Symptomatic relief of rhinorrhea associated with the common cold and allergic and nonallergic rhinitis
Usual Dosage
Nebulization:
Children ≤12 years: Asthma exacerbation, acute (*NIH Asthma Guidelines, 2007*): 250-500 mcg every 20 minutes for 3 doses, then as needed. **Note:** Should be given in combination with a short-acting beta-adrenergic agonist.
Children >12 years and Adults:
Bronchodilator for COPD: 500 mcg (one unit-dose vial) 3-4 times/day with doses 6-8 hours apart
Asthma exacerbation, acute (*NIH Asthma Guidelines, 2007*): 500 mcg every 20 minutes for 3 doses, then as needed. **Note:** Should be given in combination with a short-acting beta-adrenergic agonist.
Oral inhalation: MDI:
Children ≤12 years: Asthma exacerbation, acute (*NIH Asthma Guidelines, 2007*): 4-8 inhalations every 20 minutes as needed for up to 3 hours. **Note:** Should be given in combination with a short-acting beta-adrenergic agonist.
Children >12 years and Adults:
Bronchodilator for COPD: 2 inhalations 4 times/day, up to 12 inhalations/24 hours
Asthma exacerbation, acute (*NIH Asthma Guidelines, 2007*): 8 inhalations every 20 minutes as needed for up to 3 hours. **Note:** Should be given in combination with a short-acting beta-adrenergic agonist.

Intranasal: Nasal spray:
 Symptomatic relief of rhinorrhea associated with the common cold (safety and efficacy of use beyond 4 days in patients with the common cold have not been established):
  Children 5-11 years: 0.06%: 2 sprays in each nostril 3 times/day
  Children ≥12 years and Adults: 0.06%: 2 sprays in each nostril 3-4 times/day
 Symptomatic relief of rhinorrhea associated with allergic/nonallergic rhinitis: Children ≥6 years and Adults: 0.03%: 2 sprays in each nostril 2-3 times/day
 Symptomatic relief of rhinorrhea associated with seasonal allergic rhinitis (safety and efficacy of use beyond 3 weeks in patients with seasonal allergic rhinitis has not been established): Children ≥5 years and Adults: 0.06%: 2 sprays in each nostril 4 times/day
Dosage Forms
 Aerosol for oral inhalation:
  Atrovent® HFA: 17 mcg/actuation (12.9 g)
 Solution for nebulization: 0.02% (2.5 mL)
 Solution, intranasal [spray]:
  Atrovent®: 0.03% (30 mL); 0.06% (15 mL)

ipratropium and albuterol (i pra TROE pee um & al BYOO ter ole)
Sound-Alike/Look-Alike Issues
 Combivent® may be confused with Combivir®
Synonyms albuterol and ipratropium; salbutamol and ipratropium
U.S./Canadian Brand Names CO Ipra-Sal [Can]; Combivent® [US/Can]; DuoNeb® [US]; Gen-Combo Sterinebs [Can]; ratio-Ipra Sal UDV [Can]
Therapeutic Category Bronchodilator
Use Treatment of COPD in those patients who are currently on a regular bronchodilator who continue to have bronchospasms and require a second bronchodilator
Usual Dosage Adults:
 Aerosol for inhalation: 2 inhalations 4 times/day (maximum: 12 inhalations/24 hours)
 Solution for nebulization: Initial: 3 mL every 6 hours (maximum: 3 mL every 4 hours)
Dosage Forms
 Aerosol for oral inhalation:
  Combivent®: Ipratropium 18 mcg and albuterol 103 mcg per actuation (14.7 g) [200 metered actuations]
 Solution for nebulization: Ipratropium 0.5 mg and albuterol 2.5 mg per 3 mL (30s, 60s)
  DuoNeb®: Ipratropium 0.5 mg and albuterol 2.5 mg per 3 mL (30s, 60s)

ipratropium bromide see ipratropium on page 524
I-Prin [US-OTC] see ibuprofen on page 495
iproveratril hydrochloride see verapamil on page 974
IPV see poliovirus vaccine (inactivated) on page 764
Iquix® [US] see levofloxacin on page 557

irbesartan (ir be SAR tan)
Sound-Alike/Look-Alike Issues
 Avapro® may be confused with Anaprox®
U.S./Canadian Brand Names Avapro® [US/Can]
Therapeutic Category Angiotensin II Receptor Antagonist
Use Treatment of hypertension alone or in combination with other antihypertensives; treatment of diabetic nephropathy in patients with type 2 diabetes mellitus (noninsulin-dependent, NIDDM) and hypertension
Usual Dosage Oral:
 Hypertension:
  Children: ≥6-12 years: Initial: 75 mg once daily; may be titrated to a maximum of 150 mg once daily
  Children ≥13 years and Adults: 150 mg once daily; patients may be titrated to 300 mg once daily
  Note: Starting dose in volume-depleted patients should be 75 mg
 Nephropathy in patients with type 2 diabetes and hypertension: Adults: Target dose: 300 mg once daily
Dosage Forms
 Tablet:
  Avapro®: 75 mg, 150 mg, 300 mg

irbesartan and hydrochlorothiazide (ir be SAR tan & hye droe klor oh THYE a zide)

Sound-Alike/Look-Alike Issues
Avalide® may be confused with Avandia®

Synonyms Avapro® HCT; hydrochlorothiazide and irbesartan

U.S./Canadian Brand Names Avalide® [US/Can]

Therapeutic Category Antihypertensive Agent, Combination

Use Combination therapy for the management of hypertension; may be used as initial therapy in patients likely to need multiple drugs to achieve blood pressure goals

Note: In Canada, this combination product is approved for initial therapy in severe, essential hypertension (sitting diastolic blood pressure [DBP] ≥110 mm Hg).

Usual Dosage Oral: Adults:
Add-on therapy: Dose must be individualized. A patient who is not controlled with either agent alone may be switched to the combination product. Mean effect increases with the dose of each component. The lowest dosage available is irbesartan 150 mg/hydrochlorothiazide 12.5 mg. Dose increases should be made not more frequently than every 2-4 weeks.

Initial therapy: Irbesartan 150 mg/hydrochlorothiazide 12.5 mg once daily. If initial response is inadequate, may titrate dose after 2-4 weeks, to a maximum dose of irbesartan 300 mg/hydrochlorothiazide 25 mg once daily.

Dosage Forms
Tablet:
Avalide®: Irbesartan 150 mg and hydrochlorothiazide 12.5 mg; irbesartan 300 mg and hydrochlorothiazide 12.5 mg; irbesartan 300 mg and hydrochlorothiazide 25 mg

Ircon® [US-OTC] see ferrous fumarate *on page 397*

IRESSA® [US] see gefitinib *on page 437*

irinotecan (eye rye no TEE kan)

Synonyms camptothecin-11; CPT-11; NSC-616348

U.S./Canadian Brand Names Camptosar® [US/Can]; Irinotecan Hydrochloride Trihydrate [Can]

Therapeutic Category Antineoplastic Agent

Use Treatment of metastatic carcinoma of the colon or rectum

Usual Dosage I.V. (Refer to individual protocols): **Note:** A reduction in the starting dose by one dose level should be considered for patients ≥65 years of age, prior pelvic/abdominal radiotherapy, performance status of 2, homozygosity for UGT1A1*28 allele, or increased bilirubin (dosing for patients with a bilirubin >2 mg/dL cannot be recommended based on lack of data per manufacturer).

Single-agent therapy:
125 mg/m^2 over 90 minutes on days 1, 8, 15, and 22 of a 6-week treatment cycle
  Adjusted dose level -1: 100 mg/m^2
  Adjusted dose level -2: 75 mg/m^2
Once-every-3-week regimen: 350 mg/m^2 over 90 minutes, once every 3 weeks
  Adjusted dose level -1: 300 mg/m^2
  Adjusted dose level -2: 250 mg/m^2
Depending on the patient's ability to tolerate therapy, doses should be adjusted in increments of 25-50 mg/m^2. Irinotecan doses may range from 50-150 mg/m^2 for the weekly regimen. Patients may be dosed as low as 200 mg/m^2 (in 50 mg/m^2 decrements) for the once-every-3-week regimen.

Combination therapy with fluorouracil and leucovorin: Six-week (42-day) cycle:
Regimen 1: 125 mg/m^2 over 90 minutes on days 1, 8, 15, and 22; to be given in combination with bolus leucovorin and fluorouracil (leucovorin administered immediately following irinotecan; fluorouracil immediately following leucovorin)
  Adjusted dose level -1: 100 mg/m^2
  Adjusted dose level -2: 75 mg/m^2
Regimen 2: 180 mg/m^2 over 90 minutes on days 1, 15, and 29; to be given in combination with infusional leucovorin and bolus/infusion fluorouracil (leucovorin administered immediately following irinotecan; fluorouracil immediately following leucovorin)
  Adjusted dose level -1: 150 mg/m^2
  Adjusted dose level -2: 120 mg/m^2

Note: For all regimens: It is recommended that new courses begin only after the granulocyte count recovers to ≥1500/mm^3, the platelet count recovers to ≥100,000/mm^3, and treatment-related diarrhea has fully resolved. Treatment should be delayed 1-2 weeks to allow for recovery from treatment-related toxicities. If the patient has not recovered after a 2-week delay, consideration should be given to discontinuing irinotecan.

Dosage Forms
Injection, solution: 20 mg/mL (2 mL, 5 mL)
Camptosar®: 20 mg/mL (2 mL, 5 mL)

Irinotecan Hydrochloride Trihydrate [Can] *see* irinotecan *on page 526*

iron dextran complex (EYE ern DEKS tran KOM pleks)

Sound-Alike/Look-Alike Issues
Dexferrum® may be confused with Desferal®

U.S./Canadian Brand Names Dexferrum® [US]; Dexiron™ [Can]; INFeD® [US]; Infufer® [Can]

Therapeutic Category Electrolyte Supplement, Oral

Use Treatment of microcytic hypochromic anemia resulting from iron deficiency in patients in whom oral administration is infeasible or ineffective

Usual Dosage I.M. (Z-track method should be used for I.M. injection), I.V.:
A 0.5 mL test dose (0.25 mL in infants) should be given prior to starting iron dextran therapy; total dose should be divided into a daily schedule for I.M., total dose may be given as a single continuous infusion
Iron-deficiency anemia:
Children 5-15 kg: Should not normally be given in the first 4 months of life:
Dose (mL) = 0.0442 (desired hemoglobin - observed hemoglobin) x W + (0.26 x W)
Desired hemoglobin: Usually 12 g/dL
W = Total body weight in kg
Children >15 kg and Adults:
Dose (mL) = 0.0442 (desired hemoglobin - observed hemoglobin) x LBW + (0.26 x LBW)
Desired hemoglobin: Usually 14.8 g/dL
LBW = Lean body weight in kg
Iron replacement therapy for blood loss: Replacement iron (mg) = blood loss (mL) x hematocrit

Maximum daily dosage:
Manufacturer's labeling: **Note:** Replacement of larger estimated iron deficits may be achieved by serial administration of smaller incremental dosages. Daily dosages should be limited to:
Children:
5-15 kg: 50 mg iron (1 mL)
15-50 kg: 100 mg iron (2 mL)
Adults >50 kg: 100 mg iron (2 mL)

Dosage Forms
Injection, solution:
Dexferrum®: 50 mg/mL (1 mL, 2 mL)
INFeD®: 50 mg/mL (2 mL)

iron fumarate *see* ferrous fumarate *on page 397*
iron gluconate *see* ferrous gluconate *on page 398*
iron-polysaccharide complex *see* polysaccharide-iron complex *on page 768*

iron sucrose (EYE ern SOO krose)

U.S./Canadian Brand Names Venofer® [US/Can]

Therapeutic Category Iron Salt

Use Treatment of iron-deficiency anemia in chronic renal failure, including nondialysis-dependent patients (with or without erythropoietin therapy) and dialysis-dependent patients receiving erythropoietin therapy

Usual Dosage Doses expressed in mg of **elemental** iron. **Note:** Test dose: Product labeling does not indicate need for a test dose in product-naive patients.
I.V.: Adults: Iron-deficiency anemia in chronic renal disease:
Hemodialysis-dependent patient: 100 mg (5 mL of iron sucrose injection) administered 1-3 times/week during dialysis; administer no more than 3 times/week to a cumulative total dose of 1000 mg (10 doses); may continue to administer at lowest dose necessary to maintain target hemoglobin, hematocrit, and iron storage parameters
Peritoneal dialysis-dependent patient: Slow intravenous infusion at the following schedule: Two infusions of 300 mg each over 1 1/2 hours 14 days apart followed by a single 400 mg infusion over 2 1/2 hours 14 days later (total cumulative dose of 1000 mg in 3 divided doses)

◀ Nondialysis-dependent patient: 200 mg slow injection (over 2-5 minutes) on 5 different occasions within a 14-day period. Total cumulative dose: 1000 mg in 14-day period. **Note:** Dosage has also been administered as two infusions of 500 mg in a maximum of 250 mL 0.9% NaCl infused over 3.5-4 hours on day 1 and day 14 (limited experience)

Dosage Forms
Injection, solution [preservative free]:
Venofer®: 20 mg of elemental iron/mL (5 mL, 10 mL)

iron sulfate *see* ferrous sulfate *on page 398*
iron sulfate and vitamin C *see* ferrous sulfate and ascorbic acid *on page 399*
Isagel® [US-OTC] *see* alcohol (ethyl) *on page 41*
ISD *see* isosorbide dinitrate *on page 530*
ISDN *see* isosorbide dinitrate *on page 530*
Isentress™ [US/Can] *see* raltegravir *on page 817*
ISG *see* immune globulin (intramuscular) *on page 502*
ISMN *see* isosorbide mononitrate *on page 531*
Ismo® [US] *see* isosorbide mononitrate *on page 531*
isoamyl nitrite *see* amyl nitrite *on page 74*
isobamate *see* carisoprodol *on page 180*
Isocal® [US-OTC] *see* nutritional formula, enteral/oral *on page 689*

isocarboxazid (eye soe kar BOKS a zid)

U.S./Canadian Brand Names Marplan® [US]
Therapeutic Category Antidepressant, Monoamine Oxidase Inhibitor
Use Treatment of depression
Usual Dosage Oral: Adults: Initial: 10 mg 2-4 times/day; may increase by 10 mg/day every 2-4 days to 40 mg/day by the end of the first week (divided into 2-4 doses). After first week, may increase by up to 20 mg/week to a maximum of 60 mg/day. May take 3-6 weeks to see effects. Dose should be reduced once maximum clinical effect is seen. If no response obtained within 6 weeks, additional titration is unlikely to be beneficial. **Note:** Use caution in patients on >40 mg/day; experience is limited.
Dosage Forms
Tablet:
Marplan®: 10 mg

Isochron™ [US] *see* isosorbide dinitrate *on page 530*

isoflurane (eye soe FLURE ane)

Sound-Alike/Look-Alike Issues
isoflurane may be confused with enflurane, isoflurophate
U.S./Canadian Brand Names Forane® [US/Can]; Terrell™ [US]
Therapeutic Category General Anesthetic
Use Induction and maintenance of general anesthesia
Usual Dosage Inhalation: Adults:
Anesthesia: Minimum alveolar concentration (MAC), the concentration at which 50% of patients do not respond to surgical incision, is 1.15% (44 years of age) for isoflurane.
Induction: 1.5% to 3%
Maintenance: In nitrous oxide: 1% to 2.5%; in oxygen: 1.5% to 3.5%
Dosage Forms
Liquid, for inhalation: >99.9% (100 mL, 250 mL)
Forane®, Terrell™: >99.9% (100 mL, 250 mL)

isometheptene, acetaminophen, and dichloralphenazone *see* acetaminophen, isometheptene, and dichloralphenazone *on page 28*
isometheptene, dichloralphenazone, and acetaminophen *see* acetaminophen, isometheptene, and dichloralphenazone *on page 28*
IsonaRif™ [US] *see* rifampin and isoniazid *on page 834*

isoniazid (eye soe NYE a zid)

Synonyms INH; isonicotinic acid hydrazide
U.S./Canadian Brand Names Isotamine® [Can]; PMS-Isoniazid [Can]

Therapeutic Category Antitubercular Agent

Use Treatment of susceptible tuberculosis infections; treatment of latent tuberculosis infection (LTBI)

Usual Dosage

Usual dosage ranges: Oral, I.M.:

Infants and Children: 10-15 mg/kg/day in 1-2 divided doses (maximum: 300 mg/day) or 20-40 mg/kg given 2-3 times per week (maximum: 900 mg/dose)

Adults: 5 mg/kg/day (usual: 300 mg/day) as a single daily dose or 15 mg/kg (maximum: 900 mg/dose) given 2-3 times per week

Indication-specific dosing: Oral, I.M.: Recommendations often change due to resistant strains and newly-developed information; consult *MMWR* for current CDC recommendations. Intramuscular injection is available for patients who are unable to either take or absorb oral therapy.

Infants and Children:

Tuberculosis, active:

Daily therapy: 10-15 mg/kg/day in 1-2 divided doses (maximum: 300 mg/day)

Twice weekly or 3 times/week directly observed therapy (DOT): 20-40 mg/kg (maximum: 900 mg)

Tuberculosis, latent infection (LTBI): 10 mg/kg/day as a single dose (maximum: 300 mg/day) **or** 20-30 mg/kg (maximum: 900 mg/dose) twice weekly for 9 months

Adults: **Note:** Concomitant administration of 10-50 mg/day pyridoxine is recommended in malnourished patients or those prone to neuropathy (eg, alcoholics, patients with diabetes).

Tuberculosis, active:

Daily therapy: 5 mg/kg/day given daily (usual dose: 300 mg/day)

Twice weekly or 3 times/week directly observed therapy (DOT): 15 mg/kg (maximum: 900 mg). **Note:** CDC guidelines state that once-weekly therapy (15 mg/kg/dose) may be considered, but only after the first 2 months of initial therapy in HIV-negative patients, and only in combination with rifapentine.

Note: Treatment may be defined by the number of doses administered (eg, "six-month" therapy involves 182 doses of INH and rifampin, and 56 doses of pyrazinamide). Six months is the shortest interval of time over which these doses may be administered, assuming no interruption of therapy.

Tuberculosis, latent infection (LTBI): 300 mg/day or 900 mg twice weekly for 6-9 months in patients who do not have HIV infection (9 months is optimal, 6 months may be considered to reduce costs of therapy) and 9 months in patients who have HIV infection. Extend to 12 months of therapy if interruptions in treatment occur.

Dosage Forms

Oral solution: 50 mg/5 mL

Tablet: 100 mg, 300 mg

isoniazid and rifampin *see* rifampin and isoniazid *on page 834*

isoniazid, rifampin, and pyrazinamide *see* rifampin, isoniazid, and pyrazinamide *on page 834*

isonicotinic acid hydrazide *see* isoniazid *on page 528*

isonipecaine hydrochloride *see* meperidine *on page 603*

isophane insulin *see* insulin NPH *on page 512*

isophane insulin and regular insulin *see* insulin NPH and insulin regular *on page 512*

isophosphamide *see* ifosfamide *on page 499*

isoproterenol (eye soe proe TER e nole)

Sound-Alike/Look-Alike Issues

Isuprel® may be confused with Disophrol®, Ismelin®, Isordil®

Synonyms isoproterenol hydrochloride

U.S./Canadian Brand Names Isuprel® [US]

Therapeutic Category Adrenergic Agonist Agent

Use Ventricular arrhythmias due to AV nodal block; hemodynamically compromised bradyarrhythmias or atropine- and dopamine-resistant bradyarrhythmias (when transcutaneous/venous pacing is not available); temporary use in third-degree AV block until pacemaker insertion

Usual Dosage I.V.: Cardiac arrhythmias:

Children: Initial: 0.1 mcg/kg/minute (usual effective dose 0.2-2 mcg/kg/minute)

Adults: Initial: 2 mcg/minute; titrate to patient response (2-10 mcg/minute)

Dosage Forms

Injection, solution:

Isuprel®: 0.2 mg/mL (1:5000) (1 mL, 5 mL)

isoproterenol hydrochloride *see* isoproterenol *on page 529*
Isoptin® *(Discontinued)* *see* verapamil *on page 974*
Isoptin® SR [US/Can] *see* verapamil *on page 974*
Isopto® Atropine [US/Can] *see* atropine *on page 104*
Isopto® Carbachol [US/Can] *see* carbachol *on page 172*
Isopto® Carpine [US/Can] *see* pilocarpine *on page 753*
Isopto® Cetapred® *(Discontinued)*
Isopto® Eserine [Can] *see* physostigmine *on page 752*
Isopto® Eserine *(Discontinued)* *see* physostigmine *on page 752*
Isopto® Frin Ophthalmic Solution *(Discontinued)* *see* phenylephrine *on page 745*
Isopto® Homatropine [US] *see* homatropine *on page 475*
Isopto® Hyoscine [US] *see* scopolamine derivatives *on page 858*
Isopto® Plain Solution *(Discontinued)* *see* artificial tears *on page 95*
Isopto® Tears [US-OTC/Can] *see* hydroxypropyl methylcellulose *on page 490*
Isordil® [US] *see* isosorbide dinitrate *on page 530*

isosorbide dinitrate (eye soe SOR bide dye NYE trate)

Sound-Alike/Look-Alike Issues
    Isordil® may be confused with Inderal®, Isuprel®
Synonyms ISD; ISDN
U.S./Canadian Brand Names Apo-ISDN® [Can]; Cedocard®-SR [Can]; Coronex® [Can]; Dilatrate®-SR [US]; Isochron™ [US]; Isordil® [US]; Novo-Sorbide [Can]; PMS-Isosorbide [Can]
Therapeutic Category Vasodilator
Use Prevention and treatment of angina pectoris; for congestive heart failure; to relieve pain, dysphagia, and spasm in esophageal spasm with GE reflux
Usual Dosage Oral: Adults:
  Angina: 5-40 mg 4 times/day or 40 mg every 8-12 hours in sustained-release dosage form
    Sublingual: 2.5-5 mg every 5-10 minutes for maximum of 3 doses in 15-30 minutes; may also use prophylactically 15 minutes prior to activities which may provoke an attack
  Congestive heart failure:
    Initial dose: 20 mg 3-4 times per day
    Target dose: 120-160 mg/day in divided doses; use in combination with hydralazine
  Tolerance to nitrate effects develops with chronic exposure: Dose escalation does not overcome this effect. Tolerance can only be overcome by short periods of nitrate absence from the body. Short periods (10-12 hours) of nitrate withdrawal help minimize tolerance. General recommendations are to take the last dose of short-acting agents no later than 7 PM; administer 2-3 times/day rather than 4 times/day. Sustained release preparations could be administered at times to allow a 15- to 17-hour interval between first and last daily dose. Example: Administer sustained release at 8 AM and 2 PM for a twice daily regimen.
Dosage Forms
  Capsule, sustained release:
    Dilatrate®-SR: 40 mg
  Tablet: 5 mg, 10 mg, 20 mg, 30 mg
    Isordil®: 5 mg, 40 mg
  Tablet, extended release:
    Isochron™: 40 mg
  Tablet, sublingual: 2.5 mg, 5 mg

isosorbide dinitrate and hydralazine

(eye soe SOR bide dye NYE trate & hye DRAL a zeen)
Synonyms hydralazine and isosorbide dinitrate
U.S./Canadian Brand Names BiDil® [US]
Therapeutic Category Vasodilator
Use Treatment of heart failure, adjunct to standard therapy, in self-identified African-Americans
Usual Dosage Oral: Adults: Initial: 1 tablet 3 times/day; titrate to a maximum dose of 2 tablets 3 times/day
Dosage Forms
  Tablet:
    BiDil®: Isosorbide 20 mg and hydralazine 37.5 mg

isosorbide mononitrate (eye soe SOR bide mon oh NYE trate)

Sound-Alike/Look-Alike Issues
Imdur® may be confused with Imuran®, Inderal LA®, K-Dur®
Monoket® may be confused with Monopril®

Synonyms ISMN

U.S./Canadian Brand Names Apo-ISMN® [Can]; Imdur® [US/Can]; Ismo® [US]; Monoket® [US]; PMS-ISMN [Can]

Therapeutic Category Vasodilator

Use Long-acting metabolite of the vasodilator isosorbide dinitrate used for the prophylactic treatment of angina pectoris

Usual Dosage Oral: Adults and Geriatrics (start with lowest recommended dose):
Regular tablet: 5-20 mg twice daily with the two doses given 7 hours apart (eg, 8 AM and 3 PM) to decrease tolerance development; then titrate to 10 mg twice daily in first 2-3 days.
Extended release tablet: Initial: 30-60 mg given in morning as a single dose; titrate upward as needed, giving at least 3 days between increases; maximum daily single dose: 240 mg
Tolerance to nitrate effects develops with chronic exposure. Dose escalation does not overcome this effect. Tolerance can only be overcome by short periods of nitrate absence from the body. Short periods (10-12 hours) of nitrate withdrawal help minimize tolerance. Recommended dosage regimens incorporate this interval. General recommendations are to take the last dose of short-acting agents no later than 7 PM; administer 2 times/day rather than 4 times/day. Administer sustained release tablet once daily in the morning.

Dosage Forms
Tablet: 10 mg, 20 mg
Ismo®: 20 mg
Monoket®: 10 mg, 20 mg
Tablet, extended release: 30 mg, 60 mg, 120 mg
Imdur®: 30 mg, 60 mg, 120 mg

isosulfan blue (eye soe SUL fan bloo)

U.S./Canadian Brand Names Lymphazurin™ [US]

Therapeutic Category Contrast Agent

Use Adjunct to lymphography for visualization of the lymphatic system; sentinel node identification

Usual Dosage SubQ: Adults: Inject 0.5 mL into 3 interdigital spaces of each extremity per study; maximum: 3 mL (30 mg)

Dosage Forms
Injection, solution [preservative-free]:
Lymphazurin™: 1% (5 mL)

Isotamine® [Can] *see* isoniazid *on page 528*

isotretinoin (eye soe TRET i noyn)

Sound-Alike/Look-Alike Issues
isotretinoin may be confused with tretinoin
Accutane® may be confused with Accolate®, Accupril®

Synonyms 13-*cis*-retinoic acid

U.S./Canadian Brand Names Accutane® [US/Can]; Amnesteem™ [US]; Claravis™ [US]; Clarus™ [Can]; Isotrex® [Can]; Sotret® [US]

Therapeutic Category Retinoic Acid Derivative

Use Treatment of severe recalcitrant nodular acne unresponsive to conventional therapy

Usual Dosage Oral: Children 12-17 years and Adults: Severe recalcitrant nodular acne: 0.5-1 mg/kg/day in 2 divided doses (dosages as low as 0.05 mg/kg/day have been reported to be beneficial) for 15-20 weeks or until the total cyst count decreases by 70%, whichever is sooner. Adults with very severe disease/scarring or primarily involves the trunk may require dosage adjustment up to 2 mg/kg/day. A second course of therapy may be initiated after a period of ≥2 months off therapy.

Dosage Forms
Capsule:
Accutane®, Amnesteem™, Claravis™: 10 mg, 20 mg, 40 mg
Sotret®: 10 mg, 20 mg, 30 mg, 40 mg

Isotrex® [Can] *see* isotretinoin *on page 531*
Isovue® [US] *see* iopamidol *on page 521*
Isovue-M® [US] *see* iopamidol *on page 521*
Isovue Multipack® [US] *see* iopamidol *on page 521*

isoxsuprine (eye SOKS syoo preen)
Sound-Alike/Look-Alike Issues
Vasodilan® may be confused with Vasocidin®
Synonyms isoxsuprine hydrochloride
Therapeutic Category Vasodilator
Use Treatment of peripheral vascular diseases, such as arteriosclerosis obliterans and Raynaud disease
Usual Dosage Oral: Adults: 10-20 mg 3-4 times/day
Dosage Forms
Tablet: 10 mg, 20 mg

isoxsuprine hydrochloride *see* isoxsuprine *on page 532*

isradipine (iz RA di peen)
Sound-Alike/Look-Alike Issues
DynaCirc® may be confused with Dynabac®, Dynacin®
U.S./Canadian Brand Names DynaCirc® CR [US]; DynaCirc® [Can]
Therapeutic Category Calcium Channel Blocker
Use Treatment of hypertension
Usual Dosage Oral: Adults:
Capsule: 2.5 mg twice daily; antihypertensive response occurs in 2-3 hours; maximal response in 2-4 weeks; increase dose at 2- to 4-week intervals at 2.5-5 mg increments; usual dose range (JNC 7): 2.5-10 mg/day in 2 divided doses. **Note:** Most patients show no improvement with doses >10 mg/day except adverse reaction rate increases; therefore, maximal dose in older adults should be 10 mg/day.
Controlled release tablet: 5 mg once daily; antihypertensive response occurs in 2 hours. Adjust dose in increments of 5 mg at 2-4 week intervals. Maximum dose: 20 mg/day; adverse events are increased at doses >10 mg/day.
Dosage Forms
Capsule: 2.5 mg, 5 mg
Tablet, controlled release:
DynaCirc® CR: 5 mg, 10 mg

Istalol® [US] *see* timolol *on page 927*
Isuprel® [US] *see* isoproterenol *on page 529*
Itch-X® [US-OTC] *see* pramoxine *on page 777*

itraconazole (i tra KOE na zole)
Sound-Alike/Look-Alike Issues
Sporanox® may be confused with Suprax®
U.S./Canadian Brand Names Sporanox® [US/Can]
Therapeutic Category Antifungal Agent
Use Treatment of susceptible fungal infections in immunocompromised and immunocompetent patients including blastomycosis and histoplasmosis; indicated for aspergillosis, and onychomycosis of the toenail; treatment of onychomycosis of the fingernail without concomitant toenail infection via a pulse-type dosing regimen; has activity against *Aspergillus*, *Candida*, *Coccidioides*, *Cryptococcus*, *Sporothrix*, tinea unguium

Oral: Useful in superficial mycoses including dermatophytoses (eg, tinea capitis), pityriasis versicolor, sebopsoriasis, vaginal and chronic mucocutaneous candidiases; systemic mycoses including candidiasis, meningeal and disseminated cryptococcal infections, paracoccidioidomycosis, coccidioidomycoses; miscellaneous mycoses such as sporotrichosis, chromomycosis, leishmaniasis, fungal keratitis, alternariosis, zygomycosis
Oral solution: Treatment of oral and esophageal candidiasis
Intravenous solution: Indicated in the treatment of blastomycosis, histoplasmosis (nonmeningeal), and aspergillosis (in patients intolerant or refractory to amphotericin B therapy); empiric therapy of febrile neutropenic fever

Usual Dosage

Usual dosage ranges:

Adults: Oral, I.V.: 100-400 mg/day; doses >200 mg/day are given in 2 divided doses; length of therapy varies from 1 day to >6 months depending on the condition and mycological response

Indication-specific dosing:

Adults:

Aspergillosis, invasive (salvage therapy): Duration of therapy should be a minimum of 6-12 weeks or throughout period of immunosuppression:

Oral: 200-400 mg/day; **Note:** 2008 IDSA guidelines recommend 600 mg/day for 3 days, followed by 400 mg/day

I.V.: 200 mg twice daily for 4 doses, followed by 200 mg daily

Appropriate use: Itraconazole should **NOT** be used for voriconazole-refractory aspergillosis since the same antifungal and/or resistance mechanism(s) may be shared by both agents. Itraconazole oral solution and capsule formulations are not bioequivalent or interchangeable. Due to variable bioavailability of oral preparations, therapeutic drug monitoring advisable.

Aspergillosis, allergic (ABPA, sinusitis): Oral: 200 mg/day; may be used in conjunction with corticosteroids

Blastomycosis/histoplasmosis:

Oral: 200 mg once daily, if no obvious improvement or there is evidence of progressive fungal disease, increase the dose in 100 mg increments to a maximum of 400 mg/day; doses >200 mg/day are given in 2 divided doses; length of therapy varies from 1 day to >6 months depending on the condition and mycological response

I.V.: 200 mg twice daily for 4 doses, followed by 200 mg/day

Brain abscess: Cerebral phaeohyphomycosis (dematiaceous): Oral: 200 mg twice daily for at least 6 months with amphotericin

Candidiasis:

Oropharyngeal: Oral solution: 200 mg once daily for 1-2 weeks; in patients unresponsive or refractory to fluconazole: 100 mg twice daily (clinical response expected in 1-2 weeks)

Esophageal: Oral solution: 100-200 mg once daily for a minimum of 3 weeks; continue dosing for 2 weeks after resolution of symptoms

Coccidioides: Oral: 200 mg twice daily

Infections, life-threatening:

Oral: 200 mg 3 times/day (600 mg/day) should be given for the first 3 days of therapy

I.V.: 200 mg twice daily for 4 doses, followed by 200 mg/day

Meningitis: *Coccidioides:* Oral: 400-800 mg/day

Onychomycosis: Oral: 200 mg once daily for 12 consecutive weeks

Pneumonia: *Coccidioides:* Mild to moderate: Oral, I.V.: 200 mg twice daily

Protothecal infection: 200 mg once daily for 2 months

Sporotrichosis: Oral:

Lymphocutaneous: 100-200 mg/day for 3-6 months

Osteoarticular and pulmonary: 200 mg twice daily for 1-2 years (may use amphotericin B initially for stabilization)

Dosage Forms

Capsule: 100 mg

Sporanox®: 100 mg

Solution, oral:

Sporanox®: 100 mg/10 mL

I-Tropine® *(Discontinued)* see atropine on page 104

ivermectin (eye ver MEK tin)

U.S./Canadian Brand Names Stromectol® [US]

Therapeutic Category Antibiotic, Miscellaneous

Use Treatment of the following infections: Strongyloidiasis of the intestinal tract due to the nematode parasite *Strongyloides stercoralis*. Onchocerciasis due to the nematode parasite *Onchocerca volvulus*. Ivermectin is only active against the immature form of *Onchocerca volvulus*, and the intestinal forms of *Strongyloides stercoralis*.

Usual Dosage Oral: Children ≥15 kg and Adults:

Strongyloidiasis: 200 mcg/kg as a single dose; follow-up stool examinations

Onchocerciasis: 150 mcg/kg as a single dose; retreatment may be required every 3-12 months until the adult worms die

◀ **Dosage Forms**
  Tablet [scored]:
    Stromectol®: 3 mg

IVIG *see* immune globulin (intravenous) *on page 503*
IvyBlock® [US-OTC] *see* bentoquatam *on page 122*
Ivy-Rid® [US-OTC] *see* benzocaine *on page 124*
IvySoothe® [US-OTC] *see* hydrocortisone (topical) *on page 485*

ixabepilone (ix ab EP i lone)

Synonyms BMS-247550; NSC-710428
U.S./Canadian Brand Names Ixempra™ [US]
Therapeutic Category Antineoplastic Agent, Antimicrotubular; Antineoplastic Agent, Epothilone B Analog
Use Treatment of metastatic or locally-advanced breast cancer (refractory or resistant)
Usual Dosage Note: Premedicate with an oral H_1-antagonist (eg, diphenhydramine 50 mg) and an oral H_2-antagonist (eg, ranitidine 150-300 mg) 1 hour prior to infusion. Patients with a history of hypersensitivity should also be premedicated with corticosteroids (orally 1 hour before or I.V. 30 minutes before infusion). Body surface area (BSA) is capped at a maximum of 2.2 m^2.
I.V.: Adults: 40 mg/m^2 every 3 weeks (maximum dose: 88 mg)
Dosage Forms
Injection, powder for reconstitution:
  Ixempra™: 15 mg, 45 mg

Ixempra™ [US] *see* ixabepilone *on page 534*
Jamp® Travel Tablet [Can] *see* dimenhydrinate *on page 301*
Janimine® *(Discontinued) see* imipramine *on page 501*
Jantoven™ [US] *see* warfarin *on page 986*
Janumet™ [US] *see* sitagliptin and metformin *on page 870*
Januvia™ [US] *see* sitagliptin *on page 870*

Japanese encephalitis virus vaccine (inactivated)

(jap a NEESE en sef a LYE tis VYE rus vak SEEN, in ak ti VAY ted)
U.S./Canadian Brand Names JE-VAX® [US/Can]
Therapeutic Category Vaccine, Inactivated Virus
Use Active immunization against Japanese encephalitis
Usual Dosage U.S. recommended primary immunization schedule: SubQ:
  Children 1-3 years: Three 0.5 mL doses given on days 0, 7, and 30
  Children >3 years and Adults: Three 1 mL doses given on days 0, 7, and 30
  Booster dose: Give after 2 years, or according to current recommendation
  Abbreviated dosing schedule: Three recommended doses, given on days 0, 7, and 14 with the last dose given at least 10 days before travel. Alternately, two doses given 1 week apart provide immunity in ~80% of patients. Abbreviated schedules should be used only when necessary due to time constraints.
Dosage Forms
Injection, powder for reconstitution:
  JE-VAX®: Nakayama-NIH strain (1 mL)

Jenamicin® *(Discontinued) see* gentamicin *on page 442*
Jenest™-28 *(Discontinued) see* ethinyl estradiol and norethindrone *on page 376*
JE-VAX® [US/Can] *see* Japanese encephalitis virus vaccine (inactivated) *on page 534*
Jolessa™ [US] *see* ethinyl estradiol and levonorgestrel *on page 372*
Jolivette™ [US] *see* norethindrone *on page 679*
Junel™ [US] *see* ethinyl estradiol and norethindrone *on page 376*
Junel™ Fe [US] *see* ethinyl estradiol and norethindrone *on page 376*
Just for Kids™ [US-OTC] *see* fluoride *on page 411*
Just Tears® Solution *(Discontinued) see* artificial tears *on page 95*
Juvederm™ 24HV [US] *see* hyaluronate and derivatives *on page 476*
Juvederm™ 30 [US] *see* hyaluronate and derivatives *on page 476*
Juvederm™ 30HV [US] *see* hyaluronate and derivatives *on page 476*

K-10® [Can] *see* potassium chloride *on page 771*
Kabikinase® *(Discontinued)*
Kadian® [US/Can] *see* morphine sulfate *on page 643*
Kala® [US-OTC] *see* Lactobacillus *on page 543*
Kalcinate® *(Discontinued)* *see* calcium gluconate *on page 166*
Kaletra® [US/Can] *see* lopinavir and ritonavir *on page 574*
Kalmz [US-OTC] *see* fructose, dextrose, and phosphoric acid *on page 429*

kanamycin (kan a MYE sin)
Sound-Alike/Look-Alike Issues
    kanamycin may be confused with Garamycin®, gentamicin
Synonyms kanamycin sulfate
U.S./Canadian Brand Names Kantrex® [US/Can]
Therapeutic Category Aminoglycoside (Antibiotic)
Use Treatment of serious infections caused by susceptible strains of *E. coli, Proteus* species, *Enterobacter aerogenes, Klebsiella pneumoniae, Serratia marcescens,* and *Acinetobacter* species; second-line treatment of *Mycobacterium tuberculosis*
Usual Dosage Note: Dosing should be based on ideal body weight
    Children: Infections: I.M., I.V.: 15 mg/kg/day in divided doses every 8-12 hours
    Adults:
       Infections: I.M., I.V.: 5-7.5 mg/kg/dose in divided doses every 8-12 hours (<15 mg/kg/day)
       Intraperitoneal: After contamination in surgery: 500 mg
       Irrigating solution: 0.25%; maximum 1.5 g/day (via all administration routes)
       Aerosol: 250 mg 2-4 times/day
Dosage Forms
    Injection, solution:
       Kantrex®: 1 g/3 mL (3 mL)

kanamycin sulfate *see* kanamycin *on page 535*
Kank-A® Soft Brush™ [US-OTC] *see* benzocaine *on page 124*
Kantrex® [US/Can] *see* kanamycin *on page 535*
Kaochlor-Eff® *(Discontinued)*
Kaochlor® SF *(Discontinued)* *see* potassium chloride *on page 771*
Kaodene® *(Discontinued)*
Kaodene® NN *(Discontinued)*
Kaon-Cl-10® [US] *see* potassium chloride *on page 771*
Kao-Paverin® [US-OTC] *see* loperamide *on page 573*
Kaopectate® [US-OTC] *see* bismuth *on page 136*
Kaopectate® II *(Discontinued)* *see* loperamide *on page 573*
Kaopectate® Advanced Formula *(Discontinued)*
Kaopectate® Extra Strength [US-OTC] *see* bismuth *on page 136*
Kaopectate® Maximum Strength Caplets *(Discontinued)*
Kao-Spen® *(Discontinued)*
Kao-Tin [US-OTC] *see* bismuth *on page 136*
Kapectolin [US-OTC] *see* bismuth *on page 136*
Kapectolin® *(Discontinued)*
Karidium® *(Discontinued)* *see* fluoride *on page 411*
Karigel® *(Discontinued)* *see* fluoride *on page 411*
Karigel®-N *(Discontinued)* *see* fluoride *on page 411*
Kariva™ [US] *see* ethinyl estradiol and desogestrel *on page 369*
Kasof® *(Discontinued)* *see* docusate *on page 314*
Kaybovite-1000® *(Discontinued)* *see* cyanocobalamin *on page 254*
Kay Ciel® [US] *see* potassium chloride *on page 771*
Kayexalate® [US/Can] *see* sodium polystyrene sulfonate *on page 879*
K-Citra® [Can] *see* potassium citrate *on page 772*
KCl *see* potassium chloride *on page 771*

K-Dur® [Can] *see* potassium chloride *on page 771*
Keflex® [US] *see* cephalexin *on page 194*
Keftab® [Can] *see* cephalexin *on page 194*
Kefurox® Injection *(Discontinued)* *see* cefuroxime *on page 192*
Kefzol® *(Discontinued)* *see* cefazolin *on page 184*
K-Electrolyte® Effervescent *(Discontinued)* *see* potassium bicarbonate *on page 770*
Kelnor™ [US] *see* ethinyl estradiol and ethynodiol diacetate *on page 371*
Kemadrin® [US] *see* procyclidine *on page 789*
Kemsol® [Can] *see* dimethyl sulfoxide *on page 303*
Kenacort® Oral *(Discontinued)*
Kenaject® Injection *(Discontinued)*
Kenalog® [US/Can] *see* triamcinolone (topical) *on page 949*
Kenalog-10® [US] *see* triamcinolone (systemic) *on page 948*
Kenalog-40® [US] *see* triamcinolone (systemic) *on page 948*
Kenalog® in Orabase [Can] *see* triamcinolone (topical) *on page 949*
Kenonel® Topical *(Discontinued)*
keoxifene hydrochloride *see* raloxifene *on page 816*
Kepivance™ [US] *see* palifermin *on page 715*
Keppra® [US/Can] *see* levetiracetam *on page 554*
Kerafoam™ [US] *see* urea *on page 963*
Keralac™ [US] *see* urea *on page 963*
Keralac™ Nailstik [US] *see* urea *on page 963*
Keralyt® [US-OTC] *see* salicylic acid *on page 850*
Kerlone® [US] *see* betaxolol *on page 133*
Kerol™ [US] *see* urea *on page 963*
Kerol™ Redi-Cloths [US] *see* urea *on page 963*
Kerr Insta-Char® [US-OTC] *see* charcoal *on page 198*
Ketalar® [US/Can] *see* ketamine *on page 536*

ketamine (KEET a meen)

Sound-Alike/Look-Alike Issues
Ketalar® may be confused with Kenalog®, ketorolac
Synonyms ketamine hydrochloride
U.S./Canadian Brand Names Ketalar® [US/Can]; Ketamine Hydrochloride Injection, USP [Can]
Therapeutic Category General Anesthetic
Controlled Substance C-III
Use Induction and maintenance of general anesthesia
Usual Dosage May be used in combination with anticholinergic agents to decrease hypersalivation.
Children ≥16 years and Adults:
Induction of anesthesia:
I.M.: 6.5-13 mg/kg; usual dose to produce 12-25 minutes of anesthesia: 10 mg/kg
I.V.: 1-4.5 mg/kg; usual dose to produce 5-10 minutes of anesthesia: 2 mg/kg
I.V. infusion: 1-2 mg/kg infuse over 0.5 mg/kg/minute; may administer with diazepam to prevent emergence reactions
Maintenance of anesthesia: Supplemental doses of 1/2 to the full induction dose; may also be maintained with a continuous infusion of 0.1-5 mg/minute
Dosage Forms
Injection, solution: 50 mg/mL (10 mL); 100 mg/mL (5 mL)
Ketalar®: 10 mg/mL (20 mL); 50 mg/mL (10 mL); 100 mg/mL (5 mL)

ketamine hydrochloride *see* ketamine *on page 536*
Ketamine Hydrochloride Injection, USP [Can] *see* ketamine *on page 536*
Ketek® [US/Can] *see* telithromycin *on page 906*

ketoconazole (kee toe KOE na zole)

Sound-Alike/Look-Alike Issues
Nizoral® may be confused with Nasarel®, Neoral®, Nitrol®

U.S./Canadian Brand Names Apo-Ketoconazole® [Can]; Extina® [US]; Ketoderm® [Can]; Kuric™ [US]; Nizoral® A-D [US-OTC]; Nizoral® [US]; Novo-Ketoconazole [Can]; Xolegel™ [US/Can]

Therapeutic Category Antifungal Agent

Use
Systemic: Treatment of susceptible fungal infections, including candidiasis, oral thrush, blastomycosis, histoplasmosis, paracoccidioidomycosis, coccidioidomycosis, chromomycosis, candiduria, chronic mucocutaneous candidiasis, as well as certain recalcitrant cutaneous dermatophytoses

Topical:
Cream: Treatment of tinea corporis, tinea cruris, tinea versicolor, cutaneous candidiasis, seborrheic dermatitis
Foam, gel: Treatment of seborrheic dermatitis
Shampoo: Treatment of dandruff, seborrheic dermatitis, tinea versicolor

Usual Dosage
Oral:
Fungal infections:
Children ≥2 years: 3.3-6.6 mg/kg/day as a single dose for 1-2 weeks for candidiasis, for at least 4 weeks in recalcitrant dermatophyte infections, and for up to 6 months for other systemic mycoses
Adults: 200-400 mg/day as a single daily dose for durations as stated above
Shampoo: Seborrheic dermatitis, tinea versicolor: Children ≥12 years and Adults: Apply twice weekly for 4 weeks with at least 3 days between each shampoo
Topical:
Tinea infections: Adults: Cream: Rub gently into the affected area once daily. Duration of treatment: Tinea corporis, cruris: 2 weeks; tinea pedis: 6 weeks
Seborrheic dermatitis: Children ≥12 years and Adults:
Cream: Rub gently into the affected area twice daily for 4 weeks or until clinical response is noted
Foam: Apply to affected area twice daily for 4 weeks
Gel: Rub gently into the affected area once daily for 2 weeks

Dosage Forms
Aerosol, topical [foam]:
Extina®: 2% (50 g, 100 g)
Cream, topical: 2% (15 g, 30 g, 60 g)
Kuric™: 2%: (75 g)
Gel, topical:
Xolegel™: 2% (15 g)
Shampoo, topical: 1% (120 mL), 2% (120 mL)
Nizoral®: 2% (120 mL)
Nizoral® A-D: 1% (120 mL, 210 mL)
Tablet: 200 mg

Ketoderm® [Can] see ketoconazole on page 537
3-keto-desogestrel see etonogestrel on page 383

ketoprofen (kee toe PROE fen)

Sound-Alike/Look-Alike Issues
Oruvail® may be confused with Clinoril®, Elavil®

U.S./Canadian Brand Names Apo-Keto SR® [Can]; Apo-Keto-E® [Can]; Apo-Keto® [Can]; Novo-Keto [Can]; Novo-Keto-EC [Can]; Nu-Ketoprofen [Can]; Nu-Ketoprofen-E [Can]; Oruvail® [Can]; Rhodis SR™ [Can]; Rhodis-EC™ [Can]; Rhodis™ [Can]

Therapeutic Category Analgesic, Nonnarcotic; Nonsteroidal Antiinflammatory Drug (NSAID)

Use Acute and long-term treatment of rheumatoid arthritis and osteoarthritis; primary dysmenorrhea; mild-to-moderate pain

Usual Dosage Note: The extended release formulation is not recommended for the treatment of acute pain. Oral:
Adults:
Rheumatoid arthritis, osteoarthritis (lower doses may be used in small patients or in the elderly, or debilitated):
Regular release: 50 mg 4 times/day **or** 75 mg 3 times/day; up to a maximum of 300 mg/day

▶

◄ Extended release: 200 mg once daily
Dysmenorrhea, mild-to-moderate pain: Regular release: 25-50 mg every 6-8 hours up to a maximum of 300 mg/day
Dosage Forms
Capsule, regular release: 50 mg, 75 mg
Capsule, extended release: 200 mg

ketorolac (KEE toe role ak)

Sound-Alike/Look-Alike Issues
ketorolac may be confused with Ketalar®
Acular® may be confused with Acthar®, Ocular®
Toradol® may be confused with Foradil®, Inderal®, Tegretol®, Torecan®, traMADol, tromethamine
Synonyms ketorolac tromethamine
U.S./Canadian Brand Names Acular LS™ [US/Can]; Acular® P.F. [US]; Acular® [US/Can]; Apo-Ketorolac Injectable® [Can]; Apo-Ketorolac® [Can]; Ketorolac Tromethamine Injection, USP [Can]; Novo-Ketorolac [Can]; ratio-Ketorolac [Can]; Toradol® IM [Can]; Toradol® [Can]
Therapeutic Category Analgesic, Nonnarcotic; Nonsteroidal Antiinflammatory Drug (NSAID)
Use
Oral, injection: Short-term (≤5 days) management of moderate-to-severe acute pain requiring analgesia at the opioid level
Ophthalmic: Temporary relief of ocular itching due to seasonal allergic conjunctivitis; postoperative inflammation following cataract extraction; reduction of ocular pain and photophobia following incisional refractive surgery; reduction of ocular pain, burning, and stinging following corneal refractive surgery
Usual Dosage
Children ≥16 years and Adults (pain relief usually begins within 10 minutes with parenteral forms): **Note:** The maximum combined duration of treatment (for parenteral and oral) is 5 days; do not increase dose or frequency; supplement with low-dose opioids if needed for breakthrough pain.
I.M.: 60 mg as a single dose or 30 mg every 6 hours (maximum daily dose: 120 mg)
I.V.: 30 mg as a single dose or 30 mg every 6 hours (maximum daily dose: 120 mg)
Children ≥17 years and Adults: Oral: 20 mg, followed by 10 mg every 4-6 hours; do not exceed 40 mg/day; oral dosing is intended to be a continuation of I.M. or I.V. therapy only
Note: The maximum combined duration of treatment (for parenteral and oral) is 5 days; do not increase dose or frequency; supplement with low-dose opioids if needed for breakthrough pain. Therapy should not be initiated with oral formulation.

Ophthalmic: Children ≥3 years and Adults:
Allergic conjunctivitis (relief of ocular itching) (Acular®): Instill 1 drop (0.25 mg) 4 times/day
Inflammation following cataract extraction (Acular®): Instill 1 drop (0.25 mg) to affected eye(s) 4 times/day beginning 24 hours after surgery; continue for 2 weeks
Pain and photophobia following incisional refractive surgery (Acular® P.F.): Instill 1 drop (0.25 mg) 4 times/day to affected eye for up to 3 days
Pain following corneal refractive surgery (Acular LS™): Instill 1 drop 4 times/day as needed to affected eye for up to 4 days
Dosage Forms
Injection, solution: 15 mg/mL (1 mL); 30 mg/mL (1 mL, 2 mL, 10 mL)
Solution, ophthalmic:
Acular®: 0.5% (3 mL, 5 mL, 10 mL)
Acular LS™: 0.4% (5 mL)
Acular® P.F. [preservative free]: 0.5% (0.4 mL)
Tablet: 10 mg

ketorolac tromethamine see ketorolac on page 538
Ketorolac Tromethamine Injection, USP [Can] see ketorolac on page 538

ketotifen (kee toe TYE fen)

Synonyms ketotifen fumarate
U.S./Canadian Brand Names Alaway™ [US-OTC]; Novo-Ketotifen® [Can]; Nu-Ketotifen® [Can]; Zaditen® [Can]; Zaditor® [US-OTC/Can]
Therapeutic Category Antihistamine, H₁ Blocker, Ophthalmic
Use
Ophthalmic: Temporary prevention of eye itching due to allergic conjunctivitis

Oral (Canadian use; not approved in U.S.): Adjunctive therapy in the chronic treatment of pediatric patients ≥6 months of age with mild, atopic asthma

Usual Dosage

Ophthalmic: Allergic conjunctivitis: Children ≥3 years and Adults: Instill 1 drop into the affected eye(s) twice daily, every 8-12 hours

Oral (not approved in U.S.): Atopic asthma (**Note:** Not for acute attacks):

Children 6 months to 3 years: Initial: 0.025 mg/kg once daily or in 2 divided doses for 5 days; Maintenance: 0.05 mg/kg twice daily

Children >3 years: Initial: 0.5 mg once daily or in 2 divided doses for 5 days; Maintenance: 1 mg twice daily

Dosage Forms [CAN] = Canadian brand name

Solution, ophthalmic [drops]: 0.025% (5 mL)

Alaway™ [OTC]: 0.025% (10 mL)

Zaditor® [OTC]: 0.025% (5 mL)

Syrup: 1 mg/5 mL (250 mL) [not available in U.S.]

Novo-Ketotifen® [CAN]: 1 mg/5 mL (250 mL) [not available in U.S.]

Nu-Ketotifen® [CAN]: 1 mg/5 mL (250 mL) [not available in U.S.]

Zaditen® [CAN]: 1 mg/5 mL (250 mL) [not available in U.S.]

Tablet: 1 mg [not available in U.S.]

Novo-ketotifen® [CAN]: 1 mg [not available in U.S.]

Zaditen® [CAN]: 1 mg [not available in U.S.]

ketotifen fumarate *see* ketotifen *on page 538*

Key-E® [US-OTC] *see* vitamin E *on page 981*

Key-E® Kaps [US-OTC] *see* vitamin E *on page 981*

Keygesic [US-OTC] *see* magnesium salicylate *on page 588*

Key-Pred® *(Discontinued)*

Key-Pred-SP® *(Discontinued)*

K-G® *(Discontinued) see* potassium gluconate *on page 773*

K-Gen® Effervescent *(Discontinued) see* potassium bicarbonate *on page 770*

KI *see* potassium iodide *on page 773*

K-Ide® *(Discontinued)*

Kidkare Children's Cough and Cold [US-OTC] *see* chlorpheniramine, pseudoephedrine, and dextromethorphan *on page 212*

Kidkare Decongestant [US-OTC] *see* pseudoephedrine *on page 801*

Kidrolase® [Can] *see* asparaginase *on page 98*

Kinerase® *(Discontinued) see* hyaluronidase *on page 477*

Kineret® [US/Can] *see* anakinra *on page 75*

Kinesed® *(Discontinued) see* hyoscyamine, atropine, scopolamine, and phenobarbital *on page 493*

Kinevac® [US] *see* sincalide *on page 868*

Kinlytic™ [US] *see* urokinase *on page 965*

Kinrix™ [US] *see* diphtheria and tetanus toxoids, acellular pertussis, and poliovirus (inactivated) vaccine *on page 307*

Kionex® [US] *see* sodium polystyrene sulfonate *on page 879*

Kivexa™ [Can] *see* abacavir and lamivudine *on page 16*

Klaron® [US] *see* sulfacetamide *on page 892*

Klean-Prep® [Can] *see* polyethylene glycol-electrolyte solution *on page 766*

K-Lease® *(Discontinued) see* potassium chloride *on page 771*

Klerist-D® Tablet *(Discontinued) see* chlorpheniramine and pseudoephedrine *on page 207*

Klonopin® [US/Can] *see* clonazepam *on page 235*

Klonopin® Wafers [US] *see* clonazepam *on page 235*

K-Lor® [US/Can] *see* potassium chloride *on page 771*

Klor-Con® [US] *see* potassium chloride *on page 771*

Klor-Con® 8 [US] *see* potassium chloride *on page 771*

Klor-Con® 10 [US] *see* potassium chloride *on page 771*

Klor-Con®/25 [US] *see* potassium chloride *on page 771*

Klor-Con® M [US] *see* potassium chloride *on page 771*

Klor-Con®/EF [US] *see* potassium bicarbonate and potassium citrate *on page 770*

Klorominr® Oral *(Discontinued)* *see* chlorpheniramine *on page 205*

Klorvess® *(Discontinued)* *see* potassium chloride *on page 771*

Klorvess® Effervescent *(Discontinued)*

K-Lyte® [US] *see* potassium bicarbonate and potassium citrate *on page 770*

K-Lyte® [Can] *see* potassium citrate *on page 772*

K-Lyte/Cl® 50 *(Discontinued)* *see* potassium bicarbonate and potassium chloride *on page 770*

K-Lyte®/Cl [Can] *see* potassium chloride *on page 771*

K-Lyte/Cl® *(Discontinued)* *see* potassium bicarbonate and potassium chloride *on page 770*

K-Lyte® DS [US] *see* potassium bicarbonate and potassium citrate *on page 770*

K-Lyte® Effervescent *(Discontinued)* *see* potassium bicarbonate *on page 770*

K-Norm® *(Discontinued)* *see* potassium chloride *on page 771*

Koāte®-DVI [US] *see* antihemophilic factor (human) *on page 78*

Koāte®-HP *(Discontinued)* *see* antihemophilic factor (human) *on page 78*

Kobee [US-OTC] *see* vitamin B complex combinations *on page 981*

Koffex DM-D [Can] *see* pseudoephedrine and dextromethorphan *on page 802*

Koffex DM + Decongestant + Expectorant [Can] *see* guaifenesin, pseudoephedrine, and dextromethorphan *on page 460*

Koffex DM-Expectorant [Can] *see* guaifenesin and dextromethorphan *on page 454*

Koffex Expectorant [Can] *see* guaifenesin *on page 453*

Kogenate® [Can] *see* antihemophilic factor (recombinant) *on page 79*

Kogenate® *(Discontinued)* *see* antihemophilic factor (recombinant) *on page 79*

Kogenate® FS [US/Can] *see* antihemophilic factor (recombinant) *on page 79*

Kolephrin® [US-OTC] *see* acetaminophen, chlorpheniramine, and pseudoephedrine *on page 25*

Kolephrin® #1 [US] *see* guaifenesin and codeine *on page 454*

Kolephrin® GG/DM [US-OTC] *see* guaifenesin and dextromethorphan *on page 454*

Konakion [Can] *see* phytonadione *on page 752*

Konakion® Injection *(Discontinued)* *see* phytonadione *on page 752*

Kondon's Nasal® *(Discontinued)* *see* ephedrine *on page 343*

Konsyl® [US-OTC] *see* psyllium *on page 804*

Konsyl-D™ [US-OTC] *see* psyllium *on page 804*

Konsyl® Easy Mix™ [US-OTC] *see* psyllium *on page 804*

Konsyl® Fiber Caplets [US-OTC] *see* polycarbophil *on page 765*

Konsyl® Orange [US-OTC] *see* psyllium *on page 804*

Konsyl® Original [US-OTC] *see* psyllium *on page 804*

Kovia® [US] *see* papain and urea *on page 721*

K-Pek II [US-OTC] *see* loperamide *on page 573*

K-Pek® *(Discontinued)*

K-Phos® MF [US] *see* potassium phosphate and sodium phosphate *on page 775*

K-Phos® Neutral [US] *see* potassium phosphate and sodium phosphate *on page 775*

K-Phos® No. 2 [US] *see* potassium phosphate and sodium phosphate *on page 775*

K-Phos® Original [US] *see* potassium acid phosphate *on page 770*

KPN Prenatal [US] *see* vitamins (multiple/prenatal) *on page 983*

Kristalose® [US] *see* lactulose *on page 544*

K-Tab® [US] *see* potassium chloride *on page 771*

K-Tan [US] *see* phenylephrine and pyrilamine *on page 747*

K-Tan 4 [US] *see* phenylephrine and pyrilamine *on page 747*

kunecatechins *see* sinecatechins *on page 868*

Kuric™ [US] *see* ketoconazole *on page 537*

kutrase® *(Discontinued)* *see* pancreatin *on page 717*

Kuvan™ [US] *see* sapropterin *on page 856*

ku-zyme® *(Discontinued)* *see* pancreatin *on page 717*

ku-zyme® HP *(Discontinued)* *see* pancrelipase *on page 718*

Kwelcof® *(Discontinued)*

Kwellada-P™ [Can] *see* permethrin *on page 740*

Kytril® [US/Can] *see* granisetron *on page 452*

L-749,345 *see* ertapenem *on page 353*

L-758,298 *see* fosaprepitant *on page 426*

L-M-X™ 4 [US-OTC] *see* lidocaine *on page 561*

L-M-X™ 5 [US-OTC] *see* lidocaine *on page 561*

L 754030 *see* aprepitant *on page 90*

LA 20304a *see* gemifloxacin *on page 439*

labetalol (la BET a lole)

Sound-Alike/Look-Alike Issues
labetalol may be confused with betaxolol, Hexadrol®, lamoTRIgine
Trandate® may be confused with traMADol, Trendar®, Trental®, Tridrate®

Synonyms ibidomide hydrochloride; labetalol hydrochloride

U.S./Canadian Brand Names Apo-Labetalol® [Can]; Labetalol Hydrochloride Injection, USP [Can]; Normodyne® [Can]; Trandate® [US/Can]

Therapeutic Category Alpha-/Beta- Adrenergic Blocker

Use Treatment of mild-to-severe hypertension; I.V. for severe hypertension (eg, hypertensive emergencies)

Usual Dosage
Children: Due to limited documentation of its use, labetalol should be initiated cautiously in pediatric patients with careful dosage adjustment and blood pressure monitoring.
I.V., intermittent bolus doses of 0.3-1 mg/kg/dose have been reported.
For treatment of pediatric hypertensive emergencies, initial continuous infusions of 0.4-1 mg/kg/hour with a maximum of 3 mg/kg/hour have been used. Administration requires the use of an infusion pump.
Adults:
Oral: Initial: 100 mg twice daily, may increase as needed every 2-3 days by 100 mg until desired response is obtained; usual dose: 200-400 mg twice daily; may require up to 2.4 g/day.
Usual dose range (JNC 7): 200-800 mg/day in 2 divided doses
I.V.: 20 mg (0.25 mg/kg for an 80 kg patient) IVP over 2 minutes; may administer 40-80 mg at 10-minute intervals, up to 300 mg total dose.
I.V. infusion (acute loading): Initial: 2 mg/minute; titrate to response up to 300 mg total dose, if needed. Administration requires the use of an infusion pump.
I.V. infusion (500 mg/250 mL D_5W) rates:
1 mg/minute: 30 mL/hour
2 mg/minute: 60 mL/hour
3 mg/minute: 90 mL/hour
4 mg/minute: 120 mL/hour
5 mg/minute: 150 mL/hour
6 mg/minute: 180 mL/hour
Note: Although loading infusions are well described in the product labeling, the labeling is silent in specific clinical situations, such as in the patient who has an initial response to labetalol infusions but cannot be converted to an oral route for subsequent dosing. There is limited documentation of prolonged continuous infusions. In rare clinical situations, higher dosages (up to 6 mg/minute) have been used in the critical care setting (eg, aortic dissection). At the other extreme, continuous infusions at relatively low doses (2-6 mg/hour - note difference in units) have been used in some settings (following loading infusion in patients who are unable to be converted to oral regimens or in some cases as a continuation of outpatient oral regimens). These prolonged infusions should not be confused with loading infusions. Because of wide variation in the use of infusions, an awareness of institutional policies and practices is extremely important. Careful clarification of orders and specific infusion rates/units is required to avoid confusion. Due to the prolonged duration of action, careful monitoring should be extended for the duration of the infusion and for several hours after the infusion. Excessive administration may result in prolonged hypotension and/or bradycardia.

Dosage Forms
Injection, solution: 5 mg/mL (4 mL, 8 mL, 20 mL, 40 mL)
Trandate®: 5 mg/mL (20 mL, 40 mL)
Tablet: 100 mg, 200 mg, 300 mg
Trandate®: 100 mg, 200 mg, 300 mg

labetalol hydrochloride *see* labetalol *on page 541*

Labetalol Hydrochloride Injection, USP [Can] *see* labetalol *on page 541*

Lac-Dose [US-OTC] *see* lactase *on page 542*

Lac-Hydrin® [US] *see* lactic acid and ammonium hydroxide *on page 542*

Lac-Hydrin® Five [US-OTC] *see* lactic acid and ammonium hydroxide *on page 542*

LAClotion™ [US] *see* lactic acid and ammonium hydroxide *on page 542*

Lacril® Ophthalmic Solution *(Discontinued)* *see* artificial tears *on page 95*

Lacrisert® [US/Can] *see* hydroxypropyl cellulose *on page 490*

LaCrosse Complete [US-OTC] *see* sodium phosphates *on page 878*

Lactaid® Extra Strength *(Discontinued)* *see* lactase *on page 542*

Lactaid® Fast Act [US-OTC] *see* lactase *on page 542*

Lactaid® Original [US-OTC] *see* lactase *on page 542*

Lactaid® Ultra *(Discontinued)* *see* lactase *on page 542*

lactase (LAK tase)

U.S./Canadian Brand Names Dairyaid® [Can]; Lac-Dose [US-OTC]; Lactaid® Fast Act [US-OTC]; Lactaid® Original [US-OTC]; Lactrase® [US-OTC]

Therapeutic Category Nutritional Supplement

Use Help digest lactose in milk for patients with lactose intolerance

Usual Dosage Oral:

Capsule: 1-2 capsules taken with milk or meal; pretreat milk with 1-2 capsules/quart of milk

Liquid: 5-15 drops/quart of milk

Tablet: 1-3 tablets with meals

Dosage Forms

Caplet:

Lactaid® Original [OTC]: 3000 FCC lactase units

Lactaid® Fast Act [OTC]: 9000 FCC lactase units

Capsule:

Lactrase® [OTC]: 250 mg standardized enzyme lactase

Tablet, oral, chewable:

Lactaid® Fast Act [OTC]: 9000 FCC lactase units

Tablet, oral:

Lac-Dose [OTC]: 3000 FCC lactase units

lactic acid (LAK tik AS id)

Synonyms sodium-PCA and lactic acid

U.S./Canadian Brand Names LactiCare® [US-OTC]; Lactinol-E® [US]; Lactinol® [US]

Therapeutic Category Topical Skin Product

Use Lubricate and moisturize the skin counteracting dryness and itching

Usual Dosage Topical: Adults: Lubricant/moisturizer: Apply twice daily

Dosage Forms

Cream: 10% (120 g)

Lactinol-E®: 10% (120 g)

Lotion: 10% (360 mL)

LactiCare® [OTC]: 5% (222 mL, 340 mL)

Lactinol®: 10% (360 mL)

lactic acid and ammonium hydroxide (LAK tik AS id & a MOE nee um hye DROKS ide)

Synonyms ammonium lactate

U.S./Canadian Brand Names AmLactin® [US-OTC]; Geri-Hydrolac™ [US-OTC]; Geri-Hydrolac™-12 [US-OTC]; Lac-Hydrin® Five [US-OTC]; Lac-Hydrin® [US]; LAClotion™ [US]

Therapeutic Category Topical Skin Product

Use Treatment of moderate-to-severe xerosis and ichthyosis vulgaris

Usual Dosage Topical:

Cream: Children ≥2 years and Adults: Apply twice daily to affected area; rub in well

Lotion: Children and Adults: Apply twice daily to affected area; rub in well

Dosage Forms
Cream, topical: Lactic acid 12% with ammonium hydroxide (140 g, 280 g, 385 g)
   AmLactin® [OTC]: Lactic acid 12% with ammonium hydroxide (140 g)
   Lac-Hydrin®: Lactic acid 12% with ammonium hydroxide (280 g, 385 g)
Lotion, topical: Lactic acid 12% with ammonium hydroxide (225 g, 400 g)
   AmLactin® [OTC], Lac-Hydrin®, LAClotion™: Lactic acid 12% with ammonium hydroxide (225 g, 400 g)
   Geri-Hydrolac™ [OTC], Lac-Hydrin® Five: Lactic acid 5% with ammonium hydroxide (120 mL, 240 mL)
   Geri-Hydrolac™-12 [OTC]: Lactic acid 12% with ammonium hydroxide (120 mL, 240 mL)

LactiCare® [US-OTC] *see* lactic acid *on page 542*
Lactinex™ [US-OTC] *see* Lactobacillus *on page 543*
Lactinol® [US] *see* lactic acid *on page 542*
Lactinol-E® [US] *see* lactic acid *on page 542*

Lactobacillus (lak toe ba SIL us)

Synonyms *Lactobacillus acidophilus*; *Lactobacillus bifidus*; *Lactobacillus bulgaricus*; *Lactobacillus casei*; *Lactobacillus paracasei*; *Lactobacillus reuteri*; *Lactobacillus rhamnosus* GG

U.S./Canadian Brand Names Bacid® [US-OTC/Can]; Culturelle® [US-OTC]; Dofus [US-OTC]; Fermalac [Can]; Flora-Q™ [US-OTC]; Kala® [US-OTC]; Lactinex™ [US-OTC]; Lacto-Bifidus [US-OTC]; Lacto-Key [US-OTC]; Lacto-Pectin [US-OTC]; Lacto-TriBlend [US-OTC]; Megadophilus® [US-OTC]; MoreDophilus® [US-OTC]; Superdophilus® [US-OTC]

Therapeutic Category Gastrointestinal Agent, Miscellaneous

Use Promote normal bacterial flora of the intestinal tract

Usual Dosage Dietary supplement: Oral: Dosing varies by manufacturer; consult product labeling
Children (Culturelle®): 1 capsule daily
Adults:
   Bacid®: 2 caplets/day
   Culturelle®: 1 capsule daily; may increase to twice daily
   Flora-Q™: 1 capsule/day
   Lacto-Key 100 or 600: 1-2 capsules/day
   Lactinex™: 1 packet or 4 tablets 3-4 times/day

Dosage Forms
Capsule:
   Culturelle® [OTC]: *L. rhamnosus* GG 10 billion colony-forming units
   Dofus [OTC]: *L. acidophilus* and *L. bifidus* 10:1 ratio
   Flora-Q™ [OTC]: *L. acidophilus* and *L. paracasei* ≥8 billion colony-forming units
   Lacto-Key [OTC]:
      100: *L. acidophilus* 1 billion colony-forming units
      600: *L. acidophilus* 6 billion colony-forming units
   Lacto-Bifidus [OTC]:
      100: *L. bifidus* 1 billion colony-forming units
      600: *L. bifidus* 6 billion colony-forming units
   Lacto-Pectin [OTC]: *L. acidophilus* and *L. casei* ≥5 billion colony-forming units
   Lacto-TriBlend [OTC]:
      100: *L. acidophilus, L. bifidus,* and *L. bulgaricus* 1 billion colony-forming units
      600: *L. acidophilus, L. bifidus,* and *L. bulgaricus* 6 billion colony-forming units
   Megadophilus® [OTC], Superdophilus® [OTC]: *L. acidophilus* 2 billion units
Capsule, softgel: *L. acidophilus* 100 active units
Caplet:
   Bacid® [OTC]: *L. acidophilus 80%* and *L. bulgaricus* 10%
Granules:
   Lactinex™ [OTC]: *L. acidophilus* and *L. bulgaricus* 100 million live cells per 1 g packet (12s)
Powder:
   Lacto-TriBlend [OTC]: *L. acidophilus, L. bifidus,* and *L. bulgaricus* 10 billion colony-forming units per ¼ teaspoon
   Megadophilus® [OTC], Superdophilus® [OTC]: *L. acidophilus* 2 billion units per half-teaspoon
   MoreDophilus® [OTC]: *L. acidophilus* 12.4 billion units per teaspoon
Tablet:
   Kala® [OTC]: *L. acidophilus* 200 million units
   Lactinex™ [OTC]: *L. acidophilus* and *L. bulgaricus* 1 million live cells
Tablet, chewable: *L. reuteri* 100 million organisms
Wafer: *L. acidophilus* 90 mg and *L. bifidus* 25 mg (100s)

Lactobacillus acidophilus see Lactobacillus *on page 543*
Lactobacillus bifidus see Lactobacillus *on page 543*
Lactobacillus bulgaricus see Lactobacillus *on page 543*
Lactobacillus casei see Lactobacillus *on page 543*
Lactobacillus paracasei see Lactobacillus *on page 543*
Lactobacillus reuteri see Lactobacillus *on page 543*
Lactobacillus rhamnosus **GG** see Lactobacillus *on page 543*
Lacto-Bifidus [US-OTC] see Lactobacillus *on page 543*
lactoflavin see riboflavin *on page 832*
Lacto-Key [US-OTC] see Lactobacillus *on page 543*
Lacto-Pectin [US-OTC] see Lactobacillus *on page 543*
Lacto-TriBlend [US-OTC] see Lactobacillus *on page 543*
Lactrase® [US-OTC] see lactase *on page 542*

lactulose (LAK tyoo lose)

Sound-Alike/Look-Alike Issues
lactulose may be confused with lactose
U.S./Canadian Brand Names Acilac [Can]; Apo-Lactulose® [Can]; Constulose [US]; Enulose [US]; Generlac [US]; Kristalose® [US]; Laxilose [Can]; PMS-Lactulose [Can]
Therapeutic Category Ammonium Detoxicant; Laxative
Use Adjunct in the prevention and treatment of portal-systemic encephalopathy; treatment of chronic constipation
Usual Dosage Diarrhea may indicate overdosage and responds to dose reduction
Prevention of portal systemic encephalopathy (PSE): Oral:
Infants: 2.5-10 mL/day divided 3-4 times/day; adjust dosage to produce 2-3 stools/day
Older Children: Daily dose of 40-90 mL divided 3-4 times/day; if initial dose causes diarrhea, then reduce it immediately; adjust dosage to produce 2-3 stools/day
Constipation: Oral:
Children: 5 g/day (7.5 mL) after breakfast
Adults: 15-30 mL/day increased to 60 mL/day in 1-2 divided doses if necessary
Acute PSE: Adults:
Oral: 20-30 g (30-45 mL) every 1-2 hours to induce rapid laxation; adjust dosage daily to produce 2-3 soft stools; doses of 30-45 mL may be given hourly to cause rapid laxation, then reduce to recommended dose; usual daily dose: 60-100 g (90-150 mL) daily
Rectal administration: 200 g (300 mL) diluted with 700 mL of H_2O or NS; administer rectally via rectal balloon catheter and retain 30-60 minutes every 4-6 hours
Dosage Forms
Crystals for solution, oral:
Kristalose®: 10 g/packet (30s), 20 g/packet (30s)
Solution, oral: 10 g/15 mL
Constulose, Enulose, Generlac: 10 g/15 mL
Solution, oral/rectal: 10 g/15 mL (473 mL)

Lactulose PSE® *(Discontinued)* see lactulose *on page 544*
ladakamycin see azacitidine *on page 108*
Lagesic™ [US] see acetaminophen and phenyltoloxamine *on page 22*
L-All 12 [US] see carbetapentane and phenylephrine *on page 175*
L-AmB see amphotericin B liposomal *on page 71*
Lamictal® [US/Can] see lamotrigine *on page 545*
Lamisil® Oral [US/Can] see terbinafine (oral) *on page 910*
Lamisil® Topical [US/Can] see terbinafine (topical) *on page 910*

lamivudine (la MI vyoo deen)

Sound-Alike/Look-Alike Issues
lamiVUDine may be confused with lamoTRIgine
Epivir® may be confused with Combivir®

Synonyms 3TC

Tall-Man lamiVUDine

U.S./Canadian Brand Names 3TC® [Can]; Epivir-HBV® [US]; Epivir® [US]; Heptovir® [Can]

Therapeutic Category Antiviral Agent

Use

Epivir®: Treatment of HIV infection when antiretroviral therapy is warranted; should always be used as part of a multidrug regimen (at least three antiretroviral agents)

Epivir-HBV®: Treatment of chronic hepatitis B associated with evidence of hepatitis B viral replication and active liver inflammation

Usual Dosage Oral: **Note:** The formulation and dosage of Epivir-HBV® are not appropriate for patients infected with both HBV and HIV. Use with at least two other antiretroviral agents when treating HIV

HIV:

Neonates <30 days (AIDSinfo guidelines): 2 mg/kg/dose twice daily

Infants 1-3 months (AIDSinfo guidelines): 4 mg/kg/dose twice daily

Infants and Children 3 months to 16 years: 4 mg/kg/dose twice daily (maximum: 150 mg/dose twice daily)

Alternate weight-based dosing using scored 150 mg tablets (AIDSinfo guidelines):

14-21 kg: 75 mg/dose twice daily (150 mg/day)

22-29 kg: 75 mg in the morning, 150 mg in the evening (225 mg/day)

≥30 kg: 150 mg/dose twice daily (300 mg/day)

Adults: 150 mg twice daily or 300 mg once daily

<50 kg (AIDSinfo guidelines): 4 mg/kg/dose twice daily (maximum: 150 mg/dose twice daily)

Treatment of hepatitis B (Epivir-HBV®):

Children 2-17 years: 3 mg/kg/dose once daily (maximum: 100 mg/day)

Adults: 100 mg/day

Dosage Forms

Solution, oral:

Epivir®: 10 mg/mL

Epivir-HBV®: 5 mg/mL

Tablet:

Epivir®: 150 mg [scored], 300 mg

Epivir-HBV®: 100 mg

lamivudine, abacavir, and zidovudine *see* abacavir, lamivudine, and zidovudine *on page 16*

lamivudine and abacavir *see* abacavir and lamivudine *on page 16*

lamivudine and zidovudine *see* zidovudine and lamivudine *on page 992*

lamotrigine (la MOE tri jeen)

Sound-Alike/Look-Alike Issues

lamoTRIgine may be confused with labetalol, Lamisil®, lamiVUDine, Lomotil®, ludiomil

Lamictal® may be confused with Lamisil®, Lomotil®, ludiomil

Synonyms BW-430C; LTG

Tall-Man lamoTRIgine

U.S./Canadian Brand Names Apo-Lamotrigine® [Can]; Gen-Lamotrigine [Can]; Lamictal® [US/Can]; Novo-Lamotrigine [Can]; PMS-Lamotrigine [Can]; ratio-Lamotrigine [Can]

Therapeutic Category Anticonvulsant

Use Adjunctive therapy in the treatment of generalized seizures of Lennox-Gastaut syndrome, primary generalized tonic-clonic seizures, and partial seizures in adults and children ≥2 years of age; conversion to monotherapy in adults with partial seizures who are receiving treatment with valproic acid or a single enzyme-inducing antiepileptic drug (specifically carbamazepine, phenytoin, phenobarbital or primidone); maintenance treatment of bipolar I disorder

Usual Dosage Note: Only whole tablets should be used for dosing, round calculated dose down to the nearest whole tablet. Enzyme-inducing regimens specifically refer to those containing carbamazepine, phenytoin, phenobarbital, or primidone. Oral:

Children 2-12 years: Lennox-Gastaut (adjunctive), primary generalized tonic-clonic seizures (adjunctive), or partial seizures (adjunctive): **Note:** Children <30 kg will likely require maintenance doses to be increased as much as 50% based on clinical response regardless of regimen below:

Initial: 0.3 mg/kg/day in 1-2 divided doses for weeks 1 and 2, then increase to 0.6 mg/kg/day in 1-2 divided doses for weeks 3 and 4. Maintenance: Titrate dose to effect; after week 4, increase daily dose ▶

◄ every 1-2 weeks by 0.6 mg/kg/day; usual maintenance: 4.5-7.5 mg/kg/day in 2 divided doses; maximum: 300 mg/day in 2 divided doses

Adjustment for AED regimens **containing** valproic acid (see "Note"): Initial: 0.15 mg/kg/day in 1-2 divided doses for weeks 1 and 2, then increase to 0.3 mg/kg/day in 1-2 divided doses for weeks 3 and 4. Maintenance: Titrate dose to effect; after week 4, increase daily dose every 1-2 weeks by 0.3 mg/kg/day; usual maintenance: 1-5 mg/kg/day in 2 divided doses; maximum: 200 mg/day in 1-2 divided doses

Note: For patients >6.7 kg and <14 kg, initial dosing should be 2 mg every other day for first 2 weeks, then increased to 2 mg daily for weeks 3-4. For patients taking lamotrigine with valproic acid alone, the usual maintenance dose is 1-3 mg/kg/day in 2 divided doses

Adjustment for **enzyme-inducing** AED regimens **without** valproic acid: Initial: 0.6 mg/kg/day in 2 divided doses for weeks 1 and 2, then increase to 1.2 mg/kg/day in 2 divided doses for weeks 3 and 4. Maintenance: Titrate dose to effect; after week 4, increase daily dose every 1-2 weeks by 1.2 mg/kg/day; usual maintenance: 5-15 mg/kg/day in 2 divided doses; maximum: 400 mg/day in 2 divided doses

Children >12 years: Lennox-Gastaut (adjunctive), primary generalized tonic-clonic seizures (adjunctive), or partial seizures (adjunctive): Refer to adult dosing.

Children ≥16 years: Conversion from adjunctive therapy with valproic acid or a single enzyme-inducing AED regimen to monotherapy with lamotrigine: Refer to adult dosing.

Adults:

Lennox-Gastaut (adjunctive), primary generalized tonic-clonic seizures (adjunctive) or partial seizures (adjunctive): Initial: 25 mg/day for weeks 1 and 2, then increase to 50 mg/day for weeks 3 and 4. Maintenance: Titrate dose to effect; after week 4 increase daily dose every 1-2 weeks by 50 mg/day; usual maintenance: 225-375 mg/day in 2 divided doses

Adjustment for AED regimens **containing** valproic acid (see "Note"): Initial: 25 mg every other day for weeks 1 and 2, then increase to 25 mg every day for weeks 3 and 4. Maintenance: Titrate dose to effect; after week 4 increase daily dose every 1-2 weeks by 25-50 mg/day; usual maintenance: 100-400 mg/day in 1 or 2 divided doses

Note: For patients taking lamotrigine with valproic acid alone, the usual maintenance dose is 100-200 mg/day

Adjustment for **enzyme-inducing** AED regimens **without** valproic acid: Initial: 50 mg/day for weeks 1 and 2, then increase to 100 mg/day in 2 divided doses for weeks 3 and 4. Maintenance: titrate dose to effect; after week 4 increase daily dose every 1-2 weeks by 100 mg/day; usual maintenance: 300-500 mg/day in 2 divided doses. Doses as high as 700 mg/day have been used, though additional benefit has not been established.

Conversion to monotherapy with lamotrigine:

Conversion from adjunctive therapy with valproic acid: Initiate and titrate as per recommendations to a lamotrigine dose of 200 mg/day. Then taper valproic acid dose in decrements of not >500 mg/day at intervals of 1 week (or longer) to a valproic acid dosage of 500 mg/day; this dosage should be maintained for 1 week. The lamotrigine dosage should then be increased to 300 mg/day while valproic acid is decreased to 250 mg/day; this dosage should be maintained for 1 week. Valproic acid may then be discontinued, while the lamotrigine dose is increased by 100 mg/day at weekly intervals to achieve a lamotrigine maintenance dose of 500 mg/day.

Conversion from adjunctive therapy with carbamazepine, phenytoin, phenobarbital, or primidone: Initiate and titrate as per recommendations to a lamotrigine dose of 500 mg/day. Concomitant enzyme-inducing AED should then be withdrawn by 20% decrements each week over a 4-week period. Patients should be monitored for rash.

Conversion from adjunctive therapy with AED other than carbamazepine, phenytoin, phenobarbital, primidone or valproic acid: No specific guidelines available

Bipolar disorder:

Initial: 25 mg/day for weeks 1 and 2, then increase to 50 mg/day for weeks 3 and 4, then increase to 100 mg/day for week 5; maintenance: increase dose to 200 mg/day beginning week 6

Adjustment for regimens **containing** valproic acid: Initial: 25 mg every other day for weeks 1 and 2, then increase to 25 mg every day for weeks 3 and 4, then increase to 50 mg/day for week 5; maintenance: 100 mg/day beginning week 6

Adjustment for **enzyme-inducing** regimens **without** valproic acid: Initial: 50 mg/day for weeks 1 and 2, then increase to 100 mg/day in divided doses for weeks 3 and 4, then increase to 200 mg/day in divided doses for week 5, then increase to 300 mg/day in divided dose for week 6; maintenance: 400 mg/day in divided doses beginning week 7

Adjustment following discontinuation of psychotropic medication:

Discontinuing valproic acid with current dose of lamotrigine 100 mg/day: 150 mg/day for week 1, then increase to 200 mg/day beginning week 2

Discontinuing carbamazepine, phenytoin, phenobarbital, primidone, or rifampin with current dose of lamotrigine 400 mg/day: 400 mg/day for week 1, then decrease to 300 mg/day for week 2, then decrease to 200 mg/day beginning week 3

Discontinuing therapy: Children and Adults: Decrease dose by ~50% per week, over at least 2 weeks unless safety concerns require a more rapid withdrawal. Discontinuing carbamazepine, phenytoin, phenobarbital, or primidone should prolong the half-life of lamotrigine; discontinuing valproic acid should shorten the half-life of lamotrigine

Restarting therapy after discontinuation: If lamotrigine has been withheld for >5 half-lives, consider restarting according to initial dosing recommendations.

Dosage Forms
Tablet: 25 mg, 100 mg, 150 mg, 200 mg
Lamictal®: 25 mg, 100 mg, 150 mg, 200 mg
Tablet, combination package [each unit-dose starter kit contains]:
Lamictal® (blue kit; for patients taking valproic aid):
Tablet: Lamotrigine 25 mg (35s)
Lamictal® (green kit; for patients taking carbamazepine, phenytoin, phenobarbital, primidone, or rifampin and **not** taking valproic acid):
Tablet: Lamotrigine 25 mg (84s)
Tablet: Lamotrigine 100 mg (14s)
Lamictal® (orange kit; for patients **not** taking carbamazepine, phenytoin, phenobarbital, primidone, rifampin, or valproic acid):
Tablet: Lamotrigine 25 mg (42s)
Tablet: Lamotrigine 100 mg (7s)
Tablet, dispersible/chewable: 5 mg, 25 mg
Lamictal®: 2 mg, 5 mg, 25 mg

Lanacane® [US-OTC] *see* benzocaine *on page 124*
Lanacane® Maximum Strength [US-OTC] *see* benzocaine *on page 124*
Lanaphilic® [US-OTC] *see* urea *on page 963*

lanolin, cetyl alcohol, glycerin, petrolatum, and mineral oil
(LAN oh lin, SEE til AL koe hol, GLIS er in, pe troe LAY tum, & MIN er al oyl)
Synonyms mineral oil, petrolatum, lanolin, cetyl alcohol, and glycerin
U.S./Canadian Brand Names Lubriderm® Fragrance Free [US-OTC]; Lubriderm® [US-OTC]
Therapeutic Category Topical Skin Product
Use Treatment of dry skin
Usual Dosage Topical: Apply to skin as necessary
Dosage Forms
Lotion, topical [bottle]: 180 mL, 300 mL, 480 mL
Lubriderm® Fragrance Free [OTC], Lubriderm® [OTC]: 180 mL, 300 mL, 480 mL
Lotion, topical [tube]: 100 mL
Lubriderm® Fragrance Free [OTC], Lubriderm® [OTC]: 100 mL

Lanorinal® *(Discontinued)*
Lanoxicaps® [Can] *see* digoxin *on page 296*
Lanoxicaps® *(Discontinued)* *see* digoxin *on page 296*
Lanoxin® [US/Can] *see* digoxin *on page 296*

lanreotide (lan REE oh tide)
Sound-Alike/Look-Alike Issues
Somatuline® may be confused with somatropin, SUMAtriptan
Synonyms lanreotide acetate
U.S./Canadian Brand Names Somatuline® Autogel® [Can]; Somatuline® Depot [US]
Therapeutic Category Somatostatin Analog
Use Long-term treatment of acromegaly in patients who are not candidates for or are unresponsive to surgery and/or radiotherapy
Canadian labeling: Also approved in Canada for relief of symptoms of acromegaly

▶

◀ **Usual Dosage** SubQ: **Note: Differences in U.S. and Canadian labeled dosing:**

U.S. labeling: Adults: Acromegaly: 90 mg once every 4 weeks for 3 months; after initial 90 days of therapy, adjust dose based on clinical response of patient, growth hormone (GH) levels, and/or insulin-like growth factor 1 (IGF-1) levels as follows:
GH ≤1 ng/mL, IGF-1 normal, symptoms stable: 60 mg once every 4 weeks
GH >1-2.5 ng/mL, IGF-1 normal, symptoms stable: 90 mg once every 4 weeks
GH >2.5 ng/mL, IGF-1 elevated and/or uncontrolled symptoms: 120 mg once every 4 weeks

Canadian labeling: Children ≥16 years and Adults: Acromegaly: 90 mg once every 4 weeks for 3 months; after initial 90 days of therapy, adjust dose based on clinical response of patient, growth hormone (GH) levels, and/or insulin-like growth factor 1 (IGF-1) levels as follows:
GH = 1 ng/mL, IGF-1 normal, symptoms stable: 60 mg once every 4 weeks
GH >1-2.5 ng/mL, IGF-1 normal, symptoms stable: 90 mg once every 4 weeks
GH >2.5 ng/mL, IGF-1 elevated and/or uncontrolled symptoms: 120 mg once every 4 weeks

Dosage Forms Excipient information presented when available (limited, particularly for generics); consult specific product labeling. [CAN] = Canadian brand name
Injection, solution:
Somatuline® Autogel® [CAN]: 60 mg/ 0.3 mL (0.3 mL); 90 mg/ 0.3 mL (0.3 mL); 120 mg/0.5 mL (0.5 mL)
Somatuline® Depot®: 60 mg/0.3 mL (0.3 mL); 90 mg/0.3 mL (0.3 mL); 120 mg/0.5 mL (0.5 mL)

lanreotide acetate *see* lanreotide *on page 547*

lansoprazole (lan SOE pra zole)

Sound-Alike/Look-Alike Issues
Prevacid® may be confused with Pravachol®, Prevpac®, Prilosec®, Prinivil®
U.S./Canadian Brand Names Prevacid® SoluTab™ [US]; Prevacid® [US/Can]
Therapeutic Category Gastric Acid Secretion Inhibitor
Use Short-term treatment of active duodenal ulcers; maintenance treatment of healed duodenal ulcers; as part of a multidrug regimen for *H. pylori* eradication to reduce the risk of duodenal ulcer recurrence; short-term treatment of active benign gastric ulcer; treatment of NSAID-associated gastric ulcer; to reduce the risk of NSAID-associated gastric ulcer in patients with a history of gastric ulcer who require an NSAID; short-term treatment of symptomatic GERD; short-term treatment for all grades of erosive esophagitis; to maintain healing of erosive esophagitis; long-term treatment of pathological hypersecretory conditions, including Zollinger-Ellison syndrome
Usual Dosage Oral:
Children 1-11 years: GERD, erosive esophagitis:
≤30 kg: 15 mg once daily
>30 kg: 30 mg once daily
Note: Doses were increased in some pediatric patients if still symptomatic after 2 or more weeks of treatment (maximum dose: 30 mg twice daily)
Children 12-17 years:
Nonerosive GERD: 15 mg once daily for up to 8 weeks
Erosive esophagitis: 30 mg once daily for up to 8 weeks
Adults:
Duodenal ulcer: Short-term treatment: 15 mg once daily for 4 weeks; maintenance therapy: 15 mg once daily
Gastric ulcer: Short-term treatment: 30 mg once daily for up to 8 weeks
NSAID-associated gastric ulcer (healing): 30 mg once daily for 8 weeks; controlled studies did not extend past 8 weeks of therapy
NSAID-associated gastric ulcer (to reduce risk): 15 mg once daily for up to 12 weeks; controlled studies did not extend past 12 weeks of therapy
Symptomatic GERD: Short-term treatment: 15 mg once daily for up to 8 weeks
Erosive esophagitis: Short-term treatment: 30 mg once daily for up to 8 weeks; continued treatment for an additional 8 weeks may be considered for recurrence or for patients who do not heal after the first 8 weeks of therapy; maintenance therapy: 15 mg once daily
Hypersecretory conditions: Initial: 60 mg once daily; adjust dose based upon patient response and to reduce acid secretion to <10 mEq/hour (5 mEq/hour in patients with prior gastric surgery); doses of 90 mg twice daily have been used; administer doses >120 mg/day in divided doses
Helicobacter pylori eradication: Currently accepted recommendations (may differ from product labeling): Dose varies with regimen: 30 mg once daily or 60 mg/day in 2 divided doses; requires combination therapy with antibiotics

Dosage Forms
  Capsule, delayed release:
    Prevacid®: 15 mg, 30 mg
  Tablet, delayed release, orally disintegrating:
    Prevacid® SoluTab™: 15 mg, 30 mg

lansoprazole, amoxicillin, and clarithromycin
(lan SOE pra zole, a moks i SIL in, & kla RITH roe mye sin)

Sound-Alike/Look-Alike Issues
  Prevpac® may be confused with Prevacid®

Synonyms amoxicillin, lansoprazole, and clarithromycin; clarithromycin, lansoprazole, and amoxicillin

U.S./Canadian Brand Names Hp-PAC® [Can]; Prevpac® [US/Can]

Therapeutic Category Antibiotic, Macrolide Combination; Antibiotic, Penicillin; Gastrointestinal Agent, Miscellaneous

Use Eradication of *H. pylori* to reduce the risk of recurrent duodenal ulcer

Usual Dosage Oral: Adults: Lansoprazole 30 mg, amoxicillin 1 g, and clarithromycin 500 mg taken together twice daily for 10 or 14 days

Dosage Forms
  Combination package [each administration card contains]:
    Prevpac®:
      Capsule: Amoxicillin 500 mg (4 capsules/day)
      Capsule, delayed release (Prevacid®): Lansoprazole 30 mg (2 capsules/day)
      Tablet (Biaxin®): Clarithromycin 500 mg (2 tablets/day)

lansoprazole and naproxen (lan SOE pra zole & na PROKS en)

Sound-Alike/Look-Alike Issues
  Prevacid® may be confused with Pravachol®, Prevpac®, Prilosec®, Prinivil®

Synonyms NapraPAC™; naproxen and lansoprazole

U.S./Canadian Brand Names Prevacid® NapraPAC™ [US]

Therapeutic Category Gastric Acid Secretion Inhibitor; Nonsteroidal Antiinflammatory Drug (NSAID)

Use Reduction of the risk of NSAID-associated gastric ulcers in patients with history of gastric ulcer who require an NSAID for the treatment of rheumatoid arthritis, osteoarthritis, and ankylosing spondylitis

Usual Dosage Oral: Adults: Reduce NSAID-associated gastric ulcers during treatment for arthritis: Lansoprazole 15 mg once daily in the morning; naproxen 500 mg twice daily

Dosage Forms
  Combination package:
    Prevacid® NapraPAC™ 500 [each administration card contains]:
      Capsule, delayed release (Prevacid®): Lansoprazole 15 mg (7 capsules per card)
      Tablet (Naprosyn®): Naproxen 500 mg (14 tablets per card)

lanthanum (LAN tha num)

Synonyms lanthanum carbonate

U.S./Canadian Brand Names Fosrenol® [US/Can]

Therapeutic Category Phosphate Binder

Use Reduction of serum phosphate in patients with stage 5 chronic kidney disease (kidney failure: GFR <15 mL/minute/1.73 m^2 or dialysis)

Usual Dosage Oral: Adults: Initial: 750-1500 mg/day divided and taken with meals; typical increases of 750 mg/day every 2-3 weeks are suggested as needed to bring the serum phosphate level <6 mg/dL; usual dosage range: 1500-3000 mg; doses of up to 3750 mg have been used

Dosage Forms
  Tablet, chewable:
    Fosrenol®: 500 mg, 750 mg, 1000 mg

lanthanum carbonate *see* lanthanum *on page 549*
Lantus® [US/Can] *see* insulin glargine *on page 510*
Lantus® OptiSet® [Can] *see* insulin glargine *on page 510*
Lanvis® [Can] *see* thioguanine *on page 921*
Lapase (Discontinued) *see* pancreatin *on page 717*

lapatinib (la PA ti nib)

Sound-Alike/Look-Alike Issues
lapatinib may be confused with dasatinib, erlotinib, imatinib

Synonyms GW572016; lapatinib ditosylate; NSC-727989

U.S./Canadian Brand Names Tykerb® [US]

Therapeutic Category Antineoplastic Agent, Tyrosine Kinase Inhibitor; Epidermal Growth Factor Receptor (EGFR) Inhibitor

Use Treatment (in combination with capecitabine) of HER2/neu overexpressing advanced or metastatic breast cancer, in patients who have received prior therapy (with an anthracycline, a taxane, and trastuzumab)

Usual Dosage Details concerning dosing in combination regimens should also be consulted. **Note:** Dose reductions are likely to be needed when lapatinib is administered concomitantly with a strong CYP3A4 inhibitor (an alternate medication for CYP3A4 enzyme inhibitors should be investigated first).
Oral: Adults: 1250 mg once daily (in combination with capecitabine)

Dosage Forms
Tablet:
Tykerb®: 250 mg

lapatinib ditosylate *see* lapatinib *on page 550*
Largactil® [Can] *see* chlorpromazine *on page 213*
Lariam® [US/Can] *see* mefloquine *on page 598*

laronidase (lair OH ni days)

Synonyms recombinant α-L-iduronidase (glycosaminoglycan α-L-iduronohydrolase)

U.S./Canadian Brand Names Aldurazyme® [US/Can]

Therapeutic Category Enzyme

Use Treatment of Hurler and Hurler-Scheie forms of mucopolysaccharidosis I (MPS I); treatment of Scheie form of MPS I in patients with moderate to severe symptoms

Usual Dosage Note: Premedicate with antipyretic and/or antihistamines 1 hour prior to start of infusion.
I.V.: Children ≥5 years and Adults: 0.58 mg/kg once weekly; dose should be rounded up to the nearest whole vial

Dosage Forms
Injection, solution [preservative free]:
Aldurazyme®: 2.9 mg/5 mL (5 mL)

Lasix® [US/Can] *see* furosemide *on page 430*
Lasix® Special [Can] *see* furosemide *on page 430*
L-asparaginase *see* asparaginase *on page 98*
lassar's zinc paste *see* zinc oxide *on page 993*

latanoprost (la TA noe prost)

Sound-Alike/Look-Alike Issues
Xalatan® may be confused with Travatan®, Zarontin®

U.S./Canadian Brand Names Xalatan® [US/Can]

Therapeutic Category Prostaglandin

Use Reduction of elevated intraocular pressure in patients with open-angle glaucoma or ocular hypertension

Usual Dosage Ophthalmic: Adults: 1 drop (1.5 mcg) in the affected eye(s) once daily in the evening; do not exceed the once daily dosage because it has been shown that more frequent administration may decrease the IOP lowering effect

Note: A medication delivery device (Xal-Ease™) is available for use with Xalatan®.

Dosage Forms
Solution, ophthalmic:
Xalatan®: 0.005% (2.5 mL)

Latrodectus mactans antivenin *see* antivenin (*Latrodectus mactans*) *on page 83*
Lavacol® [US-OTC] *see* alcohol (ethyl) *on page 41*
Laxilose [Can] *see* lactulose *on page 544*

l-bunolol hydrochloride *see* levobunolol *on page 555*
L-carnitine *see* levocarnitine *on page 555*
LCD *see* coal tar *on page 240*
L-deoxythymidine *see* telbivudine *on page 906*
L-deprenyl *see* selegiline *on page 860*
LDP-341 *see* bortezomib *on page 139*
Lectopam® [Can] *see* bromazepam *(Canada only) on page 142*
Leena™ [US] *see* ethinyl estradiol and norethindrone *on page 376*

leflunomide (le FLOO noh mide)

U.S./Canadian Brand Names Apo-Leflunomide® [Can]; Arava® [US/Can]; Novo-Leflunomide [Can]
Therapeutic Category Antiinflammatory Agent
Use Treatment of active rheumatoid arthritis; indicated to reduce signs and symptoms, and to retard structural damage and improve physical function
Orphan drug: Prevention of acute and chronic rejection in recipients of solid organ transplants
Usual Dosage Oral: Adults: Rheumatoid arthritis: Initial: 100 mg/day for 3 days, followed by 20 mg/day; dosage may be decreased to 10 mg/day in patients who have difficulty tolerating the 20 mg dose. Due to the long half-life of the active metabolite, plasma levels may require a prolonged period to decline after dosage reduction.
Dosage Forms
Tablet: 10 mg, 20 mg
  Arava®: 10 mg, 20 mg

Legatrin PM® [US-OTC] *see* acetaminophen and diphenhydramine *on page 21*

lenalidomide (le na LID oh mide)

Synonyms CC-5013; IMid-3; NSC-703813
U.S./Canadian Brand Names Revlimid® [US/Can]
Therapeutic Category Angiogenesis Inhibitor; Immunosuppressant Agent; Tumor Necrosis Factor (TNF) Blocking Agent
Use Treatment of myelodysplastic syndrome (MDS) in patients with deletion 5q (del 5q) cytogenetic abnormality; treatment of multiple myeloma
Usual Dosage Oral: Adults:
Myelodysplastic syndrome (MDS): 10 mg once daily
Multiple myeloma: 25 mg once daily for 21 days of a 28-day treatment cycle (in combination with dexamethasone)
Dosage Forms
Capsule:
  Revlimid®: 5 mg, 10 mg, 15 mg, 25 mg

Lente® Iletin® II *(Discontinued)*

lepirudin (leh puh ROO din)

Synonyms lepirudin (rDNA); recombinant hirudin
U.S./Canadian Brand Names Refludan® [US/Can]
Therapeutic Category Anticoagulant (Other)
Use Indicated for anticoagulation in patients with heparin-induced thrombocytopenia (HIT) and associated thromboembolic disease in order to prevent further thromboembolic complications
Usual Dosage Note: Maximum infusion dose: Do not exceed 0.21 mg/kg/hour unless an evaluation of coagulation abnormalities limiting response has been completed.

Heparin-induced thrombocytopenia: Bolus dose: 0.4 mg/kg IVP (over 15-20 seconds), followed by continuous infusion at 0.15 mg/kg/hour (maximum initial bolus dose: 44 mg; maximum initial infusion dose: 16.5 mg/hour); bolus and infusion must be reduced in renal insufficiency
Concomitant use with thrombolytic therapy: Bolus dose: 0.2 mg/kg IVP (over 15-20 seconds), followed by continuous infusion at 0.1 mg/kg/hour

Dosing adjustments during infusions: Monitor first aPTT 4 hours after the start of the infusion. Subsequent determinations of aPTT should be obtained at least once daily during treatment. More frequent monitoring is recommended in renally- or hepatically-impaired patients. Any aPTT ratio ▶

measurement out of range (1.5-2.5) should be confirmed prior to adjusting dose, unless a clinical need for immediate reaction exists. If the aPTT is below target range, increase infusion by 20%. If the aPTT is in excess of the target range, stop infusion for 2 hours and when restarted the infusion rate should be decreased by 50%. A repeat aPTT should be obtained 4 hours after any dosing change.

Use in patients scheduled for switch to oral anticoagulants: Once platelets normalize, reduce lepirudin dose gradually to reach aPTT ratio just above 1.5 before starting warfarin therapy. Monitor PT/INR closely until results stabilize in therapeutic range. When lepirudin is discontinued, there may be a small reduction in INR.

Dosage Forms
Injection, powder for reconstitution:
Refludan®: 50 mg

lepirudin (rDNA) *see lepirudin on page 551*

Lescol® [US/Can] *see fluvastatin on page 420*

Lescol® XL [US/Can] *see fluvastatin on page 420*

Lessina™ [US] *see ethinyl estradiol and levonorgestrel on page 372*

Letairis™ [US] *see ambrisentan on page 57*

letrozole (LET roe zole)

Sound-Alike/Look-Alike Issues
Femara® may be confused with femhrt®

Synonyms CGS-20267; NSC-719345

U.S./Canadian Brand Names Femara® [US/Can]

Therapeutic Category Antineoplastic Agent, Hormone (Antiestrogen)

Use For use in postmenopausal women in the adjuvant treatment of hormone receptor positive early breast cancer, extended adjuvant treatment of early breast cancer after 5 years of tamoxifen, advanced breast cancer with disease progression following antiestrogen therapy, hormone receptor positive or hormone receptor unknown, locally-advanced, or metastatic breast cancer

Usual Dosage Oral (refer to individual protocols): Adults: Females: Breast cancer: 2.5 mg once daily

Dosage Forms
Tablet:
Femara®: 2.5 mg

leucovorin calcium (loo koe VOR in KAL see um)

Sound-Alike/Look-Alike Issues
leucovorin may be confused with Leukeran®, Leukine®, LEVOleucovorin
folinic acid may be confused with folic acid
folinic acid is an error prone synonym and should not be used

Synonyms 5-formyl tetrahydrofolate; calcium leucovorin; citrovorum factor

Therapeutic Category Folic Acid Derivative

Use Antidote for folic acid antagonists (methotrexate, trimethoprim, pyrimethamine) and rescue therapy following high-dose methotrexate; in combination with fluorouracil in the treatment of colon cancer; treatment of megaloblastic anemias when folate is deficient as in infancy, sprue, pregnancy, and nutritional deficiency when oral folate therapy is not possible

Usual Dosage
Children and Adults:
Treatment of folic acid antagonist overdosage: Oral: 5-15 mg/day
Folate-deficient megaloblastic anemia: I.M.: ≤1 mg/day
High-dose methotrexate-rescue dose: Initial: Oral, I.M., I.V.: 15 mg (~10 mg/m^2); start 24 hours after beginning methotrexate infusion; continue every 6 hours for 10 doses, until methotrexate level is <0.05 micromole/L. Adjust dose as follows:
Normal methotrexate elimination: Oral, I.M., I.V.: 15 mg every 6 hours
Delayed early methotrexate elimination: I.V.: 150 mg every 3 hours until methotrexate level is <1 micromole/L, then 15 mg every 3 hours until methotrexate level is <0.05 micromole/L
Adults:
Colorectal cancer (also refer to Combination Regimens):
I.V.: 200 mg/m^2 over at least 3 minutes (used in combination with fluorouracil 370 mg/m^2)
or
I.V.: 20 mg/m^2 (used in combination with fluorouracil 425 mg/m^2)

Dosage Forms Note: Strength expressed as base
Injection, powder for reconstitution: 50 mg, 100 mg, 200 mg, 350 mg
Injection, solution [preservative free]: 10 mg/mL (50 mL)
Tablet: 5 mg, 10 mg, 15 mg, 25 mg

Leukeran® [US/Can] *see* chlorambucil *on page 200*
Leukine® [US/Can] *see* sargramostim *on page 857*

leuprolide (loo PROE lide)

Sound-Alike/Look-Alike Issues
  Lupron® may be confused with Nuprin®
  Lupron Depot®-3 Month may be confused with Lupron Depot-Ped®
Synonyms abbott-43818; leuprolide acetate; leuprorelin acetate; TAP-144
U.S./Canadian Brand Names Eligard® [US/Can]; Lupron Depot-Ped® [US]; Lupron Depot® [US/Can]; Lupron® [US/Can]; Viadur® [Can]
Therapeutic Category Antineoplastic Agent; Luteinizing Hormone-Releasing Hormone Analog
Use Palliative treatment of advanced prostate cancer; management of endometriosis; treatment of anemia caused by uterine leiomyomata (fibroids); central precocious puberty
Usual Dosage
  Children: Precocious puberty (consider discontinuing by age 11 for females and by age 12 for males):
    SubQ (Lupron®): Initial: 50 mcg/kg/day (per manufacturer, doses of 20-45 mcg/kg/day have also been reported); titrate dose upward by 10 mcg/kg/day if down-regulation is not achieved
    I.M. (Lupron Depot-Ped®): 0.3 mg/kg/dose given every 28 days (minimum dose: 7.5 mg)
      ≤25 kg: 7.5 mg
      >25-37.5 kg: 11.25 mg
      >37.5 kg: 15 mg
      Titrate dose upward in increments of 3.75 mg every 4 weeks if down-regulation is not achieved.
  Adults:
    Advanced prostate cancer:
      SubQ:
        Eligard®: 7.5 mg monthly **or** 22.5 mg every 3 months **or** 30 mg every 4 months **or** 45 mg every 6 months
        Lupron®: 1 mg/day
        Viadur®: 65 mg implanted subcutaneously every 12 months
      I.M.:
        Lupron Depot®: 7.5 mg/dose given monthly (every 28-33 days) **or**
        Lupron Depot®-3: 22.5 mg every 3 months **or**
        Lupron Depot®-4: 30 mg every 4 months
    Endometriosis: I.M.: Initial therapy may be with leuprolide alone or in combination with norethindrone; if retreatment for an additional 6 months is necessary, norethindrone should be used. Retreatment is not recommended for longer than one additional 6-month course.
      Lupron Depot®: 3.75 mg/month for up to 6 months **or**
      Lupron Depot®-3: 11.25 mg every 3 months for up to 2 doses (6 months total duration of treatment)
    Uterine leiomyomata (fibroids): I.M. (in combination with iron):
      Lupron Depot®: 3.75 mg/month for up to 3 months **or**
      Lupron Depot®-3: 11.25 mg as a single injection
Dosage Forms
  Injection, solution: 5 mg/mL (2.8 mL)
    Lupron®: 5 mg/mL (2.8 mL)
  Injection, powder for reconstitution [depot formulation]:
    Eligard®:
      7.5 mg [released over 1 month]
      22.5 mg [released over 3 months]
      30 mg [released over 4 months]
      45 mg [released over 6 months]
    Lupron Depot®: 3.75 mg, 7.5 mg [released over 1 month]
    Lupron Depot®-3 Month: 11.25 mg, 22.5 mg [released over 3 months]
    Lupron Depot®-4 Month: 30 mg [released over 4 months]
    Lupron Depot-Ped®: 7.5 mg, 11.25 mg, 15 mg [released over 1 month]

leuprolide acetate *see* leuprolide *on page 553*

leuprorelin acetate *see* leuprolide *on page 553*
leurocristine sulfate *see* vincristine *on page 978*
Leustatin® [US/Can] *see* cladribine *on page 226*

levalbuterol (leve al BYOO ter ole)

Sound-Alike/Look-Alike Issues
  Xopenex® may be confused with Xanax®
Synonyms levalbuterol hydrochloride; levalbuterol tartrate; R-albuterol
U.S./Canadian Brand Names Xopenex HFA™ [US]; Xopenex® [US/Can]
Therapeutic Category Adrenergic Agonist Agent; Beta₂-Adrenergic Agonist Agent; Bronchodilator
Use Treatment or prevention of bronchospasm in children and adults with reversible obstructive airway disease
Usual Dosage
  Metered-dose inhaler (45 mcg/puff):
    Children 5-11 years:
      Bronchospasm, quick relief: 1-2 puffs every 4-6 hours as needed
      Exacerbation of asthma (acute, severe) *(NIH Guidelines, 2007)*: 4-8 puffs every 20 minutes for 3 doses, then every 1-4 hours as needed
    Children ≥12 years and Adults:
      Bronchospasm, quick relief: 1-2 puffs every 4-6 hours
      Exacerbation of asthma (acute, severe) *(NIH Guidelines, 2007)*: 4-8 puffs every 20 minutes for up to 4 hours, then every 1-4 hours as needed
  Solution for nebulization:
    Children: ≤4 years:
      Bronchospasm, quick relief *(NIH Guidelines, 2007)*: 0.31-1.25 mg every 4-6 hours as needed
      Exacerbation of asthma (acute, severe) *(NIH Guidelines, 2007)*: 0.075 mg/kg (minimum: 1.25 mg) every 20 minutes for 3 doses, then 0.075-0.15 mg/kg (maximum: 5 mg) every 1-4 hours as needed
    Children 5-11 years:
      Bronchospasm, quick relief: 0.31-0.63 mg every 8 hours as needed
      Exacerbation of asthma (acute severe) *(NIH Guidelines, 2007)*: 0.075 mg/kg (minimum: 1.25 mg) every 20 minutes for 3 doses, then 0.075-0.15 mg/kg (maximum: 5 mg) every 1-4 hours as needed
    Children ≥12 years and Adults:
      Bronchospasm, quick relief: 0.63-1.25 mg every 8 hours as needed
      Exacerbation of asthma (acute, severe) *(NIH Guidelines, 2007)*: 1.25-2.5 mg every 20 minutes for 3 doses, then 1.25-5 mg every 1-4 hours as needed
Dosage Forms
  Aerosol, oral:
    Xopenex®, Xopenex HFA™: 45 mcg/actuation (15 g)
  Solution for nebulization [preservative free]:
    Xopenex®, Xopenex HFA™: 0.31 mg/3 mL (24s); 0.63 mg/3 mL (24s); 1.25 mg/3 mL (24s)
  Solution for nebulization [concentrate; preservative free]:
    Xopenex®, Xopenex HFA™: 1.25 mg/0.5 mL (30s)

levalbuterol hydrochloride *see* levalbuterol *on page 554*
levalbuterol tartrate *see* levalbuterol *on page 554*
Levall™ [US] *see* carbetapentane, guaifenesin, and phenylephrine *on page 175*
Levall 5.0 *(Discontinued)*
Levall G [US] *see* guaifenesin and pseudoephedrine *on page 458*
Levaquin® [US/Can] *see* levofloxacin *on page 557*
levarterenol bitartrate *see* norepinephrine *on page 678*
Levate® [Can] *see* amitriptyline *on page 62*
Levatol® [US/Can] *see* penbutolol *on page 730*
Levbid® [US] *see* hyoscyamine *on page 492*
Levemir® [US/Can] *see* insulin detemir *on page 510*

levetiracetam (lee va tye RA se tam)

Sound-Alike/Look-Alike Issues
  Potential for dispensing errors between Keppra® and Kaletra™ (lopinavir/ritonavir)

U.S./Canadian Brand Names Apo-Levetiracetam [Can]; CO Levetiracetam [Can]; Keppra® [US/Can]; PMS-Levetiracetam [Can]

Therapeutic Category Anticonvulsant, Miscellaneous

Use Adjunctive therapy in the treatment of partial onset, myoclonic, and/or primary generalized tonic-clonic seizures

Usual Dosage

Oral:

Children 4-15 years: Partial onset seizures: 10 mg/kg/dose given twice daily; may increase every 2 weeks by 10 mg/kg/dose to a maximum of 30 mg/kg/dose twice daily

Children 6-15 years: Tonic-clonic seizures: Initial: 10 mg/kg dose given twice daily; may increase every 2 weeks by 10 mg/kg/dose to the recommended dose of 30 mg/kg twice daily. Efficacy of doses >60 mg/kg/day has not been established.

Children ≥12 years and Adults: Myoclonic seizures: Initial: 500 mg twice daily; may increase every 2 weeks by 500 mg/dose to the recommended dose of 1500 mg twice daily. Efficacy of doses >3000 mg/day has not been established.

Children ≥16 years and Adults:

Partial onset seizure: Initial: 500 mg twice daily; may increase every 2 weeks by 500 mg/dose to a maximum of 1500 mg twice daily. Doses >3000 mg/day have been used in trials; however, there is no evidence of increased benefit.

Tonic-clonic seizures: Initial: 500 mg twice daily; may increase every 2 weeks by 500 mg/dose to the recommended dose of 1500 mg twice daily. Efficacy of doses >3000 mg/day has not been established.

I.V.: Children ≥16 years and Adults: Partial onset seizure: Initial: 500 mg twice daily; may increase every 2 weeks by 500 mg/dose to a maximum of 1500 mg twice daily. Doses >3000 mg/day have been used in trials; however, there is no evidence of increased benefit.

Note: When switching from oral to I.V. formulations, the total daily dose should be the same.

Dosage Forms

Injection, solution:

Keppra®: 100 mg/mL (5 mL)

Solution, oral:

Keppra®: 100 mg/mL

Tablet:

Keppra®: 250 mg, 500 mg, 750 mg, 1000 mg

Levitra® [US/Can] *see* vardenafil *on page 971*

Levlen® [US] *see* ethinyl estradiol and levonorgestrel *on page 372*

Levlite™ [US] *see* ethinyl estradiol and levonorgestrel *on page 372*

levobunolol (lee voe BYOO noe lole)

Sound-Alike/Look-Alike Issues

levobunolol may be confused with levocabastine

Betagan® may be confused with Betadine®, Betoptic® S

Synonyms *l*-bunolol hydrochloride; levobunolol hydrochloride

U.S./Canadian Brand Names Apo-Levobunolol® [Can]; Betagan® [US/Can]; Novo-Levobunolol [Can]; Optho-Bunolol® [Can]; PMS-Levobunolol [Can]; Sandoz-Levobunolol [Can]

Therapeutic Category Beta-Adrenergic Blocker

Use To lower intraocular pressure in chronic open-angle glaucoma or ocular hypertension

Usual Dosage Ophthalmic: Adults: Instill 1 drop in the affected eye(s) 1-2 times/day

Dosage Forms

Solution, ophthalmic: 0.25% (5 mL, 10 mL); 0.5% (5 mL, 10 mL, 15 mL)

Betagan®: 0.25% (5 mL, 10 mL); 0.5% (2 mL, 5 mL, 10 mL, 15 mL)

levobunolol hydrochloride *see* levobunolol *on page 555*

levocarnitine (lee voe KAR ni teen)

Sound-Alike/Look-Alike Issues

levocarnitine may be confused with levocabastine

Synonyms L-carnitine

U.S./Canadian Brand Names Carnitor® SF [US]; Carnitor® [US/Can]

Therapeutic Category Dietary Supplement

▶

◀ **Use**
Oral: Primary systemic carnitine deficiency; acute and chronic treatment of patients with an inborn error of metabolism which results in secondary carnitine deficiency

I.V.: Acute and chronic treatment of patients with an inborn error of metabolism which results in secondary carnitine deficiency; prevention and treatment of carnitine deficiency in patients with end-stage renal disease (ESRD) who are undergoing hemodialysis.

Usual Dosage
Carnitine deficiency:
Oral:
Infants/Children: Initial: 50 mg/kg/day; titrate to 50-100 mg/kg/day in divided doses with a maximum dose of 3 g/day
Adults: 990 mg (tablet) 2-3 times/day or 1-3 g/day (solution)
I.V.: Children and Adults: 50 mg/kg/day in divided doses; titrate based on patient response. Maximum reported dose: 300 mg/kg. An equivalent loading dose may be used in patients in severe metabolic crisis.
ESRD patients on hemodialysis: I.V.: Adults: 20 mg/kg dry body weight as a slow 2- to 3-minute bolus after each dialysis session
Note: Safety and efficacy of oral carnitine have not been established in ESRD. Chronic administration of high **oral** doses to patients with severely compromised renal function or ESRD patients on dialysis may result in accumulation of **potentially toxic** metabolites.

Dosage Forms
Capsule: 250 mg
Injection, solution: 200 mg/mL (5 mL, 12.5 mL)
Carnitor®: 200 mg/mL (5 mL)
Solution, oral: 100 mg/mL
Carnitor®: 100 mg/mL
Carnitor® SF: 100 mg/mL
Tablet: 330 mg, 500 mg
Carnitor®: 330 mg

levocetirizine (LEE vo se TI ra zeen)

Sound-Alike/Look-Alike Issues
levocetirizine may be confused with cetirizine
Synonyms levocetirizine dihydrochloride
U.S./Canadian Brand Names Xyzal® [US]
Therapeutic Category Antihistamine
Use Relief of symptoms of perennial and seasonal allergic rhinitis; treatment of skin manifestations (uncomplicated) of chronic idiopathic urticaria
Usual Dosage Oral: Allergic rhinitis, chronic urticaria:
Children 6-11 years: 2.5 mg once daily (in the evening); maximum: 2.5 mg/day
Children ≥12 years and Adults: 5 mg once daily (in the evening); some patients may experience relief of symptoms with 2.5 mg once daily
Dosage Forms
Solution, oral, as dihydrochloride:
Xyzal®: 0.5 mg/mL (150 mL)
Tablet, as dihydrochloride [scored]:
Xyzal®: 5 mg

levocetirizine dihydrochloride see levocetirizine on page 556
levodopa and benserazide see benserazide and levodopa (Canada only) on page 122
levodopa and carbidopa see carbidopa and levodopa on page 177

levodopa, carbidopa, and entacapone (lee voe DOE pa, kar bi DOE pa, & en TA ka pone)

Synonyms carbidopa, levodopa, and entacapone; entacapone, carbidopa, and levodopa
U.S./Canadian Brand Names Stalevo® [US]
Therapeutic Category Anti-Parkinson Agent (Dopamine Agonist); Anti-Parkinson Agent, COMT Inhibitor
Use Treatment of idiopathic Parkinson disease
Usual Dosage Oral: Adults: Parkinson disease:
Note: All strengths of Stalevo® contain a carbidopa/levodopa ratio of 1:4 plus entacapone 200 mg.

Dose should be individualized based on therapeutic response; doses may be adjusted by changing strength or adjusting interval. Fractionated doses are not recommended and only 1 tablet should be given at each dosing interval; maximum daily dose: 8 tablets of Stalevo® 50, 100, or 150, **or** 6 tablets of Stalevo® 200.

Patients previously treated with carbidopa/levodopa immediate release tablets (ratio of 1:4):

With current entacapone therapy: May switch directly to corresponding strength of combination tablet. No data available on transferring patients from controlled release preparations or products with a 1:10 ratio of carbidopa/levodopa.

Without entacapone therapy:

If current levodopa dose is >600 mg/day: Levodopa dose reduction may be required when adding entacapone to therapy; therefore, titrate dose using individual products first (carbidopa/levodopa immediate release with a ratio of 1:4 plus entacapone 200 mg); then transfer to combination product once stabilized.

If current levodopa dose is <600 mg without dyskinesias: May transfer to corresponding dose of combination product; monitor, dose reduction of levodopa may be required.

Dosage Forms
Tablet:
Stalevo®: 50: Levodopa 50 mg, carbidopa 12.5 mg, and entacapone 200 mg; 100: Levodopa 100 mg, carbidopa 25 mg, and entacapone 200 mg; 150: Levodopa 150 mg, carbidopa 37.5 mg, and entacapone 200 mg; 200: Levodopa 200 mg, carbidopa 50 mg, and entacapone 200 mg

Levo-Dromoran® [US] *see* levorphanol *on page 559*

levofloxacin (lee voe FLOKS a sin)

Sound-Alike/Look-Alike Issues
Sound-alike/look-alike issues:
Levaquin® may be confused with Levoxyl®, Levsin/SL®, Lovenox®
Levofloxacin may be confused with levetiracetam, levodopa, levothyroxine

U.S./Canadian Brand Names Iquix® [US]; Levaquin® [US/Can]; Novo-Levofloxacin [Can]; Quixin® [US]

Therapeutic Category Antibiotic, Ophthalmic; Antibiotic, Quinolone

Use
Systemic: Treatment of community-acquired pneumonia, including multidrug resistant strains of *S. pneumoniae* (MDRSP); nosocomial pneumonia; chronic bronchitis (acute bacterial exacerbation); acute bacterial sinusitis; prostatitis, urinary tract infection (uncomplicated or complicated); acute pyelonephritis; skin or skin structure infections (uncomplicated or complicated); reduce incidence or disease progression of inhalational anthrax (postexposure)

Ophthalmic: Treatment of bacterial conjunctivitis caused by susceptible organisms (Quixin™ 0.5% ophthalmic solution); treatment of corneal ulcer caused by susceptible organisms (Iquix® 1.5% ophthalmic solution)

Usual Dosage Note: Sequential therapy (intravenous to oral) may be instituted based on prescriber's discretion.

Usual dosage range:
Children ≥1 year: Ophthalmic: 1-2 drops every 2-6 hours
Adults:
Ophthalmic: 1-2 drops every 2-6 hours
Oral, I.V.: 250-500 mg every 24 hours; severe or complicated infections: 750 mg every 24 hours

Indication-specific dosing:
Children ≥1 year and Adults: Ophthalmic:
Conjunctivitis (0.5% ophthalmic solution):
Treatment day 1 and day 2: Instill 1-2 drops into affected eye(s) every 2 hours while awake, up to 8 times/day
Treatment day 3 through day 7: Instill 1-2 drops into affected eye(s) every 4 hours while awake, up to 4 times/day
Children ≥6 years and Adults: Ophthalmic:
Corneal ulceration (1.5% ophthalmic solution): Treatment day 1 through day 3: Instill 1-2 drops into affected eye(s) every 30 minutes to 2 hours while awake and 4-6 hours after retiring.
Adults: Oral, I.V.:
Anthrax (inhalational): 500 mg every 24 hours for 60 days, beginning as soon as possible after exposure
Chronic bronchitis (acute bacterial exacerbation): 500 mg every 24 hours for at least 7 days

▶

◄ **Pneumonia:**
  Community-acquired: 500 mg every 24 hours for 7-14 days or 750 mg every 24 hours for 5 days
    (efficacy of 5-day regimen for MDRSP not established)
  Nosocomial: 750 mg every 24 hours for 7-14 days
Prostatitis (chronic bacterial): 500 mg every 24 hours for 28 days
Sinusitis (acute bacterial): 500 mg every 24 hours for 10-14 days or 750 mg every 24 hours for 5
days
Skin and skin structure infections:
  Uncomplicated: 500 mg every 24 hours for 7-10 days
  Complicated: 750 mg every 24 hours for 7-14 days
Urinary tract infections:
  Uncomplicated: 250 mg once daily for 3 days
  Complicated, including pyelonephritis: 250 mg once daily for 10 days **or** 750 mg once daily for 5 days

Dosage Forms
  Infusion [premixed in D_5W]:
    Levaquin®: 250 mg (50 mL); 500 mg (100 mL); 750 mg (150 mL)
  Injection, solution [preservative free]:
    Levaquin®: 25 mg/mL (20 mL, 30 mL)
  Solution, ophthalmic [drops]:
    Iquix®: 1.5% (5 mL)
    Quixin®: 0.5% (5 mL)
  Solution, oral:
    Levaquin®: 25 mg/mL
  Tablet, oral:
    Levaquin®: 250 mg, 500 mg, 750 mg
    Levaquin® Leva-Pak: 750 mg (5s)

levo-folinic acid *see* LEVOleucovorin *on page 558*

LEVOleucovorin
  (lee voe loo koe VOR in)
  Sound-Alike/Look-Alike Issues
    LEVOleucovorin may be confused with leucovorin calcium, Leukeran®, Leukine®
  Synonyms 6S-leucovorin; calcium levoleucovorin; L-leucovorin; levo-folinic acid; levo-leucovorin;
  levoleucovorin calcium pentahydrate; S-leucovorin
  Therapeutic Category Antidote Rescue Agent (Chemotherapy)
  Use Rescue agent after high-dose methotrexate therapy in osteosarcoma; antidote for impaired
  methotrexate elimination and for inadvertent overdosage of folic acid antagonists
  Usual Dosage Note: Levoleucovorin is dosed at **one-half** the usual dose of the racemic form (leucovorin
  calcium):
    High-dose methotrexate rescue: Children and Adults: I.V.: Usual dose: 7.5 mg (~5 mg/m^2) every 6
    hours for 10 doses, beginning 24 hours after the start of the methotrexate infusion (based on a
    methotrexate dose of 12 g/m^2 I.V. over 4 hours). Levoleucovorin (and hydration and urinary
    alkalinization) should be continued and/or adjusted until the methotrexate level is <0.05 micromolar
    (5×10^{-8} M) as follows:
    Normal methotrexate elimination (serum methotrexate levels ~10 micromolar at 24 hours post
      administration, 1 micromolar at 48 hours and <0.2 micromolar at 72 hours post infusion): 7.5 mg I.V.
      every 6 hours for 10 doses
    Delayed late methotrexate elimination (serum methotrexate levels >0.2 micromolar at 72 hours and
      >0.05 micromolar at 96 hours post methotrexate infusion): Continue 7.5 mg I.V. every 6 hours until
      methotrexate level is <0.05 micromolar
    Delayed early methotrexate elimination and/or evidence of acute renal injury (serum methotrexate level
      ≥50 micromolar at 24 hours, ≥5 micromolar at 48 hours or a doubling or more of the serum creatinine
      level at 24 hours post methotrexate infusion): 75 mg I.V. every 3 hours until methotrexate level is <1
      micromolar, followed by 7.5 mg I.V. every 3 hours until methotrexate level is <0.05 micromolar
    *Significant clinical toxicity in the presence of less severe abnormalities in methotrexate elimination or
      renal function (as described above):* Extend levoleucovorin treatment for an additional 24 hours (total
      of 14 doses) in subsequent treatment cycles.
    *Delayed methotrexate elimination due to third space fluid accumulation, renal insufficiency, or
      inadequate hydration:* May require higher levoleucovorin doses or prolonged administration.
    Methotrexate overdose (inadvertent): Children and Adults: I.V.: 7.5 mg (~5 mg/m^2) every 6 hours;
    continue until the methotrexate level is <0.01 micromolar (10^{-8} M). Initiate treatment as soon as possible

after methotrexate overdose. Increase the levoleucovorin dose to 50 mg/m² I.V. every 3 hours if the 24 hour serum creatinine has increased 50% over baseline, or if the 24-hour methotrexate level is >5 micromolar (5 x 10⁻⁶ M), or if the 48-hour methotrexate level is >0.9 micromolar (9 x 10⁻⁷ M); continue levoleucovorin until the methotrexate level is <0.01 micromolar (10⁻⁸ M). Hydration (3 L/day) and urinary alkalinization (with sodium bicarbonate) should also be maintained.

Treatment of colorectal cancer (in combination with fluorouracil; unlabeled use): Adults: I.V.: Levoleucovorin is dosed at **one-half** the usual dose of the racemic form (leucovorin)

Dosage Forms Note: Strength expressed as base
Injection, powder for reconstitution:
Fusilev™: 50 mg

levo-leucovorin *see* LEVOleucovorin *on page 558*
levoleucovorin calcium pentahydrate *see* LEVOleucovorin *on page 558*
levomepromazine *see* methotrimeprazine *(Canada only) on page 617*
levonordefrin and mepivacaine hydrochloride *see* mepivacaine and levonordefrin *on page 605*

levonorgestrel (LEE voe nor jes trel)

Synonyms LNg 20
U.S./Canadian Brand Names Mirena® [US/Can]; Norplant® Implant [Can]; Plan B® [US-RX/OTC/Can]
Therapeutic Category Contraceptive, Implant (Progestin); Contraceptive, Progestin Only
Use
Intrauterine device (IUD): Prevention of pregnancy
Oral: Emergency contraception following unprotected intercourse or possible contraceptive failure
Usual Dosage Adults: Females:
Long-term prevention of pregnancy: Intrauterine system: To be inserted into uterine cavity; should be inserted within 7 days of onset of menstruation or immediately after 1st trimester abortion; releases 20 mcg levonorgestrel/day over 5 years. May be removed and replaced with a new unit at anytime during menstrual cycle; do not leave any one system in place for >5 years
Emergency contraception: Oral tablet: One 0.75 mg tablet as soon as possible within 72 hours of unprotected sexual intercourse; a second 0.75 mg tablet should be taken 12 hours after the first dose; may be used at any time during menstrual cycle
Dosage Forms
Intrauterine device:
Mirena®: 52 mg/unit
Tablet:
Plan B®: 0.75 mg

levonorgestrel and estradiol *see* estradiol and levonorgestrel *on page 361*
levonorgestrel and ethinyl estradiol *see* ethinyl estradiol and levonorgestrel *on page 372*
Levophed® [US/Can] *see* norepinephrine *on page 678*
Levora® [US] *see* ethinyl estradiol and levonorgestrel *on page 372*

levorphanol (lee VOR fa nole)

Synonyms levorphan tartrate; levorphanol tartrate
U.S./Canadian Brand Names Levo-Dromoran® [US]
Therapeutic Category Analgesic, Narcotic
Controlled Substance C-II

Use Relief of moderate-to-severe pain; also used parenterally for preoperative sedation and an adjunct to nitrous oxide/oxygen anesthesia
Usual Dosage Adults: **Note:** These are guidelines and do not represent the maximum doses that may be required in all patients. Doses should be titrated to pain relief/prevention.
Acute pain (moderate to severe):
Oral: Initial: Opiate-naive: 2 mg every 6-8 hours as needed; patients with prior opiate exposure may require higher initial doses; usual dosage range: 2-4 mg every 6-8 hours as needed
I.M., SubQ: Initial: Opiate-naive: 1 mg every 6-8 hours as needed; patients with prior opiate exposure may require higher initial doses; usual dosage range: 1-2 mg every 6-8 hours as needed
Slow I.V.: Initial: Opiate-naive: Up to 1 mg/dose every 3-6 hours as needed; patients with prior opiate exposure may require higher initial doses
Chronic pain: Patients taking opioids chronically may become tolerant and require doses higher than the usual dosage range to maintain the desired effect. Tolerance can be managed by appropriate dose ▶

◀ titration. **There is no optimal or maximal dose for levorphanol in chronic pain. The appropriate dose is one that relieves pain throughout its dosing interval without causing unmanageable side effects.**

Premedication: I.M., SubQ: 1-2 mg/dose 60-90 minutes prior to surgery; older or debilitated patients usually require less drug

Dosage Forms

Injection, solution:

Levo-Dromoran®: 2 mg/mL (1 mL, 10 mL)

Tablet: 2 mg

Levo-Dromoran®: 2 mg

levorphanol tartrate see levorphanol on page 559

levorphan tartrate see levorphanol on page 559

Levo-T™ (Discontinued) see levothyroxine on page 560

Levothroid® [US] see levothyroxine on page 560

levothyroxine (lee voe thye ROKS een)

Sound-Alike/Look-Alike Issues

levothyroxine may be confused with liothyronine

Levoxyl® may be confused with Lanoxin®, Luvox®

Synthroid® may be confused with Symmetrel®

Synonyms L-thyroxine sodium; levothyroxine sodium; T_4

U.S./Canadian Brand Names Eltroxin® [Can]; Gen-Levothyroxine [Can]; Levothroid® [US]; Levothyroxine Sodium [Can]; Levoxyl® [US]; Synthroid® [US/Can]; Tirosint™ [US]; Unithroid® [US]

Therapeutic Category Thyroid Product

Use Replacement or supplemental therapy in hypothyroidism; pituitary TSH suppression

Usual Dosage Doses should be adjusted based on clinical response and laboratory parameters.

Oral:

Children: Hypothyroidism:

Newborns: Initial: 10-15 mcg/kg/day. Lower doses of 25 mcg/day should be considered in newborns at risk for cardiac failure. Newborns with T_4 levels <5 mcg/dL should be started at 50 mcg/day. Adjust dose at 4- to 6-week intervals.

Infants and Children: Dose based on body weight and age as listed below. Children with severe or chronic hypothyroidism should be started at 25 mcg/day; adjust dose by 25 mcg every 2-4 weeks. In older children, hyperactivity may be decreased by starting with 1/4 of the recommended dose and increasing by 1/4 dose each week until the full replacement dose is reached. Refer to adult dosing once growth and puberty are complete.

0-3 months: 10-15 mcg/kg/day

3-6 months: 8-10 mcg/kg/day

6-12 months: 6-8 mcg/kg/day

1-5 years: 5-6 mcg/kg/day

6-12 years: 4-5 mcg/kg/day

>12 years: 2-3 mcg/kg/day

Adults:

Hypothyroidism: 1.7 mcg/kg/day in otherwise healthy adults <50 years old, children in whom growth and puberty are complete, and older adults who have been recently treated for hyperthyroidism or who have been hypothyroid for only a few months. Titrate dose every 6 weeks. Average starting dose ~100 mcg; usual doses are ≤200 mcg/day; doses ≥300 mcg/day are rare (consider poor compliance, malabsorption, and/or drug interactions).

Severe hypothyroidism: Initial: 12.5-25 mcg/day; adjust dose by 25 mcg/day every 2-4 weeks as appropriate; **Note:** Oral agents are not recommended for myxedema (see I.V. dosing).

Subclinical hypothyroidism (if treated): 1 mcg/kg/day

TSH suppression:

Well-differentiated thyroid cancer: Highly individualized; Doses >2 mcg/kg/day may be needed to suppress TSH to <0.1 mU/L.

Benign nodules and nontoxic multinodular goiter: Goal TSH suppression: 0.1-0.3 mU/L

I.M., I.V.: Children, Adults: Hypothyroidism: 50% of the oral dose

I.V.: Adults: Myxedema coma or stupor: 200-500 mcg, then 100-300 mcg the next day if necessary; smaller doses should be considered in patients with cardiovascular disease

Dosage Forms
  Capsule, soft gelatin:
    Tirosint™: 13 mcg, 25 mcg, 50 mcg, 75 mcg, 100 mcg, 125 mcg, 150 mcg
  Injection, powder for reconstitution: 0.2 mg, 0.5 mg
  Tablet: 25 mcg, 50 mcg, 75 mcg, 88 mcg, 100 mcg, 112 mcg, 125 mcg, 150 mcg, 175 mcg, 200 mcg, 300 mcg
    Levothroid®: 25 mcg, 50 mcg, 75 mcg, 88 mcg, 100 mcg, 112 mcg, 125 mcg, 137 mcg, 150 mcg, 175 mcg, 200 mcg, 300 mcg
    Levoxyl®: 25 mcg, 50 mcg, 75 mcg, 88 mcg, 100 mcg, 112 mcg, 125 mcg, 137 mcg, 150 mcg, 175 mcg, 200 mcg
    Synthroid®: 25 mcg, 50 mcg, 75 mcg, 88 mcg, 100 mcg, 112 mcg, 125 mcg, 137 mcg, 150 mcg, 175 mcg, 200 mcg, 300 mcg
    Unithroid®: 25 mcg, 50 mcg, 75 mcg, 88 mcg, 100 mcg, 112 mcg, 125 mcg, 150 mcg, 175 mcg, 200 mcg, 300 mcg

Levothyroxine Sodium [Can] *see* levothyroxine *on page 560*
levothyroxine sodium *see* levothyroxine *on page 560*
Levoxyl® [US] *see* levothyroxine *on page 560*
Levsin® [US/Can] *see* hyoscyamine *on page 492*
Levsinex® [US] *see* hyoscyamine *on page 492*
Levsin/SL® [US] *see* hyoscyamine *on page 492*
Levulan® [Can] *see* aminolevulinic acid *on page 60*
Levulan® Kerastick® [US] *see* aminolevulinic acid *on page 60*
levulose, dextrose and phosphoric acid *see* fructose, dextrose, and phosphoric acid *on page 429*
Lexapro® [US] *see* escitalopram *on page 356*
Lexiscan™ [US] *see* regadenoson *on page 823*
Lexiva® [US] *see* fosamprenavir *on page 425*
Lexxel® [Can] *see* enalapril and felodipine *on page 339*
Lexxel® *(Discontinued)* *see* enalapril and felodipine *on page 339*
LFA-3/IgG(1) fusion protein, human *see* alefacept *on page 42*
LHRH *see* gonadorelin *on page 451*
***l*-hyoscyamine sulfate** *see* hyoscyamine *on page 492*
Lialda™ [US] *see* mesalamine *on page 607*
Librax® *[original formulation]* [US/Can] *see* clidinium and chlordiazepoxide *on page 229*
Librax® *[reformulation]* *(Discontinued)*
Librium® [US] *see* chlordiazepoxide *on page 201*
Lice-Enz® Shampoo *(Discontinued)*
Licide® [US-OTC] *see* pyrethrins and piperonyl butoxide *on page 806*
LidaMantle® [US] *see* lidocaine *on page 561*
Lida-Mantle® HC [US] *see* lidocaine and hydrocortisone *on page 564*
Lidemol® [Can] *see* fluocinonide *on page 410*
Lidex® [Can] *see* fluocinonide *on page 410*
Lidex® *(Discontinued)* *see* fluocinonide *on page 410*
Lidex-E® *(Discontinued)* *see* fluocinonide *on page 410*

lidocaine (LYE doe kane)

Synonyms lidocaine hydrochloride; lignocaine hydrochloride
U.S./Canadian Brand Names Anestacon® [US]; Anestafoam™ [US-OTC]; Band-Aid® Hurt-Free™ Antiseptic Wash [US-OTC]; Betacaine® [Can]; Burn Jel® [US-OTC]; Burn-O-Jel [US-OTC]; Burnamycin [US-OTC]; L-M-X™ 4 [US-OTC]; L-M-X™ 5 [US-OTC]; LidaMantle® [US]; Lidodan™ [Can]; Lidoderm® [US/Can]; LTA® 360 [US]; Premjact® [US-OTC]; Solarcaine® Aloe Extra Burn Relief [US-OTC]; Topicaine® [US-OTC]; Unburn® [US]; Xylocaine® [US]; Xylocaine® MPF [US]; Xylocaine® Viscous [US]; Xylocaine® [US/Can]; Xylocard® [Can]; Zilactin-L® [US-OTC]; Zilactin® [Can]; Zingo™ [US]
Therapeutic Category Analgesic, Topical; Antiarrhythmic Agent, Class I-B; Local Anesthetic
Use Local anesthetic and acute treatment of ventricular arrhythmias from myocardial infarction, or cardiac manipulation
  Intradermal: To provide local anesthesia prior to venipuncture or peripheral I.V. cannulation

Rectal: Temporary relief of pain and itching due to anorectal disorders

Topical: Local anesthetic for use in laser, cosmetic, and outpatient surgeries; minor burns, cuts, and abrasions of the skin

Lidoderm® Patch: Relief of allodynia (painful hypersensitivity) and chronic pain in postherpetic neuralgia

Usual Dosage

Antiarrhythmic:

Children:

I.V., I.O.: **Note:** For use in pulseless VT or VF, give after defibrillation, CPR, and epinephrine:

Loading dose: 1 mg/kg (maximum: 100 mg); follow with continuous infusion; may administer second bolus of 0.5-1 mg/kg if delay between bolus and start of infusion is >15 minutes

Continuous infusion: 20-50 mcg/kg/minute. Use 20 mcg/kg/minute in patients with shock, hepatic disease, cardiac arrest, mild CHF; moderate-to-severe CHF may require 1/2 loading dose and lower infusion rates to avoid toxicity.

E.T.: 2-3 mg/kg; flush with 5 mL of NS and follow with 5 assisted manual ventilations

Adults:

Ventricular fibrillation or pulseless ventricular tachycardia (after defibrillation, CPR, and vasopressor administration): I.V.: Initial: 1-1.5 mg/kg. Refractory ventricular tachycardia or ventricular fibrillation, a repeat 0.5-0.75 mg/kg bolus may be given every 5-10 minutes after initial dose for a maximum of 3 doses. Total dose should not exceed 3 mg/kg. Follow with continuous infusion (1-4 mg/minute) after return of perfusion. Reappearance of arrhythmia during constant infusion: 0.5 mg/kg bolus and reassessment of infusion.

E.T. (loading dose only): 2-2.5 times the recommended I.V. dose; dilute in 10 mL NS or distilled water.

Note: Absorption is greater with distilled water, but causes more adverse effects on PaO_2.

Hemodynamically stable VT: 0.5-0.75 mg/kg followed by synchronized cardioversion

Note: Decrease dose in patients with CHF, shock, or hepatic disease.

Anesthesia, topical:

Cream:

LidaMantle®: Skin irritation: Children and Adults: Apply to affected area 2-3 times/day as needed

L-M-X™ 4: Children ≥2 years and Adults: Apply 1/4 inch thick layer to intact skin. Leave on until adequate anesthetic effect is obtained. Remove cream and cleanse area before beginning procedure.

L-M-X™ 5: Relief of anorectal pain and itching: Children ≥12 years and Adults: Rectal: Apply topically to clean, dry area **or** using applicator, insert rectally, up to 6 times/day

Gel, ointment, solution: Adults: Apply to affected area ≤3 times/day as needed (maximum dose: 4.5 mg/kg, not to exceed 300 mg)

Jelly:

Children ≥10 years: Dose varies with age and weight (maximum dose: 4.5 mg/kg)

Adults (maximum dose: 30 mL [600 mg] in any 12-hour period):

Anesthesia of male urethra: 5-30 mL

Anesthesia of female urethra: 3-5 mL

Lubrication of endotracheal tube: Apply a moderate amount to external surface only

Liquid: Cold sores and fever blisters: Children ≥5 years and Adults: Apply to affected area every 6 hours as needed

Patch: Postherpetic neuralgia: Adults: Apply patch to most painful area. Up to 3 patches may be applied in a single application. Patch may remain in place for up to 12 hours in any 24-hour period.

Anesthetic, local injectable: Children and Adults: Varies with procedure, degree of anesthesia needed, vascularity of tissue, duration of anesthesia required, and physical condition of patient; maximum: 4.5 mg/kg/dose; do not repeat within 2 hours.

Dosage Forms

Aerosol, topical [foam]:

Anestafoam™: 4% (30 g)

Cream, rectal: 5% (15 g, 30 g)

L-M-X™ 5 [OTC]: 5% (15 g,30 g)

Cream, topical: 3% (30 g); 4% (5 g, 15 g, 30 g)

LidaMantle®: 3% (30 g, 85 g)

L-M-X™ 4 [OTC]: 4% (5g, 15 g,30 g)

Gel, topical:

Burn Jel® [OTC]: 2% (3.5 g, 120 g)

Burn-O-Jel [OTC]: 0.5% (90 g)

Solarcaine® Aloe Extra Burn Relief [OTC]: 0.5% (113 g, 226 g)

Topicaine® [OTC]: 4% (10 g, 30 g, 113 g)

Unburn®: 2.5% (3.5 g, 59 mL, 118 mL)

Infusion [premixed in D$_5$W]: 0.4% [4 mg/mL] (250 mL, 500 mL); 0.8% [8 mg/mL] (250 mL, 500 mL)
Injection, solution: 0.5% [5 mg/mL] (50 mL); 1% [10 mg/mL] (2 mL, 10 mL, 20 mL, 30 mL, 50 mL); 2% [20 mg/mL] (2 mL, 5 mL, 20 mL, 50 mL)
Xylocaine®: 0.5% [5 mg/mL] (50 mL); 1% [10 mg/mL] (10 mL, 20 mL, 50 mL); 2% [20 mg/mL] (1.8 mL, 10 mL, 20 mL, 50 mL)
Injection, solution: [preservative free]: 0.5% [5 mg/mL] (50 mL); 1% [10 mg/mL] (2 mL, 5 mL, 30 mL); 1.5% [15 mg/mL] (20 mL); 2% [20 mg/mL] (2 mL, 5 mL, 10 mL); 4% [40 mg/mL] (5 mL)
Xylocaine®: 10% [100 mg/mL] (5 mL)
Xylocaine® MPF: 0.5% [5 mg/mL] (50 mL); 1% [10 mg/mL] (2 mL, 5 mL, 10 mL, 30 mL); 1.5% [15 mg/mL] (10 mL, 20 mL); 2% [20 mg/mL] (2 mL, 5 mL, 10 mL); 4% [40 mg/mL] (5 mL)
Injection, solution: [premixed in D$_{7.5}$W, preservative free]: 5% (2 mL)
Jelly, topical: 2% (5 mL, 30 mL)
Anestacon®: 2% (15 mL)
Xylocaine®: 2% (5 mL, 30 mL)
Liquid, topical:
Zilactin®-L [OTC]: 2.5% (7.5 mL)
Lotion, topical: 3% (177 mL)
LidaMantle®: 3% (177 mL)
Ointment, topical: 5% (37 g, 50 g)
Powder, intradermal, as hydrochloride:
Zingo™: 0.5 mg
Solution, topical: 4% [40 mg/mL] (50 mL)
Band-Aid® Hurt-Free™ Antiseptic Wash [OTC]: 2% (180 mL)
LTA® 360: 4% [40 mg/mL] (4 mL)
Xylocaine®: 4% [40 mg/mL] (50 mL)
Solution, viscous: 2% [20 mg/mL] (20 mL, 100 mL)
Xylocaine® Viscous: 2% [20 mg/mL] (100 mL, 450 mL)
Spray, topical:
Burnamycin [OTC]: 0.5% (60 mL)
Premjact® [OTC]: 9.6% (13 mL)
Solarcaine® Aloe Extra Burn Relief [OTC]: 0.5% (127 g)
Transdermal system, topical:
Lidoderm®: 5% (30s)

lidocaine and bupivacaine (LYE doe kane & byoo PIV a kane)

Synonyms bupivacaine and lidocaine; lidocaine hydrochloride and bupivacaine hydrochloride
U.S./Canadian Brand Names Duocaine™ [US]
Therapeutic Category Local Anesthetic
Use Local or regional anesthesia in ophthalmologic surgery by peripheral nerve block techniques such as peribulbar, retrobulbar, and facial blocks; may be used with or without epinephrine
Usual Dosage Children ≥12 years and Adults: **Note:** Use lowest effective dose to limit toxic effects. Dosing based on lidocaine 1% and bupivacaine 0.375%
Retrobulbar injection: 2-5 mL; a portion of dose is injected retrobulbarly and remainder may be used to block the facial nerve
Peribulbar block: 6-12 mL
Maximum dose: 0.18 mL/kg or 12 mL; if used with epinephrine, the dose should not exceed 0.28 mL/kg or 20 mL
Dosage Forms
Injection, solution [preservative free]:
Duocaine™: Lidocaine 1% and bupivacaine 0.375% (10 mL)

lidocaine and epinephrine (LYE doe kane & ep i NEF rin)

Synonyms epinephrine and lidocaine
U.S./Canadian Brand Names LidoSite™ [US]; Lignospan® Forte [US]; Lignospan® Standard [US]; Xylocaine® MPF With Epinephrine [US]; Xylocaine® With Epinephrine [US/Can]
Therapeutic Category Local Anesthetic
Use Local infiltration anesthesia; AVS for nerve block; topical local analgesia for superficial dermatologic procedures
Usual Dosage Dosage varies with the anesthetic procedure, degree of anesthesia needed, vascularity of tissue, duration of anesthesia required, and physical condition of patient.

◄ Dental anesthesia, infiltration, or conduction block:
  Children <10 years: 20-30 mg (1-1.5 mL) of lidocaine hydrochloride as a 2% solution with epinephrine 1:100,000; maximum: 4-5 mg of lidocaine hydrochloride/kg of body weight or 100-150 mg as a single dose
  Children >10 years and Adults: Do not exceed 6.6 mg/kg body weight or 300 mg of lidocaine hydrochloride and 3 mcg (0.003 mg) of epinephrine/kg of body weight or 0.2 mg epinephrine per dental appointment. The effective anesthetic dose varies with procedure, intensity of anesthesia needed, duration of anesthesia required, and physical condition of the patient. Always use the lowest effective dose along with careful aspiration.

For most routine dental procedures, lidocaine hydrochloride 2% with epinephrine 1:100,000 is preferred. When a more pronounced hemostasis is required, a 1:50,000 epinephrine concentration should be used.

Dermatologic procedure: Children ≥5 and Adults: Topical: Place 1 transdermal patch over area requiring analgesia; attach patch to iontophoretic controller and leave on for 10 minutes. Remove patch and perform procedure within 10-20 minutes of patch removal. Do not use another patch for 30 minutes.

Dosage Forms

Injection, solution:
Generics:
  0.5% / 1:200,000: Lidocaine 0.5% and epinephrine 1:200,000 (50 mL)
  1% / 1:100,000: Lidocaine 1% and epinephrine 1:100,000 (20 mL, 30 mL, 50 mL)
  1% / 1:200,000: Lidocaine 1% and epinephrine 1:200,000 (30 mL)
  1.5% / 1:200,000: Lidocaine 1.5% and epinephrine 1:200,000 (30 mL)
  2% / 1:50,000: Lidocaine 2% and epinephrine 1:50,000 (1.8 mL)
  2% / 1:100,000: Lidocaine 2% and epinephrine 1:100,000 (1.8 mL, 30 mL, 50 mL)
  2% / 1:200,000: Lidocaine 2% and epinephrine 1:200,000 (20 mL)
Brands:
  Lignospan® Forte: 2% / 1:50,000: Lidocaine hydrochloride 2% and epinephrine 1:50,000 (1.7 mL)
  Lignospan® Standard: 2% / 1:100,000: Lidocaine hydrochloride 2% and epinephrine 1:100,000 (1.7 mL)
  Xylocaine® with Epinephrine:
    0.5% / 1:200,000: Lidocaine 0.5% and epinephrine 1:200,000 (50 mL)
    1% / 1:100,000: Lidocaine 1% and epinephrine 1:100,000 (10 mL, 20 mL, 50 mL)
    2% / 1:50,000: Lidocaine 2% and epinephrine 1:50,000 (1.8 mL)
    2% / 1:100,000: Lidocaine 2% and epinephrine 1:100,000 (1.8 mL); (10 mL, 20 mL, 50 mL)
  Xylocaine®-MPF with Epinephrine:
    1% / 1:200,000: Lidocaine 1% and epinephrine 1:200,000 (5 mL, 10 mL, 30 mL)
    1.5% / 1:200,000: Lidocaine 1.5% and epinephrine 1:200,000 (5 mL, 10 mL, 30 mL)
    2% / 1:200,000: Lidocaine 2% and epinephrine 1:200,000 (5 mL, 10 mL, 20 mL)

Transdermal system:
LidoSite™: Lidocaine 10% and epinephrine 0.1% (25s)

lidocaine and hydrocortisone (LYE doe kane & hye droe KOR ti sone)

Synonyms hydrocortisone and lidocaine

U.S./Canadian Brand Names AnaMantle HC® Forte [US]; AnaMantle® HC [US]; Lida-Mantle® HC [US]; Peranex™ HC Medi-Pad [US]; Peranex™ HC [US]; Rectacreme HC [US]; RectaGel™ HC [US]

Therapeutic Category Anesthetic/Corticosteroid

Use Topical antiinflammatory and anesthetic for skin disorders; rectal for the treatment of hemorrhoids, anal fissures, pruritus ani, or similar conditions

Usual Dosage Adults:
Topical: Apply 2-3 times/day
Rectal: One applicatorful twice daily

Dosage Forms

Cream, rectal:
  AnaMantle HC® Forte: Lidocaine 3% and hydrocortisone 1% (7 g)
  AnaMantle® HC, Rectacreme HC: Lidocaine 3% and hydrocortisone 0.5% (7 g)
  Peranex™ HC: Lidocaine 2% and hydrocortisone 2% (7 g)
  Xyralid™ RC: Lidocaine 3% and hydrocortisone % (7 g) [packaged with 7 Konsyl® psyllium packets]
Cream, topical: Lidocaine 3% and hydrocortisone 0.5% (30 g)
  Lida-Mantle® HC: Lidocaine 3% and hydrocortisone 0.5% (30 g, 85 g)
  Xyralid™: Lidocaine 3% and hydrocortisone 1% (85 g)

Gel, rectal:
AnaMantle HC®: Lidocaine 3% and hydrocortisone 2.5% (7 g)
RectaGel™ HC: Lidocaine 2.8% and hydrocortisone 0.55% (20 g)
Lotion, topical: Lidocaine 3% and hydrocortisone 0.5% (177 mL)
Lida-Mantle® HC, Xyralid™ LP: Lidocaine 3% and hydrocortisone 0.5% (177 mL)
Pad, topical:
Peranex™ HC Medi-Pad: Lidocaine 3% and hydrocortisone 1% (60s)

lidocaine and prilocaine (LYE doe kane & PRIL oh kane)

Synonyms prilocaine and lidocaine
U.S./Canadian Brand Names EMLA® [US/Can]; Oraquix® [US]
Therapeutic Category Analgesic, Topical
Use Topical anesthetic for use on normal intact skin to provide local analgesia for minor procedures such as I.V. cannulation or venipuncture; has also been used for painful procedures such as lumbar puncture and skin graft harvesting; for superficial minor surgery of genital mucous membranes and as an adjunct for local infiltration anesthesia in genital mucous membranes.
Usual Dosage Although the incidence of systemic adverse effects with EMLA® is very low, caution should be exercised, particularly when applying over large areas and leaving on for >2 hours
Children (intact skin): EMLA® should **not** be used in neonates with a gestation age <37 weeks nor in infants <12 months of age who are receiving treatment with methemoglobin-inducing agents
Dosing is based on child's age and weight:
Age 0-3 months or <5 kg: Apply a maximum of 1 g over no more than 10 cm^2 of skin; leave on for no longer than 1 hour
Age 3 months to 12 months and >5 kg: Apply no more than a maximum 2 g total over no more than 20 cm^2 of skin; leave on for no longer than 4 hours
Age 1-6 years and >10 kg: Apply no more than a maximum of 10 g total over no more than 100 cm^2 of skin; leave on for no longer than 4 hours.
Age 7-12 years and >20 kg: Apply no more than a maximum 20 g total over no more than 200 cm^2 of skin; leave on for no longer than 4 hours.
Note: If a patient greater than 3 months old does not meet the minimum weight requirement, the maximum total dose should be restricted to the corresponding maximum based on patient weight.

Adults (intact skin):
EMLA® cream and EMLA® anesthetic disc: A thick layer of EMLA® cream is applied to intact skin and covered with an occlusive dressing, or alternatively, an EMLA® anesthetic disc is applied to intact skin
Minor dermal procedures (eg, I.V. cannulation or venipuncture): Apply 2.5 g of cream (1/2 of the 5 g tube) over 20-25 cm of skin surface area, or 1 anesthetic disc (1 g over 10 cm^2) for at least 1 hour.
Note: In clinical trials, 2 sites were usually prepared in case there was a technical problem with cannulation or venipuncture at the first site.
Major dermal procedures (eg, more painful dermatological procedures involving a larger skin area such as split thickness skin graft harvesting): Apply 2 g of cream per 10 cm^2 of skin and allow to remain in contact with the skin for at least 2 hours.
Adult male genital skin (eg, pretreatment prior to local anesthetic infiltration): Apply a thick layer of cream (1 g/10 cm^2) to the skin surface for 15 minutes. Local anesthetic infiltration should be performed immediately after removal of EMLA® cream.
Note: Dermal analgesia can be expected to increase for up to 3 hours under occlusive dressing and persist for 1-2 hours after removal of the cream
Adult females: Genital mucous membranes: Minor procedures (eg, removal of condylomata acuminata, pretreatment for local anesthetic infiltration): Apply 5-10 g (thick layer) of cream for 5-10 minutes

Periodontal gel (Oraqix®): Adults: Apply on gingival margin around selected teeth using the blunt-tipped applicator included in package. Wait 30 seconds, then fill the periodontal pockets using the blunt-tipped applicator until gel becomes visible at the gingival margin. Wait another 30 seconds before starting treatment. Maximum recommended dose: One treatment session: 5 cartridges (8.5 g)
Dosage Forms
Cream, topical: Lidocaine 2.5% and prilocaine 2.5% (5 g, 30 g)
EMLA®: Lidocaine 2.5% and prilocaine 2.5% (5 g, 30 g)
Disc, topical:
EMLA®: Lidocaine 2.5% and prilocaine 2.5% per disc (2s, 10s)

lidocaine and tetracaine (LYE doe kane & TET ra kane)

Synonyms tetracaine and lidocaine
U.S./Canadian Brand Names Pliaglis™ [US]; Synera™ [US]

◀ **Therapeutic Category** Analgesic, Topical Local Anesthetic

Use Topical anesthetic for use on normal intact skin for minor procedures (eg, I.V. cannulation or venipuncture) and superficial dermatologic procedures

Usual Dosage

Topical: Cream: Adults:

Superficial dermatological procedures (eg, dermal filler injection, facial laser ablation): Apply 20-30 minutes prior to procedure

Laser-assisted tattoo removal: Apply 60 minutes prior to procedure

Note: The amount of Pliaglis™ required is determined by the size of the treatment area. Use the ruler on the carton and in the packaging to measure out the proper amount (cm length of cream). Apply evenly and thinly (~1 mm or the thickness of a dime) over the area using a flat tool (eg, spatula, tongue depressor).

If surface area of treatment site:

10 cm^2: Apply 3 cm length Pliaglis™

20 cm^2: Apply 6 cm Pliaglis™

40 cm^2: Apply 12 cm Pliaglis™

80 cm^2: Apply 24 cm Pliaglis™

100 cm^2: Apply 30 cm Pliaglis™

150 cm^2: Apply 46 cm Pliaglis™

200 cm^2: Apply 61 cm Pliaglis™

250 cm^2: Apply 76 cm Pliaglis™

300 cm^2: Apply 91 cm Pliaglis™

350 cm^2: Apply 106 cm Pliaglis™

400 cm^2: Apply 121 cm Pliaglis™

After waiting the required application time, remove the Pliaglis™ by grasping a free edge and pulling it away from the skin.

Transdermal patch: Children ≥3 years and Adults:

Venipuncture or intravenous cannulation: Prior to procedure, apply to intact skin for 20-30 minutes; **Note:** Adults can use another patch at a new location to facilitate venous access after a failed attempt; remove previous patch.

Superficial dermatological procedures: Prior to procedure, apply to intact skin for 30 minutes

Dosage Forms

Cream, topical:

Pliaglis™: Lidocaine 7% and tetracaine 7% (30 g)

Transdermal system:

Synera™: Lidocaine 70 mg and tetracaine 70 mg (10s)

lidocaine hydrochloride *see lidocaine on page 561*

lidocaine hydrochloride and bupivacaine hydrochloride *see lidocaine and bupivacaine on page 563*

Lidodan™ [Can] *see lidocaine on page 561*

Lidoderm® [US/Can] *see lidocaine on page 561*

LidoPen® I.M. Injection Auto-Injector (Discontinued) *see lidocaine on page 561*

LidoSite™ [US] *see lidocaine and epinephrine on page 563*

LID-Pack® [Can] *see bacitracin and polymyxin B on page 113*

lignocaine hydrochloride *see lidocaine on page 561*

Lignospan® Forte [US] *see lidocaine and epinephrine on page 563*

Lignospan® Standard [US] *see lidocaine and epinephrine on page 563*

Limbitrol® [US/Can] *see amitriptyline and chlordiazepoxide on page 63*

Limbitrol® DS [US] *see amitriptyline and chlordiazepoxide on page 63*

Limbrel™ [US] *see flavocoxid on page 402*

Lin-Amox [Can] *see amoxicillin on page 67*

Lin-Buspirone [Can] *see buspirone on page 153*

Lincocin® [US/Can] *see lincomycin on page 566*

lincomycin (lin koe MYE sin)

Sound-Alike/Look-Alike Issues

Lincocin® may be confused with Cleocin®, Indocin®, Minocin®

Synonyms lincomycin hydrochloride

U.S./Canadian Brand Names Lincocin® [US/Can]

Therapeutic Category Antibiotic, Lincosamide

Use Treatment of serious susceptible bacterial infections, mainly those caused by streptococci, pneumococci, and staphylococci resistant to other agents

Usual Dosage Note: Frequency may be increased if needed due to severity of infection

Children >1 month:
  I.M.: 10 mg/kg every 12-24 hours
  I.V.: 10-20 mg/kg/day in divided doses every 8-12 hours

Adults:
  I.M.: 600 mg every 12-24 hours
  I.V.: 600 mg to 1 g every 8-12 hours; maximum dose: 8 g/day
  Subconjuctival injection: 75 mg (ocular fluid levels with sufficient MICs last for at least 5 hours)

Dosage Forms
Injection, solution:
  Lincocin®: 300 mg/mL (2 mL, 10 mL)

lincomycin hydrochloride *see* lincomycin *on page 566*

lindane (LIN dane)

Synonyms benzene hexachloride; gamma benzene hexachloride; hexachlorocyclohexane

U.S./Canadian Brand Names Hexit™ [Can]; PMS-Lindane [Can]

Therapeutic Category Scabicides/Pediculicides

Use Treatment of *Sarcoptes scabiei* (scabies), *Pediculus capitis* (head lice), and *Phthirus pubis* (crab lice); FDA recommends reserving lindane as a second-line agent or with inadequate response to other therapies

Usual Dosage Topical: Children and Adults:

Scabies: Apply a thin layer of lotion and massage it on skin from the neck to the toes; after 8-12 hours, bathe and remove the drug

Head lice, crab lice: Apply shampoo to dry hair and massage into hair for 4 minutes; add small quantities of water to hair until lather forms, then rinse hair thoroughly and comb with a fine tooth comb to remove nits. Amount of shampoo needed is based on length and density of hair; most patients will require 30 mL (maximum: 60 mL).

Dosage Forms
Lotion, topical: 1% (60 mL)
Shampoo, topical: 1% (60 mL)

Linessa® [Can] *see* ethinyl estradiol and desogestrel *on page 369*

linezolid (li NE zoh lid)

Sound-Alike/Look-Alike Issues
  Zyvox® may be confused with Vioxx®, Ziox™, Zosyn®, Zovirax®

U.S./Canadian Brand Names Zyvoxam® [Can]; Zyvox® [US]

Therapeutic Category Antibiotic, Oxazolidinone

Use Treatment of vancomycin-resistant *Enterococcus faecium* (VRE) infections, nosocomial pneumonia caused by *Staphylococcus aureus* including MRSA or *Streptococcus pneumoniae* (including multidrug-resistant strains [MDRSP]), complicated and uncomplicated skin and skin structure infections (including diabetic foot infections without concomitant osteomyelitis), and community-acquired pneumonia caused by susceptible gram-positive organisms

Usual Dosage

VRE infections: Oral, I.V.:
Preterm neonates (<34 weeks gestational age): 10 mg/kg every 12 hours; neonates with a suboptimal clinical response can be advanced to 10 mg/kg every 8 hours. By day 7 of life, all neonates should receive 10 mg/kg every 8 hours.

Infants (excluding preterm neonates <1 week) and Children ≤11 years: 10 mg/kg every 8 hours for 14-28 days

Children ≥12 years and Adults: 600 mg every 12 hours for 14-28 days

▶

◀ Nosocomial pneumonia, complicated skin and skin structure infections, community-acquired pneumonia including concurrent bacteremia: Oral, I.V.:
Infants (excluding preterm neonates <1 week) and Children ≤11 years: 10 mg/kg every 8 hours for 10-14 days
Children ≥12 years and Adults: 600 mg every 12 hours for 10-14 days
Uncomplicated skin and skin structure infections: Oral:
Infants (excluding preterm neonates <1 week) and Children <5 years: 10 mg/kg every 8 hours for 10-14 days
Children 5-11 years: 10 mg/kg every 12 hours for 10-14 days
Children ≥12-18 years: 600 mg every 12 hours for 10-14 days
Adults: 400 mg every 12 hours for 10-14 days
Note: 400 mg dose is recommended in the product labeling; however, 600 mg dose is commonly employed clinically
Dosage Forms
Infusion [premixed]:
Zyvox®: 200 mg (100 mL); 600 mg (300 mL)
Powder for oral suspension:
Zyvox®: 20 mg/mL (150 mL)
Tablet:
Zyvox®: 600 mg

Lin-Fosinopril [Can] see fosinopril on page 427

Lin-Sotalol [Can] see sotalol on page 885

Lioresal® [US/Can] see baclofen on page 115

Liotec [Can] see baclofen on page 115

liothyronine (lye oh THYE roe neen)
Sound-Alike/Look-Alike Issues
liothyronine may be confused with levothyroxine
T3 is an error-prone abbreviation (mistaken as acetaminophen and codeine [ie, Tylenol® #3])
Synonyms liothyronine sodium; sodium L-triiodothyronine
U.S./Canadian Brand Names Cytomel® [US/Can]; Triostat® [US]
Therapeutic Category Thyroid Product
Use
Oral: Replacement or supplemental therapy in hypothyroidism; management of nontoxic goiter; a diagnostic aid
I.V.: Treatment of myxedema coma/precoma
Usual Dosage Doses should be adjusted based on clinical response and laboratory parameters.
Children: Congenital hypothyroidism: Oral: 5 mcg/day increase by 5 mcg every 3-4 days until the desired response is achieved. Usual maintenance dose: 20 mcg/day for infants, 50 mcg/day for children 1-3 years of age, and adult dose for children >3 years.
Adults:
Hypothyroidism: Oral: 25 mcg/day increase by increments of 12.5-25 mcg/day every 1-2 weeks to a maximum of 100 mcg/day; usual maintenance dose: 25-75 mcg/day.
Patients with cardiovascular disease: Oral: 5 mcg/day; increase by 5 mcg/day every 2 weeks
T_3 suppression test: Oral: 75-100 mcg/day for 7 days
Myxedema: Oral: Initial: 5 mcg/day; increase in increments of 5-10 mcg/day every 1-2 weeks. When 25 mcg/day is reached, dosage may be increased at intervals of 5-25 mcg/day every 1-2 weeks. Usual maintenance dose: 50-100 mcg/day.
Myxedema coma: I.V.: 25-50 mcg
Patients with known or suspected cardiovascular disease: 10-20 mcg
Note: Normally, at least 4 hours should be allowed between doses to adequately assess therapeutic response and no more than 12 hours should elapse between doses to avoid fluctuations in hormone levels. Oral therapy should be resumed as soon as the clinical situation has been stabilized and the patient is able to take oral medication. If levothyroxine rather than liothyronine sodium is used in initiating oral therapy, the physician should bear in mind that there is a delay of several days in the onset of levothyroxine activity and that I.V. therapy should be discontinued gradually.
Simple (nontoxic) goiter: Oral: Initial: 5 mcg/day; increase by 5-10 mcg every 1-2 weeks; after 25 mcg/day is reached, may increase dose by 12.5-25 mcg. Usual maintenance dose: 75 mcg/day

Dosage Forms
 Injection, solution: 10 mcg/mL (1 mL)
  Triostat®: 10 mcg/mL (1 mL)
 Tablet:
  Cytomel®: 5 mcg, 25 mcg, 50 mcg

liothyronine sodium *see liothyronine on page 568*

liotrix (LYE oh triks)

Sound-Alike/Look-Alike Issues
 liotrix may be confused with Klotrix®
 Thyrolar® may be confused with Theolair™, Thyrogen®, Thytropar®
Synonyms T$_3$/T$_4$ liotrix
U.S./Canadian Brand Names Thyrolar® [US/Can]
Therapeutic Category Thyroid Product
Use Replacement or supplemental therapy in hypothyroidism (uniform mixture of T$_4$:T$_3$ in 4:1 ratio by weight); little advantage to this product exists and cost is not justified
Usual Dosage Oral:
 Congenital hypothyroidism:
  Children (dose of T$_4$ or levothyroxine/day):
   0-6 months: 8-10 mcg/kg or 25-50 mcg/day
   6-12 months: 6-8 mcg/kg or 50-75 mcg/day
   1-5 years: 5-6 mcg/kg or 75-100 mcg/day
   6-12 years: 4-5 mcg/kg or 100-150 mcg/day
   >12 years: 2-3 mcg/kg or >150 mcg/day
 Hypothyroidism (dose of thyroid equivalent): Adults: 30 mg/day (15 mg/day if cardiovascular impairment), increasing by increments of 15 mg/day at 2- to 3-week intervals to a maximum of 180 mg/day (usual maintenance dose: 60-120 mg/day)
Dosage Forms
 Tablet:
  Thyrolar®:
   1/4 [levothyroxine 12.5 mcg and liothyronine 3.1 mcg]
   1/2 [levothyroxine 25 mcg and liothyronine 6.25 mcg]
   1 [levothyroxine 50 mcg and liothyronine 12.5 mcg]
   2 [levothyroxine 100 mcg and liothyronine 25 mcg]
   3 [levothyroxine 150 mcg and liothyronine 37.5 mcg]

lipancreatin *see pancrelipase on page 718*
Lipidil EZ® [Can] *see fenofibrate on page 393*
Lipidil Micro® [Can] *see fenofibrate on page 393*
Lipidil Supra® [Can] *see fenofibrate on page 393*
Lipitor® [US/Can] *see atorvastatin on page 102*
Lipofen™ [US] *see fenofibrate on page 393*
liposomal DAUNOrubicin *see daunorubicin citrate (liposomal) on page 269*
liposomal DOXOrubicin *see doxorubicin (liposomal) on page 323*
Liposyn® II [US/Can] *see fat emulsion on page 391*
Liposyn® III [US] *see fat emulsion on page 391*
Lipram 4500 *(Discontinued)* *see pancrelipase on page 718*
Lipram-CR *(Discontinued)* *see pancrelipase on page 718*
Lipram-PN *(Discontinued)* *see pancrelipase on page 718*
Lipram-UL *(Discontinued)* *see pancrelipase on page 718*
Liqua-Cal [US-OTC] *see calcium and vitamin D on page 162*
Liquadd™ [US] *see dextroamphetamine on page 283*
Liquaemin® *(Discontinued)* *see heparin on page 467*
Liquibid-D® [US] *see guaifenesin and phenylephrine on page 456*
Liquibid® 1200 *(Discontinued)* *see guaifenesin on page 453*
Liquibid® *(Discontinued)* *see guaifenesin on page 453*
Liquibid-PD 1200 *(Discontinued)* *see guaifenesin and phenylephrine on page 456*
Liquibid-PD *(Discontinued)* *see guaifenesin and phenylephrine on page 456*
Liqui-Char® *(Discontinued)* *see charcoal on page 198*

Liqui-Coat HD® [US] *see barium on page 116*
liquid antidote *see charcoal on page 198*
Liquid Barosperse® [US] *see barium on page 116*
Liquid Pred® (Discontinued) *see prednisone on page 782*
Liquifilm® Forte Solution (Discontinued) *see artificial tears on page 95*
Liquifilm® Tears [US-OTC] *see artificial tears on page 95*
Liquifilm® Tears Solution (Discontinued) *see artificial tears on page 95*

lisdexamfetamine (lis dex am FET a meen)

Sound-Alike/Look-Alike Issues
Vyvanse™ may be confused with Vytorin®, Glucovance®, Vivactil®

Synonyms lisdexamfetamine dimesylate; lisdexamphetamine; NRP104

U.S./Canadian Brand Names Vyvanse™ [US]

Therapeutic Category Stimulant

Controlled Substance C-II

Use Treatment of attention-deficit/hyperactivity disorder (ADHD)

Usual Dosage Oral: Individualize dosage based on patient need and response to therapy. Administer at the lowest effective dose.
Children: 6-12 years and Adults: Initial: 30 mg once daily in the morning; may increase in increments of 10 mg or 20 mg/day at weekly intervals until optimal response is obtained; maximum: 70 mg/day

Dosage Forms
Capsule:
Vyvanse™: 20 mg, 30 mg, 40 mg, 50 mg, 60 mg, 70 mg

lisdexamfetamine dimesylate *see lisdexamfetamine on page 570*
lisdexamphetamine *see lisdexamfetamine on page 570*

lisinopril (lyse IN oh pril)

Sound-Alike/Look-Alike Issues
lisinopril may be confused with fosinopril, Lioresal®, Risperdal®
Prinivil® may be confused with Plendil®, Pravachol®, Prevacid®, Prilosec®, Proventil®
Zestril® may be confused with Desyrel®, Restoril®, Vistaril®, Zetia®, Zostrix®

U.S./Canadian Brand Names Apo-Lisinopril® [Can]; CO Lisinopril [Can]; Gen-Lisinopril [Can]; Novo-Lisinopril [Can]; PMS-Lisinopril [Can]; Prinivil® [US/Can]; Ran-Lisinopril [Can]; ratio-Lisinopril [Can]; Riva-Lisinopril [Can]; Zestril® [US/Can]

Therapeutic Category Angiotensin-Converting Enzyme (ACE) Inhibitor

Use Treatment of hypertension, either alone or in combination with other antihypertensive agents; adjunctive therapy in treatment of heart failure (HF); treatment of acute myocardial infarction (MI) within 24 hours in hemodynamically-stable patients to improve survival

Usual Dosage Oral:
Hypertension:
Children ≥6 years: Initial: 0.07 mg/kg once daily (up to 5 mg); increase dose at 1- to 2-week intervals; doses >0.61 mg/kg or >40 mg have not been evaluated.
Adults: Usual dosage range (JNC 7): 10-40 mg/day
Not maintained on diuretic: Initial: 10 mg/day
Maintained on diuretic: Initial: 5 mg/day
Note: Antihypertensive effect may diminish toward the end of the dosing interval especially with doses of 10 mg/day. An increased dose may aid in extending the duration of antihypertensive effect. Doses up to 80 mg/day have been used, but do not appear to give greater effect.
Patients taking diuretics should have them discontinued 2-3 days prior to initiating lisinopril if possible. Restart diuretic after blood pressure is stable if needed. If diuretic cannot be discontinued prior to therapy, begin with 5 mg with close supervision until stable blood pressure. In patients with hyponatremia (<130 mEq/L), start dose at 2.5 mg/day
Heart failure: Adults: Initial: 2.5-5 mg once daily; then increase by no more than 10 mg increments at intervals no less than 2 weeks to a maximum daily dose of 40 mg. Usual maintenance: 5-40 mg/day as a single dose. Target dose: 20-40 mg once daily (ACC/AHA 2005 Heart Failure Guidelines)
Note: If patient has hyponatremia (serum sodium <130 meq/L) or renal impairment (Cl_{cr} <30 mL/minute or creatinine >3 mg/dL), then initial dose should be 2.5 mg/day

Acute myocardial infarction (within 24 hours in hemodynamically stable patients): 5 mg immediately, then 5 mg at 24 hours, 10 mg at 48 hours, and 10 mg every day thereafter for 6 weeks. Patients should continue to receive standard treatments such as thrombolytics, aspirin, and beta-blockers.

Dosage Forms
Tablet: 2.5 mg, 5 mg, 10 mg, 20 mg, 30 mg, 40 mg
Prinivil®: 5 mg, 10 mg, 20 mg
Zestril®: 2.5 mg, 5 mg, 10 mg, 20 mg, 30 mg, 40 mg

lisinopril and hydrochlorothiazide (lyse IN oh pril & hye droe klor oh THYE a zide)

Synonyms hydrochlorothiazide and lisinopril

U.S./Canadian Brand Names Apo-Lisinopril/Hctz [Can]; Gen-Lisinopril/Hctz [Can]; Novo-Lisinopril/Hctz [Can]; Prinzide® [US/Can]; Sandoz Lisinopril/Hctz [Can]; Zestoretic® [US/Can]

Therapeutic Category Antihypertensive Agent, Combination

Use Treatment of hypertension

Usual Dosage Oral: Adults: Dosage is individualized; see each component for appropriate dosing suggestions; doses >80 mg/day lisinopril or >50 mg/day hydrochlorothiazide are not recommended.

Dosage Forms
Tablet: 10/12.5: Lisinopril 10 mg and hydrochlorothiazide 12.5 mg; 20/12.5: Lisinopril 20 mg and hydrochlorothiazide 12.5 mg; 20/25: Lisinopril 20 mg and hydrochlorothiazide 25 mg
Prinizide®:
10/12.5: Lisinopril 10 mg and hydrochlorothiazide 12.5 mg
20/25: Lisinopril 20 mg and hydrochlorothiazide 25 mg
Zestoretic®:
10/12.5: Lisinopril 10 mg and hydrochlorothiazide 12.5 mg
20/12.5: Lisinopril 20 mg and hydrochlorothiazide 12.5 mg
20/25: Lisinopril 20 mg and hydrochlorothiazide 25 mg

lispro insulin *see* insulin lispro *on page 511*
Listermint® With Fluoride (Discontinued) *see* fluoride *on page 411*
Lithane™ [Can] *see* lithium *on page 571*
Lithane® (Discontinued) *see* lithium *on page 571*

lithium (LITH ee um)

Sound-Alike/Look-Alike Issues
Eskalith® may be confused with Estratest®
Lithobid® may be confused with Levbid®, Lithostat®

Synonyms lithium carbonate; lithium citrate

U.S./Canadian Brand Names Apo-Lithium® Carbonate SR [Can]; Apo-Lithium® Carbonate [Can]; Carbolith™ [Can]; Duralith® [Can]; Lithane™ [Can]; Lithobid® [US]; PMS-Lithium Carbonate [Can]; PMS-Lithium Citrate [Can]

Therapeutic Category Antimanic Agent

Use Management of bipolar disorders; treatment of mania in individuals with bipolar disorder (maintenance treatment prevents or diminishes intensity of subsequent episodes)

Usual Dosage Oral: Monitor serum concentrations and clinical response (efficacy and toxicity) to determine proper dose. Adults: Bipolar disorder: 900-2400 mg/day in 3-4 divided doses or 900-1800 mg/day (sustained release) in 2 divided doses

Dosage Forms
Capsule, as carbonate: 150 mg, 300 mg, 600 mg
Solution: 300 mg/5 mL
Syrup: 300 mg/5 mL
Tablet: 300 mg
Tablet, controlled release: 450 mg
Tablet, slow release: 300 mg
Lithobid®: 300 mg

lithium carbonate *see* lithium *on page 571*
lithium citrate *see* lithium *on page 571*
Lithobid® [US] *see* lithium *on page 571*
Lithonate® (Discontinued) *see* lithium *on page 571*
Lithostat® [US/Can] *see* acetohydroxamic acid *on page 29*

Lithotabs® *(Discontinued)* see lithium *on page 571*
Little Colds® Multi-Symptom Cold Formula *(Discontinued)* see acetaminophen, dextromethorphan, and phenylephrine *on page 26*
Little Fevers™ [US-OTC] see acetaminophen *on page 19*
Little Noses® Decongestant [US-OTC] see phenylephrine *on page 745*
Little Noses® Saline [US-OTC] see sodium chloride *on page 873*
Little Noses® Stuffy Nose Kit [US-OTC] see sodium chloride *on page 873*
Little Teethers® [US-OTC] see benzocaine *on page 124*
Little Tummys® Gas Relief [US-OTC] see simethicone *on page 867*
Little Tummys® Laxative [US-OTC] see senna *on page 861*
live attenuated influenza vaccine (LAIV) see influenza virus vaccine *on page 508*
live smallpox vaccine see smallpox vaccine *on page 871*
Livostin® *(Discontinued)*
L-leucovorin see LEVOleucovorin *on page 558*

l-lysine (el LYE seen)

Synonyms l-lysine hydrochloride
U.S./Canadian Brand Names Lysinyl [US-OTC]
Therapeutic Category Dietary Supplement
Use Improves utilization of vegetable proteins
Usual Dosage Oral: Adults:
  Supplement: 334-1500 mg/day
  Recurrent herpes simplex infection (dental use): 2000 mg every 4 hours until symptoms subside; begin treatment during early stage of recurrence
Dosage Forms
  Capsule: 500 mg
    Lysinyl [OTC]: 500 mg
  Powder, oral: 100% (100 g)
    Lysinyl [OTC]: 500 mg/ 1/4 teaspoon (150 g)
  Tablet: 500 mg, 1000 mg

l-lysine hydrochloride see l-lysine *on page 572*
LMD® [US] see dextran *on page 282*
L-methylfolate see methylfolate *on page 621*
LNg 20 see levonorgestrel *on page 559*
Locacorten® Vioform® [Can] see clioquinol and flumethasone *(Canada only) on page 232*
LoCHOLEST® *(Discontinued)* see cholestyramine resin *on page 215*
LoCHOLEST® Light *(Discontinued)* see cholestyramine resin *on page 215*
Locoid® [US/Can] see hydrocortisone (topical) *on page 485*
Locoid Lipocream® [US] see hydrocortisone (topical) *on page 485*
Lodine® XL *(Discontinued)* see etodolac *on page 383*
Lodine® *(Discontinued)* see etodolac *on page 383*
Lodosyn® [US] see carbidopa *on page 177*

Iodoxamide (loe DOKS a mide)

Synonyms iodoxamide tromethamine
U.S./Canadian Brand Names Alomide® [US/Can]
Therapeutic Category Mast Cell Stabilizer
Use Treatment of vernal keratoconjunctivitis, vernal conjunctivitis, and vernal keratitis
Usual Dosage Ophthalmic: Instill 1-2 drops in eye(s) 4 times/day for up to 3 months
Dosage Forms
  Solution, ophthalmic:
    Alomide®: 0.1% (10 mL)

Iodoxamide tromethamine see iodoxamide *on page 572*
Lodrane® 12D [US] see brompheniramine and pseudoephedrine *on page 144*
Lodrane® 12 Hour [US] see brompheniramine *on page 144*

Lodrane® 24 [US] *see* brompheniramine *on page 144*
Lodrane® 24D [US] *see* brompheniramine and pseudoephedrine *on page 144*
Lodrane® D [US] *see* brompheniramine and pseudoephedrine *on page 144*
Lodrane® *(Discontinued)* *see* brompheniramine and pseudoephedrine *on page 144*
Lodrane® XR [US] *see* brompheniramine *on page 144*
Loestrin® [US] *see* ethinyl estradiol and norethindrone *on page 376*
Loestrin™ 1.5/30 [Can] *see* ethinyl estradiol and norethindrone *on page 376*
Loestrin® 24 Fe [US] *see* ethinyl estradiol and norethindrone *on page 376*
Loestrin® Fe [US] *see* ethinyl estradiol and norethindrone *on page 376*
Lofibra® [US] *see* fenofibrate *on page 393*
Logen® *(Discontinued)* *see* diphenoxylate and atropine *on page 306*
LoHist-12 [US] *see* brompheniramine *on page 144*
LoHist 12D [US] *see* brompheniramine and pseudoephedrine *on page 144*
LoHist-D [US] *see* chlorpheniramine and pseudoephedrine *on page 207*
LoHist LQ [US] *see* brompheniramine and pseudoephedrine *on page 144*
LoHist PD [US] *see* brompheniramine and pseudoephedrine *on page 144*
L-OHP *see* oxaliplatin *on page 705*
LoKara™ [US] *see* desonide *on page 276*
Lomanate® *(Discontinued)* *see* diphenoxylate and atropine *on page 306*
Lomine [Can] *see* dicyclomine *on page 293*
Lomotil® [US/Can] *see* diphenoxylate and atropine *on page 306*

lomustine (loe MUS teen)

Sound-Alike/Look-Alike Issues
lomustine may be confused with carmustine
Synonyms CCNU; NSC-79037
U.S./Canadian Brand Names CeeNU® [US/Can]
Therapeutic Category Antineoplastic Agent
Use Treatment of brain tumors and Hodgkin disease
Usual Dosage Oral (refer to individual protocols):
Children: 75-150 mg/m^2 as a single dose once every 6 weeks; subsequent doses are readjusted after initial treatment according to platelet and leukocyte counts
Adults: 100-130 mg/m^2 as a single dose once every 6 weeks; readjust after initial treatment according to platelet and leukocyte counts
With compromised marrow function: Initial dose: 100 mg/m^2 as a single dose once every 6 weeks
Repeat courses should only be administered after adequate recovery: Leukocytes >4000/mm^3 and platelet counts >100,000/mm^3
Subsequent dosing adjustment based on nadir:
Leukocytes 2000-2999/mm^3, platelets 25,000-74,999/mm^3: Administer 70% of prior dose
Leukocytes <2000/mm^3, platelets <25,000/mm^3: Administer 50% of prior dose
Dosage Forms
Capsule:
CeeNU®: 10 mg, 40 mg, 100 mg
Capsule [dose pack]:
CeeNU®: 10 mg (2s); 40 mg (2s)

Loniten® 2.5 mg Tablet *(Discontinued)* *see* minoxidil *on page 636*
Lonox® [US] *see* diphenoxylate and atropine *on page 306*
Lo/Ovral® [US] *see* ethinyl estradiol and norgestrel *on page 380*
Loperacap [Can] *see* loperamide *on page 573*

loperamide (loe PER a mide)

Sound-Alike/Look-Alike Issues
Imodium® A-D may be confused with Indocin®, Ionamin®
Synonyms loperamide hydrochloride
U.S./Canadian Brand Names Apo-Loperamide® [Can]; Diamode [US-OTC]; Diarr-Eze [Can]; Dom-Loperamide [Can]; Imodium® A-D [US-OTC]; Imodium® [Can]; K-Pek II [US-OTC]; Kao-Paverin® [US-OTC]; ▶

◀ Loperacap [Can]; Novo-Loperamide [Can]; PMS-Loperamine [Can]; Rhoxal-Loperamide [Can];
Rho®-Loperamine [Can]; Riva-Loperamine [Can]; Sandoz-Loperamide [Can]

Therapeutic Category Antidiarrheal

Use Treatment of chronic diarrhea associated with inflammatory bowel disease; acute nonspecific diarrhea; increased volume of ileostomy discharge

OTC labeling: Control of symptoms of diarrhea, including traveler's diarrhea

Usual Dosage Oral:

Children:

Acute diarrhea: Initial doses (in first 24 hours):

2-5 years (13-20 kg): 1 mg 3 times/day

6-8 years (20-30 kg): 2 mg twice daily

8-12 years (>30 kg): 2 mg 3 times/day

Maintenance: After initial dosing, 0.1 mg/kg doses after each loose stool, but not exceeding initial dosage

Traveler's diarrhea:

6-8 years: 2 mg after first loose stool, followed by 1 mg after each subsequent stool (maximum dose: 4 mg/day)

9-11 years: 2 mg after first loose stool, followed by 1 mg after each subsequent stool (maximum dose: 6 mg/day)

≥12 years: See adult dosing.

Adults:

Acute diarrhea: Initial: 4 mg, followed by 2 mg after each loose stool, up to 16 mg/day

Chronic diarrhea: Initial: Follow acute diarrhea; maintenance dose should be slowly titrated downward to minimum required to control symptoms (typically, 4-8 mg/day in divided doses)

Traveler's diarrhea: Initial: 4 mg after first loose stool, followed by 2 mg after each subsequent stool (maximum dose: 8 mg/day)

Dosage Forms

Caplet: 2 mg

Diamode [OTC], Imodium® A-D [OTC], Kao-Paverin® [OTC]: 2 mg

Capsule: 2 mg

Liquid, oral: 1 mg/5 mL

Imodium® A-D [OTC]: 1 mg/5 mL

Imodium® A-D [OTC] [*new formulation*]: 1 mg/7.5 mL

Tablet: 2 mg

K-Pek II [OTC]: 2 mg

loperamide and simethicone (loe PER a mide & sye METH i kone)

Synonyms simethicone and loperamide hydrochloride

U.S./Canadian Brand Names Imodium® Advanced [US]

Therapeutic Category Antidiarrheal; Antiflatulent

Use Control of symptoms of diarrhea and gas (bloating, pressure, and cramps)

Usual Dosage Oral: Acute diarrhea (weight-based dosing is preferred):

Children:

6-8 years (48-59 lbs): 1 caplet or tablet after first loose stool, followed by 1/2 caplet/tablet with each subsequent loose stool (maximum: 2 caplets or tablets/24 hours)

9-11 years (60-95 lbs): 1 caplet or tablet after first loose stool, followed by 1/2 caplet or tablet with each subsequent loose stool (maximum: 3 caplets or tablets/24 hours)

Children >12 years and Adults: One caplet or tablet after first loose stool, followed by 1 caplet or tablet with each subsequent loose stool (maximum: 4 caplets or tablets/24 hours)

Dosage Forms

Caplet:

Imodium® Advanced: Loperamide 2 mg and simethicone 125 mg

Tablet, chewable:

Imodium® Advanced: Loperamide 2 mg and simethicone 125 mg

loperamide hydrochloride *see loperamide on page 573*

Lopid® [US/Can] *see gemfibrozil on page 439*

lopinavir and ritonavir (loe PIN a veer & rit ON uh veer)

Sound-Alike/Look-Alike Issues

Potential for dispensing errors between Kaletra™ and Keppra® (levetiracetam)

Synonyms ritonavir and lopinavir

U.S./Canadian Brand Names Kaletra® [US/Can]

Therapeutic Category Antiretroviral Agent, Nonnucleoside Reverse Transcriptase Inhibitor (NNRTI)

Use Treatment of HIV infection in combination with other antiretroviral agents

Usual Dosage Oral:

Children: Dosage based on weight, **presented based on lopinavir component** (maximum dose: Lopinavir 400 mg/ritonavir 100 mg).

14 days to 6 months: 16 mg/kg or 300 mg/m^2 twice daily

6 months to 12 years: **Note:** FDA-approved dose is approximately equivalent to lopinavir 230 mg/m^2 per dose.

7-<15 kg: 12 mg/kg twice daily

15-40 kg: 10 mg/kg twice daily

>40 kg: Lopinavir 400 mg/ritonavir 100 mg twice daily

Note: For therapy-experienced patients with suspected reduced susceptibility to lopinavir, refer to adult dosing.

Children >12 years: Therapy-naive: Lopinavir 400 mg/ritonavir 100 mg twice daily (AIDS Info guidelines).

Note: For therapy-experienced patients with suspected reduced susceptibility to lopinavir, refer to adult dosing.

Adults:

Therapy-naive: Lopinavir 800 mg/ritonavir 200 mg once daily **or** lopinavir 400 mg/ritonavir 100 mg twice daily

Note: Once-daily dosing regimen should not be used with concurrent indinavir, maraviroc, saquinavir, phenytoin, carbamazepine, or phenobarbital therapy.

Therapy-experienced: Lopinavir 400 mg/ritonavir 100 mg twice daily

Note: For therapy-experienced patients with suspected reduced susceptibility to lopinavir, clinicians may consider lopinavir 600 mg/ ritonavir 150 mg twice daily

Dosage adjustment for combination therapy:

When taken with amprenavir, efavirenz, fosamprenavir, nelfinavir, or nevirapine: **Note:** Once-daily dosing regimen should not be used

Children 14 days to 6 months: Combination therapy with these agents is not recommended due to lack of data.

Children 6 months to 12 years: Solution or tablet (**based on mg of lopinavir component**): FDA-approved dose is approximately equivalent to lopinavir 300 mg/m^2 per dose:

7-<15 kg: 13 mg/kg twice daily (**Note:** Tablets are not recommended)

15-45 kg: 11 mg/kg twice daily

>45 kg: Refer to adult dosing

Children >12 years and Adults:

Therapy-naive: Solution or tablet: Lopinavir 400 mg/ritonavir 100 mg twice daily

Therapy-experienced:

Solution: Lopinavir 533 mg/ritonavir 133 mg (6.5 mL) twice daily

Tablet: Lopinavir 600 mg/ritonavir 150 mg twice daily

When taken with maraviroc (Selzentry™): Lopinavir 400 mg/ritonavir 100 mg twice daily

When taken with saquinavir (Invirase®): Lopinavir 400 mg/ritonavir 100 mg twice daily

Dosage Forms

Solution, oral:

Kaletra®: Lopinavir 80 mg and ritonavir 20 mg per mL

Tablet:

Kaletra®:

Lopinavir 100 mg and ritonavir 25 mg

Lopinavir 200 mg and ritonavir 50 mg

Lopressor® [US/Can] *see* metoprolol *on page 626*

Lopressor HCT® [US] *see* metoprolol and hydrochlorothiazide *on page 627*

Loprox® [US/Can] *see* ciclopirox *on page 218*

Lorabid® [Can] *see* loracarbef *on page 575*

Lorabid® *(Discontinued)* *see* loracarbef *on page 575*

loracarbef (lor a KAR bef)

Sound-Alike/Look-Alike Issues

Lorabid® may be confused with Levbid®, Lopid®, Lortab®, Slo-bid™

▶

◀ **U.S./Canadian Brand Names** Lorabid® [Can]

Therapeutic Category Antibiotic, Carbacephem

Use Treatment of infections caused by susceptible organisms involving the upper and lower respiratory tract, uncomplicated skin and skin structure, and urinary tract (including uncomplicated pyelonephritis)

Usual Dosage

Usual dosage range:

Children 6 months to 12 years: Oral: 7.5-15 mg/kg twice daily

Adults: Oral: 200-400 mg every 12-24 hours

Indication-specific dosing:

Children 6 months to 12 years: Oral:

Acute otitis media: 15 mg/kg twice daily for 10 days

Pharyngitis and impetigo: 7.5-15 mg/kg twice daily for 10 days

Adults: Oral:

Bronchitis: 200-400 mg every 12 hours for 7 days

Pharyngitis/tonsillitis: 200 mg every 12 hours for 10 days

Pneumonia: 400 mg every 12 hours for 14 days

Pyelonephritis (uncomplicated): 400 mg every 12 hours for 14 days

Sinusitis: 400 mg every 12 hours for 10 days

Skin and soft tissue: 200-400 mg every 12-24 hours

Urinary tract infections (uncomplicated): 200 mg once daily for 7 days

Loradamed [US-OTC] *see* loratadine *on page 576*

loratadine (lor AT a deen)

Sound-Alike/Look-Alike Issues

Sound-alike/look-alike issues:

Claritin® may be confused with clarithromycin

U.S./Canadian Brand Names Alavert™ Allergy Relief 24-Hour [US-OTC]; Alavert™ [US-OTC]; Allergy Relief [US-OTC]; Apo-Loratadine® [Can]; Claritin® 24 Hour Allergy [US-OTC]; Claritin® Children's Allergy [US-OTC]; Claritin® Children's [US-OTC]; Claritin® Hives Relief [US-OTC]; Claritin® Kids [Can]; Claritin® [Can]; Dimetapp® ND Children's [US-OTC]; Loradamed [US-OTC]; Tavist® ND ALLERGY [US-OTC]

Therapeutic Category Antihistamine

Use Relief of nasal and nonnasal symptoms of seasonal allergic rhinitis; treatment of chronic idiopathic urticaria

Usual Dosage Oral: Seasonal allergic rhinitis, chronic idiopathic urticaria:

Children 2-5 years: 5 mg once daily

Children ≥6 years and Adults: 10 mg once daily

Dosage Forms

Solution, oral: 5 mg/5 mL (120 mL)

Syrup, oral: 1 mg/mL (120 mL)

Allergy Relief [OTC], Claritin® Children's Allergy [OTC]: 1 mg/mL (120 mL)

Claritin® Children's [OTC]: 5 mg/5 mL (60 mL, 120 mL)

Tablet, oral: 10 mg

Alavert® [OTC], Claritin® 24 Hour Allergy [OTC], Claritin® Hives Relief [OTC], Loradamed [OTC], Tavist® ND ALLERGY [OTC]: 10 mg

Tablet, chewable, oral:

Claritin® Children's Allergy [OTC]: 5 mg

Tablet, orally disintegrating, oral:

Alavert™ Allergy Relief 24-Hour [OTC], Dimetapp® ND Children's [OTC]: 10 mg

loratadine and pseudoephedrine (lor AT a deen & soo doe e FED rin)

Synonyms pseudoephedrine and loratadine

U.S./Canadian Brand Names Alavert™ Allergy and Sinus [US-OTC]; Chlor-Tripolon ND® [Can]; Claritin-D® 12 Hour Allergy & Congestion [US-OTC]; Claritin-D® 24 Hour Allergy & Congestion [US-OTC]; Claritin® Extra [Can]; Claritin® Liberator [Can]

Therapeutic Category Antihistamine/Decongestant Combination

Use Temporary relief of symptoms of seasonal allergic rhinitis, other upper respiratory allergies, or the common cold

Usual Dosage Oral: Children ≥12 years and Adults:
Claritin-D® 12 Hour Allergy & Congestion: 1 tablet every 12 hours
Alavert™ Allergy and Sinus, Claritin-D® 24 Hour: 1 tablet daily
Dosage Forms
Tablet, extended release: Loratadine 10 mg and pseudoephedrine 240 mg
  Alavert™ Allergy and Sinus [OTC]: Loratadine 5 mg and pseudoephedrine 120 mg
  Claritin-D® 12 Hour Allergy & Congestion [OTC]: Loratadine 5 mg and pseudoephedrine 120 mg
  Claritin-D® 24 Hour Allergy & Congestion [OTC]: Loratadine 10 mg and pseudoephedrine 240 mg

lorazepam (lor A ze pam)

Sound-Alike/Look-Alike Issues
  LORazepam may be confused with ALPRAZolam, clonazePAM, diazepam, temazepam
  Ativan® may be confused with Atarax®, Atgam®, Avitene®
Tall-Man LORazepam
U.S./Canadian Brand Names Apo-Lorazepam® [Can]; Ativan® [US/Can]; Lorazepam Injection, USP [Can]; Lorazepam Intensol® [US]; Novo-Lorazepam [Can]; Nu-Loraz [Can]; PHL-Lorazepam [Can]; PMS-Lorazepam [Can]; Riva-Lorazepam [Can]
Therapeutic Category Benzodiazepine
Controlled Substance C-IV
Use
Oral: Management of anxiety disorders or short-term (≤4 months) relief of the symptoms of anxiety or anxiety associated with depressive symptoms
I.V.: Status epilepticus, preanesthesia for desired amnesia
Usual Dosage
Anxiety and sedation: Adults: Oral: 1-10 mg/day in 2-3 divided doses; usual dose: 2-6 mg/day in divided doses
Insomnia: Adults: Oral: 2-4 mg at bedtime
Preoperative: Adults:
  I.M.: 0.05 mg/kg administered 2 hours before surgery (maximum: 4 mg/dose)
  I.V.: 0.044 mg/kg 15-20 minutes before surgery (usual maximum: 2 mg/dose)
Preprocedural anxiety (dental use): Adults: Oral: 1-2 mg 1 hour before procedure
Operative amnesia: Adults: I.V.: Up to 0.05 mg/kg (maximum: 4 mg/dose)
Status epilepticus: I.V.:
  Adolescents: 0.07 mg/kg slow I.V. over 2-5 minutes; maximum: 4 mg/dose; may repeat in 10-15 minutes
  Adults: 4 mg/dose slow I.V. over 2-5 minutes; may repeat in 10-15 minutes; usual maximum dose: 8 mg
Rapid tranquilization of agitated patient (administer every 30-60 minutes): Adults:
  Oral: 1-2 mg
  I.M.: 0.5-1 mg
  Average total dose for tranquilization: Oral, I.M.: 4-8 mg
Dosage Forms
Injection, solution: 2 mg/mL (1 mL, 10 mL); 4 mg/mL (1 mL, 10 mL)
  Ativan®: 2 mg/mL (1 mL, 10 mL); 4 mg/mL (1 mL, 10 mL)
Solution, oral concentrate:
  Lorazepam Intensol®: 2 mg/mL
Tablet: 0.5 mg, 1 mg, 2 mg
  Ativan®: 0.5 mg, 1 mg, 2 mg

Lorazepam Injection, USP [Can] see lorazepam on page 577
Lorazepam Intensol® [US] see lorazepam on page 577
Lorcet® 10/650 [US] see hydrocodone and acetaminophen on page 481
Lorcet®-HD (Discontinued) see hydrocodone and acetaminophen on page 481
Lorcet® Plus [US] see hydrocodone and acetaminophen on page 481
Lorsin® (Discontinued) see acetaminophen, chlorpheniramine, and pseudoephedrine on page 25
Lortab® [US] see hydrocodone and acetaminophen on page 481
Lortab® ASA (Discontinued)

losartan (loe SAR tan)

Sound-Alike/Look-Alike Issues
  losartan may be confused with valsartan
  Cozaar® may be confused with Colace®, Hyzaar®, Zocor®

▶

◀ **Synonyms** DuP 753; losartan potassium; MK594

U.S./Canadian Brand Names Cozaar® [US/Can]

Therapeutic Category Angiotensin II Receptor Antagonist

Use Treatment of hypertension (HTN); treatment of diabetic nephropathy in patients with type 2 diabetes mellitus (noninsulin-dependent, NIDDM) and a history of hypertension; stroke risk reduction in patients with HTN and left ventricular hypertrophy (LVH)

Usual Dosage Oral:

Hypertension:

Children 6-16 years:

U.S. labeling: 0.7 mg/kg once daily (maximum: 50 mg/day); doses >1.4 mg/kg (maximum: 100 mg) have not been studied

Canadian labeling:

≥20 kg to <50 kg: 25 mg once daily (maximum: 50 mg once daily)

≥50 kg: 50 mg once daily (maximum: 100 mg once daily)

Adults: Usual starting dose: 50 mg once daily; can be administered once or twice daily with total daily doses ranging from 25-100 mg

Patients receiving diuretics or with intravascular volume depletion: Usual initial dose: 25 mg once daily

Nephropathy in patients with type 2 diabetes and hypertension: Adults: Initial: 50 mg once daily; can be increased to 100 mg once daily based on blood pressure response

Stroke reduction (HTN with LVH): Adults: 50 mg once daily (maximum daily dose: 100 mg); may be used in combination with a thiazide diuretic

Dosage Forms

Tablet, oral:

Cozaar®: 25 mg, 50 mg, 100 mg

losartan and hydrochlorothiazide (loe SAR tan & hye droe klor oh THYE a zide)

Sound-Alike/Look-Alike Issues

Hyzaar® may be confused with Cozaar®

Synonyms hydrochlorothiazide and losartan

U.S./Canadian Brand Names Hyzaar® DS [Can]; Hyzaar® [US/Can]

Therapeutic Category Antihypertensive Agent, Combination

Use Treatment of hypertension; stroke risk reduction in patients with HTN and left ventricular hypertrophy (LVH)

Usual Dosage Oral: Adults: Dose is individualized (combination substituted for individual components); dose may be titrated after 2-4 weeks of therapy

Hypertension/stroke reduction in hypertension (with LVH): Usual recommended starting dose of losartan: 50 mg once daily when used as monotherapy in patients who are not volume depleted

Dosage Forms

Tablet:

Hyzaar®: 50-12.5: Losartan 50 mg and hydrochlorothiazide 12.5 mg; 100-12.5: Losartan 100 mg and hydrochlorothiazide 12.5 mg; 100-25: Losartan 100 mg and hydrochlorothiazide 25 mg

losartan potassium *see* losartan *on page 577*

Losec® [Can] *see* omeprazole *on page 697*

Losec MUPS® [Can] *see* omeprazole *on page 697*

Losopan® *(Discontinued)* *see* magaldrate and simethicone *on page 583*

Lotemax® [US/Can] *see* loteprednol *on page 578*

Lotensin® [US/Can] *see* benazepril *on page 121*

Lotensin® HCT [US] *see* benazepril and hydrochlorothiazide *on page 121*

loteprednol (loe te PRED nol)

Synonyms loteprednol etabonate

U.S./Canadian Brand Names Alrex® [US/Can]; Lotemax® [US/Can]

Therapeutic Category Corticosteroid, Ophthalmic

Use

Suspension, 0.2% (Alrex®): Temporary relief of signs and symptoms of seasonal allergic conjunctivitis

Suspension, 0.5% (Lotemax®): Inflammatory conditions (treatment of steroid-responsive inflammatory conditions of the palpebral and bulbar conjunctiva, cornea, and anterior segment of the globe such as allergic conjunctivitis, acne rosacea, superficial punctate keratitis, herpes zoster keratitis, iritis, cyclitis, selected infective conjunctivitis, when the inherent hazard of steroid use is accepted to obtain an advisable diminution in edema and inflammation) and treatment of postoperative inflammation following ocular surgery

Usual Dosage Ophthalmic: Adults:
Suspension, 0.2% (Alrex®): Instill 1 drop into affected eye(s) 4 times/day
Suspension, 0.5% (Lotemax®):
Inflammatory conditions: Apply 1-2 drops into the conjunctival sac of the affected eye(s) 4 times/day. During the initial treatment within the first week, the dosing may be increased up to 1 drop every hour. Advise patients not to discontinue therapy prematurely. If signs and symptoms fail to improve after 2 days, reevaluate the patient.
Postoperative inflammation: Apply 1-2 drops into the conjunctival sac of the operated eye(s) 4 times/day beginning 24 hours after surgery and continuing throughout the first 2 weeks of the postoperative period

Dosage Forms
Suspension, ophthalmic:
Alrex®: 0.2% (5 mL, 10 mL)
Lotemax®: 0.5% (2.5 mL, 5 mL, 10 mL, 15 mL)

loteprednol and tobramycin (loe te PRED nol & toe bra MYE sin)

Synonyms loteprednol etabonate and tobramycin; tobramycin and loteprednol etabonate
U.S./Canadian Brand Names Zylet™ [US]
Therapeutic Category Antibiotic/Corticosteroid, Ophthalmic
Use Treatment of steroid-responsive ocular inflammatory conditions where either a superficial bacterial ocular infection or the risk of a superficial bacterial ocular infection exists
Usual Dosage Ophthalmic: Adults: Instill 1-2 drops into the affected eye(s) every 4-6 hours; may increase frequency during the first 24-48 hours to every 1-2 hours. Interval should increase as signs and symptoms improve. Further evaluation should occur for use of greater than 20 mL.
Dosage Forms
Suspension, ophthalmic:
Zylet™: Loteprednol 0.5% and tobramycin 0.3% (2.5 mL, 5 mL, 10 mL)

loteprednol etabonate see loteprednol on page 578
loteprednol etabonate and tobramycin see loteprednol and tobramycin on page 579
Lotrel® [US] see amlodipine and benazepril on page 65
Lotriderm® [Can] see betamethasone and clotrimazole on page 131
Lotrimin® AF Athlete's Foot Cream [US-OTC] see clotrimazole on page 238
Lotrimin® AF Cream (Discontinued) see clotrimazole on page 238
Lotrimin® AF for Her [US-OTC] see clotrimazole on page 238
Lotrimin® AF Jock Itch Cream [US-OTC] see clotrimazole on page 238
Lotrimin® AF Jock Itch Powder Spray [US-OTC] see miconazole on page 630
Lotrimin® AF Lotion (Discontinued) see clotrimazole on page 238
Lotrimin® AF Powder/Spray [US-OTC] see miconazole on page 630
Lotrimin® AF Solution (Discontinued) see clotrimazole on page 238
Lotrimin® Ultra™ [US-OTC] see butenafine on page 156
Lotrisone® [US] see betamethasone and clotrimazole on page 131
Lotronex® [US] see alosetron on page 48

lovastatin (LOE va sta tin)

Sound-Alike/Look-Alike Issues
lovastatin may be confused with Leustatin®, Livostin®, Lotensin®
Mevacor® may be confused with Mivacron®
Synonyms mevinolin; monacolin K
U.S./Canadian Brand Names Altoprev® [US]; Apo-Lovastatin® [Can]; CO Lovastatin [Can]; Gen-Lovastatin [Can]; Mevacor® [US/Can]; Novo-Lovastatin [Can]; Nu-Lovastatin [Can]; PMS-Lovastatin [Can]; RAN™-Lovastatin [Can]; ratio-Lovastatin [Can]; Riva-Lovastatin [Can]; Sandoz-Lovastatin [Can]
Therapeutic Category HMG-CoA Reductase Inhibitor

◀ **Use**
Adjunct to dietary therapy to decrease elevated serum total and LDL-cholesterol concentrations in primary hypercholesterolemia
Primary prevention of coronary artery disease (patients without symptomatic disease with average to moderately elevated total and LDL-cholesterol and below average HDL-cholesterol); slow progression of coronary atherosclerosis in patients with coronary heart disease
Adjunct to dietary therapy in adolescent patients (10-17 years of age, females >1 year postmenarche) with heterozygous familial hypercholesterolemia having LDL >189 mg/dL, **or** LDL >160 mg/dL with positive family history of premature cardiovascular disease (CVD), **or** LDL >160 mg/dL with the presence of at least two other CVD risk factors
Usual Dosage Oral:
Adolescents 10-17 years: Immediate release tablet:
LDL reduction <20%: Initial: 10 mg/day with evening meal
LDL reduction ≥20%: Initial: 20 mg/day with evening meal
Usual range: 10-40 mg with evening meal, then adjust dose at 4-week intervals
Adults: Initial: 20 mg with evening meal, then adjust at 4-week intervals; maximum dose: 80 mg/day immediate release tablet **or** 60 mg/day extended release tablet
Dosage Forms
Tablet: 10 mg, 20 mg, 40 mg
Mevacor®: 20 mg, 40 mg
Tablet, extended release:
Altoprev®: 20 mg, 40 mg, 60 mg

lovastatin and niacin *see* niacin and lovastatin *on page 669*
Lovaza® [US] *see* omega-3-acid ethyl esters *on page 697*
Lovenox® [US/Can] *see* enoxaparin *on page 341*
Lovenox® HP [Can] *see* enoxaparin *on page 341*
Low-Ogestrel® [US] *see* ethinyl estradiol and norgestrel *on page 380*
Loxapac® IM [Can] *see* loxapine *on page 580*

loxapine (LOKS a peen)
Sound-Alike/Look-Alike Issues
Loxitane® may be confused with Lexapro®, Soriatane®
Synonyms loxapine succinate; oxilapine succinate
U.S./Canadian Brand Names Apo-Loxapine® [Can]; Loxapac® IM [Can]; Loxitane® [US]; Nu-Loxapine [Can]; PMS-Loxapine [Can]
Therapeutic Category Antipsychotic Agent, Dibenzoxazepine
Use Management of psychotic disorders
Usual Dosage Oral: Adults: 10 mg twice daily, increase dose until psychotic symptoms are controlled; usual dose range: 20-100 mg/day in divided doses 2-4 times/day; dosages >250 mg/day are not recommended
Dosage Forms
Capsule: 5 mg, 10 mg, 25 mg, 50 mg
Loxitane®: 5 mg, 10 mg, 25 mg, 50 mg

loxapine succinate *see* loxapine *on page 580*
Loxitane® [US] *see* loxapine *on page 580*
Loxitane® I.M. *(Discontinued)* *see* loxapine *on page 580*
Lozide® [Can] *see* indapamide *on page 505*
Lozi-Flur™ [US] *see* fluoride *on page 411*
Lozi-Tab® *(Discontinued)* *see* fluoride *on page 411*
Lozol® [Can] *see* indapamide *on page 505*
Lozol® *(Discontinued)* *see* indapamide *on page 505*
L-PAM *see* melphalan *on page 599*
LRH *see* gonadorelin *on page 451*
L-sarcolysin *see* melphalan *on page 599*
LTA® 360 [US] *see* lidocaine *on page 561*
LTG *see* lamotrigine *on page 545*

L-thyroxine sodium *see* levothyroxine *on page 560*
Lu-26-054 *see* escitalopram *on page 356*

lubiprostone (loo bi PROS tone)
Synonyms RU 0211; SPI 0211
U.S./Canadian Brand Names Amitiza® [US]
Therapeutic Category Gastrointestinal Agent, Miscellaneous
Use Treatment of chronic idiopathic constipation; treatment of irritable bowel syndrome with constipation in adult women
Usual Dosage Oral:
  Chronic idiopathic constipation: Adults: 24 mcg twice daily
  Irritable bowel syndrome with constipation: Females ≥18 years: 8 mcg twice daily
Dosage Forms
  Capsule, softgel:
    Amitiza®: 8 mcg, 24 mcg

Lubriderm® [US-OTC] *see* lanolin, cetyl alcohol, glycerin, petrolatum, and mineral oil *on page 547*
Lubriderm® Fragrance Free [US-OTC] *see* lanolin, cetyl alcohol, glycerin, petrolatum, and mineral oil *on page 547*
LubriTears® Solution *(Discontinued)* *see* artificial tears *on page 95*
Lucentis® [US/Can] *see* ranibizumab *on page 819*
Ludiomil® *(Discontinued)* *see* maprotiline *on page 591*
Lufyllin® [US/Can] *see* dyphylline *on page 330*
Lufyllin®-GG [US] *see* dyphylline and guaifenesin *on page 330*
Lumigan® [US/Can] *see* bimatoprost *on page 135*
Luminal® Sodium [US] *see* phenobarbital *on page 742*

lumiracoxib *(Canada only)* (loo mye ra KOX ib)
U.S./Canadian Brand Names Prexige® [Can]
Therapeutic Category Nonsteroidal Antiinflammatory Drug (NSAID), COX-2 Selective
Use Acute and chronic treatment of signs and symptoms related to osteoarthritis of the knee
Usual Dosage Oral: Adults: 100 mg once daily; (maximum: 100 mg/day); no additional therapeutic benefit is derived with increased doses
Dosage Forms [CAN] = Canadian brand name
  Tablet:
    Prexige® [CAN]: 100mg [contains lactose; not available in the U.S.]

Lumitene™ [US] *see* beta-carotene *on page 130*
Lunesta® [US] *see* eszopiclone *on page 367*
LupiCare® Dandruff [US-OTC] *see* salicylic acid *on page 850*
LupiCare® Psoriasis [US-OTC] *see* salicylic acid *on page 850*
Lupron® [US/Can] *see* leuprolide *on page 553*
Lupron Depot® [US/Can] *see* leuprolide *on page 553*
Lupron Depot-Ped® [US] *see* leuprolide *on page 553*
Luride® *(Discontinued)* *see* fluoride *on page 411*
Luride® Lozi-Tab® [US] *see* fluoride *on page 411*
Luride®-SF *(Discontinued)* *see* fluoride *on page 411*
LuSonal™ [US] *see* phenylephrine *on page 745*
Lustra® [US/Can] *see* hydroquinone *on page 488*
Lustra-AF™ [US] *see* hydroquinone *on page 488*
luteinizing hormone releasing hormone *see* gonadorelin *on page 451*
Lutera™ [US] *see* ethinyl estradiol and levonorgestrel *on page 372*
Lutrepulse™ [Can] *see* gonadorelin *on page 451*

lutropin alfa (LOO troe pin AL fa)
Synonyms r-hLH; recombinant human luteinizing hormone
U.S./Canadian Brand Names Luveris® [US]
Therapeutic Category Gonadotropin; Ovulation Stimulator

◀ **Use** Stimulation of follicular development in infertile hypogonadotropic hypogonadal (HH) women with profound luteinizing hormone (LH) deficiency; to be used in combination with follitropin alfa

Usual Dosage SubQ: Adults: Females: Infertility: 75 int. units daily until adequate follicular development is noted; maximum duration of treatment: 14 days; to be used concomitantly with follitropin alfa

Dosage Forms

Injection, powder for reconstitution:
Luveris®: 75 int. units

Luveris® [US] *see* lutropin alfa *on page 581*
Luvox® [Can] *see* fluvoxamine *on page 420*
Luvox® CR [US] *see* fluvoxamine *on page 420*
Luvox® (Discontinued) *see* fluvoxamine *on page 420*
Luxiq® [US] *see* betamethasone (topical) *on page 132*
LY139603 *see* atomoxetine *on page 102*
LY146032 *see* daptomycin *on page 267*
LY170053 *see* olanzapine *on page 694*
LY231514 *see* pemetrexed *on page 729*
LY246736 *see* alvimopan *on page 55*
LY248686 *see* duloxetine *on page 328*
LY303366 *see* anidulafungin *on page 77*
LY2148568 *see* exenatide *on page 386*
Lybrel™ [US] *see* ethinyl estradiol and levonorgestrel *on page 372*
Lycolan® Elixir (Discontinued) *see* l-lysine *on page 572*
Lyderm® [Can] *see* fluocinonide *on page 410*
LYMErix™ (Discontinued)
Lymphazurin™ [US] *see* isosulfan blue *on page 531*
lymphocyte immune globulin *see* antithymocyte globulin (equine) *on page 82*
lymphocyte mitogenic factor *see* aldesleukin *on page 42*
Lyphocin® Injection (Discontinued) *see* vancomycin *on page 969*
Lyrica® [US/Can] *see* pregabalin *on page 783*
Lysinyl [US-OTC] *see* l-lysine *on page 572*
Lysodren® [US/Can] *see* mitotane *on page 638*
M-M-R® II [US/Can] *see* measles, mumps, and rubella vaccines, combined *on page 593*
Maalox® [US-OTC] *see* aluminum hydroxide, magnesium hydroxide, and simethicone *on page 54*
Maalox® Anti-Gas (Discontinued) *see* aluminum hydroxide, magnesium hydroxide, and simethicone *on page 54*
Maalox® Anti-Gas Extra Strength (Discontinued) *see* aluminum hydroxide, magnesium hydroxide, and simethicone *on page 54*
Maalox® Extra Strength (Discontinued) *see* aluminum hydroxide and magnesium hydroxide *on page 54*
Maalox® Max [US-OTC] *see* aluminum hydroxide, magnesium hydroxide, and simethicone *on page 54*
Maalox® Plus (Discontinued) *see* aluminum hydroxide, magnesium hydroxide, and simethicone *on page 54*
Maalox® Regular Chewable [US-OTC] *see* calcium carbonate *on page 163*
Maalox® TC (Therapeutic Concentrate) (Discontinued) *see* aluminum hydroxide and magnesium hydroxide *on page 54*
Maalox® Total Stomach Relief® [US-OTC] *see* bismuth *on page 136*
MabCampath® [Can] *see* alemtuzumab *on page 43*
Macrobid® [US/Can] *see* nitrofurantoin *on page 675*
Macrodantin® [US/Can] *see* nitrofurantoin *on page 675*
Macrodex® (Discontinued) *see* dextran *on page 282*
Macugen® [US/Can] *see* pegaptanib *on page 726*

mafenide (MA fe nide)

Synonyms mafenide acetate
U.S./Canadian Brand Names Sulfamylon® [US]

Therapeutic Category Antibacterial, Topical

Use
Cream: Adjunctive antibacterial agent in the treatment of second- and third-degree burns
Solution: Adjunctive antibacterial agent for use under moist dressings over meshed autografts on excised burn wounds

Usual Dosage Topical: Children and Adults:
Cream: Apply once or twice daily with a sterile-gloved hand; apply to a thickness of approximately 1/16 inch; the burned area should be covered with cream at all times
Solution: Cover graft area with 1 layer of fine mesh gauze. Wet an 8-ply burn dressing with mafenide solution and cover graft area. Keep dressing wet using syringe or irrigation tubing every 4 hours (or as necessary), or by moistening dressing every 6-8 hours (or as necessary). Irrigation dressing should be secured with bolster dressing and wrapped as appropriate. May leave dressings in place for up to 5 days.

Dosage Forms
Cream, topical:
Sulfamylon®: 85 mg/g (60 g, 120 g, 454 g)
Powder, for topical solution, as acetate:
Sulfamylon®: 50 g/packet (5s)

mafenide acetate *see* mafenide *on page 582*

Mag 64™ [US-OTC] *see* magnesium chloride *on page 583*

magaldrate and simethicone (MAG al drate & sye METH i kone)

Sound-Alike/Look-Alike Issues
Riopan Plus® may be confused with Repan®

Synonyms simethicone and magaldrate

Therapeutic Category Antacid Antiflatulent

Use Relief of hyperacidity associated with peptic ulcer, gastritis, peptic esophagitis, and hiatal hernia which are accompanied by symptoms of gas

Usual Dosage Oral: Adults: 540-1080 mg magaldrate between meals and at bedtime

Dosage Forms
Suspension, oral: Magaldrate 540 mg and simethicone 20 mg per 5 mL

Magalox Plus® *(Discontinued)* *see* aluminum hydroxide, magnesium hydroxide, and simethicone *on page 54*

Magan® *(Discontinued)* *see* magnesium salicylate *on page 588*

Mag-Caps [US-OTC] *see* magnesium oxide *on page 587*

Mag Delay® [US-OTC] *see* magnesium chloride *on page 583*

Mag G® [US-OTC] *see* magnesium gluconate *on page 585*

MagGel™ [US-OTC] *see* magnesium oxide *on page 587*

Maginex™ [US-OTC] *see* magnesium L-aspartate hydrochloride *on page 586*

Maginex™ DS [US-OTC] *see* magnesium L-aspartate hydrochloride *on page 586*

Magnacal® [US-OTC] *see* nutritional formula, enteral/oral *on page 689*

Magnacet™ [US] *see* oxycodone and acetaminophen *on page 710*

Magnelium® [Can] *see* magnesium glucoheptonate *on page 584*

magnesia magma *see* magnesium hydroxide *on page 585*

magnesium carbonate and aluminum hydroxide *see* aluminum hydroxide and magnesium carbonate *on page 53*

magnesium chloride (mag NEE zhum KLOR ide)

U.S./Canadian Brand Names Chloromag® [US]; Mag 64™ [US-OTC]; Mag Delay® [US-OTC]; Slow-Mag® [US-OTC]

Therapeutic Category Electrolyte Supplement, Oral

Use Correction or prevention of hypomagnesemia; dietary supplement

Usual Dosage Note: Serum magnesium is poor reflection of repletional status as the majority of magnesium is intracellular; serum levels may be transiently normal for a few hours after a dose is given, therefore, aim for consistently high normal serum levels in patients with normal renal function for most efficient repletion.

◄ **Dietary supplement:** Adults: Oral (Mag 64™, Mag Delay®, Slow-Mag®): 2 tablets once daily
Parenteral nutrition supplementation: I.V. (elemental magnesium):
  Children:
    <50 kg: 0.3-0.5 mEq/kg/day
    >50 kg: 10-30 mEq/day
  Adults: 8-24 mEq/day

RDA (elemental magnesium):
  Children:
    1-3 years: 80 mg/day
    4-8 years: 130 mg/day
    9-13 years: 240 mg/day
    14-18 years:
      Female: 360 mg/day
      Pregnant female: 400 mg/day
      Male: 410 mg/day
  Adults:
    19-30 years:
      Female: 310 mg/day
      Pregnant female: 350 mg/day
      Male: 400 mg/day
    ≥31 years:
      Female: 320 mg/day
      Pregnant female: 360 mg/day
      Male: 420 mg/day

Dosage Forms
  Injection, solution: 200 mg/mL [1.97 mEq/mL] (50 mL)
    Chloromag®: 200 mg/mL [1.97 mEq/mL] (50 mL)
  Tablet [enteric coated]:
    Slow-Mag® [OTC]: Elemental magnesium 64 mg
  Tablet, extended release:
    Mag 64™ [OTC], Mag Delay® [OTC]: Magnesium chloride 535 mg

magnesium citrate (mag NEE zhum SIT rate)

Synonyms citrate of magnesia

U.S./Canadian Brand Names Citro-Mag® [Can]; Citroma® [US-OTC]

Therapeutic Category Laxative

Use Evacuation of bowel prior to certain surgical and diagnostic procedures or overdose situations

Usual Dosage Oral: Cathartic:
  Children:
    <6 years: 0.5 mL/kg up to a maximum of 200 mL repeated every 4-6 hours until stools are clear
    6-12 years: 100-150 mL
  Children ≥12 years and Adults: 1/2 to 1 full bottle (120-300 mL)

Dosage Forms
  Solution, oral: 290 mg/5 mL
    Citroma®: 290 mg/5 mL (300 mL)
  Tablet: 100 mg [as elemental magnesium]

magnesium gluceptate *see* magnesium glucoheptonate *on page 584*

magnesium glucoheptonate (mag NEE zhum gloo koh HEP toh nate)

Synonyms magnesium gluceptate

U.S./Canadian Brand Names Magnelium® [Can]; Magnolex® [Can]; Magnorol® Sirop [Can]; ratio-Magnesium [Can]

Therapeutic Category Electrolyte Supplement, Parenteral; Magnesium Salt

Use Treatment and prevention of hypomagnesemia

Usual Dosage The recommended dietary allowance (RDA) of magnesium is 4.5 mg/kg which is a total daily allowance of 350-400 mg for adult men and 280-300 mg for adult women. During pregnancy the RDA is 300 mg and during lactation the RDA is 355 mg. Average daily intakes of dietary magnesium have declined in recent years due to processing of food.

Note: Serum magnesium is poor reflection of repletional status as the majority of magnesium is intracellular; serum levels may be transiently normal for a few hours after a dose is given, therefore, aim for consistently high normal serum levels in patients with normal renal function for most efficient repletion

Hypomagnesemia: Adults: Oral: 100-600 mg (5-30 mg elemental magnesium) 1-2 times/day with food
Maintenance electrolyte requirements:
Daily requirements: 0.2-0.5 mEq/kg/24 hours or 3-10 mEq/1000 kcal/24 hours
Maximum: 8-16 mEq/24 hours

Dosage Forms [CAN] = Canadian brand name
Capsule: 20 mg, 300 mg [not available in the U.S.]
Magnelium® [CAN], Magnorol® [CAN]: 20 mg [not available in the U.S.]
Magnolex® [CAN]: 300 mg [not available in the U.S.]
Solution, oral: 100 mg/mL [not available in the U.S.]
ratio-Magnesium [CAN]: 100 mg/mL [not available in the U.S.]
Syrup: 90 mg/mL [not available in the U.S.]
Magnorol® Sirop [CAN]: 90 mg/mL [not available in the U.S.]

magnesium gluconate (mag NEE zhum GLOO koe nate)

U.S./Canadian Brand Names Almora® [US-OTC]; Mag G® [US-OTC]; Magonate® [US-OTC]; Magtrate® [US-OTC]
Therapeutic Category Electrolyte Supplement, Oral
Use Dietary supplement
Usual Dosage RDA (elemental magnesium):
Children:
1-3 years: 80 mg/day
4-8 years: 130 mg/day
9-13 years: 240 mg/day
14-18 years:
Female: 360 mg/day
Pregnant female: 400 mg/day
Male: 410 mg/day
Adults:
19-30 years:
Female: 310 mg/day
Pregnant female: 350 mg/day
Male: 400 mg/day
≥31 years:
Female: 320 mg/day
Pregnant female: 360 mg/day
Male: 420 mg/day
Dosage Forms
Solution:
Magonate® [OTC]: 1000 mg/5 mL (355 mL)
Tablet: 500 mg
Almora® [OTC], Mag G® [OTC], Magonate® [OTC], Magtrate® [OTC]: 500 mg

magnesium hydroxide (mag NEE zhum hye DROKS ide)

Synonyms magnesia magma; milk of magnesia; MOM
U.S./Canadian Brand Names Phillips'® Chews [US-OTC]; Phillips'® Milk of Magnesia [US-OTC]
Therapeutic Category Antacid; Electrolyte Supplement, Oral; Laxative
Use Short-term treatment of occasional constipation and symptoms of hyperacidity, laxative; dietary supplement
Usual Dosage Oral:
Laxative:
Liquid:
Children: Magnesium hydroxide 400 mg/5 mL: 1-3 mL/kg/day; adjust dose to induce daily bowel movement
OTC labeling:
2-5 years: Magnesium hydroxide 400 mg/5 mL: 5-15 mL/day once daily at bedtime or in divided doses

◄ 6-11 years:
Magnesium hydroxide 400 mg/5 mL: 15-30 mL/day once daily at bedtime or in divided doses
Magnesium hydroxide 800 mg/5 mL: 7.5-15 mL/day once daily at bedtime or in divided doses
Children ≥12 years and Adults:
Magnesium hydroxide 400 mg/5 mL: 30-60 mL/day once daily at bedtime or in divided doses
Magnesium hydroxide 800 mg/5 mL: 15-30 mL/day once daily at bedtime or in divided doses
Tablet: OTC labeling:
Children:
3-5 years: Magnesium hydroxide 311 mg/tablet: 2 tablets/day once daily at bedtime or in divided doses
6-11 years: Magnesium hydroxide 311 mg/tablet: 4 tablets/day once daily at bedtime or in divided doses
Children ≥12 years and Adults: Magnesium hydroxide 311 mg/tablet: 8 tablets/day once daily at bedtime or in divided doses
Antacid: OTC labeling:
Liquid: Children ≥12 years and Adults: Magnesium hydroxide 400 mg/5 mL: 5-15 mL as needed up to 4 times/day
Tablet: Children ≥12 years and Adults: Magnesium hydroxide 311 mg/tablet: 2-4 tablets every 4 hours up to 4 times/day
Dietary supplement: OTC labeling (Phillips'® Chews): Children ≥12 years and Adults: Magnesium 500 mg: 2-4 tablets/day once daily at bedtime or in divided doses
Dosage Forms
Liquid, oral: 400 mg/5 mL
Phillips'® Milk of Magnesia [OTC]: 400 mg/5 mL
Liquid, oral concentrate: 800 mg/5 mL
Phillips'® Milk of Magnesia [OTC] [concentrate]: 800 mg/5 mL
Tablet, chewable:
Phillips'® Chews [OTC]: Magnesium 500 mg
Phillips'® Milk of Magnesia [OTC]: 311 mg

magnesium hydroxide, aluminum hydroxide, and simethicone see aluminum hydroxide, magnesium hydroxide, and simethicone on page 54

magnesium hydroxide and aluminum hydroxide see aluminum hydroxide and magnesium hydroxide on page 54

magnesium hydroxide and calcium carbonate see calcium carbonate and magnesium hydroxide on page 164

magnesium hydroxide and mineral oil (mag NEE zhum hye DROKS ide & MIN er al oyl)
Synonyms Haley's M-O; MOM/mineral oil emulsion
U.S./Canadian Brand Names Phillips'® M-O [US-OTC]
Therapeutic Category Laxative
Use Short-term treatment of occasional constipation
Usual Dosage Oral: Laxative: OTC labeling:
Children 6-11 years: 20-30 mL at bedtime
Children ≥12 years and Adults: 45-60 mL at bedtime
Dosage Forms
Suspension, oral:
Phillips'® M-O [OTC]: Magnesium hydroxide 300 mg and mineral oil 1.25 mL per 5 mL

magnesium hydroxide, famotidine, and calcium carbonate see famotidine, calcium carbonate, and magnesium hydroxide on page 390

magnesium L-aspartate hydrochloride
(mag NEE zhum el as PAR tate hye droe KLOR ide)
Synonyms MAH
U.S./Canadian Brand Names Maginex™ DS [US-OTC]; Maginex™ [US-OTC]
Therapeutic Category Electrolyte Supplement, Oral

Use Dietary supplement
Usual Dosage
  RDA (elemental magnesium):
    Children:
      1-3 years: 80 mg/day
      4-8 years: 130 mg/day
      9-13 years: 240 mg/day
      14-18 years:
        Female: 360 mg/day
        Pregnant female: 400 mg/day
        Male: 410 mg/day
    Adults:
      19-30 years:
        Female: 310 mg/day
        Pregnant female: 350 mg/day
        Male: 400 mg/day
      ≥31 years:
        Female: 320 mg/day
        Pregnant female: 360 mg/day
        Male: 420 mg/day
  Dietary supplement: Adults: Oral: Magnesium-L-aspartate 1230 mg (magnesium 122 mg) up to 3 times/day
Dosage Forms
  Granules:
    Maginex™ DS [OTC]: 1230 mg/packet (30s)
  Tablet:
    Maginex™ [OTC]: 615 mg

magnesium oxide (mag NEE zhum OKS ide)

U.S./Canadian Brand Names Mag-Caps [US-OTC]; Mag-Ox® 400 [US-OTC]; MagGel™ [US-OTC]; Uro-Mag® [US-OTC]
Therapeutic Category Antacid; Electrolyte Supplement, Oral; Laxative
Use Electrolyte replacement
Usual Dosage
  RDA (elemental magnesium):
  Children:
    1-3 years: 80 mg/day
    4-8 years: 130 mg/day
    9-13 years: 240 mg/day
    14-18 years:
      Female: 360 mg/day
      Pregnant female: 400 mg/day
      Male: 410 mg/day
  Adults:
    19-30 years:
      Female: 310 mg/day
      Pregnant female: 350 mg/day
      Male: 400 mg/day
    ≥31 years:
      Female: 320 mg/day
      Pregnant female: 360 mg/day
      Male: 420 mg/day

  Dietary supplement: Adults: Oral:
    Mag-Ox 400®: 2 tablets daily with food
    Mag-Caps, Uro-Mag®: 4-5 capsules daily with food
Dosage Forms
  Capsule:
    Mag-Caps: Elemental magnesium 85 mg
    Uro-Mag® [OTC]: 140 mg

◄ **Capsule, softgel:**
MagGel™: 600 mg
Tablet: 400 mg
Mag-Ox® 400 [OTC]: 400 mg

magnesium salicylate (mag NEE zhum sa LIS i late)

U.S./Canadian Brand Names Doan's® Extra Strength [US-OTC]; Keygesic [US-OTC]; Momentum® [US-OTC]; Novasal™ [US]

Therapeutic Category Nonsteroidal Antiinflammatory Drug (NSAID)

Use Mild-to-moderate pain, fever, various inflammatory conditions; relief of pain and inflammation of rheumatoid arthritis and osteoarthritis

Usual Dosage Oral:

Children ≥12 years and Adults: Relief of mild-to-moderate pain:

Doan's® Extra Strength, Momentum®: Two caplets every 6 hours as needed (maximum: 8 caplets/24 hours)

Keygesic: One tablet every 4 hours as needed (maximum 4 tablets/24 hours)

Adults: Treatment of arthritis (Novasal™): Initial: 1 tablet 3-4 times/day. Maximum: 8 tablets/day

Dosage Forms

Caplet: 467 mg
Doan's® Extra Strength [OTC]: 467 mg
Momentum® [OTC]: 467 mg

Tablet, chelated:
Keygesic [OTC]: 650 mg

Tablet, as tetrahydrate [scored]:
Novasal™: 600 mg

magnesium sulfate (mag NEE zhum SUL fate)

Sound-Alike/Look-Alike Issues

magnesium sulfate may be confused with manganese sulfate, morphine sulfate

$MgSO_4$ is an error-prone abbreviation (mistaken as morphine sulfate)

Synonyms epsom salts

Therapeutic Category Anticonvulsant; Electrolyte Supplement, Oral; Laxative

Use Treatment and prevention of hypomagnesemia; prevention and treatment of seizures in severe preeclampsia or eclampsia, pediatric acute nephritis; torsade de pointes; treatment of cardiac arrhythmias (VT/VF) caused by hypomagnesemia; short-term treatment of constipation; soaking aid

Usual Dosage Dose represented as magnesium sulfate unless stated otherwise. **Note:** Serum magnesium is poor reflection of repletional status as the majority of magnesium is intracellular; serum levels may be transiently normal for a few hours after a dose is given, therefore, aim for consistently high normal serum levels in patients with normal renal function for most efficient repletion.

Note: 1 g of magnesium sulfate = 98.6 mg elemental magnesium = 8.12 mEq elemental magnesium

Hypomagnesemia: Note: Treatment depends on severity and clinical status:

Children: I.V., I.O.: 25-50 mg/kg/dose over 10-20 minutes (faster in cardiac arrest); maximum single dose: 2000 mg

Adults:

Mild deficiency: I.M.: 1 g every 6 hours for 4 doses, or as indicated by serum magnesium levels

Severe deficiency:

I.M.: Up to 250 mg/kg within a 4-hour period

I.V.: Severe, nonlife-threatening: 1-2 g/hour for 3-6 hours then 0.5-1 g/hour as needed to correct deficiency

Symptomatic deficiency: I.V.: 1-2 g over 5-60 minutes; maintenance infusion may be required to correct deficiency (0.5-1 g/hour).

Arrhythmia (ACLS guidelines, 2005), hypomagnesemia-induced (life-threatening): 1-2 g over 5-20 minutes (torsades with cardiac arrest) or over 5-60 minutes (symptomatic arrhythmias without cardiac arrest)

Seizures, hypomagnesemia-induced: I.V.: 2 g over 10 minutes; calcium administration may also be appropriate as many patients are also hypocalcemic.

Cathartic: Oral:

Children:

2-5 years: 2.5-5 g/kg/day in divided doses

6-11 years: 5-10 g/day in divided doses
Children ≥12 years and Adults: 10-30 g/day in divided doses

Eclampsia: Adults:
I.V.: 4-5 g infusion; followed by a 1-2 g/hour continous infusion; or may follow with I.M. doses of 4-5 g in each buttock every 4 hours. **Note:** Initial infusion may be given over 3-4 minutes if eclampsia is severe; maximum: 40 g/24 hours
ACOG Practice Bulletin 2002: 4-6 g over 15-20 minutes followed by 2 g/hour continuous infusion

Preeclampsia (severe): Adults: I.V. 4-5 g infusion; followed by a 1-2 g/hour continous infusion; or may follow with I.M. doses of 4-5 g in each buttock every 4 hours; maximum: 40 g/24 hour

Torsade de pointes: Adults: I.V.:
Pulseless: 1-2 g over 5-20 minutes
With pulse: 1-2 g over 5-60 minutes. **Note:** Slower administration preferable for stable patients.

Parenteral nutrition supplementation: I.V.:
Children:
<50 kg: 0.3-0.5 mEq elemental magnesium/kg/day
>50 kg: 10-30 mEq elemental magnesium/day
Adults: 8-24 mEq elemental magnesium/day

Soaking aid: Topical: Adults: Dissolve 2 cupfuls of powder per gallon of warm water

RDA:
Children:
1-3 years: 80 mg elemental magnesium/day
4-8 years: 130 mg elemental magnesium/day
9-13 years: 240 mg elemental magnesium/day
14-18 years:
Female: 360 mg elemental magnesium/day
Pregnant female: 400 mg elemental magnesium/day
Male: 410 mg elemental magnesium/day
Adults:
19-30 years:
Female: 310 mg elemental magnesium/day
Pregnant female: 350 mg elemental magnesium/day
Male: 400 mg elemental magnesium/day
≥31 years:
Female: 320 mg elemental magnesium/day
Pregnant female: 360 mg elemental magnesium/day
Male: 420 mg elemental magnesium/day

Dosage Forms
Infusion [premixed in D_5W]: 10 mg/mL (100 mL); 20 mg/mL (500 mL)
Infusion [premixed in water for injection]: 40 mg/mL (100 mL, 500 mL, 1000 mL); 80 mg/mL (50 mL)
Injection, solution: 500 mg/mL (2 mL, 10 mL, 20 mL, 50 mL)
Powder, oral/topical: Magnesium sulfate USP (227 g, 454 g, 480 g, 1810 g, 1920 g, 2720 g)

magnesium trisilicate and aluminum hydroxide *see* aluminum hydroxide and magnesium trisilicate *on page 54*

Magnevist® [US/Can] *see* gadopentetate dimeglumine *on page 433*

Magnolex® [Can] *see* magnesium glucoheptonate *on page 584*

Magnorol® Sirop [Can] *see* magnesium glucoheptonate *on page 584*

Magonate® [US-OTC] *see* magnesium gluconate *on page 585*

Magonate® Sport (Discontinued) *see* magnesium gluconate *on page 585*

Mag-Ox® 400 [US-OTC] *see* magnesium oxide *on page 587*

Magsal® (Discontinued) *see* magnesium salicylate *on page 588*

Magtrate® [US-OTC] *see* magnesium gluconate *on page 585*

MAH *see* magnesium L-aspartate hydrochloride *on page 586*

Majeptil® [Can] *see* thioproperazine *(Canada only) on page 922*

Malarone® [US/Can] *see* atovaquone and proguanil *on page 103*

Malarone® Pediatric [Can] *see* atovaquone and proguanil *on page 103*

malathion (mal a THYE on)

U.S./Canadian Brand Names Ovide® [US]

Therapeutic Category Scabicides/Pediculicides

Use Treatment of head lice and their ova

Usual Dosage Sprinkle Ovide® lotion on dry hair and rub gently until the scalp is thoroughly moistened; pay special attention to the back of the head and neck. Allow to dry naturally - use no heat and leave uncovered. After 8-12 hours, the hair should be washed with a nonmedicated shampoo; rinse and use a fine-toothed comb to remove dead lice and eggs. If required, repeat with second application in 7-9 days. Further treatment is generally not necessary. Other family members should be evaluated to determine if infested and if so, receive treatment.

Dosage Forms
Lotion:
Ovide®: 0.5% (59 mL)

Mallisol® *(Discontinued)* *see* povidone-iodine *on page 775*

maltodextrin (mal toe DEK strin)

U.S./Canadian Brand Names Multidex® [US-OTC]; OraRinse™ [US-OTC]

Therapeutic Category Skin and Mucous Membrane Agent

Use Topical: Treatment of infected or noninfected wounds

Usual Dosage Adults:
Oral: Management of pain due to oral lesions: OraRinse™: 1 tablespoonful, swish or gargle for ~1 minute, 4 times/day or more if needed
Topical: Wound dressing: Multidex®: After debridement and irrigation of wound, apply and cover with a nonadherent, nonocclusive dressing. May be applied to moist or dry, infected or noninfected wounds.

Dosage Forms
Gel, topical dressing:
Multidex® [OTC]: (4 mL, 7 mL, 14 mL, 85 mL)
Powder, for oral suspension:
OraRinse™ [OTC]: (19 g)
Powder, topical dressing:
Multidex®: (6 g, 12 g, 25 g, 45 g)

Mandelamine® [US/Can] *see* methenamine *on page 614*

mandrake *see* podophyllum resin *on page 764*

Manerix® [Can] *see* moclobemide *(Canada only) on page 639*

manganese *see* trace metals *on page 940*

mannitol (MAN i tole)

Sound-Alike/Look-Alike Issues
Osmitrol® may be confused with esmolol

Synonyms D-mannitol

U.S./Canadian Brand Names Osmitrol® [US/Can]; Resectisol® [US]

Therapeutic Category Diuretic, Osmotic

Use Reduction of increased intracranial pressure associated with cerebral edema; promotion of diuresis in the prevention and/or treatment of oliguria or anuria due to acute renal failure; reduction of increased intraocular pressure; promoting urinary excretion of toxic substances; genitourinary irrigant in transurethral prostatic resection or other transurethral surgical procedures

Usual Dosage
Children: I.V.:
Test dose (to assess adequate renal function): 200 mg/kg over 3-5 minutes to produce a urine flow of at least 1 mL/kg for 1-3 hours
Initial: 0.25-1 g/kg
Maintenance: 0.25-0.5 g/kg given every 4-6 hours
Adults:
I.V.:
Test dose (to assess adequate renal function): 12.5 g (200 mg/kg) over 3-5 minutes to produce a urine flow of at least 30-50 mL of urine per hour. If urine flow does not increase, a second test dose may be given. If test dose does not produce an acceptable urine output, then need to reassess management.

Initial: 0.5-1 g/kg
Maintenance: 0.25-0.5 g/kg every 4-6 hours; usual daily dose: 20-200 g/24 hours
Intracranial pressure: Cerebral edema: 0.25-1.5 g/kg/dose I.V. as a 15% to 20% solution over ≥30 minutes; maintain serum osmolality 310 to <320 mOsm/kg
Prevention of acute renal failure (oliguria): 50-100 g dose
Treatment of oliguria: 100 g dose
Preoperative for neurosurgery: 1.5-2 g/kg administered 1-1.5 hours prior to surgery
Reduction of intraocular pressure: 1.5-2 g/kg as a 15% to 20% solution; administer over 30 minutes
Topical: Transurethral irrigation: Use urogenital solution as required for irrigation

Dosage Forms
  Injection, solution: 5% [50 mg/mL] (1000 mL); 10% [100 mg/mL] (500 mL, 1000 mL); 15% [150 mg/mL] (500 mL); 20% [200 mg/mL] (150 mL, 250 mL, 500 mL); 25% [250 mg/mL] (50 mL)
    Osmitrol®: 5% [50 mg/mL] (1000 mL); 10% [100 mg/mL] (500 mL, 1000 mL); 15% [150 mg/mL] (500 mL); 20% [200 mg/mL] (250 mL, 500 mL)
  Solution, urogenital: 5% [50 mg/mL] (2000 mL, 4000 mL)
    Resectisol®: 5% [50 mg/mL] (2000 mL, 4000 mL)

mantoux *see* tuberculin tests *on page 959*
Maox® *(Discontinued)* *see* magnesium oxide *on page 587*
Mapap [US-OTC] *see* acetaminophen *on page 19*
Mapap Children's [US-OTC] *see* acetaminophen *on page 19*
Mapap Extra Strength [US-OTC] *see* acetaminophen *on page 19*
Mapap Infants [US-OTC] *see* acetaminophen *on page 19*
Mapap® Multi-Symptom Cold [US-OTC] *see* acetaminophen, dextromethorphan, and phenylephrine *on page 26*
Mapap® Sinus Congestion and Pain Daytime [US-OTC] *see* acetaminophen and phenylephrine *on page 22*
Mapap Sinus Maximum Strength [US-OTC] *see* acetaminophen and pseudoephedrine *on page 23*
Mapezine® [Can] *see* carbamazepine *on page 172*

maprotiline (ma PROE ti leen)

Sound-Alike/Look-Alike Issues
  Ludiomil® may be confused with Lamictal®, lamotrigine, Lomotil®
Synonyms maprotiline hydrochloride
U.S./Canadian Brand Names Novo-Maprotiline [Can]
Therapeutic Category Antidepressant, Tetracyclic
Use Treatment of depression and anxiety associated with depression
Usual Dosage Oral: Adults: Depression/anxiety: 75 mg/day to start, increase by 25 mg every 2 weeks up to 150-225 mg/day; given in 3 divided doses or in a single daily dose
Dosage Forms
  Tablet: 25 mg, 50 mg, 75 mg

maprotiline hydrochloride *see* maprotiline *on page 591*

maraviroc (mah RAV er rock)

Synonyms UK-427,857
U.S./Canadian Brand Names Celsentri™ [Can]; Selzentry™ [US]
Therapeutic Category Antiretroviral Agent, CCR5 Antagonist
Use Treatment of CCR5-tropic HIV-1 infection, in combination with other antiretroviral agents in treatment-experienced patients with evidence of viral replication and HIV-1 strains resistant to multiple antiretroviral therapy
Usual Dosage Oral: Adolescents ≥16 years and Adults: 300 mg twice daily
Dosage Forms
  Tablet:
    Selzentry™: 150 mg, 300 mg

Marcaine® [US/Can] *see* bupivacaine *on page 149*
Marcaine® Spinal [US] *see* bupivacaine *on page 149*

Marcaine® with Epinephrine [US] *see* bupivacaine and epinephrine *on page 150*
Margesic® H [US] *see* hydrocodone and acetaminophen *on page 481*
Marinol® [US/Can] *see* dronabinol *on page 326*
Mark 1™ *see* atropine and pralidoxime *on page 106*
Marmine® Injection *(Discontinued) see* dimenhydrinate *on page 301*
Marmine® Oral *(Discontinued) see* dimenhydrinate *on page 301*
Marplan® [US] *see* isocarboxazid *on page 528*
Marthritic® *(Discontinued) see* salsalate *on page 854*
Marvelon® [Can] *see* ethinyl estradiol and desogestrel *on page 369*
Matulane® [US/Can] *see* procarbazine *on page 788*
3M™ Avagard® *(Discontinued) see* chlorhexidine gluconate *on page 201*
Mavik® [US/Can] *see* trandolapril *on page 942*
Maxair™ Autohaler™ [US] *see* pirbuterol *on page 757*
Maxalt® [US/Can] *see* rizatriptan *on page 841*
Maxalt-MLT® [US] *see* rizatriptan *on page 841*
Maxalt RPD™ [Can] *see* rizatriptan *on page 841*
Maxaquin® *(Discontinued)*
Maxidex® [US/Can] *see* dexamethasone (ophthalmic) *on page 278*
Maxidone™ [US] *see* hydrocodone and acetaminophen *on page 481*
Maxifed® [US] *see* guaifenesin and pseudoephedrine *on page 458*
Maxifed DM [US] *see* guaifenesin, pseudoephedrine, and dextromethorphan *on page 460*
Maxifed DMX [US] *see* guaifenesin, pseudoephedrine, and dextromethorphan *on page 460*
Maxifed-G® [US] *see* guaifenesin and pseudoephedrine *on page 458*
Maxiflor® *(Discontinued) see* diflorasone *on page 295*
Maximum D3® [US] *see* cholecalciferol *on page 215*
Maximum Strength Desenex® Antifungal Cream *(Discontinued) see* miconazole *on page 630*
Maximum Strength Dex-A-Diet® *(Discontinued)*
Maximum Strength Dexatrim® *(Discontinued)*
Maxiphen DM [US] *see* guaifenesin, dextromethorphan, and phenylephrine *on page 459*
Maxipime® [US/Can] *see* cefepime *on page 185*
Maxitrol® [US/Can] *see* neomycin, polymyxin B, and dexamethasone *on page 662*
Maxi-Tuss HC® [US] *see* phenylephrine, hydrocodone, and chlorpheniramine *on page 748*
Maxi-Tuss HCG *(Discontinued)*
Maxi-Tuss HCX [US] *see* phenylephrine, hydrocodone, and chlorpheniramine *on page 748*
Maxivate® [US] *see* betamethasone (topical) *on page 132*
Maxolon® *(Discontinued) see* metoclopramide *on page 625*
Maxzide® [US] *see* hydrochlorothiazide and triamterene *on page 480*
Maxzide®-25 [US] *see* hydrochlorothiazide and triamterene *on page 480*
may apple *see* podophyllum resin *on page 764*
3M™ Cavilon™ Skin Cleanser *(Discontinued) see* benzalkonium chloride *on page 123*
MCH *see* collagen hemostat *on page 245*

m-cresyl acetate (em-KREE sil AS e tate)

U.S./Canadian Brand Names Cresylate® [US]
Therapeutic Category Otic Agent, Antiinfective
Use Provides an acid medium; for external otitis infections caused by susceptible bacteria or fungus
Usual Dosage Otic: Instill 2-4 drops as required
Dosage Forms
 Solution, otic:
  Cresylate®: 25% (15 mL)

MCT *see* medium chain triglycerides *on page 596*
MCT Oil® [US-OTC/Can] *see* medium chain triglycerides *on page 596*
MCV4 *see* meningococcal polysaccharide (Groups A / C / Y and W-135) diphtheria toxoid conjugate vaccine *on page 601*

MD-76®R [US] *see* diatrizoate meglumine and diatrizoate sodium *on page 288*

MD-Gastroview® [US] *see* diatrizoate meglumine and diatrizoate sodium *on page 288*

MDL 73,147EF *see* dolasetron *on page 316*

measles, mumps, and rubella vaccines, combined

(MEE zels, mumpz & roo BEL a VYE rus vak SEEN)

Sound-Alike/Look-Alike Issues

MMR (measles, mumps, and rubella virus vaccine) may be confused with MMRV (measles, mumps, rubella, and varicella) vaccine

Synonyms MMR; mumps, measles, and rubella vaccines, combined; rubella, measles, and mumps vaccines, combined

U.S./Canadian Brand Names M-M-R® II [US/Can]; Priorix™ [Can]

Therapeutic Category Vaccine, Live Virus

Use Measles, mumps, and rubella prophylaxis

The Advisory Committee on Immunization Practices (ACIP) recommends routine vaccination for the following:

- All children (first dose given at 12-15 months of age)
- Adults born 1957 or later (without evidence of immunity or documentation of vaccination).
- Adults at higher risk for exposure to and transmission of measles mumps and rubella should receive special consideration for vaccination. This includes international travelers, persons attending colleges and other post-high school education, persons working in healthcare facilities.

Usual Dosage SubQ:

Infants <12 months: If there is risk of exposure to measles, single-antigen measles vaccine should be administered at 6-11 months of age with a second dose (of MMR) at >12 months of age.

Children ≥12 months:

Primary immunization: 0.5 mL at 12-15 months

Revaccination: 0.5 mL at 4-6 years of age; revaccination is recommended prior to elementary school. If the second dose was not received, the schedule should be completed by the 11- to 12-year old visit. During a mumps outbreak, children ages 1-4 should consider a second dose of a live mumps virus vaccine. (Minimum interval between doses is 28 days.)

Adults:

Birth year ≥1957 without evidence of immunity: 1 or 2 doses (0.5 mL/dose); minimum interval between doses is 28 days

Routine vaccination of healthcare workers:

Birth year ≥1957 without evidence of immunity: 2 doses of a live mumps virus vaccine; minimum interval between doses is 28 days

Birth year <1957 without evidence of immunity: 1 dose of a live mumps virus vaccine.

Mumps outbreak:

Healthcare workers born <1957 without other evidence of immunity: Consider 2 doses of a live mumps virus vaccine; minimum interval between doses is 28 days

Low-risk adults: A second dose of a live mumps virus vaccine should be considered in adults who previously received 1 dose; minimum interval between doses is 28 days

Dosage Forms

Injection, powder for reconstitution [preservative free]:

M-M-R® II: Measles virus 1000 TCID50, mumps virus 20,000 $TCID_{50}$, and rubella virus 1000 $TCID_{50}$

measles, mumps, rubella, and varicella virus vaccine

(MEE zels, mumpz, roo BEL a, & var i SEL a VYE rus vak SEEN)

Synonyms MMRV; mumps, rubella, varicella, and measles vaccine; rubella, varicella, measles, and mumps vaccine; varicella, measles, mumps, and rubella vaccine

U.S./Canadian Brand Names ProQuad® [US]

Therapeutic Category Vaccine, Live (Viral)

Use To provide simultaneous active immunization against measles, mumps, rubella, and varicella

Usual Dosage SubQ: Children 12 months to 12 years: One dose (0.5 mL)

Administer on or after the first birthday, as soon as child becomes eligible for vaccination. It may be used whenever all components of the vaccine are needed in children within this age group. (Refer to current CDC Recommended Immunization Schedule)

Allow at least 1 month between administering a dose of a measles containing vaccine (eg, M-M-R® II) and ProQuad®.

◀ Allow at least 3 months between administering a varicella containing vaccine (eg, Varivax®) and ProQuad®.

Dosage Forms
Injection, powder for reconstitution [preservative free]:
ProQuad®: Measles virus ≥3.00 $\log_{10}$ $TCID_{50}$, mumps virus ≥4.3 $\log_{10}$ $TCID_{50}$, rubella virus ≥3.0 $\log_{10}$ $TCID_{50}$, and varicella virus ≥3.99 $\log_{10}$ plaque-forming units

measles virus vaccine (live) (MEE zels VYE rus vak SEEN, live)

Sound-Alike/Look-Alike Issues
Attenuvax® may be confused with Meruvax®
Synonyms more attenuated enders strain; rubeola vaccine
U.S./Canadian Brand Names Attenuvax® [US]
Therapeutic Category Vaccine, Live Virus
Use Active immunization against measles (rubeola)
Note: Trivalent measles - mumps - rubella (MMR) is the vaccine of choice if recipients are likely to be susceptible to rubella and/or mumps as well as to measles.
Usual Dosage Note: Trivalent measles - mumps - rubella (MMR) vaccine should be used unless contraindicated in adults and children ≥12 months of age.
Children ≥6 months and Adults: SubQ: 0.5 mL in outer aspect of the upper arm
Primary vaccination recommended at 12-15 months of age and repeated at 4-6 years of age. Children requiring vaccination with measles virus vaccine prior to 12 months of age (eg, during local outbreak, international travel to endemic area) should receive another dose between 12-15 months and again prior to elementary school.
Adults born in or after 1957 without documentation of live vaccine on or after first birthday, without physician-diagnosed measles, or without laboratory evidence of immunity should be vaccinated, ideally with 2 doses of vaccine separated by no less than 1 month. For those previously vaccinated with 1 dose of measles vaccine, revaccination is recommended for students entering colleges and other institutions of higher education, for healthcare workers at the time of employment, and for international travelers who visit endemic areas. Persons vaccinated between 1963 and 1967 with a killed measles vaccine, followed by live vaccine within 3 months, or with a vaccine of unknown type should be revaccinated with live measles virus vaccine.

Dosage Forms
Injection, powder for reconstitution [preservative free]:
Attenuvax®: ≥1000 $TCID_{50}$

Measurin® *(Discontinued)* *see* aspirin *on page 98*
Mebaral® [US/Can] *see* mephobarbital *on page 604*

mebendazole (me BEN da zole)

U.S./Canadian Brand Names Vermox® [Can]
Therapeutic Category Anthelmintic
Use Treatment of pinworms (*Enterobius vermicularis*), whipworms (*Trichuris trichiura*), roundworms (*Ascaris lumbricoides*), and hookworms (*Ancylostoma duodenale*)
Usual Dosage Oral: Children ≥2 years and Adults:
Pinworms: 100 mg as a single dose; may need to repeat after 2 weeks; treatment should include family members in close contact with patient
Whipworms, roundworms, hookworms: One tablet twice daily, morning and evening on 3 consecutive days; if patient is not cured within 3-4 weeks, a second course of treatment may be administered
Capillariasis: 200 mg twice daily for 20 days
Dosage Forms
Tablet, chewable: 100 mg

mecamylamine (mek a MIL a meen)

Sound-Alike/Look-Alike Issues
mecamylamine may be confused with mesalamine
Synonyms mecamylamine hydrochloride
U.S./Canadian Brand Names Inversine® [US/Can]
Therapeutic Category Ganglionic Blocking Agent

Use Treatment of moderately severe to severe hypertension and in uncomplicated malignant hypertension

Usual Dosage Oral: Adults: 2.5 mg twice daily after meals for 2 days; increased by increments of 2.5 mg at intervals ≥2 days until desired blood pressure response is achieved; average daily dose: 25 mg (usually in 3 divided doses)

Note: Reduce dosage of other antihypertensives when combined with mecamylamine with exception of thiazide diuretics which may be maintained at usual dose while decreasing mecamylamine by 50%

Dosage Forms
Tablet:
Inversine®: 2.5 mg

mecamylamine hydrochloride *see* mecamylamine *on page 594*

mecasermin (mek a SER min)

Synonyms mecasermin (rDNA origin); mecasermin rinfabate; recombinant human insulin-like growth factor-1; rhIGF-1; rhIGF-1/rhIGFBP-3

U.S./Canadian Brand Names Increlex™ [US]

Therapeutic Category Growth Hormone

Use Treatment of growth failure in children with severe primary insulin-like growth factor-1 deficiency (IGF-1 deficiency; primary IGFD), or with growth hormone (GH) gene deletions who have developed neutralizing antibodies to GH

Usual Dosage SubQ: Increlex™: Children ≥2 years: Primary IGFD: Initial: 0.04-0.08 mg/kg twice daily; if tolerated for 7 days, may increase by 0.04 mg/kg/dose (maximum dose: 0.12 mg/kg given twice daily). Must be administered within 20 minutes of a meal or snack; omit dose if patient is unable to eat. Reduce dose if hypoglycemia occurs despite adequate food intake.

Dosage Forms
Injection, solution:
Increlex™: 10 mg/mL (4 mL)

mecasermin (rDNA origin) *see* mecasermin *on page 595*
mecasermin rinfabate *see* mecasermin *on page 595*

mechlorethamine (me klor ETH a meen)

Synonyms chlorethazine; chlorethazine mustard; HN$_2$; mechlorethamine hydrochloride; mustine; nitrogen mustard; NSC-762

U.S./Canadian Brand Names Mustargen® [US/Can]

Therapeutic Category Antineoplastic Agent

Use Hodgkin disease; non-Hodgkin lymphoma; intracavitary injection for treatment of metastatic tumors; pleural and other malignant effusions; topical treatment of mycosis fungoides

Usual Dosage Refer to individual protocols.
Children and Adults: I.V.: 6 mg/m^2 on days 1 and 8 of a 28-day cycle (MOPP regimen)
Adults:
I.V.: 0.4 mg/kg **or** 12-16 mg/m^2 for one dose **or** divided into 0.1 mg/kg/day for 4 days, repeated at 4- to 6-week intervals
Intracavitary: 0.2-0.4 mg/kg (10-20 mg) as a single dose; may be repeated if fluid continues to accumulate.
Intrapericardially: 0.2-0.4 mg/kg as a single dose; may be repeated if fluid continues to accumulate.
Topical: 0.01% to 0.02% solution, lotion, or ointment

Dosage Forms
Injection, powder for reconstitution:
Mustargen®: 10 mg

mechlorethamine hydrochloride *see* mechlorethamine *on page 595*

meclizine (MEK li zeen)

Sound-Alike/Look-Alike Issues
Antivert® may be confused with Axert™

Synonyms meclizine hydrochloride; meclozine hydrochloride

U.S./Canadian Brand Names Antivert® [US]; Bonamine™ [Can]; Bonine® [US-OTC/Can]; Dramamine® Less Drowsy Formula [US-OTC]; Medi-Meclizine [US-OTC]

Therapeutic Category Antihistamine

◄ **Use** Prevention and treatment of symptoms of motion sickness; management of vertigo with diseases affecting the vestibular system

Usual Dosage Oral: Children >12 years and Adults:
Motion sickness: 12.5-25 mg 1 hour before travel, repeat dose every 12-24 hours if needed; doses up to 50 mg may be needed
Vertigo: 25-100 mg/day in divided doses

Dosage Forms
Tablet: 12.5 mg, 25 mg
Antivert®: 12.5 mg, 25 mg, 50 mg
Dramamine® Less Drowsy Formula [OTC]: 25 mg
Medi-Meclizine [OTC]: 25 mg
Tablet, chewable: 25 mg
Bonine® [OTC]: 25 mg

meclizine hydrochloride see meclizine on page 595

meclofenamate (me kloe fen AM ate)

Synonyms meclofenamate sodium
U.S./Canadian Brand Names Meclomen® [Can]
Therapeutic Category Analgesic, Nonnarcotic Nonsteroidal Antiinflammatory Drug (NSAID)
Use Treatment of inflammatory disorders, arthritis, mild-to-moderate pain, dysmenorrhea
Usual Dosage Oral: Children >14 years and Adults:
Mild-to-moderate pain: 50 mg every 4-6 hours; increases to 100 mg may be required; maximum dose: 400 mg
Rheumatoid arthritis and osteoarthritis: 50 mg every 4-6 hours; increase, over weeks, to 200-400 mg/day in 3-4 divided doses; do not exceed 400 mg/day; maximal benefit for any dose may not be seen for 2-3 weeks

Dosage Forms
Capsule: 50 mg, 100 mg

meclofenamate sodium see meclofenamate on page 596
Meclomen® [Can] see meclofenamate on page 596
meclozine hydrochloride see meclizine on page 595
Med-Diltiazem [Can] see diltiazem on page 300
Medebar® Plus [US] see barium on page 116
Medent-DM [US] see guaifenesin, pseudoephedrine, and dextromethorphan on page 460
Medent LD [US] see guaifenesin and pseudoephedrine on page 458
medicinal carbon see charcoal on page 198
medicinal charcoal see charcoal on page 198
Medicone® Suppositories [US-OTC] see phenylephrine on page 745
Medidin® Liquid (Discontinued)
Medigesic® [US] see butalbital, acetaminophen, and caffeine on page 155
Medihaler-Iso® (Discontinued) see isoproterenol on page 529
Medi-Meclizine [US-OTC] see meclizine on page 595
Medipain 5® (Discontinued) see hydrocodone and acetaminophen on page 481
Medi-Phenyl [US-OTC] see phenylephrine on page 745
Medipren® (Discontinued) see ibuprofen on page 495
Mediproxen [US-OTC] see naproxen on page 656
Medi-Quick® Topical Ointment (Discontinued) see bacitracin, neomycin, and polymyxin B on page 114
Medispaz® (Discontinued) see hyoscyamine on page 492
Medi-Synal [US-OTC] see acetaminophen and pseudoephedrine on page 23
Medi-Tuss® (Discontinued) see guaifenesin on page 453

medium chain triglycerides (mee DEE um chane trye GLIS er ides)

Synonyms MCT; triglycerides, medium chain
U.S./Canadian Brand Names MCT Oil® [US-OTC/Can]

Therapeutic Category Nutritional Supplement

Use Dietary supplement for those who cannot digest long chain fats; malabsorption associated with disorders such as pancreatic insufficiency, bile salt deficiency, short bowel syndrome, and bacterial overgrowth of the small bowel; induce ketosis as a prevention for seizures

Usual Dosage Oral:

Infants: Nutritional supplement: Initial: 0.5 mL every other feeding, then advance to every feeding, then increase in increments of 0.25-0.5 mL/feeding at intervals of 2-3 days as tolerated

Children: Seizures: About 40 mL with each meal or 50% to 70% (800-1120 kcal) of total calories (1600 kcal) as the oil will induce ketosis necessary for seizure control

Children and Adults: Cystic fibrosis: 3 tablespoons/day in divided doses

Adults: Malabsorption syndromes: 15 mL 3-4 times/day

Dosage Forms

Oil:

MCT Oil® [OTC]: 14 g/15 mL

Medralone® Injection *(Discontinued)* *see* methylprednisolone *on page 623*

Medrol® [US/Can] *see* methylprednisolone *on page 623*

medroxyprogesterone (me DROKS ee proe JES te rone)

Sound-Alike/Look-Alike Issues

medroxyPROGESTERone may be confused with hydroxyprogesterone, methylPREDNISolone, methylTESTOSTERone

Provera® may be confused with Covera®, Parlodel®, Premarin®

Synonyms acetoxymethylprogesterone; medroxyprogesterone acetate; methylacetoxyprogesterone

Tall-Man medroxy**PROGESTER**one

U.S./Canadian Brand Names Alti-MPA [Can]; Apo-Medroxy® [Can]; Depo-Prevera® [Can]; Depo-Provera® Contraceptive [US]; Depo-Provera® [US/Can]; depo-subQ provera 104™ [US]; Gen-Medroxy [Can]; Novo-Medrone [Can]; Provera-Pak [Can]; Provera® [US/Can]

Therapeutic Category Contraceptive, Progestin Only; Progestin

Use Endometrial carcinoma or renal carcinoma; secondary amenorrhea or abnormal uterine bleeding due to hormonal imbalance; reduction of endometrial hyperplasia in nonhysterectomized postmenopausal women receiving conjugated estrogens; prevention of pregnancy; management of endometriosis-associated pain

Usual Dosage

Adolescents and Adults:

Amenorrhea: Oral: 5-10 mg/day for 5-10 days

Abnormal uterine bleeding: Oral: 5-10 mg for 5-10 days starting on day 16 or 21 of cycle

Contraception:

Depo-Provera® Contraceptive: I.M.: 150 mg every 3 months

depo-subQ provera 104™: SubQ: 104 mg every 3 months (every 12-14 weeks)

Endometriosis: depo-subQ provera 104™: SubQ: 104 mg every 3 months (every 12-14 weeks)

Adults:

Endometrial or renal carcinoma (Depo-Provera®): I.M.: 400-1000 mg/week

Accompanying cyclic estrogen therapy, postmenopausal: Oral: 5-10 mg for 12-14 consecutive days each month, starting on day 1 or day 16 of the cycle; lower doses may be used if given with estrogen continuously throughout the cycle

Dosage Forms

Injection, suspension: 150 mg/mL (1 mL)

Depo-Provera®: 400 mg/mL (2.5 mL)

Depo-Provera® Contraceptive: 150 mg/mL (1 mL)

depo-subQ provera 104™: 104 mg/0.65 mL (0.65 mL)

Tablet: 2.5 mg, 5 mg, 10 mg

Provera®: 2.5 mg, 5 mg, 10 mg

medroxyprogesterone acetate *see* medroxyprogesterone *on page 597*

medroxyprogesterone and estrogens (conjugated) *see* estrogens (conjugated/equine) and medroxyprogesterone *on page 365*

medrysone (ME dri sone)

Therapeutic Category Adrenal Corticosteroid

◄ **Use** Treatment of allergic conjunctivitis, vernal conjunctivitis, episcleritis, ophthalmic epinephrine sensitivity reaction

Usual Dosage Ophthalmic: Children ≥3 years and Adults: Instill 1 drop in conjunctival sac 2-4 times/day up to every 4 hours; may use every 1-2 hours during first 1-2 days

Med-Verapamil [Can] *see verapamil on page 974*

Mefenamic-250 [Can] *see mefenamic acid on page 598*

mefenamic acid (me fe NAM ik AS id)

Sound-Alike/Look-Alike Issues
Ponstel® may be confused with Pronestyl®

U.S./Canadian Brand Names Apo-Mefenamic® [Can]; Dom-Mefenamic Acid [Can]; Mefenamic-250 [Can]; Nu-Mefenamic [Can]; PMS-Mefenamic Acid [Can]; Ponstan® [Can]; Ponstel® [US]

Therapeutic Category Analgesic, Nonnarcotic Nonsteroidal Antiinflammatory Drug (NSAID)

Use Short-term relief of mild-to-moderate pain including primary dysmenorrhea

Usual Dosage Oral: Children >14 years and Adults: 500 mg to start then 250 mg every 4 hours as needed; maximum therapy: 1 week

Dosage Forms
Capsule: 250 mg
Ponstel®: 250 mg

mefloquine (ME floe kwin)

Synonyms mefloquine hydrochloride

U.S./Canadian Brand Names Apo-Mefloquine® [Can]; Lariam® [US/Can]

Therapeutic Category Antimalarial Agent

Use Treatment of acute malarial infections and prevention of malaria

Usual Dosage Oral (dose expressed as mg of mefloquine hydrochloride):
Children ≥6 months and >5 kg:
Malaria treatment: 20-25 mg/kg in 2 divided doses, taken 6-8 hours apart (maximum: 1250 mg). If clinical improvement is not seen within 48-72 hours, an alternative therapy should be used for retreatment.
Malaria prophylaxis: 5 mg/kg/once weekly (maximum dose: 250 mg) starting 1 week before arrival in endemic area, continuing weekly during travel and for 4 weeks after leaving endemic area.
Adults:
Malaria treatment (mild-to-moderate infection): 5 tablets (1250 mg) as a single dose. If clinical improvement is not seen within 48-72 hours, an alternative therapy should be used for retreatment.
Malaria prophylaxis: 1 tablet (250 mg) weekly starting 1 week before arrival in endemic area, continuing weekly during travel and for 4 weeks after leaving endemic area

Dosage Forms
Tablet: 250 mg
Lariam®: 250 mg

mefloquine hydrochloride *see mefloquine on page 598*

Megace® [US/Can] *see megestrol on page 598*

Megace® ES [US] *see megestrol on page 598*

Megace® OS [Can] *see megestrol on page 598*

Megadophilus® [US-OTC] *see Lactobacillus on page 543*

megestrol (me JES trole)

Sound-Alike/Look-Alike Issues
Megace® may be confused with Reglan®

Synonyms 5071-1DL(6); megestrol acetate; NSC-71423

U.S./Canadian Brand Names Apo-Megestrol® [Can]; Megace® ES [US]; Megace® OS [Can]; Megace® [US/Can]; Nu-Megestrol [Can]

Therapeutic Category Antineoplastic Agent; Progestin

Use Palliative treatment of breast and endometrial carcinoma; treatment of anorexia, cachexia, or unexplained significant weight loss in patients with AIDS

Usual Dosage Oral: Adults: **Note:** Megace® ES suspension is not equivalent to other formulations on a mg-per-mg basis:

Tablet: Female (refer to individual protocols):

Breast carcinoma: 40 mg 4 times/day

Endometrial carcinoma: 40-320 mg/day in divided doses; use for 2 months to determine efficacy; maximum doses used have been up to 800 mg/day

Suspension: Male/Female: HIV-related cachexia:

Megace®: Initial dose: 800 mg/day; daily doses of 400 and 800 mg/day were found to be clinically effective

Megace® ES: 625 mg/day

Dosage Forms

Suspension, oral: 40 mg/mL

Megace®: 40 mg/mL

Megace® ES: 125 mg/mL

Tablet: 20 mg, 40 mg

megestrol acetate *see* megestrol *on page 598*

Melanex® [US] *see* hydroquinone *on page 488*

Melfiat® *(Discontinued)* *see* phendimetrazine *on page 742*

Mellaril® [Can] *see* thioridazine *on page 922*

Mellaril® (all products) *(Discontinued)* *see* thioridazine *on page 922*

Mellaril-S® *(Discontinued)* *see* thioridazine *on page 922*

meloxicam (mel OKS i kam)

U.S./Canadian Brand Names Apo-Meloxicam® [Can]; CO Meloxicam [Can]; Gen-Meloxicam [Can]; Mobicox® [Can]; Mobic® [US/Can]; Novo-Meloxicam [Can]; PMS-Meloxicam [Can]

Therapeutic Category Nonsteroidal Antiinflammatory Drug (NSAID)

Use Relief of signs and symptoms of osteoarthritis, rheumatoid arthritis, and juvenile rheumatoid arthritis (JRA)

Usual Dosage Oral:

Children ≥2 years: JRA: 0.125 mg/kg/day; maximum dose: 7.5 mg/day

Adults: Osteoarthritis, rheumatoid arthritis: Initial: 7.5 mg once daily; some patients may receive additional benefit from an increased dose of 15 mg once daily; maximum dose: 15 mg/day

Dosage Forms

Suspension: 7.5 mg/5 mL (100 mL)

Mobic®: 7.5 mg/5 mL

Tablet: 7.5 mg, 15 mg

Mobic®: 7.5 mg, 15 mg

Melpaque HP® [US] *see* hydroquinone *on page 488*

melphalan (MEL fa lan)

Sound-Alike/Look-Alike Issues

melphalan may be confused with Mephyton®, Myleran®

Alkeran® may be confused with Alferon®, Leukeran®, Myleran®

Synonyms L-PAM; L-sarcolysin; NSC-8806; phenylalanine mustard

U.S./Canadian Brand Names Alkeran® [US/Can]

Therapeutic Category Antineoplastic Agent

Use Palliative treatment of multiple myeloma and nonresectable epithelial ovarian carcinoma

Usual Dosage Refer to individual protocols.

Oral: Dose should always be adjusted to patient response and weekly blood counts: Adults:

Multiple myeloma (multiple regimens have been employed): **Note:** Response is gradual; may require repeated courses to realize benefit:

6 mg daily for 2-3 weeks initially, followed by up to 4 weeks rest, then a maintenance dose of 2 mg daily as hematologic recovery begins **or**

10 mg daily for 7-10 days; institute 2 mg daily maintenance dose after WBC >4000 cells/mm^3 and platelets >100,000 cells/mm^3 (~4-8 weeks); titrate maintenance dose to hematologic response **or**

0.15 mg/kg/day for 7 days, with a 2-6 week rest, followed by a maintenance dose of ≤0.05 mg/kg/day as hematologic recovery begins **or**

◀ 0.25 mg/kg/day for 4 days (or 0.2 mg/kg/day for 5 days); repeat at 4- to 6-week intervals as ANC and platelet counts return to normal
Ovarian carcinoma: 0.2 mg/kg/day for 5 days, repeat every 4-5 weeks.
I.V.: Adults: Multiple myeloma: 16 mg/m^2 administered at 2-week intervals for 4 doses, then administer at 4-week intervals after adequate hematologic recovery.
Dosage Forms
Injection, powder for reconstitution:
Alkeran®: 50 mg
Tablet:
Alkeran®: 2 mg

Melquin-3® [US] *see* hydroquinone *on page 488*
Melquin HP® [US] *see* hydroquinone *on page 488*

memantine (me MAN teen)
Synonyms memantine hydrochloride
U.S./Canadian Brand Names Ebixa® [Can]; Namenda™ [US]
Therapeutic Category N-Methyl-D-Aspartate Receptor Antagonist
Use Treatment of moderate-to-severe dementia of the Alzheimer type
Usual Dosage Oral: Adults:
Alzheimer disease: Initial: 5 mg/day; increase dose by 5 mg/day to a target dose of 20 mg/day; wait at least 1 week between dosage changes. Doses >5 mg/day should be given in 2 divided doses.
Suggested titration: 5 mg/day for ≥1 week; 5 mg twice daily for ≥1 week; 15 mg/day given in 5 mg and 10 mg separated doses for ≥1 week; then 10 mg twice daily
Dosage Forms
Solution, oral:
Namenda™: 2 mg/mL
Tablet:
Namenda™: 5 mg, 10 mg
Combination package [titration pack contains two separate tablet formulations]:
Namenda™: Memantine 5 mg (28s), 10 mg (21s)

memantine hydrochloride *see* memantine *on page 600*
Menactra® [US] *see* meningococcal polysaccharide (Groups A / C / Y and W-135) diphtheria toxoid conjugate vaccine *on page 601*
Menadol® *(Discontinued)* *see* ibuprofen *on page 495*
menCC *see* meningococcal group C-CRM197 conjugate vaccine *(Canada only) on page 600*
menC-CRM197 *see* meningococcal group C-CRM197 conjugate vaccine *(Canada only) on page 600*
Menest® [US/Can] *see* estrogens (esterified) *on page 365*
Meni-D® *(Discontinued)* *see* meclizine *on page 595*

meningococcal group C-CRM197 conjugate vaccine *(Canada only)*
(me NIN joe kok al groop see see ahr em wuhn nahyn tee sev uhn KON joo gate vak SEEN)
Synonyms menC-CRM197; menCC
U.S./Canadian Brand Names Menjugate® [Can]
Therapeutic Category Vaccine
Use To provide active immunization against invasive meningococcal disease caused by *N. meningitidis* serogroup C, in children ≥2 months and adults

The National Advisory Committee on Immunization (NACI) recommendations for persons considered at an increased risk for meningococcal disease:
Chemoprophylaxis and immunoprophylaxis: Selection of meningococcal vaccination to be based upon serogroup(s):
Individuals living in the same household or with close contact (eg, kissing, shared cigarettes, shared eating or drinking utensils) of infected patient
Employees and children of nursery schools or day care
Immunoprophylaxis: Selection of meningococcal vaccination to be based upon serogroup(s):
Adolescents and young adults
Laboratory workers routinely exposed to isolates of *N. meningitidis*
Military recruits

Persons traveling to or who reside in countries where *N. meningitidis* is hyperendemic or epidemic, particularly if contact with local population will be prolonged
Persons with terminal complement component deficiencies
Persons with anatomic or functional asplenia
Note: Use is also recommended during meningococcal outbreaks caused by serogroup C.
Chemoprophylaxis:
Healthcare workers with intensive unprotected contact with infected patients
Airline passengers sitting directly next to an infected patient for duration of at least 8 hours

See NACI guidelines for specific drug treatment at http://www.phac-aspc.gc.ca/naci-ccni
Usual Dosage I.M.:
Infants:
≥2-12 months: 0.5 mL as a single dose for a total of 3 doses administered at least 4 weeks apart
≥4-11 months without prior vaccination: 0.5 mL as a single dose for a total of 2 doses administered at least 4 weeks apart
Note: The NACI recommends at least 1 of the 3 sequential doses for infants ≥2-12 months be administered beyond 5 months of age.
Children ≥1 year and Adults: 0.5 mL as a single dose
Dosage Forms [CAN = Canadian brand name]
Injection, powder for reconstitution:
Menjugate® [CAN]: 10 mcg of oligosaccharide antigen group C [not available in U.S.]

meningococcal polysaccharide (Groups A / C / Y and W-135) diphtheria toxoid conjugate vaccine
(me NIN joe kok al pol i SAK a ride groops aye, see, why & dubl yoo won thur tee fyve dif THEER ee a TOKS oyds KON joo gate vak SEEN)
Synonyms MCV4; quadrivalent meningococcal conjugate vaccine
U.S./Canadian Brand Names Menactra® [US]
Therapeutic Category Vaccine
Use Provide active immunization of children and adults (2-55 years of age) against invasive meningococcal disease caused by *N. meningitidis* serogroups A, C, Y, and W-135

The ACIP recommends routine vaccination of all persons 11-18 years of age at the earliest opportunity. Adolescents should be vaccinated at the 11-12 year visit. For adolescents not previously vaccinated, vaccine should be administered prior to high school entry (~15 years of age).
The ACIP also recommends vaccination for persons at increased risk for meningococcal disease. (MCV4 is preferred for persons aged 2-55 years; MPSV4 may be used if MCV4 is not available). Persons at increased risk include:
College freshmen living in dormitories
Microbiologists routinely exposed to isolates of *N. meningitides*
Military recruits
Persons traveling to or who reside in countries where *N. meningitides* is hyperendemic or epidemic, particularly if contact with local population will be prolonged
Persons with terminal complement component deficiencies
Persons with anatomic or functional asplenia
Use is also recommended during meningococcal outbreaks caused by vaccine preventable serogroups.
Usual Dosage I.M.: Children ≥2 years and Adults ≤55 years: 0.5 mL
NOTE: Revaccination: May be indicated in patients previously vaccinated with MPSV4 who remain at increased risk for infection. The ACIP recommends the use of MCV4 for revaccination in patients 11-55 years, however use of MPSV4 is also acceptable. Consider revaccination after 3-5 years. The need for revaccination in patients previously vaccinated with MCV4 is currently under study.
Dosage Forms
Injection, solution:
Menactra®: 4 mcg each of polysaccharide antigen groups A, C, Y, and W-135 per 0.5 mL

meningococcal polysaccharide vaccine (groups A / C / Y and W-135)
(me NIN joe kok al pol i SAK a ride vak SEEN groops aye, see, why & dubl yoo won thur tee fyve)
Synonyms MPSV4; quadrivalent meningococcal conjugate vaccine
U.S./Canadian Brand Names Menomune®-A/C/Y/W-135 [US]
Therapeutic Category Vaccine, Live Bacteria

◀ **Use** Provide active immunity to meningococcal serogroups contained in the vaccine

The ACIP recommends routine vaccination for persons at increased risk for meningococcal disease. (Use of MPSV4 is recommended in children 2-10 years and adults >55 years. MCV4 is preferred for persons aged 11-55 years; MPSV4 may be used if MCV4 is not available). Persons at increased risk include:
College freshmen living in dormitories
Microbiologists routinely exposed to isolates of *N. meningitides*
Military recruits
Persons traveling to or who reside in countries where *N. meningitides* is hyperendemic or epidemic, particularly if contact with local population will be prolonged
Persons with terminal complement component deficiencies
Persons with anatomic or functional asplenia
Use is also recommended during meningococcal outbreaks caused by vaccine preventable serogroups.

Usual Dosage SubQ:
Children <2 years: Not usually recommended. Two doses (0.5 mL/dose), 3 months apart, may be considered in children 3-18 months to elicit short-term protection against serogroup A disease. A single dose may be considered in children 19-23 months.
Children ≥2 years and Adults: 0.5 mL
Note: Revaccination: May be indicated in patients previously vaccinated with MPSV4 who remain at increased risk for infection. The ACIP recommends the use of MCV4 for revaccination in patients 11-55 years, however use of MPSV4 is also acceptable.
Children first vaccinated at <4 years: Revaccinate after 2-3 years.
Adults: Not determined, consider revaccination after 3-5 years.

Dosage Forms
Injection, powder for reconstitution:
Menomune®-A/C/Y/W-135: 50 mcg each of polysaccharide antigen groups A, C, Y, and W-135

Menjugate® [Can] *see* meningococcal group C-CRM197 conjugate vaccine *(Canada only) on page 600*
Menomune®-A/C/Y/W-135 [US] *see* meningococcal polysaccharide vaccine (groups A / C / Y and W-135) *on page 601*
Menopur® [US/Can] *see* menotropins *on page 602*
Menostar® [US/Can] *see* estradiol *on page 359*

menotropins (men oh TROE pins)

Sound-Alike/Look-Alike Issues
Repronex® may be confused with Regranex®
Synonyms hMG; human menopausal gonadotropin
U.S./Canadian Brand Names Menopur® [US/Can]; Repronex® [US/Can]
Therapeutic Category Gonadotropin
Use Female:
In conjunction with hCG to induce ovulation and pregnancy in infertile females experiencing oligoanovulation or anovulation when the cause of anovulation is functional and not caused by primary ovarian failure (Repronex®)
Stimulation of multiple follicle development in ovulatory patients as part of an assisted reproductive technology (ART) (Menopur®, Repronex®)
Usual Dosage Adults:
Repronex®: I.M., SubQ:
Induction of ovulation in patients with oligoanovulation (Female): Initial: 150 int. units daily for the first 5 days of treatment. Adjustments should not be made more frequently than once every 2 days and should not exceed 75-150 int. units per adjustment. Maximum daily dose should not exceed 450 int. units and dosing beyond 12 days is not recommended. If patient's response is appropriate, hCG 5000-10,000 units should be given one day following the last dose of Repronex®. Hold dose if serum estradiol is >2000 pg/mL, if the ovaries are abnormally enlarged, or if abdominal pain occurs; the patient should also be advised to refrain from intercourse. May repeat process if follicular development is inadequate or if pregnancy does not occur.
Assisted reproductive technologies (Female): Initial (in patients who have received GnRH agonist or antagonist pituitary suppression): 225 int. units; adjustments in dose should not be made more frequently than once every 2 days and should not exceed more than 75-150 int. units per adjustment. The maximum daily doses of Repronex® given should not exceed 450 int. units and dosing beyond 12 days is not recommended. Once adequate follicular development is evident, hCG (5000-10,000 units)

should be administered to induce final follicular maturation in preparation for oocyte retrieval. Withhold treatment when ovaries are abnormally enlarged on last day of therapy (to reduce chance of developing OHSS).

Menopur®: SubQ: *Assisted reproductive technologies (ART):* Initial (in patients who have received GnRH agonist for pituitary suppression): 225 int. units; adjustments in dose should not be made more frequently than once every 2 days and should not exceed more than 150 int. units per adjustment. The maximum daily dose given should not exceed 450 int. units and dosing beyond 20 days is not recommended. Once adequate follicular development is evident, hCG should be administered to induce final follicular maturation in preparation for oocyte retrieval. Withhold treatment when ovaries are abnormally enlarged on last day of therapy (to reduce chance of developing OHSS).

Dosage Forms
Injection, powder for reconstitution:
Menopur®, Repronex®: Follicle stimulating hormone activity 75 int. units and luteinizing hormone activity 75 int. units

Mentax® [US] *see* butenafine *on page 156*
292 **MEP® [Can]** *see* meprobamate and aspirin *on page 606*

mepenzolate (me PEN zoe late)

Sound-Alike/Look-Alike Issues
Cantil® may be confused with Bentyl®
Synonyms mepenzolate bromide
U.S./Canadian Brand Names Cantil® [Can]
Therapeutic Category Anticholinergic Agent
Use Adjunctive treatment of peptic ulcer disease
Usual Dosage Oral: Adults: 25-50 mg 4 times/day with meals and at bedtime

mepenzolate bromide *see* mepenzolate *on page 603*
mepergan *see* meperidine and promethazine *on page 604*

meperidine (me PER i deen)

Sound-Alike/Look-Alike Issues
meperidine may be confused with meprobamate
Demerol® may be confused with Demulen®, Desyrel®, dicumarol, Dilaudid®, Dymelor®, Pamelor®
Synonyms isonipecaine hydrochloride; meperidine hydrochloride; pethidine hydrochloride
U.S./Canadian Brand Names Demerol® [US/Can]; Meperitab® [US]
Therapeutic Category Analgesic, Narcotic
Controlled Substance C-II
Use Management of moderate-to-severe pain; adjunct to anesthesia and preoperative sedation
Usual Dosage Note: The American Pain Society (2003) and ISMP (2007) do not recommend meperidine's use as an analgesic.

Children: Pain: Oral, I.M., I.V., SubQ: 1-1.5 mg/kg/dose every 3-4 hours as needed; 1-2 mg/kg as a single dose preoperative medication may be used; maximum 100 mg/dose (**Note:** Oral route is not recommended for acute pain.)
Adults: Pain:
Oral: Initial: Opiate-naive: 50 mg every 3-4 hours as needed; usual dosage range: 50-150 mg every 2-4 hours as needed (manufacturers recommendation; oral route is not recommended for acute pain)
I.M., SubQ: Initial: Opiate-naive: 50-75 mg every 3-4 hours as needed; patients with prior opiate exposure may require higher initial doses
Preoperatively: 50-100 mg given 30-90 minutes before the beginning of anesthesia
Note: If use in acute pain (in patients without renal or CNS disease) cannot be avoided, treatment should be limited to ≤48 hours and doses should not exceed 600 mg/24 hours.

Dosage Forms
Injection, solution [ampul]: 25 mg/0.5 mL (0.5 mL); 25 mg/mL (1 mL); 50 mg/mL (1 mL, 1.5 mL, 2 mL); 75 mg/mL (1 mL); 100 mg/mL (1 mL)
Injection, solution [prefilled syringe]: 25 mg/mL (1 mL); 50 mg/mL (1 mL); 75 mg/mL (1 mL); 100 mg/mL (1 mL)
Injection, solution [for PCA pump]: 10 mg/mL (30 mL, 50 mL, 60 mL)

▶

◄ **Injection, solution** [vial]: 25 mg/mL (1 mL); 50 mg/mL (1 mL, 30 mL); 75 mg/mL (1 mL); 100 mg/mL (1 mL, 20 mL)
Solution, oral: 50 mg/5 mL (500 mL)
Tablet: 50 mg, 100 mg
Demerol®, Meperitab®: 50 mg, 100 mg

meperidine and promethazine (me PER i deen & proe METH a zeen)
Sound-Alike/Look-Alike Issues
mepergan may be confused with meprobamate
Synonyms mepergan; promethazine and meperidine
Therapeutic Category Analgesic, Narcotic
Controlled Substance C-II
Use Management of moderate pain
Usual Dosage Oral: Adults: One capsule every 4-6 hours as needed
Dosage Forms
Capsule: Meperidine 50 mg and promethazine 25 mg

meperidine hydrochloride *see meperidine on page 603*
Meperitab® [US] *see meperidine on page 603*

mephobarbital (me foe BAR bi tal)
Sound-Alike/Look-Alike Issues
mephobarbital may be confused with methocarbamol
Mebaral® may be confused with Medrol®, Mellaril®, Tegretol®
Synonyms methylphenobarbital
U.S./Canadian Brand Names Mebaral® [US/Can]
Therapeutic Category Barbiturate
Controlled Substance C-IV
Use Sedative; treatment of grand mal and petit mal epilepsy
Usual Dosage Oral:
Epilepsy:
Children: 6-12 mg/kg/day in 2-4 divided doses
Adults: 200-600 mg/day in 2-4 divided doses
Sedation:
Children:
<5 years: 16-32 mg 3-4 times/day
>5 years: 32-64 mg 3-4 times/day
Adults: 32-100 mg 3-4 times/day
Dosage Forms
Tablet:
Mebaral®: 32 mg, 50 mg, 100 mg

Mephyton® [US/Can] *see phytonadione on page 752*

mepivacaine (me PIV a kane)
Sound-Alike/Look-Alike Issues
mepivacaine may be confused with bupivacaine
Polocaine® may be confused with prilocaine
Synonyms mepivacaine hydrochloride
U.S./Canadian Brand Names Carbocaine® [US/Can]; Polocaine® Dental [US]; Polocaine® MPF [US]; Polocaine® [US/Can]
Therapeutic Category Local Anesthetic
Use Local or regional analgesia; anesthesia by local infiltration, peripheral and central neural techniques including epidural and caudal blocks; **not** for use in spinal anesthesia
Usual Dosage
Injectable local anesthetic: Dose varies with procedure, degree of anesthesia needed, vascularity of tissue, duration of anesthesia required, and physical condition of patient. The smallest dose and concentration required to produce the desired effect should be used.

Children: Maximum dose: 5-6 mg/kg; only concentrations <2% should be used in children <3 years or <14 kg (30 lbs)

Adults: Maximum dose: 400 mg; do not exceed 1000 mg/24 hours

Cervical, brachial, intercostal, pudendal nerve block: 5-40 mL of a 1% solution (maximum: 400 mg) **or** 5-20 mL of a 2% solution (maximum: 400 mg). For pudendal block, inject 1/2 the total dose each side.

Transvaginal block (paracervical plus pudendal): Up to 30 mL (both sides) of a 1% solution (maximum: 300 mg). Inject 1/2 the total dose each side.

Paracervical block: Up to 20 mL (both sides) of a 1% solution (maximum: 200 mg). Inject 1/2 the total dose to each side. This is the maximum recommended dose per 90-minute procedure; inject slowly with 5 minutes between sides.

Caudal and epidural block (preservative free solutions only): 15-30 mL of a 1% solution (maximum: 300 mg) **or** 10-25 mL of a 1.5% solution (maximum: 375 mg) **or** 10-20 mL of a 2% solution (maximum: 400 mg)

Infiltration: Up to 40 mL of a 1% solution (maximum: 400 mg)

Therapeutic block (pain management): 1-5 mL of a 1% solution (maximum: 50 mg) **or** 1-5 mL of a 2% solution (maximum: 100 mg)

Dental anesthesia: Adults:

Single site in upper or lower jaw: 54 mg (1.8 mL) as a 3% solution

Infiltration and nerve block of entire oral cavity: 270 mg (9 mL) as a 3% solution. Manufacturer's maximum recommended dose is not more than 400 mg to normal healthy adults.

Dosage Forms

Injection, solution:

Carbocaine®: 1% (50 mL); 2% (50 mL)

Polocaine®: 1% (50 mL); 2% (50 mL)

Injection, solution [preservative free]:

Carbocaine®: 1% (30 mL); 1.5% (30 mL); 2% (20 mL); 3% (1.8 mL)

Polocaine® Dental: 3% (1.8 mL)

Polocaine® MPF: 1% (30 mL); 1.5% (30 mL); 2% (20 mL)

mepivacaine and levonordefrin (me PIV a kane & lee voe nor DEF rin)

Synonyms levonordefrin and mepivacaine hydrochloride

U.S./Canadian Brand Names Carbocaine® 2% with Neo-Cobefrin® [US]; Polocaine® 2% and Levonordefrin 1:20,000 [Can]

Therapeutic Category Local Anesthetic

Use Amide-type anesthetic used for local infiltration anesthesia; injection near nerve trunks to produce nerve block

Usual Dosage

Children <10 years: Maximum pediatric dosage must be carefully calculated on the basis of patient's weight but should not exceed 6.6 mg/kg of body weight or 180 mg of mepivacaine hydrochloride as a 2% solution with levonordefrin 1:20,000

Children >10 years and Adults:

Dental infiltration and nerve block, single site: 36 mg (1.8 mL) of mepivacaine hydrochloride as a 2% solution with levonordefrin 1:20,000

Entire oral cavity: 180 mg (9 mL) of mepivacaine hydrochloride as a 2% solution with levonordefrin 1:20,000; up to a maximum of 6.6 mg/kg of body weight but not to exceed 400 mg of mepivacaine hydrochloride per appointment. The effective anesthetic dose varies with procedure, intensity of anesthesia needed, duration of anesthesia required, and physical condition of the patient. Always use the lowest effective dose along with careful aspiration.

Dosage Forms

Injection, solution:

Carbocaine® 2% with Neo-Cobefrin®: Mepivacaine 2% and levonordefrin 1:20,000 (1.8 mL)

mepivacaine hydrochloride *see* mepivacaine *on page 604*

meprobamate (me proe BA mate)

Sound-Alike/Look-Alike Issues

meprobamate may be confused with Mepergan, meperidine

U.S./Canadian Brand Names Novo-Mepro [Can]

Therapeutic Category Antianxiety Agent, Miscellaneous

▶

◀ **Controlled Substance** C-IV
Use Management of anxiety disorders
Usual Dosage Oral: Anxiety:
  Children 6-12 years: 100-200 mg 2-3 times/day
  Adults: 400 mg 3-4 times/day, up to 2400 mg/day
Dosage Forms
  Tablet: 200 mg

meprobamate and aspirin (me proe BA mate & AS pir in)

Synonyms aspirin and meprobamate
U.S./Canadian Brand Names 292 MEP® [Can]; Equagesic® [US]
Therapeutic Category Skeletal Muscle Relaxant
Controlled Substance C-IV
Use Adjunct to the short-term treatment of pain in patients with skeletal-muscular disease exhibiting tension and/or anxiety
Usual Dosage Oral: Children ≥12 years and Adults: 1-2 tablets 3-4 times/day for up to 10 days
Dosage Forms
  Tablet:
    Equagesic®: Meprobamate 200 mg and aspirin 325 mg

Mepron® [US/Can] see atovaquone on page 103

mequinol and tretinoin (ME kwi nole & TRET i noyn)

Synonyms tretinoin and mequinol
U.S./Canadian Brand Names Solagé® [US/Can]
Therapeutic Category Retinoic Acid Derivative; Vitamin A Derivative; Vitamin, Topical
Use Treatment of solar lentigines; the efficacy of using Solagé® daily for >24 weeks has not been established
Usual Dosage Solar lentigines: Topical: Apply twice daily to solar lentigines using the applicator tip while avoiding application to the surrounding skin. Separate application by at least 8 hours or as directed by physician.
Dosage Forms
  Liquid, topical:
    Solagé®: Mequinol 2% and tretinoin 0.01% (30 mL)

mercaptopurine (mer kap toe PYOOR een)

Sound-Alike/Look-Alike Issues
  Purinethol® may be confused with propylthiouracil
  6-mercaptopurine (error-prone abbreviation)
  6-MP (error-prone abbreviation)
Synonyms NSC-755
U.S./Canadian Brand Names Purinethol® [US/Can]
Therapeutic Category Antineoplastic Agent
Use Treatment (maintenance and induction) of acute lymphoblastic leukemia (ALL)
Usual Dosage Oral (refer to individual protocols):
  Children: ALL:
    Induction: 2.5-5 mg/kg/day **or** 70-100 mg/m^2/day given once daily
    Maintenance: 1.5-2.5 mg/kg/day **or** 50-75 mg/m^2/day given once daily
  Adults: ALL:
    Induction: 2.5-5 mg/kg/day (100-200 mg)
    Maintenance: 1.5-2.5 mg/kg/day **or** 80-100 mg/m^2/day given once daily
  Note: In ALL, administration in the evening (vs morning administration) may lower the risk of relapse.
Dosage Forms
  Tablet [scored]: 50 mg
    Purinethol®: 50 mg

mercapturic acid see acetylcysteine on page 30
Meridia® [US/Can] see sibutramine on page 865

meropenem (mer oh PEN em)

Sound-Alike/Look-Alike Issues
meropenem may be confused with ertapenem, imipenem, metronidazole.

U.S./Canadian Brand Names Merrem® I.V. [US]; Merrem® [Can]

Therapeutic Category Carbapenem (Antibiotic)

Use Treatment of intraabdominal infections (complicated appendicitis and peritonitis); treatment of bacterial meningitis in pediatric patients ≥3 months of age caused by *S. pneumoniae*, *H. influenzae*, and *N. meningitidis*; treatment of complicated skin and skin structure infections caused by susceptible organisms

Usual Dosage

Usual dosage ranges:
Neonates: I.V.:
Postnatal age 0-7 days: 20 mg/kg/dose every 12 hours
Postnatal age >7 days:
Weight 1200-2000 g: 20 mg/kg/dose every 12 hours
Weight >2000 g: 20 mg/kg/dose every 8 hours
Children ≥3 months: I.V.: 30-120 mg/kg/day divided every 8 hours (maximum dose: 6 g/day)
Adults: I.V.: 1.5-6 g/day divided every 8 hours

Indication-specific dosing:
Children ≥3 months (<50 kg): I.V.:
Intraabdominal infections: 20 mg/kg every 8 hours (maximum dose: 1 g every 8 hours)
Meningitis: 40 mg/kg every 8 hours (maximum dose: 2 g every 8 hours)
Skin and skin structure infections (complicated): 10 mg/kg every 8 hours (maximum dose: 500 mg every 8 hours)
Children >50 kg and Adults: I.V.:
Cholangitis, intraabdominal infections: 1 g every 8 hours
Skin and skin structure infections (complicated): 500 mg every 8 hours; diabetic foot: 1 g every 8 hours

Dosage Forms
Injection, powder for reconstitution:
Merrem® I.V.: 500 mg, 1 g

Merrem® [Can] *see* meropenem *on page 607*

Merrem® I.V. [US] *see* meropenem *on page 607*

Mersyndol® With Codeine [Can] *see* acetaminophen, codeine, and doxylamine *(Canada only) on page 26*

Meruvax® II [US] *see* rubella virus vaccine (live) *on page 848*

mesalamine (me SAL a meen)

Sound-Alike/Look-Alike Issues
mesalamine may be confused with mecamylamine
Asacol® may be confused with Ansaid®, Os-Cal®
Lialda™ may be confused with Aldara™

Synonyms 5-aminosalicylic acid; 5-ASA; fisalamine; mesalazine

U.S./Canadian Brand Names Asacol® 800 [Can]; Asacol® [US/Can]; Canasa® [US]; Lialda™ [US]; Mesasal® [Can]; Mezavant® [Can]; Novo-5 ASA [Can]; Pendo-5 ASA [Can]; Pentasa® [US/Can]; Quintasa® [Can]; Rowasa® [US/Can]; Salofalk® [Can]

Therapeutic Category 5-Aminosalicylic Acid Derivative

Use
Oral: Treatment and maintenance of remission of mildly- to moderately-active ulcerative colitis
Rectal: Treatment of active mild-to-moderate distal ulcerative colitis, proctosigmoiditis, or proctitis

Usual Dosage Adults:
Oral:
Treatment of ulcerative colitis (usual course of therapy is 3-8 weeks):
Capsule: 1 g 4 times/day
Tablet: Initial:
Asacol®: 800 mg 3 times/day for 6 weeks
Lialda™, Mezavant®: 2.4-4.8 g once daily for up to 8 weeks

▶

◀ Maintenance of remission of ulcerative colitis:
  Capsule: 1 g 4 times/day
  Tablet (Asacol®): 1.6 g/day in divided doses; **Note:** Lialda™ and Mezavant® tablets are approved for treatment only.
Rectal:
  Retention enema: 60 mL (4 g) at bedtime, retained overnight, approximately 8 hours
  Rectal suppository (Canasa®): Insert one 1000 mg suppository in rectum daily at bedtime
  Note: Suppositories should be retained for at least 1-3 hours to achieve maximum benefit.
Note: Some patients may require rectal and oral therapy concurrently.
Dosage Forms [CAN] = Canadian brand name
  Capsule, controlled release:
  Pentasa®: 250 mg, 500 mg
  Suppository, rectal:
  Canasa®: 1000 mg
  Suspension, rectal: 4 g/60 mL (7s, 28s)
  Rowasa®: 4 g/60 mL (7s, 28s)
  Tablet, delayed release [enteric coated]:
  Asacol®: 400 mg
  Lialda™: 1.2 g
  Tablet, delayed and extended release:
  Mezavant® [CAN]: 1.2 g [not available in U.S.]

mesalazine *see mesalamine on page 607*
Mesasal® [Can] *see mesalamine on page 607*
M-Eslon® [Can] *see morphine sulfate on page 643*

mesna (MES na)
Synonyms sodium 2-mercaptoethane sulfonate
U.S./Canadian Brand Names Mesnex® [US/Can]; Uromitexan [Can]
Therapeutic Category Antidote
Use Orphan drug: Prevention of hemorrhagic cystitis induced by ifosfamide
Usual Dosage Children and Adults (refer to individual protocols):
  I.V.: Recommended dose is 60% of the ifosfamide dose given in 3 divided doses (0, 4, and 8 hours after the start of ifosfamide)
  Alternative I.V. regimens include 80% of the ifosfamide dose given in 4 divided doses (0, 3, 6, and 9 hours after the start of ifosfamide) and continuous infusions
  Oral, I.V.: Recommended dose is 100% of the ifosfamide dose, given as 20% of the ifosfamide dose I.V. at hour 0, followed by 40% of the ifosfamide dose given orally 2 and 6 hours after start of ifosfamide
Dosage Forms
  Injection, solution: 100 mg/mL (10 mL)
  Mesnex®: 100 mg/mL (10 mL)
  Tablet: 400 mg
  Mesnex®: 400 mg

Mesnex® [US/Can] *see mesna on page 608*
Mestinon® [US/Can] *see pyridostigmine on page 807*
Mestinon® Injection (Discontinued) *see pyridostigmine on page 807*
Mestinon®-SR [Can] *see pyridostigmine on page 807*
Mestinon® Timespan® [US] *see pyridostigmine on page 807*

mestranol and norethindrone (MES tra nole & nor eth IN drone)
Sound-Alike/Look-Alike Issues
  Norinyl® may be confused with Nardil®
Synonyms norethindrone and mestranol
U.S./Canadian Brand Names Necon® 1/50 [US]; Norinyl® 1+50 [US]; Ortho-Novum® 1/50 [Can]
Therapeutic Category Contraceptive, Oral

Use Prevention of pregnancy

Usual Dosage Oral: Adults: Female: Contraception:

Schedule 1 (Sunday starter): Dose begins on first Sunday after onset of menstruation; if the menstrual period starts on Sunday, take first tablet that very same day. **With a Sunday start, an additional method of contraception should be used until after the first 7 days of consecutive administration.**

For 21-tablet package: Dosage is 1 tablet daily for 21 consecutive days, followed by 7 days off of the medication; a new course begins on the 8th day after the last tablet is taken.

For 28-tablet package: Dosage is 1 tablet daily without interruption.

Schedule 2 (Day 1 starter): Dose starts on first day of menstrual cycle taking 1 tablet daily.

For 21-tablet package: Dosage is 1 tablet daily for 21 consecutive days, followed by 7 days off of the medication; a new course begins on the 8th day after the last tablet is taken.

For 28-tablet package: Dosage is 1 tablet daily without interruption.

If all doses have been taken on schedule and one menstrual period is missed, continue dosing cycle. If two consecutive menstrual periods are missed, pregnancy test is required before new dosing cycle is started.

Missed doses **monophasic formulations** (refer to package insert for complete information):

One dose missed: Take as soon as remembered or take 2 tablets next day

Two consecutive doses missed in the first 2 weeks: Take 2 tablets as soon as remembered or 2 tablets next 2 days. **An additional method of contraception should be used for 7 days after missed dose.**

Two consecutive doses missed in week 3 or three consecutive doses missed at any time: **An additional method of contraception must be used for 7 days after a missed dose:**

Schedule 1 (Sunday starter): Continue dose of 1 tablet daily until Sunday, then discard the rest of the pack, and a new pack should be started that same day.

Schedule 2 (Day 1 starter): Current pack should be discarded, and a new pack should be started that same day.

Dosage Forms

Tablet, monophasic formulations:

Necon® 1/50: Norethindrone 1 mg and mestranol 0.05 mg [21 light blue tablets and 7 white inactive tablets] (28s)

Norinyl® 1+50: Norethindrone 1 mg and mestranol 0.05 mg [21 white tablets and 7 orange inactive tablets] (28s)

metacortandralone *see* prednisolone (systemic) *on page 781*

Metadate® CD [US] *see* methylphenidate *on page 622*

Metadate® ER [US] *see* methylphenidate *on page 622*

Metadol™ [Can] *see* methadone *on page 612*

Metaglip™ [US] *see* glipizide and metformin *on page 446*

Metamucil® [US-OTC/Can] *see* psyllium *on page 804*

Metamucil® Plus Calcium [US-OTC] *see* psyllium *on page 804*

Metamucil® Smooth Texture [US-OTC] *see* psyllium *on page 804*

Metanx™ [US] *see* vitamin B complex combinations *on page 981*

metaproterenol *(met a proe TER e nol)*

Sound-Alike/Look-Alike Issues

metaproterenol may be confused with metipranolol, metoprolol

Alupent® may be confused with Atrovent®

Synonyms metaproterenol sulfate; orciprenaline sulfate

U.S./Canadian Brand Names Alupent® [US]; Apo-Orciprenaline® [Can]; ratio-Orciprenaline® [Can]; Tanta-Orciprenaline® [Can]

Therapeutic Category Adrenergic Agonist Agent

Use Bronchodilator in reversible airway obstruction due to asthma or COPD; because of its delayed onset of action (1 hour) and prolonged effect (4 or more hours), this may not be the drug of choice for assessing response to a bronchodilator

Usual Dosage

Oral:

Children:

<2 years: 0.4 mg/kg/dose given 3-4 times/day; in infants, the dose can be given every 8-12 hours

2-6 years: 1-2.6 mg/kg/day divided every 6 hours

6-9 years: 10 mg/dose 3-4 times/day

Children >9 years and Adults: 20 mg 3-4 times/day

▶

◀ Inhalation: Children >12 years and Adults: 2-3 inhalations every 3-4 hours, up to 12 inhalations in 24 hours

Nebulizer:

Infants and Children: 0.01-0.02 mL/kg of 5% solution; minimum dose: 0.1 mL; maximum dose: 0.3 mL diluted in 2-3 mL normal saline every 4-6 hours (may be given more frequently according to need)

Adolescents and Adults: 5-20 breaths of full strength 5% metaproterenol **or** 0.2 to 0.3 mL 5% metaproterenol in 2.5-3 mL normal saline until nebulized every 4-6 hours (can be given more frequently according to need)

Dosage Forms

Aerosol for oral inhalation:

Alupent®: 0.65 mg/inhalation (14 g)

Solution for nebulization [preservative free]: 0.4% [4 mg/mL] (2.5 mL); 0.6% [6 mg/mL] (2.5 mL)

Syrup: 10 mg/5 mL

Tablet: 10 mg, 20 mg

metaproterenol sulfate *see* metaproterenol *on page 609*

Metasep® *(Discontinued)*

Metastron® [US/Can] *see* strontium-89 *on page 889*

metaxalone (me TAKS a lone)

Sound-Alike/Look-Alike Issues

metaxalone may be confused with metolazone

U.S./Canadian Brand Names Skelaxin® [US/Can]

Therapeutic Category Skeletal Muscle Relaxant

Use Relief of discomfort associated with acute, painful musculoskeletal conditions

Usual Dosage Oral: Children >12 years and Adults: 800 mg 3-4 times/day

Dosage Forms

Tablet:

Skelaxin®: 800 mg

metformin (met FOR min)

Sound-Alike/Look-Alike Issues

metFORMIN may be confused with metroNIDAZOLE

Glucophage® may be confused with Glucotrol®, Glutofac®

Synonyms metformin hydrochloride

Tall-Man metFORMIN

U.S./Canadian Brand Names Alti-Metformin [Can]; Apo-Metformin® [Can]; BCI-Metformin [Can]; Fortamet® [US]; Gen-Metformin [Can]; Glucophage® XR [US]; Glucophage® [US/Can]; Glumetza™ [US/Can]; Glycon [Can]; Novo-Metformin [Can]; Nu-Metformin [Can]; PMS-Metformin [Can]; RAN™-Metformin [Can]; ratio-Metformin [Can]; Rho®-Metformin [Can]; Riomet® [US]; Sandoz-Metformin FC [Can]

Therapeutic Category Antidiabetic Agent, Oral

Use Management of type 2 diabetes mellitus (noninsulin-dependent, NIDDM) as monotherapy when hyperglycemia cannot be managed on diet alone. May be used concomitantly with a sulfonylurea or insulin to improve glycemic control.

Usual Dosage Type 2 diabetes management: **Note:** Allow 1-2 weeks between dose titrations: Generally, clinically significant responses are not seen at doses <1500 mg daily; however, a lower recommended starting dose and gradual increased dosage is recommended to minimize gastrointestinal symptoms.

Immediate release tablet or solution: Oral:

Children 10-16 years: Initial: 500 mg twice daily (given with the morning and evening meals); increases in daily dosage should be made in increments of 500 mg at weekly intervals, given in divided doses, up to a maximum of 2000 mg/day

Adults ≥17 years: Initial: 500 mg twice daily (give with the morning and evening meals) **or** 850 mg once daily; increase dosage incrementally.

Incremental dosing recommendations based on dosage form:

500 mg tablet: One tablet/day at weekly intervals

850 mg tablet: One tablet/day every other week

Oral solution: 500 mg twice daily every other week

Doses of up to 2000 mg/day may be given twice daily. If a dose >2000 mg/day is required, it may be better tolerated in three divided doses. Maximum recommended dose 2550 mg/day.

Extended release tablet: Oral: **Note:** If glycemic control is not achieved at maximum dose, may divide dose and administer twice daily.

Children ≥17 years and Adults:
Fortamet®: Initial: 1000 mg once daily; dosage may be increased by 500 mg weekly; maximum dose: 2500 mg once daily
Glucophage® XR: Initial: 500 mg once daily (with the evening meal); dosage may be increased by 500 mg weekly; maximum dose: 2000 mg once daily
Adults: Glumetza™: Initial: 1000 mg once daily; dosage may be increased by 500 mg weekly; maximum dose: 2000 mg once daily

Transfer from other antidiabetic agents: No transition period is generally necessary except when transferring from chlorpropamide. When transferring from chlorpropamide, care should be exercised during the first 2 weeks because of the prolonged retention of chlorpropamide in the body, leading to overlapping drug effects and possible hypoglycemia.

Concomitant metformin and oral sulfonylurea therapy: If patients have not responded to 4 weeks of the maximum dose of metformin monotherapy, consider a gradual addition of an oral sulfonylurea, even if prior primary or secondary failure to a sulfonylurea has occurred. Continue metformin at the maximum dose.

Failed sulfonylurea therapy: Patients with prior failure on glyburide may be treated by gradual addition of metformin. Initiate with glyburide 20 mg and metformin 500 mg daily. Metformin dosage may be increased by 500 mg/day at weekly intervals, up to a maximum metformin dose (dosage of glyburide maintained at 20 mg/day).

Concomitant metformin and insulin therapy: Initial: 500 mg metformin once daily, continue current insulin dose; increase by 500 mg metformin weekly until adequate glycemic control is achieved
Maximum daily dose: Immediate release and solution: 2550 mg metformin; Extended release: 2000-2500 mg (varies by product)
Decrease insulin dose 10% to 25% when FPG <120 mg/dL; monitor and make further adjustments as needed

Dosage Forms
Solution, oral:
Riomet®: 100 mg/mL
Tablet: 500 mg, 850 mg, 1000 mg
Glucophage®: 500 mg, 850 mg, 1000 mg
Tablet, extended release: 500 mg, 750 mg
Fortamet®: 500 mg, 1000 mg
Glucophage® XR: 500 mg
Glumetza™: 500 mg, 1000 mg

metformin and glipizide *see* glipizide and metformin *on page 446*
metformin and glyburide *see* glyburide and metformin *on page 448*
metformin and repaglinide *see* repaglinide and metformin *on page 826*
metformin and rosiglitazone *see* rosiglitazone and metformin *on page 846*
metformin and sitagliptin *see* sitagliptin and metformin *on page 870*
metformin hydrochloride *see* metformin *on page 610*
metformin hydrochloride and pioglitazone hydrochloride *see* pioglitazone and metformin *on page 755*
metformin hydrochloride and rosiglitazone maleate *see* rosiglitazone and metformin *on page 846*

methacholine (meth a KOLE leen)
Synonyms methacholine chloride
U.S./Canadian Brand Names Methacholine Omega [Can]; Provocholine® [US/Can]
Therapeutic Category Diagnostic Agent
Use Diagnosis of bronchial airway hyperactivity
Usual Dosage Before inhalation challenge, perform baseline pulmonary function tests; the patient must have an FEV_1 of at least 70% of the predicted value. The following is a suggested schedule for administration of methacholine challenge. Calculate cumulative units by multiplying number of breaths by concentration given. Total cumulative units is the sum of cumulative units for each concentration given. See table on next page.
Dosage Forms
Powder for reconstitution, for oral inhalation:
Provocholine®: 100 mg

Methacholine

Vial	Serial Concentration (mg/mL)	No. of Breaths	Cumulative Units per Concentration	Total Cumulative Units
E	0.025	5	0.125	0.125
D	0.25	5	1.25	1.375
C	2.5	5	12.5	13.88
B	10	5	50	63.88
A	25	5	125	188.88

methacholine chloride see methacholine *on page 611*

Methacholine Omega [Can] see methacholine *on page 611*

methadone (METH a done)

Sound-Alike/Look-Alike Issues

methadone may be confused with dexmethylphenidate, Mephyton®, methylphenidate, Metadate® CD, and Metadate® ER

Synonyms methadone hydrochloride

U.S./Canadian Brand Names Dolophine® [US]; Metadol™ [Can]; Methadone Diskets® [US]; Methadone Intensol™ [US]; Methadose® [US]

Therapeutic Category Analgesic, Narcotic

Controlled Substance C-II

Use Management of moderate-to-severe pain; detoxification and maintenance treatment of opioid addiction (if used for detoxification and maintenance treatment of narcotic addiction, it must be part of an FDA-approved program)

Usual Dosage Note: These are guidelines and do not represent the maximum doses that may be required in all patients. Methadone accumulates with repeated doses and dosage may need reduction after 3-5 days to prevent CNS depressant effects. Some patients may benefit from every 8-12 hour dosing interval for chronic pain management. Doses should be titrated to appropriate effects.

Adults:

Acute pain (moderate to severe):

Oral: Opioid-naive: Initial: 2.5-10 mg every 8-12 hours; more frequent administration may be required during initiation to maintain adequate analgesia. Dosage interval may range from 4-12 hours, since duration of analgesia is relatively short during the first days of therapy, but increases substantially with continued administration.

Chronic pain (opioid-tolerant): **Conversion from oral morphine to oral methadone:**

Daily oral morphine dose <100 mg: Estimated daily oral methadone dose: 20% to 30% of total daily morphine dose

Daily oral morphine dose 100-300 mg: Estimated daily oral methadone dose: 10% to 20% of total daily morphine dose

Daily oral morphine dose 300-600 mg: Estimated daily oral methadone dose: 8% to 12% of total daily morphine dose

Daily oral morphine dose 600-1000 mg: Estimated daily oral methadone dose: 5% to 10% of total daily morphine dose.

Daily oral morphine dose >1000 mg: Estimated daily oral methadone dose: <5% of total daily morphine dose.

Note: The total daily methadone dose should then be divided to reflect the intended dosing schedule.

I.V.: Manufacturers labeling: Initial: 2.5-10 mg every 8-12 hours in opioid-naive patients; titrate slowly to effect; may also be administered by SubQ or I.M. injection

Conversion from oral methadone to parenteral methadone dose: Initial dose: Parenteral:Oral ratio: 1:2 (eg, 5 mg parenteral methadone equals 10 mg oral methadone)

Detoxification: Oral:

Initial: A single dose of 20-30 mg is generally sufficient to suppress symptoms. Should not exceed 30 mg; lower doses should be considered in patients with low tolerance at initiation (eg, absence of opioids ≥5 days); an additional 5-10 mg of methadone may be provided if withdrawal symptoms have not been suppressed or if symptoms reappear after 2-4 hours; total daily dose on the first day should not exceed 40 mg, unless the program physician documents in the patient's record that 40 mg did not control opiate abstinence symptoms.

Maintenance: Titrate to a dosage which attenuates craving, blocks euphoric effects of other opiates, and tolerance to sedative effect of methadone. Usual range: 80-120 mg/day (titration should occur cautiously)

Withdrawal: Dose reductions should be <10% of the maintenance dose, every 10-14 days

Detoxification (short-term): Oral:

Initial: Titrate to ~40 mg/day in divided doses to achieve stabilization, may continue 40 mg dose for 2-3 days

Maintenance: Titrate to a dosage which prevents/attenuates euphoric effects of self-administered opioids, reduces drug craving, and withdrawal symptoms are prevented for 24 hours.

Withdrawal: Requires individualization. Decrease daily or every other day, keeping withdrawal symptoms tolerable; hospitalized patients may tolerate a 20% reduction/day; ambulatory patients may require a slower reduction

Dosage Forms

Injection, solution: 10 mg/mL (20 mL)

Solution, oral: 5 mg/5 mL, 10 mg/5 mL

Solution, oral, as hydrochloride [concentrate]: 10 mg/mL

Methadone Intensol™, Methadose®: 10 mg/mL

Tablet: 5 mg, 10 mg

Dolophine®: 5 mg, 10 mg

Methadose®: 5 mg, 10 mg [DSC]

Tablet, dispersible: 40 mg

Methadose®, Methadone Diskets®: 40 mg

Methadone Diskets® [US] *see* methadone *on page 612*

methadone hydrochloride *see* methadone *on page 612*

Methadone Intensol™ [US] *see* methadone *on page 612*

Methadose® [US] *see* methadone *on page 612*

methaminodiazepoxide hydrochloride *see* chlordiazepoxide *on page 201*

methamphetamine (meth am FET a meen)

Sound-Alike/Look-Alike Issues

Desoxyn® may be confused with digoxin

Synonyms desoxyephedrine hydrochloride; methamphetamine hydrochloride

U.S./Canadian Brand Names Desoxyn® [US/Can]

Therapeutic Category Amphetamine

Controlled Substance C-II

Use Treatment of attention-deficit/hyperactivity disorder (ADHD); exogenous obesity (short-term adjunct)

Usual Dosage Oral:

Children ≥6 years and Adults: ADHD: 5 mg 1-2 times/day; may increase by 5 mg increments at weekly intervals until optimum response is achieved, usually 20-25 mg/day

Children ≥12 years and Adults: Exogenous obesity: 5 mg 30 minutes before each meal; treatment duration should not exceed a few weeks

Dosage Forms

Tablet: 5 mg

Desoxyn®: 5 mg

methamphetamine hydrochloride *see* methamphetamine *on page 613*

methazolamide (meth a ZOE la mide)

Sound-Alike/Look-Alike Issues

methazolamide may be confused with methenamine, metolazone

Neptazane® may be confused with Nesacaine®

U.S./Canadian Brand Names Apo-Methazolamide® [Can]

Therapeutic Category Carbonic Anhydrase Inhibitor

Use Adjunctive treatment of open-angle or secondary glaucoma; short-term therapy of narrow-angle glaucoma when delay of surgery is desired

Usual Dosage Oral: Adults: 50-100 mg 2-3 times/day

Dosage Forms

Tablet: 25 mg, 50 mg

methenamine (meth EN a meen)

Sound-Alike/Look-Alike Issues
methenamine may be confused with methazolamide, methionine
Urex™ may be confused with Eurax®, Serax®

Synonyms hexamethylenetetramine; methenamine hippurate; methenamine mandelate

U.S./Canadian Brand Names Dehydral® [Can]; Hiprex® [US/Can]; Mandelamine® [US/Can]; Urasal® [Can]; Urex™ [US/Can]

Therapeutic Category Antibiotic, Miscellaneous

Use Prophylaxis or suppression of recurrent urinary tract infections; urinary tract discomfort secondary to hypermotility

Usual Dosage Oral:

Children:
>2-6 years: *Mandelate:* 50-75 mg/kg/day in 3-4 doses or 0.25 g/30 lb 4 times/day
6-12 years:
Hippurate: 0.5-1 g twice daily
Mandelate: 50-75 mg/kg/day in 3-4 doses or 0.5 g 4 times/day
Children >12 years and Adults:
Hippurate: 1 g twice daily
Mandelate: 1 g 4 times/day after meals and at bedtime

Dosage Forms
Tablet: 500 mg, 1 g
Hiprex®, Urex™: 1 g
Mandelamine®: 500 mg, 1 g

methenamine hippurate *see* methenamine *on page 614*
methenamine mandelate *see* methenamine *on page 614*
Methergine® [US/Can] *see* methylergonovine *on page 621*

methimazole (meth IM a zole)

Sound-Alike/Look-Alike Issues
methimazole may be confused with metolazone

Synonyms thiamazole

U.S./Canadian Brand Names Dom-Methimazole [Can]; Northyx™ [US]; PHL-Methimazole [Can]; Tapazole® [US/Can]

Therapeutic Category Antithyroid Agent

Use Palliative treatment of hyperthyroidism, return the hyperthyroid patient to a normal metabolic state prior to thyroidectomy, and to control thyrotoxic crisis that may accompany thyroidectomy

Usual Dosage Oral: Administer in 3 equally divided doses at approximately 8-hour intervals

Children: Initial: 0.4 mg/kg/day in 3 divided doses; maintenance: 0.2 mg/kg/day in 3 divided doses up to 30 mg/24 hours maximum
Alternatively: Initial: 0.5-0.7 mg/kg/day **or** 15-20 mg/m²/day in 3 divided doses
Maintenance: 1/3 to 2/3 of the initial dose beginning when the patient is euthyroid
Maximum: 30 mg/24 hours

Adults: Initial: 15 mg/day in 3 divided doses (approximately every 8 hours) for mild hyperthyroidism; 30-40 mg/day in moderately-severe hyperthyroidism; 60 mg/day in severe hyperthyroidism; maintenance: 5-15 mg/day (may be given as a single daily dose in many cases)

Adjust dosage as required to achieve and maintain serum T_3, T_4, and TSH levels in the normal range. An elevated T_3 may be the sole indicator of inadequate treatment. An elevated TSH indicates excessive antithyroid treatment.

Thyrotoxic crisis (recommendations vary widely and have not been evaluated in comparative trials): Dosages of 20-30 mg every 6-12 hours have been recommended for short-term initial therapy, followed by gradual reduction to a maintenance dosage (5-15 mg/day). Rectal administration has been described.

Dosage Forms
Tablet: 5 mg, 10 mg, 20 mg
Northyx™: 5 mg, 10 mg, 15 mg, 20 mg
Tapazole®: 5 mg, 10 mg

Methitest™ [US] *see* methyltestosterone *on page 624*

methocarbamol (meth oh KAR ba mole)
Sound-Alike/Look-Alike Issues
methocarbamol may be confused with mephobarbital
Robaxin® may be confused with Rubex®
U.S./Canadian Brand Names Robaxin® [US/Can]
Therapeutic Category Skeletal Muscle Relaxant
Use Treatment of muscle spasm associated with acute painful musculoskeletal conditions; supportive therapy in tetanus
Usual Dosage
Tetanus: I.V.:
Children: Recommended **only** for use in tetanus: 15 mg/kg/dose or 500 mg/m^2/dose, may repeat every 6 hours if needed; maximum dose: 1.8 g/m^2/day for 3 days only
Adults: Initial dose: 1-3 g; may repeat dose every 6 hours until oral dosing is possible; injection should not be used for more than 3 consecutive days
Muscle spasm: Children ≥16 years and Adults:
Oral: 1.5 g 4 times/day for 2-3 days (up to 8 g/day may be given in severe conditions), then decrease to 4-4.5 g/day in 3-6 divided doses
I.M., I.V.: 1 g every 8 hours if oral not possible; injection should not be used for more than 3 consecutive days. If condition persists, may repeat course of therapy after a drug-free interval of 48 hours.
Dosage Forms
Injection, solution:
Robaxin®: 100 mg/mL (10 mL)
Tablet: 500 mg, 750 mg
Robaxin®: 500 mg, 750 mg

methohexital (meth oh HEKS i tal)
Sound-Alike/Look-Alike Issues
Brevital® may be confused with Brevibloc®
Synonyms methohexital sodium
U.S./Canadian Brand Names Brevital® Sodium [US]; Brevital® [Can]
Therapeutic Category Barbiturate
Controlled Substance C-IV
Use For induction of anesthesia prior to the use of other general anesthetic agents; as an adjunct to subpotent inhalational anesthetic agents for short surgical procedures; for short surgical, diagnostic, or therapeutic procedures associated with minimal painful stimuli
Additional indications for adults: For use with other parenteral agents, usually narcotic analgesics, to supplement subpotent inhalational anesthetic agents for longer surgical procedures; as an agent to induce a hypnotic state
Usual Dosage Doses must be titrated to effect
Manufacturer's recommendations:
Infants ≥1 month and Children:
I.M.: Induction: 6.6-10 mg/kg of a 5% solution
Rectal: Induction: Usual: 25 mg/kg of a 1% solution
Alternative pediatric dosing:
Children 3-12 years:
I.M.: Preoperative: 5-10 mg/kg/dose
I.V.: Induction: 1-2 mg/kg/dose
Rectal: Preoperative/induction: 20-35 mg/kg/dose; usual: 25 mg/kg/dose; maximum dose: 500 mg/dose; give as 10% aqueous solution
Adults: I.V.: Induction: 50-120 mg to start; 20-40 mg every 4-7 minutes
Dosage Forms
Injection, powder for reconstitution:
Brevital® Sodium: 500 mg, 2.5 g

methohexital sodium see methohexital on page 615

methotrexate (meth oh TREKS ate)
Sound-Alike/Look-Alike Issues
methotrexate may be confused with metolazone, mitoxantrone
MTX is an error-prone abbreviation (mistaken as mitoxantrone)

◀ **Synonyms** amethopterin; methotrexate sodium; NSC-740

U.S./Canadian Brand Names Apo-Methotrexate® [Can]; ratio-Methotrexate [Can]; Rheumatrex® Dose Pack® [US]; Trexall™ [US]

Therapeutic Category Antineoplastic Agent

Use Treatment of trophoblastic neoplasms; leukemias; psoriasis; rheumatoid arthritis (RA), including polyarticular-course juvenile rheumatoid arthritis (JRA); breast, head and neck, and lung carcinomas; osteosarcoma; soft-tissue sarcomas; carcinoma of gastrointestinal tract, esophagus, testes; lymphomas

Usual Dosage Refer to individual protocols.

Note: Doses between 100-500 mg/m^2 **may require** leucovorin rescue. Doses >500 mg/m^2 **require** leucovorin rescue: Oral, I.M., I.V.: Leucovorin 10-15 mg/m^2 every 6 hours for 8 or 10 doses, starting 24 hours after the start of methotrexate infusion. Continue until the methotrexate level is ≤0.1 micromolar (10^7M). Some clinicians continue leucovorin until the methotrexate level is <0.05 micromolar (5×10^8M) or 0.01 micromolar (10^8M).

If the 48-hour methotrexate level is >1 micromolar (10^7M) or the 72-hour methotrexate level is >0.2 micromolar (2×10^7M): I.V., I.M, Oral: Leucovorin 100 mg/m^2 every 6 hours until the methotrexate level is ≤0.1 micromolar (10^7M). Some clinicians continue leucovorin until the methotrexate level is <0.05 micromolar (5×10^8M) or 0.01 micromolar (10^8M).

Children:

Dermatomyositis: Oral: 15-20 mg/m^2/week as a single dose once weekly **or** 0.3-1 mg/kg/dose once weekly

Juvenile rheumatoid arthritis: Oral, I.M.: 10 mg/m^2 once weekly, then 5-15 mg/m^2/week as a single dose **or** as 3 divided doses given 12 hours apart

Antineoplastic dosage range:

Oral, I.M.: 7.5-30 mg/m^2/week **or** every 2 weeks

I.V.: 10-18,000 mg/m^2 bolus dosing **or** continuous infusion over 6-42 hours

Pediatric solid tumors (high-dose): I.V.:

<12 years: 12-25 g/m^2

≥12 years: 8 g/m^2

Acute lymphocytic leukemia (intermediate-dose): I.V.: Loading: 100 mg/m^2 bolus dose, followed by 900 mg/m^2/day infusion over 23-41 hours.

Meningeal leukemia: I.T.: 10-15 mg/m^2 (maximum dose: 15 mg) **or** an age-based dosing regimen; one possible system is:

≤3 months: 3 mg/dose

4-11 months: 6 mg/dose

1 year: 8 mg/dose

2 years: 10 mg/dose

≥3 years: 12 mg/dose

Adults: I.V.: Range is wide from 30-40 mg/m^2/week to 100-12,000 mg/m^2 with leucovorin rescue

Trophoblastic neoplasms:

Oral, I.M.: 15-30 mg/day for 5 days; repeat in 7 days for 3-5 courses

I.V.: 11 mg/m^2 days 1 through 5 every 3 weeks

Head and neck cancer: Oral, I.M., I.V.: 25-50 mg/m^2 once weekly

Mycosis fungoides (cutaneous T-cell lymphoma): Oral, I.M.: Initial (early stages):

5-50 mg once weekly **or**

15-37.5 mg twice weekly

Bladder cancer: I.V.:

30 mg/m^2 day 1 and 8 every 3 weeks **or**

30 mg/m^2 day 1, 15, and 22 every 4 weeks

Breast cancer: I.V.: 30-60 mg/m^2 days 1 and 8 every 3-4 weeks

Gastric cancer: I.V.: 1500 mg/m^2 every 4 weeks

Lymphoma, non-Hodgkin: I.V.:

30 mg/m^2 days 3 and 10 every 3 weeks **or**

120 mg/m^2 day 8 and 15 every 3-4 weeks **or**

200 mg/m^2 day 8 and 15 every 3 weeks **or**

400 mg/m^2 every 4 weeks for 3 cycles **or**

1 g/m^2 every 3 weeks **or**

1.5 g/m^2 every 4 weeks

Sarcoma: I.V.: 8-12 g/m^2 weekly for 2-4 weeks

Rheumatoid arthritis: Oral: 7.5 mg once weekly **or** 2.5 mg every 12 hours for 3 doses/week, not to exceed 20 mg/week

Psoriasis:
Oral: 2.5-5 mg/dose every 12 hours for 3 doses given weekly **or**
Oral, I.M.: 10-25 mg/dose given once weekly

Dosage Forms
Injection, powder for reconstitution [preservative free]: 20 mg, 1 g
Injection, solution: 25 mg/mL (2 mL, 10 mL)
Injection, solution [preservative free]: 25 mg/mL (2 mL, 4 mL, 8 mL, 10 mL, 40 mL)
Tablet: 2.5 mg
Trexall™: 5 mg, 7.5 mg, 10 mg, 15 mg
Tablet [dose pack]: 2.5 mg (4 cards with 2, 3, 4, 5, or 6 tablets each)
Rheumatrex® Dose Pack: 2.5 mg (4 cards with 2, 3, 4, 5, or 6 tablets each)

methotrexate sodium *see* methotrexate *on page 615*

methotrimeprazine *(Canada only)* (meth oh trye MEP ra zeen)

Synonyms levomepromazine; methotrimeprazine hydrochloride
U.S./Canadian Brand Names Apo-Methoprazine® [Can]; Novo Meprazine [Can]; Nozinan® [Can]; PMS-Methotrimeprazine [Can]
Therapeutic Category Neuroleptic Agent
Use Treatment of schizophrenia or psychosis; management of pain, including pain caused by neuralgia or cancer; adjunct to general anesthesia; management of nausea and vomiting; sedation

Usual Dosage
Children >2 years:
Oral: 0.25 mg/kg/day in 2-3 divided doses; may increase gradually based on response.
Maximum dose: 40 mg/day in children <12 years
I.M.: 0.06-0.125 mg/kg/day in 1-3 divided doses
Adults:
Oral:
Anxiety, mild-moderate pain: 6-25 mg/day in 3 divided doses
Psychoses, severe pain: 50-75 mg/day in 2-3 divided doses; titrate to effect (doses up to 1000 mg/day or greater have been used in treatment of some patients with psychoses). If higher dosages are used to initiate therapy (100-200 mg/day), patients should be restricted to bed for the first few days of therapy.
Sedative: 10-25 mg at bedtime
I.M.:
Psychoses, severe pain: 75-100 mg (administered in 3-4 deep I.M. injections)
Analgesia (postoperative): 10-25 mg every 8 hours (2.5-7.5 mg every 4-6 hours is suggested postoperatively if residual effects of anesthetic may be present)
Premedication: 10-25 mg every 8 hours (final preoperative dose may be 25-50 mg administered ~1 hour prior to surgery)
I.V.: During surgical procedures/labor: 20-50 mcg/minute (some patients may require up to 100 mcg/minute)
SubQ (continuous infusion): Palliative care: 25-200 mcg/day (via syringe driver)

Dosage Forms [CAN] = Canadian brand name
Injection, solution:
Nozinan® [CAN]: 25 mg/mL (1 mL) [not available in the U.S.]
Solution, oral:
Nozinan® [CAN]: 5 mg/mL [not available in the U.S.]
Solution, oral drops:
Nozinan® [CAN]: 40 mg/mL [not available in the U.S.]
Tablet:
Apo-Methoprazine® [CAN]: 2 mg, 5 mg, 25 mg, 50 mg [not available in the U.S.]
Nozinan® [CAN]: 5 mg, 25 mg, 50 mg [not available in the U.S.]

methotrimeprazine hydrochloride *see* methotrimeprazine *(Canada only) on page 617*

methoxsalen (meth OKS a len)

Sound-Alike/Look-Alike Issues
methoxsalen soft gelatin capsules (Oxsoralen-Ultra®) may be confused with methoxsalen hard gelatin capsules (8-MOP®, Oxsoralen®); bioavailability and photosensitization onset differ between the two products. ▶

◄ **Synonyms** 8-methoxypsoralen; methoxypsoralen

U.S./Canadian Brand Names 8-MOP® [US]; Oxsoralen-Ultra® [US/Can]; Oxsoralen® [US/Can]; Ultramop™ [Can]; Uvadex® [US/Can]

Therapeutic Category Psoralen

Use

Oral: Symptomatic control of severe, recalcitrant disabling psoriasis; repigmentation of idiopathic vitiligo; palliative treatment of skin manifestations of cutaneous T-cell lymphoma (CTCL)

Topical: Repigmentation of idiopathic vitiligo

Extracorporeal: Palliative treatment of skin manifestations of CTCL

Usual Dosage Note: Refer to treatment protocols for UVA exposure guidelines.

Children >12 years and Adults: Vitiligo: Topical: Lotion is applied prior to UVA light exposure, usually no more than once weekly

Adults:

Psoriasis: Oral:

Initial: 10-70 mg 1.5-2 hours (Oxsoralen-Ultra®) or 2 hours (8-MOP®) before exposure to UVA light; dose may be repeated 2-3 times per week, based on UVA exposure; doses must be given at least 48 hours apart. Dosage is based upon patient's body weight and skin type:

<30 kg: 10 mg

30-50 kg: 20 mg

51-65 kg: 30 mg

66-80 kg: 40 mg

81-90 kg: 50 mg

91-115 kg: 60 mg

>115 kg: 70 mg

Note: Dosage may be increased (one time) by 10 mg after 15th treatment if minimal or no response.

Maintenance: When 95% psoriasis clearing achieved, may begin 1 treatment every week for at least 2 treatments; followed by 1 treatment every 2 weeks for at least 2 treatments; then every 3 weeks for at least 2 treatments then as needed to maintain response while minimizing UVA exposure.

Vitiligo:

Oral (8-MOP®): 20 mg 2-4 hours before exposure to UVA light; dose may be repeated based on erythema and tenderness of skin; do not give on 2 consecutive days

Topical (Oxsoralen®): Lotion is applied prior to UVA light exposure, usually no more than once weekly

CTCL: Extracorporeal (Uvadex®): 200 mcg injected into the photoactivation bag during the collection cycle using the UVAR® photopheresis system (consult user's guide). Treatment schedule: Two consecutive days every 4 weeks for a minimum of 7 treatment cycles, may accelerate to two consecutive days every 2 weeks if skin score worsens (eg, increases from baseline) after assessment during the fourth treatment cycle. If skin score improves by 25% after 4 consecutive weeks of accelerated therapy, may resume regular treatment schedule. Maximum: 20 accelerated therapy cycles.

Dosage Forms

Capsule:

8-MOP®, Oxsoralen-Ultra®: 10 mg

Lotion:

Oxsoralen®: 1% (30 mL)

Solution, for extracorporeal administration:

Uvadex®: 20 mcg/mL (10 mL) **[not for injection]**

methoxypsoralen *see* methoxsalen *on page 617*

8-methoxypsoralen *see* methoxsalen *on page 617*

methscopolamine (meth skoe POL a meen)

Synonyms methscopolamine bromide

U.S./Canadian Brand Names Pamine® Forte [US]; Pamine® [US/Can]

Therapeutic Category Anticholinergic Agent

Use Adjunctive therapy in the treatment of peptic ulcer

Usual Dosage Oral: Adults: 2.5 mg 30 minutes before meals or food and 2.5-5 mg at bedtime; may increase dose to 5 mg twice daily

Dosage Forms

Tablet: 2.5 mg, 5 mg

Pamine®: 2.5 mg

Pamine® Forte: 5 mg

methscopolamine and pseudoephedrine *see* pseudoephedrine and methscopolamine *on page 803*

methscopolamine bromide *see* methscopolamine *on page 618*

methscopolamine, chlorpheniramine, and pseudoephedrine *see* chlorpheniramine, pseudoephedrine, and methscopolamine *on page 213*

methscopolamine nitrate, chlorpheniramine maleate, and phenylephrine hydrochloride *see* chlorpheniramine, phenylephrine, and methscopolamine *on page 210*

methscopolamine, pseudoephedrine, and chlorpheniramine *see* chlorpheniramine, pseudoephedrine, and methscopolamine *on page 213*

methsuximide (meth SUKS i mide)

Sound-Alike/Look-Alike Issues
methsuximide may be confused with ethosuximide

U.S./Canadian Brand Names Celontin® [US/Can]

Therapeutic Category Anticonvulsant

Use Control of absence (petit mal) seizures that are refractory to other drugs

Usual Dosage Oral: Anticonvulsant:
Children: Initial: 10-15 mg/kg/day in 3-4 divided doses; increase weekly up to maximum of 30 mg/kg/day
Adults: 300 mg/day for the first week; may increase by 300 mg/day at weekly intervals up to 1.2 g/day in 2-4 divided doses/day

Dosage Forms
Capsule:
Celontin®: 150 mg, 300 mg

methyclothiazide (meth i kloe THYE a zide)

Sound-Alike/Look-Alike Issues
Enduron® may be confused with Empirin®, Imuran®, Inderal®

U.S./Canadian Brand Names Aquatensen® [Can]; Enduron® [Can]

Therapeutic Category Diuretic, Thiazide

Use Management of mild-to-moderate hypertension; treatment of edema in congestive heart failure and nephrotic syndrome

Usual Dosage Oral: Adults:
Edema: 2.5-10 mg/day
Hypertension: 2.5-5 mg/day; may add another antihypertensive if 5 mg is not adequate after a trial of 8-12 weeks of therapy

Dosage Forms
Tablet: 5 mg

methylacetoxyprogesterone *see* medroxyprogesterone *on page 597*

methylcellulose (meth il SEL yoo lose)

Sound-Alike/Look-Alike Issues
Citrucel® may be confused with Citracal®

U.S./Canadian Brand Names Citrucel® Fiber Shake [US-OTC]; Citrucel® Fiber Smoothie [US-OTC]; Citrucel® [US-OTC]

Therapeutic Category Laxative

Use Adjunct in treatment of constipation

Usual Dosage Oral:
Children 6-12 years:
Citrucel® caplet: 1 caplet up to 6 times/day; follow each dose with 8 oz of water
Citrucel® powder: Half the adult dose in 4 oz of cold water, 1-3 times/day
Children ≥12 years and Adults:
Citrucel® caplet: 2-4 caplets 1-3 times/day; follow each dose with 8 oz of water
Citrucel® powder: 1 heaping tablespoon (19 g) in 8 oz of cold water, 1-3 times/day

Dosage Forms
Caplet:
Citrucel® [OTC]: 500 mg

◀ **Powder:** 2 g/level scoop
Citrucel® Fiber Smoothie: 2 g/level scoop (275 g, 539 g)
Citrucel®: 2 g/level scoop (448 g, 840 g, 1418g, 1843 g)
Citrucel® [sugar free formulation]: 2 g/level scoop (473 g, 907g, 1190 g)
Citrucel® Fiber Shake: 2 g/level scoop (204 g, 413 g)

methylcellulose, gelatin, and pectin *see* gelatin, pectin, and methylcellulose *on page 438*

methyldopa (meth il DOE pa)

Sound-Alike/Look-Alike Issues
methyldopa may be confused with L-dopa, levodopa
Synonyms methyldopate hydrochloride
U.S./Canadian Brand Names Apo-Methyldopa® [Can]; Nu-Medopa [Can]
Therapeutic Category Alpha-Adrenergic Blocking Agent
Use Management of moderate-to-severe hypertension
Usual Dosage
Children:
Oral: Initial: 10 mg/kg/day in 2-4 divided doses; increase every 2 days as needed to maximum dose of 65 mg/kg/day; do not exceed 3 g/day.
I.V.: 5-10 mg/kg/dose every 6-8 hours up to a total dose of 65 mg/kg/24 hours or 3 g/24 hours
Adults:
Oral: Initial: 250 mg 2-3 times/day; increase every 2 days as needed (maximum dose: 3 g/day): usual dose range (JNC 7): 250-1000 mg/day in 2 divided doses
I.V.: 250-500 mg every 6-8 hours; maximum dose: 1 g every 6 hours
Dosage Forms
Injection, solution: 50 mg/mL (5 mL)
Tablet: 250 mg, 500 mg

methyldopa and hydrochlorothiazide (meth il DOE pa & hye droe klor oh THYE a zide)

Sound-Alike/Look-Alike Issues
Aldoril® may be confused with Aldoclor®, Aldomet®, Elavil®
Synonyms hydrochlorothiazide and methyldopa
U.S./Canadian Brand Names Aldoril® [US]; Apo-Methazide® [Can]
Therapeutic Category Antihypertensive Agent, Combination
Use Management of moderate-to-severe hypertension
Usual Dosage Oral: Dosage titrated on individual components, then switch to combination product; no more than methyldopa 3 g/day and/or hydrochlorothiazide 50 mg/day; maintain initial dose for first 48 hours, then decrease or increase at intervals of not less than 2 days until an adequate response is achieved
Methyldopa 250 mg and hydrochlorothiazide 15 mg: 2-3 times/day
Methyldopa 250 mg and hydrochlorothiazide 25 mg: Twice daily
Dosage Forms
Tablet: Methyldopa 250 mg and hydrochlorothiazide 15 mg; methyldopa 250 mg and hydrochlorothiazide 25 mg
Aldoril® 25: Methyldopa 250 mg and hydrochlorothiazide 25 mg

methyldopate hydrochloride *see* methyldopa *on page 620*

methylene blue (METH i leen bloo)

Therapeutic Category Antidote
Use Antidote for cyanide poisoning and drug-induced methemoglobinemia, indicator dye
Usual Dosage
Children: NADPH-methemoglobin reductase deficiency: Oral: 1-1.5 mg/kg/day (maximum: 300 mg/day) given with 5-8 mg/kg/day of ascorbic acid
Children and Adults: Methemoglobinemia: I.V.: 1-2 mg/kg or 25-50 mg/m^2 over several minutes; may be repeated in 1 hour if necessary
Adults: Genitourinary antiseptic: Oral: 65-130 mg 3 times/day with a full glass of water (maximum: 390 mg/day)
Dosage Forms
Injection, solution: 10 mg/mL (1 mL, 10 mL)

methylergometrine maleate *see* methylergonovine *on page 621*

methylergonovine (meth il er goe NOE veen)

Sound-Alike/Look-Alike Issues
methylergonovine and terbutaline parenteral dosage forms look similar. Due to their contrasting indications, use care when administering these agents.

Synonyms methylergometrine maleate; methylergonovine maleate

U.S./Canadian Brand Names Methergine® [US/Can]

Therapeutic Category Ergot Alkaloid and Derivative

Use Prevention and treatment of postpartum and postabortion hemorrhage caused by uterine atony or subinvolution

Usual Dosage Adults:
Oral: 0.2 mg 3-4 times/day in the puerperium for 2-7 days
I.M., I.V.: 0.2 mg after delivery of anterior shoulder, after delivery of placenta, or during puerperium; may be repeated as required at intervals of 2-4 hours

Dosage Forms
Injection, solution:
Methergine®: 0.2 mg/mL (1 mL)
Tablet:
Methergine®: 0.2 mg

methylergonovine maleate *see* methylergonovine *on page 621*

methylfolate (meth il FO late)

Synonyms 6(S)-5-methyltetrahydrofolate; 6(S)-5-MTHF; L-methylfolate

U.S./Canadian Brand Names Deplin™ [US]

Therapeutic Category Dietary Supplement

Use Medicinal food for management of patients with low plasma and/or low red blood cell folate

Usual Dosage Oral: Adults: One tablet (7.5 mg) daily

Dosage Forms
Tablet:
Deplin™: L-methylfolate 7.5 mg [gluten free, lactose free, sugar free, yeast free]

Methylin® [US] *see* methylphenidate *on page 622*
Methylin® ER [US] *see* methylphenidate *on page 622*
methylmorphine *see* codeine *on page 242*

methylnaltrexone (meth il nal TREKS one)

Sound-Alike/Look-Alike Issues
methylnaltrexone may be confused with naltrexone

Synonyms methylnaltrexone bromide; N-methylnaltrexone bromide

U.S./Canadian Brand Names Relistor™ [US]

Therapeutic Category Gastrointestinal Agent, Miscellaneous; Opioid Antagonist, Peripherally-Acting

Use Treatment of opioid-induced constipation in patients with advanced illness receiving palliative care with inadequate response to conventional laxative regimens

Usual Dosage SubQ: Adults: Opioid-induced constipation: Dosing is according to body weight: Administer 1 dose every other day as needed; maximum: 1 dose/24 hours
<38 kg: 0.15 mg/kg (round dose up to nearest 0.1 mL of volume)
38 to <62 kg: 8 mg
62-114 kg: 12 mg
>114 kg: 0.15 mg/kg (round dose up to nearest 0.1 mL of volume)

Dosage Forms
Injection, solution:
Relistor™: 12 mg/0.6 mL (0.6 mL) [contains edetate calcium disodium]

methylnaltrexone bromide *see* methylnaltrexone *on page 621*

methylphenidate (meth il FEN i date)

Sound-Alike/Look-Alike Issues
methylphenidate may be confused with methadone
Metadate® CD may be confused with Metadate® ER
Metadate® ER may be confused with Metadate® CD, methadone
Ritalin® may be confused with Ismelin®, Rifadin®, ritodrine

Synonyms methylphenidate hydrochloride

U.S./Canadian Brand Names Apo-Methylphenidate® SR [Can]; Apo-Methylphenidate® [Can]; Biphentin® [Can]; Concerta® [US/Can]; Daytrana™ [US]; Metadate® CD [US]; Metadate® ER [US]; Methylin® ER [US]; Methylin® [US]; PMS-Methylphenidate [Can]; Riphenidate [Can]; Ritalin-SR® [US/Can]; Ritalin® LA [US]; Ritalin® [US/Can]

Therapeutic Category Central Nervous System Stimulant, Nonamphetamine

Controlled Substance C-II

Use Treatment of attention-deficit/hyperactivity disorder (ADHD); symptomatic management of narcolepsy

Usual Dosage

ADHD:

Oral:

Immediate release products Children ≥6 years and Adults: Initial: 5 mg/dose (~0.3 mg/kg/dose) given twice daily before breakfast and lunch; increase by 5-10 mg/day (0.2 mg/kg/day) at weekly intervals; maximum dose: 60 mg/day (2 mg/kg/day). **Note:** Discontinue periodically to reevaluate or if no improvement occurs within 1 month.

Extended release products:

Children ≥6 years and Adults:

Metadate® ER, Methylin® ER, Ritalin-SR®: May be given in place of immediate release products, once the daily dose is titrated and the titrated 8-hour dosage corresponds to sustained or extended release tablet size; maximum: 60 mg/day

Metadate® CD, Ritalin® LA: Initial: 20 mg once daily; may be adjusted in 10-20 mg increments at weekly intervals; maximum: 60 mg/day

Children 6-12 years and Adolescents 13-17 years: *Concerta®:*

Patients not currently taking methylphenidate: Initial dose: 18 mg once daily in the morning

Patients currently taking methylphenidate: **Note:** Initial dose: Dosing based on current regimen and clinical judgment; suggested dosing listed below:

- Patients taking methylphenidate 5 mg 2-3 times/day **or** 20 mg/day sustained release formulation: 18 mg once every morning
- Patients taking methylphenidate 10 mg 2-3 times/day **or** 40 mg/day sustained release formulation: 36 mg once every morning
- Patients taking methylphenidate 15 mg 2-3 times/day **or** 60 mg/day sustained release formulation: 54 mg once every morning

Dose adjustment: May increase dose in increments of 18 mg; dose may be adjusted at weekly intervals. A dosage strength of 27 mg is available for situations in which a dosage between 18-36 mg is desired. Maximum dose should not exceed 2 mg/kg/day **or** 54 mg/day in children 6-12 years or 72 mg/day in children 13-17 years.

Transdermal (Daytrana™): Children ≥6 years: Initial: 10 mg patch once daily; remove up to 9 hours after application. Titrate based on response and tolerability; may increase to next transdermal dose no more frequently than every week. **Note:** Application should occur 2 hours prior to desired effect. Drug absorption may continue for a period of time after patch removal; patients converting from another formulation of methylphenidate should be initiated at 10 mg regardless of their previous dose and titrated as needed due to the differences in bioavailability of the transdermal formulation.

Narcolepsy: Oral: Adults: 10 mg 2-3 times/day, up to 60 mg/day

Dosage Forms

Capsule, extended release, oral, [bi-modal release]:

Metadate CD®: 10 mg [3 mg immediate release, 7 mg extended release]; 20 mg [6 mg immediate release, 14 mg extended release]; 30 mg [9 mg immediate release, 21 mg extended release]; 40 mg [12 mg immediate release, 28 mg extended release]; 50 mg [15 mg immediate release, 35 mg extended release]; 60 mg [18 mg immediate release, 42 mg extended release]

Ritalin LA®: 10 mg [5 mg immediate release, 5 mg extended release]; 20 mg [10 mg immediate release, 10 mg extended release]; 30 mg [15 mg immediate release, 15 mg extended release]; 40 mg [20 mg immediate release, 20 mg extended release]

Solution, oral:

Methylin®: 5 mg/5 mL, 10 mg/5 mL

Tablet: 5 mg, 10 mg, 20 mg
  Methylin®, Ritalin®: 5 mg, 10 mg, 20 mg
Tablet, chewable:
  Methylin®: 2.5 mg, 5 mg, 10 mg
Tablet, extended release: 20 mg
  Metadate® ER, Methylin® ER: 10 mg, 20 mg
Tablet, extended release [bi-modal release]:
  Concerta®: 18 mg, 27 mg, 36 mg, 54 mg
Tablet, sustained release: 20 mg
  Ritalin-SR®: 20 mg
Transdermal system [once-daily patch]:
  Daytrana™: 10 mg/9 hours (30s); 15 mg/9 hours (30s); 20 mg/9 hours (30s); 30 mg/9 hours (30s)

methylphenidate hydrochloride see methylphenidate on page 622
methylphenobarbital see mephobarbital on page 604
methylphenoxy-benzene propanamine see atomoxetine on page 102
methylphenyl isoxazolyl penicillin see oxacillin on page 705
methylphytyl napthoquinone see phytonadione on page 752

methylprednisolone (meth il pred NIS oh lone)

Sound-Alike/Look-Alike Issues
  methylPREDNISolone may be confused with medroxyPROGESTERone, predniSONE
  Depo-Medrol® may be confused with Solu-Medrol®
  Medrol® may be confused with Mebaral®
  Solu-Medrol® may be confused with Depo-Medrol®, Solu-Cortef®

Synonyms 6-α-methylprednisolone; A-methapred; methylprednisolone acetate; methylprednisolone sodium succinate

Tall-Man methyl**PREDNIS**olone

U.S./Canadian Brand Names Depo-Medrol® [US/Can]; Medrol® [US/Can]; Methylprednisolone Acetate [Can]; Solu-Medrol® [US/Can]

Therapeutic Category Adrenal Corticosteroid

Use Primarily as an antiinflammatory or immunosuppressant agent in the treatment of a variety of diseases including those of hematologic, allergic, inflammatory, neoplastic, and autoimmune origin. Prevention and treatment of graft-versus-host disease following allogeneic bone marrow transplantation.

Usual Dosage Dosing should be based on the lesser of ideal body weight or actual body weight

Only sodium succinate may be given I.V.; methylprednisolone sodium succinate is highly soluble and has a rapid effect by I.M. and I.V. routes. Methylprednisolone acetate has a low solubility and has a sustained I.M. effect.

Children:
  Antiinflammatory or immunosuppressive: Oral, I.M., I.V. (sodium succinate): 0.5-1.7 mg/kg/day **or** 5-25 mg/m²/day in divided doses every 6-12 hours; "Pulse" therapy: 15-30 mg/kg/dose over ≥30 minutes given once daily for 3 days
  Status asthmaticus: I.V. (sodium succinate): Loading dose: 2 mg/kg/dose, then 0.5-1 mg/kg/dose every 6 hours for up to 5 days
  Acute spinal cord injury: I.V. (sodium succinate): 30 mg/kg over 15 minutes, followed in 45 minutes by a continuous infusion of 5.4 mg/kg/hour for 23 hours
  Lupus nephritis: I.V. (sodium succinate): 30 mg/kg over ≥30 minutes every other day for 6 doses

Adults: **Only sodium succinate may be given I.V.;** methylprednisolone sodium succinate is highly soluble and has a rapid effect by I.M. and I.V. routes. Methylprednisolone acetate has a low solubility and has a sustained I.M. effect.
  Acute spinal cord injury: I.V. (sodium succinate): 30 mg/kg over 15 minutes, followed in 45 minutes by a continuous infusion of 5.4 mg/kg/hour for 23 hours
  Allergic conditions: Oral: Tapered-dosage schedule:
    Day 1: 24 mg on day 1 administered as 8 mg before breakfast, 4 mg after lunch, 4 mg after supper, and 8 mg at bedtime **OR** 24 mg as a single dose or divided into 2 or 3 doses upon initiation (regardless of time of day)
    Day 2: 20 mg on day 2 administered as 4 mg before breakfast, 4 mg after lunch, 4 mg after supper, and 8 mg at bedtime
    Day 3: 16 mg on day 3 administered as 4 mg before breakfast, 4 mg after lunch, 4 mg after supper, and 4 mg at bedtime

Day 4: 12 mg on day 4 administered as 4 mg before breakfast, 4 mg after lunch, and 4 mg at bedtime
Day 5: 8 mg on day 5 administered as 4 mg before breakfast and 4 mg at bedtime
Day 6: 4 mg on day 6 administered as 4 mg before breakfast
Antiinflammatory or immunosuppressive:
Oral: 2-60 mg/day in 1-4 divided doses to start, followed by gradual reduction in dosage to the lowest possible level consistent with maintaining an adequate clinical response.
I.M. (sodium succinate): 10-80 mg/day once daily
I.M. (acetate): 10-80 mg every 1-2 weeks
I.V. (sodium succinate): 10-40 mg over a period of several minutes and repeated I.V. or I.M. at intervals depending on clinical response; when high dosages are needed, give 30 mg/kg over a period ≥30 minutes and may be repeated every 4-6 hours for 48 hours.
Status asthmaticus: I.V. (sodium succinate): Loading dose: 2 mg/kg/dose, then 0.5-1 mg/kg/dose every 6 hours for up to 5 days
Lupus nephritis: High-dose "pulse" therapy: I.V. (sodium succinate): 1 g/day for 3 days
Aplastic anemia: I.V. (sodium succinate): 1 mg/kg/day or 40 mg/day (whichever dose is higher), for 4 days. After 4 days, change to oral and continue until day 10 or until symptoms of serum sickness resolve, then rapidly reduce over approximately 2 weeks.
Pneumocystis pneumonia in AIDs patients: I.V.: 30 mg twice daily for 5 days, then 30 mg once daily for 5 days, then 15 mg once daily for 11 days
Intraarticular (acetate): Administer every 1-5 weeks.
Large joints: 20-80 mg
Small joints: 4-10 mg
Intralesional (acetate): 20-60 mg every 1-5 weeks

Dosage Forms
Injection, powder for reconstitution: 40 mg, 125 mg, 500 mg, 1 g
Solu-Medrol®: 40 mg, 125 mg, 500 mg, 1 g, 2 g
Solu-Medrol®: 500 mg, 1 g
Injection, suspension: 40 mg/mL (5 mL, 10 mL); 80 mg/mL (5 mL)
Depo-Medrol®: 20 mg/mL (5 mL); 40 mg/mL (5 mL); 80 mg/mL (5 mL)
Depo-Medrol®: 40 mg/mL (1 mL); 80 mg/mL (1 mL)
Tablet: 4 mg
Medrol®: 2 mg, 4 mg, 8 mg, 16 mg, 32 mg
Tablet, dose-pack: 4 mg (21s)
Medrol® Dosepak™: 4 mg (21s)

6-α-methylprednisolone *see* methylprednisolone *on page 623*
Methylprednisolone Acetate [Can] *see* methylprednisolone *on page 623*
methylprednisolone acetate *see* methylprednisolone *on page 623*
methylprednisolone sodium succinate *see* methylprednisolone *on page 623*
4-methylpyrazole *see* fomepizole *on page 423*

methyltestosterone (meth il tes TOS te rone)

Sound-Alike/Look-Alike Issues
methylTESTOSTERone may be confused with medroxyPROGESTERone
Virilon® may be confused with Verelan®
Tall-Man methylTESTOSTERone
U.S./Canadian Brand Names Android® [US]; Methitest™ [US]; Testred® [US]; Virilon® [US]
Therapeutic Category Androgen
Controlled Substance C-III
Use
Male: Hypogonadism; delayed puberty; impotence and climacteric symptoms
Female: Palliative treatment of metastatic breast cancer
Usual Dosage Adults (buccal absorption produces twice the androgenic activity of oral tablets):
Male:
Hypogonadism, male climacteric and impotence: Oral: 10-40 mg/day
Androgen deficiency:
Oral: 10-50 mg/day
Buccal: 5-25 mg/day
Postpubertal cryptorchidism: Oral: 30 mg/day

Female:
  Breast pain/engorgement:
    Oral: 80 mg/day for 3-5 days
    Buccal: 40 mg/day for 3-5 days
  Breast cancer:
    Oral: 50-200 mg/day
    Buccal: 25-100 mg/day
Dosage Forms
  Capsule:
    Android®, Testred®, Virilon®: 10 mg
  Tablet:
    Methitest™: 10 mg

Meticorten® (Discontinued) see prednisone on page 782
Metimyd Ophthalmic Ointment (Discontinued)

metipranolol (met i PRAN oh lol)
Sound-Alike/Look-Alike Issues
  metipranolol may be confused with metaproterenol
Synonyms metipranolol hydrochloride
U.S./Canadian Brand Names OptiPranolol® [US/Can]
Therapeutic Category Beta-Adrenergic Blocker
Use Agent for lowering intraocular pressure in patients with chronic open-angle glaucoma
Usual Dosage Ophthalmic: Adults: Instill 1 drop in the affected eye(s) twice daily
Dosage Forms
  Solution, ophthalmic: 0.3% (5 mL, 10 mL)
    OptiPranolol®: 0.3% (5 mL, 10 mL)

metipranolol hydrochloride see metipranolol on page 625

metoclopramide (met oh KLOE pra mide)
Sound-Alike/Look-Alike Issues
  metoclopramide may be confused with metolazone
  Reglan® may be confused with Megace®, Regonol®, Renagel®
U.S./Canadian Brand Names Apo-Metoclop® [Can]; Metoclopramide Hydrochloride Injection [Can]; Nu-Metoclopramide [Can]; Reglan® [US]
Therapeutic Category Gastrointestinal Agent, Prokinetic
Use
  Oral: Symptomatic treatment of diabetic gastric stasis; gastroesophageal reflux
  I.V., I.M.: Symptomatic treatment of diabetic gastric stasis; postpyloric placement of enteral feeding tubes; prevention and/or treatment of nausea and vomiting associated with chemotherapy, or postsurgery; to stimulate gastric emptying and intestinal transit of barium during radiological examination
Usual Dosage
  Children:
    Postpyloric feeding tube placement: I.V.:
      <6 years: 0.1 mg/kg
      6-14 years: 2.5-5 mg
      >14 years: Refer to Adults dosing.
  Adults:
    Gastroesophageal reflux: Oral: 10-15 mg/dose up to 4 times/day 30 minutes before meals or food and at bedtime; single doses of 20 mg are occasionally needed for provoking situations. Treatment >12 weeks has not been evaluated.
    Diabetic gastric stasis:
      Oral: 10 mg 30 minutes before each meal and at bedtime
      I.M., I.V. (for severe symptoms): 10 mg over 1-2 minutes; 10 days of I.V. therapy may be necessary for best response
    Chemotherapy-induced emesis:
      I.V.: 1-2 mg/kg 30 minutes before chemotherapy and repeated every 2 hours for 2 doses, then every 3 hours for 3 doses (manufacturer labeling)
      Alternate dosing (with or without diphenhydramine):
        Moderate emetic risk chemotherapy: 0.5 mg/kg every 6 hours on days 2-4

◄

Low and minimal risk chemotherapy: 1-2 mg/kg every 3-4 hours
Breakthrough treatment: 1-2 mg/kg every 3-4 hours
Postoperative nausea and vomiting: I.M., I.V.: 10-20 mg near end of surgery
Postpyloric feeding tube placement, radiological exam: I.V.: 10 mg

Dosage Forms
Injection, solution [preservative free]: 5 mg/mL (2 mL)
Reglan®: 5 mg/mL (2 mL, 10 mL, 30 mL)
Solution, oral: 5 mg/5 mL (10 mL, 480 mL)
Tablet: 5 mg, 10 mg
Reglan®: 5 mg, 10 mg

Metoclopramide Hydrochloride Injection [Can] *see* metoclopramide *on page 625*

metolazone (me TOLE a zone)

Sound-Alike/Look-Alike Issues
metolazone may be confused with metaxalone, methazolamide, methimazole, methotrexate, metoclopramide, metoprolol, minoxidil
Zaroxolyn® may be confused with Zarontin®

U.S./Canadian Brand Names Zaroxolyn® [US/Can]

Therapeutic Category Diuretic, Miscellaneous

Use Management of mild-to-moderate hypertension; treatment of edema in congestive heart failure and nephrotic syndrome, impaired renal function

Usual Dosage Oral: Adults:
Edema: 2.5-20 mg/dose every 24 hours (ACC/AHA 2005 Heart Failure Guidelines)
Hypertension: 2.5-5 mg/dose every 24 hours

Dosage Forms
Tablet: 2.5 mg, 5 mg, 10 mg
Zaroxolyn®: 2.5 mg, 5 mg, 10 mg

Metopirone® [US] *see* metyrapone *on page 629*

metoprolol (me toe PROE lole)

Sound-Alike/Look-Alike Issues
metoprolol may be confused with metaproterenol, metolazone, misoprostol
Toprol-XL® may be confused with Tegretol®, Tegretol®-XR, Topamax®

Synonyms metoprolol succinate; metoprolol tartrate

U.S./Canadian Brand Names Apo-Metoprolol® [Can]; Betaloc® Durules® [Can]; Betaloc® [Can]; Dom-Metoprolol [Can]; Gen-Metoprolol [Can]; Lopressor® [US/Can]; Metoprolol Tartrate Injection, USP [Can]; Metoprolol-25 [Can]; Novo-Metoprolol [Can]; Nu-Metop [Can]; PHL-Metoprolol [Can]; PMS-Metoprolol [Can]; Sandoz-Metoprolol [Can]; Toprol-XL® [US/Can]

Therapeutic Category Beta-Adrenergic Blocker

Use Treatment of angina pectoris, hypertension, or hemodynamically-stable acute myocardial infarction
Extended release: Treatment of angina pectoris or hypertension; to reduce mortality/hospitalization in patients with heart failure (stable NYHA Class II or III) already receiving ACE inhibitors, diuretics, and/or digoxin

Usual Dosage
Children: Hypertension: Oral:
1-17 years: Immediate release tablet: (National High Blood Pressure Education Program Working Group on High Blood Pressure in Children and Adolescents, 2004): Initial: 1-2 mg/kg/day; maximum 6 mg/kg/day (≤200 mg/day); administer in 2 divided doses
≥6 years: Extended release tablet: Initial: 1 mg/kg once daily (maximum initial dose: 50 mg/day). Adjust dose based on patient response (maximum: 2 mg/kg/day or 200 mg/day)
Adults:
Hypertension: Oral: 100-450 mg/day in 2-3 divided doses, begin with 50 mg twice daily and increase doses at weekly intervals to desired effect; usual dosage range (JNC 7): 50-100 mg/day
Extended release: Initial: 25-100 mg/day (maximum: 400 mg/day)
Angina, SVT, MI prophylaxis: Oral: 100-450 mg/day in 2-3 divided doses, begin with 50 mg twice daily and increase doses at weekly intervals to desired effect
Extended release: Initial: 100 mg/day (maximum: 400 mg/day)

Hypertension/ventricular rate control: I.V. (in patients having nonfunctioning GI tract): Initial: 1.25-5 mg every 6-12 hours; titrate initial dose to response. Initially, low doses may be appropriate to establish response; however, up to 15 mg every 3-6 hours has been employed.

Congestive heart failure: Oral (extended release): Initial: 25 mg once daily (reduce to 12.5 mg once daily in NYHA class higher than class II); may double dosage every 2 weeks as tolerated (maximum: 200 mg/day)

Myocardial infarction (acute): I.V.: 5 mg every 2 minutes for 3 doses in early treatment of myocardial infarction; thereafter give 50 mg orally every 6 hours 15 minutes after last I.V. dose and continue for 48 hours; then administer a maintenance dose of 100 mg twice daily.

Note: Switching dosage forms:
When switching from immediate release metoprolol to extended release, the same total daily dose of metoprolol should be used.

When switching between oral and intravenous dosage forms, equivalent beta-blocking effect is achieved when doses in a 2.5:1 (Oral:I.V.) ratio is used.

Dosage Forms
Injection, solution: 1 mg/mL (5 mL)
Lopressor®: 1 mg/mL (5 mL)
Tablet: 25 mg, 50 mg, 100 mg
Lopressor®: 50 mg, 100 mg
Tablet, extended release: 25 mg, 50 mg, 100 mg, 200 mg
Toprol-XL®: 25 mg, 50 mg, 100 mg, 200 mg

Metoprolol-25 [Can] *see* metoprolol *on page 626*

metoprolol and hydrochlorothiazide (me toe PROE lole & hye droe klor oh THYE a zide)

Synonyms hydrochlorothiazide and metoprolol; hydrochlorothiazide and metoprolol tartrate; metoprolol tartrate and hydrochlorothiazide

U.S./Canadian Brand Names Lopressor HCT® [US]

Therapeutic Category Beta Blocker, Beta$_1$ Selective; Diuretic, Thiazide

Use Treatment of hypertension (not recommended for initial treatment)

Usual Dosage Oral: Adults: Hypertension: Dosage should be determined by titration of the individual agents and the combination product substituted based upon the daily requirements.

Usual dose: Metoprolol 50-100 mg and hydrochlorothiazide 25-50 mg administered daily as single or divided doses (twice daily)

Note: Hydrochlorothiazide >50 mg/day is not recommended.

Concomitant therapy: It is recommended that if an additional antihypertensive agent is required, gradual titration should occur using ¹/₂ the usual starting dose of the other agent to avoid hypotension.

Dosage Forms
Tablet: 50/25: Metoprolol 50 mg and hydrochlorothiazide 25 mg; 100/25: Metoprolol 100 mg and hydrochlorothiazide 25 mg; 100/50: Metoprolol 100 mg and hydrochlorothiazide 50 mg
Lopressor HCT®: 50/25: Metoprolol 50 mg and hydrochlorothiazide 25 mg; 100/25: Metoprolol 100 mg and hydrochlorothiazide 25 mg; 100/50: Metoprolol 100 mg and hydrochlorothiazide 50 mg

metoprolol succinate *see* metoprolol *on page 626*
metoprolol tartrate *see* metoprolol *on page 626*
metoprolol tartrate and hydrochlorothiazide *see* metoprolol and hydrochlorothiazide *on page 627*
Metoprolol Tartrate Injection, USP [Can] *see* metoprolol *on page 626*
Metreton® (Discontinued)
MetroCream® [US/Can] *see* metronidazole *on page 627*
MetroGel® [US/Can] *see* metronidazole *on page 627*
MetroGel-Vaginal® [US] *see* metronidazole *on page 627*
Metro I.V.® Injection (Discontinued) *see* metronidazole *on page 627*
MetroLotion® [US] *see* metronidazole *on page 627*

metronidazole (met roe NYE da zole)

Sound-Alike/Look-Alike Issues
metroNIDAZOLE may be confused with meropenem, metFORMIN

Synonyms metronidazole hydrochloride

◀ **Tall-Man** metroNIDAZOLE

U.S./Canadian Brand Names Apo-Metronidazole® [Can]; Flagyl ER® [US]; Flagyl® [US/Can]; Florazole® ER [Can]; MetroCream® [US/Can]; MetroGel-Vaginal® [US]; MetroGel® [US/Can]; MetroLotion® [US]; Nidagel™ [Can]; Noritate® [US/Can]; Trikacide [Can]; Vandazole™ [US]

Therapeutic Category Amebicide; Antibiotic, Miscellaneous; Antibiotic, Topical; Antiprotozoal

Use Treatment of susceptible anaerobic bacterial and protozoal infections in the following conditions: Amebiasis, symptomatic and asymptomatic trichomoniasis; skin and skin structure infections; CNS infections; intraabdominal infections (as part of combination regimen); systemic anaerobic infections; treatment of antibiotic-associated pseudomembranous colitis (AAPC), bacterial vaginosis; as part of a multidrug regimen for *H. pylori* eradication to reduce the risk of duodenal ulcer recurrence

Topical: Treatment of inflammatory lesions and erythema of rosacea

Usual Dosage

Infants and Children:

Amebiasis: Oral: 35-50 mg/kg/day in divided doses every 8 hours for 10 days

Trichomoniasis: Oral: 15-30 mg/kg/day in divided doses every 8 hours for 7 days

Anaerobic infections:

Oral: 15-35 mg/kg/day in divided doses every 8 hours

I.V.: 30 mg/kg/day in divided doses every 6 hours

Clostridium difficile (antibiotic-associated colitis): Oral: 20 mg/kg/day divided every 6 hours

Maximum dose: 2 g/day

Adults:

Anaerobic infections (diverticulitis, intraabdominal, peritonitis, cholangitis, or abscess): Oral, I.V.: 500 mg every 6-8 hours, not to exceed 4 g/day

Acne rosacea: Topical:

0.75%: Apply and rub a thin film twice daily, morning and evening, to entire affected areas after washing. Significant therapeutic results should be noticed within 3 weeks. Clinical studies have demonstrated continuing improvement through 9 weeks of therapy.

1%: Apply thin film to affected area once daily

Amebiasis: Oral: 500-750 mg every 8 hours for 5-10 days

Antibiotic-associated pseudomembranous colitis: Oral: 250-500 mg 3-4 times/day for 10-14 days

Note: Due to the emergence of a new strain of *C. difficile*, some clinicians recommend converting to oral vancomycin therapy if the patient does not show a clear clinical response after 2 days of metronidazole therapy.

Giardiasis: 500 mg twice daily for 5-7 days

Helicobacter pylori eradication: Oral: 250-500 mg with meals and at bedtime for 14 days; requires combination therapy with at least one other antibiotic and an acid-suppressing agent (proton pump inhibitor or H_2 blocker)

Bacterial vaginosis or vaginitis due to *Gardnerella, Mobiluncus*:

Oral: 500 mg twice daily (regular release) or 750 mg once daily (extended release tablet) for 7 days

Vaginal: 1 applicatorful (~37.5 mg metronidazole) intravaginally once or twice daily for 5 days; apply once in morning and evening if using twice daily, if daily, use at bedtime

Trichomoniasis: Oral: 250 mg every 8 hours for 7 days **or** 375 mg twice daily for 7 days **or** 2 g as a single dose

Dosage Forms

Capsule: 375 mg

Flagyl®: 375 mg

Cream, topical: 0.75% (45 g)

MetroCream®: 0.75% (45 g)

Noritate®: 1% (60 g)

Gel, topical: 1% (45 g)

MetroGel®: 1% (46 g, 60 g)

Gel, vaginal: 0.75% (70 g)

MetroGel-Vaginal®, Vandazole™: 0.75% (70 g)

Infusion [premixed iso-osmotic sodium chloride solution]: 500 mg (100 mL)

Lotion, topical: 0.75% (60 mL)

MetroLotion®: 0.75% (60 mL)

Tablet: 250 mg, 500 mg

Flagyl®: 250 mg, 500 mg

Tablet, extended release:

Flagyl® ER: 750 mg

metronidazole and nystatin *(Canada only)* (met roe NYE da zole & nye STAT in)

U.S./Canadian Brand Names Flagystatin® [Can]
Therapeutic Category Antifungal Agent, Vaginal; Antiprotozoal, Nitroimidazole
Use Treatment of mixed vaginal infection due to *T. vaginalis* and *C. albicans*
Usual Dosage Intravaginal: Adults:
Vaginal tablet (ovule): Insert 1 tablet/day at bedtime for 10 consecutive days. May repeat for an additional 10 days if cure is not achieved.
Vaginal cream: Insert 1 applicatorful daily at bedtime for 10 consecutive days. May repeat for an additional 10 days if cure is not achieved.
Note: If *Trichomonas vaginalis* is not completely eliminated, oral (systemic) metronidazole (250 mg twice daily for 10 days) should be administered.
Dosage Forms [CAN] = Canadian brand name
Cream, vaginal:
Flagystatin® [CAN]: Metronidazole 500 mg and nystatin 100,000 units per applicatorful (55 g) [not available in the U.S.]
Tablet, vaginal:
Flagystatin® Ovule [CAN]: Metronidazole 500 mg and nystatin 100,000 units (10s) [not available in the U.S.]

metronidazole, bismuth subcitrate potassium, and tetracycline *see* bismuth, metronidazole, and tetracycline *on page 137*

metronidazole, bismuth subsalicylate, and tetracycline *see* bismuth, metronidazole, and tetracycline *on page 137*

metronidazole hydrochloride *see* metronidazole *on page 627*

metyrapone (me TEER a pone)

Sound-Alike/Look-Alike Issues
metyrapone may be confused with metyrosine
U.S./Canadian Brand Names Metopirone® [US]
Therapeutic Category Diagnostic Agent
Use Diagnostic test for hypothalamic-pituitary ACTH function
Usual Dosage Oral:
Children: 15 mg/kg every 4 hours for 6 doses; minimum dose: 250 mg
Adults: 750 mg every 4 hours for 6 doses
Dosage Forms
Capsule:
Metopirone®: 250 mg

metyrosine (me TYE roe seen)

Sound-Alike/Look-Alike Issues
metyrosine may be confused with metyrapone
Synonyms AMPT; OGMT
U.S./Canadian Brand Names Demser® [US/Can]
Therapeutic Category Tyrosine Hydroxylase Inhibitor
Use Short-term management of pheochromocytoma before surgery, long-term management when surgery is contraindicated or when chronic malignant pheochromocytoma exists
Usual Dosage Oral: Children >12 years and Adults: Initial: 250 mg 4 times/day, increased by 250-500 mg/day up to 4 g/day; maintenance: 2-3 g/day in 4 divided doses; for preoperative preparation, administer optimum effective dosage for 5-7 days
Dosage Forms
Capsule:
Demser®: 250 mg

Mevacor® [US/Can] *see* lovastatin *on page 579*

mevinolin *see* lovastatin *on page 579*

Mexar™ *(Discontinued)* *see* sulfacetamide *on page 892*

mexiletine (meks IL e teen)

U.S./Canadian Brand Names Novo-Mexiletine [Can]
Therapeutic Category Antiarrhythmic Agent, Class I-B

◀ **Use** Management of serious ventricular arrhythmias; suppression of PVCs

Usual Dosage Oral: Adults: Initial: 200 mg every 8 hours (may load with 400 mg if necessary); adjust dose every 2-3 days; usual dose: 200-300 mg every 8 hours; maximum dose: 1.2 g/day (some patients respond to every 12-hour dosing). When switching from another antiarrhythmic, initiate a 200 mg dose 6-12 hours after stopping former agents, 3-6 hours after stopping procainamide.

Dosage Forms

Capsule: 150 mg, 200 mg, 250 mg

Mexitil® *(Discontinued)* *see* mexiletine *on page 629*

Mezavant® [Can] *see* mesalamine *on page 607*

MG 217® [US-OTC] *see* coal tar *on page 240*

MG 217® Medicated Tar [US-OTC] *see* coal tar *on page 240*

Miacalcin® [US] *see* calcitonin *on page 160*

Miacalcin® NS [Can] *see* calcitonin *on page 160*

Mi-Acid [US-OTC] *see* aluminum hydroxide, magnesium hydroxide, and simethicone *on page 54*

Mi-Acid™ Double Strength [US-OTC] *see* calcium carbonate and magnesium hydroxide *on page 164*

Mi-Acid Maximum Strength [US-OTC] *see* aluminum hydroxide, magnesium hydroxide, and simethicone *on page 54*

Micaderm® [US-OTC] *see* miconazole *on page 630*

micafungin (mi ka FUN gin)

Synonyms micafungin sodium

U.S./Canadian Brand Names Mycamine® [US/Can]

Therapeutic Category Antifungal Agent, Parental; Drug-induced Neuritis, Treatment Agent

Use Treatment of esophageal candidiasis; *Candida* prophylaxis in patients undergoing hematopoietic stem cell transplant (HSCT); treatment of candidemia, acute disseminated candidiasis, and other *Candida* infections (peritonitis and abscesses)

Usual Dosage I.V.: Adults:

Candidemia, acute disseminated candidiasis, and *Candida* peritonitis and abscesses: 100 mg daily; mean duration of therapy (from clinical trials) was 15 days (range: 10-47 days)

Esophageal candidiasis: 150 mg daily; mean duration of therapy (from clinical trials) was 15 days (range: 10-30 days)

Prophylaxis of *Candida* infection in hematopoietic stem cell transplantation: 50 mg daily

Dosage Forms

Injection, powder for reconstitution [preservative-free]:

Mycamine®: 50 mg, 100 mg [contains lactose]

micafungin sodium *see* micafungin *on page 630*

Micanol® [Can] *see* anthralin *on page 77*

Micardis® [US/Can] *see* telmisartan *on page 906*

Micardis® HCT [US] *see* telmisartan and hydrochlorothiazide *on page 906*

Micardis® Plus [Can] *see* telmisartan and hydrochlorothiazide *on page 906*

Micatin® [Can] *see* miconazole *on page 630*

Micatin® Athlete's Foot [US-OTC] *see* miconazole *on page 630*

Micatin® Jock Itch [US-OTC] *see* miconazole *on page 630*

miconazole (mi KON a zole)

Sound-Alike/Look-Alike Issues

miconazole may be confused with Micronase®, Micronor®

Lotrimin® may be confused with Lotrisone®, Otrivin®

Micatin® may be confused with Miacalcin®

Synonyms miconazole nitrate

U.S./Canadian Brand Names Aloe Vesta® 2-n-1 Antifungal [US-OTC]; Baza® Antifungal [US-OTC]; Carrington Antifungal [US-OTC]; Critic-Aid® Clear AF [US-OTC]; DermaFungal [US-OTC]; Dermagran® AF [US-OTC]; Dermazole [Can]; DiabetAid™ Antifungal Foot Bath [US-OTC]; Fungoid® Tincture [US-OTC]; Lotrimin® AF Jock Itch Powder Spray [US-OTC]; Lotrimin® AF Powder/Spray [US-OTC];

Micaderm® [US-OTC]; Micatin® Athlete's Foot [US-OTC]; Micatin® Jock Itch [US-OTC]; Micatin® [Can]; Micozole [Can]; Micro-Guard® [US-OTC]; Mitrazol™ [US-OTC]; Monistat® 1 Combination Pack [US-OTC]; Monistat® 3 Combination Pack [US-OTC]; Monistat® 3 [US-OTC/Can]; Monistat® 7 [US-OTC]; Monistat® [Can]; Neosporin® AF [US-OTC]; Podactin Cream [US-OTC]; Secura® Antifungal [US-OTC]; Zeasorb®-AF [US-OTC]

Therapeutic Category Antifungal Agent

Use Treatment of vulvovaginal candidiasis and a variety of skin and mucous membrane fungal infections

Usual Dosage

Topical: Children and Adults: **Note:** Not for OTC use in children <2 years:
  Tinea corporis: Apply twice daily for 4 weeks
  Tinea pedis: Apply twice daily for 4 weeks
    Effervescent tablet: Dissolve 1 tablet in ~1 gallon of water; soak feet for 15-30 minutes; pat dry
  Tinea cruris: Apply twice daily for 2 weeks
Vaginal: Children ≥12 years and Adults: Vulvovaginal candidiasis:
  Cream, 2%: Insert 1 applicatorful at bedtime for 7 days
  Cream, 4%: Insert 1 applicatorful at bedtime for 3 days
  Suppository, 100 mg: Insert 1 suppository at bedtime for 7 days
  Suppository, 200 mg: Insert 1 suppository at bedtime for 3 days
  Suppository, 1200 mg: Insert 1 suppository (a one-time dose); may be used at bedtime or during the day

Note: Many products are available as a combination pack, with a suppository for vaginal instillation and cream to relieve external symptoms. External cream may be used twice daily, as needed, for up to 7 days.

Dosage Forms

Combination products: Miconazole vaginal suppository 200 mg (3s) and miconazole external cream 2%
  Monistat® 1 Combination Pack: Miconazole vaginal insert 1200 mg (1) and miconazole external cream 2% (5 g) [**Note:** Do not confuse with 1-Day™ (formerly Monistat® 1) which contains tioconazole]
  Monistat® 3 Combination Pack:
    Miconazole vaginal insert 200 mg (3s) and miconazole external cream 2%
    Miconazole vaginal cream 4% and miconazole external cream 2%
  Monistat® 7 Combination Pack:
    Miconazole vaginal suppository 100 mg (7s) and miconazole external cream 2%
    Miconazole vaginal cream 2% (7 prefilled applicators) and miconazole external cream 2%
Cream, topical: 2% (15 g, 30 g, 45 g)
  Baza® Antifungal: 2% (4 g, 57 g, 142 g)
  Carrington Antifungal: 2% (150 g)
  Micaderm®, Neosporin® AF, Podactin: 2% (30 g)
  Micatin® Athlete's Foot, Micatin® Jock Itch: 2% (15 g)
  Micro-Guard®, Mitrazol™: 2% (60 g)
  Secura® Antifungal: 2% (60 g, 98 g)
Cream, vaginal [prefilled or refillable applicator]: 2% (45 g)
  Monistat® 3: 4% (15 g, 25 g)
  Monistat® 7: 2% (45 g)
Gel, topical:
  Zeasorb®-AF: 2% (24 g)
Liquid, spray, topical:
  Micatin® Athlete's Foot: 2% (90 mL)
  Neosporin AF®: 2% (105 mL)
Lotion, powder:
  Zeasorb®-AF: 2% (56 g)
Ointment, topical:
  Aloe Vesta® 2-n-1 Antifungal: 2% (60 g, 150 g)
  Critic-Aid® Clear AF: 2% (4 g, 57 g, 142 g)
  DermaFungal: 2% (113 g)
  Dermagran® AF: (113 g)
Powder, topical:
  Lotrimin® AF: 2% (160 g)
  Micro-Guard®: 2% (90 g)
  Mitrazol™: 2% (30 g)
  Zeasorb®-AF: 2% (70 g)

▶

◀ **Powder spray, topical:**
Lotrimin® AF, Lotrimin® AF Jock Itch: 2% (140 g)
Micatin® Athlete's Foot, Micatin® Jock Itch: 2% (90 g)
Neosporin® AF: 2% (85 g)
Suppository, vaginal: 100 mg (7s); 200 mg (3s)
Monistat® 3: 200 mg (3s)
Monistat® 7: 100 mg (7s)
Tablet, for solution, topical [effervescent]:
DiabetAid™ Antifungal Foot Bath: 2% (10s)
Tincture, topical:
Fungoid®: 2% (30 mL, 473 mL)

miconazole and zinc oxide (mi KON a zole & zink OKS ide)

Synonyms zinc oxide and miconazole nitrate
U.S./Canadian Brand Names Vusion® [US]
Therapeutic Category Antifungal Agent, Topical
Use Adjunctive treatment of diaper dermatitis complicated by *Candida albicans* infection
Usual Dosage Topical: Children ≥4 weeks: Diaper dermatitis: Apply to affected area with each diaper change for 7 days. Treatment should continue for 7 days, even with initial improvement. Do not use for >7 days.
Dosage Forms
Ointment, topical:
Vusion®: Miconazole 0.25% and zinc oxide 15% (60 g)

miconazole nitrate *see miconazole on page 630*
Micozole [Can] *see miconazole on page 630*
MICRhoGAM® [US] *see* Rh₀(D) immune globulin *on page 829*
microfibrillar collagen hemostat *see collagen hemostat on page 245*
Microgestin™ [US] *see ethinyl estradiol and norethindrone on page 376*
Microgestin™ Fe [US] *see ethinyl estradiol and norethindrone on page 376*
Micro-Guard® [US-OTC] *see miconazole on page 630*
microK® [US] *see potassium chloride on page 771*
microK® 10 [US] *see potassium chloride on page 771*
Micro-K Extencaps® [Can] *see potassium chloride on page 771*
Micro-K® LS *(Discontinued)* *see potassium chloride on page 771*
Microlipid™ [US-OTC] *see nutritional formula, enteral/oral on page 689*
Micronase® [US] *see glyburide on page 448*
microNefrin® *(Discontinued)* *see epinephrine on page 344*
Micronor® [Can] *see norethindrone on page 679*
Microzide™ [US] *see hydrochlorothiazide on page 479*
***Micrurus fulvius* antivenin** *see antivenin (Micrurus fulvius) on page 84*
Midamor® *(Discontinued)* *see amiloride on page 59*

midazolam (MID aye zoe lam)

Sound-Alike/Look-Alike Issues
Versed® may be confused with VePesid®, Vistaril®
Synonyms midazolam hydrochloride
U.S./Canadian Brand Names Apo-Midazolam® [Can]; Midazolam Injection [Can]
Therapeutic Category Benzodiazepine
Controlled Substance C-IV
Use Preoperative sedation and provides conscious sedation prior to diagnostic or radiographic procedures; ICU sedation (continuous infusion); intravenous anesthesia (induction); intravenous anesthesia (maintenance)
Usual Dosage The dose of midazolam needs to be individualized based on the patient's age, underlying diseases, and concurrent medications. Decrease dose (by ~30%) if narcotics or other CNS depressants are administered concomitantly. **Personnel and equipment needed for standard respiratory resuscitation should be immediately available during midazolam administration.**

Children <6 years may require higher doses and closer monitoring than older children; calculate dose on ideal body weight

Conscious sedation for procedures or preoperative sedation:

Oral: 0.25-0.5 mg/kg as a single dose preprocedure, up to a maximum of 20 mg; administer 30-45 minutes prior to procedure. Children <6 years or less cooperative patients may require as much as 1 mg/kg as a single dose; 0.25 mg/kg may suffice for children 6-16 years of age.

I.M.: 0.1-0.15 mg/kg 30-60 minutes before surgery or procedure; range 0.05-0.15 mg/kg; doses up to 0.5 mg/kg have been used in more anxious patients; maximum total dose: 10 mg

I.V.:

Infants <6 months: Limited information is available in nonintubated infants; dosing recommendations not clear; infants <6 months are at higher risk for airway obstruction and hypoventilation; titrate dose in small increments to desired effect; monitor carefully

Infants 6 months to Children 5 years: Initial: 0.05-0.1 mg/kg; titrate dose carefully; total dose of 0.6 mg/kg may be required; usual maximum total dose: 6 mg

Children 6-12 years: Initial: 0.025-0.05 mg/kg; titrate dose carefully; total doses of 0.4 mg/kg may be required; usual maximum total dose: 10 mg

Children 12-16 years: Dose as adults; usual maximum total dose: 10 mg

Conscious sedation during mechanical ventilation: Children: Loading dose: 0.05-0.2 mg/kg, followed by initial continuous infusion: 0.06-0.12 mg/kg/hour (1-2 mcg/kg/minute); titrate to the desired effect; usual range: 0.4-6 mcg/kg/minute

Adults:

Preoperative sedation:

I.M.: 0.07-0.08 mg/kg 30-60 minutes prior to surgery/procedure; usual dose: 5 mg; **Note:** Reduce dose in patients with COPD, high-risk patients, patients ≥60 years of age, and patients receiving other narcotics or CNS depressants

I.V.: 0.02-0.04 mg/kg; repeat every 5 minutes as needed to desired effect or up to 0.1-0.2 mg/kg

Conscious sedation: I.V.: Initial: 0.5-2 mg slow I.V. over at least 2 minutes; slowly titrate to effect by repeating doses every 2-3 minutes if needed; usual total dose: 2.5-5 mg

Healthy Adults <60 years: Some patients respond to doses as low as 1 mg; no more than 2.5 mg should be administered over a period of 2 minutes. Additional doses of midazolam may be administered after a 2-minute waiting period and evaluation of sedation after each dose increment. A total dose >5 mg is generally not needed. If narcotics or other CNS depressants are administered concomitantly, the midazolam dose should be reduced by 30%.

Anesthesia: I.V.:

Induction:

Unpremedicated patients: 0.3-0.35 mg/kg (up to 0.6 mg/kg in resistant cases)

Premedicated patients: 0.15-0.35 mg/kg

Maintenance: 0.05-0.3 mg/kg as needed, or continuous infusion 0.25-1.5 mcg/kg/minute

Sedation in mechanically-ventilated patients: I.V. continuous infusion: 100 mg in 250 mL D_5W or NS (if patient is fluid-restricted, may concentrate up to a maximum of 0.5 mg/mL); initial dose: 0.02-0.08 mg/kg (~1 mg to 5 mg in 70 kg adult) initially and either repeated at 5-15 minute intervals until adequate sedation is achieved or continuous infusion rates of 0.04-0.2 mg/kg/hour and titrate to reach desired level of sedation

Dosage Forms

Injection, solution: 1 mg/mL (2 mL, 5 mL, 10 mL); 5 mg/mL (1 mL, 2 mL, 5 mL, 10 mL)

Injection, solution [preservative free]: 1 mg/mL (2 mL, 5 mL); 5 mg/mL (1 mL, 2 mL)

Syrup: 2 mg/mL

midazolam hydrochloride see midazolam on page 632
midazolam hydrochloride see midazolam on page 632
Midazolam Injection [Can] see midazolam on page 632

midodrine (MI doe dreen)

Sound-Alike/Look-Alike Issues

ProAmatine® may be confused with protamine

Synonyms midodrine hydrochloride

U.S./Canadian Brand Names Amatine® [Can]; Apo-Midodrine® [Can]; ProAmatine® [US]

Therapeutic Category Alpha-Adrenergic Agonist

Use Orphan drug: Treatment of symptomatic orthostatic hypotension

Usual Dosage Oral: Adults: 10 mg 3 times/day during daytime hours (every 3-4 hours) when patient is upright (maximum: 40 mg/day)

▶

◄ **Dosage Forms**
Tablet: 2.5 mg, 5 mg, 10 mg
ProAmatine®: 2.5 mg, 5 mg, 10 mg [scored]

midodrine hydrochloride *see* midodrine *on page 633*
Midol® Cramp and Body Aches [US-OTC] *see* ibuprofen *on page 495*
Midol® Extended Relief [US] *see* naproxen *on page 656*
Midrin® [US] *see* acetaminophen, isometheptene, and dichloralphenazone *on page 28*
Mifeprex® [US] *see* mifepristone *on page 634*

mifepristone (mi FE pris tone)

Sound-Alike/Look-Alike Issues
mifepristone may be confused with misoprostol
Mifeprex® may be confused with Mirapex®
Synonyms RU-38486; RU-486
U.S./Canadian Brand Names Mifeprex® [US]
Therapeutic Category Abortifacient; Antineoplastic Agent, Hormone Antagonist; Antiprogestin
Use Medical termination of intrauterine pregnancy, through day 49 of pregnancy. Patients may need treatment with misoprostol and possibly surgery to complete therapy
Usual Dosage Oral: Adults:
Termination of pregnancy: Treatment consists of three office visits by the patient; the patient must read medication guide and sign patient agreement prior to treatment:
Day 1: 600 mg (three 200 mg tablets) taken as a single dose under physician supervision
Day 3: Patient must return to the healthcare provider 2 days following administration of mifepristone; unless abortion has occurred (confirmed using ultrasound or clinical examination): 400 mcg (two 200 mcg tablets) of misoprostol; patient may need treatment for cramps or gastrointestinal symptoms at this time
Day 14: Patient must return to the healthcare provider ~14 days after administration of mifepristone; confirm complete termination of pregnancy by ultrasound or clinical exam. Surgical termination is recommended to manage treatment failures.
Dosage Forms
Tablet:
Mifeprex®: 200 mg

Migergot [US] *see* ergotamine and caffeine *on page 352*

miglitol (MIG li tol)

U.S./Canadian Brand Names Glyset® [US/Can]
Therapeutic Category Antidiabetic Agent, Oral
Use Type 2 diabetes mellitus (noninsulin-dependent, NIDDM):
Monotherapy adjunct to diet to improve glycemic control in patients with type 2 diabetes mellitus (noninsulin-dependent, NIDDM) whose hyperglycemia cannot be managed with diet alone
Combination therapy with a sulfonylurea when diet plus either miglitol or a sulfonylurea alone do not result in adequate glycemic control. The effect of miglitol to enhance glycemic control is additive to that of sulfonylureas when used in combination.
Usual Dosage Oral: Adults: 25 mg 3 times/day with the first bite of food at each meal; the dose may be increased to 50 mg 3 times/day after 4-8 weeks; maximum recommended dose: 100 mg 3 times/day
Dosage Forms
Tablet:
Glyset®: 25 mg, 50 mg, 100 mg

miglustat (MIG loo stat)

Synonyms OGT-918
U.S./Canadian Brand Names Zavesca® [US/Can]
Therapeutic Category Enzyme Inhibitor
Use Treatment of mild-to-moderate type 1 Gaucher disease when enzyme replacement therapy is not a therapeutic option
Usual Dosage Oral: Adults: Type 1 Gaucher disease: 100 mg 3 times/day; dose may be reduced to 100 mg 1-2 times/day in patients with adverse effects (ie, tremor, GI distress)

Dosage Forms
  Capsule:
    Zavesca®: 100 mg

Migquin *(Discontinued)* see acetaminophen, isometheptene, and dichloralphenazone *on page 28*
Migranal® **[US/Can]** see dihydroergotamine *on page 299*
Migrapap® *(Discontinued)* see acetaminophen, isometheptene, and dichloralphenazone *on page 28*
Migratine [US] see acetaminophen, isometheptene, and dichloralphenazone *on page 28*
Migrazone® *(Discontinued)* see acetaminophen, isometheptene, and dichloralphenazone *on page 28*
Migrin-A *(Discontinued)* see acetaminophen, isometheptene, and dichloralphenazone *on page 28*
Mild-C® **[US-OTC]** see ascorbic acid *on page 96*
milk of magnesia see magnesium hydroxide *on page 585*
Milontin® *(Discontinued)*
Milophene® **[Can]** see clomiphene *on page 235*
Milophene® *(Discontinued)* see clomiphene *on page 235*

milrinone (MIL ri none)

Sound-Alike/Look-Alike Issues
  Primacor® may be confused with Primaxin®
Synonyms milrinone lactate
U.S./Canadian Brand Names Milrinone Lactate Injection [Can]; Primacor® [US/Can]
Therapeutic Category Cardiovascular Agent, Other
Use Short-term I.V. therapy of acutely-decompensated heart failure
Usual Dosage I.V.: Adults: Loading dose (optional): 50 mcg/kg administered over 10 minutes followed by a maintenance dose titrated according to the hemodynamic and clinical response; Maintenance dose: I.V. infusion: 0.375-0.75 mcg/kg/minute.
Dosage Forms
  Infusion [premixed in D_5W]: 200 mcg/mL (100 mL, 200 mL)
    Primacor®: 200 mcg/mL (200 mL)
  Injection, solution: 1 mg/mL (10 mL, 20 mL, 50 mL)

milrinone lactate see milrinone *on page 635*
Milrinone Lactate Injection [Can] see milrinone *on page 635*
Miltown® *(Discontinued)* see meprobamate *on page 605*
Mindal DM *(Discontinued)* see guaifenesin and dextromethorphan *on page 454*
mineral oil, petrolatum, lanolin, cetyl alcohol, and glycerin see lanolin, cetyl alcohol, glycerin, petrolatum, and mineral oil *on page 547*
Minestrin™ 1/20 [Can] see ethinyl estradiol and norethindrone *on page 376*
Mini-Gamulin® Rh *(Discontinued)*
Mini-Prenatal [US] see vitamins (multiple/prenatal) *on page 983*
Minipress® **[US/Can]** see prazosin *on page 780*
Minirin® **[Can]** see desmopressin acetate *on page 275*
Minitran™ **[US/Can]** see nitroglycerin *on page 675*
Minocin® **[Can]** see minocycline *on page 635*
Minocin® PAC [US] see minocycline *on page 635*

minocycline (mi noe SYE kleen)

Sound-Alike/Look-Alike Issues
  Dynacin® may be confused with Dyazide®, Dynabac®, DynaCirc®, Dynapen®
  Minocin® may be confused with Indocin®, Lincocin®, Minizide®, Mithracin®, niacin
Synonyms minocycline hydrochloride
U.S./Canadian Brand Names Alti-Minocycline [Can]; Apo-Minocycline® [Can]; Dynacin® [US]; Gen-Minocycline [Can]; Minocin® PAC [US]; Minocin® [Can]; myrac™ [US]; Novo-Minocycline [Can]; PMS-Minocycline [Can]; Rhoxal-minocycline [Can]; Sandoz-Minocycline [Can]; Solodyn™ [US]
Therapeutic Category Tetracycline Derivative
Use Treatment of susceptible bacterial infections of both gram-negative and gram-positive organisms; treatment of anthrax (inhalational, cutaneous, and gastrointestinal); acne; meningococcal (asymptomatic) ▶

◄ carrier state; Rickettsial diseases (including Rocky Mountain spotted fever, Q fever); nongonococcal urethritis, gonorrhea; acute intestinal amebiasis

Usual Dosage

Usual dosage range:

Children >8 years: Oral: Initial: 4 mg/kg, followed by 2 mg/kg/dose every 12 hours

Adults: Oral: Initial: 200 mg, followed by 100 mg every 12 hours (maximum: 400 mg/day)

Indication-specific dosing:

Children ≥12 years: **Acne** *(inflammatory, nonnodular, moderate to severe)* (Solodyn™): Oral:

45-59 kg: 45 mg once daily

60-90 kg: 90 mg once daily

91-136 kg: 135 mg once daily

Note: Therapy should be continued for 12 weeks. Higher doses do not confer greater efficacy, and safety of use beyond 12 weeks has not been established.

Adults: Oral:

Acne: Capsule or immediate-release tablet: 50-100 mg daily

Inflammatory, nonnodular, moderate-to-severe (Solodyn™):

45-59 kg: 45 mg once daily

60-90 kg: 90 mg once daily

91-136 kg: 135 mg once daily

Note: Therapy should be continued for 12 weeks. Higher doses do not confer greater efficacy, and safety of use beyond 12 weeks has not been established.

Chlamydial or *Ureaplasma urealyticum* infection, uncomplicated: Urethral, endocervical, or rectal: 100 mg every 12 hours for at least 7 days

Gonococcal infection, uncomplicated (males):

Without urethritis or anorectal infection: Initial: 200 mg, followed by 100 mg every 12 hours for at least 4 days (cultures 2-3 days post-therapy)

Urethritis: 100 mg every 12 hours for 5 days

Meningococcal carrier state: 100 mg every 12 hours for 5 days

***Mycobacterium marinum*:** 100 mg every 12 hours for 6-8 weeks

Nocardiosis, cutaneous (non-CNS): 100 mg every 12 hours

Syphilis: Initial: 200 mg, followed by 100 mg every 12 hours for 10-15 days

Dosage Forms

Capsule: 50 mg, 75 mg, 100 mg

Capsule, pellet filled: 50 mg, 100 mg

Minocin® PAC: 50 mg, 100 mg

Tablet: 50 mg, 75 mg, 100 mg

Dynacin®, myrac™: 50 mg, 75 mg, 100 mg

Tablet, extended release:

Solodyn™: 45 mg, 90 mg, 135 mg

minocycline hydrochloride *see minocycline on page 635*

Min-Ovral® [Can] *see ethinyl estradiol and levonorgestrel on page 372*

Minox [Can] *see minoxidil on page 636*

minoxidil (mi NOKS i dil)

Sound-Alike/Look-Alike Issues

minoxidil may be confused with metolazone, midodrine, Minipress®, Minocin®, Monopril®, Noxafil®

U.S./Canadian Brand Names Apo-Gain® [Can]; Minox [Can]; Rogaine® Extra Strength for Men [US-OTC]; Rogaine® for Men [US-OTC]; Rogaine® for Women [US-OTC]; Rogaine® [Can]

Therapeutic Category Topical Skin Product; Vasodilator

Use Management of severe hypertension (usually in combination with a diuretic and beta-blocker); treatment (topical formulation) of alopecia androgenetica in males and females

Usual Dosage

Children <12 years: Hypertension: Oral: Initial: 0.1-0.2 mg/kg once daily; maximum: 5 mg/day; increase gradually every 3 days; usual dosage range: 0.25-1 mg/kg/day in 1-2 divided doses; maximum: 50 mg/day

Children ≥12 years and Adults: Hypertension: Oral: Initial: 5 mg once daily, increase gradually every 3 days (maximum: 100 mg/day); usual dosage range (JNC 7): 2.5-80 mg/day in 1-2 divided doses

Note: Dosage adjustment is needed when added to concomitant therapy.

Adults: Alopecia: Topical: Apply twice daily; 4 months of therapy may be necessary for hair growth.

Dosage Forms
  Aerosol, topical [foam]:
    Rogaine® for Men: 5% (60 g)
  Solution, topical: 2% (60 mL); 5% (60 mL)
    Rogaine® for Women [OTC]: 2% (60 mL)
    Rogaine® Extra Strength for Men [OTC]: 5% (60 mL)
  Tablet: 2.5 mg, 10 mg

Mintab DM [US] *see* guaifenesin and dextromethorphan *on page 454*

Mint-Citalopram [Can] *see* citalopram *on page 225*

Mintezol® [US] *see* thiabendazole *on page 920*

Mintox Extra Strength [US-OTC] *see* aluminum hydroxide, magnesium hydroxide, and simethicone *on page 54*

Mintox Plus [US-OTC] *see* aluminum hydroxide, magnesium hydroxide, and simethicone *on page 54*

Mintuss DR [US] *see* chlorpheniramine, phenylephrine, and dextromethorphan *on page 209*

Mintuss G *(Discontinued)*

Mintuss HC [US] *see* phenylephrine, hydrocodone, and chlorpheniramine *on page 748*

Mintuss MS [US] *see* phenylephrine, hydrocodone, and chlorpheniramine *on page 748*

Minute-Gel® *(Discontinued)* *see* fluoride *on page 411*

Miochol®-E [US/Can] *see* acetylcholine *on page 30*

Miostat® [US/Can] *see* carbachol *on page 172*

MiraLax® [US-OTC] *see* polyethylene glycol 3350 *on page 765*

Mirapex® [US/Can] *see* pramipexole *on page 777*

Mircette® [US] *see* ethinyl estradiol and desogestrel *on page 369*

Mirena® [US/Can] *see* levonorgestrel *on page 559*

mirtazapine (mir TAZ a peen)

Sound-Alike/Look-Alike Issues
  Remeron® may be confused with Premarin®, Zemuron®

U.S./Canadian Brand Names CO Mirtazapine [Can]; Gen-Mirtazapine [Can]; Novo-Mirtazapine [Can]; PMS-Mirtazapine [Can]; ratio-Mirtazapine [Can]; Remeron SolTab® [US]; Remeron® RD [Can]; Remeron® [US/Can]; Rhoxal-mirtazapine FC [Can]; Rhoxal-mirtazapine [Can]; Riva-Mirtazapine [Can]; Sandoz-Mirtazapine FC [Can]; Sandoz-Mirtazapine [Can]

Therapeutic Category Antidepressant, Alpha-2 Antagonist

Use Treatment of depression

Usual Dosage Oral: Adults: Treatment of depression: Initial: 15 mg nightly, titrate up to 15-45 mg/day with dose increases made no more frequently than every 1-2 weeks; there is an inverse relationship between dose and sedation

Dosage Forms
  Tablet: 7.5 mg, 15 mg, 30 mg, 45 mg
    Remeron®: 15 mg, 30 mg, 45 mg
  Tablet, orally disintegrating: 15 mg, 30 mg
    Remeron SolTab®: 15 mg, 30 mg, 45 mg

misoprostol (mye soe PROST ole)

Sound-Alike/Look-Alike Issues
  misoprostol may be confused with metoprolol, mifepristone
  Cytotec® may be confused with Cytoxan®, Sytobex®

U.S./Canadian Brand Names Apo-Misoprostol® [Can]; Cytotec® [US]; Novo-Misoprostol [Can]

Therapeutic Category Prostaglandin

Use Prevention of NSAID-induced gastric ulcers; medical termination of pregnancy of ≤49 days (in conjunction with mifepristone)

Usual Dosage Oral: Adults:
  Prevention of NSAID-induced gastric ulcers: 200 mcg 4 times/day with food; if not tolerated, may decrease dose to 100 mcg 4 times/day with food or 200 mcg twice daily with food; last dose of the day should be taken at bedtime
  Medical termination of pregnancy: Refer to mifepristone monograph.

◀ **Dosage Forms**
Tablet: 100 mcg, 200 mcg
Cytotec®: 100 mcg, 200 mcg

misoprostol and diclofenac *see* diclofenac and misoprostol *on page 293*
Mito-Carn® (Discontinued) *see* levocarnitine *on page 555*

mitomycin (mye toe MYE sin)

Sound-Alike/Look-Alike Issues
mitomycin may be confused with mithramycin, mitotane, mitoxantrone
Synonyms mitomycin-C; mitomycin-X; MTC; NSC-26980
U.S./Canadian Brand Names Mutamycin® [US/Can]
Therapeutic Category Antineoplastic Agent
Use Treatment of adenocarcinoma of stomach or pancreas, bladder cancer, breast cancer, or colorectal cancer
Usual Dosage Refer to individual protocols. Adults:
Single agent therapy: I.V.: 20 mg/m^2 every 6-8 weeks
Combination therapy: I.V.: 10 mg/m^2 every 6-8 weeks
Bladder carcinoma: Intravesicular instillation (unapproved route): 20-40 mg instilled into the bladder and retained for 3 hours up to 3 times/week for up to 20 procedures per course
Dosage Forms
Injection, powder for reconstitution: 5 mg, 20 mg, 40 mg

mitomycin-X *see* mitomycin *on page 638*
mitomycin-C *see* mitomycin *on page 638*

mitotane (MYE toe tane)

Sound-Alike/Look-Alike Issues
mitotane may be confused with mitomycin
Synonyms NSC-38721; o,p'-DDD
U.S./Canadian Brand Names Lysodren® [US/Can]
Therapeutic Category Antineoplastic Agent
Use Treatment of adrenocortical carcinoma
Usual Dosage Oral: Adults: Adrenocortical carcinoma: Start at 2-6 g/day in 3-4 divided doses, then increase incrementally to 9-10 g/day in 3-4 divided doses (maximum daily dose: 18 g)
Dosage Forms
Tablet [scored]:
Lysodren®: 500 mg

mitoxantrone (mye toe ZAN trone)

Sound-Alike/Look-Alike Issues
mitoxantrone may be confused with methotrexate, mitomycin, Mutamycin®
Synonyms CL-232315; DHAD; DHAQ; dihydroxyanthracenedione dihydrochloride; mitoxantrone hydrochloride; mitozantrone; NSC-301739
U.S./Canadian Brand Names Mitoxantrone Injection® [Can]; Novantrone® [US/Can]
Therapeutic Category Antineoplastic Agent
Use Treatment of acute nonlymphocytic leukemias, prostate cancer, lymphoma, secondary progressive or relapsing-remitting multiple sclerosis (MS)
Usual Dosage Details concerning dosing in combination regimens should also be consulted. I.V. (dilute in D$_5$W or NS): Adults:
Acute leukemias:
Induction: 12 mg/m^2 once daily for 3 days; for incomplete response, may repeat at 12 mg/m^2 once daily for 2 days
Consolidation: 12 mg/m^2 once daily for 2 days, repeat in 4 weeks
Solid tumors: 12-14 mg/m^2 every 3-4 weeks **or** 2-4 mg/m^2/day for 5 days every 4 weeks
Hormone-refractory prostate cancer: 12-14 mg/m^2 every 3 weeks
Multiple sclerosis: 12 mg/m^2 every 3 months (maximum lifetime cumulative dose: 140 mg/m^2; discontinue use with LVEF <50% or clinically significant reduction in LVEF)

Dosage Forms
  Injection, solution [concentrate; preservative free]: 2 mg/mL (10 mL, 12.5 mL, 15 mL, 20 mL)
    Novantrone®: 2 mg/mL (10 mL)

mitoxantrone hydrochloride *see* mitoxantrone *on page 638*
Mitoxantrone Injection® [Can] *see* mitoxantrone *on page 638*
mitozantrone *see* mitoxantrone *on page 638*
Mitran® Oral *(Discontinued)* *see* chlordiazepoxide *on page 201*
Mitrazol™ [US-OTC] *see* miconazole *on page 630*
Mivacron® *(Discontinued)*
mivacurium *(Discontinued)*
MK-191 *see* pivampicillin *(Canada only) on page 758*
MK383 *see* tirofiban *on page 930*
MK-0431 *see* sitagliptin *on page 870*
MK462 *see* rizatriptan *on page 841*
MK 0517 *see* fosaprepitant *on page 426*
MK-0518 *see* raltegravir *on page 817*
MK594 *see* losartan *on page 577*
MK0826 *see* ertapenem *on page 353*
MK 869 *see* aprepitant *on page 90*
MLN341 *see* bortezomib *on page 139*
MMF *see* mycophenolate *on page 649*
MMR *see* measles, mumps, and rubella vaccines, combined *on page 593*
MMRV *see* measles, mumps, rubella, and varicella virus vaccine *on page 593*
Moban® [US/Can] *see* molindone *on page 640*
Mobic® [US/Can] *see* meloxicam *on page 599*
Mobicox® [Can] *see* meloxicam *on page 599*
Mobidin® *(Discontinued)* *see* magnesium salicylate *on page 588*
Mobisyl® [US-OTC] *see* trolamine *on page 957*

moclobemide *(Canada only)* (moe KLOE be mide)

U.S./Canadian Brand Names Apo-Moclobemide® [Can]; Dom-Moclobemide [Can]; Manerix® [Can]; Novo-Moclobemide [Can]; Nu-Moclobemide [Can]; PMS-Moclobemide [Can]
Therapeutic Category Antidepressant, Monoamine Oxidase Inhibitor
Use Symptomatic relief of depressive illness
Usual Dosage Oral: Adults: Initial: 300 mg/day in 2 divided doses; increase gradually to maximum of 600 mg/day; **Note:** Individual patient response may allow a reduction in daily dose in long-term therapy.
Dosage Forms [CAN] = Canadian brand name
  Tablet: 150 mg, 300 mg [not available in the U.S.]
    Alti-Moclobemide [CAN], Apo-Moclobemide® [CAN], Dom-Moclobemide® [CAN], Manerix® [CAN], Novo-Moclobemidee [CAN], Nu-Moclobemidee [CAN], PMS-Moclobemide [CAN]: 150 mg, 300 mg [not available in the U.S.]

modafinil (moe DAF i nil)

U.S./Canadian Brand Names Alertec® [Can]; Provigil® [US/Can]
Therapeutic Category Central Nervous System Stimulant, Nonamphetamine
Controlled Substance C-IV
Use Improve wakefulness in patients with excessive daytime sleepiness associated with narcolepsy and shift work sleep disorder (SWSD); adjunctive therapy for obstructive sleep apnea/hypopnea syndrome (OSAHS)
Usual Dosage Oral: Adults:
  Narcolepsy, obstructive sleep apnea/hypopnea syndrome (OSAHS): Initial: 200 mg as a single daily dose in the morning
  Shift work sleep disorder (SWSD): Initial: 200 mg as a single dose taken ~1 hour prior to start of work shift
  Note: Doses of 400 mg/day, given as a single dose, have been well tolerated, but there is no consistent evidence that this dose confers additional benefit.

◀ **Dosage Forms**
Tablet:
Provigil®: 100 mg, 200 mg

Modane® Soft *(Discontinued)* see docusate on page 314
Modecate® [Can] see fluphenazine on page 415
Modecate® Concentrate [Can] see fluphenazine on page 415
Modicon® [US] see ethinyl estradiol and norethindrone on page 376
modified Dakin's solution see sodium hypochlorite solution on page 876
Moducal® [US-OTC] see glucose polymers on page 447
Modulon® [Can] see trimebutine (Canada only) on page 952
Moduret [Can] see amiloride and hydrochlorothiazide on page 59
Moduretic® *(Discontinued)* see amiloride and hydrochlorothiazide on page 59

moexipril (mo EKS i pril)

Sound-Alike/Look-Alike Issues
 moexipril may be confused with Monopril®
Synonyms moexipril hydrochloride
U.S./Canadian Brand Names Univasc® [US]
Therapeutic Category Angiotensin-Converting Enzyme (ACE) Inhibitor
Use Treatment of hypertension, alone or in combination with thiazide diuretics
Usual Dosage Oral: Adults: Initial: 7.5 mg once daily (in patients **not** receiving diuretics), 1 hour prior to a meal **or** 3.75 mg once daily (when combined with thiazide diuretics); maintenance dose: 7.5-30 mg/day in 1 or 2 divided doses 1 hour before meals
Dosage Forms
Tablet [scored]: 7.5 mg, 15 mg
 Univasc®: 7.5 mg, 15 mg

moexipril and hydrochlorothiazide (mo EKS i pril & hye droe klor oh THYE a zide)

Synonyms hydrochlorothiazide and moexipril
U.S./Canadian Brand Names Uniretic® [US/Can]
Therapeutic Category Angiotensin-Converting Enzyme (ACE) Inhibitor; Diuretic, Thiazide
Use Treatment of hypertension; not indicated for initial treatment of hypertension
Usual Dosage Oral: Adults: 7.5-30 mg of moexipril, taken either in a single or divided dose one hour before meals; hydrochlorothiazide dose should be ≤50 mg/day
Dosage Forms
Tablet [scored]:
 7.5/12.5: Moexipril 7.5 mg and hydrochlorothiazide 12.5
 15/12.5: Moexipril 15 mg and hydrochlorothiazide 12.5
 15/25: Moexipril 15 mg and hydrochlorothiazide 25
  Uniretic®: 7.5/12.5: Moexipril 7.5 mg and hydrochlorothiazide 12.5 mg; 15/12.5: Moexipril 15 mg and hydrochlorothiazide 12.5 mg; 15/25: Moexipril 15 mg and hydrochlorothiazide 25 mg

moexipril hydrochloride see moexipril on page 640
Mogadon [Can] see nitrazepam (Canada only) on page 674
Moi-Stir® [US-OTC] see saliva substitute on page 853
Moisture® Eyes [US-OTC] see artificial tears on page 95
Moisture® Eyes PM [US-OTC] see artificial tears on page 95

molindone (moe LIN done)

Sound-Alike/Look-Alike Issues
 molindone may be confused with Mobidin®
 Moban® may be confused with Mobidin®, Modane®
Synonyms molindone hydrochloride
U.S./Canadian Brand Names Moban® [US/Can]
Therapeutic Category Antipsychotic Agent, Dihydroindoline

Use Management of schizophrenia

Usual Dosage Oral: Adults: Schizophrenia/psychoses:
Initial: 50-75 mg/day, may increase to 100 mg/day in 3-4 days; may further increase dose gradually to maximum of 225 mg/day
Maintenance: 5-15 mg (mild symptoms) or 10-25 mg (moderate symptoms) 3-4 times/day (up to 225 mg/day may be required in severe cases)

Dosage Forms
Tablet:
Moban®: 5 mg, 10 mg, 25 mg, 50 mg

molindone hydrochloride *see* molindone *on page 640*

molybdenum *see* trace metals *on page 940*

MOM *see* magnesium hydroxide *on page 585*

Momentum® [US-OTC] *see* magnesium salicylate *on page 588*

mometasone (moe MET a sone)

Sound-Alike/Look-Alike Issues
Elocon® lotion may be confused with ophthalmic solutions. Manufacturer's labeling emphasizes the product is **NOT** for use in the eyes.

Synonyms mometasone furoate

U.S./Canadian Brand Names Asmanex® Twisthaler® [US]; Elocom® [Can]; Elocon® [US]; Nasonex® [US/Can]; PMS-Mometasone [Can]; ratio-Mometasone [Can]; Taro-Mometasone [Can]

Therapeutic Category Corticosteroid, Intranasal; Corticosteroid, Topical

Use Relief of the inflammatory and pruritic manifestations of corticosteroid-responsive dermatoses (medium potency topical corticosteroid); treatment of nasal symptoms of seasonal and perennial allergic rhinitis; prevention of nasal symptoms associated with seasonal allergic rhinitis; treatment of nasal polyps in adults; maintenance treatment of asthma as prophylactic therapy or as a supplement in asthma patients requiring oral corticosteroids for the purpose of decreasing or eliminating the oral corticosteroid requirement

Usual Dosage
Oral inhalation:
Children 4-11 years: 110 mcg once daily in the evening (maximum: 110 mcg/day)
Children ≥12 years and Adults: Previous therapy:
Bronchodilators or inhaled corticosteroids: Initial: 1 inhalation (220 mcg) daily (maximum: 2 inhalations or 440 mcg/day); may be given in the evening or in divided doses twice daily
Oral corticosteroids: Initial: 440 mcg twice daily (maximum: 880 mcg/day); prednisone should be reduced no faster than 2.5 mg/day on a weekly basis, beginning after at least 1 week of mometasone furoate use
NIH Asthma Guidelines (NIH, 2007): Children ≥12 years and Adults:
"Low" dose: 220 mcg/day
"Medium" dose: 440 mcg/day
"High" dose: >440 mcg/day
Note: Maximum effects may not be evident for 1-2 weeks or longer; dose should be titrated to effect, using the lowest possible dose
Nasal spray:
Allergic rhinitis:
Children 2-11 years: 1 spray (50 mcg) in each nostril daily
Children ≥12 years and Adults: 2 sprays (100 mcg) in each nostril daily; when used for the prevention of allergic rhinitis, treatment should begin 2-4 weeks prior to pollen season
Nasal polyps: Adults: 2 sprays (100 mcg) in each nostril twice daily; 2 sprays (100 mcg) once daily may be effective in some patients
Topical: Apply sparingly, do not use occlusive dressings. Therapy should be discontinued when control is achieved; if no improvement is seen in 2 weeks, reassessment of diagnosis may be necessary.
Cream, ointment: Children ≥2 years and Adults: Apply a thin film to affected area once daily; do not use in pediatric patients for longer than 3 weeks
Lotion: Children ≥12 years and Adults: Apply a few drops to affected area once daily

Dosage Forms
Cream, topical: 0.1% (15 g, 45 g)
Elocon®: 0.1% (15 g, 45 g)
Lotion, topical: 0.1% (30 mL, 60 mL)
Elocon®: 0.1% (30 mL, 60 mL)

▶

◀ **Ointment, topical:** 0.1% (15 g, 45 g)
Elocon®: 0.1% (15 g, 45 g)
Powder for oral inhalation:
Asmanex® Twisthaler®: 110 mcg (30 units); 220 mcg (14 units, 30 units, 60 units, 120 units)
Suspension, intranasal [spray]:
Nasonex®: 50 mcg/spray (17 g)

mometasone furoate *see* mometasone *on page 641*
MOM/mineral oil emulsion *see* magnesium hydroxide and mineral oil *on page 586*
monacolin K *see* lovastatin *on page 579*
Monafed® *(Discontinued)* *see* guaifenesin *on page 453*
Monafed® DM *(Discontinued)* *see* guaifenesin and dextromethorphan *on page 454*
Monarc-M™ [US] *see* antihemophilic factor (human) *on page 78*
Monilia **skin test** *see* Candida albicans (Monilia) *on page 169*
Monistat® [Can] *see* miconazole *on page 630*
Monistat® 1 Combination Pack [US-OTC] *see* miconazole *on page 630*
Monistat® 3 [US-OTC/Can] *see* miconazole *on page 630*
Monistat® 3 Combination Pack [US-OTC] *see* miconazole *on page 630*
Monistat® 7 [US-OTC] *see* miconazole *on page 630*
Monistat-Derm® *(Discontinued)* *see* miconazole *on page 630*
Monistat i.v.™ Injection *(Discontinued)* *see* miconazole *on page 630*
Monitan® [Can] *see* acebutolol *on page 19*

monobenzone (mon oh BEN zone)
U.S./Canadian Brand Names Benoquin® [US]
Therapeutic Category Topical Skin Product
Use Final depigmentation in extensive vitiligo
Usual Dosage Topical: Children ≥12 years and Adults: Apply 2-3 times daily; once desired degree of pigmentation is obtained, may apply as needed (usually 2 times/week)
Dosage Forms
Cream, topical:
Benoquin®: 20% (35 g)

Monocaps [US-OTC] *see* vitamins (multiple/oral) *on page 983*
Monoclate-P® [US] *see* antihemophilic factor (human) *on page 78*
monoclonal antibody *see* muromonab-CD3 *on page 648*
Monocor® [Can] *see* bisoprolol *on page 138*
Monodox® [US] *see* doxycycline *on page 323*
monoethanolamine *see* ethanolamine oleate *on page 369*
Monoket® [US] *see* isosorbide mononitrate *on page 531*
MonoNessa™ [US] *see* ethinyl estradiol and norgestimate *on page 378*
Mononine® [US/Can] *see* factor IX *on page 388*
Monopril® [US/Can] *see* fosinopril *on page 427*
Monopril-HCT® [US/Can] *see* fosinopril and hydrochlorothiazide *on page 428*

montelukast (mon te LOO kast)
Sound-Alike/Look-Alike Issues
Singulair® may be confused with Sinequan®
Synonyms montelukast sodium
U.S./Canadian Brand Names Singulair® [US/Can]
Therapeutic Category Leukotriene Receptor Antagonist
Use Prophylaxis and chronic treatment of asthma; relief of symptoms of seasonal allergic rhinitis and perennial allergic rhinitis; prevention of exercise-induced bronchospasm
Usual Dosage Oral:
Children:
6-23 months: Perennial allergic rhinitis: 4 mg (oral granules) once daily

12-23 months: Asthma: 4 mg (oral granules) once daily, taken in the evening

2-5 years: Asthma, seasonal or perennial allergic rhinitis: 4 mg (chewable tablet or oral granules) once daily, taken in the evening

6-14 years: Asthma, seasonal or perennial allergic rhinitis: 5 mg (chewable tablet) once daily, taken in the evening

Children ≥15 years and Adults:

Asthma, seasonal or perennial allergic rhinitis: 10 mg/day, taken in the evening

Bronchoconstriction, exercise-induced (prevention): 10 mg at least 2 hours prior to exercise; additional doses should not be administered within 24 hours. Daily administration to prevent exercise-induced bronchoconstriction has not been evaluated.

Dosage Forms

Granules:

Singulair®: 4 mg/packet (30s)

Tablet:

Singulair®: 10 mg

Tablet, chewable:

Singulair®: 4 mg, 5 mg

montelukast sodium *see montelukast on page 642*

Monurol® [US/Can] *see fosfomycin on page 427*

8-MOP® [US] *see methoxsalen on page 617*

more attenuated enders strain *see measles virus vaccine (live) on page 594*

MoreDophilus® [US-OTC] *see Lactobacillus on page 543*

moricizine (mor I siz een)

Sound-Alike/Look-Alike Issues

Ethmozine® may be confused with Erythrocin®, erythromycin

Synonyms moricizine hydrochloride

U.S./Canadian Brand Names Ethmozine® [Can]

Therapeutic Category Antiarrhythmic Agent, Class I

Use Treatment of ventricular tachycardia and life-threatening ventricular arrhythmias

Usual Dosage Oral: Adults: 200-300 mg every 8 hours, adjust dosage at 150 mg/day at 3-day intervals.

moricizine hydrochloride *see moricizine on page 643*

morning after pill *see ethinyl estradiol and norgestrel on page 380*

Morphine HP® [Can] *see morphine sulfate on page 643*

Morphine LP® Epidural [Can] *see morphine sulfate on page 643*

morphine sulfate (MOR feen SUL fate)

Sound-Alike/Look-Alike Issues

morphine may be confused with HYDROmorphone

morphine sulfate may be confused with magnesium sulfate

Avinza® may be confused with Evista®, Invanz®

MS Contin® may be confused with Oxycontin®

MSO_4 and MS are error-prone abbreviations (mistaken as magnesium sulfate)

Roxanol™ may be confused with OxyFast®, Roxicet™, Roxicodone®

U.S./Canadian Brand Names Astramorph/PF™ [US]; Avinza® [US]; DepoDur® [US]; Doloral [Can]; Duramorph® [US]; Infumorph® [US]; Kadian® [US/Can]; M-Eslon® [Can]; M.O.S.-SR® [Can]; M.O.S.-Sulfate® [Can]; M.O.S.® 10 [Can]; M.O.S.® 20 [Can]; M.O.S.® 30 [Can]; Morphine HP® [Can]; Morphine LP® Epidural [Can]; MS Contin® [US/Can]; MS-IR® [Can]; Novo-Morphine SR [Can]; Oramorph SR® [US]; PMS-Morphine Sulfate SR [Can]; Ratio-Morphine SR [Can]; Ratio-Morphine [Can]; Roxanol™ [US]; Statex® [Can]; Zomorph® [Can]

Therapeutic Category Analgesic, Narcotic

Controlled Substance C-II

Use Relief of moderate-to-severe acute and chronic pain; relief of pain of myocardial infarction; relief of dyspnea of acute left ventricular failure and pulmonary edema; preanesthetic medication

DepoDur®: Epidural (lumbar) single-dose management of surgical pain

Infumorph®: Used in continuous microinfusion devices for intrathecal or epidural administration in treatment of intractable chronic pain

Controlled, extended, or sustained release products: Only intended/indicated for use when repeated doses for an extended period of time are required. The 100 mg and 200 mg tablets or capsules of Kadian®, MS Contin®, and morphine sulfate controlled release tablets and the 60 mg, 90 mg, and 120 mg capsules of Avinza® should only be used in opioid-tolerant patients.

Usual Dosage Note: These are guidelines and do not represent the doses that may be required in all patients. Doses and dosage intervals should be titrated to pain relief/prevention.

Children >6 months and <50 kg: Acute pain (moderate-to-severe):
Oral (immediate release formulations): 0.15-0.3 mg/kg every 3-4 hours as needed
I.M., I.V.: 0.1-0.2 mg/kg every 3-4 hours as needed
I.V. infusion: Range: 10-60 mcg/kg/hour

Adults:

Acute pain (moderate-to-severe):
Oral (immediate release formulations): Opiate-naive: Initial: 10 mg every 4 hours as needed; patients with prior opiate exposure may require higher initial doses: usual dosage range: 10-30 mg every 4 hours as needed

I.M., SubQ: **Note:** Repeated SubQ administration causes local tissue irritation, pain, and induration.
Initial: Opiate-naive: 5-10 mg every 4 hours as needed; patients with prior opiate exposure may require higher initial doses; usual dosage range: 5-20 mg every 4 hours as needed

Rectal: 10-20 mg every 3-4 hours

I.V.: Initial: Opiate-naive: 2.5-5 mg every 3-4 hours; patients with prior opiate exposure may require higher initial doses. **Note:** Repeated doses (up to every 5 minutes if needed) in small increments (eg, 1-4 mg) may be preferred to larger and less frequent doses.

Acute myocardial infarction, analgesia (ACC/AHA 2004 guidelines): Initial management: 2-4 mg, give 2-8 mg every 5-15 minutes as needed.

I.V., SubQ continuous infusion: 0.8-10 mg/hour; usual range: Up to 80 mg/hour

Patient-controlled analgesia (PCA): (Opiate-naive: Consider lower end of dosing range):
Usual concentration: 1 mg/mL
Demand dose: Usual: 1 mg; range: 0.5-2.5 mg
Lockout interval: 5-10 minutes

Intrathecal (I.T.): **Note:** Administer with extreme caution and in reduced dosage to geriatric or debilitated patients. I.T. dose is usually ¹/₁₀ that of epidural dosage.
Opioid-naive: 0.2-1 mg/dose (may provide adequate relief for 24 hours); repeat doses are **not** recommended
Continuous microinfusion (Infumorph®): Initial: 0.2-1 mg/day
Opioid-tolerant: 1-10 mg/day
Continuous microinfusion (Infumorph®): Initial: 1-10 mg/day, titrate to effect; usual maximum is ~20 mg/day

Epidural: Pain management: **Note:** Administer with extreme caution and in reduced dosage to geriatric or debilitated patients. Vigilant monitoring is particularly important in these patients.
Single-dose (Astromorph/PF™, Duramorph®): Initial: 5 mg, if pain relief not achieved in 1 hour, careful administration of 1-2 mg at intervals sufficient to assess effectiveness may be given; maximum: 10 mg/24 hours
Infusion: Bolus dose: 1-6 mg; infusion rate: 0.1-0.2 mg/hour; maximum dose: 10 mg/24 hours
Continuous microinfusion (Infumorph®):
Opioid-naive: Initial: 0.2-1 mg/day
Opioid-tolerant: Initial: 1-10 mg/day, titrate to effect; usual maximum is ~20 mg/day

Surgical anesthesia: Epidural: Single-dose (extended release, DepoDur®): Lumbar epidural only; not recommended in patients <18 years of age:
Cesarean section: 10 mg (after clamping umbilical cord)
Lower abdominal/pelvic surgery: 10-15 mg
Major orthopedic surgery of lower extremity: 15 mg
For DepoDur®: To minimize the pharmacokinetic interaction resulting in higher peak serum concentrations of morphine, administer the test dose of the local anesthetic at least 15 minutes prior to DepoDur® administration. Use of DepoDur® with epidural local anesthetics has not been studied. Other medications should not be administered into the epidural space for at least 48 hours after administration of DepoDur®.

Note: Some patients may benefit from a 20 mg dose, however, the incidence of adverse effects may be increased.

Chronic pain: Note: Patients taking opioids chronically may become tolerant and require doses higher than the usual dosage range to maintain the desired effect. Tolerance can be managed by appropriate dose titration. There is no optimal or maximal dose for morphine in chronic pain. The appropriate dose is one that relieves pain throughout its dosing interval without causing unmanageable side effects.

Oral: Controlled, extended, or sustained release formulations: A patient's morphine requirement should be established using prompt-release formulations. Conversion to long-acting products may be considered when chronic, continuous treatment is required. Higher dosages should be reserved for use only in opioid-tolerant patients.

Capsules, extended release (Avinza®): Daily dose administered once daily (for best results, administer at same time each day)

Capsules, sustained release (Kadian®): Daily dose administered once daily or in 2 divided doses daily (every 12 hours)

Tablets, controlled release (MS Contin®), sustained release (Oramorph SR®), or extended release: Daily dose divided and administered every 8 or every 12 hours

Dosage Forms [CAN] Canadian brand name

Capsule, extended release:
Avinza®: 30 mg, 60 mg, 90 mg, 120 mg
Kadian®: 10 mg, 20 mg, 30 mg, 50 mg, 60 mg, 80 mg, 100 mg, 200 mg

Infusion [premixed in D$_5$W]: 1 mg/mL (100 mL, 250 mL)

Injection, extended release liposomal suspension [lumbar epidural injection, preservative free]:
DepoDur®: 10 mg/mL (1 mL, 1.5 mL, 2 mL)

Injection, solution: 2 mg/mL (1 mL); 4 mg/mL (1 mL); 5 mg/mL (1 mL); 8 mg/mL (1 mL); 10 mg/0.7 mL (0.7 mL); 10 mg/mL (1 mL, 10 mL); 15 mg/mL (1 mL, 20 mL); 25 mg/mL (4 mL, 10 mL, 20 mL, 40 mL, 50 mL, 100 mL, 250 mL); 50 mg/mL (20 mL, 40 mL)

Injection, solution [epidural, intrathecal, or I.V. infusion; preservative free]:
Astramorph/PF™: 0.5 mg/mL (2 mL, 10 mL); 1 mg/mL (2 mL, 10 mL)
Duramorph®: 0.5 mg/mL (10 mL); 1 mg/mL (10 mL)

Injection, solution [epidural or intrathecal infusion via microinfusion device; preservative free]: 10 mg/mL (20 mL); 25 mg/mL (20 mL)
Infumorph®: 10 mg/mL (20 mL); 25 mg/mL (20 mL)

Injection, solution [I.V. infusion via PCA pump]: 0.5 mg/mL (30 mL); 1 mg/mL (30 mL, 50 mL); 2 mg/mL (30 mL); 5 mg/mL (30 mL, 50 mL)

Injection, solution [preservative free]: 0.5 mg/mL (10 mL); 1 mg/mL (10 mL); 25 mg/mL (4 mL, 10 mL, 20 mL)

Solution, oral: 10 mg/5 mL, 20 mg/5 mL, 20 mg/mL
Doloral [CAN]: 1 mg/mL; 5 mg/mL [not available in U.S.]

Solution, oral [concentrate]: 5 mg/0.25 mL; 10 mg/0.5 mL; 20 mg/mL
Roxanol™: 20 mg/mL (30 mL, 120 mL); 100 mg/5 mL (240 mL)

Suppository, rectal: 5 mg (12s), 10 mg (12s), 20 mg (12s), 30 mg (12s)

Tablet: 15 mg, 30 mg

Tablet, controlled release:
MS Contin®: 15 mg, 30 mg, 60 mg, 100 mg, 200 mg

Tablet, extended release: 15 mg, 30 mg, 60 mg, 100 mg, 200 mg

Tablet, sustained release:
Oramorph SR®: 15 mg, 30 mg, 60 mg, 100 mg

morrhuate sodium (MOR yoo ate SOW dee um)

U.S./Canadian Brand Names Scleromate® [US]

Therapeutic Category Sclerosing Agent

Use Treatment of small, uncomplicated varicose veins of the lower extremities

Usual Dosage I.V.: Adults: 50-250 mg, repeated at 5- to 7-day intervals (50-100 mg for small veins, 150-250 mg for large veins)

Dosage Forms
Injection, solution: 50 mg/mL (30 mL)
Scleromate®: 50 mg/mL (30 mL)

M.O.S.® 10 [Can] *see* morphine sulfate *on page 643*

M.O.S.® 20 [Can] *see* morphine sulfate *on page 643*

M.O.S.® 30 [Can] *see* morphine sulfate *on page 643*

Mosco® Callus & Corn Remover [US-OTC] *see* salicylic acid *on page 850*

M.O.S.-SR® [Can] *see* morphine sulfate *on page 643*

M.O.S.-Sulfate® [Can] *see* morphine sulfate *on page 643*

Motofen® *(Discontinued)* *see* difenoxin and atropine *on page 295*

Motrin® Children's [US-OTC/Can] *see* ibuprofen *on page 495*

Motrin® *(Discontinued)* *see* ibuprofen *on page 495*
Motrin® IB [US-OTC/Can] *see* ibuprofen *on page 495*
Motrin® IB Sinus *(Discontinued)* *see* pseudoephedrine and ibuprofen *on page 802*
Motrin® Infants' [US-OTC] *see* ibuprofen *on page 495*
Motrin® Junior Strength [US-OTC] *see* ibuprofen *on page 495*
Mouthkote® [US-OTC] *see* saliva substitute *on page 853*
MoviPrep® [US] *see* polyethylene glycol-electrolyte solution *on page 766*

moxifloxacin (moxs i FLOKS a sin)

Sound-Alike/Look-Alike Issues
Avelox® may be confused with Avonex®
Synonyms moxifloxacin hydrochloride
U.S./Canadian Brand Names Avelox® I.V. [US/Can]; Avelox® [US/Can]; Vigamox™ [US/Can]
Therapeutic Category Antibiotic, Quinolone
Use Treatment of mild-to-moderate community-acquired pneumonia, including multidrug-resistant *Streptococcus pneumoniae* (MDRSP); acute bacterial exacerbation of chronic bronchitis; acute bacterial sinusitis; complicated and uncomplicated skin and skin structure infections; complicated intraabdominal infections; bacterial conjunctivitis (ophthalmic formulation)
Usual Dosage
Usual dosage range:
Children ≥1 year and Adults: Ophthalmic: Instill 1 drop into affected eye(s) 3 times/day for 7 days
Adults: Oral, I.V.: 400 mg every 24 hours
Indication-specific dosing:
Children ≥1 year and Adults: Ophthalmic: **Bacterial conjunctivitis:** Instill 1 drop into affected eye(s) 3 times/day for 7 days
Adults: Oral, I.V.:
Acute bacterial sinusitis: 400 mg every 24 hours for 10 days
Chronic bronchitis, acute bacterial exacerbation: 400 mg every 24 hours for 5 days
Intraabdominal infections (complicated): 400 mg every 24 hours for 5-14 days (initiate with I.V.)
Pneumonia, community-acquired (including MDRSP): 400 mg every 24 hours for 7-14 days
Skin and skin structure infections:
Complicated: 400 mg every 24 hours for 7-21 days
Uncomplicated: 400 mg every 24 hours for 7 days
Dosage Forms
Infusion [premixed in sodium chloride 0.8%]:
Avelox® I.V.: 400 mg (250 mL)
Solution, ophthalmic:
Vigamox™: 0.5% (3 mL)
Tablet:
Avelox®: 400 mg
Avelox® ABC Pack [unit-dose pack]: 400 mg (5s)

moxifloxacin hydrochloride *see* moxifloxacin *on page 646*
4-MP *see* fomepizole *on page 423*
MPA *see* mycophenolate *on page 649*
MPA and estrogens (conjugated) *see* estrogens (conjugated/equine) and medroxyprogesterone *on page 365*
M-Prednisol® Injection *(Discontinued)* *see* methylprednisolone *on page 623*
MPSV4 *see* meningococcal polysaccharide vaccine (groups A / C / Y and W-135) *on page 601*
MS Contin® [US/Can] *see* morphine sulfate *on page 643*
MS-IR® [Can] *see* morphine sulfate *on page 643*
MTA *see* pemetrexed *on page 729*
MTC *see* mitomycin *on page 638*
Mucinex® [US-OTC] *see* guaifenesin *on page 453*
Mucinex®-D [US-OTC] *see* guaifenesin and pseudoephedrine *on page 458*
Mucinex® D Maximum Strength [US-OTC] *see* guaifenesin and pseudoephedrine *on page 458*
Mucinex®, Children's [US-OTC] *see* guaifenesin *on page 453*
Mucinex® Children's Cough [US-OTC] *see* guaifenesin and dextromethorphan *on page 454*

Mucinex®, Children's Mini-Melts™ [US-OTC] *see* guaifenesin *on page 453*
Mucinex® DM [US-OTC] *see* guaifenesin and dextromethorphan *on page 454*
Mucinex® DM Maximum Strength [US-OTC] *see* guaifenesin and dextromethorphan *on page 454*
Mucinex® Full force™ [US-OTC] *see* oxymetazoline *on page 712*
Mucinex®, Junior Mini-Melts™ [US-OTC] *see* guaifenesin *on page 453*
Mucinex® Maximum Strength [US-OTC] *see* guaifenesin *on page 453*
Mucinex® moisture smart™ [US-OTC] *see* oxymetazoline *on page 712*
Mucomyst® [Can] *see* acetylcysteine *on page 30*
Mucosil™ *(Discontinued)* *see* acetylcysteine *on page 30*
Multidex® [US-OTC] *see* maltodextrin *on page 590*
Multihance® [US] *see* gadobenate dimeglumine *on page 432*
Multihance® Multipak™ [US] *see* gadobenate dimeglumine *on page 432*
multiple vitamins *see* vitamins (multiple/oral) *on page 983*
multitargeted antifolate *see* pemetrexed *on page 729*
Multitest CMI® *(Discontinued)*
Multitrace®-4 [US] *see* trace metals *on page 940*
Multitrace®-4 Concentrate [US] *see* trace metals *on page 940*
Multitrace®-4 Neonatal [US] *see* trace metals *on page 940*
Multitrace®-4 Pediatric [US] *see* trace metals *on page 940*
Multitrace®-5 [US] *see* trace metals *on page 940*
Multitrace®-5 Concentrate [US] *see* trace metals *on page 940*
multivitamins/fluoride *see* vitamins (multiple/pediatric) *on page 983*
mumps, measles, and rubella vaccines, combined *see* measles, mumps, and rubella vaccines, combined *on page 593*
mumps, rubella, varicella, and measles vaccine *see* measles, mumps, rubella, and varicella virus vaccine *on page 593*
Mumpsvax® [US] *see* mumps virus vaccine, live, attenuated *on page 647*

mumps virus vaccine, live, attenuated
(mumpz VYE rus vak SEEN, live, a ten YOO ate ed)
U.S./Canadian Brand Names Mumpsvax® [US]
Therapeutic Category Vaccine, Live Virus
Use Mumps prophylaxis by promoting active immunity
Note: Trivalent measles-mumps-rubella (MMR) vaccine is the preferred agent for most children and many adults; persons born prior to 1957 are generally considered immune and need not be vaccinated
Usual Dosage SubQ: Children ≥12-15 months and Adults: 0.5 mL as a single dose
Dosage Forms
Injection, powder for reconstitution [preservative free]:
Mumpsvax®: $TCID_{50}$ 20,000

mupirocin (myoo PEER oh sin)
Sound-Alike/Look-Alike Issues
Bactroban® may be confused with bacitracin, baclofen, Bactrim™
Synonyms mupirocin calcium; pseudomonic acid A
U.S./Canadian Brand Names Bactroban® Nasal [US]; Bactroban® [US/Can]
Therapeutic Category Antibiotic, Topical
Use
Intranasal: Eradication of nasal colonization with MRSA in adult patients and healthcare workers
Topical: Treatment of impetigo or secondary infected traumatic skin lesions due to *S. aureus* and *S. pyogenes*
Usual Dosage
Intranasal: Children ≥12 years and Adults: Eradication of nasal MRSA: Approximately one-half of the ointment from the single-use tube should be applied into one nostril and the other half into the other nostril twice daily for 5 days

◄ Topical:
Children ≥2 months and Adults: Impetigo: Ointment: Apply to affected area 3 times/day; reevaluate after 3-5 days if no clinical response
Children ≥3 months and Adults: Secondary skin infections: Cream: Apply to affected area 3 times/day for 10 days; reevaluate after 3-5 days if no clinical response

Dosage Forms
Cream, topical:
Bactroban®: 2% (15 g, 30 g)
Ointment, intranasal, topical:
Bactroban® Nasal: 2% (1 g)
Ointment, topical: 2% (0.9 g, 22 g)
Bactroban®: 2% (22 g)

mupirocin calcium see mupirocin on page 647
Murine® Ear Wax Removal System [US-OTC] see carbamide peroxide on page 174
Murine® Tears [US-OTC] see artificial tears on page 95
Murine® Tears Plus [US-OTC] see tetrahydrozoline on page 916
Muro 128® [US-OTC] see sodium chloride on page 873
Murocel® [US-OTC] see artificial tears on page 95
Murocoll-2® [US] see phenylephrine and scopolamine on page 747

muromonab-CD3 (myoo roe MOE nab see dee three)
Synonyms monoclonal antibody; OKT3
U.S./Canadian Brand Names Orthoclone OKT® 3 [US/Can]
Therapeutic Category Immunosuppressant Agent
Use Treatment of acute allograft rejection in renal transplant patients; treatment of acute hepatic, and kidney rejection episodes resistant to conventional treatment
Usual Dosage I.V. (refer to individual protocols):
Children <30 kg: 2.5 mg/day once daily for 7-14 days
Children >30 kg: 5 mg/day once daily for 7-14 days
OR
Children <12 years: 0.1 mg/kg/day once daily for 10-14 days
Children ≥12 years and Adults: 5 mg/day once daily for 10-14 days
Dosage Forms
Injection, solution:
Orthoclone OKT® 3: 1 mg/mL (5 mL)

Muroptic-5® (Discontinued) see sodium chloride on page 873
Muse® [US] see alprostadil on page 50
Muse® Pellet [Can] see alprostadil on page 50
Mustargen® [US/Can] see mechlorethamine on page 595
mustine see mechlorethamine on page 595
Mutamycin® [US/Can] see mitomycin on page 638
M.V.I.®-12 [US] see vitamins (multiple/injectable) on page 982
M.V.I. Adult™ [US] see vitamins (multiple/injectable) on page 982
M.V.I® Pediatric [US] see vitamins (multiple/injectable) on page 982
Myadec® [US-OTC] see vitamins (multiple/oral) on page 983
Myambutol® [US] see ethambutol on page 368
Mycamine® [US/Can] see micafungin on page 630
Mycelex® [US] see clotrimazole on page 238
Mycelex®-G (Discontinued) see clotrimazole on page 238
Mycifradin® Sulfate (Discontinued) see neomycin on page 661
Mycinaire™ (Discontinued) see sodium chloride on page 873
Mycinettes® [US-OTC] see benzocaine on page 124
Mycobutin® [US/Can] see rifabutin on page 833
Mycocide® NS [US-OTC] see tolnaftate on page 934
Mycolog®-II (Discontinued) see nystatin and triamcinolone on page 690

Myco-Nail [US-OTC] *see* triacetin *on page 947*
Myconel® Topical *(Discontinued)* *see* nystatin and triamcinolone *on page 690*

mycophenolate (mye koe FEN oh late)
Synonyms MMF; MPA; mycophenolate mofetil; mycophenolate sodium; mycophenolic acid
U.S./Canadian Brand Names CellCept® [US/Can]; Myfortic® [US/Can]
Therapeutic Category Immunosuppressant Agent
Use Prophylaxis of organ rejection concomitantly with cyclosporine and corticosteroids in patients receiving allogeneic renal (CellCept®, Myfortic®), cardiac (CellCept®), or hepatic (CellCept®) transplants
Usual Dosage
Children: Renal transplant: Oral:
CellCept® suspension: 600 mg/m²/dose twice daily; maximum dose: 1 g twice daily
Alternatively, may use solid dosage forms according to BSA as follows:
BSA 1.25-1.5 m²: 750 mg capsule twice daily
BSA >1.5 m²: 1 g capsule or tablet twice daily
Myfortic®: 400 mg/m²/dose twice daily; maximum dose: 720 mg twice daily
BSA <1.19 m²: Use of this formulation is not recommended
BSA 1.19-1.58 m²: 540 mg twice daily (maximum: 1080 mg/day)
BSA >1.58 m²: 720 mg twice daily (maximum: 1440 mg/day)
Adults: **Note:** May be used I.V. for up to 14 days; transition to oral therapy as soon as tolerated.
Renal transplant:
CellCept®:
Oral: 1 g twice daily. Doses >2 g/day are not recommended.
I.V.: 1 g twice daily
Myfortic®: Oral: 720 mg twice daily (1440 mg/day)
Cardiac transplantation:
Oral (CellCept®): 1.5 g twice daily
I.V. (CellCept®): 1.5 g twice daily
Hepatic transplantation:
Oral (CellCept®): 1.5 g twice daily
I.V. (CellCept®): 1 g twice daily
Dosage Forms
Capsule:
CellCept®: 250 mg
Injection, powder for reconstitution:
CellCept®: 500 mg
Powder for oral suspension:
CellCept®: 200 mg/mL
Tablet:
CellCept®: 500 mg
Tablet, delayed release:
Myfortic®: 180 mg, 360 mg

mycophenolate mofetil *see* mycophenolate *on page 649*
mycophenolate sodium *see* mycophenolate *on page 649*
mycophenolic acid *see* mycophenolate *on page 649*
Mycostatin® [US] *see* nystatin *on page 690*
MyDex [US] *see* guaifenesin and phenylephrine *on page 456*
Mydfrin® [US/Can] *see* phenylephrine *on page 745*
Mydral™ [US] *see* tropicamide *on page 957*
Mydriacyl® [US/Can] *see* tropicamide *on page 957*
My First Flintstones® [US-OTC] *see* vitamins (multiple/pediatric) *on page 983*
Myfortic® [US/Can] *see* mycophenolate *on page 649*
MyHist-DM [US] *see* phenylephrine, pyrilamine, and dextromethorphan *on page 749*
MyKidz Iron FL™ [US-OTC] *see* vitamins (multiple/pediatric) *on page 983*
Mykrox® *(Discontinued)* *see* metolazone *on page 626*
Mylanta™ [Can] *see* aluminum hydroxide and magnesium hydroxide *on page 54*
Mylanta®-II *(Discontinued)* *see* aluminum hydroxide, magnesium hydroxide, and simethicone *on page 54*

Mylanta AR® *(Discontinued)* *see* famotidine *on page 390*

Mylanta® Children's [US-OTC] *see* calcium carbonate *on page 163*

Mylanta® Double Strength [Can] *see* aluminum hydroxide, magnesium hydroxide, and simethicone *on page 54*

Mylanta® Extra Strength [Can] *see* aluminum hydroxide, magnesium hydroxide, and simethicone *on page 54*

Mylanta® Gas Maximum Strength [US-OTC] *see* simethicone *on page 867*

Mylanta® Gelcaps® [US-OTC] *see* calcium carbonate and magnesium hydroxide *on page 164*

Mylanta® Liquid [US-OTC] *see* aluminum hydroxide, magnesium hydroxide, and simethicone *on page 54*

Mylanta® Maximum Strength Liquid [US-OTC] *see* aluminum hydroxide, magnesium hydroxide, and simethicone *on page 54*

Mylanta® Regular Strength [Can] *see* aluminum hydroxide, magnesium hydroxide, and simethicone *on page 54*

Mylanta® Supreme [US-OTC] *see* calcium carbonate and magnesium hydroxide *on page 164*

Mylanta® Ultra [US-OTC] *see* calcium carbonate and magnesium hydroxide *on page 164*

Myleran® [US/Can] *see* busulfan *on page 154*

Mylicon® Infants [US-OTC] *see* simethicone *on page 867*

Mylocel™ [US] *see* hydroxyurea *on page 490*

Mylotarg® [US/Can] *see* gemtuzumab ozogamicin *on page 439*

Myminic® Expectorant *(Discontinued)*

Myobloc® [US] *see* botulinum toxin type B *on page 141*

Myochrysine® [US/Can] *see* gold sodium thiomalate *on page 450*

Myoflex® [US-OTC/Can] *see* trolamine *on page 957*

Myotonachol® *(Discontinued)* *see* bethanechol *on page 133*

Myozyme® [US] *see* alglucosidase alfa *on page 45*

Myphetane DX [US] *see* brompheniramine, pseudoephedrine, and dextromethorphan *on page 146*

myrac™ [US] *see* minocycline *on page 635*

Mysoline® [US] *see* primidone *on page 786*

Mytelase® [US/Can] *see* ambenonium *on page 57*

Mytrex *(Discontinued)* *see* nystatin and triamcinolone *on page 690*

Mytussin® AC [US] *see* guaifenesin and codeine *on page 454*

Mytussin® DAC [US] *see* guaifenesin, pseudoephedrine, and codeine *on page 460*

N-9 *see* nonoxynol 9 *on page 677*

N-0923 *see* rotigotine *on page 847*

Na$_2$EDTA *see* edetate disodium *on page 333*

NAAK *see* atropine and pralidoxime *on page 106*

Nabi-HB® [US] *see* hepatitis B immune globulin *on page 470*

NAB-paclitaxel *see* paclitaxel (protein bound) *on page 715*

nabumetone (na BYOO me tone)

U.S./Canadian Brand Names Apo-Nabumetone® [Can]; Gen-Nabumetone [Can]; Novo-Nabumetone [Can]; Relafen® [Can]; Rhoxal-nabumetone [Can]; Sandoz-Nabumetone [Can]

Therapeutic Category Analgesic, Nonnarcotic; Nonsteroidal Antiinflammatory Drug (NSAID)

Use Management of osteoarthritis and rheumatoid arthritis

Usual Dosage Oral: Adults: 1000 mg/day; an additional 500-1000 mg may be needed in some patients to obtain more symptomatic relief; may be administered once or twice daily (maximum dose: 2000 mg/day)
Note: Patients <50 kg are less likely to require doses >1000 mg/day.

Dosage Forms
Tablet: 500 mg, 750 mg

NAC *see* acetylcysteine *on page 30*

***n*-acetyl-L-cysteine** *see* acetylcysteine *on page 30*

***n*-acetylcysteine** *see* acetylcysteine *on page 30*

n-acetyl-p-aminophenol *see* acetaminophen *on page 19*

NaCl *see* sodium chloride *on page 873*

nadolol (NAY doe lol)

Sound-Alike/Look-Alike Issues
nadolol may be confused with Mandol®
Corgard® may be confused with Cognex®

U.S./Canadian Brand Names Alti-Nadolol [Can]; Apo-Nadol® [Can]; Corgard® [US/Can]; Novo-Nadolol [Can]

Therapeutic Category Beta-Adrenergic Blocker

Use Treatment of hypertension and angina pectoris; prophylaxis of migraine headaches

Usual Dosage Oral: Adults: Initial: 40 mg/day, increase dosage gradually by 40-80 mg increments at 3- to 7-day intervals until optimum clinical response is obtained with profound slowing of heart rate; doses up to 160-240 mg/day in angina and 240-320 mg/day in hypertension may be necessary.
Hypertension: Usual dosage range (JNC 7): 40-120 mg once daily

Dosage Forms
Tablet: 20 mg, 40 mg, 80 mg
Corgard®: 20 mg, 40 mg, 80 mg

nadolol and bendroflumethiazide (NAY doe lol & ben droe floo meth EYE a zide)

Synonyms bendroflumethiazide and nadolol

U.S./Canadian Brand Names Corzide® [US]

Therapeutic Category Antihypertensive Agent, Combination; Beta-Adrenergic Blocker, Nonselective; Diuretic, Thiazide

Use Treatment of hypertension; combination product should not be used for initial therapy

Usual Dosage Oral: Adults: Treatment of hypertension: Initial: Nadolol 40 mg and bendroflumethiazide 5 mg once daily. May increase dose to nadolol 80 mg and bendroflumethiazide 5 mg once daily if needed.

Dosage Forms
Tablet: Nadolol 40 mg and bendroflumethiazide 5 mg; nadolol 80 mg and bendroflumethiazide 5 mg
Corzide® 40/5: Nadolol 40 mg and bendroflumethiazide 5 mg [scored]
Corzide® 80/5: Nadolol 80 mg and bendroflumethiazide 5 mg [scored]

nadroparin calcium *see nadroparin (Canada only) on page 651*

nadroparin *(Canada only)* (nad roe PA rin)

Synonyms nadroparin calcium

U.S./Canadian Brand Names Fraxiparine™ Forte [Can]; Fraxiparine™ [Can]

Therapeutic Category Low Molecular Weight Heparin

Use Prophylaxis of thromboembolic disorders (particularly deep venous thrombosis and pulmonary embolism) in general and orthopedic surgery; treatment of deep venous thrombosis; prevention of clotting during hemodialysis

Usual Dosage SubQ: Adults:
Prophylaxis of thromboembolic disorders in general surgery: 2850 anti-Xa int. units once daily; begin 2-4 hours before surgery and continue for 7 days
Prophylaxis of thromboembolic disorders in hip replacement: 38 anti-Xa int. units/kg 12 hours before and 12 hours after surgery, **followed by** 38 anti-Xa int. units/kg/day up to and including day 3, **then** 57 anti-Xa int. units/kg/day for up to 10 days total therapy
Treatment of thromboembolic disorders: 171 anti-Xa int. units/kg/day to a maximum of 17,100 int. units; plasma anti-Xa levels should be 1.2-1.8 anti-Xa int. units/mL 3-4 hours postinjection
Patients at increased risk of bleeding: 86 anti-Xa int. units/kg twice daily; plasma anti-Xa levels should be 0.5-1.1 anti-Xa int. units/mL 3-4 hours postinjection
Prevention of clotting during hemodialysis: Single dose of 65 anti-Xa int. units/kg into arterial line at start of each dialysis session; may give additional dose if session lasts longer than 4 hours
Patients at risk of hemorrhage: Administer 50% of dose

Dosage Forms [CAN] = Canadian brand name
Injection, solution:
Fraxiparine™ [CAN]: 9500 anti-Xa int. units/mL (0.2 mL, 0.3 mL, 0.4 mL, 0.6 mL, 0.8 mL, 1 mL) [not available in the U.S.]
Fraxiparine™ Forte [CAN]: 19,000 anti-Xa int. units/mL (0.6 mL, 0.8 mL, 1 mL) [not available in the U.S.]

nafarelin (naf a REL in)

Sound-Alike/Look-Alike Issues
nafarelin may be confused with Anafranil®, enalapril
Synonyms nafarelin acetate
U.S./Canadian Brand Names Synarel® [US/Can]
Therapeutic Category Hormone, Posterior Pituitary
Use Treatment of endometriosis, including pain and reduction of lesions; treatment of central precocious puberty (CPP; gonadotropin-dependent precocious puberty) in children of both sexes
Usual Dosage Intranasal:
Endometriosis: Adults: Female: 1 spray (200 mcg) in 1 nostril each morning and the other nostril each evening starting on days 2-4 of menstrual cycle (total: 2 sprays/day). Dose may be increased to 2 sprays (400 mcg; 1 spray in each nostril) in the morning and evening if amenorrhea is not achieved (total: 8 sprays [1600 mcg]/day). Total duration of therapy should not exceed 6 months due to decreases in bone mineral density; retreatment is not recommended by the manufacturer.
Central precocious puberty: Children: Male/Female: 2 sprays (400 mcg) into each nostril in the morning and 2 sprays (400 mcg) into each nostril in the evening (total: 8 sprays [1600 mcg]/day). If inadequate suppression, may increase dose to 3 sprays (600 mcg) into alternating nostrils 3 times/day (total: 9 sprays [1800 mcg]/day).
Dosage Forms
Solution, intranasal [spray]:
Synarel®: 2 mg/mL (8 mL)

nafarelin acetate see nafarelin *on page 652*
Nafazair® Ophthalmic (Discontinued) *see* naphazoline *on page 655*

nafcillin (naf SIL in)

Synonyms ethoxynaphthamido penicillin sodium; nafcillin sodium; sodium nafcillin
U.S./Canadian Brand Names Nallpen® [Can]; Unipen® [Can]
Therapeutic Category Penicillin
Use Treatment of infections such as osteomyelitis, septicemia, endocarditis, and CNS infections caused by susceptible strains of staphylococci species
Usual Dosage
Usual dosage range:
Neonates: I.M., I.V.:
1200-2000 g, <7 days: 50 mg/kg/day divided every 12 hours
>2000 g, <7 days: 75 mg/kg/day divided every 8 hours
1200-2000 g, ≥7 days: 75 mg/kg/day divided every 8 hours
>2000 g, ≥7 days: 100-140 mg/kg/day divided every 6 hours
Children:
I.M.: 25 mg/kg twice daily
I.V.: 50-200 mg/kg/day in divided doses every 4-6 hours (maximum: 12 g/day)
Adults:
I.M.: 500 mg every 4-6 hours
I.V.: 500-2000 mg every 4-6 hours
Indication-specific dosing:
Children:
Mild-to-moderate infections: I.M., I.V.: 50-100 mg/kg/day in divided doses every 6 hours
Severe infections: I.M., I.V.: 100-200 mg/kg/day in divided doses every 4-6 hours (maximum dose: 12 g/day)
Staphylococcal endocarditis: I.V.:
Native valve: 200 mg/kg/day in divided doses every 4-6 hours for 6 weeks
Prosthetic valve: 200 mg/kg/day in divided doses every 4-6 hours for ≥6 weeks (use with rifampin and gentamicin)
Adults: I.V.:
Endocarditis: MSSA:
Native valve: 12 g/24 hours in 4-6 divided doses for 6 weeks
Prosthetic valve: 12 g/24 hours in 6 divided doses for ≥6 weeks (use with rifampin and gentamicin)
Joint:
Bursitis, septic: 2 g every 4 hours
Prosthetic: 2 g every 4-6 hours with rifampin for 6 weeks

Staphylococcus aureus, methicillin-susceptible infections, including brain abscess, empyema, erysipelas, mastitis, myositis, orbital cellulitis, osteomyelitis, pneumonia, splenic abscess, toxic shock, urinary tract (perinephric abscess): 2 g every 4 hours

Dosage Forms
  Infusion [premixed iso-osmotic dextrose solution]: 1 g (50 mL); 2 g (100 mL)
  Injection, powder for reconstitution: 1 g, 2 g, 10 g

nafcillin sodium *see nafcillin on page 652*

naftifine (NAF ti feen)

Synonyms naftifine hydrochloride
U.S./Canadian Brand Names Naftin® [US]
Therapeutic Category Antifungal Agent
Use Topical treatment of tinea cruris (jock itch), tinea corporis (ringworm), and tinea pedis (athlete's foot)
Usual Dosage Topical: Adults: Apply cream once daily and gel twice daily (morning and evening) for up to 4 weeks
Dosage Forms
  Cream:
    Naftin®: 1% (15 g, 30 g, 60 g, 90 g)
  Gel:
    Naftin®: 1% (20 g, 40 g, 60 g, 90 g)

naftifine hydrochloride *see naftifine on page 653*
Naftin® [US] *see naftifine on page 653*
Naglazyme™ [US] *see galsulfase on page 435*
NaHCO₃ *see sodium bicarbonate on page 872*

nalbuphine (NAL byoo feen)

Sound-Alike/Look-Alike Issues
  Nubain® may be confused with Navane®, Nebcin®
Synonyms nalbuphine hydrochloride
U.S./Canadian Brand Names Nubain® [US]
Therapeutic Category Analgesic, Narcotic
Use Relief of moderate-to-severe pain; preoperative analgesia, postoperative and surgical anesthesia, and obstetrical analgesia during labor and delivery
Usual Dosage Adults:
  Pain management: I.M., I.V., SubQ: 10 mg/70 kg every 3-6 hours; maximum single dose in nonopioid-tolerant patients: 20 mg; maximum daily dose: 160 mg
  Surgical anesthesia supplement: I.V.: Induction: 0.3-3 mg/kg over 10-15 minutes; maintenance doses of 0.25-0.5 mg/kg may be given as required
Dosage Forms
  Injection, solution: 10 mg/mL (10 mL); 20 mg/mL (10 mL)
    Nubain®: 20 mg/mL (10 mL)
  Injection, solution [preservative free]: 10 mg/mL (1 mL); 20 mg/mL (1 mL)
    Nubain®: 10 mg/mL (1 mL); 20 mg/mL (1 mL)

nalbuphine hydrochloride *see nalbuphine on page 653*
Nalcrom® [Can] *see cromolyn sodium on page 251*
Naldecon® DX Adult Liquid *(Discontinued)*
Naldecon-EX® Children's Syrup *(Discontinued)*
Naldecon Senior EX® *(Discontinued) see guaifenesin on page 453*
Nalex®-A [US] *see chlorpheniramine, phenylephrine, and phenyltoloxamine on page 211*
Nalfon® [US/Can] *see fenoprofen on page 394*
Nallpen® [Can] *see nafcillin on page 652*
Nallpen® *(Discontinued) see nafcillin on page 652*
N-allylnoroxymorphine hydrochloride *see naloxone on page 654*
nalmefene *(Discontinued)*

naloxone (nal OKS one)

Sound-Alike/Look-Alike Issues
naloxone may be confused with naltrexone
Narcan® may be confused with Marcaine®, Norcuron®

Synonyms *N*-allylnoroxymorphine hydrochloride; naloxone hydrochloride

U.S./Canadian Brand Names Naloxone Hydrochloride Injection® [Can]

Therapeutic Category Antidote

Use
Complete or partial reversal of opioid depression, including respiratory depression, induced by natural and synthetic opioids, including heroin, morphine, propoxyphene, methadone, and certain mixed agonist-antagonist analgesics: nalbuphine, pentazocine, and butorphanol
Diagnosis of suspected opioid dependence or acute opioid overdose
Adjunctive agent to increase blood pressure in the management of septic shock

Usual Dosage Note: I.M., I.V. (preferred), and SubQ routes are available:
Infants and Children: Postoperative reversal: 0.01 mg/kg; may repeat every 2-3 minutes as needed based on response (adequate ventilation without significant pain)
Children:
Opioid intoxication: Respiratory depression:
I.V.:
Birth (including premature infants) to 5 years or <20 kg: Initial: 0.1 mg/kg (maximum dose: 2 mg); repeat every 2-3 minutes if needed (*Drugs for Pediatric Emergencies*, 1998)
>5 years or ≥20 kg: 2 mg/dose; if no response, repeat every 2-3 minutes (*Drugs for Pediatric Emergencies*, 1998)
Continuous infusion: I.V.: If continuous infusion is required, calculate dosage/hour based on effective intermittent dose used and duration of adequate response seen **or** use 2/3 of the initial effective naloxone bolus on an hourly basis; titrate dose (typically 0.04-0.16 mg/kg/hour for 2-5 days in children); 1/2 of the initial bolus dose should be readministered 15 minutes after initiation of the continuous infusion to prevent a drop in naloxone levels; increase infusion rate as needed to assure adequate ventilation and prevent withdrawal symptoms
Adults:
Opioid intoxication: Respiratory depression: I.V.: 0.4-2 mg; may need to repeat doses every 2-3 minutes; after reversal, may need to readminister dose(s) at a later interval (ie, 20-60 minutes) depending on type/duration of opioid. If no response is observed after 10 mg, consider other causes of respiratory depression. **Note:** Opioid-dependent patients may require lower doses (0.1 mg) titrated incrementally to avoid precipitating acute withdrawal.
Continuous infusion: I.V.: Calculate dosage/hour based on effective intermittent dose used and duration of adequate response seen **or** use 2/3 of the initial effective naloxone bolus on an hourly basis (typically 0.25-6.25 mg/hour); 1/2 of the initial bolus dose should be readministered 15 minutes after initiation of the continuous infusion to prevent a drop in naloxone levels; adjust infusion rate as needed to assure adequate ventilation and prevent withdrawal symptoms
Postoperative reversal: I.V.: 0.1-0.2 mg every 2-3 minutes until desired response (adequate ventilation and alertness without significant pain). **Note:** Repeat doses may be needed within 1-2 hour intervals depending on type, dose, and timing of the last dose of opioid administered.

Dosage Forms
Injection, solution, as hydrochloride: 0.4 mg/mL (1 mL, 10 mL)
Injection, solution, as hydrochloride [preservative free]: 0.4 mg/mL (1 mL); 1 mg/mL (2 mL)

naloxone and buprenorphine *see* buprenorphine and naloxone *on page 151*
naloxone hydrochloride *see* naloxone *on page 654*
naloxone hydrochloride and pentazocine hydrochloride *see* pentazocine *on page 735*
naloxone hydrochloride dihydrate and buprenorphine hydrochloride *see* buprenorphine and naloxone *on page 151*
Naloxone Hydrochloride Injection® [Can] *see* naloxone *on page 654*

naltrexone (nal TREKS one)

Sound-Alike/Look-Alike Issues
naltrexone may be confused with naloxone
ReVia® may be confused with Revex®

Synonyms naltrexone hydrochloride

U.S./Canadian Brand Names Depade® [US]; ReVia® [US/Can]; Vivitrol™ [US]

Therapeutic Category Antidote
Use Treatment of ethanol dependence; blockade of the effects of exogenously administered opioids
Usual Dosage Adults: Do not give until patient is opioid-free for 7-10 days as determined by urinalysis
Oral: Alcohol dependence, opioid antidote: 25 mg; if no withdrawal signs within 1 hour give another 25 mg; maintenance regimen is flexible, variable and individualized (50 mg/day to 100-150 mg 3 times/week for 12 weeks); up to 800 mg/day has been tolerated in a small number of healthy adults without an adverse effect
I.M.: Alcohol dependence: 380 mg once every 4 weeks
Dosage Forms
Injection, microspheres for suspension, extended release:
Vivitrol™: 380 mg
Tablet: 50 mg
Depade®: 25 mg, 50 mg, 100 mg
ReVia®: 50 mg

naltrexone hydrochloride *see* naltrexone *on page 654*
Namenda™ [US] *see* memantine *on page 600*

nandrolone (NAN droe lone)

Synonyms nandrolone decanoate; nandrolone phenpropionate
U.S./Canadian Brand Names Deca-Durabolin® [Can]; Durabolin® [Can]
Therapeutic Category Androgen
Controlled Substance C-III
Use Control of metastatic breast cancer; management of anemia of renal insufficiency
Usual Dosage Deep I.M. (into gluteal muscle):
Children 2-13 years (decanoate): 25-50 mg every 3-4 weeks
Adults:
Male:
Breast cancer (phenpropionate): 50-100 mg/week
Anemia of renal insufficiency (decanoate): 100-200 mg/week
Female: 50-100 mg/week
Breast cancer (phenpropionate): 50-100 mg/week
Anemia of renal insufficiency (decanoate): 50-100 mg/week

nandrolone decanoate *see* nandrolone *on page 655*
nandrolone phenpropionate *see* nandrolone *on page 655*
NAPA and NABZ *see* sodium phenylacetate and sodium benzoate *on page 877*

naphazoline (naf AZ oh leen)

Synonyms naphazoline hydrochloride
U.S./Canadian Brand Names AK-Con™ [US]; Clear eyes® for Dry Eyes and ACR Relief [US-OTC]; Clear eyes® for Dry Eyes and Redness Relief [US-OTC]; Clear eyes® Redness Relief [US-OTC]; Clear eyes® Seasonal Relief [US-OTC]; Naphcon Forte® [Can]; Naphcon® [US-OTC]; Privine® [US-OTC]; Vasocon® [Can]
Therapeutic Category Adrenergic Agonist Agent
Use Topical ocular vasoconstrictor; temporary relief of nasal congestion associated with the common cold, upper respiratory allergies or sinusitis; relief of redness of the eye due to minor irritation
Usual Dosage
Nasal: Children ≥12 years and Adults: 0.05% instill 1-2 drops or sprays every 6 hours if needed; therapy should not exceed 3 days
Ophthalmic: Adults:
0.1% (prescription): 1-2 drops into conjuctival sac every 3-4 hours as needed
0.012% or 0.025% (OTC): 1-2 drops into affected eye(s) up to 4 times a day; therapy should not exceed 3 days
Dosage Forms
Solution, intranasal drops:
Privine® [OTC]: 0.05% (25 mL)
Solution, intranasal spray:
Privine® [OTC]: 0.05% (20 mL)

Solution, ophthalmic:
AK-Con™: 0.1% (15 mL)
Clear eyes® for Dry Eyes and ACR Relief [OTC]: 0.025% (15 mL)
Clear eyes® for Dry Eyes and Redness Relief [OTC], Naphcon® [OTC]: 0.012% (15 mL)
Clear eyes® Redness Relief [OTC]: 0.012% (6 mL, 15 mL, 30 mL)
Clear eyes® Seasonal Relief [OTC]: 0.012% (15 mL, 30 mL)

naphazoline and pheniramine (naf AZ oh leen & fen NIR a meen)
Sound-Alike/Look-Alike Issues
Visine® may be confused with Visken®
Synonyms pheniramine and naphazoline
U.S./Canadian Brand Names Naphcon-A® [US-OTC/Can]; Opcon-A® [US-OTC]; Visine-A® [US-OTC]; Visine® Advanced Allergy [Can]
Therapeutic Category Antihistamine/Decongestant Combination
Use Treatment of ocular congestion, irritation, and itching
Usual Dosage Ophthalmic: Children ≥6 years and Adults: 1-2 drops up to 4 times/day
Dosage Forms
Solution, ophthalmic:
Naphcon-A®: Naphazoline 0.025% and pheniramine 0.3%
Opcon-A®: Naphazoline 0.027% and pheniramine 0.3%
Visine-A®: Naphazoline 0.025% and pheniramine 0.3%

naphazoline hydrochloride *see naphazoline on page 655*
Naphcon® [US-OTC] *see naphazoline on page 655*
Naphcon-A® [US-OTC/Can] *see naphazoline and pheniramine on page 656*
Naphcon Forte® [Can] *see naphazoline on page 655*
Naphcon Forte® Ophthalmic (Discontinued) *see naphazoline on page 655*
NapraPAC™ *see lansoprazole and naproxen on page 549*
Naprelan® [US] *see naproxen on page 656*
Naprosyn® [US/Can] *see naproxen on page 656*

naproxen (na PROKS en)
Sound-Alike/Look-Alike Issues
naproxen may be confused with Natacyn®, Nebcin®
Aleve® may be confused with Alesse®
Anaprox® may be confused with Anaspaz®, Avapro®
Naprelan® may be confused with Naprosyn®
Naprosyn® may be confused with Naprelan®, Natacyn®, Nebcin®
Synonyms naproxen sodium
U.S./Canadian Brand Names Aleve® [US-OTC]; Anaprox® DS [US/Can]; Anaprox® [US/Can]; Apo-Napro-Na DS® [Can]; Apo-Napro-Na® [Can]; Apo-Naproxen EC® [Can]; Apo-Naproxen SR® [Can]; Apo-Naproxen® [Can]; EC-Naprosyn® [US]; Gen-Naproxen EC [Can]; Mediproxen [US-OTC]; Midol® Extended Relief [US]; Naprelan® [US]; Naprosyn® [US/Can]; Naxen® EC [Can]; Naxen® [Can]; Novo-Naproc EC [Can]; Novo-Naprox Sodium DS [Can]; Novo-Naprox Sodium [Can]; Novo-Naprox SR [Can]; Novo-Naprox [Can]; Nu-Naprox [Can]; Pamprin® Maximum Strength All Day Relief [US-OTC]; PMS-Naproxen EC [Can]; Riva-Naproxen [Can]; Sab-Naproxen [Can]
Therapeutic Category Analgesic, Nonnarcotic; Antipyretic; Nonsteroidal Antiinflammatory Drug (NSAID)
Use Management of ankylosing spondylitis, osteoarthritis, and rheumatoid disorders (including juvenile rheumatoid arthritis); acute gout; mild-to-moderate pain; tendonitis, bursitis; dysmenorrhea; fever
Usual Dosage Note: Dosage expressed as naproxen base; 200 mg naproxen base is equivalent to 220 mg naproxen sodium.

Oral:
Children >2 years: Juvenile arthritis: 10 mg/kg/day in 2 divided doses
Adults:
Gout, acute: Initial: 750 mg, followed by 250 mg every 8 hours until attack subsides. **Note:** EC-Naprosyn® is not recommended.
Pain (mild to moderate), dysmenorrhea, acute tendonitis, bursitis: Initial: 500 mg, then 250 mg every 6-8 hours; maximum: 1250 mg/day naproxen base

Rheumatoid arthritis, osteoarthritis, and ankylosing spondylitis: 500-1000 mg/day in 2 divided doses; may increase to 1.5 g/day of naproxen base for limited time period

OTC labeling: Pain/fever:
Children ≥12 years and Adults ≤65 years: 200 mg naproxen base every 8-12 hours; if needed, may take 400 mg naproxen base for the initial dose; maximum: 600 mg naproxen base/24 hours
Adults >65 years: 200 mg naproxen base every 12 hours

Dosage Forms
Caplet: 220 mg
Aleve® [OTC], Midol® Extended Relief, Pamprin® Maximum Strength All Day Relief [OTC]: 220 mg
Capsule, liquid gel: 220 mg
Aleve®: 220 mg
Gelcap: 220 mg
Aleve® [OTC]: 220 mg
Suspension, oral: 125 mg/5 mL
Naprosyn®: 125 mg/5 mL
Tablet: 220 mg, 250 mg, 275 mg, 375 mg, 500 mg, 550 mg
Aleve® [OTC]: 220 mg
Anaprox®: 275 mg
Anaprox® DS: 550 mg
Mediproxen: 220 mg
Naprosyn®: 250 mg, 375 mg, 500 mg
Tablet, controlled release: 550 mg
Naprelan®: 412.5 mg, 550 mg
Tablet, delayed release: 375 mg, 500 mg
EC-Naprosyn®: 375 mg, 500 mg
Tablet, extended release: 550 mg

naproxen and lansoprazole *see* lansoprazole and naproxen *on page 549*

naproxen and pseudoephedrine (na PROKS en & soo doe e FED rin)

Synonyms naproxen sodium and pseudoephedrine; pseudoephedrine and naproxen

U.S./Canadian Brand Names Aleve® Sinus & Headache [US-OTC]; Aleve®-D Sinus & Cold [US-OTC]

Therapeutic Category Decongestant/Analgesic

Use Temporary relief of cold, sinus, and flu symptoms (including nasal congestion, sinus congestion/pressure, headache, minor body aches and pains, and fever)

Usual Dosage Oral: Children ≥12 years and Adults: Aleve® Sinus & Headache: One caplet every 12 hours (maximum dose: 2 caplets/24 hours)

Dosage Forms
Caplet, extended release:
Aleve®-D Sinus & Cold, Aleve®-D Sinus & Headache: Naproxen sodium 220 mg [equivalent to naproxen 200 mg and sodium 20 mg] and pseudoephedrine hydrochloride 120 mg

naproxen and sumatriptan *see* sumatriptan and naproxen *on page 898*

naproxen sodium *see* naproxen *on page 656*

naproxen sodium and pseudoephedrine *see* naproxen and pseudoephedrine *on page 657*

naproxen sodium and sumatriptan *see* sumatriptan and naproxen *on page 898*

naproxen sodium and sumatriptan succinate *see* sumatriptan and naproxen *on page 898*

naratriptan (NAR a trip tan)

Sound-Alike/Look-Alike Issues
Amerge® may be confused with Altace®, Amaryl®

Synonyms naratriptan hydrochloride

U.S./Canadian Brand Names Amerge® [US/Can]

Therapeutic Category Antimigraine Agent; Serotonin Agonist

Use Treatment of acute migraine headache with or without aura

Usual Dosage Oral: Adults: 1-2.5 mg at the onset of headache; it is recommended to use the lowest possible dose to minimize adverse effects. If headache returns or does not fully resolve, the dose may be repeated after 4 hours; do not exceed 5 mg in 24 hours.

▶

◄ **Dosage Forms**
Tablet:
Amerge®: 1 mg, 2.5 mg

naratriptan hydrochloride *see* naratriptan *on page 657*
Narcan® *(Discontinued) see* naloxone *on page 654*
Nardil® [US/Can] *see* phenelzine *on page 742*
Naropin® [US/Can] *see* ropivacaine *on page 844*
Nasacort® AQ [US/Can] *see* triamcinolone (inhalation, nasal) *on page 947*
Nasacort® HFA [US] *see* triamcinolone (inhalation, nasal) *on page 947*
Nasahist B® *(Discontinued) see* brompheniramine *on page 144*
NasalCrom® [US-OTC] *see* cromolyn sodium *on page 251*
Nasalide® [Can] *see* flunisolide *on page 408*
Nasal Moist® Saline [US-OTC] *see* sodium chloride *on page 873*
Nasal Spray [US-OTC] *see* sodium chloride *on page 873*
Nasarel® [US] *see* flunisolide *on page 408*
Nasatab® LA [US] *see* guaifenesin and pseudoephedrine *on page 458*
Nascobal® [US] *see* cyanocobalamin *on page 254*
Nasex-G [US] *see* guaifenesin and phenylephrine *on page 456*
Nasonex® [US/Can] *see* mometasone *on page 641*
Nasop12™ [US] *see* phenylephrine *on page 745*
Natabec® *(Discontinued)*
Natabec® FA *(Discontinued)*
Natabec® Rx *(Discontinued)*
NataCaps™ [US] *see* vitamins (multiple/prenatal) *on page 983*
NataChew™ [US] *see* vitamins (multiple/prenatal) *on page 983*
Natacyn® [US/Can] *see* natamycin *on page 658*
NataFort® [US] *see* vitamins (multiple/prenatal) *on page 983*
NatalCare® CFe 60 *(Discontinued) see* vitamins (multiple/prenatal) *on page 983*
NatalCare® GlossTabs™ [US] *see* vitamins (multiple/prenatal) *on page 983*
NatalCare® PIC [US] *see* vitamins (multiple/prenatal) *on page 983*
NatalCare® PIC Forte [US] *see* vitamins (multiple/prenatal) *on page 983*
NatalCare® Plus [US] *see* vitamins (multiple/prenatal) *on page 983*
NatalCare® Rx [US] *see* vitamins (multiple/prenatal) *on page 983*
NatalCare® Three [US] *see* vitamins (multiple/prenatal) *on page 983*
Natalins® Rx *(Discontinued)*

natalizumab (na ta LIZ u mab)

Synonyms AN100226; anti-4 alpha integrin; IgG4-kappa monoclonal antibody
U.S./Canadian Brand Names Tysabri® [US/Can]
Therapeutic Category Monoclonal Antibody, Selective Adhesion-Molecule Inhibitor
Use
U.S. labeling: Treatment of relapsing forms of multiple sclerosis; treatment of moderately- to severely-active Crohn disease
Canada labeling: Treatment of relapsing forms of multiple sclerosis
Usual Dosage I.V.: Adults:
Multiple sclerosis: 300 mg infused over 1 hour every 4 weeks
Crohn disease: 300 mg infused over 1 hour every 4 weeks; discontinue if therapeutic benefit is not observed within initial 12 weeks of therapy
Dosage Forms
Injection, solution [preservative free]:
Tysabri®: 300 mg/15 mL (15 mL)

natamycin (na ta MYE sin)

Sound-Alike/Look-Alike Issues
Natacyn® may be confused with Naprosyn®

Synonyms pimaricin
U.S./Canadian Brand Names Natacyn® [US/Can]
Therapeutic Category Antifungal Agent
Use Treatment of blepharitis, conjunctivitis, and keratitis caused by susceptible fungi (*Aspergillus*, *Candida*, *Cephalosporium*, *Fusarium*, and *Penicillium*)
Usual Dosage Ophthalmic: Adults: Instill 1 drop in conjunctival sac every 1-2 hours, after 3-4 days reduce to one drop 6-8 times/day; usual course of therapy is 2-3 weeks.
Dosage Forms
  Suspension, ophthalmic:
   Natacyn®: 5% (15 mL)

NataTab™ CFe [US] *see* vitamins (multiple/prenatal) *on page 983*
NataTab™ FA [US] *see* vitamins (multiple/prenatal) *on page 983*
NataTab™ Rx [US] *see* vitamins (multiple/prenatal) *on page 983*

nateglinide (na te GLYE nide)

U.S./Canadian Brand Names Starlix® [US/Can]
Therapeutic Category Antidiabetic Agent
Use Management of type 2 diabetes mellitus (noninsulin-dependent, NIDDM) as monotherapy when hyperglycemia cannot be managed by diet and exercise alone; in combination with metformin or a thiazolidinedione to lower blood glucose in patients whose hyperglycemia cannot be controlled by exercise, diet, or a single agent alone
Usual Dosage Oral: Adults: Management of type 2 diabetes mellitus: Initial and maintenance dose: 120 mg 3 times/day, 1-30 minutes before meals; may be given alone or in combination with metformin or a thiazolidinedione; patients close to Hb A_{1c} goal may be started at 60 mg 3 times/day
Dosage Forms
  Tablet:
   Starlix®: 60 mg, 120 mg

Natrecor® [US/Can] *see* nesiritide *on page 665*
natriuretic peptide *see* nesiritide *on page 665*
Natulan® [Can] *see* procarbazine *on page 788*
Natural Fiber Therapy [US-OTC] *see* psyllium *on page 804*
Natural Fiber Therapy Smooth Texture [US-OTC] *see* psyllium *on page 804*
natural lung surfactant *see* beractant *on page 129*
Nature's Tears® [US-OTC] *see* artificial tears *on page 95*
Nature-Throid™ [US] *see* thyroid, desiccated *on page 924*
Naus-A-Way® *(Discontinued)*
Nausea Relief [US-OTC] *see* fructose, dextrose, and phosphoric acid *on page 429*
Nauseatol [Can] *see* dimenhydrinate *on page 301*
Nausetrol® [US-OTC] *see* fructose, dextrose, and phosphoric acid *on page 429*
Navane® [US/Can] *see* thiothixene *on page 923*
Navelbine® [US/Can] *see* vinorelbine *on page 978*
Naxen® [Can] *see* naproxen *on page 656*
Naxen® EC [Can] *see* naproxen *on page 656*
Na-Zone® [US-OTC] *see* sodium chloride *on page 873*
NC-722665 *see* bicalutamide *on page 135*
n-docosanol *see* docosanol *on page 314*
Nebcin® *(Discontinued) see* tobramycin *on page 931*

nebivolol (ne BIV oh lole)

Synonyms nebivolol hydrochloride
U.S./Canadian Brand Names Bystolic™ [US]
Therapeutic Category Beta Blocker, Beta₁ Selective
Use Treatment of hypertension, alone or in combination with other agents
Usual Dosage Oral: Adults: Hypertension: Initial: 5 mg once daily; if initial response is inadequate, may be increased at 2-week intervals to a maximum dose of 40 mg once daily

▶

◀ **Dosage Forms**
  Tablet:
    Bystolic™: 2.5 mg, 5 mg, 10 mg

nebivolol hydrochloride *see* nebivolol *on page 659*
NebuPent® [US] *see* pentamidine *on page 734*
Necon® 0.5/35 [US] *see* ethinyl estradiol and norethindrone *on page 376*
Necon® 1/35 [US] *see* ethinyl estradiol and norethindrone *on page 376*
Necon® 1/50 [US] *see* mestranol and norethindrone *on page 608*
Necon® 7/7/7 [US] *see* ethinyl estradiol and norethindrone *on page 376*
Necon® 10/11 [US] *see* ethinyl estradiol and norethindrone *on page 376*

nedocromil (inhalation) (ne doe KROE mil in hil LA shun)
U.S./Canadian Brand Names Tilade® [US/Can]
Therapeutic Category Mast Cell Stabilizer
Use Maintenance therapy in patients with mild-to-moderate bronchial asthma
Usual Dosage Children >6 years and Adults: 2 inhalations 4 times/day; may reduce dosage to 2-3 times/day once desired clinical response to initial dose is observed
Dosage Forms
  Aerosol for oral inhalation:
    Tilade®: 1.75 mg/activation (16.2 g)

nedocromil (ophthalmic) (ne doe KROE mil op THAL mik)
U.S./Canadian Brand Names Alocril® [US/Can]
Therapeutic Category Mast Cell Stabilizer
Use Treatment of itching associated with allergic conjunctivitis
Usual Dosage Ophthalmic: Adults: 1-2 drops in eye(s) twice daily
Dosage Forms
  Solution, ophthalmic:
    Alocril®: 2% (5 mL)

nefazodone (nef AY zoe done)
Sound-Alike/Look-Alike Issues
    Serzone® may be confused with selegiline, Serentil®, Seroquel®, sertraline
Synonyms nefazodone hydrochloride
Therapeutic Category Antidepressant, Miscellaneous
Use Treatment of depression
Usual Dosage Oral: Adults: Depression: 200 mg/day, administered in 2 divided doses initially, with a range of 300-600 mg/day in 2 divided doses thereafter
Dosage Forms
  Tablet: 50 mg, 100 mg, 150 mg, 200 mg, 250 mg

nefazodone hydrochloride *see* nefazodone *on page 660*
NegGram® *(Discontinued)*

nelarabine (nel AY re been)
Synonyms 2-amino-6-methoxypurine arabinoside; 506U78; GW506U78
U.S./Canadian Brand Names Arranon® [US]; Atriance™ [Can]
Therapeutic Category Antineoplastic Agent, Antimetabolite
Use Treatment of relapsed or refractory T-cell acute lymphoblastic leukemia (ALL) and T-cell lymphoblastic lymphoma
Usual Dosage I.V.: T-cell ALL, T-cell lymphoblastic lymphoma:
  Children: 650 mg/m^2/day on days 1 through 5; repeat every 21 days
  Adults: 1500 mg/m^2/day on days 1, 3, and 5; repeat every 21 days
Dosage Forms [CAN] = Canadian brand name
  Injection, solution:
    Arranon®: 5 mg/mL (50 mL)
    Atriance™ [CAN]: 5 mg/ml (50 mL)

nelfinavir (nel FIN a veer)

Sound-Alike/Look-Alike Issues
nelfinavir may be confused with nevirapine
Viracept® may be confused with Viramune®

Synonyms NFV

U.S./Canadian Brand Names Viracept® [US/Can]

Therapeutic Category Antiviral Agent

Use In combination with other antiretroviral therapy in the treatment of HIV infection

Usual Dosage Oral:
Children 2-13 years: 45-55 mg/kg twice daily **or** 25-35 mg/kg 3 times/day (maximum: 2500 mg/day). If tablets are unable to be taken, use oral powder in small amount of water, milk, formula, or dietary supplements; do not use acidic food/juice or store for >6 hours.
Adults: 750 mg 3 times/day or 1250 mg twice daily with meals in combination with other antiretroviral therapies

Dosage Forms
Powder, oral:
Viracept®: 50 mg/g
Tablet:
Viracept®: 250 mg, 625 mg

Nelova™ 0.5/35E (Discontinued) *see* ethinyl estradiol and norethindrone *on page 376*

Nelova™ 1/35E (Discontinued) *see* ethinyl estradiol and norethindrone *on page 376*

Nelova™ 1/50M (Discontinued) *see* mestranol and norethindrone *on page 608*

Nelova™ 10/11 (Discontinued) *see* ethinyl estradiol and norethindrone *on page 376*

Nembutal® [US] *see* pentobarbital *on page 736*

Nembutal® Sodium [Can] *see* pentobarbital *on page 736*

NeoBenz® Micro [US] *see* benzoyl peroxide *on page 126*

NeoBenz® Micro SD [US] *see* benzoyl peroxide *on page 126*

Neo-Calglucon® (Discontinued) *see* calcium glubionate *on page 165*

Neo-Dexameth® Ophthalmic (Discontinued)

Neo DM [US] *see* chlorpheniramine, phenylephrine, and dextromethorphan *on page 209*

Neo-Durabolic® (Discontinued) *see* nandrolone *on page 655*

Neofed® (Discontinued) *see* pseudoephedrine *on page 801*

Neo-Fradin™ [US] *see* neomycin *on page 661*

Neofrin™ [US] *see* phenylephrine *on page 745*

Neomixin® Topical (Discontinued) *see* bacitracin, neomycin, and polymyxin B *on page 114*

neomycin (nee oh MYE sin)

Synonyms neomycin sulfate

U.S./Canadian Brand Names Neo-Fradin™ [US]; Neo-Rx [US]

Therapeutic Category Aminoglycoside (Antibiotic); Antibiotic, Topical

Use Orally to prepare GI tract for surgery; topically to treat minor skin infections; treatment of diarrhea caused by *E. coli*; adjunct in the treatment of hepatic encephalopathy; bladder irrigation; ocular infections

Usual Dosage
Children: Oral:
Preoperative intestinal antisepsis: 90 mg/kg/day divided every 4 hours for 2 days; or 25 mg/kg at 1 PM, 2 PM, and 11 PM on the day preceding surgery as an adjunct to mechanical cleansing of the intestine and in combination with erythromycin base
Hepatic encephalopathy: 50-100 mg/kg/day in divided doses every 6-8 hours or 2.5-7 g/m^2/day divided every 4-6 hours for 5-6 days not to exceed 12 g/day
Children and Adults: Topical: Topical solutions containing 0.1% to 1% neomycin have been used for irrigation
Adults: Oral:
Preoperative intestinal antisepsis: 1 g each hour for 4 doses then 1 g every 4 hours for 5 doses; or 1 g at 1 PM, 2 PM, and 11 PM on day preceding surgery as an adjunct to mechanical cleansing of the bowel and oral erythromycin; or 6 g/day divided every 4 hours for 2-3 days
Hepatic encephalopathy: 500-2000 mg every 6-8 hours or 4-12 g/day divided every 4-6 hours for 5-6 days

▶

◄ Chronic hepatic insufficiency: 4 g/day for an indefinite period

Dosage Forms
Powder, micronized [for prescription compounding]: (10 g, 100 g)
  Neo-Rx: (10 g, 100 g)
Solution, oral: 125 mg/5 mL
  Neo-Fradin™: 125 mg/5 mL
Tablet: 500 mg

neomycin and polymyxin B (nee oh MYE sin & pol i MIKS in bee)

Synonyms polymyxin B and neomycin
U.S./Canadian Brand Names Neosporin® G.U. Irrigant [US]; Neosporin® Irrigating Solution [Can]
Therapeutic Category Antibiotic, Topical; Genitourinary Irrigant
Use Short-term as a continuous irrigant or rinse in the urinary bladder to prevent bacteriuria and gram-negative rod septicemia associated with the use of indwelling catheters; to help prevent infection in minor cuts, scrapes, and burns
Usual Dosage Children and Adults: Bladder irrigation: **Not for injection**; add 1 mL irrigant to 1 L isotonic saline solution and connect container to the inflow of lumen of 3-way catheter. Continuous irrigant or rinse in the urinary bladder for up to a maximum of 10 days with administration rate adjusted to patient's urine output; usually no more than 1 L of irrigant is used per day.
Dosage Forms
Solution, irrigation: Neomycin 40 mg and polymyxin B 200,000 units per mL (1 mL, 20 mL)
  Neosporin® G.U. Irrigant: Neomycin 40 mg and polymyxin B 200,000 units per mL (1 mL, 20 mL)

neomycin, bacitracin, and polymyxin B see bacitracin, neomycin, and polymyxin B on page 114
neomycin, bacitracin, polymyxin B, and hydrocortisone see bacitracin, neomycin, polymyxin B, and hydrocortisone on page 114
neomycin, bacitracin, polymyxin B, and pramoxine see bacitracin, neomycin, polymyxin B, and pramoxine on page 114

neomycin, colistin, hydrocortisone, and thonzonium

(nee oh MYE sin, koe LIS tin, hye droe KOR ti sone, & thon ZOE nee um)
Synonyms colistin, neomycin, hydrocortisone, and thonzonium; hydrocortisone, neomycin, colistin, and thonzonium; thonzonium, neomycin, colistin, and hydrocortisone
U.S./Canadian Brand Names Coly-Mycin® S [US]; Cortisporin®-TC [US]
Therapeutic Category Antibiotic/Corticosteroid, Otic
Use Treatment of superficial and susceptible bacterial infections of the external auditory canal; for treatment of susceptible bacterial infections of mastoidectomy and fenestration cavities
Usual Dosage Otic:
Calibrated dropper:
  Children: 4 drops in affected ear 3-4 times/day
  Adults: 5 drops in affected ear 3-4 times/day
Dropper bottle:
  Children: 3 drops in affected ear 3-4 times/day
  Adults: 4 drops in affected ear 3-4 times/day
Note: Alternatively, a cotton wick may be inserted in the ear canal and saturated with suspension every 4 hours; wick should be replaced at least every 24 hours
Dosage Forms
Suspension, otic [drops]:
  Coly-Mycin® S: Neomycin 0.33%, colistin 0.3%, hydrocortisone 1%, and thonzonium 0.05% (5 mL)
  Cortisporin®-TC: Neomycin 0.33%, colistin 0.3%, hydrocortisone 1%, and thonzonium 0.05% (10 mL)

neomycin, polymyxin B, and dexamethasone

(nee oh MYE sin, pol i MIKS in bee, & deks a METH a sone)
Sound-Alike/Look-Alike Issues
  AK-Trol® may be confused with AKTob®
Synonyms dexamethasone, neomycin, and polymyxin B; polymyxin B, neomycin, and dexamethasone
U.S./Canadian Brand Names Dioptrol® [Can]; Maxitrol® [US/Can]; Poly-Dex™ [US]
Therapeutic Category Antibiotic/Corticosteroid, Ophthalmic
Use Steroid-responsive inflammatory ocular conditions in which a corticosteroid is indicated and where bacterial infection or a risk of bacterial infection exists

Usual Dosage Ophthalmic: Children and Adults:

Ointment: Place a small amount (~1/2") in the affected eye 3-4 times/day or apply at bedtime as an adjunct with drops

Suspension: Instill 1-2 drops into affected eye(s) every 3-4 hours; in severe disease, drops may be used hourly and tapered to discontinuation

Dosage Forms

Ointment, ophthalmic: Neomycin 3.5 mg, polymyxin B 10,000 units, and dexamethasone 0.1% per g (3.5 g)

Maxitrol®, Poly-Dex™: Neomycin 3.5 mg, polymyxin B 10,000 units, and dexamethasone 0.1% per g (3.5 g)

Suspension, ophthalmic: Neomycin 3.5 mg, polymyxin B 10,000 units, and dexamethasone 0.1% per mL (5 mL)

Maxitrol®, Poly-Dex™: Neomycin 3.5 mg, polymyxin B 10,000 units, and dexamethasone 0.1% per mL (5 mL)

neomycin, polymyxin B, and gramicidin

(nee oh MYE sin, pol i MIKS in bee, & gram i SYE din)

Synonyms gramicidin, neomycin, and polymyxin B; polymyxin B, neomycin, and gramicidin

U.S./Canadian Brand Names Neosporin® Ophthalmic Solution [US]; Neosporin® [Can]; Optimyxin Plus® [Can]

Therapeutic Category Antibiotic, Ophthalmic

Use Treatment of superficial ocular infection

Usual Dosage Ophthalmic: Children and Adults: Instill 1-2 drops 4-6 times/day or more frequently as required for severe infections

Dosage Forms

Solution, ophthalmic: Neomycin 1.75 mg, polymyxin B 10,000 units, and gramicidin 0.025 mg per mL (10 mL)

Neosporin® Ophthalmic Solution: Neomycin 1.75 mg, polymyxin B 10,000 units, and gramicidin 0.025 mg per mL (10 mL)

neomycin, polymyxin B, and hydrocortisone

(nee oh MYE sin, pol i MIKS in bee, & hye droe KOR ti sone)

Synonyms hydrocortisone, neomycin, and polymyxin B; polymyxin B, neomycin, and hydrocortisone

U.S./Canadian Brand Names Cortimyxin® [Can]; Cortisporin® Cream [US]; Cortisporin® Otic [US/Can]; PediOtic® [US]

Therapeutic Category Antibiotic/Corticosteroid, Ophthalmic; Antibiotic/Corticosteroid, Otic; Antibiotic/Corticosteroid, Topical

Use Steroid-responsive inflammatory condition for which a corticosteroid is indicated and where bacterial infection or a risk of bacterial infection exists

Usual Dosage Note: Duration of use of ophthalmic and otic preparations should be limited to 10 days unless otherwise directed by the healthcare provider.

Ophthalmic: Adults: Instill 1-2 drops 2-4 times/day, or more frequently as required for severe infections

Otic: Otic solution is used **only** for bacterial infections of external auditory canal (eg, swimmer's ear).

Children ≥2 years: Instill 3 drops into affected ear 3-4 times/day

Adults: Instill 4 drops into affected ear 3-4 times/day; otic suspension is the preferred otic preparation

Topical: Adults: Apply a thin layer 1-4 times/day. Therapy should be discontinued when control is achieved; if no improvement is seen, reassessment of diagnosis may be necessary.

Dosage Forms

Cream, topical: Neomycin 3.5 mg, polymyxin B 10,000 units, and hydrocortisone 5 mg per g (7.5 g)

Cortisporin®: Neomycin 3.5 mg, polymyxin B 10,000 units, and hydrocortisone 5 mg per g (7.5 g)

Solution, otic: Neomycin 3.5 mg, polymyxin B 10,000 units, and hydrocortisone 10 mg per mL (10 mL)

Cortisporin®: Neomycin 3.5 mg, polymyxin B 10,000 units, and hydrocortisone 10 mg per mL (10 mL)

Suspension, ophthalmic: Neomycin 3.5 mg, polymyxin B 10,000 units, and hydrocortisone 10 mg per mL (7.5 mL)

Suspension, otic: Neomycin 3.5 mg, polymyxin B 10,000 units, and hydrocortisone 10 mg per mL (10 mL)

Cortisporin®: Neomycin 3.5 mg, polymyxin B 10,000 units, and hydrocortisone 10 mg per mL (10 mL)

PediOtic®: Neomycin 3.5 mg, polymyxin B 10,000 units, and hydrocortisone 10 mg per mL (7.5 mL)

neomycin, polymyxin B, and prednisolone
(nee oh MYE sin, pol i MIKS in bee, & pred NIS oh lone)

Synonyms polymyxin B, neomycin, and prednisolone; prednisolone, neomycin, and polymyxin B

U.S./Canadian Brand Names Poly-Pred® [US]

Therapeutic Category Antibiotic/Corticosteroid, Ophthalmic

Use Steroid-responsive inflammatory ocular condition in which bacterial infection or a risk of bacterial ocular infection exists

Usual Dosage Ophthalmic: Children and Adults: Instill 1-2 drops every 3-4 hours; acute infections may require every 30-minute instillation initially with frequency of administration reduced as the infection is brought under control. To treat the lids: Instill 1-2 drops every 3-4 hours, close the eye and rub the excess on the lids and lid margins.

Dosage Forms

Suspension, ophthalmic:
Poly-Pred®: Neomycin 0.35%, polymyxin B 10,000 units per mL, and prednisolone 0.5% (5 mL)

neomycin sulfate *see* neomycin *on page 661*

neonatal trace metals *see* trace metals *on page 940*

NeoProfen® [US] *see* ibuprofen *on page 495*

Neoral® [US/Can] *see* cyclosporine *on page 257*

Neo-Rx [US] *see* neomycin *on page 661*

Neosporin® [Can] *see* neomycin, polymyxin B, and gramicidin *on page 663*

Neosporin® AF [US-OTC] *see* miconazole *on page 630*

Neosporin® G.U. Irrigant [US] *see* neomycin and polymyxin B *on page 662*

Neosporin® Irrigating Solution [Can] *see* neomycin and polymyxin B *on page 662*

Neosporin® Neo To Go® [US-OTC] *see* bacitracin, neomycin, and polymyxin B *on page 114*

Neosporin® Ophthalmic Ointment [Can] *see* bacitracin, neomycin, and polymyxin B *on page 114*

Neosporin® Ophthalmic Ointment *(Discontinued)* *see* bacitracin, neomycin, and polymyxin B *on page 114*

Neosporin® Ophthalmic Solution [US] *see* neomycin, polymyxin B, and gramicidin *on page 663*

Neosporin® + Pain Relief Ointment [US-OTC] *see* bacitracin, neomycin, polymyxin B, and pramoxine *on page 114*

Neosporin® Topical [US-OTC] *see* bacitracin, neomycin, and polymyxin B *on page 114*

neostigmine (nee oh STIG meen)

Sound-Alike/Look-Alike Issues
Prostigmin® may be confused with physostigmine

Synonyms neostigmine bromide; neostigmine methylsulfate

U.S./Canadian Brand Names Prostigmin® [US/Can]

Therapeutic Category Cholinergic Agent

Use Diagnosis and treatment of myasthenia gravis; prevention and treatment of postoperative bladder distention and urinary retention; reversal of the effects of nondepolarizing neuromuscular-blocking agents after surgery

Usual Dosage
Myasthenia gravis: Diagnosis: I.M.:
Children: 0.04 mg/kg as a single dose
Adults: 0.02 mg/kg as a single dose
Myasthenia gravis: Treatment:
Children:
Oral: 2 mg/kg/day divided every 3-4 hours
I.M., I.V., SubQ: 0.01-0.04 mg/kg every 2-4 hours
Adults:
Oral: 15 mg/dose every 3-4 hours up to 375 mg/day maximum; interval between doses must be individualized to maximal response
I.M., I.V., SubQ: 0.5-2.5 mg every 1-3 hours up to 10 mg/24 hours maximum
Reversal of nondepolarizing neuromuscular blockade after surgery in conjunction with atropine (must administer atropine several minutes prior to neostigmine): I.V.:
Infants: 0.025-0.1 mg/kg/dose
Children: 0.025-0.08 mg/kg/dose

Adults: 0.5-2.5 mg; total dose not to exceed 5 mg
Bladder atony: Adults: I.M., SubQ:
  Prevention: 0.25 mg every 4-6 hours for 2-3 days
  Treatment: 0.5-1 mg every 3 hours for 5 doses after bladder has emptied
Dosage Forms
  Injection, solution: 0.5 mg/mL (1 mL, 10 mL); 1 mg/mL (10 mL)
    Prostigmin®: 0.5 mg/mL (1 mL, 10 mL); 1 mg/mL (10 mL)
  Tablet:
    Prostigmin®: 15 mg

neostigmine bromide see neostigmine on page 664
neostigmine methylsulfate see neostigmine on page 664
NeoStrata® AHA [US-OTC] see hydroquinone on page 488
NeoStrata® HQ [Can] see hydroquinone on page 488
Neo-Synephrine® [Can] see phenylephrine on page 745
Neo-Synephrine® 12 Hour [US-OTC] see oxymetazoline on page 712
Neo-Synephrine® 12 Hour Extra Moisturizing [US-OTC] see oxymetazoline on page 712
Neo-Synephrine® Extra Strength [US-OTC] see phenylephrine on page 745
Neo-Synephrine® Injection [US] see phenylephrine on page 745
Neo-Synephrine® Mild [US-OTC] see phenylephrine on page 745
Neo-Synephrine® Ophthalmic (Discontinued) see phenylephrine on page 745
Neo-Synephrine® Regular Strength [US-OTC] see phenylephrine on page 745
Neo-Tabs® (Discontinued) see neomycin on page 661
NeoVadrin® (Discontinued)

nepafenac (ne pa FEN ak)
  U.S./Canadian Brand Names Nevanac™ [US]
  Therapeutic Category Nonsteroidal Antiinflammatory Drug (NSAID), Ophthalmic
  Use Treatment of pain and inflammation associated with cataract surgery
  Usual Dosage Ophthalmic: Children ≥10 years and Adults: Instill 1 drop into affected eye(s) 3 times/day, beginning 1 day prior to surgery, the day of surgery, and through the first 2 weeks of the postoperative period
  Dosage Forms
    Suspension, ophthalmic:
      Nevanac™: 0.1% (3 mL)

NephPlex® Rx [US] see vitamin B complex combinations on page 981
Nephro-Calci® [US-OTC] see calcium carbonate on page 163
Nephrocaps® [US] see vitamin B complex combinations on page 981
Nephro-Fer® [US-OTC] see ferrous fumarate on page 397
Nephronex® [US] see vitamin B complex combinations on page 981
Nephron FA® [US] see vitamin B complex combinations on page 981
Nephro-Vite® [US-OTC] see vitamin B complex combinations on page 981
Nephro-Vite® Rx [US] see vitamin B complex combinations on page 981
Nephrox Suspension (Discontinued) see aluminum hydroxide on page 53
Neptazane® (Discontinued) see methazolamide on page 613
nerve agent antidote kit see atropine and pralidoxime on page 106
Nervocaine® Injection (Discontinued) see lidocaine on page 561
Nesacaine® [US] see chloroprocaine on page 204
Nesacaine®-CE [Can] see chloroprocaine on page 204
Nesacaine®-MPF [US] see chloroprocaine on page 204

nesiritide (ni SIR i tide)
  Synonyms B-type natriuretic peptide (human); hBNP; natriuretic peptide
  U.S./Canadian Brand Names Natrecor® [US/Can]
  Therapeutic Category Natriuretic Peptide, B-type, Human; Vasodilator

◀ **Use** Treatment of acutely decompensated congestive heart failure (CHF) in patients with dyspnea at rest or with minimal activity

Usual Dosage I.V.: Adults: Initial: 2 mcg/kg (bolus); followed by continuous infusion at 0.01 mcg/kg/minute. **Note:** Should not be initiated at a dosage higher than initial recommended dose. There is limited experience with increasing the dose >0.01 mcg/kg/minute; in one trial, a limited number of patients received higher doses that were increased no faster than every 3 hours by 0.005 mcg/kg/minute (preceded by a bolus of 1 mcg/kg), up to a maximum of 0.03 mcg/kg/minute. Increases beyond the initial infusion rate should be limited to selected patients and accompanied by close hemodynamic and renal function monitoring.

Patients experiencing hypotension during the infusion: Infusion dose should be reduced or discontinued. Other measures to support blood pressure should be initiated (eg, I.V. fluids, Trendelenburg position). May attempt to restart at a lower dose (reduce previous infusion dose by 30% and omit bolus).

Dosage Forms
Injection, powder for reconstitution:
Natrecor®: 1.5 mg

Nestrex® *(Discontinued)* see pyridoxine *on page 808*
Netromycin® *(Discontinued)*
Neucalm-50® Injection *(Discontinued)* see hydroxyzine *on page 491*
Neulasta® [US/Can] see pegfilgrastim *on page 727*
Neuleptil® [Can] see pericyazine *(Canada only) on page 739*
Neumega® [US] see oprelvekin *on page 701*
Neupogen® [US/Can] see filgrastim *on page 401*
Neupro® *(Discontinued)* see rotigotine *on page 847*
Neuramate® *(Discontinued)* see meprobamate *on page 605*
Neurontin® [US/Can] see gabapentin *on page 431*
Neut® [US] see sodium bicarbonate *on page 872*
NeutraCare® [US] see fluoride *on page 411*
NeutraGard® [US-OTC] see fluoride *on page 411*
NeutraGard® Advanced [US] see fluoride *on page 411*
NeutraGard® Plus [US] see fluoride *on page 411*
Neutra-Phos® *(Discontinued)* see potassium phosphate and sodium phosphate *on page 775*
Neutra-Phos®-K *(Discontinued)* see potassium phosphate *on page 774*
Neutrogena® Acne Mask [US-OTC] see benzoyl peroxide *on page 126*
Neutrogena® Advanced Solutions™ [US-OTC] see salicylic acid *on page 850*
Neutrogena® Blackhead Eliminating™ 2-in-1 Foaming Pads [US-OTC] see salicylic acid *on page 850*
Neutrogena® Blackhead Eliminating™ Daily Scrub [US-OTC] see salicylic acid *on page 850*
Neutrogena® Body Clear® [US-OTC] see salicylic acid *on page 850*
Neutrogena® Clear Pore™ Oil-Controlling Astringent [US-OTC] see salicylic acid *on page 850*
Neutrogena® Oil-Free Acne Wash [US-OTC] see salicylic acid *on page 850*
Neutrogena® Oil-Free Acne Wash 60 Second Mask Scrub [US-OTC] see salicylic acid *on page 850*
Neutrogena® Oil-Free Acne Wash Cream Cleanser [US-OTC] see salicylic acid *on page 850*
Neutrogena® Oil-Free Acne Wash Foam Cleanser [US-OTC] see salicylic acid *on page 850*
Neutrogena® On The Spot® Acne Treatment [US-OTC] see benzoyl peroxide *on page 126*
Neutrogena® Rapid Clear® Acne Defense [US-OTC] see salicylic acid *on page 850*
Neutrogena® Rapid Clear® Acne Eliminating [US-OTC] see salicylic acid *on page 850*
Neutrogena® T/Gel [US-OTC] see coal tar *on page 240*
Neutrogena® T/Gel Extra Strength [US-OTC] see coal tar *on page 240*
Neutrogena® T/Gel Stubborn Itch Control [US-OTC] see coal tar *on page 240*
Nevanac™ [US] see nepafenac *on page 665*

nevirapine (ne VYE ra peen)
Sound-Alike/Look-Alike Issues
nevirapine may be confused with nelfinavir
Viramune® may be confused with Viracept®

Synonyms NVP
U.S./Canadian Brand Names Viramune® [US/Can]
Therapeutic Category Antiviral Agent
Use In combination therapy with other antiretroviral agents for the treatment of HIV-1
Usual Dosage Oral:
HIV infection:
Infants ≤2 months (AIDSinfo guidelines): Initial: 120 mg/m^2 (or 5 mg/kg/dose) once daily for the first 14 days; increase dose to 120 mg/m^2/dose twice daily for 14 days if no rash or other adverse effects occur; maintenance 200 mg/m^2/dose twice daily. **Note:** AIDSinfo guidelines suggest that dosing based on BSA provides more consistent drug exposure during childhood; studies suggest that weight-based dosing results in abrupt decrease in dose size at 8 years of age.
Infants and Children 2 months to <8 years: Initial: 4 mg/kg/dose once daily for first 14 days; increase dose to 7 mg/kg/dose every 12 hours if no rash or other adverse effects occur; maximum: 200 mg/dose every 12 hours
Children ≥8 years: Initial: 4 mg/kg/dose once daily for first 14 days; increase dose to 4 mg/kg/dose every 12 hours if no rash or other adverse effects occur; maximum: 200 mg/dose every 12 hours
Alternative pediatric dosing (AIDSinfo guidelines): Children ≥2 months: Initial 150 mg/m2/dose once daily for the first 14 days; maintenance: 150-200 mg/m^2/dose twice daily (maximum: 200 mg/dose). **Note:** Guidelines suggest that dosing based on BSA provides more consistent drug exposure during childhood; studies suggest that weight-based dosing results in abrupt decrease in dose size at 8 years of age.
Adults: Initial: 200 mg once daily for first 14 days; maintenance: 200 mg twice daily (in combination with an additional antiretroviral agent)
Note: If patient experiences a rash during the 14-day lead-in period, dose should not be increased until the rash has resolved. Discontinue if severe rash, rash with constitutional symptoms, or rash with elevated hepatic transaminases is noted. If therapy is interrupted for >7 days, restart with initial dose for 14 days. Use of prednisone to prevent nevirapine-associated rash is not recommended. Permanently discontinue if symptomatic hepatic events occur.

Prevention of maternal-fetal HIV transmission in women with no prior antiretroviral therapy (AIDS information guidelines):
Mother: 200 mg as a single dose at onset of labor. May be used in combination with zidovudine.
Infant: 2 mg/kg as a single dose at age 48-72 hours if mother received intrapartum dose of nevirapine. If mother did not receive single intrapartum dose, administer a single 2 mg/kg dose as soon as possible after birth. May be used in combination with zidovudine.

Dosage Forms
Suspension, oral:
Viramune®: 50 mg/5 mL
Tablet:
Viramune®: 200 mg

Nexavar® [US] *see* sorafenib *on page 884*
Nexium® [US/Can] *see* esomeprazole *on page 357*
Nexphen PD [US] *see* guaifenesin and phenylephrine *on page 456*
NFV *see* nelfinavir *on page 661*
N.G.A.® Topical *(Discontinued)* *see* nystatin and triamcinolone *on page 690*

niacin (NYE a sin)

Sound-Alike/Look-Alike Issues
niacin may be confused with Minocin®, Niaspan®, Nispan®
Niaspan® may be confused with niacin
Nicobid® may be confused with Nitro-Bid®
Synonyms nicotinic acid; vitamin B$_3$
U.S./Canadian Brand Names Niacin-Time® [US]; Niacor® [US]; Niaspan® [US/Can]; Slo-Niacin® [US-OTC]
Therapeutic Category Vitamin, Water Soluble
Use Adjunctive treatment of dyslipidemias (types IIa and IIb or primary hypercholesterolemia) to lower the risk of recurrent MI and/or slow progression of coronary artery disease, including combination therapy with other antidyslipidemic agents when additional triglyceride-lowering or HDL-increasing effects are desired; treatment of hypertriglyceridemia in patients at risk of pancreatitis; treatment of peripheral vascular disease and circulatory disorders; treatment of pellagra; dietary supplement

◀ **Usual Dosage Note:** Formulations of niacin (regular release versus extended release) are not interchangeable.
Children: Oral:
Pellagra: 50-100 mg/dose 3 times/day
Recommended daily allowances:
0-0.5 years: 5 mg/day
0.5-1 year: 6 mg/day
1-3 years: 9 mg/day
4-6 years: 12 mg/day
7-10 years: 13 mg/day
Children and Adolescents: Recommended daily allowances:
Male:
11-14 years: 17 mg/day
15-18 years: 20 mg/day
19-24 years: 19 mg/day
Female: 11-24 years: 15 mg/day
Adults: Oral:
Recommended daily allowances:
Male: 25-50 years: 19 mg/day; >51 years: 15 mg/day
Female: 25-50 years: 15 mg/day; >51 years: 13 mg/day
Hyperlipidemia: Usual target dose: Regular release: 1.5-6 g/day in 3 divided doses with or after meals using a dosage titration schedule. Extended release: 500 mg to 2 g once daily at bedtime.
Regular release formulation (Niacor®): Initial: 250 mg once daily (with evening meal); increase frequency and/or dose every 4-7 days to desired response or first-level therapeutic dose (1.5-2 g/day in 2-3 divided doses); after 2 months, may increase at 2- to 4-week intervals to 3 g/day in 3 divided doses (maximum dose: 6 g/day in 3 divided doses)
Extended release formulation (Niaspan®): Initial: 500 mg at bedtime for 4 weeks, then 1 g at bedtime for 4 weeks; adjust dose to response and tolerance; can increase to a maximum of 2 g/day, but only at 500 mg/day at 4-week intervals
With lovastatin: Recommended initial dose: 20 mg/day; Maximum lovastatin dose: 40 mg/day
Pellagra: 50-100 mg 3-4 times/day, maximum: 500 mg/day
Niacin deficiency: 10-20 mg/day, maximum: 100 mg/day

Dosage Forms
Capsule, extended release: 125 mg, 250 mg, 400 mg, 500 mg
Capsule, timed release: 250 mg, 500 mg
Tablet: 50 mg, 100 mg, 250 mg, 500 mg
Niacor®: 500 mg
Tablet, controlled release: 250 mg, 500 mg, 750 mg
Slo-Niacin® [OTC]: 250 mg, 500 mg, 750 mg
Tablet, extended release: 500 mg, 750 mg, 1000 mg
Niaspan®: 500 mg, 750 mg, 1000 mg
Tablet, timed release: 250 mg, 500 mg, 750 mg, 1000 mg
Niacin-Time®: 500 mg

niacinamide (nye a SIN a mide)

Sound-Alike/Look-Alike Issues
niacinamide may be confused with niCARdipine
Synonyms nicotinamide; nicotinic acid amide; vitamin B_3
U.S./Canadian Brand Names Nicomide-T™ [US]
Therapeutic Category Vitamin, Water Soluble
Use
Oral: Prophylaxis and treatment of pellagra
Topical: Improve the appearance of acne and decrease visible inflammation and irritation caused by acne medications
Usual Dosage
Pellagra: Oral:
Children: 100-300 mg/day in divided doses
Adults: 300-500 mg/day
Acne: Topical: Adults: Apply to affected area on face twice daily

Dosage Forms
Cream:
Nicomide-T™: 4% (30 g)
Gel:
Nicomide-T™: 4% (30 g)
Tablet: 100 mg, 250 mg, 500 mg

niacin and lovastatin (NYE a sin & LOE va sta tin)

Sound-Alike/Look-Alike Issues
Advicor® may be confused with Advair, Altocor™
Synonyms lovastatin and niacin
U.S./Canadian Brand Names Advicor® [US/Can]
Therapeutic Category HMG-CoA Reductase Inhibitor; Vitamin, Water Soluble
Use For use when treatment with both extended-release niacin and lovastatin is appropriate in combination with a standard cholesterol-lowering diet:
Extended-release niacin: Adjunctive treatment of dyslipidemias (types IIa and IIb or primary hypercholesterolemia) to lower the risk of recurrent MI and/or slow progression of coronary artery disease, including combination therapy with other antidyslipidemic agents when additional triglyceride-lowering or HDL-increasing effects are desired; treatment of hypertriglyceridemia in patients at risk of pancreatitis
Lovastatin: Treatment of primary hypercholesterolemia (Frederickson types IIa and IIb); primary and secondary prevention of cardiovascular disease
Usual Dosage Dosage forms are a fixed combination of niacin and lovastatin.
Oral: Adults: Lowest dose: Niacin 500 mg/lovastatin 20 mg; may increase by not more than 500 mg (niacin) at 4-week intervals (maximum dose: Niacin 2000 mg/lovastatin 40 mg daily); should be taken at bedtime with a low-fat snack. **Note:** If therapy is interrupted for >7 days, reinstitution of therapy should begin with the lowest dose followed by retitration as needed.
Not for use as initial therapy of dyslipidemias. May be substituted for equivalent dose of Niaspan®, however, manufacturer does not recommend direct substitution with other niacin products.
Dosage Forms
Tablet, variable release:
Advicor®: 500/20: Niacin 500 mg [extended release] and lovastatin 20 mg [immediate release]; 750/20: Niacin 750 mg [extended release] and lovastatin 20 mg [immediate release]; 1000/20: Niacin 1000 mg [extended release] and lovastatin 20 mg [immediate release]; 1000/40: Niacin 1000 mg [extended release] and lovastatin 40 mg [immediate release]

niacin and simvastatin (NYE a sin & sim va STAT in)

Synonyms simvastatin and niacin
U.S./Canadian Brand Names Simcor® [US]
Therapeutic Category Antilipemic Agent, HMG-CoA Reductase Inhibitor; Antilipemic Agent, Miscellaneous
Use Treatment of primary hypercholesterolemia, mixed dyslipidemia (types IIa and IIb), or hyper-triglyceridemia (type IV hyperlipidemia) in combination with standard cholesterol-lowering diet when simvastatin or niacin monotherapy is inadequate
Usual Dosage Dosage forms are a fixed combination of niacin extended release and simvastatin.
Oral: Adults:
Lowest dose (initiate in patients naïve to niacin therapy or those currently receiving niacin immediate release): Niacin 500 mg/simvastatin 20 mg once daily at bedtime with a low-fat snack; may increase by not more than 500 mg (niacin) at 4-week intervals
Maintenance dose: Niacin 1000 mg/simvastatin 20 mg to niacin 2000 mg/simvastatin 40 mg once daily (maximum: Niacin 2000 mg/simvastatin 40 mg once daily)
Note: If therapy is interrupted for >7 days, reinstitution of therapy should begin with the lowest dose followed by retitration as tolerated. Not for use as initial therapy of dyslipidemias. May be substituted for equivalent dose of niacin extended release, however, manufacturer does not recommend direct substitution with immediate release preparations.
Dosage Forms
Tablet, variable release:
Simcor®: 500/20: Niacin 500 mg [extended release] and simvastatin 20 mg [immediate release]; 750/20: Niacin 750 mg [extended release] and simvastatin 20 mg [immediate release]; 1000/20: Niacin 1000 mg [extended release] and simvastatin 20 mg [immediate release]

Niacin-Time® [US] *see* niacin *on page 667*
Niacor® [US] *see* niacin *on page 667*
Niaspan® [US/Can] *see* niacin *on page 667*
Niastase® [Can] *see* factor VIIa (recombinant) *on page 387*

nicardipine (nye KAR de peen)

Sound-Alike/Look-Alike Issues
  niCARdipine may be confused with niacinamide, NIFEdipine, niMODipine
  Cardene® may be confused with Cardizem®, Cardura®, codeine
Synonyms nicardipine hydrochloride
Tall-Man niCARdipine
U.S./Canadian Brand Names Cardene® I.V. [US]; Cardene® SR [US]; Cardene® [US]
Therapeutic Category Calcium Channel Blocker
Use Chronic stable angina (immediate release product only); management of hypertension (immediate and sustained release); parenteral only for short-term use when oral treatment is not feasible
Usual Dosage
  Adults:
  Oral:
    Immediate release: Initial: 20 mg 3 times/day; usual: 20-40 mg 3 times/day (allow 3 days between dose increases)
    Sustained release: Initial: 30 mg twice daily, titrate up to 60 mg twice daily
    Note: The total daily dose of immediate-release product may not automatically be equivalent to the daily sustained-release dose; use caution in converting.
  I.V.:
    Acute hypertension: Initial: 5 mg/hour increased by 2.5 mg/hour every 15 minutes to a maximum of 15 mg/hour; consider reduction to 3 mg/hour after response is achieved. Monitor and titrate to lowest dose necessary to maintain stable blood pressure.
    Substitution for oral therapy (approximate equivalents):
      20 mg every 8 hours oral, equivalent to 0.5 mg/hour I.V. infusion
      30 mg every 8 hours oral, equivalent to 1.2 mg/hour I.V. infusion
      40 mg every 8 hours oral, equivalent to 2.2 mg/hour I.V. infusion
Dosage Forms
  Capsule, oral: 20 mg, 30 mg
    Cardene®: 20 mg, 30 mg
  Capsule, sustained release, oral:
    Cardene® SR: 30 mg, 45 mg, 60 mg
  Infusion, premixed in iso-osmotic dextrose::
    Cardene® IV: 20 mg (200 mL)
  Infusion, premixed in iso-osmotic sodium chloride
    Cardene® IV: 20 mg (200 mL)
  Injection, solution: 2.5 mg/mL (10 mL)
    Cardene® IV: 2.5 mg/mL (10 mL)

nicardipine hydrochloride *see* nicardipine *on page 670*
N'ice® *(Discontinued)* *see* ascorbic acid *on page 96*
Nicobid® *(Discontinued)* *see* niacin *on page 667*
Nicoderm® [Can] *see* nicotine *on page 670*
NicoDerm® CQ® [US-OTC] *see* nicotine *on page 670*
Nicolar® *(Discontinued)* *see* niacin *on page 667*
Nicomide-T™ [US] *see* niacinamide *on page 668*
Nicorette® [US-OTC/Can] *see* nicotine *on page 670*
Nicorette® Plus [Can] *see* nicotine *on page 670*
nicotinamide *see* niacinamide *on page 668*

nicotine (nik oh TEEN)

Sound-Alike/Look-Alike Issues
  NicoDerm® may be confused with Nitroderm
  Nicorette® may be confused with Nordette®

U.S./Canadian Brand Names Commit® [US-OTC]; Habitrol® [Can]; NicoDerm® CQ® [US-OTC]; Nicoderm® [Can]; Nicorette® Plus [Can]; Nicorette® [US-OTC/Can]; Nicotrol® Inhaler [US]; Nicotrol® NS [US]; Nicotrol® [Can]; Thrive™ [US-OTC]

Therapeutic Category Smoking Deterrent

Use Treatment to aid smoking cessation for the relief of nicotine withdrawal symptoms (including nicotine craving)

Usual Dosage

Smoking deterrent: Patients should be advised to completely stop smoking upon initiation of therapy.

Oral:

Gum: Chew 1 piece of gum when urge to smoke, up to 24 pieces/day. Patients who smoke <25 cigarettes/day should start with 2-mg strength; patients smoking ≥25 cigarettes/day should start with the 4-mg strength. Use according to the following 12-week dosing schedule:

Weeks 1-6: Chew 1 piece of gum every 1-2 hours; to increase chances of quitting, chew at least 9 pieces/day during the first 6 weeks

Weeks 7-9: Chew 1 piece of gum every 2-4 hours

Weeks 10-12: Chew 1 piece of gum every 4-8 hours

Inhaler: Usually 6 to 16 cartridges per day; best effect was achieved by frequent continuous puffing (20 minutes); recommended duration of treatment is 3 months, after which patients may be weaned from the inhaler by gradual reduction of the daily dose over 6-12 weeks

Lozenge: Patients who smoke their first cigarette within 30 minutes of waking should use the 4 mg strength; otherwise the 2 mg strength is recommended. Use according to the following 12-week dosing schedule:

Weeks 1-6: One lozenge every 1-2 hours

Weeks 7-9: One lozenge every 2-4 hours

Weeks 10-12: One lozenge every 4-8 hours

Note: Use at least 9 lozenges/day during first 6 weeks to improve chances of quitting; do not use more than one lozenge at a time (maximum: 5 lozenges every 6 hours, 20 lozenges/day)

Topical:

Transdermal patch: Apply new patch every 24 hours to nonhairy, clean, dry skin on the upper body or upper outer arm; each patch should be applied to a different site. **Note:** Adjustment may be required during initial treatment (move to higher dose if experiencing withdrawal symptoms; lower dose if side effects are experienced).

NicoDerm CQ®:

Patients smoking ≥10 cigarettes/day: Begin with **step 1** (21 mg/day) for 6 weeks, followed by **step 2** (14 mg/day) for 2 weeks; finish with **step 3** (7 mg/day) for 2 weeks

Patients smoking <10 cigarettes/day: Begin with **step 2** (14 mg/day) for 6 weeks, followed by **step 3** (7 mg/day) for 2 weeks

Note: Patients receiving >600 mg/day of cimetidine: Decrease to the next lower patch size

Note: Benefits of use of nicotine transdermal patches beyond 3 months have not been demonstrated.

Nasal: Spray: 1-2 sprays/hour; do not exceed more than 5 doses (10 sprays) per hour [maximum: 40 doses/day (80 sprays); each dose (2 sprays) contains 1 mg of nicotine]

Dosage Forms

Gum, chewing: 2 mg (20s, 50s, 110s); 4 mg (20s, 50s, 110s)

Nicorette®: 2 mg (40s, 48s, 50s, 100s, 108s, 110s, 168s, 170s, 192s, 200s, 216s); 4 mg (40s, 48s, 50s, 100s, 108s, 110s, 168s, 170s, 192s, 200s, 216s)

Thrive™: 2 mg (40s); 4 mg (40s)

Lozenge:

Commit®: 2 mg (48s, 72s, 84s, 108s, 168s); 4 mg (48s, 72s, 84s, 108s, 168s, 192s)

Oral inhalation system:

Nicotrol® Inhaler: 10 mg cartridge [cartridge delivers 4 mg nicotine] (168s)

Solution, intranasal spray:

Nicotrol® NS: 10 mg/mL (10 mL)

Transdermal system, topical: 7 mg/24 (30s); 14 mg/24 hours (30s); 21 mg/24 hours (30s)

NicoDerm® CQ® [OTC]: 7 mg/24 hours (14s); 14 mg/24 hours (14s); 21 mg/24 hours (14s)

nicotinic acid see niacin on page 667

nicotinic acid amide see niacinamide on page 668

Nicotrol® [Can] see nicotine on page 670

Nicotrol® Inhaler [US] see nicotine on page 670

Nicotrol® NS [US] see nicotine on page 670

Nico-Vert® *(Discontinued)* see meclizine *on page 595*
Nidagel™ [Can] see metronidazole *on page 627*
Nifediac™ CC [US] see nifedipine *on page 672*
Nifedical™ XL [US] see nifedipine *on page 672*

nifedipine (nye FED i peen)

Sound-Alike/Look-Alike Issues
NIFEdipine may be confused with niCARdipine, niMODipine, nisoldipine
Procardia XL® may be confused with Cartia® XT

Tall-Man NIFEdipine

U.S./Canadian Brand Names Adalat® CC [US]; Adalat® XL® [Can]; Afeditab™ CR [US]; Apo-Nifed PA® [Can]; Apo-Nifed® [Can]; Nifediac™ CC [US]; Nifedical™ XL [US]; Novo-Nifedin [Can]; Nu-Nifed [Can]; Procardia XL® [US]; Procardia® [US/Can]

Therapeutic Category Calcium Channel Blocker

Use Angina and hypertension (sustained release only), pulmonary hypertension

Usual Dosage Oral:
Children:
Hypertrophic cardiomyopathy: 0.6-0.9 mg/kg/24 hours in 3-4 divided doses
Hypertension: Children 1-17 years: Extended release tablet: Initial: 0.25-0.5 mg/kg/day once daily or in 2 divided doses; maximum: 3 mg/kg/day up to 120 mg/day
Adults: (**Note:** When switching from immediate release to sustained release formulations, total daily dose will start the same)
Initial: 30 mg once daily as sustained release formulation, or if indicated, 10 mg 3 times/day as capsules
Usual dose: 10-30 mg 3 times/day as capsules or 30-60 mg once daily as sustained release
Maximum dose: 120-180 mg/day
Increase sustained release at 7- to 14-day intervals

Dosage Forms
Capsule, softgel: 10 mg, 20 mg
Procardia®: 10 mg
Tablet, extended release: 30 mg, 60 mg, 90 mg
Adalat® CC, Nifediac™ CC, Procardia XL®: 30 mg, 60 mg, 90 mg
Afeditab™ CR, Nifedical™ XL: 30 mg, 60 mg

Niferex® [US-OTC] see polysaccharide-iron complex *on page 768*
niftolid see flutamide *on page 416*
Nilandron® [US] see nilutamide *on page 672*

nilotinib (nye LOE ti nib)

Sound-Alike/Look-Alike Issues
nilotinib may be confused with nilutamide

Synonyms AMN107; nilotinib hydrochloride monohydrate

U.S./Canadian Brand Names Tasigna® [US]

Therapeutic Category Antineoplastic Agent, Tyrosine Kinase Inhibitor

Use Treatment of Philadelphia chromosome-positive chronic myelogenous leukemia (Ph+ CML) in chronic and accelerated phase (refractory or intolerant to prior therapy, including imatinib)

Usual Dosage Oral: Adults: 400 mg twice daily (continue treatment until disease progression or unacceptable toxicity)

Dosage Forms
Capsule:
Tasigna®: 200 mg

nilotinib hydrochloride monohydrate see nilotinib *on page 672*
Nilstat [Can] see nystatin *on page 690*
Nilstat® *(Discontinued)* see nystatin *on page 690*

nilutamide (ni LOO ta mide)

Sound-Alike/Look-Alike Issues
nilutamide may be confused with nilotinib

Synonyms NSC-684588; RU-23908

U.S./Canadian Brand Names Anandron® [Can]; Nilandron® [US]

Therapeutic Category Antineoplastic Agent

Use Treatment of metastatic prostate cancer

Usual Dosage Oral (refer to individual protocols): Adults: 300 mg daily for 30 days starting the same day or day after surgical castration, then 150 mg/day

Dosage Forms
Tablet:
Nilandron®: 150 mg

Nimbex® [US/Can] *see* cisatracurium *on page 224*

nimodipine (nye MOE di peen)

Sound-Alike/Look-Alike Issues
niMODipine may be confused with niCARdipine, NIFEdipine, nisoldipine

Tall-Man niMODipine

U.S./Canadian Brand Names Nimotop® [US/Can]

Therapeutic Category Calcium Channel Blocker

Use Spasm following subarachnoid hemorrhage from ruptured intracranial aneurysms regardless of the patients neurological condition postictus (Hunt and Hess grades I-V)

Usual Dosage Note: Capsules and contents are for oral administration **ONLY**. Oral: Adults: 60 mg every 4 hours for 21 days, start therapy within 96 hours after subarachnoid hemorrhage.

Dosage Forms
Capsule, liquid filled: 30 mg
Nimotop®: 30 mg

Nimotop® [US/Can] *see* nimodipine *on page 673*
Nipent® [US/Can] *see* pentostatin *on page 737*
Niravam™ [US] *see* alprazolam *on page 49*

nisoldipine (nye SOL di peen)

Sound-Alike/Look-Alike Issues
nisoldipine may be confused with NIFEdipine, niMODipine

U.S./Canadian Brand Names Sular® [US]

Therapeutic Category Calcium Channel Blocker

Use Management of hypertension, alone or in combination with other antihypertensive agents

Usual Dosage Oral: Adults: Initial: 17 mg once daily, then increase by 8.5 mg/week (or longer intervals) to attain adequate control of blood pressure; usual dose range: 17-34 mg once daily; doses >34 mg once daily are not recommended.

Dosage Forms
Tablet, extended release [original formulation]: 20 mg, 30 mg, 40 mg
Tablet, extended release [Geomatrix® delivery system]:
Sular®: 8.5 mg, 17 mg, 25.5 mg, 34 mg

nitalapram *see* citalopram *on page 225*

nitazoxanide (nye ta ZOX a nide)

Synonyms NTZ

U.S./Canadian Brand Names Alinia® [US]

Therapeutic Category Antiprotozoal

Use Treatment of diarrhea caused by *Cryptosporidium parvum* or *Giardia lamblia*

Usual Dosage Diarrhea caused by *Cryptosporidium parvum* or *Giardia lamblia*:
Children 1-3 years: 100 mg every 12 hours for 3 days
Children 4-11 years: 200 mg every 12 hours for 3 days
Children ≥12 years and Adults: 500 mg every 12 hours for 3 days

Dosage Forms
Powder for suspension, oral:
Alinia®: 100 mg/5 mL
Tablet:
Alinia®: 500 mg
Alinia® 3-Day Therapy Packs™ [unit-dose pack]: 500 mg (6s)

nitisinone (ni TIS i known)

U.S./Canadian Brand Names Orfadin® [US]

Therapeutic Category 4-Hydroxyphenylpyruvate Dioxygenase Inhibitor

Use Treatment of hereditary tyrosinemia type 1 (HT-1); to be used with dietary restriction of tyrosine and phenylalanine

Usual Dosage Oral: **Note:** Must be used in conjunction with a low protein diet restricted in tyrosine and phenylalanine.

Infants: See dosing for Children and Adults; infants may require maximal dose once liver function has improved

Children and Adults: Initial: 1 mg/kg/day in divided doses, given in the morning and evening, 1 hour before meals; doses do not need to be divided evenly

Dosage Forms

Capsule:

Orfadin®: 2 mg, 5 mg, 10 mg

Nitoman™ [Can] *see* tetrabenazine *(Canada only) on page 914*

Nitrazadon [Can] *see* nitrazepam *(Canada only) on page 674*

nitrazepam *(Canada only)* (nye TRA ze pam)

Synonyms nitrozepamum

U.S./Canadian Brand Names Apo-Nitrazepam® [Can]; Mogadon [Can]; Nitrazadon [Can]; Nitrazepam (Pro-Doc) [Can]; Sandoz-Nitrazepam [Can]

Therapeutic Category Benzodiazepine

Controlled Substance CDSA IV

Use Short-term management of insomnia; treatment of myoclonic seizures

Usual Dosage Oral:

Children ≤30 kg: Myoclonic seizures: 0.3-1 mg/kg/day in 3 divided doses

Adults: Insomnia: 5-10 mg at bedtime; treatment should not exceed 7-10 consecutive days; use for more than 2-3 consecutive weeks requires complete reevaluation of patient

Dosage Forms [CAN] = Canadian brand name

Tablet:

Apo-Nitrazepam® [CAN], Mogadon [CAN], Nitrazadon [CAN], Nitrazepam [CAN], Sandoz-Nitrazepam [CAN]: 5 mg, 10 mg [not available in the U.S.]

Nitrazepam (Pro-Doc) [Can] *see* nitrazepam *(Canada only) on page 674*

Nitrek® *(Discontinued)* *see* nitroglycerin *on page 675*

nitric oxide (NYE trik OKS ide)

U.S./Canadian Brand Names INOmax® [US/Can]

Therapeutic Category Vasodilator, Pulmonary

Use Treatment of term and near-term (>34 weeks) neonates with hypoxic respiratory failure associated with pulmonary hypertension; used concurrently with ventilatory support and other agents

Usual Dosage Inhalation: Neonates (up to 14 days old): 20 ppm. Treatment should be maintained up to 14 days or until the underlying oxygen desaturation has resolved and the neonate is ready to be weaned from therapy. In the CINRGI trial, patients whose oxygenation improved had their dose reduced to 5 ppm at the end of 4 hours of treatment. Doses above 20 ppm should not be used because of the risk of methemoglobinemia and elevated NO_2.

Dosage Forms

Gas, for inhalation:

INOmax®: 100 ppm [nitric oxide 0.01% and nitrogen 99.99%] (353 L, 1963 L); 800 ppm [nitric oxide 0.08% and nitrogen 99.92%] (353 L, 1963 L)

4'-nitro-3'-trifluoromethylisobutyrantide *see* flutamide *on page 416*

Nitro-Bid® [US] *see* nitroglycerin *on page 675*

Nitrodisc® Patch *(Discontinued)* *see* nitroglycerin *on page 675*

Nitro-Dur® [US/Can] *see* nitroglycerin *on page 675*

nitrofurantoin (nye troe fyoor AN toyn)

U.S./Canadian Brand Names Apo-Nitrofurantoin® [Can]; Furadantin® [US]; Macrobid® [US/Can]; Macrodantin® [US/Can]; Novo-Furantoin [Can]

Therapeutic Category Antibiotic, Miscellaneous

Use Prevention and treatment of urinary tract infections caused by susceptible strains of *E. coli, S. aureus, Enterococcus, Klebsiella,* and *Enterobacter*

Usual Dosage Oral:

Children >1 month:

UTI treatment (Furadantin®, Macrodantin®): 5-7 mg/kg/day in divided doses every 6 hours; maximum: 400 mg/day. Administer for 7 days or at least 3 days after obtaining sterile urine

UTI prophylaxis (Furadantin®, Macrodantin®): 1-2 mg/kg/day in divided doses every 12-24 hours; maximum: 100 mg/day

Children >12 years: UTI treatment (Macrobid®): 100 mg twice daily for 7 days

Adults:

UTI treatment:

Furadantin®, Macrodantin®: 50-100 mg/dose every 6 hours; administer for 7 days or at least 3 days after obtaining sterile urine

Macrobid®: 100 mg twice daily for 7 days

UTI prophylaxis (Furadantin®, Macrodantin®): 50-100 mg/dose at bedtime

Dosage Forms

Capsule, macrocrystal: 50 mg, 100 mg

Macrodantin®: 25 mg, 50 mg, 100 mg

Capsule, macrocrystal/monohydrate: 100 mg

Macrobid®: 100 mg

Suspension, oral:

Furadantin®: 25 mg/5 mL

nitrogen mustard *see* mechlorethamine *on page 595*

nitroglycerin (nye troe GLI ser in)

Sound-Alike/Look-Alike Issues

nitroglycerin may be confused with nitroprusside

Nitro-Bid® may be confused with Nicobid®

Nitrol® may be confused with Nizoral®

Nitrostat® may be confused with Nilstat®, nystatin

Synonyms glyceryl trinitrate; nitroglycerol; NTG

U.S./Canadian Brand Names Gen-Nitro [Can]; Minitran™ [US/Can]; Nitro-Bid® [US]; Nitro-Dur® [US/Can]; Nitroglycerin Injection, USP [Can]; Nitrolingual® [US]; Nitrol® [Can]; NitroQuick® [US]; Nitrostat® [US/Can]; NitroTime® [US]; Rho®-Nitro [Can]; Transderm-Nitro® [Can]; Trinipatch® 0.2 [Can]; Trinipatch® 0.4 [Can]; Trinipatch® 0.6 [Can]

Therapeutic Category Vasodilator

Use Treatment of angina pectoris; I.V. for congestive heart failure (especially when associated with acute myocardial infarction); pulmonary hypertension; hypertensive emergencies occurring perioperatively (especially during cardiovascular surgery)

Usual Dosage Note: Hemodynamic and antianginal tolerance often develop within 24-48 hours of continuous nitrate administration. Nitrate-free interval (10-12 hours/day) is recommended to avoid tolerance development; gradually decrease dose in patients receiving NTG for prolonged period to avoid withdrawal reaction.

Children: Pulmonary hypertension: Continuous infusion: Start 0.25-0.5 mcg/kg/minute and titrate by 1 mcg/kg/minute at 20- to 60-minute intervals to desired effect; usual dose: 1-3 mcg/kg/minute; maximum: 5 mcg/kg/minute

Adults:

Oral: 2.5-9 mg 2-4 times/day (up to 26 mg 4 times/day)

I.V.: 5 mcg/minute, increase by 5 mcg/minute every 3-5 minutes to 20 mcg/minute; if no response at 20 mcg/minute increase by 10 mcg/minute every 3-5 minutes, up to 200 mcg/minute

Ointment: ¹/₂" upon rising and ¹/₂" 6 hours later; the dose may be doubled and even doubled again as needed

Patch, transdermal: Initial: 0.2-0.4 mg/hour, titrate to doses of 0.4-0.8 mg/hour; tolerance is minimized by using a patch-on period of 12-14 hours and patch-off period of 10-12 hours

Sublingual: 0.2-0.6 mg every 5 minutes for maximum of 3 doses in 15 minutes; may also use prophylactically 5-10 minutes prior to activities which may provoke an attack

Translingual: 1-2 sprays into mouth under tongue every 3-5 minutes for maximum of 3 doses in 15 minutes, may also be used 5-10 minutes prior to activities which may provoke an attack prophylactically

Dosage Forms

Capsule, extended release: 2.5 mg, 6.5 mg, 9 mg
Nitro-Time®: 2.5 mg, 6.5 mg, 9 mg

Infusion [premixed in D_5W]: 25 mg (250 mL) [0.1 mg/mL]; 50 mg (250 mL) [0.2 mg/mL]; 50 mg (500 mL) [0.1 mg/mL]; 100 mg (250 mL) [0.4 mg/mL]; 200 mg (500 mL) [0.4 mg/mL]

Injection, solution: 5 mg/mL (5 mL, 10 mL)

Ointment, topical:
Nitro-Bid®: 2% [20 mg/g] (1 g, 30 g, 60 g)

Solution, translingual [spray]:
Nitrolingual®: 0.4 mg/metered spray (4.9 g, 12 g)

Tablet, sublingual: 0.3 mg, 0.4 mg, 0.6 mg
NitroQuick®, Nitrostat®, Nitro-Tab®: 0.3 mg, 0.4 mg, 0.6 mg

Transdermal system [once-daily patch]: 0.1 mg/hour (30s); 0.2 mg/hour (30s); 0.4 mg/hour (30s); 0.6 mg/hour (30s)
Minitran™: 0.1 mg/hour (30s); 0.2 mg/hour (30s); 0.4 mg/hour (30s); 0.6 mg/hour (30s)
Nitro-Dur®: 0.1 mg/hour (30s); 0.2 mg/hour (30s); 0.3 mg/hour (30s); 0.4 mg/hour (30s); 0.6 mg/hour (30s); 0.8 mg/hour (30s)

Nitroglycerin Injection, USP [Can] see nitroglycerin on page 675

nitroglycerol see nitroglycerin on page 675

Nitrol® [Can] see nitroglycerin on page 675

Nitrol® (Discontinued) see nitroglycerin on page 675

Nitrolingual® [US] see nitroglycerin on page 675

Nitrong® Oral Tablet (Discontinued) see nitroglycerin on page 675

Nitropress® [US] see nitroprusside on page 676

nitroprusside (nye troe PRUS ide)

Sound-Alike/Look-Alike Issues
nitroprusside may be confused with nitroglycerin

Synonyms nitroprusside sodium; sodium nitroferricyanide; sodium nitroprusside

U.S./Canadian Brand Names Nitropress® [US]

Therapeutic Category Vasodilator

Use Management of hypertensive crises; congestive heart failure; used for controlled hypotension to reduce bleeding during surgery

Usual Dosage Administration requires the use of an infusion pump. Average dose: 5 mcg/kg/minute.
Children: Pulmonary hypertension: I.V.: Initial: 1 mcg/kg/minute by continuous I.V. infusion; increase in increments of 1 mcg/kg/minute at intervals of 20-60 minutes; titrating to the desired response; usual dose: 3 mcg/kg/minute, rarely need >4 mcg/kg/minute; maximum: 5 mcg/kg/minute.
Adults: I.V. Initial: 0.3-0.5 mcg/kg/minute; increase in increments of 0.5 mcg/kg/minute, titrating to the desired hemodynamic effect or the appearance of headache or nausea; usual dose: 3 mcg/kg/minute; rarely need >4 mcg/kg/minute; maximum: 10 mcg/kg/minute. When administered by prolonged infusion faster than 2 mcg/kg/minute, cyanide is generated faster than an unaided patient can handle.

Dosage Forms
Injection, solution: 25 mg/mL (2 mL)
Nitropress®: 25 mg/mL (2 mL)

nitroprusside sodium see nitroprusside on page 676

NitroQuick® [US] see nitroglycerin on page 675

Nitrostat® [US/Can] see nitroglycerin on page 675

NitroTime® [US] see nitroglycerin on page 675

nitrous oxide (NYE trus OKS ide)

Therapeutic Category Anesthetic, Gas

Use Produces sedation and analgesia; principal adjunct to inhalation and intravenous general anesthesia

Usual Dosage Children and Adults:

Surgical: For sedation and analgesia: Concentrations of 25% to 50% nitrous oxide with oxygen. For general anesthesia, concentrations of 40% to 70% via mask or endotracheal tube. Minimal alveolar concentration (MAC), which can be considered the ED_{50} of inhalational anesthetics, is 105%; therefore delivery in a hyperbaric chamber is necessary to use as a complete anesthetic. When administered at 70%, reduces the MAC of other anesthetics by half.

Dental: For sedation and analgesia: Concentrations of 25% to 50% nitrous oxide with oxygen

Dosage Forms

Supplied in blue cylinders

nitrozepamum see nitrazepam *(Canada only) on page 674*

Nix® [US-OTC/Can] see permethrin *on page 740*

nizatidine (ni ZA ti deen)

Sound-Alike/Look-Alike Issues

Axid® may be confused with Ansaid®

U.S./Canadian Brand Names Apo-Nizatidine® [Can]; Axid® AR [US-OTC]; Axid® [US/Can]; Gen-Nizatidine [Can]; Novo-Nizatidine [Can]; Nu-Nizatidine [Can]; PMS-Nizatidine [Can]

Therapeutic Category Histamine H_2 Antagonist

Use Treatment and maintenance of duodenal ulcer; treatment of benign gastric ulcer; treatment of gastroesophageal reflux disease (GERD); OTC tablet used for the prevention of meal-induced heartburn, acid indigestion, and sour stomach

Usual Dosage Oral:

Children ≥12 years:

GERD: Refer to adult dosing

Meal-induced heartburn, acid indigestion and sour stomach: Refer to adult dosing

Adults:

Duodenal ulcer:

Treatment of active ulcer: 300 mg at bedtime or 150 mg twice daily

Maintenance of healed ulcer: 150 mg/day at bedtime

Gastric ulcer: 150 mg twice daily or 300 mg at bedtime

GERD: 150 mg twice daily

Meal-induced heartburn, acid indigestion, and sour stomach: 75 mg tablet [OTC] twice daily, 30 to 60 minutes prior to consuming food or beverages

Dosage Forms

Capsule: 150 mg, 300 mg

Solution, oral:

Axid®: 15 mg/mL

Tablet:

Axid® AR [OTC]: 75 mg

Nizoral® [US] see ketoconazole *on page 537*

Nizoral® A-D [US-OTC] see ketoconazole *on page 537*

N-methylhydrazine see procarbazine *on page 788*

N-methylnaltrexone bromide see methylnaltrexone *on page 621*

No Doz® Maximum Strength [US-OTC] see caffeine *on page 158*

NoHist [US] see chlorpheniramine and phenylephrine *on page 206*

NoHist-A [US] see chlorpheniramine, phenylephrine, and phenyltoloxamine *on page 211*

Nolahist® *(Discontinued)*

Nolex® LA *(Discontinued)*

Nolvadex® [Can] see tamoxifen *on page 902*

Nolvadex®-D [Can] see tamoxifen *on page 902*

Nolvadex® *(Discontinued)* see tamoxifen *on page 902*

nonoxynol 9 (non OKS i nole nine)

Sound-Alike/Look-Alike Issues

Delfen® may be confused with Delsym®

Synonyms N-9

◄ **U.S./Canadian Brand Names** Advantage-S™ [US-OTC]; Conceptrol® [US-OTC]; Delfen® [US-OTC]; Encare® [US-OTC]; Gynol II® Extra Strength [US-OTC]; Gynol II® [US-OTC]; Today® [US-OTC]; VCF™ [US-OTC]

Therapeutic Category Spermicide

Use Prevention of pregnancy

Usual Dosage Adolescents and Adults: **Note:** Prior to use, refer to specific product labeling for complete instructions.

Prevention of pregnancy: Vaginal:

Advantage-S™, Conceptrol®: Insert 1 applicatorful vaginally up to 1 hour prior to intercourse

Encare®: Unwrap and insert 1 suppository vaginally at least 10 minutes prior to intercourse; effective for 1 hour

Today® Sponge: Insert 1 sponge vaginally prior to intercourse; allow to remain in place for 6 hours after intercourse before removing; effective for use up to 24 continuous hours. Do not leave in place for >30 hours.

VCF™:

Film: Insert 1 film vaginally at least 15 minutes, but no more than 3 hours, prior to intercourse. Insert new film for each act of intercourse or if more than 3 hours have elapsed.

Foam: Insert 1 applicatorful at least 15 minutes prior to intercourse; effective for up to 1 hour

Dosage Forms

Aerosol, vaginal [foam]:
Delfen®: 12.5% (18 g) [contains benzoic acid]
VCF™: 12.5% (40 g)

Film, vaginal:
VCF™ [OTC]: 28% (3s, 6s,12s)

Gel, vaginal:
Advantage-S® [OTC]: 3.5% (1.5 g, 30 g)
Conceptrol® [OTC]: 4% (2.7 g)
Gynol II® [OTC]: 2% (85 g, 114 g)
Gynol II® Extra Strength: 3% (85.5 g)

Sponge, vaginal:
Today® [OTC]: 1 g (3s, 6s, 12s)

Suppository, vaginal:
Encare® [OTC]: 100 mg (12s, 18s)

No Pain-HP® *(Discontinued)* see capsaicin on page 171

Nora-BE™ [US] see norethindrone on page 679

noradrenaline see norepinephrine on page 678

noradrenaline acid tartrate see norepinephrine on page 678

Norcet® *(Discontinued)* see hydrocodone and acetaminophen on page 481

Norco® [US] see hydrocodone and acetaminophen on page 481

Norcuron® [Can] see vecuronium on page 973

Norcuron® *(Discontinued)* see vecuronium on page 973

nordeoxyguanosine see ganciclovir on page 435

Nordette® [US] see ethinyl estradiol and levonorgestrel on page 372

Norditropin® [US] see somatropin on page 881

Norditropin® NordiFlex® [US] see somatropin on page 881

Nordryl® Injection *(Discontinued)* see diphenhydramine on page 304

Nordryl® Oral *(Discontinued)* see diphenhydramine on page 304

Norel DM™ [US] see chlorpheniramine, phenylephrine, and dextromethorphan on page 209

norel® EX [US] see guaifenesin and phenylephrine on page 456

norelgestromin and ethinyl estradiol see ethinyl estradiol and norelgestromin on page 375

norepinephrine (nor ep i NEF rin)

Synonyms levarterenol bitartrate; noradrenaline; noradrenaline acid tartrate; norepinephrine bitartrate

U.S./Canadian Brand Names Levophed® [US/Can]

Therapeutic Category Adrenergic Agonist Agent

Use Treatment of shock which persists after adequate fluid volume replacement

Usual Dosage Administration requires the use of an infusion pump!

Note: Norepinephrine dosage is stated in terms of norepinephrine base and intravenous formulation is norepinephrine bitartrate

Norepinephrine bitartrate 2 mg = Norepinephrine base 1 mg

Continuous I.V. infusion:

Children: Initial: 0.05-0.1 mcg/kg/minute; titrate to desired effect; maximum dose: 1-2 mcg/kg/minute

Adults: Initial: 0.5-1 mcg/minute and titrate to desired response; 8-30 mcg/minute is usual range; range used in clinical trials: 0.01-3 mcg/kg/minute; ACLS dosage range: 0.5-30 mcg/minute

Dosage Forms

Injection, solution: 1 mg/mL (4 mL)

Levophed®: 1 mg/mL (4 mL)

norepinephrine bitartrate *see* norepinephrine *on page 678*

Norethin™ 1/35E *(Discontinued)* *see* ethinyl estradiol and norethindrone *on page 376*

norethindrone (nor ETH in drone)

Sound-Alike/Look-Alike Issues

Micronor® may be confused with miconazole, Micronase®

Synonyms norethindrone acetate; norethisterone

U.S./Canadian Brand Names Aygestin® [US]; Camila™ [US]; Errin™ [US]; Jolivette™ [US]; Micronor® [Can]; Nor-QD® [US]; Nora-BE™ [US]; Norlutate® [Can]; Ortho Micronor® [US]

Therapeutic Category Contraceptive, Progestin Only; Progestin

Use Treatment of amenorrhea; abnormal uterine bleeding; endometriosis; prevention of pregnancy

Usual Dosage Oral: Adolescents and Adults: Female:

Contraception: Progesterone only: Norethindrone 0.35 mg every day (no missed days)

Initial dose: Start on first day of menstrual period or the day after a miscarriage or abortion. If switching from a combined oral contraceptive, begin the day after finishing the last active combined tablet.

Missed dose: Take as soon as remembered. A backup method of contraception should be used for 48 hours if dose is taken ≥3 hours late.

Amenorrhea and abnormal uterine bleeding: Norethindrone acetate: 2.5-10 mg/day for 5-10 days during the second half of the menstrual cycle

Endometriosis: Norethindrone acetate: 5 mg/day for 14 days; increase at increments of 2.5 mg/day every 2 weeks to reach 15 mg/day; continue for 6-9 months or until breakthrough bleeding demands temporary termination

Dosage Forms

Tablet: 0.35 mg, 5 mg

Aygestin®: 5 mg

Camila™, Errin™, Jolivette™, Ortho Micronor®, Nora-BE™, Nor-QD®: 0.35 mg

norethindrone acetate *see* norethindrone *on page 679*

norethindrone acetate and ethinyl estradiol *see* ethinyl estradiol and norethindrone *on page 376*

norethindrone and estradiol *see* estradiol and norethindrone *on page 362*

norethindrone and mestranol *see* mestranol and norethindrone *on page 608*

norethisterone *see* norethindrone *on page 679*

Norflex™ [US/Can] *see* orphenadrine *on page 702*

norfloxacin (nor FLOKS a sin)

Sound-Alike/Look-Alike Issues

norfloxacin may be confused with Norflex™, Noroxin®

Noroxin® may be confused with Neurontin®, Norflex™, norfloxacin

U.S./Canadian Brand Names Apo-Norflox® [Can]; CO Norfloxacin [Can]; Norfloxacine® [Can]; Noroxin® [US/Can]; Novo-Norfloxacin [Can]; PMS-Norfloxacin [Can]; Riva-Norfloxacin [Can]

Therapeutic Category Quinolone

Use Uncomplicated and complicated urinary tract infections caused by susceptible gram-negative and gram-positive bacteria; sexually-transmitted disease (eg, uncomplicated urethral and cervical gonorrhea) caused by *N. gonorrhoeae*; prostatitis due to *E. coli*

Note: As of April 2007, the CDC no longer recommends the use of fluoroquinolones for the treatment of gonococcal disease.

◀ **Usual Dosage**
Usual dosage range:
Adults: Oral: 400 mg every 12 hours (maximum: 800 mg/day)
Indication-specific dosing:
Adults: Oral:
Prostatitis: 400 mg every 12 hours for 4-6 weeks
Uncomplicated gonorrhea: 800 mg as a single dose. **Note:** As of April 2007, the CDC no longer recommends the use of fluoroquinolones for the treatment of uncomplicated gonococcal disease.
Urinary tract infections:
Uncomplicated: 400 mg twice daily for 3-14 days
Uncomplicated due to *E. coli, K. pneumoniae, P. mirabilis*: 400 mg twice daily for 7-10 days
Complicated: 400 mg twice daily for 10-21 days
Dosage Forms
Tablet:
Noroxin®: 400 mg

Norfloxacine® [Can] *see* norfloxacin *on page 679*
Norgesic™ [Can] *see* orphenadrine, aspirin, and caffeine *on page 703*
Norgesic™ (Discontinued) *see* orphenadrine, aspirin, and caffeine *on page 703*
Norgesic™ Forte [Can] *see* orphenadrine, aspirin, and caffeine *on page 703*
Norgesic™ Forte (Discontinued) *see* orphenadrine, aspirin, and caffeine *on page 703*
norgestimate and estradiol *see* estradiol and norgestimate *on page 362*
norgestimate and ethinyl estradiol *see* ethinyl estradiol and norgestimate *on page 378*
norgestrel and ethinyl estradiol *see* ethinyl estradiol and norgestrel *on page 380*
Norinyl® 1+35 [US] *see* ethinyl estradiol and norethindrone *on page 376*
Norinyl® 1+50 [US] *see* mestranol and norethindrone *on page 608*
Noritate® [US/Can] *see* metronidazole *on page 627*
Norlutate® [Can] *see* norethindrone *on page 679*
normal human serum albumin *see* albumin *on page 38*
normal saline *see* sodium chloride *on page 873*
normal serum albumin (human) *see* albumin *on page 38*
Normiflo® (Discontinued)
Normocarb HF™ [US] *see* electrolyte solution, renal replacement *on page 336*
Normodyne® [Can] *see* labetalol *on page 541*
Noroxin® [US/Can] *see* norfloxacin *on page 679*
Norpace® [US/Can] *see* disopyramide *on page 312*
Norpace® CR [US] *see* disopyramide *on page 312*
Norplant® Implant [Can] *see* levonorgestrel *on page 559*
Norplant® Implant (Discontinued) *see* levonorgestrel *on page 559*
Norpramin® [US/Can] *see* desipramine *on page 274*
Nor-QD® [US] *see* norethindrone *on page 679*
Nortemp Children's [US-OTC] *see* acetaminophen *on page 19*
North American antisnake-bite serum *see* crotalidae polyvalent immune FAB (ovine) *on page 253*
North American coral snake antivenin *see* antivenin *(Micrurus fulvius) on page 84*
North, Central, and South American antisnake-bite serum *see* crotalidae polyvalent antivenin (equine) *on page 252*
Northyx™ [US] *see* methimazole *on page 614*
Nortrel™ [US] *see* ethinyl estradiol and norethindrone *on page 376*
Nortrel™ 7/7/7 [US] *see* ethinyl estradiol and norethindrone *on page 376*

nortriptyline (nor TRIP ti leen)
Sound-Alike/Look-Alike Issues
nortriptyline may be confused with amitriptyline, desipramine, Norpramin®
Aventyl® HCl may be confused with Bentyl®
Pamelor® may be confused with Demerol®, Dymelor®, Panlor® DC
Synonyms nortriptyline hydrochloride

U.S./Canadian Brand Names Alti-Nortriptyline [Can]; Apo-Nortriptyline® [Can]; Aventyl® [Can]; Gen-Nortriptyline [Can]; Norventyl [Can]; Novo-Nortriptyline [Can]; Nu-Nortriptyline [Can]; Pamelor® [US]; PMS-Nortriptyline [Can]

Therapeutic Category Antidepressant, Tricyclic (Secondary Amine)

Use Treatment of symptoms of depression

Usual Dosage Oral: Adults:
Depression: 25 mg 3-4 times/day up to 150 mg/day; doses may be given once daily
Myofascial pain, neuralgia, burning mouth syndrome (dental use): Initial: 10-25 mg at bedtime; dosage may be increased by 25 mg/day weekly, if tolerated; usual maintenance dose: 75 mg as a single bedtime dose or 2 divided doses

Dosage Forms
Capsule: 10 mg, 25 mg, 50 mg, 75 mg
Pamelor®: 10 mg, 25 mg, 50 mg, 75 mg
Solution:
Pamelor®: 10 mg/5 mL

nortriptyline hydrochloride *see* nortriptyline *on page 680*

Norvasc® [US/Can] *see* amlodipine *on page 63*

Norventyl [Can] *see* nortriptyline *on page 680*

Norvir® [US/Can] *see* ritonavir *on page 838*

Norvir® SEC [Can] *see* ritonavir *on page 838*

Novacet® *(Discontinued)* *see* sulfur and sulfacetamide *on page 897*

Novafed® A *(Discontinued)* *see* chlorpheniramine and pseudoephedrine *on page 207*

Novahistex® DM Decongestant [Can] *see* pseudoephedrine and dextromethorphan *on page 802*

Novahistex® DM Decongestant Expectorant [Can] *see* guaifenesin, pseudoephedrine, and dextromethorphan *on page 460*

Novahistex® Expectorant with Decongestant [Can] *see* guaifenesin and pseudoephedrine *on page 458*

Novahistine DH [US] *see* dihydrocodeine, chlorpheniramine, and phenylephrine *on page 298*

Novahistine® DM Decongestant [Can] *see* pseudoephedrine and dextromethorphan *on page 802*

Novahistine® DM Decongestant Expectorant [Can] *see* guaifenesin, pseudoephedrine, and dextromethorphan *on page 460*

Novamilor [Can] *see* amiloride and hydrochlorothiazide *on page 59*

Novamoxin® [Can] *see* amoxicillin *on page 67*

Novantrone® [US/Can] *see* mitoxantrone *on page 638*

Novarel® [US] *see* chorionic gonadotropin (human) *on page 216*

Novasal™ [US] *see* magnesium salicylate *on page 588*

Novasen [Can] *see* aspirin *on page 98*

Nove-Desmopressin [Can] *see* desmopressin acetate *on page 275*

Novo-5 ASA [Can] *see* mesalamine *on page 607*

Novo-Acebutolol [Can] *see* acebutolol *on page 19*

Novo-Alendronate [Can] *see* alendronate *on page 43*

Novo-Alprazol [Can] *see* alprazolam *on page 49*

Novo-Amiodarone [Can] *see* amiodarone *on page 61*

Novo-Ampicillin [Can] *see* ampicillin *on page 72*

Novo-Atenol [Can] *see* atenolol *on page 101*

Novo-Atenolthalidone [Can] *see* atenolol and chlorthalidone *on page 102*

Novo-Azathioprine [Can] *see* azathioprine *on page 109*

Novo-Azithromycin [Can] *see* azithromycin *on page 110*

Novo-Benzydamine [Can] *see* benzydamine *(Canada only) on page 129*

Novo-Bicalutamide [Can] *see* bicalutamide *on page 135*

Novo-Bisoprolol [Can] *see* bisoprolol *on page 138*

Novo-Bromazepam [Can] *see* bromazepam *(Canada only) on page 142*

Novo-Bupropion SR [Can] *see* bupropion *on page 152*

Novo-Buspirone [Can] *see* buspirone *on page 153*

Novocain® [US] *see* procaine *on page 787*

Novo-Captopril [Can] *see* captopril *on page 171*
Novo-Carbamaz [Can] *see* carbamazepine *on page 172*
Novo-Carvedilol [Can] *see* carvedilol *on page 181*
Novo-Cefaclor [Can] *see* cefaclor *on page 183*
Novo-Cefadroxil [Can] *see* cefadroxil *on page 184*
Novo-Chloroquine [Can] *see* chloroquine *on page 204*
Novo-Chlorpromazine [Can] *see* chlorpromazine *on page 213*
Novo-Cholamine [Can] *see* cholestyramine resin *on page 215*
Novo-Cholamine Light [Can] *see* cholestyramine resin *on page 215*
Novo-Cilazapril [Can] *see* cilazapril *(Canada only) on page 219*
Novo-Cimetidine [Can] *see* cimetidine *on page 219*
Novo-Ciprofloxacin [Can] *see* ciprofloxacin *on page 221*
Novo-Citalopram [Can] *see* citalopram *on page 225*
Novo-Clavamoxin [Can] *see* amoxicillin and clavulanate potassium *on page 68*
Novo-Clindamycin [Can] *see* clindamycin *on page 230*
Novo-Clobazam [Can] *see* clobazam *(Canada only) on page 232*
Novo-Clobetasol [Can] *see* clobetasol *on page 232*
Novo-Clonazepam [Can] *see* clonazepam *on page 235*
Novo-Clonidine [Can] *see* clonidine *on page 236*
Novo-Clopate [Can] *see* clorazepate *on page 238*
Novo-Cloxin [Can] *see* cloxacillin *(Canada only) on page 239*
Novo-Cycloprine [Can] *see* cyclobenzaprine *on page 255*
Novo-Cyproterone [Can] *see* cyproterone *(Canada only) on page 259*
Novo-Difenac [Can] *see* diclofenac *on page 292*
Novo-Difenac K [Can] *see* diclofenac *on page 292*
Novo-Difenac-SR [Can] *see* diclofenac *on page 292*
Novo-Diflunisal [Can] *see* diflunisal *on page 296*
Novo-Digoxin [Can] *see* digoxin *on page 296*
Novo-Diltazem [Can] *see* diltiazem *on page 300*
Novo-Diltazem-CD [Can] *see* diltiazem *on page 300*
Novo-Diltiazem HCl ER [Can] *see* diltiazem *on page 300*
Novo-Dimenate [Can] *see* dimenhydrinate *on page 301*
Novo-Dipam [Can] *see* diazepam *on page 289*
Novo-Divalproex [Can] *see* valproic acid and derivatives *on page 967*
Novo-Docusate Calcium [Can] *see* docusate *on page 314*
Novo-Docusate Sodium [Can] *see* docusate *on page 314*
Novo-Domperidone [Can] *see* domperidone *(Canada only) on page 317*
Novo-Doxazosin [Can] *see* doxazosin *on page 320*
Novo-Doxepin [Can] *see* doxepin *on page 321*
Novo-Doxylin [Can] *see* doxycycline *on page 323*
Novo-Enalapril [Can] *see* enalapril *on page 339*
Novo-Famotidine [Can] *see* famotidine *on page 390*
Novo-Fenofibrate [Can] *see* fenofibrate *on page 393*
Novo-Fenofibrate-S [Can] *see* fenofibrate *on page 393*
Novo-Ferrogluc [Can] *see* ferrous gluconate *on page 398*
Novo-Fluconazole [Can] *see* fluconazole *on page 405*
Novo-Flunarizine [Can] *see* flunarizine *(Canada only) on page 408*
Novo-Fluoxetine [Can] *see* fluoxetine *on page 413*
Novo-Flurprofen [Can] *see* flurbiprofen *on page 416*
Novo-Flutamide [Can] *see* flutamide *on page 416*
Novo-Fluvoxamine [Can] *see* fluvoxamine *on page 420*
Novo-Fosinopril [Can] *see* fosinopril *on page 427*
Novo-Furantoin [Can] *see* nitrofurantoin *on page 675*

Novo-Gabapentin [Can] *see* gabapentin *on page 431*
Novo-Gemfibrozil [Can] *see* gemfibrozil *on page 439*
Novo-Gesic [Can] *see* acetaminophen *on page 19*
Novo-Gliclazide [Can] *see* gliclazide *(Canada only) on page 444*
Novo-Glimepiride [Can] *see* glimepiride *on page 445*
Novo-Glyburide [Can] *see* glyburide *on page 448*
Novo-Hydrazide [Can] *see* hydrochlorothiazide *on page 479*
Novo-Hydroxyzin [Can] *see* hydroxyzine *on page 491*
Novo-Hylazin [Can] *see* hydralazine *on page 478*
Novo-Indapamide [Can] *see* indapamide *on page 505*
Novo-Ipramide [Can] *see* ipratropium *on page 524*
Novo-Keto [Can] *see* ketoprofen *on page 537*
Novo-Ketoconazole [Can] *see* ketoconazole *on page 537*
Novo-Keto-EC [Can] *see* ketoprofen *on page 537*
Novo-Ketorolac [Can] *see* ketorolac *on page 538*
Novo-Ketotifen® [Can] *see* ketotifen *on page 538*
Novo-Lamotrigine [Can] *see* lamotrigine *on page 545*
Novo-Leflunomide [Can] *see* leflunomide *on page 551*
Novo-Levobunolol [Can] *see* levobunolol *on page 555*
Novo-Levocarbidopa [Can] *see* carbidopa and levodopa *on page 177*
Novo-Levofloxacin [Can] *see* levofloxacin *on page 557*
Novo-Lexin [Can] *see* cephalexin *on page 194*
Novolin® L Insulin *(Discontinued)*
Novolin® 70/30 [US] *see* insulin NPH and insulin regular *on page 512*
Novolin® ge 10/90 [Can] *see* insulin NPH and insulin regular *on page 512*
Novolin® ge 20/80 [Can] *see* insulin NPH and insulin regular *on page 512*
Novolin® ge 30/70 [Can] *see* insulin NPH and insulin regular *on page 512*
Novolin® ge 40/60 [Can] *see* insulin NPH and insulin regular *on page 512*
Novolin® ge 50/50 [Can] *see* insulin NPH and insulin regular *on page 512*
Novolin® ge NPH [Can] *see* insulin NPH *on page 512*
Novolin® ge Toronto [Can] *see* insulin regular *on page 513*
Novolin® N [US] *see* insulin NPH *on page 512*
Novolin® R [US] *see* insulin regular *on page 513*
Novo-Lisinopril [Can] *see* lisinopril *on page 570*
Novo-Lisinopril/Hctz [Can] *see* lisinopril and hydrochlorothiazide *on page 571*
NovoLog® [US] *see* insulin aspart *on page 509*
NovoLog® Mix 70/30 [US] *see* insulin aspart protamine and insulin aspart *on page 510*
Novo-Loperamide [Can] *see* loperamide *on page 573*
Novo-Lorazepam [Can] *see* lorazepam *on page 577*
Novo-Lovastatin [Can] *see* lovastatin *on page 579*
Novo-Maprotiline [Can] *see* maprotiline *on page 591*
Novo-Medrone [Can] *see* medroxyprogesterone *on page 597*
Novo-Meloxicam [Can] *see* meloxicam *on page 599*
Novo Meprazine [Can] *see* methotrimeprazine *(Canada only) on page 617*
Novo-Mepro [Can] *see* meprobamate *on page 605*
Novo-Metformin [Can] *see* metformin *on page 610*
Novo-Methacin [Can] *see* indomethacin *on page 506*
Novo-Metoprolol [Can] *see* metoprolol *on page 626*
Novo-Mexiletine [Can] *see* mexiletine *on page 629*
Novo-Minocycline [Can] *see* minocycline *on page 635*
Novo-Mirtazapine [Can] *see* mirtazapine *on page 637*
Novo-Misoprostol [Can] *see* misoprostol *on page 637*
NovoMix® 30 [Can] *see* insulin aspart protamine and insulin aspart *on page 510*

Novo-Moclobemide [Can] *see* moclobemide *(Canada only) on page 639*
Novo-Morphine SR [Can] *see* morphine sulfate *on page 643*
Novo-Nabumetone [Can] *see* nabumetone *on page 650*
Novo-Nadolol [Can] *see* nadolol *on page 651*
Novo-Naproc EC [Can] *see* naproxen *on page 656*
Novo-Naprox [Can] *see* naproxen *on page 656*
Novo-Naprox Sodium [Can] *see* naproxen *on page 656*
Novo-Naprox Sodium DS [Can] *see* naproxen *on page 656*
Novo-Naprox SR [Can] *see* naproxen *on page 656*
Novo-Nifedin [Can] *see* nifedipine *on page 672*
Novo-Nizatidine [Can] *see* nizatidine *on page 677*
Novo Nordisk® (all products) *(Discontinued)*
Novo-Norfloxacin [Can] *see* norfloxacin *on page 679*
Novo-Nortriptyline [Can] *see* nortriptyline *on page 680*
Novo-Ofloxacin [Can] *see* ofloxacin *on page 693*
Novo-Olanzapine [Can] *see* olanzapine *on page 694*
Novo-Ondansetron [Can] *see* ondansetron *on page 698*
Novo-Oxybutynin [Can] *see* oxybutynin *on page 708*
Novo-Paroxetine [Can] *see* paroxetine *on page 724*
Novo-Pen-VK [Can] *see* penicillin V potassium *on page 734*
Novo-Peridol [Can] *see* haloperidol *on page 465*
Novo-Pheniram [Can] *see* chlorpheniramine *on page 205*
Novo-Pindol [Can] *see* pindolol *on page 754*
Novo-Pioglitazone [Can] *see* pioglitazone *on page 754*
Novo-Pirocam [Can] *see* piroxicam *on page 757*
Novo-Pramine [Can] *see* imipramine *on page 501*
Novo-Pramipexole [Can] *see* pramipexole *on page 777*
Novo-Pranol [Can] *see* propranolol *on page 796*
Novo-Pravastatin [Can] *see* pravastatin *on page 779*
Novo-Prazin [Can] *see* prazosin *on page 780*
Novo-Prednisolone [Can] *see* prednisolone (systemic) *on page 781*
Novo-Prednisone [Can] *see* prednisone *on page 782*
Novo-Profen [Can] *see* ibuprofen *on page 495*
Novo-Propamide [Can] *see* chlorpropamide *on page 214*
Novo-Purol [Can] *see* allopurinol *on page 47*
Novo-Quinidin [Can] *see* quinidine *on page 813*
Novo-Quinine [Can] *see* quinine *on page 814*
Novo-Rabeprazole EC [Can] *see* rabeprazole *on page 815*
Novo-Ramipril [Can] *see* ramipril *on page 817*
Novo-Ranidine [Can] *see* ranitidine *on page 819*
NovoRapid® [Can] *see* insulin aspart *on page 509*
Novo-Risperidone [Can] *see* risperidone *on page 837*
Novo-Rythro Estolate [Can] *see* erythromycin *on page 354*
Novo-Rythro Ethylsuccinate [Can] *see* erythromycin *on page 354*
Novo-Selegiline [Can] *see* selegiline *on page 860*
Novo-Semide [Can] *see* furosemide *on page 430*
Novo-Sertraline [Can] *see* sertraline *on page 863*
NovoSeven *(Discontinued)* *see* factor VIIa (recombinant) *on page 387*
NovoSeven® RT [US] *see* factor VIIa (recombinant) *on page 387*
Novo-Simvastatin [Can] *see* simvastatin *on page 867*
Novo-Sorbide [Can] *see* isosorbide dinitrate *on page 530*
Novo-Sotalol [Can] *see* sotalol *on page 885*
Novo-Soxazole [Can] *see* sulfisoxazole *on page 896*

Novo-Spiroton [Can] *see* spironolactone *on page 886*
Novo-Spirozine [Can] *see* hydrochlorothiazide and spironolactone *on page 480*
Novo-Sucralate [Can] *see* sucralfate *on page 890*
Novo-Sumatriptan [Can] *see* sumatriptan *on page 898*
Novo-Sundac [Can] *see* sulindac *on page 898*
Novo-Tamoxifen [Can] *see* tamoxifen *on page 902*
Novo-Tamsulosin [Can] *see* tamsulosin *on page 903*
Novo-Temazepam [Can] *see* temazepam *on page 907*
Novo-Terazosin [Can] *see* terazosin *on page 909*
Novo-Theophyl SR [Can] *see* theophylline *on page 917*
Novo-Tiaprofenic [Can] *see* tiaprofenic acid *(Canada only) on page 925*
Novo-Ticlopidine [Can] *see* ticlopidine *on page 926*
Novo-Topiramate [Can] *see* topiramate *on page 935*
Novo-Trazodone [Can] *see* trazodone *on page 944*
Novo-Triamzide [Can] *see* hydrochlorothiazide and triamterene *on page 480*
Novo-Trifluzine [Can] *see* trifluoperazine *on page 951*
Novo-Trimel [Can] *see* sulfamethoxazole and trimethoprim *on page 894*
Novo-Trimel D.S. [Can] *see* sulfamethoxazole and trimethoprim *on page 894*
Novo-Triptyn [Can] *see* amitriptyline *on page 62*
Novo-Venlafaxine XR [Can] *see* venlafaxine *on page 973*
Novo-Veramil SR [Can] *see* verapamil *on page 974*
Novo-Warfarin [Can] *see* warfarin *on page 986*
Novoxapram® [Can] *see* oxazepam *on page 706*
Novo-Zopiclone [Can] *see* zopiclone *(Canada only) on page 997*
Noxafil® [US] *see* posaconazole *on page 769*
Nozinan® [Can] *see* methotrimeprazine *(Canada only) on page 617*
NP-27® *(Discontinued)* *see* tolnaftate *on page 934*
NPH Iletin® II *(Discontinued)*
NPH Iletin® Insulin *(Discontinued)*
NPH insulin *see* insulin NPH *on page 512*
NPH insulin and regular insulin *see* insulin NPH and insulin regular *on page 512*
Nplate™ [US] *see* romiplostim *on page 843*
NRP104 *see* lisdexamfetamine *on page 570*
NRS® [US-OTC] *see* oxymetazoline *on page 712*
NSC-740 *see* methotrexate *on page 615*
NSC-750 *see* busulfan *on page 154*
NSC-752 *see* thioguanine *on page 921*
NSC-755 *see* mercaptopurine *on page 606*
NSC-762 *see* mechlorethamine *on page 595*
NSC-3053 *see* dactinomycin *on page 264*
NSC-3088 *see* chlorambucil *on page 200*
NSC-8806 *see* melphalan *on page 599*
NSC-13875 *see* altretamine *on page 53*
NSC-26271 *see* cyclophosphamide *on page 256*
NSC-26980 *see* mitomycin *on page 638*
NSC-27640 *see* floxuridine *on page 404*
NSC-38721 *see* mitotane *on page 638*
NSC-49842 *see* vinblastine *on page 977*
NSC-63878 *see* cytarabine *on page 261*
NSC-66847 *see* thalidomide *on page 917*
NSC-67574 *see* vincristine *on page 978*
NSC-71423 *see* megestrol *on page 598*
NSC-77213 *see* procarbazine *on page 788*

NSC-710428 *see* ixabepilone *on page 534*
NSC-712227 *see* doxorubicin (liposomal) *on page 323*
NSC-712807 *see* capecitabine *on page 170*
NSC-714371 *see* dalteparin *on page 264*
NSC-714692 *see* cetuximab *on page 197*
NSC-714744 *see* denileukin diftitox *on page 272*
NSC-715055 *see* gefitinib *on page 437*
NSC-715969 *see* alemtuzumab *on page 43*
NSC-716051 *see* imatinib *on page 499*
NSC-718781 *see* erlotinib *on page 353*
NSC-719344 *see* anastrozole *on page 76*
NSC-719345 *see* letrozole *on page 552*
NSC-720568 *see* gemtuzumab ozogamicin *on page 439*
NSC-721517 *see* zoledronic acid *on page 995*
NSC-721631 *see* rasburicase *on page 821*
NSC-722623 *see* ibandronate *on page 494*
NSC-722848 *see* oprelvekin *on page 701*
NSC-724223 *see* epoetin alfa *on page 347*
NSC-724577 *see* anagrelide *on page 75*
NSC-724772 *see* sorafenib *on page 884*
NSC-725961 *see* pegfilgrastim *on page 727*
NSC-727989 *see* lapatinib *on page 550*
NSC-728729 *see* infliximab *on page 507*
NSC-729969 *see* darbepoetin alfa *on page 267*
NSC-732517 *see* dasatinib *on page 268*
NSC-736511 *see* sunitinib *on page 899*
NSC-736631 *see* paclitaxel (protein bound) *on page 715*
NSC-742319 *see* panitumumab *on page 719*
NTG *see* nitroglycerin *on page 675*
NTZ *see* nitazoxanide *on page 673*
NTZ® Long Acting Nasal Solution *(Discontinued) see* oxymetazoline *on page 712*
Nu-Acebutolol [Can] *see* acebutolol *on page 19*
Nu-Acyclovir [Can] *see* acyclovir *on page 33*
Nu-Alprax [Can] *see* alprazolam *on page 49*
Nu-Amilzide [Can] *see* amiloride and hydrochlorothiazide *on page 59*
Nu-Amoxi [Can] *see* amoxicillin *on page 67*
Nu-Ampi [Can] *see* ampicillin *on page 72*
Nu-Atenol [Can] *see* atenolol *on page 101*
Nu-Baclo [Can] *see* baclofen *on page 115*
Nubain® [US] *see* nalbuphine *on page 653*
Nu-Beclomethasone [Can] *see* beclomethasone *on page 119*
Nu-Bromazepam [Can] *see* bromazepam *(Canada only) on page 142*
Nu-Buspirone [Can] *see* buspirone *on page 153*
Nu-Capto [Can] *see* captopril *on page 171*
Nu-Carbamazepine [Can] *see* carbamazepine *on page 172*
Nu-Cefaclor [Can] *see* cefaclor *on page 183*
Nu-Cephalex [Can] *see* cephalexin *on page 194*
Nu-Cimet [Can] *see* cimetidine *on page 219*
Nu-Clonazepam [Can] *see* clonazepam *on page 235*
Nu-Clonidine [Can] *see* clonidine *on page 236*
Nu-Cloxi [Can] *see* cloxacillin *(Canada only) on page 239*
Nucofed® Expectorant *(Discontinued) see* guaifenesin, pseudoephedrine, and codeine *on page 460*

Nucofed® Pediatric Expectorant *(Discontinued)* *see* guaifenesin, pseudoephedrine, and codeine *on page 460*

Nu-Cotrimox [Can] *see* sulfamethoxazole and trimethoprim *on page 894*

Nu-Cromolyn [Can] *see* cromolyn sodium *on page 251*

Nu-Cyclobenzaprine [Can] *see* cyclobenzaprine *on page 255*

Nu-Desipramine [Can] *see* desipramine *on page 274*

Nu-Diclo [Can] *see* diclofenac *on page 292*

Nu-Diclo-SR [Can] *see* diclofenac *on page 292*

Nu-Diflunisal [Can] *see* diflunisal *on page 296*

Nu-Diltiaz [Can] *see* diltiazem *on page 300*

Nu-Diltiaz-CD [Can] *see* diltiazem *on page 300*

Nu-Divalproex [Can] *see* valproic acid and derivatives *on page 967*

Nu-Domperidone [Can] *see* domperidone *(Canada only) on page 317*

Nu-Doxycycline [Can] *see* doxycycline *on page 323*

Nu-Erythromycin-S [Can] *see* erythromycin *on page 354*

Nu-Famotidine [Can] *see* famotidine *on page 390*

Nu-Fenofibrate [Can] *see* fenofibrate *on page 393*

Nu-Fluoxetine [Can] *see* fluoxetine *on page 413*

Nu-Flurprofen [Can] *see* flurbiprofen *on page 416*

Nu-Fluvoxamine [Can] *see* fluvoxamine *on page 420*

Nu-Furosemide [Can] *see* furosemide *on page 430*

Nu-Gabapentin [Can] *see* gabapentin *on page 431*

Nu-Gemfibrozil [Can] *see* gemfibrozil *on page 439*

Nu-Glyburide [Can] *see* glyburide *on page 448*

Nu-Hydral [Can] *see* hydralazine *on page 478*

Nu-Ibuprofen [Can] *see* ibuprofen *on page 495*

Nu-Indapamide [Can] *see* indapamide *on page 505*

Nu-Indo [Can] *see* indomethacin *on page 506*

Nu-Ipratropium [Can] *see* ipratropium *on page 524*

Nu-Iron® 150 [US-OTC] *see* polysaccharide-iron complex *on page 768*

Nu-Ketoprofen [Can] *see* ketoprofen *on page 537*

Nu-Ketoprofen-E [Can] *see* ketoprofen *on page 537*

Nu-Ketotifen® [Can] *see* ketotifen *on page 538*

NuLev™ *(Discontinued)* *see* hyoscyamine *on page 492*

Nu-Levocarb [Can] *see* carbidopa and levodopa *on page 177*

Nullo® [US-OTC] *see* chlorophyll *on page 203*

Nu-Loraz [Can] *see* lorazepam *on page 577*

Nu-Lovastatin [Can] *see* lovastatin *on page 579*

Nu-Loxapine [Can] *see* loxapine *on page 580*

NuLYTELY® [US] *see* polyethylene glycol-electrolyte solution *on page 766*

Nu-Medopa [Can] *see* methyldopa *on page 620*

Nu-Mefenamic [Can] *see* mefenamic acid *on page 598*

Nu-Megestrol [Can] *see* megestrol *on page 598*

Nu-Metformin [Can] *see* metformin *on page 610*

Nu-Metoclopramide [Can] *see* metoclopramide *on page 625*

Nu-Metop [Can] *see* metoprolol *on page 626*

Nu-Moclobemide [Can] *see* moclobemide *(Canada only) on page 639*

Numoisyn™ [US] *see* saliva substitute *on page 853*

Numorphan® *(Discontinued)* *see* oxymorphone *on page 713*

Numzident® *(Discontinued)* *see* benzocaine *on page 124*

Nu-Naprox [Can] *see* naproxen *on page 656*

Nu-Nifed [Can] *see* nifedipine *on page 672*

Nu-Nizatidine [Can] *see* nizatidine *on page 677*

Nu-Nortriptyline [Can] *see* nortriptyline *on page 680*
Nu-Oxybutyn [Can] *see* oxybutynin *on page 708*
Nu-Pentoxifylline SR [Can] *see* pentoxifylline *on page 737*
Nu-Pen-VK [Can] *see* penicillin V potassium *on page 734*
Nupercainal® [US-OTC] *see* dibucaine *on page 291*
Nupercainal® Hydrocortisone Cream [US-OTC] *see* hydrocortisone (rectal) *on page 484*
Nu-Pindol [Can] *see* pindolol *on page 754*
Nu-Pirox [Can] *see* piroxicam *on page 757*
Nu-Prazo [Can] *see* prazosin *on page 780*
Nuprin® *(Discontinued)* *see* ibuprofen *on page 495*
Nu-Prochlor [Can] *see* prochlorperazine *on page 788*
Nu-Propranolol [Can] *see* propranolol *on page 796*
Nuquin HP® [US] *see* hydroquinone *on page 488*
Nu-Ranit [Can] *see* ranitidine *on page 819*
Nuromax® *(Discontinued)*
Nu-Selegiline [Can] *see* selegiline *on page 860*
Nu-Sertraline [Can] *see* sertraline *on page 863*
Nu-Simvastatin [Can] *see* simvastatin *on page 867*
Nu-Sotalol [Can] *see* sotalol *on page 885*
Nu-Sucralate [Can] *see* sucralfate *on page 890*
Nu-Sundac [Can] *see* sulindac *on page 898*
Nu-Tears® [US-OTC] *see* artificial tears *on page 95*
Nu-Tears® II [US-OTC] *see* artificial tears *on page 95*
Nu-Temazepam [Can] *see* temazepam *on page 907*
Nu-Terazosin [Can] *see* terazosin *on page 909*
Nu-Tetra [Can] *see* tetracycline *on page 915*
Nu-Tiaprofenic [Can] *see* tiaprofenic acid *(Canada only) on page 925*
Nu-Ticlopidine [Can] *see* ticlopidine *on page 926*
Nu-Timolol [Can] *see* timolol *on page 927*
Nutracort® [US] *see* hydrocortisone (topical) *on page 485*
Nutralox® [US-OTC] *see* calcium carbonate *on page 163*
Nutraplus® [US-OTC] *see* urea *on page 963*
Nu-Trazodone [Can] *see* trazodone *on page 944*
Nu-Triazide [Can] *see* hydrochlorothiazide and triamterene *on page 480*
Nu-Trimipramine [Can] *see* trimipramine *on page 954*
NutriNate® [US] *see* vitamins (multiple/prenatal) *on page 983*
NutriSpire™ [US] *see* vitamins (multiple/prenatal) *on page 983*

nutritional formula, enteral/oral (noo TRISH un al FOR myoo la, EN ter al/OR al)

Synonyms dietary supplements

U.S./Canadian Brand Names Carnation Instant Breakfast® [US-OTC]; Citrotein® [US-OTC]; Criticare HN® [US-OTC]; Ensure Plus® [US-OTC]; Ensure® [US-OTC]; Isocal® [US-OTC]; Magnacal® [US-OTC]; Microlipid™ [US-OTC]; Osmolite® HN [US-OTC]; Pedialyte® [US-OTC]; Portagen® [US-OTC]; Pregestimil® [US-OTC]; Propac™ [US-OTC]; Soyalac® [US-OTC]; Vital HN® [US-OTC]; Vitaneed™ [US-OTC]; Vivonex® T.E.N. [US-OTC]; Vivonex® [US-OTC]

Therapeutic Category Nutritional Supplement

Dosage Forms
Liquid: Calcium and sodium caseinate, maltodextrin, sucrose, partially hydrogenated soy oil, soy lecithin
Powder: Amino acids, predigested carbohydrates, safflower oil

Nutropin® [US] *see* somatropin *on page 881*
Nutropin AQ® [US/Can] *see* somatropin *on page 881*
Nutropine® [Can] *see* somatropin *on page 881*
NuvaRing® [US/Can] *see* ethinyl estradiol and etonogestrel *on page 372*
Nu-Verap [Can] *see* verapamil *on page 974*

Nuvigil™ [US] *see* armodafinil *on page 94*
Nu-Zopiclone [Can] *see* zopiclone *(Canada only) on page 997*
NVP *see* nevirapine *on page 666*
Nyaderm [Can] *see* nystatin *on page 690*
Nyamyc™ [US] *see* nystatin *on page 690*
Nydrazid® *(Discontinued)* *see* isoniazid *on page 528*

nystatin (nye STAT in)

Sound-Alike/Look-Alike Issues
nystatin may be confused with Nilstat®, Nitrostat®
Nilstat® may be confused with Nitrostat®, nystatin
U.S./Canadian Brand Names Bio-Statin® [US]; Candistatin® [Can]; Mycostatin® [US]; Nilstat [Can]; Nyaderm [Can]; Nyamyc™ [US]; Nystat-Rx® [US]; Nystop® [US]; Paddock Nystatin™ [US]; Pedi-Dri® [US]; PMS-Nystatin [Can]
Therapeutic Category Antifungal Agent
Use Treatment of susceptible cutaneous, mucocutaneous, and oral cavity fungal infections normally caused by the *Candida* species
Usual Dosage
Oral candidiasis:
Suspension (swish and swallow orally):
Premature infants: 100,000 units 4 times/day
Infants: 200,000 units 4 times/day or 100,000 units to each side of mouth 4 times/day
Children and Adults: 400,000-600,000 units 4 times/day
Powder for compounding: Children and Adults: 1/8 teaspoon (500,000 units) to equal approximately 1/2 cup of water; give 4 times/day
Mucocutaneous infections: Children and Adults: Topical: Apply 2-3 times/day to affected areas; very moist topical lesions are treated best with powder
Intestinal infections: Adults: Oral: 500,000-1,000,000 units every 8 hours
Vaginal infections: Adults: Vaginal tablets: Insert 1 tablet/day at bedtime for 2 weeks
Dosage Forms
Capsule:
Bio-Statin®: 500,000 units, 1 million units
Cream: 100,000 units/g (15 g, 30 g)
Mycostatin®: 100,000 units/g (30 g)
Ointment, topical: 100,000 units/g (15 g, 30 g)
Powder, for prescription compounding: 50 million units (10 g); 150 million units (30 g); 500 million units (100 g); 2 billion units (400 g)
Nystat-Rx®: 50 million units (10 g); 150 million units (30 g); 500 million units (100 g); 1 billion units (190 g); 2 billion units (350 g)
Powder, for prescription compounding: 1 billion units (190 g); 150 million units (30 g); 2 billion units (350 g); 50 million units (10 g); 500 million units (100 g)
Bio-Statin®: 2 billion units (30 g)
Powder for suspension, oral [preservative free]:
Paddock Nystatin™: 150 million units (30 g); 2 billion units (400 g); 50 million units (10 g); 500 million units (100 g) [sugar free]
Powder, topical: 100,000 units/g (15 g, 30 g, 60 g)
Nyamyc™: 100,000 units/g (15 g, 30 g)
Nystop®: 100,000 units/g (15 g, 30 g, 60 g)
Pedi-Dri®: 100,000 units/g (56.7 g)
Suspension, oral: 100,000 units/mL
Tablet: 500,000 units
Tablet, vaginal: 100,000 units (15s)

nystatin and triamcinolone (nye STAT in & trye am SIN oh lone)

Sound-Alike/Look-Alike Issues
Mycolog®-II may be confused with Halog®
Synonyms triamcinolone and nystatin
Therapeutic Category Antifungal/Corticosteroid

Use Treatment of cutaneous candidiasis

Usual Dosage Topical: Children and Adults: Apply sparingly 2-4 times/day. Therapy should be discontinued when control is achieved; if no improvement is seen, reassessment of diagnosis may be necessary.

Dosage Forms

Cream: Nystatin 100,000 units and triamcinolone 0.1% (15 g, 30 g, 60 g)

Ointment: Nystatin 100,000 units and triamcinolone 0.1% (15 g, 30 g, 60 g)

Nystat-Rx® [US] *see* nystatin *on page 690*

Nystex® (Discontinued) *see* nystatin *on page 690*

Nystop® [US] *see* nystatin *on page 690*

Nytol® [Can] *see* diphenhydramine *on page 304*

Nytol® Extra Strength [Can] *see* diphenhydramine *on page 304*

Nytol® Quick Caps [US-OTC] *see* diphenhydramine *on page 304*

Nytol® Quick Gels [US-OTC] *see* diphenhydramine *on page 304*

NāSal™ [US-OTC] *see* sodium chloride *on page 873*

Nāsop™ (Discontinued) *see* phenylephrine *on page 745*

Nōstrilla® [US-OTC] *see* oxymetazoline *on page 712*

O-V Staticin® (Discontinued) *see* nystatin *on page 690*

Oasis® [US] *see* saliva substitute *on page 853*

Obezine® (Discontinued) *see* phendimetrazine *on page 742*

OCBZ *see* oxcarbazepine *on page 706*

Occlusal®-HP [US-OTC/Can] *see* salicylic acid *on page 850*

Ocean® [US-OTC] *see* sodium chloride *on page 873*

Ocean® for Kids [US-OTC] *see* sodium chloride *on page 873*

OCL® (Discontinued) *see* polyethylene glycol-electrolyte solution *on page 766*

Octagam® [US] *see* immune globulin (intravenous) *on page 503*

Octamide® (Discontinued) *see* metoclopramide *on page 625*

Octaplex® [Can] *see* prothrombin complex (human) [(factors II, VII, IX, X), protein C, and protein S] *(Canada only) on page 800*

Octicair® Otic (Discontinued) *see* neomycin, polymyxin B, and hydrocortisone *on page 663*

Octocaine® (Discontinued) *see* lidocaine and epinephrine *on page 563*

Octostim® [Can] *see* desmopressin acetate *on page 275*

octreotide (ok TREE oh tide)

Sound-Alike/Look-Alike Issues

Sandostatin® may be confused with Sandimmune®

Synonyms NSC-671663; octreotide acetate

U.S./Canadian Brand Names Octreotide Acetate Injection [Can]; Octreotide Acetate Omega [Can]; Sandostatin LAR® [US/Can]; Sandostatin® [US/Can]

Therapeutic Category Somatostatin Analog

Use Control of symptoms in patients with metastatic carcinoid and vasoactive intestinal peptide-secreting tumors (VIPomas); acromegaly

Usual Dosage

Carcinoid tumors: Adults:

SubQ, I.V.: Initial 2 weeks: 100-600 mcg/day in 2-4 divided doses; usual range 50-750 mcg/day (some patients may require up to 1500 mcg/day)

I.M. depot injection: Patients must be stabilized on subcutaneous octreotide for at least 2 weeks before switching to the long-acting depot. Upon switch: 20 mg I.M. intragluteally every 4 weeks for 2 months, then the dose may be modified based upon response.

Note: Patients should continue to receive their SubQ injections for the first 2 weeks at the same dose in order to maintain therapeutic levels (some patients may require 3-4 weeks of continued SubQ injections). Patients who experience periodic exacerbations of symptoms may require temporary SubQ injections in addition to depot injections (at their previous SubQ dosing regimen) until symptoms have resolved.

Dosage adjustment: See dosing adjustment for VIPomas.

VIPomas: Adults:

SubQ, I.V.: Initial 2 weeks: 200-300 mcg/day in 2-4 divided doses; titrate dose based on response/tolerance. Range: 150-750 mcg/day (doses >450 mcg/day are rarely required)

I.M. depot injection: Patients must be stabilized on subcutaneous octreotide for at least 2 weeks before switching to the long-acting depot. Upon switch: 20 mg I.M. intragluteally every 4 weeks for 2 months, then the dose may be modified based upon response.

Note: Patients receiving depot injection should continue to receive their SubQ injections for the first 2 weeks at the same dose in order to maintain therapeutic levels (some patients may require 3-4 weeks of continued SubQ injections). Patients who experience periodic exacerbations of symptoms may require temporary SubQ injections in addition to depot injections (at their previous SubQ dosing regimen) until symptoms have resolved.

Dosage adjustment for carcinoid tumors and VIPomas: After 2 months of depot injections, the dosage may be continued or modified as follows:

Increase to 30 mg I.M. every 4 weeks if symptoms are inadequately controlled

Decrease to 10 mg I.M. every 4 weeks, for a trial period, if initially responsive to 20 mg dose

Dosage >30 mg is not recommended

Acromegaly: Adults:

SubQ, I.V.: Initial: 50 mcg 3 times/day; titrate to achieve growth hormone levels <5 ng/mL or IGF-I (somatomedin C) levels <1.9 units/mL in males and <2.2 units/mL in females. Usual effective dose 100-200 mcg 3 times/day; range 300-1500 mcg/day. **Note:** Should be withdrawn yearly for a 4-week interval (8 weeks for depot injection) in patients who have received irradiation. Resume if levels increase and signs/symptoms recur.

I.M. depot injection: Patients must be stabilized on subcutaneous octreotide for at least 2 weeks before switching to the long-acting depot. Upon switch: 20 mg I.M. intragluteally every 4 weeks for 3 months, then the dose may be modified based upon response.

Dosage adjustment for acromegaly: After 3 months of depot injections, the dosage may be continued or modified as follows:

GH ≤1 ng/mL, IGF-1 normal, and symptoms controlled: Reduce octreotide LAR® to 10 mg I.M. every 4 weeks

GH ≤2.5 ng/mL, IGF-1 normal, and symptoms controlled: Maintain octreotide LAR® at 20 mg I.M. every 4 weeks

GH >2.5 ng/mL, IGF-1 elevated, and/or symptoms uncontrolled: Increase octreotide LAR® to 30 mg I.M. every 4 weeks

Note: Patients not adequately controlled at a dose of 30 mg may increase dose to 40 mg every 4 weeks. Dosages >40 mg are not recommended.

Dosage Forms

Injection, microspheres for suspension [depot formulation]:
Sandostatin LAR®: 10 mg, 20 mg, 30 mg

Injection, solution: 0.2 mg/mL (5 mL); 1 mg/mL (5 mL)
Sandostatin®: 0.2 mg/mL (5 mL); 1 mg/mL (5 mL)

Injection, solution [preservative free]: 0.05 mg/mL (1 mL); 0.1 mg/mL (1 mL); 0.5 mg/mL (1 mL)
Sandostatin®: 0.05 mg/mL (1 mL); 0.1 mg/mL (1 mL); 0.5 mg/mL (1 mL)

octreotide acetate *see* octreotide *on page 691*

Octreotide Acetate Injection [Can] *see* octreotide *on page 691*

Octreotide Acetate Omega [Can] *see* octreotide *on page 691*

OcuClear® *(Discontinued)* *see* oxymetazoline *on page 712*

OcuCoat® [US-OTC] *see* artificial tears *on page 95*

OcuCoat® PF [US-OTC] *see* artificial tears *on page 95*

Ocufen® [US/Can] *see* flurbiprofen *on page 416*

Ocuflox® [US/Can] *see* ofloxacin *on page 693*

OcuNefrin™ [US-OTC] *see* phenylephrine *on page 745*

Ocupress® *(Discontinued)* *see* carteolol *on page 181*

Ocupress® Ophthalmic [Can] *see* carteolol *on page 181*

Ocusert Pilo-20® *(Discontinued)* *see* pilocarpine *on page 753*

Ocusert Pilo-40® *(Discontinued)* *see* pilocarpine *on page 753*

Ocu-Sul® *(Discontinued)* *see* sulfacetamide *on page 892*

Ocutricin® Topical Ointment *(Discontinued)* *see* bacitracin, neomycin, and polymyxin B *on page 114*

Ocuvite® [US-OTC] *see* vitamins (multiple/oral) *on page 983*

Ocuvite® Adult [US-OTC] *see* vitamins (multiple/oral) *on page 983*
Ocuvite® Adult 50+ [US-OTC] *see* vitamins (multiple/oral) *on page 983*
Ocuvite® Extra® [US-OTC] *see* vitamins (multiple/oral) *on page 983*
Ocuvite® Lutein [US-OTC] *see* vitamins (multiple/oral) *on page 983*
O-desmethylvenlafaxine *see* desvenlafaxine *on page 277*
ODV *see* desvenlafaxine *on page 277*
Oesclim® [Can] *see* estradiol *on page 359*

ofloxacin (oh FLOKS a sin)

Sound-Alike/Look-Alike Issues
Floxin® may be confused with Flexeril®
Ocuflox® may be confused with Occlusal®-HP, Ocufen®

U.S./Canadian Brand Names Apo-Ofloxacin® [Can]; Apo-Oflox® [Can]; Floxin® [US/Can]; Novo-Ofloxacin [Can]; Ocuflox® [US/Can]; PMS-Ofloxacin [Can]

Therapeutic Category Antibiotic, Ophthalmic; Antibiotic, Otic; Quinolone

Use Quinolone antibiotic for the treatment of acute exacerbations of chronic bronchitis, community-acquired pneumonia, skin and skin structure infections (uncomplicated), urethral and cervical gonorrhea (acute, uncomplicated), urethritis and cervicitis (nongonococcal), mixed infections of the urethra and cervix, pelvic inflammatory disease (acute), cystitis (uncomplicated), urinary tract infections (complicated), prostatitis

Note: As of April 2007, the CDC no longer recommends the use of fluoroquinolones for the treatment of gonococcal disease.

Ophthalmic: Treatment of superficial ocular infections involving the conjunctiva or cornea due to strains of susceptible organisms

Otic: Otitis externa, chronic suppurative otitis media, acute otitis media

Usual Dosage

Usual dosage range:
Children ≥6 months: Otic: 5 drops daily
Children >1 year: Ophthalmic: 1-2 drops every 30 minutes to 4 hours initially, decreasing to every 4-6 hours
Children >12 years: Otic: 10 drops once or twice daily
Adults:
Ophthalmic: 1-2 drops every 30 minutes to 4 hours initially, decreasing to every 4-6 hours
Oral: 200-400 mg every 12 hours
Otic: 10 drops once or twice daily

Indication-specific dosing:
Children 6 months to 13 years: Otic: **Otitis externa:** Instill 5 drops (or the contents of 1 single-dose container) into affected ear(s) once daily for 7 days
Children 1-12 years: Otic: **Acute otitis media with tympanostomy tubes:** Instill 5 drops (or the contents of 1 single-dose container) into affected ear(s) twice daily for 10 days
Children >1 year and Adults: Ophthalmic:
Conjunctivitis: Instill 1-2 drops in affected eye(s) every 2-4 hours for the first 2 days, then use 4 times/day for an additional 5 days
Corneal ulcer: Instill 1-2 drops every 30 minutes while awake and every 4-6 hours after retiring for the first 2 days; beginning on day 3, instill 1-2 drops every hour while awake for 4-6 additional days; thereafter, 1-2 drops 4 times/day until clinical cure.
Children >12 years and Adults: Otic: **Otitis media, chronic suppurative with perforated tympanic membranes:** Instill 10 drops (or the contents of 2 single-dose containers) into affected ear twice daily for 14 days
Children ≥13 years and Adults: Otic: **Otitis externa:** Instill 10 drops (or the contents of 2 single-dose containers) into affected ear(s) once daily for 7 days
Adults: Oral:
Cervicitis/urethritis:
Nongonococcal: 300 mg every 12 hours for 7 days
Gonococcal (acute, uncomplicated): 400 mg as a single dose; **Note:** As of April 2007, the CDC no longer recommends the use of fluoroquinolones for the treatment of uncomplicated gonococcal disease.
Chronic bronchitis (acute exacerbation), community-acquired pneumonia, skin and skin structure infections (uncomplicated): 400 mg every 12 hours for 10 days

◀

Pelvic inflammatory disease (acute): 400 mg every 12 hours for 10-14 days with or without metronidazole; **Note:** The CDC recommends use only if standard cephalosporin therapy is not feasible and community prevalence of quinolone-resistant gonococcal organisms is low. Culture sensitivity must be confirmed.

Prostatitis:
Acute: 400 mg for 1 dose, then 300 mg twice daily for 10 days
Chronic: 200 mg every 12 hours for 6 weeks
UTI:
Uncomplicated: 200 mg every 12 hours for 3-7 days
Complicated: 200 mg every 12 hours for 10 days

Dosage Forms
Solution, ophthalmic [drops]: 0.3% (5 mL, 10 mL)
Ocuflox®: 0.3% (5 mL)
Solution, otic [drops]: 0.3% (5 mL, 10 mL)
Floxin®: 0.3% (5 mL, 10 mL)
Floxin® Otic Singles™: 0.3% (0.25 mL)
Tablet: 200 mg, 300 mg, 400 mg

Ogen® [US/Can] *see* estropipate *on page 366*

Ogestrel® [US] *see* ethinyl estradiol and norgestrel *on page 380*

OGMT *see* metyrosine *on page 629*

OGT-918 *see* miglustat *on page 634*

9-OH-risperidone *see* paliperidone *on page 715*

OKT3 *see* muromonab-CD3 *on page 648*

olanzapine (oh LAN za peen)

Sound-Alike/Look-Alike Issues
OLANZapine may be confused with olsalazine, QUEtiapine
Zyprexa® may be confused with Celexa™, Zyrtec®
Synonyms LY170053
Tall-Man OLANZapine
U.S./Canadian Brand Names Novo-Olanzapine [Can]; Zyprexa® Zydis® [US/Can]; Zyprexa® [US/Can]
Therapeutic Category Antipsychotic Agent
Use Treatment of the manifestations of schizophrenia; treatment of acute or mixed mania episodes associated with Bipolar I Disorder (as monotherapy or in combination with lithium or valproate); maintenance treatment of bipolar disorder; acute agitation (patients with schizophrenia or bipolar mania)
Usual Dosage Adults:
Schizophrenia: Oral: Initial: 5-10 mg once daily (increase to 10 mg once daily within 5-7 days); thereafter, adjust by 5 mg/day at 1-week intervals, up to a recommended maximum of 20 mg/day. Maintenance: 10-20 mg once daily. **Note:** Doses of 30-50 mg/day have been used; however, doses >10 mg/day have not demonstrated better efficacy, and safety and efficacy of doses >20 mg/day have not been evaluated.
Bipolar I acute mixed or manic episodes: Oral:
Monotherapy: Initial: 10-15 mg once daily; increase by 5 mg/day at intervals of not less than 24 hours. Maintenance: 5-20 mg/day; recommended maximum dose: 20 mg/day.
Combination therapy (with lithium or valproate): Initial: 10 mg once daily; dosing range: 5-20 mg/day
Agitation (acute, associated with bipolar I mania or schizophrenia): I.M.: Initial dose: 5-10 mg (a lower dose of 2.5 mg may be considered when clinical factors warrant); additional doses (2.5-10 mg) may be considered; however, 2-4 hours should be allowed between doses to evaluate response (maximum total daily dose: 30 mg, per manufacturer's recommendation)
Dosage Forms
Injection, powder for reconstitution:
Zyprexa® IntraMuscular: 10 mg
Tablet:
Zyprexa®: 2.5 mg, 5 mg, 7.5 mg, 10 mg, 15 mg, 20 mg
Tablet, orally disintegrating:
Zyprexa® Zydis®: 5 mg, 10 mg, 15 mg, 20 mg

olanzapine and fluoxetine (oh LAN za peen & floo OKS e teen)

Synonyms fluoxetine and olanzapine; olanzapine and fluoxetine hydrochloride
U.S./Canadian Brand Names Symbyax® [US]

Therapeutic Category Antidepressant, Selective Serotonin Reuptake Inhibitor; Antipsychotic Agent, Thienobenzodiaepine

Use Treatment of depressive episodes associated with bipolar disorder

Usual Dosage Oral: Adults: Depression associated with bipolar disorder: Initial: Olanzapine 3-6 mg/ fluoxetine 25 mg once daily in the evening. Dosing range: Olanzapine 6-12 mg/fluoxetine 25-50 mg. Lower doses (olanzapine 3 mg/fluoxetine 25 mg) should be used in patients predisposed to hypotension, in hepatic impairment, with combined factors for reduced metabolism (females, the elderly, nonsmokers), or enhanced sensitivity to olanzapine; use caution in dose adjustments in these patients. Safety of daily doses of olanzapine >18 mg/fluoxetine >75 mg have not been evaluated.

Dosage Forms
Capsule:
Symbyax®:
3/25: Olanzapine 3 mg and fluoxetine 25 mg
6/25: Olanzapine 6 mg and fluoxetine 25 mg
6/50: Olanzapine 6 mg and fluoxetine 50 mg
12/25: Olanzapine 12 mg and fluoxetine 25 mg
12/50: Olanzapine 12 mg and fluoxetine 50 mg

olanzapine and fluoxetine hydrochloride *see* olanzapine and fluoxetine *on page 694*

Olay® Vitamins Complete Women's [US-OTC] *see* vitamins (multiple/oral) *on page 983*

Olay® Vitamins Complete Women's 50+ [US-OTC] *see* vitamins (multiple/oral) *on page 983*

oleovitamin A *see* vitamin A *on page 979*

oleum ricini *see* castor oil *on page 183*

olmesartan (ole me SAR tan)

Synonyms olmesartan medoxomil
U.S./Canadian Brand Names Benicar® [US]
Therapeutic Category Angiotensin II Receptor Antagonist
Use Treatment of hypertension with or without concurrent use of other antihypertensive agents
Usual Dosage Oral: Adults: Initial: Usual starting dose is 20 mg once daily; if initial response is inadequate, may be increased to 40 mg once daily after 2 weeks. May administer with other antihypertensive agents if blood pressure inadequately controlled with olmesartan. Consider lower starting dose in patients with possible depletion of intravascular volume (eg, patients receiving diuretics).
Dosage Forms
Tablet:
Benicar®: 5 mg, 20 mg, 40 mg

olmesartan and amlodipine *see* amlodipine and olmesartan *on page 65*

olmesartan and hydrochlorothiazide (ole me SAR tan & hye droe klor oh THYE a zide)

Synonyms hydrochlorothiazide and olmesartan medoxomil; olmesartan medoxomil and hydrochlorothiazide
U.S./Canadian Brand Names Benicar HCT® [US]
Therapeutic Category Angiotensin II Receptor Antagonist; Diuretic, Thiazide
Use Treatment of hypertension (not recommended for initial treatment)
Usual Dosage Oral: Adults: One tablet daily; dosage must be individualized (see below). May be titrated at 2- to 4-week intervals.
Replacement therapy: May be substituted for previously titrated dosages of the individual components.
Patients not controlled with single-agent therapy: Initiate by adding the lowest available dose of the alternative component (hydrochlorothiazide 12.5 mg or olmesartan 20 mg). Titrate to effect (maximum daily hydrochlorothiazide dose: 25 mg; maximum daily olmesartan dose: 40 mg).
Dosage Forms
Tablet:
Benicar HCT®: 20/12.5: Olmesartan 20 mg and hydrochlorothiazide 12.5 mg; 40/12.5: Olmesartan 40 mg and hydrochlorothiazide 12.5 mg; 40/25: Olmesartan 40 mg and hydrochlorothiazide 25 mg

olmesartan medoxomil *see* olmesartan *on page 695*

olmesartan medoxomil and hydrochlorothiazide *see* olmesartan and hydrochlorothiazide *on page 695*

olopatadine (oh la PAT a deen)

Sound-Alike/Look-Alike Issues
Patanol® may be confused with Platinol®
Synonyms olopatadine hydrochloride
U.S./Canadian Brand Names Pataday™ [US]; Patanase® [US]; Patanol® [US/Can]
Therapeutic Category Antihistamine
Use
Nasal spray: Treatment of the symptoms of seasonal allergic rhinitis
Ophthalmic: Treatment of the signs and symptoms of allergic conjunctivitis
Usual Dosage
Intranasal (Patanase®): Children ≥12 years and Adults: 2 sprays into each nostril twice daily
Ophthalmic: Children ≥3 years and Adults:
Patanol®: Instill 1 drop into affected eye(s) twice daily (allowing 6-8 hours between doses); results from an environmental study demonstrated that olopatadine was effective when dosed twice daily for up to 6 weeks
Pataday™: Instill 1 drop into affected eye(s) once daily
Dosage Forms
Solution, intranasal [spray]:
Patanase®: 0.6% (30.5 g)
Solution, ophthalmic:
Patanol®: 0.1% (5 mL)
Pataday™: 0.2% (2.5 mL)

olopatadine hydrochloride *see olopatadine on page 696*

olsalazine (ole SAL a zeen)

Sound-Alike/Look-Alike Issues
olsalazine may be confused with OLANZapine
Dipentum® may be confused with Dilantin®
Synonyms olsalazine sodium
U.S./Canadian Brand Names Dipentum® [US/Can]
Therapeutic Category 5-Aminosalicylic Acid Derivative
Use Maintenance of remission of ulcerative colitis in patients intolerant to sulfasalazine
Usual Dosage Oral: Adults: 1 g/day in 2 divided doses
Dosage Forms
Capsule:
Dipentum®: 250 mg

olsalazine sodium *see olsalazine on page 696*
Olux® [US] *see clobetasol on page 232*
Olux-E™ [US] *see clobetasol on page 232*
Omacor® (Discontinued) *see omega-3-acid ethyl esters on page 697*

omalizumab (oh mah lye ZOO mab)

Synonyms rhuMAb-E25
U.S./Canadian Brand Names Xolair® [US/Can]
Therapeutic Category Monoclonal Antibody
Use Treatment of moderate-to-severe, persistent allergic asthma not adequately controlled with inhaled corticosteroids
Usual Dosage SubQ: Children ≥12 years and Adults: Asthma: Dose is based on pretreatment IgE serum levels and body weight. Dosing should not be adjusted based on IgE levels taken during treatment or <1 year following discontinuation of therapy; doses should be adjusted during treatment for significant changes in body weight
IgE ≥30-100 int. units/mL:
30-90 kg: 150 mg every 4 weeks
>90-150 kg: 300 mg every 4 weeks
IgE >100-200 int. units/mL:
30-90 kg: 300 mg every 4 weeks
>90-150 kg: 225 mg every 2 weeks

IgE >200-300 int. units/mL:
  30-60 kg: 300 mg every 4 weeks
  >60-90 kg: 225 mg every 2 weeks
  >90-150 kg: 300 mg every 2 weeks
IgE >300-400 int. units/mL:
  30-70 kg: 225 mg every 2 weeks
  >70-90 kg: 300 mg every 2 weeks
  >90 kg: Do not administer dose
IgE >400-500 int. units/mL:
  30-70 kg: 300 mg every 2 weeks
  >70-90 kg: 375 mg every 2 weeks
  >90 kg: Do not administer dose
IgE >500-600 int. units/mL:
  30-60 kg: 300 mg every 2 weeks
  >60-70 kg: 375 mg every 2 weeks
  >70 kg: Do not administer dose
IgE >600-700 int. units/mL:
  30-60 kg: 375 mg every 2 weeks
  >60 kg: Do not administer dose

Dosage Forms
Injection, powder for reconstitution [preservative free]:
  Xolair®: 150 mg

omega-3-acid ethyl esters (oh MEG a three AS id ETH il ES ters)

Sound-Alike/Look-Alike Issues
  Omacor® may be confused with Amicar®
Synonyms ethyl esters of omega-3 fatty acids; fish oil
U.S./Canadian Brand Names Lovaza® [US]
Therapeutic Category Antilipemic Agent, Miscellaneous
Use Lovaza®: Adjunct to diet therapy in the treatment of hypertriglyceridemia (≥500 mg/dL)
  Note: A number of OTC formulations containing omega-3 fatty acids are marketed as nutritional supplements; these do not have FDA-approved indications and may not contain the same amounts of the active ingredient.
Usual Dosage Oral: Adults: Hypertriglyceridemia: 4 g/day as a single daily dose or in 2 divided doses
Dosage Forms
Capsule:
  Lovaza®: 1 g

omeprazole (oh MEP ra zole)

Sound-Alike/Look-Alike Issues
  Prilosec® may be confused with Plendil®, Prevacid®, predniSONE, prilocaine, Prinivil®, Proventil®, Prozac®
U.S./Canadian Brand Names Apo-Omeprazole® [Can]; Losec MUPS® [Can]; Losec® [Can]; Prilosec OTC™ [US-OTC]; Prilosec® [US]; ratio-Omeprazole [Can]; Sandoz Omeprazole [Can]
Therapeutic Category Gastric Acid Secretion Inhibitor
Use Short-term (4-8 weeks) treatment of active duodenal ulcer disease or active benign gastric ulcer; treatment of heartburn and other symptoms associated with gastroesophageal reflux disease (GERD); short-term (4-8 weeks) treatment of endoscopically-diagnosed erosive esophagitis; maintenance healing of erosive esophagitis; long-term treatment of pathological hypersecretory conditions; as part of a multidrug regimen for *H. pylori* eradication to reduce the risk of duodenal ulcer recurrence

  OTC labeling: Short-term treatment of frequent, uncomplicated heartburn occurring ≥2 days/week
Usual Dosage Oral:
  Children ≥2 years: GERD or other acid-related disorders:
    <20 kg: 10 mg once daily
    ≥20 kg: 20 mg once daily
  Adults:
    Active duodenal ulcer: 20 mg/day for 4-8 weeks
    Gastric ulcers: 40 mg/day for 4-8 weeks
    Symptomatic GERD: 20 mg/day for up to 4 weeks

▶

◀ Erosive esophagitis: 20 mg/day for 4-8 weeks; maintenance of healing: 20 mg/day for up to 12 months total therapy (including treatment period of 4-8 weeks)

Helicobacter pylori eradication: Dose varies with regimen: 20 mg once daily **or** 40 mg/day as single dose or in 2 divided doses; requires combination therapy with antibiotics

Pathological hypersecretory conditions: Initial: 60 mg once daily; doses up to 120 mg 3 times/day have been administered; administer daily doses >80 mg in divided doses

Frequent heartburn (OTC labeling): 20 mg/day for 14 days; treatment may be repeated after 4 months if needed

Dosage Forms

Capsule, delayed release: 10 mg, 20 mg, 40 mg
 Prilosec®: 10 mg, 20 mg, 40 mg

Tablet, delayed release: 20 mg
 Prilosec OTC™ [OTC]: 20 mg

omeprazole and sodium bicarbonate (oh MEP ra zole & SOW dee um bye KAR bun ate)

U.S./Canadian Brand Names Zegerid® [US]

Therapeutic Category Proton Pump Inhibitor; Substituted Benzimidazole

Use Short-term (4-8 weeks) treatment of active duodenal ulcer disease or active benign gastric ulcer; treatment of heartburn and other symptoms associated with gastroesophageal reflux disease (GERD); short-term (4-8 weeks) treatment of endoscopically-diagnosed erosive esophagitis; maintenance healing of erosive esophagitis; reduction of risk of upper gastrointestinal bleeding in critically-ill patients

Usual Dosage Oral: Adults:

Active duodenal ulcer: 20 mg/day for 4-8 weeks

Gastric ulcers: 40 mg/day for 4-8 weeks

Symptomatic GERD: 20 mg/day for up to 4 weeks

Erosive esophagitis: 20 mg/day for 4-8 weeks; maintenance of healing: 20 mg/day for up to 12 months total therapy (including treatment period of 4-8 weeks)

Risk reduction of upper GI bleeding in critically-ill patients (Zegerid® powder for oral suspension):
 Loading dose: Day 1: 40 mg every 6-8 hours for two doses
 Maintenance dose: 40 mg/day for up to 14 days; therapy >14 days has not been evaluated

Dosage Forms

Capsule, immediate release:
 Zegerid®: 20 mg, 40 mg

Powder for oral suspension:
 Zegerid®: 20 mg/packet, 40 mg/packet

Omnaris™ [US/Can] *see* ciclesonide *on page 217*

Omnicef® [US/Can] *see* cefdinir *on page 185*

OMNIhist® II L.A. [US] *see* chlorpheniramine, phenylephrine, and methscopolamine *on page 210*

Omnii Gel™ [US-OTC] *see* fluoride *on page 411*

Omnipaque™ [US] *see* iohexol *on page 520*

Omnipen® *(Discontinued)* *see* ampicillin *on page 72*

Omnipen®-N *(Discontinued)* *see* ampicillin *on page 72*

Omniscan™ [US] *see* gadodiamide *on page 433*

Omnitrope™ [US] *see* somatropin *on page 881*

Oncaspar® [US] *see* pegaspargase *on page 726*

Oncet® *(Discontinued)* *see* hydrocodone and homatropine *on page 482*

Oncotice™ [Can] *see* BCG vaccine *on page 118*

Oncovin® *(Discontinued)* *see* vincristine *on page 978*

ondansetron (on DAN se tron)

Sound-Alike/Look-Alike Issues

ondansetron may be confused with dolasetron, granisetron, palonosetron

Zofran® may be confused with Zantac®, Zosyn®

Synonyms GR38032R; ondansetron hydrochloride

U.S./Canadian Brand Names Apo-Ondansetron® [Can]; Gen-Ondansetron [Can]; Novo-Ondansetron [Can]; Ondansetron Injection [Can]; Ondansetron-Omega [Can]; PHL-Ondansetron [Can]; PMS-Ondansetron [Can]; ratio-Ondansetron [Can]; Sandoz-Ondansetron [Can]; Zofran® ODT [US/Can]; Zofran® [US/Can]

Therapeutic Category Selective 5-HT$_3$ Receptor Antagonist

Use Prevention of nausea and vomiting associated with moderately- to highly-emetogenic cancer chemotherapy; radiotherapy in patients receiving total body irradiation or fractions to the abdomen; prevention of postoperative nausea and vomiting (PONV); treatment of PONV if no prophylactic dose received

Usual Dosage Note: Studies in adults have shown a single daily dose of 8-12 mg I.V. or 8-24 mg orally to be as effective as mg/kg dosing, and should be considered for **all** patients whose mg/kg dose exceeds 8-12 mg I.V.; oral solution and ODT formulations are bioequivalent to corresponding doses of tablet formulation

Children:

I.V.:

Prevention of chemotherapy-induced emesis: 6 months to 18 years: 0.15 mg/kg/dose administered 30 minutes prior to chemotherapy, 4 and 8 hours after the first dose **or** 0.45 mg/kg/day as a single dose

Prevention of postoperative nausea and vomiting: 1 month to 12 years:

≤40 kg: 0.1 mg/kg as a single dose

>40 kg: 4 mg as a single dose

Oral: Prevention of chemotherapy-induced emesis:

4-11 years: 4 mg 30 minutes before chemotherapy; repeat 4 and 8 hours after initial dose, then 4 mg every 8 hours for 1-2 days after chemotherapy completed

≥12 years: Refer to adult dosing.

Adults:

I.V.:

Prevention of chemotherapy-induced emesis:

0.15 mg/kg 3 times/day beginning 30 minutes prior to chemotherapy **or**

0.45 mg/kg once daily **or**

8-10 mg 1-2 times/day **or**

24 mg or 32 mg once daily

I.M., I.V.: Postoperative nausea and vomiting: 4 mg as a single dose approximately 30 minutes before the end of anesthesia, or as treatment if vomiting occurs after surgery

Note: Repeat doses given in response to inadequate control of nausea/vomiting from preoperative doses are generally ineffective.

Oral:

Chemotherapy-induced emesis:

Highly-emetogenic agents/single-day therapy: 24 mg given 30 minutes prior to the start of therapy

Moderately-emetogenic agents: 8 mg every 12 hours beginning 30 minutes before chemotherapy, continuously for 1-2 days after chemotherapy completed

Total body irradiation: 8 mg 1-2 hours before daily each fraction of radiotherapy

Single high-dose fraction radiotherapy to abdomen: 8 mg 1-2 hours before irradiation, then 8 mg every 8 hours after first dose for 1-2 days after completion of radiotherapy

Daily fractionated radiotherapy to abdomen: 8 mg 1-2 hours before irradiation, then 8 mg 8 hours after first dose for each day of radiotherapy

Postoperative nausea and vomiting: 16 mg given 1 hour prior to induction of anesthesia

Dosage Forms

Infusion [premixed in D$_5$W, preservative free]: 32 mg (50 mL)

Zofran®: 32 mg (50 mL)

Injection, solution: 2 mg/mL (2 mL, 20 mL)

Zofran®: 2 mg/mL (2 mL, 20 mL)

Injection, solution [preservative free]: 2 mg/mL (2 mL)

Solution, oral: 4 mg/5 mL (50 mL)

Zofran®: 4 mg/5 mL

Tablet: 4 mg; 8 mg

Zofran®: 4 mg, 8 mg

Tablet, orally disintegrating: 4 mg; 8 mg

Zofran® ODT: 4 mg, 8 mg

ondansetron hydrochloride *see* ondansetron *on page 698*

Ondansetron Injection [Can] *see* ondansetron *on page 698*

Ondansetron-Omega [Can] *see* ondansetron *on page 698*

One-A-Day® 50 Plus Formula [US-OTC] *see* vitamins (multiple/oral) *on page 983*

One-A-Day® Active Formula [US-OTC] *see* vitamins (multiple/oral) *on page 983*

One-A-Day® All Day Energy [US-OTC] *see* vitamins (multiple/oral) *on page 983*

One-A-Day® Cholesterol Plus™ [US-OTC] *see* vitamins (multiple/oral) *on page 983*
One-A-Day® Essential Formula [US-OTC] *see* vitamins (multiple/oral) *on page 983*
One-A-Day® Kids Bugs Bunny and Friends Complete [US-OTC] *see* vitamins (multiple/pediatric) *on page 983*
One-A-Day® Kids Scooby-Doo! Complete [US-OTC] *see* vitamins (multiple/pediatric) *on page 983*
One-A-Day® Kids Scooby-Doo! Plus Calcium [US-OTC] *see* vitamins (multiple/pediatric) *on page 983*
One-A-Day® Maximum Formula [US-OTC] *see* vitamins (multiple/oral) *on page 983*
One-A-Day® Men's Health Formula [US-OTC] *see* vitamins (multiple/oral) *on page 983*
One-A-Day® Scooby-Doo! Gummies [US-OTC] *see* vitamins (multiple/pediatric) *on page 983*
One-A-Day® Weight Smart [US-OTC] *see* vitamins (multiple/oral) *on page 983*
One-A-Day® Women's Formula [US-OTC] *see* vitamins (multiple/oral) *on page 983*
One Gram C [US-OTC] *see* ascorbic acid *on page 96*
ONTAK® [US] *see* denileukin diftitox *on page 272*
Onxol™ [US] *see* paclitaxel *on page 714*
Ony-Clear *(Discontinued)* *see* benzalkonium chloride *on page 123*
Opana® [US] *see* oxymorphone *on page 713*
Opana® ER [US] *see* oxymorphone *on page 713*
OPC-13013 *see* cilostazol *on page 219*
OPC-14597 *see* aripiprazole *on page 93*
OP-CCK *see* sincalide *on page 868*
Opcon-A® [US-OTC] *see* naphazoline and pheniramine *on page 656*
Opcon® Ophthalmic *(Discontinued)* *see* naphazoline *on page 655*
o,p'-DDD *see* mitotane *on page 638*
Operand® [US-OTC] *see* povidone-iodine *on page 775*
Operand® Chlorhexidine Gluconate [US-OTC] *see* chlorhexidine gluconate *on page 201*
Ophthalgan® Ophthalmic *(Discontinued)* *see* glycerin *on page 449*
Ophthetic® [US] *see* proparacaine *on page 794*
Ophthifluor® *(Discontinued)* *see* fluorescein *on page 410*
Ophthochlor® Ophthalmic *(Discontinued)* *see* chloramphenicol *on page 200*
Ophtho-Dipivefrin™ [Can] *see* dipivefrin *on page 311*
Ophtho-Tate® [Can] *see* prednisolone (ophthalmic) *on page 781*
opium and belladonna *see* belladonna and opium *on page 120*

opium tincture (OH pee um TING chur)

Sound-Alike/Look-Alike Issues
opium tincture may be confused with camphorated tincture of opium (paregoric)
DTO is an error-prone abbreviation (mistaken as Diluted Tincture of Opium; dose equivalency of paregoric)

Synonyms opium tincture, deodorized

Therapeutic Category Analgesic, Narcotic

Controlled Substance C-II

Use Treatment of diarrhea or relief of pain

Usual Dosage Oral: **Note:** Opium tincture 10% contains morphine 10 mg/mL. use caution in ordering, dispensing, and/or administering.
Children:
Diarrhea: 0.005-0.01 mL/kg/dose every 3-4 hours for a maximum of 6 doses/24 hours
Analgesia: 0.01-0.02 mL/kg/dose every 3-4 hours
Adults:
Diarrhea: 0.3-1 mL/dose every 2-6 hours to maximum of 6 mL/24 hours
Analgesia: 0.6-1.5 mL/dose every 3-4 hours

Dosage Forms
Liquid: 10%

opium tincture, deodorized *see* opium tincture *on page 700*

oprelvekin (oh PREL ve kin)

Sound-Alike/Look-Alike Issues
oprelvekin may be confused with aldesleukin, Proleukin®
Neumega® may be confused with Neulasta®, Neupogen®

Synonyms IL-11; interleukin-11; NSC-722848; recombinant human interleukin-11; recombinant interleukin-11; rhIL-11; rIL-11

U.S./Canadian Brand Names Neumega® [US]

Therapeutic Category Platelet Growth Factor

Use Prevention of severe thrombocytopenia; reduce the need for platelet transfusions following myelosuppressive chemotherapy

Usual Dosage SubQ: Administer first dose ~6-24 hours after the end of chemotherapy. Discontinue at least 48 hours before beginning the next cycle of chemotherapy.
Adults: 50 mcg/kg once daily for ~10-21 days (until postnadir platelet count ≥50,000 cells/μL)

Dosage Forms
Injection, powder for reconstitution:
Neumega®: 5 mg

Optase™ [US] see trypsin, balsam peru, and castor oil on page 958
Optho-Bunolol® [Can] see levobunolol on page 555
Opti-Clear [US-OTC] see tetrahydrozoline on page 916
Opticrom® [Can] see cromolyn sodium on page 251
Optigene® 3 *(Discontinued)* see tetrahydrozoline on page 916
OptiMARK® [US] see gadoversetamide on page 434
Optimine® *(Discontinued)*
Optimoist® Solution *(Discontinued)* see saliva substitute on page 853
Optimyxin® [Can] see bacitracin and polymyxin B on page 113
Optimyxin Plus® [Can] see neomycin, polymyxin B, and gramicidin on page 663
OptiPranolol® [US/Can] see metipranolol on page 625
Optiray® [US] see ioversol on page 523
Optivar® [US] see azelastine on page 110
Optive™ [US-OTC] see carboxymethylcellulose on page 179
Optivite® P.M.T. [US-OTC] see vitamins (multiple/oral) on page 983
Orabase® with Benzocaine [US-OTC] see benzocaine on page 124
Oracea™ [US] see doxycycline on page 323
Oracort [Can] see triamcinolone (systemic) on page 948
Oradex-C® *(Discontinued)* see dyclonine on page 330
Orajel® Baby Daytime and Nighttime [US-OTC] see benzocaine on page 124
Orajel® Baby Teething [US-OTC] see benzocaine on page 124
Orajel® Baby Teething Nighttime [US-OTC] see benzocaine on page 124
Orajel® Brace-Aid Oral Anesthetic *(Discontinued)* see benzocaine on page 124
Orajel® Denture Plus [US-OTC] see benzocaine on page 124
Orajel® Maximum Strength [US-OTC] see benzocaine on page 124
Orajel® Medicated Toothache [US-OTC] see benzocaine on page 124
Orajel® Mouth Sore [US-OTC] see benzocaine on page 124
Orajel® Multi-Action Cold Sore [US-OTC] see benzocaine on page 124
Orajel® Perioseptic® Spot Treatment [US-OTC] see carbamide peroxide on page 174
Orajel PM® Maximum Strength [US-OTC] see benzocaine on page 124
Orajel® Ultra Mouth Sore [US-OTC] see benzocaine on page 124
oral Balance® [US-OTC] see saliva substitute on page 853
Oramorph SR® [US] see morphine sulfate on page 643
Oranyl [US-OTC] see pseudoephedrine on page 801
Oranyl Plus [US-OTC] see acetaminophen and pseudoephedrine on page 23
Orap® [US/Can] see pimozide on page 753
Orapred® [US] see prednisolone (systemic) on page 781

Oraquix® [US] *see* lidocaine and prilocaine *on page 565*
OraRinse™ [US-OTC] *see* maltodextrin *on page 590*
Orasone® (Discontinued) *see* prednisone *on page 782*
Orazinc® [US-OTC] *see* zinc sulfate *on page 994*
orciprenaline sulfate *see* metaproterenol *on page 609*
Orencia® [US/Can] *see* abatacept *on page 16*
Oreton® Methyl (Discontinued) *see* methyltestosterone *on page 624*
Orfadin® [US] *see* nitisinone *on page 674*
ORG 946 *see* rocuronium *on page 842*
Orgalutran® [Can] *see* ganirelix *on page 436*
Organidin® NR [US] *see* guaifenesin *on page 453*
Orgaran® [Can] *see* danaparoid *(Canada only) on page 265*
Orgaran® (Discontinued) *see* danaparoid *(Canada only) on page 265*
ORG NC 45 *see* vecuronium *on page 973*
Orinase Diagnostic® (Discontinued) *see* tolbutamide *on page 933*
Orinase® Oral (Discontinued) *see* tolbutamide *on page 933*
ORLAAM® (Discontinued)

orlistat (OR li stat)

Sound-Alike/Look-Alike Issues
Xenical® may be confused with Xeloda®
U.S./Canadian Brand Names Alli™ [US-OTC]; Xenical® [US/Can]
Therapeutic Category Lipase Inhibitor
Use Management of obesity, including weight loss and weight management, when used in conjunction with a reduced-calorie and low-fat diet; reduce the risk of weight regain after prior weight loss; indicated for obese patients with an initial body mass index (BMI) ≥30 kg/m^2 or ≥27 kg/m^2 in the presence of other risk factors
Usual Dosage Oral:
Children ≥12 years and Adults (Xenical®): 120 mg 3 times/day with each main meal containing fat (during or up to 1 hour after the meal); omit dose if meal is occasionally missed or contains no fat.
Adults (Alli™): OTC labeling: 60 mg 3 times/day with each main meal containing fat
Dosage Forms
Capsule:
Alli™ [OTC]: 60 mg
Xenical®: 120 mg

Ormazine® (Discontinued) *see* chlorpromazine *on page 213*
Ornex® [US-OTC] *see* acetaminophen and pseudoephedrine *on page 23*
Ornex® Maximum Strength [US-OTC] *see* acetaminophen and pseudoephedrine *on page 23*
Ornidyl® Injection (Discontinued) *see* eflornithine *on page 336*
ORO-Clense [Can] *see* chlorhexidine gluconate *on page 201*
Orphenace® [Can] *see* orphenadrine *on page 702*

orphenadrine (or FEN a dreen)

Sound-Alike/Look-Alike Issues
Norflex™ may be confused with norfloxacin, Noroxin®
Synonyms orphenadrine citrate
U.S./Canadian Brand Names Norflex™ [US/Can]; Orphenace® [Can]; Rhoxal-orphendrine [Can]
Therapeutic Category Skeletal Muscle Relaxant
Use Treatment of muscle spasm associated with acute painful musculoskeletal conditions
Usual Dosage Adults:
Oral: 100 mg twice daily
I.M., I.V.: 60 mg every 12 hours
Dosage Forms
Injection, solution: 30 mg/mL (2 mL)
Norflex™: 30 mg/mL (2 mL)
Tablet, extended release: 100 mg

orphenadrine, aspirin, and caffeine (or FEN a dreen, AS pir in, & KAF een)

Sound-Alike/Look-Alike Issues
Norgesic™ Forte may be confused with Norgesic 40®

Synonyms aspirin, orphenadrine, and caffeine; caffeine, orphenadrine, and aspirin

U.S./Canadian Brand Names Norgesic™ Forte [Can]; Norgesic™ [Can]

Therapeutic Category Analgesic, Nonnarcotic; Skeletal Muscle Relaxant

Use Relief of discomfort associated with skeletal muscular conditions

Usual Dosage Oral: 1-2 tablets 3-4 times/day

Dosage Forms
Tablet: Orphenadrine 25 mg, aspirin 385 mg, and caffeine 30 mg; orphenadrine 50 mg, aspirin 770 mg, and caffeine 60 mg

orphenadrine citrate see orphenadrine on page 702

Orphengesic *(Discontinued)* see orphenadrine, aspirin, and caffeine on page 703

Orphengesic Forte *(Discontinued)* see orphenadrine, aspirin, and caffeine on page 703

Ortho® 0.5/35 [Can] see ethinyl estradiol and norethindrone on page 376

Ortho® 1/35 [Can] see ethinyl estradiol and norethindrone on page 376

Ortho® 7/7/7 [Can] see ethinyl estradiol and norethindrone on page 376

Ortho-Cept® [US/Can] see ethinyl estradiol and desogestrel on page 369

Orthoclone OKT® 3 [US/Can] see muromonab-CD3 on page 648

Ortho-Cyclen® [US] see ethinyl estradiol and norgestimate on page 378

Ortho-Est® [US] see estropipate on page 366

Ortho Evra® [US] see ethinyl estradiol and norelgestromin on page 375

Ortho Micronor® [US] see norethindrone on page 679

Ortho-Novum® [US] see ethinyl estradiol and norethindrone on page 376

Ortho-Novum® 1/50 [Can] see mestranol and norethindrone on page 608

Ortho-Novum® 1/50 *(Discontinued)* see mestranol and norethindrone on page 608

ortho prefest see estradiol and norgestimate on page 362

Ortho Tri-Cyclen® [US] see ethinyl estradiol and norgestimate on page 378

Ortho Tri-Cyclen® Lo [US] see ethinyl estradiol and norgestimate on page 378

Orthovisc® [US/Can] see hyaluronate and derivatives on page 476

Or-Tyl® Injection *(Discontinued)* see dicyclomine on page 293

Orudis® KT *(Discontinued)* see ketoprofen on page 537

Oruvail® [Can] see ketoprofen on page 537

Os-Cal® [Can] see calcium carbonate on page 163

Os-Cal® 500+D [US-OTC] see calcium and vitamin D on page 162

Os-Cal® 500 *(Discontinued)* see calcium carbonate on page 163

oseltamivir (oh sel TAM i vir)

Sound-Alike/Look-Alike Issues
Tamiflu® may be confused with Thera-Flu®

U.S./Canadian Brand Names Tamiflu® [US/Can]

Therapeutic Category Antiviral Agent, Oral

Use Treatment of uncomplicated acute illness due to influenza (A or B) infection in children ≥1 year of age and adults who have been symptomatic for no more than 2 days; prophylaxis against influenza (A or B) infection in children ≥1 year of age and adults

The Advisory Committee on Immunization Practices (ACIP) recommends that **treatment** be considered for the following:
• Persons hospitalized with laboratory confirmed influenza (may also have benefit if started >48 hours after onset of illness).
• Persons with laboratory confirmed influenza pneumonia.
• Persons with laboratory confirmed influenza and bacterial infections.
• Persons with laboratory confirmed influenza and who are at higher risk for influenza complications.
• Persons presenting for care within 48 hours of laboratory confirmed influenza onset and who want to decrease duration and/or severity of their symptoms or decrease the risk of transmission to those at high risk for complications.

◀ The ACIP recommends that **prophylaxis** be considered for the following:
   • Persons at high risk for influenza infection during the first 2 weeks following vaccination (eg, children <9 years and not previously vaccinated) if the virus is circulating in the community.
   • Persons at high risk for influenza infection, but the vaccination is contraindicated.
   • Unvaccinated family members or healthcare providers with prolonged exposure to or close contact with high-risk persons, unvaccinated persons, or infants <6 months of age.
   • Persons at high risk for influenza infection, their family members and close contacts, and healthcare workers when the circulating strain of influenza is not matched with the vaccine.
   • Persons with immune deficiency or those who may not respond to vaccination.
   • Unvaccinated staff and persons during response to an outbreak in a closed institutional setting that has patients at high risk for infection (eg, extended care facilities).

Usual Dosage Oral:
 Treatment: Initiate treatment within 2 days of onset of symptoms; duration of treatment: 5 days:
   Children: 1-12 years:
     ≤15 kg: 30 mg twice daily
     >15 kg to ≤23 kg: 45 mg twice daily
     >23 kg to ≤40 kg: 60 mg twice daily
     >40 kg: 75 mg twice daily
   Adolescents ≥13 years and Adults: 75 mg twice daily
 Prophylaxis: Initiate treatment within 2 days of contact with an infected individual; duration of treatment: 10 days
   Children: 1-12 years:
     ≤15 kg: 30 mg once daily
     >15 kg to ≤23 kg: 45 mg once daily
     >23 kg to ≤40 kg: 60 mg once daily
     >40 kg: 75 mg once daily
   Adolescents ≥13 years and Adults: 75 mg once daily. During community outbreaks, dosing is 75 mg once daily. May be used for up to 6 weeks; duration of protection lasts for length of dosing period

Dosage Forms
 Capsule:
   Tamiflu®: 30 mg, 45 mg, 75 mg
 Powder for oral suspension:
   Tamiflu®: 12 mg/mL

OSI-774 *see* erlotinib *on page 353*

Osmitrol® [US/Can] *see* mannitol *on page 590*

Osmoglyn® *(Discontinued)* *see* glycerin *on page 449*

Osmolite® HN [US-OTC] *see* nutritional formula, enteral/oral *on page 689*

OsmoPrep™ [US] *see* sodium phosphates *on page 878*

Osteocalcin® *(Discontinued)* *see* calcitonin *on page 160*

Osteocit® [Can] *see* calcium citrate *on page 165*

Ostoforte® [Can] *see* ergocalciferol *on page 350*

OTFC (oral transmucosal fentanyl citrate) *see* fentanyl *on page 394*

Otic-Care® Otic *(Discontinued)* *see* neomycin, polymyxin B, and hydrocortisone *on page 663*

Otix® [US-OTC] *see* carbamide peroxide *on page 174*

Otobiotic Otic Solution *(Discontinued)*

Otocort® Otic *(Discontinued)* *see* neomycin, polymyxin B, and hydrocortisone *on page 663*

Otosporin® Otic *(Discontinued)* *see* neomycin, polymyxin B, and hydrocortisone *on page 663*

Otrivin® *(Discontinued)*

Otrivin® Pediatric *(Discontinued)*

Outgro® [US-OTC] *see* benzocaine *on page 124*

Ovace® [US] *see* sulfacetamide *on page 892*

Ovace® Plus [US] *see* sulfacetamide *on page 892*

Ovcon® [US] *see* ethinyl estradiol and norethindrone *on page 376*

Ovide® [US] *see* malathion *on page 590*

Ovidrel® [US/Can] *see* chorionic gonadotropin (recombinant) *on page 217*

ovine corticotrophin-releasing hormone *see* corticorelin *on page 248*

Ovol® [Can] *see* simethicone *on page 867*

Ovral® [Can] *see* ethinyl estradiol and norgestrel *on page 380*
Ovral® (Discontinued) *see* ethinyl estradiol and norgestrel *on page 380*
Ovrette® (Discontinued)

oxacillin (oks a SIL in)

Synonyms methylphenyl isoxazolyl penicillin; oxacillin sodium
Therapeutic Category Penicillin
Use Treatment of infections such as osteomyelitis, septicemia, endocarditis, and CNS infections caused by susceptible strains of *Staphylococcus*
Usual Dosage
Usual dosage range:
Infants and Children: I.M., I.V.: 100-200 mg/kg/day in divided doses every 6 hours (maximum: 12 g/day)
Adults: I.M., I.V.: 250-2000 mg every 4-6 hours
Indication-specific dosing:
Children:
Arthritis (septic): I.V.: 37 mg/kg every 6 hours
Epiglottitis: I.V.: 150-200 mg/kg/day divided every 6 hours
Mild-to-moderate infections: I.M., I.V.: 100-150 mg/kg/day in divided doses every 6 hours (maximum: 4 g/day)
Severe infections: I.M., I.V.: 150-200 mg/kg/day in divided doses every 6 hours (maximum: 12 g/day)
Staphylococcal scalded-skin syndrome: I.V.: 150 mg/kg/day divided every 6 hours for 5-7 days
Adults:
Endocarditis: I.V.: 2 g every 4 hours with gentamicin
Mild-to-moderate infections: I.M., I.V.: 250-500 mg every 4-6 hours
Prosthetic joint infection: I.V.: 2 g every 4 hours with rifampin
Severe infections: I.M., I.V.: 1-2 g every 4-6 hours
Staphylococcus aureus, **methicillin-susceptible infections, including brain abscess, bursitis, erysipelas, mastitis, mastoiditis, osteomyelitis, perinephric abscess, pneumonia, pyomyositis, scalded skin syndrome, toxic shock syndrome:** I.V.: 2 g every 4 hours
Dosage Forms
Infusion [premixed iso-osmotic dextrose solution]: 1 g (50 mL); 2 g (50 mL)
Injection, powder for reconstitution: 1 g, 2 g, 10 g

oxacillin sodium *see* oxacillin *on page 705*

oxaliplatin (ox AL i pla tin)

Sound-Alike/Look-Alike Issues
oxaliplatin may be confused with Aloxi®, carboplatin
Synonyms diaminocyclohexane oxalatoplatinum; L-OHP; NSC-266046
U.S./Canadian Brand Names Eloxatin® [US]
Therapeutic Category Antineoplastic Agent, Alkylating Agent
Use Treatment of stage III colon cancer and advanced colorectal cancer
Usual Dosage Details concerning dosing in combination regimens should also be consulted.
Adults: Stage III colon cancer and colorectal cancer: I.V.: 85 mg/m^2 every 2 weeks
Dosage Forms
Injection, solution [preservative free]:
Eloxatin™: 5 mg/mL (10 mL, 20 mL, 40 mL)

Oxandrin® [US] *see* oxandrolone *on page 705*

oxandrolone (oks AN droe lone)

U.S./Canadian Brand Names Oxandrin® [US]
Therapeutic Category Androgen
Controlled Substance C-III
Use Adjunctive therapy to promote weight gain after weight loss following extensive surgery, chronic infections, or severe trauma, and in some patients who, without definite pathophysiologic reasons, fail to gain or to maintain normal weight; to offset protein catabolism with prolonged corticosteroid administration; relief of bone pain associated with osteoporosis
Usual Dosage
Children: Total daily dose: ≤0.1 mg/kg or ≤0.045 mg/lb

◀ Adults: 2.5-20 mg in divided doses 2-4 times/day based on individual response; a course of therapy of 2-4 weeks is usually adequate. This may be repeated intermittently as needed.

Dosage Forms
Tablet: 2.5 mg, 10 mg
Oxandrin®: 2.5 mg, 10 mg

oxaprozin (oks a PROE zin)

Sound-Alike/Look-Alike Issues
oxaprozin may be confused with oxazepam
Daypro® may be confused with Diupres®

U.S./Canadian Brand Names Apo-Oxaprozin® [Can]; Daypro® [US/Can]

Therapeutic Category Analgesic, Nonnarcotic; Nonsteroidal Antiinflammatory Drug (NSAID)

Use Acute and long-term use in the management of signs and symptoms of osteoarthritis and rheumatoid arthritis; juvenile rheumatoid arthritis

Usual Dosage Oral (individualize dosage to lowest effective dose to minimize adverse effects):
Children 6-16 years: Juvenile rheumatoid arthritis:
22-31 kg: 600 mg once daily
32-54 kg: 900 mg once daily
≥55 kg: 1200 mg once daily
Adults:
Osteoarthritis: 600-1200 mg once daily; patients should be titrated to lowest dose possible; patients with low body weight should start with 600 mg daily
Rheumatoid arthritis: 1200 mg once daily; a one-time loading dose of up to 1800 mg/day or 26 mg/kg (whichever is lower) may be given
Maximum doses:
Patient <50 kg: Maximum: 1200 mg/day
Patient >50 kg with normal renal/hepatic function and low risk of peptic ulcer: Maximum: 1800 mg or 26 mg/kg (whichever is lower) in divided doses

Dosage Forms
Tablet: 600 mg
Daypro®: 600 mg

oxazepam (oks A ze pam)

Sound-Alike/Look-Alike Issues
oxazepam may be confused with oxaprozin, quazepam
Serax® may be confused with Eurax®, Urex®, Zyrtec®

U.S./Canadian Brand Names Apo-Oxazepam® [Can]; Bio-Oxazepam [Can]; Novoxapram® [Can]; Oxpam® [Can]; Oxpram® [Can]; PMS-Oxazepam [Can]; Riva-Oxazepam [Can]; Serax® [US]

Therapeutic Category Anticonvulsant; Benzodiazepine

Controlled Substance C-IV

Use Treatment of anxiety; management of ethanol withdrawal

Usual Dosage Oral: Adults:
Anxiety: 10-30 mg 3-4 times/day
Ethanol withdrawal: 15-30 mg 3-4 times/day
Hypnotic: 15-30 mg

Dosage Forms
Capsule: 10 mg, 15 mg, 30 mg
Serax®: 10 mg, 15 mg, 30 mg
Tablet:
Serax®: 15 mg

oxcarbazepine (ox car BAZ e peen)

Sound-Alike/Look-Alike Issues
OXcarbazepine may be confused with carBAMazepine

Synonyms GP 47680; OCBZ

Tall-Man OXcarbazepine

U.S./Canadian Brand Names Trileptal® [US/Can]

Therapeutic Category Anticonvulsant, Miscellaneous

Use Monotherapy or adjunctive therapy in the treatment of partial seizures in adults and children ≥4 years of age with epilepsy; adjunctive therapy in the treatment of partial seizures in children ≥2 years of age with epilepsy

Usual Dosage Oral:

Children 2-3 years:
Adjunctive therapy: 8-10 mg/kg/day, not to exceed 600 mg/day, given in 2 divided daily doses. Maintenance dose should be achieved over 2 weeks, and is dependent upon patient weight.
<20 kg: Consider initiating dose at 16-20 mg/kg/day; maximum maintenance dose should be achieved over 2-4 weeks and should not exceed 60 mg/kg/day

Children 4-16 years:
Adjunctive therapy: 8-10 mg/kg/day, not to exceed 600 mg/day, given in 2 divided daily doses. Maintenance dose should be achieved over 2 weeks, and is dependent upon patient weight, according to the following:
20-29 kg: 900 mg/day in 2 divided doses
29.1-39 kg: 1200 mg/day in 2 divided doses
>39 kg: 1800 mg/day in 2 divided doses

Children 4-16 years:
Conversion to monotherapy: Oxcarbazepine 8-10 mg/kg/day in twice daily divided doses, while simultaneously initiating the reduction of the dose of the concomitant antiepileptic drug; the concomitant drug should be withdrawn over 3-6 weeks. Oxcarbazepine dose may be increased by a maximum of 10 mg/kg/day at weekly intervals. See below for recommended total daily dose by weight.
Initiation of monotherapy: Oxcarbazepine should be initiated at 8-10 mg/kg/day in twice daily divided doses; doses may be titrated by 5 mg/kg/day every third day. See below for recommended total daily dose by weight.
Range of maintenance doses by weight during monotherapy:
20 kg: 600-900 mg/day
25-30 kg: 900-1200 mg/day
35-40 kg: 900-1500 mg/day
45 kg: 1200-1500 mg/day
50-55 kg: 1200-1800 mg/day
60-65 kg: 1200-2100 mg/day
70 kg: 1500-2100 mg/day

Adults:
Adjunctive therapy: Initial: 300 mg twice daily; dose may be increased by as much as 600 mg/day at weekly intervals; recommended daily dose: 1200 mg/day in 2 divided doses. Although daily doses >1200 mg/day were somewhat more efficacious, most patients were unable to tolerate 2400 mg/day (due to CNS effects).
Conversion to monotherapy: Oxcarbazepine 600 mg/day in twice daily divided doses while simultaneously initiating the reduction of the dose of the concomitant antiepileptic drug. The concomitant dosage should be withdrawn over 3-6 weeks, while the maximum dose of oxcarbazepine should be reached in about 2-4 weeks. Recommended daily dose: 2400 mg/day.
Initiation of monotherapy: Oxcarbazepine should be initiated at a dose of 600 mg/day in twice daily divided doses; doses may be titrated upward by 300 mg/day every third day to a final dose of 1200 mg/day given in 2 daily divided doses

Dosage Forms
Suspension, oral:
Trileptal®: 300 mg/5 mL
Tablet: 150 mg, 300 mg, 600 mg
Trileptal®: 150 mg, 300 mg, 600 mg

Oxeze® Turbuhaler® [Can] *see* formoterol *on page 424*

oxiconazole (oks i KON a zole)

Synonyms oxiconazole nitrate

U.S./Canadian Brand Names Oxistat® [US/Can]

Therapeutic Category Antifungal Agent

Use Treatment of tinea pedis (athlete's foot), tinea cruris (jock itch), tinea corporis (ringworm), and tinea (pityriasis) versicolor

Usual Dosage Topical: Children and Adults:
Tinea corporis/tinea cruris: Cream, lotion: Apply to affected areas 1-2 times daily for 2 weeks

▶

Tinea pedis: Cream, lotion: Apply to affected areas 1-2 times daily for 1 month
Tinea versicolor: Cream: Apply to affected areas once daily for 2 weeks
Dosage Forms
Cream:
Oxistat®: 1% (15 g, 30 g, 60 g)
Lotion:
Oxistat®: 1% (30 mL)

oxiconazole nitrate *see* oxiconazole *on page 707*
oxidized regenerated cellulose *see* cellulose, oxidized regenerated *on page 193*
Oxilan® [US] *see* ioxilan *on page 523*
Oxilan® 300 [Can] *see* ioxilan *on page 523*
Oxilan® 350 [Can] *see* ioxilan *on page 523*
oxilapine succinate *see* loxapine *on page 580*
Oxipor® VHC [US-OTC] *see* coal tar *on page 240*
Oxistat® [US/Can] *see* oxiconazole *on page 707*
Oxpam® [Can] *see* oxazepam *on page 706*
oxpentifylline *see* pentoxifylline *on page 737*
Oxpram® [Can] *see* oxazepam *on page 706*

oxprenolol *(Canada only)* (ox PREN oh lole)
Synonyms oxprenolol hydrochloride
U.S./Canadian Brand Names Trasicor® [Can]
Therapeutic Category Beta-Adrenergic Blocker
Use Treatment of mild-or-moderate hypertension
Usual Dosage Oral: Adults:
Initial: 20 mg 3 times/day (regular-release formulation); increase by 60 mg/day (in 3 divided doses) at 1- to 2-week intervals until adequate control is obtained
Maintenance: 120-320 mg/day; do not exceed 480 mg
Dosage Forms [CAN] = Canadian brand name
Tablet:
Trasicor® [CAN]: 40 mg, 80 mg [not available in the U.S.]

oxprenolol hydrochloride *see* oxprenolol *(Canada only) on page 708*
Oxsoralen® [US/Can] *see* methoxsalen *on page 617*
Oxsoralen-Ultra® [US/Can] *see* methoxsalen *on page 617*
Oxy-5® *(Discontinued)* *see* benzoyl peroxide *on page 126*
Oxy 10® Balanced Medicated Face Wash [US-OTC] *see* benzoyl peroxide *on page 126*
Oxy 10® Balance Spot Treatment [US-OTC] *see* benzoyl peroxide *on page 126*

oxybutynin (oks i BYOO ti nin)
Sound-Alike/Look-Alike Issues
oxybutynin may be confused with OxyContin®
Ditropan® may be confused with Detrol®, diazepam, Diprivan®, dithranol
Synonyms oxybutynin chloride
U.S./Canadian Brand Names Apo-Oxybutynin® [Can]; Ditropan® XL [US/Can]; Ditropan® [US/Can]; Gen-Oxybutynin [Can]; Novo-Oxybutynin [Can]; Nu-Oxybutyn [Can]; Oxytrol® [US/Can]; PMS-Oxybutynin [Can]; Riva-Oxybutynin [Can]; Uromax® [Can]
Therapeutic Category Antispasmodic Agent, Urinary
Use Antispasmodic for neurogenic bladder (urgency, frequency, urge incontinence)
Usual Dosage
Oral:
Children:
>5 years: 5 mg twice daily, up to 5 mg 3 times/day maximum
>6 years: Extended release: 5 mg once daily; adjust dose in 5 mg increments; maximum dose: 20 mg/day
Adults: 5 mg 2-3 times/day up to 5 mg 4 times/day maximum

Extended release: Initial: 5-10 mg once daily, adjust dose in 5 mg increments at weekly intervals; maximum: 30 mg daily

Transdermal: Adults: Apply one 3.9 mg/day patch twice weekly (every 3-4 days)

Note: Should be discontinued periodically to determine whether the patient can manage without the drug and to minimize resistance to the drug

Dosage Forms
Syrup: 5 mg/5 mL
  Ditropan®: 5 mg/5 mL
Tablet: 5 mg
  Ditropan®: 5 mg
Tablet, extended release: 5 mg, 10 mg, 15 mg
  Ditropan® XL: 5 mg, 10 mg, 15 mg
Transdermal system:
  Oxytrol®: 3.9 mg/day (8s)

oxybutynin chloride *see* oxybutynin *on page 708*

oxychlorosene (oks i KLOR oh seen)

Synonyms oxychlorosene sodium
U.S./Canadian Brand Names Clorpactin® WCS-90 [US-OTC]
Therapeutic Category Antibiotic, Topical
Use Treatment of localized infections
Usual Dosage Topical (0.1% to 0.5% solutions): Apply by irrigation, instillation, spray, soaks, or wet compresses
Dosage Forms
Powder for solution:
  Clorpactin® WCS-90 [OTC]: 2 g

oxychlorosene sodium *see* oxychlorosene *on page 709*
Oxycocet® [Can] *see* oxycodone and acetaminophen *on page 710*
Oxycodan® [Can] *see* oxycodone and aspirin *on page 711*

oxycodone (oks i KOE done)

Sound-Alike/Look-Alike Issues
  OxyCODONE may be confused with HYDROcodone, OxyContin®, oxymorphone
  OxyContin® may be confused with MS Contin®, oxybutynin
  OxyFast® may be confused with Roxanol™
  Roxicodone® may be confused with Roxanol™
Synonyms dihydrohydroxycodeinone; oxycodone hydrochloride
Tall-Man oxyCODONE
U.S./Canadian Brand Names ETH-Oxydose™ [US]; Oxy.IR® [Can]; OxyContin® [US/Can]; OxyFast® [US]; OxyIR® [US]; Roxicodone® [US]; Supeudol® [Can]
Therapeutic Category Analgesic, Narcotic
Controlled Substance C-II
Use Management of moderate-to-severe pain, normally used in combination with nonopioid analgesics
  OxyContin® is indicated for around-the-clock management of moderate-to-severe pain when an analgesic is needed for an extended period of time.
Usual Dosage Oral:
Children: Immediate release:
  6-12 years: 1.25 mg every 6 hours as needed
  >12 years: 2.5 mg every 6 hours as needed
Adults:
  Immediate release: 5 mg every 6 hours as needed
  Controlled release:
    Opioid naive: 10 mg every 12 hours
    Concurrent CNS depressants: Reduce usual dose by 1/3 to 1/2
    Conversion from transdermal fentanyl: For each 25 mcg/hour transdermal dose, substitute 10 mg controlled release oxycodone every 12 hours; should be initiated 18 hours after the removal of the transdermal fentanyl patch

Currently on opioids: Use standard conversion chart to convert daily dose to oxycodone equivalent. Divide daily dose in 2 (for twice-daily dosing, usually every 12 hours) and round down to nearest dosage form.

Note: 60 mg, 80 mg, or 160 mg tablets are for use **only** in opioid-tolerant patients. Special safety considerations must be addressed when converting to OxyContin® doses ≥160 mg every 12 hours. Dietary caution must be taken when patients are initially titrated to 160 mg tablets. Using different strengths to obtain the same daily dose is equivalent (eg, four 40 mg tablets, two 80 mg tablets, one 160 mg tablet); all produce similar blood levels.

Multiplication factors for converting the daily dose of current oral opioid to the daily dose of oral oxycodone:

Current opioid mg/day dose x factor = Oxycodone mg/day dose

Codeine mg/day oral dose **x** 0.15 = Oxycodone mg/day dose
Hydrocodone mg/day oral dose **x** 0.9 = Oxycodone mg/day dose
Hydromorphone mg/day oral dose **x** 4 = Oxycodone mg/day dose
Levorphanol mg/day oral dose **x** 7.5 = Oxycodone mg/day dose
Meperidine mg/day oral dose **x** 0.1 = Oxycodone mg/day dose
Methadone mg/day oral dose **x** 1.5 = Oxycodone mg/day dose
Morphine mg/day oral dose **x** 0.5 = Oxycodone mg/day dose

Note: Divide the oxycodone mg/day dose into the appropriate dosing interval for the specific form being used.

Dosage Forms
Capsule, immediate release: 5 mg
OxyIR®: 5 mg
Liquid, oral, as hydrochloride [concentrate]:
Roxicodone®: 20 mg/mL (30 mL)
Solution, oral: 5 mg/5 mL
Roxicodone®: 5 mg/5 mL
Solution, oral [concentrate]: 20 mg/mL
ETH-Oxydose™,Oxydose®, OxyFast®: 20 mg/mL
Tablet: 5 mg, 10 mg, 15 mg, 20 mg, 30 mg
Roxicodone®: 5 mg, 15 mg, 30 mg
Tablet, controlled release: 10 mg, 20 mg, 40 mg, 80 mg, 160 mg
OxyContin®: 10 mg, 15 mg, 20 mg, 30 mg, 40 mg, 60 mg, 80 mg, 160 mg
Tablet, extended release: 10 mg, 20 mg, 40 mg

oxycodone and acetaminophen (oks i KOE done & a seet a MIN oh fen)

Sound-Alike/Look-Alike Issues
Endocet® may be confused with Indocid®
Percocet® may be confused with Fioricet®, Percodan®
Roxicet™ may be confused with Roxanol™
Tylox® may be confused with Trimox®, Tylenol®, Wymox®, Xanax®

Synonyms acetaminophen and oxycodone

U.S./Canadian Brand Names Endocet® [US/Can]; Magnacet™ [US]; Oxycocet® [Can]; Percocet® [US/Can]; Percocet®-Demi [Can]; PMS-Oxycodone-Acetaminophen [Can]; Primalev™ [US]; Roxicet™ 5/500 [US]; Roxicet™ [US]; Tylox® [US]

Therapeutic Category Analgesic, Narcotic

Controlled Substance C-II

Use Management of moderate-to-severe pain

Usual Dosage Oral: Doses should be given every 4-6 hours as needed and titrated to appropriate analgesic effects. **Note:** Initial dose is based on the **oxycodone** content; however, the maximum daily dose is based on the **acetaminophen** content.

Children: Maximum acetaminophen dose: Children <45 kg: 90 mg/kg/day; children >45 kg: 4 g/day
Mild-to-moderate pain: Initial dose, **based on oxycodone content:** 0.05-0.1 mg/kg/dose
Severe pain: Initial dose, **based on oxycodone content:** 0.3 mg/kg/dose
Adults:
Mild-to-moderate pain: Initial dose, **based on oxycodone content:** 2.5-5 mg
Severe pain: Initial dose, **based on oxycodone content:** 10-30 mg. Do not exceed acetaminophen 4 g/day.

Dosage Forms
Caplet: Oxycodone 5 mg and acetaminophen 500 mg

Roxicet™ 5/500: Oxycodone 5 mg and acetaminophen 500 mg
Capsule: Oxycodone 5 mg and acetaminophen 500 mg
Tylox®: Oxycodone 5 mg and acetaminophen 500 mg
Solution, oral: Oxycodone 5 mg and acetaminophen 325 mg per 5 mL
Roxicet™: Oxycodone 5 mg and acetaminophen 325 mg per 5 mL
Tablet:
Generics:
Oxycodone 5 mg and acetaminophen 325 mg
Oxycodone 7.5 mg and acetaminophen 325 mg
Oxycodone 7.5 mg and acetaminophen 500 mg
Oxycodone 10 mg and acetaminophen 325 mg
Oxycodone 10 mg and acetaminophen 650 mg
Brands:
Endocet®:
5/325 [scored]: Oxycodone 5 mg and acetaminophen 325 mg
7.5/325: Oxycodone 7.5 mg and acetaminophen 325 mg
7.5/500: Oxycodone 7.5 mg and acetaminophen 500 mg
10/325: Oxycodone 10 mg and acetaminophen 325 mg
10/650: Oxycodone 10 mg and acetaminophen 650 mg
Magnacet™
2.5/400: Oxycodone 2.5 mg and acetaminophen 400 mg
5/400: Oxycodone 5 mg and acetaminophen 400 mg
7.5/400: Oxycodone 7.5 mg and acetaminophen 400 mg
10/400: Oxycodone 10 mg and acetaminophen 400 mg
Percocet®:
2.5/325: Oxycodone 2.5 mg and acetaminophen 325 mg
5/325 [scored]: Oxycodone 5 mg and acetaminophen 325 mg
7.5/325: Oxycodone 7.5 mg and acetaminophen 325 mg
7.5/500: Oxycodone 7.5 mg and acetaminophen 500 mg
10/325: Oxycodone 10 mg and acetaminophen 325 mg
10/650: Oxycodone 10 mg and acetaminophen 650 mg
Primalev™:
2.5/300: Oxycodone 2.5 mg and acetaminophen 300 mg
5/300: Oxycodone 5 mg and acetaminophen 300 mg
7.5/300: Oxycodone 7.5 mg and acetaminophen 300 mg
10/300: Oxycodone 10 mg and acetaminophen 300 mg
Roxicet™ [scored]: Oxycodone 5 mg and acetaminophen 325 mg

oxycodone and aspirin (oks i KOE done & AS pir in)

Sound-Alike/Look-Alike Issues
Percodan® may be confused with Decadron®, Percocet®, Percogesic®, Periactin®
Synonyms aspirin and oxycodone
U.S./Canadian Brand Names Endodan® [US/Can]; Oxycodan® [Can]; Percodan® [US/Can]
Therapeutic Category Analgesic, Narcotic
Controlled Substance C-II
Use Management of moderate-to-severe pain
Usual Dosage Oral (based on oxycodone combined salts):
Children: Maximum oxycodone: 5 mg/dose; maximum aspirin dose should not exceed 4 g/day. Doses should be given every 6 hours as needed.
Mild-to-moderate pain: Initial dose, **based on oxycodone content:** 0.05-0.1 mg/kg/dose
Severe pain: Initial dose, **based on oxycodone content:** 0.3 mg/kg/dose
Adults: Percodan®: 1 tablet every 6 hours as needed for pain; maximum aspirin dose should not exceed 4 g/day.
Dosage Forms
Tablet: Oxycodone hydrochloride 4.5 mg, oxycodone terephthalate 0.38 mg, and aspirin 325 mg
Endodan®, Percodan®: Oxycodone hydrochloride 4.8355 mg and aspirin 325 mg

oxycodone and ibuprofen (oks i KOE done & eye byoo PROE fen)

Synonyms ibuprofen and oxycodone
U.S./Canadian Brand Names Combunox™ [US]

◀ **Therapeutic Category** Analgesic, Opioid; Nonsteroidal Antiinflammatory Drug (NSAID), Oral
Controlled Substance C-II
Use Short-term (≤7 days) management of acute, moderate-to-severe pain
Usual Dosage Oral: Adults: Pain: Take 1 tablet every 6 hours as needed (maximum: 4 tablets/24 hours); do not take for longer than 7 days
Dosage Forms
Tablet: Oxycodone 5 mg and ibuprofen 400 mg
Combunox™: 5/400: Oxycodone 5 mg and ibuprofen 400 mg

oxycodone hydrochloride *see oxycodone on page 709*
OxyContin® [US/Can] *see oxycodone on page 709*
Oxyderm™ [Can] *see benzoyl peroxide on page 126*
OxyFast® [US] *see oxycodone on page 709*
Oxy.IR® [Can] *see oxycodone on page 709*

oxymetazoline (oks i met AZ oh leen)

Sound-Alike/Look-Alike Issues
oxymetazoline may be confused with oxymetholone
Afrin® may be confused with aspirin
Visine® may be confused with Visken®
Synonyms oxymetazoline hydrochloride
U.S./Canadian Brand Names 4-Way® 12 Hour [US-OTC]; Afrin® Extra Moisturizing [US-OTC]; Afrin® Original [US-OTC]; Afrin® Severe Congestion [US-OTC]; Afrin® Sinus [US-OTC]; Claritin® Allergic Decongestant [Can]; Dristan® Long Lasting Nasal [Can]; Dristan™ 12-Hour [US-OTC]; Drixoral® Nasal [Can]; Duramist® Plus [US-OTC]; Genasal [US-OTC]; Mucinex® Full force™ [US-OTC]; Mucinex® moisture smart™ [US-OTC]; Neo-Synephrine® 12 Hour Extra Moisturizing [US-OTC]; Neo-Synephrine® 12 Hour [US-OTC]; NRS® [US-OTC]; Nōstrilla® [US-OTC]; Vicks® Early Defense™ [US-OTC]; Vicks® Sinex® 12 Hour Ultrafine Mist [US-OTC]; Visine® L.R. [US-OTC]
Therapeutic Category Adrenergic Agonist Agent
Use Adjunctive therapy of middle ear infections, associated with acute or chronic rhinitis, the common cold, sinusitis, hay fever, or other allergies
Ophthalmic: Relief of redness of eye due to minor eye irritations
Usual Dosage
Intranasal (therapy should not exceed 3 days): Children ≥6 years and Adults: 0.05% solution: Instill 2-3 sprays into each nostril twice daily
Ophthalmic: Children ≥6 years and Adults: 0.025% solution: Instill 1-2 drops in affected eye(s) every 6 hours as needed or as directed by healthcare provider
Dosage Forms
Gel, intranasal [spray]:
Vicks® Early Defense™: 0.05% (14.7 mL)
Solution, intranasal [spray]: 0.05% (15 mL, 30 mL)
Afrin® Extra Moisturizing [OTC], Afrin® Severe Congestion [OTC], Afrin® Sinus [OTC], Dristan™ 12-Hour, Duramist® Plus [OTC], Neo-Synephrine® 12 Hour [OTC], Neo-Synephrine® 12 Hour Extra Moisturizing [OTC], Nōstrilla® [OTC], Vicks Sinex® 12 Hour Ultrafine Mist [OTC], Vicks Sinex® 12 Hour [OTC], 4-Way® 12 Hour [OTC]: 0.05% (15 mL)
Afrin® Original [OTC], Genasal [OTC], NRS® [OTC]: 0.05% (15 mL, 30 mL)
Mucinex® Full force™ [OTC], Mucinex® moisture smart™ [OTC]: 0.05% (22 mL)
Solution, ophthalmic:
Visine® L.R. [OTC]: 0.025% (15 mL, 30 mL)

oxymetazoline hydrochloride *see oxymetazoline on page 712*

oxymetholone (oks i METH oh lone)

Sound-Alike/Look-Alike Issues
oxymetholone may be confused with oxymetazoline, oxymorphone
U.S./Canadian Brand Names Anadrol®-50 [US]
Therapeutic Category Anabolic Steroid

Controlled Substance C-III

Use Treatment of anemias caused by deficient red cell production

Usual Dosage Oral: Children and Adults: Erythropoietic effects: 1-5 mg/kg/day in one daily dose; usual effective dose: 1-2 mg/kg/day; give for a minimum trial of 3-6 months because response may be delayed

Dosage Forms
Tablet:
Anadrol®-50: 50 mg

oxymorphone (oks i MOR fone)

Sound-Alike/Look-Alike Issues
oxymorphone may be confused with oxycodone, oxymetholone

Synonyms oxymorphone hydrochloride

U.S./Canadian Brand Names Opana® ER [US]; Opana® [US]

Therapeutic Category Analgesic, Narcotic

Controlled Substance C-II

Use
Parenteral: Management of moderate-to-severe pain and preoperatively as a sedative and/or supplement to anesthesia
Oral, regular release: Management of moderate-to-severe pain
Oral, extended release: Management of moderate-to-severe pain in patients requiring around-the-clock opioid treatment for an extended period of time

Usual Dosage Adults: **Note:** Dosage must be individualized.
I.M., SubQ: Initial: 1-1.5 mg; may repeat every 4-6 hours as needed
Labor analgesia: I.M.: 0.5-1 mg
I.V.: Initial: 0.5 mg
Oral:
Immediate release:
Opioid-naive: 10-20 mg every 4-6 hours as needed. Initial dosages as low as 5 mg may be considered in selected patients and/or patients with renal impairment. Dosage adjustment should be based on level of analgesia, side effects, and pain intensity. Initiation of therapy with initial dose >20 mg is **not** recommended.
Currently on stable dose of parenteral oxymorphone: ~10 times the daily parenteral requirement. The calculated amount should be divided and given in 4-6 equal doses.
Currently on other opioids: Use standard conversion chart to convert daily dose to oxymorphone equivalent. Generally start with 1/2 the calculated daily oxymorphone dosage and administered in divided doses every 4-6 hours.
Extended release (Opana® ER):
Opioid-naive: Initial: 5 mg every 12 hours. Supplemental doses of immediate release oxymorphone may be used as "rescue" medication as dosage is titrated.
Note: Continued requirement for supplemental dosing may be used to titrate the dose of extended release continuous therapy. Adjust therapy incrementally, by 5-10 mg every 12 hours at intervals of every 3-7 days. Ideally, basal dosage may be titrated to generally mild pain or no pain with the regular use of fewer than 2 supplemental doses per 24 hours.
Currently on stable dose of parenteral oxymorphone: Approximately 10 times the daily parenteral requirement. The calculated amount should be given in 2 divided doses (every 12 hours).
Currently on opioids: Use conversion chart (see Note below) to convert daily dose to oxymorphone equivalent. Generally start with 1/2 the calculated daily oxymorphone dosage. Divide daily dose in 2 (for every 12-hour dosing) and round down to nearest dosage form. **Note:** Per manufacturer, the following approximate oral dosages are equivalent to oxymorphone 10 mg:
Hydrocodone 20 mg
Oxycodone 20 mg
Methadone 20 mg
Morphine 30 mg
Conversion of stable dose of immediate release oxymorphone to extended release oxymorphone: Administer 1/2 of the daily dose of immediate release oxymorphone (Opana®) as the extended release formulation (Opana® ER) every 12 hours

Dosage Forms
Injection, solution:
Opana®: 1 mg/mL (1 mL)

▶

Tablet:
Opana®: 5 mg, 10 mg
Tablet, extended release:
Opana® ER: 5 mg, 7.5 mg, 10 mg, 15 mg, 20 mg, 30 mg, 40 mg

oxymorphone hydrochloride *see* oxymorphone *on page 713*
oxytetracycline *(Discontinued)*

oxytocin (oks i TOE sin)

Sound-Alike/Look-Alike Issues
Pitocin® may be confused with Pitressin®
Synonyms pit
U.S./Canadian Brand Names Pitocin® [US/Can]; Syntocinon® [Can]
Therapeutic Category Oxytocic Agent
Use Induction of labor at term; control of postpartum bleeding; adjunctive therapy in management of abortion
Usual Dosage I.V. administration requires the use of an infusion pump. Adults:
Induction of labor: I.V.: 0.5-1 milliunits/minute; gradually increase dose in increments of 1-2 milliunits/minute until desired contraction pattern is established; dose may be decreased after desired frequency of contractions is reached and labor has progressed to 5-6 cm dilation. Infusion rates of 6 milliunits/minute provide oxytocin levels similar to those at spontaneous labor; rates >9-10 milliunits/minute are rarely required.
Postpartum bleeding:
I.M.: Total dose of 10 units after delivery
I.V.: 10-40 units by I.V. infusion in 1000 mL of intravenous fluid at a rate sufficient to control uterine atony
Adjunctive treatment of abortion: I.V.: 10-20 milliunits/minute; maximum total dose: 30 units/12 hours
Dosage Forms
Injection, solution: 10 units/mL (1 mL, 10 mL, 30 mL)
Pitocin®: 10 units/mL (1 mL, 10 mL)

Oxytrol® [US/Can] *see* oxybutynin *on page 708*
Oysco D [US-OTC] *see* calcium and vitamin D *on page 162*
Oysco 500 [US-OTC] *see* calcium carbonate *on page 163*
Oysco 500+D [US-OTC] *see* calcium and vitamin D *on page 162*
Oyst-Cal-D [US-OTC] *see* calcium and vitamin D *on page 162*
Oyst-Cal 500 [US-OTC] *see* calcium carbonate *on page 163*
Oyst-Cal-D 500 [US-OTC] *see* calcium and vitamin D *on page 162*
P2E1 *(Discontinued)*
P-V-Tussin® Syrup *(Discontinued)*
P-V Tussin Tablet *(Discontinued)*
P-071 *see* cetirizine *on page 196*
Pacerone® [US] *see* amiodarone *on page 61*
Pacis™ [Can] *see* BCG vaccine *on page 118*

paclitaxel (pac li TAKS el)

Sound-Alike/Look-Alike Issues
paclitaxel may be confused with paroxetine, Paxil®
paclitaxel (conventional) may be confused with paclitaxel (protein-bound)
Taxol® may be confused with Abraxane®, Paxil®, Taxotere®
Synonyms NSC-125973; NSC-673089
U.S./Canadian Brand Names Apo-Paclitaxel® [Can]; Onxol™ [US]; Taxol® [US/Can]
Therapeutic Category Antineoplastic Agent
Use Treatment of breast, nonsmall cell lung, and ovarian cancers; treatment of AIDS-related Kaposi sarcoma (KS)
Usual Dosage Premedication with dexamethasone (20 mg orally or I.V. at 12 and 6 hours **or** 14 and 7 hours before the dose; reduce dexamethasone dose to 10 mg orally with advanced HIV disease), diphenhydramine (50 mg I.V. 30-60 minutes prior to the dose), and cimetidine, famotidine, or ranitidine (I.V. 30-60 minutes prior to the dose) is recommended.

Adults: I.V.: Refer to individual protocols
Ovarian carcinoma: 135-175 mg/m^2 over 3 hours every 3 weeks **or**
135 mg/m^2 over 24 hours every 3 weeks **or**
50-80 mg/m^2 over 1-3 hours weekly **or**
1.4-4 mg/m^2/day continuous infusion for 14 days every 4 weeks
Metastatic breast cancer: 175-250 mg/m^2 over 3 hours every 3 weeks **or**
50-80 mg/m^2 weekly **or**
1.4-4 mg/m^2/day continuous infusion for 14 days every 4 weeks
Nonsmall cell lung carcinoma: 135 mg/m^2 over 24 hours every 3 weeks
AIDS-related Kaposi sarcoma: 135 mg/m^2 over 3 hours every 3 weeks **or**
100 mg/m^2 over 3 hours every 2 weeks

Dosage Forms
Injection, solution: 6 mg/mL (5 mL, 16.7 mL, 25 mL, 50 mL)
Onxol® : 6 mg/mL (5 mL, 25 mL, 50 mL)
Taxol®: 6 mg/mL (16.7 mL, 50 mL)

paclitaxel (protein bound) (pac li TAKS el PROE teen bownd)

Sound-Alike/Look-Alike Issues
paclitaxel (protein bound) may be confused with paclitaxel (conventional)
Abraxane® may be confused with Paxil®, Taxol®, Taxotere®

Synonyms ABI-007; albumin-bound paclitaxel; NAB-paclitaxel; NSC-736631; protein-bound paclitaxel

U.S./Canadian Brand Names Abraxane® [US]

Therapeutic Category Antineoplastic Agent, Antimicrotubular; Antineoplastic Agent, Natural Source (Plant) Derivative

Use Treatment of relapsed or refractory breast cancer

Usual Dosage I.V.: Adults: Breast cancer: 260 mg/m^2 every 3 weeks

Dosage Forms
Injection, powder for reconstitution:
Abraxane®: 100 mg

Paddock Nystatin™ [US] *see* nystatin *on page 690*
Pain-A-Lay® [US-OTC] *see* phenol *on page 743*
Pain Eze [US-OTC] *see* acetaminophen *on page 19*
Pain-Off [US-OTC] *see* acetaminophen, aspirin, and caffeine *on page 24*
Palafer® [Can] *see* ferrous fumarate *on page 397*
Palcaps *(Discontinued) see* pancrelipase *on page 718*
Palgic® [US] *see* carbinoxamine *on page 177*
Palgic®-D *(Discontinued)*
Palgic®-DS *(Discontinued)*

palifermin (pal ee FER min)

Synonyms AMJ 9701; rHu-KGF

U.S./Canadian Brand Names Kepivance™ [US]

Therapeutic Category Keratinocyte Growth Factor

Use Decrease the incidence and severity of severe oral mucositis associated with hematologic malignancies in patients receiving myelotoxic therapy requiring hematopoietic stem cell support

Usual Dosage I.V.: Adults: 60 mcg/kg/day for 3 consecutive days before and after myelotoxic therapy; total of 6 doses

Note: Administer first 3 doses prior to myelotoxic therapy, with the 3rd dose given 24-48 hours before therapy begins. The last 3 doses should be administered after myelotoxic therapy, with the first of these doses after but on the same day of hematopoietic stem cell infusion and at least 4 days after the most recent dose of palifermin.

Dosage Forms
Injection, powder for reconstitution [preservative free]:
Kepivance™: 6.25 mg

paliperidone (pal ee PER i done)

Synonyms 9-hydroxy-risperidone; 9-OH-risperidone

U.S./Canadian Brand Names Invega® [US/Can]

▶

◀ **Therapeutic Category** Antipsychotic Agent, Atypical
Use Treatment of schizophrenia
Usual Dosage Oral: Adults: Schizophrenia: Initial: 6 mg once daily in the morning; titration not required, though some may benefit from higher or lower doses. If exceeding 6 mg/day, increases of 3 mg/day are recommended no more frequently than every 5 days, up to a maximum of 12 mg/day.
Dosage Forms [CAN] = Canadian availability; not available in U.S.
Tablet, extended-release:
Invega®: 1.5 mg, 3 mg, 6 mg, 9 mg
Invega® [CAN]: 12 mg [not available in the U.S.]

palivizumab (pah li VIZ u mab)

Sound-Alike/Look-Alike Issues
Synagis® may be confused with Synalgos®-DC, Synvisc®
U.S./Canadian Brand Names Synagis® [US/Can]
Therapeutic Category Monoclonal Antibody
Use Prevention of serious lower respiratory tract disease caused by respiratory syncytial virus (RSV) in infants and children at high risk of RSV disease
Usual Dosage I.M.: Infants and Children <2 years: 15 mg/kg of body weight, monthly throughout RSV season (First dose administered prior to commencement of RSV season)
Dosage Forms
Injection, solution [preservative free]:
Synagis®: 100 mg/mL (0.5 mL, 1 mL)

Palladone™ *(Discontinued)* *see* hydromorphone *on page 486*
Palmer's® Skin Success Acne [US-OTC] *see* benzoyl peroxide *on page 126*
Palmer's® Skin Success Acne Cleanser [US-OTC] *see* salicylic acid *on page 850*
Palmer's® Skin Success Eventone® Fade Cream [US-OTC] *see* hydroquinone *on page 488*
Palmitate-A® [US-OTC] *see* vitamin A *on page 979*

palonosetron (pal oh NOE se tron)

Sound-Alike/Look-Alike Issues
palonosetron may be confused with dolasetron, granisetron, ondansetron
Aloxi® may be confused with Eloxatin®, oxaliplatin
Synonyms palonosetron hydrochloride; RS-25259; RS-25259-197
U.S./Canadian Brand Names Aloxi® [US]
Therapeutic Category Antiemetic; Selective 5-HT$_3$ Receptor Antagonist
Use Prevention of chemotherapy-associated nausea and vomiting; indicated for prevention of acute (highly-emetogenic therapy) as well as acute and delayed (moderately-emetogenic therapy) nausea and vomiting; prevention of postoperative nausea and vomiting (PONV)
Usual Dosage I.V.: Adults:
Chemotherapy-associated nausea and vomiting: 0.25 mg 30 minutes prior to the start of chemotherapy administration, day 1 of each cycle
Breakthrough: Palonosetron has not been shown to be effective in terminating nausea or vomiting once it occurs and should not be used for this purpose.
PONV: 0.075 mg immediately prior to anesthesia induction
Dosage Forms
Injection, solution:
Aloxi®: 0.05 mg/mL (1.5 mL, 5 mL)

palonosetron hydrochloride *see* palonosetron *on page 716*
2-PAM *see* pralidoxime *on page 776*
Pamelor® [US] *see* nortriptyline *on page 680*

pamidronate (pa mi DROE nate)

Sound-Alike/Look-Alike Issues
Aredia® may be confused with Adriamycin®, Meridia®
Synonyms pamidronate disodium
U.S./Canadian Brand Names Aredia® [US/Can]; Pamidronate Disodium® [Can]; Rhoxal-pamidronate [Can]

Therapeutic Category Bisphosphonate Derivative

Use Treatment of hypercalcemia associated with malignancy; treatment of osteolytic bone lesions associated with multiple myeloma or metastatic breast cancer; moderate to severe Paget disease of bone

Usual Dosage Dilute prior to administration and infuse intravenously slowly over at least 2 hours. Single doses should not exceed 90 mg. I.V.: Adults:

Hypercalcemia of malignancy:

Moderate cancer-related hypercalcemia (corrected serum calcium: 12-13.5 mg/dL): 60-90 mg, as a single dose over 2-24 hours

Severe cancer-related hypercalcemia (corrected serum calcium: >13.5 mg/dL): 90 mg, as a single dose over 2-24 hours

A period of 7 days should elapse before the use of second course; repeat infusions every 2-3 weeks have been suggested, however, could be administered every 2-3 months according to the degree and of severity of hypercalcemia and/or the type of malignancy.

Osteolytic bone lesions with multiple myeloma: 90 mg over 2-4 hours monthly

Osteolytic bone lesions with metastatic breast cancer: 90 mg over 2 hours repeated every 3-4 weeks

Paget disease: 30 mg over 4 hours daily for 3 consecutive days

Dosage Forms

Injection, powder for reconstitution: 30 mg, 90 mg

Aredia®: 30 mg, 90 mg

Injection, solution: 3 mg/mL (10 mL); 6 mg/mL (10 mL); 9 mg/mL (10 mL)

Pamidronate Disodium® [Can] *see* pamidronate *on page 716*

pamidronate disodium *see* pamidronate *on page 716*

Pamine® [US/Can] *see* methscopolamine *on page 618*

Pamine® Forte [US] *see* methscopolamine *on page 618*

p-aminoclonidine *see* apraclonidine *on page 90*

Pamprin IB® *(Discontinued)* *see* ibuprofen *on page 495*

Pamprin® Maximum Strength All Day Relief [US-OTC] *see* naproxen *on page 656*

Pan-2400™ [US-OTC] *see* pancreatin *on page 717*

Panadol® *(Discontinued)* *see* acetaminophen *on page 19*

Panafil® [US] *see* chlorophyllin, papain, and urea *on page 203*

Panafil® SE [US] *see* chlorophyllin, papain, and urea *on page 203*

Panasal® 5/500 *(Discontinued)*

Pancof® *(Discontinued)* *see* pseudoephedrine, dihydrocodeine, and chlorpheniramine *on page 803*

Pancof®-EXP [US] *see* dihydrocodeine, pseudoephedrine, and guaifenesin *on page 299*

Pancof-HC *(Discontinued)*

Pancof-XP *(Discontinued)*

Pancrease® [Can] *see* pancrelipase *on page 718*

Pancrease® MT [US/Can] *see* pancrelipase *on page 718*

pancreatin (PAN kree a tin)

Sound-Alike/Look-Alike Issues

pancreatin may be confused with Panretin®

U.S./Canadian Brand Names Hi-Vegi-Lip [US-OTC]; Pan-2400™ [US-OTC]; Veg-Pancreatin 4X [US-OTC]

Therapeutic Category Enzyme

Use Relief of functional indigestion due to enzyme deficiency or imbalance

Usual Dosage Oral: Adults: Actual dose varies with condition of patient and is usually given with each meal or snack.

Dosage Forms

Capsule: Lipase 8500 units, protease 50,000 units, amylase 50,000 units

Pan-2400™ [OTC]: Lipase 9816 units, protease 60,214 units, amylase 75,900 units

Tablet: Lipase 565 units, protease 8200 units, amylase 8200 units [pancreatin 325 mg]; lipase 2400 units, protease 30,000 units, amylase 30,000 units

Hi-Vegi-Lip [OTC]: Lipase 4800 units, protease 60,000 units, amylase 60,000 units

Veg-Pancreatin 4X [OTC]: Lipase 5500 units, protease 69,000 units, amylase 69,000 units

Pancrecarb MS® [US] *see* pancrelipase *on page 718*

pancrelipase (pan kre LYE pase)

Synonyms lipancreatin

U.S./Canadian Brand Names Cotazym® [Can]; Creon® [US/Can]; Pancrease® MT [US/Can]; Pancrease® [Can]; Pancrecarb MS® [US]; Pangestyme™ CN [US]; Pangestyme™ EC [US]; Pangestyme™ MT [US]; Pangestyme™ UL [US]; Plaretase® 8000 [US]; Ultrase® MT [US/Can]; Ultrase® [US/Can]; Viokase® [US/Can]

Therapeutic Category Enzyme

Use Replacement therapy in symptomatic treatment of malabsorption syndrome caused by pancreatic insufficiency

Usual Dosage Oral:

Powder: Actual dose depends on the condition being treated and the digestive requirements of the patient

Children <1 year: Start with 1/8 teaspoonful with feedings

Adults: 0.7 g (1/4 teaspoonful) with meals

Capsules/tablets: The following dosage recommendations are only an approximation for initial dosages. The actual dosage will depend on the condition being treated and the digestive requirements of the individual patient. Adjust dose based on body weight and stool fat content. Total daily dose reflects ~3 meals/day and 2-3 snacks/day, with half the mealtime dose given with a snack. Older patients may need less units/kg due to increased weight, but decreased ingestion of fat/kg. Maximum dose: 2500 units of lipase/kg/meal (10,000 units of lipase/kg/day)

Children:

<1 year: 2000 units of lipase with meals

1-6 years: 4000-8000 units of lipase with meals and 4000 units with snacks

7-12 years: 4000-12,000 units of lipase with meals and snacks

Adults: 4000-48,000 units of lipase with meals and snacks

Occluded feeding tubes: One tablet of Viokase® crushed with one 325 mg tablet of sodium bicarbonate (to activate the Viokase®) in 5 mL of water can be instilled into the nasogastric tube and clamped for 5 minutes; then, flushed with 50 mL of tap water

Dosage Forms

Capsule, delayed release, enteric coated granules:

Pangestyme™ CN-10: Lipase 10,000 units, protease 37,500 units, amylase 33,200 units

Pangestyme™ CN-20: Lipase 20,000 units, protease 75,000 units, amylase 66,400 units

Pangestyme™ EC: Lipase 4500 units, protease 25,000 units, and amylase 20,000 units

Pangestyme™ MT16: Lipase 16,000 units, protease 48,000 units, and amylase 48,000 units

Pangestyme™ UL 12: Lipase 12,000 units, protease 39,000 units, and amylase 39,000 units

Pangestyme™ UL 18: Lipase 18,000 units, protease 58,500 units, and amylase 58,500 units

Pangestyme™ UL 20: Lipase 20,000 units, protease 65,000 units, and amylase 65,000 units

Capsule, delayed release, enteric coated microspheres: Lipase 4500 units, protease 25,000 units, and amylase 20,000 units

Creon® 5: Lipase 5000 units, protease 18,750 units, and amylase 16,600 units

Creon® 10, Palcaps 10: Lipase 10,000 units, protease 37,500 units, and amylase 33,200 units

Creon® 20, Palcaps 20: Lipase 20,000 units, protease 75,000 units, and amylase 66,400 units

Pancrecarb MS-4®: Lipase 4000 units, protease 25,000 units, and amylase 25,000 units [buffered]

Pancrecarb MS-8®: Lipase 8000 units, protease 45,000 units, and amylase 40,000 units [buffered]

Pancrecarb MS-16®: Lipase 16,000 units, protease 52,000 units, and amylase 52,000 units [buffered]

Capsule, enteric coated microspheres: Lipase 4500 units, protease 25,000 units, and amylase 20,000 units

Ultrase®: Lipase 4500 units, protease 25,000 units, and amylase 20,000 units

Capsule, enteric coated microtablets:

Pancrease® MT 4: Lipase 4000 units, protease 12,000 units, and amylase 12,000 units

Pancrease® MT 10: Lipase 10,000 units, protease 30,000 units, and amylase 30,000 units

Pancrease® MT 16: Lipase 16,000 units, protease 48,000 units, and amylase 48,000 units

Pancrease® MT 20: Lipase 20,000 units, protease 44,000 units, and amylase 56,000 units

Capsule, enteric coated minitablets:

Ultrase® MT12: Lipase 12,000 units, protease 39,000 units, and amylase 39,000 units

Ultrase® MT18: Lipase 18,000 units, protease 58,500 units, and amylase 58,500 units

Ultrase® MT20: Lipase 20,000 units, protease 65,000 units, and amylase 65,000 units

Powder:

Viokase®: Lipase 16,800 units, protease 70,000 units, and amylase 70,000 units per 0.7 g (227 g)

Tablet: Lipase 8000 units, protease 30,000 units, and amylase 30,000 units

Plaretase™ 8000, Viokase® 8: Lipase 8000 units, protease 30,000 units, and amylase 30,000 units

Viokase® 16: Lipase 16,000 units, protease 60,000 units, and amylase 60,000 units

pancuronium (pan kyoo ROE nee um)

Sound-Alike/Look-Alike Issues
pancuronium may be confused with pipecuronium

Synonyms pancuronium bromide

U.S./Canadian Brand Names Pancuronium Bromide® [Can]

Therapeutic Category Skeletal Muscle Relaxant

Use Adjunct to general anesthesia to facilitate endotracheal intubation and to relax skeletal muscles during surgery; to facilitate mechanical ventilation in ICU patients; does not relieve pain or produce sedation

Drug of choice for neuromuscular blockade except in patients with renal failure, hepatic failure, or cardiovascular instability or in situations not suited for pancuronium's long duration of action

Usual Dosage Administer I.V.; dose to effect; doses will vary due to interpatient variability; use ideal body weight for obese patients

Surgery:

Neonates <1 month:

Test dose: 0.02 mg/kg to measure responsiveness

Initial: 0.03 mg/kg/dose repeated twice at 5- to 10-minute intervals as needed; maintenance: 0.03-0.09 mg/kg/dose every 30 minutes to 4 hours as needed

Infants >1 month, Children, and Adults: Initial: 0.06-0.1 mg/kg or 0.05 mg/kg after initial dose of succinylcholine for intubation; maintenance dose: 0.01 mg/kg 60-100 minutes after initial dose and then 0.01 mg/kg every 25-60 minutes

Pretreatment/priming: 10% of intubating dose given 3-5 minutes before initial dose

ICU: 0.05-0.1 mg/kg bolus followed by 0.8-1.7 mcg/kg/minute once initial recovery from bolus observed or 0.1-0.2 mg/kg every 1-3 hours

Dosage Forms

Injection, solution: 1 mg/mL (10 mL); 2 mg/mL (2 mL, 5 mL)

Pancuronium Bromide® [Can] *see* pancuronium *on page 719*

pancuronium bromide *see* pancuronium *on page 719*

Pandel® [US] *see* hydrocortisone (topical) *on page 485*

Panectyl® [Can] *see* trimeprazine *(Canada only) on page 953*

Pangestyme™ CN [US] *see* pancrelipase *on page 718*

Pangestyme™ EC [US] *see* pancrelipase *on page 718*

Pangestyme™ MT [US] *see* pancrelipase *on page 718*

Pangestyme™ UL [US] *see* pancrelipase *on page 718*

Panglobulin® NF *(Discontinued)* *see* immune globulin (intravenous) *on page 503*

Panhematin® [US] *see* hemin *on page 467*

panitumumab (pan i TOOM yoo mab)

Synonyms ABX-EGF; NSC-742319; rHuMAb-EGFr

U.S./Canadian Brand Names Vectibix™ [US]

Therapeutic Category Antineoplastic Agent, Monoclonal Antibody; Epidermal Growth Factor Receptor (EGFR) Inhibitor

Use Monotherapy in treatment of refractory (EGFR-expressing) metastatic colorectal cancer

Usual Dosage I.V.: Adults: Colorectal cancer: 6 mg/kg every 2 weeks

Dosing adjustment for toxicity:

Infusion reactions, mild-to-moderate (grade 1 or 2): Reduce the infusion rate by 50% for the duration of infusion

Infusion reactions, severe (grade 3 or 4): Immediately and permanently discontinue treatment

Skin toxicity (grade 3 or 4): Withhold treatment; if skin toxicity does not improve to ≤ grade 2 within 1 month, permanently discontinue. If skin toxicity improves to ≤ grade 2 within 1 month (with patient missing ≤2 doses), resume treatment at 50% of the original dose. Dose may be increased in increments of 25% of the original dose (up to 6 mg/kg) if skin toxicities do not recur. For recurrent skin toxicity, permanently discontinue.

Dosage Forms

Injection, solution [preservative free]:

Vectibix®: 20 mg/mL (5 mL, 10 mL, 20 mL)

Panixine DisperDose™ *(Discontinued)* see cephalexin *on page 194*
Panlor® DC [US] see acetaminophen, caffeine, and dihydrocodeine *on page 25*
Panlor® SS [US] see acetaminophen, caffeine, and dihydrocodeine *on page 25*
Panocaps *(Discontinued)* see pancrelipase *on page 718*
Panocaps MT *(Discontinued)* see pancrelipase *on page 718*
Panokase® 16 *(Discontinued)* see pancrelipase *on page 718*
Panokase® *(Discontinued)* see pancrelipase *on page 718*
PanOxyl® [US/Can] see benzoyl peroxide *on page 126*
PanOxyl®-AQ [US] see benzoyl peroxide *on page 126*
PanOxyl® Aqua Gel [US] see benzoyl peroxide *on page 126*
PanOxyl® Bar [US-OTC] see benzoyl peroxide *on page 126*
Panretin® [US/Can] see alitretinoin *on page 46*
Panscol® Lotion *(Discontinued)* see salicylic acid *on page 850*
Panscol® Ointment *(Discontinued)* see salicylic acid *on page 850*
Panto™ IV [Can] see pantoprazole *on page 720*
Panto-250 [US] see pantothenic acid *on page 721*
Pantoloc® [Can] see pantoprazole *on page 720*
Pantoloc® M [Can] see pantoprazole *on page 720*
Pantopon® *(Discontinued)*

pantoprazole (pan TOE pra zole)

Sound-Alike/Look-Alike Issues
Protonix® may be confused with Lotronex®, Lovenox®, protamine
U.S./Canadian Brand Names Apo-Pantoprazole [Can]; Pantoloc® M [Can]; Pantoloc® [Can]; Panto™ IV [Can]; PMS-Pantoprazole [Can]; Protonix® [US/Can]; Ran-Pantoprazole [Can]
Therapeutic Category Proton Pump Inhibitor
Use
Oral: Treatment and maintenance of healing of erosive esophagitis associated with GERD; reduction in relapse rates of daytime and nighttime heartburn symptoms in GERD; hypersecretory disorders associated with Zollinger-Ellison syndrome or other GI hypersecretory disorders
I.V.: Short-term treatment (7-10 days) of patients with gastroesophageal reflux disease (GERD) and a history of erosive esophagitis; hypersecretory disorders associated with Zollinger-Ellison syndrome or other neoplastic disorders
Usual Dosage Adults:
Oral:
Erosive esophagitis associated with GERD:
Treatment: 40 mg once daily for up to 8 weeks; an additional 8 weeks may be used in patients who have not healed after an 8-week course
Maintenance of healing: 40 mg once daily
Note: Lower doses (20 mg once daily) have been used successfully in mild GERD treatment and maintenance of healing
Hypersecretory disorders (including Zollinger-Ellison): Initial: 40 mg twice daily; adjust dose based on patient needs; doses up to 240 mg/day have been administered
I.V.:
Erosive esophagitis associated with GERD: 40 mg once daily for 7-10 days
Hypersecretory disorders: 80 mg twice daily; adjust dose based on acid output measurements; 160-240 mg/day in divided doses has been used for a limited period (up to 7 days)
Dosage Forms
Granules for suspension, delayed release, enteric coated, as sodium, oral:
Protonix®: 40 mg/packet (30s)
Injection, powder for reconstitution:
Protonix®: 40 mg
Tablet, delayed release: 20 mg, 40 mg
Protonix®: 20 mg, 40 mg
Tablet, enteric coated:
Pantoloc® M [CAN]: 40 mg [not available in the U.S.]

pantothenic acid (pan toe THEN ik AS id)

Synonyms calcium pantothenate; vitamin B_5
U.S./Canadian Brand Names Panto-250 [US]
Therapeutic Category Vitamin, Water Soluble
Use Pantothenic acid deficiency
Usual Dosage Oral: Adults: Recommended daily dose 4-7 mg/day
Dosage Forms
  Capsule:
    Panto-250: 250 mg [contains calcium 23 mg]
  Liquid: 200 mg/5 mL (240 mL)
  Tablet: 100 mg, 200 mg, 250 mg, 500 mg
  Tablet, sustained release: 500 mg

pantothenyl alcohol see dexpanthenol on page 281

papain and urea (pa PAY in & yoor EE a)

U.S./Canadian Brand Names Accuzyme® SE [US]; Accuzyme® [US]; AllanEnzyme [US]; Ethezyme™ 650 [US]; Kovia® [US]; Paptase™ [US]
Therapeutic Category Enzyme, Topical Debridement; Topical Skin Product
Use Debridement of necrotic tissue and liquefaction of slough in acute and chronic lesions such as pressure ulcers, varicose and diabetic ulcers, burns, postoperative wounds, pilonidal cyst wounds, carbuncles, and miscellaneous traumatic or infected wounds
Usual Dosage Topical: Adults: Apply with each dressing change. Daily or twice daily dressing changes are preferred, but may be every 2-3 days. Cover with dressing following application.
Ointment: Apply 1/8-inch thickness over the wound with clean applicator.
Spray: Completely cover the wound site so that the wound is not visible.
Dosage Forms
  Aerosol, topical:
    Paptase™: Papain 8.3×10^5 units/g and urea 10% (45 g)
  Emulsion, topical [spray]:
    Accuzyme® SE: Papain 8.3×10^5 units/g and urea 10% (34 mL)
  Ointment, topical:
    Accuzyme®: Papain 8.3×10^5 units/g and urea 10% (6 g, 30 g)
    AllanEnzyme 650: Papain 8.3×10^5 units/g and urea 10% (30 g)
    Kovia®: Papain 8.3×10^5 units/g and urea 10% (3.5 g) [single-dose packet]; 30 g
  Solution, topical [spray]:
    AllanEnzyme: Papain 8.3×10^5 units/g and urea 10% (33 mL)

papain, urea, and chlorophyllin see chlorophyllin, papain, and urea on page 203

papaverine (pa PAV er een)

Synonyms papaverine hydrochloride
U.S./Canadian Brand Names Para-Time SR® [US]
Therapeutic Category Vasodilator
Use Oral: Relief of peripheral and cerebral ischemia associated with arterial spasm and myocardial ischemia complicated by arrhythmias
Usual Dosage
  I.M., I.V.:
    Children: 6 mg/kg/day in 4 divided doses
    Adults: 30-65 mg (rarely up to 120 mg); may repeat every 3 hours
  Oral, sustained release: Adults: 150-300 mg every 12 hours; in difficult cases: 150 mg every 8 hours
Dosage Forms
  Capsule, sustained release: 150 mg
    Para-Time SR®: 150 mg
  Injection, solution: 30 mg/mL (2 mL, 10 mL)

papaverine hydrochloride see papaverine on page 721
Papfyll™ [US] see chlorophyllin, papain, and urea on page 203

papillomavirus (Types 6, 11, 16, 18) recombinant vaccine
(pap ih LO ma VYE rus typs six e LEV en SIX teen AYE teen ree KOM be nant vak SEEN)

Synonyms HPV Vaccine; human papillomavirus vaccine; papillomavirus vaccine, recombinant; quadrivalent human papillomavirus vaccine

U.S./Canadian Brand Names Gardasil® [US/Can]

Therapeutic Category Vaccine

Use Females: Prevention of cervical, vulvar, and vaginal cancer, genital warts, cervical adenocarcinoma *in situ*, and vulvar, vaginal, or cervical intraepithelial neoplasia caused by human papillomavirus (HPV) types 6, 11, 16, 18

The Advisory Committee on Immunization Practices (ACIP) recommends routine vaccination for females 11-12 years of age; catch-up vaccination is recommended for females 13-26 years of age

Usual Dosage I.M.: Females: Children ≥9 years and Adults ≤26 years: 0.5 mL followed by 0.5 mL at 2 and 6 months after initial dose

CDC recommended immunization schedule: Administer first dose to females at age 11-12 years; begin series in females aged 13-26 years if not previously vaccinated. Minimum interval between first and second doses is 4 weeks; the minimum interval between second and third doses is 12 weeks.

Dosage Forms

Injection, suspension [preservative free]:
Gardasil®: HPV 6 L1 protein 20 mcg, HPV 11 L1 protein 40 mcg, HPV 16 L1 protein 40 mcg, and HPV 18 L1 protein 20 mcg per 0.5 mL (0.5 mL)

papillomavirus vaccine, recombinant *see* papillomavirus (Types 6, 11, 16, 18) recombinant vaccine *on page 722*

Paptase™ [US] *see* papain and urea *on page 721*

para-aminosalicylate sodium *see* aminosalicylic acid *on page 61*

paracetamol *see* acetaminophen *on page 19*

Paraflex® (Discontinued) *see* chlorzoxazone *on page 215*

Parafon Forte® [Can] *see* chlorzoxazone *on page 215*

Parafon Forte® (Discontinued) *see* chlorzoxazone *on page 215*

Parafon Forte® DSC [US] *see* chlorzoxazone *on page 215*

Paraplatin-AQ [Can] *see* carboplatin *on page 178*

Paraplatin® (Discontinued) *see* carboplatin *on page 178*

parathyroid hormone (1-34) *see* teriparatide *on page 911*

Para-Time SR® [US] *see* papaverine *on page 721*

Parcaine™ [US] *see* proparacaine *on page 794*

Parcopa™ [US] *see* carbidopa and levodopa *on page 177*

Paredrine® (Discontinued)

paregoric (par e GOR ik)

Sound-Alike/Look-Alike Issues
paregoric may be confused with Percogesic®
camphorated tincture of opium is an error-prone synonym (mistaken as opium tincture)

Therapeutic Category Analgesic, Narcotic

Controlled Substance C-III

Use Treatment of diarrhea or relief of pain; neonatal opiate withdrawal

Usual Dosage Oral:
Neonatal opiate withdrawal: 3-6 drops every 3-6 hours as needed, or initially 0.2 mL every 3 hours; increase dosage by approximately 0.05 mL every 3 hours until withdrawal symptoms are controlled; it is rare to exceed 0.7 mL/dose. Stabilize withdrawal symptoms for 3-5 days, then gradually decrease dosage over a 2- to 4-week period.
Children: 0.25-0.5 mL/kg 1-4 times/day
Adults: 5-10 mL 1-4 times/day

Dosage Forms
Liquid, oral: Morphine equivalent 2 mg/5 mL

Paremyd® [US] *see* hydroxyamphetamine and tropicamide *on page 489*

parenteral nutrition *see* total parenteral nutrition *on page 938*

Parepectolin® (Discontinued)

paricalcitol (pah ri KAL si tole)

U.S./Canadian Brand Names Zemplar® [US/Can]

Therapeutic Category Vitamin D Analog

Use

I.V.: Prevention and treatment of secondary hyperparathyroidism associated with stage 5 chronic kidney disease (CKD)

Oral: Prevention and treatment of secondary hyperparathyroidism associated with stage 3 and 4 CKD

Usual Dosage Note: If hypercalcemia or Ca x P >75 is observed, reduce or interrupt dosing until parameters are normalized.

Secondary hyperparathyroidism associated with chronic renal failure (stage 5 CKD): Children ≥5 years and Adults: I.V.: 0.04-0.1 mcg/kg (2.8-7 mcg) given as a bolus dose no more frequently than every other day at any time during dialysis; dose may be increased by 2-4 mcg every 2-4 weeks; doses as high as 0.24 mcg/kg (16.8 mcg) have been administered safely; the dose of paricalcitol should be adjusted based on serum intact PTH (iPTH) levels, as follows:

Same or increasing iPTH level: Increase paricalcitol dose

iPTH level decreased by <30%: Increase paricalcitol dose

iPTH level decreased by >30% and <60%: Maintain paricalcitol dose

iPTH level decrease by >60%: Decrease paricalcitol dose

iPTH level 1.5-3 times upper limit of normal: Maintain paricalcitol dose

Secondary hyperparathyroidism associated with stage 3 and 4 CKD: Adults: Oral: Initial dose based on baseline iPTH:

iPTH ≤500 pg/mL: 1 mcg/day or 2 mcg 3 times/week

iPTH >500 pg/mL: 2 mcg/day or 4 mcg 3 times/week

Dosage adjustment based on iPTH level relative to baseline, adjust dose at 2-4 week intervals:

iPTH same or increased: Increase paricalcitol dose by 1 mcg/day or 2 mcg 3 times/week

iPTH decreased by <30%: Increase paricalcitol dose by 1 mcg/day or 2 mcg 3 times//week

iPTH decreased by ≥30% or ≤60%: Maintain paricalcitol dose

iPTH decreased by >60%: Decrease paricalcitol dose by 1 mcg/day* or 2 mcg 3 times/week

iPTH <60 pg/mL: Decrease paricalcitol dose by 1 mcg/day* or 2 mcg 3 times/week

*If patient is taking the lowest dose on a once-daily regimen, but further dose reduction is needed, decrease dose to 1 mcg 3 times/week. If further dose reduction is required, withhold drug as needed and restart at a lower dose. If applicable, calcium-phosphate binder dosing may also be adjusted or withheld, or switch to noncalcium-based binder

Dosage Forms

Capsule, gelatin:

Zemplar®: 1 mcg, 2 mcg, 4 mcg

Injection, solution:

Zemplar®: 2 mcg/mL (1 mL); 5 mcg/mL (1 mL, 2 mL)

Pariet® [Can] *see* rabeprazole *on page 815*

pariprazole *see* rabeprazole *on page 815*

Parlodel® [US/Can] *see* bromocriptine *on page 143*

Parlodel® SnapTabs® [US] *see* bromocriptine *on page 143*

Parnate® [US/Can] *see* tranylcypromine *on page 943*

paromomycin (par oh moe MYE sin)

Synonyms paromomycin sulfate

U.S./Canadian Brand Names Humatin® [Can]

Therapeutic Category Amebicide

Use Treatment of acute and chronic intestinal amebiasis; hepatic coma

Usual Dosage Oral:

Intestinal amebiasis: Children and Adults: 25-35 mg/kg/day in 3 divided doses for 5-10 days

Dientamoeba fragilis: Children and Adults: 25-30 mg/kg/day in 3 divided doses for 7 days

Tapeworm (fish, dog, bovine, porcine):

Children: 11 mg/kg every 15 minutes for 4 doses

Adults: 1 g every 15 minutes for 4 doses

Hepatic coma: Adults: 4 g/day in 2-4 divided doses for 5-6 days

Dwarf tapeworm: Children and Adults: 45 mg/kg/dose every day for 5-7 days

◀ **Dosage Forms**
Capsule: 250 mg

paromomycin sulfate *see paromomycin on page 723*

paroxetine (pa ROKS e teen)

Sound-Alike/Look-Alike Issues
PARoxetine may be confused with FLUoxetine, paclitaxel, pyridoxine
Paxil® may be confused with Doxil®, paclitaxel, Plavix®, Taxol®

Synonyms paroxetine hydrochloride; paroxetine mesylate

Tall-Man PARoxetine

U.S./Canadian Brand Names Apo-Paroxetine® [Can]; CO Paroxetine [Can]; Gen-Paroxetine [Can]; Novo-Paroxetine [Can]; Paxil CR® [US/Can]; Paxil® [US/Can]; Pexeva® [US]; PMS-Paroxetine [Can]; ratio-Paroxetine [Can]; Rhoxal-paroxetine [Can]; Sandoz-Paroxetine [Can]

Therapeutic Category Antidepressant, Selective Serotonin Reuptake Inhibitor

Use Treatment of major depressive disorder (MDD); treatment of panic disorder with or without agoraphobia; obsessive-compulsive disorder (OCD); social anxiety disorder (social phobia); generalized anxiety disorder (GAD); posttraumatic stress disorder (PTSD); premenstrual dysphoric disorder (PMDD)

Usual Dosage Oral: Adults:
Major depressive disorder:
Paxil®, Pexeva®: Initial: 20 mg once daily, preferably in the morning; increase if needed by 10 mg/day increments at intervals of at least 1 week; maximum dose: 50 mg/day
Paxil CR®: Initial: 25 mg once daily; increase if needed by 12.5 mg/day increments at intervals of at least 1 week; maximum dose: 62.5 mg/day
Generalized anxiety disorder (Paxil®, Pexeva®): Initial: 20 mg once daily, preferably in the morning (if dose is increased, adjust in increments of 10 mg/day at 1-week intervals); doses of 20-50 mg/day were used in clinical trials, however, no greater benefit was seen with doses >20 mg.
Obsessive-compulsive disorder (Paxil®, Pexeva™): Initial: 20 mg once daily, preferably in the morning; increase if needed by 10 mg/day increments at intervals of at least 1 week; recommended dose: 40 mg/day; range: 20-60 mg/day; maximum dose: 60 mg/day
Panic disorder:
Paxil®, Pexeva®: Initial: 10 mg once daily, preferably in the morning; increase if needed by 10 mg/day increments at intervals of at least 1 week; recommended dose: 40 mg/day; range: 10-60 mg/day; maximum dose: 60 mg/day
Paxil CR®: Initial: 12.5 mg once daily; increase if needed by 12.5 mg/day at intervals of at least 1 week; maximum dose: 75 mg/day
Premenstrual dysphoric disorder (Paxil CR®): Initial: 12.5 mg once daily in the morning; may be increased to 25 mg/day; dosing changes should occur at intervals of at least 1 week. May be given daily throughout the menstrual cycle or limited to the luteal phase.
Posttraumatic stress disorder (Paxil®): Initial: 20 mg once daily, preferably in the morning; increase if needed by 10 mg/day increments at intervals of at least 1 week; range: 20-50 mg. Limited data suggest doses of 40 mg/day were not more efficacious than 20 mg/day.
Social anxiety disorder:
Paxil®: Initial: 20 mg once daily, preferably in the morning; recommended dose: 20 mg/day; range: 20-60 mg/day; doses >20 mg may not have additional benefit
Paxil CR®: Initial: 12.5 mg once daily, preferably in the morning; may be increased by 12.5 mg/day at intervals of at least 1 week; maximum dose: 37.5 mg/day

Dosage Forms Note: Strength expressed as base:
Suspension, oral: 10 mg/5 mL
Paxil®: 10 mg/5 mL (250 mL)
Tablet: 10 mg, 20 mg, 30 mg, 40 mg
Paxil®, Pexeva®: 10 mg, 20 mg, 30 mg, 40 mg
Tablet, controlled release: 37.5 mg
Paxil CR®: 12.5 mg, 25 mg, 37.5 mg
Tablet, extended release: 12.5 mg, 25 mg

paroxetine hydrochloride *see paroxetine on page 724*
paroxetine mesylate *see paroxetine on page 724*
Partuss® LA *(Discontinued)*
Parvolex® [Can] *see acetylcysteine on page 30*
PAS *see aminosalicylic acid on page 61*

Paser® **[US]** *see* aminosalicylic acid *on page 61*
Pataday™ **[US]** *see* olopatadine *on page 696*
Patanase® **[US]** *see* olopatadine *on page 696*
Patanol® **[US/Can]** *see* olopatadine *on page 696*
Pathilon® *(Discontinued)*
Pathocil® **[Can]** *see* dicloxacillin *on page 293*
Pathocil® *(Discontinued) see* dicloxacillin *on page 293*
Pavabid® *(Discontinued) see* papaverine *on page 721*
Pavatine® *(Discontinued)*
Pavulon® *(Discontinued) see* pancuronium *on page 719*
Paxene® *(Discontinued) see* paclitaxel *on page 714*
Paxil® **[US/Can]** *see* paroxetine *on page 724*
Paxil CR® **[US/Can]** *see* paroxetine *on page 724*
PCE® **[US/Can]** *see* erythromycin *on page 354*
PCEC *see* rabies virus vaccine *on page 816*
P Chlor GG **[US]** *see* chlorpheniramine, phenylephrine, and guaifenesin *on page 210*
PCM **[US]** *see* chlorpheniramine, phenylephrine, and methscopolamine *on page 210*
PCM Allergy *(Discontinued) see* chlorpheniramine, phenylephrine, and methscopolamine *on page 210*
PCV7 *see* pneumococcal conjugate vaccine (7-valent) *on page 762*
PD-Cof **[US]** *see* chlorpheniramine, phenylephrine, and dextromethorphan *on page 209*
PD-Hist-D **[US]** *see* chlorpheniramine and phenylephrine *on page 206*
pectin, gelatin, and methylcellulose *see* gelatin, pectin, and methylcellulose *on page 438*
Pedameth® *(Discontinued)*
Pediacare® Children's Long Acting Cough Plus Cold *(Discontinued) see* pseudoephedrine and dextromethorphan *on page 802*
PediaCare® Children's Medicated Freezer Pops Long Acting Cough *(Discontinued) see* dextromethorphan *on page 284*
PediaCare® Cold and Allergy *(Discontinued) see* chlorpheniramine and pseudoephedrine *on page 207*
PediaCare® Decongestant Infants *(Discontinued) see* pseudoephedrine *on page 801*
Pediacare® Infants' Decongestant & Cough *(Discontinued) see* pseudoephedrine and dextromethorphan *on page 802*
PediaCare® Infants' Long-Acting Cough *(Discontinued) see* dextromethorphan *on page 284*
PediaCare® Multi-Symptom Cold *(Discontinued) see* chlorpheniramine, pseudoephedrine, and dextromethorphan *on page 212*
PediaCare® NightRest Cough and Cold *(Discontinued) see* chlorpheniramine, pseudoephedrine, and dextromethorphan *on page 212*
Pediacof® *(Discontinued) see* chlorpheniramine, phenylephrine, codeine, and potassium iodide *on page 212*
Pediaflor® *(Discontinued) see* fluoride *on page 411*
PediaHist DM **[US]** *see* brompheniramine, pseudoephedrine, and dextromethorphan *on page 146*
Pedialyte® **[US-OTC]** *see* nutritional formula, enteral/oral *on page 689*
PediaPatch Transdermal Patch *(Discontinued) see* salicylic acid *on page 850*
Pediapred® **[US/Can]** *see* prednisolone (systemic) *on page 781*
Pedia-Profen™ *(Discontinued) see* ibuprofen *on page 495*
Pedia Relief™ **[US-OTC]** *see* chlorpheniramine, pseudoephedrine, and dextromethorphan *on page 212*
Pedia Relief Cough and Cold **[US-OTC]** *see* pseudoephedrine and dextromethorphan *on page 802*
Pedia Relief Infants **[US-OTC]** *see* pseudoephedrine and dextromethorphan *on page 802*
Pediarix® **[US/Can]** *see* diphtheria, tetanus toxoids, acellular pertussis, hepatitis B (recombinant), and poliovirus (inactivated) vaccine *on page 308*
PediaTan™ **[US]** *see* chlorpheniramine *on page 205*
PediaTan™ D **[US]** *see* chlorpheniramine and phenylephrine *on page 206*
Pediatex™ 12 *(Discontinued) see* carbinoxamine *on page 177*
Pediatex™-D *(Discontinued)*

Pediatex™ *(Discontinued)* see carbinoxamine *on page 177*

Pediatex™ DM *(Discontinued)*

Pediatric Digoxin CSD [Can] see digoxin *on page 296*

Pediatric Triban® *(Discontinued)*

Pediatrix [Can] see acetaminophen *on page 19*

Pediazole® [Can] see erythromycin and sulfisoxazole *on page 356*

Pediazole® *(Discontinued)* see erythromycin and sulfisoxazole *on page 356*

Pedi-Boro® [US-OTC] see aluminum sulfate and calcium acetate *on page 55*

Pedi-Dri® [US] see nystatin *on page 690*

PediOtic® [US] see neomycin, polymyxin B, and hydrocortisone *on page 663*

Pedi-Pro® [US] see benzalkonium chloride *on page 123*

PedvaxHIB® [US/Can] see *Haemophilus* B conjugate vaccine *on page 464*

PEG see polyethylene glycol 3350 *on page 765*

PEG-L-asparaginase see pegaspargase *on page 726*

pegademase (bovine) (peg A de mase BOE vine)

U.S./Canadian Brand Names Adagen® [US/Can]

Therapeutic Category Enzyme

Use Orphan drug: Enzyme replacement therapy for adenosine deaminase (ADA) deficiency in patients with severe combined immunodeficiency disease (SCID) who can not benefit from bone marrow transplant; not a cure for SCID, unlike bone marrow transplants, injections must be used the rest of the child's life, therefore is not really an alternative

Usual Dosage I.M.: Children: Dose given every 7 days, 10 units/kg the first dose, 15 units/kg the second dose, and 20 units/kg the third dose; maintenance dose: 20 units/kg/week is recommended depending on patient's ADA level; maximum single dose: 30 units/kg

Dosage Forms

Injection, solution [preservative free]:

Adagen®: 250 units/mL (1.5 mL)

Peganone® [US/Can] see ethotoin *on page 381*

pegaptanib (peg AP ta nib)

Synonyms EYE001; pegaptanib sodium

U.S./Canadian Brand Names Macugen® [US/Can]

Therapeutic Category Ophthalmic Agent; Vaccine, Recombinant

Use Treatment of neovascular (wet) age-related macular degeneration (AMD)

Usual Dosage Intravitreous injection: Adults: AMD: 0.3 mg into affected eye every 6 weeks

Dosage Forms

Injection, solution [preservative free; prefilled syringe]:

Macugen®: 0.3 mg/90 μL (90 μL)

pegaptanib sodium see pegaptanib *on page 726*

pegaspargase (peg AS par jase)

Sound-Alike/Look-Alike Issues

pegaspargase may be confused with asparaginase

Synonyms NSC-644954; PEG-L-asparaginase

U.S./Canadian Brand Names Oncaspar® [US]

Therapeutic Category Antineoplastic Agent

Use Treatment of acute lymphocytic leukemia (ALL); treatment of ALL with previous hypersensitivity to native L-asparaginase

Usual Dosage Usually administered as part of a combination chemotherapy regimen.

I.M. administration is **preferred** over I.V. administration due to lower incidence of hepatotoxicity, coagulopathy, gastrointestinal, and renal disorders with I.M. administration.

Children: I.M., I.V.:

Body surface area <0.6 m²: 82.5 int. units/kg every 14 days

Body surface area ≥0.6 m²: 2500 int. units/m² every 14 days

Adults: I.M., I.V.: 2500 int. units/m² every 14 days

Hemodialysis: Significant drug removal is unlikely based on physiochemical characteristics
Peritoneal dialysis: Significant drug removal is unlikely based on physiochemical characteristics

Dosage Forms
Injection, solution [preservative free]:
Oncaspar®: 750 units/mL (5 mL)

Pegasys® [US/Can] *see* peginterferon alfa-2a *on page 727*
Pegasys [Can] *see* peginterferon alfa-2b and ribavirin *(Canada only) on page 728*
Pegasys® RBV [Can] *see* peginterferon alfa-2b and ribavirin *(Canada only) on page 728*
Pegetron™ [Can] *see* peginterferon alfa-2b and ribavirin *(Canada only) on page 728*

pegfilgrastim (peg fil GRA stim)

Sound-Alike/Look-Alike Issues
Neulasta® may be confused with Neumega® and Lunesta™
Synonyms G-CSF (PEG conjugate); granulocyte colony-stimulating factor (PEG conjugate); NSC-725961; SD/01
U.S./Canadian Brand Names Neulasta® [US/Can]
Therapeutic Category Colony-Stimulating Factor
Use To decrease the incidence of infection, by stimulation of granulocyte production, in patients with nonmyeloid malignancies receiving myelosuppressive therapy associated with a significant risk of febrile neutropenia
Usual Dosage SubQ: Adolescents >45 kg and Adults: 6 mg once per chemotherapy cycle; do not administer in the period between 14 days before and 24 hours after administration of cytotoxic chemotherapy; do not use in infants, children, and smaller adolescents weighing <45 kg
Dosage Forms
Injection, solution [preservative free]:
Neulasta®: 10 mg/mL (0.6 mL)

peginterferon alfa-2a (peg in ter FEER on AL fa too aye)

Synonyms interferon alfa-2a (PEG conjugate); pegylated interferon alfa-2a
U.S./Canadian Brand Names Pegasys® [US/Can]
Therapeutic Category Interferon
Use Treatment of chronic hepatitis C (CHC), alone or in combination with ribavirin, in patients with compensated liver disease and histological evidence of cirrhosis (Child-Pugh class A) and patients with clinically-stable HIV disease; treatment of patients with HBeAg positive and HBeAg negative chronic hepatitis B with compensated liver disease and evidence of viral replication and liver inflammation
Usual Dosage SubQ: Adults:
Chronic hepatitis C (monoinfection or coinfection with HIV):
Monotherapy: 180 mcg once weekly for 48 weeks
Combination therapy with ribavirin: Recommended dosage: 180 mcg once/week with ribavirin (Copegus®)
Duration of therapy: Monoinfection (based on genotype):
Genotype 1,4: 48 weeks
Genotype 2,3: 24 weeks
Duration of therapy: Coinfection with HIV: 48 weeks
Chronic hepatitis B: 180 mcg once weekly for 48 weeks

Dose modifications for adverse reactions/toxicity:
For moderate-to-severe adverse reactions: Initial: 135 mcg/week; may need decreased to 90 mcg/week in some cases
Based on hematologic parameters:
ANC <750/mm^3: 135 mcg/week
ANC <500/mm^3: Suspend therapy until >1000/mm^3, then restart at 90 mcg/week and monitor
Platelet count <50,000/mm^3: 90 mcg/week
Platelet count <25,000/mm^3: Discontinue therapy
Depression (severity based on DSM-IV criteria):
Mild depression: No dosage adjustment required; evaluate once weekly by visit/phone call. If depression remains stable, continue weekly visits. If depression improves, resume normal visit schedule
Moderate depression: Decrease interferon dose to 90-135 mcg once/week; evaluate once weekly with an office visit at least every other week. If depression remains stable, consider psychiatric evaluation ▶

and continue with reduced dosing. If symptoms improve and remain stable for 4 weeks, resume normal visit schedule; continue reduced dosing or return to normal dose.

Severe depression: Discontinue interferon permanently. Obtain immediate psychiatric consultation. Discontinue ribavirin if using concurrently.

Dosage Forms

Injection, solution:

Pegasys®

180 mcg/0.5 mL (0.5 mL) [prefilled syringe; contains benzyl alcohol and polysorbate 80; packaged with needles and alcohol swabs]

180 mcg/mL (1 mL) [vial; contains benzyl alcohol and polysorbate 80]

peginterferon alfa-2b (peg in ter FEER on AL fa too bee)

Sound-Alike/Look-Alike Issues

peginterferon alfa-2b may be confused with interferon alfa-2a, interferon alfa-2b, interferon alfa-n3, peginterferon alfa-2a

PegIntron™ may be confused with Intron® A

Synonyms interferon alfa-2b (PEG conjugate); pegylated interferon alfa-2b

U.S./Canadian Brand Names PegIntron™ [US/Can]

Therapeutic Category Interferon

Use Treatment of chronic hepatitis C (as monotherapy or in combination with ribavirin) in adult patients who have never received alfa interferons and have compensated liver disease

Usual Dosage SubQ: Adults:

Chronic hepatitis C: Administer dose once weekly; **Note:** Treatment duration may vary. Consult current guidelines and literature.

Monotherapy: Initial: 1 mcg/kg/week

≤45 kg: 40 mcg once weekly

46-56 kg: 50 mcg once weekly

57-72 kg: 64 mcg once weekly

73-88 kg: 80 mcg once weekly

89-106 kg: 96 mcg once weekly

107-136 kg: 120 mcg once weekly

137-160 kg: 150 mcg once weekly

Combination therapy with ribavirin: Initial: 1.5 mcg/kg/week

<40 kg: 50 mcg once weekly (with ribavirin 800 mg/day)

40-50 kg: 64 mcg once weekly (with ribavirin 800 mg/day)

51-60 kg: 80 mcg once weekly (with ribavirin 800 mg/day)

61-65 kg: 96 mcg once weekly (with ribavirin 800 mg/day)

66-75 kg: 96 mcg once weekly (with ribavirin 1000 mg/day)

76-85 kg: 120 mcg once weekly (with ribavirin 1000 mg/day)

86-105 kg: 150 mcg once weekly (with ribavirin 1200 mg/day)

>105 kg: 150 mcg once weekly (with ribavirin 1400 mg/day)

Dosage Forms

Injection, powder for reconstitution [preservative free]:

PegIntron™: 50 mcg, 80 mcg, 120 mcg, 150 mcg

PegIntron™ Redipen®: 50 mcg, 80 mcg, 120 mcg, 150 mcg

peginterferon alfa-2b and ribavirin (Canada only)

(peg in ter FEER on AL fa too bee & rye ba VYE rin)

Synonyms ribavirin and peginterferon alfa-2b

U.S./Canadian Brand Names Pegasys [Can]; Pegasys® RBV [Can]; Pegetron™ [Can]

Therapeutic Category Antiviral Agent; Interferon

Use Combination therapy for the treatment of chronic hepatitis C in patients with compensated liver disease

Usual Dosage Chronic hepatitis C:

Recommended dosage of combination therapy:

Intron® A: SubQ: 1.5 mcg/kg/week

and

Rebetol®: Oral:

≤64 kg: 800 mg/day (two 200 mg capsules in the morning and two 200 mg capsules in the evening)

64-84 kg: 1000 mg/day (two 200 mg capsules in the morning and three 200 mg capsules in the evening)

≥85 kg: 1200 mg/day (three 200 mg capsules in the morning and three 200 mg capsules in the evening)

Note: Treatment duration may vary. Consult current guidelines and literature.

Dosage Forms Combination package:
Pegasys® RBV [CAN], Pegetron™ [CAN] [not available in the U.S.]:
Injection, powder for reconstitution (Peginterferon alfa-2b): 50 mcg/0.5 mL
Capsules: Ribavirin (Rebetol®): 200 mg (56s)

Injection, powder for reconstitution (Peginterferon alfa-2b): 80 mcg/0.5 mL
Capsules: Ribavirin (Rebetol®): 200 mg (56s)

Injection, powder for reconstitution (Peginterferon alfa-2b): 100 mcg/0.5 mL
Capsules: Ribavirin (Rebetol®): 200 mg (70s)

Injection, powder for reconstitution (Peginterferon alfa-2b): 120 mcg/0.5 mL
Capsules: Ribavirin (Rebetol®): 200 mg (70s)

Injection, powder for reconstitution (Peginterferon alfa-2b): 150 mcg/0.5 mL
Capsules: Ribavirin (Rebetol®): 200 mg (84s)

PegIntron™ [US/Can] *see* peginterferon alfa-2b *on page 728*
PegLyte® [Can] *see* polyethylene glycol-electrolyte solution *on page 766*

pegvisomant (peg VI soe mant)

Synonyms B2036-PEG

U.S./Canadian Brand Names Somavert® [US/Can]

Therapeutic Category Growth Hormone Receptor Antagonist

Use Treatment of acromegaly in patients resistant to or unable to tolerate other therapies

Usual Dosage SubQ: Adults: Initial loading dose: 40 mg; maintenance dose: 10 mg once daily; doses may be adjusted by 5 mg in 4- to 6-week intervals based on IGF-I concentrations (maximum dose: 30 mg/day)

Dosage Forms
Injection, powder for reconstitution [preservative free]:
Somavert®: 10 mg, 15 mg, 20 mg

pegylated interferon alfa-2a *see* peginterferon alfa-2a *on page 727*
pegylated interferon alfa-2b *see* peginterferon alfa-2b *on page 728*
pegylated liposomal DOXOrubicin *see* doxorubicin (liposomal) *on page 323*
PE-Hist DM [US] *see* chlorpheniramine, phenylephrine, and dextromethorphan *on page 209*

pemetrexed (pem e TREKS ed)

Synonyms LY231514; MTA; multitargeted antifolate; NSC-698037; pemetrexed disodium

U.S./Canadian Brand Names Alimta® [US/Can]

Therapeutic Category Antineoplastic Agent, Antimetabolite; Antineoplastic Agent, Antimetabolite (Antifolate)

Use Treatment of malignant pleural mesothelioma; treatment of locally advanced or metastatic nonsquamous nonsmall cell lung cancer (NSCLC)

Usual Dosage I.V.: Adults: Refer to individual protocols:
Nonsmall cell lung cancer: 500 mg/m^2 on day 1 of each 21-day cycle
Malignant pleural mesothelioma: 500 mg/m^2 on day 1 of each 21-day cycle (in combination with cisplatin)
Note: Start vitamin supplements 1 week before initial dose of pemetrexed. Folic acid 350-1000 mcg/day orally (continuing for 21 days after last dose of pemetrexed) and vitamin B$_{12}$ 1000 mcg I.M. every 9 weeks. Dexamethasone 4 mg twice daily can be started the day before therapy, and continued the day of and the day after to minimize cutaneous reactions.

Dosage Forms
Injection, powder for reconstitution:
Alimta®: 100 mg, 500 mg

pemetrexed disodium *see* pemetrexed *on page 729*

pemirolast (pe MIR oh last)
U.S./Canadian Brand Names Alamast® [US/Can]
Therapeutic Category Mast Cell Stabilizer; Ophthalmic Agent, Miscellaneous
Use Prevention of itching of the eye due to allergic conjunctivitis
Usual Dosage Children >3 years and Adults: 1-2 drops instilled in affected eye(s) 4 times/day
Dosage Forms
  Solution, ophthalmic:
    Alamast®: 0.1% (10 mL)

pemoline *(Discontinued)*

penbutolol (pen BYOO toe lole)
Sound-Alike/Look-Alike Issues
  Levatol® may be confused with Lipitor®
Synonyms penbutolol sulfate
U.S./Canadian Brand Names Levatol® [US/Can]
Therapeutic Category Beta-Adrenergic Blocker
Use Treatment of mild-to-moderate arterial hypertension
Usual Dosage Oral: Adults: Initial: 20 mg once daily, full effect of a 20 or 40 mg dose is seen by the end of a 2-week period, doses of 40-80 mg have been tolerated but have shown little additional antihypertensive effects; usual dose range (JNC 7): 10-40 mg once daily
Dosage Forms
  Tablet:
    Levatol®: 20 mg

penbutolol sulfate *see* penbutolol *on page 730*

penciclovir (pen SYE kloe veer)
Sound-Alike/Look-Alike Issues
  Denavir® may be confused with indinavir
U.S./Canadian Brand Names Denavir® [US]
Therapeutic Category Antiviral Agent
Use Topical treatment of herpes simplex labialis (cold sores)
Usual Dosage Topical: Children ≥12 years and Adults: Apply cream at the first sign or symptom of cold sore (eg, tingling, swelling); apply every 2 hours during waking hours for 4 days
Dosage Forms
  Cream:
    Denavir®: 1% (1.5 g)

Pendex [US] *see* guaifenesin and phenylephrine *on page 456*
Pendo-5 ASA [Can] *see* mesalamine *on page 607*
Penetrex® *(Discontinued)*

penicillamine (pen i SIL a meen)
Sound-Alike/Look-Alike Issues
  penicillamine may be confused with penicillin
  Depen® may be confused with Endal®
Synonyms D-3-mercaptovaline; D-penicillamine; β,β-dimethylcysteine
U.S./Canadian Brand Names Cuprimine® [US/Can]; Depen® [US/Can]
Therapeutic Category Chelating Agent
Use Treatment of Wilson disease, cystinuria; adjunctive treatment of rheumatoid arthritis
Usual Dosage Oral:
Rheumatoid arthritis:
  Adults: 125-250 mg/day, may increase dose at 1- to 3-month intervals up to 1-1.5 g/day; maximum in older adults: 750 mg/day
Wilson disease (doses titrated to maintain urinary copper excretion >2 mg/day); decrease dose for surgery and during last trimester of pregnancy

Children <12 years: 20 mg/kg/day in 2-3 divided doses, round off to the nearest 250 mg dose; maximum 1 g/day

Adults: 250 mg 4 times/day (maximum in older adults: 750 mg/day)

Cystinuria: **Note:** Adjust dose to limit cystine excretion to 100-200 mg/day (<100 mg/day with history of stone formation)

Children: 30 mg/kg/day in 4 divided doses

Dosage Forms
Capsule:
Cuprimine®: 250 mg
Tablet:
Depen®: 250 mg

penicillin G benzathine (pen i SIL in jee BENZ a theen)

Sound-Alike/Look-Alike Issues
penicillin may be confused with penicillamine

Bicillin® may be confused with Wycillin®

Bicillin® C-R (penicillin G benzathine and penicillin G procaine) may be confused with Bicillin® L-A (penicillin G benzathine). Penicillin G benzathine is the only product currently approved for the treatment of syphilis. Administration of penicillin G benzathine and penicillin G procaine combination instead of Bicillin® L-A may result in inadequate treatment response.

Synonyms benzathine benzylpenicillin; benzathine penicillin G; benzylpenicillin benzathine

U.S./Canadian Brand Names Bicillin® L-A [US/Can]

Therapeutic Category Penicillin

Use Active against some gram-positive organisms, few gram-negative organisms such as *Neisseria gonorrhoeae*, and some anaerobes and spirochetes; used in the treatment of syphilis; used only for the treatment of mild to moderately severe infections caused by organisms susceptible to low concentrations of penicillin G or for prophylaxis of infections caused by these organisms

Usual Dosage Note: Administer undiluted injection; higher doses result in more sustained rather than higher levels. Use a penicillin G benzathine-penicillin G procaine combination to achieve early peak levels in acute infections.

Usual dosage range:
Children: I.M.: 25,000-50,000 units/kg as a single dose (maximum: 2.4 million units)
Adults: I.M.: 1.2-2.4 million units as a single dose

Indication-specific dosing:
Neonates >1200 g: I.M.:
  Congenital syphilis (asymptomatic): 50,000 units/kg as a single dose
Infants and Children: I.M.:
  Group A streptococcal upper respiratory infection: 25,000-50,000 units/kg as a single dose (maximum: 1.2 million units)
  Prophylaxis of recurrent rheumatic fever: 25,000-50,000 units/kg every 3-4 weeks (maximum: 1.2 million units/dose)
  Syphilis:
    Early: 50,000 units/kg as a single injection (maximum: 2.4 million units)
    More than 1-year duration: 50,000 units/kg every week for 3 doses (maximum: 2.4 million units/dose)
Adults: I.M.:
  Group A streptococcal upper respiratory infection: 1.2 million units as a single dose
  Prophylaxis of recurrent rheumatic fever: 1.2 million units every 3-4 weeks or 600,000 units twice monthly
  Syphilis:
    Early: 2.4 million units as a single dose in 2 injection sites
    More than 1-year duration: 2.4 million units in 2 injection sites once weekly for 3 doses
    Neurosyphilis: Not indicated as single-drug therapy, but may be given once weekly for 3 weeks following I.V. treatment; refer to Penicillin G Parenteral/Aqueous monograph for dosing

Dosage Forms
Injection, suspension [prefilled syringe]:
Bicillin® L-A: 600,000 units/mL (1 mL, 2 mL, 4 mL)

penicillin G benzathine and penicillin G procaine
(pen i SIL in jee BENZ a theen & pen i SIL in jee PROE kane)

Sound-Alike/Look-Alike Issues
penicillin may be confused with penicillamine

▶

◀ Bicillin® may be confused with Wycillin®

Bicillin® C-R (penicillin G benzathine and penicillin G procaine) may be confused with Bicillin® L-A (penicillin G benzathine). Penicillin G benzathine is the only product currently approved for the treatment of syphilis. Administration of penicillin G benzathine and penicillin G procaine combination instead of Bicillin® L-A may result in inadequate treatment response.

Synonyms penicillin G procaine and benzathine combined

U.S./Canadian Brand Names Bicillin® C-R 900/300 [US]; Bicillin® C-R [US]

Therapeutic Category Penicillin

Use May be used in specific situations in the treatment of streptococcal infections

Usual Dosage

Usual dosage range and indication-specific dosing:

Streptococcal infections:

Children: I.M.:

<14 kg: 600,000 units in a single dose

14-27 kg: 900,000 units to 1.2 million units in a single dose

Children >27 kg and Adults: 2.4 million units in a single dose

Dosage Forms

Injection, suspension [prefilled syringe]:

Bicillin® C-R: 1,200,000 units: Penicillin G benzathine 600,000 units and penicillin G procaine 600,000 units per 2 mL (2 mL)

Bicillin® C-R 900/300: 1,200,000 units: Penicillin G benzathine 900,000 units and penicillin G procaine 300,000 units per 2 mL (2 mL)

penicillin G (parenteral/aqueous) (pen i SIL in jee, pa REN ter al, AYE kwee us)

Sound-Alike/Look-Alike Issues

penicillin may be confused with penicillamine

Synonyms benzylpenicillin potassium; benzylpenicillin sodium; crystalline penicillin; penicillin G potassium; penicillin G sodium

U.S./Canadian Brand Names Pfizerpen® [US/Can]

Therapeutic Category Penicillin

Use Treatment of infections (including sepsis, pneumonia, pericarditis, endocarditis, meningitis, anthrax) caused by susceptible organisms; active against some gram-positive organisms, generally not *Staphylococcus aureus*; some gram-negative organisms such as *Neisseria gonorrhoeae*, and some anaerobes and spirochetes

Usual Dosage

Usual dosage range:

Infants >1 month and Children: I.M., I.V.: 100,000-400,000 units/kg/day in divided doses every 4-6 hours (maximum dose: 24 million units/day)

Adults: I.M., I.V.: 2-30 million units/day in divided doses every 4-6 hours depending on sensitivity of the organism and severity of the infection

Indication-specific dosing:

Infants >1 month and Children:

Meningitis (gonococcal): I.V.: 250,000 units/kg/day in 4 divided doses

Moderate infections: I.M., I.V.: 100,000-250,000 units/kg/day in 4 divided doses

Severe infections: I.M., I.V.: 250,000-400,000 units/kg/day in divided doses every 4-6 hours (maximum dose: 24 million units/day)

Syphilis (congenital): Infants: I.V.: 50,000 units/kg every 4-6 hours for 10 days

Adults:

Actinomyces species: I.V.: 10-20 million units/day in divided doses every 4-6 hours for 4-6 weeks

Clostridium perfringens: I.V.: 24 million units/day in divided doses every 4-6 hours with clindamycin

Corynebacterium diphtheriae: I.V.: 2-3 million units/day in divided doses every 4-6 hours for 10-12 days

Erysipelas: I.V.: 1-2 million units every 4-6 hours

Erysipelothrix: I.V.: 2-4 million units every 4 hours

Fascial space infections: I.V.: 2-4 million units every 4-6 hours with metronidazole

Leptospirosis: I.V.: 1.5 million units every 6 hours for 7 days

Listeria: I.V.: 15-20 million units/day in divided doses every 4-6 hours for 2 weeks (meningitis) or 4 weeks (endocarditis)

Lyme disease (meningitis): I.V.: 20 million units/day in divided doses

Neurosyphilis: I.V.: 18-24 million units/day in divided doses every 4 hours (or by continuous infusion) for 10-14 days

Streptococcus:

Brain abscess: I.V.: 18-24 million units/day in divided doses every 4 hours with metronidazole

Endocarditis or osteomyelitis: I.V.: 3-4 million units every 4 hours for at least 4 weeks

Pregnancy (prophylaxis GBS): I.V.: 5-6 million units x 1 dose, then 2.5-3 million units every 4 hours until delivery

Skin and soft tissue: I.V.: 3-4 million units every 4 hours for 10 days

Toxic shock: I.V.: 24 million units/day in divided doses with clindamycin

Streptococcal pneumonia: I.V.: 2-3 million units every 4 hours

Whipple disease: I.V.: 2 million units every 4 hours for 2 weeks, followed by oral trimethoprim/sulfamethoxazole or doxycycline for 1 year

Relapse or CNS involvement: 4 million units every 4 hours for 4 weeks

Dosage Forms

Infusion, as potassium [premixed iso-osmotic dextrose solution, frozen]: 1 million units (50 mL), 2 million units (50 mL), 3 million units (50 mL)

Injection, powder for reconstitution: 5 million units, 20 million units

Pfizerpen®: 5 million units, 20 million units

penicillin G potassium *see* penicillin G (parenteral/aqueous) *on page 732*

penicillin G procaine (pen i SIL in jee PROE kane)

Sound-Alike/Look-Alike Issues

penicillin G procaine may be confused with penicillin V potassium

Wycillin® may be confused with Bicillin®

Synonyms APPG; aqueous procaine penicillin G; procaine benzylpenicillin; procaine penicillin G

U.S./Canadian Brand Names Pfizerpen-AS® [Can]; Wycillin® [Can]

Therapeutic Category Penicillin

Use Treatment of moderately-severe infections due to *Treponema pallidum* and other penicillin G-sensitive microorganisms that are susceptible to low, but prolonged serum penicillin concentrations; anthrax due to *Bacillus anthracis* (postexposure) to reduce the incidence or progression of disease following exposure to aerolized *Bacillus anthracis*

Usual Dosage

Usual dosage range:

Infants and Children: I.M.: 25,000-50,000 units/kg/day in divided doses 1-2 times/day; (maximum: 4.8 million units/day)

Adults: I.M.: 0.6-4.8 million units/day in divided doses every 12-24 hours

Indication-specific dosing:

Children: I.M.:

Anthrax, inhalational (postexposure prophylaxis): 25,000 units/kg every 12 hours (maximum: 1,200,000 units every 12 hours); see "Note" in Adults dosing

Syphilis (congenital): 50,000 units/kg/day for 10 days; if more than 1 day of therapy is missed, the entire course should be restarted

Adults: I.M.:

Anthrax:

Inhalational (postexposure prophylaxis): 1,200,000 units every 12 hours

Note: Overall treatment duration should be 60 days. Available safety data suggest continued administration of penicillin G procaine for longer than 2 weeks may incur additional risk for adverse reactions. Clinicians may consider switching to effective alternative treatment for completion of therapy beyond 2 weeks.

Cutaneous (treatment): 600,000-1,200,000 units/day; alternative therapy is recommended in severe cutaneous or other forms of anthrax infection

Endocarditis caused by susceptible viridans *Streptococcus* (when used in conjunction with an aminoglycoside): 1.2 million units every 6 hours for 2-4 weeks

Gonorrhea (uncomplicated): 4.8 million units as a single dose divided in 2 sites given 30 minutes after probenecid 1 g orally

Neurosyphilis: 2.4 million units/day with 500 mg probenecid by mouth 4 times/day for 10-14 days; **Note: Penicillin G aqueous I.V. is the preferred agent**

Whipple disease: 1.2 million units/day (with streptomycin) for 10-14 days, followed by oral trimethoprim/sulfamethoxazole or doxycycline for 1 year

▶

◀ **Dosage Forms**
   Injection, suspension: 600,000 units/mL (1 mL, 2 mL)

penicillin G procaine and benzathine combined see penicillin G benzathine and penicillin G procaine on page 731

penicillin G sodium see penicillin G (parenteral/aqueous) on page 732

penicillin V potassium (pen i SIL in vee poe TASS ee um)

Sound-Alike/Look-Alike Issues
   penicillin V procaine may be confused with penicillin G potassium

Synonyms pen VK; phenoxymethyl penicillin

U.S./Canadian Brand Names Apo-Pen VK® [Can]; Novo-Pen-VK [Can]; Nu-Pen-VK [Can]

Therapeutic Category Penicillin

Use Treatment of infections caused by susceptible organisms involving the respiratory tract, otitis media, sinusitis, skin, and urinary tract; prophylaxis in rheumatic fever

Usual Dosage
   Usual dosage range:
      Children <12 years: Oral: 25-50 mg/kg/day in divided doses every 6-8 hours (maximum dose: 3 g/day)
      Children ≥12 years and Adults: Oral: 125-500 mg every 6-8 hours
   Indication-specific dosing:
      Children: Oral:
         Pharyngitis (streptococcal): 250 mg 2-3 times/day for 10 days
         Prophylaxis of pneumococcal infections:
            Children <5 years: 125 mg twice daily
            Children ≥5 years: 250 mg twice daily
         Prophylaxis of recurrent rheumatic fever:
            Children <5 years: 125 mg twice daily
            Children ≥5 years: 250 mg twice daily
      Adults: Oral:
         Acintomycosis:
            Mild: 2-4 g/day in 4 divided doses for 8 weeks
            Surgical: 2-4 g/day in 4 divided doses for 6-12 months (after I.V. penicillin G therapy of 4-6 weeks)
         Erysipelas: 500 mg 4 times/day
         Periodontal infections: 250-500 mg every 6 hours for 5-7 days
            Note: Efficacy of antimicrobial therapy in periapical abscess is questionable; the American Academy of Periodontology recommends use of antibiotic therapy only when systemic symptoms (eg, fever, lymphadenopathy) are present or in immunocompromised patients.
         Pharyngitis (streptococcal): 500 mg 3-4 times/day for 10 days
         Prophylaxis of pneumococcal or recurrent rheumatic fever infections: 250 mg twice daily

Dosage Forms 250 mg = 400,000 units
   Powder for oral solution: 125 mg/5 mL, 250 mg/5 mL
   Tablet: 250 mg, 500 mg

penicilloyl-polylysine see benzylpenicilloyl-polylysine on page 129

Penlac® [US/Can] see ciclopirox on page 218

Pennsaid® [Can] see diclofenac on page 292

Pentacarinat® Injection (Discontinued) see pentamidine on page 734

Pentacel® [US] see diphtheria and tetanus toxoids, acellular pertussis, poliovirus (inactivated) and Haemophilus b conjugate vaccine on page 308

pentahydrate see sodium thiosulfate on page 880

Pentam-300® [US] see pentamidine on page 734

pentamidine (pen TAM i deen)

Synonyms pentamidine isethionate

U.S./Canadian Brand Names NebuPent® [US]; Pentam-300® [US]; Pentamidine Isetionate for Injection [Can]

Therapeutic Category Antiprotozoal

Use Treatment and prevention of pneumonia caused by *Pneumocystis carinii* (PCP)

Usual Dosage

Children:
Treatment of PCP pneumonia: I.M., I.V. (I.V. preferred): 4 mg/kg/day once daily for 10-14 days
Prevention of PCP pneumonia:
I.M., I.V.: 4 mg/kg monthly or every 2 weeks
Inhalation (aerosolized pentamidine in children ≥5 years): 300 mg/dose given every 3-4 weeks via Respirgard® II inhaler (8 mg/kg dose has also been used in children <5 years)
Adults:
Treatment: I.M., I.V. (I.V. preferred): 4 mg/kg/day once daily for 14-21 days
Prevention: Inhalation: 300 mg every 4 weeks via Respirgard® II nebulizer

Dosage Forms

Injection, powder for reconstitution: [preservative free]:
Pentam-300®: 300 mg
Powder for nebulization: [preservative free]:
NebuPent®: 300 mg

pentamidine isethionate *see* pentamidine *on page 734*
Pentamidine Isetionate for Injection [Can] *see* pentamidine *on page 734*
Pentamycetin® [Can] *see* chloramphenicol *on page 200*
Pentasa® [US/Can] *see* mesalamine *on page 607*
pentasodium colistin methanesulfonate *see* colistimethate *on page 245*
Pentaspan® [US/Can] *see* pentastarch *on page 735*

pentastarch (PEN ta starch)

U.S./Canadian Brand Names Pentaspan® [US/Can]

Therapeutic Category Blood Modifiers

Use Orphan drug: Adjunct in leukapheresis to improve harvesting and increase yield of leukocytes by centrifugal means

Usual Dosage 250-700 mL to which citrate anticoagulant has been added is administered by adding to the input line of the centrifugation apparatus at a ratio of 1:8-1:13 to venous whole blood

Dosage Forms

Infusion [premixed in NS]:
Pentaspan®: 10% (500 mL)

Penta-Triamterene HCTZ [Can] *see* hydrochlorothiazide and triamterene *on page 480*
pentavalent human-bovine reassortant rotavirus vaccine (PRV) *see* rotavirus vaccine *on page 847*

pentazocine (pen TAZ oh seen)

Synonyms naloxone hydrochloride and pentazocine hydrochloride; pentazocine hydrochloride; pentazocine hydrochloride and naloxone hydrochloride; pentazocine lactate

U.S./Canadian Brand Names Talwin® NX [US]; Talwin® [US/Can]

Therapeutic Category Analgesic, Narcotic

Controlled Substance C-IV

Use Relief of moderate-to-severe pain; has also been used as a sedative prior to surgery and as a supplement to surgical anesthesia

Usual Dosage

Preoperative/preanesthetic: Children 1-16 years: I.M.: 0.5 mg/kg
Analgesia:
Children: I.M.:
5-8 years: 15 mg
8-14 years: 30 mg
Children >12 years and Adults: Oral: 50 mg every 3-4 hours; may increase to 100 mg/dose if needed, but should not exceed 600 mg/day
Adults:
I.M., SubQ: 30-60 mg every 3-4 hours; do not exceed 60 mg/dose (maximum: 360 mg/day)
I.V.: 30 mg every 3-4 hours; do not exceed 30 mg/dose (maximum: 360 mg/day)

◀ **Dosage Forms**
Injection, solution:
  Talwin®: 30 mg/mL (1 mL, 10 mL)
  Tablet: Pentazocine 50 mg and naloxone 0.5 mg
  Talwin® Nx: Pentazocine 50 mg and naloxone 0.5 mg

pentazocine and acetaminophen (pen TAZ oh seen & a seet a MIN oh fen)

Sound-Alike/Look-Alike Issues
  Talacen® may be confused with Tegison®, Timoptic®, Tinactin®
Synonyms acetaminophen and pentazocine; pentazocine hydrochloride and acetaminophen
U.S./Canadian Brand Names Talacen® [US]
Therapeutic Category Analgesic Combination (Opioid)
Controlled Substance C-IV
Use Relief of mild-to-moderate pain
Usual Dosage Oral: Adults: Analgesic: 1 caplet every 4 hours, up to a maximum of 6 caplets
Dosage Forms
  Caplet: Pentazocine 25 mg and acetaminophen 650 mg
    Talacen®: Pentazocine 25 mg and acetaminophen 650 mg
  Tablet: Pentazocine 25 mg and acetaminophen 650 mg

pentazocine hydrochloride *see pentazocine on page 735*
pentazocine hydrochloride and acetaminophen *see pentazocine and acetaminophen on page 736*
pentazocine hydrochloride and naloxone hydrochloride *see pentazocine on page 735*
pentazocine lactate *see pentazocine on page 735*
pentetate calcium trisodium *see diethylene triamine penta-acetic acid on page 294*
pentetate zinc trisodium *see diethylene triamine penta-acetic acid on page 294*
Penthrane® *(Discontinued)*

pentobarbital (pen toe BAR bi tal)

Sound-Alike/Look-Alike Issues
  PENTobarbital may be confused with PHENobarbital
  Nembutal® may be confused with Myambutol®
Synonyms pentobarbital sodium
Tall-Man PENTobarbital
U.S./Canadian Brand Names Nembutal® Sodium [Can]; Nembutal® [US]
Therapeutic Category Barbiturate
Controlled Substance C-II
Use Sedative/hypnotic; preanesthetic; high-dose barbiturate coma for treatment of increased intracranial pressure or status epilepticus unresponsive to other therapy
Usual Dosage
  Children:
    Hypnotic: I.M.: 2-6 mg/kg; maximum: 100 mg/dose
    Preoperative/preprocedure sedation: ≥6 months:
      Note: Limited information is available for infants <6 months of age.
      I.M.: 2-6 mg/kg; maximum: 100 mg/dose
      I.V.: 1-3 mg/kg to a maximum of 100 mg until asleep
    Conscious sedation prior to a procedure: Children 5-12 years: I.V.: 2 mg/kg 5-10 minutes before procedures, may repeat one time
  Adolescents: Conscious sedation: I.V.: 100 mg prior to a procedure
  Children and Adults: Barbiturate coma in head injury patients: I.V.: Loading dose: 5-10 mg/kg given slowly over 1-2 hours; monitor blood pressure and respiratory rate; Maintenance infusion: Initial: 1 mg/kg/hour; may increase to 2-3 mg/kg/hour; maintain burst suppression on EEG
  Status epilepticus: I.V.: **Note:** Intubation required; monitor hemodynamics
    Children: Loading dose: 5-15 mg/kg given slowly over 1-2 hours; maintenance infusion: 0.5-5 mg/kg/hour
    Adults: Loading dose: 10-20 mg/kg given slowly over 1-2 hours; maintenance infusion: 0.5-3 mg/kg/hour

Adults:
Hypnotic:
I.M.: 150-200 mg
I.V.: Initial: 100 mg, may repeat every 1-3 minutes up to 200-500 mg total dose
Preoperative sedation: I.M.: 150-200 mg

Dosage Forms
Injection, solution:
Nembutal®: 50 mg/mL (20 mL, 50 mL)

pentobarbital sodium *see* pentobarbital *on page 736*

pentosan polysulfate sodium (PEN toe san pol i SUL fate SOW dee um)

Sound-Alike/Look-Alike Issues
pentosan may be confused with pentostatin
Elmiron® may be confused with Imuran®

Synonyms PPS

U.S./Canadian Brand Names Elmiron® [US/Can]

Therapeutic Category Analgesic, Urinary

Use Orphan drug: Relief of bladder pain or discomfort due to interstitial cystitis

Usual Dosage Oral: Adults: 100 mg 3 times/day taken with water 1 hour before or 2 hours after meals Patients should be evaluated at 3 months and may be continued an additional 3 months if there has been no improvement and if there are no therapy-limiting side effects. **The risks and benefits of continued use beyond 6 months in patients who have not responded is not yet known**.

Dosage Forms
Capsule:
Elmiron®: 100 mg

pentostatin (pen toe STAT in)

Sound-Alike/Look-Alike Issues
pentostatin may be confused with pentosan

Synonyms 2'-deoxycoformycin; CL-825; co-vidarabine; dCF; deoxycoformycin; NSC-218321

U.S./Canadian Brand Names Nipent® [US/Can]

Therapeutic Category Antineoplastic Agent

Use Treatment of hairy cell leukemia; non-Hodgkin lymphoma, cutaneous T-cell lymphoma

Usual Dosage Refractory hairy cell leukemia: Adults (refer to individual protocols):
4 mg/m^2 every other week **or**
4 mg/m^2 weekly for 3 weeks, then every 2 weeks **or**
5 mg/m^2 daily for 3 days every 3 weeks

Dosage Forms
Injection, powder for reconstitution [preservative free]: 10 mg
Nipent®: 10 mg

Pentothal® [US/Can] *see* thiopental *on page 921*
Pentothal® Sodium Rectal Suspension (Discontinued) *see* thiopental *on page 921*

pentoxifylline (pen toks IF i lin)

Sound-Alike/Look-Alike Issues
pentoxifylline may be confused with tamoxifen
Trental® may be confused with Bentyl®, Tegretol®, Trandate®

Synonyms oxpentifylline

U.S./Canadian Brand Names Albert® Pentoxifylline [Can]; Apo-Pentoxifylline SR® [Can]; Nu-Pentoxifylline SR [Can]; Pentoxil® [US]; ratio-Pentoxifylline [Can]; Trental® [US/Can]

Therapeutic Category Blood Viscosity Reducer Agent

Use Treatment of intermittent claudication on the basis of chronic occlusive arterial disease of the limbs; may improve function and symptoms, but not intended to replace more definitive therapy

Usual Dosage Oral: Adults: 400 mg 3 times/day with meals; maximal therapeutic benefit may take 2-4 weeks to develop; recommended to maintain therapy for at least 8 weeks. May reduce to 400 mg twice daily if GI or CNS side effects occur.

◄ **Dosage Forms**
Tablet, controlled release:
Trental®: 400 mg
Tablet, extended release: 400 mg
Pentoxil®: 400 mg

Pentoxil® [US] *see* pentoxifylline *on page 737*
Pen.Vee® K *(Discontinued)* *see* penicillin V potassium *on page 734*
pen VK *see* penicillin V potassium *on page 734*
Pepcid® [US/Can] *see* famotidine *on page 390*
Pepcid® AC [US-OTC/Can] *see* famotidine *on page 390*
Pepcid® AC Maximum Strength [US-OTC] *see* famotidine *on page 390*
Pepcid® Complete [US-OTC/Can] *see* famotidine, calcium carbonate, and magnesium hydroxide *on page 390*
Pepcid® I.V. [Can] *see* famotidine *on page 390*
Pepcid RPD® *(Discontinued)* *see* famotidine *on page 390*
Peptic Relief [US-OTC] *see* bismuth *on page 136*
Pepto-Bismol® [US-OTC] *see* bismuth *on page 136*
Pepto-Bismol® Maximum Strength [US-OTC] *see* bismuth *on page 136*
Pepto® Diarrhea Control *(Discontinued)* *see* loperamide *on page 573*
Pepto Relief [US-OTC] *see* bismuth *on page 136*
Peranex™ HC [US] *see* lidocaine and hydrocortisone *on page 564*
Peranex™ HC Medi-Pad [US] *see* lidocaine and hydrocortisone *on page 564*
Perchloracap® *(Discontinued)*
Percocet® [US/Can] *see* oxycodone and acetaminophen *on page 710*
Percocet®-Demi [Can] *see* oxycodone and acetaminophen *on page 710*
Percodan® [US/Can] *see* oxycodone and aspirin *on page 711*
Percodan®-Demi *(Discontinued)* *see* oxycodone and aspirin *on page 711*
Percogesic® [US-OTC] *see* acetaminophen and phenyltoloxamine *on page 22*
Percogesic® Extra Strength [US-OTC] *see* acetaminophen and diphenhydramine *on page 21*
Percolone® *(Discontinued)* *see* oxycodone *on page 709*
Perdiem® Overnight Relief [US-OTC] *see* senna *on page 861*
Perfectoderm® Gel *(Discontinued)* *see* benzoyl peroxide *on page 126*

perflutren lipid microspheres (per FLOO tren LIP id MIKE roe sfeers)

U.S./Canadian Brand Names Definity® [US/Can]
Therapeutic Category Diagnostic Agent
Use Opacification of left ventricular chamber and improvement of delineation of the left ventricular endocardial border in patients with suboptimal echocardiograms
Usual Dosage Adults: Dose should be given following baseline noncontrast echocardiography. Imaging should begin immediately following dose and compared to noncontrast image. Mechanical index for the ultrasound device should be set at ≤0.8. **Note:** Maximum dose is either two I.V. bolus doses or one single I.V. infusion.
I.V. bolus: 10 microliters (µL)/kg of activated product, followed by 10 mL saline flush; may repeat in 30 minutes if needed
I.V. infusion: Initial: 4 mL/minute (or 240 mL/hour) of prepared infusion; titrate to achieve optimal image; maximum rate: 10 mL/minute (or 600 mL/hour)
Dosage Forms
Injection, solution [preservative free]:
Definity®: OFP 6.52 mg/mL and lipid blend 0.75 mg/mL (2 mL)

Perforomist™ [US] *see* formoterol *on page 424*
Pergonal® *(Discontinued)* *see* menotropins *on page 602*
Periactin® *(Discontinued)* *see* cyproheptadine *on page 259*
Peri-Colace® [US-OTC] *see* docusate and senna *on page 315*

pericyazine *(Canada only)* (per ee CYE ah zeen)
U.S./Canadian Brand Names Neuleptil® [Can]
Therapeutic Category Phenothiazine Derivative
Use Adjunctive therapy in selected psychotic patients to control prevailing hostility, impulsivity, or aggression
Usual Dosage Oral:
Children >5 years: 2.5-10 mg in the morning, followed by 5-30 mg in the evening. In general, lower dosage should be used on initiation and gradually increased based on effect and tolerance.
Adults: 5-20 mg in the morning, followed by 10-40 mg in the evening. In dividing doses, it is suggested that the larger dose should be administered in the evening. In general, lower dosage should be used on initiation and gradually increased based on effect and tolerance.
Dosage Forms [CAN] = Canadian brand name
Capsule:
Neuleptil® [CAN]: 5 mg, 10 mg, 20 mg [not available in the U.S.]
Solution, oral drops:
Neuleptil® [CAN]: 10 mg/mL [not available in the U.S.]

Peridex® [US] *see* chlorhexidine gluconate *on page 201*
Peridex® Oral Rinse [Can] *see* chlorhexidine gluconate *on page 201*
Peridol [Can] *see* haloperidol *on page 465*
perindopril and indapamide *see* perindopril erbumine and indapamide *(Canada only) on page 739*

perindopril erbumine (per IN doe pril er BYOO meen)
U.S./Canadian Brand Names Aceon® [US]; Apo-Perindopril® [Can]; Coversyl® [Can]
Therapeutic Category Miscellaneous Product
Use Treatment of hypertension; reduction of cardiovascular mortality or nonfatal myocardial infarction in patients with stable coronary artery disease
Usual Dosage Oral: Adults:
Essential hypertension: Initial: 4 mg/day but may be titrated to response; usual range: 4-8 mg/day (may be given in 2 divided doses); increase at 1- to 2-week intervals (maximum: 16 mg/day)
Concomitant therapy with diuretics: To reduce the risk of hypotension, discontinue diuretic, if possible, 2-3 days prior to initiating perindopril. If unable to stop diuretic, initiate perindopril at 2-4 mg/day and monitor blood pressure closely for the first 2 weeks of therapy, and after any dose adjustment of perindopril or diuretic.
Stable coronary artery disease: Initial: 4 mg once daily for 2 weeks; increase as tolerated to 8 mg once daily.
Dosage Forms
Tablet:
Aceon®: 2 mg, 4 mg, 8 mg

perindopril erbumine and indapamide *(Canada only)*
(per IN doe pril er BYOO meen & in DAP a mide)
Synonyms indapamide and perindopril erbumine; perindopril and indapamide
U.S./Canadian Brand Names Coversyl® Plus [Can]
Therapeutic Category Angiotensin-Converting Enzyme (ACE) Inhibitor; Antihypertensive Agent, Combination; Diuretic, Thiazide-Related
Use Treatment of hypertension; not indicated for initial treatment of hypertension
Usual Dosage Note: Not for initial therapy. Titration of individual components to an appropriate clinical response is required prior to converting to an equivalent dose of the combination product.
Oral: Adults: Hypertension: Usual maintenance dose: Perindopril 4 mg/indapamide 1.25 mg once daily
Dosage Forms [CAN] = Canadian brand name
Tablet:
Coversyl® Plus [CAN]: Perindopril erbumine 4 mg and indapamide 1.25 mg [not available in the U.S.]

PerioChip® [US] *see* chlorhexidine gluconate *on page 201*
PerioGard® [US] *see* chlorhexidine gluconate *on page 201*
PerioMed™ [US] *see* fluoride *on page 411*
Periostat® [US/Can] *see* doxycycline *on page 323*
Perlane® [US] *see* hyaluronate and derivatives *on page 476*

permethrin (per METH rin)

U.S./Canadian Brand Names A200® Lice [US-OTC]; Acticin® [US]; Elimite® [US]; Kwellada-P™ [Can]; Nix® [US-OTC/Can]; Rid® Spray [US-OTC]

Therapeutic Category Scabicides/Pediculicides

Use Single-application treatment of infestation with *Pediculus humanus capitis* (head louse) and its nits or *Sarcoptes scabiei* (scabies); indicated for prophylactic use during epidemics of lice

Usual Dosage Topical:

Head lice: Children >2 months and Adults: After hair has been washed with shampoo, rinsed with water, and towel dried, apply a sufficient volume of topical liquid (lotion or cream rinse) to saturate the hair and scalp. Leave on hair for 10 minutes before rinsing off with water; remove remaining nits; may repeat in 1 week if lice or nits still present.

Scabies: Apply cream from head to toe; leave on for 8-14 hours before washing off with water; for infants, also apply on the hairline, neck, scalp, temple, and forehead; may reapply in 1 week if live mites appear Permethrin 5% cream was shown to be safe and effective when applied to an infant <1 month of age with neonatal scabies; time of application was limited to 6 hours before rinsing with soap and water

Dosage Forms

Cream, topical: 5% (60 g)
Acticin®, Elimite®: 5% (60 g)
Lotion, topical: 1% (59 mL)
Liquid, topical [creme rinse formulation]: 1% (60 mL)
Nix® [OTC]: 1% (60 mL)
Solution, spray [for bedding and furniture]:
A200® Lice [OTC]: 0.5% (180 mL)
Nix® [OTC]: 0.25% (148 mL)
Rid® [OTC]: 0.5% (150 mL)

Permitil® Oral *(Discontinued)* *see* fluphenazine *on page 415*
Peroxin A5® *(Discontinued)* *see* benzoyl peroxide *on page 126*
Peroxin A10® *(Discontinued)* *see* benzoyl peroxide *on page 126*

perphenazine (per FEN a zeen)

Sound-Alike/Look-Alike Issues
Trilafon® may be confused with Tri-Levlen®

U.S./Canadian Brand Names Apo-Perphenazine® [Can]

Therapeutic Category Phenothiazine Derivative

Use Treatment of schizophrenia; severe nausea and vomiting

Usual Dosage Oral: Adults:

Schizophrenia/psychoses:
Nonhospitalized: Initial: 4-8 mg 3 times/day; reduce dose as soon as possible to minimum effective dosage (maximum: 64 mg/day)
Hospitalized: 8-16 mg 2-4 times/day (maximum: 64 mg/day)
Nausea/vomiting: 8-16 mg/day in divided doses (maximum: 24 mg/day)

Dosage Forms
Tablet: 2 mg, 4 mg, 8 mg, 16 mg

perphenazine and amitriptyline hydrochloride *see* amitriptyline and perphenazine *on page 63*
Persa-Gel® *(Discontinued)* *see* benzoyl peroxide *on page 126*
Persantine® [US/Can] *see* dipyridamole *on page 311*
Pertussin® CS *(Discontinued)* *see* dextromethorphan *on page 284*
Pertussin® ES *(Discontinued)* *see* dextromethorphan *on page 284*
pertussis, acellular (adsorbed) *see* diphtheria and tetanus toxoids, acellular pertussis, poliovirus (inactivated) and *Haemophilus* b conjugate vaccine *on page 308*
pethidine hydrochloride *see* meperidine *on page 603*
Pexeva® [US] *see* paroxetine *on page 724*
Pexicam® [Can] *see* piroxicam *on page 757*
PFA *see* foscarnet *on page 427*
Pfizerpen® [US/Can] *see* penicillin G (parenteral/aqueous) *on page 732*
Pfizerpen-AS® [Can] *see* penicillin G procaine *on page 733*

PGE₁ *see* alprostadil *on page 50*
PGE₂ *see* dinoprostone *on page 303*
PGI₂ *see* epoprostenol *on page 349*
PGX *see* epoprostenol *on page 349*
Phanasin® [US-OTC] *see* guaifenesin *on page 453*
Phanasin® Diabetic Choice [US-OTC] *see* guaifenesin *on page 453*
Phanatuss® DM [US-OTC] *see* guaifenesin and dextromethorphan *on page 454*
Phanatuss® HC *(Discontinued)*
Pharmaflur® [US] *see* fluoride *on page 411*
Pharmaflur® 1.1 [US] *see* fluoride *on page 411*
Pharmorubicin® [Can] *see* epirubicin *on page 346*
Phazyme™ [Can] *see* simethicone *on page 867*
Phazyme® *(Discontinued) see* simethicone *on page 867*
Phazyme® Ultra Strength [US-OTC] *see* simethicone *on page 867*
Phenabid® [US] *see* chlorpheniramine and phenylephrine *on page 206*
Phenabid DM® [US] *see* chlorpheniramine, phenylephrine, and dextromethorphan *on page 209*
Phenadex® Senior *(Discontinued) see* guaifenesin and dextromethorphan *on page 454*
Phenadoz™ [US] *see* promethazine *on page 791*
Phenagesic [US-OTC] *see* acetaminophen and phenyltoloxamine *on page 22*
Phenameth® DM *(Discontinued) see* promethazine and dextromethorphan *on page 792*
Phenaphen® *(Discontinued) see* acetaminophen *on page 19*
Phenaseptic [US-OTC] *see* phenol *on page 743*
PhenaVent™ D *(Discontinued) see* guaifenesin and phenylephrine *on page 456*
PhenaVent™ *(Discontinued) see* guaifenesin and phenylephrine *on page 456*
PhenaVent™ LA *(Discontinued) see* guaifenesin and phenylephrine *on page 456*
PhenaVent™ Ped *(Discontinued) see* guaifenesin and phenylephrine *on page 456*
Phenazine® Injection *(Discontinued) see* promethazine *on page 791*
Phenazo™ [Can] *see* phenazopyridine *on page 741*

phenazopyridine (fen az oh PEER i deen)

Sound-Alike/Look-Alike Issues
phenazopyridine may be confused with phenoxybenzamine
Pyridium® may be confused with Dyrenium®, Perdiem®, pyridoxine, pyrithione
Synonyms phenazopyridine hydrochloride; phenylazo diamino pyridine hydrochloride
U.S./Canadian Brand Names AZO-Gesic® [US-OTC]; AZO-Standard® Maximum Strength [US-OTC]; AZO-Standard® [US-OTC]; Baridium® [US-OTC]; Phenazo™ [Can]; Prodium® [US-OTC]; Pyridium® [US]; ReAzo [US-OTC]; UTI Relief® [US-OTC]
Therapeutic Category Analgesic, Urinary
Use Symptomatic relief of urinary burning, itching, frequency and urgency in association with urinary tract infection or following urologic procedures
Usual Dosage Oral:
Children: 12 mg/kg/day in 3 divided doses administered after meals for 2 days
Adults: 100-200 mg 3 times/day after meals for 2 days when used concomitantly with an antibacterial agent
Dosage Forms
Tablet: 100 mg, 200 mg
AZO-Gesic® [OTC], Prodium® [OTC], ReAzo [OTC]: 95 mg
AZO-Standard® [OTC]: 95 mg [gluten free]
AZO Standard® Maximum Strength [OTC]: 97.5 mg [gluten free]
Baridium® [OTC], UTI Relief® [OTC]: 97.2 mg
Pyridium®: 100 mg, 200 mg

phenazopyridine hydrochloride *see* phenazopyridine *on page 741*
Phencarb GG [US] *see* carbetapentane, guaifenesin, and phenylephrine *on page 175*

phendimetrazine (fen dye ME tra zeen)

Sound-Alike/Look-Alike Issues
Bontril PDM® may be confused with Bentyl®
Synonyms phendimetrazine tartrate
U.S./Canadian Brand Names Bontril PDM® [US]; Bontril® Slow-Release [US]; Bontril® [Can]; Plegine® [Can]; Statobex® [Can]
Therapeutic Category Anorexiant
Controlled Substance C-III
Use Short-term (few weeks) adjunct in exogenous obesity
Usual Dosage Oral: Adults:
Capsule: 105 mg once daily in the morning before breakfast
Tablet: 17.5-35 mg 2 or 3 times daily, 1 hour before meals (maximum: 70 mg 3 times/day)
Dosage Forms
Capsule, slow release: 105 mg
Bontril® Slow Release: 105 mg
Tablet: 35 mg
Bontril PDM®: 35 mg

phendimetrazine tartrate *see* phendimetrazine *on page 742*
Phendry® Oral *(Discontinued)* *see* diphenhydramine *on page 304*

phenelzine (FEN el zeen)

Sound-Alike/Look-Alike Issues
phenelzine may be confused with phenytoin
Nardil® may be confused with Norinyl®
Synonyms phenelzine sulfate
U.S./Canadian Brand Names Nardil® [US/Can]
Therapeutic Category Antidepressant, Monoamine Oxidase Inhibitor
Use Symptomatic treatment of atypical, nonendogenous, or neurotic depression
Usual Dosage Oral: Adults: Depression: 15 mg 3 times/day; may increase to 60-90 mg/day during early phase of treatment, then reduce dose for maintenance therapy slowly after maximum benefit is obtained; takes 2-4 weeks for a significant response to occur
Dosage Forms
Tablet:
Nardil®: 15 mg

phenelzine sulfate *see* phenelzine *on page 742*
Phenerbel-S® *(Discontinued)*
Phenergan® [US/Can] *see* promethazine *on page 791*
Phenergan® VC With Codeine *(Discontinued)* *see* promethazine, phenylephrine, and codeine *on page 792*
Phenergan® With Dextromethorphan *(Discontinued)* *see* promethazine and dextromethorphan *on page 792*
pheniramine and naphazoline *see* naphazoline and pheniramine *on page 656*

phenobarbital (fee noe BAR bi tal)

Sound-Alike/Look-Alike Issues
PHENobarbital may be confused with PENTobarbital
Luminal® may be confused with Tuinal®
Synonyms phenobarbital sodium; phenobarbitone; phenylethylmalonylurea
Tall-Man PHENobarbital
U.S./Canadian Brand Names Luminal® Sodium [US]; PMS-Phenobarbital [Can]
Therapeutic Category Anticonvulsant; Barbiturate
Controlled Substance C-IV
Use Management of generalized tonic-clonic (grand mal) and partial seizures; sedative
Usual Dosage
Children:
Sedation: Oral: 2 mg/kg 3 times/day

Hypnotic: I.M., I.V., SubQ: 3-5 mg/kg at bedtime
Preoperative sedation: Oral, I.M., I.V.: 1-3 mg/kg 1-1.5 hours before procedure
Adults:
Sedation: Oral, I.M.: 30-120 mg/day in 2-3 divided doses
Hypnotic: Oral, I.M., I.V., SubQ: 100-320 mg at bedtime
Preoperative sedation: I.M.: 100-200 mg 1-1.5 hours before procedure

Anticonvulsant: Status epilepticus: **Loading dose:** I.V.:
Infants and Children: 10-20 mg/kg in a single or divided dose; in select patients may administer additional 5 mg/kg/dose every 15-30 minutes until seizure is controlled or a total dose of 40 mg/kg is reached
Adults: 300-800 mg initially followed by 120-240 mg/dose at 20-minute intervals until seizures are controlled or a total dose of 1-2 g
Anticonvulsant maintenance dose: Oral, I.V.:
Infants: 5-8 mg/kg/day in 1-2 divided doses
Children:
1-5 years: 6-8 mg/kg/day in 1-2 divided doses
5-12 years: 4-6 mg/kg/day in 1-2 divided doses
Children >12 years and Adults: 1-3 mg/kg/day in divided doses or 50-100 mg 2-3 times/day
Dosage Forms
Elixir: 20 mg/5 mL
Injection, solution: 65 mg/mL (1 mL); 130 mg/mL (1 mL)
Luminal® Sodium: 60 mg/mL (1 mL); 130 mg/mL (1 mL)
Tablet: 15 mg, 30 mg, 60 mg, 100 mg

phenobarbital, belladonna, and ergotamine tartrate see belladonna, phenobarbital, and ergot-amine on page 120
phenobarbital, hyoscyamine, atropine, and scopolamine see hyoscyamine, atropine, scopol-amine, and phenobarbital on page 493
phenobarbital sodium see phenobarbital on page 742
phenobarbitone see phenobarbital on page 742

phenol (FEE nol)
Sound-Alike/Look-Alike Issues
Cēpastat® may be confused with Capastat®
Synonyms carbolic acid
U.S./Canadian Brand Names Castellani Paint Modified [US-OTC]; Cheracol® [US-OTC]; Chloraseptic® Gargle [US-OTC]; Chloraseptic® Mouth Pain [US-OTC]; Chloraseptic® Pocket Pump [US-OTC]; Chloraseptic® Spray for Kids [US-OTC]; Chloraseptic® Spray [US-OTC]; Cēpastat® Extra Strength [US-OTC]; Cēpastat® [US-OTC]; P & S™ Liquid Phenol [Can]; Pain-A-Lay® [US-OTC]; Phenaseptic [US-OTC]; Phenol EZ® [US-OTC]; Ulcerease® [US-OTC]; Vicks® Formula 44® Sore Throat [US-OTC]
Therapeutic Category Pharmaceutical Aid
Use Relief of sore throat pain, mouth, gum, and throat irritations; antiseptic; topical anesthetic
Usual Dosage Oral:
Sore throat:
Children 2-12 years:
Chloraseptic®: Three sprays onto throat or affected area; may repeat every 2 hours
Chloraseptic® Spray for Kids: Five sprays onto throat or affected area; may repeat every 2 hours
Children >3 years (Ulcerease®): Refer to adult dosing.
Children 6-12 years:
Cēpastat®: Up to 1 lozenge every 2 hours as needed (maximum: 18 lozenges/24 hours)
Cēpastat® Extra Strength: Up to 1 lozenge every 2 hours as needed (maximum: 10 lozenges/24 hours)
Pain-A-Lay® Gargle: Using gauze pad, apply 10 mL to affected area, or gargle or swish for 15 seconds, then expectorate
Children ≥12 years and Adults:
Cēpastat® Extra Strength, Cēpastat®: Up to 2 lozenges every 2 hours as needed
Cheracol®, Pain-A-Lay® Spray: Spray directly in throat; rinse for 15 seconds then expectorate; may repeat every 2 hours
Chloraseptic®: Five sprays onto throat or affected area; may repeat every 2 hours
Chloraseptic® Gargle, Chloraseptic® Mouth Pain, Pain-A-Lay® Gargle, Ulcerease®: Gargle or swish for 15 seconds, then expectorate; may repeat every 2 hours

◀ Topical: Antiseptic: Adults: Castellani Paint Modified: Apply small amount to affected area 1-3 times/day

Dosage Forms
Lozenge, oral:
Cēpastat® [OTC]: 14.5 mg (18s)
Cēpastat® Extra Strength [OTC]: 29 mg (18s)
Solution, oral [gargle]:
Chloraseptic® [OTC]: 1.4% (296 mL)
Pain-A-Lay® [OTC]: 1.4% (240 mL, 540 mL)
Ulcerease® [OTC]: 0.6% (180 mL)
Solution, oral [spray]:
Cheracol [OTC], Chloraseptic® [OTC], Pain-A-Lay® [OTC], Phenaseptic [OTC], Vicks® Formula 44®
Sore Throat [OTC]: 1.4% (180 mL)
Chloraseptic® for Kids [OTC]: 0.5% (177 mL)
Chloraseptic® Mouth Pain [OTC]: 1.4% (30 mL)
Chloraseptic® Pocket Pump [OTC]: 1.4% (20 mL)
Solution, topical:
Castellani Paint Modified [OTC]: Phenol 1.5% (30 mL)
Castellani Paint Modified [OTC] [colorless]: Phenol 1.5% (30 mL)
Swabs, topical:
Phenol EZ® [OTC]: 89% (30s) [~0.2 mL]

phenol and camphor see camphor and phenol on page 168
Phenol EZ® [US-OTC] see phenol on page 743
phenoptin see sapropterin on page 856
Phenoxine® (Discontinued)

phenoxybenzamine (fen oks ee BEN za meen)

Sound-Alike/Look-Alike Issues
phenoxybenzamine may be confused with phenazopyridine
Synonyms phenoxybenzamine hydrochloride
U.S./Canadian Brand Names Dibenzyline® [US/Can]
Therapeutic Category Alpha-Adrenergic Blocking Agent
Use Symptomatic management of pheochromocytoma
Usual Dosage Oral: Adults: Pheochromocytoma, hypertension: Initial: 10 mg twice daily; increase by 10 mg every other day until optimal blood pressure response is achieved; usual range: 20-40 mg 2-3 times/day. Doses up to 240 mg/day have been reported.
Dosage Forms
Capsule:
Dibenzyline®: 10 mg

phenoxybenzamine hydrochloride see phenoxybenzamine on page 744
phenoxymethyl penicillin see penicillin V potassium on page 734

phentermine (FEN ter meen)

Sound-Alike/Look-Alike Issues
phentermine may be confused with phentolamine, phenytoin
Ionamin® may be confused with Imodium®
Synonyms phentermine hydrochloride
U.S./Canadian Brand Names Adipex-P® [US]; Ionamin® [US/Can]
Therapeutic Category Anorexiant
Controlled Substance C-IV
Use Short-term (few weeks) adjunct in exogenous obesity
Usual Dosage Oral: Children >16 years and Adults: Obesity:
Phentermine hydrochloride: 18.75-37.5 mg/day
Phentermine resin: 15-30 mg/day
Dosage Forms
Capsule: 15 mg, 30 mg, 37.5 mg
Adipex-P®: 37.5 mg
Capsule, resin complex:
Ionamin®: 15 mg

Tablet: 37.5 mg
Adipex-P®: 37.5 mg

phentermine hydrochloride *see phentermine on page 744*

phentolamine (fen TOLE a meen)

Sound-Alike/Look-Alike Issues
phentolamine may be confused with phentermine, Ventolin®

Synonyms phentolamine mesylate

U.S./Canadian Brand Names Regitine® [Can]; Rogitine® [Can]

Therapeutic Category Alpha-Adrenergic Blocking Agent; Diagnostic Agent

Use Diagnosis of pheochromocytoma and treatment of hypertension associated with pheochromocytoma or other forms of hypertension caused by excess sympathomimetic amines; as treatment of dermal necrosis after extravasation of drugs with alpha-adrenergic effects (norepinephrine, dopamine, epinephrine)
OraVerse™: Reversal of soft tissue anesthesia and the associated functional deficits resulting from a local dental anesthetic containing a vasoconstrictor

Usual Dosage
Treatment of alpha-adrenergic drug extravasation: SubQ:
Children: 0.1-0.2 mg/kg diluted in 10 mL 0.9% sodium chloride infiltrated into area of extravasation within 12 hours
Adults: Infiltrate area with small amount of solution made by diluting 5-10 mg in 10 mL 0.9% sodium chloride within 12 hours of extravasation; do not exceed 0.1-0.2 mg/kg or 5 mg total
If dose is effective, normal skin color should return to the blanched area within 1 hour
Diagnosis of pheochromocytoma: I.M., I.V.:
Children: 0.05-0.1 mg/kg/dose, maximum single dose: 5 mg
Adults: 5 mg
Surgery for pheochromocytoma: Hypertension: I.M., I.V.:
Children: 0.05-0.1 mg/kg/dose given 1-2 hours before procedure; repeat as needed every 2-4 hours until hypertension is controlled; maximum single dose: 5 mg
Adults: 5 mg given 1-2 hours before procedure and repeated as needed every 2-4 hours
Hypertensive crisis: Adults: 5-20 mg

Dosage Forms
Injection, powder for reconstitution: 5 mg
Injection, solution [preservative free]:
OraVerse™: 0.4 mg/1.7 mL [dental cartridge]

phentolamine mesylate *see phentolamine on page 745*
phenylalanine mustard *see melphalan on page 599*
phenylazo diamino pyridine hydrochloride *see phenazopyridine on page 741*
Phenyldrine® *(Discontinued)*

phenylephrine (fen il EF rin)

Sound-Alike/Look-Alike Issues
Mydfrin® may be confused with Midrin®

Synonyms phenylephrine hydrochloride; phenylephrine tannate

U.S./Canadian Brand Names 4 Way® Fast Acting [US-OTC]; 4 Way® Menthol [US-OTC]; 4 Way® No Drip [US-OTC]; AK-Dilate® [US]; Altafrin [US]; Anu-Med [US-OTC]; Dimetapp® Toddler's [US-OTC]; Dionephrine® [Can]; Formulation R™ [US-OTC]; Little Noses® Decongestant [US-OTC]; LuSonal™ [US]; Medi-Phenyl [US-OTC]; Medicone® Suppositories [US-OTC]; Mydfrin® [US/Can]; Nasop12™ [US]; Neo-Synephrine® Extra Strength [US-OTC]; Neo-Synephrine® Injection [US]; Neo-Synephrine® Mild [US-OTC]; Neo-Synephrine® Regular Strength [US-OTC]; Neo-Synephrine® [Can]; Neofrin™ [US]; OcuNefrin™ [US-OTC]; Preparation H® [US-OTC]; Rectacaine [US-OTC]; Rhinall [US-OTC]; Sudafed PE™ [US-OTC]; Triaminic® Thin Strips® Cold [US-OTC]; Tronolane® Suppository [US-OTC]; Tur-bi-kal® [US-OTC]; Vicks® Sinex® Nasal Spray [US-OTC]; Vicks® Sinex® UltraFine Mist [US-OTC]

Therapeutic Category Adrenergic Agonist Agent

Use Treatment of hypotension, vascular failure in shock; as a vasoconstrictor in regional analgesia; as a mydriatic in ophthalmic procedures and treatment of wide-angle glaucoma; supraventricular tachycardia

For OTC use as symptomatic relief of nasal and nasopharyngeal mucosal congestion, treatment of hemorrhoids, relief of redness of the eye due to irritation

◀ **Usual Dosage**
Hemorrhoids: Children ≥12 years and Adults: Rectal:
  Cream/ointment: Apply to clean dry area, up to 4 times/day; may be used externally or inserted rectally using applicator.
  Suppository: Insert 1 suppository rectally, up to 4 times/day
Hypotension/shock:
  Children:
    I.V. bolus: 5-20 mcg/kg/dose every 10-15 minutes as needed
    I.V. infusion: 0.1-0.5 mcg/kg/minute
  Adults:
    I.V. bolus: 0.1-0.5 mg/dose every 10-15 minutes as needed (initial dose should not exceed 0.5 mg)
    I.V. infusion: Initial dose: 100-180 mcg/minute; when blood pressure is stabilized, maintenance rate: 40-60 mcg/minute; rates up to 360 mcg/minute have been reported; dosing range: 0.4-9.1 mcg/kg/minute
Nasal decongestant:
  Children:
    2-6 years:
      Intranasal: Instill 1 drop every 2-4 hours of 0.125% solution as needed. (**Note:** Therapy should not exceed 3 continuous days.)
      Oral: Tannate salt: 1.87-3.75 mg every 12 hours
    6-12 years:
      Intranasal: Instill 1-2 sprays or instill 1-2 drops every 4 hours of 0.25% solution as needed. (**Note:** Therapy should not exceed 3 continuous days.)
      Oral:
        Hydrochloride salt: 10 mg every 4 hours
        Tannate salt: 3.75-7.5 mg every 12 hours
    Children >12 years and Adults:
      Intranasal: Instill 1-2 sprays or instill 1-2 drops every 4 hours of 0.25% to 0.5% solution as needed; 1% solution may be used in adult in cases of extreme nasal congestion; do not use nasal solutions more than 3 days
      Oral:
        Hydrochloride salt: 10-20 mg every 4 hours
        Tannate salt: 7.5-15 mg every 12 hours
  Ocular procedures:
    Infants <1 year: Instill 1 drop of 2.5% 15-30 minutes before procedures
    Children and Adults: Instill 1 drop of 2.5% or 10% solution, may repeat in 10-60 minutes as needed
  Ophthalmic irritation (OTC formulation for relief of eye redness): Adults: Instill 1-2 drops 0.12% solution into affected eye, up to 4 times/day; do not use for >72 hours
  Paroxysmal supraventricular tachycardia: I.V.:
    Children: 5-10 mcg/kg/dose over 20-30 seconds
    Adults: 0.25-0.5 mg/dose over 20-30 seconds
Dosage Forms
Cream, rectal:
  Formulation R™ [OTC]: 0.25% (54 g)
Filmstrip, orally disintegrating:
  Sudafed PE™ [OTC]: 10 mg (5s, 10s)
  Triaminic® Thin Strips® Cold [OTC]: 2.5 mg
Injection, solution: 1% [10 mg/mL] (1 mL, 5 mL, 10 mL)
  Neo-Synephrine®: 1% (1 mL)
Liquid, oral:
  LuSonal™: 7.5 mg/5 mL
Liquid, oral [drops]:
  Dimetapp® Toddler's [OTC]: 1.25 mg/0.8 mL
Ointment, rectal:
  Formulation R™ [OTC], Preparation H® [OTC]: 0.25% (30 g, 60 g)
  Rectacaine [OTC]: 0.25% (30 g)
Solution, intranasal [drops]:
  Little Noses® Decongestant [OTC]: 0.125% (15 mL)
  Neo-Synephrine® Extra Strength [OTC]: 1% (15 mL)
  Neo-Synephrine® Regular Strength [OTC]: 0.5% (15 mL)
  Rhinall [OTC]: 0.25% (30 mL)
  Tur-bi-kal® [OTC]: 0.17% (30 mL)

Solution, intranasal [spray]:
4 Way® Fast Acting [OTC]: 1% (15 mL, 30 mL) [contains benzalkonium chloride]
4 Way® Menthol [OTC], 4 Way® No Drip [OTC], Neo-Synephrine® Extra Strength [OTC]: 1% (15 mL)
Neo-Synephrine® Mild [OTC]: 0.25% (15 mL)
Neo-Synephrine® Regular Strength [OTC], Vicks® Sinex® [OTC], Vicks® Sinex® UltraFine Mist [OTC]:
0.5% (15 mL)
Rhinall [OTC]: 0.25% (40 mL)
Solution, ophthalmic: 2.5% (2 mL, 3 mL, 5 mL, 15 mL)
AK-Dilate®: 2.5% (2 mL, 15 mL); 10% (5 mL)
Altrafrin: 0.12% (15 mL) [OTC]; 2.5% (15 mL); 10% (5 mL)
Mydfrin® [OTC]: 2.5% (3 mL, 5 mL)
Neofrin™: 2.5% (15 mL); 10% (15 mL)
OcuNefrin™ [OTC]: 0.12% (15 mL)
Suppository, rectal: 0.25% (12s)
Anu-Med [OTC]: 0.25% (12s)
Formulation R™ [OTC], Preparation H® [OTC]: 0.25% (12s, 24s, 48s)
Medicone® [OTC], Tronolane® [OTC]: 0.25% (12s, 24s)
Rectacaine [OTC]: 0.25% (12s)
Tablet: 10 mg
Medi-Phenyl [OTC]: 5 mg
Sudafed PE™ [OTC]: 10 mg
Tablet, chewable:
Nasop12™: 10 mg

Phenylephrine CM [US] *see* chlorpheniramine, phenylephrine, and methscopolamine *on page 210*
phenylephrine, acetaminophen, and dextromethorphan *see* acetaminophen, dextromethorphan, and phenylephrine *on page 26*
phenylephrine and chlorpheniramine *see* chlorpheniramine and phenylephrine *on page 206*
phenylephrine and cyclopentolate *see* cyclopentolate and phenylephrine *on page 256*
phenylephrine and promethazine *see* promethazine and phenylephrine *on page 792*

phenylephrine and pyrilamine (fen il EF rin & peer IL a meen)

Synonyms pyrilamine tannate and phenylephrine tannate
U.S./Canadian Brand Names Aldex®D [US]; Deconsal® CT [US]; K-Tan 4 [US]; K-Tan [US]; Pyrilafen Tannate-12™ [US]; Ry-T 12 [US]; Ryna-12 S™ [US]; Ryna-12™ [US]; Rynesa 12S™ [US]; V-Tann™ [US]
Therapeutic Category Antihistamine; Antihistamine/Decongestant Combination; Sympathomimetic
Use Symptomatic relief of nasal congestion and discharge associated with the common cold, sinusitis, allergic rhinitis, and other respiratory tract conditions
Usual Dosage Oral: Relief of cough, congestion:
Children 2-6 years: 2.5 mL of the suspension or 1/2 tablet every 12 hours
Children 6-12 years: 5 mL of the suspension or 1/2 to 1 tablet every 12 hours
Children >12 years and Adults: 5-10 mL of the suspension or 1-2 tablets every 12 hours
Dosage Forms
Suspension:
Aldex®D: Phenylephrine 5 mg and pyrilamine 16 mg
K-Tan 4, Pyrilafen Tannate-12™, Ryna-12 S™, Rynesa 12S™, Ry-T 12: Phenylephrine 5 mg and pyrilamine 30 mg per 5 mL
V-Tann™: Phenylephrine 12.5 mg and pyrilamine 30 mg per 5 mL
Tablet:
K-Tan, Ryna-12™: Phenylephrine 25 mg and pyrilamine 60 mg
Tablet, chewable:
Deconsal® CT: Phenylephrine 10 mg and pyrilamine 16 mg

phenylephrine and scopolamine (fen il EF rin & skoe POL a meen)

Sound-Alike/Look-Alike Issues
Murocoll-2® may be confused with Murocel®
Synonyms scopolamine and phenylephrine
U.S./Canadian Brand Names Murocoll-2® [US]
Therapeutic Category Anticholinergic/Adrenergic Agonist

◀ **Use** Mydriasis, cycloplegia, and to break posterior synechiae in iritis

Usual Dosage Ophthalmic: Instill 1-2 drops into eye(s); repeat in 5 minutes

Dosage Forms

  Solution, ophthalmic:

    Murocoll-2®: Phenylephrine 10% and scopolamine 0.3% (5 mL)

phenylephrine and zinc sulfate *(Canada only)* (fen il EF rin & zingk SUL fate)

Synonyms zinc sulfate and phenylephrine

U.S./Canadian Brand Names Zincfrin® [Can]

Therapeutic Category Adrenergic Agonist Agent

Use Soothe, moisturize, and remove redness due to minor eye irritation

Usual Dosage Ophthalmic: Instill 1-2 drops in eye(s) 2-4 times/day as needed

Dosage Forms

  Solution, ophthalmic:

    Zincfrin® [OTC; CAN]: Phenylephrine 0.12% and zinc sulfate 0.25% (15 mL)

phenylephrine, chlorpheniramine, and carbetapentane *see* carbetapentane, phenylephrine, and chlorpheniramine *on page 176*

phenylephrine, chlorpheniramine, and dextromethorphan *see* chlorpheniramine, phenylephrine, and dextromethorphan *on page 209*

phenylephrine, chlorpheniramine, and dihydrocodeine *see* dihydrocodeine, chlorpheniramine, and phenylephrine *on page 298*

phenylephrine, chlorpheniramine, and guaifenesin *see* chlorpheniramine, phenylephrine, and guaifenesin *on page 210*

phenylephrine, chlorpheniramine, and phenyltoloxamine *see* chlorpheniramine, phenylephrine, and phenyltoloxamine *on page 211*

phenylephrine, chlorpheniramine, codeine, and potassium iodide *see* chlorpheniramine, phenylephrine, codeine, and potassium iodide *on page 212*

phenylephrine, dextromethorphan, and acetaminophen *see* acetaminophen, dextromethorphan, and phenylephrine *on page 26*

phenylephrine, ephedrine, chlorpheniramine, and carbetapentane *see* chlorpheniramine, ephedrine, phenylephrine, and carbetapentane *on page 208*

phenylephrine hydrochloride *see* phenylephrine *on page 745*

phenylephrine hydrochloride and acetaminophen *see* acetaminophen and phenylephrine *on page 22*

phenylephrine hydrochloride and guaifenesin *see* guaifenesin and phenylephrine *on page 456*

phenylephrine hydrochloride, carbetapentane citrate, and guaifenesin *see* carbetapentane, guaifenesin, and phenylephrine *on page 175*

phenylephrine hydrochloride, chlorpheniramine maleate, dextromethorphan hydrobromide, and guaifenesin *see* dextromethorphan, chlorpheniramine, phenylephrine, and guaifenesin *on page 285*

phenylephrine hydrochloride, guaifenesin, and dextromethorphan hydrobromide *see* guaifenesin, dextromethorphan, and phenylephrine *on page 459*

phenylephrine hydrochloride, hydrocodone bitartrate, and chlorpheniramine maleate *see* phenylephrine, hydrocodone, and chlorpheniramine *on page 748*

phenylephrine, hydrocodone, and chlorpheniramine

(fen il EF rin, hye droe KOE done, & klor fen IR a meen)

Synonyms chlorpheniramine, phenylephrine, and hydrocodone; dihydrocodeine bitartrate, phenylephrine hydrochloride, and chlorpheniramine maleate; hydrocodone, phenylephrine, and chlorpheniramine; phenylephrine hydrochloride, hydrocodone bitartrate, and chlorpheniramine maleate

U.S./Canadian Brand Names B-Tuss™ [US]; Coughtuss [US]; Cytuss HC [US]; De-Chlor HC [US]; DroTuss-CP [US]; ED-TLC [US]; ED-Tuss HC [US]; Histinex® HC [US]; Hydro PC II Plus [US]; Hydro-PC II [US]; Hydron CP [US]; Maxi-Tuss HCX [US]; Maxi-Tuss HC® [US]; Mintuss HC [US]; Mintuss MS [US]; PolyTussin HD [US]; Relacon-HC [US]; Rindal HD Plus [US]; Triant-HC™ [US]

Therapeutic Category Antihistamine; Antihistamine/Decongestant/Antitussive; Antitussive; Decongestant

Controlled Substance C-III

Use Symptomatic relief of cough and congestion associated with the common cold, sinusitis, or acute upper respiratory tract infections

Usual Dosage Oral:

Children 6-12 years:

Histinex® HC, Cytuss HC: 5 mL every 4 hours (maximum: 20 mL/24 hours)

Maxi-Tuss HC®, Maxi-Tuss HCX: 2.5 mL every 4 hours (maximum: 15 mL/24 hours)

Adults:

Histinex® HC, Cytuss HC: 10 mL every 4 hours (maximum: 40 mL/24 hours)

Maxi-Tuss HC®, Maxi-Tuss HCX: 5 mL every 4 hours (maximum: 30 mL/24 hours)

Dosage Forms

Liquid:

B-Tuss™: Phenylephrine 5 mg, hydrocodone 5 mg, and chlorpheniramine 2 mg per 5 mL

Coughtuss, DroTuss-CP: Phenylephrine 5 mg, hydrocodone 5 mg, and chlorpheniramine 2 mg per 5 mL

De-Chlor HC: Phenylephrine 10 mg, hydrocodone 2.5 mg, and chlorpheniramine 2 mg per 5 mL

ED-Tuss HC: Phenylephrine 10 mg, hydrocodone 3.5 mg, and chlorpheniramine 4 mg per 5 mL

ED-TLC: Phenylephrine 5 mg, hydrocodone 1.67 mg, and chlorpheniramine 2 mg per 5 mL

Hydro PC II Plus: Phenylephrine 7.5 mg, hydrocodone 3.5 mg, and chlorpheniramine 2 mg per 5 mL

Hydron CP: Phenylephrine 10 mg, hydrocodone 5 mg, and chlorpheniramine 2 mg per 5 mL

Maxi-Tuss HCX: Phenylephrine 12 mg, hydrocodone 6 mg and chlorpheniramine 2 mg per 5 mL

Relacon-HC: Phenylephrine 10 mg, hydrocodone 3.5 mg, and chlorpheniramine 2.5 mg per 5 mL

Triant-HC™: Phenylephrine 5 mg, hydrocodone 1.67 mg, and chlorpheniramine 2 mg per 5 mL

Syrup:

Cytuss HC, Histinex® HC: Phenylephrine 5 mg, hydrocodone 2.5 mg, and chlorpheniramine 2 mg per 5 mL

Hydro-PC II: Phenylephrine 7.5 mg, hydrocodone 2 mg, and chlorpheniramine 2 mg per 5 mL

Maxi-Tuss HC®, Mintuss HD: Phenylephrine 10 mg, hydrocodone 2.5 mg, and chlorpheniramine 4 mg per 5 mL

Mintuss HC: Phenylephrine 10 mg, hydrocodone 2.5 mg, and chlorpheniramine 2 mg per 5 mL

Mintuss MS: Phenylephrine 10 mg, hydrocodone 5 mg, and chlorpheniramine 2 mg per 5 mL

PolyTussin HD: Phenylephrine 5 mg, hydrocodone 6 mg, and chlorpheniramine 2 mg per 5 mL

Rindal HD Plus: Phenylephrine 7.5 mg, hydrocodone 3.5 mg, and chlorpheniramine 2 mg per 5 mL

phenylephrine, promethazine, and codeine *see promethazine, phenylephrine, and codeine* *on page 792*

phenylephrine, pyrilamine, and dextromethorphan

(fen il EF rin, peer IL a meen, & deks troe meth OR fan)

Synonyms dextromethorphan tannate, pyrilamine tannate, and phenylephrine tannate; pyrilamine maleate, dextromethorphan hydrobromide, and phenylephrine hydrochloride

U.S./Canadian Brand Names Aldex® DM [US]; AllanVan-DM [US]; Codal-DM [US-OTC]; codimal® DM [US-OTC]; Codituss DM [US-OTC]; MyHist-DM [US]; Poly-Hist DM [US]; Tannate-V-DM [US]; Viravan®-DM [US]

Therapeutic Category Antihistamine; Antihistamine/Decongestant/Antitussive; Antitussive; Sympathomimetic

Use Symptomatic relief of cough, nasal congestion, and discharge associated with the common cold, sinusitis, allergic rhinitis, and other respiratory tract conditions

Usual Dosage Oral: Relief of cough, congestion:

Children 2-6 years (Viravan®-DM): 2.5 mL of the suspension or 1/2 tablet every 12 hours

Children 6-12 years:

codimal® DM: 5 mL every 4 hours; maximum: 30 mL/24 hours

Viravan®-DM: 5 mL of the suspension or 1/2 to 1 tablet every 12 hours

Children >12 years and Adults:

codimal® DM: 10 mL every 4 hours; maximum: 60 mL/24 hours

Viravan®-DM: 5-10 mL of the suspension or 1-2 tablets every 12 hours

Dosage Forms

Liquid:

MyHist-DM: Phenylephrine 7.5 mg, pyrilamine 12.5 mg, and dextromethorphan 15 mg per 5 mL

▶

◀ **Suspension:**
AllanVan-DM, Tannate-V-DM, Viravan®-DM: Phenylephrine 12.5 mg, pyrilamine 30 mg, and dextromethorphan 25 mg per 5 mL
Aldex® DM: Phenylephrine 5 mg, pyrilamine 16 mg, and dextromethorphan 15 mg per 5 mL
Syrup:
Codal-DM [OTC], Codimal® DM [OTC], Codituss DM [OTC]: Phenylephrine 5 mg, pyrilamine 8.33 mg, and dextromethorphan 10 mg
Poly Hist DM: Phenylephrine 7.5 mg, pyrilamine 8.33 mg, and dextromethorphan 10 mg
Tablet, chewable [scored]:
Deconsal® DM: Phenylephrine 10 mg, pyrilamine 16 mg, and dextromethorphan 15 mg
Viravan®-DM: Phenylephrine 25 mg, pyrilamine 30 mg, and dextromethorphan 25 mg

phenylephrine tannate see phenylephrine on page 745

phenylephrine tannate and carbetapentane tannate see carbetapentane and phenylephrine on page 175

phenylephrine tannate, carbetapentane tannate, and pyrilamine tannate see carbetapentane, phenylephrine, and pyrilamine on page 176

phenylephrine tannate, chlorpheniramine tannate, and methscopolamine nitrate see chlorpheniramine, phenylephrine, and methscopolamine on page 210

phenylethylmalonylurea see phenobarbital on page 742

Phenylfenesin® L.A. *(Discontinued)*

Phenylgesic [US-OTC] see acetaminophen and phenyltoloxamine on page 22

phenyltoloxamine, chlorpheniramine, and phenylephrine see chlorpheniramine, phenylephrine, and phenyltoloxamine on page 211

phenyltoloxamine citrate and acetaminophen see acetaminophen and phenyltoloxamine on page 22

Phenytek® [US] see phenytoin on page 750

phenytoin (FEN i toyn)

Sound-Alike/Look-Alike Issues
phenytoin may be confused with phenelzine, phentermine
Dilantin® may be confused with Dilaudid®, diltiazem, Dipentum®

Synonyms diphenylhydantoin; DPH; phenytoin sodium; phenytoin sodium, extended; phenytoin sodium, prompt

U.S./Canadian Brand Names Dilantin® [US/Can]; Phenytek® [US]

Therapeutic Category Antiarrhythmic Agent, Class I-B; Hydantoin

Use Management of generalized tonic-clonic (grand mal), complex partial seizures; prevention of seizures following head trauma/neurosurgery

Usual Dosage
Status epilepticus: I.V.:
Infants and Children: Loading dose: 15-20 mg/kg in a single or divided dose; maintenance dose: Initial: 5 mg/kg/day in 2 divided doses; usual doses:
6 months to 3 years: 8-10 mg/kg/day
4-6 years: 7.5-9 mg/kg/day
7-9 years: 7-8 mg/kg/day
10-16 years: 6-7 mg/kg/day, some patients may require every 8 hours dosing
Adults: Loading dose: Manufacturer recommends 10-15 mg/kg, however, 15-20 mg/kg is generally recommended; maximum rate: 50 mg/minute
Anticonvulsant: Children and Adults: Oral:
Loading dose: 15-20 mg/kg; based on phenytoin serum concentrations and recent dosing history; administer oral loading dose in 3 divided doses given every 2-4 hours to decrease GI adverse effects and to ensure complete oral absorption; maintenance dose: same as I.V.
Neurosurgery (prophylactic): 100-200 mg at approximately 4-hour intervals during surgery and during the immediate postoperative period

Dosage Forms
Capsule, extended release: 100 mg
Dilantin®: 30 mg, 100 mg
Phenytek®: 200 mg, 300 mg
Capsule, prompt release: 100 mg
Injection, solution: 50 mg/mL (2 mL, 5 mL)

Suspension, oral: 100 mg/4 mL, 125 mg/5 mL
   Dilantin®: 125 mg/5 mL
Tablet, chewable:
   Dilantin®: 50 mg

phenytoin sodium *see* phenytoin *on page 750*
phenytoin sodium, extended *see* phenytoin *on page 750*
phenytoin sodium, prompt *see* phenytoin *on page 750*
Pherazine® VC With Codeine *(Discontinued)* *see* promethazine, phenylephrine, and codeine *on page 792*
Pherazine® With Codeine *(Discontinued)* *see* promethazine and codeine *on page 791*
Pherazine® With DM *(Discontinued)* *see* promethazine and dextromethorphan *on page 792*
Phillips'® M-O [US-OTC] *see* magnesium hydroxide and mineral oil *on page 586*
Phillips'® Chews [US-OTC] *see* magnesium hydroxide *on page 585*
Phillips'® Milk of Magnesia [US-OTC] *see* magnesium hydroxide *on page 585*
Phillips'® Stool Softener Laxative [US-OTC] *see* docusate *on page 314*
pHisoHex® [US/Can] *see* hexachlorophene *on page 473*
PHL-Alendronate [Can] *see* alendronate *on page 43*
PHL-Alendronate-FC [Can] *see* alendronate *on page 43*
PHL-Amiodarone [Can] *see* amiodarone *on page 61*
PHL-Amoxicillin [Can] *see* amoxicillin *on page 67*
PHL-Anagrelide [Can] *see* anagrelide *on page 75*
PHL-Azithromycin [Can] *see* azithromycin *on page 110*
PHL-Bicalutamide [Can] *see* bicalutamide *on page 135*
PHL-Carbamazepine [Can] *see* carbamazepine *on page 172*
PHL-Ciprofloxacin [Can] *see* ciprofloxacin *on page 221*
PHL-Citalopram [Can] *see* citalopram *on page 225*
PHL-Divalproex [Can] *see* valproic acid and derivatives *on page 967*
PHL-Domperidone [Can] *see* domperidone *(Canada only)* *on page 317*
Phlemex [US] *see* guaifenesin and dextromethorphan *on page 454*
PHL-Fenofibrate Supra [Can] *see* fenofibrate *on page 393*
PHL-Fluconazole [Can] *see* fluconazole *on page 405*
PHL-Fluoxetine [Can] *see* fluoxetine *on page 413*
PHL-Lorazepam [Can] *see* lorazepam *on page 577*
PHL-Methimazole [Can] *see* methimazole *on page 614*
PHL-Metoprolol [Can] *see* metoprolol *on page 626*
PHL-Ondansetron [Can] *see* ondansetron *on page 698*
PHL-Risperidone [Can] *see* risperidone *on page 837*
PHL-Sertraline [Can] *see* sertraline *on page 863*
PHL-Simvastatin [Can] *see* simvastatin *on page 867*
PHL-Sumatriptan [Can] *see* sumatriptan *on page 898*
PHL-Temazepam [Can] *see* temazepam *on page 907*
PHL-Topiramate [Can] *see* topiramate *on page 935*
PHL-Ursodiol C [Can] *see* ursodiol *on page 965*
PHL-Valproic Acid [Can] *see* valproic acid and derivatives *on page 967*
PHL-Valproic Acid E.C. [Can] *see* valproic acid and derivatives *on page 967*
PHL-Verapamil [Can] *see* verapamil *on page 974*
Phos-Flur® [US] *see* fluoride *on page 411*
Phos-Flur® Rinse [US-OTC] *see* fluoride *on page 411*
PhosLo® [US/Can] *see* calcium acetate *on page 162*
Phos-NaK [US] *see* potassium phosphate and sodium phosphate *on page 775*
Phospha 250™ Neutral [US] *see* potassium phosphate and sodium phosphate *on page 775*
phosphate, potassium *see* potassium phosphate *on page 774*
Phospholine Iodide® [US] *see* echothiophate iodide *on page 331*
phosphonoformate *see* foscarnet *on page 427*

phosphonoformic acid *see* foscarnet *on page 427*

phosphorated carbohydrate solution *see* fructose, dextrose, and phosphoric acid *on page 429*

phosphoric acid, levulose and dextrose *see* fructose, dextrose, and phosphoric acid *on page 429*

Photofrin® [US/Can] *see* porfimer *on page 769*

Phoxal-timolol [Can] *see* timolol *on page 927*

Phrenilin® [US] *see* butalbital and acetaminophen *on page 155*

Phrenilin® Forte [US] *see* butalbital and acetaminophen *on page 155*

Phrenilin® with Caffeine and Codeine [US] *see* butalbital, acetaminophen, caffeine, and codeine *on page 155*

p-hydroxyampicillin *see* amoxicillin *on page 67*

Phyllocontin® [Can] *see* aminophylline *on page 60*

Phyllocontin®-350 [Can] *see* aminophylline *on page 60*

phylloquinone *see* phytonadione *on page 752*

physostigmine (fye zoe STIG meen)

Sound-Alike/Look-Alike Issues
physostigmine may be confused with Prostigmin®, pyridostigmine

Synonyms eserine salicylate; physostigmine salicylate; physostigmine sulfate

U.S./Canadian Brand Names Eserine® [Can]; Isopto® Eserine [Can]

Therapeutic Category Cholinesterase Inhibitor

Use Reverse toxic, life-threatening delirium caused by atropine, diphenhydramine, dimenhydrinate, *Atropa belladonna* (deadly nightshade), or jimsonweed (*Datura* spp)

Usual Dosage Reversal of toxic anticholinergic effects: **Note:** Administer slowly over 5 minutes to prevent respiratory distress and seizures. Continuous infusions of physostigmine should never be used.
Children: **Note:** Reserve for life-threatening situations only: I.V.: 0.01-0.03 mg/kg/dose; may repeat after 5-10 minutes to a maximum total dose of 2 mg or until response occurs or adverse cholinergic effects occur
Adults: I.M., I.V.: 0.5-2 mg to start, repeat every 20 minutes until response occurs or adverse effect occurs; repeat 1-4 mg every 30-60 minutes as life-threatening symptoms recur

Dosage Forms
Injection, solution: 1 mg/mL (2 mL)

physostigmine salicylate *see* physostigmine *on page 752*

physostigmine sulfate *see* physostigmine *on page 752*

phytomenadione *see* phytonadione *on page 752*

phytonadione (fye toe na DYE one)

Sound-Alike/Look-Alike Issues
Mephyton® may be confused with melphalan, methadone

Synonyms methylphytyl napthoquinone; phylloquinone; phytomenadione; vitamin K_1

U.S./Canadian Brand Names AquaMEPHYTON® [Can]; Konakion [Can]; Mephyton® [US/Can]

Therapeutic Category Vitamin, Fat Soluble

Use Prevention and treatment of hypoprothrombinemia caused by coumarin derivative-induced or other drug-induced vitamin K deficiency, hypoprothrombinemia caused by malabsorption or inability to synthesize vitamin K; hemorrhagic disease of the newborn

Usual Dosage Note: According to the manufacturer, SubQ is the preferred parenteral route; I.M. route should be avoided due to the risk of hematoma formation; I.V. route should be restricted for emergency use only. The American College of Chest Physicians recommends the I.V. route in patients with serious or life-threatening bleeding secondary to use of vitamin K antagonists.
Adequate intake:
Children:
1-3 years: 30 mcg/day
4-8 years: 55 mcg/day
9-13 years: 60 mcg/day
14-18 years: 75 mcg/day
Adults: Males: 120 mcg/day; Females: 90 mcg/day

Dosage Forms
Injection, aqueous colloidal: 2 mg/mL (0.5 mL); 10 mg/mL (1 mL)

Tablet: 100 mcg [OTC]
Mephyton®: 5 mg

α₁-PI *see* alpha₁-proteinase inhibitor *on page 48*
pidorubicin *see* epirubicin *on page 346*
pidorubicin hydrochloride *see* epirubicin *on page 346*
Pilagan® Ophthalmic *(Discontinued)* *see* pilocarpine *on page 753*

pilocarpine (pye loe KAR peen)

Sound-Alike/Look-Alike Issues
Isopto® Carpine may be confused with Isopto® Carbachol
Salagen® may be confused with Salacid®, selegiline
Synonyms pilocarpine hydrochloride
U.S./Canadian Brand Names Diocarpine [Can]; Isopto® Carpine [US/Can]; Pilopine HS® [US/Can]; Salagen® [US/Can]
Therapeutic Category Cholinergic Agent
Use
Ophthalmic: Management of chronic simple glaucoma, chronic and acute angle-closure glaucoma
Oral: Symptomatic treatment of xerostomia caused by salivary gland hypofunction resulting from radiotherapy for cancer of the head and neck or Sjögren syndrome
Usual Dosage Adults:
Ophthalmic: Glaucoma:
Solution: Instill 1-2 drops up to 6 times/day; adjust the concentration and frequency as required to control elevated intraocular pressure
Gel: Instill 0.5" ribbon into lower conjunctival sac once daily at bedtime
Oral: Xerostomia:
Following head and neck cancer: 5 mg 3 times/day, titration up to 10 mg 3 times/day may be considered for patients who have not responded adequately; do not exceed 2 tablets/dose
Sjögren's syndrome: 5 mg 4 times/day
Dosage Forms
Gel, ophthalmic:
Pilopine HS®: 4% (4 g)
Solution, ophthalmic: 0.5% (15 mL); 1% (2 mL, 15 mL); 2% (2 mL, 15 mL); 3% (15 mL); 4% (2 mL, 15 mL); 6% (15 mL)
Isopto® Carpine: 1% (15 mL); 2% (15 mL); 4% (15 mL)
Tablet: 5 mg, 7.5 mg
Salagen®: 5 mg, 7.5 mg

pilocarpine hydrochloride *see* pilocarpine *on page 753*
Pilopine HS® [US/Can] *see* pilocarpine *on page 753*
Pilostat® Ophthalmic *(Discontinued)* *see* pilocarpine *on page 753*
pimaricin *see* natamycin *on page 658*

pimecrolimus (pim e KROE li mus)

U.S./Canadian Brand Names Elidel® [US/Can]
Therapeutic Category Immunosuppressant Agent; Topical Skin Product
Use Short-term and intermittent long-term treatment of mild-to-moderate atopic dermatitis in patients not responsive to conventional therapy or when conventional therapy is not appropriate
Usual Dosage Topical: Children ≥2 years and Adults: Apply thin layer to affected area twice daily; rub in gently and completely. **Note:** Limit application to involved areas. Continue as long as signs and symptoms persist; discontinue if resolution occurs; reevaluate if symptoms persist >6 weeks.
Dosage Forms
Cream, topical:
Elidel®: 1% (30 g, 60 g, 100 g)

pimozide (PI moe zide)

U.S./Canadian Brand Names Apo-Pimozide® [Can]; Orap® [US/Can]
Therapeutic Category Neuroleptic Agent

◀ **Use** Suppression of severe motor and phonic tics in patients with Tourette disorder who have failed to respond satisfactorily to standard treatment

Usual Dosage Oral: **Note:** An ECG should be performed baseline and periodically thereafter, especially during dosage adjustment:

Children ≤12 years: Tourette disorder: Initial: 0.05 mg/kg preferably once at bedtime; may be increased every third day; usual range: 2-4 mg/day; do not exceed 10 mg/day (0.2 mg/kg/day)

Children >12 years and Adults: Tourette disorder: Initial: 1-2 mg/day in divided doses, then increase dosage as needed every other day; range is usually 7-16 mg/day, maximum dose: 10 mg/day or 0.2 mg/kg/day are not generally recommended

Note: Sudden unexpected deaths have occurred in patients taking doses >10 mg. Therefore, dosages exceeding 10 mg/day are generally not recommended.

Dosage Forms
Tablet:
Orap®: 1 mg, 2 mg

Pin-X® [US-OTC] *see pyrantel pamoate on page 806*
pinaverium bromide *see pinaverium (Canada only) on page 754*

pinaverium *(Canada only)* (pin ah VEER ee um)

Synonyms pinaverium bromide
U.S./Canadian Brand Names Dicetel® [Can]
Therapeutic Category Calcium Antagonist; Gastrointestinal Agent, Miscellaneous
Use Treatment and relief of symptoms associated with irritable bowel syndrome (IBS); treatment of symptoms related to functional disorders of the biliary tract
Usual Dosage Oral: Adults: 50 mg 3 times/day; in exceptional cases, the dosage may be increased up to 100 mg 3 times/day (maximum dose: 300 mg/day). Tablets should be taken with a full glass of water during a meal/snack.
Dosage Forms [CAN] = Canadian brand name
Tablet:
Dicetel® [CAN]: 50 mg, 100 mg [not available in the U.S.]

pindolol (PIN doe lole)

Sound-Alike/Look-Alike Issues
pindolol may be confused with Parlodel®, Plendil®
Visken® may be confused with Visine®
U.S./Canadian Brand Names Apo-Pindol® [Can]; Gen-Pindolol [Can]; Novo-Pindol [Can]; Nu-Pindol [Can]; PMS-Pindolol [Can]; Visken® [Can]
Therapeutic Category Beta-Adrenergic Blocker
Use Treatment of hypertension, alone or in combination with other agents
Usual Dosage Oral: Adults: Hypertension: Initial: 5 mg twice daily, increase as necessary by 10 mg/day every 3-4 weeks (maximum daily dose: 60 mg); usual dose range (JNC 7): 10-40 mg twice daily
Dosage Forms
Tablet: 5 mg, 10 mg

pink bismuth *see bismuth on page 136*
Pin-Rid® *(Discontinued)* *see pyrantel pamoate on page 806*

pioglitazone (pye oh GLI ta zone)

Sound-Alike/Look-Alike Issues
Actos® may be confused with Actidose®, Actonel®
U.S./Canadian Brand Names Actos® [US/Can]; Apo-Pioglitazone [Can]; CO Pioglitazone [Can]; Gen-Pioglitazone [Can]; Novo-Pioglitazone [Can]; PMS-Pioglitazone [Can]; ratio-Pioglitazone [Can]; Sandoz-Pioglitazone [Can]; SPEF-Pioglitazone [Can]
Therapeutic Category Antidiabetic Agent; Thiazolidinedione Derivative
Use
Type 2 diabetes mellitus (noninsulin-dependent, NIDDM), monotherapy: Adjunct to diet and exercise, to improve glycemic control
Type 2 diabetes mellitus (noninsulin-dependent, NIDDM), combination therapy with sulfonylurea, metformin, or insulin: When diet, exercise, and a single agent alone does not result in adequate glycemic control

Usual Dosage Oral:
Adults:
Monotherapy: Initial: 15-30 mg once daily; if response is inadequate, the dosage may be increased in increments up to 45 mg once daily; maximum recommended dose: 45 mg once daily
Combination therapy: Maximum recommended dose: 45 mg/day
With sulfonylureas: Initial: 15-30 mg once daily; dose of sulfonylurea should be reduced if the patient reports hypoglycemia
With metformin: Initial: 15-30 mg once daily; it is unlikely that the dose of metformin will need to be reduced due to hypoglycemia
With insulin: Initial: 15-30 mg once daily; dose of insulin should be reduced by 10% to 25% if the patient reports hypoglycemia or if the plasma glucose falls to <100 mg/dL.
Dosage adjustment in patients with CHF (NYHA Class II) in mono- or combination therapy: Initial: 15 mg once daily; may be increased after several months of treatment, with close attention to heart failure symptoms

Dosage Forms
Tablet:
Actos®: 15 mg, 30 mg, 45 mg

pioglitazone and glimepiride (pye oh GLI ta zone & GLYE me pye ride)

Synonyms glimepiride and pioglitazone; glimepiride and pioglitazone hydrochloride
U.S./Canadian Brand Names Duetact™ [US]
Therapeutic Category Antidiabetic Agent, Sulfonylurea; Antidiabetic Agent, Thiazolidinedione; Hypoglycemic Agent, Oral
Use Management of type 2 diabetes mellitus (noninsulin-dependent, NIDDM) as an adjunct to diet and exercise
Usual Dosage Oral: Type 2 diabetes mellitus:
Adults: Initial dose should be based on current dose of pioglitazone and/or sulfonylurea.
Patients inadequately controlled on **glimepiride** alone: Initial dose: 30 mg/2 mg or 30 mg/4 mg once daily
Patients inadequately controlled on **pioglitazone** alone: Initial dose: 30 mg/2 mg once daily
Patients with systolic dysfunction (eg, NYHA Class I and II): Initiate only after patient has been safely titrated to 30 mg of pioglitazone. Initial dose: 30 mg/2 mg or 30 mg/4 mg once daily.
Note: No exact dosing relationship exists between glimepiride and other sulfonlyureas. Dosing should be limited to less than or equal to the maximum initial dose of glimepiride (2 mg). When converting patients from other sulfonylureas with longer half lives (eg, chlorpropamide) to glimepiride, observe patient carefully for 1-2 weeks due to overlapping hypoglycemic effects.
Dosing adjustment: Dosage may be increased up to max dose and formulation strengths available; tablet should not be given more than once daily; see individual agents for frequency of adjustments. Dosage adjustments in patients with systolic dysfunction should be done carefully and patient monitored for symptoms of worsening heart failure.
Maximum dose: Pioglitazone 45 mg/glimepiride 8 mg daily

Dosage Forms
Tablet:
Duetact™: 30 mg/2 mg: Pioglitazone 30 mg and glimepiride 2 mg; 30 mg/4 mg: Pioglitazone 30 mg and glimepiride 4 mg

pioglitazone and metformin (pye oh GLI ta zone & met FOR min)

Synonyms metformin hydrochloride and pioglitazone hydrochloride
U.S./Canadian Brand Names Actoplus Met™ [US]
Therapeutic Category Antidiabetic Agent, Biguanide; Antidiabetic Agent, Thiazolidinedione
Use Management of type 2 diabetes mellitus (noninsulin-dependent, NIDDM)
Usual Dosage Oral: Type 2 diabetes mellitus:
Adults: Initial dose should be based on current dose of pioglitazone and/or metformin; daily dose should be divided and given with meals
Patients inadequately controlled on **metformin alone**: Initial dose: Pioglitazone 15-30 mg/day plus current dose of metformin
Patients inadequately controlled on **pioglitazone alone**: Initial dose: Metformin 1000-1700 mg/day plus current dose of pioglitazone
Note: When switching from combination pioglitazone and metformin as separate tablets: Use current dose.

◄ **Dosing adjustment:** Doses may be increased as increments of pioglitazone 15 mg and/or metformin 500-850 mg, up to the maximum dose; doses should be titrated gradually. Guidelines for frequency of adjustment (adapted from rosiglitazone/metformin combination labeling):
After a change in the **metformin** dosage, titration can be done after 1-2 weeks
After a change in the **pioglitazone** dosage, titration can be done after 8-12 weeks
Maximum dose: Pioglitazone 45 mg/metformin 2550 mg daily

Dosage Forms
Tablet:
Actoplus Met™: 15/500: Pioglitazone 15 mg and metformin 500 mg; 15/850: Pioglitazone 15 mg and metformin 850 mg

piperacillin (pi PER a sil in)

Synonyms piperacillin sodium
U.S./Canadian Brand Names Piperacillin for Injection, USP [Can]
Therapeutic Category Penicillin
Use Treatment of susceptible infections such as septicemia, acute and chronic respiratory tract infections, skin and soft tissue infections, and urinary tract infections due to susceptible strains of *Pseudomonas*, *Proteus*, and *Escherichia coli* and *Enterobacter*; active against some streptococci and some anaerobic bacteria; febrile neutropenia (as part of combination regimen)
Usual Dosage
Usual dosage range:
Neonates: I.M., I.V.: 100 mg/kg every 12 hours
Infants and Children: I.M., I.V.: 200-300 mg/kg/day in divided doses every 4-6 hours
Adults: I.M., I.V.: 2-4 g/dose every 4-6 hours (maximum: 24 g/day)
Indication-specific dosing:
Children: I.M., I.V.: **Cystic fibrosis:** 350-500 mg/kg/day in divided doses every 4-6 hours
Adults:
Burn wound sepsis: I.V.: 4 g every 4 hours with vancomycin and amikacin
Cholangitis, acute: I.V.: 4 g every 6 hours
Keratitis *(Pseudomonas):* Ophthalmic: 6-12 mg/mL every 15-60 minutes around the clock for 24-72 hours, then slow reduction
Malignant otitis externa: I.V.: 4-6 g every 4-6 hours with tobramycin
Moderate infections: I.M., I.V.: 2-3 g/dose every 6-12 hours (maximum: 2 g I.M./site)
Prosthetic joint *(Pseudomonas):* I.V.: 3 g every 6 hours with aminoglycoside
***Pseudomonas*infections:** I.V.: 4 g every 4 hours
Severe infections: I.M., I.V.: 3-4 g/dose every 4-6 hours (maximum: 24 g/24 hours)
Urinary tract infections: I.V.: 2-3 g/dose every 6-12 hours
Uncomplicated gonorrhea: I.M.: 2 g in a single dose accompanied by 1 g probenecid 30 minutes prior to injection
Dosage Forms
Injection, powder for reconstitution: 2 g, 3 g, 4 g, 40 g

piperacillin and tazobactam sodium (pi PER a sil in & ta zoe BAK tam SOW dee um)

Sound-Alike/Look-Alike Issues
Zosyn® may be confused with Zofran®, Zyvox®
Synonyms piperacillin sodium and tazobactam sodium; tazobactam and piperacillin
U.S./Canadian Brand Names Tazocin® [Can]; Zosyn® [US]
Therapeutic Category Penicillin
Use Treatment of moderate-to-severe infections caused by susceptible organisms, including infections of the lower respiratory tract (community-acquired pneumonia, nosocomial pneumonia); urinary tract; uncomplicated and complicated skin and skin structures; gynecologic (endometritis, pelvic inflammatory disease); bone and joint infections; intraabdominal infections (appendicitis with rupture/abscess, peritonitis); and septicemia. Tazobactam expands activity of piperacillin to include beta-lactamase producing strains of *S. aureus*, *H. influenzae*, *Bacteroides*, and other gram-negative bacteria.
Usual Dosage
Usual dosage range:
Children: I.V.:
2-8 months: 80 mg of piperacillin component/kg every 8 hours
≥9 months and ≤40 kg: 100 mg of piperacillin component/kg every 8 hours
Adults: I.V.: 3.375 g every 6 hours **or** 4.5 g every 6-8 hours; maximum: 18 g/day

Indication-specific dosing: I.V.:
  Children: **Note:** Dosing based on piperacillin component:
  Appendicitis, peritonitis:
    2-8 months: 80 mg/kg every 8 hours
    ≥9 months and ≤40 kg: 100 mg/kg every 8 hours
    >40 kg: refer to Adult dosing
  Adults:
  Diverticulitis, intraabdominal abscess, peritonitis: I.V.: 3.375 g every 6 hours; **Note:** Some clinicians use 4.5 g every 8 hours for empiric coverage since the %time>MIC is similar between the regimens for most pathogens; however, this regimen is NOT recommended for nosocomial pneumonia or *Pseudomonas* coverage.
  Pneumonia (nosocomial): I.V.: 4.5 g every 6 hours for 7-14 days (when used empirically, combination with an aminoglycoside or antipseudomonal fluoroquinolone is recommended; consider discontinuation of additional agent if *P. aeruginosa* is not isolated)
  Severe infections: I.V.: 3.375 g every 6 hours for 7-10 days; **Note:** Some clinicians use 4.5 g every 8 hours for empiric coverage since the %time>MIC is similar between the regimens for most pathogens; however, this regimen is NOT recommended for nosocomial pneumonia or *Pseudomonas* coverage.

Dosage Forms 8:1 ratio of piperacillin sodium/tazobactam sodium
  Infusion [premixed iso-osmotic solution, frozen]:
    Zosyn®
    2.25 g: Piperacillin 2 g and tazobactam 0.25 g (50 mL)
    3.375 g: Piperacillin 3 g and tazobactam 0.375 g (50 mL)
    4.5 g: Piperacillin 4 g and tazobactam 0.5 g (50 mL)
  Injection, powder for reconstitution:
    Zosyn®
    2.25 g: Piperacillin 2 g and tazobactam 0.25 g
    3.375 g: Piperacillin 3 g and tazobactam 0.375 g
    4.5 g: Piperacillin 4 g and tazobactam 0.5 g
    40.5 g: Piperacillin 36 g and tazobactam 4.5 g

Piperacillin for Injection, USP [Can] *see* piperacillin *on page 756*

piperacillin sodium *see* piperacillin *on page 756*

piperacillin sodium and tazobactam sodium *see* piperacillin and tazobactam sodium *on page 756*

piperazine estrone sulfate *see* estropipate *on page 366*

piperonyl butoxide and pyrethrins *see* pyrethrins and piperonyl butoxide *on page 806*

Pipracil® *(Discontinued)* *see* piperacillin *on page 756*

pirbuterol (peer BYOO ter ole)

Synonyms pirbuterol acetate
U.S./Canadian Brand Names Maxair™ Autohaler™ [US]
Therapeutic Category Adrenergic Agonist Agent
Use Prevention and treatment of reversible bronchospasm including asthma
Usual Dosage Children ≥12 years and Adults: 2 inhalations every 4-6 hours for prevention; two inhalations at an interval of at least 1-3 minutes, followed by a third inhalation in treatment of bronchospasm, not to exceed 12 inhalations/day
Dosage Forms
  Aerosol for oral inhalation:
    Maxair™ Autohaler™: 200 mcg/actuation (14 g)

pirbuterol acetate *see* pirbuterol *on page 757*

piroxicam (peer OKS i kam)

U.S./Canadian Brand Names Apo-Piroxicam® [Can]; Feldene® [US]; Gen-Piroxicam [Can]; Novo-Pirocam [Can]; Nu-Pirox [Can]; Pexicam® [Can]
Therapeutic Category Analgesic, Nonnarcotic; Nonsteroidal Antiinflammatory Drug (NSAID)
Use Symptomatic treatment of acute and chronic rheumatoid arthritis and osteoarthritis
Usual Dosage Oral: Adults: 10-20 mg/day once daily; although associated with increase in GI adverse effects, doses >20 mg/day have been used (ie, 30-40 mg/day)
Dosage Forms
  Capsule: 10 mg, 20 mg
    Feldene®: 10 mg, 20 mg

p-isobutylhydratropic acid *see* ibuprofen *on page 495*
pit *see* oxytocin *on page 714*
Pitocin® [US/Can] *see* oxytocin *on page 714*
Pitrex [Can] *see* tolnaftate *on page 934*
pit viper antivenin *see* crotalidae polyvalent antivenin (equine) *on page 252*
pivampicilin *see* pivampicillin *(Canada only) on page 758*

pivampicillin *(Canada only)* (piv am pi SIL in)

Synonyms MK-191; pivampicilin
U.S./Canadian Brand Names Pondocillin® [Can]
Therapeutic Category Penicillin
Use Treatment of susceptible bacterial infections (nonbeta-lactamase-producing organisms); susceptible bacterial infections caused by streptococci, pneumococci, nonpenicillinase-producing staphylococci, *H. influenzae, N. gonorrhoeae, E. coli, P. mirabilis, Listeria, Salmonella, Shigella, Enterobacter,* and *Klebsiella*
Usual Dosage Oral:
  Infants and Children: Bacterial infections: Oral suspension:
    Infants <3 months: Use of pivampicillin in this age group should be avoided
    Infants 3-12 months: Dosage range: 40-60 mg/kg/day in 2 divided doses
    Children ≤10 years: Dosage range: 25-35 mg/kg/day, not to exceed recommended daily adult dose of 500 mg twice daily
    Alternatively: Children:
      1-3 years: 175 mg twice daily
      4-6 years: 262.5 mg twice daily
      7-10 years: 350 mg twice daily
    Children >10 years and Adults: Usual dose: 500 mg (tablet) or 525 mg (suspension) twice daily; dosage may be doubled in severe infections
    Gonococcal urethritis: 1.5 g as a single dose with 1 g probenecid concurrently
Dosage Forms [CAN] = Canadian brand name
  Powder for oral suspension:
    Pondocillin® [CAN]: 175 mg/5 mL (100 mL, 150 mL, 200 mL) [not available in the U.S.]
  Tablet:
    Pondocillin® [CAN]: 500 mg [equivalent to 377 mg ampicillin; not available in the U.S.]

pix carbonis *see* coal tar *on page 240*

pizotifen *(Canada only)* (pi ZOE ti fen)

Synonyms pizotifen malate
U.S./Canadian Brand Names Sandomigran DS® [Can]; Sandomigran® [Can]
Therapeutic Category Antimigraine Agent
Use Migraine prophylaxis
Usual Dosage Oral: Children ≥12 years and Adults: Migraine prophylaxis: Initial: 0.5 mg at bedtime; increase gradually to 0.5 mg 3 times/day; usual dosage range: 1-6 mg/day
  Note: Therapeutic response may require several weeks of therapy. Do not discontinue abruptly (reduce gradually over 2-week period).
Dosage Forms [CAN] = Canadian brand name
  Tablet:
    Sandomigran® [CAN]: 0.5 mg [not available in the U.S.]
  Tablet, double strength:
    Sandomigran® DS [CAN]: 1 mg [not available in the U.S.]

pizotifen malate *see* pizotifen *(Canada only) on page 758*
Plan B® [US-RX/OTC/Can] *see* levonorgestrel *on page 559*
plantago seed *see* psyllium *on page 804*
plantain seed *see* psyllium *on page 804*
Plaquase® *(Discontinued) see* collagenase *on page 245*
Plaquenil® [US/Can] *see* hydroxychloroquine *on page 489*

Plaretase® 8000 [US] *see* pancrelipase *on page 718*
Plasbumin® [US] *see* albumin *on page 38*
Plasbumin®-5 [Can] *see* albumin *on page 38*
Plasbumin®-25 [Can] *see* albumin *on page 38*
Plasmanate® [US] *see* plasma protein fraction *on page 759*
Plasma-Plex® *(Discontinued)* *see* plasma protein fraction *on page 759*

plasma protein fraction (PLAS mah PROE teen FRAK shun)

U.S./Canadian Brand Names Plasmanate® [US]
Therapeutic Category Blood Product Derivative
Use Plasma volume expansion and maintenance of cardiac output in the treatment of certain types of shock or impending shock
Usual Dosage I.V.: Adults: Usual minimum dose: 250-500 mL; adjust dose based on response
Dosage Forms
  Injection, solution [human, preservative free]:
    Plasmanate®: 5% (50 mL, 250 mL)

Plasmatein® *(Discontinued)* *see* plasma protein fraction *on page 759*
Platinol®-AQ *(Discontinued)* *see* cisplatin *on page 224*
Plavix® [US/Can] *see* clopidogrel *on page 237*
Plegine® [Can] *see* phendimetrazine *on page 742*
Plegine® *(Discontinued)* *see* phendimetrazine *on page 742*
Plenaxis™ *(Discontinued)*
Plendil® [US/Can] *see* felodipine *on page 392*
Pletal® [US/Can] *see* cilostazol *on page 219*
Plexion® [US] *see* sulfur and sulfacetamide *on page 897*
Plexion SCT® [US] *see* sulfur and sulfacetamide *on page 897*
Plexion TS® *(Discontinued)* *see* sulfur and sulfacetamide *on page 897*
Pliaglis™ [US] *see* lidocaine and tetracaine *on page 565*
PMPA *see* tenofovir *on page 909*
PMS-Alendronate [Can] *see* alendronate *on page 43*
PMS-Alendronate-FC [Can] *see* alendronate *on page 43*
PMS-Amantadine [Can] *see* amantadine *on page 56*
PMS-Amiodarone [Can] *see* amiodarone *on page 61*
PMS-Amitriptyline [Can] *see* amitriptyline *on page 62*
PMS-Amoxicillin [Can] *see* amoxicillin *on page 67*
PMS-Anagrelide [Can] *see* anagrelide *on page 75*
PMS-Atenolol [Can] *see* atenolol *on page 101*
PMS-Azithromycin [Can] *see* azithromycin *on page 110*
PMS-Baclofen [Can] *see* baclofen *on page 115*
PMS-Benzydamine [Can] *see* benzydamine *(Canada only)* *on page 129*
PMS-Bethanechol [Can] *see* bethanechol *on page 133*
PMS-Bezafibrate [Can] *see* bezafibrate *(Canada only)* *on page 134*
PMS-Bicalutamide [Can] *see* bicalutamide *on page 135*
PMS-Bisoprolol [Can] *see* bisoprolol *on page 138*
PMS-Brimonidine Tartrate [Can] *see* brimonidine *on page 142*
PMS-Bromocriptine [Can] *see* bromocriptine *on page 143*
PMS-Buspirone [Can] *see* buspirone *on page 153*
PMS-Butorphanol [Can] *see* butorphanol *on page 157*
PMS-Captopril [Can] *see* captopril *on page 171*
PMS-Carbamazepine [Can] *see* carbamazepine *on page 172*
PMS-Carvedilol [Can] *see* carvedilol *on page 181*
PMS-Cefaclor [Can] *see* cefaclor *on page 183*
PMS-Chloral Hydrate [Can] *see* chloral hydrate *on page 199*
PMS-Cholestyramine [Can] *see* cholestyramine resin *on page 215*

PMS-Cilazapril [Can] *see* cilazapril *(Canada only) on page 219*
PMS-Cimetidine [Can] *see* cimetidine *on page 219*
PMS-Ciprofloxacin [Can] *see* ciprofloxacin *on page 221*
PMS-Citalopram [Can] *see* citalopram *on page 225*
PMS-Clarithromycin [Can] *see* clarithromycin *on page 227*
PMS-Clindamycin [Can] *see* clindamycin *on page 230*
PMS-Clobazam [Can] *see* clobazam *(Canada only) on page 232*
PMS-Clonazepam [Can] *see* clonazepam *on page 235*
PMS-Deferoxamine [Can] *see* deferoxamine *on page 271*
PMS-Desipramine [Can] *see* desipramine *on page 274*
PMS-Desmopressin [Can] *see* desmopressin acetate *on page 275*
PMS-Desonide [Can] *see* desonide *on page 276*
PMS-Dexamethasone [Can] *see* dexamethasone (systemic) *on page 278*
PMS-Diclofenac [Can] *see* diclofenac *on page 292*
PMS-Diclofenac SR [Can] *see* diclofenac *on page 292*
PMS-Diphenhydramine [Can] *see* diphenhydramine *on page 304*
PMS-Dipivefrin [Can] *see* dipivefrin *on page 311*
PMS-Docusate Calcium [Can] *see* docusate *on page 314*
PMS-Docusate Sodium [Can] *see* docusate *on page 314*
PMS-Domperidone [Can] *see* domperidone *(Canada only) on page 317*
PMS-Enalapril [Can] *see* enalapril *on page 339*
PMS-Erythromycin [Can] *see* erythromycin *on page 354*
PMS-Famciclovir [Can] *see* famciclovir *on page 389*
PMS-Fenofibrate Micro [Can] *see* fenofibrate *on page 393*
PMS-Fenofibrate Supra [Can] *see* fenofibrate *on page 393*
PMS-Fluconazole [Can] *see* fluconazole *on page 405*
PMS-Flunisolide [Can] *see* flunisolide *on page 408*
PMS-Fluorometholone [Can] *see* fluorometholone *on page 412*
PMS-Fluoxetine [Can] *see* fluoxetine *on page 413*
PMS-Fluphenazine Decanoate [Can] *see* fluphenazine *on page 415*
PMS-Fluvoxamine [Can] *see* fluvoxamine *on page 420*
PMS-Fosinopril [Can] *see* fosinopril *on page 427*
PMS-Furosemide [Can] *see* furosemide *on page 430*
PMS-Gabapentin [Can] *see* gabapentin *on page 431*
PMS-Gemfibrozil [Can] *see* gemfibrozil *on page 439*
PMS-Gliclazide [Can] *see* gliclazide *(Canada only) on page 444*
PMS-Glimepiride [Can] *see* glimepiride *on page 445*
PMS-Glyburide [Can] *see* glyburide *on page 448*
PMS-Haloperidol LA [Can] *see* haloperidol *on page 465*
PMS-Hydrochlorothiazide [Can] *see* hydrochlorothiazide *on page 479*
PMS-Hydromorphone [Can] *see* hydromorphone *on page 486*
PMS-Hydroxyzine [Can] *see* hydroxyzine *on page 491*
PMS-Indapamide [Can] *see* indapamide *on page 505*
PMS-Ipratropium [Can] *see* ipratropium *on page 524*
PMS-ISMN [Can] *see* isosorbide mononitrate *on page 531*
PMS-Isoniazid [Can] *see* isoniazid *on page 528*
PMS-Isosorbide [Can] *see* isosorbide dinitrate *on page 530*
PMS-Lactulose [Can] *see* lactulose *on page 544*
PMS-Lamotrigine [Can] *see* lamotrigine *on page 545*
PMS-Levetiracetam [Can] *see* levetiracetam *on page 554*
PMS-Levobunolol [Can] *see* levobunolol *on page 555*
PMS-Lindane [Can] *see* lindane *on page 567*
PMS-Lisinopril [Can] *see* lisinopril *on page 570*

PMS-Lithium Carbonate [Can] *see* lithium *on page 571*
PMS-Lithium Citrate [Can] *see* lithium *on page 571*
PMS-Loperamine [Can] *see* loperamide *on page 573*
PMS-Lorazepam [Can] *see* lorazepam *on page 577*
PMS-Lovastatin [Can] *see* lovastatin *on page 579*
PMS-Loxapine [Can] *see* loxapine *on page 580*
PMS-Mefenamic Acid [Can] *see* mefenamic acid *on page 598*
PMS-Meloxicam [Can] *see* meloxicam *on page 599*
PMS-Metformin [Can] *see* metformin *on page 610*
PMS-Methotrimeprazine [Can] *see* methotrimeprazine *(Canada only) on page 617*
PMS-Methylphenidate [Can] *see* methylphenidate *on page 622*
PMS-Metoprolol [Can] *see* metoprolol *on page 626*
PMS-Minocycline [Can] *see* minocycline *on page 635*
PMS-Mirtazapine [Can] *see* mirtazapine *on page 637*
PMS-Moclobemide [Can] *see* moclobemide *(Canada only) on page 639*
PMS-Mometasone [Can] *see* mometasone *on page 641*
PMS-Morphine Sulfate SR [Can] *see* morphine sulfate *on page 643*
PMS-Naproxen EC [Can] *see* naproxen *on page 656*
PMS-Nizatidine [Can] *see* nizatidine *on page 677*
PMS-Norfloxacin [Can] *see* norfloxacin *on page 679*
PMS-Nortriptyline [Can] *see* nortriptyline *on page 680*
PMS-Nystatin [Can] *see* nystatin *on page 690*
PMS-Ofloxacin [Can] *see* ofloxacin *on page 693*
PMS-Ondansetron [Can] *see* ondansetron *on page 698*
PMS-Oxazepam [Can] *see* oxazepam *on page 706*
PMS-Oxybutynin [Can] *see* oxybutynin *on page 708*
PMS-Oxycodone-Acetaminophen [Can] *see* oxycodone and acetaminophen *on page 710*
PMS-Pantoprazole [Can] *see* pantoprazole *on page 720*
PMS-Paroxetine [Can] *see* paroxetine *on page 724*
PMS-Phenobarbital [Can] *see* phenobarbital *on page 742*
PMS-Pindolol [Can] *see* pindolol *on page 754*
PMS-Pioglitazone [Can] *see* pioglitazone *on page 754*
PMS-Polytrimethoprim [Can] *see* trimethoprim and polymyxin B *on page 954*
PMS-Pramipexole [Can] *see* pramipexole *on page 777*
PMS-Pravastatin [Can] *see* pravastatin *on page 779*
PMS-Procyclidine [Can] *see* procyclidine *on page 789*
PMS-Promethazine [Can] *see* promethazine *on page 791*
PMS-Propafenone [Can] *see* propafenone *on page 793*
PMS-Propranolol [Can] *see* propranolol *on page 796*
PMS-Pseudoephedrine [Can] *see* pseudoephedrine *on page 801*
PMS-Ranitidine [Can] *see* ranitidine *on page 819*
PMS-Risperidone ODT [Can] *see* risperidone *on page 837*
PMS-Salbutamol [Can] *see* albuterol *on page 39*
PMS-Sertraline [Can] *see* sertraline *on page 863*
PMS-Simvastatin [Can] *see* simvastatin *on page 867*
PMS-Sodium Polystyrene Sulfonate [Can] *see* sodium polystyrene sulfonate *on page 879*
PMS-Sotalol [Can] *see* sotalol *on page 885*
PMS-Sucralate [Can] *see* sucralfate *on page 890*
PMS-Sumatriptan [Can] *see* sumatriptan *on page 898*
PMS-Temazepam [Can] *see* temazepam *on page 907*
PMS-Terazosin [Can] *see* terazosin *on page 909*
PMS-Theophylline [Can] *see* theophylline *on page 917*
PMS-Tiaprofenic [Can] *see* tiaprofenic acid *(Canada only) on page 925*

PMS-Timolol [Can] *see* timolol *on page 927*
PMS-Tobramycin [Can] *see* tobramycin *on page 931*
PMS-Topiramate [Can] *see* topiramate *on page 935*
PMS-Trazodone [Can] *see* trazodone *on page 944*
PMS-Trifluoperazine [Can] *see* trifluoperazine *on page 951*
PMS-Ursodiol C [Can] *see* ursodiol *on page 965*
PMS-Valproic Acid [Can] *see* valproic acid and derivatives *on page 967*
PMS-Valproic Acid E.C. [Can] *see* valproic acid and derivatives *on page 967*
PMS-Venlafaxine XR [Can] *see* venlafaxine *on page 973*
PMS-Verapamil SR [Can] *see* verapamil *on page 974*
PMS-Yohimbine [Can] *see* yohimbine *on page 988*
PMS-Zopiclone [Can] *see* zopiclone *(Canada only) on page 997*
PN *see* total parenteral nutrition *on page 938*
Pneumo 23™ [Can] *see* pneumococcal polysaccharide vaccine (polyvalent) *on page 763*
pneumococcal 7-valent conjugate vaccine *see* pneumococcal conjugate vaccine (7-valent) *on page 762*

pneumococcal conjugate vaccine (7-valent)
(noo moe KOK al KON ju gate vak SEEN, seven vay lent)

Sound-Alike/Look-Alike Issues
  Prevnar® may be confused with PREVEN®

Synonyms diphtheria CRM$_{197}$ protein; PCV7; pneumococcal 7-valent conjugate vaccine

U.S./Canadian Brand Names Prevnar® [US/Can]

Therapeutic Category Vaccine

Use Immunization of infants and toddlers against *Streptococcus pneumoniae* infection caused by serotypes included in the vaccine

  Advisory Committee on Immunization Practices (ACIP) guidelines also recommend PCV7 for use in:
  All children 2-23 months
  Children ≥2-59 months with cochlear implants
  Children ages 24-59 months with: Sickle cell disease (including other sickle cell hemoglobinopathies, asplenia, splenic dysfunction), HIV infection, immunocompromising conditions (congenital immuno-deficiencies, renal failure, nephrotic syndrome, diseases associated with immunosuppressive or radiation therapy, solid organ transplant), chronic illnesses (cardiac disease, cerebrospinal fluid leaks, diabetes mellitus, pulmonary disease excluding asthma unless on high dose corticosteroids)
  Consider use in all children 24-59 months with priority given to:
  Children 24-35 months
  Children 24-59 months who are of Alaska native, American Indian, or African-American descent
  Children 24-59 months who attend group day care centers

Usual Dosage I.M.:
  Infants: 2-6 months: 0.5 mL at approximately 2-month intervals for 3 consecutive doses, followed by a fourth dose of 0.5 mL at 12-15 months of age; first dose may be given as young as 6 weeks of age, but is typically given at 2 months of age. In case of a moderate shortage of vaccine, defer the fourth dose until shortage is resolved; in case of a severe shortage of vaccine, defer third and fourth doses until shortage is resolved.
  Previously unvaccinated older infants and children:
    7-11 months: 0.5 mL for a total of 3 doses; 2 doses at least 4 weeks apart, followed by a third dose after the 1-year birthday (12-15 months), separated from the second dose by at least 2 months. In case of a severe shortage of vaccine, defer the third dose until shortage is resolved.
    12-23 months: 0.5 mL for a total of 2 doses, separated by at least 2 months. In case of a severe shortage of vaccine, defer the second dose until shortage is resolved.
    24-59 months:
      Healthy Children: 0.5 mL as a single dose. In case of a severe shortage of vaccine, defer dosing until shortage is resolved.
      Children with sickle cell disease, asplenia, HIV infection, chronic illness or immunocompromising conditions (not including bone marrow transplants - results pending; use PPV23 [pneumococcal polysaccharide vaccine, polyvalent] at 12- and 24-months until studies are complete): 0.5 mL for a total of 2 doses, separated by 2 months

Previously vaccinated children with a lapse in vaccine administration:
7-11 months: Previously received 1 or 2 doses PCV7: 0.5 mL dose at 7-11 months of age, followed by a second dose ≥2 months later at 12-15 months of age
12-23 months:
Previously received 1 dose before 12 months of age: 0.5 mL dose, followed by a second dose ≥2 months later
Previously received 2 doses before age 12 months: 0.5 mL dose ≥2 months after the most recent dose
24-59 months: Any incomplete schedule: 0.5 mL as a single dose; **Note:** Patients with chronic diseases or immunosuppressing conditions should receive 2 doses ≥2 months apart

Dosage Forms
Injection, suspension:
Prevnar®: 2 mcg of each saccharide for serotypes 4, 9V, 14, 18C, 19F, and 23F, and 4 mcg of serotype 6B per 0.5 mL (0.5 mL)

pneumococcal polysaccharide vaccine (polyvalent)
(noo moe KOK al pol i SAK a ride vak SEEN, pol i VAY lent)
Synonyms 23-valent pneumococcal polysaccharide vaccine; 23PS; PPV23
U.S./Canadian Brand Names Pneumo 23™ [Can]; Pneumovax® 23 [US/Can]
Therapeutic Category Vaccine, Inactivated Bacteria
Use Children ≥2 years of age and adults who are at increased risk of pneumococcal disease and its complications because of underlying health conditions (including patients with cochlear implants); routine use in older adults >50 years of age, including all those ≥65 years
Current Advisory Committee on Immunization Practices (ACIP) guidelines recommend **pneumococcal 7-valent conjugate vaccine (PCV7)** be used for children 2-23 months of age and, in certain situations, children up to 59 months of age
Usual Dosage I.M., SubQ:
Children >2 years and Adults: 0.5 mL
Previously vaccinated with PCV7 vaccine: Children ≥2 years and Adults:
With sickle cell disease, asplenia, immunocompromised or HIV infection: 0.5 mL at ≥2 years of age and ≥2 months after last dose of PCV7; revaccination with PPV23 should be given ≥5 years for children >10 years of age and every 3-5 years for children ≤10 years of age; revaccination should not be administered <3 years after the previous PPV23 dose
With chronic illness: 0.5 mL at ≥2 years of age and ≥2 months after last dose of PCV7; revaccination with PPV23 is not recommended
Following bone marrow transplant (use of PCV7 under study): Administer one dose PPV23 at 12- and 24-months following BMT

Revaccination should be considered:
1. If ≥6 years since initial vaccination has elapsed, or
2. In patients who received 14-valent pneumococcal vaccine and are at highest risk (asplenic) for fatal infection or
3. At ≥6 years in patients with nephrotic syndrome, renal failure, or transplant recipients, or
4. 3-5 years in children with nephrotic syndrome, asplenia, or sickle cell disease

Pneumomist® *(Discontinued)* *see* guaifenesin *on page 453*
Pneumotussin® *(Discontinued)*
Pneumovax® 23 [US/Can] *see* pneumococcal polysaccharide vaccine (polyvalent) *on page 763*
PNU-140690E *see* tipranavir *on page 930*
Pnu-Imune® 23 *(Discontinued)*
Podactin Cream [US-OTC] *see* miconazole *on page 630*
Podactin Powder [US-OTC] *see* tolnaftate *on page 934*
Pod-Ben-25® *(Discontinued)* *see* podophyllum resin *on page 764*
Podocon-25® [US] *see* podophyllum resin *on page 764*
Podofilm® [Can] *see* podophyllum resin *on page 764*

podofilox (poe DOF il oks)
U.S./Canadian Brand Names Condyline™ [Can]; Condylox® [US]; Wartec® [Can]
Therapeutic Category Keratolytic Agent

Use Treatment of external genital warts

Usual Dosage Topical: Adults: Apply twice daily (morning and evening) for 3 consecutive days, then withhold use for 4 consecutive days; this cycle may be repeated up to 4 times until there is no visible wart tissue

Dosage Forms
  Gel:
    Condylox®: 0.5% (3.5 g)
  Solution, topical: 0.5% (3.5 mL)
    Condylox®: 0.5% (3.5 mL)

Podofin® *(Discontinued)* *see* podophyllum resin *on page 764*
podophyllin *see* podophyllum resin *on page 764*

podophyllum resin (po DOF fil um REZ in)

Synonyms mandrake; may apple; podophyllin

U.S./Canadian Brand Names Podocon-25® [US]; Podofilm® [Can]

Therapeutic Category Keratolytic Agent

Use Topical treatment of benign growths including external genital and perianal warts, papillomas, fibroids; compound benzoin tincture generally is used as the medium for topical application

Usual Dosage Topical:

Children and Adults: 10% to 25% solution in compound benzoin tincture; apply drug to dry surface, use 1 drop at a time allowing drying between drops until area is covered; total volume should be limited to <0.5 mL per treatment session

Condylomata acuminatum: 25% solution is applied daily; use a 10% solution when applied to or near mucous membranes

Verrucae: 25% solution is applied 3-5 times/day directly to the wart

Dosage Forms
  Liquid, topical:
    Podocon-25®: 25% (15 mL)

Point-Two® *(Discontinued)* *see* fluoride *on page 411*
Poladex® *(Discontinued)* *see* dexchlorpheniramine *on page 280*
Polaramine® *(Discontinued)* *see* dexchlorpheniramine *on page 280*
poliovirus, inactivated (IPV) *see* diphtheria and tetanus toxoids, acellular pertussis, and poliovirus (inactivated) vaccine *on page 307*
poliovirus, inactivated (IPV) *see* diphtheria and tetanus toxoids, acellular pertussis, poliovirus (inactivated) and *Haemophilus* b conjugate vaccine *on page 308*

poliovirus vaccine (inactivated) (POE lee oh VYE rus vak SEEN, in ak ti VAY ted)

Synonyms enhanced-potency inactivated poliovirus vaccine; IPV; salk vaccine

U.S./Canadian Brand Names IPOL® [US/Can]

Therapeutic Category Vaccine, Live Virus and Inactivated Virus

Use Active immunization against poliomyelitis caused by poliovirus types 1, 2 and 3. Routine immunization of adults in the United States is generally not recommended. Adults with previous wild poliovirus disease, who have never been immunized, or those who are incompletely immunized may receive inactivated poliovirus vaccine if they fall into one of the following categories:
- Travelers to regions or countries where poliomyelitis is endemic or epidemic
- Healthcare workers in close contact with patients who may be excreting poliovirus
- Laboratory workers handling specimens that may contain poliovirus
- Members of communities or specific population groups with diseases caused by wild poliovirus
- Incompletely vaccinated or unvaccinated adults in a household or with other close contact with children receiving oral poliovirus (may be at increased risk of vaccine associated paralytic poliomyelitis)

Usual Dosage I.M., SubQ:

Children:

Primary immunization: Administer three 0.5 mL doses, preferably 8 or more weeks apart, at 2,4, and 6-18 months of age. First dose may be given as early as 6 weeks of age. Do not administer more frequently than 4 weeks apart.

Booster dose: 0.5 mL at 4-6 years of age

Adults:
Previously unvaccinated: Two 0.5 mL doses administered at 1- to 2-month intervals, followed by a third dose 6-12 months later. If <3 months, but at least 2 months are available before protection is needed, 3 doses may be administered at least 1 month apart. If administration must be completed within 1-2 months, give 2 doses at least 1 month apart. If <1 month is available, give 1 dose.
Incompletely vaccinated: Adults with at least 1 previous dose of OPV, <3 doses of IPV, or a combination of OPV and IPV equaling <3 doses, administer at least one 0.5 mL dose of IPV. Additional doses to complete the series may be given if time permits.
Completely vaccinated: One 0.5 mL dose

Dosage Forms
Injection, suspension:
IPOL®: Type 1 poliovirus 40 D antigen units, type 2 poliovirus 8 D antigen units, and type 3 poliovirus 32 D antigen units per 0.5 mL (0.5 mL, 5 mL)

Polocaine® [US/Can] see mepivacaine on page 604
Polocaine® 2% and Levonordefrin 1:20,000 [Can] see mepivacaine and levonordefrin on page 605
Polocaine® Dental [US] see mepivacaine on page 604
Polocaine® MPF [US] see mepivacaine on page 604

polycarbophil (pol i KAR boe fil)
U.S./Canadian Brand Names Equalactin® [US-OTC]; Fiber-Lax® [US-OTC]; Fiber-Tabs™ [US-OTC]; FiberCon® [US-OTC]; Konsyl® Fiber Caplets [US-OTC]
Therapeutic Category Gastrointestinal Agent, Miscellaneous; Laxative
Use Treatment of constipation or diarrhea
Usual Dosage Oral: General dosing guidelines (OTC labeling):
Children 6-12 years: 625 mg calcium polycarbophil 1-4 times/day
Children ≥12 years and Adults: 1250 mg calcium polycarbophil 1-4 times/day
Dosage Forms
Caplet: Calcium polycarbophil 625 mg [equivalent to polycarbophil 500 mg]
FiberCon® [OTC], Konsyl® Fiber [OTC]: Calcium polycarbophil 625 mg
Captab:
Fiber-Lax® [OTC]: Calcium polycarbophil 625 mg
Tablet: Calcium polycarbophil 625 mg
Fiber-Tabs™: Calcium polycarbophil 625 mg
Tablet, chewable:
Equalactin® [OTC]: Calcium polycarbophil 625 mg

Polycitra® [US] see citric acid, sodium citrate, and potassium citrate on page 226
Polycitra®-K [US] see potassium citrate and citric acid on page 772
Polycitra®-LC [US] see citric acid, sodium citrate, and potassium citrate on page 226
Polycose® [US-OTC] see glucose polymers on page 447
Poly-Dex™ [US] see neomycin, polymyxin B, and dexamethasone on page 662

polyethylene glycol 3350 (pol i ETH i leen GLY kol 3350)
Sound-Alike/Look-Alike Issues
MiraLax® may be confused with Mirapex®
Synonyms PEG
U.S./Canadian Brand Names GlycoLax® [US]; MiraLax® [US-OTC]
Therapeutic Category Laxative, Osmotic
Use Treatment of occasional constipation in adults
Usual Dosage Oral: Adults: Occasional constipation: 17 g of powder (~1 heaping tablespoon) dissolved in 8 oz of water, once daily; do not use for >2 weeks.
Dosage Forms
Powder, for oral solution: PEG 3350 17 g/packet (12s); PEG 3350 255 g (14 oz); PEG 3350 527 g (26 oz)
GlycoLax™: PEG 3350 527 g (24 oz)
MiraLax® [OTC]: PEG 3350 255 g (14 oz)

polyethylene glycol-electrolyte solution

(pol i ETH i leen GLY kol ee LEK troe lite soe LOO shun)

Sound-Alike/Look-Alike Issues

GoLYTELY® may be confused with NuLYTELY®

NuLYTELY® may be confused with GoLYTELY®

Synonyms electrolyte lavage solution

U.S./Canadian Brand Names Colyte® [US/Can]; GoLYTELY® [US]; Klean-Prep® [Can]; MoviPrep® [US]; NuLYTELY® [US]; PegLyte® [Can]; TriLyte® [US]

Therapeutic Category Laxative

Use Bowel cleansing prior to GI examination

Usual Dosage

Oral:

Children ≥6 months: Bowel cleansing prior to GI exam (CoLyte®, GoLYTELY®, NuLYTELY®, TriLyte®): 25 mL/kg/hour (some studies have used up to 40 mL/kg/hour) for 4-10 hours (until rectal effluent is clear). Maximum total dose: 4 L. **Note:** The solution may be given via nasogastric tube to patients who are unwilling or unable to drink the solution. Patients <2 years should be monitored closely.

Adults: Bowel cleansing prior to GI exam:

CoLyte®, GoLYTELY®, NuLYTELY®, TriLyte®: 240 mL (8 oz) every 10 minutes, until 4 L are consumed or the rectal effluent is clear; rapid drinking of each portion is preferred to drinking small amounts continuously. Ideally, patients should fast for ~3-4 hours prior to administration; absolutely no solid food for at least 2 hours before the solution is given. **Note:** The solution may be given via nasogastric tube to patients who are unwilling or unable to drink the solution.

MoviPrep®: Administer 2 L total with an additional 1 L of clear fluid prior to colonoscopy as follows:

Split dose: Evening before colonoscopy: 240 mL (8 oz) every 15 minutes until 1 L is consumed. Then drink 16 oz of clear liquid. On the morning of the colonoscopy, repeat process with second liter over 1 hour and then drink 16 oz of clear liquid at least 1 hour before the procedure.

Full dose: Evening before colonoscopy (~6 PM): 240 mL (8 oz every 15 minutes) until 1 L is consumed; 90 minutes later (~7:30 PM), repeat dose. Then drink 32 oz of clear liquid.

Nasogastric tube (CoLyte®, GoLYTELY®, NuLYTELY®, TriLyte®):

Bowel cleansing prior to GI exam:

Children ≥6 months: 25 mL/kg/hour until rectal effluent is clear.

Adults: Bowel cleansing prior to GI exam: 20-30 mL/minute (1.2-1.8 L/hour); the first bowel movement should occur ~1 hour after the start of administration.

Dosage Forms

Powder, for oral solution: PEG 3350 240 g, sodium sulfate 22.72 g, sodium bicarbonate 6.72 g, sodium chloride 5.84 g, and potassium 2.98 g

Colyte®: PEG 3350 240 g, sodium sulfate 22.72 g, sodium bicarbonate 6.72 g, sodium chloride 5.84 g, and potassium 2.98 g

GoLYTELY®:

PEG 3350 236 g, sodium sulfate 22.74 g, sodium bicarbonate 6.74 g, sodium chloride 5.86 g, and potassium2.97 g

PEG 3350 227.1 g, sodium sulfate 21.5 g, sodium bicarbonate 6.36 g, sodium chloride 5.53 g, and potassium 2.82 g per packet (1s)

MoviPrep®: Pouch A: PEG 3350 100g, sodium sulfate 7.5 g, sodium chloride 2.69 g, potassium chloride 1.015 g; Pouch B: Ascorbic acid 4.7 g, sodium ascorbate 5.9 g

NuLYTELY®: PEG 3350 420 g, sodium bicarbonate 5.72 g, sodium chloride 11.2 g, and potassium 1.48

TriLyte®: PEG 3350 420 g, sodium bicarbonate 5.72 g, sodium chloride 11.2 g, and potassium 1.48

polyethylene glycol-electrolyte solution and bisacodyl

(pol i ETH i leen GLY kol ee LEK troe lite soe LOO shun & bis a KOE dil)

Synonyms electrolyte lavage solution

U.S./Canadian Brand Names HalfLytely® and Bisacodyl [US]

Therapeutic Category Laxative, Bowel Evacuant; Laxative, Stimulant

Use Bowel cleansing prior to colonoscopy

Usual Dosage Oral: Adults: Bowel cleansing:

Bisacodyl: 4 tablets as a single dose. After bowel movement or 6 hours (whichever occurs first), initiate polyethylene glycol-electrolyte solution

Polyethylene glycol-electrolyte solution: 8 ounces every 10 minutes until 2 L are consumed

Dosage Forms
Kit [each kit contains]:
HalfLytely® and Bisacodyl:
Powder for oral solution (HalfLytely®): PEG 3350 210 g, sodium bicarbonate 2.86 g, sodium chloride 5.6 g, potassium 0.74 g
Tablet, delayed release (Bisacodyl): 5 mg (2s)

Polygam® S/D *(Discontinued)* see immune globulin (intravenous) *on page 503*
Poly-Hist DM [US] see phenylephrine, pyrilamine, and dextromethorphan *on page 749*
Poly-Histine-D® Capsule *(Discontinued)*
Poly-Iron 150 [US-OTC] see polysaccharide-iron complex *on page 768*

polymyxin B (pol i MIKS in bee)

Synonyms polymyxin B sulfate
U.S./Canadian Brand Names Poly-Rx [US]
Therapeutic Category Antibiotic, Irrigation; Antibiotic, Miscellaneous
Use Treatment of acute infections caused by susceptible strains of *Pseudomonas aeruginosa*; used occasionally for gut decontamination; parenteral use of polymyxin B has mainly been replaced by less toxic antibiotics, reserved for life-threatening infections caused by organisms resistant to the preferred drugs (eg, pseudomonal meningitis - intrathecal administration)
Usual Dosage
Otic (in combination with other drugs): 1-2 drops, 3-4 times/day; should be used sparingly to avoid accumulation of excess debris
Infants <2 years:
I.M.: Up to 40,000 units/kg/day divided every 6 hours (not routinely recommended due to pain at injection sites)
I.V.: Up to 40,000 units/kg/day divided every 12 hours
Intrathecal: 20,000 units/day for 3-4 days, then 25,000 units every other day for at least 2 weeks after CSF cultures are negative and CSF (glucose) has returned to within normal limits
Children ≥2 years and Adults:
I.M.: 25,000-30,000 units/kg/day divided every 4-6 hours (not routinely recommended due to pain at injection sites)
I.V.: 15,000-25,000 units/kg/day divided every 12 hours
Intrathecal: 50,000 units/day for 3-4 days, then every other day for at least 2 weeks after CSF cultures are negative and CSF (glucose) has returned to within normal limits
Total daily dose should not exceed 2,000,000 units/day
Bladder irrigation: Continuous irrigant or rinse in the urinary bladder for up to 10 days using 20 mg (equal to 200,000 units) added to 1 L of normal saline; usually no more than 1 L of irrigant is used per day unless urine flow rate is high; administration rate is adjusted to patient's urine output
Topical irrigation or topical solution: 500,000 units/L of normal saline; topical irrigation should not exceed 2 million units/day in adults
Gut sterilization: Oral: 15,000-25,000 units/kg/day in divided doses every 6 hours
Clostridium difficile enteritis: Oral: 25,000 units every 6 hours for 10 days
Ophthalmic: A concentration of 0.1% to 0.25% is administered as 1-3 drops every hour, then increasing the interval as response indicates to 1-2 drops 4-6 times/day
Dosage Forms
Injection, powder for reconstitution: 500,000 units
Powder [for prescription compounding]:
Poly-Rx: 100 million units (13 g)

polymyxin B and bacitracin see bacitracin and polymyxin B *on page 113*
polymyxin B and neomycin see neomycin and polymyxin B *on page 662*
polymyxin B and trimethoprim see trimethoprim and polymyxin B *on page 954*
polymyxin B, bacitracin, and neomycin see bacitracin, neomycin, and polymyxin B *on page 114*
polymyxin B, bacitracin, neomycin, and hydrocortisone see bacitracin, neomycin, polymyxin B, and hydrocortisone *on page 114*
polymyxin B, neomycin, and dexamethasone see neomycin, polymyxin B, and dexamethasone *on page 662*
polymyxin B, neomycin, and gramicidin see neomycin, polymyxin B, and gramicidin *on page 663*

polymyxin B, neomycin, and hydrocortisone *see* neomycin, polymyxin B, and hydrocortisone *on page 663*

polymyxin B, neomycin, and prednisolone *see* neomycin, polymyxin B, and prednisolone *on page 664*

polymyxin B, neomycin, bacitracin, and pramoxine *see* bacitracin, neomycin, polymyxin B, and pramoxine *on page 114*

polymyxin B sulfate *see* polymyxin B *on page 767*

polyphenols *see* sinecatechins *on page 868*

polyphenon E *see* sinecatechins *on page 868*

Poly-Pred® [US] *see* neomycin, polymyxin B, and prednisolone *on page 664*

Poly-Rx [US] *see* polymyxin B *on page 767*

polysaccharide-iron complex (pol i SAK a ride-EYE ern KOM pleks)

Sound-Alike/Look-Alike Issues
Niferex® may be confused with Nephrox®

Synonyms iron-polysaccharide complex

U.S./Canadian Brand Names Ferrex 150 [US-OTC]; Niferex® [US-OTC]; Nu-Iron® 150 [US-OTC]; Poly-Iron 150 [US-OTC]; ProFe [US-OTC]

Therapeutic Category Electrolyte Supplement, Oral

Use Prevention and treatment of iron-deficiency anemias

Usual Dosage
Children ≥6 years: Tablets/elixir: 50-100 mg/day; may be given in divided doses
Adults:
Elixir: 50-100 mg twice daily
Capsules: 150-300 mg/day

Dosage Forms
Capsule: Elemental iron 150 mg
Ferrex 150 [OTC], Nu-Iron® 150 [OTC], Poly-Iron 150 [OTC]: Elemental iron 150 mg
Niferex®: Elemental iron 60 mg
ProFe: Elemental iron 180 mg
Elixir:
Niferex® [OTC]: Elemental iron 100 mg/5 mL

Polysporin® [US-OTC] *see* bacitracin and polymyxin B *on page 113*

Polytar® *(Discontinued)* *see* coal tar *on page 240*

Polytrim® [US/Can] *see* trimethoprim and polymyxin B *on page 954*

Poly Tussin DM [US] *see* chlorpheniramine, phenylephrine, and dextromethorphan *on page 209*

PolyTussin HD [US] *see* phenylephrine, hydrocodone, and chlorpheniramine *on page 748*

Poly-Vi-Flor® *(Discontinued)* *see* vitamins (multiple/pediatric) *on page 983*

Poly-Vi-Flor® With Iron [US] *see* vitamins (multiple/pediatric) *on page 983*

polyvinyl alcohol *see* artificial tears *on page 95*

polyvinylpyrrolidone with iodine *see* povidone-iodine *on page 775*

Poly-Vi-Sol® [US-OTC] *see* vitamins (multiple/pediatric) *on page 983*

Poly-Vi-Sol® with Iron [US-OTC] *see* vitamins (multiple/pediatric) *on page 983*

Pondocillin® [Can] *see* pivampicillin *(Canada only)* *on page 758*

Ponstan® [Can] *see* mefenamic acid *on page 598*

Ponstel® [US] *see* mefenamic acid *on page 598*

Pontocaine® [US/Can] *see* tetracaine *on page 914*

Pontocaine® Niphanoid® [US] *see* tetracaine *on page 914*

poractant alfa (por AKT ant AL fa)

U.S./Canadian Brand Names Curosurf® [US/Can]

Therapeutic Category Lung Surfactant

Use Orphan drug: Treatment and prevention of respiratory distress syndrome (RDS) in premature infants

Usual Dosage Intratracheal use **only:** Premature infant with RDS: Initial dose is 2.5 mL/kg of birth weight. Up to 2 subsequent doses of 1.25 mL/kg birth weight can be administered at 12-hour intervals if needed in infants who continue to require mechanical ventilation and supplemental oxygen.

Dosage Forms
Suspension, intratracheal [preservative free; porcine derived]:
Curosurf®: 80 mg/mL

Porcelana® Sunscreen *(Discontinued)* *see* hydroquinone *on page 488*

porfimer (POR fi mer)

Synonyms CL-184116; dihematoporphyrin ether; porfimer sodium
U.S./Canadian Brand Names Photofrin® [US/Can]
Therapeutic Category Antineoplastic Agent
Use Adjunct to laser light therapy for obstructing esophageal cancer, obstructing endobronchial nonsmall cell lung cancer (NSCLC), ablation of high-grade dysplasia in Barrett esophagus
Usual Dosage I.V. (refer to individual protocols): Adults: 2 mg/kg, followed by exposure to the appropriate laser light; repeat courses must be separated by at least 30 days (esophageal or endobronchial cancer) or 90 days (Barrett esophagus) for a maximum of 3 courses
Dosage Forms
Injection, powder for reconstitution:
Photofrin®: 75 mg

porfimer sodium *see* porfimer *on page 769*
Portagen® [US-OTC] *see* nutritional formula, enteral/oral *on page 689*
Portia™ [US] *see* ethinyl estradiol and levonorgestrel *on page 372*

posaconazole (poe sa KON a zole)

Sound-Alike/Look-Alike Issues
Noxafil® may be confused with minoxidil
Synonyms SCH 56592
U.S./Canadian Brand Names Noxafil® [US]; Spriafil® [Can]
Therapeutic Category Antifungal Agent, Oral
Use Prophylaxis of invasive *Aspergillus* and *Candida* infections in severely-immunocompromised patients [eg, hematopoietic stem cell transplant (HSCT) recipients with graft-versus-host disease (GVHD) or those with prolonged neutropenia secondary to chemotherapy for hematologic malignancies]; treatment of oropharyngeal candidiasis (including patients refractory to itraconazole and/or fluconazole)
Usual Dosage Oral: Children ≥13 years and Adults:
Aspergillosis, invasive: *Prophylaxis:* 200 mg 3 times/day
Candidal infections:
Prophylaxis: 200 mg 3 times/day
Treatment of oropharyngeal infection: Initial: 100 mg twice daily for 1 day; maintenance: 100 mg once daily for 13 days
Treatment of refractory oropharyngeal infection: 400 mg twice daily
Dosage Forms
Suspension, oral:
Noxafil®: 40 mg/mL

Post Peel Healing Balm [US-OTC] *see* hydrocortisone (topical) *on page 485*
Posture® [US-OTC] *see* calcium phosphate (tribasic) *on page 167*
Potasalan® *(Discontinued)* *see* potassium chloride *on page 771*

potassium acetate (poe TASS ee um AS e tate)

Therapeutic Category Electrolyte Supplement, Oral
Use Potassium deficiency; to avoid chloride when high concentration of potassium is needed, source of bicarbonate
Usual Dosage I.V. doses should be incorporated into the patient's maintenance I.V. fluids, intermittent I.V. potassium administration should be reserved for severe depletion situations and requires ECG monitoring; doses listed as mEq of potassium

Children:
Treatment of hypokalemia: I.V.: 2-5 mEq/kg/day
I.V. intermittent infusion (must be diluted prior to administration): 0.5-1 mEq/kg/dose (maximum: 30 mEq/dose) to infuse at 0.3-0.5 mEq/kg/hour (maximum: 1 mEq/kg/hour)

▶

◄ **Note:** Use caution in premature neonates; potassium acetate for injection contains aluminum.
Adults:
Treatment of hypokalemia: I.V.: 40-100 mEq/day
I.V. intermittent infusion (must be diluted prior to administration): 5-10 mEq/dose (maximum: 40 mEq/
dose) to infuse over 2-3 hours (maximum: 40 mEq over 1 hour)
Note: Continuous cardiac monitor recommended for rates >0.5 mEq/hour
Potassium dosage/rate of infusion guidelines:
Serum potassium >2.5 mEq/L: Maximum infusion rate: 10 mEq/hour; maximum concentration: 40 mEq/
L; maximum 24-hour dose: 200 mEq
Serum potassium <2.5 mEq/L: Maximum infusion rate: 40 mEq/hour; maximum concentration: 80 mEq/
L; maximum 24-hour dose: 400 mEq
Dosage Forms
Injection, solution: 2 mEq/mL (20 mL, 50 mL, 100 mL) [contains aluminum]
Injection, solution [concentrate]: 4 mEq/mL (50 mL) [contains aluminum]

potassium acid phosphate (poe TASS ee um AS id FOS fate)
U.S./Canadian Brand Names K-Phos® Original [US]
Therapeutic Category Urinary Acidifying Agent
Use Acidifies urine and lowers urinary calcium concentration; reduces odor and rash caused by
ammoniacal urine; increases the antibacterial activity of methenamine
Usual Dosage Oral: Adults: 1000 mg dissolved in 6-8 oz of water 4 times/day with meals and at bedtime;
for best results, soak tablets in water for 2-5 minutes, then stir and swallow
Dosage Forms
Tablet [scored]:
K-Phos® Original: 500 mg

potassium bicarbonate (poe TASS ee um bye KAR bun ate)
Therapeutic Category Electrolyte Supplement, Oral
Use Potassium deficiency, hypokalemia
Usual Dosage Oral:
Children: 1-4 mEq/kg/day
Adults: 25 mEq 2-4 times/day
Dosage Forms
Tablet for oral solution, effervescent: Potassium 25 mEq

potassium bicarbonate and potassium chloride
(poe TASS ee um bye KAR bun ate & poe TASS ee um KLOR ide)
Synonyms potassium bicarbonate and potassium chloride (effervescent)
Therapeutic Category Electrolyte Supplement, Oral
Use Treatment or prevention of hypokalemia
Usual Dosage Oral:
Children: 1-4 mEq/kg/24 hours in divided doses as required to maintain normal serum potassium
Adults:
Prevention: 16-24 mEq/day in 2-4 divided doses
Treatment: 40-100 mEq/day in 2-4 divided doses
Dosage Forms
Tablet for solution, oral [effervescent]: Potassium chloride 25 mEq

potassium bicarbonate and potassium chloride (effervescent) *see* potassium bicarbonate and
potassium chloride *on page 770*

potassium bicarbonate and potassium citrate
(poe TASS ee um bye KAR bun ate & poe TASS ee um SIT rate)
Sound-Alike/Look-Alike Issues
Klor-Con® may be confused with Klaron®, K-Lor®
Synonyms potassium bicarbonate and potassium citrate (effervescent)
U.S./Canadian Brand Names Effer-K™ [US]; K-Lyte® DS [US]; K-Lyte® [US]; Klor-Con®/EF [US]
Therapeutic Category Electrolyte Supplement, Oral

Use Treatment or prevention of hypokalemia

Usual Dosage Oral:

Children: 1-4 mEq/kg/24 hours in divided doses as required to maintain normal serum potassium

Adults:

Prevention: 16-24 mEq/day in 2-4 divided doses

Treatment: 40-100 mEq/day in 2-4 divided doses

Dosage Forms

Tablet, effervescent:

Effer-K™, Klor-Con®/EF, K-Lyte®: Potassium 25 mEq

K-Lyte® DS: Potassium 50 mEq

potassium bicarbonate and potassium citrate (effervescent) *see* potassium bicarbonate and potassium citrate *on page 770*

potassium chloride (poe TASS ee um KLOR ide)

Sound-Alike/Look-Alike Issues

Kaon-Cl-10® may be confused with kaolin

KCl may be confused with HCl

K-Lor® may be confused with Klor-Con®

Klor-Con® may be confused with Klaron®, K-Lor®

microK® may be confused with Micronase®

Synonyms KCl

U.S./Canadian Brand Names Apo-K® [Can]; K-10® [Can]; K-Dur® [Can]; K-Lor® [US/Can]; K-Lyte®/Cl [Can]; K-Tab® [US]; Kaon-Cl-10® [US]; Kay Ciel® [US]; Klor-Con® 10 [US]; Klor-Con® 8 [US]; Klor-Con® M [US]; Klor-Con® [US]; Klor-Con®/25 [US]; Micro-K Extencaps® [Can]; microK® 10 [US]; microK® [US]; Roychlor® [Can]; Slo-Pot [Can]; Slow-K® [Can]

Therapeutic Category Electrolyte Supplement, Oral

Use Treatment or prevention of hypokalemia

Usual Dosage I.V. doses should be incorporated into the patient's maintenance I.V. fluids; intermittent I.V. potassium administration should be reserved for severe depletion situations in patients undergoing ECG monitoring. Doses expressed as mEq of potassium.

Normal daily requirements: Oral, I.V.:

Children: 1-2 mEq/kg/day

Adults: 40-80 mEq/day

Prevention of hypokalemia: Oral:

Children: 1-2 mEq/kg/day in 1-2 divided doses

Adults: 20-40 mEq/day in 1-2 divided doses

Treatment of hypokalemia: Children:

Oral: 1-2 mEq/kg initially, then as needed based on frequently obtained lab values. If deficits are severe or ongoing losses are great, I.V. route should be considered.

I.V. intermittent infusion: 0.5-1 mEq/kg/dose (maximum dose: 40 mEq). If infusion exceeds 0.5 mEq/kg/ hour, physician should be at bedside and patient should have continuous ECG monitoring; repeat as needed based on frequently obtained lab values.

Treatment of hypokalemia: Adults:

Oral:

Asymptomatic, mild hypokalemia: Usual dosage range: 40-100 mEq/day divided in 2-5 doses; generally recommended to limit doses to 20-25 mEq/dose to avoid GI discomfort.

Mild-to-moderate hypokalemia: Some clinicians may administer up to 120-240 mEq/day divided in 3-4 doses; limit doses to 40-60 mEq/dose. If deficits are severe or ongoing losses are great, I.V. route should be considered.

I.V. intermittent infusion: Peripheral or central line: ≤10 mEq/hour; repeat as needed based on frequently obtained lab values; central line infusion and continuous ECG monitoring highly recommended for infusions >10 mEq/hour.

Potassium dosage/rate of infusion general guidelines (per product labeling): **Note:** High variability exists in dosing/infusion rate recommendations; therapy guided by patient condition and specific institutional guidelines.

Serum potassium >2.5 mEq/L: Maximum infusion rate: 10 mEq/hour; maximum concentration: 40 mEq/L; maximum 24-hour dose: 200 mEq

Serum potassium <2 mEq/L and symptomatic (excluding emergency treatment of cardiac arrest): Maximum infusion rate (central line only): 40 mEq/hour in presence of continuous ECG monitoring and frequent lab monitoring; In selected situations, patients may require up to 400 mEq/24 hours. ▶

◀ **Dosage Forms**
  Capsule, extended release, microencapsulated: 10 mEq [750 mg]
    microK®: 8 mEq [600 mg]
    microK® 10: 10 mEq [750 mg]
  Infusion [premixed in D_5W]: 20 mEq (1000 mL); 30 mEq (1000 mL); 40 mEq (1000 mL)
  Infusion [premixed in D_5W and LR]: 20 mEq (1000 mL); 30 mEq (1000 mL); 40 mEq (1000 mL)
  Infusion [premixed in D_5W and sodium chloride 0.2%]: 5 mEq (250 mL); 10 mEq (500 mL, 1000 mL); 20 mEq (1000 mL); 30 mEq (1000 mL); 40 mEq (1000 mL)
  Infusion [premixed in D_5W and sodium chloride 0.225%]: 10 mEq (500 mL, 1000 mL); 20 mEq (1000 mL); 30 mEq (1000 mL); 40 mEq (1000 mL)
  Infusion [premixed in D_5W and sodium chloride 0.3%]: 10 mEq (500 mL); 20 mEq (1000 mL)
  Infusion [premixed in D_5W and sodium chloride 0.33%]: 10 mEq (500 mL); 20 mEq (1000 mL)
  Infusion [premixed in D_5W and sodium chloride 0.45%]: 10 mEq (500 mL, 1000 mL); 20 mEq (1000 mL); 30 mEq (1000 mL); 40 mEq (1000 mL)
  Infusion [premixed in D_5W and NS]: 20 mEq (1000 mL); 40 mEq (1000 mL)
  Infusion [premixed in $D_{10}W$ and sodium chloride 0.2%]: 5 mEq (250 mL)
  Infusion [premixed in sodium chloride 0.45%]: 20 mEq (1000 mL); 40 mEq (1000 mL)
  Infusion [premixed in NS]: 20 mEq (1000 mL); 40 mEq (1000 mL)
  Infusion [premixed in SWFI; highly concentrated]: 10 mEq (50 mL, 100 mL); 20 mEq (50 mL, 100 mL); 30 mEq (100 mL); 40 mEq (100 mL)
  Injection, solution [concentrate]: 2 mEq/mL (5 mL, 10 mL, 15 mL, 20 mL, 30 mL, 250 mL, 500 mL)
  Powder, for oral solution: 20 mEq/packet
    K-Lor™, Klor-Con®: 20 mEq/packet
    Klor-Con®/25: 25 mEq/packet
  Solution, oral: 20 mEq/15 mL, 40 mEq/15 mL
  Tablet, extended release: 8 mEq [600 mg]; 10 mEq [750 mg]; 20 mEq [1500 mg]
    K-Tab®, Kaon-Cl®: 10 mEq
  Tablet, extended release, microencapsulated: 10 mEq, 20 mEq
    Klor-Con® M10: 10 mEq
    Klor-Con® M15: 15 mEq
    Klor-Con® M20: 20 mEq
  Tablet, extended release, wax matrix: 8 mEq, 10 mEq
    Klor-Con® 8: 8 mEq [600 mg]
    Klor-Con® 10: 10 mEq)750 mg]

potassium citrate (poe TASS ee um SIT rate)
  Sound-Alike/Look-Alike Issues
    Urocit®-K may be confused with Urised®
  U.S./Canadian Brand Names K-Citra® [Can]; K-Lyte® [Can]; Urocit®-K [US]
  Therapeutic Category Alkalinizing Agent
  Use Prevention of uric acid nephrolithiasis; prevention of calcium renal stones in patients with hypocitraturia; urinary alkalinizer when sodium citrate is contraindicated
  Usual Dosage Oral: Adults: 10-20 mEq 3 times/day with meals up to 100 mEq/day
  Dosage Forms
    Tablet: 540 mg [5 mEq]; 1080 mg [10 mEq]
      Urocit®-K: 540 mg [5 mEq]; 1080 mg [10 mEq]
    Tablet, extended release: 540 mg [5 mEq]; 1080 mg [10 mEq]

potassium citrate and citric acid (poe TASS ee um SIT rate & SI trik AS id)
  Synonyms citric acid and potassium citrate
  U.S./Canadian Brand Names Cytra-K [US]; Polycitra®-K [US]
  Therapeutic Category Alkalinizing Agent
  Use Treatment of metabolic acidosis; alkalinizing agent in conditions where long-term maintenance of an alkaline urine is desirable
  Usual Dosage Urine alkalizing agent:
  Children: Solution: 5-15 mL after meals and at bedtime; adjust dose based on urinary pH
  Adults:
    Powder: One packet dissolved in water after meals and at bedtime; adjust dose to urinary pH
    Solution: 15-30 mL after meals and at bedtime; adjust dose based on urinary pH

Dosage Forms Equivalent to potassium 2 mEq/mL and bicarbonate 2 mEq/mL
  Powder for solution, oral:
    Cytra-K: Potassium citrate 3300 mg and citric acid 1002 mg per packet (100s)
    Polycitra®-K: Potassium citrate 3300 mg and citric acid 1002 mg per packet (100s)
  Solution:
    Cytra-K: Potassium citrate 1100 mg and citric acid 334 mg per 5 mL
    Polycitra®-K: Potassium citrate 1100 mg and citric acid 334 mg per 5 mL

potassium citrate, citric acid, and sodium citrate *see* citric acid, sodium citrate, and potassium citrate *on page 226*

potassium gluconate (poe TASS ee um GLOO coe nate)

Therapeutic Category Electrolyte Supplement, Oral

Use Treatment or prevention of hypokalemia

Usual Dosage Oral (doses listed as mEq of potassium):
  Normal daily requirement:
    Children: 2-3 mEq/kg/day
    Adults: 40-80 mEq/day
  Prevention of hypokalemia during diuretic therapy:
    Children: 1-2 mEq/kg/day in 1-2 divided doses
    Adults: 16-24 mEq/day in 1-2 divided doses
  Treatment of hypokalemia:
    Children: 2-5 mEq/kg/day in 2-4 divided doses
    Adults: 40-100 mEq/day in 2-4 divided doses

Dosage Forms
  Caplet: 595 mg
  Capsule: 99 mg
  Tablet: 99 mg, 550 mg, 595 mg
  Tablet, timed release: 95 mg

potassium iodide (poe TASS ee um EYE oh dide)

Sound-Alike/Look-Alike Issues
  potassium iodide products, including saturated solution of potassium iodide (SSKI®) may be confused with potassium iodide and iodine (Strong Iodide Solution or Lugol's solution)

Synonyms KI

U.S./Canadian Brand Names Iosat™ [US-OTC]; SSKI® [US]; ThyroSafe™ [US-OTC]; ThyroShield™ [US-OTC]

Therapeutic Category Antithyroid Agent; Expectorant

Use Expectorant for the symptomatic treatment of chronic pulmonary diseases complicated by mucous; reduce thyroid vascularity prior to thyroidectomy and management of thyrotoxic crisis; block thyroidal uptake of radioactive isotopes of iodine in a radiation emergency or other exposure to radioactive iodine

Usual Dosage Oral:
  Adults: RDA: 150 mcg (iodine)
  Expectorant: Adults: SSKI®: 300-600 mg 3-4 times/day
  Preoperative thyroidectomy: Children and Adults: 50-250 mg (1-5 drops SSKI®) 3 times/day; administer for 10 days before surgery
  To reduce risk of thyroid cancer following nuclear accident (Iosat™, ThyroSafe™, ThyroShield™): Dosing should continue until risk of exposure has passed or other measures are implemented:
    Children (see adult dose for children >68 kg):
      Infants <1 month: 16.25 mg once daily
      1 month to 3 years: 32.5 mg once daily
      3-18 years: 65 mg once daily
    Children >68 kg and Adults (including pregnant/lactating women): 130 mg once daily
  Thyrotoxic crisis:
    Infants <1 year: 150-250 mg (3-5 drops SSKI®) 3 times/day
    Children and Adults: 300-500 mg (6-10 drops SSKI®) 3 times/day

Dosage Forms
  Solution, oral:
    SSKI®: 1 g/mL
    ThyroShield™ [OTC]: 65 mg/mL

▶

◄ **Tablet:**
Iosat™ [OTC]: 130 mg
ThyroSafe™ [OTC]: 65 mg

potassium iodide, chlorpheniramine, phenylephrine, and codeine see chlorpheniramine, phenylephrine, codeine, and potassium iodide on page 212

potassium phosphate (poe TASS ee um FOS fate)

Sound-Alike/Look-Alike Issues
Neutra-Phos®-K may be confused with K-Phos Neutral®

Synonyms phosphate, potassium

Therapeutic Category Electrolyte Supplement, Oral

Use Treatment and prevention of hypophosphatemia or hypokalemia

Usual Dosage
Oral:
Normal Requirements Elemental Phosphorus:
0-6 months: 240 mg
6-12 months: 360 mg
1-10 years: 800 mg
>10 years: 1200 mg
Pregnancy/lactation: Additional 400 mg/day
Adults: 800 mg

Oral Maintenance:
Children <4 years: 1 capsule (250 mg phosphorus/8 mmol) 4 times/day; dilute as instructed
Children >4 years and Adults: 1-2 capsules (250-500 mg phosphorus/8-16 mmol) 4 times/day; dilute as instructed

I.V.: Doses listed as mmol of phosphate. **Caution: With orders for I.V. phosphate, there is considerable confusion associated with the use of millimoles (mmol) versus milliequivalents (mEq) to express the phosphate requirement.** The most reliable method of ordering I.V. phosphate is by millimoles, then specifying the potassium or sodium salt.

Acute treatment of hypophosphatemia: It is recommended that repletion of severe hypophosphatemia be done I.V. because large doses of oral phosphate may cause diarrhea and intestinal absorption may be unreliable. Intermittent I.V. infusion should be reserved for severe depletion situations; requires continuous cardiac monitoring. Guidelines differ based on degree of illness, need/use of TPN, and severity of hypophosphatemia. If potassium >4.0 mEq/L consider phosphate replacement strategy without potassium (eg, sodium phosphates). Obese patients and/or severe renal impairment were excluded from phosphate supplement trials.

Children and Adults: **Note:** There are no prospective studies of parenteral phosphate replacement in children. The following weight-based guidelines for adult dosing may be cautiously employed in pediatric patients.

General replacement guidelines:
Low dose: 0.08 mmol/kg over 6 hours; use if losses are recent and uncomplicated
Intermediate dose: 0.16-0.24 mmol/kg over 4-6 hours; use if serum phosphorus level 0.5-1 mg/dL (0.16-0.32 mmoles/L)
Note: The initial dose may be increased by 25% to 50% if the patient is symptomatic secondary to hypophosphatemia and lowered by 25% to 50% if the patient is hypercalcemic.
Patients receiving TPN; supplemental dose:
Low dose: 0.16 mmol/kg over 4-6 hours; use if serum phosphorus level 2.3-3 mg/dL (0.73-0.96 mmoles/L)
Intermediate dose: 0.32 mmol/kg over 4-6 hours; use if serum phosphorus level 1.6-2.2 mg/dL (0.51-0.72 mmoles/L)
High dose: 0.64 mmol/kg over 8-12 hours; use if serum phosphorus <1.5 mg/dL (<0.5 mmoles/L)
Critically-ill adult trauma patients receiving TPN:
Low dose: 0.32 mmol/kg over 4-6 hours; use if serum phosphorus level 2.3-3 mg/dL (0.73-0.96 mmoles/L)
Intermediate dose: 0.64 mmol/kg over 4-6 hours; use if serum phosphorus level 1.6-2.2 mg/dL (0.51-0.72 mmoles/L)
High dose: 1 mmol/kg over 8-12 hours; use if serum phosphorus <1.5 mg/dL (<0.5 mmoles/L)

Maintenance: I.V. solutions: Doses may be incorporated into the patient's maintenance I.V. fluids.

Children: 0.5-1.5 mmol/kg/24 hours I.V. or 2-3 mmol/kg/24 hours orally in divided doses
Adults: 15-30 mmol/24 hours I.V. or 50-150 mmol/24 hours orally in divided doses

Dosage Forms
Injection, solution: Potassium 4.4 mEq and phosphorus 3 mmol per mL (5 mL, 15 mL, 50 mL)

potassium phosphate and sodium phosphate
(poe TASS ee um FOS fate & SOW dee um FOS fate)

Sound-Alike/Look-Alike Issues
K-Phos® Neutral may be confused with Neutra-Phos-K®

Synonyms sodium phosphate and potassium phosphate

U.S./Canadian Brand Names K-Phos® MF [US]; K-Phos® Neutral [US]; K-Phos® No. 2 [US]; Phos-NaK [US]; Phospha 250™ Neutral [US]; Uro-KP-Neutral® [US]

Therapeutic Category Electrolyte Supplement, Oral

Use Treatment of conditions associated with excessive renal phosphate loss or inadequate GI absorption of phosphate; to acidify the urine to lower calcium concentrations; to increase the antibacterial activity of methenamine; reduce odor and rash caused by ammonia in urine

Usual Dosage All dosage forms to be mixed in 6-8 oz of water prior to administration
Children ≥4 years: Elemental phosphorus 250 mg 4 times/day after meals and at bedtime
Adults: Elemental phosphorus 250-500 mg 4 times/day after meals and at bedtime

Dosage Forms
Caplet:
Uro-KP-Neutral®: Dipotassium phosphate, disodium phosphate, and monobasic sodium phosphate
Powder, for oral solution:
Phos-NaK: Dibasic potassium phosphate, monobasic potassium phosphate, dibasic sodium phosphate, and monosodium phosphate per packet (100s)
Tablet:
K-Phos® MF: Potassium phosphate 155 mg and sodium phosphate 350 mg
K-Phos® Neutral: Monobasic potassium phosphate 155 mg, dibasic sodium phosphate 852 mg, and monobasic sodium phosphate 130 mg
K-Phos® No. 2: Potassium phosphate 305 mg and sodium phosphate 700 mg
Phospha 250™ Neutral: Monobasic potassium phosphate 155 mg, dibasic sodium phosphate 852 mg, and monobasic sodium phosphate 130 mg

Povidine™ [US-OTC] see povidone-iodine *on page 775*

povidone-iodine (POE vi done EYE oh dyne)

Sound-Alike/Look-Alike Issues
Betadine® may be confused with Betagan®, betaine

Synonyms polyvinylpyrrolidone with iodine; PVP-I

U.S./Canadian Brand Names Betadine® Ophthalmic [US]; Betadine® [US-OTC/Can]; Operand® [US-OTC]; Povidine™ [US-OTC]; Proviodine [Can]; Summer's Eve® Medicated Douche [US-OTC]; Vagi-Gard® [US-OTC]

Therapeutic Category Antibacterial, Topical

Use External antiseptic with broad microbicidal spectrum for the prevention or treatment of topical infections associated with surgery, burns, minor cuts/scrapes; relief of minor vaginal irritation

Usual Dosage
Antiseptic: Apply topically to affected area as needed. Ophthalmic solution may be used to irrigate the eye or applied to area around the eye such as skin, eyelashes, or lid margins.
Surgical scrub: Topical: Apply solution to wet skin or hands, scrub for ~5 minutes, rinse; refer to product labeling for specific procedure-related instructions.
Vaginal irritation: Douche: Insert 0.3% solution vaginally once daily for 5-7 days

Dosage Forms
Gel, topical: 10% (120 g)
Operand® [OTC]: 10% (120 g)
Liquid, topical [prep-swab ampule]: 10% (0.65 mL)
Ointment, topical: 10% (1 g)
Povidine™ [OTC]: 10% (30 g)
Pad [prep pads]: 10% (200s)
Betadine® SwabAids [OTC]: 10% (100s)
Solution, ophthalmic: 5% (30 mL)
Betadine® [OTC]: 5% (30 mL)

◀ **Solution, perineal** [concentrate]:
 Operand® [OTC]: 10% (240 mL)
Solution, topical: 10% (22 mL, 60 mL, 90 mL, 240 mL, 480 mL, 3840 mL)
 Betadine® [OTC]: 10% (15 mL, 120 mL, 240 mL, 480 mL, 960 mL, 3840 mL)
 Operand® [OTC]: 10% (60 mL, 120 mL, 240 mL, 480 mL, 960 mL, 3840 mL)
 Povidine™ [OTC}: 10% (240 mL)
Solution, topical [cleanser]:
 Betadine® Skin Cleanser [OTC]: 7.5% (120 mL)
Solution, topical [paint sponge]: 10% (50s)
Solution, topical [paint]: 10% (60 mL, 90 mL, 120 mL)
Solution, topical [surgical scrub]: 7.5% (60 mL, 120 mL)
 Betadine® Surgical Scrub [OTC]: 7.5% (120 mL, 480 mL, 960 mL, 3840 mL)
 Operand® [OTC]: 7.5% (60 mL, 120 mL, 240 mL, 480 mL, 960 mL, 3840 mL)
Solution, topical [spray]: 10% (60 mL)
 Betadine® [OTC]: 5% (90 mL)
 Operand® [OTC]: 10% (59 mL)
Solution, topical [surgical scrub sponge]: 10% (50s)
Solution, vaginal [concentrate, douche]:
 Operand® [OTC]: 10% (240 mL)
 Vagi-Gard® [OTC]: 10% (180 mL, 240 mL)
Solution, vaginal [douche]:
 Summer's Eve® Medicated Douche [OTC]: 0.3% (135 mL) [contains sodium benzoate]
Solution [concentrate, whirlpool]:
 Operand® [OTC]: 10% (3840 mL)
Swabsticks: 10% (25s, 50s, 1000s)
 Betadine® [OTC]: 10% (50s, 200s)
Swabsticks [gel saturated]: 10% (50s)
Swabsticks, topical [surgical scrub]: 7.5% (25s, 50s, 1000s)

PPD *see* tuberculin tests *on page 959*
PPL *see* benzylpenicilloyl-polylysine *on page 129*
PPS *see* pentosan polysulfate sodium *on page 737*
PPV23 *see* pneumococcal polysaccharide vaccine (polyvalent) *on page 763*
Pradax™ [Can] *see* dabigatran etexilate *(Canada only) on page 262*

pralidoxime (pra li DOKS eem)

Sound-Alike/Look-Alike Issues
 pralidoxime may be confused with pramoxine, pyridoxine
 Protopam® may be confused with Proloprim®, protamine, Protropin®
Synonyms 2-PAM; 2-pyridine aldoxime methochloride; pralidoxime chloride
U.S./Canadian Brand Names Protopam® [US/Can]
Therapeutic Category Antidote
Use Reverse muscle paralysis caused by toxic exposure to organophosphate anticholinesterase pesticides and chemicals; control of overdose of anticholinesterase medications used to treat myasthenia gravis (ambenonium, neostigmine, pyridostigmine)
Usual Dosage
 Organic phosphorus poisoning (use in conjunction with atropine; atropine effects should be established before pralidoxime is administered): I.V. (may be given I.M. or SubQ if I.V. is not feasible):
 Children: 20-50 mg/kg/dose; repeat in 1-2 hours if muscle weakness has not been relieved, then at 8- to 12-hour intervals if cholinergic signs recur
 Adults: Initial: 30 mg/kg over 20 minutes, maintenance: I.V. infusion: 4-8 mg/kg/hour
 Treatment of acetylcholinesterase inhibitor toxicity: Adults: I.V.: Initial: 1-2 g followed by increments of 250 mg every 5 minutes until response is observed
Dosage Forms
Injection, powder for reconstitution:
 Protopam®: 1 g
Injection, solution: 300 mg/mL (2 mL)

pralidoxime and atropine *see* atropine and pralidoxime *on page 106*
pralidoxime chloride *see* pralidoxime *on page 776*

Pramet® FA *(Discontinued)*
Pramilet® FA *(Discontinued)*

pramipexole (pra mi PEKS ole)
Sound-Alike/Look-Alike Issues
Mirapex® may be confused with Mifeprex®, MiraLax™
U.S./Canadian Brand Names Apo-Pramipexole [Can]; Mirapex® [US/Can]; Novo-Pramipexole [Can]; PMS-Pramipexole [Can]
Therapeutic Category Anti-Parkinson Agent (Dopamine Agonist)
Use Treatment of the signs and symptoms of idiopathic Parkinson disease; treatment of moderate-to-severe primary Restless Legs Syndrome (RLS)
Usual Dosage Oral: Adults:
Parkinson disease: Initial: 0.375 mg/day given in 3 divided doses, increase gradually by 0.125 mg/dose every 5-7 days; range: 1.5-4.5 mg/day
Restless legs syndrome: Initial: 0.125 mg once daily 2-3 hours before bedtime. Dose may be doubled every 4-7 days up to 0.5 mg/day. Maximum dose: 0.5 mg/day (manufacturer's recommendation).
Note: Most patients require <0.5 mg/day, but higher doses have been used (2 mg/day). If augmentation occurs, dose earlier in the day.
Dosage Forms [CAN] = Canadian product
Tablet: 0.25 mg [CAN; generic not available in U.S.], 0.5 mg [CAN; generic not available in U.S.], 1 mg [CAN; generic not available in U.S.], 1.5 mg [CAN; generic not available in U.S.]
Mirapex®: 0.125 mg, 0.25 mg, 0.5 mg, 0.75 mg, 1 mg, 1.5 mg

pramlintide (PRAM lin tide)
Synonyms pramlintide acetate
U.S./Canadian Brand Names Symlin® [US]
Therapeutic Category Antidiabetic Agent
Use
Adjunctive treatment with mealtime insulin in type 1 diabetes mellitus (insulin-dependent, IDDM) patients who have failed to achieve desired glucose control despite optimal insulin therapy
Adjunctive treatment with mealtime insulin in type 2 diabetes mellitus (noninsulin-dependent, NIDDM) patients who have failed to achieve desired glucose control despite optimal insulin therapy, with or without concurrent sulfonylurea and/or metformin
Usual Dosage SubQ: Adults: **Note:** When initiating pramlintide, reduce current insulin dose (including rapidly- and mixed-acting preparations) by 50% to avoid hypoglycemia.
Type 1 diabetes mellitus (insulin-dependent, IDDM): Initial: 15 mcg immediately prior to meals; titrate in 15 mcg increments every 3 days (if no significant nausea occurs) to target dose of 30-60 mcg (consider discontinuation if intolerant of 30 mcg dose)
Type 2 diabetes mellitus (noninsulin-dependent, NIDDM): Initial: 60 mcg immediately prior to meals; after 3-7 days, increase to 120 mcg prior to meals if no significant nausea occurs (if nausea occurs at 120 mcg dose, reduce to 60 mcg)
If pramlintide is discontinued for any reason, restart therapy with same initial titration protocol.
Dosage Forms
Injection, solution:
Symlin®: 600 mcg/mL (5 mL); 1000 mcg/mL (1.5 mL); 1000 mcg/mL (2.7 mL)

pramlintide acetate *see pramlintide on page 777*
Pramosone® [US] *see pramoxine and hydrocortisone on page 778*
Pramox® HC [Can] *see pramoxine and hydrocortisone on page 778*

pramoxine (pra MOKS een)
Sound-Alike/Look-Alike Issues
pramoxine may be confused with pralidoxime
Anusol® may be confused with Anusol-HC®, Aplisol®, Aquasol®
Synonyms pramoxine hydrochloride
U.S./Canadian Brand Names Anusol® Ointment [US-OTC]; Caladryl® Clear [US-OTC]; CalaMycin® Cool and Clear [US-OTC]; Callergy Clear [US-OTC]; Curasore [US-OTC]; Itch-X® [US-OTC]; Prax® [US-OTC]; ProctoFoam® NS [US-OTC]; Sarna® Sensitive [US-OTC]; Soothing Care™ Itch Relief [US-OTC];

◄ Summer's Eve® Anti-Itch Maximum Strength [US-OTC]; Tronolane® Cream [US-OTC]; Tucks® Hemorrhoidal [US-OTC]

Therapeutic Category Local Anesthetic

Use Temporary relief of pain and itching associated with anogenital pruritus or irritation; dermatosis, minor burns, or hemorrhoids

Usual Dosage Topical: Adults: Apply as directed, usually every 3-4 hours to affected area (maximum adult dose: 200 mg)

Dosage Forms

Aerosol, topical [foam]:
ProctoFoam® NS [OTC]: 1% (15 g)

Cloth:
Summer's Eve® Anti-Itch Maximum Strength [OTC]: 1% (12s)

Cream, topical:
Tronolane® [OTC]: 1% (30 g, 60 g)

Gel, topical:
Itch-X® [OTC]: 1% (35.4 g)
Summer's Eve® Anti-Itch Maximum Strength [OTC]: 1% (30 mL)

Liquid, topical:
Curasore® [OTC]: 1% (15 mL)

Lotion, topical:
Caladryl® Clear [OTC]: 1% (177 mL)
Callergy Clear [OTC]: 1% (180 mL)
Prax® [OTC]: 1% (15 mL, 120 mL, 240 mL)
Sarna® Sensitive: 1% (222 mL)

Ointment, rectal:
Anusol® [OTC], Tucks® Hemorrhoidal [OTC]: 1% (30 g)

Solution, topical [spray]:
CalaMycin® Cool and Clear [OTC], Itch-X® [OTC]: 1% (60 mL)
Soothing Care™ Itch Relief: 1% (74 mL)

pramoxine and hydrocortisone (pra MOKS een & hye droe KOR ti sone)

Sound-Alike/Look-Alike Issues
Pramosone® may be confused with predniSONE

Synonyms hydrocortisone and pramoxine; pramoxine hydrochloride and hydrocortisone acetate

U.S./Canadian Brand Names Analpram-HC® [US]; Epifoam® [US]; Pramosone® [US]; Pramox® HC [Can]; ProctoFoam®-HC [US/Can]

Therapeutic Category Anesthetic/Corticosteroid

Use Relief of inflammatory and pruritic manifestations of corticosteroid-responsive dermatoses

Usual Dosage Topical/rectal: Apply to affected areas 3-4 times/day

Dosage Forms

Cream, topical:
Analpram-HC®: Pramoxine 1% and hydrocortisone 1% (4 g, 30 g); pramoxine 1% and hydrocortisone 2.5% (4 g, 30 g)
Pramosone®: Pramoxine 1% and hydrocortisone 1% (30 g, 60 g); pramoxine 1% and hydrocortisone 2.5% (30 g, 60 g)

Foam, rectal:
ProctoFoam®-HC: Pramoxine 1% and hydrocortisone 1% (10 g)

Foam, topical:
Epifoam®: Pramoxine 1% and hydrocortisone 1% (10 g)

Lotion, topical:
Analpram-HC®: Pramoxine 1% and hydrocortisone 2.5% (60 mL)
Pramosone®: Pramoxine 1% and hydrocortisone 1% (60 mL, 120 mL, 240 mL); pramoxine 1% and hydrocortisone 2.5% (60 mL, 120 mL)

Ointment, topical:
Pramosone®: Pramoxine 1% and hydrocortisone 1% (30 g); pramoxine 1% and hydrocortisone 2.5% (30 g)

pramoxine hydrochloride *see* pramoxine *on page 777*

pramoxine hydrochloride and hydrocortisone acetate *see* pramoxine and hydrocortisone *on page 778*

pramoxine, neomycin, bacitracin, and polymyxin B *see* bacitracin, neomycin, polymyxin B, and pramoxine *on page 114*
Prandase® [Can] *see* acarbose *on page 18*
PrandiMet™ [US] *see* repaglinide and metformin *on page 826*
Prandin® [US/Can] *see* repaglinide *on page 825*
Prascion® [US] *see* sulfur and sulfacetamide *on page 897*
Prascion® AV [US] *see* sulfur and sulfacetamide *on page 897*
Prascion® FC [US] *see* sulfur and sulfacetamide *on page 897*
Prascion® RA [US] *see* sulfur and sulfacetamide *on page 897*
Prascion® TS [US] *see* sulfur and sulfacetamide *on page 897*
Pravachol® [US/Can] *see* pravastatin *on page 779*

pravastatin (prav a STAT in)

Sound-Alike/Look-Alike Issues
Pravachol® may be confused with Prevacid®, Prinivil®, propranolol
Synonyms pravastatin sodium
U.S./Canadian Brand Names Apo-Pravastatin® [Can]; CO Pravastatin [Can]; Novo-Pravastatin [Can]; PMS-Pravastatin [Can]; Pravachol® [US/Can]; ratio-Pravastatin [Can]; Riva-Pravastatin [Can]; Sandoz-Pravastatin [Can]
Therapeutic Category HMG-CoA Reductase Inhibitor
Use Use with dietary therapy for the following:
Primary prevention of coronary events: In hypercholesterolemic patients without established coronary heart disease to reduce cardiovascular morbidity (myocardial infarction, coronary revascularization procedures) and mortality.
Secondary prevention of cardiovascular events in patients with established coronary heart disease: To slow the progression of coronary atherosclerosis; to reduce cardiovascular morbidity (myocardial infarction, coronary vascular procedures) and to reduce mortality; to reduce the risk of stroke and transient ischemic attacks
Hyperlipidemias: Reduce elevations in total cholesterol, LDL-C, apolipoprotein B, and triglycerides (elevations of 1 or more components are present in Fredrickson type IIa, IIb, III, and IV hyperlipidemias)
Heterozygous familial hypercholesterolemia (HeFH): In pediatric patients, 8-18 years of age, with HeFH having LDL-C ≥190 mg/dL **or** LDL ≥160 mg/dL with positive family history of premature cardiovascular disease (CVD) or 2 or more CVD risk factors in the pediatric patient
Usual Dosage Oral: **Note:** Doses should be individualized according to the baseline LDL-cholesterol levels, the recommended goal of therapy, and patient response; adjustments should be made at intervals of 4 weeks or more; doses may need adjusted based on concomitant medications
Children: HeFH:
8-13 years: 20 mg/day
14-18 years: 40 mg/day
Dosage adjustment for pravastatin based on concomitant cyclosporine: Refer to adult dosing section
Adults: Hyperlipidemias, primary prevention of coronary events, secondary prevention of cardiovascular events: Initial: 40 mg once daily; titrate dosage to response; usual range: 10-80 mg; (maximum dose: 80 mg once daily)
Dosage adjustment for pravastatin based on concomitant cyclosporine: Initial: 10 mg/day, titrate with caution (maximum dose: 20 mg/day)
Dosage Forms
Tablet: 10 mg, 20 mg, 40 mg, 80 mg
Pravachol®: 10 mg, 40 mg, 80 mg

pravastatin sodium *see* pravastatin *on page 779*
Pravigard™ PAC (Discontinued)
Prax® [US-OTC] *see* pramoxine *on page 777*

praziquantel (pray zi KWON tel)

U.S./Canadian Brand Names Biltricide® [US/Can]
Therapeutic Category Anthelmintic
Use All stages of schistosomiasis caused by all *Schistosoma* species pathogenic to humans; clonorchiasis and opisthorchiasis

Usual Dosage Oral: Children >4 years and Adults:
Schistosomiasis: 20 mg/kg/dose 2-3 times/day for 1 day at 4- to 6-hour intervals
Clonorchiasis/opisthorchiasis: 3 doses of 25 mg/kg as a 1-day treatment
Dosage Forms
Tablet [tri-scored]:
Biltricide®: 600 mg

prazosin (PRAZ oh sin)

Sound-Alike/Look-Alike Issues
prazosin may be confused with predniSONE
Synonyms furazosin; prazosin hydrochloride
U.S./Canadian Brand Names Apo-Prazo® [Can]; Minipress® [US/Can]; Novo-Prazin [Can]; Nu-Prazo
[Can]
Therapeutic Category Alpha-Adrenergic Blocking Agent
Use Treatment of hypertension
Usual Dosage Oral: Adults:
Hypertension: Initial: 1 mg/dose 2-3 times/day; usual maintenance dose: 3-15 mg/day in divided doses
2-4 times/day; maximum daily dose: 20 mg
Hypertensive urgency: 10-20 mg once, may repeat in 30 minutes
Dosage Forms
Capsule: 1 mg, 2 mg, 5 mg
Minipress®: 1 mg, 2 mg, 5 mg

prazosin hydrochloride *see* prazosin *on page 780*
PreCare® [US] *see* vitamins (multiple/prenatal) *on page 983*
PreCare® Conceive™ [US] *see* vitamins (multiple/prenatal) *on page 983*
PreCare Premier™ [US] *see* vitamins (multiple/prenatal) *on page 983*
PreCare® Prenatal [US] *see* vitamins (multiple/prenatal) *on page 983*
Precedex™ [US/Can] *see* dexmedetomidine *on page 280*
Precose® [US] *see* acarbose *on page 18*
Pred Forte® [US/Can] *see* prednisolone (ophthalmic) *on page 781*
Pred-G® [US] *see* prednisolone and gentamicin *on page 780*
Pred Mild® [US/Can] *see* prednisolone (ophthalmic) *on page 781*

prednicarbate (pred ni KAR bate)

Sound-Alike/Look-Alike Issues
Dermatop® may be confused with Dimetapp®
U.S./Canadian Brand Names Dermatop® [US/Can]
Therapeutic Category Corticosteroid, Topical
Use Relief of the inflammatory and pruritic manifestations of corticosteroid-responsive dermatoses
(medium potency topical corticosteroid)
Usual Dosage Topical: Adults: Apply a thin film to affected area twice daily. Therapy should be
discontinued when control is achieved; if no improvement is seen, reassessment of diagnosis may be
necessary.
Dosage Forms
Cream: 0.1% (15 g, 60 g)
Dermatop®: 0.1% (60 g)
Ointment: 0.1% (15 g, 60 g)
Dermatop®: 0.1% (60 g)

Prednicen-M® *(Discontinued)* *see* prednisone *on page 782*
prednisolone acetate *see* prednisolone (systemic) *on page 781*
prednisolone acetate, ophthalmic *see* prednisolone (ophthalmic) *on page 781*

prednisolone and gentamicin (pred NIS oh lone & jen ta MYE sin)

Synonyms gentamicin and prednisolone
U.S./Canadian Brand Names Pred-G® [US]
Therapeutic Category Antibiotic/Corticosteroid, Ophthalmic

Use Treatment of steroid responsive inflammatory conditions and superficial ocular infections due to microorganisms susceptible to gentamicin

Usual Dosage Ophthalmic: Children and Adults:

Ointment: Apply 1/2 inch ribbon in the conjunctival sac 1-3 times/day

Suspension: 1 drop 2-4 times/day; during the initial 24-48 hours, the dosing frequency may be increased if necessary up to 1 drop every hour

Dosage Forms

Ointment, ophthalmic:

Pred-G®: Prednisolone 0.6% and gentamicin 0.3% (3.5 g)

Suspension, ophthalmic:

Pred-G®: Prednisolone 1% and gentamicin 0.3% (5 mL, 10 mL)

prednisolone and sulfacetamide *see* sulfacetamide and prednisolone *on page 893*

prednisolone, neomycin, and polymyxin B *see* neomycin, polymyxin B, and prednisolone *on page 664*

prednisolone (ophthalmic) (pred NISS oh lone op THAL mik)

Sound-Alike/Look-Alike Issues

prednisoLONE may be confused with predniSONE

Synonyms prednisolone acetate, ophthalmic; prednisolone sodium phosphate, ophthalmic

Tall-Man prednisoLONE (ophthalmic)

U.S./Canadian Brand Names AK-Pred® [US]; Econopred® Plus [US]; Inflamase® Mild [Can]; Ophtho-Tate® [Can]; Pred Forte® [US/Can]; Pred Mild® [US/Can]

Therapeutic Category Adrenal Corticosteroid

Use Treatment of palpebral and bulbar conjunctivitis; corneal injury from chemical, radiation, thermal burns, or foreign body penetration

Usual Dosage Ophthalmic suspension/solution: Children and Adults: Conjunctivitis, corneal injury: Instill 1-2 drops into conjunctival sac every hour during day, every 2 hours at night until favorable response is obtained, then use 1 drop every 4 hours.

Dosage Forms

Solution, ophthalmic: 1% (5 mL, 10 mL, 15 mL)

Suspension, ophthalmic: 1% (5 mL, 10 mL, 15 mL)

Econopred® Plus: 1% (5 mL, 10 mL)

Pred Forte®: 1% (1 mL, 5 mL, 10 mL, 15 mL)

Pred Mild®: 0.12% (5 mL, 10 mL)

prednisolone sodium phosphate *see* prednisolone (systemic) *on page 781*

prednisolone sodium phosphate, ophthalmic *see* prednisolone (ophthalmic) *on page 781*

prednisolone (systemic) (pred NISS oh lone sis TEM ik)

Sound-Alike/Look-Alike Issues

prednisoLONE may be confused with predniSONE

Pediapred® may be confused with Pediazole®

Synonyms deltahydrocortisone; metacortandralone; prednisolone acetate; prednisolone sodium phosphate

Tall-Man prednisoLONE (systemic)

U.S./Canadian Brand Names Bubbli-Pred™ [US]; Diopred® [Can]; Hydeltra T.B.A.® [Can]; Novo-Prednisolone [Can]; Orapred® [US]; Pediapred® [US/Can]; Prelone® [US]; Sab-Prenase [Can]

Therapeutic Category Adrenal Corticosteroid

Use Treatment of endocrine disorders, rheumatic disorders, collagen diseases, dermatologic diseases, allergic states, ophthalmic diseases, respiratory diseases, hematologic disorders, neoplastic diseases, edematous states, and gastrointestinal diseases; resolution of acute exacerbations of multiple sclerosis

Usual Dosage Dose depends upon condition being treated and response of patient; dosage for infants and children should be based on severity of the disease and response of the patient rather than on strict adherence to dosage indicated by age, weight, or body surface area. Consider alternate day therapy for long-term therapy. Discontinuation of long-term therapy requires gradual withdrawal by tapering the dose. Patients undergoing unusual stress while receiving corticosteroids, should receive increased doses prior to, during, and after the stressful situation.

◀ Children: Oral:
Acute asthma: 1-2 mg/kg/day in divided doses 1-2 times/day for 3-5 days
Antiinflammatory or immunosuppressive dose: 0.1-2 mg/kg/day in divided doses 1-4 times/day
Nephrotic syndrome:
Initial (first 3 episodes): 2 mg/kg/day **or** 60 mg/m^2/day (maximum: 80 mg/day) in divided doses 3-4 times/day until urine is protein free for 3 consecutive days (maximum: 28 days); followed by 1-1.5 mg/kg/dose **or** 40 mg/m^2/dose given every other day for 4 weeks
Maintenance (long-term maintenance dose for frequent relapses): 0.5-1 mg/kg/dose given every other day for 3-6 months
Adults: Oral:
Usual range: 5-60 mg/day
Multiple sclerosis: 200 mg/day for 1 week followed by 80 mg every other day for 1 month
Rheumatoid arthritis: Initial: 5-7.5 mg/day; adjust dose as necessary

Dosage Forms
Solution, oral: Prednisolone 15 mg/5 mL
Solution, oral: Prednisolone 5 mg/5 mL
Orapred®: 20 mg/5 mL
Pediapred®: 6.7 mg/5 mL
Syrup: 5 mg/5 m, 15 mg/5 mL
Prelone®: 15 mg/5 mL
Tablet: 5 mg
Tablet, orally disintegrating:
Orapred ODT™: 10 mg, 15 mg, 30 mg [grape flavor]

prednisone (PRED ni sone)

Sound-Alike/Look-Alike Issues
predniSONE may be confused with methylPREDNISolone, Pramosone®, prazosin, prednisoLONE, Prilosec®, primidone, promethazine

Synonyms deltacortisone; deltadehydrocortisone

Tall-Man predni**SONE**

U.S./Canadian Brand Names Apo-Prednisone® [Can]; Novo-Prednisone [Can]; PredniSONE Intensol™ [US]; Sterapred® DS [US]; Sterapred® [US]; Winpred™ [Can]

Therapeutic Category Adrenal Corticosteroid

Use Treatment of a variety of diseases, including:
Allergic states (including adjunctive treatment of anaphylaxis)
Autoimmune disorders (including systemic lupus erythematosus [SLE])
Collagen diseases
Dermatologic conditions/diseases
Edematous states (including nephrotic syndrome)
Endocrine disorders
Gastrointestinal diseases
Hematologic disorders (including idiopathic thrombocytopenia purpura [ITP])
Multiple sclerosis exacerbations
Neoplastic diseases
Ophthalmic diseases
Respiratory diseases (including acute asthma exacerbation)
Rheumatic disorders (including rheumatoid arthritis)
Trichinosis with neurologic or myocardial involvement
Tuberculous meningitis

Usual Dosage Oral: Dose depends upon condition being treated and response of patient; dosage for infants and children should be based on severity of the disease and response of the patient rather than on strict adherence to dosage indicated by age, weight, or body surface area. Consider alternate day therapy for long-term therapy. Discontinuation of long-term therapy requires gradual withdrawal by tapering the dose.

Children:
Antiinflammatory or immunosuppressive dose: 0.05-2 mg/kg/day divided 1-4 times/day
Acute asthma: 1-2 mg/kg/day in divided doses 1-2 times/day for 3-5 days
Alternatively (for 3- to 5-day "burst"):
<1 year: 10 mg every 12 hours
1-4 years: 20 mg every 12 hours
5-13 years: 30 mg every 12 hours

>13 years: 40 mg every 12 hours
Asthma long-term therapy (alternative dosing by age):
  <1 year: 10 mg every other day
  1-4 years: 20 mg every other day
  5-13 years: 30 mg every other day
  >13 years: 40 mg every other day
Nephrotic syndrome:
  Initial (first 3 episodes): 2 mg/kg/day **or** 60 mg/m^2/day (maximum: 80 mg/day) in divided doses 3-4 times/day until urine is protein free for 3 consecutive days (maximum: 28 days); followed by 1-1.5 mg/kg/dose **or** 40 mg/m^2/dose given every other day for 4 weeks
  Maintenance dose (long-term maintenance dose for frequent relapses): 0.5-1 mg/kg/dose given every other day for 3-6 months
Children and Adults: Physiologic replacement: 4-5 mg/m^2/day
Children ≥5 years and Adults: Asthma:
  Moderate persistent: Inhaled corticosteroid (medium dose) or inhaled corticosteroid (low-medium dose) with a long-acting bronchodilator
  Severe persistent: Inhaled corticosteroid (high dose) and corticosteroid tablets or syrup long term: 2 mg/kg/day, generally not to exceed 60 mg/day
Adults:
  Immunosuppression/chemotherapy adjunct: Range: 5-60 mg/day in divided doses 1-4 times/day
  Allergic reaction (contact dermatitis):
    Day 1: 30 mg divided as 10 mg before breakfast, 5 mg at lunch, 5 mg at dinner, 10 mg at bedtime
    Day 2: 5 mg at breakfast, 5 mg at lunch, 5 mg at dinner, 10 mg at bedtime
    Day 3: 5 mg 4 times/day (with meals and at bedtime)
    Day 4: 5 mg 3 times/day (breakfast, lunch, bedtime)
    Day 5: 5 mg 2 times/day (breakfast, bedtime)
    Day 6: 5 mg before breakfast
  Pneumocystis carinii pneumonia (PCP):
    40 mg twice daily for 5 days **followed by**
    40 mg once daily for 5 days **followed by**
    20 mg once daily for 11 days or until antimicrobial regimen is completed
  Thyrotoxicosis: Oral: 60 mg/day
  Chemotherapy (refer to individual protocols): Oral: Range: 20 mg/day to 100 mg/m^2/day
  Rheumatoid arthritis: Oral: Use lowest possible daily dose (often ≤7.5 mg/day)
  Idiopathic thrombocytopenia purpura (ITP): Oral: 60 mg daily for 4-6 weeks, gradually tapered over several weeks
  Systemic lupus erythematosus (SLE): Oral:
    Acute: 1-2 mg/kg/day in 2-3 divided doses
    Maintenance: Reduce to lowest possible dose, usually <1 mg/kg/day as single dose (morning)
Dosage Forms
  Solution, oral: 1 mg/mL
  Solution, oral [concentrate]:
    PredniSONE Intensol™: 5 mg/mL
  Tablet: 1 mg, 2.5 mg, 5 mg, 10 mg, 20 mg, 50 mg
    Sterapred®: 5 mg
    Sterapred® DS: 10 mg

PredniSONE Intensol™ [US] *see* prednisone *on page 782*
Prefest™ [US] *see* estradiol and norgestimate *on page 362*
Prefrin™ (Discontinued) *see* phenylephrine *on page 745*

pregabalin (pre GAB a lin)

Synonyms CI-1008; S-(+)-3-isobutylgaba
U.S./Canadian Brand Names Lyrica® [US/Can]
Therapeutic Category Analgesic, Miscellaneous; Anticonvulsant, Miscellaneous
Controlled Substance C-V
Use Management of pain associated with diabetic peripheral neuropathy; management of postherpetic neuralgia; adjunctive therapy for partial-onset seizure disorder in adults; management of fibromyalgia
Usual Dosage Oral: Adults:
  Fibromyalgia: Initial: 150 mg/day in divided doses (75 mg 2 times/day); may be increased to 300 mg/day (150 mg 2 times/day) within 1 week based on tolerability and effect; may be further increased to 450 mg/day

◄ (225 mg 2 times/day). Maximum dose: 450 mg/day (dosages up to 600 mg/day were evaluated with no significant additional benefit and an increase in adverse effects)

Neuropathic pain (diabetes-associated): Initial: 150 mg/day in divided doses (50 mg 3 times/day); may be increased within 1 week based on tolerability and effect; maximum dose: 300 mg/day (dosages up to 600 mg/day were evaluated with no significant additional benefit and an increase in adverse effects)

Postherpetic neuralgia: Initial: 150 mg/day in divided doses (75 mg 2 times/day or 50 mg 3 times/day); may be increased to 300 mg/day within 1 week based on tolerability and effect; further titration (to 600 mg/day) after 2-4 weeks may be considered in patients who do not experience sufficient relief of pain provided they are able to tolerate pregabalin. Maximum dose: 600 mg/day

Partial-onset seizures (adjunctive therapy): Initial: 150 mg per day in divided doses (75 mg 2 times/day or 50 mg 3 times/day); may be increased based on tolerability and effect (optimal titration schedule has not been defined). Maximum dose: 600 mg/day

Discontinuing therapy: Pregabalin should not be abruptly discontinued; taper dosage over at least 1 week

Dosage Forms

Capsule:

Lyrica®: 25 mg, 50 mg, 75 mg, 100 mg, 150 mg, 200 mg, 225 mg, 300 mg

Pregestimil® [US-OTC] see nutritional formula, enteral/oral on page 689

pregnenedione see progesterone on page 790

Pregnyl® [US/Can] see chorionic gonadotropin (human) on page 216

Prelone® [US] see prednisolone (systemic) on page 781

Prelu-2® (Discontinued) see phendimetrazine on page 742

Premarin® [US/Can] see estrogens (conjugated/equine) on page 364

Premarin® With Methyltestosterone (Discontinued)

Premjact® [US-OTC] see lidocaine on page 561

Premphase® [US/Can] see estrogens (conjugated/equine) and medroxyprogesterone on page 365

Premplus® [Can] see estrogens (conjugated/equine) and medroxyprogesterone on page 365

Prempro™ [US/Can] see estrogens (conjugated/equine) and medroxyprogesterone on page 365

Prenatal AD [US] see vitamins (multiple/prenatal) on page 983

Prenatal H [US] see vitamins (multiple/prenatal) on page 983

Prenatal MR 90 Fe™ [US] see vitamins (multiple/prenatal) on page 983

Prenatal MTR with Selenium [US] see vitamins (multiple/prenatal) on page 983

Prenatal Plus [US] see vitamins (multiple/prenatal) on page 983

Prenatal Rx 1 [US] see vitamins (multiple/prenatal) on page 983

Prenatal U [US] see vitamins (multiple/prenatal) on page 983

prenatal vitamins see vitamins (multiple/prenatal) on page 983

Prenatal Z [US] see vitamins (multiple/prenatal) on page 983

Prenate DHA™ [US] see vitamins (multiple/prenatal) on page 983

Prenate Elite™ [US] see vitamins (multiple/prenatal) on page 983

Preparation H® [US-OTC] see phenylephrine on page 745

Preparation H® Cleansing Pads [Can] see witch hazel on page 987

Preparation H® Hydrocortisone [US-OTC] see hydrocortisone (rectal) on page 484

Preparation H® Medicated Wipes [US-OTC] see witch hazel on page 987

Prepcat [US] see barium on page 116

Pre-Pen® (Discontinued) see benzylpenicilloyl-polylysine on page 129

Prepidil® [US/Can] see dinoprostone on page 303

Prescription Strength Desenex® (Discontinued) see miconazole on page 630

Preservative-Free Cosopt® [Can] see dorzolamide and timolol on page 319

PreserVision® AREDS [US-OTC] see vitamins (multiple/oral) on page 983

PreserVision® Lutein [US-OTC] see vitamins (multiple/oral) on page 983

Pressyn® [Can] see vasopressin on page 972

Pressyn® AR [Can] see vasopressin on page 972

Pretz® [US-OTC] see sodium chloride on page 873

Pretz-D® [US-OTC] see ephedrine on page 343

Prevacare® [US-OTC] see alcohol (ethyl) on page 41

Prevacid® [US/Can] see lansoprazole on page 548

prilocaine (PRIL oh kane)

Sound-Alike/Look-Alike Issues
    prilocaine may be confused with Polocaine®, Prilosec®
U.S./Canadian Brand Names Citanest® Plain Dental [US]; Citanest® Plain [Can]
Therapeutic Category Local Anesthetic
Usual Dosage
    Children <10 years: Doses >40 mg (1 mL) as a 4% solution per procedure rarely needed
    Children >10 years and Adults: Dental anesthesia, infiltration, or conduction block: Initial: 40-80 mg (1-2 mL) as a 4% solution; up to a maximum of 400 mg (10 mL) as a 4% solution within a 2-hour period. Manufacturer's maximum recommended dose is not more than 600 mg to normal healthy adults. The effective anesthetic dose varies with procedure, intensity of anesthesia needed, duration of anesthesia required and physical condition of the patient. Always use the lowest effective dose along with careful aspiration.
    Note: Adult and children doses of prilocaine hydrochloride cited from USP Dispensing Information (USP DI), 17th ed, The United States Pharmacopeial Convention, Inc, Rockville, MD, 1997, 139.
Dosage Forms
    Injection, solution:
        Citanest® Plain Dental: Prilocaine 4% (1.8 mL)

primaquine (PRIM a kween)

Sound-Alike/Look-Alike Issues
    Sound-alike/look-alike issues:
        Primaquine may be confused with primidone
Synonyms primaquine phosphate; prymaccone
Therapeutic Category Aminoquinoline (Antimalarial)
Use Prevention of relapse of *P. vivax* malaria
Usual Dosage Oral: Dosage expressed as mg of base (15 mg base = 26.3 mg primaquine phosphate): Treatment of malaria (decrease risk of delayed primary attacks and prevent relapse):
    Children: 0.3 mg base/kg/day once daily for 14 days (not to exceed 15 mg/day) or 0.9 mg base/kg once weekly for 8 weeks not to exceed 45 mg base/week
    Adults: 15 mg/day (base) once daily for 14 days or 45 mg base once weekly for 8 weeks
    CDC treatment recommendations: Begin therapy during last 2 weeks of, or following a course of, suppression with chloroquine or a comparable drug

Note: A second course (30 mg/day) for 14 days may be required in patients with relapse. Higher initial doses (30 mg/day) have also been used following exposure in S.E. Asia or Somalia.

Dosage Forms
Tablet: 26.3 mg

primaquine phosphate see primaquine on page 785
Primatene® Mist [US-OTC] see epinephrine on page 344
Primaxin® [US/Can] see imipenem and cilastatin on page 500
Primaxin® I.V. [Can] see imipenem and cilastatin on page 500

primidone (PRI mi done)

Sound-Alike/Look-Alike Issues
primidone may be confused with predniSONE
Synonyms desoxyphenobarbital; primaclone
U.S./Canadian Brand Names Apo-Primidone® [Can]; Mysoline® [US]
Therapeutic Category Anticonvulsant; Barbiturate
Use Management of grand mal, psychomotor, and focal seizures
Usual Dosage Oral:
Children <8 years: Initial: 50-125 mg/day given at bedtime; increase by 50-125 mg/day increments every 3-7 days; usual dose: 10-25 mg/kg/day in divided doses 3-4 times/day
Children ≥8 years and Adults: Initial: 125-250 mg/day at bedtime; increase by 125-250 mg/day every 3-7 days; usual dose: 750-1500 mg/day in divided doses 3-4 times/day with maximum dosage of 2 g/day
Dosage Forms [CAN] = Canadian brand name
Tablet: 50 mg [U.S. only], 125 [CAN only], 250 mg
Mysoline®: 50 mg, 250 mg

Primsol® [US] see trimethoprim on page 953
Prinivil® [US/Can] see lisinopril on page 570
Prinzide® [US/Can] see lisinopril and hydrochlorothiazide on page 571
Priorix™ [Can] see measles, mumps, and rubella vaccines, combined on page 593
Priscoline® (Discontinued)
PrismaSol [US] see electrolyte solution, renal replacement on page 336
pristinamycin see quinupristin and dalfopristin on page 814
Pristiq™ [US] see desvenlafaxine on page 277
Privigen™ [US] see immune globulin (intravenous) on page 503
Privine® [US-OTC] see naphazoline on page 655
ProAir™ HFA [US] see albuterol on page 39
ProAmatine® [US] see midodrine on page 633
Pro-Banthine® (Discontinued) see propantheline on page 793

probenecid (proe BEN e sid)

Sound-Alike/Look-Alike Issues
probenecid may be confused with Procanbid®
U.S./Canadian Brand Names Benuryl™ [Can]
Therapeutic Category Uricosuric Agent
Use Prevention of hyperuricemia associated with gout or gouty arthritis; prolongation and elevation of beta-lactam plasma levels
Usual Dosage Oral:
Children:
<2 years: Contraindicated
2-14 years: Prolong penicillin serum levels: Initial: 25 mg/kg, then 40 mg/kg/day given 4 times/day (maximum: 500 mg/dose)
Gonorrhea: >45 kg: Refer to adult guidelines
Adults:
Hyperuricemia with gout: 250 mg twice daily for one week; increase to 250-500 mg/day; may increase by 500 mg/month, if needed, to maximum of 2-3 g/day (dosages may be increased by 500 mg every 6 months if serum urate concentrations are controlled)
Prolong penicillin serum levels: 500 mg 4 times/day

Gonorrhea: CDC guidelines (alternative regimen): Probenecid 1 g orally with cefoxitin 2 g I.M.

Pelvic inflammatory disease: CDC guidelines: Cefoxitin 2 g I.M. plus probenecid 1 g orally as a single dose

Neurosyphilis: CDC guidelines (alternative regimen): Procaine penicillin 2.4 million units/day I.M. plus probenecid 500 mg 4 times/day; both administered for 10-14 days

Dosage Forms
Tablet: 500 mg

probenecid and colchicine *see* colchicine and probenecid *on page 244*
Pro-Bionate® *(Discontinued)*

procainamide (pro KANE a mide)

Sound-Alike/Look-Alike Issues
Procanbid® may be confused with probenecid
Pronestyl® may be confused with Ponstel®
PCA is an error-prone abbreviation (mistaken as patient controlled analgesia)

Synonyms procainamide hydrochloride; procaine amide hydrochloride

U.S./Canadian Brand Names Apo-Procainamide® [Can]; Procainamide Hydrochloride Injection, USP [Can]; Procan® SR [Can]; Pronestyl®-SR [Can]

Therapeutic Category Antiarrhythmic Agent, Class I-A

Use Treatment of ventricular tachycardia (VT), premature ventricular contractions, paroxysmal atrial tachycardia (PSVT), and atrial fibrillation (AF); prevent recurrence of ventricular tachycardia, paroxysmal supraventricular tachycardia, atrial fibrillation or flutter

Usual Dosage Must be titrated to patient's response

Children:
Oral: 15-50 mg/kg/24 hours divided every 3-6 hours
I.M.: 50 mg/kg/24 hours divided into doses of $1/8$ to $1/4$ every 3-6 hours in divided doses until oral therapy is possible
I.V. (infusion requires use of an infusion pump):
Load: 3-6 mg/kg/dose over 5 minutes not to exceed 100 mg/dose; may repeat every 5-10 minutes to maximum of 15 mg/kg/load
Maintenance as continuous I.V. infusion: 20-80 mcg/kg/minute; maximum: 2 g/24 hours
Possible VT (pulses and poor perfusion) [PALS 2005 Guidelines]: I.V.; I.O.: 15 mg/kg over 30-60 minutes

Adults:
Oral: Usual dose: 50 mg/kg/24 hours: maximum: 5 g/24 hours
Immediate release formulation: 250-500 mg/dose every 3-6 hours
Extended release formulation: 500 mg to 1 g every 6 hours
I.M.: 0.5-1 g every 4-8 hours until oral therapy is possible
I.V. (infusion requires use of an infusion pump):
Loading dose: 15-18 mg/kg administered as slow infusion over 25-30 minutes **or** 100-200 mg/dose repeated every 5 minutes as needed to a total dose of 1 g. Reduce loading dose to 12 mg/kg in severe renal or cardiac impairment.
Maintenance dose: 1-4 mg/minute by continuous infusion. Maintenance infusions should be reduced by one-third in patients with moderate renal or cardiac impairment and by two-thirds in patients with severe renal or cardiac impairment.
ACLS guidelines: Infuse 20 mg/minute until arrhythmia is controlled, hypotension occurs, QRS complex widens by 50% of its original width, or total of 17 mg/kg is given.

Dosage Forms
Injection, solution: 100 mg/mL (10 mL); 500 mg/mL (2 mL)

procainamide hydrochloride *see* procainamide *on page 787*
Procainamide Hydrochloride Injection, USP [Can] *see* procainamide *on page 787*

procaine (PROE kane)

Synonyms procaine hydrochloride
U.S./Canadian Brand Names Novocain® [US]
Therapeutic Category Local Anesthetic

▶

◀ **Use** Produces spinal anesthesia

Usual Dosage Dose varies with procedure, desired depth, and duration of anesthesia, desired muscle relaxation, vascularity of tissues, physical condition, and age of patient

Adults: Spinal analgesia: Extent of anesthesia:

Perineum: Total dose: 50 mg; Procaine 10%: 0.5 mL with 0.5 mL diluent

Perineum and lower extremities: Total dose: 100 mg; Procaine 10%: 1 mL with 1 mL diluent

Up to costal margin: Total dose: 200 mg; Procaine 10%: 2 mL with 1 mL diluent

Dosage Forms

Injection, solution:

Novocain®: 10% (2 mL)

procaine amide hydrochloride *see* procainamide *on page 787*

procaine benzylpenicillin *see* penicillin G procaine *on page 733*

procaine hydrochloride *see* procaine *on page 787*

procaine penicillin G *see* penicillin G procaine *on page 733*

Pro-Cal-Sof® *(Discontinued)* *see* docusate *on page 314*

Procanbid® *(Discontinued)* *see* procainamide *on page 787*

Procan® SR [Can] *see* procainamide *on page 787*

procarbazine (proe KAR ba zeen)

Sound-Alike/Look-Alike Issues

procarbazine may be confused with dacarbazine

Matulane® may be confused with Modane®

Synonyms benzmethyzin; N-methylhydrazine; NSC-77213; procarbazine hydrochloride

U.S./Canadian Brand Names Matulane® [US/Can]; Natulan® [Can]

Therapeutic Category Antineoplastic Agent

Use Treatment of Hodgkin disease

Usual Dosage Refer to individual protocols. Manufacturer states that the dose is based on patient's ideal weight if the patient is obese or has abnormal fluid retention. Other studies suggest that ideal body weight may not be necessary. Oral (may be given as a single daily dose or in 2-3 divided doses):

Children:

BMT aplastic anemia conditioning regimen: 12.5 mg/kg/day every other day for 4 doses

Hodgkin disease: MOPP/IC-MOPP regimens: 100 mg/m^2/day for 14 days and repeated every 4 weeks

Neuroblastoma and medulloblastoma: Doses as high as 100-200 mg/m^2/day once daily have been used

Adults: Initial: 2-4 mg/kg/day in single or divided doses for 7 days then increase dose to 4-6 mg/kg/day until response is obtained or leukocyte count decreased <4000/mm^3 or the platelet count decreased <100,000/mm^3; maintenance: 1-2 mg/kg/day

Dosage Forms

Capsule:

Matulane®: 50 mg

procarbazine hydrochloride *see* procarbazine *on page 788*

Procardia® [US/Can] *see* nifedipine *on page 672*

Procardia XL® [US] *see* nifedipine *on page 672*

procetofene *see* fenofibrate *on page 393*

Prochieve® [US] *see* progesterone *on page 790*

prochlorperazine (proe klor PER a zeen)

Sound-Alike/Look-Alike Issues

prochlorperazine may be confused with chlorproMAZINE

Compazine® may be confused with Copaxone®, Coumadin®

CPZ (occasional abbreviation for Compazine®) is an error-prone abbreviation (mistaken as chlorpromazine)

Synonyms chlormeprazine; prochlorperazine edisylate; prochlorperazine maleate

U.S./Canadian Brand Names Apo-Prochlorperazine® [Can]; Compazine® [Can]; Compro™ [US]; Nu-Prochlor [Can]; Stemetil® [Can]

Therapeutic Category Phenothiazine Derivative

Use Management of nausea and vomiting; psychotic disorders including schizophrenia; anxiety

Usual Dosage

Antiemetic: Children (therapy >1 day usually not required): **Note:** Not recommended for use in children <9 kg or <2 years:

Oral, rectal: >9 kg: 0.4 mg/kg/24 hours in 3-4 divided doses; **or**

9-13 kg: 2.5 mg every 12-24 hours as needed; maximum: 7.5 mg/day

13.1-17 kg: 2.5 mg every 8-12 hours as needed; maximum: 10 mg/day

17.1-37 kg: 2.5 mg every 8 hours or 5 mg every 12 hours as needed; maximum: 15 mg/day

I.M.: 0.13 mg/kg/dose; change to oral as soon as possible

Antiemetic: Adults:

Oral (tablet): 5-10 mg 3-4 times/day; usual maximum: 40 mg/day; larger doses may rarely be required

I.M. (deep): 5-10 mg every 3-4 hours; usual maximum: 40 mg/day

I.V.: 2.5-10 mg; maximum 10 mg/dose or 40 mg/day; may repeat dose every 3-4 hours as needed

Rectal: 25 mg twice daily

Surgical nausea/vomiting: Adults: **Note:** Should not exceed 40 mg/day

I.M.: 5-10 mg 1-2 hours before induction or to control symptoms during or after surgery; may repeat once if necessary

I.V. (administer slow IVP <5 mg/minute): 5-10 mg 15-30 minutes before induction or to control symptoms during or after surgery; may repeat once if necessary

Antipsychotic:

Children 2-12 years (not recommended in children <9 kg or <2 years):

Oral, rectal: 2.5 mg 2-3 times/day; do not give more than 10 mg the first day; increase dosage as needed to maximum daily dose of 20 mg for 2-5 years and 25 mg for 6-12 years

I.M.: 0.13 mg/kg/dose; change to oral as soon as possible

Adults:

Oral: 5-10 mg 3-4 times/day; titrate dose slowly every 2-3 days; doses up to 150 mg/day may be required in some patients for treatment of severe disturbances

I.M.: Initial: 10-20 mg; if necessary repeat initial dose every 1-4 hours to gain control; more than 3-4 doses are rarely needed. If parenteral administration is still required; give 10-20 mg every 4-6 hours; change to oral as soon as possible.

Nonpsychotic anxiety: Oral (tablet): Adults: Usual dose: 15-20 mg/day in divided doses; do not give doses >20 mg/day or for longer than 12 weeks

Dosage Forms

Injection, solution: 5 mg/mL (2 mL, 10 mL)

Suppository, rectal: 25 mg (12s)

Compro™: 25 mg (12s)

Tablet: 5 mg, 10 mg

prochlorperazine edisylate *see* prochlorperazine *on page 788*

prochlorperazine maleate *see* prochlorperazine *on page 788*

Procrit® [US] *see* epoetin alfa *on page 347*

Proctocort® [US] *see* hydrocortisone (rectal) *on page 484*

ProctoCream® HC [US] *see* hydrocortisone (rectal) *on page 484*

proctofene *see* fenofibrate *on page 393*

ProctoFoam®-HC [US/Can] *see* pramoxine and hydrocortisone *on page 778*

ProctoFoam® NS [US-OTC] *see* pramoxine *on page 777*

Procto-Kit™ [US] *see* hydrocortisone (rectal) *on page 484*

Procto-Pak™ [US] *see* hydrocortisone (rectal) *on page 484*

Proctosert [US] *see* hydrocortisone (rectal) *on page 484*

Proctosol-HC® [US] *see* hydrocortisone (rectal) *on page 484*

Proctozone-HC™ [US] *see* hydrocortisone (rectal) *on page 484*

procyclidine (proe SYE kli deen)

Sound-Alike/Look-Alike Issues

Kemadrin® may be confused with Coumadin®

Synonyms procyclidine hydrochloride

U.S./Canadian Brand Names Kemadrin® [US]; PMS-Procyclidine [Can]

Therapeutic Category Anti-Parkinson Agent; Anticholinergic Agent

◀ **Use** Relieves symptoms of parkinsonian syndrome and drug-induced extrapyramidal symptoms

Usual Dosage Oral: Adults: 2.5 mg 3 times/day after meals; if tolerated, gradually increase dose, maximum of 20 mg/day if necessary

procyclidine hydrochloride *see procyclidine on page 789*

Procytox® [Can] *see cyclophosphamide on page 256*

Prodium® [US-OTC] *see phenazopyridine on page 741*

Pro Doc Limitee Bromazepam [Can] *see bromazepam (Canada only) on page 142*

Profasi® HP [Can] *see chorionic gonadotropin (human) on page 216*

ProFe [US-OTC] *see polysaccharide-iron complex on page 768*

Profen II DM® [US] *see guaifenesin, pseudoephedrine, and dextromethorphan on page 460*

Profen Forte™ DM [US] *see guaifenesin, pseudoephedrine, and dextromethorphan on page 460*

Profen LA® *(Discontinued)*

Profilnine® SD [US] *see factor IX complex (human) on page 389*

Proflavanol C™ [Can] *see ascorbic acid on page 96*

progesterone (proe JES ter one)

Synonyms pregnenedione; progestin

U.S./Canadian Brand Names Crinone® [US/Can]; Endometrin® [US]; First™-Progesterone VGS [US]; Prochieve® [US]; Prometrium® [US/Can]

Therapeutic Category Progestin

Use

Oral: Prevention of endometrial hyperplasia in nonhysterectomized, postmenopausal women who are receiving conjugated estrogen tablets; secondary amenorrhea

I.M.: Amenorrhea; abnormal uterine bleeding due to hormonal imbalance

Intravaginal gel: Part of assisted reproductive technology (ART) for infertile women with progesterone deficiency; secondary amenorrhea

Vaginal tablet: Part of ART for infertile women with progesterone deficiency

Usual Dosage Adults:

I.M.: Females:

Amenorrhea: 5-10 mg/day for 6-8 consecutive days

Functional uterine bleeding: 5-10 mg/day for 6 doses

Oral: Females:

Prevention of endometrial hyperplasia (in postmenopausal women with a uterus who are receiving daily conjugated estrogen tablets): 200 mg as a single daily dose every evening for 12 days sequentially per 28-day cycle

Amenorrhea: 400 mg every evening for 10 days

Intravaginal gel: Females:

ART in women who require progesterone supplementation: 90 mg (8% gel) once daily; if pregnancy occurs, may continue treatment for up to 10-12 weeks

ART in women with partial or complete ovarian failure: 90 mg (8% gel) intravaginally twice daily; if pregnancy occurs, may continue up to 10-12 weeks

Secondary amenorrhea: 45 mg (4% gel) intravaginally every other day for up to 6 doses; women who fail to respond may be increased to 90 mg (8% gel) every other day for up to 6 doses

Intravaginal tablet: Females: ART: 100 mg 2-3 times daily starting at oocyte retrieval and continuing for up to 10 weeks.

Dosage Forms

Capsule:

Prometrium®: 100 mg, 200 mg

Gel, vaginal:

Crinone®: 8% (1.45 g) [90 mg/dose; contains palm oil; 6 or 18 prefilled applicators]

Prochieve®: 4% (1.45 mg) [45 mg/dose; contains palm oil; 6 prefilled applicators]; 8% (1.45 g) [90 mg/dose; contains palm oil; 6 or 18 prefilled applicators]

Injection, oil: 50 mg/mL (10 mL)

Powder, for prescription compounding [micronized]: Progesterone USP (10 g, 25 g, 100 g, 1000 g)

Powder, for prescription compounding [wettable]: Progesterone USP (10 g, 25 g, 100 g, 1000 g)

First™-Progesterone VGS 25: Progesterone USP (0.75 g)

First™-Progesterone VGS 50: Progesterone USP (1.5 g)

First™-Progesterone VGS 100: Progesterone USP (3 g)

First™-Progesterone VGS 200: Progesterone USP (6 g)

First™-Progesterone VGS 400: Progesterone USP (12 g)
Tablet, vaginal:
Endometrin®: 100 mg (21s)

progestin *see progesterone on page 790*
Proglycem® [US/Can] *see diazoxide on page 290*
Prograf® [US/Can] *see tacrolimus on page 901*
proguanil and atovaquone *see atovaquone and proguanil on page 103*
ProHance® [US] *see gadoteridol on page 434*
ProHIBiT® *(Discontinued)*
Prolastin® [US/Can] *see alpha₁-proteinase inhibitor on page 48*
Proleukin® [US/Can] *see aldesleukin on page 42*
Prolex®-D *(Discontinued)* *see guaifenesin and phenylephrine on page 456*
Prolex®-PD *(Discontinued)* *see guaifenesin and phenylephrine on page 456*
Prolixin® *(Discontinued)* *see fluphenazine on page 415*
Prolixin Enanthate® *(Discontinued)* *see fluphenazine on page 415*
Prolopa® [Can] *see benserazide and levodopa (Canada only) on page 122*
Promacet [US] *see butalbital and acetaminophen on page 155*
Prometa® *(Discontinued)*

promethazine (proe METH a zeen)

Sound-Alike/Look-Alike Issues
promethazine may be confused with chlorproMAZINE, predniSONE, promazine
Phenergan® may be confused with Phenaphen®, Phrenilin®, Theragran®
Synonyms promethazine hydrochloride
U.S./Canadian Brand Names Bioniche Promethazine [Can]; Histantil [Can]; Phenadoz™ [US]; Phenergan® [US/Can]; PMS-Promethazine [Can]; Promethegan™ [US]
Therapeutic Category Antiemetic; Phenothiazine Derivative
Use Symptomatic treatment of various allergic conditions; antiemetic; motion sickness; sedative; postoperative pain (adjunctive therapy); anesthetic (adjunctive therapy); anaphylactic reactions (adjunctive therapy)
Usual Dosage
Children ≥2 years:
Allergic conditions: Oral, rectal: 0.1 mg/kg/dose (maximum: 12.5 mg) every 6 hours during the day and 0.5 mg/kg/dose (maximum: 25 mg) at bedtime as needed
Antiemetic: Oral, I.M., I.V., rectal: 0.25-1 mg/kg 4-6 times/day as needed (maximum: 25 mg/dose)
Motion sickness: Oral, rectal: 0.5 mg/kg/dose 30 minutes to 1 hour before departure, then every 12 hours as needed (maximum dose: 25 mg twice daily)
Sedation: Oral, I.M., I.V., rectal: 0.5-1 mg/kg/dose every 6 hours as needed (maximum: 50 mg/dose)
Adults:
Allergic conditions (including allergic reactions to blood or plasma):
Oral, rectal: 25 mg at bedtime **or** 12.5 mg before meals and at bedtime (range: 6.25-12.5 mg 3 times/day)
I.M., I.V.: 25 mg, may repeat in 2 hours when necessary; switch to oral route as soon as feasible
Antiemetic: Oral, I.M., I.V., rectal: 12.5-25 mg every 4-6 hours as needed
Motion sickness: Oral, rectal: 25 mg 30-60 minutes before departure, then every 12 hours as needed
Sedation: Oral, I.M., I.V., rectal: 12.5-50 mg/dose
Dosage Forms
Injection, solution: 25 mg/mL (1 mL); 50 mg/mL (1 mL)
Phenergan®: 25 mg/mL (1 mL); 50 mg/mL (1 mL)
Suppository, rectal: 12.5 mg, 25 mg, 50 mg
Phenadoz™: 12.5 mg, 25 mg
Promethegan™: 12.5 mg, 25 mg, 50 mg
Syrup: 6.25 mg/5 mL
Tablet: 12.5 mg, 25 mg, 50 mg

promethazine and codeine (proe METH a zeen & KOE deen)

Synonyms codeine and promethazine
Therapeutic Category Antihistamine/Antitussive

Controlled Substance C-V

Use Temporary relief of coughs and upper respiratory symptoms associated with allergy or the common cold

Usual Dosage Oral:

Children <16 years: **Note:** Use of promethazine/codeine combination is contraindicated in children <16 years of age

Children ≥16 years and Adults: 5 mL every 4-6 hours (maximum 30 mL/24 hours)

Dosage Forms

Syrup: Promethazine 6.25 mg and codeine 10 mg per 5 mL

promethazine and dextromethorphan (proe METH a zeen & deks troe meth OR fan)

Synonyms dextromethorphan and promethazine

Therapeutic Category Antihistamine/Antitussive

Use Temporary relief of coughs and upper respiratory symptoms associated with allergy or the common cold

Usual Dosage Oral:

Children:

<2 years: Use of promethazine is contraindicated

2-6 years: 1.25-2.5 mL every 4-6 hours up to 10 mL in 24 hours

6-12 years: 2.5-5 mL every 4-6 hours up to 20 mL in 24 hours

Adults: 5 mL every 4-6 hours up to 30 mL in 24 hours

Dosage Forms

Syrup: Promethazine 6.25 mg and dextromethorphan 15 mg per 5 mL

promethazine and meperidine see meperidine and promethazine on page 604

promethazine and phenylephrine (proe METH a zeen & fen il EF rin)

Synonyms phenylephrine and promethazine

Therapeutic Category Antihistamine/Decongestant Combination

Use Temporary relief of upper respiratory symptoms associated with allergy or the common cold

Usual Dosage Oral:

Children:

<2 years: Use of promethazine is contraindicated

2-6 years: 1.25-2.5 mL every 4-6 hours, not to exceed 7.5 mL in 24 hours

6-12 years: 2.5-5 mL every 4-6 hours, not to exceed 30 mL in 24 hours

Children >12 years and Adults: 5 mL every 4-6 hours, not to exceed 30 mL in 24 hours

Dosage Forms

Syrup: Promethazine 6.25 mg and phenylephrine 5 mg per 5 mL

promethazine hydrochloride see promethazine on page 791

promethazine, phenylephrine, and codeine

(proe METH a zeen, fen il EF rin, & KOE deen)

Synonyms codeine, promethazine, and phenylephrine; phenylephrine, promethazine, and codeine

Therapeutic Category Antihistamine/Decongestant/Antitussive

Controlled Substance C-V

Use Temporary relief of coughs and upper respiratory symptoms including nasal congestion associated with allergy or the common cold

Usual Dosage Oral:

Children <16 years: **Note:** Use of promethazine/codeine combination is contraindicated in children <16 years of age

Children ≥16 years and Adults: 5 mL every 4-6 hours, not to exceed 30 mL/24 hours

Dosage Forms

Syrup: Promethazine 6.25 mg, phenylephrine 5 mg, and codeine 10 mg per 5 mL

Promethegan™ [US] see promethazine on page 791

Promethist® With Codeine (Discontinued) see promethazine, phenylephrine, and codeine on page 792

Prometh® VC Plain Liquid (Discontinued) see promethazine and phenylephrine on page 792

Prometh® VC With Codeine *(Discontinued)* *see* promethazine, phenylephrine, and codeine *on page 792*

Prometrium® [US/Can] *see* progesterone *on page 790*

Promit® *(Discontinued)* *see* dextran 1 *on page 282*

Pronestyl® *(Discontinued)* *see* procainamide *on page 787*

Pronestyl®-SR [Can] *see* procainamide *on page 787*

Pronto® Complete Lice Removal System [US-OTC] *see* pyrethrins and piperonyl butoxide *on page 806*

Pronto® Lice Control [Can] *see* pyrethrins and piperonyl butoxide *on page 806*

Pronto® Plus Hair and Scalp Masque *(Discontinued)* *see* pyrethrins and piperonyl butoxide *on page 806*

Pronto® Plus Lice Egg Remover Kit [US-OTC] *see* benzalkonium chloride *on page 123*

Pronto® Plus Lice Killing Mousse Plus Vitamin E [US-OTC] *see* pyrethrins and piperonyl butoxide *on page 806*

Pronto® Plus Lice Killing Mousse Shampoo Plus Natural Extracts and Oils [US-OTC] *see* pyrethrins and piperonyl butoxide *on page 806*

Pronto® Plus Warm Oil Treatment and Conditioner [US-OTC] *see* pyrethrins and piperonyl butoxide *on page 806*

Propac™ [US-OTC] *see* nutritional formula, enteral/oral *on page 689*

Propacet® *(Discontinued)* *see* propoxyphene and acetaminophen *on page 795*

Propaderm® [Can] *see* beclomethasone *on page 119*

propafenone (pro PAF en one)

Synonyms propafenone hydrochloride

U.S./Canadian Brand Names Apo-Propafenone® [Can]; PMS-Propafenone [Can]; Rythmol® Gen-Propafenone [Can]; Rythmol® SR [US]; Rythmol® [US]

Therapeutic Category Antiarrhythmic Agent, Class I-C

Use Treatment of life-threatening ventricular arrhythmias
Rythmol® SR: Maintenance of normal sinus rhythm in patients with symptomatic atrial fibrillation

Usual Dosage Oral: Adults: **Note:** Patients who exhibit significant widening of QRS complex or second- or third-degree AV block may need dose reduction.
Ventricular arrhythmias:
  Immediate release tablet: Initial: 150 mg every 8 hours, increase at 3- to 4-day intervals up to 300 mg every 8 hours.
  Extended release capsule: Initial: 225 mg every 12 hours; dosage increase may be made at a minimum of 5-day intervals; may increase to 325 mg every 12 hours; if further increase is necessary, may increase to 425 mg every 12 hours

Dosage Forms
Capsule, extended release:
  Rythmol® SR: 225 mg, 325 mg, 425 mg
  Tablet: 150 mg, 225 mg, 300 mg
  Rythmol®: 150 mg, 225 mg, 300 mg

propafenone hydrochloride *see* propafenone *on page 793*

Propagest® *(Discontinued)*

propantheline (proe PAN the leen)

Synonyms propantheline bromide

Therapeutic Category Anticholinergic Agent

Use Adjunctive treatment of peptic ulcer, irritable bowel syndrome, pancreatitis, ureteral and urinary bladder spasm; reduce duodenal motility during diagnostic radiologic procedures

Usual Dosage Oral:
Antisecretory:
  Children: 1-2 mg/kg/day in 3-4 divided doses
  Adults: 15 mg 3 times/day before meals or food and 30 mg at bedtime
Antispasmodic:
  Children: 2-3 mg/kg/day in divided doses every 4-6 hours and at bedtime
  Adults: 15 mg 3 times/day before meals or food and 30 mg at bedtime

Dosage Forms
Tablet: 15 mg

propantheline bromide see propantheline on page 793

proparacaine (proe PAR a kane)

Sound-Alike/Look-Alike Issues
proparacaine may be confused with propoxyphene
Synonyms proparacaine hydrochloride; proxymetacaine
U.S./Canadian Brand Names Alcaine® [US/Can]; Diocaine® [Can]; Ophthetic® [US]; Parcaine™ [US]
Therapeutic Category Local Anesthetic
Use Anesthesia for tonometry, gonioscopy; suture removal from cornea; removal of corneal foreign body; cataract extraction, glaucoma surgery; short operative procedure involving the cornea and conjunctiva
Usual Dosage Children and Adults:
Ophthalmic surgery: Instill 1 drop of 0.5% solution in eye every 5-10 minutes for 5-7 doses
Tonometry, gonioscopy, suture removal: Instill 1-2 drops of 0.5% solution in eye just prior to procedure
Dosage Forms
Solution, ophthalmic: 0.5% (15 mL)
Alcaine®, Ophthetic®, Parcaine™: 0.5% (15 mL)

proparacaine and fluorescein (proe PAR a kane & FLURE e seen)

Synonyms fluorescein and proparacaine
U.S./Canadian Brand Names Flucaine® [US]
Therapeutic Category Diagnostic Agent; Local Anesthetic
Use Anesthesia for tonometry, gonioscopy; suture removal from cornea; removal of corneal foreign body; cataract extraction, glaucoma surgery
Usual Dosage
Ophthalmic surgery: Children and Adults: Instill 1 drop in each eye every 5-10 minutes for 5-7 doses
Tonometry, gonioscopy, suture removal: Adults: Instill 1-2 drops in each eye just prior to procedure
Dosage Forms
Solution, ophthalmic: Proparacaine 0.5% and fluorescein 0.25% (5 mL)
Flucaine®: Proparacaine 0.5% and fluorescein 0.25% (5 mL)

proparacaine hydrochloride see proparacaine on page 794
Propecia® [US/Can] see finasteride on page 401
Propine® [US/Can] see dipivefrin on page 311
Proplex® T (Discontinued) see factor IX complex (human) on page 389

propofol (PROE po fole)

Sound-Alike/Look-Alike Issues
Diprivan® may be confused with Diflucan®, Ditropan®
U.S./Canadian Brand Names Diprivan® [US/Can]
Therapeutic Category General Anesthetic
Use Induction of anesthesia for inpatient or outpatient surgery in patients ≥3 years of age; maintenance of anesthesia for inpatient or outpatient surgery in patients >2 months of age; in adults, for induction and maintenance of monitored anesthesia care sedation during procedures; sedation in intubated, mechanically-ventilated ICU patients
Usual Dosage Dosage must be individualized based on total body weight and titrated to the desired clinical effect; wait at least 3-5 minutes between dosage adjustments to clinically assess drug effects; smaller doses are required when used with narcotics; the following are general dosing guidelines:

General anesthesia:
Induction: I.V.:
Children (healthy) 3-16 years, ASA-PS 1 or 2: 2.5-3.5 mg/kg over 20-30 seconds; use a lower dose for children ASA-PS 3 or 4
Adults (healthy), ASA-PS 1 or 2, <55 years: 2-2.5 mg/kg (~40 mg every 10 seconds until onset of induction)
Cardiac anesthesia: 0.5-1.5 mg/kg (~20 mg every 10 seconds until onset of induction)
Neurosurgical patients: 1-2 mg/kg (~20 mg every 10 seconds until onset of induction)

Maintenance: I.V. infusion:
Children (healthy) 2 months to 16 years, ASA-PS 1 or 2: Initial: 200-300 mcg/kg/minute; after 30 minutes, if clinical signs of light anesthesia are absent, decrease the infusion rate; usual infusion rate: 125-150 mcg/kg/minute (range: 125-300 mcg/kg/minute); children ≤5 years may require larger infusion rates compared to older children
Adults (healthy), ASA-PS 1 or 2, <55 years: Initial: 100-200 mcg/kg/minute for 10-15 minutes; decrease by 30% to 50% during first 30 minutes of maintenance; usual infusion rate: 50-100 mcg/kg/minute to optimize recovery time
Cardiac anesthesia:
Low-dose propofol with primary opioid: 50-100 mcg/kg/minute (see manufacturer's labeling)
Primary propofol with secondary opioid: 100-150 mcg/kg/minute
Neurosurgical patients: 100-200 mcg/kg/minute
Maintenance: I.V. intermittent bolus: Adults (healthy), ASA-PS 1 or 2, <55 years: 25-50 mg increments as needed

Monitored anesthesia care sedation:
Initiation: Adults (healthy), ASA-PS 1 or 2, <55 years: Slow I.V. infusion: 100-150 mcg/kg/minute for 3-5 minutes **or** slow injection: 0.5 mg/kg over 3-5 minutes
Maintenance: Adults (healthy), ASA-PS 1 or 2, <55 years: I.V. infusion using variable rates (preferred over intermittent boluses): 25-75 mcg/kg/minute **or** incremental bolus doses: 10 mg or 20 mg

ICU sedation in intubated mechanically-ventilated patients: Avoid rapid bolus injection; individualize dose and titrate to response. Continuous infusion: Initial: 5 mcg/kg/minute; increase by 5-10 mcg/kg/minute every 5-10 minutes until desired sedation level is achieved; usual maintenance: 5-80 mcg/kg/minute; use 80% of healthy adult dose in elderly, debilitated, and ASA-PS 3 or 4 patients; reduce dose after adequate sedation established and adjust to response (eg, evaluate frequently to use minimum dose for sedation). Daily interruption with retitration is recommended to minimize prolonged sedative effects.

Dosage Forms
Injection, emulsion: 10 mg/mL (20 mL, 50 mL, 100 mL)
Diprivan®: 10 mg/mL (20 mL, 50 mL, 100 mL)

Propoxacet-N® *(Discontinued)* see propoxyphene and acetaminophen on page 795

propoxyphene (proe POKS i feen)
Sound-Alike/Look-Alike Issues
propoxyphene may be confused with proparacaine
Darvon® may be confused with Devrom®, Diovan®
Darvon-N® may be confused with Darvocet-N®
Synonyms dextropropoxyphene; propoxyphene hydrochloride; propoxyphene napsylate
U.S./Canadian Brand Names 642® Tablet [Can]; Darvon-N® [US/Can]; Darvon® [US]
Therapeutic Category Analgesic, Narcotic
Controlled Substance C-IV
Use Management of mild-to-moderate pain
Usual Dosage Oral: Adults:
Hydrochloride: 65 mg every 3-4 hours as needed for pain; maximum: 390 mg/day
Napsylate: 100 mg every 4 hours as needed for pain; maximum: 600 mg/day
Dosage Forms
Capsule: 65 mg
Darvon®: 65 mg
Tablet:
Darvon-N®: 100 mg

propoxyphene and acetaminophen (proe POKS i feen & a seet a MIN oh fen)
Sound-Alike/Look-Alike Issues
Darvocet-N® may be confused with Darvon-N®
Synonyms acetaminophen and propoxyphene; propoxyphene hydrochloride and acetaminophen; propoxyphene napsylate and acetaminophen
U.S./Canadian Brand Names Balacet 325™ [US]; Darvocet A500® [US]; Darvocet-N® 100 [US/Can]; Darvocet-N® 50 [US/Can]
Therapeutic Category Analgesic, Narcotic

◄ **Controlled Substance** C-IV

Use Management of mild-to-moderate pain

Usual Dosage Oral: Adults:

Darvocet A500®, Darvocet-N® 100: 1 tablet every 4 hours as needed; maximum: 600 mg propoxyphene napsilate/day

Darvocet-N® 50: 1-2 tablets every 4 hours as needed; maximum: 600 mg propoxyphene napsylate/day

Propoxyphene hydrochloride 65 mg and acetaminophen 650 mg: 1 tablet every 4 hours as needed; maximum: 390 mg/day propoxyphene hydrochloride, 4 g/day acetaminophen)

Note: Dosage of acetaminophen should not exceed 4 g/day (6 tablets of Darvocet-N® 100); possibly less in patients with ethanol

Dosage Forms

Tablet:

65/650: Propoxyphene 65 mg and acetaminophen 650 mg; 100/500: Propoxyphene 100 mg and acetaminophen 500 mg; 100/650: Propoxyphene 100 mg and acetaminophen 650 mg

Balacet 325™: Propoxyphene 100 mg and acetaminophen 325 mg

Darvocet A500®: Propoxyphene 100 mg and acetaminophen 500 mg

Darvocet-N® 50: Propoxyphene 50 mg and acetaminophen 325 mg

Darvocet-N® 100: Propoxyphene 100 mg and acetaminophen 650 mg

propoxyphene, aspirin, and caffeine (proe POKS i feen, AS pir in, & KAF een)

Sound-Alike/Look-Alike Issues

Darvon® may be confused with Devrom®, Diovan®

Synonyms aspirin, caffeine, and propoxyphene; caffeine, propoxyphene, and aspirin; propoxyphene hydrochloride, aspirin, and caffeine

Therapeutic Category Analgesic Combination (Narcotic)

Controlled Substance C-IV

Use Treatment of mild-to-moderate pain

Usual Dosage Oral: Adults: Pain: One capsule (providing propoxyphene 65 mg) every 4 hours as needed; maximum propoxyphene 390 mg/day. This will also provide aspirin 389 mg and caffeine 32.4 mg per capsule.

propoxyphene hydrochloride *see* propoxyphene *on page 795*

propoxyphene hydrochloride and acetaminophen *see* propoxyphene and acetaminophen *on page 795*

propoxyphene hydrochloride, aspirin, and caffeine *see* propoxyphene, aspirin, and caffeine *on page 796*

propoxyphene napsylate *see* propoxyphene *on page 795*

propoxyphene napsylate and acetaminophen *see* propoxyphene and acetaminophen *on page 795*

propranolol (proe PRAN oh lole)

Sound-Alike/Look-Alike Issues

propranolol may be confused with Pravachol®, Propulsid®

Inderal® may be confused with Adderall®, Enduron®, Enduronyl®, Imdur®, Imuran®, Inderide®, Isordil®, Toradol®

Inderal® 40 may be confused with Enduronyl® Forte

Synonyms propranolol hydrochloride

U.S./Canadian Brand Names Apo-Propranolol® [Can]; Dom-Propranolol [Can]; Inderal® LA [US/Can]; Inderal® [US/Can]; InnoPran XL™ [US]; Novo-Pranol [Can]; Nu-Propranolol [Can]; PMS-Propranolol [Can]; Propranolol Hydrochloride Injection, USP [Can]

Therapeutic Category Antiarrhythmic Agent, Class II; Beta-Adrenergic Blocker

Use Management of hypertension; angina pectoris; pheochromocytoma; essential tremor; supraventricular arrhythmias (such as atrial fibrillation and flutter, AV nodal reentrant tachycardias), ventricular tachycardias (catecholamine-induced arrhythmias, digoxin toxicity); prevention of myocardial infarction; migraine headache prophylaxis; symptomatic treatment of hypertrophic subaortic stenosis (hypertrophic obstructive cardiomyopathy)

Usual Dosage

Essential tremor: Oral: Adults: 40 mg twice daily initially; maintenance doses: Usually 120-320 mg/day

Hypertension: Oral: Adults: Initial: 40 mg twice daily; increase dosage every 3-7 days; usual dose: 120-240 mg divided in 2-3 doses/day; maximum daily dose: 640 mg; usual dosage range (JNC 7): 40-160 mg/day in 2 divided doses

Extended release formulations:

Inderal® LA: Initial: 80 mg once daily; usual maintenance: 120-160 mg once daily; maximum daily dose: 640 mg; usual dosage range (JNC 7): 60-180 mg/day once daily

InnoPran XL™: Initial: 80 mg once daily at bedtime; if initial response is inadequate, may be increased at 2-3 week intervals to a maximum dose of 120 mg

Hypertrophic subaortic stenosis: Oral: Adults: 20-40 mg 3-4 times/day

Inderal® LA: 80-160 mg once daily

Migraine headache prophylaxis: Oral: Adults: Initial: 80 mg/day divided every 6-8 hours; increase by 20-40 mg/dose every 3-4 weeks to a maximum of 160-240 mg/day given in divided doses every 6-8 hours; if satisfactory response not achieved within 6 weeks of starting therapy, drug should be withdrawn gradually over several weeks

Inderal® LA: Initial: 80 mg once daily; effective dose range: 160-240 mg once daily

Post-MI mortality reduction: Oral: Adults: Initial: 40 mg 3 times/day; usual dosage range: 180-240 mg/day in 3-4 divided doses

Pheochromocytoma: Oral: Adults: 30-60 mg/day in divided doses

Stable angina: Oral: Adults: 80-320 mg/day in doses divided 2-4 times/day

Inderal® LA: Initial: 80 mg once daily; maximum dose: 320 mg once daily

Tachyarrhythmias:

Oral: Adults: 10-30 mg/dose every 6-8 hours

I.V.: Adults: 1-3 mg/dose slow IVP; repeat every 2-5 minutes up to a total of 5 mg; titrate initial dose to desired response

or

0.1 mg/kg divided into 3 equal doses given at 2-3 minute intervals. May repeat total dose in 2 minutes if necessary (ACLS guidelines, 2005)

Note: Once response achieved or maximum dose administered, additional doses should not be given for at least 4 hours.

Dosage Forms

Capsule, extended release: 60 mg, 80 mg, 120 mg, 160 mg

InnoPran XL™: 80 mg, 120 mg

Capsule, sustained release:

Inderal® LA: 60 mg, 80 mg, 120 mg, 160 mg

Injection, solution: 1 mg/mL (1 mL)

Inderal®: 1 mg/mL (1 mL)

Solution, oral: 4 mg/mL, 8 mg/mL

Tablet: 10 mg, 20 mg, 40 mg, 80 mg

Inderal®: 10 mg, 20 mg, 40 mg

propranolol and hydrochlorothiazide (proe PRAN oh lole & hye droe klor oh THYE a zide)

Sound-Alike/Look-Alike Issues

Inderide® may be confused with Inderal®

Synonyms hydrochlorothiazide and propranolol

U.S./Canadian Brand Names Inderide® [US]

Therapeutic Category Antihypertensive Agent, Combination

Use Management of hypertension

Usual Dosage Oral: Adults: Hypertension: Dose is individualized; typical dosages of **hydrochlorothiazide**: 12.5-50 mg/day; initial dose of **propranolol**: 80 mg/day

Daily dose of tablet form should be divided into 2 daily doses; may be used to maximum dosage of up to 160 mg of propranolol; higher dosages would result in higher than optimal thiazide dosages.

Dosage Forms

Tablet: Propranolol 40 mg and hydrochlorothiazide 25 mg; propranolol 80 mg and hydrochlorothiazide 25 mg

Inderide®: 40/25: Propranolol 40 mg and hydrochlorothiazide 25 mg

propranolol hydrochloride *see* propranolol *on page 796*

Propranolol Hydrochloride Injection, USP [Can] *see* propranolol *on page 796*

Proprinal [US-OTC] *see* ibuprofen *on page 495*

Proprinal® Cold and Sinus [US-OTC] *see* pseudoephedrine and ibuprofen *on page 802*

Propulsid® [US] *see* cisapride *on page 223*

propylene glycol diacetate, acetic acid, and hydrocortisone *see* acetic acid, propylene glycol diacetate, and hydrocortisone *on page 29*

propylhexedrine (proe pil HEKS e dreen)

U.S./Canadian Brand Names Benzedrex® [US-OTC]

Therapeutic Category Adrenergic Agonist Agent

Use Topical nasal decongestant

Usual Dosage Nasal: Children 6-12 years and Adults: Two inhalations in each nostril, not more frequently than every 2 hours

Dosage Forms

Inhaler, nasal:

Benzedrex® [OTC]: 0.4-0.5 mg/inhalation (1s)

2-propylpentanoic acid *see* valproic acid and derivatives *on page 967*

propylthiouracil (proe pil thye oh YOOR a sil)

Sound-Alike/Look-Alike Issues

propylthiouracil may be confused with Purinethol®

PTU is an error-prone abbreviation (mistaken as mercaptopurine [Purinethol®; 6-MP])

U.S./Canadian Brand Names Propyl-Thyracil® [Can]

Therapeutic Category Antithyroid Agent

Use Palliative treatment of hyperthyroidism as an adjunct to ameliorate hyperthyroidism in preparation for surgical treatment or radioactive iodine therapy; management of thyrotoxic crisis

Usual Dosage Oral: Administer in 3 equally divided doses at approximately 8-hour intervals. Adjust dosage to maintain T_3, T_4, and TSH levels in normal range; elevated T_3 may be sole indicator of inadequate treatment. Elevated TSH indicates excessive antithyroid treatment.

Children: Initial: 5-7 mg/kg/day **or** 150-200 mg/m^2/day in divided doses every 8 hours

or

6-10 years: 50-150 mg/day

>10 years: 150-300 mg/day

Maintenance: Determined by patient response **or** 1/3 to 2/3 of the initial dose in divided doses every 8-12 hours. This usually begins after 2 months on an effective initial dose.

Adults: Initial: 300-400 mg/day in divided doses every 6-8 hours. In patients with severe hyperthyroidism, very large goiters, or both, the initial dosage is usually 400 mg/day; an occasional patient will require 600-900 mg/day; maintenance: 100-150 mg/day in divided doses every 8-12 hours

Thyrotoxic crisis (recommendations vary widely and have not been evaluated in comparative trials): Dosages of 200-300 mg every 4-6 hours have been recommended for short-term initial therapy (until initial response), followed by gradual reduction to a maintenance dosage (100-150 mg/day in divided doses).

Dosage Forms

Tablet: 50 mg

Propyl-Thyracil® [Can] *see* propylthiouracil *on page 798*

2-propylvaleric acid *see* valproic acid and derivatives *on page 967*

ProQuad® [US] *see* measles, mumps, rubella, and varicella virus vaccine *on page 593*

Proquin® XR [US] *see* ciprofloxacin *on page 221*

Proscar® [US/Can] *see* finasteride *on page 401*

ProSom® *(Discontinued)* *see* estazolam *on page 359*

prostacyclin *see* epoprostenol *on page 349*

prostacyclin PGI$_2$ *see* iloprost *on page 499*

prostaglandin E$_1$ *see* alprostadil *on page 50*

prostaglandin E$_2$ *see* dinoprostone *on page 303*

prostaglandin F$_2$ *see* carboprost tromethamine *on page 178*

ProStep® Patch *(Discontinued)* *see* nicotine *on page 670*

Prostigmin® [US/Can] *see* neostigmine *on page 664*

Prostin E$_2$® [US/Can] *see* dinoprostone *on page 303*

Prostin F$_2$ Alpha® *(Discontinued)*

Prostin® VR [Can] *see* alprostadil *on page 50*

Prostin VR Pediatric® [US] *see* alprostadil *on page 50*

protamine sulfate (PROE ta meen SUL fate)

Sound-Alike/Look-Alike Issues
protamine may be confused with ProAmatine®, protamine, Protopam®, Protropin®
Therapeutic Category Antidote
Use Treatment of heparin overdosage; neutralize heparin during surgery or dialysis procedures
Usual Dosage
Heparin neutralization: I.V.: Protamine dosage is determined by the dosage of heparin; 1 mg of protamine neutralizes 90 USP units of heparin (lung) and 115 USP units of heparin (intestinal); maximum dose: 50 mg
Heparin overdosage, following intravenous administration: I.V.: Since blood heparin concentrations decrease rapidly **after** administration, adjust the protamine dosage depending upon the duration of time since heparin administration.
Note: Excessive protamine doses may worsen bleeding potential.
Dosage Forms
Injection, solution [preservative free]: 10 mg/mL (5 mL, 25 mL)

Protection Plus® [US-OTC] *see* alcohol (ethyl) *on page 41*
protein C *see* protein C concentrate (human) *on page 799*
protein C (activated), human, recombinant *see* drotrecogin alfa *on page 327*
protein-bound paclitaxel *see* paclitaxel (protein bound) *on page 715*

protein C concentrate (human) (PROE teen cee KON suhn trate HYU man)

Sound-Alike/Look-Alike Issues
protein C concentrate (human) may be confused with activated protein C (human, recombinant) which refers to drotrecogin alfa
Ceprotin may be confused with aprotinin, Cipro®
Synonyms protein C
U.S./Canadian Brand Names Ceprotin [US]
Therapeutic Category Anticoagulant
Use Replacement therapy for severe congenital protein C deficiency for the prevention and/or treatment of venous thromboembolism and purpura fulminans
Usual Dosage Patient variables (including age, clinical condition, and plasma levels of protein C) will influence dosing and duration of therapy. Individualize dosing based on protein C activity and patient pharmacokinetic profile. Dosing is dependent on the severity of protein C deficiency, age of patient, clinical condition, and patient's level of protein C. The frequency, duration, and dose should be individualized.

I.V.: Children and Adults: Severe congenital protein C deficiency:
Acute episode/short-term prophylaxis: Initial dose: 100-120 int. units/kg (for determination of recovery and half-life)
Subsequent 3 doses: 60-80 int. units/kg every 6 hours (adjust to maintain peak protein C activity of 100%)
Maintenance dose: 45-60 int. units/kg every 6 or 12 hours (adjust to maintain recommended maintenance trough protein C activity levels >25%)
Long-term prophylaxis: Maintenance dose: 45-60 int. units/kg every 12 hours (recommended maintenance trough protein C activity levels >25%)

Note: Maintain target peak protein C activity of 100% during acute episodes and short-term prophylaxis. Maintain trough levels of protein C activity >25%. Higher peak levels of protein C may be necessary in prophylactic therapy of patients at increased risk for thrombosis (eg, infection, trauma, surgical intervention).
Dosage Forms
Injection, powder for reconstitution:
Ceprotin: ~500 int. units, ~1000 int. units

Protenate® *(Discontinued)* *see* plasma protein fraction *on page 759*
Prothazine-DC® *(Discontinued)* *see* promethazine and codeine *on page 791*
prothrombin complex concentrate *see* factor IX complex (human) *on page 389*

prothrombin complex concentrate *see* prothrombin complex (human) [(factors II, VII, IX, X), protein C, and protein S] *(Canada only) on page 800*

prothrombin complex (human) [(factors II, VII, IX, X), protein C, and protein S] *(Canada only)*

(PRO throm bin KOM pleks HYU man FAK ters too SEV en nyne ten PROE teen cee & PROE teen ess)

Synonyms prothrombin complex concentrate

U.S./Canadian Brand Names Octaplex® [Can]

Therapeutic Category Hemostatic Agent

Use Prophylaxis (perioperative) and treatment of bleeding due to acquired deficiency (eg, overdose of vitamin K antagonist) of one or more of the prothrombin complex coagulation factors II, VII, IX, and X, when rapid correction of factor deficiency is necessary

Usual Dosage

Dosing should be individualized based on severity of disorder, extent and location of bleeding, and clinical status of patient. Maximum dose not to exceed 120 mL.

I.V. Adolescents ≥17 years and Adults: Approximate doses required for normalization of INR (≤1.2 within 1 hour):

Initial INR: 2-2.5: Administer 0.9-1.3 mL/kg

2.5-3: Administer 1.3-1.6 mL/kg

3-3.5: Administer 1.6-1.9 mL/kg

>3.5: Administer >1.9 mL/kg

With the correction of vitamin K antagonist-induced impairment of hemostasis in patients who have been treated concomitantly with an appropriate vitamin K dose, repeat dosing with PCC is usually not necessary.

Dosage Forms

Injection, powder for reconstitution:

Octaplex®: Human coagulation factor II: 11-38 int. units/mL; factor VII: 9-24 int. units/mL; factor IX: 20-31 int. units/mL; factor X: 18-30 int. units/mL: protein C: 7-31 int. units/mL; protein S: 7-32 int. units/mL (20 mL)

Protilase® *(Discontinued)* *see* pancrelipase *on page 718*

Protonix® [US/Can] *see* pantoprazole *on page 720*

Protopam® [US/Can] *see* pralidoxime *on page 776*

Protopic® [US/Can] *see* tacrolimus *on page 901*

Protostat® Oral *(Discontinued)* *see* metronidazole *on page 627*

protriptyline (proe TRIP ti leen)

Sound-Alike/Look-Alike Issues

Vivactil® may be confused with Vyvanse™

Synonyms protriptyline hydrochloride

U.S./Canadian Brand Names Vivactil® [US]

Therapeutic Category Antidepressant, Tricyclic (Secondary Amine)

Use Treatment of depression

Usual Dosage Oral:

Adolescents: 15-20 mg/day

Adults: 15-60 mg/day in 3-4 divided doses

Dosage Forms

Tablet:

Vivactil®: 5 mg, 10 mg

protriptyline hydrochloride *see* protriptyline *on page 800*

Protuss®-DM *(Discontinued)* *see* guaifenesin, pseudoephedrine, and dextromethorphan *on page 460*

Proventil® *(Discontinued)* *see* albuterol *on page 39*

Proventil® HFA [US] *see* albuterol *on page 39*

Proventil® Inhaler *(Discontinued)* *see* albuterol *on page 39*

Proventil® Solution *(Discontinued)* *see* albuterol *on page 39*

Proventil® Tablet *(Discontinued)* *see* albuterol *on page 39*

Provera® [US/Can] *see* medroxyprogesterone *on page 597*

Provera-Pak [Can] *see* medroxyprogesterone *on page 597*
Provigil® [US/Can] *see* modafinil *on page 639*
Proviodine [Can] *see* povidone-iodine *on page 775*
Provisc® [US] *see* hyaluronate and derivatives *on page 476*
Provocholine® [US/Can] *see* methacholine *on page 611*
proxymetacaine *see* proparacaine *on page 794*
Prozac® [US/Can] *see* fluoxetine *on page 413*
Prozac® Weekly™ [US] *see* fluoxetine *on page 413*
PRP-OMP *see* Haemophilus B conjugate vaccine *on page 464*
PRP-T *see* Haemophilus B conjugate vaccine *on page 464*
Prudoxin™ [US] *see* doxepin *on page 321*
prussian blue *see* ferric hexacyanoferrate *on page 397*
prymaccone *see* primaquine *on page 785*
P&S® [US-OTC] *see* salicylic acid *on page 850*
23PS *see* pneumococcal polysaccharide vaccine (polyvalent) *on page 763*
PS-341 *see* bortezomib *on page 139*
Pseudacarb™ [US] *see* carbetapentane and pseudoephedrine *on page 175*

pseudoephedrine (soo doe e FED rin)

Sound-Alike/Look-Alike Issues
Dimetapp® may be confused with Dermatop®, Dimetabs®, Dimetane®
Sudafed® may be confused with Sufenta®
Synonyms *d*-isoephedrine hydrochloride; pseudoephedrine hydrochloride; pseudoephedrine sulfate
U.S./Canadian Brand Names Balminil Decongestant [Can]; Benylin® D for Infants [Can]; Contac® Cold 12 Hour Relief Non Drowsy [Can]; Drixoral® ND [Can]; Eltor® [Can]; Genaphed® [US-OTC]; Kidkare Decongestant [US-OTC]; Oranyl [US-OTC]; PMS-Pseudoephedrine [Can]; Pseudofrin [Can]; Robidrine® [Can]; Silfedrine Children's [US-OTC]; Sudafed® 12 Hour [US-OTC]; Sudafed® 24 Hour [US-OTC]; Sudafed® Children's [US-OTC]; Sudafed® Decongestant [Can]; Sudafed® Maximum Strength Nasal Decongestant [US-OTC]; Sudo-Tab® [US-OTC]; SudoGest [US-OTC]; Unifed [US-OTC]
Therapeutic Category Adrenergic Agonist Agent
Use Temporary symptomatic relief of nasal congestion due to common cold, upper respiratory allergies, and sinusitis; also promotes nasal or sinus drainage
Usual Dosage Oral: General dosing guidelines:
Children:
<2 years: 4 mg/kg/day in divided doses every 6 hours
2-5 years: 15 mg every 4-6 hours; maximum: 60 mg/24 hours
6-12 years: 30 mg every 4-6 hours; maximum: 120 mg/24 hours
Adults: 30-60 mg every 4-6 hours, sustained release: 120 mg every 12 hours; maximum: 240 mg/24 hours
Dosage Forms
Caplet, extended release:
Sudafed® 12 Hour [OTC]: 120 mg
Liquid: 30 mg/5 mL
Silfedrine Children's [OTC], Sudafed® Children's [OTC]: 15 mg/5 mL
Unifed [OTC]: 30 mg/5 mL
Liquid, oral [drops]:
Kidkare Decongestant [OTC]: 7.5 mg/0.8 mL
Syrup: 30 mg/5 mL
Tablet: 30 mg, 60 mg
Genaphed® [OTC], Oranyl [OTC], Sudafed® [OTC], Sudo-Tab® [OTC]: 30 mg
SudoGest [OTC]: 30 mg, 60 mg
Tablet, chewable:
Sudafed® Children's [OTC]: 15 mg
Tablet, extended release:
Sudafed® 24 Hour [OTC]: 240 mg

pseudoephedrine, acetaminophen, and chlorpheniramine *see* acetaminophen, chlorpheniramine, and pseudoephedrine *on page 25*

pseudoephedrine, acetaminophen, and dextromethorphan *see* acetaminophen, dextromethorphan, and pseudoephedrine *on page 27*

pseudoephedrine and acetaminophen *see* acetaminophen and pseudoephedrine *on page 23*

pseudoephedrine and brompheniramine *see* brompheniramine and pseudoephedrine *on page 144*

pseudoephedrine and carbetapentane *see* carbetapentane and pseudoephedrine *on page 175*

pseudoephedrine and chlorpheniramine *see* chlorpheniramine and pseudoephedrine *on page 207*

pseudoephedrine and desloratadine *see* desloratadine and pseudoephedrine *on page 275*

pseudoephedrine and dexbrompheniramine *see* dexbrompheniramine and pseudoephedrine *on page 279*

pseudoephedrine and dextromethorphan (soo doe e FED rin & deks troe meth OR fan)

Synonyms dextromethorphan and pseudoephedrine

U.S./Canadian Brand Names Balminil DM D [Can]; Benylin® DM-D [Can]; Koffex DM-D [Can]; Novahistex® DM Decongestant [Can]; Novahistine® DM Decongestant [Can]; Pedia Relief Cough and Cold [US-OTC]; Pedia Relief Infants [US-OTC]; Robitussin® Childrens Cough & Cold [Can]; Sudafed® Children's Cold & Cough [US-OTC]; SudoGest Children's [US-OTC]

Therapeutic Category Antitussive/Decongestant

Use Temporary symptomatic relief of nasal congestion and cough due to common cold, hay fever, upper respiratory allergies

Usual Dosage Relief of nasal congestion and cough: Oral:
General dosing guidelines base on pseudoephedrine component:
 Children 2-6 years: 15 mg every 4-6 hours (maximum: 60 mg/24 hours)
 Children 6-12 years: 30 mg every 4-6 hours (maximum: 120 mg/24 hours)
 Children ≥12 years and Adults: 60 mg every 4-6 hours (maximum: 240 mg/24 hours)

Product-specific dosing:
 Children 2-6 years (Sudafed® Children's Cold & Cough): 5 mL every 4 hours (maximum: 20 mL/24 hours)
 Children 6-12 years (Sudafed® Children's Cold & Cough): 10 mL every 4 hours (maximum: 40 mL/24 hours)
 Children ≥12 years and Adults (Sudafed® Children's Cold & Cough): 20 mL every 4 hours (maximum: 80 mL/24 hours)

Dosage Forms
Liquid:
 Sudafed® Children's Cold & Cough [OTC]: Pseudoephedrine 15 mg and dextromethorphan 5 mg per 5 mL
Liquid, oral [drops]:
 Pedia Relief Infants [OTC]: Pseudoephedrine 7.5 mg and dextromethorphan 2.5 mg per 0.8 mL
Syrup:
 Pedia Relief Cough and Cold [OTC]: Pseudoephedrine 15 mg and dextromethorphan 7.5 mg per 5 mL
 SudoGest Children's [OTC]: Pseudoephedrine 15 mg and dextromethorphan 5 mg per 5 mL

pseudoephedrine and diphenhydramine *see* diphenhydramine and pseudoephedrine *on page 306*

pseudoephedrine and fexofenadine *see* fexofenadine and pseudoephedrine *on page 399*

pseudoephedrine and guaifenesin *see* guaifenesin and pseudoephedrine *on page 458*

pseudoephedrine and ibuprofen (soo doe e FED rin & eye byoo PROE fen)

Synonyms ibuprofen and pseudoephedrine

U.S./Canadian Brand Names Advil® Cold & Sinus [US-OTC/Can]; Children's Advil® Cold [Can]; Proprinal® Cold and Sinus [US-OTC]; Sudafed® Sinus Advance [Can]

Therapeutic Category Decongestant/Analgesic

Use For temporary relief of cold, sinus, and flu symptoms (including nasal congestion, headache, sore throat, minor body aches and pains, and fever)

Usual Dosage OTC labeling: Oral:
Children: Ibuprofen 100 mg and pseudoephedrine 15 mg per 5 mL: May repeat dose every 6 hours (maximum: 4 doses/24 hours); dose should be based on weight when possible. Contact healthcare provider if symptoms have not improved within 3 days (2 days if treating sore throat accompanied by fever).
 2-5 years or 11 to <22 kg (24-47 pounds): 5 mL
 6-11 years or 22-43 kg (48-95 pounds): 10 mL

Children ≥12 years and Adults: Ibuprofen 200 mg and pseudoephedrine 30 mg per dose: One dose every 4-6 hours as needed; may increase to 2 doses if necessary (maximum: 6 doses/24 hours). Contact healthcare provider if symptoms have not improved within 7 days when treating cold symptoms or within 3 days when treating fever.

Dosage Forms
Caplet:
Advil® Cold and Sinus [OTC], Proprinal® Cold and Sinus [OTC]: Pseudoephedrine 30 mg and ibuprofen 200 mg
Capsule, liquid filled:
Advil® Cold and Sinus [OTC]: Pseudoephedrine 30 mg and ibuprofen 200 mg

pseudoephedrine and loratadine *see* loratadine and pseudoephedrine *on page 576*

pseudoephedrine and methscopolamine (soo doe e FED rin & meth skoe POL a meen)

Synonyms methscopolamine and pseudoephedrine; pseudoephedrine hydrochloride and methscopolamine nitrate

U.S./Canadian Brand Names AlleRx™-D [US]; Amdry-D [US]; Extendryl PSE [US]

Therapeutic Category Decongestant/Anticholingeric Combination

Use Relief of symptoms of allergic rhinitis, vasomotor rhinitis, sinusitis, and the common cold

Usual Dosage Oral: Children ≥12 years and Adults (Allerx™-D, Amdry-D): One tablet every 12 hours (maximum: 2 tablets/24 hours)

Dosage Forms
Tablet: Pseudoephedrine hydrochloride 120 mg and methscopolamine nitrate 2.5 mg
Allerx™-D, Amdry-D: Pseudoephedrine 120 mg and methscopolamine 2.5 mg
Tablet, extended release:
Extendryl PSE: Pseudoephedrine 120 mg and methscopolamine 2.5 mg

pseudoephedrine and naproxen *see* naproxen and pseudoephedrine *on page 657*

pseudoephedrine and triprolidine *see* triprolidine and pseudoephedrine *on page 955*

pseudoephedrine, chlorpheniramine, and acetaminophen *see* acetaminophen, chlorpheniramine, and pseudoephedrine *on page 25*

pseudoephedrine, chlorpheniramine, and codeine *see* chlorpheniramine, pseudoephedrine, and codeine *on page 212*

pseudoephedrine, chlorpheniramine, and dextromethorphan *see* chlorpheniramine, pseudoephedrine, and dextromethorphan *on page 212*

pseudoephedrine, chlorpheniramine, and dihydrocodeine *see* pseudoephedrine, dihydrocodeine, and chlorpheniramine *on page 803*

pseudoephedrine, chlorpheniramine, and ibuprofen *see* ibuprofen, pseudoephedrine, and chlorpheniramine *on page 497*

pseudoephedrine, codeine, and triprolidine *see* triprolidine, pseudoephedrine, and codeine *(Canada only) on page 955*

pseudoephedrine, dextromethorphan, and acetaminophen *see* acetaminophen, dextromethorphan, and pseudoephedrine *on page 27*

pseudoephedrine, dextromethorphan, and guaifenesin *see* guaifenesin, pseudoephedrine, and dextromethorphan *on page 460*

pseudoephedrine, dihydrocodeine, and chlorpheniramine
(soo doe e FED rin, dye hye droe KOE deen, & klor fen IR a meen)

Synonyms chlorpheniramine, pseudoephedrine, and dihydrocodeine; dihydrocodeine bitartrate, pseudoephedrine hydrochloride, and chlorpheniramine maleate; pseudoephedrine, chlorpheniramine, and dihydrocodeine

U.S./Canadian Brand Names Coldcough [US]; DiHydro-CP [US]

Therapeutic Category Antihistamine/Decongestant/Antitussive

Controlled Substance C-III

Use Temporary relief of cough, congestion, and sneezing due to colds, respiratory infections, or hay fever

Usual Dosage Oral:
Children:
2-6 years: 1.25-2.5 mL every 4-6 hours; do not exceed 4 doses in 24 hours
6-12 years: 2.5-5 mL every 4-6 hours; do not exceed 4 doses in 24 hours
Children >12 years and Adults: 5-10 mL every 4-6 hours; do not exceed 4 doses in 24 hours

▶

◄ **Dosage Forms**
Syrup:
Coldcough, DiHydro-CP: Pseudoephedrine 15 mg, dihydrocodeine 7.5 mg, and chlorpheniramine 2 mg per 5 mL

pseudoephedrine, guaifenesin, and codeine *see* guaifenesin, pseudoephedrine, and codeine *on page 460*

pseudoephedrine hydrochloride *see* pseudoephedrine *on page 801*

pseudoephedrine hydrochloride and acrivastine *see* acrivastine and pseudoephedrine *on page 31*

pseudoephedrine hydrochloride and cetirizine hydrochloride *see* cetirizine and pseudoephedrine *on page 196*

pseudoephedrine hydrochloride and methscopolamine nitrate *see* pseudoephedrine and methscopolamine *on page 803*

pseudoephedrine hydrochloride, guaifenesin, and dihydrocodeine bitartrate *see* dihydrocodeine, pseudoephedrine, and guaifenesin *on page 299*

pseudoephedrine hydrochloride, methscopolamine nitrate, and chlorpheniramine maleate *see* chlorpheniramine, pseudoephedrine, and methscopolamine *on page 213*

pseudoephedrine, hydrocodone, and carbinoxamine *see* hydrocodone, carbinoxamine, and pseudoephedrine *on page 483*

pseudoephedrine, hydrocodone, and chlorpheniramine *(Discontinued)*

pseudoephedrine, methscopolamine, and chlorpheniramine *see* chlorpheniramine, pseudoephedrine, and methscopolamine *on page 213*

pseudoephedrine sulfate *see* pseudoephedrine *on page 801*

pseudoephedrine tannate and dexchlorpheniramine tannate *see* dexchlorpheniramine and pseudoephedrine *on page 280*

pseudoephedrine tannate, dextromethorphan tannate, and brompheniramine tannate *see* brompheniramine, pseudoephedrine, and dextromethorphan *on page 146*

pseudoephedrine, triprolidine, and codeine *see* triprolidine, pseudoephedrine, and codeine *(Canada only) on page 955*

Pseudofrin [Can] *see* pseudoephedrine *on page 801*

Pseudo-Gest Plus® Tablet *(Discontinued)* *see* chlorpheniramine and pseudoephedrine *on page 207*

Pseudo GG TR [US] *see* guaifenesin and pseudoephedrine *on page 458*

Pseudo Max [US] *see* guaifenesin and pseudoephedrine *on page 458*

Pseudo Max DMX [US] *see* guaifenesin, pseudoephedrine, and dextromethorphan *on page 460*

pseudomonic acid A *see* mupirocin *on page 647*

Pseudovent™ 400 *(Discontinued)* *see* guaifenesin and pseudoephedrine *on page 458*

Pseudovent™ *(Discontinued)* *see* guaifenesin and pseudoephedrine *on page 458*

Pseudovent™ DM *(Discontinued)* *see* guaifenesin, pseudoephedrine, and dextromethorphan *on page 460*

Pseudovent™-Ped *(Discontinued)* *see* guaifenesin and pseudoephedrine *on page 458*

P & S™ Liquid Phenol [Can] *see* phenol *on page 743*

Psorcon® [Can] *see* diflorasone *on page 295*

Psorcon® *(Discontinued)* *see* diflorasone *on page 295*

Psorcon® e™ *(Discontinued)* *see* diflorasone *on page 295*

Psoriatec™ [US] *see* anthralin *on page 77*

PsoriGel® *(Discontinued)* *see* coal tar *on page 240*

Psorion® Topical *(Discontinued)*

psyllium (SIL i yum)

Sound-Alike/Look-Alike Issues
Fiberall® may be confused with Feverall®
Hydrocil® may be confused with Hydrocet®

Synonyms plantago seed; plantain seed; psyllium husk; psyllium hydrophilic mucilloid

U.S./Canadian Brand Names Bulk-K [US-OTC]; Fiberall® [US]; Fibro-Lax [US-OTC]; Fibro-XL [US-OTC]; Genfiber™ [US-OTC]; Hydrocil® Instant [US-OTC]; Konsyl-D™ [US-OTC]; Konsyl® Easy Mix™

[US-OTC]; Konsyl® Orange [US-OTC]; Konsyl® Original [US-OTC]; Konsyl® [US-OTC]; Metamucil® Plus Calcium [US-OTC]; Metamucil® Smooth Texture [US-OTC]; Metamucil® [US-OTC/Can]; Natural Fiber Therapy Smooth Texture [US-OTC]; Natural Fiber Therapy [US-OTC]; Reguloid® [US-OTC]

Therapeutic Category Laxative

Use OTC labeling: Dietary fiber supplement; treatment of occasional constipation; reduce risk of coronary heart disease (CHD)

Usual Dosage Oral: General dosing guidelines; consult specific product labeling.

Adequate intake for total fiber: Note: The definition of "fiber" varies; however, the soluble fiber in psyllium is only one type of fiber which makes up the daily recommended intake of total fiber.

Children 1-3 years: 19 g/day
Children 4-8 years: 25 g/day
Children 9-13 years: Male: 31 g/day; Female: 26 g/day
Children 14-18 years: Male: 38 g/day; Female: 26 g/day
Adults 19-50 years: Male: 38 g/day; Female: 25 g/day
Adults ≥51 years: Male: 30 g/day; Female: 21 g/day
Pregnancy: 28 g/day
Lactation: 29 g/day

Constipation:

Children 6-11 years: Psyllium: 1.25-15 g per day in divided doses
Children ≥12 years and Adults: Psyllium: 2.5-30 g per day in divided doses

Reduce risk of CHD: Children ≥12 years and Adults: Soluble fiber ≥7 g (psyllium seed husk ≥10.2 g) per day

Dosage Forms

Capsule:

Fibro XL [OTC]: 0.675 g
Genfiber™ [OTC], Konsyl® [OTC], Metamucil® [OTC], Metamucil® Plus Calcium [OTC], Reguloid [OTC]: 0.52 g

Powder:

Bulk-K [OTC], Fibro-Lax [OTC]: 4.7 g/teaspoon
Fiberall®: 0.05 g/tablespoon
Genfiber™ [OTC], Konsyl-D® [OTC], Konsyl® Orange [OTC], Metamucil® [OTC], Metamucil® Smooth Texture [OTC], Natural Fiber Therapy Smooth Texture [OTC], Reguloid® [OTC]: 3.4 g/teaspoon
Genfiber™ [OTC], Konsyl® Orange [OTC], Metamucil® [OTC], Metamucil® Smooth Texture [OTC], Natural Fiber Therapy [OTC], Reguloid® [OTC]: 3.4 g/tablespoon
Hydrocil® Instant: [OTC]: 3.5 g/packet, 3.5 g/teaspoon
Konsyl-D® [OTC], Konsyl® Orange [OTC]: 3.4 g/packet
Konsyl® Original [OTC], Konsyl® Easy Mix [OTC]: 6 g/packet, 6 g/teaspoon
Metamucil® Smooth Texture [OTC]: 3.3 g/teaspoon, 3.4 g/packet

Wafers:

Metamucil® [OTC]: 3.4 g/2 wafers

psyllium husk *see* psyllium *on page 804*
psyllium hydrophilic mucilloid *see* psyllium *on page 804*
P-Tann D [US] *see* chlorpheniramine and phenylephrine *on page 206*
pteroylglutamic acid *see* folic acid *on page 421*
Pulmicort® [Can] *see* budesonide *on page 147*
Pulmicort Flexhaler™ [US] *see* budesonide *on page 147*
Pulmicort Respules® [US] *see* budesonide *on page 147*
Pulmicort Turbuhaler® *(Discontinued)* *see* budesonide *on page 147*
Pulmophylline [Can] *see* theophylline *on page 917*
Pulmozyme® [US/Can] *see* dornase alfa *on page 319*
Puralube® Tears [US-OTC] *see* artificial tears *on page 95*
Puregon® [Can] *see* follitropin beta *on page 423*
Purell® [US-OTC] *see* alcohol (ethyl) *on page 41*
Purell® 2 in 1 [US-OTC] *see* alcohol (ethyl) *on page 41*
Purell® with Aloe [US-OTC] *see* alcohol (ethyl) *on page 41*
purified chick embryo cell *see* rabies virus vaccine *on page 816*
Purinethol® [US/Can] *see* mercaptopurine *on page 606*

PVP-I *see* povidone-iodine *on page 775*

Pylera™ [US] *see* bismuth, metronidazole, and tetracycline *on page 137*

pyrantel pamoate (pi RAN tel PAM oh ate)

U.S./Canadian Brand Names Combantrin™ [Can]; Pin-X® [US-OTC]; Reese's® Pinworm Medicine [US-OTC]

Therapeutic Category Anthelmintic

Use Treatment of pinworms (*Enterobius vermicularis*) and roundworms (*Ascaris lumbricoides*)

Usual Dosage Oral: Children and Adults (purgation is not required prior to use): **Note:** Dose is expressed as pyrantel base: Roundworm, pinworm, or trichostrongyliasis: 11 mg/kg administered as a single dose; maximum dose: 1 g. (**Note:** For pinworm infection, dosage should be repeated in 2 weeks and all family members should be treated).

Dosage Forms

Caplet:

Reese's® Pinworm Medicine [OTC]: 180 mg

Suspension, oral:

Pin-X® [OTC], Reese's® Pinworm Medicine [OTC]: 144 mg/mL

Tablet:

Pin-X® [OTC]: 720.5 mg

pyrazinamide (peer a ZIN a mide)

Synonyms pyrazinoic acid amide

U.S./Canadian Brand Names Tebrazid™ [Can]

Therapeutic Category Antitubercular Agent

Use Adjunctive treatment of tuberculosis in combination with other antituberculosis agents

Usual Dosage Oral: Treatment of tuberculosis:

Note: Used as part of a multidrug regimen. Treatment regimens consist of an initial 2-month phase, followed by a continuation phase of 4 or 7 additional months; frequency of dosing may differ depending on phase of therapy.

Children:

Daily therapy: 15-30 mg/kg/day (maximum: 2 g/day)

Twice weekly directly observed therapy (DOT): 50 mg/kg/dose (maximum: 4 g/dose)

Adults (dosing is based on lean body weight):

Daily therapy: 15-30 mg/kg/day

40-55 kg: 1000 mg

56-75 kg: 1500 mg

76-90 kg: 2000 mg (maximum dose regardless of weight)

Twice weekly directly observed therapy (DOT): 50 mg/kg

40-55 kg: 2000 mg

56-75 kg: 3000 mg

76-90 kg: 4000 mg (maximum dose regardless of weight)

Three times/week DOT: 25-30 mg/kg (maximum: 2.5 g)

40-55 kg: 1500 mg

56-75 kg: 2500 mg

76-90 kg: 3000 mg (maximum dose regardless of weight)

Dosage Forms

Tablet: 500 mg

pyrazinamide, rifampin, and isoniazid *see* rifampin, isoniazid, and pyrazinamide *on page 834*

pyrazinoic acid amide *see* pyrazinamide *on page 806*

pyrethrins and piperonyl butoxide (pye RE thrins & pi PER oh nil byo TOKS ide)

Synonyms piperonyl butoxide and pyrethrins

U.S./Canadian Brand Names A-200® Lice Treatment Kit [US-OTC]; A-200® Maximum Strength [US-OTC]; Licide® [US-OTC]; Pronto® Complete Lice Removal System [US-OTC]; Pronto® Lice Control [Can]; Pronto® Plus Lice Killing Mousse Plus Vitamin E [US-OTC]; Pronto® Plus Lice Killing Mousse Shampoo Plus Natural Extracts and Oils [US-OTC]; Pronto® Plus Warm Oil Treatment and Conditioner [US-OTC]; R & C™ II [Can]; R & C™ Shampoo/Conditioner [Can]; RID® Maximum Strength [US-OTC]; RID® Mousse [Can]; Tisit® Blue Gel [US-OTC]; Tisit® [US-OTC]

Therapeutic Category Scabicides/Pediculicides

Use Treatment of *Pediculus humanus* infestations (head lice, body lice, pubic lice, and their eggs)

Usual Dosage Application of pyrethrins:

Topical products:

Apply enough solution to completely wet infested area, including hair

Allow to remain on area for 10 minutes

Wash and rinse with large amounts of warm water.

Use fine-toothed comb to remove lice and eggs from hair

Shampoo hair to restore body and luster

Treatment may be repeated if necessary once in a 24-hour period

Repeat treatment in 7-10 days to kill newly hatched lice

Note: Keep out of eyes when rinsing hair; protect eyes with a washcloth or towel

Solution for furniture, bedding: Spray on entire area to be treated; allow to dry before use. Intended for use on items which cannot be laundered or dry cleaned. **Not for use on humans or animals.**

Dosage Forms

Gel, topical:

Tisit® Blue Gel [OTC]: Pyrethrins 0.33% and piperonyl butoxide 3% (30 g)

Kit:

A-200® Lice Treatment Kit [OTC]:

Shampoo: Pyrethrins 0.33% and piperonyl butoxide 4% (120 mL)

Solution: Permethrin 0.5% (180 mL)

Pronto® Complete Lice Removal System [OTC]:

Shampoo: Pyrethrins 0.33% and piperonyl butoxide 4% (60 mL)

Solution, topical: Benzalkonium chloride 0.1% (60 mL)

Liquid, topical:

Tisit® [OTC]: Pyrethrins 0.33% and piperonyl butoxide 2% (60 mL, 120 mL)

Oil, topical:

Pronto® Plus Warm Oil Treatment and Conditioner [OTC]: Pyrethrins 0.33% and piperonyl butoxide 4% (36 mL)

Shampoo: Pyrethrins 0.33% and piperonyl butoxide 4% (60 mL, 120 mL)

A-200® Maximum Strength [OTC], Tisit® [OTC]: Pyrethrins 0.33% and piperonyl butoxide 4% (60 mL, 120 mL)

Licide® [OTC], Pronto® Plus Lice Killing Mousse Shampoo Plus Vitamin E: Pyrethrins 0.33% and piperonyl butoxide 4% (120 mL)

Pronto® Plus Lice Killing Mousse Shampoo Plus Natural Extracts and Oils: Pyrethrins 0.33% and piperonyl butoxide 4% (60 mL)

Pronto® Plus Lice Killing Mousse Shampoo Plus Vitamin E: Pyrethrins 0.33% and piperonyl butoxide 4% (120 mL)

RID® Maximum Strength [OTC]: Pyrethrins 0.33% and piperonyl butoxide 4% (60 mL, 120 mL, 180 mL, 240 mL)

Solution:

Tisit® [OTC]: Pyrethrins 0.4% and piperonyl butoxide 2% (150 mL)

Pyri-500 [US-OTC] *see* pyridoxine *on page 808*

2-pyridine aldoxime methochloride *see* pralidoxime *on page 776*

Pyridium® [US] *see* phenazopyridine *on page 741*

pyridostigmine (peer id oh STIG meen)

Sound-Alike/Look-Alike Issues

pyridostigmine may be confused with physostigmine

Mestinon® may be confused with Metatensin®

Regonol® may be confused with Reglan®, Renagel®

Synonyms pyridostigmine bromide

U.S./Canadian Brand Names Mestinon® Timespan® [US]; Mestinon® [US/Can]; Mestinon®-SR [Can]; Regonol® [US]

Therapeutic Category Cholinergic Agent

Use Symptomatic treatment of myasthenia gravis; antidote for nondepolarizing neuromuscular blockers

Military use: Pretreatment for soman nerve gas exposure

Usual Dosage

Myasthenia gravis:

Oral:

Children: 7 mg/kg/24 hours divided into 5-6 doses

▶

Adults: Highly individualized dosing ranges: 60-1500 mg/day, usually 600 mg/day divided into 5-6 doses, spaced to provide maximum relief
Sustained release formulation: Highly individualized dosing ranges: 180-540 mg once or twice daily (doses separated by at least 6 hours); **Note:** Most clinicians reserve sustained release dosage form for bedtime dose only.
I.M., slow I.V. push:
Children: 0.05-0.15 mg/kg/dose
Adults: To supplement oral dosage pre- and postoperatively during labor and postpartum, during myasthenic crisis, or when oral therapy is impractical: ~1/30th of oral dose; observe patient closely for cholinergic reactions
or
I.V. infusion: Initial: 2 mg/hour with gradual titration in increments of 0.5-1 mg/hour, up to a maximum rate of 4 mg/hour
Pretreatment for soman nerve gas exposure (military use): Oral: Adults: 30 mg every 8 hours beginning several hours prior to exposure; discontinue at first sign of nerve agent exposure, then begin atropine and pralidoxime
Reversal of nondepolarizing muscle relaxants: **Note:** Atropine sulfate (0.6-1.2 mg) I.V. immediately prior to pyridostigmine to minimize side effects: I.V.:
Children: Dosing range: 0.1-0.25 mg/kg/dose*
Adults: 0.1-0.25 mg/kg/dose; 10-20 mg is usually sufficient*
*Full recovery usually occurs ≤15 minutes, but ≥30 minutes may be required
Dosage Forms
Injection, solution:
Regonol®: 5 mg/mL (2 mL)
Syrup:
Mestinon®: 60 mg/5 mL
Tablet: 60 mg
Mestinon®: 60 mg
Tablet, sustained release:
Mestinon® Timespan®: 180 mg

pyridostigmine bromide see pyridostigmine on page 807

pyridoxine (peer i DOKS een)
Sound-Alike/Look-Alike Issues
pyridoxine may be confused with paroxetine, pralidoxime, Pyridium®
Synonyms pyridoxine hydrochloride; vitamin B_6
U.S./Canadian Brand Names Aminoxin [US-OTC]; Pyri-500 [US-OTC]
Therapeutic Category Vitamin, Water Soluble
Use Prevention and treatment of vitamin B_6 deficiency, pyridoxine-dependent seizures in infants
Usual Dosage
Recommended daily allowance (RDA):
Children:
1-3 years: 0.9 mg
4-6 years: 1.3 mg
7-10 years: 1.6 mg
Adults:
Male: 1.7-2.0 mg
Female: 1.4-1.6 mg
Pyridoxine-dependent Infants:
Oral: 2-100 mg/day
I.M., I.V., SubQ: 10-100 mg
Dietary deficiency: Oral:
Children: 5-25 mg/24 hours for 3 weeks, then 1.5-2.5 mg/day in multiple vitamin product
Adults: 10-20 mg/day for 3 weeks
Drug-induced neuritis (eg, isoniazid, hydralazine, penicillamine, cycloserine): Oral:
Children:
Treatment: 10-50 mg/24 hours
Prophylaxis: 1-2 mg/kg/24 hours
Adults:
Treatment: 100-200 mg/24 hours
Prophylaxis: 25-100 mg/24 hours

Dosage Forms
Capsule: 50 mg, 250 mg
  Aminoxin [OTC]: 20 mg
Injection, solution:100 mg/mL (1 mL)
Liquid, oral: 200 mg/5 mL (120 mL)
Tablet: 25 mg, 50 mg, 100 mg, 250 mg, 500 mg
Tablet, sustained release:
  Pyri-500 [OTC]: 500 mg

pyridoxine and doxylamine *see* doxylamine and pyridoxine *(Canada only) on page 325*

pyridoxine, folic acid, and cyanocobalamin *see* folic acid, cyanocobalamin, and pyridoxine *on page 422*

pyridoxine hydrochloride *see* pyridoxine *on page 808*

Pyrilafen Tannate-12™ [US] *see* phenylephrine and pyrilamine *on page 747*

pyrilamine maleate, dextromethorphan hydrobromide, and phenylephrine hydrochloride *see* phenylephrine, pyrilamine, and dextromethorphan *on page 749*

pyrilamine, phenylephrine, and carbetapentane *see* carbetapentane, phenylephrine, and pyrilamine *on page 176*

pyrilamine tannate and phenylephrine tannate *see* phenylephrine and pyrilamine *on page 747*

pyrimethamine (peer i METH a meen)
Sound-Alike/Look-Alike Issues
  Daraprim® may be confused with Dantrium®, Daranide®
U.S./Canadian Brand Names Daraprim® [US/Can]
Therapeutic Category Folic Acid Antagonist (Antimalarial)
Use Prophylaxis of malaria due to susceptible strains of plasmodia; used in conjunction with quinine and sulfadiazine for the treatment of uncomplicated attacks of chloroquine-resistant *P. falciparum* malaria; used in conjunction with fast-acting schizonticide to initiate transmission control and suppression cure; synergistic combination with sulfonamide in treatment of toxoplasmosis
Usual Dosage
  Malaria chemoprophylaxis (for areas where chloroquine-resistant *P. falciparum* exists): Begin prophylaxis 2 weeks before entering endemic area:
    Children: 0.5 mg/kg once weekly; not to exceed 25 mg/dose
    or
    Children:
      <4 years: 6.25 mg once weekly
      4-10 years: 12.5 mg once weekly
    Children >10 years and Adults: 25 mg once weekly
    Dosage should be continued for all age groups for at least 6-10 weeks after leaving endemic areas
  Chloroquine-resistant *P. falciparum* malaria (when used in conjunction with quinine and sulfadiazine):
    Children:
      <10 kg: 6.25 mg/day once daily for 3 days
      10-20 kg: 12.5 mg/day once daily for 3 days
      20-40 kg: 25 mg/day once daily for 3 days
    Adults: 25 mg twice daily for 3 days
  Toxoplasmosis:
    Infants (congenital toxoplasmosis): Oral: 1 mg/kg once daily for 6 months with sulfadiazine then every other month with sulfa, alternating with spiramycin.
    Children: Loading dose: 2 mg/kg/day divided into 2 equal daily doses for 1-3 days (maximum: 100 mg/day) followed by 1 mg/kg/day divided into 2 doses for 4 weeks; maximum: 25 mg/day
      With sulfadiazine or trisulfapyrimidines: 2 mg/kg/day divided every 12 hours for 3 days, followed by 1 mg/kg/day once daily or divided twice daily for 4 weeks given with trisulfapyrimidines or sulfadiazine
    Adults: 50-75 mg/day together with 1-4 g of a sulfonamide for 1-3 weeks depending on patient's tolerance and response, then reduce dose by 50% and continue for 4-5 weeks **or** 25-50 mg/day for 3-4 weeks
  Prophylaxis for first episode of *Toxoplasma gondii*:
    Children ≥1 month of age: 1 mg/kg/day once daily with dapsone, plus oral folinic acid 5 mg every 3 days
    Adolescents and Adults: 50 mg once weekly with dapsone, plus oral folinic acid 25 mg once weekly

◀ Prophylaxis to prevent recurrence of *Toxoplasma gondii*:
Children ≥1 month of age: 1 mg/kg/day once daily given with sulfadiazine or clindamycin, plus oral folinic acid 5 mg every 3 days
Adolescents and Adults: 25-50 mg once daily in combination with sulfadiazine or clindamycin, plus oral folinic acid 10-25 mg daily; atovaquone plus oral folinic acid has also been used in combination with pyrimethamine.

Dosage Forms
Tablet:
Daraprim®: 25 mg

pyrimethamine and sulfadoxine *see* sulfadoxine and pyrimethamine *on page 894*

pyrithione zinc (peer i THYE one zingk)

Sound-Alike/Look-Alike Issues
pyrithione may be confused with Pyridium®

U.S./Canadian Brand Names BetaMed [US-OTC]; Denorex® Daily Protection [US-OTC]; DermaZinc™ [US-OTC]; DHS™ Zinc [US-OTC]; Head & Shoulders® Citrus Breeze 2-in-1 [US-OTC]; Head & Shoulders® Citrus Breeze [US-OTC]; Head & Shoulders® Classic Clean 2-In-1 [US-OTC]; Head & Shoulders® Classic Clean [US-OTC]; Head & Shoulders® Dry Scalp Care 2-in-1 [US-OTC]; Head & Shoulders® Dry Scalp Care [US-OTC]; Head & Shoulders® Extra Volume [US-OTC]; Head & Shoulders® intensive solutions 2-in-1 [US-OTC]; Head & Shoulders® intensive solutions for dry/damaged hair [US-OTC]; Head & Shoulders® intensive solutions for fine/oily hair [US-OTC]; Head & Shoulders® intensive solutions for normal hair [US-OTC]; Head & Shoulders® Ocean Lift 2-in-1 [US-OTC]; Head & Shoulders® Ocean Lift [US-OTC]; Head & Shoulders® Refresh 2-in-1 [US-OTC]; Head & Shoulders® Refresh [US-OTC]; Head & Shoulders® Restoring Shine 2-in-1 [US-OTC]; Head & Shoulders® Restoring Shine [US-OTC]; Head & Shoulders® Sensitive Care 2-in-1 [US-OTC]; Head & Shoulders® Sensitive Care [US-OTC]; Head & Shoulders® Smooth & Silky 2-In-1 [US-OTC]; Head & Shoulders® Smooth & Silky [US-OTC]; Selsun® Salon™ 2-in-1 [US-OTC]; Selsun® Salon™ Classic [US-OTC]; Selsun® Salon™ Moisturizing [US-OTC]; Selsun® Salon™ Volumizing [US-OTC]; Skin Care™ [US-OTC]; T/Gel® Daily Control 2 in 1 [US-OTC]; T/Gel® Daily Control [US-OTC]; Zincon® [US-OTC]; ZNP® Bar [US-OTC]

Therapeutic Category Antiseborrheic Agent, Topical

Use Relieves the itching, irritation, and scalp flaking associated with dandruff and/or seborrheal dermatitis

Usual Dosage Adults: Products should be used at least twice weekly for best results, but may be used with each washing.
Bar: May be used on body and or scalp; wet area, massage in, and rinse.
Shampoo: Should be applied to wet hair and massaged into scalp; rinse. May be followed with conditioner

Dosage Forms
Conditioner, topical:
Head & Shoulders® Classic Clean [OTC], Head & Shoulders® Dry Scalp Care [OTC]: 0.5% (400 mL)
Cream, topical:
DermaZinc™ [OTC]: 0.25% (120 g)
Lotion, topical:
Skin Care™ [OTC]: 0.25% (120 mL)
Shampoo, topical:
BetaMed [OTC]: 2% (480 mL)
Denorex® Daily Protection [OTC]: 2% (120 mL, 360 mL) [alcohol free]
DermaZinc™ [OTC]: 2% (240 mL)
DHS™ Zinc [OTC]: 2% (240 mL, 360 mL)
Head & Shoulders® Citrus Breeze [OTC], Head & Shoulders® Extra Volume [OTC], Head & Shoulders® Sensitive Care [OTC], Head & Shoulders® Ocean Lift [OTC], Head & Shoulders® Restoring Shine [OTC]: 1% (420 mL, 700 mL)
Head & Shoulders® Classic Clean [OTC]: 1% (50 mL, 420 mL, 700 mL, 1000 mL, 1200 mL)
Head & Shoulders® Dry Scalp Care [OTC]: 1% (340 mL, 420 mL, 700 mL, 1200 mL)
Head & Shoulders® intensive solutions for dry/damaged hair [OTC], Head & Shoulders® intensive solutions for fine/oily hair [OTC], Head & Shoulders® intensive solutions for normal hair [OTC]: 2% (251 mL)
Head & Shoulders® Refresh [OTC]: 1% (420 mL, 700 mL, 1000 mL, 1200 mL)
Head & Shoulders® Smooth & Silky [OTC]: 1% (420 mL)

Selsun® Salon™ Classic [OTC], Selsun® Salon™ Moisturizing [OTC], Selsun® Salon™ Volumizing [OTC]: 1% (384 mL)
T/Gel® Daily Control [OTC]: 1% (250 mL)
Zincon® [OTC]: 1% (120 mL, 240 mL)
Shampoo, topical [with conditioner]:
Head & Shoulders® Citrus Breeze 2-in-1 [OTC], Head & Shoulders® Refresh 2-in-1 [OTC], Head & Shoulders® Restoring Shine 2-in-1 [OTC]: 1% (420 mL)
Head & Shoulders® Classic Clean 2-in-1 [OTC], Head & Shoulders® Dry Scalp Care 2-in-1 [OTC], Head & Shoulders® Smooth and Silky 2-in-1 [OTC], Head & Shoulders® Ocean Lift 2-in-1 [OTC], Head & Shoulders® Sensitive Care 2-in-1 [OTC]: 1% (420 mL, 700 mL)
Head & Shoulders® intensive solutions 2-in-1 [OTC]: 2% (251 mL)
Selsun® Salon™ 2-in-1 [OTC]: 1% (384 mL)
T/Gel® Daily Control 2 in 1 [OTC]: 1% (250 mL)
Soap, topical:
DermaZinc™ [OTC]: 2% (112.5 g)
ZNP® [OTC]) 2% (119 g) [bar]
Solution, topical [spray/drops]:
DermaZinc™ [OTC]: 0.25% (120 mL)

QDALL® AR [US] *see* chlorpheniramine *on page 205*
QDALL® (Discontinued) *see* chlorpheniramine and pseudoephedrine *on page 207*
quadrivalent human papillomavirus vaccine *see* papillomavirus (Types 6, 11, 16, 18) recombinant vaccine *on page 722*
quadrivalent meningococcal conjugate vaccine *see* meningococcal polysaccharide (Groups A / C / Y and W-135) diphtheria toxoid conjugate vaccine *on page 601*
quadrivalent meningococcal conjugate vaccine *see* meningococcal polysaccharide vaccine (groups A / C / Y and W-135) *on page 601*
Quad Tann® [US] *see* chlorpheniramine, ephedrine, phenylephrine, and carbetapentane *on page 208*
Quad Tann® Pediatric [US] *see* chlorpheniramine, ephedrine, phenylephrine, and carbetapentane *on page 208*
Qualaquin™ [US] *see* quinine *on page 814*
Quartuss™ [US] *see* dextromethorphan, chlorpheniramine, phenylephrine, and guaifenesin *on page 285*
Quasense™ [US] *see* ethinyl estradiol and levonorgestrel *on page 372*
quaternium-18 bentonite *see* bentoquatam *on page 122*

quazepam (KWAZ e pam)
Sound-Alike/Look-Alike Issues
quazepam may be confused with oxazepam
U.S./Canadian Brand Names Doral® [US/Can]
Therapeutic Category Benzodiazepine
Controlled Substance C-IV
Use Treatment of insomnia
Usual Dosage Oral: Adults: Initial: 15 mg at bedtime, in some patients the dose may be reduced to 7.5 mg after a few nights
Dosage Forms
Tablet:
Doral®: 15 mg

Quelicin® [US/Can] *see* succinylcholine *on page 890*
Queltuss® (Discontinued) *see* guaifenesin and dextromethorphan *on page 454*
Questran® [US/Can] *see* cholestyramine resin *on page 215*
Questran® Light [US] *see* cholestyramine resin *on page 215*
Questran® Light Sugar Free [Can] *see* cholestyramine resin *on page 215*

quetiapine (kwe TYE a peen)
Sound-Alike/Look-Alike Issues
QUEtiapine may be confused with OLANZapine
Seroquel® may be confused with Serentil®, Serzone®, Sinequan®
Synonyms quetiapine fumarate

◀ **Tall-Man** QUEtiapine

U.S./Canadian Brand Names Seroquel® XR [US/Can]; Seroquel® [US/Can]

Therapeutic Category Antipsychotic Agent

Use Treatment of schizophrenia; treatment of acute manic episodes associated with bipolar disorder (as monotherapy or in combination with lithium or divalproex); maintenance treatment of bipolar disorder (in combination with lithium or divalproex); treatment of depressive episodes associated with bipolar disorder

Usual Dosage Oral: Adults:

Bipolar disorder:

Depression: Immediate release tablet: Initial: 50 mg/day the first day; increase to 100 mg/day on day 2, further increasing by 100 mg/day each day to a target of 300 mg/day by day 4. Further increases up to 600 mg/day by day 8 have been evaluated in clinical trials, but no additional antidepressant efficacy was noted.

Mania: Immediate release tablet: Initial: 50 mg twice daily on day 1, increase dose in increments of 100 mg/day to 200 mg twice daily on day 4; may increase to a target dose of 800 mg/day by day 6 at increments ≤200 mg/day. Usual dosage range: 400-800 mg/day.

Schizophrenia/psychoses:

Immediate release tablet: Initial: 25 mg twice daily; increase in increments of 25-50 mg 2-3 times/day on the second and third day, if tolerated, to a target dose of 300-400 mg/day in 2-3 divided doses by day 4. Make further adjustments as needed at intervals of at least 2 days in adjustments of 25-50 mg twice daily. Usual maintenance range: 300-800 mg/day.

Extended release tablet: Initial: 300 mg once daily; increase in increments of up to 300 mg/day (in intervals of ≥1 day). For dosage requirements <200 mg during initial titration, the immediate release formulation should be used. Usual maintenance range: 400-800 mg/day.

Note: Dose reductions should be attempted periodically to establish lowest effective dose in patients with psychosis. Patients being restarted after 1 week of no drug need to be titrated as above.

Dosage Forms

Tablet:

Seroquel®: 25 mg, 50 mg, 100 mg, 200 mg, 300 mg, 400 mg

Tablet, extended release:

Seroquel® XR: 50 mg [CAN] (not available in U.S.), 200 mg, 300 mg, 400 mg

quietiapine fumarate see quietiapine on page 811

Quibron® (Discontinued) see theophylline and guaifenesin on page 919

Quibron®-T (Discontinued) see theophylline on page 917

Quibron®-T/SR (Discontinued) see theophylline on page 917

Quiess® Injection (Discontinued) see hydroxyzine on page 491

Quinaglute® Dura-Tabs® (Discontinued) see quinidine on page 813

quinagolide (Discontinued)

Quinalan® (Discontinued) see quinidine on page 813

quinalbarbitone sodium see secobarbital on page 859

quinapril (KWIN a pril)

Sound-Alike/Look-Alike Issues

Accupril® may be confused with Accolate®, Accutane®, AcipHex®, Monopril®

Synonyms quinapril hydrochloride

U.S./Canadian Brand Names Accupril® [US/Can]; GD-Quinapril [Can]

Therapeutic Category Angiotensin-Converting Enzyme (ACE) Inhibitor

Use Treatment of hypertension; treatment of heart failure

Usual Dosage Oral: Adults:

Hypertension: Initial: 10-20 mg once daily, adjust according to blood pressure response at peak and trough blood levels; initial dose may be reduced to 5 mg in patients receiving diuretic therapy if the diuretic is continued; usual dose range (JNC 7): 10-40 mg once daily

Heart failure: Initial: 5 mg once or twice daily, titrated at weekly intervals to 20-40 mg daily in 2 divided doses; target dose (heart failure): 20 mg twice daily (ACC/AHA 2005 Heart Failure Guidelines)

Dosage Forms

Tablet: 5 mg, 10 mg, 20 mg, 40 mg

Accupril®: 5 mg, 10 mg, 20 mg, 40 mg

quinapril and hydrochlorothiazide (KWIN a pril & hye droe klor oh THYE a zide)

Synonyms hydrochlorothiazide and quinapril

U.S./Canadian Brand Names Accuretic® [US/Can]; Quinaretic [US]

Therapeutic Category Antihypertensive Agent, Combination

Use Treatment of hypertension (not for initial therapy)

Usual Dosage Oral: Adults: Initial:

Patients who have failed quinapril monotherapy:
Quinapril 10 mg/hydrochlorothiazide 12.5 mg **or**
Quinapril 20 mg/hydrochlorothiazide 12.5 mg once daily

Patients with adequate blood pressure control on hydrochlorothiazide 25 mg/day, but significant potassium loss:
Quinapril 10 mg/hydrochlorothiazide 12.5 mg **or**
Quinapril 20 mg/hydrochlorothiazide 12.5 mg once daily

Note: Clinical trials of quinapril/hydrochlorothiazide combinations used quinapril doses of 2.5-40 mg/day and hydrochlorothiazide doses of 6.25-25 mg/day.

Dosage Forms

Tablet: 10/12.5: Quinapril 10 mg and hydrochlorothiazide 12.5 mg; 20/12.5: Quinapril 20 mg and hydrochlorothiazide 12.5 mg; 20/25: Quinapril 20 mg and hydrochlorothiazide 25 mg

Accuretic®, Quinaretic: 10/12.5: Quinapril 10 mg and hydrochlorothiazide 12.5 mg; 20/12.5: Quinapril 20 mg and hydrochlorothiazide 12.5 mg; 20/25: Quinapril 20 mg and hydrochlorothiazide 25 mg

quinapril hydrochloride see quinapril on page 812

Quinaretic [US] see quinapril and hydrochlorothiazide on page 813

Quinate® [Can] see quinidine on page 813

Quin B Strong [US-OTC] see vitamin B complex combinations on page 981

Quin B Strong with C and Zinc [US-OTC] see vitamin B complex combinations on page 981

quinidine (KWIN i deen)

Sound-Alike/Look-Alike Issues

quiNIDine may be confused with cloNIDine, quiNINE, Quinora®

Synonyms quinidine gluconate; quinidine polygalacturonate; quinidine sulfate

Tall-Man quiNIDine

U.S./Canadian Brand Names Apo-Quinidine® [Can]; BioQuin® Durules™ [Can]; Novo-Quinidin [Can]; Quinate® [Can]

Therapeutic Category Antiarrhythmic Agent, Class I-A

Use Prophylaxis after cardioversion of atrial fibrillation and/or flutter to maintain normal sinus rhythm; prevent recurrence of paroxysmal supraventricular tachycardia, paroxysmal AV junctional rhythm, paroxysmal ventricular tachycardia, paroxysmal atrial fibrillation, and atrial or ventricular premature contractions; has activity against *Plasmodium falciparum* malaria

Usual Dosage Dosage expressed in terms of the salt: 267 mg of quinidine gluconate = 200 mg of quinidine sulfate.

Children: Test dose for idiosyncratic reaction (sulfate, oral or gluconate, I.M.): 2 mg/kg or 60 mg/m^2

Oral (quinidine sulfate): 15-60 mg/kg/day in 4-5 divided doses or 6 mg/kg every 4-6 hours; usual 30 mg/kg/day or 900 mg/m^2/day given in 5 daily doses

I.V. **not** recommended (quinidine gluconate): 2-10 mg/kg/dose given at a rate ≤10 mg/minute every 3-6 hours as needed

Adults: Test dose: Oral, I.M.: 200 mg administered several hours before full dosage (to determine possibility of idiosyncratic reaction)

Oral (for malaria):

Sulfate: 100-600 mg/dose every 4-6 hours; begin at 200 mg/dose and titrate to desired effect (maximum daily dose: 3-4 g)

Gluconate: 324-972 mg every 8-12 hours

I.M.: 400 mg/dose every 2-6 hours; initial dose: 600 mg (gluconate)

I.V.: 200-400 mg/dose diluted and given at a rate ≤10 mg/minute; may require as much as 500-750 mg

Dosage Forms

Injection, solution: 80 mg/mL (10 mL)

Tablet: 200 mg, 300 mg

Tablet, extended release: 300 mg, 324 mg

quinidine gluconate *see* quinidine *on page 813*
quinidine polygalacturonate *see* quinidine *on page 813*
quinidine sulfate *see* quinidine *on page 813*

quinine (KWYE nine)

Sound-Alike/Look-Alike Issues
quiNINE may be confused with quiNIDine
Synonyms quinine sulfate
Tall-Man quiNINE
U.S./Canadian Brand Names Apo-Quinine® [Can]; Novo-Quinine [Can]; Qualaquin™ [US]; Quinine-Odan™ [Can]
Therapeutic Category Antimalarial Agent
Use In conjunction with other antimalarial agents, treatment of uncomplicated chloroquine-resistant *P. falciparum* malaria
Usual Dosage Note: Actual duration of treatment for malaria may be dependent upon the geographic region or pathogen. Oral:
Children: Treatment of chloroquine-resistant malaria (CDC guidelines): 30 mg/kg/day in divided doses every 8 hours for 3-7 days with tetracycline, doxycycline, or clindamycin (consider risk versus benefit of using tetracycline or doxycycline in children <8 years of age)
Adults: Treatment of chloroquine-resistant malaria: 648 mg every 8 hours for 7 days with tetracycline, doxycycline, or clindamycin
Dosage Forms
Capsule:
Qualaquin™: 324 mg

Quinine-Odan™ [Can] *see* quinine *on page 814*
quinine sulfate *see* quinine *on page 814*
quinol *see* hydroquinone *on page 488*
Quinora® *(Discontinued) see* quinidine *on page 813*
Quintabs [US-OTC] *see* vitamins (multiple/oral) *on page 983*
Quintabs-M [US-OTC] *see* vitamins (multiple/oral) *on page 983*
Quintasa® [Can] *see* mesalamine *on page 607*

quinupristin and dalfopristin (kwi NYOO pris tin & dal FOE pris tin)

Synonyms pristinamycin; RP-59500
U.S./Canadian Brand Names Synercid® [US/Can]
Therapeutic Category Antibiotic, Streptogramin
Use Treatment of serious or life-threatening infections associated with vancomycin-resistant *Enterococcus faecium* bacteremia; treatment of complicated skin and skin structure infections caused by methcillin-susceptible *Staphylococcus aureus* or *Streptococcus pyogenes*

Has been studied in the treatment of a variety of infections caused by *Enterococcus faecium* (not *E. fecalis*) including vancomycin-resistant strains. May also be effective in the treatment of serious infections caused by *Staphylococcus* species including those resistant to methicillin.
Usual Dosage I.V.:
Children (limited information): Dosages similar to adult dosing have been used in the treatment of complicated skin/soft tissue infections and infections caused by vancomycin-resistant *Enterococcus faecium*
CNS shunt infection due to vancomycin-resistant *Enterococcus faecium*: 7.5 mg/kg/dose every 8 hours; concurrent intrathecal doses of 1-2 mg/day have been administered for up to 68 days
Adults:
Vancomycin-resistant *Enterococcus faecium*: 7.5 mg/kg every 8 hours
Complicated skin and skin structure infection: 7.5 mg/kg every 12 hours
Dosage Forms
Injection, powder for reconstitution:
Synercid®: 500 mg: Quinupristin 150 mg and dalfopristin 350 mg

Quixin® [US] *see* levofloxacin *on page 557*
QVAR® [US/Can] *see* beclomethasone *on page 119*

R 14-15 *see* erlotinib *on page 353*
R & C™ II [Can] *see* pyrethrins and piperonyl butoxide *on page 806*
R & C® Lice *(Discontinued)* *see* permethrin *on page 740*
R & C™ Shampoo/Conditioner [Can] *see* pyrethrins and piperonyl butoxide *on page 806*
RabAvert® [US/Can] *see* rabies virus vaccine *on page 816*

rabeprazole (ra BEP ra zole)

Sound-Alike/Look-Alike Issues
rabeprazole may be confused with aripiprazole,donepezil, lansoprazole, omeprazole, raloxifene
AcipHex® may be confused with Acephen®, Accupril®, Aricept®, pHisoHex®
Synonyms pariprazole
U.S./Canadian Brand Names AcipHex® [US/Can]; Novo-Rabeprazole EC [Can]; Pariet® [Can]; Ran-Rabeprazole [Can]
Therapeutic Category Gastric Acid Secretion Inhibitor
Use Short-term (4-8 weeks) treatment and maintenance of erosive or ulcerative gastroesophageal reflux disease (GERD); symptomatic GERD; short-term (up to 4 weeks) treatment of duodenal ulcers; long-term treatment of pathological hypersecretory conditions, including Zollinger-Ellison syndrome; *H. pylori* eradication (in combination with amoxicillin and clarithromycin)
Canadian labeling: Additional uses (not in U.S. labeling): Treatment of nonerosive reflux disease (NERD); treatment of gastric ulcers
Usual Dosage Oral:
Children ≥12 years: *U.S. labeling:* Short-term treatment of GERD: 20 mg once daily for ≤8 weeks
Adults >18 years:
Erosive/ulcerative GERD: Treatment: 20 mg once daily for 4-8 weeks; if inadequate response, may repeat up to an additional 8 weeks; maintenance: 20 mg once daily
Canadian labeling: 20 mg once daily for 4 weeks; if inadequate response, may repeat for an additional 4 weeks (lack of symptom control after 4 weeks warrants further evaluation); maintenance: 10 mg once daily (maximum: 20 mg once daily)
Symptomatic GERD: Treatment: 20 mg once daily for 4 weeks; if inadequate response, may repeat for an additional 4 weeks
Canadian labeling: 10 mg once daily (maximum: 20 mg once daily) for 4 weeks; lack of symptom control after 4 weeks warrants further evaluation
Duodenal ulcer: 20 mg/day before breakfast for 4 weeks; additional therapy may be required for some patients
Gastric ulcers (*Canadian labeling*): 20 mg once daily up to 6 weeks; additional therapy may be required for some patients
H. pylori eradication: 20 mg twice daily for 7 days; to be administered with amoxicillin 1000 mg and clarithromycin 500 mg, also given twice daily for 7 days.
Hypersecretory conditions: 60 mg once daily; dose may need to be adjusted as necessary. Doses as high as 100 mg once daily and 60 mg twice daily have been used, and continued as long as necessary (up to 1 year in some patients).
NERD (*Canadian labeling*): Treatment: 10 mg (maximum: 20 mg once daily) for 4 weeks; lack of symptom control after 4 weeks warrants further evaluation
Dosage Forms [CAN] = Canadian brand name
Tablet, delayed release, enteric coated:
AcipHex®: 20 mg
Pariet® [CAN]: 10 mg, 20 mg

rabies immune globulin (human) (RAY beez i MYUN GLOB yoo lin, HYU man)

Synonyms RIG
U.S./Canadian Brand Names HyperRAB™ S/D [US/Can]; Imogam® Rabies Pasteurized [Can]; Imogam® Rabies-HT [US]
Therapeutic Category Immune Globulin
Use Part of postexposure prophylaxis of persons with rabies exposure who lack a history of pre-exposure or postexposure prophylaxis with rabies vaccine or a recently documented neutralizing antibody response to previous rabies vaccination; although it is preferable to administer RIG with the first dose of vaccine, it can be given up to 8 days after vaccination
Usual Dosage Children and Adults: Postexposure prophylaxis: Local wound infiltration: 20 units/kg in a single dose, RIG should always be administered as part of rabies vaccine (HDCV) regimen as soon as ▶

possible (after the first dose of vaccine, up to 8 days). If anatomically feasible, the full rabies immune globulin dose should be infiltrated around and into the wound(s); remaining volume should be administered I.M. at a site distant from the vaccine administration site. If rabies vaccine was initiated without rabies immune globulin, rabies immune globulin may be administered through the seventh day after the first vaccine dose.

Note: Persons known to have an adequate titer or who have been completely immunized with rabies vaccine should not receive RIG, only booster doses of HDCV

Dosage Forms

Injection, solution [preservative free]:

HyperRAB™ S/D, Imogam® Rabies-HT: 150 int. units/mL (2 mL, 10 mL)

rabies virus vaccine (RAY beez VYE rus vak SEEN)

Synonyms HDCV; human diploid cell cultures rabies vaccine; PCEC; purified chick embryo cell

U.S./Canadian Brand Names Imovax® Rabies [US/Can]; RabAvert® [US/Can]

Therapeutic Category Vaccine, Inactivated Virus

Use Pre-exposure immunization: Vaccinate persons with greater than usual risk due to occupation or avocation including veterinarians, rangers, animal handlers, certain laboratory workers, and persons living in or visiting countries for longer than 1 month where rabies is a constant threat.

Postexposure prophylaxis: If a bite from a carrier animal is unprovoked, if it is not captured and rabies is present in that species and area, administer rabies immune globulin (RIG) and the vaccine as indicated

Usual Dosage

Pre-exposure prophylaxis: 1 mL I.M. on days 0, 7, and 21 to 28. **Note:** Prolonging the interval between doses does not interfere with immunity achieved after the concluding dose of the basic series.

Postexposure prophylaxis: All postexposure treatment should begin with immediate cleansing of the wound with soap and water

Persons not previously immunized as above: I.M.: 5 doses (1 mL each) on days 0, 3, 7, 14, 28. In addition, patients should receive rabies immune globulin 20 units/kg body weight, half infiltrated at bite site if possible, remainder I.M.)

Persons who have previously received postexposure prophylaxis with rabies vaccine, received a recommended I.M. pre-exposure series of rabies vaccine or have a previously documented rabies antibody titer considered adequate: 1 mL of either vaccine I.M. only on days 0 and 3; do not administer RIG

Booster (for occupational or other continuing risk): 1 mL I.M. every 2-5 years or based on antibody titers

Dosage Forms

Injection, powder for reconstitution:

Imovax® Rabies: 2.5 int. units [HDCV]

RabAvert®: 2.5 int. units [PCEC]

racepinephrine see epinephrine on page 344

Radiogardase™ [US] see ferric hexacyanoferrate on page 397

rAHF see antihemophilic factor (recombinant) on page 79

R-albuterol see levalbuterol on page 554

Ralivia™ ER [Can] see tramadol on page 941

Ralix [US] see chlorpheniramine, phenylephrine, and methscopolamine on page 210

raloxifene (ral OKS i feen)

Sound-Alike/Look-Alike Issues

Evista® may be confused with Avinza™

Synonyms keoxifene hydrochloride; NSC-706725; raloxifene hydrochloride

U.S./Canadian Brand Names Evista® [US/Can]

Therapeutic Category Selective Estrogen Receptor Modulator (SERM)

Use Prevention and treatment of osteoporosis in postmenopausal women; risk reduction for invasive breast cancer in postmenopausal women with osteoporosis and in postmenopausal women with high risk for invasive breast cancer

Usual Dosage Oral: Adults: Females:

Osteoporosis: 60 mg/day

Invasive breast cancer risk reduction: 60 mg/day

Dosage Forms
Tablet:
Evista®: 60 mg

raloxifene hydrochloride *see raloxifene on page 816*

raltegravir (ral TEG ra vir)
Synonyms MK-0518
U.S./Canadian Brand Names Isentress™ [US/Can]
Therapeutic Category Antiretroviral Agent, Integrase Inhibitor
Use Treatment of HIV-1 infection in combination with other antiretroviral agents in treatment-experienced patients with virus that shows multidrug resistance and active replication
Usual Dosage Oral: Adolescents ≥16 years and Adults: 400 mg twice daily
Dosage Forms
Tablet:
Isentress™: 400 mg

raltitrexed *(Canada only)* (ral ti TREX ed)
Synonyms ICI-D1694; NSC-639186; raltitrexed disodium; ZD1694
U.S./Canadian Brand Names Tomudex® [Can]
Therapeutic Category Antineoplastic Agent
Use Treatment of advanced colorectal neoplasms
Usual Dosage I.V. (refer to individual protocols): 3 mg/m^2 every 3 weeks
Dosage Forms
Injection, powder for reconstitution:
2 mg [not available in the U.S.; investigational]

raltitrexed disodium *see raltitrexed (Canada only) on page 817*

ramelteon (ra MEL tee on)
Sound-Alike/Look-Alike Issues
Rozerem™ may be confused with Razadyne™
Synonyms TAK-375
U.S./Canadian Brand Names Rozerem™ [US]
Therapeutic Category Hypnotic, Nonbenzodiazepine
Use Treatment of insomnia characterized by difficulty with sleep onset
Usual Dosage Oral: Adults: One 8 mg tablet within 30 minutes of bedtime
Dosage Forms
Tablet:
Rozerem™: 8 mg

ramipril (RA mi pril)
Sound-Alike/Look-Alike Issues
ramipril may be confused with enalapril, Monopril®
Altace® may be confused with alteplase, Amaryl®, Amerge®, Artane®
U.S./Canadian Brand Names Altace® [US/Can]; Apo-Ramipril® [Can]; CO Ramipril [Can]; Novo-Ramipril [Can]; ratio-Ramipril [Can]; Sandoz-Ramipril [Can]
Therapeutic Category Angiotensin-Converting Enzyme (ACE) Inhibitor
Use Treatment of hypertension, alone or in combination with thiazide diuretics; treatment of left ventricular dysfunction after MI; to reduce risk of MI, stroke, and death in patients at increased risk for these events
Usual Dosage Oral: Adults:
Hypertension: 2.5-5 mg once daily, maximum: 20 mg/day
Reduction in risk of MI, stroke, and death from cardiovascular causes: Initial: 2.5 mg once daily for 1 week, then 5 mg once daily for the next 3 weeks, then increase as tolerated to 10 mg once daily (may be given as divided dose)
Heart failure postmyocardial infarction: Initial: 2.5 mg twice daily titrated upward, if possible, to 5 mg twice daily.

◄ **Note:** The dose of any concomitant diuretic should be reduced. If the diuretic cannot be discontinued, initiate therapy with 1.25 mg. After the initial dose, the patient should be monitored carefully until blood pressure has stabilized.

Dosage Forms
Capsule: 1.25 mg, 2.5 mg, 5 mg, 10 mg
    Altace®: 1.25 mg, 2.5 mg, 5 mg, 10 mg
Tablet:
    Altace®: 1.25 mg, 2.5 mg, 5 mg, 10 mg

ramipril and felodipine *(Canada only)* (RA mi pril & fe LOE di peen)

Synonyms felodipine and ramipril; ramipril and felodipine ER

U.S./Canadian Brand Names Altace® Plus Felodipine [Can]

Therapeutic Category Antihypertensive Agent, Combination

Use Treatment of hypertension when combination therapy is appropriate (not for initial therapy)

Usual Dosage Oral: **Note:** Not for initial therapy; titration of individual agents to an appropriate clinical response is required before patient is converted over to an equivalent dose of the combination product. Adults (dose is individualized): Ramipril 2.5-10 mg and felodipine ER 2.5-10 mg once daily; adjust dose no more frequently than every 2 weeks

Dosage Forms [CAN] = Canadian brand name
Tablet, variable release:
    Altace® Plus Felodipine 2.5/2.5 [CAN]: Ramipril 2.5 mg [immediate release] and felodipine 2.5 mg [extended release] [not available in the U.S.]
    Altace® Plus Felodipine 5/5 [CAN]: Ramipril 5 mg [immediate release] and felodipine 5 mg [extended release] [not available in the U.S.]

ramipril and felodipine ER *see* ramipril and felodipine *(Canada only) on page 818*

ramipril and hydrochlorothiazide *(Canada only)*
(RA mi pril & hye droe klor oh THYE a zide)

Sound-Alike/Look-Alike Issues
    Altace® HCT may be confused with alteplase, Artane®, Altace®

Synonyms hydrochlorothiazide and ramipril

U.S./Canadian Brand Names Altace® HCT [Can]

Therapeutic Category Angiotensin-Converting Enzyme (ACE) Inhibitor; Antihypertensive Agent, Combination; Diuretic, Thiazide

Use Treatment of essential hypertension (not for initial therapy)

Usual Dosage Oral: Adults: **Note:** Not for initial therapy; titration of individual agents to an appropriate clinical response is required before patient is converted over to an equivalent dose of the combination product.
    Usual dosage: Ramipril 2.5 mg/hydrochlorothiazide 12.5 mg once daily; titrate to maximum ramipril 10 mg/hydrochlorothiazide 50 mg once daily

Dosage Forms
Tablet:
    Altace® HCT 2.5/12.5 [CAN]: Ramipril 2.5 mg and hydrochlorothiazide 12.5 mg [not available in the U.S.]
    Altace® HCT 5/12.5 [CAN]: Ramipril 5 mg and hydrochlorothiazide 12.5 mg [not available in the U.S.]
    Altace® HCT 5/25 [CAN]: Ramipril 5 mg and hydrochlorothiazide 25 mg [not available in the U.S.]
    Altace® HCT 10/12.5 [CAN]: Ramipril 10 mg and hydrochlorothiazide 12.5 mg [not available in the U.S.]
    Altace® HCT 10/25 [CAN]: Ramipril 10 mg and hydrochlorothiazide 25 mg [not available in the U.S.]

RAN™-Atenolol [Can] *see* atenolol *on page 101*

RAN™-Carvedilol [Can] *see* carvedilol *on page 181*

Ran-Cefprozil [Can] *see* cefprozil *on page 188*

RAN™-Ciprofloxacin [Can] *see* ciprofloxacin *on page 221*

RAN™-Citalopram [Can] *see* citalopram *on page 225*

RAN™-Domperidone [Can] *see* domperidone *(Canada only) on page 317*

Ranexa® [US] *see* ranolazine *on page 820*

RAN™-Fentanyl Transdermal System [Can] *see* fentanyl *on page 394*

RAN-Fosinopril [Can] *see* fosinopril *on page 427*

ranibizumab (ra ni BIZ oo mab)

Synonyms rhuFabV2

U.S./Canadian Brand Names Lucentis® [US/Can]

Therapeutic Category Monoclonal Antibody; Ophthalmic Agent; Vascular Endothelial Growth Factor (VEGF) Inhibitor

Use Treatment of neovascular (wet) age-related macular degeneration (AMD)

Usual Dosage Intravitreal: Adults:

Age-related macular degeneration (AMD): 0.5 mg (0.05 mL) once a month. **Note:** Frequency may be reduced after the first 4 injections to once every 3 months if monthly injections are not feasible; however, this regimen has reportedly resulted in a ~5 letter (1 line) loss of visual acuity over 9 months, as compared to monthly dosing.

Canadian labeling: AMD: 0.5 mg (0.05 mL) once a month. Frequency may be reduced after the first 3 injections to once every 3 months if monthly injections are not feasible.

Dosage Forms [CAN] = Canadian product availability

Injection, solution [preservative free]:

Lucentis®: 10 mg/mL (0.2 mL)

Lucentis® [CAN]: 10 mg/mL (0.3 mL)

Raniclor™ [US] *see* cefaclor *on page 183*

ranitidine (ra NI ti deen)

Sound-Alike/Look-Alike Issues

ranitidine may be confused with amantadine, rimantadine

Zantac® may be confused with Xanax®, Zarontin®, Zofran®, Zyrtec®

Synonyms ranitidine hydrochloride

U.S./Canadian Brand Names Acid Reducer Maximum Strength Non Prescription [Can]; Acid Reducer [Can]; Alti-Ranitidine [Can]; Apo-Ranitidine® [Can]; BCI-Ranitidine [Can]; CO Ranitidine [Can]; Dom-Ranitidine [Can]; Gen-Ranidine [Can]; Novo-Ranidine [Can]; Nu-Ranit [Can]; PMS-Ranitidine [Can]; Ranitidine Injection, USP [Can]; Ratio-Ranitidine [Can]; Rhoxal-ranitidine [Can]; Riva-Ranitidine [Can]; Sandoz-Ranitidine [Can]; ScheinPharm Ranitidine [Can]; Zantac 150™ [US-OTC]; Zantac 75® [US-OTC/Can]; Zantac Maximum Strength Non-Prescription [Can]; Zantac® EFFERdose® [US]; Zantac® [US/Can]

Therapeutic Category Histamine H_2 Antagonist

Use

Zantac®: Short-term and maintenance therapy of duodenal ulcer, gastric ulcer, gastroesophageal reflux, active benign ulcer, erosive esophagitis, and pathological hypersecretory conditions; as part of a multidrug regimen for *H. pylori* eradication to reduce the risk of duodenal ulcer recurrence

Zantac 75® [OTC]: Relief of heartburn, acid indigestion, and sour stomach

Usual Dosage

Children 1 month to 16 years:

Duodenal and gastric ulcer:

Oral:

Treatment: 2-4 mg/kg/day divided twice daily; maximum treatment dose: 300 mg/day

Maintenance: 2-4 mg/kg once daily; maximum maintenance dose: 150 mg/day

I.V.: 2-4 mg/kg/day divided every 6-8 hours; maximum: 200 mg/day

GERD and erosive esophagitis: Oral: 5-10 mg/kg/day divided twice daily; maximum: GERD: 300 mg/day, erosive esophagitis: 600 mg/day

Children ≥12 years: Prevention of heartburn: Oral: Zantac 75® [OTC]: 75 mg 30-60 minutes before eating food or drinking beverages which cause heartburn; maximum: 150 mg/24 hours; do not use for more than 14 days

Adults:

Duodenal ulcer: Oral: Treatment: 150 mg twice daily, or 300 mg once daily after the evening meal or at bedtime; maintenance: 150 mg once daily at bedtime

Helicobacter pylori eradication: 150 mg twice daily; requires combination therapy

Pathological hypersecretory conditions:

Oral: 150 mg twice daily; adjust dose or frequency as clinically indicated; doses of up to 6 g/day have been used

I.V.: Continuous infusion for Zollinger-Ellison: 1 mg/kg/hour; measure gastric acid output at 4 hours, if >10 mEq or if patient is symptomatic, increase dose in increments of 0.5 mg/kg/hour; doses of up to 2.5 mg/kg/hour have been used

Gastric ulcer, benign: Oral: 150 mg twice daily; maintenance: 150 mg once daily at bedtime

◄ Erosive esophagitis: Oral: Treatment: 150 mg 4 times/day; maintenance: 150 mg twice daily
Prevention of heartburn: Oral: Zantac 75® [OTC]: 75 mg 30-60 minutes before eating food or drinking beverages which cause heartburn; maximum: 150 mg in 24 hours; do not use for more than 14 days
Patients not able to take oral medication:
I.M.: 50 mg every 6-8 hours
I.V.: Intermittent bolus or infusion: 50 mg every 6-8 hours
Continuous I.V. infusion: 6.25 mg/hour

Dosage Forms
Capsule: 150 mg, 300 mg
Infusion [premixed in NaCl 0.45%; preservative free]: 50 mg (50 mL)
Zantac®: 50 mg (50 mL)
Injection, solution: 25 mg/mL (2 mL, 6 mL)
Zantac®: 25 mg/mL (2 mL, 6 mL, 40 mL)
Syrup: 15 mg/mL
Zantac®: 15 mg/mL
Tablet: 75 mg [OTC], 150 mg, 300 mg
Zantac®: 150 mg, 300 mg
Zantac 75® [OTC]: 75 mg
Zantac 150™ [OTC]: 150 mg
Tablet, effervescent:
Zantac® EFFERdose®: 25 mg

ranitidine hydrochloride *see* ranitidine *on page 819*
Ranitidine Injection, USP [Can] *see* ranitidine *on page 819*
Ran-Lisinopril [Can] *see* lisinopril *on page 570*
RAN™-Lovastatin [Can] *see* lovastatin *on page 579*
RAN™-Metformin [Can] *see* metformin *on page 610*

ranolazine (ra NOE la zeen)
Sound-Alike/Look-Alike Issues
Ranexa® may be confused with Celexa®
U.S./Canadian Brand Names Ranexa® [US]
Therapeutic Category Cardiovascular Agent, Miscellaneous
Use Treatment of refractory chronic angina in combination with amlodipine, beta-blockers, or nitrates
Usual Dosage Oral: Adults: Chronic angina: Initial: 500 mg twice daily; maximum recommended dose: 1000 mg twice daily
Dosage Forms
Tablet, extended release:
Ranexa®: 500 mg, 1000 mg

Ran-Pantoprazole [Can] *see* pantoprazole *on page 720*
Ran-Rabeprazole [Can] *see* rabeprazole *on page 815*
Ran-Risperidone [Can] *see* risperidone *on page 837*
Ran-Tamsulosin [Can] *see* tamsulosin *on page 903*
RAN™-Zopiclone [Can] *see* zopiclone *(Canada only) on page 997*
Rapamune® [US/Can] *see* sirolimus *on page 869*
Raphon [US-OTC] *see* epinephrine *on page 344*
Raplon® *(Discontinued)*
Raptiva® [US] *see* efalizumab *on page 335*

rasagiline (ra SA ji leen)
Sound-Alike/Look-Alike Issues
Azilect® may be confused with Aricept®
Synonyms AGN 1135; rasagiline mesylate; TVP-1012
U.S./Canadian Brand Names Azilect® [US]
Therapeutic Category Anti-Parkinson Agent, MAO Type B Inhibitor
Use Initial monotherapy or as adjunct to levodopa in the treatment of idiopathic Parkinson disease
Usual Dosage Oral: Adults: Parkinson disease:
Monotherapy: 1 mg once daily

Adjunctive therapy with levodopa: Initial: 0.5 mg once daily; may increase to 1 mg once daily based on response and tolerability

Note: When added to existing levodopa therapy, a dose reduction of levodopa may be required to avoid exacerbation of dyskinesias; typical dose reductions of ~9% to 13% were employed in clinical trials

Dosage Forms
Tablet:
Azilect®: 0.5 mg, 1 mg

rasagiline mesylate *see* rasagiline *on page 820*

rasabuicase (ras BYOOR i kayse)

Synonyms NSC-721631; recombinant urate oxidase
U.S./Canadian Brand Names Elitek™ [US]; Fasturtec® [Can]
Therapeutic Category Enzyme
Use Initial management of uric acid levels in pediatric patients with leukemia, lymphoma, and solid tumor malignancies receiving anticancer therapy expected to result in tumor lysis and elevation of plasma uric acid

Usual Dosage I.V.:
Children: Management of uric acid levels: 0.15 mg/kg or 0.2 mg/kg once daily for 5 days (manufacturer-recommended duration); begin chemotherapy 4-24 hours after the first dose
Limited data suggest that a single prechemotherapy dose (versus multiple-day administration) may be sufficiently efficacious. Monitoring electrolytes, hydration status, and uric acid concentrations are necessary to identify the need for additional doses. Other clinical manifestations of tumor lysis syndrome (eg, hyperphosphatemia, hypocalcemia, and hyperkalemia) may occur.

Dosage Forms
Injection, powder for reconstitution:
Elitek™: 1.5 mg, 7.5 mg

Rasilez® [Can] *see* aliskiren *on page 45*
rATG *see* antithymocyte globulin (rabbit) *on page 83*
ratio-Aclavulanate [Can] *see* amoxicillin and clavulanate potassium *on page 68*
ratio-Acyclovir [Can] *see* acyclovir *on page 33*
ratio-Alendronate [Can] *see* alendronate *on page 43*
ratio-Amcinonide [Can] *see* amcinonide *on page 57*
Ratio-Amiodarone [Can] *see* amiodarone *on page 61*
Ratio-Amiodarone I.V. [Can] *see* amiodarone *on page 61*
ratio-Azithromycin [Can] *see* azithromycin *on page 110*
ratio-Benzydamine [Can] *see* benzydamine *(Canada only) on page 129*
ratio-Bicalutamide [Can] *see* bicalutamide *on page 135*
ratio-Brimonidine [Can] *see* brimonidine *on page 142*
ratio-Buspirone [Can] *see* buspirone *on page 153*
ratio-Carvedilol [Can] *see* carvedilol *on page 181*
ratio-Cefuroxime [Can] *see* cefuroxime *on page 192*
ratio-Ciprofloxacin [Can] *see* ciprofloxacin *on page 221*
ratio-Citalopram [Can] *see* citalopram *on page 225*
ratio-Clarithromycin [Can] *see* clarithromycin *on page 227*
ratio-Clindamycin [Can] *see* clindamycin *on page 230*
ratio-Clobazam [Can] *see* clobazam *(Canada only) on page 232*
ratio-Cotridin [Can] *see* triprolidine, pseudoephedrine, and codeine *(Canada only) on page 955*
ratio-Diltiazem CD [Can] *see* diltiazem *on page 300*
ratio-Domperidone [Can] *see* domperidone *(Canada only) on page 317*
ratio-Emtec [Can] *see* acetaminophen and codeine *on page 20*
ratio-Enalapril [Can] *see* enalapril *on page 339*
ratio-Famotidine [Can] *see* famotidine *on page 390*
ratio-Fenofibrate MC [Can] *see* fenofibrate *on page 393*
ratio-Fentanyl [Can] *see* fentanyl *on page 394*
ratio-Fluoxetine [Can] *see* fluoxetine *on page 413*

ratio-Fosinopril [Can] *see* fosinopril *on page 427*
ratio-Glimepiride [Can] *see* glimepiride *on page 445*
ratio-Glyburide [Can] *see* glyburide *on page 448*
ratio-Inspra-Sal [Can] *see* albuterol *on page 39*
ratio-Ipra Sal UDV [Can] *see* ipratropium and albuterol *on page 525*
ratio-Ketorolac [Can] *see* ketorolac *on page 538*
ratio-Lamotrigine [Can] *see* lamotrigine *on page 545*
ratio-Lenoltec [Can] *see* acetaminophen and codeine *on page 20*
ratio-Lisinopril [Can] *see* lisinopril *on page 570*
ratio-Lovastatin [Can] *see* lovastatin *on page 579*
ratio-Magnesium [Can] *see* magnesium glucoheptonate *on page 584*
ratio-Metformin [Can] *see* metformin *on page 610*
ratio-Methotrexate [Can] *see* methotrexate *on page 615*
ratio-Mirtazapine [Can] *see* mirtazapine *on page 637*
ratio-Mometasone [Can] *see* mometasone *on page 641*
Ratio-Morphine [Can] *see* morphine sulfate *on page 643*
Ratio-Morphine SR [Can] *see* morphine sulfate *on page 643*
ratio-Omeprazole [Can] *see* omeprazole *on page 697*
ratio-Ondansetron [Can] *see* ondansetron *on page 698*
ratio-Orciprenaline® [Can] *see* metaproterenol *on page 609*
ratio-Paroxetine [Can] *see* paroxetine *on page 724*
ratio-Pentoxifylline [Can] *see* pentoxifylline *on page 737*
ratio-Pioglitazone [Can] *see* pioglitazone *on page 754*
ratio-Pravastatin [Can] *see* pravastatin *on page 779*
ratio-Ramipril [Can] *see* ramipril *on page 817*
Ratio-Ranitidine [Can] *see* ranitidine *on page 819*
Ratio-Risperidone [Can] *see* risperidone *on page 837*
ratio-Salbutamol [Can] *see* albuterol *on page 39*
ratio-Sertraline [Can] *see* sertraline *on page 863*
ratio-Simvastatin [Can] *see* simvastatin *on page 867*
ratio-Sumatriptan [Can] *see* sumatriptan *on page 898*
ratio-Tamsulosin [Can] *see* tamsulosin *on page 903*
ratio-Temazepam [Can] *see* temazepam *on page 907*
ratio-Theo-Bronc [Can] *see* theophylline *on page 917*
ratio-Topiramate [Can] *see* topiramate *on page 935*
ratio-Trazodone [Can] *see* trazodone *on page 944*
ratio-Valproic [Can] *see* valproic acid and derivatives *on page 967*
ratio-Valproic ECC [Can] *see* valproic acid and derivatives *on page 967*
ratio-Venlafaxine XR [Can] *see* venlafaxine *on page 973*
Ratio-Zopiclone [Can] *see* zopiclone *(Canada only) on page 997*
Raudixin® *(Discontinued)*
Rauverid® *(Discontinued)*
Razadyne™ [US] *see* galantamine *on page 434*
Razadyne™ ER [US] *see* galantamine *on page 434*
6R-BH4 *see* sapropterin *on page 856*
Reactine™ [Can] *see* cetirizine *on page 196*
Reactine® Allergy and Sinus [Can] *see* cetirizine and pseudoephedrine *on page 196*
Readi-Cat® [US] *see* barium *on page 116*
Readi-Cat® 2 [US] *see* barium *on page 116*
Rea-Lo® [US-OTC] *see* urea *on page 963*
ReAzo [US-OTC] *see* phenazopyridine *on page 741*
Rebetol® [US] *see* ribavirin *on page 831*
Rebetron® [US] *see* interferon alfa-2b and ribavirin *on page 516*

Rebif® [US/Can] *see* interferon beta-1a *on page 517*
Reclast® [US] *see* zoledronic acid *on page 995*
Reclipsen™ [US] *see* ethinyl estradiol and desogestrel *on page 369*
recombinant α-L-iduronidase (glycosaminoglycan α-L-iduronohydrolase) *see* laronidase *on page 550*
recombinant hirudin *see* lepirudin *on page 551*
recombinant human deoxyribonuclease *see* dornase alfa *on page 319*
recombinant human insulin-like growth factor-1 *see* mecasermin *on page 595*
recombinant human interleukin-11 *see* oprelvekin *on page 701*
recombinant human luteinizing hormone *see* lutropin alfa *on page 581*
recombinant human parathyroid hormone (1-34) *see* teriparatide *on page 911*
recombinant human platelet-derived growth factor B *see* becaplermin *on page 119*
recombinant human thyrotropin *see* thyrotropin alpha *on page 924*
recombinant interleukin-11 *see* oprelvekin *on page 701*
recombinant N-acetylgalactosamine 4-sulfatase *see* galsulfase *on page 435*
recombinant plasminogen activator *see* reteplase *on page 827*
recombinant urate oxidase *see* rasburicase *on page 821*
Recombinate [US/Can] *see* antihemophilic factor (recombinant) *on page 79*
Recombivax HB® [US/Can] *see* hepatitis B vaccine *on page 471*
Recothrom™ [US] *see* thrombin (topical) *on page 923*
Rectacaine [US-OTC] *see* phenylephrine *on page 745*
Rectacreme HC [US] *see* lidocaine and hydrocortisone *on page 564*
RectaGel™ HC [US] *see* lidocaine and hydrocortisone *on page 564*
Red Cross™ Canker Sore [US-OTC] *see* benzocaine *on page 124*
Redisol® (Discontinued) *see* cyanocobalamin *on page 254*
Reese's® Pinworm Medicine [US-OTC] *see* pyrantel pamoate *on page 806*
ReFacto® [US/Can] *see* antihemophilic factor (recombinant) *on page 79*
Refenesen™ [US-OTC] *see* guaifenesin *on page 453*
Refenesen™ 400 [US-OTC] *see* guaifenesin *on page 453*
Refenesen™ DM [US-OTC] *see* guaifenesin and dextromethorphan *on page 454*
Refenesen™ PE [US-OTC] *see* guaifenesin and phenylephrine *on page 456*
Refenesen Plus [US-OTC] *see* guaifenesin and pseudoephedrine *on page 458*
Refludan® [US/Can] *see* lepirudin *on page 551*
Refresh® [US-OTC] *see* artificial tears *on page 95*
Refresh Liquigel® [US-OTC] *see* carboxymethylcellulose *on page 179*
Refresh Plus® [US-OTC] *see* artificial tears *on page 95*
Refresh Plus® [US-OTC/Can] *see* carboxymethylcellulose *on page 179*
Refresh Tears® [US-OTC] *see* artificial tears *on page 95*
Refresh Tears® [US-OTC/Can] *see* carboxymethylcellulose *on page 179*

regadenoson (re ga DEN of son)
    Synonyms CVT-3146
    U.S./Canadian Brand Names Lexiscan™ [US]
    Therapeutic Category Diagnostic Agent
    Use Radionuclide myocardial perfusion imaging (MPI) in patients unable to undergo adequate exercise stress testing
    Usual Dosage I.V.: Adults: 0.4 mg (5 mL) over ~10 seconds, followed immediately by a 5 mL saline flush. Wait 10-20 seconds, then administer the radionuclide myocardial perfusion imaging agent.
    Dosage Forms
      Injection, solution [preservative free]:
        Lexiscan™ 0.08 mg/mL (5 mL)

Regitine® [Can] *see* phentolamine *on page 745*
Regitine® (Discontinued) *see* phentolamine *on page 745*
Reglan® [US] *see* metoclopramide *on page 625*
Reglan® Syrup (Discontinued) *see* metoclopramide *on page 625*

Regonol® [US] *see* pyridostigmine *on page 807*
Regranex® [US/Can] *see* becaplermin *on page 119*
Regular Iletin® II *(Discontinued)*
regular insulin *see* insulin regular *on page 513*
Regulax SS® *(Discontinued)* *see* docusate *on page 314*
Regulex® [Can] *see* docusate *on page 314*
Reguloid® [US-OTC] *see* psyllium *on page 804*
Rejuva-A® [Can] *see* tretinoin (topical) *on page 946*
Relacon-DM NR [US] *see* guaifenesin, pseudoephedrine, and dextromethorphan *on page 460*
Relacon-HC [US] *see* phenylephrine, hydrocodone, and chlorpheniramine *on page 748*
Relafen® [Can] *see* nabumetone *on page 650*
Relafen® *(Discontinued)* *see* nabumetone *on page 650*
Relenza® [US/Can] *see* zanamivir *on page 989*
Relief® *(Discontinued)* *see* phenylephrine *on page 745*
Relief® Ophthalmic Solution *(Discontinued)* *see* phenylephrine *on page 745*
Relistor™ [US] *see* methylnaltrexone *on page 621*
Relpax® [US/Can] *see* eletriptan *on page 337*
Remeron® [US/Can] *see* mirtazapine *on page 637*
Remeron® RD [Can] *see* mirtazapine *on page 637*
Remeron SolTab® [US] *see* mirtazapine *on page 637*
Reme-T™ [US-OTC] *see* coal tar *on page 240*
Remicade® [US/Can] *see* infliximab *on page 507*

remifentanil (rem i FEN ta nil)

Sound-Alike/Look-Alike Issues
remifentanil may be confused with alfentanil
Synonyms GI87084B
U.S./Canadian Brand Names Ultiva® [US/Can]
Therapeutic Category Analgesic, Narcotic
Controlled Substance C-II
Use Analgesic for use during the induction and maintenance of general anesthesia; for continued analgesia into the immediate postoperative period; analgesic component of monitored anesthesia
Usual Dosage I.V. continuous infusion: Dose should be based on ideal body weight (IBW) in obese patients (>30% over IBW).
Children birth to 2 months: Maintenance of anesthesia with nitrous oxide (70%): 0.4 mcg/kg/minute (range: 0.4-1 mcg/kg/minute); supplemental bolus dose of 1 mcg/kg may be administered, smaller bolus dose may be required with potent inhalation agents, potent neuraxial anesthesia, significant comorbidities, significant fluid shifts, or without atropine pretreatment. Clearance in neonates is highly variable; dose should be carefully titrated.
Children 1-12 years: Maintenance of anesthesia with halothane, sevoflurane, or isoflurane: 0.25 mcg/kg/minute (range: 0.05-1.3 mcg/kg/minute); supplemental bolus dose of 1 mcg/kg may be administered every 2-5 minutes. Consider increasing concomitant anesthetics with infusion rate >1 mcg/kg/minute. Infusion rate can be titrated upward in increments up to 50% or titrated downward in decrements of 25% to 50%. May titrate every 2-5 minutes.
Adults:
Induction of anesthesia: 0.5-1 mcg/kg/minute; if endotracheal intubation is to occur in <8 minutes, an initial dose of 1 mcg/kg may be given over 30-60 seconds
Coronary bypass surgery: 1 mcg/kg/minute
Maintenance of anesthesia: **Note:** Supplemental bolus dose of 1 mcg/kg may be administered every 2-5 minutes. Consider increasing concomitant anesthetics with infusion rate >1 mcg/kg/minute. Infusion rate can be titrated upward in increments of 25% to 100% or downward in decrements of 25% to 50%. May titrate every 2-5 minutes.
With nitrous oxide (66%): 0.4 mcg/kg/minute (range: 0.1-2 mcg/kg/minute)
With isoflurane: 0.25 mcg/kg/minute (range: 0.05-2 mcg/kg/minute)
With propofol: 0.25 mcg/kg/minute (range: 0.05-2 mcg/kg/minute)
Coronary bypass surgery: 1 mcg/kg/minute (range: 0.125-4 mcg/kg/minute); supplemental dose: 0.5-1 mcg/kg

Continuation as an analgesic in immediate postoperative period: 0.1 mcg/kg/minute (range: 0.025-0.2 mcg/kg/minute). Infusion rate may be adjusted every 5 minutes in increments of 0.025 mcg/kg/minute. Bolus doses are not recommended. Infusion rates >0.2 mcg/kg/minute are associated with respiratory depression.

Coronary bypass surgery, continuation as an analgesic into the ICU: 1 mcg/kg/minute (range: 0.05-1 mcg/kg/minute)

Analgesic component of monitored anesthesia care: **Note:** Supplemental oxygen is recommended:
Single I.V. dose given 90 seconds prior to local anesthetic:
Remifentanil alone: 1 mcg/kg over 30-60 seconds
With midazolam: 0.5 mcg/kg over 30-60 seconds
Continuous infusion beginning 5 minutes prior to local anesthetic:
Remifentanil alone: 0.1 mcg/kg minute
With midazolam: 0.05 mcg/kg/minute
Continuous infusion given after local anesthetic:
Remifentanil alone: 0.05 mcg/kg/minute (range: 0.025-0.2 mcg/kg/minute)
With midazolam: 0.025 mcg/kg/minute (range: 0.025-0.2 mcg/kg/minute)
Note: Following local or anesthetic block, infusion rate should be decreased to 0.05 mcg/kg/minute; rate adjustments of 0.025 mcg/kg/minute may be done at 5-minute intervals

Dosage Forms
Injection, powder for reconstitution:
Ultiva®: 1 mg, 2 mg, 5 mg

Reminyl® [Can] see galantamine on page 434
Reminyl® (Discontinued) see galantamine on page 434
Reminyl® ER [Can] see galantamine on page 434
Remodulin® [US/Can] see treprostinil on page 945
Renacidin® [US] see citric acid, magnesium carbonate, and glucono-delta-lactone on page 225
Renagel® [US/Can] see sevelamer on page 864
Renal Caps [US] see vitamin B complex combinations on page 981
renal replacement solution see electrolyte solution, renal replacement on page 336
Rena-Vite [US-OTC] see vitamin B complex combinations on page 981
Rena-Vite RX [US] see vitamin B complex combinations on page 981
Renedil® [Can] see felodipine on page 392
Reno-30® [US] see diatrizoate meglumine on page 288
Reno-60® [US] see diatrizoate meglumine on page 288
RenoCal-76® (Discontinued) see diatrizoate meglumine and diatrizoate sodium on page 288
Reno-Dip® [US] see diatrizoate meglumine on page 288
Renografin®-60 [US] see diatrizoate meglumine and diatrizoate sodium on page 288
Renoquid® (Discontinued)
Renova® [US] see tretinoin (topical) on page 946
Renvela® [US] see sevelamer on page 864
ReoPro® [US/Can] see abciximab on page 17

repaglinide (re PAG li nide)

Sound-Alike/Look-Alike Issues
Prandin® may be confused with Avandia®

U.S./Canadian Brand Names GlucoNorm® [Can]; Prandin® [US/Can]

Therapeutic Category Hypoglycemic Agent, Oral

Use Management of type 2 diabetes mellitus (noninsulin-dependent, NIDDM); may be used in combination with metformin or thiazolidinediones

Usual Dosage Oral: Adults: Should be taken within 15 minutes of the meal, but time may vary from immediately preceding the meal to as long as 30 minutes before the meal

Initial: For patients not previously treated or whose Hb A_{1c} is <8%, the starting dose is 0.5 mg before each meal. For patients previously treated with blood glucose-lowering agents whose Hb A_{1c} is ≥8%, the initial dose is 1 or 2 mg before each meal.
Dose adjustment: Determine dosing adjustments by blood glucose response, usually fasting blood glucose. Double the preprandial dose up to 4 mg until satisfactory blood glucose response is achieved. At least 1 week should elapse to assess response after each dose adjustment. ▶

Dose range: 0.5-4 mg taken with meals. Repaglinide may be dosed preprandial 2, 3, or 4 times/day in response to changes in the patient's meal pattern. Maximum recommended daily dose: 16 mg.

Patients receiving other oral hypoglycemic agents: When repaglinide is used to replace therapy with other oral hypoglycemic agents, it may be started the day after the final dose is given. Observe patients carefully for hypoglycemia because of potential overlapping of drug effects. When transferred from longer half-life sulfonylureas (eg, chlorpropamide), close monitoring may be indicated for up to ≥1 week.

Combination therapy: If repaglinide monotherapy does not result in adequate glycemic control, metformin or a thiazolidinedione may be added. Or, if metformin or thiazolidinedione therapy does not provide adequate control, repaglinide may be added. The starting dose and dose adjustments for combination therapy are the same as repaglinide monotherapy. Carefully adjust the dose of each drug to determine the minimal dose required to achieve the desired pharmacologic effect. Failure to do so could result in an increase in the incidence of hypoglycemic episodes. Use appropriate monitoring of FPG and Hb A_{1c} measurements to ensure that the patient is not subjected to excessive drug exposure or increased probability of secondary drug failure. If glucose is not achieved after a suitable trial of combination therapy, consider discontinuing these drugs and using insulin.

Dosage Forms
Tablet:
Prandin®: 0.5 mg, 1 mg, 2 mg

repaglinide and metformin (re PAG li nide & met FOR min)

Sound-Alike/Look-Alike Issues
PrandiMet™ may be confused with Avandamet®, Prandin®

Synonyms metformin and repaglinide; repaglinide and metformin hydrochloride

U.S./Canadian Brand Names PrandiMet™ [US]

Therapeutic Category Antidiabetic Agent, Biguanide; Antidiabetic Agent, Meglitinide Derivative; Hypoglycemic Agent, Oral

Use Management of type 2 diabetes mellitus (noninsulin-dependent, NIDDM), as an adjunct to diet and exercise, in patients currently receiving or not adequately controlled on metformin and/or a meglitinide

Usual Dosage Oral: Adults: Type 2 diabetes mellitus:
Patients currently taking repaglinide and metformin: Initial doses should be based on (but not exceeding) the patient's current doses of repaglinide and metformin; daily doses should be divided and given 2-3 times daily with meals (maximum single dose: 4 mg/dose [repaglinide], 1000 mg/dose [metformin]; maximum daily dose: 10 mg/day [repaglinide], 2500 mg/day [metformin])
Patients inadequately controlled on metformin alone: Initial dose: repaglinide 1 mg/ metformin 500 mg twice daily with meals. Titrate slowly to reduce the risk of repaglinide-induced hypoglycemia.
Patients inadequately controlled on a meglitinide alone: Initial dose: metformin 500 mg twice daily plus repaglinide at a dose similar to (but not exceeding) the patient's current dose. Titrate slowly to reduce the risk of metformin-induced gastrointestinal adverse effects.

Dosage Forms
Tablet:
PrandiMet™: 1/500: Repaglinide 1 mg and metformin hydrochloride 500 mg; 2/500: Repaglinide 2 mg and metformin hydrochloride 500 mg

Rescon GG [US-OTC] *see* guaifenesin and phenylephrine *on page 456*
Rescon-Jr® [US] *see* chlorpheniramine and phenylephrine *on page 206*
Rescriptor® [US/Can] *see* delavirdine *on page 271*
Rescula® *(Discontinued)*
Resectisol® [US] *see* mannitol *on page 590*

reserpine (re SER peen)

Sound-Alike/Look-Alike Issues
  reserpine may be confused with Risperdal®, risperidone
Therapeutic Category Rauwolfia Alkaloid
Use Management of mild-to-moderate hypertension; treatment of agitated psychotic states (schizophrenia)
Usual Dosage Note: When used for management of hypertension, full antihypertensive effects may take as long as 3 weeks.
Oral:
  Children: Hypertension: 0.01-0.02 mg/kg/24 hours divided every 12 hours; maximum dose: 0.25 mg/day (not recommended in children)
  Adults: Hypertension:
    Manufacturer's labeling: Initial: 0.5 mg/day for 1-2 weeks; maintenance: 0.1-0.25 mg/day
    Note: Clinically, the need for a "loading" period (as recommended by the manufacturer) is not well supported, and alternative dosing is preferred.
      Usual dose range (JNC 7): 0.05-0.25 mg once daily; 0.1 mg every other day may be given to achieve 0.05 mg once daily
Dosage Forms
  Tablet: 0.1 mg, 0.25 mg

Respa®-1ˢᵗ [US] *see* guaifenesin and pseudoephedrine *on page 458*
Respa-DM® [US] *see* guaifenesin and dextromethorphan *on page 454*
Respa-GF® *(Discontinued)* *see* guaifenesin *on page 453*
Respahist® [US] *see* brompheniramine and pseudoephedrine *on page 144*
Respaire®-60 SR *(Discontinued)* *see* guaifenesin and pseudoephedrine *on page 458*
Respaire®-120 SR *(Discontinued)* *see* guaifenesin and pseudoephedrine *on page 458*
Respa® PE *(Discontinued)* *see* guaifenesin and phenylephrine *on page 456*
Respbid® *(Discontinued)* *see* theophylline *on page 917*
Respi-Tann™ [US] *see* carbetapentane and pseudoephedrine *on page 175*
Resporal® *(Discontinued)* *see* dexbrompheniramine and pseudoephedrine *on page 279*
Restall® *(Discontinued)* *see* hydroxyzine *on page 491*
Restasis® [US] *see* cyclosporine *on page 257*
Restoril® [US/Can] *see* temazepam *on page 907*
Restylane® [US] *see* hyaluronate and derivatives *on page 476*

retapamulin (re te PAM ue lin)

U.S./Canadian Brand Names Altabax™ [US]
Therapeutic Category Antibiotic, Pleuromutilin; Antibiotic, Topical
Use Treatment of impetigo caused by susceptible strains of *S. pyogenes* or methicillin-susceptible *S. aureus*
Usual Dosage Topical: Impetigo:
  Children ≥9 months: Apply to affected area twice daily for 5 days. Total treatment area should not exceed 2% of total body surface area.
  Adults: Apply to affected area twice daily for 5 days. Total treatment area should not exceed 100 cm² total body surface area.
Dosage Forms
  Ointment, topical:
    Altabax™: 1% (5 g, 10 g, 15 g)

Retavase® [US/Can] *see* reteplase *on page 827*

reteplase (RE ta plase)

Synonyms r-PA; recombinant plasminogen activator
U.S./Canadian Brand Names Retavase® [US/Can]

◄ **Therapeutic Category** Fibrinolytic Agent

Use Management of acute myocardial infarction (AMI); improvement of ventricular function; reduction of the incidence of CHF and the reduction of mortality following AMI

Usual Dosage Adults: 10 units I.V. over 2 minutes, followed by a second dose 30 minutes later of 10 units I.V. over 2 minutes

Withhold second dose if serious bleeding or anaphylaxis occurs

Dosage Forms

Injection, powder for reconstitution [preservative free]:

Retavase®: 10.4 units

Retin-A® [US/Can] *see* tretinoin (topical) *on page 946*

Retin-A® Micro [US/Can] *see* tretinoin (topical) *on page 946*

retinoic acid *see* tretinoin (topical) *on page 946*

Retinova® [Can] *see* tretinoin (topical) *on page 946*

Retisert® [US] *see* fluocinolone *on page 409*

Retrovir® [US/Can] *see* zidovudine *on page 991*

Revatio® [US] *see* sildenafil *on page 865*

Revex® *(Discontinued)*

ReVia® [US/Can] *see* naltrexone *on page 654*

Revitalose C-1000® [Can] *see* ascorbic acid *on page 96*

Revlimid® [US/Can] *see* lenalidomide *on page 551*

Rexigen Forte® *(Discontinued) see* phendimetrazine *on page 742*

Reyataz® [US/Can] *see* atazanavir *on page 100*

Rezulin® *(Discontinued)*

rFSH-alpha *see* follitropin alfa *on page 422*

rFSH-beta *see* follitropin beta *on page 423*

rFVIIa *see* factor VIIa (recombinant) *on page 387*

R-Gel® *(Discontinued) see* capsaicin *on page 171*

R-Gene® [US] *see* arginine *on page 93*

rGM-CSF *see* sargramostim *on page 857*

rhASB *see* galsulfase *on page 435*

r-hCG *see* chorionic gonadotropin (recombinant) *on page 217*

rhDNase *see* dornase alfa *on page 319*

Rheaban® *(Discontinued)*

Rheomacrodex® *(Discontinued) see* dextran *on page 282*

Rheumatrex® Dose Pack® [US] *see* methotrexate *on page 615*

rhFSH-alpha *see* follitropin alfa *on page 422*

rhFSH-beta *see* follitropin beta *on page 423*

rhGAA *see* alglucosidase alfa *on page 45*

r-h α-GAL *see* agalsidase beta *on page 37*

RhIG *see* Rh$_o$(D) immune globulin *on page 829*

rhIGF-1 *see* mecasermin *on page 595*

rhIGF-1/rhIGFBP-3 *see* mecasermin *on page 595*

rhIL-11 *see* oprelvekin *on page 701*

Rhinacon A [US] *see* chlorpheniramine, phenylephrine, and phenyltoloxamine *on page 211*

Rhinalar® [Can] *see* flunisolide *on page 408*

Rhinall [US-OTC] *see* phenylephrine *on page 745*

Rhinocort® Aqua® [US/Can] *see* budesonide *on page 147*

Rhinocort® Nasal Inhaler *(Discontinued) see* budesonide *on page 147*

Rhinocort® Turbuhaler® [Can] *see* budesonide *on page 147*

RhinoFlex™ [US] *see* acetaminophen and phenyltoloxamine *on page 22*

RhinoFlex 650 [US] *see* acetaminophen and phenyltoloxamine *on page 22*

r-hLH *see* lutropin alfa *on page 581*

Rho(D) immune globulin (human) *see* Rh$_o$(D) immune globulin *on page 829*

Rho®-Clonazepam [Can] *see* clonazepam *on page 235*
Rhodacine® [Can] *see* indomethacin *on page 506*

Rhₒ(D) immune globulin (ar aych oh (dee) i MYUN GLOB yoo lin)

Synonyms RhIG; Rho(D) immune globulin (human); RhoIGIV; RhoIVIM

U.S./Canadian Brand Names HyperRHO™ S/D Full Dose [US]; HyperRHO™ S/D Mini Dose [US]; MICRhoGAM® [US]; RhoGAM® [US]; Rhophylac® [US]; WinRho® SDF [US/Can]

Therapeutic Category Immune Globulin

Use

Suppression of Rh isoimmunization: Use in the following situations when an Rhₒ(D)-negative individual is exposed to Rhₒ(D)-positive blood: During delivery of an Rhₒ(D)-positive infant; abortion; amniocentesis; chorionic villus sampling; ruptured tubal pregnancy; abdominal trauma; hydatidiform mole; transplacental hemorrhage. Used when the mother is Rhₒ(D) negative, the father of the child is either Rhₒ(D) positive or Rhₒ(D) unknown, the baby is either Rhₒ(D) positive or Rhₒ(D) unknown.

Transfusion: Suppression of Rh isoimmunization in Rhₒ(D)-negative individuals transfused with Rhₒ(D) antigen-positive RBCs or blood components containing Rhₒ(D) antigen-positive RBCs

Treatment of idiopathic thrombocytopenic purpura (ITP): Used in the following nonsplenectomized Rhₒ(D) positive individuals: Children with acute or chronic ITP, adults with chronic ITP, children and adults with ITP secondary to HIV infection

Usual Dosage

ITP: Children and Adults:

Rhophylac®: I.V.: 50 mcg/kg

WinRho® SDF: I.V.:

Initial: 50 mcg/kg as a single injection, or can be given as a divided dose on separate days. If hemoglobin is <10 g/dL: Dose should be reduced to 25-40 mcg/kg.

Subsequent dosing: 25-60 mcg/kg can be used if required to elevate platelet count

Maintenance dosing if patient **did respond** to initial dosing: 25-60 mcg/kg based on platelet and hemoglobin levels

Maintenance dosing if patient **did not respond** to initial dosing:

Hemoglobin 8-10 g/dL: Redose between 25-40 mcg/kg

Hemoglobin >10 g/dL: Redose between 50-60 mcg/kg

Hemoglobin <8 g/dL: Use with caution

Rhₒ(D) suppression: Adults: **Note:** One "full dose" (300 mcg) provides enough antibody to prevent Rh sensitization if the volume of RBC entering the circulation is ≤15 mL. When >15 mL is suspected, a fetal red cell count should be performed to determine the appropriate dose.

Pregnancy:

Antepartum prophylaxis: In general, dose is given at 28 weeks. If given early in pregnancy, administer every 12 weeks to ensure adequate levels of passively acquired anti-Rh

HyperRHO™ S/D Full Dose, RhoGAM®: I.M.: 300 mcg

Rhophylac®, WinRho® SDF: I.M., I.V.: 300 mcg

Postpartum prophylaxis: In general, dose is administered as soon as possible after delivery, preferably within 72 hours. Can be given up to 28 days following delivery

HyperRHO™ S/D Full Dose, RhoGAM®: I.M.: 300 mcg

Rhophylac®: I.M., I.V.: 300 mcg

WinRho® SDF: I.M., I.V.: 120 mcg

Threatened abortion, any time during pregnancy (with continuation of pregnancy):

HyperRHO™ S/D Full Dose, RhoGAM®: I.M.: 300 mcg; administer as soon as possible

Rhophylac®, WinRho® SDF: I.M., I.V.: 300 mcg; administer as soon as possible

Abortion, miscarriage, termination of ectopic pregnancy:

RhoGAM®: I.M.: ≥13 weeks gestation: 300 mcg.

HyperRHO™ S/D Mini Dose, MICRhoGAM®: <13 weeks gestation: I.M.: 50 mcg

Rhophylac®: I.M., I.V.: 300 mcg

WinRho® SDF: I.M., I.V.: After 34 weeks gestation: 120 mcg; administer immediately or within 72 hours

Amniocentesis, chorionic villus sampling:

HyperRHO™ S/D Full Dose, RhoGAM®: I.M.: At 15-18 weeks gestation or during the 3rd trimester: 300 mcg. If dose is given between 13-18 weeks, repeat at 26-28 weeks and within 72 hours of delivery.

Rhophylac®: I.M., I.V.: 300 mcg

WinRho® SDF: I.M., I.V.: Before 34 weeks gestation: 300 mcg; administer immediately, repeat dose every 12 weeks during pregnancy; After 34 weeks gestation: 120 mcg, administered immediately or within 72 hours

Excessive fetomaternal hemorrhage (>15 mL): Rhophylac®: I.M., I.V.: 300 mcg within 72 hours plus 20 mcg/mL fetal RBCs in excess of 15 mL if excess transplacental bleeding is quantified **or** 300 mcg/dose if bleeding cannot be quantified

Abdominal trauma, manipulation:

HyperRHO™ S/D Full Dose, RhoGAM®: I.M.: 2nd or 3rd trimester: 300 mcg. If dose is given between 13-18 weeks, repeat at 26-28 weeks and within 72 hours of delivery

Rhophylac®: I.M., I.V.: 300 mcg within 72 hours

WinRho® SDF: I.M./I.V.: After 34 weeks gestation: 120 mcg; administer immediately or within 72 hours

Transfusion:

Children and Adults: WinRho® SDF: Administer within 72 hours after exposure of incompatible blood transfusions or massive fetal hemorrhage.

I.V.: Calculate dose as follows; administer 600 mcg every 8 hours until the total dose is administered:

Exposure to $Rh_o(D)$ positive whole blood: 9 mcg/mL blood

Exposure to $Rh_o(D)$ positive red blood cells: 18 mcg/mL cells

I.M.: Calculate dose as follows; administer 1200 mcg every 12 hours until the total dose is administered:

Exposure to $Rh_o(D)$ positive whole blood: 12 mcg/mL blood

Exposure to $Rh_o(D)$ positive red blood cells: 24 mcg/mL cells

Adults:

HyperRHO™ S/D Full Dose, RhoGAM®: I.M.: Multiply the volume of Rh positive whole blood administered by the hematocrit of the donor unit to equal the volume of RBCs transfused. The volume of RBCs is then divided by 15 mL, providing the number of 300 mcg doses (vials/syringes) to administer. If the dose calculated results in a fraction, round up to the next higher whole 300 mcg dose (vial/syringe).

Rhophylac®: I.M., I.V.: 20 mcg/2 mL transfused blood or 20 mcg/mL erythrocyte concentrate

Dosage Forms

Injection, solution [preservative free]:

HyperRHO™ S/D Full Dose, RhoGAM®: 300 mcg [I.M. use only]

HyperRHO™ S/D Mini Dose, MICRhoGAM®: 50 mcg [I.M. use only]

WinRho® SDF:

300 mcg/~1.3 mL (~1.3 mL)

500 mcg/~2.2 mL (~2.2 mL)

1000 mcg/~4.4 mL (~4.4 mL)

3000 mcg/~13 mL (~13 mL)

Rhodis™ [Can] see ketoprofen on page 537

Rhodis-EC™ [Can] see ketoprofen on page 537

Rhodis SR™ [Can] see ketoprofen on page 537

RhoGAM® [US] see $Rh_o(D)$ immune globulin on page 829

RhoIGIV see $Rh_o(D)$ immune globulin on page 829

RhoIVIM see $Rh_o(D)$ immune globulin on page 829

Rho®-Loperamine [Can] see loperamide on page 573

Rho®-Metformin [Can] see metformin on page 610

Rho®-Nitro [Can] see nitroglycerin on page 675

Rhophylac® [US] see $Rh_o(D)$ immune globulin on page 829

Rho®-Sotalol [Can] see sotalol on page 885

Rhotral [Can] see acebutolol on page 19

Rhotrimine® [Can] see trimipramine on page 954

Rhovane® [Can] see zopiclone (Canada only) on page 997

Rhoxal-acebutolol [Can] see acebutolol on page 19

Rhoxal-atenolol [Can] see atenolol on page 101

Rhoxal-cyclosporine [Can] see cyclosporine on page 257

Rhoxal-diltiazem CD [Can] see diltiazem on page 300

Rhoxal-diltiazem SR [Can] see diltiazem on page 300

Rhoxal-diltiazem T [Can] see diltiazem on page 300

Rhoxal-fluoxetine [Can] see fluoxetine on page 413

Rhoxal-fluvoxamine [Can] see fluvoxamine on page 420

Rhoxal-glimepiride [Can] see glimepiride on page 445

Rhoxal-Loperamide [Can] see loperamide on page 573
Rhoxal-minocycline [Can] see minocycline on page 635
Rhoxal-mirtazapine [Can] see mirtazapine on page 637
Rhoxal-mirtazapine FC [Can] see mirtazapine on page 637
Rhoxal-nabumetone [Can] see nabumetone on page 650
Rhoxal-orphendrine [Can] see orphenadrine on page 702
Rhoxal-pamidronate [Can] see pamidronate on page 716
Rhoxal-paroxetine [Can] see paroxetine on page 724
Rhoxal-ranitidine [Can] see ranitidine on page 819
Rhoxal-salbutamol [Can] see albuterol on page 39
Rhoxal-Sertraline [Can] see sertraline on page 863
Rhoxal-sumatriptan [Can] see sumatriptan on page 898
Rhoxal-ticlopidine [Can] see ticlopidine on page 926
Rhoxal-valproic [Can] see valproic acid and derivatives on page 967
Rhoxal-zopiclone [Can] see zopiclone (Canada only) on page 997
rhPTH(1-34) see teriparatide on page 911
Rh-TSH see thyrotropin alpha on page 924
rHuEPO-α see epoetin alfa on page 347
rhuFabV2 see ranibizumab on page 819
rHu-KGF see palifermin on page 715
Rhulicaine® (Discontinued) see benzocaine on page 124
rhuMAb-E25 see omalizumab on page 696
rHuMAb-EGFr see panitumumab on page 719
rhuMAb-VEGF see bevacizumab on page 134
RibaPak™ [US] see ribavirin on page 831
Ribasphere™ [US] see ribavirin on page 831

ribavirin (rye ba VYE rin)

Sound-Alike/Look-Alike Issues
ribavirin may be confused with riboflavin

Synonyms RTCA; tribavirin

U.S./Canadian Brand Names Copegus® [US]; Rebetol® [US]; RibaPak™ [US]; Ribasphere™ [US]; Virazole® [US/Can]

Therapeutic Category Antiviral Agent

Use
Inhalation: Treatment of patients with respiratory syncytial virus (RSV) infections; specially indicated for treatment of severe lower respiratory tract RSV infections in patients with an underlying compromising condition (prematurity, bronchopulmonary dysplasia and other chronic lung conditions, congenital heart disease, immunodeficiency, immunosuppression), and recent transplant recipients

Oral capsule:
In combination with interferon alfa-2b (Intron® A) injection for the treatment of chronic hepatitis C in patients with compensated liver disease who have relapsed after alpha interferon therapy or were previously untreated with alpha interferons
In combination with peginterferon alfa-2b (PEG-Intron®) injection for the treatment of chronic hepatitis C in patients with compensated liver disease who were previously untreated with alpha interferons

Oral solution: In combination with interferon alfa 2b (Intron® A) injection for the treatment of chronic hepatitis C in patients with compensated liver disease who were previously untreated with alpha interferons or patients who have relapsed after alpha interferon therapy

Oral tablet: In combination with peginterferon alfa-2a (Pegasys®) injection for the treatment of chronic hepatitis C in patients with compensated liver disease who were previously untreated with alpha interferons (includes patients with histological evidence of cirrhosis [Child-Pugh class A] and patients with clinically-stable HIV disease)

Usual Dosage
Aerosol inhalation: Infants and Children: Use with Viratek® small particle aerosol generator (SPAG-2) at a concentration of 20 mg/mL (6 g reconstituted with 300 mL of sterile water without preservatives). Continuous aerosol administration: 12-18 hours/day for 3 days, up to 7 days in length

Oral capsule or solution: Children ≥3 years: Chronic hepatitis C (in combination with interferon alfa-2b): Rebetol®: Oral: **Note:** Oral solution should be used in children 3-5 years of age, children ≤25 kg, or those unable to swallow capsules.
Capsule/solution: 15 mg/kg/day in 2 divided doses (morning and evening)
Capsule dosing recommendations:
  25-36 kg: 400 mg/day (200 mg morning and evening)
  37-49 kg: 600 mg/day (200 mg in the morning and 400 mg in the evening)
  50-61 kg: 800 mg/day (400 mg in the morning and evening)
  >61 kg: Refer to adult dosing
  Note: Treatment duration may vary. Consult current guidelines and literature.
Oral capsule (Rebetol®, Ribasphere®): Adults:
Chronic hepatitis C (in combination with interferon alfa-2b):
  ≤75 kg: 400 mg in the morning, then 600 mg in the evening
  >75 kg: 600 mg in the morning, then 600 mg in the evening
Chronic hepatitis C (in combination with peginterferon alfa-2b): 400 mg twice daily
  Note: Treatment duration may vary. Consult current guidelines and literature.
Oral tablet (Copegus®, in combination with peginterferon alfa-2b): Adults: Chronic hepatitis C:
Monoinfection, genotype 1,4:
  <75kg: 1000 mg/day in 2 divided doses
  ≥75kg: 1200 mg/day in 2 divided doses
Monoinfection, genotype 2,3: 800 mg/day in 2 divided doses
Coinfection with HIV: 800 mg/day in 2 divided doses
  Note: Treatment duration may vary. Consult current guidelines and literature.
Dosage Forms
Capsule: 200 mg
  Rebetol®, Ribasphere®: 200 mg
Combination package [dose pack]:
  RibaPak™ 400/600 [each package contains]:
    Tablet: 400 mg (7s)
    Tablet: 600 mg (2s)
Powder for solution [for nebulization]:
  Virazole®: 6 g
Solution, oral:
  Rebetol®: 40 mg/mL
Tablet: 200 mg
  Copegus®: 200 mg
  Ribasphere®: 200 mg, 400 mg, 600 mg
Tablet [dose pack]:
  RibaPak™: 400 mg (14s), 600 mg (14s)

ribavirin and interferon alfa-2b combination pack *see* interferon alfa-2b and ribavirin *on page 516*
ribavirin and peginterferon alfa-2b *see* peginterferon alfa-2b and ribavirin *(Canada only) on page 728*
Ribo-100 [US] *see* riboflavin *on page 832*

riboflavin (RYE boe flay vin)

Sound-Alike/Look-Alike Issues
  riboflavin may be confused with ribavirin
Synonyms lactoflavin; vitamin B_2; vitamin G
U.S./Canadian Brand Names Ribo-100 [US]
Therapeutic Category Vitamin, Water Soluble
Use Prevention of riboflavin deficiency and treatment of ariboflavinosis
Usual Dosage Oral:
  Riboflavin deficiency:
    Children: 2.5-10 mg/day in divided doses
    Adults: 5-30 mg/day in divided doses
  Recommended daily allowance:
    Children: 0.4-1.8 mg
    Adults: 1.2-1.7 mg
Dosage Forms
  Tablet: 25 mg, 50 mg, 100 mg
    Ribo-100: 100 mg

Rid-A-Pain Dental [US-OTC] *see* benzocaine *on page 124*
Ridaura® [US/Can] *see* auranofin *on page 107*
RID® *(Discontinued)* *see* pyrethrins and piperonyl butoxide *on page 806*
RID® Maximum Strength [US-OTC] *see* pyrethrins and piperonyl butoxide *on page 806*
RID® Mousse [Can] *see* pyrethrins and piperonyl butoxide *on page 806*
Rid® Spray [US-OTC] *see* permethrin *on page 740*

rifabutin (rif a BYOO tin)

Sound-Alike/Look-Alike Issues
  rifabutin may be confused with rifampin
Synonyms ansamycin
U.S./Canadian Brand Names Mycobutin® [US/Can]
Therapeutic Category Antibiotic, Miscellaneous
Use Prevention of disseminated *Mycobacterium avium* complex (MAC) in patients with advanced HIV infection
Usual Dosage Oral: Prophylaxis:
  Children >1 year: 5 mg/kg daily; higher dosages have been used in limited trials
  Adults: 300 mg once daily (alone or in combination with azithromycin)
Dosage Forms
  Capsule:
  Mycobutin®: 150 mg

Rifadin® [US/Can] *see* rifampin *on page 833*
Rifamate® [US/Can] *see* rifampin and isoniazid *on page 834*
rifampicin *see* rifampin *on page 833*

rifampin (rif AM pin)

Sound-Alike/Look-Alike Issues
  rifampin may be confused with rifabutin, Rifamate®, rifapentine, rifaximin
  Rifadin® may be confused with Ritalin®
Synonyms rifampicin
U.S./Canadian Brand Names Rifadin® [US/Can]; Rofact™ [Can]
Therapeutic Category Antibiotic, Miscellaneous
Use Management of active tuberculosis in combination with other agents; elimination of meningococci from the nasopharynx in asymptomatic carriers
Usual Dosage
  Usual dosage ranges: Oral, I.V.:
  Infants and Children: 10-20 mg/kg/day as a single dose or in 2 divided doses; maximum: 600 mg/day
  Adults: 600 mg once or twice daily
  Indication-specific dosing: Oral, I.V.:
  Tuberculosis, active: Note: A four-drug regimen (isoniazid, rifampin, pyrazinamide, and ethambutol) is preferred for the initial, empiric treatment of TB. When the drug susceptibility results are available, the regimen should be altered as appropriate.
  Infants and Children <12 years:
  Daily therapy: 10-20 mg/kg/day usually as a single dose (maximum: 600 mg/day)
  Twice weekly directly observed therapy (DOT): 10-20 mg/kg (maximum: 600 mg)
  Adults:
  Daily therapy: 10 mg/kg/day (maximum: 600 mg/day)
  Twice weekly directly observed therapy (DOT): 10 mg/kg (maximum: 600 mg); 3 times/week: 10 mg/kg (maximum: 600 mg)
  Tuberculosis, latent infection (LTBI): As an alternative to isoniazid:
  Children: 10-20 mg/kg/day (maximum: 600 mg/day) for 6 months
  Adults: 10 mg/kg/day (maximum: 600 mg/day) for 4 months. **Note:** Combination with pyrazinamide should not generally be offered (*MMWR*, Aug 8, 2003).
Dosage Forms
  Capsule: 150 mg, 300 mg
  Rifadin®: 150 mg, 300 mg
  Injection, powder for reconstitution: 600 mg
  Rifadin®: 600 mg

rifampin and isoniazid (rif AM pin & eye soe NYE a zid)

Sound-Alike/Look-Alike Issues
Rifamate® may be confused with rifampin

Synonyms isoniazid and rifampin

U.S./Canadian Brand Names IsonaRif™ [US]; Rifamate® [US/Can]

Therapeutic Category Antibiotic, Miscellaneous

Use Management of active tuberculosis; see individual agents for additional information

Usual Dosage Oral: 2 capsules/day

Dosage Forms
Capsule:
IsonaRif™, Rifamate®: 300/150: Rifampin 300 mg and isoniazid 150 mg

rifampin, isoniazid, and pyrazinamide
(rif AM pin, eye soe NYE a zid, & peer a ZIN a mide)

Sound-Alike/Look-Alike Issues
Rifater® may be confused with Rifadin®

Synonyms isoniazid, rifampin, and pyrazinamide; pyrazinamide, rifampin, and isoniazid

U.S./Canadian Brand Names Rifater® [US/Can]

Therapeutic Category Antibiotic, Miscellaneous

Use Initial phase, short-course treatment of pulmonary tuberculosis; see individual agents for additional information

Usual Dosage Oral: Adults: Patients weighing:
≤44 kg: 4 tablets
45-54 kg: 5 tablets
≥55 kg: 6 tablets
Doses should be administered in a single daily dose

Dosage Forms
Tablet:
Rifater®: Rifampin 120 mg, isoniazid 50 mg, and pyrazinamide 300 mg

rifapentine (rif a PEN teen)

Sound-Alike/Look-Alike Issues
rifapentine may be confused with rifampin

U.S./Canadian Brand Names Priftin® [US/Can]

Therapeutic Category Antitubercular Agent

Use Treatment of pulmonary tuberculosis; rifapentine must always be used in conjunction with at least one other antituberculosis drug to which the isolate is susceptible; it may also be necessary to add a third agent (either streptomycin or ethambutol) until susceptibility is known.

Usual Dosage
Children: No dosing information available
Adults: **Rifapentine should not be used alone**; initial phase should include a 3- to 4-drug regimen
Intensive phase (initial 2 months) of short-term therapy: 600 mg (four 150 mg tablets) given twice weekly (with an interval of not less than 72 hours between doses); following the intensive phase, treatment should continue with rifapentine 600 mg once weekly for 4 months in combination with INH or appropriate agent for susceptible organisms

Dosage Forms
Tablet:
Priftin®: 150 mg

Rifater® [US/Can] *see* rifampin, isoniazid, and pyrazinamide *on page 834*

rifaximin (rif AX i min)

Sound-Alike/Look-Alike Issues
rifaximin may be confused with rifampin

U.S./Canadian Brand Names Xifaxan™ [US]

Therapeutic Category Antibiotic, Miscellaneous

Use Treatment of traveler's diarrhea caused by noninvasive strains of *E. coli*

Usual Dosage Oral: Children ≥12 years and Adults: Traveler's diarrhea: 200 mg 3 times/day for 3 days

Dosage Forms
Tablet:
Xifaxan™: 200 mg

rIFN-A *see* interferon alfa-2a *on page 514*
rIFN beta-1a *see* interferon beta-1a *on page 517*
rIFN beta-1b *see* interferon beta-1b *on page 518*
RIG *see* rabies immune globulin (human) *on page 815*
rIL-11 *see* oprelvekin *on page 701*

rilonacept (ri LON a sept)

U.S./Canadian Brand Names Arcalyst™ [US]

Therapeutic Category Interleukin-1 Inhibitor

Use Orphan drug: Treatment of cryopyrin-associated periodic syndromes (CAPS) including familial cold autoinflammatory syndrome (FCAS) and Muckle-Wells syndrome (MWS)

Usual Dosage SubQ: Cryopyrin-associated periodic syndromes:
Children ≥12 years: Loading dose 4.4 mg/kg (maximum dose: 320 mg) given as 1-2 separate injections (maximum: 2 mL/injection) on the same day, followed by 2.2 mg/kg (maximum dose: 160 mg) once weekly. **Note:** Do not administer more frequently than once weekly.
Adults: Loading dose 320 mg given as 2 separate injections (160 mg each) on the same day at 2 different sites, followed a week later by 160 mg, then once weekly. **Note:** Do not administer more frequently than once weekly.

Dosage Forms
Injection, powder for reconstitution:
Arcalyst™: 220 mg

Rilutek® [US/Can] *see* riluzole *on page 835*

riluzole (RIL yoo zole)

Synonyms 2-amino-6-trifluoromethoxy-benzothiazole; RP-54274

U.S./Canadian Brand Names Rilutek® [US/Can]

Therapeutic Category Miscellaneous Product

Use Treatment of amyotrophic lateral sclerosis (ALS); riluzole can extend survival or time to tracheostomy

Usual Dosage Oral: Adults: 50 mg every 12 hours; no increased benefit can be expected from higher daily doses, but adverse events are increased
Dosage adjustment in smoking: Cigarette smoking is known to induce CYP1A2; patients who smoke cigarettes would be expected to eliminate riluzole faster. There is no information, however, on the effect of, or need for, dosage adjustment in these patients.
Dosage adjustment in special populations: Females and Japanese patients may possess a lower metabolic capacity to eliminate riluzole compared with male and Caucasian subjects, respectively

Dosage Forms
Tablet:
Rilutek®: 50 mg

rimantadine (ri MAN ta deen)

Sound-Alike/Look-Alike Issues
rimantadine may be confused with amantadine, ranitidine, Rimactane®
Flumadine® may be confused with fludarabine, flunisolide, flutamide

Synonyms rimantadine hydrochloride

U.S./Canadian Brand Names Flumadine® [US/Can]

Therapeutic Category Antiviral Agent

Use Prophylaxis (adults and children >1 year of age) and treatment (adults) of influenza A viral infection (per manufacturer labeling; also refer to current ACIP guidelines for recommendations during current flu season)

Note: In certain circumstances, the ACIP recommends use of rimantadine in combination with oseltamivir for the treatment or prophylaxis of influenza A infection when resistance to oseltamivir is suspected.

◀ **Usual Dosage** Oral:
Prophylaxis:
Children 1-10 years: 5 mg/kg/day; maximum: 150 mg/day
Children >10 years and Adults: 100 mg twice daily
Treatment: Adults: 100 mg twice daily
Dosage Forms
Tablet: 100 mg
Flumadine®: 100 mg

rimantadine hydrochloride see rimantadine on page 835

rimexolone (ri MEKS oh lone)
Sound-Alike/Look-Alike Issues
Vexol® may be confused with VoSol®
U.S./Canadian Brand Names Vexol® [US/Can]
Therapeutic Category Adrenal Corticosteroid
Use Treatment of inflammation after ocular surgery and the treatment of anterior uveitis
Usual Dosage Ophthalmic: Adults: Instill 1 drop in conjunctival sac 2-4 times/day up to every 4 hours; may use every 1-2 hours during first 1-2 days
Dosage Forms
Suspension, ophthalmic:
Vexol®: 1% (5 mL, 10 mL)

Rimso®-50 [US/Can] see dimethyl sulfoxide on page 303
Rinate™ Pediatric [US] see chlorpheniramine and phenylephrine on page 206
Rindal HD Plus [US] see phenylephrine, hydrocodone, and chlorpheniramine on page 748
Rindal HPD *(Discontinued)*
Riobin® *(Discontinued)* see riboflavin on page 832
Riomet® [US] see metformin on page 610
Riopan® Plus *(Discontinued)* see magaldrate and simethicone on page 583
Riopan® Plus Double Strength *(Discontinued)* see magaldrate and simethicone on page 583
Riphenidate [Can] see methylphenidate on page 622

risedronate (ris ED roe nate)
Sound-Alike/Look-Alike Issues
Actonel® may be confused with Actos®
Synonyms risedronate sodium
U.S./Canadian Brand Names Actonel® [US/Can]
Therapeutic Category Bisphosphonate Derivative
Use Treatment of Paget disease of the bone; treatment and prevention of glucocorticoid-induced osteoporosis; treatment and prevention of osteoporosis in postmenopausal women; treatment of osteoporosis in men
Usual Dosage Oral: Adults:
Paget disease of bone: 30 mg once daily for 2 months
Retreatment may be considered (following post-treatment observation of at least 2 months) if relapse occurs, or if treatment fails to normalize serum alkaline phosphatase. For retreatment, the dose and duration of therapy are the same as for initial treatment. No data are available on more than one course of retreatment.
Osteoporosis (postmenopausal) prevention and treatment: 5 mg once daily **or** 35 mg once weekly **or** one 75 mg tablet taken on 2 consecutive days once a month (total of 2 tablets/month) **or** 150 mg once a month
Osteoporosis (male) treatment: 35 mg once weekly
Osteoporosis (glucocorticoid-induced) prevention and treatment: 5 mg once daily
Dosage Forms
Tablet:
Actonel®: 5 mg, 30 mg, 35 mg, 75 mg, 150 mg

risedronate and calcium (ris ED roe nate & KAL see um)

Sound-Alike/Look-Alike Issues
Actonel® may be confused with Actos®
Synonyms calcium and risedronate; risedronate sodium and calcium carbonate
U.S./Canadian Brand Names Actonel® and Calcium [US]
Therapeutic Category Bisphosphonate Derivative; Calcium Salt
Use Treatment and prevention of osteoporosis in postmenopausal women
Usual Dosage Oral: Adults: Osteoporosis in postmenopausal females:
Risedronate: 35 mg once weekly on day 1 of 7-day treatment cycle
Calcium carbonate: 1250 mg (elemental calcium 500 mg) once daily on days 2 through 7 of 7-day treatment cycle
Dosage Forms
Combination package [each package contains]:
Actonel® and Calcium:
Tablet (Actonel®): Risedronate 35 mg (4s)
Tablet: Calcium 1250 mg (24s)

risedronate sodium *see* risedronate *on page 836*
risedronate sodium and calcium carbonate *see* risedronate and calcium *on page 837*
Risperdal® [US/Can] *see* risperidone *on page 837*
Risperdal® M-Tab® [US/Can] *see* risperidone *on page 837*
Risperdal® Consta® [US/Can] *see* risperidone *on page 837*

risperidone (ris PER i done)

Sound-Alike/Look-Alike Issues
risperidone may be confused with reserpine
Risperdal® may be confused with lisinopril, reserpine
U.S./Canadian Brand Names Apo-Risperidone® [Can]; CO Risperidone [Can]; Dom-Risperidone [Can]; Gen-Risperidone [Can]; Novo-Risperidone [Can]; PHL-Risperidone [Can]; PMS-Risperidone ODT [Can]; Ran-Risperidone [Can]; Ratio-Risperidone [Can]; Risperdal® Consta® [US/Can]; Risperdal® M-Tab® [US/Can]; Risperdal® [US/Can]; Riva-Risperidone [Can]; Sandoz Risperidone [Can]
Therapeutic Category Antipsychotic Agent, Benzisoxazole
Use Treatment of schizophrenia; treatment of acute mania or mixed episodes associated with bipolar I disorder (as monotherapy in children or adults, or in combination with lithium or valproate in adults); treatment of irritability/aggression associated with autistic disorder
Usual Dosage
Oral:
Children ≥5 years and Adolescents: Autism:
<15 kg: Use with caution; specific dosing recommendations not available
<20 kg: Initial: 0.25 mg/day; may increase dose to 0.5 mg/day after ≥4 days, maintain dose for ≥14 days. In patients not achieving sufficient clinical response, may increase dose by 0.25 mg/day in ≥2-week intervals. Therapeutic effect reached plateau at 1 mg/day in clinical trials. Following clinical response, consider gradually lowering dose. May be administered once daily or in divided doses twice daily.
≥20 kg: Initial: 0.5 mg/day; may increase dose to 1 mg/day after ≥4 days, maintain dose for ≥14 days. In patients not achieving sufficient clinical response, may increase dose by 0.5 mg/day in ≥2-week intervals. Therapeutic effect reached plateau at 2.5 mg/day (3 mg/day in children >45 kg) in clinical trials. Following clinical response, consider gradually lowering dose. May be administered once daily or in divided doses twice daily.
Children and Adolescents:
Schizophrenia: Adolescents 13-17 years: Initial: 0.5 mg once daily; dose may be adjusted in increments of 0.5-1 mg/day at intervals ≥24 hours to a dose of 3 mg/day. Doses ranging from 1-6 mg/day have been evaluated, however, doses >3 mg/day do not confer additional benefit and are associated with increased adverse events.
Bipolar disorder: Children and Adolescents 10-17 years: Initial: 0.5 mg once daily; dose may be adjusted in increments of 0.5-1 mg/day at intervals ≥24 hours to a dose of 2.5 mg/day. Doses ranging from 0.5-6 mg/day have been evaluated, however doses >2.5 mg/day do not confer additional benefit and are associated with increased adverse events.

▶

◀ Adults:

Schizophrenia:

Initial: 1 mg twice daily; may be increased by 1-2 mg/day at intervals ≥24 hours to a target dose of 6 mg/day; usual range: 4-8 mg/day; may be given as a single daily dose once maintenance dose is achieved; daily dosages >6 mg do not appear to confer any additional benefit, and the incidence of extrapyramidal symptoms is higher than with lower doses. Further dose adjustments should be made in increments/decrements of 1-2 mg/day on a weekly basis. Dose range studied in clinical trials: 4-16 mg/day.

Maintenance: Target dose: 4 mg once daily (range 2-8 mg/day)

Bipolar mania:

Initial: 2-3 mg once daily; if needed, adjust dose by 1 mg/day in intervals ≥24 hours; dosing range: 1-6 mg/day

Maintenance: No dosing recommendation available for treatment >3 weeks duration.

I.M.: Adults: Schizophrenia (Risperdal® Consta®): 25 mg every 2 weeks; some patients may benefit from larger doses; maximum dose not to exceed 50 mg every 2 weeks. Dosage adjustments should not be made more frequently than every 4 weeks. A lower initial dose of 12.5 mg may be appropriate in some patients.

Note: Oral risperidone (or other antipsychotic) should be administered with the initial injection of Risperdal® Consta® and continued for 3 weeks (then discontinued) to maintain adequate therapeutic plasma concentrations prior to main release phase of risperidone from injection site. When switching from depot administration to a short-acting formulation, administer short-acting agent in place of the next regularly-scheduled depot injection.

Dosage Forms

Injection, microspheres for reconstitution, extended release:

Risperdal® Consta®: 12.5 mg, 25 mg, 37.5 mg, 50 mg

Solution, oral:

Risperdal®: 1 mg/mL

Tablet: 0.25 mg, 0.5 mg, 1 mg, 2 mg, 3 mg, 4 mg

Risperdal®: 0.25 mg, 0.5 mg, 1 mg, 2 mg, 3 mg, 4 mg

Tablet, orally disintegrating:

Risperdal® M-Tabs®: 0.5 mg, 1 mg, 2 mg, 3 mg, 4 mg

Ritalin® [US/Can] see methylphenidate on page 622

Ritalin® LA [US] see methylphenidate on page 622

Ritalin-SR® [US/Can] see methylphenidate on page 622

ritonavir (ri TOE na veer)

Sound-Alike/Look-Alike Issues

ritonavir may be confused with Retrovir®

Norvir® may be confused with Norvasc®

U.S./Canadian Brand Names Norvir® SEC [Can]; Norvir® [US/Can]

Therapeutic Category Antiviral Agent

Use Treatment of HIV infection; should always be used as part of a multidrug regimen (at least three antiretroviral agents); may be used as a pharmacokinetic "booster" for other protease inhibitors

Usual Dosage Oral: Treatment of HIV infection:

Children >1 month: 350-400 mg/m^2 twice daily (maximum dose: 600 mg twice daily). Initiate dose at 250 mg/m^2 twice daily; titrate dose upward every 2-3 days by 50 mg/m^2 twice daily.

Adults: 600 mg twice daily; dose escalation tends to avoid nausea that many patients experience upon initiation of full dosing. Escalate the dose as follows: 300 mg twice daily for 1 day, 400 mg twice daily for 2 days, 500 mg twice daily for 1 day, then 600 mg twice daily. Ritonavir may be better tolerated when used in combination with other antiretrovirals by initiating the drug alone and subsequently adding the second agent within 2 weeks.

Pharmacokinetic "booster" in combination with other protease inhibitors: 100-400 mg/day

Refer to individual monographs; specific dosage recommendations often require adjustment of both agents.

Note: Dosage adjustments for ritonavir when administered in combination therapy:

Amprenavir: Adjustments necessary for each agent:

Amprenavir 1200 mg with ritonavir 200 mg once daily **or**

Amprenavir 600 mg with ritonavir 100 mg twice daily

Amprenavir plus efavirenz (3-drug regimen): Amprenavir 1200 mg twice daily plus ritonavir 200 mg twice daily plus efavirenz at standard dose

Indinavir: Adjustments necessary for both agents:
   Indinavir 800 mg twice daily plus ritonavir 100-200 mg twice daily **or**
   Indinavir 400 mg twice daily plus ritonavir 400 mg twice daily
Nelfinavir: Ritonavir 400 mg twice daily
Rifabutin: Decrease rifabutin dose to 150 mg every other day
Saquinavir: Ritonavir 400 mg twice daily

Dosage Forms
Capsule, soft gelatin:
   Norvir®: 100 mg
Solution:
   Norvir®: 80 mg/mL

ritonavir and lopinavir *see lopinavir and ritonavir on page 574*
Rituxan® [US/Can] *see rituximab on page 839*

rituximab (ri TUK si mab)

Sound-Alike/Look-Alike Issues
   riTUXimab may be confused with inFLIXimab
   Rituxan® may be confused with Remicade®
Synonyms anti-CD20 monoclonal antibody; C2B8 monoclonal antibody; IDEC-C2B8; NSC-687451
Tall-Man riTUXimab
U.S./Canadian Brand Names Rituxan® [US/Can]
Therapeutic Category Antineoplastic Agent
Use Treatment of low-grade or follicular CD20-positive, B-cell non-Hodgkin lymphoma (NHL); treatment of diffuse large B-cell CD20-positive NHL; treatment of moderately- to severely-active rheumatoid arthritis (RA) in combination with methotrexate
Usual Dosage Note: Pretreatment with acetaminophen and an antihistamine is recommended.
   Adults: I.V. infusion (refer to individual protocols):
      NHL (relapsed/refractory, low-grade or follicular CD20-positive, B-cell): 375 mg/m^2 once weekly for 4 or 8 doses
         Retreatment following disease progression: 375 mg/m^2 once weekly for 4 doses
      NHL (diffuse large B-cell): 375 mg/m^2 given on day 1 of each chemotherapy cycle for up to 8 doses
      NHL (follicular, CD20-positive, B-cell, previously untreated): 375 mg/m^2 given on day 1 of each chemotherapy cycle for up to 8 doses
      NHL (nonprogressing, low-grade, CD20-positive, B-cell, after first line CVP): 375 mg/m^2 once weekly for 4 doses every 6 months for up to 4 cycles (initiate after 6-8 cycles of chemotherapy are completed)
      Rheumatoid arthritis: 1000 mg on days 1 and 15 in combination with methotrexate
      Note: Premedication with a corticosteroid (eg, methylprednisolone 100 mg I.V.) 30 minutes prior to each rituximab dose is recommended. In clinical trials, patients received oral corticosteroids on a tapering schedule from baseline through day 16.
      Combination therapy with ibritumomab: 250 mg/m^2 I.V. day 1; repeat in 7-9 days with ibritumomab (also see Ibritumomab monograph):
Dosage Forms
Injection, solution [preservative free]:
   Rituxan®: 10 mg/mL (10 mL, 50 mL)

Riva-Alendronate [Can] *see alendronate on page 43*
Riva-Atenolol [Can] *see atenolol on page 101*
Riva-Buspirone [Can] *see buspirone on page 153*
Riva-Ciprofloxacin [Can] *see ciprofloxacin on page 221*
Riva-Citalopram [Can] *see citalopram on page 225*
Riva-Clindamycin [Can] *see clindamycin on page 230*
Riva-Diclofenac [Can] *see diclofenac on page 292*
Riva-Diclofenac-K [Can] *see diclofenac on page 292*
Riva-Dicyclomine [Can] *see dicyclomine on page 293*
Riva-Enalapril [Can] *see enalapril on page 339*
Riva-Famotidine [Can] *see famotidine on page 390*
Riva-Fluconazole [Can] *see fluconazole on page 405*
Riva-Fluoxetine [Can] *see fluoxetine on page 413*

Riva-Fosinopril [Can] see fosinopril on page 427
Riva-Lisinopril [Can] see lisinopril on page 570
Riva-Loperamine [Can] see loperamide on page 573
Riva-Lorazepam [Can] see lorazepam on page 577
Riva-Lovastatin [Can] see lovastatin on page 579
Riva-Mirtazapine [Can] see mirtazapine on page 637
Riva-Naproxen [Can] see naproxen on page 656
Rivanase AQ [Can] see beclomethasone on page 119
Riva-Norfloxacin [Can] see norfloxacin on page 679
Riva-Oxazepam [Can] see oxazepam on page 706
Riva-Oxybutynin [Can] see oxybutynin on page 708
Riva-Pravastatin [Can] see pravastatin on page 779
Riva-Ranitidine [Can] see ranitidine on page 819
Riva-Risperidone [Can] see risperidone on page 837
Riva-Sertraline [Can] see sertraline on page 863
Riva-Simvastatin [Can] see simvastatin on page 867
Rivasol [Can] see zinc sulfate on page 994
Riva-Sotalol [Can] see sotalol on page 885

rivastigmine (ri va STIG meen)

Synonyms ENA 713; rivastigmine tartrate; SDZ ENA 713
U.S./Canadian Brand Names Exelon® [US/Can]
Therapeutic Category Acetylcholinesterase Inhibitor; Cholinergic Agent
Use Treatment of mild-to-moderate dementia associated with Alzheimer disease or Parkinson disease
Usual Dosage Adults:
Oral: **Note:** Exelon® oral solution and capsules are bioequivalent.
Mild-to-moderate Alzheimer dementia: Initial: 1.5 mg twice daily; may increase by 3 mg/day (1.5 mg/dose) every 2 weeks based on tolerability (maximum recommended dose: 6 mg twice daily)
Note: If GI adverse events occur, discontinue treatment for several doses then restart at the same or next lower dosage level; antiemetics have been used to control GI symptoms. If treatment is interrupted for longer than several days, restart the treatment at the lowest dose and titrate as previously described.
Mild-to-moderate Parkinson-related dementia: Initial: 1.5 mg twice daily; may increase by 3 mg/day (1.5 mg/dose) every 4 weeks based on tolerability (maximum recommended dose: 6 mg twice daily)
Transdermal patch: Mild-to-moderate Alzheimer- or Parkinson-related dementia:
Initial: 4.6 mg/24 hours; if well tolerated, may be increased (after at least 4 weeks) to 9.5 mg/24 hours (recommended effective dose)
Maintenance: 9.5 mg/24 hours (maximum dose: 9.5 mg/24 hours)
Note: If intolerance is noted (nausea, vomiting), patch should be removed and treatment interrupted for several days and restarted at the same or lower dosage. If interrupted for more than several days, reinitiate at lowest dosage and increase to maintenance dose after 4 weeks.
Conversion from oral therapy: If oral daily dose <6 mg, switch to 4.6 mg/24 hours patch; if oral daily dose 6-12 mg, switch to 9.5 mg/24 hours patch. Apply patch on the next day following last oral dose.
Dosage Forms
Capsule:
Exelon®: 1.5 mg, 3 mg, 4.5 mg, 6 mg
Solution, oral:
Exelon®: 2 mg/mL
Transdermal system [once-daily patch]:
Exelon®: 4.6 mg/24hours (30s); 9.5 mg/24hours (30s)

rivastigmine tartrate see rivastigmine on page 840
Riva-Sumatriptan [Can] see sumatriptan on page 898
Riva-Verapamil SR [Can] see verapamil on page 974
Riva-Zide [Can] see hydrochlorothiazide and triamterene on page 480
Riva-Zopiclone [Can] see zopiclone (Canada only) on page 997
Rivotril® [Can] see clonazepam on page 235

rizatriptan (rye za TRIP tan)

Synonyms MK462

U.S./Canadian Brand Names Maxalt RPD™ [Can]; Maxalt-MLT® [US]; Maxalt® [US/Can]

Therapeutic Category Antimigraine Agent; Serotonin Agonist

Use Acute treatment of migraine with or without aura

Usual Dosage Note: In patients with risk factors for coronary artery disease, following adequate evaluation to establish the absence of coronary artery disease, the initial dose should be administered in a setting where response may be evaluated (physician's office or similarly staffed setting). ECG monitoring may be considered.

Oral: 5-10 mg, repeat after 2 hours if significant relief is not attained; maximum: 30 mg in a 24-hour period (use 5 mg dose in patients receiving propranolol with a maximum of 15 mg in 24 hours)

Note: For orally-disintegrating tablets (Maxalt-MLT®): Patient should be instructed to place tablet on tongue and allow to dissolve. Dissolved tablet will be swallowed with saliva.

Dosage Forms

Tablet:
Maxalt®: 5 mg, 10 mg

Tablet, orally disintegrating:
Maxalt-MLT®: 5 mg, 10 mg

rLFN-α2 *see* interferon alfa-2b *on page 515*

R-modafinil *see* armodafinil *on page 94*

RMS® *(Discontinued)* *see* morphine sulfate *on page 643*

Ro 5488 *see* tretinoin (oral) *on page 946*

Robafen® AC [US] *see* guaifenesin and codeine *on page 454*

Robafen® CF *(Discontinued)*

Robafen DM [US-OTC] *see* guaifenesin and dextromethorphan *on page 454*

Robafen DM Clear [US-OTC] *see* guaifenesin and dextromethorphan *on page 454*

Robaxin® [US/Can] *see* methocarbamol *on page 615*

Robidrine® [Can] *see* pseudoephedrine *on page 801*

Robinul® [US] *see* glycopyrrolate *on page 449*

Robinul® Forte [US] *see* glycopyrrolate *on page 449*

Robitussin® [US-OTC/Can] *see* guaifenesin *on page 453*

Robitussin® A-C *(Discontinued)* *see* guaifenesin and codeine *on page 454*

Robitussin® Childrens Cough & Cold [Can] *see* pseudoephedrine and dextromethorphan *on page 802*

Robitussin® Cold and Cough CF [US-OTC] *see* guaifenesin, dextromethorphan, and phenylephrine *on page 459*

Robitussin® Cough and Allergy [US-OTC] *see* chlorpheniramine, phenylephrine, and dextromethorphan *on page 209*

Robitussin® Cough and Cold [US-OTC/Can] *see* guaifenesin, pseudoephedrine, and dextromethorphan *on page 460*

Robitussin® Cough and Cold CF [US-OTC] *see* guaifenesin, pseudoephedrine, and dextromethorphan *on page 460*

Robitussin® Cough and Cold Infant CF [US-OTC] *see* guaifenesin, pseudoephedrine, and dextromethorphan *on page 460*

Robitussin® Cough and Cold Nighttime [US-OTC] *see* chlorpheniramine, phenylephrine, and dextromethorphan *on page 209*

Robitussin® Cough and Congestion [US-OTC] *see* guaifenesin and dextromethorphan *on page 454*

Robitussin® CoughGels™ [US-OTC] *see* dextromethorphan *on page 284*

Robitussin®-DAC *(Discontinued)* *see* guaifenesin, pseudoephedrine, and codeine *on page 460*

Robitussin® DM [US-OTC/Can] *see* guaifenesin and dextromethorphan *on page 454*

Robitussin® DM Infant *(Discontinued)* *see* guaifenesin and dextromethorphan *on page 454*

Robitussin® Maximum Strength Cough [US-OTC] *see* dextromethorphan *on page 284*

Robitussin® Maximum Strength Cough & Cold *(Discontinued)* *see* pseudoephedrine and dextromethorphan *on page 802*

Robitussin® Pediatric Cold and Cough CF [US-OTC] *see* guaifenesin, dextromethorphan, and phenylephrine *on page 459*

Robitussin® Pediatric Cough [US-OTC] *see* dextromethorphan *on page 284*

Robitussin® Pediatric Cough and Cold Nighttime [US-OTC] *see* chlorpheniramine, phenylephrine, and dextromethorphan *on page 209*

Robitussin® Pediatric Cough & Cold *(Discontinued)* *see* pseudoephedrine and dextromethorphan *on page 802*

Robitussin® Pediatric Night Relief *(Discontinued)* *see* chlorpheniramine, pseudoephedrine, and dextromethorphan *on page 212*

Robitussin-PE® *(Discontinued)* *see* guaifenesin and pseudoephedrine *on page 458*

Robitussin® Severe Congestion *(Discontinued)* *see* guaifenesin and pseudoephedrine *on page 458*

Robitussin® Sugar Free Cough [US-OTC] *see* guaifenesin and dextromethorphan *on page 454*

Rocaltrol® [US/Can] *see* calcitriol *on page 160*

Rocephin® [US/Can] *see* ceftriaxone *on page 190*

rocuronium (roe kyoor OH nee um)

Sound-Alike/Look-Alike Issues
Zemuron® may be confused with Remeron®

Synonyms ORG 946; rocuronium bromide

U.S./Canadian Brand Names Zemuron® [US/Can]

Therapeutic Category Skeletal Muscle Relaxant

Use Adjunct to general anesthesia to facilitate both rapid sequence and routine endotracheal intubation and to relax skeletal muscles during surgery; to facilitate mechanical ventilation in ICU patients

Usual Dosage Administer I.V.; dose to effect; doses will vary due to interpatient variability; use ideal body weight for obese patients

Children ≥3 months:

Initial: 0.6 mg/kg under halothane anesthesia produce excellent to good intubating conditions within 1 minute and will provide a median time of 41 minutes of clinical relaxation in children 3 months to 1 year of age, and 27 minutes in children 1-12 years

Maintenance: 0.075-0.125 mg/kg administered upon return of T_1 to 25% of control provides clinical relaxation for 7-10 minutes

Adults:

Tracheal intubation: I.V.:

Initial: 0.6 mg/kg is expected to provide approximately 31 minutes of clinical relaxation under opioid/nitrous oxide/oxygen anesthesia with neuromuscular block sufficient for intubation attained in 1-2 minutes; lower doses (0.45 mg/kg) may be used to provide 22 minutes of clinical relaxation with median time to neuromuscular block of 1-3 minutes; maximum blockade is achieved in <4 minutes

Maximum: 0.9-1.2 mg/kg may be given during surgery under opioid/nitrous oxide/oxygen anesthesia without adverse cardiovascular effects and is expected to provide 58-67 minutes of clinical relaxation; neuromuscular blockade sufficient for intubation is achieved in <2 minutes with maximum blockade in <3 minutes

Maintenance: 0.1, 0.15, and 0.2 mg/kg administered at 25% recovery of control T_1 (defined as 3 twitches of train-of-four) provides a median of 12, 17, and 24 minutes of clinical duration under anesthesia

Rapid sequence intubation: 0.6-1.2 mg/kg in appropriately premedicated and anesthetized patients with excellent or good intubating conditions within 2 minutes

Continuous infusion: Initial: 0.01-0.012 mg/kg/minute only after early evidence of spontaneous recovery of neuromuscular function is evident; infusion rates have ranged from 4-16 mcg/kg/minute

ICU: 10 mcg/kg/minute; adjust dose to maintain appropriate degree of neuromuscular blockade (eg, 1 or 2 twitches on train-of-four)

Dosage Forms

Injection, solution:
Zemuron®: 10 mg/mL (5 mL, 10 mL)

rocuronium bromide *see* rocuronium *on page 842*

Rofact™ [Can] *see* rifampin *on page 833*

Roferon-A® [Can] *see* interferon alfa-2a *on page 514*

Roferon-A® *(Discontinued)* *see* interferon alfa-2a *on page 514*

Rogaine® [Can] *see* minoxidil *on page 636*
Rogaine® Extra Strength for Men [US-OTC] *see* minoxidil *on page 636*
Rogaine® for Men [US-OTC] *see* minoxidil *on page 636*
Rogaine® for Women [US-OTC] *see* minoxidil *on page 636*
Rogitine® [Can] *see* phentolamine *on page 745*
Rolaids® [US-OTC] *see* calcium carbonate and magnesium hydroxide *on page 164*
Rolaids® Extra Strength [US-OTC] *see* calcium carbonate and magnesium hydroxide *on page 164*
Rolaids® Softchews [US-OTC] *see* calcium carbonate *on page 163*
Rolatuss® Plain Liquid *(Discontinued)* *see* chlorpheniramine and phenylephrine *on page 206*
Romazicon® [US/Can] *see* flumazenil *on page 407*
Romilar® AC [US] *see* guaifenesin and codeine *on page 454*

romiplostim (roe mi PLOE stim)

Synonyms AMG 531
U.S./Canadian Brand Names Nplate™ [US]
Therapeutic Category Colony-Stimulating Factor; Thrombopoietic Agent
Use Treatment of thrombocytopenia in patients with chronic immune (idiopathic) thrombocytopenia purpura (ITP) who have had insufficient response to corticosteroids, immune globulin, or splenectomy
Usual Dosage Note: Initial dose is based on actual body weight. Discontinue if platelet count does not respond to a level that avoids clinically important bleeding after 4 weeks at the maximum recommended dose.
SubQ: Adults: ITP: Initial: 1 mcg/kg once weekly; adjust dose by 1 mcg/kg/week to achieve platelet count ≥50,000/mm^3 and to reduce the risk of bleeding; Maximum: 10 mcg/kg (median dose needed to achieve response in clinical trials: 2 mcg/kg)
Dosage Forms
Injection, powder for reconstitution:
Nplate™: 250 mcg, 500 mcg

Romycin® [US] *see* erythromycin *on page 354*
Rondec® [US] *see* chlorpheniramine and phenylephrine *on page 206*
Rondec®-DM [US] *see* chlorpheniramine, phenylephrine, and dextromethorphan *on page 209*
Rondec®-DM Drops *(Discontinued)*
Rondec®-DM Syrup *(Discontinued)* *see* brompheniramine, pseudoephedrine, and dextromethorphan *on page 146*
Rondec® Drops *(Discontinued)*
Rondec® Syrup *(Discontinued)* *see* brompheniramine and pseudoephedrine *on page 144*
Rondomycin® Capsule *(Discontinued)*

ropinirole (roe PIN i role)

Sound-Alike/Look-Alike Issues
ropinirole may be confused with ropivacaine
Requip® may be confused with Reglan®
Synonyms ropinirole hydrochloride
U.S./Canadian Brand Names Requip® XL™ [US]; Requip® [US/Can]
Therapeutic Category Anti-Parkinson Agent (Dopamine Agonist)
Use Treatment of idiopathic Parkinson disease; in patients with early Parkinson disease who were not receiving concomitant levodopa therapy as well as in patients with advanced disease on concomitant levodopa; treatment of moderate-to-severe primary restless legs syndrome (RLS)
Usual Dosage Oral: Adults:
Parkinson disease:
Immediate release tablet: The dosage should be increased to achieve a maximum therapeutic effect, balanced against the principal side effects of nausea, dizziness, somnolence and dyskinesia. Recommended starting dose is 0.25 mg 3 times/day; based on individual patient response, the dosage should be titrated with weekly increments as described below:
• Week 1: 0.25 mg 3 times/day; total daily dose: 0.75 mg
• Week 2: 0.5 mg 3 times/day; total daily dose: 1.5 mg
• Week 3: 0.75 mg 3 times/day; total daily dose: 2.25 mg
• Week 4: 1 mg 3 times/day; total daily dose: 3 mg

◄

Note: After week 4, if necessary, daily dosage may be increased by 1.5 mg/day on a weekly basis up to a dose of 9 mg/day, and then by up to 3 mg/day weekly to a total of 24 mg/day

Parkinson disease discontinuation taper: Ropinirole should be gradually tapered over 7 days as follows: reduce frequency of administration from 3 times daily to twice daily for 4 days, then reduce to once daily for remaining 3 days.

Extended release tablet: Initial: 2 mg once daily for 1-2 weeks, followed by increases of 2 mg/day at weekly or longer intervals based on therapeutic response and tolerability (maximum: 24 mg/day); Note: When discontinuing gradually taper over 7 days.

Restless legs syndrome: Immediate release tablets: Initial: 0.25 mg once daily 1-3 hours before bedtime. Dose may be increased after 2 days to 0.5 mg daily, and after 7 days to 1 mg daily. Dose may be further titrated upward in 0.5 mg increments every week until reaching a daily dose of 3 mg during week 6. If symptoms persist or reappear, the daily dose may be increased to a maximum of 4 mg beginning week 7.

Note: Doses up to 4 mg per day may be discontinued without tapering.

Converting from ropinirole immediate release tablets to ropinirole extended release tablets: Choose a once daily extended release dose that most closely matches current immediate release daily dose.

Dosage Forms
Tablet: 0.25 mg, 0.5 mg, 1 mg, 2 mg, 3 mg, 4 mg, 5 mg
Requip®: 0.25 mg, 0.5 mg, 1 mg, 2 mg, 3 mg, 4 mg, 5 mg
Tablet, extended-release:
Requip® XL™: 2 mg, 4 mg, 8 mg

ropinirole hydrochloride *see* ropinirole *on page 843*

ropivacaine (roe PIV a kane)

Sound-Alike/Look-Alike Issues
ropivacaine may be confused with bupivacaine, ropinirole
Synonyms ropivacaine hydrochloride
U.S./Canadian Brand Names Naropin® [US/Can]
Therapeutic Category Local Anesthetic
Use Local anesthetic for use in surgery, postoperative pain management, and obstetrical procedures when local or regional anesthesia is needed
Usual Dosage Dose varies with procedure, onset and depth of anesthesia desired, vascularity of tissues, duration of anesthesia, and condition of patient: Adults:

Surgical anesthesia:
Lumbar epidural: 15-30 mL of 0.5% to 1% solution
Lumbar epidural block for cesarean section:
20-30 mL dose of 0.5% solution
15-20 mL dose of 0.75% solution
Thoracic epidural block: 5-15 mL dose of 0.5% to 0.75% solution
Major nerve block:
35-50 mL dose of 0.5% solution (175-250 mg)
10-40 mL dose of 0.75% solution (75-300 mg)
Field block: 1-40 mL dose of 0.5% solution (5-200 mg)
Labor pain management: Lumbar epidural: Initial: 10-20 mL 0.2% solution; continuous infusion dose: 6-14 mL/hour of 0.2% solution with incremental injections of 10-15 mL/hour of 0.2% solution
Postoperative pain management:
Lumbar or thoracic epidural: Continuous infusion dose: 6-14 mL/hour of 0.2% solution
Infiltration/minor nerve block:
1-100 mL dose of 0.2% solution
1-40 mL dose of 0.5% solution
Dosage Forms
Infusion:
Naropin®: 2 mg/mL (100 mL, 200 mL)
Injection, solution [preservative free]:
Naropin®: 2 mg/mL (10 mL, 20 mL); 5 mg/mL (20 mL, 30 mL); 7.5 mg/mL (20 mL); 10 mg/mL (10 mL, 20 mL)

ropivacaine hydrochloride *see* ropivacaine *on page 844*
Rosac® [US] *see* sulfur and sulfacetamide *on page 897*

Rosanil® [US] *see* sulfur and sulfacetamide *on page 897*

rosiglitazone (roh si GLI ta zone)

Sound-Alike/Look-Alike Issues
Avandia® may be confused with Avalide®, Coumadin®, Prandin®

U.S./Canadian Brand Names Avandia® [US/Can]

Therapeutic Category Hypoglycemic Agent, Oral; Thiazolidinedione Derivative

Use Type 2 diabetes mellitus (noninsulin-dependent, NIDDM):
Monotherapy: Improve glycemic control as an adjunct to diet and exercise
Note: Canadian labeling approves use as monotherapy only when metformin is contraindicated or not tolerated.
Combination therapy: **Note:** Use when diet, exercise, and a single agent do not result in adequate glycemic control.
U.S. labeling: In combination with a sulfonylurea, metformin, or sulfonylurea plus metformin
Canadian labeling: In combination with metformin or with a sulfonylurea only when metformin use is contraindicated or not tolerated

Usual Dosage Oral:
Adults: **Note:** All patients should be initiated at the lowest recommended dose.
Monotherapy: Initial: 4 mg daily as a single daily dose or in divided doses twice daily. If response is inadequate after 8-12 weeks of treatment, the dosage may be increased to 8 mg daily as a single daily dose or in divided doses twice daily. In clinical trials, the 4 mg twice-daily regimen resulted in the greatest reduction in fasting plasma glucose and Hb A$_{1c}$.
Combination therapy: When adding rosiglitazone to existing therapy, continue current dose(s) of previous agents:
U.S. labeling: With sulfonylureas or metformin (or sulfonylurea plus metformin): Initial: 4 mg daily as a single daily dose or in divided doses twice daily. If response is inadequate after 8-12 weeks of treatment, the dosage may be increased to 8 mg daily as a single daily dose or in divided doses twice daily. Reduce dose of sulfonylurea if hypoglycemia occurs. It is unlikely that the dose of metformin will need to be reduced due to hypoglycemia.
Canadian labeling:
With metformin: Initial: 4 mg daily as a single daily dose or in divided doses twice daily. If response is inadequate after 8-12 weeks of treatment, the dosage may be increased to 8 mg daily as a single daily dose or in divided doses twice daily.
With a sulfonylurea: 4 mg daily as a single daily dose or in divided doses twice daily. Dose should not exceed 4 mg daily when using in combination with a sulfonylurea. Reduce dose of sulfonylurea if hypoglycemia occurs.

Dosage Forms
Tablet:
Avandia®: 2 mg, 4 mg, 8 mg

rosiglitazone and glimepiride (roh si GLI ta zone & GLYE me pye ride)

Synonyms glimepiride and rosiglitazone maleate

U.S./Canadian Brand Names Avandaryl™ [US]

Therapeutic Category Antidiabetic Agent, Sulfonylurea; Antidiabetic Agent, Thiazolidinedione

Use Management of type 2 diabetes mellitus (noninsulin-dependent, NIDDM) as an adjunct to diet and exercise

Usual Dosage Oral: Adults: Type 2 diabetes mellitus:
Initial: Rosiglitazone 4 mg and glimepiride 1 mg once daily **or** rosiglitazone 4 mg and glimepiride 2 mg once daily (for patients previously treated with sulfonylurea or thiazolidinedione monotherapy)
Patients switching from combination rosiglitazone and glimepiride as separate tablets: Use current dose
Maximum:
U.S. labeling: Rosiglitazone 8 mg and glimepiride 4 mg once daily
Canadian labeling: Rosiglitazone 4 mg and glimepiride 4 mg once daily
Titration:
Dose adjustment in patients previously on sulfonylurea monotherapy: May take 2 weeks to observe decreased blood glucose and 2-3 months to see full effects of rosiglitazone component. If not adequately controlled after 8-12 weeks, increase daily dose of rosiglitazone component.
Maximum:
U.S. labeling: Rosiglitazone 8 mg and glimepiride 4 mg once daily
Canadian labeling: Rosiglitazone 4 mg and glimepiride 4 mg once daily

◀ Titration:

Dose adjustment in patients previously on thiazolidinedione monotherapy: If not adequately controlled after 1-2 weeks, increase daily dose of glimepiride component in ≤2 mg increments in 1-2 week intervals.

Maximum:
U.S. labeling: Rosiglitazone 8 mg and glimepiride 4 mg once daily
Canadian labeling: Rosiglitazone 4 mg and glimepiride 4 mg once daily

Dosage Forms
Tablet:
Avandaryl™: 4 mg/1 mg: Rosiglitazone 4 mg and glimepiride 1 mg; 4 mg/2 mg: Rosiglitazone 4 mg and glimepiride 2 mg; 4 mg/4 mg: Rosiglitazone 4 mg and glimepiride 4 mg; 8 mg/2 mg: Rosiglitazone 8 mg and glimepiride 2 mg; 8 mg/4 mg: Rosiglitazone 8 mg and glimepiride 4 mg

rosiglitazone and metformin (roh si GLI ta zone & met FOR min)

Sound-Alike/Look-Alike Issues
Avandamet® may be confused with Anzemet®

Synonyms metformin and rosiglitazone; metformin hydrochloride and rosiglitazone maleate; rosiglitazone maleate and metformin hydrochloride

U.S./Canadian Brand Names Avandamet® [US/Can]

Therapeutic Category Antidiabetic Agent (Biguanide); Antidiabetic Agent (Thiazolidinedione)

Use Management of type 2 diabetes mellitus (noninsulin-dependent, NIDDM) as an adjunct to diet and exercise in patients where dual rosiglitazone and metformin therapy is appropriate

Usual Dosage Oral:
Adults: Type 2 diabetes mellitus: Daily dose should be divided and given with meals:
First-line therapy (drug-naive patients): Initial: Rosiglitazone 2 mg and metformin 500 mg once or twice daily; may increase by 2 mg/500 mg per day after 4 weeks to a maximum of 8 mg/2000 mg per day.
Second-line therapy:
Patients inadequately controlled on **metformin alone**: Initial dose: Rosiglitazone 4 mg/day plus current dose of metformin
Patients inadequately controlled on **rosiglitazone alone**: Initial dose: Metformin 1000 mg/day plus current dose of rosiglitazone
Note: When switching from combination rosiglitazone and metformin as separate tablets: Use current dose
Dose adjustment: Doses may be increased as increments of rosiglitazone 4 mg and/or metformin 500 mg, up to the maximum dose; doses should be titrated gradually.
After a change in the metformin dosage, titration can be done after 1-2 weeks
After a change in the rosiglitazone dosage, titration can be done after 8-12 weeks
Maximum dose: Rosiglitazone 8 mg/metformin 2000 mg daily

Dosage Forms
Tablet:
Avandamet®: 2/500: Rosiglitazone 2 mg and metformin 500 mg
Avandamet®: 4/500: Rosiglitazone 4 mg and metformin 500 mg
Avandamet®: 2/1000: Rosiglitazone 2 mg and metformin 1000 mg
Avandamet®: 4/1000: Rosiglitazone 4 mg and metformin 1000 mg

rosiglitazone maleate and metformin hydrochloride *see* rosiglitazone and metformin *on page 846*

Rosula® [US] *see* sulfur and sulfacetamide *on page 897*

Rosula® Clarifying [US] *see* sulfur and sulfacetamide *on page 897*

Rosula® NS [US] *see* sulfacetamide *on page 892*

rosuvastatin (roe soo va STAT in)

Synonyms rosuvastatin calcium

U.S./Canadian Brand Names Crestor® [US/Can]

Therapeutic Category Antilipemic Agent, HMG-CoA Reductase Inhibitor

Use Used with dietary therapy for hyperlipidemias to reduce elevations in total cholesterol (TC), LDL-C, apolipoprotein B, and triglycerides (TG) in patients with primary hypercholesterolemia (elevations of 1 or more components are present in Fredrickson type IIa, IIb, and IV hyperlipidemias); treatment of homozygous familial hypercholesterolemia (FH); to slow progression of atherosclerosis as an adjunct to diet to lower TC and LDL-C

Usual Dosage Oral: Adults:

Hyperlipidemia, mixed dyslipidemia, hypertriglyceridemia, slowing progression of atherosclerosis:

Initial dose:

General dosing: 10 mg once daily; 20 mg once daily may be used in patients with severe hyperlipidemia (LDL >190 mg/dL) and aggressive lipid targets

Conservative dosing: Patients requiring less aggressive treatment or predisposed to myopathy (including patients of Asian descent): 5 mg once daily

Titration: After 2 weeks, may be increased by 5-10 mg once daily; dosing range: 5-40 mg/day (maximum dose: 40 mg once daily)

Note: The 40 mg dose should be reserved for patients who have not achieved goal cholesterol levels on a dose of 20 mg/day, including patients switched from another HMG-CoA reductase inhibitor.

Homozygous familial hypercholesterolemia (FH): Initial: 20 mg once daily (maximum dose: 40 mg/day)

Dosage Forms

Tablet:

Crestor®: 5 mg, 10 mg, 20 mg, 40 mg

rosuvastatin calcium *see* rosuvastatin *on page 846*

Rotarix® [US] *see* rotavirus vaccine *on page 847*

RotaShield® *(Discontinued)*

RotaTeq® [US] *see* rotavirus vaccine *on page 847*

rotavirus vaccine (ROE ta vye rus vak SEEN)

Synonyms human rotavirus vaccine, attenuated (HRV); pentavalent human-bovine reassortant rotavirus vaccine (PRV); rotavirus vaccine, pentavalent; RV1 (RotaTeq®); RV5 (Rotarix®)

U.S./Canadian Brand Names Rotarix® [US]; RotaTeq® [US]

Therapeutic Category Vaccine

Use Prevention of rotavirus gastroenteritis in infants and children

The Advisory Committee on Immunization Practices (ACIP) recommends routine vaccination of all infants.

Usual Dosage Oral:

Infants 6-24 weeks of age: Rotarix®: A total of two 1mL doses, the first dose given at 6 weeks of age. The first and second dose should be separated by ≥4 weeks. The 2-dose series should be completed by 24 weeks of age.

Infants 6-32 weeks: RotaTeq®: A total of three 2 mL doses given at 2-, 4-, and 6 months of age; the first given at 6-12 weeks of age, followed by subsequent doses at 4- to 10-week intervals. Routine administration of the first dose at >12 weeks of age is not recommended (insufficient data). Administer all doses by 32 weeks of age. Infants who have had rotavirus gastroenteritis before getting the full course of vaccine should still initiate or complete the 3-dose schedule; initial infection provides only partial immunity.

Note: The ACIP Provisional Recommendations for vaccination recommend completing the vaccine series with the same product whenever possible. If continuing with same product will cause vaccination to be deferred, or if product used previously is unknown, vaccination should be completed with the product available. If RotaTeq® was used in any previous doses, or if the specific product used was unknown, a total of 3 doses should be given.

Dosage Forms

Powder, for suspension, oral [preservative free; human derived]:

Rotarix®: G1P[8] $\geq 10^6$ infectious units per 1 mL [oral applicator contains natural latex/natural rubber]

Suspension, oral [preservative free]:

RotaTeq®: G1 ≥ 2.2 10^6 infectious units, G2 ≥ 2.8 10^6 infectious units, G3 ≥ 2.2 10^6 infectious units, G4 ≥ 2 10^6 infectious units, and P1 [8] ≥ 2.3 10^6 infectious units per 2 mL (2 mL)

rotavirus vaccine, pentavalent *see* rotavirus vaccine *on page 847*

rotigotine (roe TIG oh teen)

Sound-Alike/Look-Alike Issues

Neupro® may be confused with Neupogen®

Synonyms N-0923

Therapeutic Category Anti-Parkinson Agent (Dopamine Agonist)

▶

◀ **Use** Treatment of the signs and symptoms of early-stage idiopathic Parkinson disease

Usual Dosage Topical: Transdermal: Adults: Initial: Apply 2 mg/24 hours patch once daily; may increase by 2 mg/24 hours weekly, based on clinical response and tolerability (maximum: 6 mg/24 hours)

Dosage reductions or discontinuation: Decrease by 2 mg/24 hours every other day

Note: In clinical trials, the lowest effective dose was 4 mg/24 hours and doses >6 mg/24 hours did not provide any additional therapeutic benefit and increased incidence of adverse effects

Rowasa® [US/Can] *see* mesalamine *on page 607*

Roxanol™ [US] *see* morphine sulfate *on page 643*

Roxanol SR™ Oral *(Discontinued)* *see* morphine sulfate *on page 643*

Roxanol™-T *(Discontinued)* *see* morphine sulfate *on page 643*

Roxicet™ [US] *see* oxycodone and acetaminophen *on page 710*

Roxicet™ 5/500 [US] *see* oxycodone and acetaminophen *on page 710*

Roxicodone® [US] *see* oxycodone *on page 709*

Roxiprin® *(Discontinued)* *see* oxycodone and aspirin *on page 711*

Roychlor® [Can] *see* potassium chloride *on page 771*

Rozerem™ [US] *see* ramelteon *on page 817*

RP-6976 *see* docetaxel *on page 313*

RP-54274 *see* riluzole *on page 835*

RP-59500 *see* quinupristin and dalfopristin *on page 814*

r-PA *see* reteplase *on page 827*

rPDGF-BB *see* becaplermin *on page 119*

(R,R)-formoterol L-tartrate *see* arformoterol *on page 92*

RS-25259 *see* palonosetron *on page 716*

RS-25259-197 *see* palonosetron *on page 716*

R-Tanna [US] *see* chlorpheniramine and phenylephrine *on page 206*

R-Tanna Pediatric [US] *see* chlorpheniramine and phenylephrine *on page 206*

RTCA *see* ribavirin *on page 831*

RU 0211 *see* lubiprostone *on page 581*

RU-486 *see* mifepristone *on page 634*

RU-23908 *see* nilutamide *on page 672*

RU-38486 *see* mifepristone *on page 634*

rubella, measles, and mumps vaccines, combined *see* measles, mumps, and rubella vaccines, combined *on page 593*

rubella, varicella, measles, and mumps vaccine *see* measles, mumps, rubella, and varicella virus vaccine *on page 593*

rubella virus vaccine (live) (rue BEL a VYE rus vak SEEN, live)

Sound-Alike/Look-Alike Issues

Meruvax® II may be confused with Attenuvax®

Synonyms German measles vaccine

U.S./Canadian Brand Names Meruvax® II [US]

Therapeutic Category Vaccine, Live Virus

Use Selective active immunization against rubella

Note: Trivalent measles - mumps - rubella (MMR) vaccine is the preferred immunizing agent for most children and many adults.

Usual Dosage SubQ: Children ≥12 months and Adults: 0.5 mL

Primary immunization is recommended at 12-15 months; revaccination with MMR-II at 4-6 years of age is recommended prior to elementary school. Previously unvaccinated children of susceptible pregnant women should be vaccinated.

Adults without documentation of immunity: Vaccination is recommended for students entering colleges and other institutions of higher education, for military personal, for healthcare workers, for international travelers who visit endemic areas, and to women of childbearing potential. Do not administer to women who may become pregnant within 4 weeks of receiving vaccine; administer following completion or termination of pregnancy

Dosage Forms
Injection, powder for reconstitution [preservative free]:
Meruvax® II: ≥1000 $TCID_{50}$ (Wistar RA 27/3 Strain)

rubeola vaccine *see* measles virus vaccine (live) *on page 594*
Rubex® *(Discontinued) see* doxorubicin *on page 322*
rubidomycin hydrochloride *see* daunorubicin hydrochloride *on page 269*
Rubramin-PC® *(Discontinued) see* cyanocobalamin *on page 254*
Rulox [US-OTC] *see* aluminum hydroxide and magnesium hydroxide *on page 54*
Rulox No. 1 *(Discontinued) see* aluminum hydroxide and magnesium hydroxide *on page 54*
Ru-Tuss DM [US] *see* guaifenesin, pseudoephedrine, and dextromethorphan *on page 460*
Rutuss Jr [US] *see* guaifenesin and pseudoephedrine *on page 458*
Ru-Tuss® Liquid *(Discontinued) see* chlorpheniramine and phenylephrine *on page 206*
Ru-Vert-M® *(Discontinued) see* meclizine *on page 595*
RV1 (RotaTeq®) *see* rotavirus vaccine *on page 847*
RV5 (Rotarix®) *see* rotavirus vaccine *on page 847*
Rylosol [Can] *see* sotalol *on page 885*
Rymed® *(Discontinued) see* guaifenesin and pseudoephedrine *on page 458*
Rymed-TR® *(Discontinued)*
Ryna-12™ [US] *see* phenylephrine and pyrilamine *on page 747*
Ryna-12 S™ [US] *see* phenylephrine and pyrilamine *on page 747*
Ryna-C® *(Discontinued) see* chlorpheniramine, pseudoephedrine, and codeine *on page 212*
Ryna® *(Discontinued) see* chlorpheniramine, pseudoephedrine, and codeine *on page 212*
Rynatan® [US] *see* chlorpheniramine and phenylephrine *on page 206*
Rynatan® Pediatric [US] *see* chlorpheniramine and phenylephrine *on page 206*
Rynatuss® [US] *see* chlorpheniramine, ephedrine, phenylephrine, and carbetapentane *on page 208*
Rynatuss® Pediatric *(Discontinued) see* chlorpheniramine, ephedrine, phenylephrine, and carbetapentane *on page 208*
Rynesa 12S™ [US] *see* phenylephrine and pyrilamine *on page 747*
Ry-T 12 [US] *see* phenylephrine and pyrilamine *on page 747*
Rythmodan® [Can] *see* disopyramide *on page 312*
Rythmodan®-LA [Can] *see* disopyramide *on page 312*
Rythmol® [US] *see* propafenone *on page 793*
Rythmol® Gen-Propafenone [Can] *see* propafenone *on page 793*
Rythmol® SR [US] *see* propafenone *on page 793*
Rēv-Eyes™ *(Discontinued)*
S2® [US-OTC] *see* epinephrine *on page 344*
S-(+)-3-isobutylgaba *see* pregabalin *on page 783*
6(S)-5-methyltetrahydrofolate *see* methylfolate *on page 621*
6(S)-5-MTHF *see* methylfolate *on page 621*
S-4661 *see* doripenem *on page 318*
Sab-Diclofenac [Can] *see* diclofenac *on page 292*
SAB-Dimenhydrinate [Can] *see* dimenhydrinate *on page 301*
SAB-Gentamicin [Can] *see* gentamicin *on page 442*
Sab-Naproxen [Can] *see* naproxen *on page 656*
Sab-Prenase [Can] *see* prednisolone (systemic) *on page 781*
Sabril® [Can] *see* vigabatrin *(Canada only) on page 977*
SAB-Trifluridine [Can] *see* trifluridine *on page 952*

Saccharomyces boulardii (sak roe MYE sees boo LAR dee)

Synonyms *S. boulardii*; *Saccharomyces boulardii lyo*
U.S./Canadian Brand Names Florastor® Kids [US-OTC]; Florastor® [US-OTC]
Therapeutic Category Dietary Supplement; Probiotic

◄ **Use** Promote maintenance of normal microflora in the gastrointestinal tract; used in management of bloating, gas, and diarrhea, particularly to decrease the incidence of diarrhea associated with antibiotic use

Usual Dosage Oral: Dietary supplement: Dosing varies by manufacturer; consult product labeling.
Children (Florastor® Kids): 250 mg twice daily
Adults (Florastor®): 250 mg twice daily

Dosage Forms
Capsule, oral:
Florastor®: *S. boulardii lyo* 250 mg
Powder, oral:
Florastor® Kids: *S. boulardii lyo* 250 mg/packet (10s)

Saccharomyces boulardii lyo see Saccharomyces boulardii on page 849

sacrosidase (sak ROE si dase)
U.S./Canadian Brand Names Sucraid® [US/Can]
Therapeutic Category Enzyme
Use Orphan drug: Oral replacement therapy in sucrase deficiency, as seen in congenital sucrase-isomaltase deficiency (CSID)
Usual Dosage Oral:
Infants ≥5 months and Children <15 kg: 8500 int. units (1 mL) per meal or snack
Children >15 kg and Adults: 17,000 int. units (2 mL) per meal or snack
Doses should be diluted with 2-4 oz of water, milk, or formula with each meal or snack. Approximately one-half of the dose may be taken before, and the remainder of a dose taken at the completion of each meal or snack.
Dosage Forms
Solution, oral:
Sucraid®: 8500 int. units per mL

Safe Tussin® DM [US-OTC] see guaifenesin and dextromethorphan on page 454
SAHA see vorinostat on page 985
Saizen® [US/Can] see somatropin on page 881
SalAc® [US-OTC] see salicylic acid on page 850
Sal-Acid® [US-OTC] see salicylic acid on page 850
Salacid® Ointment (Discontinued) see salicylic acid on page 850
Salactic® [US-OTC] see salicylic acid on page 850
Salagen® [US/Can] see pilocarpine on page 753
Salazopyrin® [Can] see sulfasalazine on page 896
Salazopyrin En-Tabs® [Can] see sulfasalazine on page 896
Salbu-2 [Can] see albuterol on page 39
Salbu-4 [Can] see albuterol on page 39
salbutamol see albuterol on page 39
salbutamol and ipratropium see ipratropium and albuterol on page 525
salbutamol sulphate see albuterol on page 39
Saleto-200® (Discontinued) see ibuprofen on page 495
Saleto-400® (Discontinued) see ibuprofen on page 495
Salex® [US] see salicylic acid on page 850
Salflex® [Can] see salsalate on page 854
Salgesic® (Discontinued) see salsalate on page 854
salicylazosulfapyridine see sulfasalazine on page 896

salicylic acid (sal i SIL ik AS id)
Sound-Alike/Look-Alike Issues
Occlusal®-HP may be confused with Ocuflox®
U.S./Canadian Brand Names Akurza [US]; Beta Sal® [US-OTC]; Compound W® One-Step Wart Remover for Feet [US-OTC]; Compound W® One-Step Wart Remover for Kids [US-OTC]; Compound W® One-Step Wart Remover [US-OTC]; Compound W® [US-OTC]; Dermarest® Psoriasis Medicated Moisturizer [US-OTC]; Dermarest® Psoriasis Medicated Scalp Treatment [US-OTC]; Dermarest®

Psoriasis Medicated Shampoo/Conditioner [US-OTC]; Dermarest® Psoriasis Medicated Skin Treatment [US-OTC]; Dermarest® Psoriasis Overnight Treatment [US-OTC]; DHS™ Sal [US-OTC]; DuoFilm® [Can]; Duoforte® 27 [Can]; Freezone® [US-OTC]; Fung-O® [US-OTC]; Gordofilm® [US-OTC]; Hydrisalic™ [US-OTC]; Ionil Plus® [US-OTC]; Ionil® [US-OTC]; Keralyt® [US-OTC]; LupiCare® Dandruff [US-OTC]; LupiCare® Psoriasis [US-OTC]; Mosco® Callus & Corn Remover [US-OTC]; Neutrogena® Advanced Solutions™ [US-OTC]; Neutrogena® Blackhead Eliminating™ 2-in-1 Foaming Pads [US-OTC]; Neutrogena® Blackhead Eliminating™ Daily Scrub [US-OTC]; Neutrogena® Body Clear® [US-OTC]; Neutrogena® Clear Pore™ Oil-Controlling Astringent [US-OTC]; Neutrogena® Oil-Free Acne Wash 60 Second Mask Scrub [US-OTC]; Neutrogena® Oil-Free Acne Wash Cream Cleanser [US-OTC]; Neutrogena® Oil-Free Acne Wash Foam Cleanser [US-OTC]; Neutrogena® Oil-Free Acne Wash [US-OTC]; Neutrogena® Rapid Clear® Acne Defense [US-OTC]; Neutrogena® Rapid Clear® Acne Eliminating [US-OTC]; Occlusal®-HP [US-OTC/Can]; P&S® [US-OTC]; Palmer's® Skin Success Acne Cleanser [US-OTC]; Sal-Acid® [US-OTC]; Sal-Plant® [US-OTC]; Salactic® [US-OTC]; SalAc® [US-OTC]; Salex® [US]; Salitop™ [US]; Sebcur® [Can]; Soluver® Plus [Can]; Soluver® [Can]; Stridex® Essential Care® [US-OTC]; Stridex® Facewipes To Go® [US-OTC]; Stridex® Maximum Strength [US-OTC]; Stridex® Sensitive Skin [US-OTC]; Tinamed® Corn and Callus Remover [US-OTC]; Tinamed® Wart Remover [US-OTC]; Trans-Plantar® [Can]; Trans-Ver-Sal® [US-OTC/Can]; Wart-Off® Maximum Strength [US-OTC]

Therapeutic Category Keratolytic Agent

Use Topically for its keratolytic effect in controlling seborrheic dermatitis or psoriasis of body and scalp, dandruff, and other scaling dermatoses; also used to remove warts, corns, and calluses; acne

Usual Dosage Children and Adults (consult specific product labeling for use in children <12 years):
Acne:
Cream, cloth, foam, or liquid cleansers (2%): Use to cleanse skin once or twice daily. Massage gently into skin, work into lather and rinse thoroughly. Cloths should be wet with water prior to using and disposed of (not flushed) after use.
Gel (0.5% or 2%): Apply small amount to face in the morning or evening; if peeling occurs, may be used every other day. Some products may be labeled for OTC use up to 3 or 4 times per day. Apply to clean, dry skin
Pads (0.5% or 2%): Use pad to cover affected area with thin layer of salicylic acid one to three times a day. Apply to clean, dry skin. Do not leave pad on skin.
Patch (2%): At bedtime, after washing face, allow skin to dry at least 5 minutes. Apply patch directly over pimple being treated. Remove in the morning.
Shower/bath gels or soap (2%): Use once daily in shower or bath to massage over skin prone to acne. Rinse well.
Callus, corns, or warts:
Gel or liquid (17%): Apply to each wart and allow to dry. May repeat once or twice daily, up to 12 weeks. Apply to clean dry area.
Gel (6%): Apply to affected area once daily, generally used at night and rinsed off in the morning.
Plaster or transdermal patch (40%): Apply directly over affected area, leave in place for 48 hours. Some products may be cut to fit area or secured with adhesive strips. May repeat procedure for up to 12 weeks. Apply to clean, dry skin
Transdermal patch (15%): Apply directly over affected area at bedtime, leave in place overnight and remove in the morning. Patch should be trimmed to cover affected area. May repeat daily for up to 12 weeks.
Dandruff, psoriasis, or seborrheic dermatitis:
Cream (2.5%): Apply to affected area 3-4 times daily. Apply to clean, dry skin. Some products may be left in place overnight.
Ointment (3%): Apply to scales or plaques on skin up to 4 times per day (not for scalp or face)
Shampoo (1.8% to 3%): Massage into wet hair or affected area; leave in place for several minutes; rinse thoroughly. Labeled for OTC use 2-3 times a week, or as directed by healthcare provider. Some products may be left in place overnight.

Dosage Forms
Bar, topical [soap]: 2%
Cloth, topical:
Neutrogena® Oil-Free Acne Wash [OTC]: 2% (30s)
Cream, topical: 6% (400 g)
Akurza: 6% (340 g)
LupiCare™ Psoriasis [OTC]: 2% (227 g)
Neutrogena® Oil-Free Acne Wash Cream Cleanser [OTC]: 2% (200 mL)
Salex®: 6% (454 g)
Salitop™: 6% (400 g)

Gel, topical:
Compound W® [OTC]: 17.6% (7 g)
Dermarest® Psoriasis Medicated Scalp Treatment [OTC], Dermarest® Psoriasis Medicated Skin Treatment [OTC]: 3% (118 mL)
Dermarest® Psoriasis Overnight Treatment [OTC]: 3% (56.7 g)
Hydrisalic® [OTC]: 6% (28 g)
Keralyt® [OTC]: 3% (30 g); 6% (40 g)
Neutrogena® Oil-Free Acne Wash [OTC]: 2% (177 mL)
Neutrogena® Rapid Clear® Acne Eliminating [OTC]: 2% (15 mL)
Sal-Plant® [OTC]: 17% (14 g)
Gel, topical [peel]:
Neutrogena® Advanced Solutions™ [OTC]: 2% (40 g)
Liquid, topical: 17% (14.8 mL)
Compound W® [OTC], Mosco® Callus & Corn Remover [OTC]: 17.6% (9 mL)
Freezone® [OTC]: 17.6% (9.3 mL)
Fung-O® [OTC], Salactic® [OTC], Tinamed® Corn and Callus Remover [OTC], Tinamed® Wart Remover [OTC]: 17% (15 mL)
Gordofilm [OTC]: 16.7% (15 mL)
Neutrogena® Blackhead Eliminating™ Daily Scrub [OTC]: 2% (125 mL)
Neutrogena® Clear Pore™ Oil-Controlling Astringent [OTC]: 2% (236 mL)
Occlusal®-HP [OTC]: 17% (10 mL)
Palmer's® Skin Success Acne Cleanser [OTC]: 0.5% (240 mL)
Wart-Off® Maximum Strength [OTC]: 17% (13 mL)
Liquid, topical [body scrub with microbeads]:
Neutrogena® Body Clear® [OTC]: 2% (250 mL)
Liquid, topical [body wash]:
Neutrogena® Body Clear® [OTC]: 2% (250 mL)
Liquid, topical [cleanser]:
SalAc® [OTC]: 2% (177 mL)
Liquid, topical [foam]:
Neutrogena® Oil-Free Acne Wash Foam Cleanser [OTC]: 2% (150 mL)
Liquid, topical [mask/wash]:
Neutrogena® Oil-Free Acne Wash 60 Second Mask Scrub [OTC]: 1% (170 g)
Lotion, topical: 6% (414 mL, 420 mL)
Akurza: 6% (355 mL)
Dermarest® Psoriasis Medicated Moisturizer [OTC]: 2% (118 mL)
Neutrogena® Rapid Clear® Acne Defense [OTC]: 2% (50 mL)
Salex®: 6% (237 mL)
Salitop™: 6% (414 mL)
Pad, topical:
Neutrogena® Blackhead Eliminating™ 2-in-1 Foaming Pads [OTC]: 0.5% (28s)
Stridex® Essential Care® [OTC]: 1% (55s)
Stridex® Facewipes To Go™ [OTC]: 0.5% (32s)
Stridex® Maximum Strength [OTC]: 2% (55s, 90s)
Stridex® Sensitive Skin [OTC]: 0.5% (55s, 90s)
Patch, topical:
Compound W® One-Step Wart Remover for Feet [OTC]: 40% (20s)
Compound W® One-Step Wart Remover [OTC]: 40% (14s)
Compound W® One-Step Wart Remover for Kids [OTC]: 40% (12s)
Trans-Ver-Sal® [OTC]: 15% (10s, 25s)
Trans-Ver-Sal® [OTC]: 15% (15s, 40s)
Trans-Ver-Sal® [OTC]: 15% (12s, 40s)
Plaster, topical:
Sal-Acid® [OTC]: 40% (14s)
Shampoo, topical: 6% (177 mL)
Aliclen™, Salex®: 6% (177 mL)
Beta Sal® [OTC]: 3% (480 mL)
DHS™ Sal [OTC]: 3% (120 mL)
Ionil Plus® [OTC]: 2% (240 mL)
Ionil® [OTC]: 2% (120 mL)
LupiCare® Dandruff [OTC], LupiCare® Psoriasis [OTC]: 2% (237 mL)
P&S® [OTC]: 2% (118 mL, 236 mL)

Shampoo/conditioner, topical:
Dermarest® Psoriasis Medicated Shampoo/Conditioner [OTC]: 3% (236 mL)

salicylic acid and coal tar *see* coal tar and salicylic acid *on page 241*
salicylsalicylic acid *see* salsalate *on page 854*
Saline Mist [US-OTC] *see* sodium chloride *on page 873*
SalineX® (Discontinued) *see* sodium chloride *on page 873*
Salitop™ [US] *see* salicylic acid *on page 850*
Salivart® [US-OTC] *see* saliva substitute *on page 853*

saliva substitute (sa LYE va SUB stee tute)

Synonyms artificial saliva
U.S./Canadian Brand Names Aquoral™ [US]; Caphosol® [US]; Entertainer's Secret® [US-OTC]; Moi-Stir® [US-OTC]; Mouthkote® [US-OTC]; Numoisyn™ [US]; Oasis® [US]; oral Balance® [US-OTC]; Saliva Substitute® [US-OTC]; Salivart® [US-OTC]; SalivaSure™ [US-OTC]
Therapeutic Category Gastrointestinal Agent, Miscellaneous
Use Relief of dry mouth and throat in xerostomia or hyposalivation; adjunct to standard oral care in relief of symptoms associated with chemotherapy or radiation therapy-induced mucositis
Usual Dosage Adults: Use as needed or product-specific dosing:
Caphosol®:
 Mucositis symptoms: Swish and spit 4-10 doses per day (begin at onset of chemo- or radiation therapy)
 Xerostomia: Swish and spit 2-10 doses per day
Numoisyn™ liquid: Use 2 mL as needed
Numoisyn™ lozenges: Dissolve 1 slowly; maximum 16 lozenges/day
Oasis® mouthwash: Rinse mouth with ~30 mL twice daily or as needed; do not swallow
Oasis® spray: 1-2 sprays as needed; maximum 60 sprays/day
oral Balance®: Use after meals, at bedtime and as needed
Dosage Forms
Liquid:
 Numoisyn™: Water, sorbitol, linseed extract, *Chondrus crispus*, methylparaben, sodium benzoate, potassium sorbate, dipotassium phosphate, propylparaben
 Oral Balance® [OTC]: Water, starch, sunflower oil, propylene glycol, xylitol, glycerine, purified milk extract
Lozenge:
 Numoisyn™: Sorbitol 0.3 g/lozenge, polyethylene glycol, malic acid, sodium citrate, calcium phosphate dibasic, hydrogenated cottonseed oil, citric acid, magnesium stearate, silicon dioxide
 SalivaSure™: Xylitol, citric acid, apple acid, sodium citrate dihydrate, sodium carboxymethylcellulose, dibasic calcium phosphate, silica colloidal, magnesium stearate, stearic acid
Solution, oral:
 Caphosol: Dibasic sodium phosphate 0.032%, monobasic sodium phosphate 0.009%, calcium chloride 0.052%, sodium chloride 0.569%, purified water
 Entertainer's Secret®: Sodium carboxymethylcellulose, aloe vera gel, glycerin (60 mL)
Solution, oral [mouthwash/gargle]:
 Oasis®: Water, glycerin, sorbitol, poloxamer 338, PEG-60, hydrogenated castor oil, copovidone, sodium benzoate, carboxymethycellulose
Solution, oral [preservative free; spray]:
 Salivart® [OTC]: Water, sodium carboxymethylcellulose, sorbitol, sodium chloride, potassium chloride, calcium chloride, magnesium chloride, potassium phosphate
Solution, oral [spray]:
 Aquoral™: Oxidized glycerol triesters and silicon dioxide
 Moi-Stir® [OTC]: Water, sorbitol, sodium carboxymethylcellulose, methylparaben, propylparaben, potassium chloride, dibasic sodium phosphate, calcium chloride, magnesium chloride, sodium chloride
 Mouthkote® [OTC]: Water, xylitol, sorbitol, yerba santa, citric acid, ascorbic acid, sodium saccharin, sodium benzoate
 Oasis®: Glycerin, cetylpyridinium, copovidone

Saliva Substitute® [US-OTC] *see* saliva substitute *on page 853*
SalivaSure™ [US-OTC] *see* saliva substitute *on page 853*
salk vaccine *see* poliovirus vaccine (inactivated) *on page 764*

salmeterol (sal ME te role)

Sound-Alike/Look-Alike Issues
 salmeterol may be confused with salbutamol
 Serevent® may be confused with Serentil®
Synonyms salmeterol xinafoate
U.S./Canadian Brand Names Serevent® Diskhaler® Disk [Can]; Serevent® Diskus® [US/Can]
Therapeutic Category Adrenergic Agonist Agent
Use Maintenance treatment of asthma; prevention of bronchospasm with reversible obstructive airway disease, including patients with symptoms of nocturnal asthma; prevention of exercise-induced bronchospasm; maintenance treatment of bronchospasm associated with COPD
Usual Dosage Inhalation, powder (50 mcg/inhalation):
 Asthma, maintenance and prevention: Children ≥4 years and Adults: One inhalation twice daily (~12 hours apart); maximum: 1 inhalation twice daily
 Exercise-induced asthma, prevention: Children ≥4 years and Adults: One inhalation at least 30 minutes prior to exercise; additional doses should not be used for 12 hours; should not be used in individuals already receiving salmeterol twice daily
 COPD maintenance: Adults: One inhalation twice daily (~12 hours apart); maximum: 1 inhalation twice daily
Dosage Forms [CAN] = Canadian brand name
 Powder for oral inhalation:
 Serevent® Diskus®: 50 mcg (28s, 60s)
 Serevent® Diskhaler® Disk [CAN]: 50 mcg (60s)

salmeterol and fluticasone see fluticasone and salmeterol on page 417
salmeterol xinafoate see salmeterol on page 854

Salmonella typhi Vi capsular polysaccharide vaccine (Canada only)
(sal mo NEL la TI fi vi CAP su lar po le SAK ar ide VAK seen)
U.S./Canadian Brand Names Typherix™ [Can]
Therapeutic Category Vaccine
Use For active immunization against typhoid fever in persons 2 years of age and older.
Usual Dosage One dose administered I.M. ensures protection for at least 3 years. The vaccine must be given at least 2 weeks prior to travel to endemic areas.
Dosage Forms Injection: Vi polysaccharide vaccine of S. typhi 25 mcg (0.5 mL)

Salmonine® (Discontinued) see calcitonin on page 160
Salofalk® [Can] see mesalamine on page 607
Sal-Plant® [US-OTC] see salicylic acid on page 850

salsalate (SAL sa late)

Sound-Alike/Look-Alike Issues
 salsalate may be confused with sucralfate, sulfasalazine
Synonyms disalicylic acid; salicylsalicylic acid
U.S./Canadian Brand Names Amigesic® [Can]; Salflex® [Can]
Therapeutic Category Analgesic, Nonnarcotic; Antipyretic; Nonsteroidal Antiinflammatory Drug (NSAID)
Use Treatment of minor pain or fever; arthritis
Usual Dosage Oral: Adults: 3 g/day in 2-3 divided doses
Dosage Forms
 Tablet: 500 mg, 750 mg

Salsitab® (Discontinued) see salsalate on page 854
salt see sodium chloride on page 873
salt-poor albumin see albumin on page 38
Sal-Tropine™ [US] see atropine on page 104
Sanctura® [US] see trospium on page 958
Sanctura® XR [US] see trospium on page 958
Sandimmune® [US] see cyclosporine on page 257
Sandimmune® I.V. [Can] see cyclosporine on page 257

Sandomigran® [Can] see pizotifen *(Canada only) on page 758*
Sandomigran DS® [Can] see pizotifen *(Canada only) on page 758*
Sandostatin® [US/Can] see octreotide *on page 691*
Sandostatin LAR® [US/Can] see octreotide *on page 691*
Sandoz-Acebutolol [Can] see acebutolol *on page 19*
Sandoz Alendronate [Can] see alendronate *on page 43*
Sandoz-Amiodarone [Can] see amiodarone *on page 61*
Sandoz-Anagrelide [Can] see anagrelide *on page 75*
Sandoz-Atenolol [Can] see atenolol *on page 101*
Sandoz-Azithromycin [Can] see azithromycin *on page 110*
Sandoz-Betaxolol [Can] see betaxolol *on page 133*
Sandoz-Bicalutamide [Can] see bicalutamide *on page 135*
Sandoz-Bisoprolol [Can] see bisoprolol *on page 138*
Sandoz-Brimonidine [Can] see brimonidine *on page 142*
Sandoz-Carbamazepine [Can] see carbamazepine *on page 172*
Sandoz-Cefprozil [Can] see cefprozil *on page 188*
Sandoz-Ciprofloxacin [Can] see ciprofloxacin *on page 221*
Sandoz-Citalopram [Can] see citalopram *on page 225*
Sandoz-Clonazepam [Can] see clonazepam *on page 235*
Sandoz-Cyclosporine [Can] see cyclosporine *on page 257*
Sandoz-Diclofenac [Can] see diclofenac *on page 292*
Sandoz-Diltiazem CD [Can] see diltiazem *on page 300*
Sandoz-Diltiazem T [Can] see diltiazem *on page 300*
Sandoz-Enalapril [Can] see enalapril *on page 339*
Sandoz-Estradiol Derm 50 [Can] see estradiol *on page 359*
Sandoz-Estradiol Derm 75 [Can] see estradiol *on page 359*
Sandoz-Estradiol Derm 100 [Can] see estradiol *on page 359*
Sandoz-Famciclovir [Can] see famciclovir *on page 389*
Sandoz Fenofibrate S [Can] see fenofibrate *on page 393*
Sandoz-Fluoxetine [Can] see fluoxetine *on page 413*
Sandoz-Fluvoxamine [Can] see fluvoxamine *on page 420*
Sandoz-Gliclazide [Can] see gliclazide *(Canada only) on page 444*
Sandoz-Glimepiride [Can] see glimepiride *on page 445*
Sandoz-Glyburide [Can] see glyburide *on page 448*
Sandoz-Levobunolol [Can] see levobunolol *on page 555*
Sandoz Lisinopril/Hctz [Can] see lisinopril and hydrochlorothiazide *on page 571*
Sandoz-Loperamide [Can] see loperamide *on page 573*
Sandoz-Lovastatin [Can] see lovastatin *on page 579*
Sandoz-Metformin FC [Can] see metformin *on page 610*
Sandoz-Metoprolol [Can] see metoprolol *on page 626*
Sandoz-Minocycline [Can] see minocycline *on page 635*
Sandoz-Mirtazapine [Can] see mirtazapine *on page 637*
Sandoz-Mirtazapine FC [Can] see mirtazapine *on page 637*
Sandoz-Nabumetone [Can] see nabumetone *on page 650*
Sandoz-Nitrazepam [Can] see nitrazepam *(Canada only) on page 674*
Sandoz Omeprazole [Can] see omeprazole *on page 697*
Sandoz-Ondansetron [Can] see ondansetron *on page 698*
Sandoz-Paroxetine [Can] see paroxetine *on page 724*
Sandoz-Pioglitazone [Can] see pioglitazone *on page 754*
Sandoz-Pravastatin [Can] see pravastatin *on page 779*
Sandoz-Ramipril [Can] see ramipril *on page 817*
Sandoz-Ranitidine [Can] see ranitidine *on page 819*
Sandoz Risperidone [Can] see risperidone *on page 837*

Sandoz-Sertraline [Can] *see* sertraline *on page 863*
Sandoz-Simvastatin [Can] *see* simvastatin *on page 867*
Sandoz-Sumatriptan [Can] *see* sumatriptan *on page 898*
Sandoz-Tamsulosin [Can] *see* tamsulosin *on page 903*
Sandoz-Ticlopidine [Can] *see* ticlopidine *on page 926*
Sandoz-Timolol [Can] *see* timolol *on page 927*
Sandoz-Tobramycin [Can] *see* tobramycin *on page 931*
Sandoz-Topiramate [Can] *see* topiramate *on page 935*
Sandoz-Trifluridine [Can] *see* trifluridine *on page 952*
Sandoz-Valporic [Can] *see* valproic acid and derivatives *on page 967*
Sandoz-Zopiclone [Can] *see* zopiclone *(Canada only) on page 997*
SangCya™ *(Discontinued) see* cyclosporine *on page 257*
Sani-Supp® [US-OTC] *see* glycerin *on page 449*
Sans Acne® [Can] *see* erythromycin *on page 354*
Santyl® [US] *see* collagenase *on page 245*

sapropterin (sap roe TER in)
Sound-Alike/Look-Alike Issues
  sapropterin may be confused with cyproterone
Synonyms 6R-BH4; phenoptin; sapropterin dihydrochloride
U.S./Canadian Brand Names Kuvan™ [US]
Therapeutic Category Enzyme Cofactor
Use Adjunct to dietary management in the treatment of tetrahydrobiopterin (BH4) responsive phenylketonuria (PKU)
Usual Dosage Oral: Children ≥4 years and Adults: PKU: Initial: 10 mg/kg once daily; adjust after 1 month based on blood phenylalanine levels (if phenylalanine levels do not decrease from baseline, increase dose to 20 mg/kg once daily); discontinue if phenylalanine levels do not decrease after 1 month of treatment at 20 mg/kg/day (nonresponder). Maintenance range: 5-20 mg/kg once daily
Dosage Forms
  Tablet:
  Kuvan™: 100 mg

sapropterin dihydrochloride *see* sapropterin *on page 856*

saquinavir (sa KWIN a veer)
Sound-Alike/Look-Alike Issues
  saquinavir may be confused with Sinequan®
Synonyms saquinavir mesylate
U.S./Canadian Brand Names Invirase® [US/Can]
Therapeutic Category Antiviral Agent
Use Treatment of HIV infection; used in combination with at least two other antiretroviral agents
Usual Dosage Oral:
  Children >16 years and Adults (Invirase®): 1000 mg (five 200 mg capsules or two 500 mg tablets) twice daily given in combination with ritonavir 100 mg twice daily. This combination should be given together and within 2 hours after a full meal in combination with a nucleoside analog. **Note:** Saquinavir (Invirase®) should not be used in "unboosted regimens."
  Dosage adjustments when administered in combination therapy: Lopinavir and ritonavir (Kaletra™): Invirase® 1000 mg twice daily
Dosage Forms
  Capsule:
  Invirase®: 200 mg
  Tablet:
  Invirase®: 500 mg

saquinavir mesylate *see* saquinavir *on page 856*

Sarafem® [US] *see* fluoxetine *on page 413*

sargramostim (sar GRAM oh stim)

Sound-Alike/Look-Alike Issues
Leukine® may be confused with Leukeran®, leucovorin

Synonyms GM-CSF; granulocyte-macrophage colony-stimulating factor; NSC-613795; rGM-CSF

U.S./Canadian Brand Names Leukine® [US/Can]

Therapeutic Category Colony-Stimulating Factor

Use

Acute myelogenous leukemia (AML) following induction chemotherapy in older adults (≥55 years of age) to shorten time to neutrophil recovery and to reduce the incidence of severe and life-threatening infections and infections resulting in death

Bone marrow transplant (allogeneic or autologous) failure or engraftment delay

Myeloid reconstitution after allogeneic bone marrow transplantation

Myeloid reconstitution after autologous bone marrow transplantation: Non-Hodgkin lymphoma (NHL), acute lymphoblastic leukemia (ALL), Hodgkin lymphoma

Peripheral stem cell transplantation: Mobilization and myeloid reconstitution following autologous peripheral stem cell transplantation

Usual Dosage Adults: I.V. infusion over ≥2 hours or SubQ: **Rounding the dose to the nearest vial size enhances patient convenience and reduces costs without clinical detriment**

Myeloid reconstitution after allogeneic or autologous bone marrow transplant: I.V.: 250 mcg/m^2/day (over 2 hours), begin 2-4 hours after the marrow infusion and ≥24 hours after chemotherapy or radiotherapy, when the post marrow infusion ANC is <500 cells/mm^3, and continue until ANC >1500 cells/mm^3 for 3 consecutive days

If a severe adverse reaction occurs, reduce dose by 50% or temporarily discontinue the dose until the reaction abates

If blast cells appear or progression of the underlying disease occurs, discontinue treatment

If ANC >20,000 cells/mm^3, interrupt treatment or reduce the dose by 50%

Neutrophil recovery following chemotherapy in AML: I.V.: 250 mcg/m^2/day (over 4 hours) starting approximately on day 11 or 4 days following the completion of induction chemotherapy, if day 10 bone marrow is hypoplastic with <5% blasts

If a second cycle of chemotherapy is necessary, administer ~4 days after the completion of chemotherapy if the bone marrow is hypoplastic with <5% blasts

Continue sargramostim until ANC is >1500 cells/mm^3 for 3 consecutive days or a maximum of 42 days

Discontinue sargramostim immediately if leukemic regrowth occurs

If a severe adverse reaction occurs, reduce the dose by 50% or temporarily discontinue the dose until the reaction abates

If ANC >20,000 cells/mm^3, interrupt treatment or reduce the dose by 50%

Mobilization of peripheral blood progenitor cells: I.V., SubQ: 250 mcg/m^2/day I.V. over 24 hours or SubQ once daily

Continue the same dose through the period of PBPC collection

The optimal schedule for PBPC collection has not been established (usually begun by day 5 and performed daily until protocol specified targets are achieved)

If WBC >50,000 cells/mm^3, reduce the dose by 50%

If adequate numbers of progenitor cells are not collected, consider other mobilization therapy

Postperipheral blood progenitor cell transplantation: I.V., SubQ: 250 mcg/m^2/day I.V. over 24 hours or SubQ once daily beginning immediately following infusion of progenitor cells and continuing until ANC is >1500 cells/mm^3 for 3 consecutive days is attained

BMT failure or engraftment delay: I.V.: 250 mcg/m^2/day over 2 hours for 14 days

May be repeated after 7 days off therapy if engraftment has not occurred

If engraftment still has not occurred, a third course of 500 mcg/m^2/day for 14 days may be tried after another 7 days off therapy; if there is still no improvement, it is unlikely that further dose escalation will be beneficial

If a severe adverse reaction occurs, reduce the dose by 50% or temporarily discontinue the dose until the reaction abates

If blast cells appear or disease progression occurs, discontinue treatment

If ANC >20,000 cells/mm^3, interrupt treatment or reduce the dose by 50%

Dosage Forms

Injection, powder for reconstitution:
Leukine®: 250 mcg

Injection, solution:
Leukine®: 500 mcg/mL (1 mL)

Sarna® HC [Can] *see* hydrocortisone (topical) *on page 485*

Sarna® Sensitive [US-OTC] *see* pramoxine *on page 777*

Sarnol®-HC [US-OTC] *see* hydrocortisone (topical) *on page 485*

Sativex® [Can] *see* tetrahydrocannabinol and cannabidiol *(Canada only) on page 915*

SB-265805 *see* gemifloxacin *on page 439*

S. boulardii *see Saccharomyces boulardii on page 849*

SC 33428 *see* idarubicin *on page 498*

SCH 13521 *see* flutamide *on page 416*

SCH 56592 *see* posaconazole *on page 769*

ScheinPharm Ranitidine [Can] *see* ranitidine *on page 819*

SCIG *see* immune globulin (subcutaneous) *on page 504*

S-citalopram *see* escitalopram *on page 356*

Scleromate® [US] *see* morrhuate sodium *on page 645*

Sclerosol® [US] *see* talc (sterile) *on page 902*

Scopace™ [US] *see* scopolamine derivatives *on page 858*

scopolamine and phenylephrine *see* phenylephrine and scopolamine *on page 747*

scopolamine base *see* scopolamine derivatives *on page 858*

scopolamine butylbromide *see* scopolamine derivatives *on page 858*

scopolamine derivatives (skoe POL a meen dah RIV ah tives)

Synonyms hyoscine butylbromide; hyoscine hydrobromide; scopolamine base; scopolamine butylbromide; scopolamine hydrobromide

U.S./Canadian Brand Names Buscopan® [Can]; Isopto® Hyoscine [US]; Scopace™ [US]; Transderm Scōp® [US]; Transderm-V® [Can]

Therapeutic Category Anticholinergic Agent

Use

Scopolamine base:
Transdermal: Prevention of nausea/vomiting associated with motion sickness and recovery from anesthesia and surgery

Scopolamine hydrobromide:
Injection: Preoperative medication to produce amnesia, sedation, tranquilization, antiemetic effects, and decrease salivary and respiratory secretions
Ophthalmic: Produce cycloplegia and mydriasis; treatment of iridocyclitis
Oral: Symptomatic treatment of postencephalitic parkinsonism and paralysis agitans; in spastic states; inhibits excessive motility and hypertonus of the gastrointestinal tract in such conditions as the irritable colon syndrome, mild dysentery, diverticulitis, pylorospasm, and cardiospasm

Scopolamine butylbromide [not available in the U.S.]:
Oral/injection: Treatment of smooth muscle spasm of the genitourinary or gastrointestinal tract; injection may also be used to prior to radiological/diagnostic procedures to prevent spasm

Usual Dosage Note: Scopolamine (hyoscine) hydrobromide should not be interchanged with scopolamine butylbromide formulations. Dosages are not equivalent.

Scopolamine base: Transdermal patch: Adults:
Preoperative: Apply 1 patch to hairless area behind ear the night before surgery or 1 hour prior to cesarean section (apply no sooner than 1 hour before surgery to minimize newborn exposure); remove 24 hours after surgery
Motion sickness: Apply 1 patch behind the ear at least 4 hours prior to exposure and every 3 days as needed; effective if applied as soon as 2-3 hours before anticipated need, best if 12 hours before

Scopolamine hydrobromide:
Antiemetic: SubQ:
Children: 0.006 mg/kg
Adults: 0.6-1 mg
Preoperative: I.M., I.V., SubQ:
Children 6 months to 3 years: 0.1-0.15 mg
Children 3-6 years: 0.2-0.3 mg
Adults: 0.3-0.65 mg
Sedation, tranquilization: I.M., I.V., SubQ: Adults: 0.6 mg 3-4 times/day

Refraction: Ophthalmic:
  Children: Instill 1 drop of 0.25% to eye(s) twice daily for 2 days before procedure
  Adults: Instill 1-2 drops of 0.25% to eye(s) 1 hour before procedure
Iridocyclitis: Ophthalmic:
  Children: Instill 1 drop of 0.25% to eye(s) up to 3 times/day
  Adults: Instill 1-2 drops of 0.25% to eye(s) up to 4 times/day
Parkinsonism, spasticity, motion sickness: Adults: Oral: 0.4-0.8 mg. May repeat every 8-12 hours as needed; the dosage may be cautiously increased in parkinsonism and spastic states. For motion sickness, administration at least 1 hour before exposure is recommended.

Scopolamine butylbromide:
Gastrointestinal/genitourinary spasm (Buscopan® [CAN]; not available in the U.S.): Adults:
  Oral: 10-20 mg daily (1-2 tablets); maximum: 6 tablets/day
  I.M., I.V., SubQ: 10-20 mg; maximum: 100 mg/day. Intramuscular injections should be administered 10-15 minutes prior to radiological/diagnostic procedures
Dosage Forms [CAN] = Canadian brand name
  Injection, solution: 0.4 mg/mL (1 mL)
    Buscopan® [CAN]: 20 mg/mL [not available in the U.S.]
  Solution, ophthalmic:
    Isopto® Hyoscine: 0.25% (5 mL)
  Tablet:
    Buscopan® [CAN]: 10 mg [not available in the U.S.]
  Tablet, soluble:
    Scopace™: 0.4 mg
  Transdermal system:
    Transderm Scōp®: 1.5 mg (4s, 10s, 24s)

scopolamine hydrobromide *see* scopolamine derivatives *on page 858*

scopolamine, hyoscyamine, atropine, and phenobarbital *see* hyoscyamine, atropine, scopolamine, and phenobarbital *on page 493*

Scot-Tussin DM® Cough Chasers *(Discontinued) see* dextromethorphan *on page 284*

Scot-Tussin® Expectorant [US-OTC] *see* guaifenesin *on page 453*

Scot-Tussin® Senior [US-OTC] *see* guaifenesin and dextromethorphan *on page 454*

SD/01 *see* pegfilgrastim *on page 727*

SDX-105 *see* bendamustine *on page 122*

SDZ ENA 713 *see* rivastigmine *on page 840*

Seasonale® [US/Can] *see* ethinyl estradiol and levonorgestrel *on page 372*

Seasonique™ [US] *see* ethinyl estradiol and levonorgestrel *on page 372*

Seba-Gel™ [US] *see* benzoyl peroxide *on page 126*

Sebcur® [Can] *see* salicylic acid *on page 850*

Sebcur/T® [Can] *see* coal tar and salicylic acid *on page 241*

Sebivo® [Can] *see* telbivudine *on page 906*

Sebizon® *(Discontinued) see* sulfacetamide *on page 892*

Seb-Prev™ [US] *see* sulfacetamide *on page 892*

secobarbital (see koe BAR bi tal)

Sound-Alike/Look-Alike Issues
  Seconal® may be confused with Sectral®
Synonyms quinalbarbitone sodium; secobarbital sodium
U.S./Canadian Brand Names Seconal® [US]
Therapeutic Category Barbiturate
Controlled Substance C-II
Use Preanesthetic agent; short-term treatment of insomnia
Usual Dosage Oral:
  Children:
    Preoperative sedation: 2-6 mg/kg (maximum dose: 100 mg/dose) 1-2 hours before procedure
    Sedation: 6 mg/kg/day divided every 8 hours
  Adults:
    Hypnotic: Usual: 100 mg/dose at bedtime; range 100-200 mg/dose
    Preoperative sedation: 100-300 mg 1-2 hours before procedure

◄ **Dosage Forms**
Capsule:
Seconal®: 100 mg

secobarbital sodium *see secobarbital on page 859*
Seconal® [US] *see secobarbital on page 859*
Secran® (Discontinued)
SecreFlo™ [US] *see secretin on page 860*

secretin (SEE kr tin)

Synonyms secretin, human; secretin, porcine
U.S./Canadian Brand Names ChiRhoStim® [US]; SecreFlo™ [US]
Therapeutic Category Diagnostic Agent
Use Secretin-stimulation testing to aid in diagnosis of pancreatic exocrine dysfunction; diagnosis of gastrinoma (Zollinger-Ellison syndrome); facilitation of endoscopic retrograde cholangiopancreatography (ERCP) visualization
Usual Dosage I.V.: Adults: **Note:** A test dose of 0.1 mL (0.2-0.4 mcg) is injected to test for possible allergy. Dosing may be completed if no reaction occurs after 1 minute.
Diagnosis of pancreatic dysfunction, facilitation of ERCP: 0.2 mcg/kg over 1 minute
Diagnosis of gastrinoma: 0.4 mcg/kg over 1 minute
Dosage Forms
Injection, powder for reconstitution [human derived]:
ChiRhoStim®: 16 mcg

secretin, human *see secretin on page 860*
secretin, porcine *see secretin on page 860*
Sectral® [US/Can] *see acebutolol on page 19*
Secura® Antifungal [US-OTC] *see miconazole on page 630*
Sedapap® [US] *see butalbital and acetaminophen on page 155*
Selax® [Can] *see docusate on page 314*
Select™ 1/35 [Can] *see ethinyl estradiol and norethindrone on page 376*

selegiline (se LE ji leen)

Sound-Alike/Look-Alike Issues
selegiline may be confused with Salagen®, Serentil®, sertraline, Serzone®, Stelazine®
Eldepryl® may be confused with Elavil®, enalapril
Zelapar™ may be confused with zaleplon, Zemplar®
Synonyms deprenyl; L-deprenyl; selegiline hydrochloride
U.S./Canadian Brand Names Apo-Selegiline® [Can]; Eldepryl® [US]; Emsam® [US]; Gen-Selegiline [Can]; Novo-Selegiline [Can]; Nu-Selegiline [Can]; Zelapar™ [US]
Therapeutic Category Anti-Parkinson Agent; Dopaminergic Agent (Anti-Parkinson)
Use Adjunct in the management of parkinsonian patients in which levodopa/carbidopa therapy is deteriorating (oral products); treatment of major depressive disorder (transdermal product)
Usual Dosage Adults:
Parkinson disease:
Capsule/tablet: 5 mg twice daily with breakfast and lunch or 10 mg in the morning
Orally disintegrating tablet (Zelapar™): Initial 1.25 mg daily for at least 6 weeks; may increase to 2.5 mg daily based on clinical response (maximum: 2.5 mg daily)
Depression: Transdermal (Emsam®): Initial: 6 mg/24 hours once daily; may titrate based on clinical response in increments of 3 mg/day every 2 weeks up to a maximum of 12 mg/24 hours
Dosage Forms
Capsule, oral: 5 mg
Eldepryl®: 5 mg
Tablet, oral: 5 mg
Tablet, orally-disintegrating:
Zelapar™: 1.25 mg

Transdermal system, topical [once-daily patch]:
Emsam®: 6 mg/24 hours (30s) [20 cm^2, total selegiline 20 mg]; 9 mg/24 hours (30s) [30 cm^2, total selegiline 30 mg]; 12 mg/24 hours (30s) [40 cm^2, total selegiline 40 mg]

selegiline hydrochloride *see selegiline on page 860*
selenium *see trace metals on page 940*

selenium sulfide (se LEE nee um SUL fide)

U.S./Canadian Brand Names Dandrex [US-OTC]; Head & Shoulders® Intensive Treatment [US-OTC]; Selseb® [US]; Selsun blue® 2-in-1 Treatment [US-OTC]; Selsun blue® Daily Treatment [US-OTC]; Selsun blue® Medicated Treatment [US-OTC]; Selsun blue® Moisturizing Treatment [US-OTC]; Tersi [US]; Versel® [Can]

Therapeutic Category Antiseborrheic Agent, Topical

Use Treatment of itching and flaking of the scalp associated with dandruff, to control scalp seborrheic dermatitis; treatment of tinea versicolor

Usual Dosage Topical:
Dandruff, seborrhea: Massage 5-10 mL into wet scalp, leave on scalp 2-3 minutes, rinse thoroughly
Tinea versicolor: Apply the 2.5% lotion to affected area and lather with small amounts of water; leave on skin for 10 minutes, then rinse thoroughly; apply every day for 7 days

Dosage Forms
Aerosol, topical [foam]:
Tersi: 2.25% (70 g)
Lotion, topical: 2.5% (120 mL)
Shampoo, topical: 1% (210 mL)
Dandrex [OTC]: 1% (240 mL)
Head & Shoulders® Intensive Treatment [OTC]: 1% (420 mL)
Selseb®: 2.5% (180 mL)
Selsun blue® Daily Treatment [OTC], Selsun blue® Moisturizing Treatment [OTC], Selsun blue® 2-in-1-Treatment [OTC]: 1% (207 mL, 325 mL)
Selsun blue® Medicated Treatment [OTC]: 1% (120 mL, 207 mL, 325 mL)

Selfemra™ [US] *see fluoxetine on page 413*
Selpak® (Discontinued) *see selegiline on page 860*
Selseb® [US] *see selenium sulfide on page 861*
Selsun blue® 2-in-1 Treatment [US-OTC] *see selenium sulfide on page 861*
Selsun blue® Daily Treatment [US-OTC] *see selenium sulfide on page 861*
Selsun blue® Medicated Treatment [US-OTC] *see selenium sulfide on page 861*
Selsun blue® Moisturizing Treatment [US-OTC] *see selenium sulfide on page 861*
Selsun Gold® for Women (Discontinued) *see selenium sulfide on page 861*
Selsun® Salon™ 2-in-1 [US-OTC] *see pyrithione zinc on page 810*
Selsun® Salon™ Classic [US-OTC] *see pyrithione zinc on page 810*
Selsun® Salon™ Moisturizing [US-OTC] *see pyrithione zinc on page 810*
Selsun® Salon™ Volumizing [US-OTC] *see pyrithione zinc on page 810*
Selzentry™ [US] *see maraviroc on page 591*
Semprex®-D [US] *see acrivastine and pseudoephedrine on page 31*
Senatec HC (Discontinued) *see lidocaine and hydrocortisone on page 564*
Senexon [US-OTC] *see senna on page 861*
Senilezol [US] *see vitamin B complex combinations on page 981*

senna (SEN na)

Sound-Alike/Look-Alike Issues
Perdiem® may be confused with Pyridium®
Senexon may be confused with Cenestin®
Senokot® may be confused with Depakote®

U.S./Canadian Brand Names Black-Draught Tablets [US-OTC]; Evac-U-Gen [US-OTC]; ex-lax® Maximum Strength [US-OTC]; ex-lax® [US-OTC]; Fletcher's® [US-OTC]; Little Tummys® Laxative [US-OTC]; Perdiem® Overnight Relief [US-OTC]; Senexon [US-OTC]; Senna-Gen® [US-OTC]; SenokotXTRA® [US-OTC]; Senokot® [US-OTC]

Therapeutic Category Laxative

▶

◀ **Use** Short-term treatment of constipation; evacuate the colon for bowel or rectal examinations

Usual Dosage Oral:

Constipation: OTC ranges:

Children:

2-6 years:

Sennosides: Initial: 3.75 mg once daily (maximum: 15 mg/day, divided twice daily)

Senna concentrate: 33.3 mg/mL: 5-10 mL up to twice daily

6-12 years:

Sennosides: Initial: 8.6 mg once daily (maximum: 50 mg/day, divided twice daily)

Senna concentrate: 33.3 mg/mL: 10-30 mL up to twice daily

Children ≥12 years and Adults: Sennosides 15 mg once daily (maximum: 70-100 mg/day, divided twice daily)

Dosage Forms

Liquid:

Senexon [OTC]: Sennosides 8.8 mg/5 mL

Liquid [concentrate]:

Fletcher's® [OTC]: Senna concentrate 33.3 mg/mL

Liquid [concentrate; drops]:

Little Tummys® Laxative [OTC]: Sennosides 8.8 mg/1 mL

Syrup: Sennosides 8.8 mg/5 mL

Tablet: Sennosides 8.6 mg

ex-lax® [OTC], Perdiem® Overnight Relief [OTC]: Sennosides USP 15 mg

ex-lax® Maximum Strength [OTC]: Sennosides USP 25 mg

Senokot® [OTC], Senexon® [OTC], Senna-Gen® [OTC]: Sennosides 8.6 mg

SenokotXTRA® [OTC]: Sennosides 17 mg

Tablet, chewable:

Black-Draught™ [OTC]: Sennosides 10 mg

Evac-U-Gen [OTC]: Sennosides 10 mg

ex-lax® [OTC]: Sennosides USP 15 mg

senna and docusate see docusate and senna on page 315

Senna-Gen® [US-OTC] see senna on page 861

senna-S see docusate and senna on page 315

Senokot® [US-OTC] see senna on page 861

Senokot-S® [US-OTC] see docusate and senna on page 315

SenokotXTRA® [US-OTC] see senna on page 861

SenoSol™-X (Discontinued) see senna on page 861

SenoSol™ (Discontinued) see senna on page 861

SenoSol™-SS [US-OTC] see docusate and senna on page 315

Sensipar® [US/Can] see cinacalcet on page 220

Sensorcaine® [US/Can] see bupivacaine on page 149

Sensorcaine®-MPF [US] see bupivacaine on page 149

Sensorcaine®-MPF Spinal [US] see bupivacaine on page 149

Sensorcaine®-MPF with Epinephrine [US] see bupivacaine and epinephrine on page 150

Sensorcaine® with Epinephrine [US/Can] see bupivacaine and epinephrine on page 150

Sepasoothe® [US] see benzocaine on page 124

Septanest® N [Can] see articaine and epinephrine on page 95

Septanest® SP [Can] see articaine and epinephrine on page 95

Septa® Topical Ointment (Discontinued) see bacitracin, neomycin, and polymyxin B on page 114

Septisol® (Discontinued) see hexachlorophene on page 473

Septocaine® with epinephrine 1:100,000 [US] see articaine and epinephrine on page 95

Septocaine® with epinephrine 1:200,000 [US] see articaine and epinephrine on page 95

Septra® [US] see sulfamethoxazole and trimethoprim on page 894

Septra® DS [US] see sulfamethoxazole and trimethoprim on page 894

Septra® Injection [Can] see sulfamethoxazole and trimethoprim on page 894

Serax® [US] see oxazepam on page 706

Serc® [Can] see betahistine (Canada only) on page 130

Serevent® (Discontinued) see salmeterol on page 854

Serevent® Diskhaler® Disk [Can] *see* salmeterol *on page 854*
Serevent® Diskus® [US/Can] *see* salmeterol *on page 854*

sermorelin acetate (ser moe REL in AS e tate)
U.S./Canadian Brand Names Geref® Diagnostic [US]
Therapeutic Category Diagnostic Agent
Use Geref® Diagnostic: For evaluation of the ability of the pituitary gland to secrete growth hormone (GH)
Usual Dosage I.V.: Children and Adults: Diagnostic: 1 mcg/kg as a single dose in the morning following an overnight fast
Note: Response to diagnostic test may be decreased in patients >40 years
Dosage Forms
Injection, powder for reconstitution:
Geref® Diagnostic: 50 mcg

Seromycin® [US] *see* cycloserine *on page 257*
Serophene® [US/Can] *see* clomiphene *on page 235*
Seroquel® [US/Can] *see* quetiapine *on page 811*
Seroquel® XR [US/Can] *see* quetiapine *on page 811*
Serostim® [US/Can] *see* somatropin *on page 881*
Serpalan® *(Discontinued)* *see* reserpine *on page 827*
Serpatabs® *(Discontinued)* *see* reserpine *on page 827*

sertaconazole (ser ta KOE na zole)
Synonyms sertaconazole nitrate
U.S./Canadian Brand Names Ertaczo® [US]
Therapeutic Category Antifungal Agent, Topical
Use Topical treatment of tinea pedis (athlete's foot)
Usual Dosage Topical: Children ≥12 years and Adults: Apply between toes and to surrounding healthy skin twice daily for 4 weeks
Dosage Forms
Cream, topical:
Ertaczo®: 2% (30 g, 60 g)

sertaconazole nitrate *see* sertaconazole *on page 863*

sertraline (SER tra leen)
Sound-Alike/Look-Alike Issues
sertraline may be confused with selegiline, Serentil®
Zoloft® may be confused with Zocor®
Synonyms sertraline hydrochloride
U.S./Canadian Brand Names Apo-Sertraline® [Can]; CO Sertraline [Can]; Dom-Sertraline [Can]; Gen-Sertraline [Can]; GMD-Sertraline [Can]; Novo-Sertraline [Can]; Nu-Sertraline [Can]; PHL-Sertraline [Can]; PMS-Sertraline [Can]; ratio-Sertraline [Can]; Rhoxal-Sertraline [Can]; Riva-Sertraline [Can]; Sandoz-Sertraline [Can]; Zoloft® [US/Can]
Therapeutic Category Antidepressant, Selective Serotonin Reuptake Inhibitor
Use Treatment of major depression; obsessive-compulsive disorder (OCD); panic disorder; posttraumatic stress disorder (PTSD); premenstrual dysphoric disorder (PMDD); social anxiety disorder
Usual Dosage Oral:
Children and Adolescents: Obsessive-compulsive disorder:
6-12 years: Initial: 25 mg once daily
13-17 years: Initial: 50 mg once daily
Note: May increase daily dose, at intervals of not less than 1 week, to a maximum of 200 mg/day. If somnolence is noted, give at bedtime.
Adults:
Depression/obsessive-compulsive disorder: Oral: Initial: 50 mg/day (see "Note" above)
Panic disorder, posttraumatic stress disorder, social anxiety disorder: Initial: 25 mg once daily; increase to 50 mg once daily after 1 week (see "Note" above)
Premenstrual dysphoric disorder: 50 mg/day either daily throughout menstrual cycle **or** limited to the luteal phase of menstrual cycle, depending on physician assessment. Patients not responding to ▶

◄ 50 mg/day may benefit from dose increases (50 mg increments per menstrual cycle) up to 150 mg/day when dosing throughout menstrual cycle **or** up to 100 mg day when dosing during luteal phase only. If a 100 mg/day dose has been established with luteal phase dosing, a 50 mg/day titration step for 3 days should be utilized at the beginning of each luteal phase dosing period.

Dosage Forms
 Solution, oral [concentrate]: 20 mg/mL (60 mL)
  Zoloft®: 20 mg/mL
 Tablet: 25 mg, 50 mg, 100 mg
  Zoloft®: 25 mg, 50 mg, 100 mg

sertraline hydrochloride *see* sertraline *on page 863*
Serzone® *(Discontinued) see* nefazodone *on page 660*

sevelamer (se VEL a mer)

Sound-Alike/Look-Alike Issues
 Renagel® may be confused with Reglan®, Regonol®, Renal Caps, Renvela®
 Renvela® may be confused with Reglan®, Regonol®, Renagel®, Renal Caps
Synonyms sevelamer carbonate; sevelamer hydrochloride
U.S./Canadian Brand Names Renagel® [US/Can]; Renvela® [US]
Therapeutic Category Phosphate Binder
Use Reduction or control of serum phosphorous in patients with chronic kidney disease on hemodialysis
Usual Dosage Oral: **Note:** The dosing of sevelamer carbonate and sevelamer hydrochloride are expected to be similar, when switching from one product to another, the same dose (on a mg-per-mg basis) should be utilized.
 Adults: Patients not taking a phosphate binder: 800-1600 mg 3 times/day with meals; the initial dose may be based on serum phosphorous levels:
  >5.5 mg/dL to <7.5 mg/dL: 800 mg 3 times/day
  ≥7.5 mg/dL to <9.0 mg/dL: 1200-1600 mg 3 times/day
  ≥9.0 mg/dL: 1600 mg 3 times/day
 Maintenance dose adjustment based on serum phosphorous concentration (goal range of 3.5-5.5 mg/dL; maximum dose studied was equivalent to 13 g/day [sevelamer hydrochloride] or 14 g/day [sevelamer carbonate]):
  >5.5 mg/dL: Increase by 1 tablet per meal at 2-week intervals
  3.5-5.5 mg/dL: Maintain current dose
  <3.5 mg/dL: Decrease by 1 tablet per meal
 Dosage adjustment when switching between phosphate binder products: 667 mg of calcium acetate is equivalent to 800 mg sevelamer (carbonate or hydrochloride)
Dosage Forms
 Tablet:
  Renagel®: 400 mg, 800 mg
  Renvela®: 800 mg

sevelamer carbonate *see* sevelamer *on page 864*
sevelamer hydrochloride *see* sevelamer *on page 864*

sevoflurane (see voe FLOO rane)

Sound-Alike/Look-Alike Issues
 Ultane® may be confused with Ultram®
U.S./Canadian Brand Names Sevorane® AF [Can]; Sojourn™ [US]; Ultane® [US]
Therapeutic Category General Anesthetic
Use Induction and maintenance of general anesthesia
Usual Dosage Minimum alveolar concentration (MAC), the concentration that abolishes movement in response to a noxious stimulus (surgical incision) in 50% of patients, is 2.6% (25 years of age) for sevoflurane. Surgical levels of anesthesia are generally achieved with concentrations from 0.5% to 3%; the concentration at which amnesia and loss of awareness occur is 0.6%.
 Minimum alveolar concentrations (MAC) values for surgical levels of anesthesia:
  0 to 1 month old full-term neonates: Sevoflurane in oxygen: 3.3%
  1 to <6 months: Sevoflurane in oxygen: 3%
  6 months to <3 years:
   Sevoflurane in oxygen: 2.8%

Sevoflurane in 60% N₂0/40% oxygen: 2%
3-12 years: Sevoflurane in oxygen: 2.5%
25 years:
  Sevoflurane in oxygen: 2.6%
  Sevoflurane in 65% N₂0/35% oxygen: 1.4%
40 years:
  Sevoflurane in oxygen: 2.1%
  Sevoflurane in 65% N₂0/35% oxygen: 1.1%
60 years:
  Sevoflurane in oxygen: 1.7%
  Sevoflurane in 65% N₂0/35% oxygen: 0.9%
80 years:
  Sevoflurane in oxygen: 1.4%
  Sevoflurane in 65% N₂0/35% oxygen: 0.7%

Dosage Forms
  Liquid for inhalation: 100% (250 mL)
    Sojourn™, Ultane®: 100% (250 mL)

Sevorane® AF [Can] *see* sevoflurane *on page 864*
shingles vaccine *see* zoster vaccine *on page 997*
Shur-Seal® *(Discontinued)* *see* nonoxynol 9 *on page 677*
Sibelium® [Can] *see* flunarizine *(Canada only) on page 408*

sibutramine (si BYOO tra meen)

Sound-Alike/Look-Alike Issues
  Meridia® may be confused with Aredia®
Synonyms sibutramine hydrochloride monohydrate
U.S./Canadian Brand Names Meridia® [US/Can]
Therapeutic Category Anorexiant
Controlled Substance C-IV
Use Management of obesity
Usual Dosage Children ≥16 years and Adults:
  Initial: 10 mg once daily; after 4 weeks may titrate up to 15 mg once daily as needed and tolerated (may be used for up to 2 years, per manufacturer labeling)
  Maintenance: 5-15 mg once daily
Dosage Forms
  Capsule:
    Meridia®: 5 mg, 10 mg, 15 mg

sibutramine hydrochloride monohydrate *see* sibutramine *on page 865*
Silace [US-OTC] *see* docusate *on page 314*
Siladryl® Allergy [US-OTC] *see* diphenhydramine *on page 304*
Silafed® [US-OTC] *see* triprolidine and pseudoephedrine *on page 955*
Silain® *(Discontinued)* *see* simethicone *on page 867*
Silaminic® Expectorant *(Discontinued)*
Silapap® Children's [US-OTC] *see* acetaminophen *on page 19*
Silapap® Infants [US-OTC] *see* acetaminophen *on page 19*
Sildec *(Discontinued)*
Sildec-DM *(Discontinued)*
Sildec PE [US] *see* chlorpheniramine and phenylephrine *on page 206*
Sildec PE-DM [US] *see* chlorpheniramine, phenylephrine, and dextromethorphan *on page 209*
Sildec Syrup [US] *see* brompheniramine and pseudoephedrine *on page 144*

sildenafil (sil DEN a fil)

Sound-Alike/Look-Alike Issues
  Revatio® may be confused with ReVia®
  Viagra® may be confused with Allegra®, Vaniqa™
Synonyms UK92480

◀ **U.S./Canadian Brand Names** Revatio® [US]; Viagra® [US/Can]

Therapeutic Category Phosphodiesterase (Type 5) Enzyme Inhibitor

Use

Revatio®: Treatment of pulmonary arterial hypertension (WHO Group I)

Viagra®: Treatment of erectile dysfunction (ED)

Usual Dosage Oral: Adults:

Erectile dysfunction (Viagra®): For most patients, the recommended dose is 25-50 mg taken as needed, approximately 1 hour before sexual activity. However, sildenafil may be taken anywhere from 30 minutes to 4 hours before sexual activity. Based on effectiveness and tolerance, the dose may be increased to a maximum recommended dose of 100 mg or decreased to 25 mg. The maximum recommended dosing frequency is once daily.

Pulmonary arterial hypertension (Revatio®): 20 mg 3 times/day, taken 4-6 hours apart

Dosage Forms

Tablet:

Revatio®: 20 mg

Viagra®: 25 mg, 50 mg, 100 mg

Sildicon-E® *(Discontinued)*

Silexin [US-OTC] *see* guaifenesin and dextromethorphan *on page 454*

Silfedrine Children's [US-OTC] *see* pseudoephedrine *on page 801*

Silphen® [US-OTC] *see* diphenhydramine *on page 304*

Silphen DM® [US-OTC] *see* dextromethorphan *on page 284*

Sil-Tex [US] *see* guaifenesin and phenylephrine *on page 456*

Siltussin-CF® *(Discontinued)*

Siltussin DAS [US-OTC] *see* guaifenesin *on page 453*

Siltussin DM [US-OTC] *see* guaifenesin and dextromethorphan *on page 454*

Siltussin DM DAS [US-OTC] *see* guaifenesin and dextromethorphan *on page 454*

Siltussin SA [US-OTC] *see* guaifenesin *on page 453*

Silvadene® [US] *see* silver sulfadiazine *on page 866*

silver nitrate (SIL ver NYE trate)

Synonyms AgNO₃

Therapeutic Category Topical Skin Product

Use Cauterization of wounds and sluggish ulcers, removal of granulation tissue and warts; aseptic prophylaxis of burns

Usual Dosage Children and Adults:

Sticks: Apply to mucous membranes and other moist skin surfaces only on area to be treated 2-3 times/week for 2-3 weeks

Topical solution: Apply a cotton applicator dipped in solution on the affected area 2-3 times/week for 2-3 weeks

Dosage Forms

Applicator sticks, topical: Silver nitrate 75% and potassium 25% (6", 12", 18")

Solution, topical: 0.5% (960 mL); 10% (30 mL); 25% (30 mL); 50% (30 mL)

silver sulfadiazine (SIL ver sul fa DYE a zeen)

U.S./Canadian Brand Names Flamazine® [Can]; Silvadene® [US]; SSD® AF [US]; SSD® [US]; Thermazene® [US]

Therapeutic Category Antibacterial, Topical

Use Prevention and treatment of infection in second and third degree burns

Usual Dosage Topical: Children and Adults: Apply once or twice daily with a sterile-gloved hand; apply to a thickness of 1/16"; burned area should be covered with cream at all times

Dosage Forms

Cream, topical: 1% (25 g, 50 g, 85 g, 400 g)

Silvadene®, Thermazene®: 1% (20 g, 50 g, 85 g, 400 g, 1000 g)

SSD®: 1% (25 g, 50 g, 85 g, 400 g)

SSD® AF: 1% (50 g, 400 g)

Simcor® [US] *see* niacin and simvastatin *on page 669*

simethicone (sye METH i kone)

Sound-Alike/Look-Alike Issues
simethicone may be confused with cimetidine
Mylanta® may be confused with Mynatal®
Mylicon® may be confused with Modicon®, Myleran®
Phazyme® may be confused with Pherazine®

Synonyms activated dimethicone; activated methylpolysiloxane

U.S./Canadian Brand Names Equalizer Gas Relief [US-OTC]; Gas-X® Extra Strength [US-OTC]; Gas-X® Infant [US-OTC]; Gas-X® Maximum Strength [US-OTC]; Gas-X® Thin Strips™ [US-OTC]; Gas-X® [US-OTC]; Gas-X®, Children's Tongue Twisters™ [US-OTC]; Genasyme® [US-OTC]; Infantaire Gas Drops [US-OTC]; Little Tummys® Gas Relief [US-OTC]; Mylanta® Gas Maximum Strength [US-OTC]; Mylicon® Infants [US-OTC]; Ovol® [Can]; Phazyme® Ultra Strength [US-OTC]; Phazyme™ [Can]

Therapeutic Category Antiflatulent

Use Postoperative gas pain or for use in endoscopic examination; relief of bloating, pressure, and discomfort of gas

Usual Dosage Oral:
Infants and Children <2 years or <11 kg: 20 mg 4 times/day, as needed
Children >2 years or >11 kg: 40 mg 4 times/day, as needed
Children >12 years and Adults: 40-360 mg after meals and at bedtime, as needed

Dosage Forms
Softgels: 125 mg
Gas-X® Extra Strength [OTC], Mylanta® Gas Maximum Strength [OTC]: 125 mg
Gas-X® Maximum Strength [OTC]: 166 mg
Phazyme® Ultra Strength [OTC]: 180 mg
Strips, oral:
Gas-X®, Children's Tongue Twisters™ [OTC]: 40 mg (16s)
Gas-X® Thin Strips™ [OTC]: 62.5 mg (18s, 32s)
Suspension, oral [drops]: 40 mg/0.6 mL
Equalizer Gas Relief [OTC], Gas-X® Infant [OTC], Genasyme® [OTC], Infantaire Gas [OTC], Little Tummys® Gas Relief [OTC], Mylicon® Infants [OTC]: 40 mg/0.6 mL
Tablet, chewable: 80 mg, 125 mg
Gas-X® [OTC], Genasyme® [OTC]: 80 mg
Gas-X® Extra Strength [OTC], Mylanta® Gas Maximum Strength [OTC]: 125 mg

simethicone, aluminum hydroxide, and magnesium hydroxide see aluminum hydroxide, magnesium hydroxide, and simethicone on page 54

simethicone and calcium carbonate see calcium carbonate and simethicone on page 164

simethicone and loperamide hydrochloride see loperamide and simethicone on page 574

simethicone and magaldrate see magaldrate and simethicone on page 583

Similac® Glucose [US] see dextrose on page 286

Simply Cough® (Discontinued) see dextromethorphan on page 284

Simply Saline® [US-OTC] see sodium chloride on page 873

Simply Saline® Baby [US-OTC] see sodium chloride on page 873

Simply Saline® Nasal Moist® [US-OTC] see sodium chloride on page 873

Simply Sleep® [US-OTC/Can] see diphenhydramine on page 304

Simply Stuffy™ (Discontinued) see pseudoephedrine on page 801

Simuc (Discontinued) see guaifenesin and phenylephrine on page 456

Simuc-DM [US] see guaifenesin and dextromethorphan on page 454

Simulect® [US/Can] see basiliximab on page 117

simvastatin (sim va STAT in)

Sound-Alike/Look-Alike Issues
Zocor® may be confused with Cozaar®, Yocon®, Zoloft®

U.S./Canadian Brand Names Apo-Simvastatin® [Can]; CO Simvastatin [Can]; Dom-Simvastatin [Can]; Gen-Simvastatin [Can]; Novo-Simvastatin [Can]; Nu-Simvastatin [Can]; PHL-Simvastatin [Can]; PMS-Simvastatin [Can]; ratio-Simvastatin [Can]; Riva-Simvastatin [Can]; Sandoz-Simvastatin [Can]; Taro-Simvastatin [Can]; Zocor® [US/Can]

Therapeutic Category HMG-CoA Reductase Inhibitor

▶

◀ **Use** Used with dietary therapy for the following:

Secondary prevention of cardiovascular events in hypercholesterolemic patients with established coronary heart disease (CHD) or at high risk for CHD: To reduce cardiovascular morbidity (myocardial infarction, coronary revascularization procedures) and mortality; to reduce the risk of stroke and transient ischemic attacks

Hyperlipidemias: To reduce elevations in total cholesterol, LDL-C, apolipoprotein B, and triglycerides, and increase HDL-C in patients with primary hypercholesterolemia (elevations of 1 or more components are present in Fredrickson type IIa, IIb, III, and IV hyperlipidemias); treatment of homozygous familial hypercholesterolemia

Heterozygous familial hypercholesterolemia (HeFH): In adolescent patients (10-17 years of age, females >1 year postmenarche) with HeFH having LDL-C ≥190 mg/dL **or** LDL ≥160 mg/dL with positive family history of premature cardiovascular disease (CVD), or 2 or more CVD risk factors in the adolescent patient

Usual Dosage Oral: **Note:** Doses should be individualized according to the baseline LDL-cholesterol levels, the recommended goal of therapy, and the patient's response; adjustments should be made at intervals of 4 weeks or more; doses may need adjusted based on concomitant medications

Children 10-17 years (females >1 year postmenarche): HeFH: 10 mg once daily in the evening; range: 10-40 mg/day (maximum: 40 mg/day)

Adults:

Homozygous familial hypercholesterolemia: 40 mg once daily in the evening **or** 80 mg/day (given as 20 mg, 20 mg, and 40 mg evening dose)

Prevention of cardiovascular events, hyperlipidemias: 20-40 mg once daily in the evening; range: 5-80 mg/day

Patients requiring only moderate reduction of LDL-cholesterol may be started at 10 mg once daily

Patients requiring reduction of >45% in low-density lipoprotein (LDL) cholesterol may be started at 40 mg once daily in the evening

Patients with CHD or at high risk for CHD: Dosing should be started at 40 mg once daily in the evening; simvastatin should be started simultaneously with diet therapy.

Dosage Forms

Tablet: 5 mg, 10 mg, 20 mg, 40 mg, 80 mg

Zocor®: 10 mg, 20 mg, 40 mg, 80 mg

Simvastatin and Ezetimibe *see ezetimibe and simvastatin on page 387*

simvastatin and niacin *see niacin and simvastatin on page 669*

Sina-12X [US] *see guaifenesin and phenylephrine on page 456*

sincalide (SIN ka lide)

Synonyms C8-CCK; OP-CCK

U.S./Canadian Brand Names Kinevac® [US]

Therapeutic Category Diagnostic Agent

Use Postevacuation cholecystography; gallbladder bile sampling; stimulate pancreatic secretion for analysis; accelerate the transit of barium through the small bowel

Usual Dosage Adults:

Contraction of gallbladder:

I.V.: 0.02 mcg/kg over 30-60 seconds; may repeat in 15 minutes with a 0.04 mcg/kg dose

Infusion: 0.12 mcg/kg in 100 mL of NS; administer over 50 minutes

I.M.: 0.1 mcg/kg

Pancreatic function: I.V.: 0.02 mcg/kg over 30 minutes

Accelerate barium transit through small bowel:

I.V.: 0.04 mcg/kg over 30-60 seconds; if movement of barium has not occurred in 30 minutes, may repeat dose

Infusion: 0.12 mcg/kg in 30 mL of NS; administer over 30 minutes

Dosage Forms

Injection, powder for reconstitution:

Kinevac®: 5 mcg

Sine-Aid® IB *(Discontinued)* *see pseudoephedrine and ibuprofen on page 802*

sinecatechins (sin e KAT e kins)

Synonyms catechins; green tea extract; kunecatechins; polyphenols; polyphenon E

U.S./Canadian Brand Names Veregen™ [US]

Therapeutic Category Immunomodulator, Topical; Topical Skin Product

Use Treatment of external genital and perianal warts secondary to *Condylomata acuminata*

Usual Dosage Topical: Adults: Apply a thin layer (~0.5 cm strand) 3 times/day to all external genital and perianal warts until all warts have been cleared (maximum duration: 16 weeks)

Dosage Forms

Ointment, topical:

Veregen®: 15% (15 g)

Sinemet® [US/Can] *see* carbidopa and levodopa *on page 177*

Sinemet® CR [US/Can] *see* carbidopa and levodopa *on page 177*

Sinequan® [Can] *see* doxepin *on page 321*

Sinequan® *(Discontinued) see* doxepin *on page 321*

Singulair® [US/Can] *see* montelukast *on page 642*

Sinografin® [US] *see* diatrizoate meglumine and iodipamide meglumine *on page 289*

Sinubid® *(Discontinued)*

Sinufed® Timecelles® *(Discontinued) see* guaifenesin and pseudoephedrine *on page 458*

Sinumed® *(Discontinued) see* acetaminophen, chlorpheniramine, and pseudoephedrine *on page 25*

Sinumist®-SR Capsulets® *(Discontinued) see* guaifenesin *on page 453*

Sinus-Relief *(Discontinued) see* acetaminophen and pseudoephedrine *on page 23*

Sinutab® Non Drowsy [Can] *see* acetaminophen and pseudoephedrine *on page 23*

Sinutab® Non-Drying [US-OTC] *see* guaifenesin and pseudoephedrine *on page 458*

Sinutab® Sinus [US-OTC] *see* acetaminophen and phenylephrine *on page 22*

Sinutab® Sinus & Allergy [Can] *see* acetaminophen, chlorpheniramine, and pseudoephedrine *on page 25*

Sinutab® Sinus Allergy Maximum Strength [US-OTC] *see* acetaminophen, chlorpheniramine, and pseudoephedrine *on page 25*

SINUtuss® DM [US] *see* guaifenesin, dextromethorphan, and phenylephrine *on page 459*

SINUvent® PE [US] *see* guaifenesin and phenylephrine *on page 456*

Sirdalud® *(Discontinued) see* tizanidine *on page 931*

sirolimus (sir OH li mus)

Sound-Alike/Look-Alike Issues

sirolimus may be confused with tacrolimus, temsirolimus

U.S./Canadian Brand Names Rapamune® [US/Can]

Therapeutic Category Immunosuppressant Agent

Use Prophylaxis of organ rejection in patients receiving renal transplants, in combination with corticosteroids and cyclosporine (cyclosporine may be withdrawn in low-to-moderate immunological risk patients after 2-4 months, in conjunction with an increase in sirolimus dosage; in high-risk patients, use in combination with cyclosporine and corticosteroids is recommended for the first year)

Usual Dosage Oral:

Combination therapy with cyclosporine: Doses should be taken 4 hours after cyclosporine, and should be taken consistently either with or without food.

Low- to moderate-risk renal transplant patients: Children ≥13 years and Adults: Dosing by body weight:

<40 kg: Loading dose: 3 mg/m^2 on day 1, followed by maintenance dosing of 1 mg/m^2 once daily

≥40 kg: Loading dose: 6 mg on day 1; maintenance: 2 mg once daily

High-risk renal transplant patients: Adults: Loading dose: Up to 15 mg on day 1; maintenance: 5 mg/day; obtain trough concentration between days 5-7 and adjust accordingly. Continue concurrent cyclosporine/sirolimus therapy for 1 year following transplantation. Further adjustment of the regimen must be based on clinical status.

◄ **Dosage adjustment:** Sirolimus dosages should be adjusted to maintain trough concentrations within desired range based on risk and concomitant therapy. Maximum daily dose: 40 mg. Dosage should be adjusted at intervals of 7-14 days to account for the long half-life of sirolimus. In general, dose proportionality may be assumed. New sirolimus dose **equals** current dose **multiplied by** (target concentration/current concentration). **Note:** If large dose increase is required, consider loading dose calculated as:

Loading dose **equals** (new maintenance dose **minus** current maintenance dose) **multiplied by** 3
Maximum dose in 1 day: 40 mg; if required dose is >40 mg (due to loading dose), divide over 2 days.
Serum concentrations should not be used as the sole basis for dosage adjustment (monitor clinical signs/symptoms, tissue biopsy, and laboratory parameters).

Maintenance therapy after withdrawal of cyclosporine: Cyclosporine withdrawal is not recommended in high immunological risk patients. Following 2-4 months of combined therapy, withdrawal of cyclosporine may be considered in low-to-moderate risk patients. Cyclosporine should be discontinued over 4-8 weeks, and a necessary increase in the dosage of sirolimus (up to fourfold) should be anticipated due to removal of metabolic inhibition by cyclosporine and to maintain adequate immunosuppressive effects. Dose-adjusted trough target concentrations are typically 16-24 ng/mL for the first year post-transplant and 12-20 ng/mL thereafter (measured by chromatographic methodology).

Dosage Forms
Solution, oral:
Rapamune®: 1 mg/mL
Tablet:
Rapamune®: 1 mg, 2 mg

sitagliptin (sit a GLIP tin)

Sound-Alike/Look-Alike Issues
sitaGLIPtin may be confused with SUMAtriptan
Januvia™ may be confused with Jantoven™

Synonyms MK-0431; sitagliptin phosphate

Tall-Man sita**GLIP**tin

U.S./Canadian Brand Names Januvia™ [US]

Therapeutic Category Antidiabetic Agent, Dipeptidyl Peptidase IV (DPP-IV) Inhibitor

Use Management of type 2 diabetes mellitus (noninsulin-dependent, NIDDM) as an adjunct to diet and exercise as monotherapy or in combination therapy with other antidiabetic agents

Usual Dosage Oral: Adults: Type 2 diabetes: 100 mg once daily

Dosage Forms
Tablet:
Januvia™: 25 mg, 50 mg, 100 mg

sitagliptin and metformin (sit a GLIP tin & met FOR min)

Sound-Alike/Look-Alike Issues
Janumet™ may be confused with Jantoven™

Synonyms metformin and sitagliptin; sitagliptin phosphate and metformin hydrochloride

U.S./Canadian Brand Names Janumet™ [US]

Therapeutic Category Antidiabetic Agent, Biguanide; Antidiabetic Agent, Dipeptidyl Peptidase IV (DPP-IV) Inhibitor; Hypoglycemic Agent, Oral

Use Management of type 2 diabetes mellitus (noninsulin-dependent, NIDDM) in patients not adequately controlled on metformin or sitagliptin monotherapy and as an adjunct to diet and exercise

Usual Dosage Oral: Type 2 diabetes mellitus:

Adults: Initial doses should be based on current dose of sitagliptin and metformin; daily doses should be divided and given twice daily with meals. Maximum: Sitagliptin 100 mg/metformin 2000 mg daily

Patients inadequately controlled on metformin alone: Initial dose: Sitagliptin 100 mg/day plus current dose of metformin. **Note:** Per manufacturer labeling, patients currently receiving metformin 850 mg twice daily should receive an initial dose of sitagliptin 50 mg and metformin 1000 mg twice daily

Patients inadequately controlled on sitagliptin alone: Initial dose: Metformin 1000 mg/day plus sitagliptin 100 mg/day. **Note:** Patients currently receiving a renally adjusted dose of sitagliptin should not be switched to combination product.

Dosing adjustment: Metformin component may be gradually increased up to the maximum dose. Maximum dose: Sitagliptin 100 mg/metformin 2000 mg daily

Dosage Forms
Tablet:
Janumet™:
50/500: Sitagliptin 50 mg and metformin 500 mg
50/1000: Sitagliptin 50 mg and metformin 1000 mg

sitagliptin phosphate *see* sitagliptin *on page 870*
sitagliptin phosphate and metformin hydrochloride *see* sitagliptin and metformin *on page 870*

sitaxsentan *(Canada only)* (sye TACKS en tan)

Sound-Alike/Look-Alike Issues
Thelin™ may be confused with Theolair™
Synonyms sitaxsentan sodium
U.S./Canadian Brand Names Thelin™ [Can]
Therapeutic Category Endothelin Antagonist
Use Treatment of primary pulmonary arterial hypertension (PAH) or pulmonary hypertension secondary to connective tissue disease, in World Health Organization (WHO) class III patients unresponsive to conventional therapy; treatment of PAH in WHO class II patients who are unresponsive to conventional therapy and have no alternative treatment options
Usual Dosage Oral: Adults: 100 mg once daily. (**Note:** Doses above 100 mg/day are not recommended; higher doses have not been shown to provide additional benefit and may increase risk of hepatic toxicity).
Dosage Forms CAN = Canadian brand name
Tablet:
Thelin™ [CAN]: 100 mg [not available in U.S.]

sitaxsentan sodium *see* sitaxsentan *(Canada only) on page 871*
Skeeter Stik [US-OTC] *see* benzocaine *on page 124*
Skelaxin® [US/Can] *see* metaxalone *on page 610*
Skelid® [US] *see* tiludronate *on page 927*
SKF 104864 *see* topotecan *on page 936*
SKF 104864-A *see* topotecan *on page 936*
Skin Care™ [US-OTC] *see* pyrithione zinc *on page 810*
Sleep-ettes D [US-OTC] *see* diphenhydramine *on page 304*
Sleep-eze 3® Oral *(Discontinued)* *see* diphenhydramine *on page 304*
Sleepinal® [US-OTC] *see* diphenhydramine *on page 304*
Sleepwell 2-nite® *(Discontinued)* *see* diphenhydramine *on page 304*
S-leucovorin *see* LEVOleucovorin *on page 558*
6S-leucovorin *see* LEVOleucovorin *on page 558*
Slim-Mint® *(Discontinued)* *see* benzocaine *on page 124*
Slo-bid™ *(Discontinued)* *see* theophylline *on page 917*
Slo-Niacin® [US-OTC] *see* niacin *on page 667*
Slo-Phyllin® (all products) *(Discontinued)* *see* theophylline *on page 917*
Slo-Phyllin® GG *(Discontinued)* *see* theophylline and guaifenesin *on page 919*
Slo-Pot [Can] *see* potassium chloride *on page 771*
Slow FE® [US-OTC] *see* ferrous sulfate *on page 398*
Slow-K® [Can] *see* potassium chloride *on page 771*
Slow-K® *(Discontinued)* *see* potassium chloride *on page 771*
Slow-Mag® [US-OTC] *see* magnesium chloride *on page 583*

smallpox vaccine (SMAL poks vak SEEN)

Synonyms dried smallpox vaccine; live smallpox vaccine; vaccinia vaccine
U.S./Canadian Brand Names ACAM2000™ [US]
Therapeutic Category Vaccine
Use Active immunization against vaccinia virus, the causative agent of smallpox in persons determined to be at risk for smallpox infection. The ACIP recommends vaccination of laboratory workers at risk of exposure from cultures or contaminated animals which may be a source of vaccinia or related Orthopoxviruses capable of causing infections in humans (monkeypox, cowpox, or variola). The ACIP ▶

◀ also recommends that consideration be given for vaccination in healthcare workers having contact with clinical specimens, contaminated material, or patients receiving vaccinia or recombinant vaccinia viruses. ACIP recommends revaccination every 10 years. The Armed Forces recommend vaccination of certain personnel categories. Recommendations for use in response to bioterrorism are regularly updated by the CDC, and may be found at www.cdc.gov.

Usual Dosage Not for I.M., I.V., or SubQ injection: Vaccination by scarification (multiple-puncture technique) only: **Note:** A trace of blood should appear at vaccination site after 15-20 seconds; if no trace of blood is visible, an additional 3 insertions should be made using the same needle, without reinserting the needle into the vaccine bottle.

Dosage Forms

Injection, powder for reconstitution [purified monkey cell source]:
ACAM2000™: 1-5 x 10^8 plaque-forming units per mL

smelling salts *see* ammonia spirit (aromatic) *on page 66*

SMZ-TMP *see* sulfamethoxazole and trimethoprim *on page 894*

snake antivenin *see* crotalidae polyvalent immune FAB (ovine) *on page 253*

snake (pit vipers) antivenin *see* crotalidae polyvalent antivenin (equine) *on page 252*

Snaplets-EX® *(Discontinued)*

(+)-(S)-N-methyl-γ-(1-naphthyloxy)-2-thiophenepropylamine hydrochloride *see* duloxetine *on page 328*

sodium 2-mercaptoethane sulfonate *see* mesna *on page 608*

sodium 4-hydroxybutyrate *see* sodium oxybate *on page 877*

sodium L-triiodothyronine *see* liothyronine *on page 568*

sodium acetate (SOW dee um AS e tate)

Therapeutic Category Alkalinizing Agent; Electrolyte Supplement, Oral

Use Sodium source in large volume I.V. fluids to prevent or correct hyponatremia in patients with restricted intake; used to counter acidosis through conversion to bicarbonate

Usual Dosage Sodium acetate is metabolized to bicarbonate on an equimolar basis outside the liver; administer in large volume I.V. fluids as a sodium source. Refer to sodium bicarbonate monograph. Maintenance electrolyte requirements of sodium in parenteral nutrition solutions:
Daily requirements: 3-4 mEq/kg/24 hours or 25-40 mEq/1000 kcal/24 hours
Maximum: 100-150 mEq/24 hours

Dosage Forms

Injection, solution [concentrate]: 2 mEq/mL (20 mL, 50 mL, 100 mL, 250 mL); 4 mEq/mL (50 mL, 100 mL)

sodium acid carbonate *see* sodium bicarbonate *on page 872*

sodium aurothiomalate *see* gold sodium thiomalate *on page 450*

sodium benzoate and caffeine *see* caffeine *on page 158*

sodium benzoate and sodium phenylacetate *see* sodium phenylacetate and sodium benzoate *on page 877*

sodium bicarbonate (SOW dee um bye KAR bun ate)

Synonyms baking soda; $NaHCO_3$; sodium acid carbonate; sodium hydrogen carbonate

U.S./Canadian Brand Names Brioschi® [US-OTC]; Neut® [US]

Therapeutic Category Alkalinizing Agent; Antacid Electrolyte Supplement, Oral

Use Management of metabolic acidosis; gastric hyperacidity; as an alkalinization agent for the urine; treatment of hyperkalemia; management of overdose of certain drugs, including tricyclic antidepressants and aspirin

Usual Dosage

Cardiac arrest: **Routine use of NaHCO₃ is not recommended and should be given only after adequate alveolar ventilation has been established and effective cardiac compressions are provided**
Infants and Children: I.V.: 0.5-1 mEq/kg/dose repeated every 10 minutes or as indicated by arterial blood gases; rate of infusion should not exceed 10 mEq/minute; neonates and children <2 years of age should receive 4.2% (0.5 mEq/mL) solution
Adults: I.V.: Initial: 1 mEq/kg/dose one time; maintenance: 0.5 mEq/kg/dose every 10 minutes or as indicated by arterial blood gases

Metabolic acidosis: Infants, Children, and Adults: Dosage should be based on the following formula if blood gases and pH measurements are available:

HCO_3^- (mEq) = 0.3 x weight (kg) x base deficit (mEq/L)

Administer ½ dose initially, then remaining ½ dose over the next 24 hours; monitor pH, serum HCO_3^-, and clinical status

Note: If acid-base status is not available: Dose for older Children and Adults: 2-5 mEq/kg I.V. infusion over 4-8 hours; subsequent doses should be based on patient's acid-base status

Chronic renal failure: Oral: Initiate when plasma HCO_3^- <15 mEq/L

Children: 1-3 mEq/kg/day

Adults: Start with 20-36 mEq/day in divided doses, titrate to bicarbonate level of 18-20 mEq/L

Hyperkalemia: Adults: I.V.: 1 mEq/kg over 5 minutes

Renal tubular acidosis: Oral:

Distal:

Children: 2-3 mEq/kg/day

Adults: 0.5-2 mEq/kg/day in 4-5 divided doses

Proximal: Children and Adults: Initial: 5-10 mEq/kg/day; maintenance: Increase as required to maintain serum bicarbonate in the normal range

Urine alkalinization: Oral:

Children: 1-10 mEq (84-840 mg)/kg/day in divided doses every 4-6 hours; dose should be titrated to desired urinary pH

Adults: Initial: 48 mEq (4 g), then 12-24 mEq (1-2 g) every 4 hours; dose should be titrated to desired urinary pH; doses up to 16 g/day (200 mEq) in patients <60 years and 8 g (100 mEq) in patients >60 years

Antacid: Adults: Oral: 325 mg to 2 g 1-4 times/day

Dosage Forms

Granules, for solution, oral [effervescent]:

Brioschi® [OTC]: 2.69 g/packet, 2.69 g/capful

Infusion [premixed in water for injection]: 5% (500 mL)

Injection, solution:

4.2% (10 mL) [5 mEq/10 mL]

7.5% (50 mL) [8.92 mEq/10 mL]

8.4% (10 mL, 50 mL) [10 mEq/10 mL]

Neut®: 4% (5 mL) [2.4 mEq/5 mL]

Powder: Sodium bicarbonate USP (120 g, 480 g)

Tablet: 325 mg [3.8 mEq]; 650 mg [7.6 mEq]

sodium chloride (SOW dee um KLOR ide)

Synonyms NaCl; normal saline; salt

U.S./Canadian Brand Names 4-Way® Saline Moisturizing Mist [US-OTC]; Altachlore [US-OTC]; Altamist [US-OTC]; Ayr® Allergy Sinus [US-OTC]; Ayr® Baby Saline [US-OTC]; Ayr® Saline No-Drip [US-OTC]; Ayr® Saline [US-OTC]; Breathe Free® [US-OTC]; Deep Sea [US-OTC]; Entsol® [US-OTC]; Humist® for Kids [US-OTC]; Humist® [US-OTC]; Hyper-Sal™ [US]; Little Noses® Saline [US-OTC]; Little Noses® Stuffy Nose Kit [US-OTC]; Muro 128® [US-OTC]; Na-Zone® [US-OTC]; Nasal Moist® Saline [US-OTC]; Nasal Spray [US-OTC]; NāSal™ [US-OTC]; Ocean® for Kids [US-OTC]; Ocean® [US-OTC]; Pretz® [US-OTC]; Saline Mist [US-OTC]; Simply Saline® Baby [US-OTC]; Simply Saline® Nasal Moist® [US-OTC]; Simply Saline® [US-OTC]; Syrex [US]; Wound Wash Saline™ [US-OTC]

Therapeutic Category Electrolyte Supplement, Oral; Lubricant, Ocular

Use

Parenteral: Restores sodium ion in patients with restricted oral intake (especially hyponatremia states or low salt syndrome). In general, parenteral saline uses:

Bacteriostatic sodium chloride: Dilution or dissolving drugs for I.M., I.V., or SubQ injections

Concentrated sodium chloride: Additive for parenteral fluid therapy

Hypertonic sodium chloride: For severe hyponatremia and hypochloremia

Hypotonic sodium chloride: Hydrating solution

Normal saline: Restores water/sodium losses

Pharmaceutical aid/diluent for infusion of compatible drug additives

Ophthalmic: Reduces corneal edema

Inhalation: Restores moisture to pulmonary system; loosens and thins congestion caused by colds or allergies; diluent for bronchodilator solutions that require dilution before inhalation

Intranasal: Restores moisture to nasal membranes

Irrigation: Wound cleansing, irrigation, and flushing

▶

◀ **Usual Dosage**

Children: I.V.: Hypertonic solutions (>0.9%) should only be used for the initial treatment of acute serious symptomatic hyponatremia; maintenance: 3-4 mEq/kg/day; maximum: 100-150 mEq/day; dosage varies widely depending on clinical condition

Replacement: Determined by laboratory determinations mEq

Sodium deficiency (mEq/kg) = [% dehydration (L/kg)/100 x 70 (mEq/L)] + [0.6 (L/kg) x (140 - serum sodium) (mEq/L)]

Children ≥2 years and Adults:

Intranasal: 2-3 sprays in each nostril as needed

Irrigation: Spray affected area

Children and Adults: Inhalation: Bronchodilator diluent: 1-3 sprays (1-3 mL) to dilute bronchodilator solution in nebulizer prior to administration

Adults:

GU irrigant: 1-3 L/day by intermittent irrigation

Replacement I.V.: Determined by laboratory determinations mEq

Sodium deficiency (mEq/kg) = [% dehydration (L/kg)/100 x 70 (mEq/L)] + [0.6 (L/kg) x (140 - serum sodium) (mEq/L)]

To correct acute, serious hyponatremia: mEq sodium = [desired sodium (mEq/L) - actual sodium (mEq/L)] x [0.6 x wt (kg)]; for acute correction use 125 mEq/L as the desired serum sodium; acutely correct serum sodium in 5 mEq/L/dose increments; more gradual correction in increments of 10 mEq/L/day is indicated in the asymptomatic patient

Chloride maintenance electrolyte requirement in parenteral nutrition: 2-4 mEq/kg/24 hours or 25-40 mEq/1000 kcals/24 hours; maximum: 100-150 mEq/24 hours

Sodium maintenance electrolyte requirement in parenteral nutrition: 3-4 mEq/kg/24 hours or 25-40 mEq/1000 kcals/24 hours; maximum: 100-150 mEq/24 hours.

Ophthalmic:

Ointment: Apply once daily or more often

Solution: Instill 1-2 drops into affected eye(s) every 3-4 hours

Dosage Forms

Aerosol, intranasal [spray; preservative free]:

Entsol® [OTC]: 3% (100 mL)

Gel, intranasal:

Ayr® Saline [OTC]: <0.5% (14 g)

Entsol® [OTC]: 3% (20 g)

Simply Saline® Nasal Moist®: 0.65% (30 g) [contains aloe]

Gel, intranasal [spray]:

Ayr® Saline No-Drip [OTC]: <0.5% (22 mL)

Injection, solution: 0.45% (25 mL, 50 mL, 100 mL, 250 mL, 500 mL, 1000 mL); 0.9% (25 mL, 50 mL, 100 mL, 150 mL, 250 mL, 500 mL, 1000 mL, 1 g); 3% (500 mL); 5% (500 mL)

Injection, solution [preservative free]: 0.9% (2 mL, 3 mL, 5 mL, 10 mL, 20 mL, 50 mL, 100 mL)

Injection, solution [I.V. flush]: 0.9% (10 mL)

Injection, solution [I.V. flush; preservative free]: 0.9% (1 mL, 2 mL, 2.5 mL, 3 mL, 5 mL, 10 mL)

Syrex: 0.9% (2.5 mL, 3 mL, 5 mL, 10 mL)

Injection, solution [bacteriostatic]: 0.9% (10 mL, 20 mL, 30 mL)

Injection, solution [concentrate]: 14.6% (40 mL); 23.4% (100 mL, 250 mL)

Injection, solution [concentrate; preservative free]: 14.6% (20 mL, 40 mL); 23.4% (30 mL, 100 mL, 200 mL)

Ointment, ophthalmic: 5% (3.5 g)

Altachlore [OTC]: 5% (3.5 g)

Ointment, ophthalmic [preservative free]:

Muro 128®: 5% (3.5 g)

Powder for solution, intranasal [preservative free]:

Entsol® [OTC]: 3% (10.5 g)

Solution for blood processing [not for injection]: 0.9% (3000 mL)

Solution for inhalation [preservative free]: 0.9% (3 mL, 5 mL, 15 mL); 3% (15 mL)

Solution for inhalation [hypertonic; preservative free]: 10% (15 mL)

Solution for inhalation [hypotonic; preservative free]: 0.45% (5 mL)

Solution for injection [I.V. flush; preservative free]: 0.9% (2.5 mL, 5 mL, 10 mL)

Solution for irrigation: 0.45% (2000 mL); 0.9% (250 mL, 500 mL, 1000 mL, 1500 mL, 2000 mL, 3000 mL, 4000 mL, 5000 mL)

Solution for irrigation [preservative free]: 0.45% (2000 mL); 0.9% (250 mL, 500 mL, 1000 mL, 1500 mL, 2000 mL, 3000 mL)

Solution for irrigation [slush solution]: 0.9% (1000 mL)
Solution for nebulization [preservative free]:
  Hyper-Sal™: 7% (4 mL)
Solution, intranasal [preservative free]:
  Simply Saline®: 3% (44 mL)
Solution, intranasal [drops]:
  Humist®: 0.65% (45 mL)
  Humist® for Kids: 0.65% (30 mL)
  Ayr® Saline [OTC]: 0.65% (50 mL)
  NāSal™ [OTC]: 0.65% (15 mL)
Solution, intranasal [drops, mist, spray]:
  Ocean® [OTC]: 0.65% (45 mL, 473 mL)
  Ocean® for Kids [OTC]: 0.65% (37.5 mL)
Solution, intranasal [drops, spray]:
  Ayr® Baby Saline [OTC]: 0.65% (30 mL)
  Little Noses® Saline: 0.65% (30 mL)
  Little Noses® Stuffy Nose Kit: 0.65% (15 mL)
Solution, intranasal [irrigation]:
  Pretz® [OTC]: 0.75% (237 mL, 960 mL)
Solution, intranasal [mist]:
  Ayr® Allergy Sinus [OTC]: 2.65% (50 mL)
  Ayr® Saline [OTC]: 0.65% (50 mL)
  Entsol® [OTC]: 3% (30 mL)
  Saline Mist [OTC]: 0.65% (45 mL)
  4-Way® Moisturizing Mist: 0.74% (29.6 mL)
Solution, intranasal [mist, preservative free]:
  Simply Saline®: 0.9% (44 mL, 90 mL)
  Simply Saline® Baby: 0.9% (45 mL)
Solution, intranasal [nasal wash; preservative free]:
  Entsol® [OTC]: 3% (240 mL)
Solution, intranasal [spray]:
  Altamist [OTC], Na-Zone® [OTC]: 0.65% (60 mL)
  Breathe Free® [OTC]: 0.65% (44.3 mL)
  Deep Sea [OTC], Nasal Moist® Saline [OTC], Nasal Spray [OTC]: 0.65% (45 mL)
  NāSal™ [OTC]: 0.65% (30 mL)
Solution, intranasal [spray, isotonic, buffered]:
  Pretz® [OTC]: 0.75% (50 mL)
Solution, ophthalmic: 5% (15 mL)
Solution, ophthalmic [drops]: 5% (15 mL)
  Altachlore [OTC]: 5% (15 mL, 30 mL)
  Muro 128®: 2% (15 mL); 5% (15 mL, 30 mL)
Solution, topical [preservative free]:
  Wound Wash Saline™: 0.9% (90 mL, 210 mL)
Swab, intranasal:
  Ayr® Saline [OTC]: <0.5% (20)
Tablet for solution, topical: 1000 mg

sodium chondroitin sulfate and sodium hyaluronate
(SOW de um kon DROY tin SUL fate & SOW de um hye al yoor ON ate)

Synonyms chondroitin sulfate and sodium hyaluronate; sodium hyaluronate and chondroitin sulfate

U.S./Canadian Brand Names DisCoVisc® [US]; Viscoat® [US]

Therapeutic Category Ophthalmic Agent, Viscoelastic

Use Ophthalmic surgical aid in the anterior segment during cataract extraction and intraocular lens implantation

Usual Dosage Ophthalmic: Adults: Carefully introduce (using a 27-gauge cannula) into anterior chamber during surgery

Dosage Forms
Injection, solution, intraocular:
  DisCoVisc™: Sodium chondroitin sulfate ≤4% and sodium hyaluronate ≤1.7% (0.5 mL, 1 mL)
  Viscoat®: Sodium chondroitin sulfate ≤4% and sodium hyaluronate ≤3% (0.5 mL, 0.75 mL)

sodium citrate, citric acid, and potassium citrate *see* citric acid, sodium citrate, and potassium citrate *on page 226*

Sodium Diuril® [US] *see* chlorothiazide *on page 205*

sodium edetate *see* edetate disodium *on page 333*

sodium etidronate *see* etidronate disodium *on page 382*

sodium ferric gluconate *see* ferric gluconate *on page 397*

sodium fluorescein *see* fluorescein *on page 410*

sodium fluoride *see* fluoride *on page 411*

sodium fusidate *see* fusidic acid *(Canada only) on page 431*

sodium hyaluronate *see* hyaluronate and derivatives *on page 476*

sodium hyaluronate and chondroitin sulfate *see* sodium chondroitin sulfate and sodium hyaluronate *on page 875*

sodium hydrogen carbonate *see* sodium bicarbonate *on page 872*

sodium hypochlorite solution (SOW dee um hye poe KLOR ite soe LOO shun)

Synonyms modified Dakin's solution

U.S./Canadian Brand Names Dakin's Solution [US]; Di-Dak-Sol [US]

Therapeutic Category Disinfectant

Use Treatment of athlete's foot (0.5%); wound irrigation (0.5%); disinfection of utensils and equipment (5%)

Usual Dosage Topical irrigation

Dosage Forms
  Solution, topical:
    Dakin's: 0.125% (480 mL); 0.25% (480 mL); 0.5% (480 mL, 3840 mL)
    Di-Dak-Sol: 0.0125% (480 mL)

sodium hyposulfate *see* sodium thiosulfate *on page 880*

sodium lactate (SOW dee um LAK tate)

Therapeutic Category Alkalinizing Agent

Use Source of bicarbonate for prevention and treatment of mild-to-moderate metabolic acidosis

Usual Dosage Dosage depends on degree of acidosis

Dosage Forms
  Infusion: 18.7 g (1000 mL)
  Injection, solution [concentrate; preservative free]: 560 mg/mL (10 mL)

sodium nafcillin *see* nafcillin *on page 652*

sodium nitrite, sodium thiosulfate, and amyl nitrite
(SOW dee um NYE trite, SOW dee um thye oh SUL fate, & AM il NYE trite)

Synonyms amyl nitrite, sodium thiosulfate, and sodium nitrite; cyanide antidote kit; sodium thiosulfate, sodium nitrite, and amyl nitrite

U.S./Canadian Brand Names Cyanide Antidote Package [US]

Therapeutic Category Antidote

Use Treatment of cyanide poisoning

Usual Dosage Cyanide poisoning:
  Children: 0.3 mL ampul of amyl nitrite is crushed every minute and vapor is inhaled for 15-30 seconds until an I.V. sodium nitrite infusion is available. Following administration of sodium nitrite I.V. 10 mg/kg (0.33 mL/kg or 6-8 mL/m^2 of a 3% solution; maximum: 10 mL), inject sodium thiosulfate I.V. 7 g/m^2 (maximum: 12.5 g) over ~10 minutes, if needed; injection of both may be repeated at 1/2 the original dose.
  Adults: 0.3 mL ampul of amyl nitrite is crushed every minute and vapor is inhaled for 15-30 seconds until an I.V. sodium nitrite infusion is available. Following administration of 300 mg or 10 mg/kg I.V. sodium nitrite, inject 12.5 g sodium thiosulfate I.V. (over ~10 minutes), if needed; injection of both may be repeated at 1/2 the original dose.

Dosage Forms Kit [each kit contains]:
  Cyanide Antidote Package:
    Injection, solution:
      Sodium nitrite 300 mg/10 mL (2)

Sodium thiosulfate 12.5 g/50 mL (2)
Inhalant: Amyl nitrite 0.3 mL (12)

sodium nitroferricyanide *see* nitroprusside *on page 676*
sodium nitroprusside *see* nitroprusside *on page 676*

sodium oxybate (SOW dee um ox i BATE)

Synonyms 4-hydroxybutyrate; gamma hydroxybutyric acid; GHB; sodium 4-hydroxybutyrate
U.S./Canadian Brand Names Xyrem® [US/Can]
Therapeutic Category Central Nervous System Depressant
Controlled Substance C-I (illicit use); C-III (medical use)
Use Treatment of cataplexy and daytime sleepiness in patients with narcolepsy
Usual Dosage Oral: Children ≥16 years and Adults: Narcolepsy: Initial: 4.5 g/day, in 2 equal doses; first dose to be given at bedtime after the patient is in bed, and second dose to be given 2.5-4 hours later. Dose may be increased or adjusted in 2-week intervals; average dose: 6-9 g/day (maximum: 9 g/day)
Dosage Forms
Solution, oral:
Xyrem®: 500 mg/mL

sodium PAS *see* aminosalicylic acid *on page 61*
sodium-PCA and lactic acid *see* lactic acid *on page 542*

sodium phenylacetate and sodium benzoate

(SOW dee um fen il AS e tate & SOW dee um BENZ oh ate)
Synonyms NAPA and NABZ; sodium benzoate and sodium phenylacetate
U.S./Canadian Brand Names Ammonul® [US]
Therapeutic Category Ammonium Detoxicant
Use Adjunct to treatment of acute hyperammonemia and encephalopathy in patients with urea cycle disorders involving partial or complete deficiencies of carbamyl-phosphate synthetase (CPS), ornithine transcarbamoylase (OTC), argininosuccinate lysase (ASL), or argininosuccinate synthetase (ASS); for use with hemodialysis in acute neonatal hyperammonemic coma, moderate-to-severe hyperammonemic encephalopathy and hyperammonemia which fails to respond to initial therapy
Usual Dosage Administer as a loading dose over 90-120 minutes, followed by an equivalent maintenance infusion given over 24 hours. Dosage based on weight and specific enzyme deficiency; therapy should continue until ammonia levels are in normal range.
≤20 kg:
CPS and OTC deficiency: Ammonul® 2.5 mL/kg and arginine 10% 2 mL/kg (provides sodium phenylacetate 250 mg/kg, sodium benzoate 250 mg/kg, and arginine hydrochloride 200 mg/kg).
ASS and ASL deficiency: Ammonul® 2.5 mL/kg and arginine 10% 6 mL/kg (provides sodium phenylacetate 250 mg/kg, sodium benzoate 250 mg/kg, and arginine hydrochloride 600 mg/kg)
Note: Pending a specific diagnosis in infants, the bolus and maintenance dose of arginine should be 6 mL/kg. If ASS or ASL are excluded as diagnostic possibilities, reduce dose of arginine to 2 mL/kg/day.
>20 kg:
CPS and OTC deficiency: Ammonul® 55 mL/m^2 and arginine 10% 2 mL/kg (provides sodium phenylacetate 5.5 g/m^2, sodium benzoate 5.5 g/m^2, and arginine hydrochloride 200 mg/kg)
ASS and ASL deficiency: Ammonul® 55 mL/m^2 and arginine 10% 6 mL/kg (provides sodium phenylacetate 5.5 g/m^2, sodium benzoate 5.5 g/m^2, and arginine hydrochloride 600 mg/kg)
Dosage Forms
Injection, solution [concentrate]:
Ammonul®: Sodium phenylacetate 100 mg and sodium benzoate 100 mg per 1 mL (50 mL)

sodium phenylbutyrate (SOW dee um fen il BYOO ti rate)

Synonyms ammonapse
U.S./Canadian Brand Names Buphenyl® [US]
Therapeutic Category Miscellaneous Product
Use Adjunctive therapy in the chronic management of patients with urea cycle disorder involving deficiencies of carbamoylphosphate synthetase, ornithine transcarbamylase, or argininosuccinic acid synthetase

◀ **Usual Dosage** Oral: Management of urea cycle disorders:
   Children <20 kg: Powder: 450-600 mg/kg/day, administered in equally divided amounts with each meal or feeding, 3-6 times daily (maximum dose: 20 g/day)
   Children ≥20 kg and Adults: Powder or tablet: 9.9-13 g/m^2/day, administered in equally divided amounts with each meal or feeding, 3-6 times daily (maximum dose: 20 g/day)

Dosage Forms
   Powder, for oral solution:
   Buphenyl®: 3 g/level teaspoon
   Tablet:
   Buphenyl®: 500 mg

sodium phosphate and potassium phosphate *see* potassium phosphate and sodium phosphate *on page 775*

sodium phosphates (SOW dee um FOS fates)
Sound-Alike/Look-Alike Issues
   Visicol® may be confused with VESIcare®
U.S./Canadian Brand Names Fleet® Enema Extra® [US-OTC]; Fleet® Enema for Children [US-OTC]; Fleet® Enema [US-OTC/Can]; Fleet® Phospho-soda® EZ-Prep™ [US-OTC]; Fleet® Phospho-Soda® Oral Laxative [Can]; Fleet® Phospho-soda® [US-OTC]; LaCrosse Complete [US-OTC]; OsmoPrep™ [US]; Visicol® [US]
Therapeutic Category Electrolyte Supplement, Oral; Laxative
Use
   Oral, rectal: Short-term treatment of constipation and to evacuate the colon for rectal and bowel exams
   I.V.: Source of phosphate in large volume I.V. fluids and parenteral nutrition; treatment and prevention of hypophosphatemia
Usual Dosage
   Normal requirements elemental phosphorus: Oral:
   0-6 months: Adequate intake: 100 mg/day
   6-12 months: Adequate intake: 275 mg/day
   1-3 years: RDA: 460 mg
   4-8 years: RDA: 500 mg
   9-18 years: RDA: 1250 mg
   ≥19 years: RDA: 700 mg

Hypophosphatemia: It is difficult to provide concrete guidelines for the treatment of severe hypophosphatemia because the extent of total body deficits and response to therapy are difficult to predict. Aggressive doses of phosphate may result in a transient serum elevation followed by redistribution into intracellular compartments or bone tissue. Intermittent I.V. infusion should be reserved for severe depletion situations (<1 mg/dL in adults); large doses of oral phosphate may cause diarrhea and intestinal absorption may be unreliable. I.V. solutions should be infused slowly. Use caution when mixing with calcium and magnesium, precipitate may form. The following dosages are empiric guidelines. **Note:** 1 mmol phosphate = 31 mg phosphorus; 1 mg phosphorus = 0.032 mmol phosphate

Hypophosphatemia treatment: Doses listed as mmol of phosphate:
Intermittent I.V. infusion: Acute repletion or replacement:
   Children:
     Low dose: 0.08 mmol/kg over 6 hours; use if losses are recent and uncomplicated
     Intermediate dose: 0.16-0.24 mmol/kg over 4-6 hours; use if serum phosphorus level 0.5-1 mg/dL
     High dose: 0.36 mmol/kg over 6 hours; use if serum phosphorus <0.5 mg/dL
   Adults: Varying dosages: 0.15-0.3 mmol/kg/dose over 12 hours; may repeat as needed to achieve desired serum level **or**
     15 mmol/dose over 2 hours; use if serum phosphorus <2 mg/dL **or**
     Low dose: 0.16 mmol/kg over 4-6 hours; use if serum phosphorus level 2.3-3 mg/dL
     Intermediate dose: 0.32 mmol/kg over 4-6 hours; use if serum phosphorus level 1.6-2.2 mg/dL
     High dose: 0.64 mmol/kg over 8-12 hours; use if serum phosphorus <1.5 mg/dL
   Oral: Adults: 0.5-1 g elemental phosphorus 2-3 times/day may be used when serum phosphorus level is 1-2.5 mg/dL
Maintenance: Doses listed as mmol of phosphate:
   Children:
     Oral: 2-3 mmol/kg/day in divided doses
     I.V.: 0.5-1.5 mmol/kg/day

Adults:
Oral: 50-150 mmol/day in divided doses
I.V.: 50-70 mmol/day

Laxative (Fleet®): Rectal:
Children 2-<5 years: One-half contents of one 2.25 oz pediatric enema
Children 5-12 years: Contents of one 2.25 oz pediatric enema, may repeat
Children ≥12 years and Adults: Contents of one 4.5 oz enema as a single dose, may repeat

Laxative (Fleet® Phospho-Soda®): Oral: Take on an empty stomach; dilute dose with 8 ounces cool water, then follow dose with 8 ounces water; **do not repeat dose within 24 hours**
Children 5-9 years: 7.5 mL as a single dose; maximum daily dose: 7.5 mL
Children 10-12 years: 15 mL as a single dose; maximum daily dose: 15 mL
Children ≥12 years and Adults: 15 mL as a single dose; maximum daily dose: 45 mL

Bowel cleansing prior to colonoscopy: Adults: **Note:** Each dose should be taken with a minimum of 8 ounces of clear liquids. Do not repeat treatment within 7 days. Do not use additional agents, especially sodium phosphate products.
Fleet® Phospho-Soda®: Oral: Prior to procedure (timing of doses determined by prescriber): One dose is equal to 45 mL (2 doses are recommended): Each dose is diluted as follows:
Mix 45 mL with 120 mL clear liquid; drink, then follow with at least 240 mL of clear liquid; **or**
Mix 15 mL with 240 mL clear liquid; drink, then follow with 240 mL clear liquid; repeat every 10 minutes for a total of 45 mL
Visicol®: Oral: Adults: A total of 40 tablets divided as follows:
Evening before colonoscopy: 3 tablets every 15 minutes for 6 doses, then 2 additional tablets in 15 minutes (total of 20 tablets)
3-5 hours prior to colonoscopy: 3 tablets every 15 minutes for 6 doses, then 2 additional tablets in 15 minutes (total of 20 tablets)
OsmoPrep™: A total of 32 tablets divided as follows:
Evening before colonoscopy: 4 tablets every 15 minutes for 5 doses (total of 20 tablets)
3-5 hours prior to colonoscopy: 4 tablets every 15 minutes for 3 doses (total of 12 tablets)

Dosage Forms
Kit:
Fleet® Phospho-soda® EZ-Prep™ [OTC]:
Solution, oral: Monobasic sodium phosphate 2.4 g and dibasic sodium phosphate 0.9 g per 5 mL (30 mL)
Solution, oral: Monobasic sodium phosphate 2.4 g and dibasic sodium phosphate 0.9 g per 5 mL (45 mL)
Injection, solution [concentrate; preservative free]: Phosphorus 3 mmol and sodium 4 mEq per 1 mL (5 mL, 15 mL, 50 mL)
Solution, oral: Monobasic sodium phosphate 2.4 g and dibasic sodium phosphate 0.9 g per 5 mL (45 mL)
Fleet® Phospho-soda® [OTC]: Monobasic sodium phosphate 2.4 g and dibasic sodium phosphate 0.9 g per 5 mL (45 mL)
Solution, rectal [enema]: Monobasic sodium phosphate 19 g and dibasic sodium phosphate 7 g per 118 mL delivered dose (133 mL)
Fleet® Enema [OTC], LaCrosse Complete [OTC]: Monobasic sodium phosphate 19 g and dibasic sodium phosphate 7 g per 118 mL delivered dose (133 mL)
Fleet® Enema Extra® [OTC]: Monobasic sodium phosphate 19 g and dibasic sodium phosphate 7 g per 197 mL delivered dose (230 mL)
Fleet® Enema for Children [OTC]: Monobasic sodium phosphate 9.5 g and dibasic sodium phosphate 3.5 g per 59 mL delivered dose (66 mL)
Tablet, oral [scored]:
OsmoPrep™, Visicol®: Monobasic sodium phosphate 1.102 g and dibasic sodium phosphate 0.398 g

sodium polystyrene sulfonate (SOW dee um pol ee STYE reen SUL fon ate)

Sound-Alike/Look-Alike Issues
Kayexalate® may be confused with Kaopectate®
U.S./Canadian Brand Names Kayexalate® [US/Can]; Kionex® [US]; PMS-Sodium Polystyrene Sulfonate [Can]; SPS® [US]
Therapeutic Category Antidote

◀ **Use** Treatment of hyperkalemia
Usual Dosage
Children:
Oral: 1 g/kg/dose every 6 hours
Rectal: 1 g/kg/dose every 2-6 hours (In small children and infants, employ lower doses by using the practical exchange ratio of 1 mEq K$^+$/g of resin as the basis for calculation)
Adults: Hyperkalemia:
Oral: 15 g 1-4 times/day
Rectal: 30-50 g every 6 hours
Dosage Forms
Powder for suspension, oral/rectal: 15 g/4 level teaspoons
Kayexalate®, Kionex®: 15 g/4 level teaspoons
Suspension, oral/rectal: 15 g/60 mL
SPS®: 15 g/60 mL

sodium sulfacetamide *see* sulfacetamide *on page 892*
sodium sulfacetamide and sulfur *see* sulfur and sulfacetamide *on page 897*

sodium tetradecyl (SOW dee um tetra DEK il)

Synonyms sodium tetradecyl sulfate
U.S./Canadian Brand Names Sotradecol® [US]; Trombovar® [Can]
Therapeutic Category Sclerosing Agent
Use Treatment of small, uncomplicated varicose veins of the lower extremities
Usual Dosage I.V.: Test dose: 0.5 mL given several hours prior to administration of larger dose; 0.5-2 mL (preferred maximum: 1 mL) in each vein, maximum: 10 mL per treatment session; 3% solution reserved for large varices
Dosage Forms
Injection:
Sotradecol®: 1% (2 mL); 3% (2 mL)

sodium tetradecyl sulfate *see* sodium tetradecyl *on page 880*

sodium thiosulfate (SOW dee um thye oh SUL fate)

Synonyms disodium thiosulfate pentahydrate; pentahydrate; sodium hyposulfate; sodium thiosulphate; thiosulfuric acid disodium salt
U.S./Canadian Brand Names Versiclear™ [US]
Therapeutic Category Antidote; Antifungal Agent
Use
Parenteral: Used alone or with sodium nitrite or amyl nitrite in cyanide poisoning; reduce the risk of nephrotoxicity associated with cisplatin therapy
Topical: Treatment of tinea versicolor
Usual Dosage
Cyanide and nitroprusside antidote: I.V.:
Children <25 kg: 50 mg/kg after receiving 4.5-10 mg/kg sodium nitrite; a half dose of each may be repeated if necessary
Children >25 kg and Adults: 12.5 g after 300 mg of sodium nitrite; a half dose of each may be repeated if necessary
Cyanide poisoning: I.V.: Dose should be based on determination as with nitrite, at rate of 2.5-5 mL/minute to maximum of 50 mL.
Cisplatin rescue should be given before or during cisplatin administration: I.V. infusion (in sterile water): 12 g/m^2 over 6 hours or 9 g/m^2 I.V. push followed by 1.2 g/m^2 continuous infusion for 6 hours
Tinea versicolor: Children and Adults: Topical: 20% to 25% solution: Apply a thin layer to affected areas twice daily
Dosage Forms
Injection, solution [preservative free]: 100 mg/mL (10 mL); 250 mg/mL (50 mL)
Versiclear™: 100 mg/mL (10 mL); 250 mg/mL (50 mL)
Lotion:
Versiclear™: Sodium thiosulfate 25% and salicylic acid 1% (120 mL)

sodium thiosulfate, sodium nitrite, and amyl nitrite *see* sodium nitrite, sodium thiosulfate, and amyl nitrite *on page 876*

sodium thiosulphate *see* sodium thiosulfate *on page 880*
Soflax™ [Can] *see* docusate *on page 314*
Sofra-Tulle® [Can] *see* framycetin *(Canada only) on page 428*
Sojourn™ [US] *see* sevoflurane *on page 864*
Solagé® [US/Can] *see* mequinol and tretinoin *on page 606*
Solaquin® [US-OTC/Can] *see* hydroquinone *on page 488*
Solaquin Forte® [US/Can] *see* hydroquinone *on page 488*
Solaraze® [US] *see* diclofenac *on page 292*
Solarcaine® Aloe Extra Burn Relief [US-OTC] *see* lidocaine *on page 561*
Solfoton® *(Discontinued)* *see* phenobarbital *on page 742*
Solia™ [US] *see* ethinyl estradiol and desogestrel *on page 369*

solifenacin (sol i FEN a sin)

Sound-Alike/Look-Alike Issues
  VESIcare® may be confused with Visicol®
Synonyms solifenacin succinate; YM905
U.S./Canadian Brand Names VESIcare® [US]
Therapeutic Category Anticholinergic Agent
Use Treatment of overactive bladder with symptoms of urinary frequency, urgency, or urge incontinence
Usual Dosage Oral: Adults: 5 mg/day; if tolerated, may increase to 10 mg/day
Dosage Forms
  Tablet:
    VESIcare®: 5 mg, 10 mg

solifenacin succinate *see* solifenacin *on page 881*
Soliris™ [US] *see* eculizumab *on page 332*
Solodyn™ [US] *see* minocycline *on page 635*
Soltamox™ *(Discontinued)* *see* tamoxifen *on page 902*
soluble fluorescein *see* fluorescein *on page 410*
Solu-Cortef® [US/Can] *see* hydrocortisone (systemic) *on page 484*
Solugel® [Can] *see* benzoyl peroxide *on page 126*
Solu-Medrol® [US/Can] *see* methylprednisolone *on page 623*
Soluver® [Can] *see* salicylic acid *on page 850*
Soluver® Plus [Can] *see* salicylic acid *on page 850*
Soma® [US/Can] *see* carisoprodol *on page 180*
Soma® Compound [US] *see* carisoprodol and aspirin *on page 180*
Soma® Compound w/Codeine *(Discontinued)* *see* carisoprodol, aspirin, and codeine *on page 180*

somatostatin *(Canada only)* (soe mat oh STA tin)

Therapeutic Category Variceal Bleeding (Acute) Agent
Use For the symptomatic treatment of acute bleeding from esophageal varices. Other treatment options for long-term management of the condition may be considered if necessary, once initial control has been established.
Usual Dosage Slow 250 mcg I.V. bolus injection over 3 to 5 minutes, followed by a continuous infusion at a rate of 250 mcg/hour until bleeding from the varices has stopped (usually within 12-24 hours). Once bleeding has been controlled, it is recommended that the infusion be continued for at least another 48 to 72 hours, or out to a maximum of 120 hours to prevent recurrent bleeding.
Dosage Forms
  Injection: 250 mcg, 3 mg

somatrem *see* somatropin *on page 881*

somatropin (soe ma TROE pin)

Sound-Alike/Look-Alike Issues
  somatropin may be confused with somatrem, sumatriptan
  somatrem may be confused with somatropin
Synonyms hGH; human growth hormone; somatrem

◀ **U.S./Canadian Brand Names** Genotropin Miniquick® [US]; Genotropin® [US]; Humatrope® [US/Can]; Norditropin® NordiFlex® [US]; Norditropin® [US]; Nutropin AQ® [US/Can]; Nutropine® [Can]; Nutropin® [US]; Omnitrope™ [US]; Saizen® [US/Can]; Serostim® [US/Can]; Tev-Tropin® [US]; Zorbtive® [US]

Therapeutic Category Growth Hormone

Use

Children:

Treatment of growth failure due to inadequate endogenous growth hormone secretion (Genotropin®, Humatrope®, Norditropin®, Nutropin®, Nutropin AQ®, Omnitrope™, Saizen®, Tev-Tropin®)

Treatment of short stature associated with Turner syndrome (Genotropin®, Humatrope®, Norditropin®, Nutropin®, Nutropin AQ®)

Treatment of Prader-Willi syndrome (Genotropin®)

Treatment of growth failure associated with chronic renal insufficiency (CRI) up until the time of renal transplantation (Nutropin®, Nutropin AQ®)

Treatment of growth failure in children born small for gestational age who fail to manifest catch-up growth by 2 years of age (Genotropin®)

Treatment of idiopathic short stature (nongrowth hormone-deficient short stature) defined by height standard deviation score (SDS) less than or equal to -2.25 and growth rate not likely to attain normal adult height (Genotropin®, Humatrope®, Nutropin®, Nutropin AQ®)

Treatment of short stature or growth failure associated with short stature homeobox gene (SHOX) deficiency (Humatrope®)

Treatment of short stature associated with Noonan syndrome (Norditropin®)

Adults:

HIV patients with wasting or cachexia with concomitant antiviral therapy (Serostim®)

Replacement of endogenous growth hormone in patients with adult growth hormone deficiency who meet both of the following criteria (Genotropin®, Humatrope®, Norditropin®, Nutropin®, Nutropin AQ®, Omnitrope™, Saizen®):

Biochemical diagnosis of adult growth hormone deficiency by means of a subnormal response to a standard growth hormone stimulation test (peak growth hormone ≤5 mcg/L). Confirmatory testing may not be required in patients with congenital/genetic growth hormone deficiency or multiple pituitary hormone deficiencies due to organic diseases.

and

Adult-onset: Patients who have adult growth hormone deficiency whether alone or with multiple hormone deficiencies (hypopituitarism) as a result of pituitary disease, hypothalamic disease, surgery, radiation therapy, or trauma

or

Childhood-onset: Patients who were growth hormone deficient during childhood, confirmed as an adult before replacement therapy is initiated

Treatment of short-bowel syndrome (Zorbtive®)

Usual Dosage

Children (individualize dose):

Chronic renal insufficiency (CRI): Nutropin®, Nutropin® AQ: SubQ: Weekly dosage: 0.35 mg/kg divided into daily injections; continue until the time of renal transplantation

Dosage recommendations in patients treated for CRI who require dialysis:

Hemodialysis: Administer dose at night prior to bedtime or at least 3-4 hours after hemodialysis to prevent hematoma formation from heparin

CCPD: Administer dose in the morning following dialysis

CAPD: Administer dose in the evening at the time of overnight exchange

Growth hormone deficiency:

Genotropin®, Omnitrope™: SubQ: Weekly dosage: 0.16-0.24 mg/kg divided into 6-7 daily doses

Humatrope®: I.M., SubQ: Weekly dosage: 0.18 mg/kg; maximum replacement dose: 0.3 mg/kg/week; dosing should be divided into equal doses given 3 times/week on alternating days, 6 times/week, or daily

Norditropin®: SubQ: 0.024-0.034 mg/kg/day, 6-7 times/week

Nutropin®, Nutropin® AQ: SubQ: Weekly dosage: 0.3 mg/kg divided into daily doses; pubertal patients: ≤0.7 mg/kg/week divided daily

Tev-Tropin®: SubQ: Up to 0.1 mg/kg administered 3 times/week

Saizen®: I.M., SubQ: 0.18 mg/kg/week in divided doses administered daily **or** as 0.06 mg/kg/dose administered 3 times/week **or** as 0.03 mg/kg/dose administered 6 times/week

Note: Therapy should be discontinued when patient has reached satisfactory adult height, when epiphyses have fused, or when the patient ceases to respond. Growth of 5 cm/year or more is expected, if growth rate does not exceed 2.5 cm in a 6-month period, double the dose for the next 6 months; if there is still no satisfactory response, discontinue therapy

Idiopathic short stature:
Humatrope®: SubQ: Weekly dosage: 0.37 mg/kg divided into equal doses 6-7 times per week
Nutropin®, Nutropin AQ®: SubQ: Weekly dosage: Up to 0.3 mg/kg divided into daily doses
Noonan syndrome: Norditropin®: SubQ: Up to 0.066 mg/kg/day
Prader-Willi syndrome: Genotropin®: SubQ: Weekly dosage: 0.24 mg/kg divided into 6-7 doses
SHOX deficiency: Humatrope®: SubQ: 0.35 mg/kg/week divided into equal daily doses
Small for gestational age: Genotropin®: SubQ: Weekly dosage: 0.48 mg/kg divided into 6-7 doses
Turner syndrome:
Genotropin®: SubQ: Weekly dosage: 0.33 mg/kg divided into 6-7 doses
Humatrope®, Nutropin®, Nutropin® AQ: SubQ: Weekly dosage: ≤0.375 mg/kg divided into equal doses 3-7 times per week
Norditropin®: Up to 0.067 mg/kg/day

Adults:
Growth hormone deficiency: Adjust dose based on individual requirements: To minimize adverse events in older or overweight patients, reduced dosages may be necessary. During therapy, dosage should be decreased if required by the occurrence of side effects or excessive IGF-I levels.
Norditropin®: SubQ: Initial dose ≤0.004 mg/kg/day; after 6 weeks of therapy, may increase dose up to 0.016 mg/kg/day
Nutropin®, Nutropin® AQ: SubQ: ≤0.006 mg/kg/day; dose may be increased up to a maximum of 0.025 mg/kg/day in patients <35 years of age, or up to a maximum of 0.0125 mg/kg/day in patients ≥35 years of age
Humatrope®: SubQ: ≤0.006 mg/kg/day; dose may be increased up to a maximum of 0.0125 mg/kg/day
Genotropin®, Omnitrope™: SubQ: Weekly dosage: ≤0.04 mg/kg divided into 6-7 daily doses; dose may be increased at 4- to 8-week intervals to a maximum of 0.08 mg/kg/week
Saizen®: SubQ: ≤0.005 mg/kg/day; dose may be increased to not more than 0.01 mg/kg/day after 4 weeks
Alternate dosing (growth hormone deficiency): SubQ: Initial: 0.2 mg/day (range: 0.15-0.3 mg/day); may increase every 1-2 months by 0.1-0.2 mg/day
Dosage adjustment with estrogen supplementation (growth hormone deficiency): Larger doses of somatropin may be needed for women taking oral estrogen replacement products; dosing not affected by topical products
HIV patients with wasting or cachexia: Serostim®: SubQ: 0.1 mg/kg once daily at bedtime (maximum: 6 mg/day). Alternately, patients at risk for side effects may be started at 0.1 mg/kg every other day. Patients who continue to lose weight after 12 weeks should be re-evaluated for opportunistic infections or other clinical events; rotate injection sites to avoid lipodystrophy Adjust dose if needed to manage side effects.
Daily dose based on body weight:
<35 kg: 0.1 mg/kg
35-45 kg: 4 mg
45-55 kg: 5 mg
>55 kg: 6 mg
Short-bowel syndrome (Zorbtive®): SubQ: 0.1 mg/kg once daily for 4 weeks (maximum: 8 mg/day)
Fluid retention (moderate) or arthralgias: Treat symptomatically or reduce dose by 50%
Severe toxicity: Discontinue therapy for up to 5 days; when symptoms resolve, restart at 50% of dose. If severe toxicity recurs or does not disappear within 5 days after discontinuation, permanently discontinue treatment.

Dosage Forms
Injection, powder for reconstitution [rDNA origin]:
Genotropin®: 5.8 mg [~15 int. units/mL]; 13.8 mg [~36 int. units/mL]
Genotropin Miniquick® [preservative free]: 0.2 mg, 0.4 mg, 0.6 mg, 0.8 mg, 1 mg, 1.2 mg, 1.4 mg, 1.6 mg, 1.8 mg, 2 mg
Humatrope®: 5 mg [15 int. units], 6 mg [18 int. units], 12 mg [36 int. units], 24 mg [72 int. units]
Nutropin®: 5 mg [~15 int. units]; 10 mg [~30 int. units]
Omnitrope™: 5.8 mg [~17.4 int. units]
Saizen®: 5 mg [~15 int. units]; 8.8 mg [~26.4 int. units]
Serostim®: 4 mg [~12 int. units]; 5 mg [15 int. units]; 6 mg [18 int. units]; 8.8 mg [~26.4 int. units]
Tev-Tropin®: 5 mg [15 int. units/mL]
Zorbtive®: 8.8 mg [~26.4 int. units]

◀ **Injection, solution** [rDNA origin]:
Norditropin®: 5 mg/1.5 mL (1.5 mL); 15 mg/1.5 mL (1.5 mL)
Norditropin® NordiFlex®: 5 mg/1.5 mL (1.5 mL); 10 mg/1.5 mL (1.5 mL); 15 mg/1.5 mL (1.5 mL)
Nutropin AQ®: 5 mg/mL [~15 int. units/mL] (2 mL)
Omnitrope™: 5 mg/1.5 mL (1.5 mL)

Somatuline® Autogel® [Can] see lanreotide on page 547
Somatuline® Depot [US] see lanreotide on page 547
Somavert® [US/Can] see pegvisomant on page 729
Sominex® [US-OTC] see diphenhydramine on page 304
Sominex® Maximum Strength [US-OTC] see diphenhydramine on page 304
Somnote® [US] see chloral hydrate on page 199
Som Pam [Can] see flurazepam on page 416
Sonata® [US] see zaleplon on page 989
Soothe® [US-OTC] see artificial tears on page 95
Soothing Care™ Itch Relief [US-OTC] see pramoxine on page 777

sorafenib (sor AF e nib)

Sound-Alike/Look-Alike Issues
Nexavar® may be confused with Nexium®
Synonyms BAY 43-9006; NSC-724772; sorafenib tosylate
U.S./Canadian Brand Names Nexavar® [US]
Therapeutic Category Antineoplastic Agent, Tyrosine Kinase Inhibitor; Vascular Endothelial Growth Factor (VEGF) Inhibitor
Use Treatment of advanced renal cell cancer (RCC), unresectable hepatocellular cancer (HCC)
Usual Dosage Oral: Adults:
Advanced renal cell carcinoma: 400 mg twice daily
Hepatocellular cancer: 400 mg twice daily
Dosage Forms
Tablet:
Nexavar®: 200 mg

sorafenib tosylate see sorafenib on page 884

sorbitol (SOR bi tole)

Therapeutic Category Genitourinary Irrigant; Laxative
Use Genitourinary irrigant in transurethral prostatic resection or other transurethral resection or other transurethral surgical procedures; diuretic; humectant; sweetening agent; hyperosmotic laxative; facilitate the passage of sodium polystyrene sulfonate through the intestinal tract
Usual Dosage Hyperosmotic laxative (as single dose, at infrequent intervals):
Children 2-11 years:
Oral: 2 mL/kg (as 70% solution)
Rectal enema: 30-60 mL as 25% to 30% solution
Children >12 years and Adults:
Oral: 30-150 mL (as 70% solution)
Rectal enema: 120 mL as 25% to 30% solution
Adjunct to sodium polystyrene sulfonate: 15 mL as 70% solution orally until diarrhea occurs (10-20 mL/2 hours) or 20-100 mL as an oral vehicle for the sodium polystyrene sulfonate resin
When administered with charcoal:
Oral:
Children: 4.3 mL/kg of 35% sorbitol with 1 g/kg of activated charcoal
Adults: 4.3 mL/kg of 70% sorbitol with 1 g/kg of activated charcoal every 4 hours until first stool containing charcoal is passed
Topical: 3% to 3.3% as transurethral surgical procedure irrigation
Dosage Forms
Solution, genitourinary irrigation: 3% (3000 mL, 5000 mL); 3.3% (2000 mL, 4000 mL)
Solution, oral: 70%

Sorbitrate® (Discontinued) see isosorbide dinitrate on page 530
Soriatane® [Can] see acitretin on page 31
Soriatane® CK Convenience Kit™ [US] see acitretin on page 31
Soriatane® (Discontinued) see acitretin on page 31

Sorine® [US] *see* sotalol *on page 885*
Sotacor® [Can] *see* sotalol *on page 885*

sotalol (SOE ta lole)

Sound-Alike/Look-Alike Issues
sotalol may be confused with Stadol®
Betapace® may be confused with Betapace AF®
Betapace AF® may be confused with Betapace®

Synonyms sotalol hydrochloride

U.S./Canadian Brand Names Alti-Sotalol [Can]; Apo-Sotalol® [Can]; Betapace AF® [US/Can]; Betapace® [US]; CO Sotalol [Can]; Gen-Sotalol [Can]; Lin-Sotalol [Can]; Novo-Sotalol [Can]; Nu-Sotalol [Can]; PMS-Sotalol [Can]; Rho®-Sotalol [Can]; Riva-Sotalol [Can]; Rylosol [Can]; Sorine® [US]; Sotacor® [Can]

Therapeutic Category Antiarrhythmic Agent, Class II; Antiarrhythmic Agent, Class III; Beta-Adrenergic Blocker, Nonselective

Use Treatment of documented ventricular arrhythmias (ie, sustained ventricular tachycardia), that in the judgment of the physician are life-threatening; maintenance of normal sinus rhythm in patients with symptomatic atrial fibrillation and atrial flutter who are currently in sinus rhythm. Manufacturer states substitutions should not be made for Betapace AF® since Betapace AF® is distributed with a patient package insert specific for atrial fibrillation/flutter.

Usual Dosage Sotalol should be initiated and doses increased in a hospital with facilities for cardiac rhythm monitoring and assessment. Proarrhythmic events can occur after initiation of therapy and with each upward dosage adjustment.

Children: Oral: The safety and efficacy of sotalol in children have not been established
 Note: Dosing per manufacturer, based on pediatric pharmacokinetic data; wait at least 36 hours between dosage adjustments to allow monitoring of QT intervals
  ≤2 years: Dosage should be adjusted (decreased) by plotting of the child's age on a logarithmic scale; refer to manufacturer's package labeling.
  >2 years: Initial: 90 mg/m^2/day in 3 divided doses; may be incrementally increased to a maximum of 180 mg/m^2/day
Adults: Oral:
 Ventricular arrhythmias (Betapace®, Sorine®):
  Initial: 80 mg twice daily
  Dose may be increased gradually to 240-320 mg/day; allow 3 days between dosing increments in order to attain steady-state plasma concentrations and to allow monitoring of QT intervals
  Most patients respond to a total daily dose of 160-320 mg/day in 2-3 divided doses.
  Some patients, with life-threatening refractory ventricular arrhythmias, may require doses as high as 480-640 mg/day; however, these doses should only be prescribed when the potential benefit outweighs the increased of adverse events.
 Atrial fibrillation or atrial flutter (Betapace AF®): Initial: 80 mg twice daily
  If the initial dose does not reduce the frequency of relapses of atrial fibrillation/flutter and is tolerated without excessive QT prolongation (not >520 msec) after 3 days, the dose may be increased to 120 mg twice daily. This may be further increased to 160 mg twice daily if response is inadequate and QT prolongation is not excessive.

Dosage Forms
 Tablet: 80 mg, 80 mg [artrial fibrillation], 120 mg, 120 mg [artrial fibrillation], 160 mg, 160 mg [artrial fibrillation], 240 mg
 Betapace®: 80 mg, 120 mg, 160 mg, 240 mg
 Betapace AF®: 80 mg, 120 mg, 160 mg [artrial fibrillation]
 Sorine®: 80 mg, 120 mg, 160 mg, 240 mg

sotalol hydrochloride *see* sotalol *on page 885*
Sotradecol® [US] *see* sodium tetradecyl *on page 880*
Sotret® [US] *see* isotretinoin *on page 531*
SourceCF® [US-OTC] *see* vitamins (multiple/pediatric) *on page 983*
SourceCF® Softgels [US] *see* vitamins (multiple/oral) *on page 983*
Soyacal® *(Discontinued) see* fat emulsion *on page 391*
Soyalac® [US-OTC] *see* nutritional formula, enteral/oral *on page 689*
SPA *see* albumin *on page 38*

Spacol *(Discontinued)* *see* hyoscyamine *on page 492*
Spacol T/S *(Discontinued)* *see* hyoscyamine *on page 492*
Span-FF® *(Discontinued)* *see* ferrous fumarate *on page 397*
Spasmolin® *(Discontinued)* *see* hyoscyamine, atropine, scopolamine, and phenobarbital *on page 493*
Spastrin® *(Discontinued)* *see* belladonna, phenobarbital, and ergotamine *on page 120*
SPD417 *see* carbamazepine *on page 172*
Spectazole® *(Discontinued)* *see* econazole *on page 332*
Spec-T® *(Discontinued)* *see* benzocaine *on page 124*

spectinomycin (spek ti noe MYE sin)

Sound-Alike/Look-Alike Issues
Trobicin® may be confused with tobramycin
Synonyms spectinomycin hydrochloride
Therapeutic Category Antibiotic, Miscellaneous
Use Treatment of uncomplicated gonorrhea
Usual Dosage I.M.:
Children:
<45 kg: 40 mg/kg/dose 1 time (ceftriaxone preferred)
≥45 kg: Refer to adult dosing.
Children >8 years who are allergic to PCNS/cephalosporins may be treated with oral tetracycline
Adults:
Uncomplicated urethral, cervical, pharyngeal, or rectal gonorrhea: 2 g deep I.M. or 4 g where antibiotic resistance is prevalent 1 time; 4 g (10 mL) dose should be given as two 5 mL injections, followed by adequate chlamydial treatment (doxycycline 100 mg twice daily for 7 days)
Disseminated gonococcal infection: 2 g every 12 hours

spectinomycin hydrochloride *see* spectinomycin *on page 886*
Spectracef® [US] *see* cefditoren *on page 185*
Spectrocin Plus™ *(Discontinued)* *see* bacitracin, neomycin, polymyxin B, and pramoxine *on page 114*
SPEF-Pioglitazone [Can] *see* pioglitazone *on page 754*
SPI 0211 *see* lubiprostone *on page 581*
Spiriva® [Can] *see* tiotropium *on page 929*
Spiriva® HandiHaler® [US] *see* tiotropium *on page 929*
Spironazide® *(Discontinued)* *see* hydrochlorothiazide and spironolactone *on page 480*

spironolactone (speer on oh LAK tone)

Sound-Alike/Look-Alike Issues
Aldactone® may be confused with Aldactazide®
U.S./Canadian Brand Names Aldactone® [US/Can]; Novo-Spiroton [Can]
Therapeutic Category Diuretic, Potassium Sparing
Use Management of edema associated with excessive aldosterone excretion; hypertension; congestive heart failure; primary hyperaldosteronism; hypokalemia; cirrhosis of liver accompanied by edema or ascites
Usual Dosage To reduce delay in onset of effect, a loading dose of 2 or 3 times the daily dose may be administered on the first day of therapy. Oral: Adults:
Edema, hypokalemia: 25-200 mg/day in 1-2 divided doses
Hypertension (JNC 7): 25-50 mg/day in 1-2 divided doses
Diagnosis of primary aldosteronism: 100-400 mg/day in 1-2 divided doses
CHF, severe (with ACE inhibitor and a loop diuretic ± digoxin): 12.5-25 mg/day; maximum daily dose: 50 mg (higher doses may occasionallly be used). In the RALES trial, 25 mg every other day was the lowest maintenance dose possible.
Note: If potassium >5.4 mEq/L, consider dosage reduction.
Dosage Forms
Tablet: 25 mg, 50 mg, 100 mg
Aldactone®: 25 mg, 50 mg, 100 mg

spironolactone and hydrochlorothiazide *see* hydrochlorothiazide and spironolactone *on page 480*

Spirozide® *(Discontinued)* *see* hydrochlorothiazide and spironolactone *on page 480*
Sporanox® [US/Can] *see* itraconazole *on page 532*
Sportscreme® [US-OTC] *see* trolamine *on page 957*
SPP100 *see* aliskiren *on page 45*
Sprayzoin™ [US-OTC] *see* benzoin *on page 126*
Spriafil® [Can] *see* posaconazole *on page 769*
Sprintec™ [US] *see* ethinyl estradiol and norgestimate *on page 378*
Sprycel® [US/Can] *see* dasatinib *on page 268*
SPS® [US] *see* sodium polystyrene sulfonate *on page 879*
SRC® Expectorant *(Discontinued)*
Sronyx™ [US] *see* ethinyl estradiol and levonorgestrel *on page 372*
SSD® [US] *see* silver sulfadiazine *on page 866*
SSD® AF [US] *see* silver sulfadiazine *on page 866*
SSKI® [US] *see* potassium iodide *on page 773*
S.T. 37® [US-OTC] *see* hexylresorcinol *on page 474*
Stadol® *(Discontinued)* *see* butorphanol *on page 157*
Stadol® NS *(Discontinued)* *see* butorphanol *on page 157*
Staflex [US] *see* acetaminophen and phenyltoloxamine *on page 22*
Stagesic® [US] *see* hydrocodone and acetaminophen *on page 481*
Stalevo® [US] *see* levodopa, carbidopa, and entacapone *on page 556*
StanGard® [US] *see* fluoride *on page 411*
StanGard® Perio [US] *see* fluoride *on page 411*
stannous fluoride *see* fluoride *on page 411*
stanozolol *(Discontinued)*
Starlix® [US/Can] *see* nateglinide *on page 659*
Statex® [Can] *see* morphine sulfate *on page 643*
Staticin® *(Discontinued)* *see* erythromycin *on page 354*
Statobex® [Can] *see* phendimetrazine *on page 742*
Statuss™ DM [US] *see* chlorpheniramine, phenylephrine, and dextromethorphan *on page 209*

stavudine (STAV yoo deen)

Sound-Alike/Look-Alike Issues
   Zerit® may be confused with Ziac®
Synonyms d4T
U.S./Canadian Brand Names Zerit® [US/Can]
Therapeutic Category Antiviral Agent
Use Treatment of HIV infection in combination with other antiretroviral agents
Usual Dosage Oral:
   Newborns (Birth to 13 days): 0.5 mg/kg every 12 hours
   Children:
      >14 days and <30 kg: 1 mg/kg every 12 hours
      ≥30 kg: Refer to Adults dosing
   Adults:
      ≥60 kg: 40 mg every 12 hours
      <60 kg: 30 mg every 12 hours
Dosage Forms
   Capsule:
      Zerit®: 15 mg, 20 mg, 30 mg, 40 mg
   Powder for solution, oral:
      Zerit®: 1 mg/mL

Stavzor™ [US] *see* valproic acid and derivatives *on page 967*
Stelazine® *(Discontinued)* *see* trifluoperazine *on page 951*
Stemetil® [Can] *see* prochlorperazine *on page 788*
Sterapred® [US] *see* prednisone *on page 782*
Sterapred® DS [US] *see* prednisone *on page 782*

sterile talc *see* talc (sterile) *on page 902*
Sterile Talc Powder™ [US] *see* talc (sterile) *on page 902*
STI571 *see* imatinib *on page 499*
Stieprox® [Can] *see* ciclopirox *on page 218*
Stimate® [US] *see* desmopressin acetate *on page 275*
Sting-Kill [US-OTC] *see* benzocaine *on page 124*
St. Joseph® Adult Aspirin [US-OTC] *see* aspirin *on page 98*
St. Joseph® Cough Suppressant *(Discontinued)* *see* dextromethorphan *on page 284*
St. Joseph® Measured Dose Nasal Solution *(Discontinued)* *see* phenylephrine *on page 745*
Stop® [US] *see* fluoride *on page 411*
Strattera® [US/Can] *see* atomoxetine *on page 102*
Streptase® *(Discontinued)*
streptokinase *(Discontinued)*

streptomycin (strep toe MYE sin)
Sound-Alike/Look-Alike Issues
streptomycin may be confused with streptozocin
Synonyms streptomycin sulfate
Therapeutic Category Antibiotic, Aminoglycoside; Antitubercular Agent
Use Part of combination therapy of active tuberculosis; used in combination with other agents for treatment of streptococcal or enterococcal endocarditis, mycobacterial infections, plague, tularemia, and brucellosis
Usual Dosage Note: For I.M. administration; I.V. use is not recommended
Usual dosage range:
Children: 20-40 mg/kg/day (maximum: 1 g)
Adults: 15-30 mg/kg/day or 1-2 g/day
Indication-specific dosing:
Children: **Tuberculosis:** I.M.:
Daily therapy: 20-40 mg/kg/day (maximum: 1 g/day)
Directly observed therapy (DOT): Twice weekly: 25-30 mg/kg (maximum: 1.5 g)
Directly observed therapy (DOT): 3 times/week: 25-30 mg/kg (maximum: 1.5 g)
Adults: I.M.:
Brucellosis: 1 g/day for 14-21 days (with doxycycline, 100 mg twice daily for 6 weeks)
Endocarditis:
Enterococcal: 1 g every 12 hours for 2 weeks, 500 mg every 12 hours for 4 weeks in combination with penicillin
Streptococcal: 1 g every 12 hours for 1 week, 500 mg every 12 hours for 1 week
***Mycobacterium avium* complex:** Adjunct therapy (with macrolide, rifamycin, and ethambutol): 15 mg/kg 3 times/week for first 2-3 months for severe disease
Plague: 15 mg/kg (or 1 g) every 12 hours until the patient is afebrile for at least 3 days
Tuberculosis:
Daily therapy: 15 mg/kg/day (maximum: 1 g)
Directly observed therapy (DOT): Twice weekly: 25-30 mg/kg (maximum: 1.5 g)
Directly observed therapy (DOT): 3 times/week: 25-30 mg/kg (maximum: 1.5 g)
Tularemia: 10-15 mg/kg every 12 hours (maximum: 2 g/day) for 7-10 days or until patient is afebrile for 5-7 days
Dosage Forms
Injection, powder for reconstitution: 1 g

streptomycin sulfate *see* streptomycin *on page 888*

streptozocin (strep toe ZOE sin)
Sound-Alike/Look-Alike Issues
streptozocin may be confused with streptomycin
Synonyms NSC-85998
U.S./Canadian Brand Names Zanosar® [US/Can]
Therapeutic Category Antineoplastic Agent
Use Treatment of metastatic islet cell carcinoma of the pancreas, carcinoid tumor and syndrome, Hodgkin disease, palliative treatment of colorectal cancer

Usual Dosage I.V. (refer to individual protocols): Children and Adults:

Single agent therapy: 1-1.5 g/m^2 weekly for 6 weeks followed by a 4-week rest period

Combination therapy: 0.5-1 g/m^2 for 5 consecutive days followed by a 4- to 6-week rest period

Dosage Forms

Injection, powder for reconstitution:

Zanosar®: 1 g

Stresstabs® High Potency Advanced [US-OTC] *see* vitamin B complex combinations *on page 981*

Stresstabs® High Potency Energy [US-OTC] *see* vitamin B complex combinations *on page 981*

Stresstabs® High Potency Weight [US-OTC] *see* vitamin B complex combinations *on page 981*

Striant® [US] *see* testosterone *on page 912*

Stridex® Essential Care® [US-OTC] *see* salicylic acid *on page 850*

Stridex® Facewipes To Go® [US-OTC] *see* salicylic acid *on page 850*

Stridex® Maximum Strength [US-OTC] *see* salicylic acid *on page 850*

Stridex® Sensitive Skin [US-OTC] *see* salicylic acid *on page 850*

Strifon Forte® [Can] *see* chlorzoxazone *on page 215*

Stromectol® [US] *see* ivermectin *on page 533*

StrongStart™ [US] *see* vitamins (multiple/prenatal) *on page 983*

strontium-89 chloride *see* strontium-89 *on page 889*

strontium-89 (STRON shee um atey nine)

Synonyms strontium-89 chloride

U.S./Canadian Brand Names Metastron® [US/Can]

Therapeutic Category Radiopharmaceutical

Use Relief of bone pain in patients with skeletal metastases

Usual Dosage I.V.: Adults: 148 megabecquerel (4 millicurie) administered by slow I.V. injection over 1-2 minutes or 1.5-2.2 megabecquerel (40-60 microcurie)/kg; repeated doses are generally not recommended at intervals <90 days; measure the patient dose by a suitable radioactivity calibration system immediately prior to administration

Dosage Forms

Injection, solution [preservative free]:

Metastron®: 10.9-22.6 mg/mL (4 mL) [148 megabecquerel, 4 millicurie per vial]

Strovite® Advance [US] *see* vitamins (multiple/oral) *on page 983*

Strovite (Discontinued) *see* vitamin B complex combinations *on page 981*

Strovite® Forte [US] *see* vitamins (multiple/oral) *on page 983*

Stuartnatal® Plus 3™ [OTC] (Discontinued) *see* vitamins (multiple/prenatal) *on page 983*

Stuart Prenatal® [US-OTC] *see* vitamins (multiple/prenatal) *on page 983*

SU11248 *see* sunitinib *on page 899*

suberoylanilide hydroxamic acid *see* vorinostat *on page 985*

Sublimaze® [US] *see* fentanyl *on page 394*

Suboxone® [US] *see* buprenorphine and naloxone *on page 151*

Subutex® [US/Can] *see* buprenorphine *on page 151*

succimer (SUKS si mer)

Synonyms DMSA

U.S./Canadian Brand Names Chemet® [US/Can]

Therapeutic Category Chelating Agent

Use Treatment of lead poisoning in children with serum lead levels >45 mcg/dL

Usual Dosage Note: For the treatment of high blood lead levels in children, the CDC recommends chelation treatment when blood lead levels are >45 mcg/dL (CDC, 2002). Children with blood lead levels >70 mcg/dL or symptomatic lead poisoning should be treated with parenteral agents (AAP, 2005). In adults, available guidelines recommend chelation therapy with blood lead levels >50 mcg/dL and significant symptoms; chelation therapy may also be indicated with blood lead levels ≥100 mcg/dL and/or symptoms.

Children: Oral: 10 mg/kg/dose (or 350 mg/m^2/dose) every 8 hours for 5 days followed by 10 mg/kg/dose (or 350 mg/m^2/dose) every 12 hours for 14 days. Maximum: 500 mg/dose. For children <5 years of age, dose should be based on mg/m^2; dosing by mg/kg may be suboptimal.

Adults (mild symptoms or blood lead levels 70-100 mg/dL; unlabeled use): 10 mg/kg/dose (or 350 mg/m^2/dose) every 8 hours for 5 days, followed by 10 mg/kg/dose (or 350 mg/m^2/dose) every 12 hours for 14 days; Maximum: 500 mg/dose

Note: Treatment courses may be repeated, but 2-week intervals between courses is generally recommended.

Dosage Forms
Capsule:
Chemet®: 100 mg

succinylcholine (suks in il KOE leen)

Synonyms succinylcholine chloride; suxamethonium chloride

U.S./Canadian Brand Names Anectine® [US]; Quelicin® [US/Can]

Therapeutic Category Skeletal Muscle Relaxant

Use Adjunct to general anesthesia to facilitate both rapid sequence and routine endotracheal intubation and to relax skeletal muscles during surgery; to reduce the intensity of muscle contractions of pharmacologically- or electrically-induced convulsions; does not relieve pain or produce sedation

Usual Dosage I.M., I.V.: Dose to effect; doses will vary due to interpatient variability; use ideal body weight for obese patients

I.M.: Children and Adults: Up to 3-4 mg/kg, total dose should not exceed 150 mg

I.V.:

Children: **Note:** Because of the risk of malignant hyperthermia, use of continuous infusions is not recommended in infants and children.

Smaller Children: Intermittent: Initial: 2 mg/kg/dose one time; maintenance: 0.3-0.6 mg/kg/dose every 5-10 minutes as needed

Older Children and Adolescents: Intermittent: Initial: 1 mg/kg/dose one time; maintenance: 0.3-0.6 mg/kg every 5-10 minutes as needed

Adults: Initial:

Short surgical procedures: 0.6 mg/kg (range 0.3-1.1 mg/kg)

Long surgical procedures:

Continuous infusion: 2.5-4.3 mg/minute; adjust dose based on response

Intermittent: Initial: 0.3-1.1 mg/kg; maintenance: 0.04-0.07 mg/kg/dose as required

Note: Initial dose of succinylcholine must be increased when nondepolarizing agent pretreatment used because of the antagonism between succinylcholine and nondepolarizing neuromuscular-blocking agents.

Dosage Forms
Injection, solution:
Anectine®: 20 mg/mL (10 mL)
Quelicin®: 20 mg/mL (10 mL)
Injection, solution [preservative free]:
Quelicin®: 100 mg/mL (10 mL)

succinylcholine chloride *see succinylcholine on page 890*
Suclor™ [US] *see chlorpheniramine and pseudoephedrine on page 207*
Sucraid® [US/Can] *see sacrosidase on page 850*

sucralfate (soo KRAL fate)

Sound-Alike/Look-Alike Issues
sucralfate may be confused with salsalate
Carafate® may be confused with Cafergot®

Synonyms aluminum sucrose sulfate, basic

U.S./Canadian Brand Names Carafate® [US]; Novo-Sucralate [Can]; Nu-Sucralate [Can]; PMS-Sucralate [Can]; Sulcrate® Suspension Plus [Can]; Sulcrate® [Can]

Therapeutic Category Gastrointestinal Agent, Gastric or Duodenal Ulcer Treatment

Use Short-term (≤8 weeks) management of duodenal ulcers; maintenance therapy for duodenal ulcers

Usual Dosage Oral: Adults: Duodenal ulcer:

Treatment: 1 g 4 times/day on an empty stomach and at bedtime for 4-8 weeks, or alternatively 2 g twice daily; treatment is recommended for 4-8 weeks in adults

Maintenance: Prophylaxis: 1 g twice daily

Dosage Forms
Suspension, oral: 1 g/10 mL (10 mL)
Carafate®: 1 g/10 mL
Tablet: 1 g
Carafate®: 1 g

Sucrets® [US-OTC] *see* dyclonine *on page 330*
Sucrets® Cough Calmers (Discontinued) *see* dextromethorphan *on page 284*
Sucrets® Original [US-OTC] *see* hexylresorcinol *on page 474*
Sudafed® 12 Hour [US-OTC] *see* pseudoephedrine *on page 801*
Sudafed® 24 Hour [US-OTC] *see* pseudoephedrine *on page 801*
Sudafed® Children's [US-OTC] *see* pseudoephedrine *on page 801*
Sudafed® Children's Cold & Cough [US-OTC] *see* pseudoephedrine and dextromethorphan *on page 802*
Sudafed® Cold & Cough Extra Strength [Can] *see* acetaminophen, dextromethorphan, and pseudoephedrine *on page 27*
Sudafed® Decongestant [Can] *see* pseudoephedrine *on page 801*
Sudafed® Head Cold and Sinus Extra Strength [Can] *see* acetaminophen and pseudoephedrine *on page 23*
Sudafed® Maximum Strength Nasal Decongestant [US-OTC] *see* pseudoephedrine *on page 801*
Sudafed® Maximum Strength Sinus Nighttime (Discontinued) *see* triprolidine and pseudoephedrine *on page 955*
Sudafed® Multi-Symptom Sinus and Cold [US-OTC] *see* acetaminophen and pseudoephedrine *on page 23*
Sudafed® Non-Drying Sinus (Discontinued) *see* guaifenesin and pseudoephedrine *on page 458*
Sudafed PE™ [US-OTC] *see* phenylephrine *on page 745*
Sudafed PE® Sinus & Allergy [US-OTC] *see* chlorpheniramine and phenylephrine *on page 206*
Sudafed PE® Sinus Headache [US-OTC] *see* acetaminophen and phenylephrine *on page 22*
Sudafed® Sinus Advance [Can] *see* pseudoephedrine and ibuprofen *on page 802*
Sudafed® Sinus & Allergy [US-OTC] *see* chlorpheniramine and pseudoephedrine *on page 207*
SudaHist® [US] *see* chlorpheniramine and pseudoephedrine *on page 207*
Sudal® 12 [US] *see* chlorpheniramine and pseudoephedrine *on page 207*
SudaTex-DM [US] *see* guaifenesin, pseudoephedrine, and dextromethorphan *on page 460*
SudaTex-G [US] *see* guaifenesin and pseudoephedrine *on page 458*
Sudex® (Discontinued) *see* guaifenesin and pseudoephedrine *on page 458*
SudoGest [US-OTC] *see* pseudoephedrine *on page 801*
SudoGest Children's [US-OTC] *see* pseudoephedrine and dextromethorphan *on page 802*
Sudo-Tab® [US-OTC] *see* pseudoephedrine *on page 801*
Sufedrin® (Discontinued) *see* pseudoephedrine *on page 801*
Sufenta® [US/Can] *see* sufentanil *on page 891*

sufentanil (soo FEN ta nil)

Sound-Alike/Look-Alike Issues
SUFentanil may be confused with alfentanil, fentaNYL
Sufenta® may be confused with Alfenta®, Sudafed®, Survanta®
Synonyms sufentanil citrate
Tall-Man SUFentanil
U.S./Canadian Brand Names Sufentanil Citrate Injection, USP [Can]; Sufenta® [US/Can]
Therapeutic Category Analgesic, Narcotic; General Anesthetic
Controlled Substance C-II
Use Analgesic supplement in maintenance of balanced general anesthesia; primary anesthetic for induction and maintenance of anesthesia in patients undergoing major surgical procedures; epidural anesthetic in conjunction with bupivacaine in labor and delivery

◄ **Usual Dosage**
I.V.:

 Children 2-12 years: Induction: 10-25 mcg/kg (10-15 mcg/kg most common dose) with 100% O_2; Maintenance: Up to 1-2 mcg/kg total dose

 Adults: Dose should be based on body weight. **Note:** In obese patients (eg, >20% above ideal body weight), use lean body weight to determine dosage.
 Surgical analgesia (surgery 1-2 hours long): Total dose: 1-2 mcg/kg; ≥75% of dose administered prior to intubation; administered with N_2O/O_2; Maintenance: 5-20 mcg as needed. Total dose should not exceed 1 mcg/kg/hour of expected surgical time.
 Epidural: Adults: Analgesia: Labor and delivery: 10-15 mcg with 10 mL bupivacaine 0.125% with/without epinephrine. May repeat at ≥1-hour interval for 2 additional doses.

Dosage Forms
 Injection, solution [preservative free]: 50 mcg/mL (1 mL, 2 mL, 5 mL)
 Sufenta®: 50 mcg/mL (1 mL, 2 mL, 5 mL)

sufentanil citrate see sufentanil on page 891
Sufentanil Citrate Injection, USP [Can] see sufentanil on page 891
Sular® [US] see nisoldipine on page 673
sulbactam and ampicillin see ampicillin and sulbactam on page 73

sulconazole (sul KON a zole)

Synonyms sulconazole nitrate
U.S./Canadian Brand Names Exelderm® [US/Can]
Therapeutic Category Antifungal Agent
Use Treatment of superficial fungal infections of the skin, including tinea cruris (jock itch), tinea corporis (ringworm), tinea versicolor, and possibly tinea pedis (athlete's foot, cream only)
Usual Dosage Topical: Adults: Apply a small amount to the affected area and gently massage once or twice daily for 3 weeks (tinea cruris, tinea corporis, tinea versicolor) to 4 weeks (tinea pedis).
Dosage Forms
 Cream:
 Exelderm®: 1% (15 g, 30 g, 60 g)
 Solution, topical:
 Exelderm®: 1% (30 mL)

sulconazole nitrate see sulconazole on page 892
Sulcrate® [Can] see sucralfate on page 890
Sulcrate® Suspension Plus [Can] see sucralfate on page 890

sulfabenzamide, sulfacetamide, and sulfathiazole
(sul fa BENZ a mide, sul fa SEE ta mide, & sul fa THYE a zole)
Synonyms triple sulfa
U.S./Canadian Brand Names V.V.S.® [US]
Therapeutic Category Antibiotic, Vaginal
Use Treatment of *Haemophilus vaginalis* vaginitis
Usual Dosage Intravaginal: Adults: Female: Cream: Insert one applicatorful into vagina twice daily for 4-6 days; dosage may then be decreased to 1/2 to 1/4 of an applicatorful twice daily
Dosage Forms
 Cream, vaginal: Sulfabenzamide 3.7%, sulfacetamide 2.86%, and sulfathiazole 3.42% (78 g with applicator)
 V.V.S.®: Sulfabenzamide 3.7%, sulfacetamide 2.86%, and sulfathiazole 3.42% (78 g with applicator)

sulfacetamide (sul fa SEE ta mide)

Sound-Alike/Look-Alike Issues
 Bleph®-10 may be confused with Blephamide®
 Klaron® may be confused with Klor-Con®
Synonyms sodium sulfacetamide; sulfacetamide sodium
U.S./Canadian Brand Names Bleph®-10 [US]; Carmol® Scalp Treatment [US]; Cetamide™ [Can]; Diosulf™ [Can]; Klaron® [US]; Ovace® Plus [US]; Ovace® [US]; Rosula® NS [US]; Seb-Prev™ [US]
Therapeutic Category Antibiotic, Ophthalmic

Use
Ophthalmic: Treatment and prophylaxis of conjunctivitis due to susceptible organisms; corneal ulcers; adjunctive treatment with systemic sulfonamides for therapy of trachoma
Dermatologic: Scaling dermatosis (seborrheic); bacterial infections of the skin; acne vulgaris

Usual Dosage
Children >2 months and Adults: Ophthalmic:
Ointment: Apply to lower conjunctival sac 1-4 times/day and at bedtime
Solution: Instill 1-2 drops several times daily up to every 2-3 hours in lower conjunctival sac during waking hours and less frequently at night; increase dosing interval as condition responds. Usual duration of treatment: 7-10 days
Trachoma: Instill 2 drops into the conjunctival sac every 2 hours; must be used in conjunction with systemic therapy
Children >12 years and Adults: Topical:
Acne: Apply thin film to affected area twice daily
Seborrheic dermatitis: Apply at bedtime and allow to remain overnight; in severe cases, may apply twice daily. Duration of therapy is usually 8-10 applications; dosing interval may be increased as eruption subsides. Applications once or twice weekly, or every other week may be used to prevent eruptions.
Secondary cutaneous bacterial infections: Apply 2-4 times/day until infection clears

Dosage Forms
Aerosol, topical:
Ovace®: 10% (100 g)
Cream, topical:
Seb-Prev™: 10% (30 g, 60 g)
Gel, topical:
Seb-Prev™: 10% (30 g, 60 g)
Lotion, topical: 10% (120 mL)
Carmol® Scalp Treatment: 10% (85 g)
Klaron®: 10% (120 mL)
Lotion, topical [wash]:
Ovace®: 10% (180 mL, 360 mL)
Lotion, topical [emulsion-based wash]:
Ovace® Plus: 10% (180 mL, 360 mL)
Pad, topical:
Rosula® NS: 10% (30s)
Soap, topical [wash]:
Seb-Prev™: 10% (170 mL, 340 mL)
Solution, ophthalmic [drops]: 10% (15 mL)
Bleph®-10: 10% (5 mL)
Suspension, topical: 10% (118 mL)

sulfacetamide and prednisolone (sul fa SEE ta mide & pred NIS oh lone)

Sound-Alike/Look-Alike Issues
Blephamide® may be confused with Bleph®-10
Synonyms prednisolone and sulfacetamide
U.S./Canadian Brand Names Blephamide® [US/Can]; Dioptimyd® [Can]
Therapeutic Category Antibiotic/Corticosteroid, Ophthalmic
Use Steroid-responsive inflammatory ocular conditions where infection is present or there is a risk of infection; ophthalmic suspension may be used as an otic preparation
Usual Dosage Ophthalmic: Children ≥6 years and Adults:
Ointment: Apply to lower conjunctival sac 1-4 times/day
Solution, suspension: Instill 1-3 drops every 2-3 hours while awake
Dosage Forms
Ointment, ophthalmic:
Blephamide®: Sulfacetamide 10% and prednisolone 0.2% (3.5 g)
Solution, ophthalmic: Sulfacetamide 10% and prednisolone 0.25% (5 mL, 10 mL)
Suspension, ophthalmic:
Blephamide®: Sulfacetamide 10% and prednisolone 0.2% (5 mL, 10 mL)

sulfacetamide and sulfur see sulfur and sulfacetamide on page 897
sulfacetamide sodium see sulfacetamide on page 892
sulfacetamide sodium and fluorometholone *(Discontinued)*

Sulfacet-R® [US/Can] *see* sulfur and sulfacetamide *on page 897*

sulfadiazine (sul fa DYE a zeen)

Sound-Alike/Look-Alike Issues
sulfaDIAZINE may be confused with sulfasalazine, sulfiSOXAZOLE
Tall-Man sulfADIAZINE
Therapeutic Category Sulfonamide
Use Treatment of urinary tract infections and nocardiosis; adjunctive treatment in toxoplasmosis; uncomplicated attack of malaria
Usual Dosage Oral:
Asymptomatic meningococcal carriers:
Infants 1-12 months: 500 mg once daily for 2 days
Children 1-12 years: 500 mg twice daily for 2 days
Adults: 1 g twice daily for 2 days
Congenital toxoplasmosis:
Newborns and Children <2 months: 100 mg/kg/day divided every 6 hours in conjunction with pyrimethamine 1 mg/kg/day once daily and supplemental folinic acid 5 mg every 3 days for 6 months
Children >2 months: 25-50 mg/kg/dose 4 times/day
Nocardiosis: 4-8 g/day for a minimum of 6 weeks
Toxoplasmosis:
Children >2 months: Loading dose: 75 mg/kg; maintenance dose: 120-150 mg/kg/day, maximum dose: 6 g/day; divided every 4-6 hours in conjunction with pyrimethamine 2 mg/kg/day divided every 12 hours for 3 days followed by 1 mg/kg/day once daily with supplemental folinic acid
Adults: 2-6 g/day in divided doses every 6 hours in conjunction with pyrimethamine 50-75 mg/day and with supplemental folinic acid
Dosage Forms
Tablet: 500 mg

sulfadoxine and pyrimethamine (sul fa DOKS een & peer i METH a meen)

Synonyms pyrimethamine and sulfadoxine
U.S./Canadian Brand Names Fansidar® [US]
Therapeutic Category Antimalarial Agent
Use Treatment of *Plasmodium falciparum* malaria in patients in whom chloroquine resistance is suspected; malaria prophylaxis for travelers to areas where chloroquine-resistant malaria is endemic
Usual Dosage Oral: Children and Adults:
Treatment of acute attack of malaria: A single dose of the following number of Fansidar® tablets is used in sequence with quinine or alone:
2-11 months: 1/4 tablet
1-3 years: 1/2 tablet
4-8 years: 1 tablet
9-14 years: 2 tablets
>14 years: 3 tablets
Malaria prophylaxis: A single dose should be carried for self-treatment in the event of febrile illness when medical attention is not immediately available:
2-11 months: 1/4 tablet
1-3 years: 1/2 tablet
4-8 years: 1 tablet
9-14 years: 2 tablets
>14 years and Adults: 3 tablets
Dosage Forms
Tablet:
Fansidar®: Sulfadoxine 500 mg and pyrimethamine 25 mg

Sulfa-Gyn® (Discontinued) *see* sulfabenzamide, sulfacetamide, and sulfathiazole *on page 892*
Sulfamethoprim® (Discontinued)

sulfamethoxazole and trimethoprim (sul fa meth OKS a zole & trye METH oh prim)

Sound-Alike/Look-Alike Issues
Bactrim™ may be confused with bacitracin, Bactine®, Bactroban®
co-trimoxazole may be confused with clotrimazole

Septra® may be confused with Ceptaz®, Sectral®

Septra® DS may be confused with Semprex®-D

Synonyms co-trimoxazole; SMZ-TMP; TMP-SMZ; trimethoprim and sulfamethoxazole

U.S./Canadian Brand Names Apo-Sulfatrim® DS [Can]; Apo-Sulfatrim® Pediatric [Can]; Apo-Sulfatrim® [Can]; Bactrim™ DS [US]; Bactrim™ [US]; Novo-Trimel D.S. [Can]; Novo-Trimel [Can]; Nu-Cotrimox [Can]; Septra® DS [US]; Septra® Injection [Can]; Septra® [US]; Sulfatrim® [US]

Therapeutic Category Sulfonamide

Use

Oral treatment of urinary tract infections due to *E. coli*, *Klebsiella* and *Enterobacter* sp, *M. morganii*, *P. mirabilis* and *P. vulgaris*; acute otitis media in children; acute exacerbations of chronic bronchitis in adults due to susceptible strains of *H. influenzae* or *S. pneumoniae*; treatment and prophylaxis of *Pneumocystis jiroveci* pneumonitis (PCP); traveler's diarrhea due to enterotoxigenic *E. coli*; treatment of enteritis caused by *Shigella flexneri* or *Shigella sonnei*

I.V. treatment or severe or complicated infections when oral therapy is not feasible, for documented PCP, empiric treatment of PCP in immune compromised patients; treatment of documented or suspected shigellosis, typhoid fever, *Nocardia asteroides* infection, or other infections caused by susceptible bacteria

Usual Dosage Dosage recommendations are based on the trimethoprim component. Double-strength tablets are equivalent to sulfamethoxazole 800 mg and trimethoprim 160 mg.

Usual dosage ranges:

Children >2 months:

Mild-to-moderate infections: Oral: 8-12 mg TMP/kg/day in divided doses every 12 hours

Serious infection:

  Oral: 20 mg TMP/kg/day in divided doses every 6 hours

  I.V.: 8-12 mg TMP/kg/day in divided doses every 6 hours

Adults:

  Oral: One double strength tablet (sulfamethoxazole 800 mg; trimethoprim 160 mg) every 12-24 hours

  I.V.: 8-20 mg TMP/kg/day divided every 6-12 hours

Indication-specifc dosing:

Children >2 months:

Acute otitis media: Oral: 8 mg TMP/kg/day in divided doses every 12 hours for 10 days. **Note:** Recommended by the American Academy of Pediatrics as an alternative agent in penicillin-allergic patients at a dose of 6-10 mg TMP/kg/day (AOM guidelines, 2004).

Urinary tract infection:

Treatment:

  Oral: 6-12 mg TMP/kg/day in divided doses every 12 hours

  I.V.: 8-10 mg TMP/kg/day in divided doses every 6, 8, or 12 hours for up to 14 days with serious infections

Prophylaxis: Oral: 2 mg TMP/kg/dose daily or 5 mg TMP/kg/dose twice weekly

Pneumocystis jiroveci:

Treatment: Oral, I.V.: 15-20 mg TMP/kg/day in divided doses every 6-8 hours

Prophylaxis: Oral, 150 mg TMP/m^2/day in divided doses every 12 hours for 3 days/week; dose should not exceed trimethoprim 320 mg and sulfamethoxazole 1600 mg daily

Alternative prophylaxis dosing schedules include:

  150 mg TMP/m^2/day as a single daily dose 3 times/week on consecutive days

or

  150 mg TMP/m^2/day in divided doses every 12 hours administered 7 days/week

or

  150 mg TMP/m^2/day in divided doses every 12 hours administered 3 times/week on alternate days

Shigellosis:

Oral: 8 mg TMP/kg/day in divided doses every 12 hours for 5 days

I.V.: 8-10 mg TMP/kg/day in divided doses every 6, 8, or 12 hours for up to 5 days

Adults:

Urinary tract infection:

Oral: One double-strength tablet every 12 hours

  Duration of therapy: Uncomplicated: 3-5 days; Complicated: 7-10 days

    Pyelonephritis: 14 days

    Prostatitis: Acute: 2 weeks; Chronic: 2-3 months

I.V.: 8-10 mg TMP/kg/day in divided doses every 6, 8, or 12 hours for up to 14 days with severe infections

Chronic bronchitis (acute): Oral: One double-strength tablet every 12 hours for 10-14 days

◄ **Meningitis (bacterial):** I.V.: 10-20 mg TMP/kg/day in divided doses every 6-12 hours
Shigellosis:
　Oral: One double strength tablet every 12 hours for 5 days
　I.V.: 8-10 mg TMP/kg/day in divided doses every 6, 8, or 12 hours for up to 5 days
Traveler's diarrhea: Oral: One double strength tablet every 12 hours for 5 days
Sepsis: I.V.: 20 TMP/kg/day divided every 6 hours
Pneumocystis jiroveci:
　Prophylaxis: Oral: 1 double strength tablet daily or 3 times/week
　Treatment: Oral, I.V.: 15-20 mg TMP/kg/day in 3-4 divided doses
Dosage Forms The 5:1 ratio (SMX:TMP) remains constant in all dosage forms.
　Injection, solution: Sulfamethoxazole 80 mg and trimethoprim 16 mg per mL (5 mL, 10 mL, 30 mL)
　Suspension, oral: Sulfamethoxazole 200 mg and trimethoprim 40 mg per 5 mL
　Sulfatrim®: Sulfamethoxazole 200 mg and trimethoprim 40 mg per 5 mL
　Tablet: Sulfamethoxazole 400 mg and trimethoprim 80 mg
　Bactrim™, Septra®: Sulfamethoxazole 400 mg and trimethoprim 80 mg
　Tablet, double strength: Sulfamethoxazole 800 mg and trimethoprim 160 mg
　Bactrim™ DS, Septra® DS: Sulfamethoxazole 800 mg and trimethoprim 160 mg

Sulfamylon® [US] *see mafenide on page 582*

sulfasalazine (sul fa SAL a zeen)
Sound-Alike/Look-Alike Issues
　sulfasalazine may be confused with salsalate, sulfaDIAZINE, sulfiSOXAZOLE
　Azulfidine® may be confused with Augmentin®, azaTHIOprine
Synonyms salicylazosulfapyridine
U.S./Canadian Brand Names Alti-Sulfasalazine [Can]; Azulfidine® EN-tabs® [US]; Azulfidine® [US]; Salazopyrin En-Tabs® [Can]; Salazopyrin® [Can]; Sulfazine EC [US]; Sulfazine [US]
Therapeutic Category 5-Aminosalicylic Acid Derivative
Use Management of ulcerative colitis; enteric coated tablets are also used for rheumatoid arthritis (including juvenile rheumatoid arthritis) in patients who inadequately respond to analgesics and NSAIDs
Usual Dosage Oral:
　Children ≥2 years: Ulcerative colitis: Initial: 40-60 mg/kg/day in 3-6 divided doses; maintenance dose: 20-30 mg/kg/day in 4 divided doses
　Children ≥6 years: Juvenile rheumatoid arthritis: Enteric coated tablet: 30-50 mg/kg/day in 2 divided doses; Initial: Begin with 1/4 to 1/3 of expected maintenance dose; increase weekly; maximum: 2 g/day typically
　Adults:
　　Ulcerative colitis: Initial: 1 g 3-4 times/day, 2 g/day maintenance in divided doses; may initiate therapy with 0.5-1 g/day
　　Rheumatoid arthritis: Enteric coated tablet: Initial: 0.5-1 g/day; increase weekly to maintenance dose of 2 g/day in 2 divided doses; maximum: 3 g/day (if response to 2 g/day is inadequate after 12 weeks of treatment)
Dosage Forms
　Tablet: 500 mg
　Azulfidine®, Sulfazine: 500 mg
　Tablet, delayed release, enteric coated: 500 mg
　Azulfidine® EN-tabs®, Sulfazine EC: 500 mg

Sulfatol® [US] *see sulfur and sulfacetamide on page 897*
Sulfatol®-M [US] *see sulfur and sulfacetamide on page 897*
Sulfatrim® [US] *see sulfamethoxazole and trimethoprim on page 894*
Sulfa-Trip® *(Discontinued)* *see sulfabenzamide, sulfacetamide, and sulfathiazole on page 892*
Sulfazine [US] *see sulfasalazine on page 896*
Sulfazine EC [US] *see sulfasalazine on page 896*
sulfinpyrazone *(Discontinued)*

sulfisoxazole (sul fi SOKS a zole)
Sound-Alike/Look-Alike Issues
　sulfiSOXAZOLE may be confused with sulfaDIAZINE, sulfamethoxazole, sulfasalazine
　Gantrisin® may be confused with Gastrosed™

Synonyms sulfisoxazole acetyl; sulphafurazole
Tall-Man sulfiSOXAZOLE
U.S./Canadian Brand Names Gantrisin® [US]; Novo-Soxazole [Can]; Sulfizole® [Can]
Therapeutic Category Sulfonamide
Use Treatment of urinary tract infections, otitis media, *Chlamydia*; nocardiosis
Usual Dosage Oral: Not for use in patients <2 months of age:
Children >2 months: Initial: 75 mg/kg, followed by 120-150 mg/kg/day in divided doses every 4-6 hours; not to exceed 6 g/day
Adults: Initial: 2-4 g, then 4-8 g/day in divided doses every 4-6 hours
Dosage Forms
Suspension, oral [pediatric]:
Gantrisin®: 500 mg/5 mL

sulfisoxazole acetyl *see* sulfisoxazole *on page 896*
sulfisoxazole and erythromycin *see* erythromycin and sulfisoxazole *on page 356*
Sulfizole® [Can] *see* sulfisoxazole *on page 896*

sulfur and sulfacetamide (SUL fur & sul fa SEE ta mide)

Synonyms sodium sulfacetamide and sulfur; sulfacetamide and sulfur; sulfur and sulfacetamide sodium
U.S./Canadian Brand Names AVAR™-e [US]; Clarifoam™ EF [US]; Clenia™ [US]; Plexion SCT® [US]; Plexion® [US]; Prascion® AV [US]; Prascion® FC [US]; Prascion® RA [US]; Prascion® TS [US]; Prascion® [US]; Rosac® [US]; Rosanil® [US]; Rosula® Clarifying [US]; Rosula® [US]; Sulfacet-R® [US/Can]; Sulfatol® [US]; Sulfatol®-M [US]; Suphera™ [US]
Therapeutic Category Antiseborrheic Agent, Topical
Use Aid in the treatment of acne vulgaris, acne rosacea, and seborrheic dermatitis
Usual Dosage Topical: Children ≥12 years and Adults: Apply in a thin film 1-3 times/day. Cleansing products should be used 1-2 times/day.
Dosage Forms
Aerosol, topical [foam]:
Clarifoam™ EF: Sulfur 5% and sulfacetamide 10% (60 g)
Cleanser, topical:
AVAR™: Sulfur 5% and sulfacetamide 10% (228 g)
Plexion®, Prascion®: Sulfur 5% and sulfacetamide 10% (170 g, 340 g)
Prascion® AV: Sulfur 5% and sulfacetamide 10% (227 g)
Rosanil®: Sulfur 5% and sulfacetamide 10% (170 g, 390 g)
Rosula®: Sulfur 5% and sulfacetamide 10% (355 mL)
Cleanser, topical [emulsion-based]:
Sulfatol®: Sulfur 5% and sulfacetamide 10% (355 mL)
Cream, topical:
AVAR™-e, AVAR™-e Green, Prascion® RA, Rosac®: Sulfur 5% and sulfacetamide 10% (45 g)
Clenia™: Sulfur 5% and sulfacetamide sodium 10% (28 g)
Plexion SCT®: Sulfur 5% and sulfacetamide sodium 10% (120 g)
Suphera™: Sulfur 5% and sulfacetamide sodium 10% (113 g)
Gel, topical:
AVAR™, Rosula®: Sulfur 5% and sulfacetamide 10% (45 g)
Gel, topical [emulsion-based]:
Sulfatol®: Sulfur 5% and sulfacetamide 10% (45 mL)
Lotion, topical: Sulfur 5% and sulfacetamide 10% (25 g, 30 g, 45 g, 60 g)
Sulfacaet-R®, Sulfatol®-M: Sulfur 5% and sulfacetamide 10% (25 g)
Pad, topical [cleansing cloth]:
Plexion®, Prascion®: Sulfur 5% and sulfacetamide 10% (30s, 60s)
Suspension, topical: Sulfur 5% and sulfacetamide 10% (30 g)
Prascion® TS: Sulfur 5% and sulfacetamide 10% (30 g)
Wash, topical: Sulfur 5% and sulfacetamide 10% (170 g, 340 g)
Rosac®: Sulfur 1% and sulfacetamide sodium 10% (170 g)
Clenia™, Zetacet®: Sulfur 5% and sulfacetamide 10% (170 g, 340 g)
Wash, topical [emulsion-based]:
Rosula® Clarifying: Sulfur 4% and sulfacetamide 10% (473 mL)

sulfur and sulfacetamide sodium *see* sulfur and sulfacetamide *on page 897*

sulindac (SUL in dak)

Sound-Alike/Look-Alike Issues
Clinoril® may be confused with Cleocin®, Clozaril®, Oruvail®

U.S./Canadian Brand Names Apo-Sulin® [Can]; Clinoril® [US]; Novo-Sundac [Can]; Nu-Sundac [Can]

Therapeutic Category Analgesic, Nonnarcotic; Nonsteroidal Antiinflammatory Drug (NSAID)

Use Management of inflammatory diseases including osteoarthritis, rheumatoid arthritis, acute gouty arthritis, ankylosing spondylitis, acute painful shoulder (bursitis/tendonitis)

Usual Dosage Oral: Adults: **Note:** Maximum daily dose: 400 mg
Osteoarthritis, rheumatoid arthritis, ankylosing spondylitis: 150 mg twice daily
Acute painful shoulder (bursitis/tendonitis): 200 mg twice daily; usual treatment: 7-14 days
Acute gouty arthritis: 200 mg twice daily; usual treatment: 7 days

Dosage Forms
Tablet: 150 mg, 200 mg
Clinoril®: 200 mg

sulphafurazole *see sulfisoxazole on page 896*

Sultrin™ *(Discontinued)* *see sulfabenzamide, sulfacetamide, and sulfathiazole on page 892*

sumatriptan (soo ma TRIP tan)

Sound-Alike/Look-Alike Issues
SUMAtriptan may be confused with sitaGLIPtin, somatropin, zolmitriptan

Synonyms sumatriptan succinate

Tall-Man SUMAtriptan

U.S./Canadian Brand Names Apo-Sumatriptan® [Can]; CO Sumatriptan [Can]; Dom-Sumatriptan [Can]; Gen-Sumatriptan [Can]; Imitrex® DF [Can]; Imitrex® Nasal Spray [Can]; Imitrex® [US/Can]; Novo-Sumatriptan [Can]; PHL-Sumatriptan [Can]; PMS-Sumatriptan [Can]; ratio-Sumatriptan [Can]; Rhoxal-sumatriptan [Can]; Riva-Sumatriptan [Can]; Sandoz-Sumatriptan [Can]; Sumatryx [Can]

Therapeutic Category Antimigraine Agent

Use
Oral, SubQ: Acute treatment of migraine with or without aura
SubQ: Acute treatment of cluster headache episodes

Usual Dosage Adults:
Oral: A single dose of 25 mg, 50 mg, or 100 mg (taken with fluids). If a satisfactory response has not been obtained at 2 hours, a second dose may be administered. Results from clinical trials show that initial doses of 50 mg and 100 mg are more effective than doses of 25 mg, and that 100 mg doses do not provide a greater effect than 50 mg and may have increased incidence of side effects. Although doses of up to 300 mg/day have been studied, the total daily dose should not exceed 200 mg. The safety of treating an average of >4 headaches in a 30-day period have not been established.
Intranasal: A single dose of 5 mg, 10 mg, or 20 mg administered in one nostril. A 10 mg dose may be achieved by administering a single 5 mg dose in each nostril. If headache returns, the dose may be repeated once after 2 hours, not to exceed a total daily dose of 40 mg. The safety of treating an average of >4 headaches in a 30-day period has not been established.
SubQ: Up to 6 mg; if side effects are dose-limiting, lower doses may be used. A second injection may be administered at least 1 hour after the initial dose, but not more than 2 injections in a 24-hour period.

Dosage Forms
Injection, solution:
Imitrex®: 8 mg/mL (0.5 mL); 12 mg/mL (0.5 mL)
Solution, intranasal [spray]:
Imitrex®: 5 mg/0.1 mL device (6s); 20 mg/0.1 mL device (6s)
Tablet:
Imitrex®: 25 mg, 50 mg, 100 mg

sumatriptan and naproxen (soo ma TRIP tan & na PROKS en)

Sound-Alike/Look-Alike Issues
naproxen may be confused with Natacyn®, Nebcin®, neomycin, niacin
SUMAtriptan may be confused with somatropin, zolmitriptan
Treximet™ may be confused with Trexall™

Synonyms naproxen and sumatriptan; naproxen sodium and sumatriptan; naproxen sodium and sumatriptan succinate; sumatriptan succinate and naproxen; sumatriptan succinate and naproxen sodium

U.S./Canadian Brand Names Treximet™ [US]

Therapeutic Category Antimigraine Agent; Nonsteroidal Antiinflammatory Drug (NSAID); Serotonin 5-HT$_{1B, 1D}$ Receptor Agonist

Use Acute treatment of migraine with or without aura

Usual Dosage Oral: Adults: 1 tablet (sumatriptan 85 mg and naproxen 500 mg). If a satisfactory response has not been obtained at 2 hours, a second dose may be administered (maximum: 2 tablets/24 hours). **Note:** The safety of treating an average of >5 migraine headaches in a 30-day period has not been established.

Dosage Forms
Tablet:
Treximet™ 85/500: Sumatriptan 85 mg and naproxen sodium 500 mg

sumatriptan succinate *see* sumatriptan *on page 898*
sumatriptan succinate and naproxen *see* sumatriptan and naproxen *on page 898*
sumatriptan succinate and naproxen sodium *see* sumatriptan and naproxen *on page 898*
Sumatryx [Can] *see* sumatriptan *on page 898*
Summer's Eve® Anti-Itch Maximum Strength [US-OTC] *see* pramoxine *on page 777*
Summer's Eve® Medicated Douche [US-OTC] *see* povidone-iodine *on page 775*
Summer's Eve® SpecialCare™ Medicated Anti-Itch Cream *(Discontinued)* *see* hydrocortisone (topical) *on page 485*
Sumycin® *(Discontinued)* *see* tetracycline *on page 915*
Sun-Benz® [Can] *see* benzydamine *(Canada only) on page 129*

sunitinib (su NIT e nib)

Synonyms NSC736511; SU11248; sunitinib maleate

U.S./Canadian Brand Names Sutent® [US/Can]

Therapeutic Category Antineoplastic Agent, Tyrosine Kinase Inhibitor; Vascular Endothelial Growth Factor (VEGF) Inhibitor

Use Treatment of gastrointestinal stromal tumor (GIST) following failure of or intolerance to imatinib; treatment of advanced renal cell cancer (RCC)

Usual Dosage Oral: Adults: Gastrointestinal stromal tumor, renal cell cancer: 50 mg once daily for 4 weeks of a 6-week treatment cycle (4 weeks on, 2 weeks off). **Note:** Dosage modifications should be done in increments of 12.5 mg; individualize based on safety and tolerability.

Dosage Forms
Capsule:
Sutent®: 12.5 mg, 25 mg, 50 mg

sunitinib maleate *see* sunitinib *on page 899*
Supartz™ [US] *see* hyaluronate and derivatives *on page 476*
Super Dec B 100 [US-OTC] *see* vitamin B complex combinations *on page 981*
Superdophilus® [US-OTC] *see* Lactobacillus *on page 543*
Superplex-T™ [US-OTC] *see* vitamin B complex combinations *on page 981*
Super Quints 50 [US-OTC] *see* vitamin B complex combinations *on page 981*
Supeudol® [Can] *see* oxycodone *on page 709*
Suphera™ [US] *see* sulfur and sulfacetamide *on page 897*
Suplasyn® [Can] *see* hyaluronate and derivatives *on page 476*
Suppress® *(Discontinued)* *see* dextromethorphan *on page 284*
Suprane® [US/Can] *see* desflurane *on page 274*
Suprefact® [Can] *see* buserelin acetate *(Canada only) on page 153*
Suprefact® Depot [Can] *see* buserelin acetate *(Canada only) on page 153*
Surbex-T® [US-OTC] *see* vitamin B complex combinations *on page 981*
Surfak® [US-OTC] *see* docusate *on page 314*
Surgam® [Can] *see* tiaprofenic acid *(Canada only) on page 925*
Surgicel® [US] *see* cellulose, oxidized regenerated *on page 193*

Surgicel® Fibrillar [US] *see* cellulose, oxidized regenerated *on page 193*
Surgicel® NuKnit [US] *see* cellulose, oxidized regenerated *on page 193*
Surmontil® [US/Can] *see* trimipramine *on page 954*
Survanta® [US/Can] *see* beractant *on page 129*
Sus-Phrine® *(Discontinued)* *see* epinephrine *on page 344*
Sustaire® *(Discontinued)* *see* theophylline *on page 917*
Sustiva® [US/Can] *see* efavirenz *on page 335*
SuTan [US] *see* dexchlorpheniramine and pseudoephedrine *on page 280*
Sutent® [US/Can] *see* sunitinib *on page 899*
Su-Tuss DM [US] *see* guaifenesin and dextromethorphan *on page 454*
Su-Tuss®-HD *(Discontinued)*
suxamethonium chloride *see* succinylcholine *on page 890*
Sween Cream® [US-OTC] *see* vitamin A and vitamin D *on page 980*
Symadine® *(Discontinued)*
Symax SL [US] *see* hyoscyamine *on page 492*
Symax SR [US] *see* hyoscyamine *on page 492*
Symbicort® [US/Can] *see* budesonide and formoterol *on page 148*
Symbyax® [US] *see* olanzapine and fluoxetine *on page 694*
Symlin® [US] *see* pramlintide *on page 777*
Symmetrel® [US/Can] *see* amantadine *on page 56*
SymTan™ *(Discontinued)*
synacthen *see* cosyntropin *on page 250*
Synagis® [US/Can] *see* palivizumab *on page 716*
Synalar® [Can] *see* fluocinolone *on page 409*
Synalar® *(Discontinued)* *see* fluocinolone *on page 409*
Synalar-HP® Topical *(Discontinued)* *see* fluocinolone *on page 409*
Synalgos®-DC [US] *see* dihydrocodeine, aspirin, and caffeine *on page 298*
Synarel® [US/Can] *see* nafarelin *on page 652*
Syn-Diltiazem® [Can] *see* diltiazem *on page 300*
Synemol® Topical *(Discontinued)* *see* fluocinolone *on page 409*
Synera™ [US] *see* lidocaine and tetracaine *on page 565*
Synercid® [US/Can] *see* quinupristin and dalfopristin *on page 814*
Synphasic® [Can] *see* ethinyl estradiol and norethindrone *on page 376*
Syntest D.S. *(Discontinued)* *see* estrogens (esterified) and methyltestosterone *on page 366*
Syntest H.S. *(Discontinued)* *see* estrogens (esterified) and methyltestosterone *on page 366*
Synthroid® [US/Can] *see* levothyroxine *on page 560*
Syntocinon® [Can] *see* oxytocin *on page 714*
Synvisc® [US] *see* hyaluronate and derivatives *on page 476*
Syprine® [US/Can] *see* trientine *on page 951*
Syrex [US] *see* sodium chloride *on page 873*
SyringeAvitene™ [US] *see* collagen hemostat *on page 245*
syrup of ipecac *see* ipecac syrup *on page 524*
Systane® [US-OTC] *see* artificial tears *on page 95*
Systane® Free [US-OTC] *see* artificial tears *on page 95*
Sytobex® *(Discontinued)* *see* cyanocobalamin *on page 254*
T_3/T_4 liotrix *see* liotrix *on page 569*
T_4 *see* levothyroxine *on page 560*
T-20 *see* enfuvirtide *on page 340*
642® Tablet [Can] *see* propoxyphene *on page 795*
Tabloid® [US] *see* thioguanine *on page 921*
Tac™-40 Injection *(Discontinued)*
Taclonex® [US] *see* calcipotriene and betamethasone *on page 159*
Taclonex Scalp® [US] *see* calcipotriene and betamethasone *on page 159*

tacrine (TAK reen)

Sound-Alike/Look-Alike Issues
Cognex® may be confused with Corgard®

Synonyms tacrine hydrochloride; tetrahydroaminoacrine; THA

U.S./Canadian Brand Names Cognex® [US]

Therapeutic Category Acetylcholinesterase Inhibitor; Cholinergic Agent

Use Treatment of mild-to-moderate dementia of the Alzheimer type

Usual Dosage Adults: Initial: 10 mg 4 times/day; may increase by 40 mg/day adjusted every 6 weeks; maximum: 160 mg/day; best administered separate from meal times.
Dose adjustment based upon transaminase elevations:
ALT ≤3 times ULN*: Continue titration
ALT >3 to ≤5 times ULN*: Decrease dose by 40 mg/day, resume when ALT returns to normal
ALT >5 times ULN*: Stop treatment, may rechallenge upon return of ALT to normal
*ULN = upper limit of normal
Patients with clinical jaundice confirmed by elevated total bilirubin (>3 mg/dL) should not be rechallenged with tacrine

Dosage Forms
Capsule:
Cognex®: 10 mg, 20 mg, 30 mg, 40 mg

tacrine hydrochloride *see* tacrine *on page 901*

tacrolimus (ta KROE li mus)

Sound-Alike/Look-Alike Issues
tacrolimus may be confused with sirolimus, temsirolimus
Prograf® may be confused with Gengraf®, Prozac®

Synonyms FK506

U.S./Canadian Brand Names Advagraf™ [Can]; Prograf® [US/Can]; Protopic® [US/Can]

Therapeutic Category Immunosuppressant Agent

Use
Oral/injection: Potent immunosuppressive drug used in heart, kidney, or liver transplant recipients
Topical: Moderate-to-severe atopic dermatitis in patients not responsive to conventional therapy or when conventional therapy is not appropriate

Usual Dosage
Oral:
Children: **Notes:** Patients without preexisting renal or hepatic dysfunction have required (and tolerated) higher doses than adults to achieve similar blood concentrations. It is recommended that therapy be initiated at high end of the recommended adult I.V. and oral dosing ranges; dosage adjustments may be required. If switching from I.V. to oral, the oral dose should be started 8-12 hours after stopping the infusion. Adjunctive therapy with corticosteroids is recommended early post-transplant.
Liver transplant: Initial dose: 0.15-0.20 mg/kg/day in 2 divided doses, given every 12 hours; begin oral dose no sooner than 6 hours post-transplant
Adults: **Notes:** If switching from I.V. to oral, the oral dose should be started 8-12 hours after stopping the infusion. Adjunctive therapy with corticosteroids is recommended early post-transplant.
Heart transplant: Initial dose: 0.075 mg/kg/day in 2 divided doses, given every 12 hours; begin oral dose no sooner than 6 hours post-transplant
Kidney transplant: Initial dose: 0.2 mg/kg/day in 2 divided doses, given every 12 hours; initial dose may be given within 24 hours of transplant, but should be delayed until renal function has recovered; African-American patients may require larger doses to maintain trough concentration
Liver transplant: Initial dose: 0.1-0.15 mg/kg/day in 2 divided doses, given every 12 hours; begin oral dose no sooner than 6 hours post-transplant

I.V.: Children and Adults: **Note:** I.V. route should only be used in patients not able to take oral medications and continued only until oral medication can be tolerated; anaphylaxis has been reported. Begin no sooner than 6 hours post-transplant; adjunctive therapy with corticosteroids is recommended.
Heart transplant: Initial dose: 0.01 mg/kg/day as a continuous infusion
Kidney, liver transplant: Initial dose: 0.03-0.05 mg/kg/day as a continuous infusion
Prevention of graft-vs-host disease: 0.03 mg/kg/day as continuous infusion

Topical: Children ≥2 years and Adults: Atopic dermatitis (moderate to severe): Apply minimum amount of 0.03% or 0.1% ointment to affected area twice daily; rub in gently and completely. Discontinue use when ▶

symptoms have cleared. If no improvement within 6 weeks, patients should be reexamined to confirm diagnosis.

Dosage Forms
Capsule:
Prograf®: 0.5 mg, 1 mg, 5 mg
Injection, solution:
Prograf®: 5 mg/mL (1 mL)
Ointment, topical:
Protopic®: 0.03% (30 g, 60 g, 100 g); 0.1% (30 g, 60 g, 100 g)

tadalafil (tah DA la fil)

Sound-Alike/Look-Alike Issues
Sound-alike/look-alike issues:
Tadalafil may be confused with sildenafil, vardenafil
Synonyms GF196960
U.S./Canadian Brand Names Cialis® [US/Can]
Therapeutic Category Phosphodiesterase (Type 5) Enzyme Inhibitor
Use Treatment of erectile dysfunction (ED)
Usual Dosage Oral: Erectile dysfunction:
Adults:
As-needed dosing: 10 mg at least 30 minutes prior to anticipated sexual activity (dosing range: 5-20 mg); to be given as one single dose and not given more than once daily. **Note:** Erectile function may be improved for up to 36 hours following a single dose; adjust dose.
Once-daily dosing: 2.5 mg once daily. Dosing range: 2.5-5 mg/day
Dosage Forms
Tablet:
Cialis®: 2.5 mg, 5 mg, 10 mg, 20 mg

Tagamet® *(Discontinued) see* cimetidine *on page 219*
Tagamet® HB [Can] *see* cimetidine *on page 219*
Tagamet® HB 200 [US-OTC] *see* cimetidine *on page 219*
TAK-375 *see* ramelteon *on page 817*
Talacen® [US] *see* pentazocine and acetaminophen *on page 736*
talc *see* talc (sterile) *on page 902*
talc for pleurodesis *see* talc (sterile) *on page 902*

talc (sterile) (talk STARE il)

Synonyms intrapleural talc; sterile talc; talc; talc for pleurodesis
U.S./Canadian Brand Names Sclerosol® [US]; Sterile Talc Powder™ [US]
Therapeutic Category Sclerosing Agent
Use Prevention of recurrence of malignant pleural effusion in symptomatic patients
Usual Dosage Adults: Pleural effusion:
Intrapleural aerosol: 4-8 g (1-2 cans) as a single dose
Intrapleural instillation: 5 g
Dosage Forms
Aerosol, intrapleural [powder]:
Sclerosol®: 4 g
Powder, intrapleural:
Sterile Talc Powder™: Talc USP 5 g

Talwin® [US/Can] *see* pentazocine *on page 735*
Talwin® NX [US] *see* pentazocine *on page 735*
Tambocor™ [US/Can] *see* flecainide *on page 403*
Tamiflu® [US/Can] *see* oseltamivir *on page 703*
Tamofen® [Can] *see* tamoxifen *on page 902*

tamoxifen (ta MOKS i fen)

Sound-Alike/Look-Alike Issues
tamoxifen may be confused with pentoxifylline, Tambocor™

Synonyms ICI-46474; tamoxifen citrate

U.S./Canadian Brand Names Apo-Tamox® [Can]; Gen-Tamoxifen [Can]; Nolvadex® [Can]; Nolvadex®-D [Can]; Novo-Tamoxifen [Can]; Tamofen® [Can]

Therapeutic Category Antineoplastic Agent

Use Treatment of metastatic (female and male) breast cancer; adjuvant treatment of breast cancer; reduce risk of invasive breast cancer in women with ductal carcinoma *in situ* (DCIS); reduce the incidence of breast cancer in women at high risk

Usual Dosage Oral (refer to individual protocols): Adults:
Breast cancer treatment:
  Metastatic (males and females) or adjuvant therapy (females): 20-40 mg/day; daily doses >20 mg should be given in 2 divided doses (morning and evening); doses >20 mg/day are not more effective in adjuvant therapy
  DCIS (females): 20 mg once daily for 5 years
  Breast cancer risk reduction (pre- and postmenopausal high-risk females): 20 mg/day for 5 years

Dosage Forms
Tablet: 10 mg, 20 mg

tamoxifen citrate *see* tamoxifen *on page 902*

tamsulosin (tam SOO loe sin)

Sound-Alike/Look-Alike Issues
  tamsulosin may be confused with tacrolimus, tamoxifen, terazosin
  Flomax® may be confused with Flonase®, Flovent®, Foltx®, Fosamax®, Volmax®

Synonyms tamsulosin hydrochloride

U.S./Canadian Brand Names Flomax® CR [Can]; Flomax® [US/Can]; Gen-Tamsulosin [Can]; Novo-Tamsulosin [Can]; Ran-Tamsulosin [Can]; ratio-Tamsulosin [Can]; Sandoz-Tamsulosin [Can]

Therapeutic Category Alpha-Adrenergic Blocking Agent

Use Treatment of signs and symptoms of benign prostatic hyperplasia (BPH)

Usual Dosage Oral: Adults: BPH: 0.4 mg once daily ~30 minutes after the same meal each day; dose may be increased after 2-4 weeks to 0.8 mg once daily in patients who fail to respond. If therapy is interrupted for several days, restart with 0.4 mg once daily.

Dosage Forms
Capsule:
  Flomax®: 0.4 mg

tamsulosin hydrochloride *see* tamsulosin *on page 903*

Tanac® [US-OTC] *see* benzocaine *on page 124*

TanaCof-XR [US] *see* brompheniramine *on page 144*

Tanafed® (Discontinued) *see* chlorpheniramine and pseudoephedrine *on page 207*

Tanafed DMX™ [US] *see* chlorpheniramine, pseudoephedrine, and dextromethorphan *on page 212*

Tandem® OB [US] *see* vitamins (multiple/prenatal) *on page 983*

Tannate-V-DM [US] *see* phenylephrine, pyrilamine, and dextromethorphan *on page 749*

Tannate 12 S [US] *see* carbetapentane and chlorpheniramine *on page 174*

Tannate PD-DM [US] *see* chlorpheniramine, pseudoephedrine, and dextromethorphan *on page 212*

Tannate Pediatric [US] *see* chlorpheniramine and phenylephrine *on page 206*

Tannic-12 (Discontinued) *see* carbetapentane and chlorpheniramine *on page 174*

Tannic-12 S [US] *see* carbetapentane and chlorpheniramine *on page 174*

Tannihist-12 D (Discontinued) *see* carbetapentane, phenylephrine, and pyrilamine *on page 176*

Tannihist-12 RF (Discontinued) *see* carbetapentane and chlorpheniramine *on page 174*

Tanta-Orciprenaline® [Can] *see* metaproterenol *on page 609*

Tantum® [Can] *see* benzydamine *(Canada only) on page 129*

TAP-144 *see* leuprolide *on page 553*

Tapazole® [US/Can] *see* methimazole *on page 614*

Tarabine® PFS (Discontinued) *see* cytarabine *on page 261*

Tarceva® [US/Can] *see* erlotinib *on page 353*

Targel® [Can] *see* coal tar *on page 240*

Targretin® [US/Can] *see* bexarotene *on page 134*

Tarka® [US/Can] *see* trandolapril and verapamil *on page 942*
Taro-Amcinonide [Can] *see* amcinonide *on page 57*
Taro-Carbamazepine Chewable [Can] *see* carbamazepine *on page 172*
Taro-Ciprofloxacin [Can] *see* ciprofloxacin *on page 221*
Taro-Clindamycin [Can] *see* clindamycin *on page 230*
Taro-Clobetasol [Can] *see* clobetasol *on page 232*
Taro-Desoximetasone [Can] *see* desoximetasone *on page 277*
Taro-Enalapril [Can] *see* enalapril *on page 339*
Taro-Fluconazole [Can] *see* fluconazole *on page 405*
Taro-Mometasone [Can] *see* mometasone *on page 641*
Taro-Simvastatin [Can] *see* simvastatin *on page 867*
Taro-Sone® [Can] *see* betamethasone (topical) *on page 132*
Taro-Warfarin [Can] *see* warfarin *on page 986*
Tarsum® [US-OTC] *see* coal tar and salicylic acid *on page 241*
Tasigna® [US] *see* nilotinib *on page 672*
Tasmar® [US] *see* tolcapone *on page 934*
Tavist® Allergy [US-OTC] *see* clemastine *on page 228*
Tavist® ND ALLERGY [US-OTC] *see* loratadine *on page 576*
Taxol® [US/Can] *see* paclitaxel *on page 714*
Taxotere® [US/Can] *see* docetaxel *on page 313*

tazarotene (taz AR oh teen)

U.S./Canadian Brand Names Avage™ [US]; Tazorac® [US/Can]
Therapeutic Category Keratolytic Agent
Use Topical treatment of facial acne vulgaris; topical treatment of stable plaque psoriasis of up to 20% body surface area involvement; mitigation (palliation) of facial skin wrinkling, facial mottled hyper-/hypopigmentation, and benign facial lentigines
Usual Dosage Topical: **Note:** In patients experiencing excessive pruritus, burning, skin redness, or peeling, discontinue until integrity of the skin is restored, or reduce dosing to an interval the patient is able to tolerate.
Children ≥12 years and Adults:
Acne: Tazorac® cream/gel 0.1%: Cleanse the face gently. After the skin is dry, apply a thin film of tazarotene (2 mg/cm^2) once daily, in the evening, to the skin where the acne lesions appear; use enough to cover the entire affected area
Psoriasis: Tazorac® gel 0.05% or 0.1%: Apply once daily, in the evening, to psoriatic lesions using enough (2 mg/cm^2) to cover only the lesion with a thin film to no more than 20% of body surface area. If a bath or shower is taken prior to application, dry the skin before applying. Unaffected skin may be more susceptible to irritation, avoid application to these areas.
Children ≥17 years and Adults: Palliation of fine facial wrinkles, facial mottled hyper/hypopigmentation, benign facial lentigines: Avage™: Apply a pea-sized amount once daily to clean dry face at bedtime; lightly cover entire face including eyelids if desired. Emollients or moisturizers may be applied before or after; if applied before tazarotene, ensure cream or lotion has absorbed into the skin and has dried completely.
Adults: Psoriasis: Tazorac® cream 0.05% or 0.1%: Apply once daily, in the evening, to psoriatic lesions using enough (2 mg/cm^2) to cover only the lesion with a thin film to no more than 20% of body surface area. If a bath or shower is taken prior to application, dry the skin before applying. Unaffected skin may be more susceptible to irritation, avoid application to these areas.
Dosage Forms
Cream:
Avage™: 0.1% (30 g)
Tazorac®: 0.05% (30 g, 60 g); 0.1% (30 g, 60 g)
Gel:
Tazorac®: 0.05% (30 g, 100 g); 0.1% (30 g, 100 g)

Tazicef® [US] *see* ceftazidime *on page 189*
tazobactam and piperacillin *see* piperacillin and tazobactam sodium *on page 756*
Tazocin® [Can] *see* piperacillin and tazobactam sodium *on page 756*
Tazorac® [US/Can] *see* tazarotene *on page 904*

Taztia XT™ [US] *see* diltiazem *on page 300*

TB skin test *see* tuberculin tests *on page 959*

3TC® [Can] *see* lamivudine *on page 544*

3TC *see* lamivudine *on page 544*

3TC, abacavir, and zidovudine *see* abacavir, lamivudine, and zidovudine *on page 16*

T-cell growth factor *see* aldesleukin *on page 42*

TCGF *see* aldesleukin *on page 42*

TCN *see* tetracycline *on page 915*

Td *see* diphtheria and tetanus toxoid *on page 306*

Td Adsorbed [Can] *see* diphtheria and tetanus toxoid *on page 306*

Tdap *see* diphtheria, tetanus toxoids, and acellular pertussis vaccine *on page 309*

TDF *see* tenofovir *on page 909*

Teardrops® [Can] *see* artificial tears *on page 95*

Tear Drop® Solution *(Discontinued)* *see* artificial tears *on page 95*

TearGard® Ophthalmic Solution *(Discontinued)* *see* artificial tears *on page 95*

Teargen® [US-OTC] *see* artificial tears *on page 95*

Teargen® II [US-OTC] *see* artificial tears *on page 95*

Tearisol® [US-OTC] *see* artificial tears *on page 95*

Tearisol® [US-OTC] *see* hydroxypropyl methylcellulose *on page 490*

Tears Again® [US-OTC] *see* artificial tears *on page 95*

Tears Again® MC [US-OTC] *see* hydroxypropyl methylcellulose *on page 490*

Tears Again® Gel Drops™ [US-OTC] *see* carboxymethylcellulose *on page 179*

Tears Again® Night and Day™ [US-OTC] *see* carboxymethylcellulose *on page 179*

Tears Naturale® [US-OTC] *see* artificial tears *on page 95*

Tears Naturale® II [US-OTC] *see* artificial tears *on page 95*

Tears Naturale® Free [US-OTC] *see* artificial tears *on page 95*

Tears Plus® [US-OTC] *see* artificial tears *on page 95*

Tears Renewed® [US-OTC] *see* artificial tears *on page 95*

TEAS *see* trolamine *on page 957*

Tebrazid™ [Can] *see* pyrazinamide *on page 806*

Tecnal C 1/2 [Can] *see* butalbital, aspirin, caffeine, and codeine *on page 156*

Tecnal C 1/4 [Can] *see* butalbital, aspirin, caffeine, and codeine *on page 156*

tegaserod (teg a SER od)

Synonyms HTF919; tegaserod maleate

U.S./Canadian Brand Names Zelnorm® [US]

Therapeutic Category Serotonin 5-HT$_4$ Receptor Agonist

Use Emergency treatment of irritable bowel syndrome with constipation (IBS-C) and chronic idiopathic constipation (CIC) in women (<55 years of age) in which no alternative therapy exists

Usual Dosage Oral: Adults (<55 years of age): Females:

IBS with constipation: 6 mg twice daily, before meals, for 4-6 weeks; may consider continuing treatment for an additional 4-6 weeks in patients who respond initially

Chronic idiopathic constipation: 6 mg twice daily, before meals; the need for continued therapy should be reassessed periodically

Dosage Forms

Tablet:

Zelnorm®: 2 mg, 6 mg

tegaserod maleate *see* tegaserod *on page 905*

Tega-Vert® Oral *(Discontinued)* *see* dimenhydrinate *on page 301*

Tegretol® [US/Can] *see* carbamazepine *on page 172*

Tegretol®-XR [US] *see* carbamazepine *on page 172*

Tekturna® [US] *see* aliskiren *on page 45*

Tekturna HCT® [US] *see* aliskiren and hydrochlorothiazide *on page 45*

Telachlor® Oral *(Discontinued)* *see* chlorpheniramine *on page 205*

Teladar® Topical *(Discontinued)*

telbivudine (tel BI vyoo deen)
Synonyms L-deoxythymidine
U.S./Canadian Brand Names Sebivo® [Can]; Tyzeka™ [US]
Therapeutic Category Antiretroviral Agent, Reverse Transcriptase Inhibitor (Nucleoside)
Use Treatment of chronic hepatitis B with evidence of viral replication and either persistent transaminase elevations or histologically-active disease
Usual Dosage Oral: Adolescents ≥16 years and Adults: Chronic hepatitis B: 600 mg once daily
Dosage Forms
Tablet:
Tyzeka™: 600 mg

Teldrin® HBP [US-OTC] *see* chlorpheniramine *on page 205*
Teldrin® Oral *(Discontinued)* *see* chlorpheniramine *on page 205*

telithromycin (tel ith roe MYE sin)
Synonyms HMR 3647
U.S./Canadian Brand Names Ketek® [US/Can]
Therapeutic Category Antibiotic, Ketolide
Use Treatment of community-acquired pneumonia (mild-to-moderate) caused by susceptible strains of *Streptococcus pneumoniae* (including multidrug-resistant isolates), *Haemophilus influenzae*, *Chlamydophila pneumoniae*, *Moraxella catarrhalis*, and *Mycoplasma pneumoniae*
Usual Dosage Oral: Adults: Community-acquired pneumonia: 800 mg once daily for 7-10 days
Dosage Forms
Tablet:
Ketek®: 300 mg [not available in Canada], 400 mg

telmisartan (tel mi SAR tan)
U.S./Canadian Brand Names Micardis® [US/Can]
Therapeutic Category Angiotensin II Receptor Antagonist
Use Treatment of hypertension; may be used alone or in combination with other antihypertensive agents
Usual Dosage Oral: Adults: Initial: 40 mg once daily; usual maintenance dose range: 20-80 mg/day. Patients with volume depletion should be initiated on the lower dosage with close supervision.
Dosage Forms
Tablet:
Micardis®: 20 mg, 40 mg, 80 mg

telmisartan and hydrochlorothiazide (tel mi SAR tan & hye droe klor oh THYE a zide)
Synonyms hydrochlorothiazide and telmisartan
U.S./Canadian Brand Names Micardis® HCT [US]; Micardis® Plus [Can]
Therapeutic Category Antihypertensive Agent, Combination
Use Treatment of hypertension; combination product should not be used for initial therapy
Usual Dosage Oral: Adults: Replacement therapy: Combination product can be substituted for individual titrated agents. Initiation of combination therapy when monotherapy has failed to achieve desired effects:
Patients currently on telmisartan: Initial dose if blood pressure is not currently controlled on monotherapy of 80 mg telmisartan: Telmisartan 80 mg/hydrochlorothiazide 12.5 mg once daily; may titrate up to telmisartan 160 mg/hydrochlorothiazide 25 mg if needed
Patients currently on HCTZ: Initial dose if blood pressure is not currently controlled on monotherapy of 25 mg once daily: Telmisartan 80 mg/hydrochlorothiazide 12.5 mg once daily or telmisartan 80 mg/hydrochlorothiazide 25 mg once daily; may titrate up to telmisartan 160 mg/hydrochlorothiazide 25 mg if blood pressure remains uncontrolled after 2-4 weeks of therapy. Patients who develop hypokalemia may be switched to telmisartan 80 mg/hydrochlorothiazide 12.5 mg.
Dosage Forms [CAN]: Canadian brand name
Tablet:
Micardis® HCT: 40/12.5: Telmisartan 40 mg and hydrochlorothiazide 12.5 mg; 80/12.5: Telmisartan 80 mg and hydrochlorothiazide 12.5 mg; 80/25: Telmisartan 80 mg and hydrochlorothiazide 25 mg

Micardis® Plus [CAN]: 80/25: Telmisartan 80 mg and hydrochlorothiazide 25 mg [not available in the U.S.]

Telzir® [Can] *see* fosamprenavir *on page 425*

temazepam (te MAZ e pam)

Sound-Alike/Look-Alike Issues
temazepam may be confused with flurazepam, LORazepam
Restoril® may be confused with Vistaril®, Zestril®

U.S./Canadian Brand Names Apo-Temazepam® [Can]; CO Temazepam [Can]; Dom-Temazepam [Can]; Gen-Temazepam [Can]; Novo-Temazepam [Can]; Nu-Temazepam [Can]; PHL-Temazepam [Can]; PMS-Temazepam [Can]; ratio-Temazepam [Can]; Restoril® [US/Can]

Therapeutic Category Benzodiazepine

Controlled Substance C-IV

Use Short-term treatment of insomnia

Usual Dosage Oral: Adults: 15-30 mg at bedtime

Dosage Forms
Capsule: 15 mg, 22.5 mg, 30 mg
Restoril®: 7.5 mg, 15 mg, 22.5 mg, 30 mg

Temodal® [Can] *see* temozolomide *on page 907*
Temodar® [US/Can] *see* temozolomide *on page 907*
Temovate® [US] *see* clobetasol *on page 232*
Temovate E® [US] *see* clobetasol *on page 232*

temozolomide (te moe ZOE loe mide)

Synonyms NSC-362856; TMZ

U.S./Canadian Brand Names Temodal® [Can]; Temodar® [US/Can]

Therapeutic Category Antineoplastic Agent, Alkylating Agent

Use Treatment of adult patients with refractory anaplastic astrocytoma; newly-diagnosed glioblastoma multiforme

Usual Dosage Oral (refer to individual protocols): Adults:
Anaplastic astrocytoma (refractory): Initial dose: 150 mg/m^2/day for 5 days; repeat every 28 days. Subsequent doses of 100-200 mg/m^2/day for 5 days per treatment cycle; based upon hematologic tolerance.
ANC <1000/mm^3 or platelets <50,000/mm^3 on day 22 or day 29 (day 1 of next cycle): Postpone therapy until ANC >1500/mm^3 and platelets >100,000/mm^3; reduce dose by 50 mg/m^2/day for subsequent cycle
ANC 1000-1500/mm^3 or platelets 50,000-100,000/mm^3 on day 22 or day 29 (day 1 of next cycle): Postpone therapy until ANC >1500/mm^3 and platelets >100,000/mm^3; maintain initial dose
ANC >1500/mm^3 and platelets >100,000/mm^3 on day 22 or day 29 (day 1 of next cycle): Increase dose to or maintain dose at 200 mg/m^2/day for 5 days for subsequent cycle

Glioblastoma multiforme (high-grade glioma):
Concomitant phase: 75 mg/m^2/day for 42 days with radiotherapy (60Gy administered in 30 fractions). **Note:** PCP prophylaxis is required during concomitant phase and should continue in patients who develop lymphocytopenia until recovery (common toxicity criteria [CTC] ≤1). Obtain weekly CBC.
ANC ≥1500/mm^3, platelet count ≥100,000/mm^3, and nonhematologic CTC ≤grade 1 (excludes alopecia, nausea/vomiting): Temodar® 75 mg/m^2/day may be continued throughout the 42-day concomitant period up to 49 days
Dosage modification:
ANC ≥500/mm^3 but <1500/mm^3 or platelet count ≥10,000/mm^3 but <100,000/mm^3 or nonhematologic CTC grade 2 (excludes alopecia, nausea/vomiting): Interrupt therapy
ANC <500/mm^3 or platelet count <10,000/mm^3 or nonhematologic CTC grade 3/4 (excludes alopecia, nausea/vomiting): Discontinue therapy
Maintenance phase (consists of 6 treatment cycles): Begin 4 weeks after concomitant phase completion. **Note:** Each subsequent cycle is 28 days (consisting of 5 days of drug treatment followed by 23 days without treatment). Draw CBC within 48 hours of day 22; hold next cycle and do weekly CBC until ANC >1500/mm^3 and platelet count >100,000/mm^3; dosing modification should be based on lowest blood counts and worst nonhematologic toxicity during the previous cycle.
Cycle 1: 150 mg/m^2/day for 5 days; repeat every 28 days

Dosage modification for next cycle:

ANC <1000/mm^3, platelet count <50,000/mm^3, or nonhematologic CTC grade 3 (excludes for alopecia, nausea/vomiting) during previous cycle: Decrease dose by 50 mg/m^2/day for 5 days, unless dose has already been lowered to 100 mg/m^2/day, then discontinue therapy.

If dose reduction <100 mg/m^2/day is required or nonhematologic CTC grade 4 (excludes for alopecia, nausea/vomiting), or if the same grade 3 nonhematologic toxicity occurs after dose reduction: Discontinue therapy

Cycle 2: 200 mg/m^2/day for 5 days every 28 days, unless prior toxicity, then refer to Dosage Modifications under "Cycle 1" and give adjusted dose for 5 days

Cycles 3-6: Continue with previous cycle's dose for 5 days every 28 days unless toxicity has occurred then, refer to Dosage Modifications under "Cycle 1" and give adjusted dose for 5 days

Dosage Forms

Capsule:

Temodar®: 5 mg, 20 mg, 100 mg, 140 mg, 180 mg, 250 mg

Tempra® [Can] *see* acetaminophen *on page 19*

Tempra® (Discontinued) *see* acetaminophen *on page 19*

temsirolimus (tem sir OH li mus)

Sound-Alike/Look-Alike Issues

temsirolimus may be confused with sirolimus, tacrolimus

Synonyms CCI-779; NSC-683864

U.S./Canadian Brand Names Torisel™ [US/Can]

Therapeutic Category Antineoplastic Agent, mTOR Kinase Inhibitor

Use Treatment of advanced renal cell cancer (RCC)

Usual Dosage Note: For infusion reaction prophylaxis, premedicate with diphenhydramine 25-50 mg I.V. 30 minutes prior to infusion.

I.V.: Adults: RCC: 25 mg weekly

Dosage Forms

Injection, solution [concentrate]:

Torisel®: 25 mg/mL

tenecteplase (ten EK te plase)

Sound-Alike/Look-Alike Issues

TNKase® may be confused with t-PA

TNK (occasional abbreviation for TNKase™) is an error-prone abbreviation (mistaken as TPA)

U.S./Canadian Brand Names TNKase® [US/Can]

Therapeutic Category Thrombolytic Agent

Use Thrombolytic agent used in the management of acute myocardial infarction for the lysis of thrombi in the coronary vasculature to restore perfusion and reduce mortality.

Usual Dosage I.V.:

Adults: Recommended total dose should not exceed 50 mg and is based on patient's weight; administer as a bolus over 5 seconds

If patient's weight:

<60 kg, dose: 30 mg

≥60 to <70 kg, dose: 35 mg

≥70 to <80 kg, dose: 40 mg

≥80 to <90 kg, dose: 45 mg

≥90 kg, dose: 50 mg

All patients received 150-325 mg of aspirin as soon as possible and then daily. Intravenous heparin was initiated as soon as possible and aPTT was maintained between 50-70 seconds.

Dosage Forms

Injection, powder for reconstitution, recombinant:

TNKase®: 50 mg

Tenex® [US/Can] *see* guanfacine *on page 462*

teniposide (ten i POE side)

Sound-Alike/Look-Alike Issues

teniposide may be confused with etoposide

Synonyms EPT; VM-26
U.S./Canadian Brand Names Vumon® [US/Can]
Therapeutic Category Antineoplastic Agent
Use Treatment of acute lymphocytic leukemia, small-cell lung cancer
Usual Dosage I.V.:
Children: 130 mg/m^2/week, increasing to 150 mg/m^2 after 3 weeks and up to 180 mg/m^2 after 6 weeks
Acute lymphoblastic leukemia (ALL): 165 mg/m^2 twice weekly for 8-9 doses **or** 250 mg/m^2 weekly for 4-8 weeks
Adults: 50-180 mg/m^2 once or twice weekly for 4-6 weeks or 20-60 mg/m^2/day for 5 days
Small cell lung cancer: 80-90 mg/m^2/day for 5 days every 4-6 weeks
Dosage Forms
Injection, solution:
Vumon®: 10 mg/mL (5 mL)

Ten-K® _(Discontinued)_ _see_ potassium chloride _on page 771_

tenofovir (te NOE fo veer)

Synonyms PMPA; TDF; tenofovir disoproxil fumarate
U.S./Canadian Brand Names Viread® [US/Can]
Therapeutic Category Antiretroviral Agent, Reverse Transcriptase Inhibitor (Nucleotide)
Use Management of HIV infections in combination with at least two other antiretroviral agents; treatment of chronic hepatitis B virus (HBV)
Usual Dosage Oral: Adults: HIV infection: 300 mg once daily
Dosage Forms
Tablet:
Viread®: 300 mg

tenofovir and emtricitabine _see_ emtricitabine and tenofovir _on page 338_
tenofovir disoproxil fumarate _see_ tenofovir _on page 909_
tenofovir disoproxil fumarate, efavirenz, and emtricitabine _see_ efavirenz, emtricitabine, and tenofovir _on page 335_
Tenolin [Can] _see_ atenolol _on page 101_
Tenoretic® [US/Can] _see_ atenolol and chlorthalidone _on page 102_
Tenormin® [US/Can] _see_ atenolol _on page 101_
Tensilon® [Can] _see_ edrophonium _(Canada only)_ _on page 334_
Tenuate® [Can] _see_ diethylpropion _on page 295_
Tenuate® _(Discontinued)_ _see_ diethylpropion _on page 295_
Tenuate® Dospan® [Can] _see_ diethylpropion _on page 295_
Tenuate® Dospan® _(Discontinued)_ _see_ diethylpropion _on page 295_
Tequin® _(Discontinued)_ _see_ gatifloxacin _on page 436_
Tera-Gel™ [US-OTC] _see_ coal tar _on page 240_
Terazol® [Can] _see_ terconazole _on page 911_
Terazol® 3 [US] _see_ terconazole _on page 911_
Terazol® 7 [US] _see_ terconazole _on page 911_

terazosin (ter AY zoe sin)

U.S./Canadian Brand Names Alti-Terazosin [Can]; Apo-Terazosin® [Can]; Hytrin® [Can]; Novo-Terazosin [Can]; Nu-Terazosin [Can]; PMS-Terazosin [Can]
Therapeutic Category Alpha-Adrenergic Blocking Agent
Use Management of mild-to-moderate hypertension; alone or in combination with other agents such as diuretics or beta-blockers; benign prostate hyperplasia (BPH)
Usual Dosage Oral: Adults:
Hypertension: Initial: 1 mg at bedtime; slowly increase dose to achieve desired blood pressure, up to 20 mg/day; usual dose range (JNC 7): 1-20 mg once daily
Dosage reduction may be needed when adding a diuretic or other antihypertensive agent; if drug is discontinued for greater than several days, consider beginning with initial dose and retitrate as needed; dosage may be given on a twice daily regimen if response is diminished at 24 hours and hypotensive is observed at 2-4 hours following a dose

▶

◄ Benign prostatic hyperplasia: Initial: 1 mg at bedtime, increasing as needed; most patients require 10 mg/day; if no response after 4-6 weeks of 10 mg/day, may increase to 20 mg/day

Dosage Forms
Capsule: 1 mg, 2 mg, 5 mg, 10 mg

terbinafine (oral) (TER bin a feen OR al)

Sound-Alike/Look-Alike Issues
terbinafine may be confused with terbutaline
Lamisil® may be confused with Lamictal®, Lomotil®

U.S./Canadian Brand Names Lamisil® Oral [US/Can]

Therapeutic Category Antifungal Agent

Use Treatment of onychomycosis infections of the toenail or fingernail

Usual Dosage Oral: Adults:
Fingernail onychomycosis: 250 mg once daily for 6 weeks
Toenail onychomycosis: 250 mg once daily for 12 weeks

Dosage Forms
Tablet: 250 mg
Lamisil®: 250 mg

terbinafine (topical) (TER bin a feen TOP i kal)

Sound-Alike/Look-Alike Issues
terbinafine may be confused with terbutaline
Lamisil® may be confused with Lamictal®, Lomotil®

U.S./Canadian Brand Names Lamisil® Topical [US/Can]

Therapeutic Category Antifungal Agent

Use Topical antifungal for the treatment of tinea pedis (athlete's foot), tinea cruris (jock itch), and tinea corporis (ring worm); tinea versicolor (lotion)

Usual Dosage Topical: Adults:
Athlete's foot: Apply to affected area twice daily for at least 1 week, not to exceed 4 weeks
Ringworm and jock itch: Apply to affected area once or twice daily for at least 1 week, not to exceed 4 weeks

Dosage Forms
Cream: 1% (12 g, 24 g)
Lamisil® AT™: 1% (12 g)
Solution [topical spray]:
Lamisil® AT™ [OTC]: 1% (30 mL)

terbutaline (ter BYOO ta leen)

Sound-Alike/Look-Alike Issues
terbutaline may be confused with terbinafine, TOLBUTamide

U.S./Canadian Brand Names Bricanyl® [Can]

Therapeutic Category Adrenergic Agonist Agent

Use Bronchodilator in reversible airway obstruction and bronchial asthma

Usual Dosage
Children <12 years: Bronchoconstriction:
Oral: Initial: 0.05 mg/kg/dose 3 times/day, increased gradually as required; maximum: 0.15 mg/kg/dose 3-4 times/day or a total of 5 mg/24 hours
SubQ: 0.005-0.01 mg/kg/dose to a maximum of 0.3 mg/dose; may repeat in 15-20 minutes
Children ≥6 years and Adults: Bronchospasm (acute): Inhalation (Bricanyl® [CAN] MDI: 500 mcg/puff, *not labeled for use in the U.S.*): One puff as needed; may repeat with 1 inhalation (after 5 minutes); more than 6 inhalations should not be necessary in any 24 hour period. **Note:** If a previously effective dosage regimen fails to provide the usual relief, or the effects of a dose last for >3 hours, medical advice should be sought immediately; this is a sign of seriously worsening asthma that requires reassessment of therapy.
Children >12 years and Adults: Bronchoconstriction:
Oral:
12-15 years: 2.5 mg every 6 hours 3 times/day; not to exceed 7.5 mg in 24 hours
>15 years: 5 mg/dose every 6 hours 3 times/day; if side effects occur, reduce dose to 2.5 mg every 6 hours; not to exceed 15 mg in 24 hours

SubQ: 0.25 mg/dose; may repeat in 15-30 minutes (maximum: 0.5 mg/4-hour period)
Dosage Forms [CAN] = Canadian brand name
Injection, solution: 1 mg/mL (1 mL)
Powder for oral inhalation:
Bricanyl® Turbuhaler [CAN]: 500 mcg/actuation [50 or 200 metered actuations] [not available in the U.S.]
Tablet: 2.5 mg, 5 mg

terconazole (ter KONE a zole)
Sound-Alike/Look-Alike Issues
terconazole may be confused with tioconazole
Synonyms triaconazole
U.S./Canadian Brand Names Terazol® 3 [US]; Terazol® 7 [US]; Terazol® [Can]; Zazole™ [US]
Therapeutic Category Antifungal Agent
Use Local treatment of vulvovaginal candidiasis
Usual Dosage Adults: Female:
Terazol® 3, Zazole™ 0.8% vaginal cream: Insert 1 applicatorful intravaginally at bedtime for 3 consecutive days
Terazol® 7, Zazole™ 0.4% vaginal cream: Insert 1 applicatorful intravaginally at bedtime for 7 consecutive days
Terazol® 3 vaginal suppository: Insert 1 suppository intravaginally at bedtime for 3 consecutive days
Dosage Forms
Cream, vaginal: 0.4% (45 g); 0.8% (20 g)
Terazol® 7, Zazole™: 0.4% (45 g)
Terazol® 3, Zazole™: 0.8% (20 g)
Suppository, vaginal:
Terazol® 3: 80 mg (3s)

Terfluzine [Can] see trifluoperazine on page 951

teriparatide (ter i PAR a tide)
Synonyms parathyroid hormone (1-34); recombinant human parathyroid hormone (1-34); rhPTH(1-34)
U.S./Canadian Brand Names Forteo® [US/Can]
Therapeutic Category Diagnostic Agent
Use Treatment of osteoporosis in postmenopausal women at high risk of fracture; treatment of primary or hypogonadal osteoporosis in men at high risk of fracture
Usual Dosage SubQ: Adults: 20 mcg once daily; **Note:** Initial administration should occur under circumstances in which the patient may sit or lie down, in the event of orthostasis.
Dosage Forms
Injection, solution:
Forteo®: 250 mcg/mL (3 mL)

terpin hydrate *(Discontinued)*
Terra-Cortril® Ophthalmic Suspension *(Discontinued)*
Terramycin® I.M. *(Discontinued)*
Terramycin® Oral *(Discontinued)*
Terrell™ [US] see isoflurane on page 528
Tersi [US] see selenium sulfide on page 861
Tesamone® Injection *(Discontinued)* see testosterone on page 912
Teslac® [Can] see testolactone on page 912
Teslac® *(Discontinued)* see testolactone on page 912
TESPA see thiotepa on page 922
Tessalon® [US/Can] see benzonatate on page 126
Testim® [US] see testosterone on page 912
Testoderm® *(Discontinued)* see testosterone on page 912
Testoderm® TTS *(Discontinued)* see testosterone on page 912
Testoderm® With Adhesive *(Discontinued)* see testosterone on page 912

testolactone (tes toe LAK tone)

Sound-Alike/Look-Alike Issues
testolactone may be confused with testosterone

U.S./Canadian Brand Names Teslac® [Can]

Therapeutic Category Androgen

Controlled Substance C-III

Use Palliative treatment of advanced or disseminated breast carcinoma

Usual Dosage Oral: Adults: Females: 250 mg 4 times/day for at least 3 months; desired response may take as long as 3 months

Testomar® *(Discontinued) see* yohimbine *on page 988*

Testopel® [US] *see* testosterone *on page 912*

Testopel® Pellet *(Discontinued) see* testosterone *on page 912*

testosterone (tes TOS ter one)

Sound-Alike/Look-Alike Issues
testosterone may be confused with testolactone
Testoderm® may be confused with Estraderm®

Synonyms testosterone cypionate; testosterone enanthate

U.S./Canadian Brand Names Andriol® [Can]; Androderm® [US/Can]; AndroGel® [US/Can]; Andropository [Can]; Delatestryl® [US/Can]; Depotest® 100 [Can]; Depo®-Testosterone [US]; Everone® 200 [Can]; First® Testosterone MC [US]; First® Testosterone [US]; Striant® [US]; Testim® [US]; Testopel® [US]; Virilon® IM [Can]

Therapeutic Category Androgen

Controlled Substance C-III

Use

Injection: Androgen replacement therapy in the treatment of delayed male puberty; male hypogonadism (primary or hypogonadotropic); inoperable metastatic female breast cancer (enanthate only)

Pellet: Androgen replacement therapy in the treatment of delayed male puberty; male hypogonadism (primary or hypogonadotropic)

Topical (buccal system, gel, transdermal system): Male hypogonadism (primary or hypogonadotropic)

Capsule (not available in U.S.): Androgen replacement therapy in the treatment of delayed male puberty; male hypogonadism (primary or hypogonadotropic); replacement therapy in impotence or for male climacteric symptoms due to androgen deficiency

Usual Dosage

Adolescents and Adults: Male:

I.M.:

Hypogonadism: Testosterone enanthate or testosterone cypionate: 50-400 mg every 2-4 weeks (FDA-approved dosing range); 75-100 mg/week or 150-200 mg every 2 weeks (per practice guidelines)

Delayed puberty: Testosterone enanthate: 50-200 mg every 2-4 weeks for a limited duration

Pellet (for subcutaneous implantation): Delayed male puberty, male hypogonadism: 150-450 mg every 3-6 months

Oral: Delayed puberty, hypogonadism, or hypogonadotropic hypogonadism: Capsule (Andriol®; not available in U.S.): Initial: 120-160 mg/day in 2 divided doses for 2-3 weeks; adjust according to individual response; usual maintenance dose: 40-120 mg/day (in divided doses)

Adults:

I.M.: Females: Inoperable metastatic breast cancer: Testosterone enanthate: 200-400 mg every 2-4 weeks

Topical: Primary male hypogonadism **or** hypogonadotropic hypogonadism:

Buccal: 30 mg twice daily (every 12 hours) applied to the gum region above the incisor tooth

Transdermal system: Androderm®: Initial: Apply 5 mg/day once nightly to clean, dry area on the back, abdomen, upper arms, or thighs (do **not** apply to scrotum); dosing range: 2.5-7.5 mg/day; in nonvirilized patients, dose may be initiated at 2.5 mg/day

Gel: AndroGel®, Testim®: 5 g (to deliver 50 mg of testosterone with 5 mg systemically absorbed) applied once daily (preferably in the morning) to clean, dry, intact skin of the shoulder and upper arms. AndroGel® may also be applied to the abdomen. Dosage may be increased to a maximum of 10 g (100 mg). **Do not apply testosterone gel to the genitals.**

Dose adjustment based on testosterone levels:

Less than normal range: Increase dose from 5 g to 7.5 g to 10 g

Greater than normal range: Decrease dose. Discontinue if consistently above normal at 5 g/day

Dosage Forms [CAN] = Canadian brand name
  Capsule, gelatin:
    Andriol™ [CAN]: 40 mg (10s) [not available in the U.S.]
  Gel, topical:
    AndroGel®: 1.25 g/actuation (75 g); 2.5 g (30s); 5 g (30s)
    Testim®: 5 g (30s)
  Implant, subcutaneous:
    Testopel®: 75 mg (10s, 100s)
  Injection, in oil: 100 mg/mL (10 mL); 200 mg/mL (1 mL, 5 mL, 10 mL)
    Depo®-Testosterone: 100 mg/mL (10 mL); 200 mg/mL (1 mL, 10 mL)
    Delatestryl®: 200 mg/mL (1 mL, 5 mL)
  Kit [for prescription compounding; testosterone 2%]:
    First®-Testosterone:
      Injection, in oil: Testosterone 100 mg/mL (12 mL)
      Ointment: White petrolatum (48 g)
    First®-Testosterone MC:
      Injection, in oil: Testosterone 100 mg/mL (12 mL)
      Cream: Moisturizing cream (48 g)
  Mucoadhesive, for buccal application [buccal system]:
    Striant®: 30 mg (10s)
  Transdermal system:
    Androderm®: 2.5 mg/day (60s); 5 mg/day (30s)

testosterone cypionate *see* testosterone *on page 912*

testosterone enanthate *see* testosterone *on page 912*

Testred® [US] *see* methyltestosterone *on page 624*

tetanus and diphtheria toxoid *see* diphtheria and tetanus toxoid *on page 306*

tetanus immune globulin (human) (TET a nus i MYUN GLOB yoo lin HYU man)

Synonyms TIG

U.S./Canadian Brand Names HyperTET™ S/D [US/Can]

Therapeutic Category Immune Globulin

Use Passive immunization against tetanus; tetanus immune globulin is preferred over tetanus antitoxin for treatment of active tetanus; part of the management of an unclean, wound in a person whose history of previous receipt of tetanus toxoid is unknown or who has received less than three doses of tetanus toxoid

Usual Dosage I.M.:
  Prophylaxis of tetanus:
    Children: 4 units/kg; some recommend administering 250 units to small children
    Adults: 250 units
  Treatment of tetanus:
    Children: 500-3000 units; some should infiltrate locally around the wound
    Adults: 3000-6000 units

Dosage Forms
  Injection, solution [preservative free]:
    HyperTET™ S/D: 250 units/mL (1 mL)

tetanus toxoid *see* diphtheria and tetanus toxoids, acellular pertussis, poliovirus (inactivated) and *Haemophilus* b conjugate vaccine *on page 308*

tetanus toxoid (adsorbed) (TET a nus TOKS oyd, ad SORBED)

Sound-Alike/Look-Alike Issues
  Tetanus toxoid products may be confused with influenza virus vaccine and tuberculin products. Medication errors have occurred when tetanus toxoid products have been inadvertently administered instead of tuberculin skin tests (PPD) and influenza virus vaccine. These products are refrigerated and often stored in close proximity to each other.

Therapeutic Category Toxoid

Use Active immunization against tetanus when combination antigen preparations are not indicated. **Note:** Tetanus and diphtheria toxoids for adult use (Td) is the preferred immunizing agent for most adults and for children after their seventh birthday. Young children should receive trivalent DTaP (diphtheria/tetanus/acellular pertussis), as part of their childhood immunization program, unless pertussis is contraindicated, then DT is warranted.

▶

◄ **Usual Dosage** I.M.: Children ≥7 years and Adults:
Primary immunization: 0.5 mL; repeat 0.5 mL at 4-8 weeks after first dose and at 6-12 months after second dose
Routine booster dose: Recommended every 10 years
Note: In most patients, Td is the recommended product for primary immunization, booster doses, and tetanus immunization in wound management (refer to diphtheria and tetanus toxoid monograph)
Dosage Forms
Injection, suspension:
Tetanus 5 Lf units per 0.5 mL (0.5 mL)

tetanus toxoid (fluid) (TET a nus TOKS oyd FLOO id)
Sound-Alike/Look-Alike Issues
Tetanus toxoid products may be confused with influenza virus vaccine and tuberculin products. Medication errors have occurred when tetanus toxoid products have been inadvertently administered instead of tuberculin skin tests (PPD) and influenza virus vaccine. These products are refrigerated and often stored in close proximity to each other.
Synonyms tetanus toxoid plain
Therapeutic Category Toxoid
Use Indicated as booster dose in the active immunization against tetanus in the rare adult or child who is allergic to the aluminum adjuvant (a product containing adsorbed tetanus toxoid is preferred); not indicated for primary immunization
Usual Dosage Booster doses: I.M., SubQ: 0.5 mL every 10 years

tetanus toxoid plain *see* tetanus toxoid (fluid) *on page 914*
tetanus toxoid, reduced diphtheria toxoid, and acellular pertussis, adsorbed *see* diphtheria, tetanus toxoids, and acellular pertussis vaccine *on page 309*

tetrabenazine *(Canada only)* (tet ra BEN a zeen)
U.S./Canadian Brand Names Nitoman™ [Can]
Therapeutic Category Monoamine Depleting Agent
Use Treatment of hyperkinetic movement disorders, including Huntington chorea, hemiballismus, senile chorea, Tourette syndrome, and tardive dyskinesia
Usual Dosage Oral:
Children (limited data): Consider initiation at 1/2 recommended adult dosage; must be titrated slowly to individualize dosage
Adults: Initial: 12.5 mg twice daily (may be given 3 times/day); may be increased by 12.5 mg/day every 3-5 days; should be titrated slowly to maximal tolerated and effective dose (dose is individualized)
Usual maximum tolerated dosage: 25 mg 3 times/day; maximum recommended dose: 200 mg/day
Note: If there is no improvement at the maximum tolerated dose after 7 days, improvement is unlikely; discontinuation should be considered.
Dosage Forms [CAN] = Canadian brand name
Tablet:
Nitoman™ [CAN]: 25 mg [not available in the U.S.]
Xenazine®: 12.5 mg, 25 mg

tetracaine (TET ra kane)
Synonyms amethocaine hydrochloride; tetracaine hydrochloride
U.S./Canadian Brand Names Ametop™ [Can]; Pontocaine® Niphanoid® [US]; Pontocaine® [US/Can]
Therapeutic Category Local Anesthetic
Use Spinal anesthesia; local anesthesia in the eye for various diagnostic and examination purposes; topically applied to nose and throat for various diagnostic procedures
Usual Dosage Adults:
Ophthalmic: Short-term anesthesia of the eye: 0.5% solution: Instill 1-2 drops; prolonged use (especially for at-home self-medication) is not recommended
Injection: Spinal anesthesia: **Note:** Dosage varies with the anesthetic procedure, the degree of anesthesia required, and the individual patient response; it is administered by subarachnoid injection for spinal anesthesia.
Perineal anesthesia: 5 mg
Perineal and lower extremities: 10 mg

Anesthesia extending up to costal margin: 15 mg; doses up to 20 mg may be given, but are reserved for exceptional cases
Low spinal anesthesia (saddle block): 2-5 mg
Topical mucous membranes (rhinolaryngology): Used as a 0.25% or 0.5% solution by direct application or nebulization; total dose should not exceed 20 mg

Dosage Forms
Injection, powder for reconstitution [preservative free]:
Pontocaine® Niphanoid®: 20 mg
Injection, solution: 1% [10 mg/mL] (2 mL)
Pontocaine®: 1% [10 mg/mL] (2 mL)
Solution, ophthalmic: 0.5% [5 mg/mL] (2 mL, 15 mL)
Solution, topical:
Pontocaine®: 2% [20 mg/mL] (30 mL, 118 mL)

tetracaine and lidocaine see lidocaine and tetracaine on page 565
tetracaine, benzocaine, and butamben see benzocaine, butamben, and tetracaine on page 126
tetracaine hydrochloride see tetracaine on page 914
Tetracap® *(Discontinued)* see tetracycline on page 915
tetracosactide see cosyntropin on page 250

tetracycline (tet ra SYE kleen)

Sound-Alike/Look-Alike Issues
tetracycline may be confused with tetradecyl sulfate
achromycin may be confused with actinomycin, Adriamycin PFS®
Synonyms achromycin; TCN; tetracycline hydrochloride
U.S./Canadian Brand Names Apo-Tetra® [Can]; Nu-Tetra [Can]
Therapeutic Category Antibiotic, Ophthalmic; Antibiotic, Topical; Tetracycline Derivative
Use Treatment of susceptible bacterial infections of both gram-positive and gram-negative organisms; also infections due to *Mycoplasma*, *Chlamydia*, and *Rickettsia*; indicated for acne, exacerbations of chronic bronchitis, and treatment of gonorrhea and syphilis in patients who are allergic to penicillin; as part of a multidrug regimen for *H. pylori* eradication to reduce the risk of duodenal ulcer recurrence
Usual Dosage
Usual dosage range:
Children >8 years: Oral: 25-50 mg/kg/day in divided doses every 6 hours
Adults: Oral: 250-500 mg/dose every 6 hours
Indication-specific dosing:
Adults: Oral:
Acne: 250-500 twice daily
Chronic bronchitis, acute exacerbation: 500 mg 4 times/day
Erlichiosis: 500 mg 4 times/day for 7-14 days
Peptic ulcer disease: Eradication of *Helicobacter pylori*: 500 mg 2-4 times/day depending on regimen; requires combination therapy with at least one other antibiotic and an acid-suppressing agent (proton pump inhibitor or H_2 blocker)
Periodontitis: 250 mg every 6 hours until improvement (usually 10 days)
Vibrio cholerae: 500 mg 4 times/day for 3 days
Dosage Forms
Capsule: 250 mg, 500 mg

tetracycline hydrochloride see tetracycline on page 915
tetracycline, metronidazole, and bismuth subcitrate potassium see bismuth, metronidazole, and tetracycline on page 137
tetracycline, metronidazole, and bismuth subsalicylate see bismuth, metronidazole, and tetracycline on page 137
tetrahydroaminoacrine see tacrine on page 901
tetrahydrocannabinol see dronabinol on page 326

tetrahydrocannabinol and cannabidiol *(Canada only)*

(TET ra hye droe can NAB e nol & can nab e DYE ol)
Synonyms cannabidiol and tetrahydrocannabinol; delta-9-tetrahydrocannabinol and cannabinol; GW-1000-02; THC and CBD

◀ **U.S./Canadian Brand Names** Sativex® [Can]
Therapeutic Category Analgesic, Miscellaneous
Controlled Substance CDSA-II
Use Adjunctive treatment of neuropathic pain in multiple sclerosis; adjunctive treatment of moderate-to-severe pain in advanced cancer
Usual Dosage Buccal spray: Adults: Neuropathic pain (MS), cancer pain: Initial: One spray every 4 hours to a maximum of 4 sprays on first day
  Titration and individualization: Dosage is self-titrated by the patient. In the treatment of MS, the mean daily dosage after titration in clinical trials was 5 sprays per day. The usual maximum dose is 12 sprays per day although some patients may require and tolerate a higher number of sprays per day. In the treatment of cancer pain, the mean daily dosage after titration was 8 sprays per day. Dosage should be adjusted as necessary, based on effect and tolerance. Sprays should be evenly distributed over the course of the day during initial titration. If adverse reactions, including intoxication-type symptoms, are noted the dosage should be suspended until resolution of the symptoms; a dosage reduction or extension of the interval between doses may be used to avoid a recurrence of symptoms. Retitration may be required in the event of adverse reactions and/or worsening of symptoms.
Dosage Forms [CAN] = Canadian brand name
  Solution, buccal [spray]:
    Sativex® [CAN]: Delta-9 tetrahydrocannabinol 27 mg/mL and cannabidiol 25 mg/mL (5.5 mL) [not available in the U.S.]

tetrahydrozoline (tet ra hye DROZ a leen)

Sound-Alike/Look-Alike Issues
  Visine® may be confused with Visken®
Synonyms tetrahydrozoline hydrochloride; tetryzoline
U.S./Canadian Brand Names Geneye [US-OTC]; Murine® Tears Plus [US-OTC]; Opti-Clear [US-OTC]; Tyzine® Pediatric [US]; Tyzine® [US]; Visine® Advanced Relief [US-OTC]; Visine® Original [US-OTC]
Therapeutic Category Adrenergic Agonist Agent
Use Symptomatic relief of nasal congestion and conjunctival congestion
Usual Dosage
  Nasal congestion: Intranasal:
    Children 2-6 years: Instill 2-3 drops of 0.05% solution every 4-6 hours as needed, no more frequent than every 3 hours
    Children >6 years and Adults: Instill 2-4 drops or 3-4 sprays of 0.1% solution every 3-4 hours as needed, no more frequent than every 3 hours
  Conjunctival congestion: Ophthalmic: Adults: Instill 1-2 drops in each eye 2-4 times/day
Dosage Forms
  Solution, intranasal:
    Tyzine®: 0.1% (30 mL)
    Tyzine® Pediatric: 0.05% (15 mL)
  Solution, intranasal [spray]:
    Tyzine®: 0.1% (15 mL)
  Solution, ophthalmic: 0.05% (15 mL)
    Geneye [OTC], Opti-Clear [OTC]: 0.05% (15 mL)
    Murine® Tears Plus [OTC], Visine® Original [OTC]: 0.05% (15 mL, 30 mL)
    Visine® Advanced Relief [OTC]: 0.05% (30 mL)

Texacort® [US] *see* hydrocortisone (topical) *on page 485*
TG *see* thioguanine *on page 921*
T/Gel® Daily Control [US-OTC] *see* pyrithione zinc *on page 810*
T/Gel® Daily Control 2 in 1 [US-OTC] *see* pyrithione zinc *on page 810*
T-Gen® *(Discontinued)* *see* trimethobenzamide *on page 953*
THA *see* tacrine *on page 901*

thalidomide (tha LI doe mide)

Sound-Alike/Look-Alike Issues
thalidomide may be confused with flutamide
Synonyms NSC-66847
U.S./Canadian Brand Names Thalomid® [US/Can]
Therapeutic Category Immunosuppressant Agent
Use Treatment of multiple myeloma; treatment and maintenance of cutaneous manifestations of erythema nodosum leprosum (ENL)
Usual Dosage Oral:
Multiple myeloma: 200 mg once daily (with dexamethasone 40 mg daily on days 1-4, 9-12, and 17-20 of a 28-day treatment cycle)
Cutaneous ENL:
Initial: 100-300 mg/day taken once daily at bedtime with water (at least 1 hour after evening meal)
Patients weighing <50 kg: Initiate at lower end of the dosing range
Severe cutaneous reaction or patients previously requiring high dose may be initiated at 400 mg/day; doses may be divided, but taken 1 hour after meals
Maintenance: Dosing should continue until active reaction subsides (usually at least 2 weeks), then tapered in 50 mg decrements every 2-4 weeks
Patients who flare during tapering or with a history or requiring prolonged maintenance should be maintained on the minimum dosage necessary to control the reaction. Efforts to taper should be repeated every 3-6 months, in increments of 50 mg every 2-4 weeks.
Dosage Forms
Capsule:
Thalomid®: 50 mg, 100 mg, 200 mg

Thalitone® [US] *see* chlorthalidone *on page 214*
Thalomid® [US/Can] *see* thalidomide *on page 917*
THAM® [US] *see* tromethamine *on page 957*
THC *see* dronabinol *on page 326*
THC and CBD *see* tetrahydrocannabinol and cannabidiol *(Canada only) on page 915*
Thelin™ [Can] *see* sitaxsentan *(Canada only) on page 871*
Theo-X® *(Discontinued)* *see* theophylline *on page 917*
Theo-24® [US] *see* theophylline *on page 917*
Theobid® *(Discontinued)* *see* theophylline *on page 917*
TheoCap™ [US] *see* theophylline *on page 917*
Theochron™ [US] *see* theophylline *on page 917*
Theochron® SR [Can] *see* theophylline *on page 917*
Theoclear-80® *(Discontinued)* *see* theophylline *on page 917*
Theoclear®-L.A. *(Discontinued)* *see* theophylline *on page 917*
Theo-Dur® (all products) *(Discontinued)* *see* theophylline *on page 917*
Theolair™ [Can] *see* theophylline *on page 917*
Theolair-SR® *(Discontinued)* *see* theophylline *on page 917*
Theolate *(Discontinued)* *see* theophylline and guaifenesin *on page 919*

theophylline (thee OFF i lin)

Sound-Alike/Look-Alike Issues
Theolair™ may be confused with Thiola®, Thyrolar®
Synonyms theophylline anhydrous

◄ **U.S./Canadian Brand Names** Apo-Theo LA® [Can]; Elixophyllin® [US]; Novo-Theophyl SR [Can]; PMS-Theophylline [Can]; Pulmophylline [Can]; ratio-Theo-Bronc [Can]; Theo-24® [US]; TheoCap™ [US]; Theochron® SR [Can]; Theochron™ [US]; Theolair™ [Can]; Uniphyl® SRT [Can]; Uniphyl® [US]

Therapeutic Category Theophylline Derivative

Use Treatment of symptoms and reversible airway obstruction due to chronic asthma, chronic bronchitis, or COPD

Usual Dosage Use ideal body weight for obese patients

I.V.: Initial: Maintenance infusion rates:

Children:

6 weeks to 6 months: 0.5 mg/kg/hour
6 months to 1 year: 0.6-0.7 mg/kg/hour

Children >1 year and Adults:

Acute bronchospasm: Approximate I.V. theophylline dosage for treatment of acute bronchospasm: **Note:** Equivalent hydrous aminophylline dosage is indicated in parentheses.

Infants 6 weeks to 6 months: 0.5 mg/kg/hour for next 12 hours

Children 6 months to 1 year: 0.6-0.7 mg/kg/hour for next 12 hours

Children 1-9 years: 0.95 mg/kg/hour (1.2 mg/kg/hour) for next 12 hours; 0.79 mg/kg/hour (1 mg/kg/hour) after 12 hours

Children 9-16 years and young adult smokers: 0.79 mg/kg/hour (1 mg/kg/hour) for next 12 hours; 0.63 mg/kg/hour (0.8 mg/kg/hour) after 12 hours

Healthy, nonsmoking adults: 0.55 mg/kg/hour (0.7 mg/kg/hour) for next 12 hours; 0.39 mg/kg/hour (0.5 mg/kg/hour) after 12 hours

Older patients and patients with cor pulmonale: 0.47 mg/kg/hour (0.6 mg/kg/hour) for next 12 hours; 0.24 mg/kg/hour (0.3 mg/kg/hour) after 12 hours

Patients with congestive heart failure or liver failure: 0.39 mg/kg/hour (0.5 mg/kg/hour) for next 12 hours; 0.08-0.16 mg/kg/hour (0.1-0.2 mg/kg/hour) after 12 hours

Approximate I.V. maintenance dosages are based upon continuous infusions; bolus dosing (often used in children <6 months of age) may be determined by multiplying the hourly infusion rate by 24 hours and dividing by the desired number of doses/day. See the following: Maintenance dose for acute symptoms:

Premature infant or newborn to 6 weeks (for apnea/bradycardia):
Oral theophylline: 4 mg/kg/day
I.V. aminophylline: 5 mg/kg/day
6 weeks to 6 months:
Oral theophylline: 10 mg/kg/day
I.V. aminophylline: 12 mg/kg/day or continuous I.V. infusion[1]
Infants 6 months to 1 year:
Oral theophylline: 12-18 mg/kg/day
I.V. aminophylline: 15 mg/kg/day or continuous I.V. infusion[1]
Children 1-9 years:
Oral theophylline: 20-24 mg/kg/day
I.V. aminophylline: 1 mg/kg/hour
Children 9-12 years, and adolescent daily smokers of cigarettes or marijuana, and otherwise healthy adult smokers <50 years:
Oral theophylline: 16 mg/kg/day
I.V. aminophylline: 0.9 mg/kg/hour
Adolescents 12-16 years (nonsmokers):
Oral theophylline: 13 mg/kg/day
I.V. aminophylline: 0.7 mg/kg/hour
Otherwise healthy nonsmoking adults:
Oral theophylline: 10 mg/kg/day (not to exceed 900 mg/day)
I.V. aminophylline: 0.5 mg/kg/hour
Cardiac decompensation, cor pulmonale, and/or liver dysfunction:
Oral theophylline: 5 mg/kg/day (not to exceed 400 mg/day)
I.V. aminophylline: 0.25 mg/kg/hour

[1]For continuous I.V. infusion, divide total daily dose by 24 = mg/kg/hour.

Oral theophylline: Initial dosage recommendation: Loading dose (to achieve a serum level of about 10 mcg/mL; loading doses should be given using a rapidly absorbed oral product **not** a sustained release product):

If no theophylline has been administered in the previous 24 hours: 4-6 mg/kg theophylline

If theophylline has been administered in the previous 24 hours: administer 1/2 loading dose or 2-3 mg/kg theophylline can be given in emergencies when serum levels are not available

On the average, for every 1 mg/kg theophylline given, blood levels will rise 2 mcg/mL

Ideally, defer the loading dose if a serum theophylline concentration can be obtained rapidly. However, if this is not possible, exercise clinical judgment. If the patient is not experiencing theophylline toxicity, this is unlikely to result in dangerous adverse effects.

Oral theophylline dosage for bronchial asthma (by age):

<1 year:

Initial 3 days and second 3 days: 0.2 x (age in weeks) + 5 = mg/kg/24 hours of theophylline

Steady-state maintenance: 0.3 x (age in weeks) + 8 = mg/kg/24 hours of theophylline

1-9 years:

Initial 3 days: 16 mg/kg/24 hours of theophylline, up to a maximum of 400 mg/24 hours

Second 3 days: 20 mg/kg/24 hours of theophylline

Steady-state maintenance: 22 mg/kg/24 hours of theophylline

9-12 years:

Initial 3 days: 16 mg/kg/24 hours of theophylline, up to a maximum of 400 mg/24 hours

Second 3 days: 16 mg/kg/24 hours of theophylline, up to a maximum of 600 mg/24 hours

Steady-state maintenance: 20 mg/kg/24 hours of theophylline, up to a maximum of 800 mg/24 hours

12-16 years:

Initial 3 days: 16 mg/kg/24 hours of theophylline, up to a maximum of 400 mg/24 hours

Second 3 days: 16 mg/kg/24 hours of theophylline, up to a maximum of 600 mg/24 hours

Steady-state maintenance: 18 mg/kg/24 hours of theophylline, up to a maximum of 900 mg/24 hours

Adults:

Initial 3 days: 400 mg/24 hours

Second 3 days: 600 mg/24 hours

Steady-state maintenance: 900 mg/24 hours

Increasing dose: The dosage may be increased in approximately 25% increments at 2- to 3-day intervals so long as the drug is tolerated or until the maximum dose is reached

Maintenance dose: In children and healthy adults, a slow-release product can be used; the total daily dose can be divided every 8-12 hours

Dosage Forms

Capsule, extended release:

TheoCap™: 125 mg, 200 mg [12 hour]

Theo-24®: 100 mg, 200 mg, 300 mg, 400 mg [24 hours]

Elixir:

Elixophyllin®: 80 mg/15 mL (473 mL)

Infusion [premixed in D_5W]: 200 mg (50 mL, 100 mL); 400 mg (250 mL, 500 mL); 800 mg (250 mL, 500 mL, 1000 mL)

Tablet, controlled release:

Uniphyl®: 400 mg, 600 mg [24 hours]

Tablet, extended release: 100 mg, 200 mg, 300 mg, 400 mg, 450 mg, 600 mg

Theochron™: 100 mg, 200 mg, 300 mg, 450 mg [12-24 hours]

theophylline and guaifenesin (thee OFF i lin & gwye FEN e sin)

Synonyms guaifenesin and theophylline

U.S./Canadian Brand Names Elixophyllin-GG® [US]

Therapeutic Category Theophylline Derivative

Use Symptomatic treatment of bronchospasm associated with bronchial asthma, chronic bronchitis, and pulmonary emphysema

Usual Dosage Oral: Adults: 16 mg/kg/day or 400 mg theophylline/day, in divided doses, every 6-8 hours

Dosage Forms

Liquid:

Elixophyllin-GG®: Theophylline 100 mg and guaifenesin 100 mg per 15 mL

theophylline anhydrous see theophylline *on page 917*

theophylline ethylenediamine *see* aminophylline *on page 60*

Theo-Sav® (Discontinued) see theophylline *on page 917*

Theospan®-SR *(Discontinued)* see theophylline on page 917
Theostat-80® *(Discontinued)* see theophylline on page 917
Theovent® *(Discontinued)* see theophylline on page 917
Therabid® *(Discontinued)*
TheraCys® [US] see BCG vaccine on page 118
Thera-Flur® *(Discontinued)* see fluoride on page 411
Thera-Flur-N® *(Discontinued)* see fluoride on page 411
Thera-Flu® Severe Cold Non-Drowsy *(Discontinued)* see acetaminophen, dextromethorphan, and pseudoephedrine on page 27
Theragran-M® Advanced Formula *(Discontinued)* see vitamins (multiple/oral) on page 983
Theragran® Heart Right™ *(Discontinued)* see vitamins (multiple/oral) on page 983
TheraPatch® Warm *(Discontinued)* see capsaicin on page 171
therapeutic multivitamins see vitamins (multiple/oral) on page 983
Theratears® [US] see carboxymethylcellulose on page 179
Thermazene® [US] see silver sulfadiazine on page 866

thiabendazole (thye a BEN da zole)

Synonyms tiabendazole
U.S./Canadian Brand Names Mintezol® [US]
Therapeutic Category Anthelmintic
Use Treatment of strongyloidiasis, cutaneous larva migrans, visceral larva migrans, dracunculiasis, trichinosis, and mixed helminthic infections
Usual Dosage Purgation is not required prior to use; drinking of fruit juice aids in expulsion of worms by removing the mucous to which the intestinal tapeworms attach themselves.

Children and Adults:
Oral: 50 mg/kg/day divided every 12 hours (if >68 kg: 1.5 g/dose); maximum dose: 3 g/day
Treatment duration:
Strongyloidiasis, ascariasis, uncinariasis: For 2 consecutive days
Cutaneous larva migrans: For 2 consecutive days; if active lesions are still present 2 days after completion, a second course of treatment is recommended.
Visceral larva migrans: For 7 consecutive days
Trichinosis: For 2-4 consecutive days; optimal dosage not established
Dracunculosis: 50-75 mg/kg/day divided every 12 hours for 3 days

Dosage Forms
Tablet, chewable:
Mintezol®: 500 mg

thiamazole see methimazole on page 614

thiamine (THYE a min)

Sound-Alike/Look-Alike Issues
thiamine may be confused with Tenormin®, Thorazine®
Synonyms aneurine hydrochloride; thiamine hydrochloride; thiaminium chloride hydrochloride; vitamin B₁
U.S./Canadian Brand Names Betaxin® [Can]
Therapeutic Category Vitamin, Water Soluble
Use Treatment of thiamine deficiency including beriberi, Wernicke encephalopathy, Korsakoff syndrome, neuritis associated with pregnancy, or in alcoholic patients; dietary supplement
Usual Dosage
Adequate Intake:
0-6 months: 0.2 mg/day
7-12 months: 0.3 mg/day
Recommended daily intake:
1-3 years: 0.5 mg
4-8 years: 0.6 mg
9-13 years: 0.9 mg
14-18 years: Female: 1 mg; Male: 1.2 mg
≥19 years: Female: 1.1 mg; Male: 1.2 mg
Pregnancy, lactation: 1.4 mg

Parenteral nutrition supplementation:
Infants: 1.2 mg/day
Adults: 6 mg/day; may be increased to 25-50 mg/day with history of alcohol abuse
Thiamine deficiency (beriberi):
Children: 10-25 mg/dose I.M. or I.V. daily (if critically ill), or 10-50 mg/dose orally every day for 2 weeks, then 5-10 mg/dose orally daily for 1 month
Adults: 5-30 mg/dose I.M. or I.V. 3 times/day (if critically ill); then orally 5-30 mg/day in single or divided doses 3 times/day for 1 month
Alcohol withdrawal syndrome: Adults: 100 mg/day I.M. or I.V. for several days, followed by 50-100 mg/day orally
Wernicke encephalopathy: Adults: Treatment: Initial: 100 mg I.V., then 50-100 mg/day I.M. or I.V. until consuming a regular, balanced diet. Larger doses may be needed in patients with alcohol abuse.
Dosage Forms
Injection, solution: 100 mg/mL (2 mL)
Tablet: 50 mg, 100 mg, 250 mg, 500 mg

thiamine hydrochloride *see* thiamine *on page 920*
thiaminium chloride hydrochloride *see* thiamine *on page 920*

thioguanine (thye oh GWAH neen)
Sound-Alike/Look-Alike Issues
6-thioguanine and 6-TG are error-prone abbreviations (associated with six-fold overdoses of thioguanine)
Synonyms 2-amino-6-mercaptopurine; NSC-752; TG; tioguanine
U.S./Canadian Brand Names Lanvis® [Can]; Tabloid® [US]
Therapeutic Category Antineoplastic Agent
Use Treatment of acute myelogenous (nonlymphocytic) leukemia; treatment of chronic myelogenous leukemia and granulocytic leukemia
Usual Dosage Total daily dose can be given at one time. Oral (refer to individual protocols):
Infants and Children <3 years: Combination drug therapy for acute nonlymphocytic leukemia: 3.3 mg/kg/day in divided doses twice daily for 4 days
Children and Adults: 2-3 mg/kg/day calculated to nearest 20 mg or 75-200 mg/m^2/day in 1-2 divided doses for 5-7 days or until remission is attained
Dosage Forms
Tablet [scored]:
Tabloid®: 40 mg

Thiola® [US/Can] *see* tiopronin *on page 929*

thiopental (thye oh PEN tal)
Synonyms thiopental sodium
U.S./Canadian Brand Names Pentothal® [US/Can]
Therapeutic Category Barbiturate
Controlled Substance C-III
Use Induction of anesthesia; adjunct for intubation in head injury patients; control of convulsive states; treatment of elevated intracranial pressure
Usual Dosage I.V.:
Induction anesthesia:
Infants: 5-8 mg/kg
Children 1-12 years: 5-6 mg/kg
Adults: 3-5 mg/kg
Maintenance anesthesia:
Children: 1 mg/kg as needed
Adults: 25-100 mg as needed
Increased intracranial pressure: Children and Adults: 1.5-5 mg/kg/dose; repeat as needed to control intracranial pressure
Seizures:
Children: 2-3 mg/kg/dose; repeat as needed
Adults: 75-250 mg/dose; repeat as needed

◀ **Dosage Forms**
Injection, powder for reconstitution:
Pentothal®: 250 mg, 400 mg, 500 mg, 1 g

thiopental sodium *see* thiopental *on page 921*
thiophosphoramide *see* thiotepa *on page 922*
Thioplex® (Discontinued) *see* thiotepa *on page 922*

thioproperazine (Canada only) (thye oh pro PER a zeen)

U.S./Canadian Brand Names Majeptil® [Can]
Therapeutic Category Neuroleptic Agent
Use All types of acute and chronic schizophrenia, including those which did not respond to the usual neuroleptics; manic syndromes.
Usual Dosage Initial treatment: Adults: It is recommended to start treatment at a low dosage of about 5 mg/day in a single dose or in divided doses. This initial dosage is gradually increased by the same amount every 2-3 days until the usual effective dosage of 30-40 mg/day is reached. In some cases, higher dosages of 90 mg or more per day, are necessary to control the psychotic manifestations.
Children >10 years of age: Start treatment with a daily dosage of 1-3 mg following the method of treatment described for adults
Maintenance therapy: Adults and Children: Dosage should be reduced gradually to the lowest effective level, which may be as low as a few mg per day and maintained as long as necessary
Dosage Forms
Tablet, as mesylate: 10 mg

thioridazine (thye oh RID a zeen)

Sound-Alike/Look-Alike Issues
thioridazine may be confused with thiothixene, Thorazine®
Mellaril® may be confused with Elavil®, Mebaral®
Synonyms thioridazine hydrochloride
U.S./Canadian Brand Names Mellaril® [Can]
Therapeutic Category Phenothiazine Derivative
Use Management of schizophrenic patients who fail to respond adequately to treatment with other antipsychotic drugs, either because of insufficient effectiveness or the inability to achieve an effective dose due to intolerable adverse effects from those medications
Usual Dosage Oral: Adults: Schizophrenia/psychoses: Initial: 50-100 mg 3 times/day with gradual increments as needed and tolerated; maximum: 800 mg/day in 2-4 divided doses
Dosage Forms
Tablet: 10 mg, 25 mg, 50 mg, 100 mg

thioridazine hydrochloride *see* thioridazine *on page 922*
thiosulfuric acid disodium salt *see* sodium thiosulfate *on page 880*

thiotepa (thye oh TEP a)

Synonyms TESPA; thiophosphoramide; triethylenethiophosphoramide; TSPA
Therapeutic Category Antineoplastic Agent
Use Treatment of superficial tumors of the bladder; palliative treatment of adenocarcinoma of breast or ovary; lymphomas and sarcomas; controlling intracavitary effusions caused by metastatic tumors; I.T. use: CNS leukemia/lymphoma, CNS metastases
Usual Dosage Refer to individual protocols.
Children: Sarcomas: I.V.: 25-65 mg/m^2 as a single dose every 21 days
Adults:
I.M., I.V., SubQ: 30-60 mg/m^2 once weekly
I.V.: 0.3-0.4 mg/kg by rapid I.V. administration every 1-4 weeks, **or** 0.2 mg/kg or 6-8 mg/m^2/day for 4-5 days every 2-4 weeks
High-dose therapy for bone marrow transplant: I.V.: 500 mg/m^2, up to 900 mg/m^2
I.M.: 15-30 mg in various schedules have been given
Intracavitary: 0.6-0.8 mg/kg or 30-60 mg weekly
Intrapericardial: 15-30 mg
Intrathecal: 10-15 mg or 5-11.5 mg/m^2

Dosage Forms
Injection, powder for reconstitution: 15 mg, 30 mg

thiothixene (thye oh THIKS een)

Sound-Alike/Look-Alike Issues
thiothixene may be confused with thioridazine
Navane® may be confused with Norvasc®, Nubain®

Synonyms tiotixene

U.S./Canadian Brand Names Navane® [US/Can]

Therapeutic Category Thioxanthene Derivative

Use Management of schizophrenia

Usual Dosage Oral: Adults:
Mild-to-moderate psychosis: 2 mg 3 times/day, up to 20-30 mg/day; more severe psychosis: Initial: 5 mg 2 times/day, may increase gradually, if necessary; maximum: 60 mg/day
Rapid tranquilization of the agitated patient (administered every 30-60 minutes): 5-10 mg; average total dose for tranquilization: 15-30 mg

Dosage Forms
Capsule: 1 mg, 2 mg, 5 mg, 10 mg
Navane®: 2 mg, 5 mg, 10 mg, 20 mg

thonzonium, neomycin, colistin, and hydrocortisone *see* neomycin, colistin, hydrocortisone, and thonzonium *on page 662*

Thorazine® *(Discontinued)* *see* chlorpromazine *on page 213*

Thorets [US-OTC] *see* benzocaine *on page 124*

Thrive™ [US-OTC] *see* nicotine *on page 670*

Thrombate III® [US/Can] *see* antithrombin III *on page 82*

Thrombinar® *(Discontinued)* *see* thrombin (topical) *on page 923*

Thrombin-JMI® [US] *see* thrombin (topical) *on page 923*

Thrombin-JMI® Epistaxis Kit [US] *see* thrombin (topical) *on page 923*

Thrombin-JMI® Spray Kit [US] *see* thrombin (topical) *on page 923*

Thrombin-JMI® Syringe Spray Kit [US] *see* thrombin (topical) *on page 923*

thrombin (topical) (THROM bin, TOP i kal)

U.S./Canadian Brand Names Evithrom™ [US]; Recothrom™ [US]; Thrombin-JMI® Epistaxis Kit [US]; Thrombin-JMI® Spray Kit [US]; Thrombin-JMI® Syringe Spray Kit [US]; Thrombin-JMI® [US]

Therapeutic Category Hemostatic Agent

Use Hemostasis whenever minor bleeding from capillaries and small venules is accessible

Usual Dosage Children and Adults: **Note:** For topical use only; do not administer intravenously or intraarterially.
Evithrom™: Dose depends on area to be treated; up to 10 mL was used with absorbable gelatin sponge in clinical studies
Recothrom™: Dose depends on area to be treated
Thrombin-JMI®:
Solution: Use 1000-2000 units/mL of solution where bleeding is profuse; use 100 units/mL for bleeding from skin or mucosal surfaces
Powder: May apply powder directly to the site of bleeding or on oozing surfaces

Dosage Forms
Powder for reconstitution, topical:
Thrombin-JMI®: 5000 units, 20,000 units
Thrombin-JMI® Epistaxis kit: 5000 units
Thrombin-JMI® Spray Kit, Thrombin-JMI® Syringe Spray Kit: 20,000 units
Powder for reconstitution, topical [preservative free]:
Recothrom™: 5000 int. units; 20,000 int. units
Solution, topical:
Evithrom™: 800-1200 int. units/mL (2 mL, 5 mL, 20 mL)

Thrombostat® *(Discontinued)* *see* thrombin (topical) *on page 923*

thymocyte stimulating factor *see* aldesleukin *on page 42*

Thymoglobulin® [US] *see* antithymocyte globulin (rabbit) *on page 83*

Thyrar® *(Discontinued)* *see* thyroid, desiccated *on page 924*
Thyrel® TRH *(Discontinued)*
Thyro-Block® *(Discontinued)* *see* potassium iodide *on page 773*
Thyrogen® [US/Can] *see* thyrotropin alpha *on page 924*

thyroid, desiccated (THYE roid DES i kay tid)

Synonyms desiccated thyroid; thyroid extract; thyroid USP
U.S./Canadian Brand Names Armour® Thyroid [US]; Nature-Throid™ [US]; Westhroid™ [US]
Therapeutic Category Thyroid Product
Use Replacement or supplemental therapy in hypothyroidism; pituitary TSH suppressants (thyroid nodules, thyroiditis, multinodular goiter, thyroid cancer), thyrotoxicosis, diagnostic suppression tests
Usual Dosage Oral:
Children: Recommended pediatric dosage for congenital hypothyroidism:
0-6 months: 15-30 mg/day; 4.8-6 mg/kg/day
6-12 months: 30-45 mg/day; 3.6-4.8 mg/kg/day
1-5 years: 45-60 mg/day; 3-3.6 mg/kg/day
6-12 years: 60-90 mg/day; 2.4-3 mg/kg/day
>12 years: >90 mg/day; 1.2-1.8 mg/kg/day
Adults: Initial: 15-30 mg; increase with 15 mg increments every 2-4 weeks; use 15 mg in patients with cardiovascular disease or myxedema. Maintenance dose: Usually 60-120 mg/day; monitor TSH and clinical symptoms.
Thyroid cancer: Requires larger amounts than replacement therapy
Dosage Forms
Tablet: 30 mg, 32.5 mg, 60 mg, 65 mg, 120 mg, 130 mg, 180 mg
Armour® Thyroid: 15 mg, 30 mg, 60 mg, 90 mg, 120 mg, 180 mg, 240 mg, 300 mg
Nature-Throid™: 16.25 mg, 32.5 mg, 65 mg, 130 mg, 195 mg
Westhroid™: 32.5 mg, 65 mg, 130 mg

thyroid extract *see* thyroid, desiccated *on page 924*
Thyroid Strong® *(Discontinued)* *see* thyroid, desiccated *on page 924*
thyroid USP *see* thyroid, desiccated *on page 924*
Thyrolar® [US/Can] *see* liotrix *on page 569*
ThyroSafe™ [US-OTC] *see* potassium iodide *on page 773*
ThyroShield™ [US-OTC] *see* potassium iodide *on page 773*

thyrotropin alpha (thye roe TROH pin AL fa)

Sound-Alike/Look-Alike Issues
Thyrogen® may be confused with Thyrolar®
Synonyms human thyroid stimulating hormone; recombinant human thyrotropin; Rh-TSH; TSH
U.S./Canadian Brand Names Thyrogen® [US/Can]
Therapeutic Category Diagnostic Agent
Use As an adjunctive diagnostic tool for serum thyroglobulin (Tg) testing; adjunctive treatment for radioiodine ablation of thyroid tissue remnants after total or near-total thyroidectomy in patients with well-differentiated thyroid cancer without evidence of metastatic disease
Potential clinical uses include: Patients with an undetectable Tg on thyroid hormone suppressive therapy to exclude the diagnosis of residual or recurrent thyroid cancer, patients requiring serum Tg testing and radioiodine imaging who are unwilling to undergo thyroid hormone withdrawal testing and whose treating physician believes that use of a less sensitive test is justified, patients who are either unable to mount an adequate endogenous TSH response to thyroid hormone withdrawal or in whom withdrawal is medically contraindicated, and patients without evidence of metastatic disease to ablate thyroid remnants (in combination with radioiodine [I^{131}]) following near-total thyroidectomy.
Usual Dosage I.M.: Children >16 years and Adults: Radioiodine imaging or ablation: 0.9 mg, followed 24 hours later by a second 0.9 mg dose
For radioiodine imaging or remnant ablation, radioiodine administration should be given 24 hours following the second thyrotropin injection. Diagnostic scanning should be performed 48 hours after radioiodine administration (72 hours after the second thyrotropin injection). Post-therapy scanning may be delayed (additional days) to allow decline of background activity.
For serum Tg testing, serum Tg should be obtained 72 hours after final injection of thyrotropin.

Dosage Forms Injection, powder for reconstitution:
Thyrogen®: 1.1 mg

tiabendazole *see* thiabendazole *on page 920*

tiagabine (tye AG a been)

Sound-Alike/Look-Alike Issues
tiaGABine may be confused with tiZANidine
Synonyms tiagabine hydrochloride
Tall-Man tiaGABine
U.S./Canadian Brand Names Gabitril® [US/Can]
Therapeutic Category Anticonvulsant
Use Adjunctive therapy in adults and children ≥12 years of age in the treatment of partial seizures
Usual Dosage Oral (administer with food):
Patients receiving enzyme-inducing AED regimens:
Children 12-18 years: 4 mg once daily for 1 week; may increase to 8 mg daily in 2 divided doses for 1 week; then may increase by 4-8 mg weekly to response or up to 32 mg daily in 2-4 divided doses
Adults: 4 mg once daily for 1 week; may increase by 4-8 mg weekly to response or up to 56 mg daily in 2-4 divided doses; usual maintenance: 32-56 mg/day
Patients **not** receiving enzyme-inducing AED regimens: The estimated plasma concentrations of tiagabine in patients not taking enzyme-inducing medications is twice that of patients receiving enzyme-inducing AEDs. Lower doses are required; slower titration may be necessary.
Dosage Forms
Tablet:
Gabitril®: 2 mg, 4 mg, 12 mg, 16 mg

tiagabine hydrochloride *see* tiagabine *on page 925*
Tiamate® *(Discontinued)* *see* diltiazem *on page 300*
Tiamol® [Can] *see* fluocinonide *on page 410*
Tiaprofenic-200 [Can] *see* tiaprofenic acid *(Canada only)* *on page 925*
Tiaprofenic-300 [Can] *see* tiaprofenic acid *(Canada only)* *on page 925*

tiaprofenic acid *(Canada only)* (tye ah PRO fen ik AS id)

U.S./Canadian Brand Names Apo-Tiaprofenic® [Can]; Dom-Tiaprofenic® [Can]; Novo-Tiaprofenic [Can]; Nu-Tiaprofenic [Can]; PMS-Tiaprofenic [Can]; Surgam® [Can]; Tiaprofenic-200 [Can]; Tiaprofenic-300 [Can]
Therapeutic Category Nonsteroidal Antiinflammatory Drug (NSAID)
Use Relief of signs and symptoms of rheumatoid arthritis and osteoarthritis (degenerative joint disease)
Usual Dosage Oral: Adults:
Rheumatoid arthritis:
Tablet: Usual initial and maintenance dose: 600 mg/day in 3 divided doses; some patients may do well on 300 mg twice daily; maximum daily dose: 600 mg
Sustained release capsule: Initial and maintenance dose: 2 sustained release capsules of 300 mg once daily
Osteoarthritis:
Tablet: Usual initial and maintenance dose: 600 mg/day in 2 or 3 divided doses; in rare instances patients may be maintained on 300 mg/day in divided doses; maximum daily dose: 600 mg
Sustained release capsule: Initial and maintenance dose: 2 sustained release capsules of 300 mg once daily
Dosage Forms [CAN] = Canadian brand name
Capsule, sustained release: 300 mg [not available in the U.S.]
Tablet: 200 mg, 300 mg
Apo-Tiaprofenic® [CAN], Novo-Tiaprofenic [CAN], Nu-Tiaprofenic [CAN], PMS-Tiaprofenic: 200 mg, 300 mg [not available in the U.S.]
Albert® Tiafen [CAN], Dom-Tiaprofenic® [CAN], Surgam® [CAN]: 300 mg [not available in the U.S.]

Tiazac® [US/Can] *see* diltiazem *on page 300*
Tiazac® XC [Can] *see* diltiazem *on page 300*

ticarcillin and clavulanate potassium (tye kar SIL in & klav yoo LAN ate poe TASS ee um)

Synonyms ticarcillin and clavulanic acid

U.S./Canadian Brand Names Timentin® [US/Can]

Therapeutic Category Penicillin

Use Treatment of lower respiratory tract, urinary tract, skin and skin structures, bone and joint, gynecologic (endometritis) and intraabdominal (peritonitis) infections, and septicemia caused by susceptible organisms. Clavulanate expands activity of ticarcillin to include beta-lactamase producing strains of *S. aureus*, *H. influenzae*, *Bacteroides* species, and some other gram-negative bacilli

Usual Dosage Note: Timentin® (ticarcillin/clavulanate) is a combination product; each 3.1 g dosage form contains 3 g ticarcillin disodium and 0.1 g clavulanic acid.

Usual dosage range:
Children and Adults <60 kg: I.V.: 200-300 mg of ticarcillin component/kg/day in divided doses every 4-6 hours
Children ≥60 kg and Adults: I.V.: 3.1 g (ticarcillin 3 g plus clavulanic acid 0.1 g) every 4-6 hours (maximum: 24 g of ticarcillin component/day)

Indication-specific dosing:
Children: I.V.:
  Bite wounds (animal): 200 mg of ticarcillin component/kg/day in divided doses
  Neutropenic fever: 75 mg of ticarcillin component/kg every 6 hours (maximum: 3.1 g/dose)
  Pneumonia (nosocomial): 300 mg of ticarcillin component/kg/day in 4 divided doses (maximum: 18-24 g of ticarcillin component/day)
Children ≥60 kg and Adults: I.V.:
  Amnionitis, cholangitis, diverticulitis, endometritis, epididymo-orchitis, mastoiditis, orbital cellulitis, peritonitis, pneumonia (aspiration): 3.1 g every 6 hours
  Liver abscess, parafascial space infections, septic thrombophlebitis: 3.1 g every 4 hours
  ***Pseudomonas* infections:** 3.1 g every 4 hours
  Urinary tract infections: 3.1 g every 6-8 hours

Dosage Forms
Infusion [premixed, frozen]:
Timentin®: Ticarcillin 3 g and clavulanic acid 0.1 g (100 mL)
Injection, powder for reconstitution:
Timentin®: Ticarcillin 3 g and clavulanic acid 0.1 g (3.1 g, 31 g)

ticarcillin and clavulanic acid *see* ticarcillin and clavulanate potassium *on page 926*
ticarcillin *(Discontinued)*
Ticar® *(Discontinued)*
TICE® BCG [US] *see* BCG vaccine *on page 118*
Ticlid® [US/Can] *see* ticlopidine *on page 926*

ticlopidine (tye KLOE pi deen)

Synonyms ticlopidine hydrochloride

U.S./Canadian Brand Names Alti-Ticlopidine [Can]; Apo-Ticlopidine® [Can]; Gen-Ticlopidine [Can]; Novo-Ticlopidine [Can]; Nu-Ticlopidine [Can]; Rhoxal-ticlopidine [Can]; Sandoz-Ticlopidine [Can]; Ticlid® [US/Can]

Therapeutic Category Antiplatelet Agent

Use Platelet aggregation inhibitor that reduces the risk of thrombotic stroke in patients who have had a stroke or stroke precursors. **Note:** Due to its association with life-threatening hematologic disorders, ticlopidine should be reserved for patients who are intolerant to aspirin, or who have failed aspirin therapy. Adjunctive therapy (with aspirin) following successful coronary stent implantation to reduce the incidence of subacute stent thrombosis.

Usual Dosage Oral: Adults:
Stroke prevention: 250 mg twice daily with food
Coronary artery stenting (initiate after successful implantation): 250 mg twice daily with food (in combination with antiplatelet doses of aspirin) for up to 30 days

Dosage Forms
Tablet: 250 mg
Ticlid®: 250 mg

ticlopidine hydrochloride *see* ticlopidine *on page 926*
Ticon® *(Discontinued)* *see* trimethobenzamide *on page 953*

TIG *see* tetanus immune globulin (human) *on page 913*
Tigan® [US/Can] *see* trimethobenzamide *on page 953*

tigecycline (tye ge SYE kleen)
Synonyms GAR-936
U.S./Canadian Brand Names Tygacil® [US]
Therapeutic Category Antibiotic, Glycylcycline
Use Treatment of complicated skin and skin structure infections caused by susceptible organisms, including methicillin-resistant *Staphylococcus aureus* and vancomycin-sensitive *Enterococcus faecalis*; treatment of complicated intraabdominal infections
Usual Dosage I.V.: Adults:
Initial: 100 mg as a single dose
Maintenance dose: 50 mg every 12 hours
Recommended duration of therapy: Intraabdominal infections or complicated skin/skin structure infections: 5-14 days.
Dosage Forms
Injection, powder for reconstitution:
Tygacil®: 50 mg

Tikosyn® [US/Can] *see* dofetilide *on page 315*
Tilade® [US/Can] *see* nedocromil (inhalation) *on page 660*
Tilia™ Fe [US] *see* ethinyl estradiol and norethindrone *on page 376*

tiludronate (tye LOO droe nate)
Synonyms tiludronate disodium
U.S./Canadian Brand Names Skelid® [US]
Therapeutic Category Bisphosphonate Derivative
Use Treatment of Paget disease of the bone (osteitis deformans) in patients who have a level of serum alkaline phosphatase (SAP) at least twice the upper limit of normal, or who are symptomatic, or who are at risk for future complications of their disease
Usual Dosage Oral: Adults: 400 mg (2 tablets of tiludronic acid) daily for a period of 3 months; allow an interval of 3 months to assess response
Dosage Forms
Tablet:
Skelid®: 200 mg

tiludronate disodium *see* tiludronate *on page 927*
Tim-AK [Can] *see* timolol *on page 927*
Time-C [US-OTC] *see* ascorbic acid *on page 96*
Time-C-Bio [US-OTC] *see* ascorbic acid *on page 96*
Timecelles® *(Discontinued)* *see* ascorbic acid *on page 96*
Timentin® [US/Can] *see* ticarcillin and clavulanate potassium *on page 926*

timolol (TIM oh lol)
Sound-Alike/Look-Alike Issues
timolol may be confused with atenolol, Tylenol®
Timoptic® may be confused with Talacen®, Viroptic®
Synonyms timolol hemihydrate; timolol maleate
U.S./Canadian Brand Names Alti-Timolol [Can]; Apo-Timol® [Can]; Apo-Timop® [Can]; Betimol® [US]; Gen-Timolol [Can]; Istalol® [US]; Nu-Timolol [Can]; Phoxal-timolol [Can]; PMS-Timolol [Can]; Sandoz-Timolol [Can]; Tim-AK [Can]; Timolol GFS [US]; Timoptic-XE® [US/Can]; Timoptic® in OcuDose® [US]; Timoptic® [US/Can]
Therapeutic Category Beta-Adrenergic Blocker
Use
Ophthalmic: Treatment of elevated intraocular pressure such as glaucoma or ocular hypertension
Oral: Treatment of hypertension and angina; to reduce mortality following myocardial infarction; prophylaxis of migraine

▶

◀ **Usual Dosage**
Ophthalmic:
Children and Adults:
Solution: Initial: Instill 1 drop (0.25% solution) into affected eye(s) twice daily; increase to 0.5% solution if response not adequate; decrease to 1 drop/day if controlled; do not exceed 1 drop twice daily of 0.5% solution
Gel-forming solution (Timolol GFS, Timoptic-XE®): Instill 1 drop (either 0.25% or 0.5% solution) once daily
Adults: Solution (Istalol®): Instill 1 drop (0.5% solution) once daily in the morning
Oral: Adults:
Hypertension: Initial: 10 mg twice daily, increase gradually every 7 days, usual dosage: 20-40 mg/day in 2 divided doses; maximum: 60 mg/day
Prevention of myocardial infarction: 10 mg twice daily initiated within 1-4 weeks after infarction
Migraine headache: Initial: 10 mg twice daily, increase to maximum of 30 mg/day
Dosage Forms
Gel-forming solution, ophthalmic: 0.25% (5 mL); 0.5% (2.5 mL, 5 mL)
Timolol GFS: 0.25% (2.5 mL, 5 mL); 0.5% (2.5 mL, 5 mL)
Timoptic-XE®: 0.25% (5 mL); 0.5% (5 mL)
Solution, ophthalmic: 0.25% (5 mL, 10 mL, 15 mL); 0.5% (5 mL, 10 mL, 15 mL)
Betimol®: 0.25% (5 mL); 0.5% (5 mL, 10 mL, 15 mL)
Istalol®: 0.5% (10 mL)
Timoptic®: 0.25% (5 mL); 0.5% (5 mL, 10 mL)
Solution, ophthalmic [preservative free]: 0.25% (0.2 mL); 0.5% (0.2 mL)
Timoptic® in OcuDose®: 0.25% (0.2 mL); 0.5% (0.2 mL)
Tablet: 5 mg, 10 mg, 20 mg

timolol and brimonidine *see* brimonidine and timolol *on page 142*
timolol and dorzolamide *see* dorzolamide and timolol *on page 319*
Timolol GFS [US] *see* timolol *on page 927*
timolol hemihydrate *see* timolol *on page 927*
timolol maleate *see* timolol *on page 927*
Timoptic® [US/Can] *see* timolol *on page 927*
Timoptic® in OcuDose® [US] *see* timolol *on page 927*
Timoptic-XE® [US/Can] *see* timolol *on page 927*
Tinactin® Antifungal [US-OTC] *see* tolnaftate *on page 934*
Tinactin® Antifungal Deodorant [US-OTC] *see* tolnaftate *on page 934*
Tinactin® Antifungal Jock Itch [US-OTC] *see* tolnaftate *on page 934*
Tinaderm [US-OTC] *see* tolnaftate *on page 934*
Tinamed® Corn and Callus Remover [US-OTC] *see* salicylic acid *on page 850*
Tinamed® Wart Remover [US-OTC] *see* salicylic acid *on page 850*
TinBen® *(Discontinued)* *see* benzoin *on page 126*
Tindamax® [US] *see* tinidazole *on page 928*
Ting® Cream [US-OTC] *see* tolnaftate *on page 934*
Ting® Spray Liquid [US-OTC] *see* tolnaftate *on page 934*

tinidazole (tye NI da zole)
U.S./Canadian Brand Names Tindamax® [US]
Therapeutic Category Amebicide; Antibiotic, Miscellaneous; Antiprotozoal, Nitroimidazole
Use Treatment of trichomoniasis caused by *T. vaginalis*; treatment of giardiasis caused by *G. duodenalis* (*G. lamblia*); treatment of intestinal amebiasis and amebic liver abscess caused by *E. histolytica*; treatment of bacterial vaginosis caused by *Bacteroides* spp, *Gardnerella vaginalis*, and *Prevotella* spp in nonpregnant females
Usual Dosage Oral:
Children >3 years:
Amebiasis, intestinal: 50 mg/kg/day for 3 days (maximum dose: 2 g/day)
Amebiasis, liver abscess: 50 mg/kg/day for 3-5 days (maximum dose: 2 g/day)
Giardiasis: 50 mg/kg as a single dose (maximum dose: 2 g)
Adults:
Amebiasis, intestinal: 2 g/day for 3 days

Amebiasis, liver abscess: 2 g/day for 3-5 days
Bacterial vaginosis: 2 g/day for 2 days or 1 g/day for 5 days
Giardiasis: 2 g as a single dose
Trichomoniasis: 2 g as a single dose; sexual partners should be treated at the same time
Dosage Forms
  Tablet [scored]:
    Tindamax®: 250 mg, 500 mg

Tinver® *(Discontinued)* *see* sodium thiosulfate *on page 880*

tinzaparin (tin ZA pa rin)
Synonyms tinzaparin sodium
U.S./Canadian Brand Names Innohep® [US/Can]
Therapeutic Category Anticoagulant (Other)
Use Treatment of acute symptomatic deep vein thrombosis, with or without pulmonary embolism, in conjunction with warfarin sodium
Usual Dosage SubQ:
  Adults: 175 anti-Xa int. units/kg of body weight once daily. Warfarin sodium should be started when appropriate. Administer tinzaparin for at least 6 days and until patient is adequately anticoagulated with warfarin.
  Note: To calculate the volume of solution to administer per dose: Volume to be administered (mL) = patient weight (kg) x 0.00875 mL/kg (may be rounded off to the nearest 0.05 mL)
Dosage Forms
  Injection, solution:,
    Innohep®: 20,000 anti-Xa int. units/mL (2 mL)

tinzaparin sodium *see* tinzaparin *on page 929*

tioconazole (tye oh KONE a zole)
Sound-Alike/Look-Alike Issues
  tioconazole may be confused with terconazole
U.S./Canadian Brand Names 1-Day™ [US-OTC]; Vagistat®-1 [US-OTC]
Therapeutic Category Antifungal Agent
Use Local treatment of vulvovaginal candidiasis
Usual Dosage Adults: Vaginal: Insert 1 applicatorful in vagina, just prior to bedtime, as a single dose
Dosage Forms
  Ointment, vaginal:
    1-Day™ [OTC], Vagistat®-1 [OTC]: 6.5% (4.6 g)

tioguanine *see* thioguanine *on page 921*

tiopronin (tye oh PROE nin)
Sound-Alike/Look-Alike Issues
  Thiola® may be confused with Theolair™
U.S./Canadian Brand Names Thiola® [US/Can]
Therapeutic Category Urinary Tract Product
Use Prevention of kidney stone (cystine) formation in patients with severe homozygous cystinuric who have urinary cystine >500 mg/day who are resistant to treatment with high fluid intake, alkali, and diet modification, or who have had adverse reactions to penicillamine
Usual Dosage Adults: Initial dose is 800 mg/day, average dose is 1000 mg/day
Dosage Forms
  Tablet:
    Thiola®: 100 mg

tiotixene *see* thiothixene *on page 923*

tiotropium (ty oh TRO pee um)
Sound-Alike/Look-Alike Issues
  Spiriva® may be confused with Inspra™
Synonyms tiotropium bromide monohydrate

▶

◄ **U.S./Canadian Brand Names** Spiriva® HandiHaler® [US]; Spiriva® [Can]
Therapeutic Category Anticholinergic Agent
Use Maintenance treatment of bronchospasm associated with COPD (bronchitis and emphysema)
Usual Dosage Oral inhalation: Adults: Contents of 1 capsule (18 mcg) inhaled once daily using HandiHaler® device
Dosage Forms
 Powder for oral inhalation [capsule]:
  Spiriva® HandiHaler®: 18 mcg/capsule (5s, 30s, 90s)

tiotropium bromide monohydrate *see* tiotropium *on page 929*

tipranavir (tip RA na veer)
 Synonyms PNU-140690E; TPV
 U.S./Canadian Brand Names Aptivus® [US/Can]
 Therapeutic Category Antiretroviral Agent, Protease Inhibitor
 Use Treatment of HIV-1 infections in combination with ritonavir and other antiretroviral agents; limited to highly treatment-experienced or multiprotease inhibitor-resistant patients.
 Usual Dosage Oral:
  Children ≥2 years: 14 mg/kg or 375 mg/m^2 (maximum: 500 mg/dose) twice daily. **Note:** Coadministration with ritonavir (6 mg/kg or 150 mg/m^2 [maximum 200 mg/dose] twice daily) is required.
   If intolerance or toxicity develops and virus is not resistant to multiple protease inhibitors: May decrease dose to 12 mg/kg or 290 mg/m^2 twice daily. **Note:** Coadministration with ritonavir (5 mg/kg or 115 mg/m^2 twice daily) is required.
  Adults: 500 mg twice daily with a high-fat meal. **Note:** Coadministration with ritonavir (200 mg twice daily) is required.
 Dosage Forms
  Capsule, soft gelatin:
   Aptivus®: 250 mg
  Solution:
   Aptivus®: 100 mg/mL (95 mL)

TipTapToe *(Discontinued) see* tolnaftate *on page 934*

tirofiban (tye roe FYE ban)
 Sound-Alike/Look-Alike Issues
  Aggrastat® may be confused with Aggrenox®, argatroban
 Synonyms MK383; tirofiban hydrochloride
 U.S./Canadian Brand Names Aggrastat® [US/Can]
 Therapeutic Category Antiplatelet Agent
 Use In combination with heparin, is indicated for the treatment of acute coronary syndrome, including patients who are to be managed medically and those undergoing PTCA or atherectomy. In this setting, it has been shown to decrease the rate of a combined endpoint of death, new myocardial infarction or refractory ischemia/repeat cardiac procedure.
 Usual Dosage I.V.: Adults: Initial rate of 0.4 mcg/kg/minute for 30 minutes and then continued at 0.1 mcg/kg/minute; dosing should be continued through angiography and for 12-24 hours after angioplasty or atherectomy.
 Dosage Forms
  Infusion [premixed in sodium chloride]:
   Aggrastat®: 50 mcg/mL (100 mL, 250 mL)

tirofiban hydrochloride *see* tirofiban *on page 930*
Tirosint™ [US] *see* levothyroxine *on page 560*
Tisit® [US-OTC] *see* pyrethrins and piperonyl butoxide *on page 806*
Tisit® Blue Gel [US-OTC] *see* pyrethrins and piperonyl butoxide *on page 806*
Tisseel® VH [US/Can] *see* fibrin sealant kit *on page 400*
Titralac™ [US-OTC] *see* calcium carbonate *on page 163*
Titralac® Plus [US-OTC] *see* calcium carbonate and simethicone *on page 164*
Ti-U-Lac® H [Can] *see* urea and hydrocortisone *on page 964*

tizanidine (tye ZAN i deen)

Sound-Alike/Look-Alike Issues
   tiZANidine may be confused with tiaGABine
Tall-Man ti**ZAN**idine
U.S./Canadian Brand Names Apo-Tizanidine® [Can]; Gen-Tizanidine [Can]; Zanaflex Capsules™ [US]; Zanaflex® [US/Can]
Therapeutic Category Alpha$_2$-Adrenergic Agonist Agent
Use Skeletal muscle relaxant used for treatment of muscle spasticity
Usual Dosage Adults: 2-4 mg 3 times/day
   Usual initial dose: 4 mg, may increase by 2-4 mg as needed for satisfactory reduction of muscle tone every 6-8 hours to a maximum of 3 doses in any 24-hour period
   Maximum: 36 mg/day
Dosage Forms
   Capsule:
   Zanaflex Capsules™: 2 mg, 4 mg, 6 mg
   Tablet: 2 mg, 4 mg
   Zanaflex®: 4 mg [scored]

TMC-114 *see* darunavir *on page 268*
TMC125 *see* etravirine *on page 385*
TMP *see* trimethoprim *on page 953*
TMP-SMZ *see* sulfamethoxazole and trimethoprim *on page 894*
TMZ *see* temozolomide *on page 907*
T.N. Dickinson's® Hazelets [US-OTC] *see* witch hazel *on page 987*
TNKase® [US/Can] *see* tenecteplase *on page 908*
TOBI® [US/Can] *see* tobramycin *on page 931*
TobraDex® [US/Can] *see* tobramycin and dexamethasone *on page 932*

tobramycin (toe bra MYE sin)

Sound-Alike/Look-Alike Issues
   tobramycin may be confused with Trobicin®
   AKTob® may be confused with AK-Trol®
   Nebcin® may be confused with Inapsine®, Naprosyn®, Nubain®
   Tobrex® may be confused with TobraDex®
Synonyms tobramycin sulfate
U.S./Canadian Brand Names AKTob® [US]; PMS-Tobramycin [Can]; Sandoz-Tobramycin [Can]; TOBI® [US/Can]; Tobramycin Injection, USP [Can]; Tobrex® [US/Can]
Therapeutic Category Aminoglycoside (Antibiotic); Antibiotic, Ophthalmic
Use Treatment of documented or suspected infections caused by susceptible gram-negative bacilli including *Pseudomonas aeruginosa*; topically used to treat superficial ophthalmic infections caused by susceptible bacteria. Tobramycin solution for inhalation is indicated for the management of cystic fibrosis patients (>6 years of age) with *Pseudomonas aeruginosa*.
Usual Dosage Note: Dosage individualization is **critical** because of the low therapeutic index.
   Use of ideal body weight (IBW) for determining the mg/kg/dose appears to be more accurate than dosing on the basis of total body weight (TBW). In morbid obesity, dosage requirement may best be estimated using a dosing weight of IBW + 0.4 (TBW - IBW).
   Initial and periodic plasma drug levels (eg, peak and trough with conventional dosing) should be determined, particularly in critically-ill patients with serious infections or in disease states known to significantly alter aminoglycoside pharmacokinetics (eg, cystic fibrosis, burns, or major surgery).

   Usual dosage range:
   Infants and Children <5 years: I.M., I.V.: 2.5 mg/kg/dose every 8 hours
   Children ≥5 years: I.M., I.V.: 2-2.5 mg/kg/dose every 8 hours
      Note: Higher individual doses and/or more frequent intervals (eg, every 6 hours) may be required in selected clinical situations (cystic fibrosis) or serum levels document the need.
   Children and Adults:
      Inhalation: TOBI®: Children ≥6 years and Adults: 300 mg every 12 hours (do not administer doses <6 hours apart); administer in repeated cycles of 28 days on drug followed by 28 days off drug.
      Intrathecal: 4-8 mg/day

Ophthalmic: Children ≥2 months and Adults:
  Ointment: Instill ½" (1.25 cm) 2-3 times/day every 3-4 hours
  Solution: Instill 1-2 drops every 2-4 hours, up to 2 drops every hour for severe infections
Topical: Apply 3-4 times/day to affected area
Adults: I.M., I.V.:
  Conventional: 1-2.5 mg/kg/dose every 8-12 hours; to ensure adequate peak concentrations early in therapy, higher initial dosage may be considered in selected patients when extracellular water is increased (edema, septic shock, postsurgical, and/or trauma)
  Once-daily: 4-7 mg/kg/dose once daily; some clinicians recommend this approach for all patients with normal renal function; this dose is at least as efficacious with similar, if not less, toxicity than conventional dosing.

Indication-specific dosing:
Neonates:
Meningitis: I.M., I.V.:
  0-7 days: <2000 g: 2.5 mg/kg every 18-24 hours; >2000 g: 2.5 mg/kg every 12 hours
  8-28 days: <2000 g: 2.5 mg/kg every 8-12 hours; >2000 g: 2.5 mg/kg every 8 hours
Children:
Cystic fibrosis:
  I.M., I.V.: 2.5-3.3 mg/kg every 6-8 hours; **Note:** Some patients may require larger or more frequent doses if serum levels document the need (eg, cystic fibrosis or febrile granulocytopenic patients).
  Inhalation: See adult dosing.
Adults:
I.M., I.V.:
  Brucellosis: 240 mg (I.M.) daily or 5 mg/kg (I.V.) daily for 7 days; either regimen recommended in combination with doxycycline
  Cholangitis: 4-6 mg/kg once daily with ampicillin
  Diverticulitis, complicated: 1.5-2 mg/kg every 8 hours (with ampicillin and metronidazole)
  Infective endocarditis or synergy (for gram-positive infections): I.M., I.V.: 1 mg/kg every 8 hours (with ampicillin)
  Meningitis *(Enterococcus or Pseudomonas aeruginosa):* I.V.: Loading dose: 2 mg/kg, then 1.7 mg/kg/dose every 8 hours (administered with another bacteriocidal drug)
  Pelvic inflammatory disease: Loading dose: 2 mg/kg, then 1.5 mg/kg every 8 hours **or** 4.5 mg/kg once daily
  Plague *(Yersinia pestis):* Treatment: 5 mg/kg/day, followed by postexposure prophylaxis with doxycycline
  Pneumonia, hospital- or ventilator-associated: 7 mg/kg/day (with antipseudomonal beta-lactam or carbapenem)
  Prophylaxis against endocarditis (dental, oral, upper respiratory procedures, GI/GU procedures): 1.5 mg/kg with ampicillin (50 mg/kg) 30 minutes prior to procedure. **Note:** AHA guidelines now recommend prophylaxis only in patients undergoing invasive procedures and in whom underlying cardiac conditions may predispose to a higher risk of adverse outcomes should infection occur. As of April 2007, routine prophylaxis no longer recommended by the AHA.
  Tularemia: 5 mg/kg/day divided every 8 hours for 1-2 weeks
  Urinary tract infection: 1.5 mg/kg/dose every 8 hours
Inhalation: **Cystic fibrosis:** TOBI®: 300 mg every 12 hours (do not administer doses <6 hours apart); administer in repeated cycles of 28 days on drug followed by 28 days off drug.

Dosage Forms
Infusion [premixed in NS]: 60 mg (50 mL); 80 mg (100 mL)
Injection, powder for reconstitution: 1.2 g
Injection, solution: 10 mg/mL (2 mL, 8 mL); 40 mg/mL (2 mL, 30 mL, 50 mL)
Ointment, ophthalmic:
  Tobrex®: 0.3% (3.5 g)
Solution for nebulization [preservative free]:
  TOBI®: 60 mg/mL (5 mL)
Solution, ophthalmic: 0.3% (5 mL)
  AKTob®, Tobrex®: 0.3% (5 mL)

tobramycin and dexamethasone (toe bra MYE sin & deks a METH a sone)

Sound-Alike/Look-Alike Issues
  TobraDex® may be confused with Tobrex®
Synonyms dexamethasone and tobramycin

U.S./Canadian Brand Names TobraDex® [US/Can]

Therapeutic Category Antibiotic/Corticosteroid, Ophthalmic

Use Treatment of external ocular infection caused by susceptible gram-negative bacteria and steroid responsive inflammatory conditions of the palpebral and bulbar conjunctiva, lid, cornea, and anterior segment of the globe

Usual Dosage Ophthalmic: Children and Adults: Instill 1-2 drops of solution every 4 hours; apply ointment 2-3 times/day; for severe infections apply ointment every 3-4 hours, or solution 2 drops every 30-60 minutes initially, then reduce to less frequent intervals

Dosage Forms

Ointment, ophthalmic:
TobraDex®: Tobramycin 0.3% and dexamethasone 0.1% (3.5 g)

Suspension, ophthalmic:
TobraDex®: Tobramycin 0.3% and dexamethasone 0.1% (2.5 mL, 5 mL, 10 mL)

tobramycin and loteprednol etabonate see loteprednol and tobramycin *on page 579*

Tobramycin Injection, USP [Can] see tobramycin *on page 931*

tobramycin sulfate see tobramycin *on page 931*

Tobrex® [US/Can] see tobramycin *on page 931*

tocophersolan *(Discontinued)*

Today® [US-OTC] see nonoxynol 9 *on page 677*

Tofranil® [US/Can] see imipramine *on page 501*

Tofranil-PM® [US] see imipramine *on page 501*

tolazamide (tole AZ a mide)

Sound-Alike/Look-Alike Issues
TOLAZamide may be confused with tolazoline, TOLBUTamide
Tolinase® may be confused with Orinase®

Tall-Man TOLAZamide

U.S./Canadian Brand Names Tolinase® [Can]

Therapeutic Category Antidiabetic Agent, Oral

Use Adjunct to diet for the management of mild to moderately severe, stable, type 2 diabetes mellitus (noninsulin-dependent, NIDDM)

Usual Dosage Oral: Doses >500 mg/day should be given in 2 divided doses: Adults:
Initial: 100-250 mg/day with breakfast or the first main meal of the day
Fasting blood sugar <200 mg/dL: 100 mg/day
Fasting blood sugar >200 mg/dL: 250 mg/day
Patient is malnourished, underweight, elderly, or not eating properly: 100 mg/day
Adjust dose in increments of 100-250 mg/day at weekly intervals to response; maximum daily dose: 1 g (doses >1 g/day are not likely to improve control)

Conversion from insulin to tolazamide
<20 units day = 100 mg/day
21- <40 units/day = 250 mg/day
≥40 units/day = 250 mg/day and 50% of insulin dose

Dosage Forms
Tablet: 250 mg, 500 mg

tolbutamide (tole BYOO ta mide)

Sound-Alike/Look-Alike Issues
TOLBUTamide may be confused with terbutaline, TOLAZamide
Orinase® may be confused with Orabase®, Ornex®, Tolinase®

Synonyms tolbutamide sodium

Tall-Man TOLBUTamide

U.S./Canadian Brand Names Apo-Tolbutamide® [Can]

Therapeutic Category Antidiabetic Agent, Oral

Use Adjunct to diet for the management of type 2 diabetes mellitus (noninsulin-dependent, NIDDM)

Usual Dosage Note: Divided doses may improve gastrointestinal tolerance
Oral: Adults: Initial: 1-2 g/day as a single dose in the morning or in divided doses throughout the day. Maintenance dose: 0.25-3 g/day; however, a maintenance dose >2 g/day is seldom required.

▶

◀ **Dosage Forms**
Tablet: 500 mg

tolbutamide sodium *see* tolbutamide *on page 933*

tolcapone (TOLE ka pone)

U.S./Canadian Brand Names Tasmar® [US]
Therapeutic Category Anti-Parkinson Agent
Use Adjunct to levodopa and carbidopa for the treatment of signs and symptoms of idiopathic Parkinson disease in patients with motor fluctuations not responsive to other therapies
Usual Dosage Note: If clinical improvement is not observed after 3 weeks of therapy (regardless of dose), tolcapone treatment should be discontinued.
Oral: Adults: Initial: 100 mg 3 times/day; may increase as tolerated to 200 mg 3 times/day. **Note:** Levodopa dose may need to be decreased upon initiation of tolcapone (average reduction in clinical trials was 30%). As many as 70% of patients receiving levodopa doses >600 mg daily required levodopa dosage reduction in clinical trials. Patients with moderate-to-severe dyskinesia prior to initiation are also more likely to require dosage reduction.
Dosage Forms
Tablet:
Tasmar®: 100 mg, 200 mg

Tolectin® DS (Discontinued) *see* tolmetin *on page 934*
Tolinase® [Can] *see* tolazamide *on page 933*
Tolinase® (Discontinued) *see* tolazamide *on page 933*

tolmetin (TOLE met in)

Synonyms tolmetin sodium
Therapeutic Category Analgesic, Nonnarcotic; Nonsteroidal Antiinflammatory Drug (NSAID)
Use Treatment of rheumatoid arthritis and osteoarthritis, juvenile rheumatoid arthritis
Usual Dosage Oral:
Children ≥2 years: JRA: Initial: 20 mg/kg/day in 3-4 divided doses, then 15-30 mg/kg/day in 3-4 divided doses (maximum dose: 30 mg/kg/day)
Adults: RA, osteoarthritis: 400 mg 3 times/day; usual dose: 600 mg to 1.8 g/day; maximum: 1.8 g/day
Dosage Forms
Capsule: 400 mg
Tablet: 200 mg, 600 mg

tolmetin sodium *see* tolmetin *on page 934*

tolnaftate (tole NAF tate)

Sound-Alike/Look-Alike Issues
tolnaftate may be confused with Tornalate®
Tinactin® may be confused with Talacen®
U.S./Canadian Brand Names Blis-To-Sol® [US-OTC]; FungiGuard [US-OTC]; Mycocide® NS [US-OTC]; Pitrex [Can]; Podactin Powder [US-OTC]; Tinactin® Antifungal Deodorant [US-OTC]; Tinactin® Antifungal Jock Itch [US-OTC]; Tinactin® Antifungal [US-OTC]; Tinaderm [US-OTC]; Ting® Cream [US-OTC]; Ting® Spray Liquid [US-OTC]
Therapeutic Category Antifungal Agent
Use Treatment of tinea pedis, tinea cruris, tinea corporis
Usual Dosage Topical: Children ≥2 years and Adults: Wash and dry affected area; spray aerosol or apply 1-3 drops of solution or a small amount of cream, or powder and rub into the affected areas 2 times/day
Note: May use for up to 4 weeks for tinea pedis or tinea corporis, and up to 2 weeks for tinea cruris
Dosage Forms
Aerosol, topical [spray]:
Tinactin® Antifungal [OTC]: 1% (150 g)
Ting®: 1% (128 g)
Aerosol, topical [powder, spray]:
Tinactin® Antifungal Deodorant [OTC], Tinactin® Antifungal [OTC], Tinactin® Antifungal Jock Itch [OTC]: 1% (133 g)

Cream, topical: 1% (15 g, 30 g)
FungiGuard [OTC], Tinactin® Antifungal Jock Itch [OTC], Ting® [OTC]: 1% (15 g)
Tinactin® Antifungal [OTC]: 1% (15 g, 30 g)
Liquid, topical:
Blis-To-Sol® [OTC]: 1% (30 mL, 55 mL)
FungiGuard [OTC]: 1% (30 mL)
Liquid, topical [spray]:
Tinactin® Antifungal [OTC]: 1% (59 mL)
Powder, topical: 1% (45 g)
Podactin [OTC]: 1% (45 g)
Tinactin® Antifungal [OTC]: 1% (108 g)
Solution, topical: 1% (10 mL)
Mycocide® NS [OTC]: 1% (30 mL)
Tinaderm [OTC]: 1% (10 mL)

tolterodine (tole TER oh deen)

Sound-Alike/Look-Alike Issues
Detrol® may be confused with Ditropan®
Synonyms tolterodine tartrate
U.S./Canadian Brand Names Detrol® LA [US/Can]; Detrol® [US/Can]; Unidet® [Can]
Therapeutic Category Anticholinergic Agent
Use Treatment of patients with an overactive bladder with symptoms of urinary frequency, urgency, or urge incontinence
Usual Dosage Oral: Adults: Treatment of overactive bladder:
Immediate release tablet: 2 mg twice daily; the dose may be lowered to 1 mg twice daily based on individual response and tolerability
Extended release capsule: 4 mg once a day; dose may be lowered to 2 mg daily based on individual response and tolerability
Dosage Forms
Capsule, extended release:
Detrol® LA: 2 mg, 4 mg
Tablet:
Detrol®: 1 mg, 2 mg

tolterodine tartrate *see* tolterodine *on page 935*
Tomocat® [US] *see* barium *on page 116*
Tomocat® 1000 [US] *see* barium *on page 116*
tomoxetine *see* atomoxetine *on page 102*
Tomudex® [Can] *see* raltitrexed *(Canada only) on page 817*
Tomycine® *(Discontinued)* *see* tobramycin *on page 931*
Tonocard® *(Discontinued)*
Tonojug [US] *see* barium *on page 116*
Tonopaque [US] *see* barium *on page 116*
Topamax® [US/Can] *see* topiramate *on page 935*
Topamax® 200 mg Tablet *(Discontinued)* *see* topiramate *on page 935*
Topicaine® [US-OTC] *see* lidocaine *on page 561*
Topicort® [US/Can] *see* desoximetasone *on page 277*
Topicort®-LP [US] *see* desoximetasone *on page 277*
Topicycline® Topical *(Discontinued)* *see* tetracycline *on page 915*
Topilene® [Can] *see* betamethasone (topical) *on page 132*

topiramate (toe PYRE a mate)

Sound-Alike/Look-Alike Issues
Topamax® may be confused with Tegretol®, Tegretol®-XR, Toprol-XL®
U.S./Canadian Brand Names Apo-Topiramate [Can]; Co-Topiramate [Can]; Dom-Topiramate [Can]; Gen-Topiramate [Can]; Novo-Topiramate [Can]; PHL-Topiramate [Can]; PMS-Topiramate [Can]; ratio-Topiramate [Can]; Sandoz-Topiramate [Can]; Topamax® [US/Can]
Therapeutic Category Anticonvulsant

▶

◀ **Use** Monotherapy or adjunctive therapy for partial onset seizures and primary generalized tonic-clonic seizures; adjunctive treatment of seizures associated with Lennox-Gastaut syndrome; prophylaxis of migraine headache

Usual Dosage Oral: **Note:** Do not abruptly discontinue therapy; taper dosage gradually to prevent rebound effects. (In clinical trials, adult doses were withdrawn by decreasing in weekly intervals of 50-100 mg/day gradually over 2-8 weeks for seizure treatment, and by decreasing in weekly intervals by 25-50 mg/day for migraine prophylaxis.)

Epilepsy, monotherapy: Children ≥10 years and Adults: Partial onset seizure and primary generalized tonic-clonic seizure: Initial: 25 mg twice daily; may increase weekly by 50 mg/day up to 100 mg twice daily (week 4 dose); thereafter, may further increase weekly by 100 mg/day up to the recommended maximum of 200 mg twice daily.

Epilepsy, adjunctive therapy:

Children 2-16 years:

Partial onset seizure or seizure associated with Lennox-Gastaut syndrome: Initial dose titration should begin at 25 mg (or less, based on a range of 1-3 mg/kg/day) nightly for the first week; dosage may be increased in increments of 1-3 mg/kg/day (administered in 2 divided doses) at 1- or 2-week intervals to a total daily dose of 5-9 mg/kg/day

Primary generalized tonic-clonic seizure: Use initial dose listed above, but use slower initial titration rate; titrate to recommended maintenance dose by the end of 8 weeks

Adolescents ≥17 years and Adults:

Partial onset seizures: Initial: 25-50 mg/day (given in 2 divided doses) for 1 week; increase at weekly intervals by 25-50 mg/day until response; usual maintenance dose: 100-200 mg twice daily. Doses >1600 mg/day have not been studied.

Primary generalized tonic-clonic seizures: Use initial dose as listed above for partial onset seizures, but use slower initial titration rate; titrate upwards to recommended dose by the end of 8 weeks; usual maintenance dose: 200 mg twice daily. Doses >1600 mg/day have not been studied.

Adults: Migraine prophylaxis: Initial: 25 mg/day (in the evening), titrated at weekly intervals in 25 mg increments, up to the recommended total daily dose of 100 mg/day given in 2 divided doses

Dosage Forms

Capsule, sprinkle:

Topamax®: 15 mg, 25 mg

Tablet:

Topamax®: 25 mg, 50 mg, 100 mg, 200 mg

Topisone® [Can] *see* betamethasone (topical) *on page 132*

Toposar® [US] *see* etoposide *on page 384*

topotecan (toe poe TEE kan)

Sound-Alike/Look-Alike Issues

Hycamtin® may be confused with Hycomine®, Mycamine®

Synonyms hycamptamine; NSC-609699; SKF 104864; SKF 104864-A; topotecan hydrochloride

U.S./Canadian Brand Names Hycamtin® [US/Can]

Therapeutic Category Antineoplastic Agent

Use Treatment of ovarian cancer and small cell lung cancer; cervical cancer (in combination with cisplatin)

Usual Dosage Adults (refer to individual protocols): **Note:** Baseline neutrophil count should be >1500/mm^3; retreatment neutrophil count should be >1000/mm^3; baseline and retreatment platelet count should be >100,000/mm^3; (also, for oral topotecan, retreatment hemoglobin should be ≥9 g/dL):

Small cell lung cancer:

IVPB: 1.5 mg/m^2/day for 5 days; repeated every 21 days

Oral: 2.3 mg/m^2/day for 5 days; repeated every 21 days (round dose to the nearest 0.25 mg); if patient vomits after dose is administered, do not give a replacement dose.

Metastatic ovarian cancer: IVPB: 1.5 mg/m^2/day for 5 days; repeated every 21 days

Cervical cancer: IVPB: 0.75 mg/m^2/day for 3 days (followed by cisplatin 50 mg/m^2 on day 1 only, [with hydration]); repeated every 21 days

Dosage Forms

Capsule:

Hycamtin®: 0.25 mg, 1 mg

Injection, powder for reconstitution:

Hycamtin®: 4 mg

topotecan hydrochloride *see* topotecan *on page 936*

Toprol-XL® [US/Can] *see* metoprolol *on page 626*
Topsyn® [Can] *see* fluocinonide *on page 410*
Toradol® [Can] *see* ketorolac *on page 538*
Toradol® IM [Can] *see* ketorolac *on page 538*

toremifene (tore EM i feen)
Synonyms FC1157a; toremifene citrate
U.S./Canadian Brand Names Fareston® [US/Can]
Therapeutic Category Antineoplastic Agent
Use Treatment of postmenopausal metastatic breast cancer (estrogen receptor positive or estrogen receptor status unknown)
Usual Dosage Oral: Adults: 60 mg once daily, generally continued until disease progression is observed
Dosage Forms
Tablet:
Fareston®: 60 mg

toremifene citrate *see* toremifene *on page 937*
Torisel™ [US/Can] *see* temsirolimus *on page 908*

torsemide (TORE se mide)
Sound-Alike/Look-Alike Issues
torsemide may be confused with furosemide
Demadex® may be confused with Denorex®
U.S./Canadian Brand Names Demadex® [US]
Therapeutic Category Diuretic, Loop
Use Management of edema associated with congestive heart failure and hepatic or renal disease; used alone or in combination with antihypertensives in treatment of hypertension; I.V. form is indicated when rapid onset is desired
Usual Dosage Oral, I.V.: Adults:
Congestive heart failure: 10-20 mg once daily; may increase gradually for chronic treatment by doubling dose until the diuretic response is apparent (for acute treatment, I.V. dose may be repeated every 2 hours with double the dose as needed). **Note:** ACC/AHA 2005 guidelines for chronic heart failure recommend a maximum daily oral dose of 200 mg; maximum single I.V. dose of 100-200 mg
Continuous I.V. infusion: 20 mg I.V. load then 5-20 mg/hour
Chronic renal failure: 20 mg once daily; increase as described above
Hepatic cirrhosis: 5-10 mg once daily with an aldosterone antagonist or a potassium-sparing diuretic; increase as described above
Hypertension: 2.5-5 mg once daily; increase to 10 mg after 4-6 weeks if an adequate hypotensive response is not apparent; if still not effective, an additional antihypertensive agent may be added
Dosage Forms
Injection, solution:
Demadex®: 10 mg/mL
Tablet: 5 mg, 10 mg, 20 mg, 100 mg
Demadex®: 5 mg, 10 mg, 20 mg, 100 mg [scpred]

tositumomab I-131 *see* tositumomab and iodine I 131 tositumomab *on page 937*

tositumomab and iodine I 131 tositumomab
(toe si TYOO mo mab & EYE oh dyne eye one THUR tee one toe si TYOO mo mab)
Synonyms 131 I anti-B1 antibody; 131 I-anti-B1 monoclonal antibody; anti-CD20-murine monoclonal antibody I-131; B1; B1 antibody; iodine I 131 tositumomab and tositumomab; tositumomab I-131
U.S./Canadian Brand Names Bexxar® [US]
Therapeutic Category Antineoplastic Agent, Monoclonal Antibody; Radiopharmaceutical
Use Treatment of relapsed or refractory CD20 positive, low-grade, follicular, or transformed non-Hodgkin lymphoma
Usual Dosage I.V.: Adults: Dosing consists of four components administered in 2 steps. Thyroid protective agents (SSKI, Lugol's solution or potassium iodide), acetaminophen and diphenhydramine should be given prior to or with treatment.

◀ Step 1: Dosimetric step (Day 0):
Tositumomab 450 mg in NS 50 mL administered over 60 minutes
Iodine I 131 tositumomab (containing I-131 5.0 mCi and tositumomab 35 mg) in NS 30 mL administered over 20 minutes
Note: Whole body dosimetry and biodistribution should be determined on Day 0; days 2, 3, or 4; and day 6 or 7 prior to administration of Step 2. If biodistribution is not acceptable, do not administer the therapeutic step. On day 6 or 7, calculate the patient specific activity of iodine I 131 tositumomab to deliver 75 cGy TBD or 65 cGy TBD (in mCi).
Step 2: Therapeutic step (Day 7):
Tositumomab 450 mg in NS 50 mL administered over 60 minutes
Iodine I 131 tositumomab:
Platelets ≥150,000/mm^3: Iodine I 131 calculated to deliver 75 cGy total body irradiation and tositumomab 35 mg over 20 minutes
Platelets ≥100,000/mm^3 and <150,000/mm^3: Iodine I 131 calculated to deliver 65 cGy total body irradiation and tositumomab 35 mg over 20 minutes
Dosage Forms
Kit [dosimetric package]:
Bexxar®: Tositumomab 225 mg/16.1 mL [2 vials], tositumomab 35 mg/2.5 mL [1 vial], and iodine I 131 tositumomab 0.1 mg/mL and 0.61mCi/mL (20 mL) [1 vial]
Kit [therapeutic package]:
Bexxar®: Tositumomab 225 mg/16.1 mL [2 vials], tositumomab 35 mg/2.5 mL [1 vial], and iodine I 131 tositumomab 1.1 mg/mL and 5.6 mCi/mL (20 mL) [1 or 2 vials]

Totacillin® *(Discontinued)* see ampicillin on page 72

total parenteral nutrition (TOE tal par EN ter al noo TRISH un)
Synonyms hyperal; hyperalimentation; parenteral nutrition; PN; TPN
Therapeutic Category Caloric Agent; Intravenous Nutritional Therapy
Use Infusion of nutrient solutions into the bloodstream to support nutritional needs during a time when patient is unable to absorb nutrients via the gastrointestinal tract, cannot take adequate nutrition orally or enterally, or have had (or are expected to have) inadequate oral intake for 7-14 days
Usual Dosage PN is a highly-individualized therapy. The following general guidelines may be used in the estimation of needs. Electrolytes, vitamins, and trace minerals should be added to TPN mixtures based on patients individualized needs.

Neonates: I.V.: **Note:** When indicated for premature neonates, start on day 1 of life if possible.
Total calories:
Term: 85-105 kcal/kg/day
Preterm (stable): 90-120 kcal/kg/day
Fluid:
<1.5 kg: 130-150 mL/kg/day
1.5-2 kg: 110-130 mL/kg/day
2-10 kg: 100 mL/kg/day
Carbohydrate (dextrose): 40% to 50% of caloric intake; advance as tolerated
Term: Initial: 6-8 mg/kg/minute; goal: 10-14 mg/kg/minute
Premature: Initial: 6 mg/kg/minute; goal: 10-13 mg/kg/minute
Protein (amino acids):
Term: Initial: 2.5 g/kg/day; goal: 3 g/kg/day
Extremely (<1000 g) and very (<1500 g) low-birth-weight (stable): Initial: 1-1.5 g/kg/day; goal: 3.5-3.85 g/kg/day to promote utero growth rates.
Sepsis, hypoxia: Initial: 1 g/kg/day; goal: 3-3.85 g/kg/day
Fat:
Term: Initial: 0.5-1 g/kg/day (maximum: 3 g/kg/day); administer over 24 hours
Preterm: Initial: 0.25-0.5 g/kg/day (maximum: 3 g/kg/day or 1 g/kg/day if on phototherapy); administer over 24 hours
Note: Monitor triglycerides while receiving intralipids. If triglycerides >200 mg/dL, stop infusion and restart at 0.5-1g/kg/day
Heparin: 1 unit/mL of parenteral nutrition fluids should be added to enhance clearance of lipid emulsions

Children: I.V.: **Note:** Give within 5-7 days if unable to meet needs orally or with enteral nutrition:
Total calories:
<6 months: 85-105 kcal/kg/day
6-12 months: 80-100 kcal/kg/day

1-7 years: 75-90 kcal/kg/day
7-12 years: 50-75 kcal/kg/day
12-18 years: 30-50 kcal/kg/day
Fluid:
2-10 kg: 100 mL/kg
>10-20 kg: 1000 mL for 10 kg plus 50 mL/kg for each kg >10
>20 kg: 1500 mL for 10 kg plus 20 mL/kg for each kg >20
Carbohydrate (dextrose): 40% to 50% of caloric intake
<1 year: Initial: 6-8 mg/kg/minute; goal: 10-14 mg/kg/minute
1-10 years: Initial: 10% to 12.5%; daily increase: 5% increments (maximum: 15 mg/kg/minute)
>10 years: Initial: 10% to 15%; daily increase: 5% increments (maximum: 8.5 mg/kg/minute)
Protein (amino acids):
1-12 months: Initial: 2-3 g/kg/day; daily increase: 1 g/kg/day (maximum: 3 g/kg/day)
1-10 years: Initial: 1-2 g/kg/day; daily increase: 1 g/kg/day (maximum: 2-2.5 g/kg/day)
>10 years: Initial: 0.8-1.5 g/kg/day; daily increase: 1 g/kg/day (maximum: 1.5-2 g/kg/day)
Fat: Initial: 1 g/kg/day; daily increase: 1 g/kg/day (maximum: 3 g/kg/day); **Note:** Monitor triglycerides while receiving intralipids.

Adults: I.V.:
Total calories: Calculate using Harris-Benedict equation or based on stress level as indicated below:
Harris-Benedict Equation (BEE):
Females: 655.1 + [(9.56 x W) + (1.85 x H) - (4.68 x A)]
Males: 66.47 + [(13.75 x W) + (5 x H) - (6.76 x A)]
Then multiply BEE x (activity factor) x (stress factor)
W = weight in kg; H = height in cm; A = age in years
Activity factor = 1.2 sedentary, 1.3 normal activity, 1.4 active, 1.5 very active
Stress factor = 1.5 for trauma, stressed, or surgical patients and underweight (to promote weight gain); 2.0 for severe burn patients
Stress level:
Normal/mild stress level: 20-25 kcal/kg/day
Moderate stress level: 25-30 kcal/kg/day
Severe stress level: 30-40 kcal/kg/day
Pregnant women in second or third trimester: Add an additional 300 kcal/day
Fluid: mL/day = 30-40 mL/kg
Carbohydrate (dextrose):
5 g/kg/day or 3.5 mg/kg/minute (maximum rate: 4-7 mg/kg/minute)
Minimum recommended amount: 400 calories/day or 100 g/day
Protein (amino acids):
Maintenance: 0.8-1 g/kg/day
Normal/mild stress level: 1-1.2 g/kg/day
Moderate stress level: 1.2-1.5 g/kg/day
Severe stress level: 1.5-2 g/kg/day
Burn patients (severe): Increase protein until significant wound healing achieved
Solid organ transplant: Perioperative: 1.5-2 g/kg/day
Renal failure:
Acute (severely malnourished or hypercatabolic): 1.5-1.8 g/kg/day
Chronic, with dialysis: 1.2-1.3 g/kg/day
Chronic, without dialysis: 0.6-0.8 g/kg/day
Continuous hemofiltration: ≥1 g/kg/day
Hepatic failure:
Acute management when other treatments have failed:
With encephalopathy: 0.6-1 g/kg/day
Without encephalopathy: 1-1.5 g/kg/day
Chronic encephalopathy: Use branch chain amino acid enriched diets only if unresponsive to pharmacotherapy
Pregnant women in second or third trimester: Add an additional 10-14 g/day
Fat:
Initial: 20% to 40 % of total calories (maximum: 60% of total calories or 2.5 g/kg/day); **Note:** Monitor triglycerides while receiving intralipids.
Safe for use in pregnancy
I.V. lipids are safe in adults with pancreatitis if triglyceride levels <400 mg/dL
Dosage Forms TPN is usually compounded from optimal combinations of macronutrients (water, protein, dextrose, and lipids) and micronutrients (electrolytes, trace elements, and vitamins) to meet the specific ▶

◀ nutritional requirements of a patient. Individual hospitals may have designated standard TPN formulas. There are a few commercially-available amino acids with electrolytes solutions; however, these products may not meet an individual's specific nutrition requirements.

Totect™ [US] *see dexrazoxane on page 281*

Touro® CC [US] *see guaifenesin, pseudoephedrine, and dextromethorphan on page 460*

Touro® CC-LD [US] *see guaifenesin, pseudoephedrine, and dextromethorphan on page 460*

Touro® Allergy [US] *see brompheniramine and pseudoephedrine on page 144*

Touro® DM [US] *see guaifenesin and dextromethorphan on page 454*

Touro Ex® *(Discontinued)* *see guaifenesin on page 453*

Touro® HC *(Discontinued)*

Touro LA® [US] *see guaifenesin and pseudoephedrine on page 458*

tPA *see alteplase on page 51*

TPN *see total parenteral nutrition on page 938*

TPV *see tipranavir on page 930*

tRA *see tretinoin (oral) on page 946*

4 Trace Elements [US] *see trace metals on page 940*

Trace Elements 4 Pediatric [US] *see trace metals on page 940*

trace metals (trase MET als)

Synonyms chromium; copper; iodine; manganese; molybdenum; neonatal trace metals; selenium; zinc

U.S./Canadian Brand Names 4 Trace Elements [US]; Multitrace®-4 Concentrate [US]; Multitrace®-4 Neonatal [US]; Multitrace®-4 Pediatric [US]; Multitrace®-4 [US]; Multitrace®-5 Concentrate [US]; Multitrace®-5 [US]; Trace Elements 4 Pediatric [US]

Therapeutic Category Trace Element

Use Prevention and correction of trace metal deficiencies

Usual Dosage Recommended daily parenteral dosage:
  Chromium:[1]
    Infants: 0.2 mcg/kg
    Children: 0.2 mcg/kg (maximum: 5 mcg)
    Adults: 10-15 mcg
  Copper:[2]
    Infants: 20 mcg/kg
    Children: 20 mcg/kg (maximum: 300 mcg)
    Adults: 0.5-1.5 mg
  Manganese:[2,3]
    Infants: 1 mcg/kg
    Children: 1 mcg/kg (maximum: 50 mcg)
    Adults: 150-800 mcg
  Molybdenum:[1,4]
    Infants: 0.25 mcg/kg
    Children: 0.25 mcg/kg (maximum: 5 mcg)
    Adults: 20-120 mcg
  Selenium:[1,4]
    Infants: 2 mcg/kg
    Children: 2 mcg/kg (maximum: 30 mcg)
    Adults: 20-40 mcg
  Zinc:
    Infants, preterm: 400 mcg/kg
    Infants, term <3 months: 250 mcg/kg
    Infants, term >3 months: 100 mcg/kg
    Children: 50 mcg/kg (maximum: 5 mg)
    Adults: 2.5-4 mg
[1]Omit in patients with renal dysfunction.
[2]Omit in patients with obstructive jaundice.
[3]Current available commercial products are not in appropriate ratios to maintain this recommendation; doses of up to 10 mcg/kg have been used.
[4]Indicated for use in long-term parenteral nutrition patients.

Dosage Forms
Injection, solution [combination products]:
  Multitrace®-4: Chromium 4 mcg, copper 0.4 mg, manganese 0.1 mg, and zinc 1 mg per 1 mL (10 mL)
  Multitrace®-4 Concentrate: Chromium 10 mcg, copper 1 mg, manganese 0.5 mg, and zinc 5 mg per 1 mL (1 mL, 10 mL)
  Multitrace®-4 Neonatal: Chromium 0.85 mcg, copper 0.1 mg, manganese 0.025 mg, and zinc 1.5 mg per 1 mL (2 mL)
  Multitrace®-5: Chromium 4 mcg, copper 0.4 mg, manganese 0.1 mg, selenium 20 mcg, and zinc 1 mg per 1 mL (10 mL)
  Multitrace®-5 Concentrate: Chromium 10 mcg, copper 1 mg, manganese 0.5 mg, selenium 60 mcg, and zinc 5 mg per 1 mL (1 mL, 10 mL)
  Trace Elements 4 Pediatric: Chromium 1 mcg, copper 0.1 mg, manganese 0.03 mg, and zinc 0.5 mg per 1 mL (10 mL)
Injection, solution [combination products, preservative free]:
  4 Trace Elements: Chromium 2 mcg, copper 0.2 mg, manganese 0.16 mg, and zinc 0.8 mg per 1 mL (5 mL, 50 mL)
  Multitrace®-4 Pediatric: Chromium 1 mcg, copper 0.1 mg, manganese 0.025 mg, and zinc 1 mg per 1 mL (3 mL)

Tracleer® [US/Can] *see* bosentan *on page 140*
Tramacet [Can] *see* acetaminophen and tramadol *on page 24*

tramadol (TRA ma dole)

Sound-Alike/Look-Alike Issues
  traMADol may be confused with Toradol®, Trandate®, traZODone, Voltaren®
  Ultram® may be confused with Ultane®, Ultracet®, Voltaren®
Synonyms tramadol hydrochloride
Tall-Man traMADol
U.S./Canadian Brand Names Ralivia™ ER [Can]; Tridural™ [Can]; Ultram® ER [US]; Ultram® [US]; Zytram® XL [Can]
Therapeutic Category Analgesic, Nonnarcotic
Use Relief of moderate to moderately-severe pain
Usual Dosage Moderate-to-severe chronic pain: Oral: Adults:
  Immediate release formulation: 50-100 mg every 4-6 hours (not to exceed 400 mg/day)
    For patients not requiring rapid onset of effect, tolerability may be improved by starting dose at 25 mg/day and titrating dose by 25 mg every 3 days, until reaching 25 mg 4 times/day. The total daily dose may then be increased by 50 mg every 3 days as tolerated, to reach dose of 50 mg 4 times/day. After titration, 50-100 mg may be given every 4-6 hours as needed up to a maximum 400 mg/day.
  Extended release formulations:
    Ultram® ER: Patients not currently on immediate release: 100 mg once daily; titrate every 5 days (maximum: 300 mg/day); Patients currently on immediate release: Calculate 24-hour immediate release total and initiate total daily dose (round dose to the next lowest 100 mg increment); titrate (maximum: 300 mg/day)
    Ralivia™ ER (Canadian labeling, not available in U.S.): 100 mg once daily; titrate every 5 days as needed based on clinical response and severity of pain (maximum: 300 mg/day)
    Tridural™ (Canadian labeling, not available in U.S.): 100 mg once daily; titrate by 100 mg/day every 2 days as needed based on clinical response and severity of pain (maximum: 300 mg/day)
    Zytram® XL (Canadian labeling, not available in U.S.): 150 mg once daily; if pain relief is not achieved may titrate by increasing dosage incrementally, with sufficient time to evaluate effect of increased dosage; generally not more often than every 7 days (maximum: 400 mg/day)
Dosage Forms [CAN] = Canadian brand name
  Tablet: 50 mg
    Ultram®: 50 mg
  Tablet, extended release:
    Ultram® ER: 100 mg, 200 mg, 300 mg
    Ralivia™ ER [CAN]: 100 mg, 200 mg, 300 mg [not available in the U.S.]
    Tridural™ [CAN]: 100 mg, 200 mg, 300 mg [not available in the U.S.]
    Zytram® XL [CAN]: 150 mg, 200 mg, 300 mg, 400 mg

tramadol hydrochloride *see* tramadol *on page 941*
tramadol hydrochloride and acetaminophen *see* acetaminophen and tramadol *on page 24*

Trandate® [US/Can] *see* labetalol *on page 541*

trandolapril (tran DOE la pril)

U.S./Canadian Brand Names Mavik® [US/Can]

Therapeutic Category Angiotensin-Converting Enzyme (ACE) Inhibitor

Use Treatment of hypertension alone or in combination with other antihypertensive agents; treatment of heart failure or left ventricular dysfunction after myocardial infarction

Usual Dosage Oral: Adults:

Hypertension: Initial dose in patients not receiving a diuretic: 1 mg/day (2 mg/day in black patients). Adjust dosage according to the blood pressure response. Make dosage adjustments at intervals of ≥1 week. Most patients have required dosages of 2-4 mg/day. There is a little experience with doses >8 mg/day. Patients inadequately treated with once daily dosing at 4 mg may be treated with twice daily dosing. If blood pressure is not adequately controlled with trandolapril monotherapy, a diuretic may be added.

Usual dose range (JNC 7): 1-4 mg once daily

Heart failure postmyocardial infarction or left ventricular dysfunction postmyocardial infarction: Initial: 1 mg/day; titrate patients (as tolerated) towards the target dose of 4 mg/day. If a 4 mg dose is not tolerated, patients can continue therapy with the greatest tolerated dose.

Dosage Forms

Tablet: 1 mg, 2 mg, 4 mg

Mavik®: 1 mg, 2 mg, 4 mg

trandolapril and verapamil (tran DOE la pril & ver AP a mil)

Synonyms verapamil and trandolapril

U.S./Canadian Brand Names Tarka® [US/Can]

Therapeutic Category Antihypertensive Agent, Combination

Use Treatment of hypertension; however, not indicated for initial treatment of hypertension

Usual Dosage Dose is individualized.

Dosage Forms

Tablet, variable release:

Tarka®:

1/240: Trandolapril 1 mg [immediate release] and verapamil 240 mg [sustained release]

2/180: Trandolapril 2 mg [immediate release] and verapamil 180 mg [sustained release]

2/240: Trandolapril 2 mg [immediate release] and verapamil 240 mg [sustained release]

4/240: Trandolapril 4 mg [immediate release] and verapamil 240 mg [sustained release]

tranexamic acid (tran eks AM ik AS id)

Sound-Alike/Look-Alike Issues

Cyklokapron® may be confused with cycloSPORINE

U.S./Canadian Brand Names Cyklokapron® [US/Can]; Tranexamic Acid Injection BP [Can]

Therapeutic Category Antihemophilic Agent

Use Short-term use (2-8 days) in hemophilia patients during and following tooth extraction to reduce or prevent hemorrhage

Usual Dosage I.V.: Children and Adults: 10 mg/kg immediately before surgery, then 25 mg/kg/dose orally 3-4 times/day for 2-8 days

Alternatively:

Oral: 25 mg/kg 3-4 times/day beginning 1 day prior to surgery

I.V.: 10 mg/kg 3-4 times/day in patients who are unable to take oral

Dosage Forms

Injection, solution:

Cyklokapron®: 100 mg/mL (10 mL)

Tablet:

Cyklokapron®: 500 mg [not available in the U.S.; available from manufacturer for select cases]

Tranexamic Acid Injection BP [Can] *see* tranexamic acid *on page 942*

transamine sulphate *see* tranylcypromine *on page 943*

Transderm-V® [Can] *see* scopolamine derivatives *on page 858*

Transdermal-NTG® Patch *(Discontinued)* *see* nitroglycerin *on page 675*

Transderm-Nitro® [Can] *see* nitroglycerin *on page 675*

Transderm Scōp® [US] *see* scopolamine derivatives *on page 858*
Trans-Plantar® [Can] *see* salicylic acid *on page 850*
Trans-Plantar® Transdermal Patch *(Discontinued)* *see* salicylic acid *on page 850*
***trans*-retinoic acid** *see* tretinoin (topical) *on page 946*
Trans-Ver-Sal® [US-OTC/Can] *see* salicylic acid *on page 850*
Tranxene® SD™ [US] *see* clorazepate *on page 238*
Tranxene® SD™-Half Strength [US] *see* clorazepate *on page 238*
Tranxene® T-Tab® [US] *see* clorazepate *on page 238*

tranylcypromine (tran il SIP roe meen)

Synonyms transamine sulphate; tranylcypromine sulfate
U.S./Canadian Brand Names Parnate® [US/Can]
Therapeutic Category Antidepressant, Monoamine Oxidase Inhibitor
Use Treatment of major depressive episode without melancholia
Usual Dosage Oral: Adults: 10 mg twice daily, increase by 10 mg increments at 1- to 3-week intervals; maximum: 60 mg/day; usual effective dose: 30 mg/day
Dosage Forms
Tablet:
Parnate®: 10 mg

tranylcypromine sulfate *see* tranylcypromine *on page 943*
Trasicor® [Can] *see* oxprenolol *(Canada only) on page 708*

trastuzumab (tras TU zoo mab)

Synonyms NSC-688097
U.S./Canadian Brand Names Herceptin® [US/Can]
Therapeutic Category Antineoplastic Agent
Use Adjuvant treatment of HER-2 overexpressing breast cancer; treatment of HER-2 overexpressing metastatic breast cancer
Usual Dosage Details concerning dosing in combination regimens should also be consulted. Adults: I.V. infusion:
Adjuvant treatment of breast cancer:
With concurrent paclitaxel or docetaxel:
Initial loading dose: 4 mg/kg infused over 90 minutes
Maintenance dose: 2 mg/kg infused over 30 minutes weekly for total of 12 weeks, followed 1 week later (when concurrent chemotherapy completed) by 6 mg/kg infused over 30-60 minutes every 3 weeks for total therapy duration of 52 weeks
With concurrent docetaxel/carboplatin:
Initial loading dose: 4 mg/kg infused over 90 minutes
Maintenance dose: 2 mg/kg infused over 30 minutes weekly for total of 18 weeks, followed 1 week later (when concurrent chemotherapy completed) by 6 mg/kg infused over 30-60 minutes every 3 weeks for total therapy duration of 52 weeks
Following completion of anthracycline-based chemotherapy:
Initial loading dose: 8 mg/kg infused over 90 minutes
Maintenance dose: 6 mg/kg infused over 30 minutes every 3 weeks for total therapy duration of 52 weeks
Metastatic breast cancer (either as a single agent or in combination with paclitaxel):
Initial loading dose: 4 mg/kg infused over 90 minutes
Maintenance dose: 2 mg/kg infused over 30 minutes weekly until disease progression
Dosage Forms
Injection, powder for reconstitution:
Herceptin®: 440 mg

Trasylol® [US/Can] *see* aprotinin *on page 91*
Travatan® [US/Can] *see* travoprost *on page 944*
Travatan® Z [US] *see* travoprost *on page 944*

traveler's diarrhea and cholera vaccine *(Canada only)*
(TRAV uh lerz dahy uh REE uh & KOL er uh vak SEEN)

Synonyms *Vibrio cholera* and enterotoxigenic *Escherichia coli vaccine*; cholera and traveler's diarrhea vaccine; enterotoxigenic *Escherichia coli* and *Vibrio cholera* vaccine; traveller's diarrhea vaccine and cholera

U.S./Canadian Brand Names Dukoral™ [Can]

Therapeutic Category Vaccine

Use Protection against traveler's diarrhea and/or cholera in adults and children ≥2 years of age who will be visiting areas where there is a risk of contacting traveler's diarrhea caused by enterotoxigenic *E. coli* (ETEC) or cholera caused by *V. cholerae* O1 (classical and El Tor biotypes)

Usual Dosage Oral:
Cholera:
Primary immunization:
Children 2-6 years: 3 doses given at intervals of ≥1 week and completed at least 1 week prior to trip to endemic/epidemic areas; restart treatment if interval between doses >6 weeks
Children ≥6 years and Adults: 2 doses given at intervals of ≥1 week and completed at least 1 week prior to trip to endemic/epidemic areas; restart treatment if interval between doses >6 weeks
Booster:
Children 2-6 years: 1 dose after 6 months have elapsed since vaccination
Children ≥6 years and Adults: 1 dose after 2 years have elapsed since vaccination
ETEC:
Primary immunization: Children ≥2 years and Adults: 2 doses given at intervals of ≥1 week; restart treatment if interval between doses >6 weeks
Booster: Children ≥2 years and Adults:
Continued risk: 1 dose every 3 months
Renewed protection: 1 dose may be given if last booster or original immunization was <5 years ago (if >5 years, revaccinate)

Dosage Forms [CAN] = Canadian brand name
Suspension [vial]:
Dukoral™ [CAN]: 2.5 x 10^{10} of each of the following *Vibrio cholerae* O1 strains: Inaba classic (heat inactived), Inaba El Tor (formalin inactivated), Ogawa classic (heat inactivated), Ogawa classic (formalin inactivated), and 1 mg recombinant cholera toxin B subunit (rCTB) (3 mL) [not available in the U.S.]

traveller's diarrhea vaccine and cholera *see* traveler's diarrhea and cholera vaccine *(Canada only)* on page 944

travoprost (TRA voe prost)
Sound-Alike/Look-Alike Issues
Travatan® may be confused with Xalatan®

U.S./Canadian Brand Names Travatan® Z [US]; Travatan® [US/Can]

Therapeutic Category Prostaglandin, Ophthalmic

Use Reduction of elevated intraocular pressure in patients with open-angle glaucoma or ocular hypertension who are intolerant of the other IOP-lowering medications or insufficiently responsive (failed to achieve target IOP determined after multiple measurements over time) to another IOP-lowering medication

Usual Dosage Ophthalmic: Adults: Glaucoma (open angle) or ocular hypertension: Instill 1 drop into affected eye(s) once daily in the evening; do not exceed once-daily dosing (may decrease IOP-lowering effect). If used with other topical ophthalmic agents, separate administration by at least 5 minutes.

Dosage Forms
Solution, ophthalmic:
Travatan®: 0.004% (2.5 mL, 5 mL)
Travatan® Z: 0.004% (2.5 mL, 5 mL)

trazodone (TRAZ oh done)
Sound-Alike/Look-Alike Issues
traZODone may be confused with traMADol
Desyrel® may be confused with Demerol®, Delsym®, Zestril®

Synonyms trazodone hydrochloride

Tall-Man traZODone

U.S./Canadian Brand Names Alti-Trazodone [Can]; Apo-Trazodone D® [Can]; Apo-Trazodone® [Can]; Desyrel® [Can]; Gen-Trazodone [Can]; Novo-Trazodone [Can]; Nu-Trazodone [Can]; PMS-Trazodone [Can]; ratio-Trazodone [Can]; Trazorel® [Can]

Therapeutic Category Antidepressant, Triazolopyridine

Use Treatment of depression

Usual Dosage Oral: Therapeutic effects may take up to 6 weeks to occur; therapy is normally maintained for 6-12 months after optimum response is reached to prevent recurrence of depression

Adults: Depression: Initial: 150 mg/day in 3 divided doses (may increase by 50 mg/day every 3-7 days); maximum: 600 mg/day

Dosage Forms

Tablet, as hydrochloride: 50 mg, 100 mg, 150 mg, 300 mg

trazodone hydrochloride see trazodone on page 944

Trazorel® [Can] see trazodone on page 944

Treanda® [US] see bendamustine on page 122

Trecator® [US/Can] see ethionamide on page 380

Trelstar® [Can] see triptorelin on page 956

Trelstar® Depot [US/Can] see triptorelin on page 956

Trelstar® LA [US/Can] see triptorelin on page 956

Trendar® (Discontinued) see ibuprofen on page 495

Trental® [US/Can] see pentoxifylline on page 737

treprostinil (tre PROST in il)

Synonyms treprostinil sodium

U.S./Canadian Brand Names Remodulin® [US/Can]

Therapeutic Category Vasodilator

Use Treatment of pulmonary arterial hypertension (PAH) in patients with NYHA Class II-IV symptoms to decrease exercise-associated symptoms; to diminish clinical deterioration when transitioning from epoprostenol (I.V.)

Usual Dosage Note: Prior to initiation, patients should be carefully evaluated for ability to administer treprostinil and care for the infusion system outside of inpatient setting. Immediate access to backup pump, infusion sets, and medication is essential to prevent treatment interruptions.

Adults: PAH: SubQ or I.V. infusion:

Initial: New to prostacyclin therapy: 1.25 ng/kg/minute continuous; if dose cannot be tolerated due to systemic effects, reduce to 0.625 ng/kg/minute. Increase at rate not >1.25 ng/kg/minute per week for first 4 weeks, and not >2.5 ng/kg/minute per week for remainder of therapy. Limited experience with doses >40 ng/kg/minute. **Note:** Dose must be carefully and individually titrated (symptom improvement with minimal adverse effects). Avoid abrupt withdrawal. If infusion is restarted within a few hours of discontinuation, the same dose rate may be used. Interruptions for longer periods may require retitration.

Transitioning from epoprostenol (see below): SubQ (preferred) or I.V. infusion: **Note:** Transition should occur in a hospital setting to follow response (eg, walking distance, sign/symptoms of disease progression). May take 24-48 hours to transition. Transition is accomplished by initiating the infusion of treprostinil, and increasing it while simultaneously reducing the dose of intravenous epoprostenol. During transition, increases in PAH symptoms should be first treated with an increase in treprostinil dose. Occurrence of prostacyclin associated side effects should be treated by decreasing the dose of epoprostenol.

Transitioning From I.V. epoprostenol to SubQ (preferred) or I.V. treprostinil

Step 1:
Epoprostenol: Maintain current dose
Treprostinil: Initiate at 10% initial epoprostenol dose

Step 2:
Epoprostenol: Decrease dose to 80% of starting dose
Treprostinil: Increase to 30% initial epoprostenol dose

Step 3:
Epoprostenol: Decrease dose to 60% of starting dose
Treprostinil: Increase to 50% initial epoprostenol dose

▶

◀ *Step 4:*
   Epoprostenol: Decrease dose to 40% of starting dose
   Treprostinil: Increase to 70% initial epoprostenol dose
Step 5:
   Epoprostenol: Decrease dose to 20% of starting dose
   Treprostinil: Increase to 90% initial epoprostenol dose
Step 6:
   Epoprostenol: Decrease dose to 5% of starting dose
   Treprostinil: Increase to 110% initial epoprostenol dose
Step 7:
   Epoprostenol: Discontinue
   Treprostinil: Maintain current dose plus additional 5% to 10% as needed
Dosage Forms
   Injection, solution:
   Remodulin®: 1 mg/mL (20 mL); 2.5 mg/mL (20 mL); 5 mg/mL (20 mL); 10 mg/mL (20 mL)

treprostinil sodium *see* treprostinil *on page 945*
Tretin-X™ [US] *see* tretinoin (topical) *on page 946*
tretinoin and clindamycin *see* clindamycin and tretinoin *on page 231*
tretinoin and mequinol *see* mequinol and tretinoin *on page 606*
tretinoin, fluocinolone acetonide, and hydroquinone *see* fluocinolone, hydroquinone, and
   tretinoin *on page 409*

tretinoin (oral) (TRET i noyn, oral)
Sound-Alike/Look-Alike Issues
   tretinoin may be confused with isotretinoin, trientine
Synonyms all-*trans*-retinoic acid; ATRA; NSC-122758; Ro 5488; tRA
U.S./Canadian Brand Names Vesanoid® [US/Can]
Therapeutic Category Antineoplastic Agent
Use Induction of remission in patients with acute promyelocytic leukemia (APL), French American British
   (FAB) classification M3 (including the M3 variant)
Usual Dosage Oral: Children and Adults:
   Remission induction: 45 mg/m²/day in 2-3 divided doses for up to 30 days after complete remission
   (maximum duration of treatment: 90 days)
   Remission maintenance: 45-200 mg/m²/day in 2-3 divided doses for up to 12 months.
Dosage Forms
   Capsule: 10 mg
   Vesanoid®: 10 mg

tretinoin (topical) (TRET i noyn TOP i kal)
Sound-Alike/Look-Alike Issues
   tretinoin may be confused with isotretinoin, trientine
Synonyms *trans*-retinoic acid; retinoic acid; vitamin A acid
U.S./Canadian Brand Names Atralin™ [US]; Avita® [US]; Rejuva-A® [Can]; Renova® [US]; Retin-A®
   Micro [US/Can]; Retin-A® [US/Can]; Retinova® [Can]; Tretin-X™ [US]
Therapeutic Category Retinoic Acid Derivative
Use Treatment of acne vulgaris; photodamaged skin; palliation of fine wrinkles, mottled hyperpigmentation,
   and tactile roughness of facial skin as part of a comprehensive skin care and sun avoidance program
Usual Dosage Topical:
   Children >12 years and Adults: Acne vulgaris: Begin therapy with a weaker formulation of tretinoin
   (0.025% cream, 0.04% microsphere gel, or 0.01% gel) and increase the concentration as tolerated;
   apply once daily to acne lesions before retiring or on alternate days; if stinging or irritation develop,
   decrease frequency of application
   Adults ≥18: Palliation of fine wrinkles, mottled hyperpigmentation, and tactile roughness of facial skin:
   Pea-sized amount of the 0.02% or 0.05% cream applied to entire face once daily in the evening
Dosage Forms
   Cream, topical: 0.025% (20 g, 45 g); 0.05% (20 g, 45 g); 0.1% (20 g, 45 g)
   Avita®: 0.025% (20 g, 45 g)
   Renova®: 0.02% (40 g, 60 g)
   Retin-A®: 0.025% (20 g, 45 g); 0.05% (20 g, 45 g); 0.1% (20 g, 45 g)

Tretin-X™: 0.025% (35 g); 0.05% (35 g); 0.1% (35 g)
Gel, topical: 0.01% (15 g, 45 g); 0.025% (15 g, 45 g)
Atralin™: 0.05% (45 g)
Avita®: 0.025% (20 g, 45 g)
Retin-A®: 0.01% (15 g, 45 g); 0.025% (15 g, 45 g)
Tretin-X™: 0.025% (35 g); 0.01% (35 g)
Gel, topical [microsphere gel]:
Retin-A® Micro: 0.04% (20 g, 45 g, 50 g); 0.1% (20 g, 45 g, 50 g)

Trexall™ [US] *see* methotrexate *on page 615*
Treximet™ [US] *see* sumatriptan and naproxen *on page 898*

triacetin (trye a SEE tin)

Sound-Alike/Look-Alike Issues
triacetin may be confused with Triacin®
Synonyms glycerol triacetate
U.S./Canadian Brand Names Myco-Nail [US-OTC]
Therapeutic Category Antifungal Agent
Use Fungistat for athlete's foot and other superficial fungal infections
Usual Dosage Apply twice daily, cleanse areas with dilute alcohol or mild soap and water before application; continue treatment for 7 days after symptoms have disappeared
Dosage Forms
Liquid, topical:
Myco-Nail [OTC]: 25% (30 mL)

Triacin-C® (Discontinued) *see* triprolidine, pseudoephedrine, and codeine *(Canada only) on page 955*
triaconazole *see* terconazole *on page 911*
Triaderm [Can] *see* triamcinolone (topical) *on page 949*
Triafed® (Discontinued) *see* triprolidine and pseudoephedrine *on page 955*
Triall™ [US] *see* chlorpheniramine, phenylephrine, and methscopolamine *on page 210*
triamcinolone acetonide, parenteral *see* triamcinolone (systemic) *on page 948*
triamcinolone and nystatin *see* nystatin and triamcinolone *on page 690*
triamcinolone diacetate, oral *see* triamcinolone (systemic) *on page 948*
triamcinolone diacetate, parenteral *see* triamcinolone (systemic) *on page 948*
triamcinolone hexacetonide *see* triamcinolone (systemic) *on page 948*

triamcinolone (inhalation, nasal) (trye am SIN oh lone in hil LA shun, NAY sal)

Sound-Alike/Look-Alike Issues
Nasacort® may be confused with NasalCrom®
U.S./Canadian Brand Names Nasacort® AQ [US/Can]; Nasacort® HFA [US]; Tri-Nasal® [US/Can]
Therapeutic Category Adrenal Corticosteroid
Use Nasal inhalation: Management of seasonal and perennial allergic rhinitis in patients ≥6 years of age
Usual Dosage Intranasal: Perennial allergic rhinitis, seasonal allergic rhinitis:
Nasal spray:
Children 6-11 years: 110 mcg/day as 1 spray in each nostril once daily.
Children ≥12 years and Adults: 220 mcg/day as 2 sprays in each nostril once daily
Nasal inhaler:
Children 6-11 years: Initial: 220 mcg/day as 2 sprays in each nostril once daily
Children ≥12 years and Adults: Initial: 220 mcg/day as 2 sprays in each nostril once daily; may increase dose to 440 mcg/day (given once daily or divided and given 2 or 4 times/day)
Dosage Forms
Solution, intranasal:
Tri-Nasal®: 50 mcg/inhalation (15 mL)
Suspension, intranasal:
Nasacort® AQ: 55 mcg/inhalation (16.5 g)

triamcinolone (inhalation, oral) (trye am SIN oh lone in hil LA shun, OR al)

Sound-Alike/Look-Alike Issues
TAC (occasional abbreviation for triamcinolone) is an error-prone abbreviation (mistaken as tetracaine-adrenaline-cocaine)

U.S./Canadian Brand Names Azmacort® [US]

Therapeutic Category Adrenal Corticosteroid

Use Oral inhalation: Control of bronchial asthma and related bronchospastic conditions

Usual Dosage Oral inhalation: Asthma:
Children 6-12 years: 100-200 mcg 3-4 times/day **or** 200-400 mcg twice daily; maximum dose: 1200 mcg/day

Children >12 years and Adults: 200 mcg 3-4 times/day **or** 400 mcg twice daily; maximum dose: 1600 mcg/day

Dosage Forms
Aerosol for oral inhalation:
Azmacort®: 100 mcg per actuation (20 g)

triamcinolone, oral see triamcinolone (systemic) on page 948

triamcinolone (systemic) (trye am SIN oh lone sis TEM ik)

Sound-Alike/Look-Alike Issues
Kenalog® may be confused with Ketalar®

Synonyms triamcinolone acetonide, parenteral; triamcinolone diacetate, oral; triamcinolone diacetate, parenteral; triamcinolone hexacetonide; triamcinolone, oral

U.S./Canadian Brand Names Aristospan® [US/Can]; Kenalog-10® [US]; Kenalog-40® [US]; Oracort [Can]

Therapeutic Category Adrenal Corticosteroid

Use Systemic: Adrenocortical insufficiency, rheumatic disorders, allergic states, respiratory diseases, systemic lupus erythematosus (SLE), and other diseases requiring antiinflammatory or immunosuppressive effects

Usual Dosage The lowest possible dose should be used to control the condition; when dose reduction is possible, the dose should be reduced gradually. Parenteral dose is usually 1/3 to 1/2 the oral dose given every 12 hours. In life-threatening situations, parenteral doses larger than the oral dose may be needed.

Injection:
Acetonide:
Intraarticular, intrabursal, tendon sheaths: Adults: Initial: Smaller joints: 2.5-5 mg, larger joints: 5-15 mg
Intradermal: Adults: Initial: 1 mg
I.M.: Range: 2.5-60 mg/day
Children 6-12 years: Initial: 40 mg
Children >12 years and Adults: Initial: 60 mg
Hexacetonide: Adults:
Intralesional, sublesional: Up to 0.5 mg/square inch of affected skin
Intraarticular: Range: 2-20 mg

Oral: Adults:
Acute rheumatic carditis: Initial: 20-60 mg/day; reduce dose during maintenance therapy
Acute seasonal or perennial allergic rhinitis: 8-12 mg/day
Adrenocortical insufficiency: Range 4-12 mg/day
Bronchial asthma: 8-16 mg/day
Dermatological disorders, contact/atopic dermatitis: Initial: 8-16 mg/day
Ophthalmic disorders: 12-40 mg/day
Rheumatic disorders: Range: 8-16 mg/day
SLE: Initial: 20-32 mg/day, some patients may need initial doses ≥48 mg; reduce dose during maintenance therapy

Dosage Forms
Injection, suspension:
Kenalog-10®: 10 mg/mL (5 mL) [not for I.V. or I.M. use]
Kenalog-40®: 40 mg/mL (1 mL, 5 mL, 10 mL) [not for I.V. or intradermal use]
Injection, suspension:
Aristospan®: 5 mg/mL (5 mL); 20 mg/mL (1 mL, 5 mL) [not for I.V. use]

triamcinolone (topical) (trye am SIN oh lone TOP i kal)

Sound-Alike/Look-Alike Issues
Kenalog® may be confused with Ketalar®

U.S./Canadian Brand Names Aristocort® A [US]; Kenalog® in Orabase [Can]; Kenalog® [US/Can]; Triaderm [Can]; Triderm® [US]

Therapeutic Category Corticosteroid, Topical

Use
Oral topical: Adjunctive treatment and temporary relief of symptoms associated with oral inflammatory lesions and ulcerative lesions resulting from trauma
Topical: Inflammatory dermatoses responsive to steroids

Usual Dosage
Oral topical: Oral inflammatory lesions/ulcers: Press a small dab (about 1/4 inch) to the lesion until a thin film develops. A larger quantity may be required for coverage of some lesions. For optimal results use only enough to coat the lesion with a thin film; do not rub in.
Topical:
Cream, Ointment: Apply thin film to affected areas 2-4 times/day
Spray: Apply to affected area 3-4 times/day

Dosage Forms
Aerosol, topical:
Kenalog®: 0.2 mg/2-second spray (63 g)
Cream: 0.025% (15 g, 80 g, 454 g); 0.1% (15 g, 80 g, 454 g, 2270 g); 0.5% (15 g)
Triderm®: 0.1% (30 g, 85 g)
Lotion: 0.025% (60 mL); 0.1% (60 mL)
Ointment, topical: 0.025% (15 g, 80 g, 454 g); 0.1% (15 g, 80 g, 454 g); 0.5% (15 g)
Paste, oral, topical: 0.1% (5 g)

Triaminic® Cold & Allergy [Can] see chlorpheniramine and pseudoephedrine *on page 207*
Triaminic® Cold and Allergy [US-OTC] see chlorpheniramine and phenylephrine *on page 206*
Triaminic® Cold and Cough *(Discontinued)* see chlorpheniramine, pseudoephedrine, and dextromethorphan *on page 212*
Triaminic® Cough and Sore Throat Formula *(Discontinued)* see acetaminophen, dextromethorphan, and pseudoephedrine *on page 27*
Triaminic® Cough *(Discontinued)* see pseudoephedrine and dextromethorphan *on page 802*
Triaminic® Cough & Nasal Congestion *(Discontinued)* see pseudoephedrine and dextromethorphan *on page 802*
Triaminic® Expectorant *(Discontinued)*
Triaminic® Infant Thin Strips® Decongestant *(Discontinued)* see phenylephrine *on page 745*
Triaminic® Night Time Cough and Cold *(Discontinued)* see chlorpheniramine, pseudoephedrine, and dextromethorphan *on page 212*
Triaminic® Thin Strips® Cold [US-OTC] see phenylephrine *on page 745*
Triaminic® Thin Strips™ Cough and Runny Nose [US-OTC] see diphenhydramine *on page 304*
Triaminic® Thin Strips™ Long Acting Cough [US-OTC] see dextromethorphan *on page 284*
Triamonide® Injection *(Discontinued)*

triamterene (trye AM ter een)

Sound-Alike/Look-Alike Issues
triamterene may be confused with trimipramine
Dyrenium® may be confused with Pyridium®

U.S./Canadian Brand Names Dyrenium® [US]

Therapeutic Category Diuretic, Potassium Sparing

Use Alone or in combination with other diuretics in treatment of edema and hypertension; decreases potassium excretion caused by kaliuretic diuretics

Usual Dosage Oral: Adults: Hypertension, edema: 100-300 mg/day in 1-2 divided doses; maximum dose: 300 mg/day; usual dosage range (JNC 7): 50-100 mg/day

Dosage Forms
Capsule:
Dyrenium®: 50 mg, 100 mg

triamterene and hydrochlorothiazide see hydrochlorothiazide and triamterene *on page 480*

Triant-HC™ [US] *see* phenylephrine, hydrocodone, and chlorpheniramine *on page 748*
Triapin® *(Discontinued)*
Triatec-8 [Can] *see* acetaminophen and codeine *on page 20*
Triatec-8 Strong [Can] *see* acetaminophen and codeine *on page 20*
Triatec-30 [Can] *see* acetaminophen and codeine *on page 20*
Triavil® *(Discontinued) see* amitriptyline and perphenazine *on page 63*
Triaz® [US] *see* benzoyl peroxide *on page 126*
Triaz® Cleanser [US] *see* benzoyl peroxide *on page 126*

triazolam (trye AY zoe lam)

Sound-Alike/Look-Alike Issues
triazolam may be confused with alPRAZolam
Halcion® may be confused with halcinonide, Haldol®
U.S./Canadian Brand Names Apo-Triazo® [Can]; Gen-Triazolam [Can]; Halcion® [US/Can]
Therapeutic Category Benzodiazepine
Controlled Substance C-IV
Use Short-term treatment of insomnia
Usual Dosage Oral (onset of action is rapid, patient should be in bed when taking medication): Adults: Insomnia (short-term): 0.125-0.25 mg at bedtime (maximum dose: 0.5 mg/day)
Preprocedure sedation (dental): 0.25 mg taken the evening before oral surgery; or 0.25 mg 1 hour before procedure
Dosage Forms
Tablet: 0.125 mg, 0.25 mg
Halcion®: 0.25 mg

tribavirin *see* ribavirin *on page 831*
Tri Biozene [US-OTC] *see* bacitracin, neomycin, polymyxin B, and pramoxine *on page 114*
tricalcium phosphate *see* calcium phosphate (tribasic) *on page 167*
Tricardio B [US] *see* folic acid, cyanocobalamin, and pyridoxine *on page 422*
Tri-Chlor® [US] *see* trichloroacetic acid *on page 950*
Trichlor Fresh Pac™ [US] *see* trichloroacetic acid *on page 950*
trichloroacetaldehyde monohydrate *see* chloral hydrate *on page 199*

trichloroacetic acid (trye klor oh a SEE tik AS id)

U.S./Canadian Brand Names Tri-Chlor® [US]; Trichlor Fresh Pac™ [US]
Therapeutic Category Keratolytic Agent
Use Chemical used in compounding agents for the treatment of warts, skin resurfacing (chemical peels)
Usual Dosage Topical: Apply to verruca, cover with bandage for 5-6 days, remove verruca, reapply as needed
Dosage Forms
Liquid: 80%
Tri-Chlor®: 80%
Powder for reconstitution, topical: 10% (28 mL); 15% (28 mL); 20% (28 mL); 25% (28 mL); 30% (28 mL); 35% (28 mL); 40% (28 mL); 50% (28 mL)
Trichlor Fresh Pac™: 10% (28 mL); 15% (28 mL); 20% (28 mL); 25% (28 mL); 30% (28 mL); 35% (28 mL); 40% (28 mL); 50% (28 mL)

trichloromonofluoromethane and dichlorodifluoromethane *see* dichlorodifluoromethane and trichloromonofluoromethane *on page 291*

Trichophyton skin test (trye koe FYE ton skin test)

Therapeutic Category Diagnostic Agent
Use Assess cell-mediated immunity
Usual Dosage 0.1 mL intradermally, examine reaction site in 24-48 hours; induration of ≥5 mm in diameter is a positive reaction
Dosage Forms
Injection, solution: 1:200 (2 mL)

Tricitrates [US] *see* citric acid, sodium citrate, and potassium citrate *on page 226*

Tri-Clear® Expectorant *(Discontinued)*

TriCor® [US/Can] *see* fenofibrate *on page 393*

tricosal *see* choline magnesium trisalicylate *on page 216*

Tri-Cyclen® [Can] *see* ethinyl estradiol and norgestimate *on page 378*

Tri-Cyclen® Lo [Can] *see* ethinyl estradiol and norgestimate *on page 378*

Triderm® [US] *see* triamcinolone (topical) *on page 949*

Tridil® Injection *(Discontinued) see* nitroglycerin *on page 675*

Tridione® *(Discontinued)*

Tridural™ [Can] *see* tramadol *on page 941*

trien *see* trientine *on page 951*

trientine (TRYE en teen)

Sound-Alike/Look-Alike Issues
trientine may be confused with Trental®, tretinoin

Synonyms 2,2,2-tetramine; trien; trientine hydrochloride; triethylene tetramine dihydrochloride

U.S./Canadian Brand Names Syprine® [US/Can]

Therapeutic Category Chelating Agent

Use Treatment of Wilson disease in patients intolerant to penicillamine

Usual Dosage Oral (administer on an empty stomach):
Children <12 years: 500-750 mg/day in divided doses 2-4 times/day; maximum: 1.5 g/day. The practice guideline suggests 20 mg/kg/day rounded off to the nearest 250 mg, given in 2-3 divided doses
Children ≥12 years and Adults: 750-1250 mg/day in divided doses 2-4 times/day; maximum dose: 2 g/day. The practice guideline suggests typical doses of 750-1500 mg/day in 2-3 divided doses with maintenance therapy of 750-1000 mg/day

Dosage Forms
Capsule:
Syprine®: 250 mg

trientine hydrochloride *see* trientine *on page 951*

triethanolamine salicylate *see* trolamine *on page 957*

triethylene tetramine dihydrochloride *see* trientine *on page 951*

triethylenethiophosphoramide *see* thiotepa *on page 922*

Trifed-C® *(Discontinued) see* triprolidine, pseudoephedrine, and codeine *(Canada only) on page 955*

trifluoperazine (trye floo oh PER a zeen)

Sound-Alike/Look-Alike Issues
trifluoperazine may be confused with triflupromazine, trihexyphenidyl
Stelazine® may be confused with selegiline

Synonyms trifluoperazine hydrochloride

U.S./Canadian Brand Names Apo-Trifluoperazine® [Can]; Novo-Trifluzine [Can]; PMS-Trifluoperazine [Can]; Terfluzine [Can]

Therapeutic Category Phenothiazine Derivative

Use Treatment of schizophrenia

Usual Dosage Oral:
Children 6-12 years: Schizophrenia/psychoses: Hospitalized or well-supervised patients: Initial: 1 mg 1-2 times/day, gradually increase until symptoms are controlled or adverse effects become troublesome; maximum: 15 mg/day
Adults:
Schizophrenia/psychoses:
Outpatients: 1-2 mg twice daily
Hospitalized or well-supervised patients: Initial: 2-5 mg twice daily with optimum response in the 15-20 mg/day range; do not exceed 40 mg/day
Nonpsychotic anxiety: 1-2 mg twice daily; maximum: 6 mg/day; therapy for anxiety should not exceed 12 weeks; do not exceed 6 mg/day for longer than 12 weeks when treating anxiety; agitation, jitteriness, or insomnia may be confused with original neurotic or psychotic symptoms

Dosage Forms
Tablet: 1 mg, 2 mg, 5 mg, 10 mg

trifluoperazine hydrochloride *see* trifluoperazine *on page 951*
trifluorothymidine *see* trifluridine *on page 952*

trifluridine (trye FLURE i deen)

Sound-Alike/Look-Alike Issues
Viroptic® may be confused with Timoptic®
Synonyms F_3T; trifluorothymidine
U.S./Canadian Brand Names SAB-Trifluridine [Can]; Sandoz-Trifluridine [Can]; Viroptic® [US/Can]
Therapeutic Category Antiviral Agent
Use Treatment of primary keratoconjunctivitis and recurrent epithelial keratitis caused by herpes simplex virus types I and II
Usual Dosage Adults: Instill 1 drop into affected eye every 2 hours while awake, to a maximum of 9 drops/day, until reepithelialization of corneal ulcer occurs; then use 1 drop every 4 hours for another 7 days; do **not** exceed 21 days of treatment; if improvement has not taken place in 7-14 days, consider another form of therapy
Dosage Forms
Solution, ophthalmic: 1% (7.5 mL)
Viroptic®: 1% (7.5 mL)

Triglide™ [US] *see* fenofibrate *on page 393*
triglycerides, medium chain *see* medium chain triglycerides *on page 596*

trihexyphenidyl (trye heks ee FEN i dil)

Sound-Alike/Look-Alike Issues
trihexyphenidyl may be confused with trifluoperazine
Artane® may be confused with Altace®, Anturane®, Aramine®
Synonyms benzhexol hydrochloride; trihexyphenidyl hydrochloride
U.S./Canadian Brand Names Apo-Trihex® [Can]
Therapeutic Category Anti-Parkinson Agent; Anticholinergic Agent
Use Adjunctive treatment of Parkinson disease; treatment of drug-induced extrapyramidal symptoms
Usual Dosage Oral: Adults: Initial: 1-2 mg/day, increase by 2 mg increments at intervals of 3-5 days; usual dose: 5-15 mg/day in 3-4 divided doses
Dosage Forms
Elixir: 2 mg/5 mL
Tablet: 2 mg, 5 mg

trihexyphenidyl hydrochloride *see* trihexyphenidyl *on page 952*
TriHIBit® [US] *see* diphtheria, tetanus toxoids, and acellular pertussis vaccine and *Haemophilus influenzae* b conjugate vaccine *on page 310*
Trikacide [Can] *see* metronidazole *on page 627*
Trikof-D® *(Discontinued)* *see* guaifenesin, pseudoephedrine, and dextromethorphan *on page 460*
Tri-Kort® Injection *(Discontinued)*
Trilafon® *(Discontinued)* *see* perphenazine *on page 740*
Trileptal® [US/Can] *see* oxcarbazepine *on page 706*
Tri-Levlen® *(Discontinued)* *see* ethinyl estradiol and levonorgestrel *on page 372*
Trilisate® *(Discontinued)* *see* choline magnesium trisalicylate *on page 216*
Trilog® Injection *(Discontinued)*
Trilone® Injection *(Discontinued)*
Tri-Luma™ [US] *see* fluocinolone, hydroquinone, and tretinoin *on page 409*
TriLyte® [US] *see* polyethylene glycol-electrolyte solution *on page 766*
Trimazide® *(Discontinued)* *see* trimethobenzamide *on page 953*

trimebutine *(Canada only)* (trye me BYOO teen)

Synonyms trimebutine maleate
U.S./Canadian Brand Names Apo-Trimebutine® [Can]; Modulon® [Can]
Therapeutic Category Antispasmodic Agent, Gastrointestinal

Use Treatment and relief of symptoms associated with irritable bowel syndrome (IBS) (spastic colon). In postoperative paralytic ileus in order to accelerate the resumption of the intestinal transit following abdominal surgery.

Usual Dosage Oral: Children ≥12 years and Adults: 200 mg 3 times/day before meals

Dosage Forms [CAN] = Canadian brand name

Tablet:
Apo-Trimebutine® [CAN], Modulon® [CAN]: 100 mg, 200 mg [not available in the U.S.]

trimebutine maleate *see* trimebutine *(Canada only) on page 952*

trimeprazine *(Canada only)* (trye MEP re zeen)

U.S./Canadian Brand Names Panectyl® [Can]

Therapeutic Category Antihistamine

Use Perennial and seasonal allergic rhinitis and other allergic symptoms including urticaria

Usual Dosage Oral:
Children:
6 months to 3 years: 1.25 mg at bedtime or 3 times/day if needed
>3 years: 2.5 mg at bedtime or 3 times/day if needed
>6 years: Sustained release: 5 mg/day
Adults: 2.5 mg 4 times/day (5 mg every 12-hour sustained release)

Dosage Forms
Tablet, as tartrate: 2.5 mg, 5 mg

trimethadione *(Discontinued)*

trimethobenzamide (trye meth oh BEN za mide)

Sound-Alike/Look-Alike Issues
trimethobenzamide may be confused with metoclopramide, trimethoprim
Tigan® may be confused with Tiazac®, Ticar®, Ticlid®

Synonyms trimethobenzamide hydrochloride

U.S./Canadian Brand Names Tigan® [US/Can]

Therapeutic Category Anticholinergic Agent; Antiemetic

Use Treatment of postoperative nausea and vomiting; treatment of nausea associated with gastroenteritis

Usual Dosage
Children >40 kg: Oral: 300 mg 3-4 times/day
Adults:
Oral: 300 mg 3-4 times/day
I.M.: 200 mg 3-4 times/day
Postoperative nausea and vomiting (PONV): I.M.: 200 mg, followed 1 hour later by a second 200 mg dose

Dosage Forms
Capsule: 300 mg
Tigan®: 300 mg
Injection, solution: 100 mg/mL (2 mL)
Tigan®: 100 mg/mL (20 mL)
Injection, solution [preservative free]:
Tigan®: 100 mg/mL (2 mL)

trimethobenzamide hydrochloride *see* trimethobenzamide *on page 953*

trimethoprim (trye METH oh prim)

Sound-Alike/Look-Alike Issues
trimethoprim may be confused with trimethaphan

Synonyms TMP

U.S./Canadian Brand Names Apo-Trimethoprim® [Can]; Primsol® [US]

Therapeutic Category Antibiotic, Miscellaneous

Use Treatment of urinary tract infections due to susceptible strains of *E. coli, P. mirabilis, K. pneumoniae, Enterobacter* sp and coagulase-negative *Staphylococcus* including *S. saprophyticus*; acute otitis media in children; acute exacerbations of chronic bronchitis in adults; in combination with other agents for ▶

◀ treatment of toxoplasmosis, *Pneumocystis carinii*; treatment of superficial ocular infections involving the conjunctiva and cornea

Usual Dosage Oral:

Children: 4 mg/kg/day in divided doses every 12 hours

Adults: 100 mg every 12 hours or 200 mg every 24 hours for 10 days; longer treatment periods may be necessary for prostatitis (ie, 4-16 weeks); in the treatment of *Pneumocystis carinii* pneumonia; dose may be as high as 15-20 mg/kg/day in 3-4 divided doses

Dosage Forms

Solution, oral:

Primsol®: 50 mg/5 mL

Tablet: 100 mg

trimethoprim and polymyxin B (trye METH oh prim & pol i MIKS in bee)

Synonyms polymyxin B and trimethoprim

U.S./Canadian Brand Names PMS-Polytrimethoprim [Can]; Polytrim® [US/Can]

Therapeutic Category Antibiotic, Ophthalmic

Use Treatment of surface ocular bacterial conjunctivitis and blepharoconjunctivitis

Usual Dosage Instill 1-2 drops in eye(s) every 4-6 hours

Dosage Forms

Solution, ophthalmic: Trimethoprim 1 mg and polymyxin B 10,000 units per mL (10 mL)

Polytrim®: Trimethoprim 1 mg and polymyxin B 10,000 units per mL (10 mL)

trimethoprim and sulfamethoxazole *see* sulfamethoxazole and trimethoprim *on page 894*

trimipramine (trye MI pra meen)

Sound-Alike/Look-Alike Issues

trimipramine may be confused with triamterene, trimeprazine

Synonyms trimipramine maleate

U.S./Canadian Brand Names Apo-Trimip® [Can]; Nu-Trimipramine [Can]; Rhotrimine® [Can]; Surmontil® [US/Can]

Therapeutic Category Antidepressant, Tricyclic (Tertiary Amine)

Use Treatment of depression

Usual Dosage Oral: Adults: 50-150 mg/day as a single bedtime dose up to a maximum of 200 mg/day outpatient and 300 mg/day inpatient

Dosage Forms

Capsule:

Surmontil®: 25 mg, 50 mg, 100 mg

trimipramine maleate *see* trimipramine *on page 954*

Trimox® *(Discontinued)* *see* amoxicillin *on page 67*

Trimpex® *(Discontinued)* *see* trimethoprim *on page 953*

Tri-Nasal® [US/Can] *see* triamcinolone (inhalation, nasal) *on page 947*

Trinate [US] *see* vitamins (multiple/prenatal) *on page 983*

TriNessa™ [US] *see* ethinyl estradiol and norgestimate *on page 378*

Trinipatch® 0.2 [Can] *see* nitroglycerin *on page 675*

Trinipatch® 0.4 [Can] *see* nitroglycerin *on page 675*

Trinipatch® 0.6 [Can] *see* nitroglycerin *on page 675*

Tri-Norinyl® [US] *see* ethinyl estradiol and norethindrone *on page 376*

Trinsicon® *(Discontinued)* *see* vitamin B complex combinations *on page 981*

Triofed® Syrup *(Discontinued)* *see* triprolidine and pseudoephedrine *on page 955*

Trionate® *(Discontinued)* *see* carbetapentane and chlorpheniramine *on page 174*

Triostat® [US] *see* liothyronine *on page 568*

Tripedia® [US] *see* diphtheria, tetanus toxoids, and acellular pertussis vaccine *on page 309*

Triphasil® [US/Can] *see* ethinyl estradiol and levonorgestrel *on page 372*

Triphenyl® Expectorant *(Discontinued)*

triple antibiotic *see* bacitracin, neomycin, and polymyxin B *on page 114*

triple sulfa *see* sulfabenzamide, sulfacetamide, and sulfathiazole *on page 892*

Triposed® Syrup *(Discontinued)* see triprolidine and pseudoephedrine *on page 955*
Tri-Previfem™ [US] *see* ethinyl estradiol and norgestimate *on page 378*

triprolidine and pseudoephedrine (trye PROE li deen & soo doe e FED rin)

Sound-Alike/Look-Alike Issues
Aprodine® may be confused with Aphrodyne®
Synonyms pseudoephedrine and triprolidine
U.S./Canadian Brand Names Actifed® [Can]; Allerfrim® [US-OTC]; Aprodine® [US-OTC]; Genac® [US-OTC]; Silafed® [US-OTC]; Zymine®-D [US]
Therapeutic Category Antihistamine/Decongestant Combination
Use Temporary relief of nasal congestion, decongest sinus openings, running nose, sneezing, itching of nose or throat and itchy, watery eyes due to common cold, hay fever, or other upper respiratory allergies
Usual Dosage Oral:
Liquid (Zymine®-D):
Children:
2-4 years: 1.25 mL every 4-6 hours (maximum pseudoephedrine: 60 mg/24 hours)
4-6 years: 2.5 mL every 4-6 hours (maximum pseudoephedrine: 60 mg/24 hours)
6-12 years: 2.5-5 mL every 4-6 hours (maximum pseudoephedrine: 120 mg/24 hours)
Children ≥12 years and Adults: 5-10 mL every 4-6 hours (maximum pseudoephedrine: 240 mg/24 hours)
Syrup (Allerfrim®, Aprodine®):
Children 6-12 years: 5 mL every 4-6 hours; do not exceed 4 doses in 24 hours
Children >12 years and Adults: 10 mL every 4-6 hours; do not exceed 4 doses in 24 hours
Tablet (Aprodine®):
Children 6-12 years: 1/2 tablet every 4-6 hours; do not exceed 4 doses in 24 hours
Children >12 years and Adults: One tablet every 4-6 hours; do not exceed 4 doses in 24 hours
Dosage Forms
Liquid:
Zymine®-D: Triprolidine 1.25 mg and pseudoephedrine 45 mg per 5 mL
Syrup:
Allerfrim [OTC], Aprodine® [OTC], Silafed® [OTC]: Triprolidine 1.25 mg and pseudoephedrine 30 mg per 5 mL
Tablet:
Allerfrim [OTC], Aprodine® [OTC], Genac® [OTC], Sudafed® Maximum Strength Sinus Nighttime [OTC]: Triprolidine 2.5 mg and pseudoephedrine 60 mg

triprolidine, codeine, and pseudoephedrine *see* triprolidine, pseudoephedrine, and codeine *(Canada only) on page 955*

triprolidine, pseudoephedrine, and codeine *(Canada only)*
(trye PROE li deen, soo doe e FED rin, & KOE deen)
Sound-Alike/Look-Alike Issues
Triacin-C® may be confused with triacetin
Synonyms codeine, pseudoephedrine, and triprolidine; codeine, triprolidine, and pseudoephedrine; pseudoephedrine, codeine, and triprolidine; pseudoephedrine, triprolidine, and codeine; triprolidine, codeine, and pseudoephedrine
U.S./Canadian Brand Names CoActifed® [Can]; Covan® [Can]; ratio-Cotridin [Can]
Therapeutic Category Antihistamine/Decongestant/Antitussive
Controlled Substance C-V (CDSA-I)
Use Symptomatic relief of upper respiratory symptoms and cough
Usual Dosage Oral:
Children:
2-6 years: 2.5 mL 4 times/day
7-12 years: 5 mL 4 times/day **or** 1/2 tablet 4 times/day
Children >12 years and Adults: 10 mL 4 times/day **or** 1 tablet 4 times/day
Dosage Forms [CAN] = Canadian brand name
Syrup:
CoActifed® [CAN], ratio-Cotridin [CAN]: Triprolidine 2 mg, pseudoephedrine 30 mg, and codeine 10 mg per 5 mL (100 mL, 2000 mL) [not available in the U.S.]

▶

TRIPROLIDINE, PSEUDOEPHEDRINE, AND CODEINE *(CANADA ONLY)*

◄ CoVan® [CAN]: Triprolidine 2 mg, pseudoephedrine 30 mg, and codeine 10 mg per 5 mL (500 mL) [not available in the U.S.]
Tablet:
CoActifed® [CAN]: Triprolidine 4 mg, pseudoephedrine 60 mg, and codeine 20 mg (50s) [not available in the U.S.]

Tri-Pseudo® *(Discontinued)* *see* triprolidine and pseudoephedrine *on page 955*
TripTone® [US-OTC] *see* dimenhydrinate *on page 301*
triptoraline *see* triptorelin *on page 956*

triptorelin (trip toe REL in)

Synonyms AY-25650; CL-118,532; D-Trp(6)-LHRH; triptoraline; triptorelin pamoate; tryptoreline
U.S./Canadian Brand Names Trelstar® Depot [US/Can]; Trelstar® LA [US/Can]; Trelstar® [Can]
Therapeutic Category Luteinizing Hormone-Releasing Hormone Analog
Use Palliative treatment of advanced prostate cancer as an alternative to orchiectomy or estrogen administration
Usual Dosage I.M.: Adults: Prostate cancer:
Trelstar® Depot: 3.75 mg once every 28 days
Trelstar® LA: 11.25 mg once every 84 days
Dosage Forms
Injection, powder for reconstitution:
Trelstar® Depot: 3.75 mg
Trelstar® LA: 11.25 mg

triptorelin pamoate *see* triptorelin *on page 956*
Triquilar® [Can] *see* ethinyl estradiol and levonorgestrel *on page 372*
tris buffer *see* tromethamine *on page 957*
Trisenox® [US] *see* arsenic trioxide *on page 94*
tris(hydroxymethyl)aminomethane *see* tromethamine *on page 957*
trisodium calcium diethylenetriaminepentaacetate (Ca-DTPA) *see* diethylene triamine penta-acetic acid *on page 294*
Tri-Sprintec™ [US] *see* ethinyl estradiol and norgestimate *on page 378*
Tri-Statin® II Topical *(Discontinued)* *see* nystatin and triamcinolone *on page 690*
Tristoject® Injection *(Discontinued)*
Trisudex® *(Discontinued)* *see* triprolidine and pseudoephedrine *on page 955*
Tri-Sudo® *(Discontinued)* *see* triprolidine and pseudoephedrine *on page 955*
Trital DM [US] *see* chlorpheniramine, phenylephrine, and dextromethorphan *on page 209*
Tri-Tannate Plus® *(Discontinued)* *see* chlorpheniramine, ephedrine, phenylephrine, and carbeta-pentane *on page 208*
TriTuss® [US] *see* guaifenesin, dextromethorphan, and phenylephrine *on page 459*
TriTuss® ER [US] *see* guaifenesin, dextromethorphan, and phenylephrine *on page 459*
Trivagizole-3® [Can] *see* clotrimazole *on page 238*
Trivagizole-3® *(Discontinued)* *see* clotrimazole *on page 238*
trivalent inactivated influenza vaccine (TIV) *see* influenza virus vaccine *on page 508*
Tri-Vent™ DM *(Discontinued)* *see* guaifenesin, pseudoephedrine, and dextromethorphan *on page 460*
Tri-Vent™ DPC *(Discontinued)* *see* chlorpheniramine, phenylephrine, and dextromethorphan *on page 209*
Tri-Vent™ HC *(Discontinued)* *see* hydrocodone, carbinoxamine, and pseudoephedrine *on page 483*
Tri-Vi-Sol® [US-OTC] *see* vitamins (multiple/pediatric) *on page 983*
Tri-Vi-Sol® with Iron [US-OTC] *see* vitamins (multiple/pediatric) *on page 983*
Trivora® [US] *see* ethinyl estradiol and levonorgestrel *on page 372*
Trizivir® [US] *see* abacavir, lamivudine, and zidovudine *on page 16*
Trobicin® *(Discontinued)* *see* spectinomycin *on page 886*
Trocaine® [US-OTC] *see* benzocaine *on page 124*
Trocal® *(Discontinued)* *see* dextromethorphan *on page 284*

trolamine (TROLE a meen)

Sound-Alike/Look-Alike Issues
Myoflex® may be confused with Mycelex®

Synonyms TEAS; triethanolamine salicylate; trolamine salicylate

U.S./Canadian Brand Names Antiphlogistine Rub A-535 No Odour [Can]; Aspercreme® [US-OTC]; Flex-Power [US-OTC]; Mobisyl® [US-OTC]; Myoflex® [US-OTC/Can]; Sportscreme® [US-OTC]

Therapeutic Category Analgesic, Topical

Use Relief of pain of muscular aches, rheumatism, neuralgia, sprains, arthritis on intact skin

Usual Dosage Topical: Apply to area as needed

Dosage Forms
Cream, topical: 10% (90 g)
  Aspercreme® [OTC]: 10% (35 g, 85 g, 142 g)
  Flex-Power [OTC]: 10% (57 g, 113 g)
  Mobisyl® [OTC]: 10% (100 g, 227 g)
  Myoflex® [OTC]: 10% (57 g, 113 g)
  Sportscreme® [OTC]: 10% (35 g, 85 g)
Lotion, topical: 10% (180 mL)
  Aspercreme® [OTC]: 10% (180 mL)

trolamine salicylate *see* trolamine *on page 957*
Trombovar® [Can] *see* sodium tetradecyl *on page 880*

tromethamine (troe METH a meen)

Sound-Alike/Look-Alike Issues
tromethamine may be confused with TrophAmine®

Synonyms tris buffer; tris(hydroxymethyl)aminomethane

U.S./Canadian Brand Names THAM® [US]

Therapeutic Category Alkalinizing Agent

Use Correction of metabolic acidosis associated with cardiac bypass surgery or cardiac arrest; to correct excess acidity of stored blood that is preserved with acid citrate dextrose (ACD); indicated in infants needing alkalinization after receiving maximum sodium bicarbonate (8-10 mEq/kg/24 hours)

Usual Dosage
Neonates and Infants: Metabolic acidosis associated with RDS: Initial: Approximately 1 mL/kg for each pH unit below 7.4; additional doses determined by changes in PaO_2, pH, and pCO_2; **Note:** Although THAM® solution does not raise pCO_2 when treating metabolic acidosis with concurrent respiratory acidosis, bicarbonate may be preferred because the osmotic effects of THAM® are greater.

Adults: Dose depends on buffer base deficit; when deficit is known: tromethamine (mL of 0.3 M solution) = body weight (kg) x base deficit (mEq/L) x 1.1
Metabolic acidosis with cardiac arrest:
  I.V.: 3.6-10.8 g (111-333 mL); additional amounts may be required to control acidosis after arrest reversed
  Open chest: Intraventricular: 2-6 g (62-185 mL). **Note:** Do not inject into cardiac muscle
Acidosis associated with cardiac bypass surgery: Average dose: 9 mL/kg (2.7 mEq/kg); 500 mL is adequate for most adults; maximum dose: 500 mg/kg in ≤1 hour
Excess acidity of acid citrate dextrose (ACD) blood in coronary artery surgery: 15-77 mL of 0.3 molar solution added to each 500 mL of blood

Dosage Forms
Injection, solution:
  THAM®: 18 g [0.3 molar] (500 mL)

Tronolane® Cream [US-OTC] *see* pramoxine *on page 777*
Tronolane® Suppository [US-OTC] *see* phenylephrine *on page 745*
Tropicacyl® [US] *see* tropicamide *on page 957*

tropicamide (troe PIK a mide)

Synonyms bistropamide

U.S./Canadian Brand Names Diotrope® [Can]; Mydral™ [US]; Mydriacyl® [US/Can]; Tropicacyl® [US]

Therapeutic Category Anticholinergic Agent

▶

◄ **Use** Short-acting mydriatic used in diagnostic procedures; as well as preoperatively and postoperatively; treatment of some cases of acute iritis, iridocyclitis, and keratitis

Usual Dosage Ophthalmic: Children and Adults (individuals with heavily pigmented eyes may require larger doses):

Cycloplegia: Instill 1-2 drops (1%); may repeat in 5 minutes

Exam must be performed within 30 minutes after the repeat dose; if the patient is not examined within 20-30 minutes, instill an additional drop

Mydriasis: Instill 1-2 drops (0.5%) 15-20 minutes before exam; may repeat every 30 minutes as needed

Dosage Forms

Solution, ophthalmic [drops]: 0.5% (15 mL); 1% (2 mL, 3 mL, 15 mL)

Mydriacyl®: 1% (3 mL, 15 mL)

Mydral™, Tropicacyl®: 0.5% (15 mL); 1% (15 mL)

tropicamide and hydroxyamphetamine *see* hydroxyamphetamine and tropicamide *on page 489*

Trosec [Can] *see* trospium *on page 958*

trospium (TROSE pee um)

Synonyms trospium chloride

U.S./Canadian Brand Names Sanctura® XR [US]; Sanctura® [US]; Trosec [Can]

Therapeutic Category Anticholinergic Agent

Use Treatment of overactive bladder with symptoms of urgency, incontinence, and urinary frequency

Usual Dosage Oral: Adults: Immediate release formulation: 20 mg twice daily; extended release formulation: 60 mg once daily

Dosage Forms

Capsule, extended release:

Sanctura® XR: 60 mg

Tablet:

Sanctura®: 20 mg

trospium chloride *see* trospium *on page 958*

Trovan® *(Discontinued)*

Truphylline® *(Discontinued)* *see* aminophylline *on page 60*

Trusopt® [US/Can] *see* dorzolamide *on page 319*

Truvada® [US/Can] *see* emtricitabine and tenofovir *on page 338*

trypsin, balsam peru, and castor oil (TRIP sin, BAL sam pe RUE, & KAS tor oyl)

Sound-Alike/Look-Alike Issues

Granulex® may be confused with Regranex®

Synonyms balsam peru, trypsin, and castor oil; castor oil, trypsin, and balsam peru

U.S./Canadian Brand Names Allanderm-T™ [US]; Granulex® [US]; Optase™ [US]; Xenaderm™ [US]

Therapeutic Category Protectant, Topical

Use Treatment of decubitus ulcers, varicose ulcers, debridement of eschar, dehiscent wounds and sunburn; promote wound healing; reduce odor from necrotic wounds

Usual Dosage Topical: Apply a minimum of twice daily or as often as necessary

Dosage Forms

Aerosol, topical: Trypsin 0.12 mg, balsam Peru 87 mg, and castor oil 788 mg per gram (120 g)

Granulex®: Trypsin 0.12 mg, balsam Peru 87 mg, and castor oil 788 mg per gram (60 g, 120 g)

Gel, topical:

Optase™: Trypsin 0.12 mg, balsam Peru 87 mg, and castor oil 788 mg per gram (95 g)

Ointment, topical:

Allanderm-T™, Xenaderm™: Trypsin 90 USP units, balsam Peru 87 mg, and castor oil 788 mg per gram (30 g, 60 g)

tryptoreline *see* triptorelin *on page 956*

Trysul® *(Discontinued)* *see* sulfabenzamide, sulfacetamide, and sulfathiazole *on page 892*

TSH *see* thyrotropin alpha *on page 924*

TSPA *see* thiotepa *on page 922*

TST *see* tuberculin tests *on page 959*

T-Stat® *(Discontinued)* *see* erythromycin *on page 354*

tuberculin purified protein derivative *see* tuberculin tests *on page 959*
tuberculin skin test *see* tuberculin tests *on page 959*

tuberculin tests (too BER kyoo lin tests)

Sound-Alike/Look-Alike Issues
Aplisol® may be confused with Anusol®, A.P.L.®, Aplitest®, Atropisol®
Tuberculin products may be confused with tetanus toxoid products and influenza virus vaccine. Medication errors have occurred when tuberculin skin tests (PPD) have been inadvertently administered instead of tetanus toxoid products and influenza virus vaccine. These products are refrigerated and often stored in close proximity to each other.
Synonyms mantoux; PPD; TB skin test; TST; tuberculin purified protein derivative; tuberculin skin test
U.S./Canadian Brand Names Aplisol® [US]; Tubersol® [US]
Therapeutic Category Diagnostic Agent
Use Skin test in diagnosis of tuberculosis
Usual Dosage Children and Adults: Intradermal: 0.1 mL

TST interpretation: Criteria for positive TST read at 48-72 hours (see Note below for healthcare workers):
Induration ≥5 mm: Persons with HIV infection (or risk factors for HIV infection, but unknown status), recent close contact to person with known active TB, persons with chest x-ray consistent with healed TB, persons who are immunosuppressed
Induration ≥10 mm: Persons with clinical conditions which increase risk of TB infection, recent immigrants, I.V. drug users, residents and employees of high-risk settings, children <4 years of age
Induration ≥15 mm: Persons who do not meet any of the above criteria (no risk factors for TB)
Note: A two-step test is recommended when testing will be performed at regular intervals (eg, for healthcare workers). If the first test is negative, a second TST should be administered 1-3 weeks after the first test was read.

TST interpretation (CDC guidelines) in a healthcare setting:
Baseline test: ≥10 mm is positive (either first or second step)
Serial testing without known exposure: Increase of ≥10 mm is positive
Known exposure:
≥5 mm is positive in patients with baseline of 0 mm
≥10 mm is positive in patients with negative baseline or previous screening result of ≥0 mm
Read test at 48-72 hours following placement. Test results with 0 mm induration or measured induration less than the defined cutoff point are considered to signify absence of infection with *M. tuberculosis*. Test results should be documented in millimeters even if classified as negative. Erythema and redness of skin are not indicative of a positive test result.

Dosage Forms
Injection, solution:
Aplisol®, Tubersol®: 5 TU/0.1 mL (1 mL, 5 mL)

Tubersol® [US] *see* tuberculin tests *on page 959*
Tucks® [US-OTC] *see* witch hazel *on page 987*
Tucks® Anti-Itch [US-OTC] *see* hydrocortisone (rectal) *on page 484*
Tucks® Hemorrhoidal [US-OTC] *see* pramoxine *on page 777*
Tuinal® *(Discontinued)*
Tums® [US-OTC] *see* calcium carbonate *on page 163*
Tums® E-X [US-OTC] *see* calcium carbonate *on page 163*
Tums® Extra Strength Sugar Free [US-OTC] *see* calcium carbonate *on page 163*
Tums® Smoothies™ [US-OTC] *see* calcium carbonate *on page 163*
Tums® Ultra [US-OTC] *see* calcium carbonate *on page 163*
Tur-bi-kal® [US-OTC] *see* phenylephrine *on page 745*
Tusal® *(Discontinued)*
Tusibron® *(Discontinued)* *see* guaifenesin *on page 453*
Tusibron-DM® *(Discontinued)* *see* guaifenesin and dextromethorphan *on page 454*
Tusnel-DM Pediatric® [US] *see* guaifenesin, pseudoephedrine, and dextromethorphan *on page 460*
Tusnel Liquid® [US] *see* guaifenesin, pseudoephedrine, and dextromethorphan *on page 460*
Tusnel Pediatric® [US] *see* guaifenesin, pseudoephedrine, and dextromethorphan *on page 460*

Tussafed® *(Discontinued)*

Tussafed® HC *(Discontinued)*

Tussafed® HCG *(Discontinued)*

Tussafin® Expectorant *(Discontinued)*

Tussend® Expectorant *(Discontinued)*

Tussend® Syrup *(Discontinued)*

Tussend® Tablet *(Discontinued)*

Tussi-12® [US] *see* carbetapentane and chlorpheniramine *on page 174*

Tussi-12® D [US] *see* carbetapentane, phenylephrine, and pyrilamine *on page 176*

Tussi-12® DS [US] *see* carbetapentane, phenylephrine, and pyrilamine *on page 176*

Tussi-12 S™ [US] *see* carbetapentane and chlorpheniramine *on page 174*

Tussigon® [US] *see* hydrocodone and homatropine *on page 482*

TussiNate™ *(Discontinued)*

Tussionex® [US] *see* hydrocodone and chlorpheniramine *on page 482*

Tussi-Organidin® DM NR [US] *see* guaifenesin and dextromethorphan *on page 454*

Tussi-Organidin® DM-S NR [US] *see* guaifenesin and dextromethorphan *on page 454*

Tussi-Organidin® NR [US] *see* guaifenesin and codeine *on page 454*

Tussi-Organidin® S-NR [US] *see* guaifenesin and codeine *on page 454*

Tussizone-12 RF™ [US] *see* carbetapentane and chlorpheniramine *on page 174*

Tuss-LA® *(Discontinued)* *see* guaifenesin and pseudoephedrine *on page 458*

Tusso-C™ [US] *see* guaifenesin and codeine *on page 454*

Tusso-DF® *(Discontinued)*

Tusso™-DMR [US] *see* guaifenesin, dextromethorphan, and phenylephrine *on page 459*

Tussplex™ DM [US] *see* chlorpheniramine, phenylephrine, and dextromethorphan *on page 209*

Tustan 12S™ [US] *see* carbetapentane and chlorpheniramine *on page 174*

T-Vites [US-OTC] *see* vitamins (multiple/oral) *on page 983*

TVP-1012 *see* rasagiline *on page 820*

Twelve Resin-K [US] *see* cyanocobalamin *on page 254*

Twilite® [US-OTC] *see* diphenhydramine *on page 304*

Twinject™ [US/Can] *see* epinephrine *on page 344*

Twin-K® *(Discontinued)*

Twinrix® [US/Can] *see* hepatitis A inactivated and hepatitis B (recombinant) vaccine *on page 469*

Two-Dyne® *(Discontinued)*

Ty21a vaccine *see* typhoid vaccine *on page 961*

Tycolene [US-OTC] *see* acetaminophen *on page 19*

Tycolene Maximum Strength [US-OTC] *see* acetaminophen *on page 19*

Tygacil® [US] *see* tigecycline *on page 927*

Tykerb® [US] *see* lapatinib *on page 550*

Tylenol® [US-OTC/Can] *see* acetaminophen *on page 19*

Tylenol® 8 Hour [US-OTC] *see* acetaminophen *on page 19*

Tylenol® Allergy Sinus [Can] *see* acetaminophen, chlorpheniramine, and pseudoephedrine *on page 25*

Tylenol® Allergy Sinus *(Discontinued)* *see* acetaminophen, chlorpheniramine, and pseudoephedrine *on page 25*

Tylenol® Arthritis Pain [US-OTC] *see* acetaminophen *on page 19*

Tylenol® Children's [US-OTC] *see* acetaminophen *on page 19*

Tylenol® Children's Plus Cold Nighttime *(Discontinued)* *see* acetaminophen, chlorpheniramine, and pseudoephedrine *on page 25*

Tylenol® Children's with Flavor Creator [US-OTC] *see* acetaminophen *on page 19*

Tylenol® Cold Day Non-Drowsy [US-OTC] *see* acetaminophen, dextromethorphan, and pseudoephedrine *on page 27*

Tylenol® Cold Daytime [Can] *see* acetaminophen, dextromethorphan, and pseudoephedrine *on page 27*

Tylenol® Cold Daytime, Children's [US-OTC] *see* acetaminophen and pseudoephedrine *on page 23*

Tylenol® Cold Head Congestion Daytime [US-OTC] *see* acetaminophen, dextromethorphan, and phenylephrine *on page 26*

Tylenol® Cold, Infants *(Discontinued)* *see* acetaminophen and pseudoephedrine *on page 23*

Tylenol® Cold Multi-Symptom Daytime [US-OTC] *see* acetaminophen, dextromethorphan, and phenylephrine *on page 26*

Tylenol® Decongestant [Can] *see* acetaminophen and pseudoephedrine *on page 23*

Tylenol® Elixir with Codeine [Can] *see* acetaminophen and codeine *on page 20*

Tylenol® Extra Strength [US-OTC] *see* acetaminophen *on page 19*

Tylenol® Flu Non-Drowsy Maximum Strength [US-OTC] *see* acetaminophen, dextromethorphan, and pseudoephedrine *on page 27*

Tylenol® Infants [US-OTC] *see* acetaminophen *on page 19*

Tylenol® Junior [US-OTC] *see* acetaminophen *on page 19*

Tylenol® No. 1 [Can] *see* acetaminophen and codeine *on page 20*

Tylenol® No. 1 Forte [Can] *see* acetaminophen and codeine *on page 20*

Tylenol® No. 2 with Codeine [Can] *see* acetaminophen and codeine *on page 20*

Tylenol® No. 3 with Codeine [Can] *see* acetaminophen and codeine *on page 20*

Tylenol® No. 4 with Codeine [Can] *see* acetaminophen and codeine *on page 20*

Tylenol® Plus Infants Cold & Cough *(Discontinued)* *see* acetaminophen, dextromethorphan, and phenylephrine *on page 26*

Tylenol® PM [US-OTC] *see* acetaminophen and diphenhydramine *on page 21*

Tylenol® Severe Allergy [US-OTC] *see* acetaminophen and diphenhydramine *on page 21*

Tylenol® Sinus [Can] *see* acetaminophen and pseudoephedrine *on page 23*

Tylenol® Sinus Congestion & Pain Daytime [US-OTC] *see* acetaminophen and phenylephrine *on page 22*

Tylenol® Sinus Daytime [US-OTC] *see* acetaminophen and pseudoephedrine *on page 23*

Tylenol® With Codeine [US] *see* acetaminophen and codeine *on page 20*

Tylenol® with Codeine (Elixir) *(Discontinued)* *see* acetaminophen and codeine *on page 20*

Tylox® [US] *see* oxycodone and acetaminophen *on page 710*

Typherix™ [Can] *see* Salmonella typhi Vi capsular polysaccharide vaccine *(Canada only) on page 854*

Typhim Vi® [US/Can] *see* typhoid vaccine *on page 961*

typhoid vaccine (TYE foid vak SEEN)

Synonyms Ty21a vaccine; typhoid vaccine live oral Ty21a; Vi vaccine

U.S./Canadian Brand Names Typhim Vi® [US/Can]; Vivotif® [US/Can]

Therapeutic Category Vaccine, Inactivated Bacteria

Use Active immunization against typhoid fever caused by *Salmonella typhi*

Not for routine vaccination. In the United States and Canada, use should be limited to:
- Travelers to areas with a prolonged risk of exposure to *S. typhi*
- Persons with intimate exposure to a *S. typhi* carrier
- Laboratory technicians with exposure to *S. typhi*
- Travelers with achlorhydria or hypochlorhydria (Canadian recommendation)

Usual Dosage Immunization:

Oral: Children ≥6 years and Adults:

Primary immunization: One capsule on alternate days (day 1, 3, 5, and 7) for a total of 4 doses; all doses should be complete at least 1 week prior to potential exposure

Booster immunization: Repeat full course of primary immunization every 5 years

I.M.: Children ≥2 years and Adults: 0.5 mL given at least 2 weeks prior to expected exposure

Reimmunization:

Typhim Vi®: 0.5 mL; optimal schedule has not been established; a single dose every 2 years is currently recommended for repeated or continued exposure

Typherix®: 0.5 mL every 3 years

Dosage Forms [CAN] = Canadian brand name

Capsule, enteric coated:

Vivotif®: Viable *S. typhi* Ty21a 2-6.8 x 10^9 colony-forming units and nonviable *S. typhi* Ty21a 5-50 x 10^9 bacterial cells [contains lactose 100-180 mg/capsule and sucrose 26-130 mg/capsule]

◄ **Injection, solution:**
Typherix® [CAN]: Vi capsular polysaccharide 25 mcg/0.5 mL (0.5 mL) [derived from *S. typhi* Ty2 strain] [not available in U.S.]
Typhim Vi®: Purified Vi capsular polysaccharide 25 mcg/0.5 mL (0.5 mL, 10 mL) [derived from *S. typhi* Ty2 strain]

typhoid vaccine live oral Ty21a *see* typhoid vaccine *on page 961*
Tyrodone® Liquid *(Discontinued)*
Tysabri® [US/Can] *see* natalizumab *on page 658*
Tyzeka™ [US] *see* telbivudine *on page 906*
Tyzine® [US] *see* tetrahydrozoline *on page 916*
Tyzine® Pediatric [US] *see* tetrahydrozoline *on page 916*
506U78 *see* nelarabine *on page 660*
U-90152S *see* delavirdine *on page 271*
UAD Otic® *(Discontinued) see* neomycin, polymyxin B, and hydrocortisone *on page 663*
UCB-P071 *see* cetirizine *on page 196*
UK *see* urokinase *on page 965*
UK-88,525 *see* darifenacin *on page 268*
UK-427,857 *see* maraviroc *on page 591*
UK92480 *see* sildenafil *on page 865*
UK109496 *see* voriconazole *on page 984*
Ulcerease® [US-OTC] *see* phenol *on page 743*
Ulcidine [Can] *see* famotidine *on page 390*
ULR-LA® *(Discontinued)*
Ultane® [US] *see* sevoflurane *on page 864*
Ultiva® [US/Can] *see* remifentanil *on page 824*
Ultracaine® D-S [Can] *see* articaine and epinephrine *on page 95*
Ultracaine® D-S Forte [Can] *see* articaine and epinephrine *on page 95*
Ultracaps MT *(Discontinued) see* pancrelipase *on page 718*
Ultracet™ [US] *see* acetaminophen and tramadol *on page 24*
Ultra Freeda Iron Free [US-OTC] *see* vitamins (multiple/oral) *on page 983*
Ultra Freeda with Iron [US-OTC] *see* vitamins (multiple/oral) *on page 983*
Ultram® [US] *see* tramadol *on page 941*
Ultram® ER [US] *see* tramadol *on page 941*
Ultra Mide® [US-OTC] *see* urea *on page 963*
UltraMide 25™ [Can] *see* urea *on page 963*
Ultramop™ [Can] *see* methoxsalen *on page 617*
Ultra NatalCare® [US] *see* vitamins (multiple/prenatal) *on page 983*
Ultraprin [US-OTC] *see* ibuprofen *on page 495*
Ultraquin™ [Can] *see* hydroquinone *on page 488*
Ultrase® [US/Can] *see* pancrelipase *on page 718*
Ultrase® MT [US/Can] *see* pancrelipase *on page 718*
Ultra Tears® [US-OTC] *see* artificial tears *on page 95*
Ultravate® [US/Can] *see* halobetasol *on page 465*
Ultravist® [US] *see* iopromide *on page 521*
Umecta® [US] *see* urea *on page 963*
Unasyn® [US/Can] *see* ampicillin and sulbactam *on page 73*
Unburn® [US] *see* lidocaine *on page 561*

undecylenic acid and derivatives (un de sil EN ik AS id & dah RIV ah tivs)

Synonyms zinc undecylenate
U.S./Canadian Brand Names Fungi-Nail® [US-OTC]
Therapeutic Category Antifungal Agent

Use Treatment of athlete's foot (tinea pedis); ringworm (except nails and scalp)

Usual Dosage Topical: Children ≥2 years and Adults: Apply twice daily to affected area for 4 weeks; apply to clean, dry area

Dosage Forms
  Solution, topical:
    Fungi-Nail® [OTC]: Undecylenic acid 25% (29.57 mL)

Unguentine® *(Discontinued)* *see benzocaine on page 124*
Uni-Bent® Cough Syrup *(Discontinued)* *see diphenhydramine on page 304*
Unicap M® [US-OTC] *see vitamins (multiple/oral) on page 983*
Unicap Sr® [US-OTC] *see vitamins (multiple/oral) on page 983*
Unicap T™ [US-OTC] *see vitamins (multiple/oral) on page 983*
Uni-Cenna *(Discontinued)* *see senna on page 861*
Uni-Cof *(Discontinued)* *see pseudoephedrine, dihydrocodeine, and chlorpheniramine on page 803*
Unidet® [Can] *see tolterodine on page 935*
Uni-Dur® *(Discontinued)* *see theophylline on page 917*
Unifed [US-OTC] *see pseudoephedrine on page 801*
Unipen® [Can] *see nafcillin on page 652*
Uniphyl® [US] *see theophylline on page 917*
Uniphyl® SRT [Can] *see theophylline on page 917*
Uni-Pro® *(Discontinued)* *see ibuprofen on page 495*
Uniretic® [US/Can] *see moexipril and hydrochlorothiazide on page 640*
Unisom® Maximum Strength SleepGels® [US-OTC] *see diphenhydramine on page 304*
Unisom® SleepTabs® [US-OTC] *see doxylamine on page 325*
Unithroid® [US] *see levothyroxine on page 560*
Unitrol® *(Discontinued)*
Uni-tussin® *(Discontinued)* *see guaifenesin on page 453*
Uni-tussin® DM *(Discontinued)* *see guaifenesin and dextromethorphan on page 454*
Univasc® [US] *see moexipril on page 640*
unna's boot *see zinc gelatin on page 993*
unna's paste *see zinc gelatin on page 993*
Urabeth® *(Discontinued)* *see bethanechol on page 133*
Urasal® [Can] *see methenamine on page 614*

urea (yoor EE a)

Synonyms carbamide

U.S./Canadian Brand Names Aquacare® [US-OTC]; Aquaphilic® With Carbamide [US-OTC]; Carmol® 10 [US-OTC]; Carmol® 20 [US-OTC]; Carmol® 40 [US]; Carmol® Deep Cleaning [US]; Cerovel™ [US]; DPM™ [US-OTC]; Gormel® [US-OTC]; Hydro 40™ [US]; Kerafoam™ [US]; Keralac™ Nailstik [US]; Keralac™ [US]; Kerol™ Redi-Cloths [US]; Kerol™ [US]; Lanaphilic® [US-OTC]; Nutraplus® [US-OTC]; Rea-Lo® [US-OTC]; Ultra Mide® [US-OTC]; UltraMide 25™ [Can]; Umecta® [US]; Ureacin® [US-OTC]; Uremol® [Can]; Urisec® [Can]; Vanamide™ [US]

Therapeutic Category Diuretic, Osmotic; Topical Skin Product

Use Keratolytic agent to soften nails or skin; OTC: Moisturizer for dry, rough skin

Usual Dosage Topical: Adults: Hyperkeratotic conditions, dry skin: Apply 1-3 times/day

Dosage Forms
  Aerosol, topical [foam]:
    Hydro 40™: 40% (70 g)
    Kerafoam™: 30% (60 g)
  Cloth, topical:
    Kerol™ Redi-Cloths: 42% (30s)
  Cream, topical: 40% (30 g, 85 g, 199 g)
    Aquacare® [OTC]: 10% (75 g)
    Carmol® 20 [OTC]: 20% (90 g)
    Carmol® 40: 40% (30 g, 90 g, 210 g)
    Cerovel™: 40% (133 g)
    DPM™ [OTC]: 20% (118 g)

Gormel® [OTC]: 20% (75 g, 120 g, 454 g, 2270 g)
Keralac™: 50% (142 g, 255 g)
Nutraplus® [OTC]: 10% (90 g, 454 g)
Rea-Lo® [OTC]: 30% (60 g, 240 g)
Ureacin®-20 [OTC]: 20% (120 g)
Vanamide™: 40% (85 g, 199 g)
Emulsion, topical:
Umecta®: 40% (120 mL, 480 mL)
Gel: 40% (15 mL)
Carmol® 40: 40% (15 mL)
Cerovel™: 40% (25 mL)
Keralac™: 50% (18 mL)
Lotion, topical: 40% (240 mL)
Aquacare® [OTC]: 10% (240 mL)
Carmol® 10 [OTC]: 10% (180 mL)
Carmol® 40: 40% (240 mL)
Cerovel™: 40% (325 mL)
Keralac™: 35% (207 mL, 325 mL)
Nutraplus® [OTC]: 10% (240 mL, 480 mL)
Ultra Mide® [OTC]: 25% (120 mL, 240 mL)
Ureacin®-10 [OTC]: 10% (240 mL)
Ointment, topical:
Aquaphilic® with Carbamide [OTC]: 10% (180 g, 480 g); 20% (480 g)
Keralac™: 50% (90 g)
Lanaphilic® [OTC]: 10% (454 g); 20% (454 g)
Shampoo, topical:
Carmol® Deep Cleaning: 10% (240 mL)
Solution, topical:
Keralac™ Nailstick: 50% (2.4 mL)
Suspension, topical: 50% (284 g)
Kerol™: 50% (284 g)
Umecta®: 40% (18 mL, 300 mL)

urea and hydrocortisone (yoor EE a & hye droe KOR ti sone)

Synonyms hydrocortisone and urea
U.S./Canadian Brand Names Carmol-HC® [US]; Ti-U-Lac® H [Can]; Uremol® HC [Can]
Therapeutic Category Corticosteroid, Topical
Use Inflammation of corticosteroid-responsive dermatoses
Usual Dosage Apply thin film and rub in well 1-4 times/day. Therapy should be discontinued when control is achieved; if no improvement is seen, reassessment of diagnosis may be necessary.
Dosage Forms
Cream:
Carmol-HC®: Urea 10% and hydrocortisone 1% (30 g)

urea, chlorophyllin, and papain *see* chlorophyllin, papain, and urea *on page 203*
Ureacin® [US-OTC] *see* urea *on page 963*
urea peroxide *see* carbamide peroxide *on page 174*
Urecholine® [US] *see* bethanechol *on page 133*
Uremol® [Can] *see* urea *on page 963*
Uremol® HC [Can] *see* urea and hydrocortisone *on page 964*
Urex™ [US/Can] *see* methenamine *on page 614*
Urisec® [Can] *see* urea *on page 963*
Urispas® [US/Can] *see* flavoxate *on page 402*
Uristat® *(Discontinued)* *see* phenazopyridine *on page 741*
Urocit®-K [US] *see* potassium citrate *on page 772*
Urodine® *(Discontinued)* *see* phenazopyridine *on page 741*

urofollitropin (yoor oh fol li TROE pin)

Synonyms follicle-stimulating hormone, human; FSH; hFSH
U.S./Canadian Brand Names Bravelle® [US/Can]; Fertinorm® H.P. [Can]

Therapeutic Category Gonadotropin; Ovulation Stimulator

Use Ovulation induction in patients who previously received pituitary suppression; development of multiple follicles with Assisted Reproductive Technologies (ART)

Usual Dosage Note: Dose should be individualized. Use the lowest dose consistent with the expectation of good results. Over the course of treatment, doses may vary depending on individual patient response.
Adults: Female:
Ovulation induction: I.M., SubQ: Initial: 150 int. units daily for the first 5 days of treatment. Dose adjustments ≤75-150 int. units can be made every ≥2 days; maximum daily dose: 450 int. units; treatment >12 days is not recommended. If response to follitropin is appropriate, hCG is given 1 day following the last dose. Withhold hCG if serum estradiol is >2000 pg/mL, if the ovaries are abnormally enlarged, or if abdominal pain occurs.
ART: SubQ: 225 int. units daily for the first 5 days; dose may be adjusted based on patient response, but adjustments should not be made more frequently than once every 2 days; maximum adjustment: 75-150 int. units; maximum daily dose: 450 int. units; maximum duration of treatment: 12 days. When a sufficient number of follicles of adequate size are present, the final maturation of the follicles is induced by administering hCG. Withhold hCG in cases where the ovaries are abnormally enlarged on the last day of therapy.

Dosage Forms
Injection, powder for reconstitution [human origin]:
Bravelle®: 75 int. units

urokinase (ur oh KYE nase)

Synonyms UK

U.S./Canadian Brand Names Kinlytic™ [US]

Therapeutic Category Thrombolytic Agent

Use Thrombolytic agent for the lysis of acute massive pulmonary emboli or pulmonary emboli with unstable hemodynamics

Usual Dosage I.V.: Adults: Acute pulmonary embolism: Loading: 4400 int. units/kg over 10 minutes; maintenance: 4400 int. units/kg/hour for 12 hours. Following infusion, anticoagulation treatment is recommended to prevent recurrent thrombosis. Do not start anticoagulation until aPTT has decreased to less than twice the normal control value. If heparin is used, do not administer loading dose. Treatment should be followed with oral anticoagulants.

Dosage Forms
Injection, powder for reconstitution:
Kinlytic™: 250,000 int. units

Uro-KP-Neutral® [US] *see* potassium phosphate and sodium phosphate *on page 775*

Urolene Blue® *(Discontinued)* *see* methylene blue *on page 620*

Uro-Mag® [US-OTC] *see* magnesium oxide *on page 587*

Uromax® [Can] *see* oxybutynin *on page 708*

Uromitexan [Can] *see* mesna *on page 608*

Uroplus® DS *(Discontinued)*

Uroplus® SS *(Discontinued)*

Uroxatral® [US] *see* alfuzosin *on page 44*

Urso® [Can] *see* ursodiol *on page 965*

Urso 250™ [US] *see* ursodiol *on page 965*

ursodeoxycholic acid *see* ursodiol *on page 965*

ursodiol (ur soe DYE ol)

Synonyms ursodeoxycholic acid

U.S./Canadian Brand Names Actigall® [US]; DOM-Ursodiol C [Can]; PHL-Ursodiol C [Can]; PMS-Ursodiol C [Can]; Urso 250™ [US]; Urso Forte™ [US]; Urso® DS [Can]; Urso® [Can]

Therapeutic Category Gallstone Dissolution Agent

Use Actigall®: Gallbladder stone dissolution; prevention of gallstones in obese patients experiencing rapid weight loss; Urso®: Primary biliary cirrhosis

◀ **Usual Dosage** Oral: Adults:

Gallstone dissolution: 8-10 mg/kg/day in 2-3 divided doses; use beyond 24 months is not established; obtain ultrasound images at 6-month intervals for the first year of therapy; 30% of patients have stone recurrence after dissolution

Gallstone prevention: 300 mg twice daily

Primary biliary cirrhosis: 13-15 mg/kg/day in 2-4 divided doses (with food)

Dosage Forms

Capsule: 300 mg

Actigall®: 300 mg

Tablet:

Urso 250™: 250 mg

Urso Forte™: 500 mg

Urso® DS [Can] *see* ursodiol *on page 965*

Urso Forte™ [US] *see* ursodiol *on page 965*

UTI Relief® [US-OTC] *see* phenazopyridine *on page 741*

Utradol™ [Can] *see* etodolac *on page 383*

Uvadex® [US/Can] *see* methoxsalen *on page 617*

vaccinia immune globulin (intravenous)

(vax IN ee a i MYUN GLOB yoo lin IN tra VEE nus)

Synonyms VIGIV

U.S./Canadian Brand Names CNJ-016™ [US]

Therapeutic Category Immune Globulin

Use Treatment of infectious complications of smallpox (vaccinia virus) vaccination, such as eczema vaccinatum, progressive vaccinia, and severe generalized vaccinia; treatment of vaccinia infections in individuals with concurrent skin conditions or accidental virus exposure to eyes (except vaccinia keratitis), mouth, or other areas where viral infection would pose significant risk

Usual Dosage I.V.: Adults:

CNJ-016™ (Cangene product): 6000 units/kg; 9000 units/kg may be considered if patient does not respond to initial dose.

DynPort product: Total dose: 2 mL/kg (100 mg/kg); higher doses (200-500 mg/kg) may be considered if patient does not respond to initial recommended dose (sucrose-related renal impairment is worsened at doses ≥400 mg/kg)

Dosage Forms Injection, solution [preservative free; solvent-detergent treated]:

CNJ-016™: Cangene product: ≥50,000 units/15 mL (15 mL)

DynPort product: 50 mg/mL (50 mL)

vaccinia vaccine *see* smallpox vaccine *on page 871*

Vagifem® [US/Can] *see* estradiol *on page 359*

Vagi-Gard® [US-OTC] *see* povidone-iodine *on page 775*

Vagistat®-1 [US-OTC] *see* tioconazole *on page 929*

Vagitrol® *(Discontinued)*

valacyclovir (val ay SYE kloe veer)

Sound-Alike/Look-Alike Issues

valacyclovir may be confused with valganciclovir

Valtrex® may be confused with Valcyte™

Synonyms valacyclovir hydrochloride

U.S./Canadian Brand Names Valtrex® [US/Can]

Therapeutic Category Antiviral Agent

Use Treatment of herpes zoster (shingles) in immunocompetent patients; treatment of first-episode and recurrent genital herpes; suppression of recurrent genital herpes and reduction of heterosexual transmission of genital herpes in immunocompetent patients; suppression of genital herpes in HIV-infected individuals; treatment of herpes labialis (cold sores)

Usual Dosage Oral:

Adolescents and Adults: Herpes labialis (cold sores): 2 g twice daily for 1 day (separate doses by ~12 hours)

Adults:
Herpes zoster (shingles): 1 g 3 times/day for 7 days
Genital herpes:
  Initial episode: 1 g twice daily for 10 days
  Recurrent episode: 500 mg twice daily for 3 days
  Reduction of transmission: 500 mg once daily (source partner)
  Suppressive therapy:
    Immunocompetent patients: 1000 mg once daily (500 mg once daily in patients with <9 recurrences per year)
    HIV-infected patients (CD4 ≥100 cells/mm^3): 500 mg twice daily

Dosage Forms
  Caplet:
    Valtrex®: 500 mg, 1000 mg

valacyclovir hydrochloride *see valacyclovir on page 966*
Valcyte™ [US/Can] *see valganciclovir on page 967*
23-valent pneumococcal polysaccharide vaccine *see pneumococcal polysaccharide vaccine (polyvalent) on page 763*

valganciclovir (val gan SYE kloh veer)

Sound-Alike/Look-Alike Issues
  valganciclovir may be confused with valacyclovir
  Valcyte™ may be confused with Valium®, Valtrex®
Synonyms valganciclovir hydrochloride
U.S./Canadian Brand Names Valcyte™ [US/Can]
Therapeutic Category Antiviral Agent
Use Treatment of cytomegalovirus (CMV) retinitis in patients with acquired immunodeficiency syndrome (AIDS); prevention of CMV disease in high-risk patients (donor CMV positive/recipient CMV negative) undergoing kidney, heart, or kidney/pancreas transplantation
Usual Dosage Oral: Adults:
  CMV retinitis:
    Induction: 900 mg twice daily for 21 days (with food)
    Maintenance: Following induction treatment, or for patients with inactive CMV retinitis who require maintenance therapy: Recommended dose: 900 mg once daily (with food)
  Prevention of CMV disease following transplantation: 900 mg once daily (with food) beginning within 10 days of transplantation; continue therapy until 100 days posttransplantation
Dosage Forms
  Tablet:
    Valcyte™: 450 mg

valganciclovir hydrochloride *see valganciclovir on page 967*
Valisone® Scalp Lotion [Can] *see betamethasone (topical) on page 132*
Valisone® Topical *(Discontinued)*
Valium® [US/Can] *see diazepam on page 289*
Valorin [US-OTC] *see acetaminophen on page 19*
Valorin Extra [US-OTC] *see acetaminophen on page 19*
valproate semisodium *see valproic acid and derivatives on page 967*
valproate sodium *see valproic acid and derivatives on page 967*
valproic acid *see valproic acid and derivatives on page 967*

valproic acid and derivatives (val PROE ik AS id & dah RIV ah tives)

Sound-Alike/Look-Alike Issues
  Depakene® may be confused with Depakote®
  Depakote® may be confused with Depakene®, Depakote® ER, Senokot®
Synonyms 2-propylpentanoic acid; 2-propylvaleric acid; dipropylacetic acid; divalproex sodium; DPA; valproate semisodium; valproate sodium; valproic acid
U.S./Canadian Brand Names Alti-Divalproex [Can]; Apo-Divalproex® [Can]; Apo-Valproic® [Can]; Depacon® [US]; Depakene® [US/Can]; Depakote® ER [US]; Depakote® Sprinkle [US]; Depakote® [US]; Dom-Divalproex [Can]; Epival® I.V. [Can]; Gen-Divalproex [Can]; Novo-Divalproex [Can]; Nu-Divalproex

▶

◄ [Can]; PHL-Divalproex [Can]; PHL-Valproic Acid E.C. [Can]; PHL-Valproic Acid [Can]; PMS-Valproic Acid E.C. [Can]; PMS-Valproic Acid [Can]; ratio-Valproic ECC [Can]; ratio-Valproic [Can]; Rhoxal-valproic [Can]; Sandoz-Valporic [Can]; Stavzor™ [US]

Therapeutic Category Anticonvulsant

Use

Depacon®, Depakene®, Depakote®, Depakote® ER, Depakote® Sprinkle, Stavzor™: Monotherapy and adjunctive therapy in the treatment of patients with complex partial seizures; monotherapy and adjunctive therapy of simple and complex absence seizures; adjunctive therapy in patients with multiple seizure types that include absence seizures

Depakote®, Depakote® ER, Stavzor™: Mania associated with bipolar disorder; migraine prophylaxis

Usual Dosage

Seizure disorders: **Note:** Administer doses >250 mg/day in divided doses.

Oral:

Simple and complex absence seizures: Children and Adults: Initial: 15 mg/kg/day; increase by 5-10 mg/kg/day at weekly intervals until therapeutic levels are achieved; maximum: 60 mg/kg/day. Larger maintenance doses may be required in younger children.

Complex partial seizures: Children ≥10 years and Adults: Initial: 10-15 mg/kg/day; increase by 5-10 mg/kg/day at weekly intervals until therapeutic levels are achieved; maximum: 60 mg/kg/day. Larger maintenance doses may be required in younger children.

Note: Regular release and delayed release formulations are usually given in 2-4 divided doses/day; extended release formulation (Depakote® ER) is usually given once daily. Conversion to Depakote® ER from a stable dose of Depakote® may require an increase in the total daily dose between 8% and 20% to maintain similar serum concentrations. Depakote® ER is not recommended for use in children <10 years of age.

I.V.: Administer as a 60-minute infusion (≤20 mg/minute) with the same frequency as oral products; switch patient to oral products as soon as possible. Rapid infusions ≤45 mg/kg over 5-10 minutes (1.5-6 mg/kg/minute) were generally well tolerated in a clinical trial.

Mania: Adults: Oral:

Depakote® tablet: Initial: 750 mg/day in divided doses; dose should be adjusted as rapidly as possible to desired clinical effect; maximum recommended dosage: 60 mg/kg/day

Depakote® ER: Initial: 25 mg/kg/day given once daily; dose should be adjusted as rapidly as possible to desired clinical effect; maximum recommended dose: 60 mg/kg/day.

Migraine prophylaxis: Children ≥16 years and Adults: Oral:

Depakote® tablet: 250 mg twice daily; adjust dose based on patient response, up to 1000 mg/day

Depakote® ER: 500 mg once daily for 7 days, then increase to 1000 mg once daily; adjust dose based on patient response; usual dosage range 500-1000 mg/day

Dosage Forms Strength expressed as valproic acid.

Capsule, softgel: 250 mg

Depakene®: 250 mg

Capsule, softgel, delayed release:

Stavzor™: 125 mg, 250 mg, 500 mg

Capsule, sprinkles:

Depakote® Sprinkle: 125 mg

Injection, solution: 100 mg/mL (5 mL)

Depacon®: 100 mg/mL (5 mL)

Syrup: 250 mg/5 mL

Depakene®: 250 mg/5 mL

Tablet, delayed release: 125 mg, 250 mg, 500 mg

Depakote®: 125 mg, 250 mg, 500 mg

Tablet, delayed release, enteric coated: 125 mg, 250 mg, 500 mg

Tablet, extended release:

Depakote® ER: 250 mg, 500 mg

valsartan (val SAR tan)

Sound-Alike/Look-Alike Issues

valsartan may be confused with losartan, Valstar™

Diovan® may be confused with Darvon®, Dioval®, Zyban®

U.S./Canadian Brand Names Diovan® [US/Can]

Therapeutic Category Angiotensin II Receptor Antagonist

Use Alone or in combination with other antihypertensive agents in the treatment of essential hypertension; reduction of cardiovascular mortality in patients with left ventricular dysfunction postmyocardial infarction; treatment of heart failure (NYHA Class II-IV)

Usual Dosage Oral:

Hypertension:

Children 6-16 years: Initial: 1.3 mg/kg once daily (maximum: 40 mg/day); dose may be increased to achieve desired effect; doses >2.7 mg/kg (maximum: 160 mg) have not been studied

Adults: Initial: 80 mg or 160 mg once daily (in patients who are not volume depleted); dose may be increased to achieve desired effect; maximum recommended dose: 320 mg/day

Heart failure: Adults: Initial: 40 mg twice daily; titrate dose to 80-160 mg twice daily, as tolerated; maximum daily dose: 320 mg

Left ventricular dysfunction after MI: Adults: Initial: 20 mg twice daily; titrate dose to target of 160 mg twice daily as tolerated; may initiate ≥12 hours following MI

Dosage Forms

Tablet:

Diovan®: 40 mg, 80 mg, 160 mg, 320 mg

valsartan and amlodipine *see* amlodipine and valsartan *on page 65*

valsartan and hydrochlorothiazide (val SAR tan & hye droe klor oh THYE a zide)

Sound-Alike/Look-Alike Issues

Diovan® may be confused with Darvon®, Dioval®, Zyban®

Synonyms hydrochlorothiazide and valsartan

U.S./Canadian Brand Names Diovan HCT® [US/Can]

Therapeutic Category Antihypertensive Agent, Combination

Use Treatment of hypertension

Usual Dosage Oral: Adults: Dose is individualized (combination substituted for individual components); dose may be titrated after 3-4 weeks of therapy.

Usual recommended starting dose of valsartan: 80 mg or 160 mg once daily (maximum: 320 mg/day) when used as monotherapy in patients who are not volume depleted

Usual recommended starting dose of hydrochlorothiazide: 12.5-25 mg once daily (maximum: 25 mg/day)

Dosage Forms

Tablet:

Diovan HCT®: 80 mg/12.5 mg: Valsartan 80 mg and hydrochlorothiazide 12.5 mg; 160 mg/12.5 mg: Valsartan 160 mg and hydrochlorothiazide 12.5 mg; 160 mg/25 mg: Valsartan 160 mg and hydrochlorothiazide 25 mg; 320 mg/12.5 mg: Valsartan 320 mg and hydrochlorothiazide 12.5 mg; 320 mg/25 mg: Valsartan 320 mg and hydrochlorothiazide 25 mg

Valstar® *(Discontinued)*

Valtrex® [US/Can] *see* valacyclovir *on page 966*

Vamate® Oral *(Discontinued) see* hydroxyzine *on page 491*

Vanamide™ [US] *see* urea *on page 963*

Vanatrip® *(Discontinued) see* amitriptyline *on page 62*

Vancenase® AQ 84 mcg *(Discontinued) see* beclomethasone *on page 119*

Vancenase® Pockethaler® *(Discontinued) see* beclomethasone *on page 119*

Vanceril® AEM [Can] *see* beclomethasone *on page 119*

Vanceril® *(Discontinued) see* beclomethasone *on page 119*

Vancocin® [US/Can] *see* vancomycin *on page 969*

vancomycin (van koe MYE sin)

Sound-Alike/Look-Alike Issues

vancomycin may be confused with clindamycin, vecuronium

I.V. vancomycin may be confused with Invanz®

Synonyms vancomycin hydrochloride

U.S./Canadian Brand Names Vancocin® [US/Can]

Therapeutic Category Antibiotic, Miscellaneous

◀ **Use** Treatment of patients with infections caused by staphylococcal species and streptococcal species; used orally for staphylococcal enterocolitis or for antibiotic-associated pseudomembranous colitis produced by *C. difficile*

Usual Dosage

Usual dosage range:
Infants >1 month and Children: I.V.: 10-15 mg/kg every 6 hours
Adults:
   I.V.: 2-3 g/day (20-45 mg/kg/day) in divided doses every 6-12 hours; maximum 3 g/day; **Note:** Dose requires adjustment in renal impairment
   Oral: 500-1000 mg/day in divided doses every 6 hours

Indication-specific dosing:
Infants >1 month and Children:
  Colitis (*C. difficile*): Oral: 40 mg/kg/day in divided doses added to fluids
  Meningitis/CNS infection:
   I.V.: 15 mg/kg every 6 hours
   Intrathecal: 5-20 mg/day
  Prophylaxis against infective endocarditis: I.V.:
   Dental, oral, or upper respiratory tract surgery: 20 mg/kg 1 hour prior to the procedure. **Note:** American Heart Association (AHA) guidelines now recommend prophylaxis only in patients undergoing invasive procedures and in whom underlying cardiac conditions may predispose to a higher risk of adverse outcomes should infection occur.
   GI/GU procedure: 20 mg/kg plus gentamicin 2 mg/kg 1 hour prior to surgery. **Note:** As of April 2007, routine prophylaxis no longer recommended by the AHA.
  Susceptible gram-positive infections: I.V.: 10 mg/kg every 6 hours
Adults:
  Catheter-related infections: Antibiotic lock technique: 2 mg/mL in SWFI/NS or D_5W; instill 3-5 mL into catheter port as a flush solution instead of heparin lock (**Note:** Do not mix with any other solutions.)
  Hospital-acquired pneumonia (HAP): I.V.: 15 mg/kg/dose every 12 hours (American Thoracic Society [ATS] 2005 guidelines)
  Meningitis (*Pneumococcus* or *Staphylococcus*)
   I.V.: 30-45 mg/kg/day in divided doses every 8-12 hours **or** 500-750 mg every 6 hours (with third-generation cephalosporin for PCN-resistant *Streptococcus pneumoniae*); maximum dose: 2-3 g/day
   Intrathecal: Up to 20 mg/day
  Prophylaxis against infective endocarditis: I.V.:
   Dental, oral, or upper respiratory tract surgery: 1 g 1 hour before surgery. **Note:** AHA guidelines now recommend prophylaxis only in patients undergoing invasive procedures and in whom underlying cardiac conditions may predispose to a higher risk of adverse outcomes should infection occur
   GI/GU procedure: 1 g plus 1.5 mg/kg gentamicin 1 hour prior to surgery. **Note:** As of April 2007, routine prophylaxis no longer recommended by the AHA.
  Susceptible gram-positive infections: I.V.: 15-20 mg/kg/dose (usual: 750-1500 mg) every 12 hours

Dosage Forms

Capsule:
  Vancocin®: 125 mg, 250 mg
Infusion [premixed in iso-osmotic dextrose]:
  Vancocin®: 500 mg (100 mL); 1 g (200 mL)
Injection, powder for reconstitution: 500 mg, 1 g, 5 g, 10 g

vancomycin hydrochloride *see vancomycin on page 969*

Vandazole™ [US] *see metronidazole on page 627*

Vanex Forte™-D (*Discontinued*) *see chlorpheniramine, phenylephrine, and methscopolamine on page 210*

Vanex-HD® (*Discontinued*) *see phenylephrine, hydrocodone, and chlorpheniramine on page 748*

Vaniqa™ [US/Can] *see eflornithine on page 336*

Vanos™ [US] *see fluocinonide on page 410*

Vanoxide® (*Discontinued*) *see benzoyl peroxide on page 126*

Vanoxide-HC® [US/Can] *see benzoyl peroxide and hydrocortisone on page 128*

Vanquish® Extra Strength Pain Reliever [US-OTC] *see acetaminophen, aspirin, and caffeine on page 24*

Vansil™ (*Discontinued*)

Vantin® [US/Can] *see cefpodoxime on page 188*

Vaponefrin® *(Discontinued) see* epinephrine *on page 344*
Vaprisol® [US] *see* conivaptan *on page 247*
VAQTA® [US/Can] *see* hepatitis A vaccine *on page 469*

vardenafil (var DEN a fil)

Sound-Alike/Look-Alike Issues
Levitra® may be confused with Lexiva®
Synonyms vardenafil hydrochloride
U.S./Canadian Brand Names Levitra® [US/Can]
Therapeutic Category Phosphodiesterase (Type 5) Enzyme Inhibitor
Use Treatment of erectile dysfunction (ED)
Usual Dosage Oral: Adults: Erectile dysfunction: 10 mg 60 minutes prior to sexual activity; dosing range:
5-20 mg; to be given as one single dose and not given more than once daily
Dosage Forms
Tablet:
Levitra®: 2.5 mg, 5 mg, 10 mg, 20 mg

vardenafil hydrochloride *see* vardenafil *on page 971*

varenicline (var e NI kleen)

Synonyms varenicline tartrate
U.S./Canadian Brand Names Champix® [Can]; Chantix® [US]
Therapeutic Category Partial Nicotine Agonist
Use Treatment to aid in smoking cessation
Usual Dosage Oral: Adults:
Initial:
Days 1-3: 0.5 mg once daily
Days 4-7: 0.5 mg twice daily
Maintenance (≥ Day 8): 1 mg twice daily
Note: Start 1 week before target quit date. Patients who cannot tolerate adverse events may require
temporary reduction in dose. If patient successfully quits smoking during the 12 weeks, may continue for
another 12 weeks to help maintain success. If not successful in first 12 weeks, then stop medication and
reassess factors contributing to failure.
Dosage Forms
Tablet:
Chantix®: 0.5 mg, 1 mg
Combination package, oral [dose-pack]:
Chantix®:
Tablet, oral: 0.5 mg (11)
Tablet, oral: 1 mg (42)

varenicline tartrate *see* varenicline *on page 971*
Varibar® Honey [US] *see* barium *on page 116*
Varibar® Nectar [US] *see* barium *on page 116*
Varibar® Pudding [US] *see* barium *on page 116*
Varibar® Thin Honey [US] *see* barium *on page 116*
Varibar® Thin Liquid [US] *see* barium *on page 116*
varicella, measles, mumps, and rubella vaccine *see* measles, mumps, rubella, and varicella virus
vaccine *on page 593*

varicella virus vaccine (var i SEL a VYE rus vak SEEN)

Sound-Alike/Look-Alike Issues
varicella virus vaccine has been given in error (instead of the indicated varicella immune globulin) to
pregnant women exposed to varicella
Synonyms chickenpox vaccine; varicella-zoster virus (VZV) vaccine (varicella); VZV vaccine (varicella)
U.S./Canadian Brand Names Varilrix® [Can]; Varivax® III [Can]; Varivax® [US]
Therapeutic Category Vaccine, Live Virus

▶

◀ **Use** Immunization against varicella in children ≥12 months of age and adults
The ACIP recommends vaccination for all children, adolescents, and adults who do not have evidence of immunity. Vaccination is especially important for:
- Persons with close contact to those at high risk for severe disease
- Persons living or working in environments where transmission is likely (teachers, child-care workers, residents and staff of institutional settings)
- Persons in environments where transmission has been reported
- Nonpregnant women of childbearing age
- Adolescents and adults in households with children
- International travelers

Postexposure prophylaxis: Vaccination within 3 days (possibly 5 days) after exposure to rash is effective in preventing illness or modifying severity of disease

Usual Dosage SubQ:
Children 12 months to 12 years: 0.5 mL; a second dose may be administered ≥3 months later
Note: The ACIP recommends the routine childhood vaccination be 2 doses, with the first dose administered at 12-15 months of age. School age children should receive the second dose at 4-6 years of age, but it may be administered earlier provided ≥3 months have elapsed after the first dose. All children and adolescents who received only 1 dose of vaccine should receive a second dose.
Children ≥13 years to Adults: 2 doses of 0.5 mL separated by 4-8 weeks

Dosage Forms [CAN] = Canadian brand name
Injection, powder for reconstitution [preservative free]:
Varivax®: 1350 plaque-forming units (PFU)
Varivax® III [CAN]: 1350 plaque-forming units (PFU) [not available in the U.S.]
Injection, powder for reconstitution:
Valrilix® [CAN]: $10^{3.3}$ plaque-forming units (PFU) [not available in the U.S.]

varicella-zoster immune globulin (human)
(var i SEL a- ZOS ter i MYUN GLOB yoo lin HYU man)

Sound-Alike/Look-Alike Issues
varicella virus vaccine has been given in error (instead of the indicated varicella immune globulin) to pregnant women exposed to varicella.

Synonyms VZIG

U.S./Canadian Brand Names VariZIG™ [Can]

Therapeutic Category Immune Globulin

Use In pregnant women, for the prevention or reduction in severity of maternal infection within 4 days of exposure to the varicella zoster virus.

Usual Dosage I.M., I.V.: Adults: Prevention or reduction of maternal infection: 125 int. units/10 kg (minimum dose: 125 int. units; maximum dose: 625 int. units). Administer within 96 hours of exposure.

Dosage Forms [CAN = Canadian brand name]
Injection, powder for reconstitution [preservative free]:
VariZIG™ [CAN]: 125 int. units [package with diluent] [available in the U.S under expanded access protocol]

varicella-zoster virus (VZV) vaccine (varicella) *see* varicella virus vaccine *on page 971*
varicella-zoster (VZV) vaccine (zoster) *see* zoster vaccine *on page 997*
Varilrix® [Can] *see* varicella virus vaccine *on page 971*
Varivax® [US] *see* varicella virus vaccine *on page 971*
Varivax® III [Can] *see* varicella virus vaccine *on page 971*
VariZIG™ [Can] *see* varicella-zoster immune globulin (human) *on page 972*
Vaseretic® [US/Can] *see* enalapril and hydrochlorothiazide *on page 339*
VasoClear® *(Discontinued)* *see* naphazoline *on page 655*
Vasocon® [Can] *see* naphazoline *on page 655*
Vasocon®-A *(Discontinued)*
Vasocon Regular® Ophthalmic *(Discontinued)* *see* naphazoline *on page 655*
Vasodilan® *(Discontinued)* *see* isoxsuprine *on page 532*

vasopressin (vay soe PRES in)
Synonyms 8-arginine vasopressin; ADH; antidiuretic hormone
U.S./Canadian Brand Names Pressyn® AR [Can]; Pressyn® [Can]

Therapeutic Category Hormone, Posterior Pituitary

Use Treatment of diabetes insipidus; differential diagnosis of diabetes insipidus

Usual Dosage

Diabetes insipidus: **Note:** Highly variable dosage; titrated based on serum and urine sodium and osmolality in addition to fluid balance and urine output; vasopressin rarely used for this indication; other therapies are available.

I.M., SubQ:

Children: 2.5-10 units 2-4 times/day as needed

Adults: 5-10 units 2-3 times/day as needed

Dosage Forms

Injection, solution: 20 units/mL (0.5 mL, 1 mL, 10 mL)

Vasotec® [US/Can] *see* enalapril *on page 339*

Vasotec® I.V. [Can] *see* enalapril *on page 339*

Vasovist® [Can] *see* gadofosveset *(Canada only) on page 433*

Vaxigrip® [Can] *see* influenza virus vaccine *on page 508*

VCF™ [US-OTC] *see* nonoxynol 9 *on page 677*

Vectibix™ [US] *see* panitumumab *on page 719*

Vectrin® *(Discontinued)* *see* minocycline *on page 635*

vecuronium (vek ue ROE nee um)

Sound-Alike/Look-Alike Issues

vecuronium may be confused with vancomycin

Norcuron® may be confused with Narcan®

Synonyms ORG NC 45

U.S./Canadian Brand Names Norcuron® [Can]

Therapeutic Category Skeletal Muscle Relaxant

Use Adjunct to general anesthesia to facilitate endotracheal intubation and to relax skeletal muscles during surgery; to facilitate mechanical ventilation in ICU patients; does not relieve pain or produce sedation

Usual Dosage Administer I.V.; dose to effect; doses will vary due to interpatient variability; use ideal body weight for obese patients

Surgery:

Neonates: 0.1 mg/kg/dose; maintenance: 0.03-0.15 mg/kg every 1-2 hours as needed

Infants >7 weeks to 1 year: Initial: 0.08-0.1 mg/kg/dose; maintenance: 0.05-0.1 mg/kg every 60 minutes as needed

Children >1 year and Adults: Initial: 0.08-0.1 mg/kg or 0.04-0.06 mg/kg after initial dose of succinylcholine for intubation; maintenance: 0.01-0.015 mg/kg 25-40 minutes after initial dose, then 0.01-0.015 mg/kg every 12-15 minutes (higher doses will allow less frequent maintenance doses); may be administered as a continuous infusion at 0.8-2 mcg/kg/minute

Pretreatment/priming: Adults: 10% of intubating dose given 3-5 minutes before initial dose

ICU: Adults: 0.05-0.1 mg/kg bolus followed by 0.8-1.7 mcg/kg/minute once initial recovery from bolus observed or 0.1-0.2 mg/kg/dose every 1 hour

Note: Children (1-10 years) may require slightly higher initial doses and slightly more frequent supplementation; infants >7 weeks to 1 year may be more sensitive to vecuronium and have a longer recovery time

Dosage Forms

Injection, powder for reconstitution: 10 mg, 20 mg

Veg-Pancreatin 4X [US-OTC] *see* pancreatin *on page 717*

Velban® *(Discontinued)* *see* vinblastine *on page 977*

Velcade® [US/Can] *see* bortezomib *on page 139*

Velivet™ [US] *see* ethinyl estradiol and desogestrel *on page 369*

Velosulin® BR (Buffered) *(Discontinued)*

venlafaxine (ven la FAX een)

U.S./Canadian Brand Names Co-Venlafaxine XR [Can]; Effexor XR® [US/Can]; Effexor® [US]; Novo-Venlafaxine XR [Can]; PMS-Venlafaxine XR [Can]; ratio-Venlafaxine XR [Can]

▶

◀ **Therapeutic Category** Antidepressant, Phenethylamine

Use Treatment of major depressive disorder, generalized anxiety disorder (GAD), social anxiety disorder (social phobia), panic disorder

Usual Dosage Oral: Adults:

Depression:

Immediate release tablets: 75 mg/day, administered in 2 or 3 divided doses, taken with food; dose may be increased in 75 mg/day increments at intervals of at least 4 days, up to 225-375 mg/day

Extended release capsules: 75 mg once daily taken with food; for some new patients, it may be desirable to start at 37.5 mg/day for 4-7 days before increasing to 75 mg once daily; dose may be increased by up to 75 mg/day increments every 4 days as tolerated, up to a recommended maximum of 225 mg/day

Generalized anxiety disorder, social anxiety disorder: Extended release capsules: 75 mg once daily taken with food; for some new patients, it may be desirable to start at 37.5 mg/day for 4-7 days before increasing to 75 mg once daily; dose may be increased by up to 75 mg/day increments every 4 days as tolerated, up to a maximum of 225 mg/day

Panic disorder: Extended release capsules: 37.5 mg once daily for 1 week; may increase to 75 mg daily, with subsequent weekly increases of 75 mg/day up to a maximum of 225 mg/day.

Note: When discontinuing this medication after more than 1 week of treatment, it is generally recommended that the dose be tapered. If venlafaxine is used for 6 weeks or longer, the dose should be tapered over 2 weeks when discontinuing its use.

Dosage Forms

Capsule, extended release:

Effexor XR®: 37.5 mg, 75 mg, 150 mg

Tablet: 25 mg, 37.5 mg, 50 mg, 75 mg, 100 mg

Effexor®: 25 mg, 37.5 mg, 50 mg, 75 mg, 100 mg

Venofer® [US/Can] *see* iron sucrose *on page 527*

Venoglobulin®-I *(Discontinued) see* immune globulin (intravenous) *on page 503*

Venoglobulin®-S *(Discontinued) see* immune globulin (intravenous) *on page 503*

Ventavis® [US] *see* iloprost *on page 499*

Ventolin® [Can] *see* albuterol *on page 39*

Ventolin® *(Discontinued) see* albuterol *on page 39*

Ventolin® Diskus [Can] *see* albuterol *on page 39*

Ventolin® HFA [US/Can] *see* albuterol *on page 39*

Ventolin® Inhaler Aerosol *(Discontinued) see* albuterol *on page 39*

Ventolin® I.V. Infusion [Can] *see* albuterol *on page 39*

Ventrodisk [Can] *see* albuterol *on page 39*

VePesid® [Can] *see* etoposide *on page 384*

VePesid® *(Discontinued) see* etoposide *on page 384*

Veracolate [US-OTC] *see* bisacodyl *on page 136*

verapamil (ver AP a mil)

Sound-Alike/Look-Alike Issues

verapamil may be confused with Verelan®

Calan® may be confused with Colace®

Covera-HS® may be confused with Provera®

Isoptin® may be confused with Isopto® Tears

Verelan® may be confused with verapamil, Virilon®, Voltaren®

Synonyms iproveratril hydrochloride; verapamil hydrochloride

U.S./Canadian Brand Names Apo-Verap® SR [Can]; Apo-Verap® [Can]; Calan® SR [US]; Calan® [US/Can]; Chronovera® [Can]; Covera-HS® [US/Can]; Covera® [Can]; Dom-Verapamil SR [Can]; Gen-Verapamil SR [Can]; Gen-Verapamil [Can]; Isoptin® SR [US/Can]; Med-Verapamil [Can]; Novo-Veramil SR [Can]; Nu-Verap [Can]; PHL-Verapamil [Can]; PMS-Verapamil SR [Can]; Riva-Verapamil SR [Can]; Verapamil Hydrochloride Injection, USP [Can]; Verelan SRC [Can]; Verelan® PM [US]; Verelan® [US]

Therapeutic Category Antiarrhythmic Agent, Class IV; Calcium Channel Blocker

Use Orally for treatment of angina pectoris (vasospastic, chronic stable, unstable) and hypertension; I.V. for supraventricular tachyarrhythmias (PSVT, atrial fibrillation, atrial flutter)

Usual Dosage

Children: SVT: I.V.:

<1 year: 0.1-0.2 mg/kg over 2 minutes; repeat every 30 minutes as needed

1-15 years: 0.1-0.3 mg/kg over 2 minutes; maximum: 5 mg/dose, may repeat dose in 15 minutes if adequate response not achieved; maximum for second dose: 10 mg/dose

Adults:

SVT: I.V.: 2.5-5 mg (over 2 minutes); second dose of 5-10 mg (~0.15 mg/kg) may be given 15-30 minutes after the initial dose if patient tolerates, but does not respond to initial dose; maximum total dose: 20 mg

Angina: Oral: Initial dose: 80-120 mg 3 times/day (elderly or small stature: 40 mg 3 times/day); range: 240-480 mg/day in 3-4 divided doses

Hypertension: Oral:

Immediate release: 80 mg 3 times/day; usual dose range (JNC 7): 80-320 mg/day in 2 divided doses

Sustained release: 240 mg/day; usual dose range (JNC 7): 120-360 mg/day in 1-2 divided doses; 120 mg/day in the elderly or small patients (no evidence of additional benefit in doses >360 mg/day).

Extended release:

Covera-HS®: Usual dose range (JNC 7): 120-360 mg once daily (once-daily dosing is recommended at bedtime)

Verelan® PM: Usual dose range: 200-400 mg once daily at bedtime

Dosage Forms

Caplet, sustained release: 120 mg, 180 mg, 240 mg

Calan® SR: 120 mg, 180 mg, 240 mg

Capsule, extended release: 120 mg, 180 mg, 240 mg

Capsule, extended release, controlled onset: 100 mg, 200 mg, 300 mg

Verelan® PM: 100 mg, 200 mg, 300 mg

Capsule, sustained release: 120 mg, 180 mg, 240 mg, 360 mg

Verelan®: 120 mg, 180 mg, 240 mg, 360 mg

Injection, solution: 2.5 mg/mL (2 mL, 4 mL)

Tablet: 40 mg, 80 mg, 120 mg

Calan®: 40 mg, 80 mg, 120 mg

Tablet, extended release: 120 mg, 180 mg, 240 mg

Tablet, extended release, controlled onset:

Covera-HS®: 180 mg, 240 mg

Tablet, sustained release: 120 mg, 180 mg, 240 mg

Isoptin® SR: 120 mg, 180 mg, 240 mg

verapamil and trandolapril *see* trandolapril and verapamil *on page 942*

verapamil hydrochloride *see* verapamil *on page 974*

Verapamil Hydrochloride Injection, USP [Can] *see* verapamil *on page 974*

Verazinc® Oral *(Discontinued)* *see* zinc sulfate *on page 994*

Verdeso™ [US] *see* desonide *on page 276*

Veregen™ [US] *see* sinecatechins *on page 868*

Verelan® [US] *see* verapamil *on page 974*

Verelan® PM [US] *see* verapamil *on page 974*

Verelan SRC [Can] *see* verapamil *on page 974*

Vergogel® Gel *(Discontinued)* *see* salicylic acid *on page 850*

Vergon® *(Discontinued)* *see* meclizine *on page 595*

Vermox® [Can] *see* mebendazole *on page 594*

Vermox® *(Discontinued)* *see* mebendazole *on page 594*

Versed® *(Discontinued)* *see* midazolam *on page 632*

Versel® [Can] *see* selenium sulfide *on page 861*

Versiclear™ [US] *see* sodium thiosulfate *on page 880*

verteporfin (ver te POR fin)

U.S./Canadian Brand Names Visudyne® [US/Can]

Therapeutic Category Ophthalmic Agent

Use Treatment of predominantly classic subfoveal choroidal neovascularization due to macular degeneration, presumed ocular histoplasmosis, or pathologic myopia

Usual Dosage Therapy is a two-step process; first the infusion of verteporfin, then the activation of verteporfin with a nonthermal diode laser.

Adults: I.V.: 6 mg/m^2 body surface area

Note: Treatment in more than one eye: Patients who have lesions in both eyes should be evaluated and treatment should first be done to the more aggressive lesion. Following safe and acceptable treatment, the second eye can be treated one week later. Patients who have had previous verteporfin therapy, with an acceptable safety profile, may then have both eyes treated concurrently. Treat the more aggressive lesion followed immediately with the second eye. The light treatment to the second eye should begin no later than 20 minutes from the start of the infusion.

Dosage Forms

Injection, powder for reconstitution:

Visudyne®: 15 mg

Verukan® Solution (Discontinued) see salicylic acid on page 850

Vesanoid® [US/Can] see tretinoin (oral) on page 946

VESIcare® [US] see solifenacin on page 881

Vexol® [US/Can] see rimexolone on page 836

VFEND® [US/Can] see voriconazole on page 984

Viactiv® flavor glides [US-OTC] see vitamins (multiple/oral) on page 983

Viactiv® Multivitamin [US-OTC] see vitamins (multiple/oral) on page 983

Viadur® [Can] see leuprolide on page 553

Viadur® (Discontinued) see leuprolide on page 553

Viagra® [US/Can] see sildenafil on page 865

Vibramycin® [US] see doxycycline on page 323

Vibramycin® I.V. (Discontinued) see doxycycline on page 323

Vibra-Tabs® [US/Can] see doxycycline on page 323

***Vibrio cholera* and enterotoxigenic *Escherichia coli* vaccine** see traveler's diarrhea and cholera vaccine (Canada only) on page 944

Vicks® 44® Cough Relief [US-OTC] see dextromethorphan on page 284

Vicks® 44D Cough & Head Congestion (Discontinued) see pseudoephedrine and dextromethorphan on page 802

Vicks® 44E [US-OTC] see guaifenesin and dextromethorphan on page 454

Vicks® 44® Non-Drowsy Cold & Cough Liqui-Caps (Discontinued) see pseudoephedrine and dextromethorphan on page 802

Vicks® Casero™ Chest Congestion Relief [US-OTC] see guaifenesin on page 453

Vicks® Children's Chloraseptic® (Discontinued) see benzocaine on page 124

Vicks® Children's NyQuil® (Discontinued) see chlorpheniramine, pseudoephedrine, and dextromethorphan on page 212

Vicks® Chloraseptic® Sore Throat (Discontinued) see benzocaine on page 124

Vicks® DayQuil® Cold/Flu Multi-Symptom Relief [US-OTC] see acetaminophen, dextromethorphan, and phenylephrine on page 26

Vicks® DayQuil® Multi-Symptom Cold and Flu (Discontinued) see acetaminophen, dextromethorphan, and pseudoephedrine on page 27

Vicks® DayQuil® Sinus Pressure & Congestion Relief (Discontinued)

Vicks® Early Defense™ [US-OTC] see oxymetazoline on page 712

Vicks® Formula 44® (Discontinued) see dextromethorphan on page 284

Vicks® Formula 44® Pediatric Formula (Discontinued) see dextromethorphan on page 284

Vicks® Formula 44® Sore Throat [US-OTC] see phenol on page 743

Vicks® Pediatric 44®m (Discontinued) see chlorpheniramine, pseudoephedrine, and dextromethorphan on page 212

Vicks® Pediatric Formula 44E [US-OTC] see guaifenesin and dextromethorphan on page 454

Vicks® Sinex® 12 Hour [US-OTC] see oxymetazoline on page 712

Vicks® Sinex® 12 Hour Ultrafine Mist [US-OTC] see oxymetazoline on page 712

Vicks® Sinex® Nasal Spray [US-OTC] see phenylephrine on page 745

Vicks® Sinex® UltraFine Mist [US-OTC] see phenylephrine on page 745

Vicks® Vitamin C [US-OTC] see ascorbic acid on page 96

Vicodin® [US] see hydrocodone and acetaminophen on page 481

Vicodin® ES [US] *see* hydrocodone and acetaminophen *on page 481*
Vicodin® HP [US] *see* hydrocodone and acetaminophen *on page 481*
Vicoprofen® [US/Can] *see* hydrocodone and ibuprofen *on page 483*
Vi-Daylin® ADC *(Discontinued) see* vitamins (multiple/pediatric) *on page 983*
Vi-Daylin® ADC + Iron *(Discontinued) see* vitamins (multiple/pediatric) *on page 983*
Vi-Daylin® Drops *(Discontinued) see* vitamins (multiple/pediatric) *on page 983*
Vi-Daylin®/F ADC *(Discontinued) see* vitamins (multiple/pediatric) *on page 983*
Vi-Daylin®/F ADC + Iron *(Discontinued) see* vitamins (multiple/pediatric) *on page 983*
Vi-Daylin®/F *(Discontinued) see* vitamins (multiple/pediatric) *on page 983*
Vi-Daylin®/F + Iron *(Discontinued) see* vitamins (multiple/pediatric) *on page 983*
Vi-Daylin® + Iron Drops *(Discontinued) see* vitamins (multiple/pediatric) *on page 983*
Vi-Daylin® + Iron Liquid *(Discontinued) see* vitamins (multiple/oral) *on page 983*
Vi-Daylin® Liquid *(Discontinued) see* vitamins (multiple/oral) *on page 983*
Vidaza® [US] *see* azacitidine *on page 108*
Videx® [US/Can] *see* didanosine *on page 294*
Videx® EC [US/Can] *see* didanosine *on page 294*

vigabatrin *(Canada only)* (vye GA ba trin)

U.S./Canadian Brand Names Sabril® [Can]
Therapeutic Category Anticonvulsant
Use Active management of partial or secondary generalized seizures not controlled by usual treatments; treatment of infantile spasms
Usual Dosage Oral:
  Children: **Note:** Administer daily dose in 2 divided doses, especially in the higher dosage ranges:
    Adjunctive treatment of seizures: Initial: 40 mg/kg/day; maintenance dosages based on patient weight:
      10-15 kg: 0.5-1 g/day
      16-30 kg: 1-1.5 g/day
      31-50 kg: 1.5-3 g/day
      >50 kg: 2-3 g/day
    Infantile spasms: 50-100 mg/kg/day, depending on severity of symptoms; higher doses (up to 150 mg/kg/day) have been used in some cases.
  Adults: Adjunctive treatment of seizures: Initial: 1 g/day (severe manifestations may require 2 g/day); dose may be given as a single daily dose or divided into 2 equal doses. Increase daily dose by 0.5 g based on response and tolerability. Optimal dose range: 2-3 g/day (maximum dose: 3 g/day)
Dosage Forms [CAN] = Canadian brand name
  Powder for oral suspension [sachets]:
    Sabril® [CAN]: 0.5 g [not available in the U.S.]
  Tablet:
    Sabril® [CAN]: 500 mg [not available in the U.S.]

Vigamox™ [US/Can] *see* moxifloxacin *on page 646*
VIGIV *see* vaccinia immune globulin (intravenous) *on page 966*

vinblastine (vin BLAS teen)

Sound-Alike/Look-Alike Issues
  vinBLAStine may be confused with vinCRIStine, vinorelbine
Synonyms NSC-49842; vinblastine sulfate; VLB
Tall-Man vin**BLAS**tine
Therapeutic Category Antineoplastic Agent
Use Treatment of Hodgkin and non-Hodgkin lymphoma, testicular, lung, head and neck, breast, and renal carcinomas, Mycosis fungoides, Kaposi sarcoma, histiocytosis, choriocarcinoma, and idiopathic thrombocytopenic purpura
Usual Dosage I.V. (refer to individual protocols): Children and Adults: 4-20 mg/m^2 (0.1-0.5 mg/kg) every 7-10 days **or** 5-day continuous infusion of 1.5-2 mg/m^2/day **or** 0.1-0.5 mg/kg/week
Dosage Forms
  Injection, powder for reconstitution: 10 mg
  Injection, solution: 1 mg/mL (10 mL)

vinblastine sulfate *see* vinblastine *on page 977*
Vincasar PFS® [US/Can] *see* vincristine *on page 978*

vincristine (vin KRIS teen)

Sound-Alike/Look-Alike Issues
vinCRIStine may be confused with vinBLAStine
Oncovin® may be confused with Ancobon®
Synonyms leurocristine sulfate; NSC-67574; vincristine sulfate
Tall-Man vinCRIStine
U.S./Canadian Brand Names Vincasar PFS® [US/Can]
Therapeutic Category Antineoplastic Agent
Use Treatment of leukemias, Hodgkin disease, non-Hodgkin lymphomas, Wilms tumor, neuroblastoma, rhabdomyosarcoma
Usual Dosage Note: Doses are often capped at 2 mg; however, this may reduce the efficacy of the therapy and may not be advisable. Refer to individual protocols; orders for single doses >2.5 mg or >5 mg/treatment cycle should be verified with the specific treatment regimen and/or an experienced oncologist prior to dispensing. I.V.:

Children ≤10 kg or BSA <1 m^2: Initial therapy: 0.05 mg/kg once weekly then titrate dose
Children >10 kg or BSA ≥1 m^2: 1-2 mg/m^2, may repeat once weekly for 3-6 weeks; maximum single dose: 2 mg
Neuroblastoma: I.V. continuous infusion with doxorubicin: 1 mg/m^2/day for 72 hours
Adults: 0.4-1.4 mg/m^2, may repeat every week **or**
0.4-0.5 mg/day continuous infusion for 4 days every 4 weeks **or**
0.25-0.5 mg/m^2/day for 5 days every 4 weeks
Dosage Forms
Injection, solution [preservative free]:
Vincasar PFS®: 1 mg/mL (1 mL, 2 mL)

vincristine sulfate *see* vincristine *on page 978*

vinorelbine (vi NOR el been)

Sound-Alike/Look-Alike Issues
vinorelbine may be confused with vinBLAStine
Synonyms dihydroxydeoxynorvinkaleukoblastine; vinorelbine tartrate
U.S./Canadian Brand Names Navelbine® [US/Can]; Vinorelbine Injection, USP [Can]; Vinorelbine Tartrate for Injection [Can]
Therapeutic Category Antineoplastic Agent
Use Treatment of nonsmall-cell lung cancer (NSCLC)
Usual Dosage Details concerning dosing in combination regimens should also be consulted.
I.V.: Adults: NSCLC:
Single-agent therapy: 30 mg/m^2/dose every 7 days
Combination therapy with cisplatin: 25-30 mg/m^2/dose every 7 days (in combination with cisplatin)
Dosage Forms
Injection, solution [preservative free]: 10 mg/mL (1 mL, 5 mL)
Navelbine®: 10 mg/mL (1 mL, 5 mL)

Vinorelbine Injection, USP [Can] *see* vinorelbine *on page 978*
vinorelbine tartrate *see* vinorelbine *on page 978*
Vinorelbine Tartrate for Injection [Can] *see* vinorelbine *on page 978*
Viokase® [US/Can] *see* pancrelipase *on page 718*
viosterol *see* ergocalciferol *on page 350*
Vioxx® *(Discontinued)*
Viracept® [US/Can] *see* nelfinavir *on page 661*
Viramune® [US/Can] *see* nevirapine *on page 666*
Viravan® *(Discontinued)* *see* phenylephrine and pyrilamine *on page 747*
Viravan®-DM [US] *see* phenylephrine, pyrilamine, and dextromethorphan *on page 749*
Virazole® [US/Can] *see* ribavirin *on page 831*
Viread® [US/Can] *see* tenofovir *on page 909*

Virilon® [US] *see* methyltestosterone *on page 624*
Virilon® IM [Can] *see* testosterone *on page 912*
Viroptic® [US/Can] *see* trifluridine *on page 952*
Viscoat® [US] *see* sodium chondroitin sulfate and sodium hyaluronate *on page 875*
Visicol® [US] *see* sodium phosphates *on page 878*
Visine-A® [US-OTC] *see* naphazoline and pheniramine *on page 656*
Visine® Advanced Allergy [Can] *see* naphazoline and pheniramine *on page 656*
Visine® Advanced Relief [US-OTC] *see* tetrahydrozoline *on page 916*
Visine® L.R. [US-OTC] *see* oxymetazoline *on page 712*
Visine® Original [US-OTC] *see* tetrahydrozoline *on page 916*
Visipaque™ [US] *see* iodixanol *on page 519*
Visken® [Can] *see* pindolol *on page 754*
Visken® (Discontinued) *see* pindolol *on page 754*
Vistacon-50® Injection (Discontinued) *see* hydroxyzine *on page 491*
Vistaquel® Injection (Discontinued) *see* hydroxyzine *on page 491*
Vistaril® [US/Can] *see* hydroxyzine *on page 491*
Vistazine® Injection (Discontinued) *see* hydroxyzine *on page 491*
Vistide® [US] *see* cidofovir *on page 218*
Visudyne® [US/Can] *see* verteporfin *on page 975*
Vita-C® [US-OTC] *see* ascorbic acid *on page 96*
Vitaball® [US-OTC] *see* vitamins (multiple/pediatric) *on page 983*
Vitaball® Minis [US-OTC] *see* vitamins (multiple/pediatric) *on page 983*
Vitaball® Wild 'N Fruity [US-OTC] *see* vitamins (multiple/pediatric) *on page 983*
VitaCarn® Oral (Discontinued) *see* levocarnitine *on page 555*
Vitacon Forte [US] *see* vitamins (multiple/oral) *on page 983*
Vitafol [US] *see* vitamin B complex combinations *on page 981*
Vital HN® [US-OTC] *see* nutritional formula, enteral/oral *on page 689*
vitamin C *see* ascorbic acid *on page 96*
vitamin D$_2$ *see* ergocalciferol *on page 350*
vitamin D$_3$ and alendronate *see* alendronate and cholecalciferol *on page 43*
vitamin D and calcium carbonate *see* calcium and vitamin D *on page 162*

vitamin A (VYE ta min aye)

Sound-Alike/Look-Alike Issues
Aquasol® may be confused with Anusol®
Synonyms oleovitamin A
U.S./Canadian Brand Names Aquasol A® [US]; Palmitate-A® [US-OTC]
Therapeutic Category Vitamin, Fat Soluble
Use Treatment and prevention of vitamin A deficiency; parenteral (I.M.) route is indicated when oral administration is not feasible or when absorption is insufficient (malabsorption syndrome)
Usual Dosage
RDA:
  <1 year: 375 mcg
  1-3 years: 400 mcg
  4-6 years: 500 mcg*
  7-10 years: 700 mcg*
  >10 years: 800-1000 mcg*
  Male: 1000 mcg
  Female: 800 mcg
  * mcg retinol equivalent (0.3 mcg retinol = 1 unit vitamin A)
Vitamin A supplementation in measles (recommendation of the World Health Organization): Children: Oral: Administer as a single dose; repeat the next day and at 4 weeks for children with ophthalmologic evidence of vitamin A deficiency:
  6 months to 1 year: 100,000 units
  >1 year: 200,000 units

◀ **Note:** Use of vitamin A in measles is recommended only for patients 6 months to 2 years of age hospitalized with measles and its complications **or** patients >6 months of age who have any of the following risk factors and who are not already receiving vitamin A: immunodeficiency, ophthalmologic evidence of vitamin A deficiency including night blindness, Bitot spots or evidence of xerophthalmia, impaired intestinal absorption, moderate-to-severe malnutrition including that associated with eating disorders, or recent immigration from areas where high mortality rates from measles have been observed

Note: Monitor patients closely; dosages >25,000 units/kg have been associated with toxicity

Severe deficiency with xerophthalmia: Oral:
  Children 1-8 years: 5000-10,000 units/kg/day for 5 days or until recovery occurs
  Children >8 years and Adults: 500,000 units/day for 3 days, then 50,000 units/day for 14 days, then 10,000-20,000 units/day for 2 months

Deficiency (without corneal changes): Oral:
  Infants <1 year: 100,000 units every 4-6 months
  Children 1-8 years: 200,000 units every 4-6 months
  Children >8 years and Adults: 100,000 units/day for 3 days then 50,000 units/day for 14 days

Deficiency: I.M.: **Note:** I.M. route is indicated when oral administration is not feasible or when absorption is insufficient (malabsorption syndrome):
  Infants: 7500-15,000 units/day for 10 days
  Children 1-8 years: 17,500-35,000 units/day for 10 days
  Children >8 years and Adults: 100,000 units/day for 3 days, followed by 50,000 units/day for 2 weeks
  Note: Follow-up therapy with an oral therapeutic multivitamin (containing additional vitamin A) is recommended:
    Low Birth Weight Infants: Additional vitamin A is recommended, however, no dosage amount has been established
    Children ≤8 years: 5000-10,000 units/day
    Children >8 years and Adults: 10,000-20,000 units/day

Malabsorption syndrome (prophylaxis): Children >8 years and Adults: Oral: 10,000-50,000 units/day of water miscible product

Dietary supplement: Oral:
  Infants up to 6 months: 1500 units/day
  Children:
    6 months to 3 years: 1500-2000 units/day
    4-6 years: 2500 units/day
    7-10 years: 3300-3500 units/day
  Children >10 years and Adults: 4000-5000 units/day

Dosage Forms
Capsule [softgel]: 10,000 units; 25,000 units
Injection, solution:
  Aquasol A®: 50,000 units/mL (2 mL)
Tablet:
  Palmitate-A® [OTC]: 5000 units, 15,000 units

vitamin A acid *see* tretinoin (topical) *on page 946*

vitamin A and vitamin D (VYE ta min aye & VYE ta min dee)

Synonyms cod liver oil
U.S./Canadian Brand Names A and D® Original [US-OTC]; Baza® Clear [US-OTC]; Sween Cream® [US-OTC]
Therapeutic Category Protectant, Topical
Use Temporary relief of discomfort due to chapped skin, diaper rash, minor burns, abrasions, as well as irritations associated with ostomy skin care
Usual Dosage Topical: Apply locally with gentle massage as needed
Dosage Forms
Capsule, softgel: Vitamin A 1250 int. units and vitamin D 135 int. units; vitamin A 1250 int. units and vitamin D 130 int. units; vitamin A 5,000 int. units and vitamin D 400 int. units; vitamin A 10,000 int. units and vitamin D 400 int. units; vitamin A 10,000 int. units and vitamin D 5000 int. units; vitamin A 25,000 int. units and vitamin D 1000 int. units
Cream:
  Sween Cream® [OTC]: 2 g, 57 g, 85 g, 142 g, 184 g, 339 g

Ointment: 0.9 g, 5 g, 60 g, 120 g, 454 g
A and D® Original [OTC]: 45 g, 120 g, 454 g
Baza® Clear [OTC]: 50 g, 150 g, 240 g
Tablet: Vitamin A 10,000 int. units and vitamin D 400 int. units

vitamin B₁ *see* thiamine *on page 920*
vitamin B₂ *see* riboflavin *on page 832*
vitamin B₃ *see* niacin *on page 667*
vitamin B₃ *see* niacinamide *on page 668*
vitamin B₅ *see* pantothenic acid *on page 721*
vitamin B₆ *see* pyridoxine *on page 808*
vitamin B₁₂ *see* cyanocobalamin *on page 254*

vitamin B complex combinations (VYE ta min bee KOM pleks kom bi NAY shuns)

Sound-Alike/Look-Alike Issues
Nephrocaps® may be confused with Nephro-Calci®
Renal Caps may be confused with Renagel®, Renvela®
Surbex® may be confused with Sebex®, Suprax®, Surfak®
Synonyms B complex combinations; B vitamin combinations
U.S./Canadian Brand Names Allbee® C-800 + Iron [US-OTC]; Allbee® C-800 [US-OTC]; Allbee® with C [US-OTC]; Apatate® [US-OTC]; DexFol™ [US]; Gevrabon® [US-OTC]; Kobee [US-OTC]; Metanx™ [US]; NephPlex® Rx [US]; Nephro-Vite® Rx [US]; Nephro-Vite® [US-OTC]; Nephrocaps® [US]; Nephron FA® [US]; Nephronex® [US]; Quin B Strong with C and Zinc [US-OTC]; Quin B Strong [US-OTC]; Rena-Vite RX [US]; Rena-Vite [US-OTC]; Renal Caps [US]; Senilezol [US]; Stresstabs® High Potency Advanced [US-OTC]; Stresstabs® High Potency Energy [US-OTC]; Stresstabs® High Potency Weight [US-OTC]; Super Dec B 100 [US-OTC]; Super Quints 50 [US-OTC]; Superplex-T™ [US-OTC]; Surbex-T® [US-OTC]; Vitafol [US]; Z-Bec® [US-OTC]
Therapeutic Category Vitamin, Water Soluble
Use Supplement for use in the wasting syndrome in chronic renal failure, uremia, impaired metabolic functions of the kidney, dialysis; labeled for OTC use as a dietary supplement
Usual Dosage Oral: Adults:
Dietary supplement: One tablet daily
Apatate® liquid: One teaspoonful daily, 1 hour prior to mid-day meal
Gevrabon® liquid: Two tablespoonsful (30 mL) once daily; shake well before use
Renal patients: One tablet or capsule daily between meals; take after treatment if on dialysis
Nephron FA®: Two tablets once daily, between meals
Dosage Forms Content varies depending on product used. For more detailed information on ingredients in these and other multivitamins, please refer to package labeling.

Vitamin D3 [US-OTC] *see* cholecalciferol *on page 215*

vitamin E (VYE ta min ee)

Sound-Alike/Look-Alike Issues
Aquasol E® may be confused with Anusol®
Synonyms d-alpha tocopherol; dl-alpha tocopherol
U.S./Canadian Brand Names Alph-E [US-OTC]; Alph-E-Mixed [US-OTC]; Aquasol E® [US-OTC]; Aquavit-E® [US-OTC]; d-Alpha-Gems™ [US-OTC]; E-Gems Elite® [US-OTC]; E-Gems Plus® [US-OTC]; E-Gems® [US-OTC]; Ester-E™ [US-OTC]; Gamma E-Gems® [US-OTC]; Gamma-E Plus® [US-OTC]; High Gamma Vitamin E Complete™ [US-OTC]; Key-E® Kaps [US-OTC]; Key-E® [US-OTC]
Therapeutic Category Vitamin, Fat Soluble; Vitamin, Topical
Use Dietary supplement
Usual Dosage Vitamin E may be expressed as alpha-tocopherol equivalents (ATE), which refer to the biologically active (R) stereoisomer content. Oral:
Recommended daily allowance (RDA):
Infants (adequate intake; RDA not establshed):
≤6 months: 4 mg
7-12 months: 6 mg
Children:
1-3 years: 6 mg; upper limit of intake should not exceed 200 mg/day
4-8 years: 7 mg; upper limit of intake should not exceed 300 mg/day
9-13 years: 11 mg; upper limit of intake should not exceed 600 mg/day

◀ 14-18 years: 15 mg; upper limit of intake should not exceed 800 mg/day
Adults: 15 mg; upper limit of intake should not exceed 1000 mg/day
Pregnant female:
≤18 years: 15 mg; upper level of intake should not exceed 800 mg/day
19-50 years: 15 mg; upper level of intake should not exceed 1000 mg/day
Lactating female:
≤18 years: 19 mg; upper level of intake should not exceed 800 mg/day
19-50 years: 19 mg; upper level of intake should not exceed 1000 mg/day
Vitamin E deficiency:
Children (with malabsorption syndrome): 1 unit/kg/day of water miscible vitamin E (to raise plasma tocopherol concentrations to the normal range within 2 months and to maintain normal plasma concentrations)
Adults: 60-75 units/day
Prevention of vitamin E deficiency: Adults: 30 units/day
Cystic fibrosis, beta-thalassemia, sickle cell anemia may require higher daily maintenance doses:
Children:
Cystic fibrosis: 100-400 units/day
Beta-thalassemia: 750 units/day
Adults: Sickle cell: 450 units/day

Dosage Forms
Capsule: 400 int. units, 1000 int. units
Key-E® Kaps [OTC]: 200 int. units, 400 int. units
Capsule, softgel: 200 int. units, 400 int. units, 600 int. units, 1000 int. units
Alph-E [OTC], Aqua Gem E® [OTC]: 200 int. units, 400 int. units
Alph-E-Mixed [OTC]: 200 int. units, 400 int. units, 1000 int. units
d-Alpha-Gems™ [OTC], E-Gems Elite® [OTC], Ester-E™ [OTC]: 400 int. units
E-Gems® [OTC]: 30 int. units, 100 int. units, 200 int. units, 400 int. units, 600 int. units, 800 int. units, 1000 int. units, 1200 int. units
E-Gems Plus® [OTC]: 200 int. units, 400 int. units, 800 int. units
Gamma E-Gems® [OTC]: 90 int. units
Gamma-E Plus [OTC], High Gamma Vitamin E Complete™ [OTC]: 200 int. units
Cream: 50 int. units/g (60 g), 100 int. units/g (60 g), 1000 int. units/120 g (120 g), 30,000 int. units/57 g (57g)
Key-E® [OTC]: 30 int. units/g (60 g, 120 g, 600 g)
Lip balm:
E-Gem® Lip Care: 1000 int. units/tube
Oil, oral/topical: 100 int. units/0.25 mL, 1150 units/0.25 mL, 28,000 int. units/30 mL
Alph-E [OTC]: 28,000 int. units/30 mL
E-Gems® [OTC]: 100 units/10 drops
Ointment, topical:
Key-E® [OTC]: 30 units/g (60 g, 120 g, 480 g)
Powder:
Key-E® [OTC]: 700 int. units per 1/4 teaspoon
Solution, oral drops: 15 int. units/0.3 mL
Aquasol E® [OTC], Aquavit-E [OTC]: 15 int. units/0.3 mL
Suppository, rectal/vaginal:
Key-E® [OTC]: 30 int. units (12s, 24s)
Tablet: 100 int. units, 200 int. units, 400 int. units, 500 int. units
Key-E® [OTC]: 200 int. units, 400 int. units

vitamin G *see* riboflavin *on page 832*
vitamin K₁ *see* phytonadione *on page 752*

vitamins (multiple/injectable) (VYE ta mins, MUL ti pul/in JEK ti bal)

U.S./Canadian Brand Names Infuvite® Adult [US]; Infuvite® Pediatric [US]; M.V.I. Adult™ [US]; M.V.I.®-12 [US]; M.V.I® Pediatric [US]
Therapeutic Category Vitamin
Use Nutritional supplement in patients receiving parenteral nutrition or requiring intravenous administration
Usual Dosage I.V.: Not for direct infusion
Children: ≥3 kg to 11 years: Pediatric formulation: 5 mL/day added to TPN or ≥100 mL of appropriate solution

Children >11 years and Adults: Adult formulation: 10 mL/day added to TPN or ≥500 mL of appropriate solution

Dosage Forms Content varies depending on product used. For more detailed information on ingredients in these and other multivitamins, please refer to package labeling.

vitamins (multiple/oral) (VYE ta mins, MUL ti pul/OR al)

Sound-Alike/Look-Alike Issues

Theragran® may be confused with Phenergan®

Synonyms multiple vitamins; therapeutic multivitamins; vitamins, multiple (oral); vitamins, multiple (therapeutic); vitamins, multiple with iron

U.S./Canadian Brand Names Androvite® [US-OTC]; Centamin [US-OTC]; Centrum® Performance™ [US-OTC]; Centrum® Silver® [US-OTC]; Centrum® [US-OTC]; Diatx®Zn [US]; Drinkables® Multi-Vitamins [US-OTC]; Encora™ [US]; Freedavite [US-OTC]; Geri-Freeda [US-OTC]; Geriation [US-OTC]; Geritol Complete® [US-OTC]; Geritol Extend® [US-OTC]; Geritol® Tonic [US-OTC]; Glutofac®-MX [US]; Glutofac®-ZX [US]; Gynovite® Plus [US-OTC]; Hemocyte Plus® [US]; Hi-Kovite [US-OTC]; Iberet® [US-OTC]; Iberet®-500 [US-OTC]; Monocaps [US-OTC]; Myadec® [US-OTC]; Ocuvite® Adult 50+ [US-OTC]; Ocuvite® Adult [US-OTC]; Ocuvite® Extra® [US-OTC]; Ocuvite® Lutein [US-OTC]; Ocuvite® [US-OTC]; Olay® Vitamins Complete Women's 50+ [US-OTC]; Olay® Vitamins Complete Women's [US-OTC]; One-A-Day® 50 Plus Formula [US-OTC]; One-A-Day® Active Formula [US-OTC]; One-A-Day® All Day Energy [US-OTC]; One-A-Day® Cholesterol Plus™ [US-OTC]; One-A-Day® Essential Formula [US-OTC]; One-A-Day® Maximum Formula [US-OTC]; One-A-Day® Men's Health Formula [US-OTC]; One-A-Day® Weight Smart [US-OTC]; One-A-Day® Women's Formula [US-OTC]; Optivite® P.M.T. [US-OTC]; PreserVision® AREDS [US-OTC]; PreserVision® Lutein [US-OTC]; Quintabs [US-OTC]; Quintabs-M [US-OTC]; Replace with Iron [US-OTC]; Replace [US-OTC]; Repliva 21/7™ [US]; SourceCF® Softgels [US]; Strovite® Advance [US]; Strovite® Forte [US]; T-Vites [US-OTC]; Ultra Freeda Iron Free [US-OTC]; Ultra Freeda with Iron [US-OTC]; Unicap M® [US-OTC]; Unicap Sr® [US-OTC]; Unicap T™ [US-OTC]; Viactiv® flavor glides [US-OTC]; Viactiv® Multivitamin [US-OTC]; Vitacon Forte [US]; Xtramins [US-OTC]

Therapeutic Category Vitamin

Use Prevention/treatment of vitamin and mineral deficiencies; labeled for OTC use as a dietary supplement

Usual Dosage Oral: Adults: Daily dose of adult preparations varies by product. Generally, 1 tablet or capsule or 5-15 mL of liquid per day. Consult package labeling. Prescription doses may be higher for burn or cystic fibrosis patients.

Dosage Forms Content varies depending on product used. For more detailed information on ingredients in these and other multivitamins, please refer to package labeling.

vitamins, multiple (oral) see vitamins (multiple/oral) on page 983

vitamins (multiple/pediatric) (VYE ta mins, MUL ti pul/pe de AT rik)

Synonyms children's vitamins; multivitamins/fluoride

U.S./Canadian Brand Names ADEKs [US-OTC]; AquADEKs™ [US-OTC]; Centrum Kids® Complete [US-OTC]; Centrum Kids® Dora the Explorer™ Complete [US-OTC]; Centrum Kids® Rugrats® Complete [US-OTC]; Centrum Kids® SpongeBob™ SquarePants Complete [US-OTC]; Flintstones® Complete [US-OTC]; Flintstones® Plus Iron [US-OTC]; Flintstones™ Gummies [US-OTC]; Flintstones™ Plus Immunity Support [US-OTC]; Flintstones™ Sour Gummies [US-OTC]; My First Flintstones® [US-OTC]; MyKidz Iron FL™ [US-OTC]; One-A-Day® Kids Bugs Bunny and Friends Complete [US-OTC]; One-A-Day® Kids Scooby-Doo! Complete [US-OTC]; One-A-Day® Kids Scooby-Doo! Plus Calcium [US-OTC]; One-A-Day® Scooby-Doo! Gummies [US-OTC]; Poly-Vi-Flor® With Iron [US]; Poly-Vi-Sol® with Iron [US-OTC]; Poly-Vi-Sol® [US-OTC]; SourceCF® [US-OTC]; Tri-Vi-Sol® with Iron [US-OTC]; Tri-Vi-Sol® [US-OTC]; Vitaball® Minis [US-OTC]; Vitaball® Wild 'N Fruity [US-OTC]; Vitaball® [US-OTC]

Therapeutic Category Vitamin

Use Prevention/treatment of vitamin deficiency; products containing fluoride are used to prevent dental caries; labeled for OTC use as a dietary supplement

Usual Dosage Daily dose varies by product; refer to package insert for specific product labeling

Dosage Forms Content varies depending on product used. For more detailed information on ingredients in these and other multivitamins, please refer to package labeling.

vitamins (multiple/prenatal) (VYE ta mins, MUL ti pul/pree NAY tal)

Sound-Alike/Look-Alike Issues

PreCare® may be confused with Precose®

◄ **Synonyms** prenatal vitamins

U.S./Canadian Brand Names A-Free Prenatal [US]; Advanced NatalCare® [US]; Advanced-RF NatalCare® [US]; Aminate Fe-90 [US]; Cal-Nate™ [US]; CareNatal™ DHA [US]; CitraNatal™ 90 DHA [US]; CitraNatal™ DHA [US]; CitraNatal™ Rx [US]; Daily Prenatal [US]; Duet® DHA^ec [US]; Duet® [US]; Duet™ DHA [US]; Icar™ Prenatal [US]; KPN Prenatal [US]; Mini-Prenatal [US]; NataCaps™ [US]; NataChew™ [US]; NataFort® [US]; NatalCare® GlossTabs™ [US]; NatalCare® PIC Forte [US]; NatalCare® PIC [US]; NatalCare® Plus [US]; NatalCare® Rx [US]; NatalCare® Three [US]; NataTab™ CFe [US]; NataTab™ FA [US]; NataTab™ Rx [US]; NutriNate® [US]; NutriSpire™ [US]; PreCare Premier™ [US]; PreCare® Conceive™ [US]; PreCare® Prenatal [US]; PreCare® [US]; Prenatal AD [US]; Prenatal H [US]; Prenatal MR 90 Fe™ [US]; Prenatal MTR with Selenium [US]; Prenatal Plus [US]; Prenatal Rx 1 [US]; Prenatal U [US]; Prenatal Z [US]; Prenate DHA™ [US]; Prenate Elite™ [US]; PrimaCare® One [US]; PrimaCare® [US]; StrongStart™ [US]; Stuart Prenatal® [US-OTC]; Tandem® OB [US]; Trinate [US]; Ultra NatalCare® [US]

Therapeutic Category Vitamin

Use Nutritional supplement for use prior to conception, during pregnancy, and postnatal (in lactating and nonlactating women)

Usual Dosage Oral: Adults:

Capsule, tablet: One daily

Powder: 4 teaspoonfuls/day; given once daily or in divided doses; mix 1 teaspoonful in 1 ounce of water

Dosage Forms Content varies depending on product used. For more detailed information on ingredients in these and other multivitamins, please refer to package labeling.

vitamins, multiple (therapeutic) *see* vitamins (multiple/oral) *on page 983*
vitamins, multiple with iron *see* vitamins (multiple/oral) *on page 983*
Vitaneed™ [US-OTC] *see* nutritional formula, enteral/oral *on page 689*
Vitelle™ Irospan® (Discontinued) *see* ferrous sulfate and ascorbic acid *on page 399*
Vitrase® [US] *see* hyaluronidase *on page 477*
Vitrasert® [US/Can] *see* ganciclovir *on page 435*
Vitrax® [US] *see* hyaluronate and derivatives *on page 476*
Vitussin (Discontinued)
Vivacaine™ [US] *see* bupivacaine and epinephrine *on page 150*
Vi vaccine *see* typhoid vaccine *on page 961*
Vivactil® [US] *see* protriptyline *on page 800*
Viva-Drops® [US-OTC] *see* artificial tears *on page 95*
Vivaglobin® [US] *see* immune globulin (subcutaneous) *on page 504*
Vivarin® [US-OTC] *see* caffeine *on page 158*
Vivelle® (Discontinued) *see* estradiol *on page 359*
Vivelle-Dot® [US] *see* estradiol *on page 359*
Vivitrol™ [US] *see* naltrexone *on page 654*
Vivonex® [US-OTC] *see* nutritional formula, enteral/oral *on page 689*
Vivonex® T.E.N. [US-OTC] *see* nutritional formula, enteral/oral *on page 689*
Vivotif® [US/Can] *see* typhoid vaccine *on page 961*
VLB *see* vinblastine *on page 977*
VM-26 *see* teniposide *on page 908*
Volmax® (Discontinued) *see* albuterol *on page 39*
Voltaren® [US/Can] *see* diclofenac *on page 292*
Voltaren® Gel [US] *see* diclofenac *on page 292*
Voltaren Ophtha® [Can] *see* diclofenac *on page 292*
Voltaren Ophthalmic® [US] *see* diclofenac *on page 292*
Voltaren Rapide® [Can] *see* diclofenac *on page 292*
Voltaren®-XR [US] *see* diclofenac *on page 292*
VoLumen™ [US] *see* barium *on page 116*
Voluven® [Can] *see* hetastarch *on page 473*

voriconazole (vor i KOE na zole)

Synonyms UK109496
U.S./Canadian Brand Names VFEND® [US/Can]

Therapeutic Category Antifungal Agent

Use Treatment of invasive aspergillosis; treatment of esophageal candidiasis; treatment of candidemia (in nonneutropenic patients); treatment of disseminated *Candida* infections of the skin and viscera; treatment of serious fungal infections caused by *Scedosporium apiospermum* and *Fusarium* spp (including *Fusarium solani*) in patients intolerant of, or refractory to, other therapy

Usual Dosage

Usual dosage ranges:
Children ≥12 years and Adults:
Oral: 100-300 mg every 12 hours
I.V.: 6 mg/kg every 12 hours for 2 doses; followed by maintenance dose of 4 mg/kg every 12 hours
Indication-specific dosing: Children ≥12 years and Adults:
Aspergillosis, invasive, including disseminated and extrapulmonary infection: Duration of therapy should be a minimum of 6-12 weeks or throughout period of immunosuppression:
I.V.: Initial: Loading dose: 6 mg/kg every 12 hours for 2 doses; followed by maintenance dose of 4 mg/kg every 12 hours
Oral: May consider oral therapy in place of I.V. with dosing of 4 mg/kg (rounded up to convenient tablet dosage form) every 12 hours; however, I.V. administration is preferred in serious infections since comparative efficacy with the oral formulation has not been established.
Scedosporiosis, fusariosis: I.V.: Initial: Loading dose: 6 mg/kg every 12 hours for 2 doses; followed by maintenance dose of 4 mg/kg every 12 hours
Candidemia and other deep tissue *Candida* infections: I.V.: Initial: Loading dose 6 mg/kg every 12 hours for 2 doses; followed by maintenance dose of 3-4 mg/kg every 12 hours
Endophthalmitis, fungal: I.V.: 6 mg/kg every 12 hours for 2 doses, then 200 mg orally twice daily
Esophageal candidiasis: Oral:
Patients <40 kg: 100 mg every 12 hours; maximum: 300 mg/day
Patients ≥40 kg: 200 mg every 12 hours; maximum: 600 mg/day
Note: Treatment should continue for a minimum of 14 days, and for at least 7 days following resolution of symptoms.
Conversion to oral dosing:
Patients <40 kg: 100 mg every 12 hours; increase to 150 mg every 12 hours in patients who fail to respond adequately
Patients ≥40 kg: 200 mg every 12 hours; increase to 300 mg every 12 hours in patients who fail to respond adequately

Dosage Forms
Injection, powder for reconstitution:
VFEND®: 200 mg
Powder for oral suspension:
VFEND®: 200 mg/5 mL
Tablet:
VFEND®: 50 mg, 200 mg

vorinostat (vor IN oh stat)

Synonyms NSC-701852; SAHA; suberoylanilide hydroxamic acid

U.S./Canadian Brand Names Zolinza™ [US]

Therapeutic Category Antineoplastic Agent, Histone Deacetylase Inhibitor

Use Treatment of progressive, persistent, or recurrent cutaneous T-cell lymphoma (CTCL)

Usual Dosage Oral: Adults: Cutaneous T-cell lymphoma: 400 mg once daily
Dosage adjustment for intolerance: Reduce dose to 300 mg once daily; may further reduce to 300 mg daily for 5 consecutive days per week
In clinical trials, **dose reductions** were instituted for the following adverse events: Increased serum creatinine, decreased appetite, hypokalemia, leukopenia, nausea, neutropenia, thrombocytopenia, and vomiting. Vorinostat was **discontinued** for the following adverse events: Anemia, angioneurotic edema, weakness, chest pain, exfoliative dermatitis, DVT, ischemic stroke, lethargy, pulmonary embolism, and spinal cord injury.

Dosage Forms
Capsule:
Zolinza™: 100 mg

VoSol® (Discontinued) see acetic acid *on page 29*

VoSol® HC [US] see acetic acid, propylene glycol diacetate, and hydrocortisone *on page 29*

VoSpire ER® [US] *see albuterol on page 39*

VP-16 *see etoposide on page 384*

VP-16-213 *see etoposide on page 384*

V-Tann™ [US] *see phenylephrine and pyrilamine on page 747*

Vumon® [US/Can] *see teniposide on page 908*

Vusion® [US] *see miconazole and zinc oxide on page 632*

V.V.S.® [US] *see sulfabenzamide, sulfacetamide, and sulfathiazole on page 892*

vWF:RCof *see antihemophilic factor/von Willebrand factor complex (human) on page 80*

Vytone® [US] *see iodoquinol and hydrocortisone on page 520*

Vytorin® [US] *see ezetimibe and simvastatin on page 387*

Vyvanse™ [US] *see lisdexamfetamine on page 570*

VZIG *see varicella-zoster immune globulin (human) on page 972*

VZV vaccine (varicella) *see varicella virus vaccine on page 971*

VZV vaccine (zoster) *see zoster vaccine on page 997*

warfarin (WAR far in)

Sound-Alike/Look-Alike Issues
Coumadin® may be confused with Avandia®, Cardura®, Compazine®, Kemadrin®
Jantoven™ may be confused with Janumet™, Januvia™

Synonyms warfarin sodium

U.S./Canadian Brand Names Apo-Warfarin® [Can]; Coumadin® [US/Can]; Gen-Warfarin [Can]; Jantoven™ [US]; Novo-Warfarin [Can]; Taro-Warfarin [Can]

Therapeutic Category Anticoagulant (Other)

Use Prophylaxis and treatment of thromboembolic disorders (eg, venous, pulmonary) and embolic complications arising from atrial fibrillation or cardiac valve replacement; adjunct to reduce risk of systemic embolism (eg, recurrent MI, stroke) after myocardial infarction

Usual Dosage Note: New labeling identifies genetic factors which may increase patient sensitivity to warfarin. Specifically, genetic variations in the proteins CYP2C9 and VKORC1, responsible for warfarin's primary metabolism and pharmacodynamic activity, respectively, have been identified as predisposing factors associated with decreased dose requirement and increased bleeding risk. A genotyping test is available, and may provide important guidance on initiation of anticoagulant therapy.

Oral: Adults: Initial dosing must be individualized. Consider the patient (hepatic function, cardiac function, age, nutritional status, concurrent therapy, risk of bleeding) in addition to prior dose response (if available) and the clinical situation. Start 2-5 mg daily for 2 days **or** 5-10 mg daily for 1-2 days. Adjust dose according to INR results; usual maintenance dose ranges from 2-10 mg daily (individual patients may require loading and maintenance doses outside these general guidelines).

Note: Lower starting doses may be required for patients with hepatic impairment, poor nutrition, CHF, elderly, high risk of bleeding, or patients who are debilitated, or those with reduced function genomic variants of the catabolic enzymes CYP2C9 (*2 or *3 alleles) or VKORC1 (-1639 polymorphism). Higher initial doses may be reasonable in selected patients (ie, receiving enzyme-inducing agents and with low risk of bleeding).

I.V.: Adults: 2-5 mg/day administered as a slow bolus injection

Dosage Forms
Injection, powder for reconstitution:
Coumadin®: 5 mg
Tablet: 1 mg, 2 mg, 2.5 mg, 3 mg, 4 mg, 5 mg, 6 mg, 7.5 mg, 10 mg
Coumadin®, Jantoven®: 1 mg, 2 mg, 2.5 mg, 3 mg, 4 mg, 5 mg, 6 mg, 7.5 mg, 10 mg

warfarin sodium *see warfarin on page 986*

Wartec® [Can] *see podofilox on page 763*

Wart-Off® Maximum Strength [US-OTC] *see salicylic acid on page 850*

4-Way® 12 Hour [US-OTC] *see oxymetazoline on page 712*

4 Way® Fast Acting [US-OTC] *see phenylephrine on page 745*

4 Way® Menthol [US-OTC] *see phenylephrine on page 745*

4 Way® No Drip [US-OTC] *see phenylephrine on page 745*

4-Way® Saline Moisturizing Mist [US-OTC] *see sodium chloride on page 873*

WelChol® [US/Can] *see colesevelam on page 244*

Wellbutrin® [US/Can] *see bupropion on page 152*

Wellbutrin XL™ [US/Can] *see* bupropion *on page 152*
Wellbutrin SR® [US] *see* bupropion *on page 152*
Wellcovorin® *(Discontinued) see* leucovorin calcium *on page 552*
Westcort® [US/Can] *see* hydrocortisone (topical) *on page 485*
Westhroid™ [US] *see* thyroid, desiccated *on page 924*
40 Winks® *(Discontinued) see* diphenhydramine *on page 304*
Winpred™ [Can] *see* prednisone *on page 782*
WinRho SD® *(Discontinued)*
WinRho® SDF [US/Can] *see* Rho(D) immune globulin *on page 829*
Winstrol® *(Discontinued)*

witch hazel (witch HAY zel)

Synonyms hamamelis water
U.S./Canadian Brand Names Dickinson's® Witch Hazel [US-OTC]; Preparation H® Cleansing Pads [Can]; Preparation H® Medicated Wipes [US-OTC]; T.N. Dickinson's® Hazelets [US-OTC]; Tucks® [US-OTC]
Therapeutic Category Astringent
Use After-stool wipe to remove most causes of local irritation; temporary management of vulvitis, pruritus ani and vulva; help relieve the discomfort of simple hemorrhoids, anorectal surgical wounds, and episiotomies
Usual Dosage Apply to anorectal area as needed
Dosage Forms
  Liquid, topical: 100% (120 mL, 480 mL)
    Dickinson's® Witch Hazel [OTC]: 100% (60 mL, 240 mL, 480 mL)
  Pads: 50% (100s)
    Dickinson's® Witch Hazel [OTC]: 50% (20s, 50s, 100s)
    Preparation H® Medicated Wipes [OTC]: 50% (8s, 48s)
    T.N. Dickinson's® Hazelets [OTC]: 50% (50s, 60s)
    Tucks® [OTC]: 50% (12s, 40s, 100s)

Wolfina® *(Discontinued)*
Wound Wash Saline™ [US-OTC] *see* sodium chloride *on page 873*
WR-2721 *see* amifostine *on page 58*
WR-139007 *see* dacarbazine *on page 263*
WR-139013 *see* chlorambucil *on page 200*
WR-139021 *see* carmustine *on page 180*
Wycillin® [Can] *see* penicillin G procaine *on page 733*
Wycillin *(Discontinued) see* penicillin G procaine *on page 733*
Wydase® *(Discontinued) see* hyaluronidase *on page 477*
Wygesic® *(Discontinued) see* propoxyphene and acetaminophen *on page 795*
Wymox® *(Discontinued) see* amoxicillin *on page 67*
Wytensin® [Can] *see* guanabenz *on page 462*
Wytensin® *(Discontinued) see* guanabenz *on page 462*
Xalatan® [US/Can] *see* latanoprost *on page 550*
Xanax® [US/Can] *see* alprazolam *on page 49*
Xanax TS™ [Can] *see* alprazolam *on page 49*
Xanax XR® [US] *see* alprazolam *on page 49*
Xatral [Can] *see* alfuzosin *on page 44*
Xeloda® [US/Can] *see* capecitabine *on page 170*
Xenaderm™ [US] *see* trypsin, balsam peru, and castor oil *on page 958*
Xenical® [US/Can] *see* orlistat *on page 702*
Xerac AC™ [US] *see* aluminum chloride hexahydrate *on page 53*
Xibrom™ [US] *see* bromfenac *on page 143*
Xifaxan™ [US] *see* rifaximin *on page 834*
Xigris® [US/Can] *see* drotrecogin alfa *on page 327*
XiraTuss™ *(Discontinued) see* carbetapentane, phenylephrine, and chlorpheniramine *on page 176*

Xodol® 5/300 [US] *see* hydrocodone and acetaminophen *on page 481*
Xodol® 7.5/300 [US] *see* hydrocodone and acetaminophen *on page 481*
Xodol® 10/300 [US] *see* hydrocodone and acetaminophen *on page 481*
Xolair® [US/Can] *see* omalizumab *on page 696*
Xolegel™ [US/Can] *see* ketoconazole *on page 537*
Xopenex® [US/Can] *see* levalbuterol *on page 554*
Xopenex HFA™ [US] *see* levalbuterol *on page 554*
XPECT™ [US-OTC] *see* guaifenesin *on page 453*
Xpect-HC™ *(Discontinued)*
XPECT-PE™ *(Discontinued) see* guaifenesin and phenylephrine *on page 456*
X-Prep® *(Discontinued) see* senna *on page 861*
X-Seb T® Pearl [US-OTC] *see* coal tar and salicylic acid *on page 241*
X-Seb T® Plus [US-OTC] *see* coal tar and salicylic acid *on page 241*
Xtramins [US-OTC] *see* vitamins (multiple/oral) *on page 983*
Xylocaine® [US/Can] *see* lidocaine *on page 561*
Xylocaine® MPF [US] *see* lidocaine *on page 561*
Xylocaine® MPF With Epinephrine [US] *see* lidocaine and epinephrine *on page 563*
Xylocaine® Viscous [US] *see* lidocaine *on page 561*
Xylocaine® With Epinephrine [US/Can] *see* lidocaine and epinephrine *on page 563*
Xylocard® [Can] *see* lidocaine *on page 561*
Xyrem® [US/Can] *see* sodium oxybate *on page 877*
Xyzal® [US] *see* levocetirizine *on page 556*
Y-90 ibritumomab *see* ibritumomab *on page 495*
Y-90 zevalin *see* ibritumomab *on page 495*
Yasmin® [US/Can] *see* ethinyl estradiol and drospirenone *on page 370*
Yaz [US] *see* ethinyl estradiol and drospirenone *on page 370*

yellow fever vaccine (YEL oh FEE ver vak SEEN)

U.S./Canadian Brand Names YF-VAX® [US/Can]
Therapeutic Category Vaccine, Live Virus
Use Induction of active immunity against yellow fever virus, primarily among persons traveling or living in areas where yellow fever infection exists and laboratory workers who may be exposed to the virus; vaccination may also be required for some international travelers
Usual Dosage SubQ: Children ≥9 months (per manufacturer) and Adults: One dose (0.5 mL) ≥10 days before travel; Booster: Every 10 years for those at continued risk of exposure
Dosage Forms
Injection, powder for reconstitution [17D-204 strain]:
  YF-VAX®: ≥4.74 Log_{10} plaque-forming units (PFU) per 0.5 mL dose

YF-VAX® [US/Can] *see* yellow fever vaccine *on page 988*
YM087 *see* conivaptan *on page 247*
YM905 *see* solifenacin *on page 881*
YM-08310 *see* amifostine *on page 58*
Yocon® [US/Can] *see* yohimbine *on page 988*
Yodoxin® [US] *see* iodoquinol *on page 520*

yohimbine (yo HIM bine)

Sound-Alike/Look-Alike Issues
  Aphrodyne® may be confused with Aprodine®
  Yocon® may be confused with Zocor®
Synonyms yohimbine hydrochloride
U.S./Canadian Brand Names PMS-Yohimbine [Can]; Yocon® [US/Can]
Therapeutic Category Miscellaneous Product

Usual Dosage Oral: Adults:
Male erectile impotence: 5.4 mg tablet 3 times/day have been used. If side effects occur, reduce to 1/2 tablet (2.7 mg) 3 times/day followed by gradual increases to 1 tablet 3 times/day. Results of therapy >10 weeks are not known.
Orthostatic hypotension: Doses of 12.5 mg/day have been utilized; however, more research is necessary

Dosage Forms
Tablet: 5.4 mg

yohimbine hydrochloride *see* yohimbine *on page 988*
Yohimex™ *(Discontinued)* *see* yohimbine *on page 988*
Yutopar® Injection *(Discontinued)*
Z4942 *see* ifosfamide *on page 499*
Zaditen® [Can] *see* ketotifen *on page 538*
Zaditor® [US-OTC/Can] *see* ketotifen *on page 538*

zafirlukast (za FIR loo kast)

Sound-Alike/Look-Alike Issues
Accolate® may be confused with Accupril®, Accutane®, Aclovate®
Synonyms ICI-204,219
U.S./Canadian Brand Names Accolate® [US/Can]
Therapeutic Category Leukotriene Receptor Antagonist
Use Prophylaxis and chronic treatment of asthma in adults and children ≥5 years of age
Usual Dosage Oral:
Children 5-11 years: 10 mg twice daily
Children ≥12 years and Adults: 20 mg twice daily
Dosage Forms
Tablet:
Accolate®: 10 mg, 20 mg

Zagam® *(Discontinued)*

zaleplon (ZAL e plon)

U.S./Canadian Brand Names Sonata® [US]
Therapeutic Category Hypnotic, Nonbenzodiazepine (Pyrazolopyrimidine)
Controlled Substance C-IV
Use Short-term (7-10 days) treatment of insomnia (has been demonstrated to be effective for up to 5 weeks in controlled trial)
Usual Dosage Oral: Adults: 10 mg at bedtime (range: 5-20 mg); has been used for up to 5 weeks of treatment in controlled trial setting
Dosage Forms
Capsule: 5 mg, 10 mg
Sonata®: 5 mg, 10 mg

Zanaflex® [US/Can] *see* tizanidine *on page 931*
Zanaflex Capsules™ [US] *see* tizanidine *on page 931*

zanamivir (za NA mi veer)

U.S./Canadian Brand Names Relenza® [US/Can]
Therapeutic Category Antiviral Agent, Inhalation Therapy
Use Treatment of uncomplicated acute illness due to influenza virus A and B in patients who have been symptomatic for no more than 2 days; prophylaxis against influenza virus A and B

The Advisory Committee on Immunization Practices (ACIP) recommends that **treatment** be considered for the following:
• Persons hospitalized with laboratory confirmed influenza (may also have benefit if started >48 hours after onset of illness).
• Persons with laboratory confirmed influenza pneumonia.
• Persons with laboratory confirmed influenza and bacterial infections.
• Persons with laboratory confirmed influenza and who are at higher risk for influenza complications.

◄ • Persons presenting for care within 48 hours of laboratory confirmed influenza onset and who want to decrease duration and/or severity of their symptoms or decrease the risk of transmission to those at high risk for complications.

The ACIP recommends that **prophylaxis** be considered for the following:
- Persons at high risk for influenza infection during the first 2 weeks following vaccination (eg, children <9 years and not previously vaccinated) if the virus is circulating in the community.
- Persons at high risk for influenza infection, but the vaccination is contraindicated.
- Unvaccinated family members or healthcare providers with prolonged exposure to or close contact with high-risk persons, unvaccinated persons, or infants <6 months of age.
- Persons at high risk for influenza infection, their family members and close contacts, and healthcare workers when the circulating strain of influenza is not matched with the vaccine.
- Persons with immune deficiency or those who may not respond to vaccination.
- Unvaccinated staff and persons during response to an outbreak in a closed institutional setting that has patients at high risk for infection (eg, extended care facilities).

Usual Dosage Oral inhalation:
Children ≥5 years and Adults: Prophylaxis (household setting): Two inhalations (10 mg) once daily for 10 days. Begin within 1 1/2 days following onset of signs or symptoms of index case.
Children ≥7 years and Adults: Treatment: Two inhalations (10 mg total) twice daily for 5 days. Doses on first day should be separated by at least 2 hours; on subsequent days, doses should be spaced by ~12 hours. Begin within 2 days of signs or symptoms.
Adolescents and Adults: Prophylaxis (community outbreak): Two inhalations (10 mg) once daily for 28 days. Begin within 5 days of outbreak.

Dosage Forms
Powder for oral inhalation:
Relenza®: 5 mg/blister (20s)

Zanosar® [US/Can] see streptozocin on page 888
Zantac® [US/Can] see ranitidine on page 819
Zantac 75® [US-OTC/Can] see ranitidine on page 819
Zantac 150™ [US-OTC] see ranitidine on page 819
Zantac® EFFERdose® [US] see ranitidine on page 819
Zantac Maximum Strength Non-Prescription [Can] see ranitidine on page 819
Zantryl® (Discontinued) see phentermine on page 744
Zapzyt® [US-OTC] see benzoyl peroxide on page 126
Zarontin® [US/Can] see ethosuximide on page 381
Zaroxolyn® [US/Can] see metolazone on page 626
Zartan® (Discontinued) see cephalexin on page 194
Zavesca® [US/Can] see miglustat on page 634
Zazole™ [US] see terconazole on page 911
Z-Bec® [US-OTC] see vitamin B complex combinations on page 981
Z-chlopenthixol see zuclopenthixol (Canada only) on page 997
Z-Cof™ 12DM [US] see guaifenesin, pseudoephedrine, and dextromethorphan on page 460
Z-Cof HC (Discontinued) see phenylephrine, hydrocodone, and chlorpheniramine on page 748
Z-Cof LA™ [US] see guaifenesin and dextromethorphan on page 454
ZD1033 see anastrozole on page 76
ZD1694 see raltitrexed (Canada only) on page 817
ZD1839 see gefitinib on page 437
ZDV see zidovudine on page 991
ZDV, abacavir, and lamivudine see abacavir, lamivudine, and zidovudine on page 16
Zeasorb®-AF [US-OTC] see miconazole on page 630
Zebeta® [US/Can] see bisoprolol on page 138
Zebutal™ [US] see butalbital, acetaminophen, and caffeine on page 155
Zefazone® (Discontinued)
Zegerid® [US] see omeprazole and sodium bicarbonate on page 698
Zelapar™ [US] see selegiline on page 860
Zeldox® [Can] see ziprasidone on page 994
Zelnorm® [US] see tegaserod on page 905

Zemaira® [US] *see* alpha₁-proteinase inhibitor *on page 48*
Zemplar® [US/Can] *see* paricalcitol *on page 723*
Zemuron® [US/Can] *see* rocuronium *on page 842*
Zenapax® [US/Can] *see* daclizumab *on page 263*
Zenchent™ [US] *see* ethinyl estradiol and norethindrone *on page 376*
zeneca 182,780 *see* fulvestrant *on page 430*
Zephiran® [US-OTC] *see* benzalkonium chloride *on page 123*
Zephrex LA® *(Discontinued)* *see* guaifenesin and pseudoephedrine *on page 458*
Zerit® [US/Can] *see* stavudine *on page 887*
ZerLor™ [US] *see* acetaminophen, caffeine, and dihydrocodeine *on page 25*
Zestoretic® [US/Can] *see* lisinopril and hydrochlorothiazide *on page 571*
Zestril® [US/Can] *see* lisinopril *on page 570*
Zetar® [US-OTC] *see* coal tar *on page 240*
Zetia® [US] *see* ezetimibe *on page 387*
Zevalin® [US/Can] *see* ibritumomab *on page 495*
Ziac® [US/Can] *see* bisoprolol and hydrochlorothiazide *on page 138*
Ziagen® [US/Can] *see* abacavir *on page 16*
Ziana™ [US] *see* clindamycin and tretinoin *on page 231*

ziconotide (zi KOE no tide)

U.S./Canadian Brand Names Prialt® [US]
Therapeutic Category Analgesic, Nonnarcotic; Calcium Channel Blocker, N-Type
Use Management of severe chronic pain in patients requiring intrathecal (I.T.) therapy and who are intolerant or refractory to other therapies
Usual Dosage I.T.: Adults: Chronic pain: Initial dose: ≤2.4 mcg/day (0.1 mcg/hour)
Dose may be titrated by ≤2.4 mcg/day (0.1 mcg/hour) at intervals ≤2-3 times/week to a maximum dose of 19.2 mcg/day (0.8 mcg/hour) by day 21; average dose at day 21: 6.9 mcg/day (0.29 mcg/hour). A faster titration should be used only if the urgent need for analgesia outweighs the possible risk to patient safety.
Dosage Forms
Injection, solution [preservative free]:
Prialt®: 25 mcg/mL (20 mL); 100 mcg/mL (1 mL, 5 mL)

zidovudine (zye DOE vyoo deen)

Sound-Alike/Look-Alike Issues
azidothymidine may be confused with azaTHIOprine, aztreonam
Retrovir® may be confused with ritonavir
AZT is an error-prone abbreviation (mistaken as azathioprine, aztreonam)
Synonyms azidothymidine; compound S; ZDV
U.S./Canadian Brand Names Apo-Zidovudine® [Can]; AZT™ [Can]; Retrovir® [US/Can]
Therapeutic Category Antiviral Agent
Use Treatment of HIV infection in combination with at least two other antiretroviral agents; prevention of maternal/fetal HIV transmission as monotherapy
Usual Dosage
Prevention of maternal-fetal HIV transmission:
Neonatal: **Note:** Dosing should begin 6-12 hours after birth and continue for the first 6 weeks of life.
Oral:
Full-term infants: 2 mg/kg/dose every 6 hours
Infants ≥30 weeks and <35 weeks gestation at birth: 2 mg/kg/dose every 12 hours; at 2 weeks of age, advance to 2 mg/kg/dose every 8 hours
Infants <30 weeks gestation at birth: 2 mg/kg/dose every 12 hours; at 4 weeks of age, advance to 2 mg/kg/dose every 8 hours
I.V.: Infants unable to receive oral dosing:
Full term: 1.5 mg/kg/dose every 6 hours
Infants ≥30 weeks and <35 weeks gestation at birth: 1.5 mg/kg/dose every 12 hours; at 2 weeks of age, advance to 1.5 mg/kg/dose every 8 hours

Infants <30 weeks gestation at birth: 1.5 mg/kg/dose every 12 hours; at 4 weeks of age, advance to 1.5 mg/kg/dose every 8 hours

Maternal: Oral (per AIDSinfo guidelines): 100 mg 5 times/day **or** 200 mg 3 times/day **or** 300 mg twice daily. Begin at 14-34 weeks gestation and continue until start of labor.

During labor and delivery, administer zidovudine I.V. at 2 mg/kg as loading dose followed by a continuous I.V. infusion of 1 mg/kg/hour until the umbilical cord is clamped

Treatment of HIV infection:

Children 6 weeks to 12 years:

Oral: 160 mg/m^2/dose every 8 hours (maximum: 200 mg every 8 hours); some Working Group members use a dose of 180 mg/m^2 to 240 mg/m^2 every 12 hours when using in drug combinations with other antiretroviral compounds, but data on this dosing in children is limited

I.V. continuous infusion: 20 mg/m^2/hour

I.V. intermittent infusion: 120 mg/m^2/dose every 6 hours

Adults:

Oral: 300 mg twice daily or 200 mg 3 times/day

I.V.: 1 mg/kg/dose administered every 4 hours around-the-clock (5-6 doses/day)

Dosage Forms
Capsule:
Retrovir®: 100 mg
Injection, solution [preservative free]:
Retrovir®: 10 mg/mL (20 mL)
Syrup:
Retrovir®: 50 mg/5 mL
Tablet: 300 mg
Retrovir®: 300 mg

zidovudine, abacavir, and lamivudine *see* abacavir, lamivudine, and zidovudine *on page 16*

zidovudine and lamivudine (zye DOE vyoo deen & la MI vyoo deen)

Sound-Alike/Look-Alike Issues
Combivir® may be confused with Combivent®, Epivir®

AZT is an error-prone abbreviation (mistaken as azaTHIOprine, aztreonam)

Synonyms lamivudine and zidovudine

U.S./Canadian Brand Names Combivir® [US/Can]

Therapeutic Category Antiviral Agent

Use Treatment of HIV infection when therapy is warranted based on clinical and/or immunological evidence of disease progression

Usual Dosage Oral: Children ≥12 years and Adults: One tablet twice daily

Note: Because this is a fixed-dose combination product, avoid use in patients requiring dosage reduction including children <12 years of age, renally-impaired patients with a creatinine clearance ≤50 mL/minute, hepatic impairment, or those patients experiencing dose-limiting adverse effects.

Dosage Forms
Tablet:
Combivir®: Zidovudine 300 mg and lamivudine 150 mg

Zilactin® [Can] *see* lidocaine *on page 561*
Zilactin-L® [US-OTC] *see* lidocaine *on page 561*
Zilactin®-B [US-OTC/Can] *see* benzocaine *on page 124*
Zilactin Baby® [Can] *see* benzocaine *on page 124*
Zilactin Toothache and Gum Pain® [US-OTC] *see* benzocaine *on page 124*

zileuton (zye LOO ton)

U.S./Canadian Brand Names Zyflo CR™ [US]

Therapeutic Category 5-Lipoxygenase Inhibitor

Use Prophylaxis and chronic treatment of asthma in children ≥12 years of age and adults

Usual Dosage Oral: Children ≥12 years and Adults: Zyflo CR™: 1200 mg twice daily.

Dosage Forms
Tablet, extended release:
Zyflo CR™: 600 mg

Zinacef® [US/Can] *see* cefuroxime *on page 192*
zinc *see* trace metals *on page 940*
Zincate® [US] *see* zinc sulfate *on page 994*

zinc chloride (zink KLOR ide)

Therapeutic Category Trace Element
Use Cofactor for replacement therapy to different enzymes; helps maintain normal growth rates, normal skin hydration, and senses of taste and smell
Usual Dosage Clinical response may not occur for up to 6-8 weeks
  Supplemental to I.V. solutions:
    Premature Infants <1500 g, up to 3 kg: 300 mcg/kg/day
    Infants (full term) and Children ≤5 years: 100 mcg/kg/day
    Adults:
      Stable with fluid loss from small bowel: 12.2 mg zinc/L TPN or 17.1 mg zinc/kg (added to 1000 mL I.V. fluids) of stool or ileostomy output
      Metabolically stable: 2.5-4 mg/day; add 2 mg/day for acute catabolic states
Dosage Forms
  Injection, solution [preservative free]: 1 mg/mL (10 mL, 50 mL)

zinc diethylenetriaminepentaacetate (Zn-DTPA) *see* diethylene triamine penta-acetic acid *on page 294*
Zincfrin® [Can] *see* phenylephrine and zinc sulfate *(Canada only) on page 748*

zinc gelatin (zink JEL ah tin)

Synonyms dome paste bandage; unna's boot; unna's paste; zinc gelatin boot
U.S./Canadian Brand Names Gelucast® [US]
Therapeutic Category Protectant, Topical
Use As a protectant and to support varicosities and similar lesions of the lower limbs
Usual Dosage Topical: Apply externally as an occlusive boot
Dosage Forms
  Bandage: 3" x 10 yards; 4" x 10 yards
    Gelucast®: 3" x 10 yards; 4" x 10 yards

zinc gelatin boot *see* zinc gelatin *on page 993*
Zincofax® [Can] *see* zinc oxide *on page 993*
Zincon® [US-OTC] *see* pyrithione zinc *on page 810*

zinc oxide (zink OKS ide)

Synonyms base ointment; lassar's zinc paste
U.S./Canadian Brand Names Ammens® Medicated Deodorant [US-OTC]; Balmex® [US-OTC]; Boudreaux's® Butt Paste [US-OTC]; Critic-Aid Skin Care® [US-OTC]; Desitin® Creamy [US-OTC]; Desitin® [US-OTC]; Zincofax® [Can]
Therapeutic Category Topical Skin Product
Use Protective coating for mild skin irritations and abrasions; soothing and protective ointment to promote healing of chapped skin, diaper rash
Usual Dosage Topical: Infants, Children, and Adults: Apply as required for affected areas several times daily
Dosage Forms
  Cream:
    Balmex® [OTC]: 11.3% (60 g, 120 g, 480 g)
  Ointment, topical: 20% (30 g, 60 g, 454 g); 40% (120 g)
    Desitin® [OTC]: 40% (30 g, 60 g, 90 g, 120 g, 270 g, 480 g)
    Desitin® Creamy [OTC]: 10% (60 g, 120 g)
  Paste, topical:
    Boudreaux's® Butt Paste [OTC]: 16% (30 g, 60 g, 120 g, 480 g)
    Critic-Aid Skin Care® [OTC]: 20% (71 g, 170 g)
  Powder, topical:
    Ammens® Medicated Deodorant [OTC]: 9.1% (187.5 g, 330 g)

zinc oxide and miconazole nitrate *see* miconazole and zinc oxide *on page 632*

zinc sulfate (zink SUL fate)

Sound-Alike/Look-Alike Issues
$ZnSO_4$ is an error-prone abbreviation (mistaken as morphine sulfate)

U.S./Canadian Brand Names Anuzinc [Can]; Orazinc® [US-OTC]; Rivasol [Can]; Zincate® [US]

Therapeutic Category Electrolyte Supplement, Oral

Use Zinc supplement (oral and parenteral); may improve wound healing in those who are deficient

Usual Dosage
RDA: Oral:
  Birth to 6 months: 3 mg elemental zinc/day
  6-12 months: 5 mg elemental zinc/day
  1-10 years: 10 mg elemental zinc/day
  ≥11 years: 15 mg elemental zinc/day
Zinc deficiency: Oral:
  Infants and Children: 0.5-1 mg elemental zinc/kg/day divided 1-3 times/day; somewhat larger quantities may be needed if there is impaired intestinal absorption or an excessive loss of zinc
  Adults: 110-220 mg zinc sulfate (25-50 mg elemental zinc)/dose 3 times/day
Parenteral TPN: I.V.:
  Infants (premature, birth weight <1500 g up to 3 kg): 300 mcg/kg/day
  Infants (full-term) and Children ≤5 years: 100 mcg/kg/day
  Adults:
    Acute metabolic states: 4.5-6 mg/day
    Metabolically stable: 2.5-4 mg/day
    Stable with fluid loss from the small bowel: 12.2 mg zinc/L of TPN solution, or an additional 17.1 mg zinc (added to 1000 mL I.V. fluids) per kg of stool or ileostomy output

Dosage Forms
Capsule: 220 mg
  Orazinc® [OTC], Zincate®: 220 mg
Injection, solution [preservative free]: 1 mg elemental zinc/mL (10 mL); 5 mg elemental zinc/mL (5 mL)
Tablet: 110 mg
  Orazinc® [OTC]: 110 mg

zinc sulfate and phenylephrine see phenylephrine and zinc sulfate (Canada only) on page 748
zinc undecylenate see undecylenic acid and derivatives on page 962
Zinecard® [US/Can] see dexrazoxane on page 281
Zingo™ [US] see lidocaine on page 561
Ziox™ [US] see chlorophyllin, papain, and urea on page 203
Ziox 405™ [US] see chlorophyllin, papain, and urea on page 203

ziprasidone (zi PRAS i done)

Synonyms ziprasidone hydrochloride; ziprasidone mesylate

U.S./Canadian Brand Names Geodon® [US]; Zeldox® [Can]

Therapeutic Category Antipsychotic Agent

Use Treatment of schizophrenia; treatment of acute manic or mixed episodes associated with bipolar disorder with or without psychosis; acute agitation in patients with schizophrenia

Usual Dosage Adults:
Bipolar mania: Oral: Initial: 40 mg twice daily (with food)
  Adjustment: May increase to 60 or 80 mg twice daily on second day of treatment; average dose 40-80 mg twice daily
Schizophrenia: Oral: Initial: 20 mg twice daily (with food)
  Adjustment: Increases (if indicated) should be made no more frequently than every 2 days; ordinarily patients should be observed for improvement over several weeks before adjusting the dose
  Maintenance: Range 20-100 mg twice daily; however, dosages >80 mg twice daily are generally not recommended
Acute agitation (schizophrenia): I.M.: 10 mg every 2 hours **or** 20 mg every 4 hours; maximum: 40 mg/day; oral therapy should replace I.M. administration as soon as possible

Dosage Forms
Capsule:
  Geodon®: 20 mg, 40 mg, 60 mg, 80 mg

Injection, powder for reconstitution:
Geodon®: 20 mg

ziprasidone hydrochloride *see* ziprasidone *on page 994*
ziprasidone mesylate *see* ziprasidone *on page 994*
Zithromax® [US/Can] *see* azithromycin *on page 110*
Zithromax® TRI-PAK™ *see* azithromycin *on page 110*
Zithromax® Z-PAK® *see* azithromycin *on page 110*
ZM-182,780 *see* fulvestrant *on page 430*
Zmax™ [US] *see* azithromycin *on page 110*
Zn-DTPA *see* diethylene triamine penta-acetic acid *on page 294*
ZNP® Bar [US-OTC] *see* pyrithione zinc *on page 810*
Zocor® [US/Can] *see* simvastatin *on page 867*
Zoderm® [US] *see* benzoyl peroxide *on page 126*
Zoderm® Hydrating Wash™ [US] *see* benzoyl peroxide *on page 126*
Zofran® [US/Can] *see* ondansetron *on page 698*
Zofran® ODT [US/Can] *see* ondansetron *on page 698*
Zoladex® [US/Can] *see* goserelin *on page 451*
Zoladex® LA [Can] *see* goserelin *on page 451*
zoledronate *see* zoledronic acid *on page 995*

zoledronic acid (zoe le DRON ik AS id)

Sound-Alike/Look-Alike Issues
Zometa® may be confused with Zofran® , Zoladex®
Synonyms CGP-42446; NSC-721517; zoledronate
U.S./Canadian Brand Names Aclasta® [Can]; Reclast® [US]; Zometa® [US/Can]
Therapeutic Category Bisphosphonate Derivative
Use Treatment of hypercalcemia of malignancy, multiple myeloma, bone metastases of solid tumors, Paget disease of bone, postmenopausal osteoporosis
Usual Dosage I.V.: Adults: **Note:** Patients treated for multiple myeloma, osteoporosis, and Paget disease should receive a daily calcium supplement and multivitamin containing vitamin D (if dietary intake is inadequate).
Hypercalcemia of malignancy (albumin-corrected serum calcium ≥ 12 mg/dL) (Zometa®): 4 mg (maximum) given as a single dose. Wait at least 7 days before considering retreatment. Dosage adjustment may be needed in patients with decreased renal function following treatment.
Multiple myeloma or metastatic bone lesions from solid tumors (Zometa®): 4 mg every 3-4 weeks
Osteoporosis (Reclast®, Aclasta® [CAN]): 5 mg infused over at least 15 minutes every 12 months
Paget disease (Reclast®, Aclasta® [CAN]): 5 mg infused over at least 15 minutes. **Note:** Data concerning retreatment is not available, but may be considered.
Dosage Forms [CAN] = Canadian brand name
Infusion, solution [premixed]:
Aclasta® [CAN]): 5 mg (100 mL) [not available in the U.S.]
Relcast®: 5 mg (100 mL)
Injection, solution:
Zometa®: 4 mg/5 mL (5 mL)

Zolicef® (Discontinued) *see* cefazolin *on page 184*
Zolinza™ [US] *see* vorinostat *on page 985*

zolmitriptan (zohl mi TRIP tan)

Sound-Alike/Look-Alike Issues
zolmitriptan may be confused with SUMAtriptan
Synonyms 311C90
U.S./Canadian Brand Names Zomig-ZMT® [US]; Zomig® Nasal Spray [Can]; Zomig® Rapimelt [Can]; Zomig® [US/Can]
Therapeutic Category Antimigraine Agent; Serotonin Agonist

◄ **Use** Acute treatment of migraine with or without aura

Usual Dosage Oral: Adults: Migraine:

Tablet: Initial: ≤2.5 mg at the onset of migraine headache; may break 2.5 mg tablet in half

Orally-disintegrating tablet: Initial: 2.5 mg at the onset of migraine headache

Nasal spray: Initial: 1 spray (5 mg) at the onset of migraine headache

Note: Use the lowest possible dose to minimize adverse events. If the headache returns, the dose may be repeated after 2 hours; do not exceed 10 mg within a 24-hour period. Controlled trials have not established the effectiveness of a second dose if the initial one was ineffective

Dosage Forms

Solution, intranasal [spray]:

Zomig®: 5 mg/0.1 mL (0.1 mL)

Tablet:

Zomig®: 2.5 mg, 5 mg

Tablet, orally disintegrating

Zomig-ZMT®: 2.5 mg, 5 mg

Zoloft® [US/Can] *see* sertraline *on page 863*

zolpidem (zole PI dem)

Sound-Alike/Look-Alike Issues

Ambien® may be confused with Ambi 10®

Synonyms zolpidem tartrate

U.S./Canadian Brand Names Ambien CR® [US]; Ambien® [US]

Therapeutic Category Hypnotic, Nonbarbiturate

Controlled Substance C-IV

Use

Ambien®: Short-term treatment of insomnia (with difficulty of sleep onset)

Ambien CR®: Treatment of insomnia (with difficulty of sleep onset and/or sleep maintenance)

Usual Dosage Oral: Adults:

Ambien®: 10 mg immediately before bedtime; maximum dose: 10 mg

Ambien CR®: 12.5 mg immediately before bedtime

Dosage Forms

Tablet: 5 mg, 10 mg

Ambien®: 5 mg, 10 mg

Tablet, extended release:

Ambien CR®: 6.25 mg, 12.5 mg

zolpidem tartrate *see* zolpidem *on page 996*

Zometa® [US/Can] *see* zoledronic acid *on page 995*

Zomig® [US/Can] *see* zolmitriptan *on page 995*

Zomig® Nasal Spray [Can] *see* zolmitriptan *on page 995*

Zomig® Rapimelt [Can] *see* zolmitriptan *on page 995*

Zomig-ZMT® [US] *see* zolmitriptan *on page 995*

Zomorph® [Can] *see* morphine sulfate *on page 643*

Zonalon® [US/Can] *see* doxepin *on page 321*

Zonegran® [US/Can] *see* zonisamide *on page 996*

zonisamide (zoe NIS a mide)

U.S./Canadian Brand Names Zonegran® [US/Can]

Therapeutic Category Anticonvulsant, Sulfonamide

Use Adjunct treatment of partial seizures in children >16 years of age and adults with epilepsy

Usual Dosage Oral: Children >16 years and Adults: Adjunctive treatment of partial seizures: Initial: 100 mg/day; dose may be increased to 200 mg/day after 2 weeks. Further dosage increases to 300 mg/day and 400 mg/day can then be made with a minimum of 2 weeks between adjustments, in order to reach steady state at each dosage level. Doses of up to 600 mg/day have been studied, however, there is no evidence of increased response with doses above 400 mg/day.

Dosage Forms

Capsule: 25 mg, 50 mg, 100 mg

Zonegran®: 25 mg, 100 mg

zopiclone *(Canada only)* (ZOE pi clone)

U.S./Canadian Brand Names Apo-Zopiclone® [Can]; CO Zopiclone [Can]; Dom-Zopiclone [Can]; Gen-Zopiclone [Can]; Imovane® [Can]; Novo-Zopiclone [Can]; Nu-Zopiclone [Can]; PMS-Zopiclone [Can]; RAN™-Zopiclone [Can]; Ratio-Zopiclone [Can]; Rhovane® [Can]; Rhoxal-zopiclone [Can]; Riva-Zopiclone [Can]; Sandoz-Zopiclone [Can]

Therapeutic Category Hypnotic

Use Symptomatic relief of transient and short-term insomnia

Usual Dosage Administer just before bedtime: Oral: Adults: 5-7.5 mg
Patients with chronic respiratory insufficiency: 3.75 mg; may increase up to 7.5 mg with caution in appropriate cases

Dosage Forms [CAN] = Canadian brand name
Tablet: 5 mg, 7.5 mg [not available in the U.S.]
Apo-Zopiclone® [CAN], Gen-Zopiclone [CAN], Imovane® [CAN], Novo-Zopiclone [CAN], Nu-Zopiclone [CAN], PMS-Zopiclone [CAN], Rhovane® [CAN], Rhoxal-zopiclone [CAN]: 5 mg, 7.5 mg

Zorbtive® [US] *see* somatropin *on page 881*
Zorcaine™ [US/Can] *see* articaine and epinephrine *on page 95*
ZORprin® [US] *see* aspirin *on page 98*
Zostavax® [US] *see* zoster vaccine *on page 997*

zoster vaccine (ZOS ter vak SEEN)

Synonyms shingles vaccine; varicella-zoster (VZV) vaccine (zoster); VZV vaccine (zoster)
U.S./Canadian Brand Names Zostavax® [US]
Therapeutic Category Vaccine
Use Prevention of herpes zoster (shingles) in patients ≥60 years of age
The Advisory Committee on Immunization Practices (ACIP) recommends routine vaccination of all patients ≥60 years of age, including:
• Patients who report a previous episode of zoster.
• Patients with chronic medical conditions (eg, chronic renal failure, diabetes mellitus, rheumatoid arthritis, chronic pulmonary disease) unless those conditions are contraindications.
• Residents of nursing homes and other long-term care facilities ≥60 years of age, without contraindications.

Usual Dosage SubQ: Adults ≥60 years: 0.65 mL administered as a single dose; there is no data to support readministration of the vaccine

Dosage Forms
Injection, powder for reconstitution [preservative free]
Zostavax®: 19,400 plaque-forming units (PFU)

Zostrix® [US-OTC/Can] *see* capsaicin *on page 171*
Zostrix®-HP [US-OTC/Can] *see* capsaicin *on page 171*
Zosyn® [US] *see* piperacillin and tazobactam sodium *on page 756*
Zovia® [US] *see* ethinyl estradiol and ethynodiol diacetate *on page 371*
Zovirax® [US/Can] *see* acyclovir *on page 33*
Ztuss™ Tablet *(Discontinued)*
Ztuss™ ZT *(Discontinued)*
zuclopenthixol acetate *see* zuclopenthixol *(Canada only) on page 997*

zuclopenthixol *(Canada only)* (zoo kloe pen THIX ol)

Synonyms Z-chlopenthixol; zuclopenthixol acetate; zuclopenthixol decanoate; zuclopenthixol dihydrochloride
U.S./Canadian Brand Names Clopixol-Acuphase® [Can]; Clopixol® Depot [Can]; Clopixol® [Can]
Therapeutic Category Antipsychotic Agent
Use Management of schizophrenia; acetate injection is intended for short-term acute treatment; decanoate injection is for long-term management; dihydrochloride tablets may be used in either phase
Usual Dosage Adults:
Oral: Zuclopenthixol dihydrochloride: Initial: 20-30 mg/day in 2-3 divided doses; usual maintenance dose: 20-40 mg/day; maximum daily dose: 100 mg

▶

◀ I.M.:
Zuclopenthixol acetate: 50-150 mg; may be repeated in 2-3 days; no more than 4 injections should be given in the course of treatment; maximum dose during course of treatment: 400 mg (maximum treatment period: 2 weeks)
Transfer of patients from I.M. acetate to oral (tablets):
50 mg = 20 mg daily
100 mg = 40 mg daily
150 mg = 60 mg daily
Zuclopenthixol decanoate: 100 mg by deep I.M. injection; additional I.M. doses of 100-200 mg may be given over the following 1-4 weeks; maximum weekly dose: 600 mg; usual maintenance dose: 150-300 mg every 2 weeks
Transfer of patients from oral (tablets) to I.M. decanoate (depot):
≤20 mg daily = 100 mg every 2 weeks
25-40 mg daily = 200 mg every 2 weeks
50-75 mg daily = 300 mg every 2 weeks
>75 mg/day = 400 mg every 2 weeks
Transfer of patients from I.M. acetate to I.M. decanoate (depot):
50 mg every 2-3 days = 100 mg every 2 weeks
100 mg every 2-3 days = 200 mg every 2 weeks
150 mg every 2-3 days = 300 mg every 2 weeks
Dosage Forms [CAN] = Canadian brand name
Injection:
Clopixol Acuphase® [CAN]: 50 mg/mL [zuclopenthixol 42.5 mg/mL] (1 mL, 2 mL) [not available in the U.S.]
Clopixol® Depot [CAN]: 200 mg/mL [zuclopenthixol 144.4 mg/mL] (10 mL) [not available in the U.S.]
Tablet:
Clopixol® [CAN]: 10 mg, 25 mg, 40 mg [not available in the U.S.]

zuclopenthixol decanoate *see* zuclopenthixol *(Canada only) on page 997*
zuclopenthixol dihydrochloride *see* zuclopenthixol *(Canada only) on page 997*
Zyban® [US/Can] *see* bupropion *on page 152*
Zydone® [US] *see* hydrocodone and acetaminophen *on page 481*
Zyflo CR™ [US] *see* zileuton *on page 992*
Zyflo® *(Discontinued)* *see* zileuton *on page 992*
Zylet™ [US] *see* loteprednol and tobramycin *on page 579*
Zyloprim® [US/Can] *see* allopurinol *on page 47*
Zymar® [US/Can] *see* gatifloxacin *on page 436*
Zymase® *(Discontinued)* *see* pancrelipase *on page 718*
Zym-Fluconazole [Can] *see* fluconazole *on page 405*
Zymine®-D [US] *see* triprolidine and pseudoephedrine *on page 955*
Zyprexa® [US/Can] *see* olanzapine *on page 694*
Zyprexa® Zydis® [US/Can] *see* olanzapine *on page 694*
Zyrtec® [US-OTC] *see* cetirizine *on page 196*
Zyrtec-D 12 Hour® *(Discontinued)* *see* cetirizine and pseudoephedrine *on page 196*
Zyrtec® Allergy [US-OTC] *see* cetirizine *on page 196*
Zyrtec®, Children's Allergy [US-OTC] *see* cetirizine *on page 196*
Zyrtec®, Children's Hives Relief [US-OTC] *see* cetirizine *on page 196*
Zytram® XL [Can] *see* tramadol *on page 941*
Zytrec-D® Allergy & Congestion [US-OTC] *see* cetirizine and pseudoephedrine *on page 196*
Zyvox® [US] *see* linezolid *on page 567*
Zyvoxam® [Can] *see* linezolid *on page 567*

CHEMOTHERAPY REGIMENS

5 + 2

Use Leukemia, acute myeloid (induction)

Regimen
Cytarabine: I.V.: 100-200 mg/m^2/day continuous infusion days 1 to 5
[total dose/cycle = 500-1000 mg/m^2]
with
Daunorubicin: I.V.: 45 mg/m^2/day days 1 and 2
[total dose/cycle = 90 mg/m^2]

7 + 3 (Daunorubicin)

Use Leukemia, acute myeloid (induction)

Regimen
Cytarabine: I.V.: 100 mg/m^2/day continuous infusion days 1 to 7
[total dose/cycle = 700 mg/m^2]
Daunorubicin: I.V.: 45 mg/m^2/day days 1, 2, and 3
[total dose/cycle = 135 mg/m^2]
Administer one cycle only

7 + 3 (Idarubicin)

Use Leukemia, acute myeloid (induction)

Regimen
Cytarabine: I.V.: 100-200 mg/m^2/day continuous infusion days 1 to 7
[total dose/cycle = 700 - 1400 mg/m^2]
Idarubicin: I.V.: 12 mg/m^2/day days 1, 2, and 3
[total dose/cycle = 36 mg/m^2]
Administer one cycle only

7 + 3 (Mitoxantrone)

Use Leukemia, acute myeloid (induction)

Regimen
Cytarabine: I.V.: 100-200 mg/m^2/day continuous infusion days 1 to 7
[total dose/cycle = 700-1400 mg/m^2]
Mitoxantrone: I.V.: 12 mg/m^2/day days 1, 2, and 3
[total dose/cycle = 36 mg/m^2]
Administer one cycle only

7 + 3 + 7

Use Leukemia, acute myeloid

Regimen
Cytarabine: I.V.: 100 mg/m^2/day continuous infusion days 1 to 7
[total dose/cycle = 700 mg/m^2]
Daunorubicin: I.V.: 50 mg/m^2/day days 1, 2, and 3
[total dose/cycle = 150 mg/m^2]
Etoposide: I.V.: 75 mg/m^2/day days 1 to 7
[total dose/cycle = 525 mg/m^2]
Repeat cycle every 21 days; up to 3 cycles may be given based on individual response

8 in 1 (Brain Tumors)

Use Brain tumors

Regimen NOTE: Multiple variations are listed below.
Variation 1:
Methylprednisolone: I.V.: 300 mg/m^2 every 6 hours day 1 (3 doses)
[total dose/cycle = 900 mg/m^2]
Vincristine: I.V.: 1.5 mg/m^2 (maximum 2 mg) day 1
Lomustine: Oral: 75 mg/m^2 day 1
Procarbazine: Oral: 75 mg/m^2 day 1; 1 hour after methylprednisolone and vincristine
Hydroxyurea: Oral: 3000 mg/m^2 day 1; 2 hours after methylprednisolone and vincristine
Cisplatin: I.V.: 90 mg/m^2 day 1; 3 hours after methylprednisolone and vincristine
Cytarabine: I.V.: 300 mg/m^2 day 1; 9 hours after methylprednisolone and vincristine
Dacarbazine: I.V.: 150 mg/m^2 day 1; 12 hours after methylprednisolone and vincristine
Repeat cycle every 14 days

Variation 2:
  Methylprednisolone: I.V.: 300 mg/m² every 6 hours day 1 (3 doses)
    [total dose/cycle = 900 mg/m²]
  Vincristine: I.V.: 1.5 mg/m² (maximum 2 mg) day 1
  Lomustine: Oral: 75 mg/m² day 1
  Procarbazine: Oral: 75 mg/m² day 1; 1 hour after methylprednisolone and vincristine
  Hydroxyurea: Oral: 3000 mg/m² day 1; 2 hours after methylprednisolone and vincristine
  Cisplatin: I.V.: 60 mg/m² day 1; 3 hours after methylprednisolone and vincristine
  Cytarabine: I.V.: 300 mg/m² day 1; 9 hours after methylprednisolone and vincristine
  Cyclophosphamide: I.V.: 300 mg/m² day 1; 12 hours after methylprednisolone and vincristine
  Repeat cycle every 14 days

8 in 1 (Retinoblastoma)

Use Retinoblastoma
Regimen
  Vincristine: I.V.: 1.5 mg/m² day 1
  Methylprednisolone: I.V.: 300 mg/m² day 1
  Lomustine: Oral: 75 mg/m² day 1
  Procarbazine: Oral: 75 mg/m² day 1
  Hydroxyurea: Oral: 1500 mg/m² day 1
  Cisplatin: I.V.: 60 mg/m² day 1
  Cytarabine: I.V.: 300 mg/m² day 1
  Repeat cycle every 28 days

AAV (DD)

Use Wilms tumor
Regimen
  Dactinomycin: I.V.: 15 mcg/kg/day days 1 to 5 of weeks 0, 13, 26, 39, 52, and 65
    [total dose/cycle = 450 mcg/kg]
  Doxorubicin: I.V.: 20 mg/m²/day days 1, 2, and 3 of weeks 6, 19, 32, 45, and 58
    [total dose/cycle = 300 mg/m²]
  Vincristine: I.V.: 1.5 mg/m² day 1 of weeks 0-10, 13, 14, 26, 27, 39, 40, 52, 53, 65, and 66
    [total dose/cycle = 31.5 mg/m²]

ABVD

Use Lymphoma, Hodgkin disease
Regimen
  Doxorubicin: I.V.: 25 mg/m²/day days 1 and 15
    [total dose/cycle = 50 mg/m²]
  Bleomycin: I.V.: 10 units/m²/day days 1 and 15
    [total dose/cycle = 20 units/m²]
  Vinblastine: I.V.: 6 mg/m²/day days 1 and 15
    [total dose/cycle = 12 mg/m²]
  Dacarbazine: I.V.: 375 mg/m²/day days 1 and 15
    [total dose/cycle = 750 mg/m²]
  Repeat cycle every 28 days

AC

Use Breast cancer
Regimen NOTE: Multiple variations are listed below.
  Variation 1: AC (conventional):
  Doxorubicin: I.V.: 60 mg/m² day 1
    [total dose/cycle = 60 mg/m²]
  Cyclophosphamide: I.V.: 600 mg/m² day 1
    [total dose/cycle = 600 mg/m²]
  Repeat cycle every 21 days
  Variation 2:
  Cyclophosphamide: Oral: 200 mg/m²/day days 3 to 6
    [total dose/cycle = 800 mg/m²]
  Doxorubicin: I.V.: 40 mg/m² day 1
    [total dose/cycle = 40 mg/m²]
  Repeat cycle every 3 weeks for 3 cycles, then every 4 weeks

ACAV (J)

Use Wilms tumor

Regimen

Dactinomycin: I.V.: 15 mcg/kg/day days 1 to 5 of weeks 0, 13, 26, 39, 52, and 65
[total dose/cycle = 450 mcg/kg]
Cyclophosphamide: I.V.: 10 mg/kg/day days 1, 2, and 3 of weeks 0, 6, 13, 19, 26, 32, 39, 45, 52, 58, and 65
[total dose/cycle = 330 mg/kg]
Doxorubicin: I.V.: 20 mg/m^2/day days 1, 2, and 3 of weeks 6, 19, 32, 45, and 58
[total dose/cycle = 300 mg/m^2]
Vincristine: I.V.: 1.5 mg/m^2 day 1 of weeks 0-10, 13, 14, 19, 20, 26, 27, 32, 33, 39, 40, 45, 52, 53, 56, 57, 65, and 66
[total dose/cycle = 42 mg/m^2]

AC/Paclitaxel (Sequential)

Use Breast cancer

Regimen

Variation 1: AC + Paclitaxel (conventional):
Doxorubicin: I.V.: 60 mg/m^2 day 1
[total dose/cycle = 60 mg/m^2]
Cyclophosphamide: I.V.: 600 mg/m^2 day 1
[total dose/cycle = 600 mg/m^2]
Repeat cycle every 21 days for 4 cycles
followed by
Paclitaxel: I.V.: 175 mg/m^2 day 1
[total dose/cycle = 175 mg/m^2]
Repeat cycle every 21 days for 4 cycles
Variation 2: AC + Paclitaxel (dose dense):
Doxorubicin: I.V.: 60 mg/m^2 day 1
[total dose/cycle = 60 mg/m^2]
Cyclophosphamide: I.V.: 600 mg/m^2 day 1
[total dose/cycle = 600 mg/m^2]
Filgrastim: SubQ: 5 mcg/kg/day days 3 to 10
[total dose/cycle = 40 mcg/kg]
Repeat cycle every 14 days for 4 cycles
followed by
Paclitaxel: I.V.: 175 mg/m^2 day 1
[total dose/cycle = 175 mg/m^2]
Filgrastim: SubQ: 5 mcg/kg/day days 3 to 10
[total dose/cycle = 40 mcg/kg]
Repeat cycle every 14 days for 4 cycles

AC-Paclitaxel-Trastuzumab

Use Breast cancer

Regimen NOTE: Multiple variations are listed below.

Variation 1:
Doxorubicin: I.V.: 60 mg/m^2 day 1
[total dose/cycle = 60 mg/m^2]
Cyclophosphamide: I.V.: 600 mg/m^2 day 1
[total dose/cycle = 600 mg/m^2]
Repeat cycle every 21 days for 4 cycles
followed by
Paclitaxel: I.V.: 175 mg/m^2 day 1
[total dose/cycle = 175 mg/m^2]
Trastuzumab: I.V.: 4 mg/kg (loading dose) day 1 (cycle 1 only)
[total dose/cycle = 4 mg/kg]
followed by I.V.: 2 mg/kg/day days 8 and 15 (cycle 1)
[total dose/cycle = 4 mg/kg]
then I.V.: 2 mg/kg/day days 1, 8, and 15 (cycles 2, 3, and 4)
[total dose/cycle = 6 mg/kg]
Repeat cycle every 21 days for 4 cycles
followed by
Trastuzumab: I.V.: 2 mg/kg weekly for 40 weeks

Variation 2:
  Doxorubicin: I.V.: 60 mg/m^2 day 1
    [total dose/cycle = 60 mg/m^2]
  Cyclophosphamide: I.V.: 600 mg/m^2 day 1
    [total dose/cycle = 600 mg/m^2]
  Repeat cycle every 21 days for 4 cycles
  followed by
  Paclitaxel: I.V.: 80 mg/m^{2}day 1 week 13
    [total dose/cycle = 80 mg/m^2]
  Trastuzumab: I.V.: 4 mg/kg (loading dose) day 1 week 13 only
    [total dose/cycle = 4 mg/kg]
  followed by
  Paclitaxel: I.V.: 80 mg/m^2 weekly
    [total dose/cycle = 80 mg/m^2]
  Trastuzumab: I.V.: 2 mg/kg /weekly
    [total dose/cycle = 2 mg/kg]
  Repeat cycle every week for 11 cycles
  followed by
  Trastuzumab: I.V.: 2 mg/kg /weekly for 40 weeks

AD

Use Soft tissue sarcoma
Regimen
  Doxorubicin: I.V.: 60 mg/m^2/day day 1
    [total dose/cycle = 60 mg/m^2]
  Dacarbazine: I.V.: 250 mg/m^2/day days 1 to 5
    [total dose/cycle = 1250 mg/m^2]
  Repeat cycle every 21 days

AI

Use Soft tissue sarcoma
Regimen NOTE: Multiple variations are listed below.
  Variation 1:
  Doxorubicin: I.V.: 25 mg/m^2/day continuous infusion days 1, 2, and 3
    [total dose/cycle = 75 mg/m^2]
  Ifosfamide: I.V.: 2 g/m^2/day days 1 to 5
    [total dose/cycle = 10 g/m^2]
  Mesna: I.V.: 400 mg/m^2 day 1
    followed by I.V.: 1200 mg/m^2/day continuous infusion days 1 to 5
      [total dose/cycle = 6400 mg/m^2]
  Repeat cycle every 3 weeks
  Variation 2:
  Doxorubicin: I.V.: 30 mg/m^2/day continuous infusion days 1, 2, and 3
    [total dose/cycle = 90 mg/m^2]
  Ifosfamide: I.V.: 2.5 g/m^2 /day days 1 to 4
    [total dose/cycle = 10 g/m^2]
  Mesna: I.V.: 500 mg/m^2 day 1
    followed by I.V.: 1500 mg/m^2/day continuous infusion days 1 to 4
      [total dose/cycle = 6500 mg/m^2]
  Filgrastim: SubQ: 5 mcg/kg/day days 5 through ANC recovery
  Repeat cycle every 3 weeks

AP

Use Endometrial cancer
Regimen
  Doxorubicin: I.V.: 60 mg/m^2 day 1
    [total dose/cycle = 60 mg/m^2]
  Cisplatin: I.V.: 60 mg/m^2 day 1
    [total dose/cycle = 60 mg/m^2]
  Repeat cycle every 21-28 days

AT

Use Breast cancer

Regimen NOTE: Multiple variations are listed below.
Variation 1:
Doxorubicin: I.V.: 50 mg/m^2 day 1
[total dose/cycle = 50 mg/m^2]
Docetaxel: I.V.: 75 mg/m^2 day 1
[total dose/cycle = 75 mg/m^2]
Repeat cycle every 3 weeks
Variation 2:
Doxorubicin: I.V.: 60 mg/m^2 day 1
[total dose/cycle = 60 mg/m^2]
Docetaxel: I.V.: 60 mg/m^2
[total dose/cycle = 60 mg/m^2]
Repeat cycle every 3 weeks
Variation 3:
Doxorubicin: I.V.: 50 mg/m^2 day 1
[total dose/cycle = 50 mg/m^2]
Docetaxel: I.V.: 75 mg/m^2 day 1
[total dose/cycle = 75 mg/m^2]
Repeat cycle every 14 days
Variation 4:
Doxorubicin: I.V.: 50 mg/m^2 day 1
[total dose/cycle = 50 mg/m^2]
Docetaxel: I.V.: 60 mg/m^2 day 1
[total dose/cycle = 60 mg/m^2]
Repeat cycle every 3 weeks
Variation 5:
Doxorubicin: I.V.: 50 mg/m^2 day 1
[total dose/cycle = 50 mg/m^2]
Docetaxel: I.V.: 60 mg/m^2 day 1
[total dose/cycle = 60 mg/m^2]
Repeat cycle every 3-4 weeks
Variation 6:
Doxorubicin: I.V.: 56 mg/m^2 day 1
[total dose/cycle = 56 mg/m^2]
Docetaxel: I.V.: 75 mg/m^2 day 1
[total dose/cycle = 75 mg/m^2]
Repeat cycle every 3 weeks
Variation 7:
Doxorubicin: I.V.: 50 mg/m^2 day 1
[total dose/cycle = 50 mg/m^2]
Docetaxel: I.V.: 75 mg/m^2 day 2
[total dose/cycle = 75 mg/m^2]
Repeat cycle every 4 weeks

AVD

Use Wilms tumor

Regimen
Dactinomycin: I.V.: 15 mcg/kg/day days 1 to 5 of weeks 0, 13, 26, 39, 52, and 65
[total dose/cycle = 450 mcg/kg]
Doxorubicin: I.V.: 60 mg/m^2/day day 1 of weeks 6, 19, 32, 45, and 58
[total dose/cycle = 300 mg/m^2]
Vincristine: I.V.: 1.5 mg/m^2 day 1 of weeks 1 to 8, 13, 14, 26, 27, 39, 40, 52, 53, 65, and 66
[total dose/cycle = 27 mg/m^2]

AV (EE)

Use Wilms tumor

Regimen
Dactinomycin: I.V.: 15 mcg/kg/day days 1 to 5 of weeks 0, 5, 13, and 26
[total dose/cycle = 300 mcg/kg]
Vincristine: I.V.: 1.5 mg/m^2/dose day 1 of weeks 1 to 10, and days 1 and 5 of weeks 13 and 26
[total dose/cycle = 21 mg/m^2]

AV (K)

Use Wilms tumor

Regimen
Dactinomycin: I.V.: 15 mcg/kg/day days 1 to 5 of weeks 0, 5, 13, 22, 31, 40, 49, and 58
[total dose/cycle = 600 mcg/kg]
Vincristine: I.V.: 1.5 mg/m^2/dose day 1 of weeks 0-10, 15-20, 24-29, 33-38, 42-47, 51-56, and 60-65
[total dose/cycle = 70.5 mg/m^2]

AV (L)

Use Wilms tumor

Regimen
Dactinomycin: I.V.: 15 mcg/kg/day days 1 to 5 of weeks 0 and 5
[total dose/cycle = 150 mcg/kg]
Vincristine: I.V.: 1.5 mg/m^2 day 1 of weeks 0-10
[total dose/cycle = 16.5 mg/m^2]

AV (Wilms Tumor)

Use Wilms tumor

Regimen
Dactinomycin: I.V.: 15 mcg/kg/day days 1 to 5 of weeks 0, 13, 26, 39, 52, and 65
[total dose/cycle = 450 mcg/kg]
Vincristine: I.V.: 1.5 mg/m^2/dose day 1 of weeks 1 to 8, 13, 14, 26, 27, 39, 40, 52, 53, 65, and 66
[total dose/cycle = 27 mg/m^2]

BEACOPP

Use Lymphoma, Hodgkin disease

Regimen
Bleomycin: I.V.: 10 units/m^2 day 8
[total dose/cycle = 10 units/m^2]
Etoposide: I.V.: 100 mg/m^2/day days 1, 2 and 3
[total dose/cycle = 300 mg/m^2]
Doxorubicin: I.V.: 25 mg/m^2 day 1
[total dose/cycle = 25 mg/m^2]
Cyclophosphamide: I.V.: 650 mg/m^2 day 1
[total dose/cycle = 650 mg/m^2]
Vincristine: I.V.: 1.4 mg/m^2 (maximum 2 mg) day 8
[total dose/cycle = 1.4 mg/m^2; maximum 2 mg]
Procarbazine: Oral: 100 mg/m^2/day days 1 to 7
[total dose/cycle = 700 mg/m^2]
Prednisone: Oral: 40 mg/m^2/day days 1 to 14
[total dose/cycle = 560 mg/m^2]
Repeat cycle every 21 days

Bendamustine-Rituximab

Use Lymphoma, non-Hodgkin (Mantle cell or low-grade NHL)

Regimen
Pretreatment:
Rituximab: I.V.: 375 mg/m^2 1 week before the start of cycle 1
[total dose/pretreatment = 375 mg/m^2]
Cycles:
Rituximab: I.V.: 375 mg/m^2 day 1
[total dose/cycle = 375 mg/m^2]
Bendamustine: I.V.: 90 mg/m^2 days 2 and 3
[total dose/cycle = 180 mg/m^2]
Repeat cycle every 4 weeks for up to 4 cycles
Post-Treatment:
Rituximab: I.V.: 375 mg/m^2 4 weeks after the last cycle
[total dose/post-treatment = 375 mg/m^2]

BEP (Ovarian Cancer)

Use Ovarian cancer

Regimen
Bleomycin: I.V.: 20 units/m^2 (maximum 30 units) day 1
  [total dose/cycle = 20 units/m^2]
Etoposide: I.V.: 75 mg/m^2/day days 1 to 5
  [total dose/cycle = 375 mg/m^2]
  or 75 mg/m^2/day days 1 to 4 (if received prior radiation therapy)
    [total dose/cycle = 300 mg/m^2]
Cisplatin: I.V.: 20 mg/m^2/day days 1 to 5
  [total dose/cycle = 100 mg/m^2]
Repeat cycle every 3 weeks for 4 cycles

BEP (Ovarian Cancer, Testicular Cancer)

Use Ovarian cancer; Testicular cancer

Regimen
Bleomycin: I.V.: 30 units/day days 2, 9, and 16
  [total dose/cycle = 90 units]
Etoposide: I.V.: 100 mg/m^2/day days 1 to 5
  [total dose/cycle = 500 mg/m^2]
  or 120 mg/m^2/day days 1, 2, and 3
    [total dose/cycle = 360 mg/m^2]
Cisplatin: I.V.: 20 mg/m^2/day days 1 to 5
  [total dose/cycle = 100 mg/m^2]
Repeat cycle every 21 days

BEP (Testicular Cancer)

Use Testicular cancer

Regimen NOTE: Multiple variations are listed below.
Variation 1:
  Bleomycin: I.V.: 30 units/day days 2, 9, and 16
    [total dose/cycle = 90 units]
  Etoposide: I.V.: 100 mg/m^2/day days 1 to 5
    [total dose/cycle = 500 mg/m^2]
  Cisplatin: I.V.: 20 mg/m^2/day days 1 to 5
    [total dose/cycle = 100 mg/m^2]
  Repeat cycle every 21 days
Variation 2:
  Bleomycin: I.V.: 30 units once weekly
    [total dose/cycle = 90 units]
  Etoposide: I.V.: 120 mg/m^2/day days 1, 3, and 5
    [total dose/cycle = 360 mg/m^2]
  Cisplatin: I.V.: 20 mg/m^2/day days 1 to 5
    [total dose/cycle = 100 mg/m^2]
  Repeat cycle every 21 days
Variation 3:
  Bleomycin: I.V.: 30 units/day days 1, 8, and 15
    [total dose/cycle = 90 units]
  Etoposide: I.V.: 165 mg/m^2/day days 1, 2, and 3
    [total dose/cycle = 495 mg/m^2]
  Cisplatin: I.V.: 50 mg/m^2/day days 1 and 2
    [total dose/cycle = 100 mg/m^2]
  Repeat cycle every 21 days

Bevacizumab-Capecitabine

Use Breast cancer

Regimen
Capecitabine: Oral: 1250 mg/m^2 twice daily days 1 to 14
  [total dose/cycle = 35,000 mg/m^2]
Bevacizumab: I.V.: 15 mg/kg/day day 1
  [total dose/cycle = 15 mg/kg]
Repeat cycle every 21 days for up to 35 cycles

Bevacizumab-Fluorouracil-Leucovorin

Use Colorectal cancer

Regimen
Bevacizumab: I.V.: 5 mg/kg/day days 1, 15, 29, and 43
[total dose/cycle = 20 mg/kg]
Leucovorin: I.V.: 500 mg/m^2/day days 1, 8, 15, 22, 29, and 36
[total dose/cycle = 3000 mg/m^2]
Fluorouracil: I.V.: 500 mg/m^2/day days 1, 8, 15, 22, 29, and 36
[total dose/cycle = 3000 mg/m^2]
Repeat cycle every 56 days

Bevacizumab-Interferon Alfa-2a

Use Renal cell cancer

Regimen
Interferon Alfa-2a: SubQ: 9 million units 3 times/week
[total dose/cycle = 54 million units]
Bevacizumab: I.V.: 10 mg/kg/day day 1
[total dose/cycle = 10 mg/kg]
Repeat cycle every 14 days for up to 1 year or until disease progression

Bevacizumab-Irinotecan-Fluorouracil-Leucovorin

Use Colorectal cancer

Regimen
Bevacizumab: I.V.: 5 mg/kg/day days 1, 15, and 29
[total dose/cycle = 15 mg/kg]
Irinotecan: I.V.: 125 mg/m^2/day days 1, 8, 15, and 22
[total dose/cycle = 500 mg/m^2]
Fluorouracil: I.V.: 500 mg/m^2/day days 1, 8, 15, and 22
[total dose/cycle = 2000 mg/m^2]
Leucovorin: I.V.: 20 mg/m^2/day days 1, 8, 15, and 22
[total dose/cycle = 80 mg/m^2]
Repeat cycle every 42 days

Bevacizumab-Irinotecan (Glioblastoma)

Use Brain tumors

Regimen Note: Patients receiving concurrent antiepileptic enzyme-inducing drugs received an increased dose of irinotecan (340 mg/m^2/dose).
Bevacizumab: I.V.: 10 mg/kg day 1
[total dose/cycle = 10 mg/kg]
Irinotecan: I.V.: 125 mg/m^2 day 1
[total dose/cycle = 125 mg/m^2]
Repeat cycle every 14 days

Bevacizumab-Oxaliplatin-Fluorouracil-Leucovorin

Use Colorectal cancer

Regimen
Bevacizumab: I.V.: 10 mg/kg day 1
[total dose/cycle = 10 mg/kg]
Oxaliplatin: I.V.: 85 mg/m^2 day 1
[total dose/cycle = 85 mg/m^2]
Leucovorin: I.V.: 200 mg/m^2/day days 1 and 2
[total dose/cycle = 400 mg/m^2]
Fluorouracil: I.V. bolus: 400 mg/m^2/day days 1 and 2
followed by I.V.: 600 mg/m^2 continuous infusion over 22 hours days 1 and 2
[total dose/cycle = 2000 mg/m^2]
Repeat cycle every 14 days

Bicalutamide + LHRH-A

Use Prostate cancer

Regimen
Bicalutamide: Oral: 50 mg/day
[total dose/cycle = 50 mg]
with
Goserelin acetate: SubQ: 3.6 mg day 1
[total dose/cycle = 3.6 mg]
or
Leuprolide depot: I.M.: 7.5 mg day 1
[total dose/cycle = 7.5 mg]
Repeat cycle every 28 days

BIP

Use Cervical cancer

Regimen
Bleomycin: I.V.: 30 units continuous infusion day 1
[total dose/cycle = 30 units]
Cisplatin: I.V.: 50 mg/m^2 day 2
[total dose/cycle = 50 mg/m^2]
Ifosfamide: I.V.: 5 g/m^2 continuous infusion day 2
[total dose/cycle = 5 g/m^2]
Mesna: I.V.: 6 g/m^2 continuous infusion over 36 hours day 2 (start with ifosfamide)
[total dose/cycle = 6 g/m^2]
Repeat cycle every 21 days

BOLD

Use Melanoma

Regimen
Dacarbazine: I.V.: 200 mg/m^2/day days 1 to 5
[total dose/cycle = 1000 mg/m^2]
Vincristine: I.V.: 1 mg/m^2/day days 1 and 4
[total dose/cycle = 2 mg/m^2]
Bleomycin: I.V.: 15 units/day days 2 and 5
[total dose/cycle = 30 units]
Lomustine: Oral: 80 mg day 1
[total dose/cycle = 80 mg]
Repeat cycle every 4 weeks

BOLD + Interferon

Use Melanoma

Regimen NOTE: Multiple variations are listed below.
Variation 1:
Bleomycin: I.V.: 15 units/day days 2 and 5
[total dose/cycle = 30 units]
Vincristine: I.V.: 1 mg/m^2/day days 1 and 4
[total dose/cycle = 2 mg/m^2]
Lomustine: Oral: 80 mg day 1
[total dose/cycle = 80 mg]
Dacarbazine: I.V.: 200 mg/m^2/day days 1 to 5
[total dose/cycle = 1000 mg/m^2]
Interferon Alfa-2b: SubQ: 3 million units/day days 8 to 49 (cycles 1 and 2)
[total dose through day 49 = 126 million units]
followed by SubQ: 6 million units 3 times/week (beginning day 50 and subsequent cycles)
[total dose/cycle = 72 million units]
Repeat cycle every 4 weeks
Variation 2:
Bleomycin: I.V.: 30 units day 1
[total dose/cycle = 30 units]
Vincristine: I.V.: 2 mg day 1
[total dose/cycle = 2 mg]

Lomustine: Oral: 80 mg day 1
[total dose/cycle = 80 mg]
Dacarbazine: I.V.: 700 mg/m^2 day 1
[total dose/cycle = 700 mg/m^2]
Interferon Alfa-2b: SubQ: 3 million units 3 times/week
[total dose/cycle = 36 million units]
Repeat cycle every 4 weeks
Variation 3:
Bleomycin: I.V.: 15 units/day days 2 and 5
[total dose/cycle = 30 units]
Vincristine: I.V.: 1-2 mg/day days 1 and 4
[total dose/cycle = 2-4 mg]
Lomustine: Oral: 80 mg day 1
[total dose/cycle = 80 mg]
Dacarbazine: I.V.: 200 mg/m^2/day days 1 to 5
[total dose/cycle = 1000 mg/m^2]
Interferon Alfa-2b: SubQ: 6 million units 3 times/week, for 6 doses, starting day 8
[total dose/cycle = 36 million units]
Repeat cycle every 4 weeks
Variation 4:
Bleomycin: I.V.: 15 units/day days 2 and 5
[total dose/cycle = 30 units]
Vincristine: I.V.: 1 mg/m^2/day (maximum 2 mg/dose) days 1 and 4
[total dose/cycle = 2 mg/m^2]
Lomustine: Oral: 80 mg day 1
[total dose/cycle = 80 mg]
Dacarbazine: I.V.: 200 mg/m^2/day days 1 to 5
[total dose/cycle = 1000 mg/m^2]
Interferon Alfa-2b: SubQ: 3 million units/day days 8, 10, 12, 15, 17, and 19
[total dose/cycle = 18 million units]
Repeat cycle every 4 weeks

BOLD (Melanoma)

Use Melanoma

Regimen NOTE: Multiple variations are listed below.
Variation 1:
Bleomycin: SubQ: 7.5 units/day days 1 and 4 (cycle 1 only)
followed by SubQ: 15 units/day days 1 and 4 (subsequent cycles)
[total dose/cycle = 45 units; maximum total dose (all cycles) = 400 units]
Vincristine: I.V.: 1 mg/m^2/day days 1 and 5
[total dose/cycle = 2 mg/m^2]
Lomustine: Oral: 80 mg/m^2 (maximum 150 mg/dose) day 1
[total dose/cycle = 80 mg/m^2]
Dacarbazine: I.V.: 200 mg/m^2/day (maximum 400 mg/dose) days 1 to 5
[total dose/cycle = 1000 mg/m^2; maximum 2000 mg]
Repeat cycle every 4-6 weeks
Variation 2:
Bleomycin: I.V.: 15 units/day days 1 and 4
[total dose/cycle = 30 units]
Vincristine: I.V.: 1 mg/m^2/day days 1 and 5
[total dose/cycle = 2 mg/m^2]
Lomustine: Oral: 80 mg/m^2 (maximum 150 mg/dose) day 1
[total dose/cycle = 80 mg/m^2]
Dacarbazine: I.V.: 200 mg/m^2/day days 1 to 5
[total dose/cycle = 1000 mg/m^2]
Repeat cycle every 4 weeks
Variation 3:
Bleomycin: I.V.: 15 units/day days 1 and 4
[total dose/cycle = 30 units]
Vincristine: I.V.: 1 mg/m^2 day 1
[total dose/cycle = 1 mg/m^2]
Lomustine: Oral: 80 mg/m^2 day 3 (odd numbered cycles)
[total dose/cycle = 80 mg/m^2; every other cycle]

Dacarbazine: I.V.: 200 mg/m^2/day days 1 to 5
[total dose/cycle = 1000 mg/m^2]
Repeat cycle every 4 weeks

Bortezomib-Dexamethasone

Use Multiple myeloma

Regimen NOTE: Multiple variations are listed below.
  Variation 1:
   Cycles 1 and 2:
    Bortezomib: I.V.: 1.3 mg/m^2/day days 1, 4, 8, and 11
     [total dose/cycle = 5.2 mg/m^2]
    Dexamethasone: Oral: 40 mg/day days 1 to 4 and days 9 to 12
     [total dose/cycle = 320 mg]
    Treatment cycle is 21 days
   Cycles 3 and 4:
    Bortezomib: I.V.: 1.3 mg/m^2/day days 1, 4, 8, and 11
     [total dose/cycle = 5.2 mg/m^2]
    Dexamethasone: Oral: 40 mg/day days 1 to 4
     [total dose/cycle = 160 mg]
    Treatment cycle is 21 days
  Variation 2:
   Cycles 1 and 2:
    Bortezomib: I.V.: 1.3 mg/m^2/day days 1, 4, 8, and 11
     [total dose/cycle = 5.2 mg/m^2]
    Treatment cycle is 21 days
   Cycles 3 through 6 (begin dexamethasone after cycle 2 if partial response not achieved or after cycle 4 if complete response not achieved):
    Bortezomib: I.V.: 1.3 mg/m^2/day days 1, 4, 8, and 11
     [total dose/cycle = 5.2 mg/m^2]
    Dexamethasone: Oral: 40 mg/day days 1 and 2
     [total dose/cycle = 80 mg]
    Treatment cycle is 21 days (for up to a total of 6 cycles)

Bortezomib-Doxorubicin-Dexamethasone

Use Multiple myeloma

Regimen NOTE: Multiple variations are listed below.
  Variation 1:
   Cycle 1:
    Bortezomib: I.V.: 1.3 mg/m^2/day days 1, 4, 8, and 11
     [total dose/cycle = 5.2 mg/m^2]
    Dexamethasone: Oral: 40 mg/day days 1 to 4, 8 to 11, and 15 to 18
     [total dose/cycle = 480 mg]
    Doxorubicin: I.V.: 4.5 or 9 mg/m^2/day days 1 to 4
     [total dose/cycle = 18-36 mg/m^2]
    Treatment cycle is 21 days
   Cycles 2-4:
    Bortezomib: I.V.: 1.3 mg/m^2/day days 1, 4, 8, and 11
     [total dose/cycle = 5.2 mg/m^2]
    Dexamethasone: Oral: 40 mg/day days 1 to 4
     [total dose/cycle = 160 mg]
    Doxorubicin: I.V.: 4.5 or 9 mg/m^2/day days 1 to 4
     [total dose/cycle = 18-36 mg/m^2]
    Treatment cycle is 21 days
  Variation 2:
   Cycle 1:
    Bortezomib: I.V.: 1 mg/m^2/day days 1, 4, 8, and 11
     [total dose/cycle = 4 mg/m^2]
    Dexamethasone: Oral: 40 mg/day days 1 to 4, 8 to 11, and 15 to 18
     [total dose/cycle = 480 mg]
    Doxorubicin: I.V.: 9 mg/m^2/day days 1 to 4
     [total dose/cycle = 36 mg/m^2]
    Treatment cycle is 21 days

Cycles 2-4:
   Bortezomib: I.V.: 1 mg/m^2/day days 1, 4, 8, and 11
      [total dose/cycle = 4 mg/m^2]
   Dexamethasone: Oral: 40 mg/day days 1 to 4
      [total dose/cycle = 160 mg]
   Doxorubicin: I.V.: 9 mg/m^2/day days 1 to 4
      [total dose/cycle = 36 mg/m^2]
   Treatment cycle is 21 days
Variation 3:
   Bortezomib: I.V.: 1.3 mg/m^2/day days 1, 4, 8, and 11
      [total dose/cycle = 5.2 mg/m^2]
   Dexamethasone: Oral: 40 mg/day days 1 to 4
      [total dose/cycle = 160 mg]
   Doxorubicin: I.V.: 20 mg/m^2/day days 1 and 4
      [total dose/cycle = 40 mg/m^2]
   Repeat cycle every 28 days for up to 6 cycles

Bortezomib-Doxorubicin (Liposomal)

Use Multiple myeloma
Regimen
   Bortezomib: I.V.: 1.3 mg/m^2/day days 1, 4, 8, and 11
      [total dose/cycle = 5.2 mg/m^2]
   Doxorubicin (liposomal): I.V.: 30 mg/m^2 day 4
      [total dose/cycle = 30 mg/m^2]
   Repeat cycle every 21 days for up to 8 cycles

Bortezomib-Doxorubicin (Liposomal)-Dexamethasone

Use Multiple myeloma
Regimen
   Bortezomib: I.V.: 1.3 mg/m^2/day days 1, 4, 8, and 11
      [total dose/cycle = 5.2 mg/m^2]
   Doxorubicin (Liposomal): I.V.: 30 mg/m^2/day day 1
      [total dose/cycle = 30 mg/m^2]
   Dexamethasone: Oral: 40 mg/day days 1 to 4
      [total dose/cycle = 160 mg]
   Repeat cycle every 28 days for up to 6 cycles

Bortezomib-Melphalan-Prednisone

Use Multiple myeloma
Regimen NOTE: Multiple variations are listed below.
Variation 1:
   Bortezomib: I.V.: 1.3 mg/m^2/day days 1, 4, 8, 11, 22, 25, 29, and 32
      [total dose/cycle = 10.4 mg/m^2]
   Melphalan: Oral: 9 mg/m^2/day days 1 to 4
      [total dose/cycle = 36 mg/m^2]
   Prednisone: Oral: 60 mg/m^2/day days 1 to 4
      [total dose/cycle = 240 mg/m^2]
   Repeat cycle every 42 days for 4 cycles
   followed by
   Bortezomib: I.V.: 1.3 mg/m^2/day days 1, 8, 22, and 29
      [total dose/cycle = 5.2 mg/m^2]
   Melphalan: Oral: 9 mg/m^2/day days 1 to 4
      [total dose/cycle = 36 mg/m^2]
   Prednisone: Oral: 60 mg/m^2/day days 1 to 4
      [total dose/cycle = 240 mg/m^2]
   Repeat cycle every 42 days for 5 cycles
Variation 2:
   Bortezomib: I.V.: 1-1.3 mg/m^2/day days 1, 4, 8, 11, 22, 25, 29, and 32
      [total dose/cycle = 8-10.4 mg/m^2]
   Melphalan: Oral: 9 mg/m^2/day days 1 to 4
      [total dose/cycle = 36 mg/m^2]

◀ Prednisone: Oral: 60 mg/m^2/day days 1 to 4
  [total dose/cycle = 240 mg/m^2]
Repeat cycle every 42 days for 4 cycles
followed by
Bortezomib: I.V.: 1-1.3 mg/m^2/day days 1, 8, 15, and 22
  [total dose/cycle = 4-5.2 mg/m^2]
Melphalan: Oral: 9 mg/m^2/day days 1 to 4
  [total dose/cycle = 36 mg/m^2]
Prednisone: Oral: 60 mg/m^2/day days 1 to 4
  [total dose/cycle = 240 mg/m^2]
Repeat cycle every 35 days for 5 cycles

Bortezomib-Melphalan-Prednisone-Thalidomide

Use Multiple myeloma
Regimen
Bortezomib: I.V.: 1-1.3 mg/m^2/day days 1, 4, 15, and 22
  [total dose/cycle = 4-5.2 mg/m^2]
Melphalan: Oral: 6 mg/m^2/day days 1 to 5
  [total dose/cycle = 30 mg/m^2]
Prednisone: Oral: 60 mg/m^2/day days 1 to 5
  [total dose/cycle = 300 mg/m^2]
Thalidomide: Oral: 50 mg/day days 1 to 35
  [total dose/cycle = 1750 mg]
Repeat cycle every 35 days for 6 cycles

CA

Use Leukemia, acute myeloid
Regimen
Cytarabine: I.V.: 3000 mg/m^2 every 12 hours days 1 and 2 (4 doses)
  [total dose/cycle = 12,000 mg/m^2]
Asparaginase: I.M.: 6000 units/m^2 at hour 42
  [total dose/cycle = 6000 units/m^2]
Repeat cycle every 7 days for 2 or 3 cycles

CABO

Use Head and neck cancer
Regimen
Cisplatin: I.V.: 50 mg/m^2 day 4
  [total dose/cycle = 50 mg/m^2]
Methotrexate: I.V.: 40 mg/m^2/day days 1 and 15
  [total dose/cycle = 80 mg/m^2]
Bleomycin: I.V.: 10 units/day days 1, 8, and 15
  [total dose/cycle = 30 units]
Vincristine: I.V.: 2 mg/day days 1, 8, and 15
  [total dose/cycle = 6 mg]
Repeat cycle every 21 days

CAD/MOPP/ABV

Use Lymphoma, Hodgkin disease
Regimen
CAD:
  Lomustine: Oral: 100 mg/m^2 day 1
    [total dose/cycle = 100 mg/m^2]
  Melphalan: Oral: 6 mg/m^2/day days 1 to 4
    [total dose/cycle = 24 mg/m^2]
  Vindesine: I.V.: 3 mg/m^2/day day 1 and 8
    [total dose/cycle = 6 mg/m^2]
MOPP:
  Mechlorethamine: I.V.: 6 mg/m^2/day days 1 and 8
    [total dose/cycle = 12 mg/m^2]
  Vincristine: I.V.: 1.4 mg/m^2/day days 1 and 8
    [total dose/cycle = 2.8 mg/m^2]

Procarbazine: Oral: 100 mg/m^2/day days 1 to 14
[total dose/cycle = 1400 mg/m^2]
Prednisone: Oral: 40 mg/m^2/day days 1 to 14
[total dose/cycle = 560 mg/m^2]
ABV:
Doxorubicin: I.V.: 25 mg/m^2/day days 1 and 14
[total dose/cycle = 50 mg/m^2]
Bleomycin: SubQ: 6 units/m^2/day days 1 and 14
[total dose/cycle = 12 units/m^2]
Vinblastine: I.V.: 2 mg/m^2 continuous infusion days 4 to 12 and 18 to 26
[total dose/cycle = 36 mg/m^2]
CAD is administered first, then MOPP begins on day 29 or day 37 following CAD. ABV is administered on day 29 following MOPP; CAD recycles on day 29 following ABV.

CAF

Use Breast cancer
Regimen NOTE: Multiple variations are listed below.
Variation 1:
Cyclophosphamide: Oral: 100 mg/m^2/day days 1 to 14
[total dose/cycle = 1400 mg/m^2]
Doxorubicin: I.V.: 30 mg/m^2/day days 1 and 8
[total dose/cycle = 60 mg/m^2]
Fluorouracil: I.V.: 500 mg/m^2/day days 1 and 8
[total dose/cycle = 1000 mg/m^2]
Repeat cycle every 28 days
Variation 2:
Cyclophosphamide: Oral: 100 mg/m^2/day days 1 to 14
[total dose/cycle = 1400 mg/m^2]
Doxorubicin: I.V.: 25 mg/m^2/day days 1 and 8
[total dose/cycle = 50 mg/m^2]
Fluorouracil: I.V.: 500 mg/m^2/day days 1 and 8
[total dose/cycle = 1000 mg/m^2]
Repeat cycle every 28 days

CAP

Use Bladder cancer
Regimen
Cyclophosphamide: I.V.: 400 mg/m^2 day 1
[total dose = 400 mg/m^2]
Doxorubicin: I.V.: 40 mg/m^2 day 1
[total dose = 40 mg/m^2]
Cisplatin: I.V.: 60 mg/m^2 day 1
[total dose = 60 mg/m^2]
Repeat cycle every 21 days

Capecitabine + Docetaxel (Breast Cancer)

Use Breast cancer
Regimen NOTE: Multiple variations are listed below.
Variation 1:
Capecitabine: Oral: 1250 mg/m^2 twice daily days 1 to 14
[total dose/cycle = 35,000 mg/m^2]
Docetaxel: I.V.: 75 mg/m^2 day 1
[total dose/cycle = 75 mg/m^2]
Repeat cycle every 3 weeks
Variation 2:
Capecitabine: Oral: 1000 mg/m^2 twice daily days 2 to 15
[total dose/cycle = 28,000 mg/m^2]
Docetaxel: I.V.: 75 mg/m^2 day 1
[total dose/cycle = 75 mg/m^2]
Repeat cycle every 3 weeks
Variation 3:
Capecitabine: Oral: 937.5 mg/m^2 twice daily days 2 to 15
[total dose/cycle = 26,250 mg/m^2]

▶

Docetaxel: I.V.: 60 mg/m^2 day 1
[total dose/cycle = 60 mg/m^2]
Repeat cycle every 3 weeks

Capecitabine + Docetaxel (Gastric Cancer)

Use Gastric cancer

Regimen NOTE: Multiple variations are listed below
Variation 1:
Capecitabine: Oral: 1000 mg/m^2 twice daily days 1 to 14
[total dose/cycle = 28,000 mg/m^2]
Docetaxel: I.V.: 75 mg/m^2 day 1
[total dose/cycle = 75 mg/m^2]
Repeat cycle every 3 weeks
Variation 2:
Capecitabine: Oral: 1000 mg/m^2 twice daily days 1 to 14
[total dose/cycle = 28,000 mg/m^2]
Docetaxel: I.V.: 36 mg/m^2 days 1 and 8
[total dose/cycle = 72 mg/m^2]
Repeat cycle every 3 weeks

Capecitabine + Docetaxel (Nonsmall Cell Lung Cancer)

Use Lung cancer, nonsmall cell

Regimen NOTE: Multiple variations are listed below
Variation 1:
Capecitabine: Oral: 1000 mg/m^2 twice daily days 1 to 14
[total dose/cycle = 28,000 mg/m^2]
Docetaxel: I.V.: 36 mg/m^2 days 1 and 8
[total dose/cycle = 72 mg/m^2]
Repeat cycle every 3 weeks
Variation 2:
Capecitabine: Oral: 625 mg/m^2 twice daily days 5 to 18
[total dose/cycle = 17,500 mg/m^2]
Docetaxel: I.V.: 36 mg/m^2 days 1, 8, and 15
[total dose/cycle = 108 mg/m^2]
Repeat cycle every 4 weeks

Capecitabine + Lapatinib

Use Breast cancer

Regimen
Capecitabine: Oral: 1000 mg/m^2 twice daily days 1 to 14
[total dose/cycle = 28,000 mg/m^2]
Lapatinib: Oral: 1250 mg/day days 1 to 21
[total dose/cycle = 26,250 mg]
Repeat cycle every 3 weeks

Capecitabine-Trastuzumab

Use Breast cancer

Regimen NOTE: Multiple variations are listed below.
Variation 1:
Cycle 1:
Capecitabine: Oral: 1250 mg/m^2 twice daily days 1 to 14
[total dose/cycle 1 = 35,000 mg/m^2]
Trastuzumab: I.V.: 4 mg/kg (loading dose) day 1 cycle 1
followed by I.V.: 2 mg/kg/day days 8 and 15 cycle 1
[total dose/cycle 1 = 8 mg/kg]
Treatment cycle is 21 days
Subsequent cycles:
Capecitabine: Oral: 1250 mg/m^2 twice daily days 1 to 14
[total dose/cycle = 35,000 mg/m^2]
Trastuzumab: I.V.: 2 mg/kg/day days 1, 8, and 15
[total dose/cycle = 6 mg/kg]
Repeat cycle every 21 days

Variation 2:
  Cycle 1:
    Capecitabine: Oral: 1250 mg/m^2 twice daily days 1 to 14
      [total dose/cycle 1 = 35,000 mg/m^2]
    Trastuzumab: I.V.: 8 mg/kg (loading dose) day 1 cycle 1
      [total dose/cycle 1 = 8 mg/kg]
    Treatment cycle is 21 days
  Subsequent cycles:
    Capecitabine: Oral: 1250 mg/m^2 twice daily days 1 to 14
      [total dose/cycle = 35,000 mg/m^2]
    Trastuzumab: I.V.: 6 mg/kg day 1
      [total dose/cycle = 6 mg/kg]
    Repeat cycle every 21 days

Carboplatin-Cetuximab

Use Head and neck cancer

Regimen
  Cycle 1:
    Cetuximab: I.V.: 400 mg/m^2 (loading dose) day 1 (week 1, cycle 1 only)
      [total loading dose = 400 mg/m^2]
      followed by I.V.: 250 mg/m^2/day days 8 and 15
        [total dose/cycle 1 = 900 mg/m^2]
    Carboplatin: I.V.: AUC 5 day 1
      [total dose/cycle = AUC = 5]
    Treatment cycle is 3 weeks
  Subsequent cycles:
    Cetuximab: I.V.: 250 mg/m^2/day days 1, 8, and 15
      [total dose/cycle = 750 mg/m^2]
    Carboplatin: I.V.: AUC 5 day 1
      [total dose/cycle = AUC = 5]
    Repeat cycle every 3 weeks

Carbo-Tax (Adenocarcinoma)

Use Adenocarcinoma, unknown primary

Regimen
  Paclitaxel: I.V.: 135 mg/m^2 infused over 24 hours day 1,
    [total dose = 135 mg/m^2]
  followed by
  Carboplatin: I.V.: Target AUC 7.5
    [total dose = AUC = 7.5]
  Repeat cycle every 21 days

Carbo-Tax (Nonsmall Cell Lung Cancer)

Use Lung cancer, nonsmall cell

Regimen
  Paclitaxel: I.V.: 135-215 mg/m^2 infused over 24 hours day 1
    [total dose/cycle = 135-215 mg/m^2]
    or I.V.: 175 mg/m^2 infused over 3 hours day 1
      [total dose/cycle = 175 mg/m^2]
  followed by
  Carboplatin: I.V.: Target AUC 7.5
    [total dose/cycle = AUC = 7.5]
  Repeat cycle every 21 days

Carbo-Tax (Ovarian Cancer)

Use Ovarian cancer

Regimen NOTE: Multiple variations are listed below.
  Variation 1:
    Paclitaxel: I.V.: 135 mg/m^2 infused over 24 hours day 1
      [total dose/cycle = 135 mg/m^2]
      or I.V.: 175 mg/m^2 infused over 3 hours day 1
        [total dose/cycle = 175 mg/m^2]

◀ **followed by**
  Carboplatin: I.V.: Target AUC 5
    [total dose/cycle = AUC = 5]
  Repeat cycle every 21 days
  Variation 2:
  Paclitaxel: I.V.: 175 mg/m^2 day 1
    [total dose/cycle = 175 mg/m^2]
  Carboplatin: I.V.: AUC 7.5 day 1
    [total dose/cycle = AUC = 7.5]
  Repeat cycle every 21 days
  Variation 3:
  Paclitaxel: I.V.: 185 mg/m^2 day 1
    [total dose/cycle = 185 mg/m^2]
  Carboplatin: I.V.: AUC 6 day 1
    [total dose/cycle = AUC = 6]
  Repeat cycle every 21 days

CaT (Nonsmall Cell Lung Cancer)

Use Lung cancer, nonsmall cell
Regimen NOTE: Multiple variations are listed below.
  Variation 1:
  Paclitaxel: I.V.: 175 mg/m^2 day 1
    [total dose/cycle = 175 mg/m^2]
      or 135 mg/m^2 continuous infusion day 1
        [total dose/cycle = 135 mg/m^2]
  Carboplatin: I.V.: AUC 7.5 day 1 or 2
    [total dose/cycle = AUC = 7.5]
  Repeat cycle every 21 days
  Variation 2:
  Paclitaxel: I.V.: 225 mg/m^2 day 1
    [total dose/cycle = 225 mg/m^2]
  Carboplatin: I.V.: AUC 6 day 1
    [total dose/cycle = AUC = 6]
  Repeat cycle every 21 days

CaT (Ovarian Cancer)

Use Ovarian cancer
Regimen
  Paclitaxel: I.V.: 175 mg/m^2 day 1
    [total dose/cycle = 175 mg/m^2]
      or 135 mg/m^2 continuous infusion day 1
        [total dose/cycle = 135 mg/m^2]
  Carboplatin: I.V.: AUC 7.5 day 1 or 2
    [total dose/cycle = AUC = 7.5]
  Repeat cycle every 21 days

CAVE

Use Lung cancer, small cell
Regimen
  Cyclophosphamide: I.V.: 750 mg/m^2 day 1
    [total dose/cycle = 750 mg/m^2]
  Doxorubicin: I.V.: 50 mg/m^2 day 1
    [total dose/cycle = 50 mg/m^2]
  Vincristine: I.V.: 1.4 mg/m^2 (maximum 2 mg) day 1
    [total dose/cycle = 1.4 mg/m^2]
  Etoposide: I.V.: 60-100 mg/m^2/day days 1, 2, and 3
    [total dose/cycle = 180-300 mg/m^2]
  Repeat cycle every 21 days

CAV-P/VP

Use Neuroblastoma

Regimen

Course 1, 2, 4, and 6:
  Cyclophosphamide: I.V.: 70 mg/kg/day days 1 and 2
  [total dose/cycle = 140 mg/kg]
  Doxorubicin: I.V.: 25 mg/m^2/day continuous infusion days 1, 2, and 3
  [total dose/cycle = 75 mg/m^2]
  Vincristine: I.V.: 0.033 mg/kg/day continuous infusion days 1, 2, and 3
  [total dose/cycle = 0.099 mg/kg]
  Vincristine: I.V.: 1.5 mg/m^2 day 9
  [total dose/cycle = 1.5 mg/m^2]
Course 3, 5, and 7:
  Etoposide: I.V.: 200 mg/m^2/day days 1, 2, and 3
  [total dose/cycle = 600 mg/m^2]
  Cisplatin: I.V.: 50 mg/m^2/day days 1 to 4
  [total dose/cycle = 200 mg/m^2]

CC

Use Ovarian cancer

Regimen

Carboplatin: I.V.: Target AUC 5-7.5 day 1
[total dose/cycle = AUC = 5-7.5]
Cyclophosphamide: I.V.: 600 mg/m^2 day 1
[total dose/cycle = 600 mg/m^2]
Repeat cycle every 28 days

CCCDE (Retinoblastoma)

Use Retinoblastoma

Regimen

Cyclophosphamide: I.V.: 150 mg/m^2/day days 1 to 7
[total dose/cycle = 1050 mg/m^2]
Cyclophosphamide: Oral: 150 mg/m^2/day days 22 to 28 and 43 to 49
[total dose/cycle = 2100 mg/m^2]
Doxorubicin: I.V.: 35 mg/m^2/day days 10 and 52
[total dose/cycle = 70 mg/m^2]
Cisplatin: I.V.: 90 mg/m^2/day days 8, 50, and 71
[total dose/cycle = 270 mg/m^2]
Etoposide: I.V.: 150 mg/m^2/day continuous infusion days 29 to 31 and 73 to 75
[total dose/cycle = 900 mg/m^2]

CCDDT (Neuroblastoma)

Use Neuroblastoma

Regimen

Cyclophosphamide: I.V.: 40 mg/kg/day days 1 and 2
[total dose/cycle = 80 mg/kg]
Cisplatin: I.V.: 20 mg/m^2/day days 1 to 5
[total dose/cycle = 100 mg/m^2]
Teniposide: I.V.: 100 mg/m^2 day 7
[total dose/cycle = 100 mg/m^2]
Doxorubicin: I.V.: 60 mg/m^2 day 1
[total dose/cycle = 60 mg/m^2]
Dacarbazine: I.V.: 250 mg/m^2/day days 1 to 5
[total dose/cycle = 1250 mg/m^2]
Repeat cycle every 21-28 days

CCDT (Melanoma)

Use Melanoma

Regimen

Dacarbazine: I.V.: 220 mg/m^2/day days 1, 2, and 3, every 21 to 28 days
[total dose/cycle = 660 mg/m^2]

Carmustine: I.V.: 150 mg/m^2 day 1, every 42 to 56 days
[total dose/cycle = 150 mg/m^2]
Cisplatin: I.V.: 25 mg/m^2/day days 1, 2, and 3, every 21 to 28 days
[total dose/cycle = 75 mg/m^2]
Tamoxifen: Oral: 20 mg/day (use of tamoxifen is optional)

CCT (Neuroblastoma)

Use Neuroblastoma
Regimen
Cyclophosphamide: I.V.: 40 mg/kg/day days 1 and 2
[total dose/cycle = 80 mg/kg]
Cisplatin: I.V.: 20 mg/m^2/day days 22 to 26
[total dose/cycle = 100 mg/m^2]
Teniposide: I.V.: 100 mg/m^2 day 28
[total dose/cycle = 100 mg/m^2]
Repeat every 42 days for 3 cycles

CDDP/VP-16

Use Brain tumors
Regimen
Cisplatin: I.V.: 90 mg/m^2 day 1
[total dose/cycle = 90 mg/m^2]
Etoposide: I.V.: 150 mg/m^2/day days 3 and 4
[total dose/cycle = 300 mg/m^2]
Repeat cycle every 21 days

CE-CAdO

Use Neuroblastoma
Regimen
Carboplatin: I.V.: 160 mg/m^2/day days 1 to 5
[total dose/cycle = 800 mg/m^2]
Etoposide: I.V.: 100 mg/m^2/day days 1 to 5
[total dose/cycle = 500 mg/m^2]
or
Carboplatin: I.V.: 200 mg/m^2/day days 1, 2, and 3
[total dose/cycle = 600 mg/m^2]
Etoposide: I.V.: 150 mg/m^2/day days 1, 2, and 3
[total dose/cycle = 450 mg/m^2]
and
Cyclophosphamide: I.V.: 300 mg/m^2/day days 1 to 5
[total dose/cycle = 1500 mg/m^2]
Doxorubicin: I.V.: 60 mg/m^2 day 5
[total dose/cycle = 60 mg/m^2]
Vincristine: I.V.: 1.5 mg/m^2/day days 1 and 5
[total dose/cycle = 3 mg/m^2]
Repeat cycle every 21 days

CEF

Use Breast cancer
Regimen
Cyclophosphamide: Oral: 75 mg/m^2/day days 1 to 14
[total dose/cycle = 1050 mg/m^2]
Epirubicin: I.V.: 60 mg/m^2/day days 1 and 8
[total dose/cycle = 120 mg/m^2]
Fluorouracil: I.V.: 500 mg/m^2/day days 1 and 8
[total dose/cycle = 1000 mg/m^2]
Repeat cycle every 28 days

CE (Neuroblastoma)

Use Neuroblastoma

Regimen
Carboplatin: I.V.: 500 mg/m^2/day days 1 and 2
  [total dose/cycle = 1000 mg/m^2]
Etoposide: I.V.: 100 mg/m^2/day days 1, 2, and 3
  [total dose/cycle = 300 mg/m^2]
Repeat cycle every 21-28 days

CEPP(B)

Use Lymphoma, non-Hodgkin

Regimen
Cyclophosphamide: I.V.: 600-650 mg/m^2/day days 1 and 8
  [total dose/cycle = 1200-1300 mg/m^2]
Etoposide: I.V.: 70-85 mg/m^2/day days 1, 2, and 3
  [total dose/cycle = 210-255 mg/m^2]
Procarbazine: Oral: 60 mg/m^2/day days 1 to 10
  [total dose/cycle = 600 mg/m^2]
Prednisone: Oral: 60 mg/m^2/day days 1 to 10
  [total dose/cycle = 600 mg/m^2]
Bleomycin: I.V.: 15 units/m^2/day days 1 and 15 (Bleomycin is sometimes omitted)
  [total dose/cycle = 30 units/m^2]
Repeat cycle every 28 days

CE (Retinoblastoma)

Use Retinoblastoma

Regimen
Etoposide: I.V.: 100 mg/m^2/day days 1 to 5
  [total dose/cycle = 500 mg/m^2]
Carboplatin: I.V.: 160 mg/m^2/day days 1 to 5
  [total dose/cycle = 800 mg/m^2]
Repeat cycle every 21 days

Cetuximab-FOLFOX4

Use Colorectal cancer

Regimen
Cycle 1:
  Cetuximab: I.V.: 400 mg/m^2 (loading dose) day 1 (week 1, cycle 1 only)
    followed by I.V.: 250 mg/m^2/day day 8
      [total dose/cycle 1 = 650 mg/m^2]
  Oxaliplatin: I.V.: 85 mg/m^2 (over 2 hours) day 1
    [total dose/cycle = 85 mg/m^2]
  Leucovorin: I.V.: 200 mg/m^2/day (over 2 hours) days 1 and 2
    [total dose/cycle = 400 mg/m^2]
  Fluorouracil: I.V. bolus: 400 mg/m^2/day days 1 and 2
    followed by I.V.: 600 mg/m^2 continuous infusion (over 22 hours) days 1 and 2
      [total dose/cycle = 2000 mg/m^2]
  Note: Bolus fluorouracil and continuous infusion are both given on each day.
  Treatment cycle is 14 days
Subsequent cycles:
  Cetuximab: I.V.: 250 mg/m^2/day days 1 and 8
    [total dose/cycle = 500 mg/m^2]
  Oxaliplatin: I.V.: 85 mg/m^2 day 1
    [total dose/cycle = 85 mg/m^2]
  Leucovorin: I.V.: 200 mg/m^2/day (over 2 hours) days 1 and 2
    [total dose/cycle = 400 mg/m^2]
  Fluorouracil: I.V. bolus: 400 mg/m^2/day days 1 and 2
    followed by I.V.: 600 mg/m^2 continuous infusion (over 22 hours) days 1 and 2
      [total dose/cycle = 2000 mg/m^2]
  Note: Bolus fluorouracil and continuous infusion are both given on each day.
  Repeat cycle every 14 days

Cetuximab-Irinotecan

Use Colorectal cancer

Regimen NOTE: Multiple variations are listed below.

Variation 1:

Cycle 1:

Cetuximab: I.V.: 400 mg/m^2 (loading dose) day 1 (week 1, cycle 1 only)
[total loading dose = 400 mg/m^2]
followed by I.V.: 250 mg/m^2/day days 8, 15, 22, 29, and 36
[total dose/cycle 1 = 1650 mg/m^2]
Irinotecan: I.V.: 125 mg/m^2/day days 1, 8, 15, and 22
[total dose/cycle = 500 mg/m^2]

Subsequent cycles:

Cetuximab: I.V.: 250 mg/m^2/day days 1, 8, 15, 22, 29, and 36
[total dose/cycle = 1500 mg/m^2]
Irinotecan: I.V.: 125 mg/m^2/day days 1, 8, 15, and 22
[total dose/cycle = 500 mg/m^2]
Repeat cycle every 42 days

Variation 2:

Cycle 1:

Cetuximab: I.V.: 400 mg/m^2 (loading dose) day 1 (week 1, cycle 1 only)
[total loading dose = 400 mg/m^2]
followed by I.V.: 250 mg/m^2/day days 8 and 15 (cycle 1)
[total dose/cycle 1 = 900 mg/m^2]
Irinotecan: I.V.: 350 mg/m^2 day 1
[total dose/cycle = 350 mg/m^2]

Subsequent cycles:

Cetuximab: I.V.: 250 mg/m^2/day days 1, 8, and 15
[total dose/cycle = 750 mg/m^2]
Irinotecan: I.V.: 350 mg/m^2 day 1
[total dose/cycle = 350 mg/m^2]
Repeat cycle every 21 days

CEV

Use Rhabdomyosarcoma

Regimen

Carboplatin: I.V.: 500 mg/m^2 day 1
[total dose/cycle = 500 mg/m^2]
Epirubicin: I.V.: 150 mg/m^2 day 1
[total dose/cycle = 150 mg/m^2]
Vincristine: I.V.: 1.5 mg/m^2/day days 1 and 7
[total dose/cycle = 3 mg/m^2]
Repeat cycle every 21 days

CF

Use Head and neck cancer

Regimen NOTE: Multiple variations are listed below.

Variation 1:

Cisplatin: I.V.: 100 mg/m^2 day 1
[total dose/cycle = 100 mg/m^2]
Fluorouracil: I.V.: 1000 mg/m^2/day continuous infusion days 1 to 4
[total dose/cycle = 4000 mg/m^2]
Repeat cycle every 3 or 4 weeks

Variation 2:

Cisplatin: I.V.: 100 mg/m^2 day 1
[total dose/cycle = 100 mg/m^2]
Fluorouracil: I.V.: 1000 mg/m^2/day continuous infusion days 1 to 5
[total dose/cycle = 5000 mg/m^2]
Repeat cycle every 3 or 4 weeks

Variation 3:

Cisplatin: I.V.: 60 mg/m^2 day 1
[total dose/cycle = 60 mg/m^2]

Fluorouracil: I.V.: 800 mg/m^2/day continuous infusion days 1 to 5
[total dose/cycle = 4000 mg/m^2]
Repeat cycle every 14 days
Variation 4:
Cisplatin: I.V.: 20 mg/m^2/day days 1 to 5
[total dose/cycle = 100 mg/m^2]
Fluorouracil: I.V.: 200 mg/m^2/day days 1 to 5
[total dose/cycle = 1000 mg/m^2]
Repeat cycle every 3 weeks
Variation 5:
Cisplatin: I.V.: 80 mg/m^2 continuous infusion day 1
[total dose/cycle = 80 mg/m^2]
Fluorouracil: I.V.: 800 mg/m^2/day continuous infusion days 2 to 6
[total dose/cycle = 4000 mg/m^2]
Repeat cycle every 3 weeks
Variation 6:
Cisplatin: I.V.: 75 mg/m^2 day 1
[total dose/cycle = 75 mg/m^2]
Fluorouracil: I.V.: 1000 mg/m^2/day continuous infusion days 1 to 4
[total dose/cycle = 4000 mg/m^2]
Repeat cycle every 4 weeks
Variation 7:
Cisplatin: I.V.: 120 mg/m^2 day 1
[total dose/cycle = 120 mg/m^2]
Fluorouracil: I.V.: 1000 mg/m^2/day continuous infusion days 1 to 5
[total dose/cycle = 5000 mg/m^2]
Repeat cycle every 3 weeks
Variation 8:
Cisplatin: I.V.: 25 mg/m^2/day continuous infusion days 1 to 4
[total dose/cycle = 100 mg/m^2]
Fluorouracil: I.V.: 1000 mg/m^2/day days 1 to 4
[total dose/cycle = 4000 mg/m^2]
Repeat cycle every 3 weeks
Variation 9:
Fluorouracil: I.V.: 350 mg/m^2/day continuous infusion days 1 to 5
[total dose/cycle = 1750 mg/m^2]
Cisplatin: I.V.: 50 mg/m^2 day 6
[total dose/cycle = 50 mg/m^2]
Repeat cycle every 3 weeks
Variation 10:
Cisplatin: I.V.: 5 mg/m^2/day continuous infusion days 1 to 14
[total dose/cycle = 70 mg/m^2]
Fluorouracil: I.V.: 200 mg/m^2/day continuous infusion days 1 to 14
[total dose/cycle = 2800 mg/m^2]
With concurrent radiation therapy, cycle does not repeat

CFP

Use Breast cancer
Regimen
Cyclophosphamide: I.V.: 150 mg/m^2/day days 1 to 5
[total dose/cycle = 750 mg/m^2]
Fluorouracil: I.V.: 300 mg/m^2/day days 1 to 5
[total dose/cycle = 1500 mg/m^2]
Prednisone: Oral: 30 mg/day days 1 to 14 (cycle 1 only)
followed by Oral: 20 mg/day days 15 to 21 (cycle 1 only)
followed by Oral: 10 mg daily thereafter as maintenance
[total dose/cycle = 700 mg in cycle 1; 350 mg in subsequent cycles]
Repeat cycle every 35 days

CHAMOCA (Modified Bagshawe Regimen)

Use Gestational trophoblastic tumor

Regimen NOTE: Multiple variations are listed below.

Variation 1:

Hydroxyurea: Oral: 500 mg every 6 hours, for 4 doses, day 1 (start at 6 AM)
[total dose/cycle = 2000 mg]

Dactinomycin: I.V.: 0.2 mg/day days 1, 2, and 3 (give at 7 PM)
followed by I.V.: 0.5 mg/day days 4 and 5 (give at 7 PM)
[total dose/cycle = 1.6 mg]

Cyclophosphamide: I.V.: 500 mg/m^2/day days 3 and 8 (give at 7 PM)
[total dose/cycle = 1000 mg/m^2]

Vincristine: I.V.: 1 mg/m^2 (maximum 2 mg) day 2 (give at 7 AM)
[total dose/cycle = 1 mg/m^2; maximum 2 mg]

Methotrexate: I.V. bolus: 100 mg/m^2 day 2 (give at 7 PM)
followed by I.V.: 200 mg/m^2 continuous infusion over 12 hours day 2
[total dose/cycle = 300 mg/m^2]

Leucovorin: I.M.: 14 mg every 6 hours, for 6 doses, days 3, 4, and 5 (begin at 7 PM on day 3; start 24 hours after the start of methotrexate)
[total dose/cycle = 84 mg]

Doxorubicin: I.V.: 30 mg/m^2 day 8 (give at 7 PM)
[total dose/cycle = 30 mg/m^2]

Repeat cycle every 18 days or as toxicity permits (cycle may be repeated 10 days after last treatment)

Variation 2:

Hydroxyurea: Oral: 500 mg every 12 hours, for 4 doses, days 1 and 2 (usually started in early morning)
[total dose/cycle = 2000 mg]

Dactinomycin: I.V.: 10 mcg/kg/day days 5, 6, and 7
[total dose/cycle = 30 mcg/kg]

Vincristine: I.V.: 1 mg/m^2 day 3
[total dose/cycle = 1 mg/m^2]

Methotrexate: I.V. bolus: 100 mg/m^2 day 3
followed by I.V.: 200 mg/m^2 continuous infusion over 12 hours day 3
[total dose/cycle = 300 mg/m^2]

Leucovorin: I.M.: 10 mg/m^2 every 12 hours, for 4 doses, days 4 and 5 (start 24 hours after the start of methotrexate)
[total dose/cycle = 40 mg/m^2]

Cyclophosphamide: I.V.: 600 mg/m^2 day 5
[total dose/cycle = 600 mg/m^2]

Doxorubicin: I.V.: 30 mg/m^2 day 10
[total dose/cycle = 30 mg/m^2]

Repeat cycle every 3 weeks

Variation 3:

Hydroxyurea: Oral: 500 mg every 12 hours, for 4 doses, days 1 and 2 (usually started in early morning)
[total dose/cycle = 2000 mg/m^2]

Vincristine: I.V.: 1 mg/m^2 day 3
[total dose/cycle = 1 mg/m^2]

Methotrexate: I.V. bolus: 100 mg/m^2 day 3
followed by I.V.: 200 mg/m^2 continuous infusion over 12 hours day 3
[total dose/cycle = 300 mg/m^2]

Leucovorin: I.M.: 14 mg every 6 hours, for 6 doses, days 4, 5, and 6 (start 24 hours after start of methotrexate)
[total dose/cycle = 84 mg]

Dactinomycin: I.V.: 0.2 mg/day days 2, 3, and 4
followed by I.V.: 0.5 mg/day days 5 and 6
[total dose/cycle = 1.6 mg]

Cyclophosphamide: I.V.: 500 mg/m^2 day 4
[total dose/cycle = 500 mg/m^2]

Doxorubicin: I.V.: 30 mg/m^2 day 9
[total dose/cycle = 30 mg/m^2]

Melphalan: I.V.: 6 mg/m^2 day 9
[total dose/cycle = 6 mg/m^2]

Repeat cycle approximately every 3 weeks

Variation 4:
Hydroxyurea: Oral: 500 mg 4 times/day, for 4 doses, day 1
[total dose/cycle = 2000 mg/m^2]
Vincristine: I.V.: 1 mg/m^2 day 2
[total dose/cycle = 1 mg/m^2]
Methotrexate: I.V. bolus: 100 mg/m^2 day 2
followed by I.V.: 200 mg/m^2 continuous infusion over 12 hours day 2
[total dose/cycle = 300 mg/m^2]
Leucovorin: I.M.: 14 mg every 6 hours, for 6 doses, days 3, 4, and 5 (start 24 hours after the start of methotrexate)
[total dose/cycle = 84 mg]
Dactinomycin: I.V.: 0.2 mg days 1, 2, and 3, then 0.5 mg days 4 and 5
[total dose/cycle = 1.6 mg]
Cyclophosphamide: I.V.: 500 mg/m^2 day 3
[total dose/cycle = 500 mg/m^2]
Cyclophosphamide: I.V.: 300 mg/m^2 on day 8
[total dose/cycle = 300 mg/m^2]
Doxorubicin: I.V.: 30 mg/m^2 day 8
[total dose/cycle = 30 mg/m^2]
Repeat cycle approximately every 3 weeks

CHAMOMA (Bagshawe Regimen)

Use Gestational trophoblastic tumor

Regimen
Hydroxyurea: Oral: 500 mg every 12 hours, for 4 doses, days 1 and 2
[total dose/cycle = 2000 mg]
Vincristine: I.V.: 1 mg/m^2 day 3
[total dose/cycle = 1 mg/m^2]
Methotrexate: I.V. bolus: 100 mg/m^2 day 3
followed by I.V.: 200 mg/m^2 continuous infusion over 12 hours day 3
[total dose/cycle = 300 mg/m^2]
Leucovorin: I.M.: 12 mg/m^2 every 12 hours, for 4 doses, days 4 and 5 (start 12 hours after the end of methotrexate infusion)
[total dose/cycle = 48 mg/m^2]
Dactinomycin: I.V.: 10 mcg/kg/day days 5, 6, and 7
[total dose/cycle = 30 mcg/kg]
Cyclophosphamide: I.V.: 600 mg/m^2 day 5
[total dose/cycle = 600 mg/m^2]
Doxorubicin: I.V.: 30 mg/m^2 day 10
[total dose/cycle = 30 mg/m^2]
Melphalan: I.V.: 6 mg/m^2 day 10
[total dose/cycle = 6 mg/m^2]
Repeat cycle approximately every 3 weeks

ChlVPP

Use Lymphoma, Hodgkin disease

Regimen
Chlorambucil: Oral: 6 mg/m^2/day (maximum 10 mg) days 1 to 14
[total dose/cycle = 84 mg/m^2]
Vinblastine: I.V.: 6 mg/m^2/day (maximum 10 mg) days 1 and 8
[total dose/cycle = 12 mg/m^2]
Procarbazine: Oral: 100 mg/m^2/day (maximum 150 mg) days 1 to 14
[total dose/cycle = 1400 mg/m^2]
Prednisone: Oral: 40-50 mg/day days 1 to 14
[total dose/cycle = 560-700 mg]
Repeat cycle every 28 days

CHL + PRED

Use Leukemia, chronic lymphocytic

Regimen
Chlorambucil: Oral: 0.4 mg/kg/day for 1 day every other week; increase initial dose of 0.4 mg/kg by 0.1 mg/kg every 2 weeks until toxicity or disease control is achieved
Prednisone: Oral: 100 mg/day for 2 days every other week

CHOP

Use Lymphoma, non-Hodgkin

Regimen NOTE: Multiple variations are listed below.

Variation 1:

Cyclophosphamide: I.V.: 750 mg/m^2 day 1
[total dose/cycle = 750 mg/m^2]
Doxorubicin: I.V.: 50 mg/m^2 day 1
[total dose/cycle = 50 mg/m^2]
Vincristine: I.V.: 1.4 mg/m^2 (maximum 2 mg) day 1
[total dose/cycle = 1.4 mg/m^2]
Prednisone: Oral: 100 mg/day days 1 to 5
[total dose/cycle = 500 mg]
  or 50 mg/m^2/day days 1 to 5
  [total dose/cycle = 250 mg/m^2]
    or 100 mg/m^2/day days 1 to 5
    [total dose/cycle = 500 mg/m^2]
Repeat cycle every 21 days

Variation 2:

Cyclophosphamide: I.V.: 750 mg/m^2 day 1
[total dose/cycle = 750 mg/m^2]
Doxorubicin: I.V.: 50 mg/m^2 day 1
[total dose/cycle = 50 mg/m^2]
Vincristine: I.V.: 2 mg day 1
[total dose/cycle = 2 mg]
Prednisone: Oral: 75 mg/day days 1 to 5
[total dose/cycle = 375 mg]
Repeat cycle every 21 days

Variation 3:

Cyclophosphamide: I.V.: 750 mg/m^2/day days 1 and 8
[total dose/cycle = 1500 mg/m^2]
Doxorubicin: I.V.: 25 mg/m^2/day days 1 and 8
[total dose/cycle = 50 mg/m^2]
Vincristine: I.V.: 1.4 mg/m^2/day (maximum 2 mg) days 1 and 8
[total dose/cycle = 2.8 mg/m^2]
Prednisone: Oral: 50 mg/m^2/day days 1 to 8
[total dose/cycle = 400 mg/m^2]
Repeat cycle every 28 days

Variation 4 - "mini-CHOP":

Cyclophosphamide: I.V.: 250 mg/m^2/day days 1, 8, and 15
[total dose/cycle = 750 mg/m^2]
Doxorubicin: I.V.: 16.7 mg/m^2/day days 1, 8, and 15
[total dose/cycle = 50.1 mg/m^2]
Vincristine: I.V.: 0.67 mg/day days 1, 8, and 15
[total dose/cycle = 2.01 mg]
Prednisone: Oral: 75 mg/day days 1 to 5
[total dose/cycle = 375 mg]
Repeat cycle every 21 days

CI (Neuroblastoma)

Use Neuroblastoma

Regimen

Ifosfamide: I.V.: 1500 mg/m^2/day days 1, 2, and 3
[total dose/cycle = 4500 mg/m^2]
Mesna: I.V.: 500 mg/m^2 every 3 hours, for 3 doses each day, days 1, 2, and 3
[total dose/cycle = 4500 mg/m^2]
Carboplatin: I.V.: 400 mg/m^2 day 4
[total dose/cycle = 400 mg/m^2]
Repeat cycle every 21-28 days

CISCA

Use Bladder cancer

Regimen
Cyclophosphamide: I.V.: 650 mg/m^2 day 1
[total dose = 650 mg/m^2]
Doxorubicin: I.V.: 50 mg/m^2 day 1
[total dose = 50 mg/m^2]
Cisplatin: I.V.: 100 mg/m^2 day 2
[total dose = 100 mg/m^2]
Repeat cycle every 21-28 days

Cisplatin-Cetuximab

Use Head and neck cancer

Regimen NOTE: Multiple variations are listed below.
Variation 1:
Cycle 1:
Cetuximab: I.V.: 400 mg/m^2 (loading dose) day 1 (week 1, cycle 1 only)
[total loading dose = 400 mg/m^2]
followed by I.V.: 250 mg/m^2/day days 8, 15, and 22
[total dose/cycle 1 = 1150 mg/m^2]
Cisplatin: I.V.: 100 mg/m^2 day 1
[total dose/cycle = 100 mg/m^2]
Treatment cycle is 4 weeks
Subsequent cycles:
Cetuximab: I.V.: 250 mg/m^2/day days 1, 8, 15, and 22
[total dose/cycle = 1000 mg/m^2]
Cisplatin: I.V.: 100 mg/m^2 day 1
[total dose/cycle = 100 mg/m^2]
Repeat cycle every 4 weeks
Variation 2:
Cycle 1:
Cetuximab: I.V.: 400 mg/m^2 (loading dose) day 1 (week 1, cycle 1 only)
[total loading dose = 400 mg/m^2]
followed by I.V.: 250 mg/m^2/day days 8 and 15
[total dose/cycle 1 = 900 mg/m^2]
Cisplatin: I.V.: 75-100 mg/m^2 day 1
[total dose/cycle = 75-100 mg/m^2]
Treatment cycle is 3 weeks
Subsequent cycles:
Cetuximab: I.V.: 250 mg/m^2/day days 1, 8, and 15
[total dose/cycle = 750 mg/m^2]
Cisplatin: I.V.: 75-100 mg/m^2 day 1
[total dose/cycle = 75-100 mg/m^2]
Repeat cycle every 3 weeks

Cisplatin-Dacarbazine-Carmustine (Melanoma)

Use Melanoma

Regimen NOTE: Multiple variations are listed below.
Variation 1:
Cisplatin: I.V.: 25 mg/m^2/day days 1, 2, and 3
[total dose/cycle = 75 mg/m^2]
Dacarbazine: I.V.: 220 mg/m^2/day days 1, 2, and 3
[total dose/cycle = 660 mg/m^2]
Carmustine: I.V.: 150 mg/m^2 day 1 (every other cycle **[odd cycles]**)
[total dose/**odd** cycles = 150 mg/m^2]
Repeat cycle every 21 days
Variation 2:
Carmustine: I.V.: 150 mg/m^2 day 1
[total dose/cycle = 150 mg/m^2]
Cisplatin: I.V.: 25 mg/m^2/day days 1, 2, 3, 22, 23, and 24
[total dose/cycle = 150 mg/m^2]

Dacarbazine: I.V.: 220 mg/m^2/day days 1, 2, 3, 22, 23, and 24
[total dose/cycle = 1320 mg/m^2]
Repeat cycle every 42 days

Cisplatin-Dacarbazine-Interferon Alfa-2b-Aldesleukin

Use Melanoma

Regimen

Cisplatin: I.V.: 25 mg/m^2/day days 1, 2, and 3
[total dose/cycle = 75 mg/m^2]
Dacarbazine: 250 mg/m^2/day days 1, 2, and 3
[total dose/cycle = 750 mg/m^2]
Interferon Alfa-2b: SubQ: 5 million units/m^2/day days 6, 8, 10, 13, and 15
[total dose/cycle = 25 million units/m^2]
Aldesleukin: I.V.: 18 million units/m^2/day days 6, 7, 8, 9, 10, 13, 14, and 15
[total dose/cycle = 144 million units/m^2]
Repeat cycle every 28 days

Cisplatin-Docetaxel

Use Bladder cancer

Regimen

Cisplatin: I.V.: 30 mg/m^2 day 1
[total dose/cycle = 30 mg/m^2]
Docetaxel: I.V.: 40 mg/m^2 day 4
[total dose/cycle = 40 mg/m^2]
Repeat cycle weekly for 8 weeks

Cisplatin-Etoposide (Nonsmall Cell Lung Cancer)

Use Lung cancer, nonsmall cell

Regimen NOTE: Multiple variations are listed below.

Variation 1:
Cisplatin: I.V.: 80 mg/m^2/day day 1
[total dose/cycle = 80 mg/m^2]
Etoposide: I.V.: 100 mg/m^2/day days 1, 2, and 3
[total dose/cycle = 300 mg/m^2]
Repeat cycle every 21 days for a total of 4 cycles
Variation 2:
Cisplatin: I.V.: 100 mg/m^2/day day 1
[total dose/cycle = 100 mg/m^2]
Etoposide: I.V.: 100 mg/m^2/day days 1, 2, and 3
[total dose/cycle = 300 mg/m^2]
Repeat cycle every 28 days for a total of 3 cycles
Variation 3:
Cisplatin: I.V.: 100 mg/m^2/day day 1
[total dose/cycle = 100 mg/m^2]
Etoposide: I.V.: 100 mg/m^2/day days 1, 2, and 3
[total dose/cycle = 300 mg/m^2]
Repeat cycle every 28 days for a total of 4 cycles
Variation 4:
Cisplatin: I.V.: 120 mg/m^2/day days 1, 29, and 71
[total dose/treatment = 360 mg/m^2]
Etoposide: I.V.: 100 mg/m^2/day days 1, 2, 3, 29, 30, 31, 71, 72, and 73
[total dose/treatment = 900 mg/m^2]
Variation 5:
Cisplatin: I.V.: 75 mg/m^2/day day 1
[total dose/cycle = 75 mg/m^2]
Etoposide: I.V.: 100 mg/m^2/day days 1, 2, and 3
[total dose/cycle = 300 mg/m^2]
Repeat cycle every 21 days for up to 10 cycles

Cisplatin-Fluorouracil

Use Cervical cancer

Regimen NOTE: Multiple variations are listed below.
Variation 1:
  Cisplatin: I.V.: 75 mg/m^2 day 1
   [total dose/cycle = 75 mg/m^2]
  Fluorouracil: I.V.: 1000 mg/m^2/day continuous infusion days 1 to 4 (96 hours)
   [total dose/cycle = 4000 mg/m^2]
  Repeat cycle every 21 days
Variation 2:
  Cisplatin: I.V.: 50 mg/m^2 day 1 starting 4 hours before radiotherapy
   [total dose/cycle = 50 mg/m^2]
  Fluorouracil: I.V.: 1000 mg/m^2/day continuous infusion days 2 to 5 (96 hours)
   [total dose/cycle = 4000 mg/m^2]
  Repeat cycle every 28 days

Cisplatin-Paclitaxel (Intraperitoneal Regimen)

Use Ovarian cancer

Regimen Note: I.P. therapies administered in 2 liters warmed saline
  Paclitaxel: I.V.: 135 mg/m^2 continuous infusion (over 24 hours) day 1
   [total dose/cycle = 135 mg/m^2]
  Cisplatin: I.P.: 100 mg/m^2 day 2
   [total dose/cycle = 100 mg/m^2]
  Paclitaxel: I.P.: 60 mg/m^2 day 8
   [total dose/cycle = 60 mg/m^2]
  Repeat cycle every 21 days for 6 cycles

Cisplatin-Pemetrexed

Use Malignant pleural mesothelioma

Regimen
  Pemetrexed: I.V.: 500 mg/m^2 infused over 10 minutes day 1
   [total dose/cycle = 500 mg/m^2]
  Cisplatin: I.V.: 75 mg/m^2 infused over 2 hours day 1 (start 30 minutes after pemetrexed)
   [total dose/cycle = 75 mg/m^2]
  Repeat cycle every 21 days

CVD

Use Melanoma

Regimen NOTE: Multiple variations are listed below.
Variation 1:
  Cisplatin: I.V.: 20 mg/m^2/day days 2 to 5
   [total dose/cycle = 80 mg/m^2]
  Vinblastine: I.V.: 1.6 mg/m^2/day days 1 to 5
   [total dose/cycle = 8 mg/m^2]
  Dacarbazine: I.V.: 800 mg/m^2 day 1
   [total dose/cycle = 800 mg/m^2]
  Repeat cycle every 21 days
Variation 2:
  Cisplatin: I.V.: 20 mg/m^2/day days 1 to 4
   [total dose/cycle = 80 mg/m^2]
  Vinblastine: I.V.: 2 mg/m^2/day days 1 to 4
   [total dose/cycle = 8 mg/m^2]
  Dacarbazine: I.V.: 800 mg/m^2 day 1
   [total dose/cycle = 800 mg/m^2]
  Repeat cycle every 21 days

Cisplatin-Vinblastine (Nonsmall Cell Lung Cancer)

Use Lung cancer, nonsmall cell

Regimen NOTE: Multiple variations are listed below.
Variation 1:
  Cisplatin: I.V.: 80 mg/m^2/day days 1, 22, 43, and 64
   [total dose/treatment = 320 mg/m^2]

◄ Vinblastine: I.V.: 4 mg/m^2/day days 1, 8, 15, 22, 29, 43, and 57
  [total dose/treatment = 28 mg/m^2]
Variation 2:
 Cisplatin: I.V.: 100 mg/m^2/day days 1, 29, and 57
  [total dose/treatment = 300 mg/m^2]
 Vinblastine: I.V.: 4 mg/m^2/day days 1, 8, 15, 22, 29, 43, and 57
  [total dose/treatment = 28 mg/m^2]
Variation 3:
 Cisplatin: I.V.: 100 mg/m^2/day days 1, 29, 57, and 85
  [total dose/treatment = 400 mg/m^2]
 Vinblastine: I.V.: 4 mg/m^2/day days 1, 8, 15, 22, 29, 43, 57, 71, and 85
  [total dose/treatment = 36 mg/m^2]
Variation 4:
 Cisplatin: I.V.: 120 mg/m^2/day days 1, 29, and 71
  [total dose/treatment = 360 mg/m^2]
 Vinblastine: I.V.: 4 mg/m^2/day days 1, 8, 15, 22, 29, 43, 57, and 71
  [total dose/treatment = 32 mg/m^2]

Cisplatin-Vinorelbine

Use Cervical cancer

Regimen
 Cisplatin: I.V.: 80 mg/m^2 day 1
  [total dose/cycle = 80 mg/m^2]
 Vinorelbine: I.V.: 25 mg/m^2/day days 1 and 8
  [total dose/cycle = 50 mg/m^2]
 Repeat cycle every 21 days

CMF

Use Breast cancer

Regimen NOTE: Multiple variations are listed below.
 Variation 1:
 Methotrexate: I.V.: 40 mg/m^2/day days 1 and 8
  [total dose/cycle = 80 mg/m^2]
 Fluorouracil: I.V.: 600 mg/m^2/day days 1 and 8
  [total dose/cycle = 1200 mg/m^2]
 Cyclophosphamide: Oral: 100 mg/m^2/day days 1 to 14
  [total dose/cycle = 1400 mg/m^2]
 Repeat cycle every 28 days
 Variation 2 (>60 years of age):
 Methotrexate: I.V.: 30 mg/m^2/day days 1 and 8
  [total dose/cycle = 60 mg/m^2]
 Fluorouracil: I.V.: 400 mg/m^2/day days 1 and 8
  [total dose/cycle = 800 mg/m^2]
 Cyclophosphamide: Oral: 100 mg/m^2/day days 1 to 14
  [total dose/cycle = 1400 mg/m^2]
 Repeat cycle every 28 days

CMF-IV

Use Breast cancer

Regimen
 Cyclophosphamide: I.V.: 600 mg/m^2 day 1
  [total dose/cycle = 600 mg/m^2]
 Methotrexate: I.V.: 40 mg/m^2 day 1
  [total dose/cycle = 40 mg/m^2]
 Fluorouracil: I.V.: 600 mg/m^2 day 1
  [total dose/cycle = 600 mg/m^2]
 Repeat cycle every 21 or 28 days

CMFP

Use Breast cancer

Regimen

Cyclophosphamide: Oral: 100 mg/m^2/day days 1 to 14
  [total dose = 1400 mg/m^2]
Methotrexate: I.V.: 30 or 40 mg/m^2/day days 1 and 8
  [total dose = 60 or 80 mg/m^2]
Fluorouracil: I.V.: 400 or 600 mg/m^2/day days 1 and 8
  [total dose = 800 or 1200 mg/m^2]
Prednisone: Oral: 40 mg/m^2/day days 1 to 14
  [total dose = 560 mg/m^2]
Repeat cycle every 28 days

CMFVP (Cooper Regimen, VPCMF)

Use Breast cancer

Regimen

Cyclophosphamide: Oral: 2 mg/kg/day days 1 to 252
  [total dose/cycle = 504 mg/kg]
Methotrexate: I.V.: 0.7 mg/kg day 1, weeks 1 to 8, 10, 12, 14, 16, 18, 20, 22, 24, 26, 28, 30, 32, 34, and 36
  [total dose/cycle = 15.4 mg/kg]
Fluorouracil: I.V.: 12 mg/kg day 1, weeks 1 to 8, 10, 12, 14, 16, 18, 20, 22, 24, 26, 28, 30, 32, 34, and 36
  [total dose/cycle = 264 mg/kg]
Vincristine: I.V.: 0.035 mg/kg (maximum 2 mg) day 1, weeks 1 to 5, 8, 12, 16, 20, 24, 28, 32, and 36
  [total dose/cycle = 0.455 mg/kg]
Prednisone: Oral: 0.75 mg/kg/day days 1 to 10, taper off over next 40 days
Administer one cycle only

CMV

Use Bladder cancer

Regimen

Cisplatin: I.V.: 100 mg/m^2 infused over 4 hours (start at least 12 hours after methotrexate) day 2
  [total dose = 100 mg/m^2]
Methotrexate: I.V.: 30 mg/m^2/day days 1 and 8
  [total dose = 60 mg/m^2]
Vinblastine: I.V.: 4 mg/m^2/day days 1 and 8
  [total dose = 8 mg/m^2]
Repeat cycle every 21 days

CNF

Use Breast cancer

Regimen NOTE: Multiple variations are listed below.

Variation 1:
  Cyclophosphamide: I.V.: 500 mg/m^2 day 1
    [total dose/cycle = 500 mg/m^2]
  Mitoxantrone: I.V.: 10 mg/m^2 day 1
    [total dose/cycle = 10 mg/m^2]
  Fluorouracil: I.V.: 500 mg/m^2 day 1
    [total dose/cycle = 500 mg/m^2]
  Repeat cycle every 21 days
Variation 2:
  Cyclophosphamide: I.V.: 500-600 mg/m^2 day 1
    [total dose/cycle = 500-600 mg/m^2]
  Fluorouracil: I.V.: 500-600 mg/m^2 day 1
    [total dose/cycle = 500-600 mg/m^2]
  Mitoxantrone: I.V.: 10-12 mg/m^2 day 1
    [total dose/cycle = 10-12 mg/m^2]
  Repeat cycle every 21 days

CNOP

Use Lymphoma, non-Hodgkin

Regimen
Cyclophosphamide: I.V.: 750 mg/m^2 day 1
  [total dose/cycle = 750 mg/m^2]
Mitoxantrone: I.V.: 10 mg/m^2 day 1
  [total dose/cycle = 10 mg/m^2]
Vincristine: I.V.: 1.4 mg/m^2 day 1
  [total dose/cycle = 1.4 mg/m^2]
Prednisone: Oral: 50 mg/m^2/day days 1 to 5
  [total dose/cycle = 250 mg/m^2]
Repeat cycle every 21 days

CO

Use Retinoblastoma

Regimen
Cyclophosphamide: I.V.: 10 mg/kg/day days 1, 2, and 3
  [total dose/cycle = 30 mg/kg]
Vincristine: I.V.: 1.5 mg/m^2 day 1
  [total dose/cycle = 1.5 mg/m^2]
Repeat cycle every 21 days

CODOX-M

Use Lymphoma, non-Hodgkin

Regimen
Cytarabine: I.T.: 70 mg/day days 1 and 3
  [total dose/cycle = 140 mg]
Cyclophosphamide: I.V.: 800 mg/m^2 day 1, then 200 mg/m^2/day days 2 to 5
  [total dose/cycle = 1600 mg/m^2]
Vincristine: I.V.: 1.5 mg/m^2/day days 1 and 8 (cycle 1); days 1, 8, and 15 (cycle 3)
  [total dose/cycle = 3-4.5 mg/m^2]
Doxorubicin: I.V.: 40 mg/m^2 day 1
  [total dose/cycle = 40 mg/m^2]
Methotrexate:
  I.T.: 12 mg day 15
    [total dose/cycle = 12 mg]
  I.V.: 1200 mg/m^2 loading dose then 240 mg/m^2/hour for 23 hours day 10
    [total dose/cycle = 6720 mg/m^2]
Leucovorin: I.V.: 192 mg/m^2 day 11 then 12 mg/m^2 every 6 hours until methotrexate level <5 X 10^{-8}M (begin
  36 hours after the start of methotrexate infusion)
Sargramostim: SubQ: 7.5 mcg/kg/day day 13 until ANC >1000 cells/mm^3
Repeat cycle when ANC >1000 cells/mm^3

CODOX-M/IVAC

Use Lymphoma, non-Hodgkin (Burkitt)

Regimen
CODOX-M
Cyclophosphamide: I.V.: 800 mg/m^2/day days 1 and 2
  [total dose/cycle = 1600 mg/m^2]
Vincristine: I.V.: 1.4 mg/m^2/day (maximum 2 mg) days 1 and 10
  [total dose/cycle = 2.8 mg/m^2; maximum 4 mg/cycle]
Doxorubicin: I.V.: 50 mg/m^2 day 1
  [total dose/cycle = 50 mg/m^2]
Methotrexate: I.V.: 3 g/m^2 day 10
  [total dose/cycle = 3 g/m^2]
Leucovorin: I.V.: 200 mg/m^2 day 11
  followed by Oral, I.V.: 15 mg/m^2 every 6 hours until methotrexate level <0.1 Mmol/L
Cytarabine: I.T.: 50 mg/day days 1 and 3
  [total dose/cycle = 100 mg]
Methotrexate: I.T.: 12 mg day 1
  [total dose/cycle = 12 mg]

Filgrastim: SubQ: Dose not specified, days 3 to 8 and day 12 until ANC >1000 cells/mm^3
Cycle alternates with IVAC (cycles begin when ANC >1000 cells/mm^3)
Note: Hydrocortisone 50 mg may be added to intrathecal therapy to reduce the incidence of side effects/chemical arachnoiditis.

IVAC
Ifosfamide: I.V.: 1500 mg/m^2/day days 1 to 5
[total dose/cycle = 7500 mg/m^2]
Mesna: I.V.: 1500 mg/m^2/day (in divided doses) days 1 to 5
[total dose/cycle = 7500 mg/m^2]
Etoposide: I.V.: 60 mg/m^2/day days 1 to 5
[total dose/cycle = 300 mg/m^2]
Cytarabine: I.V.: 2 g/m^2 every 12 hours, for 4 doses, days 1 and 2
[total dose/cycle = 8 g/m^2]
Methotrexate: I.T.: 12 mg day 5
[total dose/cycle = 12 mg]
Filgrastim: SubQ: Dose not specified, day 6 until ANC >1000 cells/mm^3
Cycle alternates with CODOX-M (cycles begin when ANC >1000 cells/mm^3)
Note: Hydrocortisone 50 mg may be added to intrathecal therapy to reduce the incidence of side effects/chemical arachnoiditis.

COMLA

Use Lymphoma, non-Hodgkin

Regimen
Cyclophosphamide: I.V.: 1500 mg/m^2 day 1
[total dose/cycle = 1500 mg/m^2]
Vincristine: I.V.: 1.4 mg/m^2/day (maximum 2 mg) days 1, 8, and 15
[total dose/cycle = 4.2 mg/m^2]
Methotrexate: I.V.: 120 mg/m^2/day days 22, 29, 36, 43, 50, 57, 64, and 71
[total dose/cycle = 960 mg/m^2]
Leucovorin: Oral: 25 mg/m^2 every 6 hours for 4 doses (beginning 24 hours after each methotrexate dose)
[total dose/cycle = 800 mg/m^2]
Cytarabine: I.V.: 300 mg/m^2/day days 22, 29, 36, 43, 50, 57, 64, and 71
[total dose/cycle = 2400 mg/m^2]
Repeat cycle every 85 days

COMP

Use Lymphoma, Hodgkin disease; Lymphoma, non-Hodgkin disease

Regimen
Cyclophosphamide: I.V.: 1200 mg/m^2 day 1, cycle 1
[total dose/cycle = 1200 mg/m^2]
followed by I.V.: 1000 mg/m^2 day 1 on subsequent cycles
[total dose/cycle = 1000 mg/m^2]
Vincristine: I.V.: 2 mg/m^2/day (maximum 2 mg) days 3, 10, 17, 24, cycle 1
[total dose/cycle = 8 mg/m^2]
followed by I.V.: 1.5 mg/m^2/day days 1 and 4, on subsequent cycles
[total dose/cycle = 3 mg/m^2]
Methotrexate: I.V.: 300 mg/m^2 day 12
[total dose/cycle = 300 mg/m^2]
Prednisone: Oral: 60 mg/m^2/day (maximum 60 mg) days 3 to 30 then taper over next 7 days, cycle 1
[total dose/cycle = 1680 mg/m^2 + taper over next 7 days]
followed by Oral: 60 mg/m^2 (maximum 60 mg) days 1 to 5, on subsequent cycles
[total dose/cycle = 300 mg/m^2]
Maintenance cycles repeat every 28 days

COP-BLAM

Use Lymphoma, non-Hodgkin

Regimen
Cyclophosphamide: I.V.: 400 mg/m^2 day 1
[total dose/cycle = 400 mg/m^2]
Vincristine: I.V.: 1 mg/m^2 day 1
[total dose/cycle = 1 mg/m^2]
Prednisone: Oral: 40 mg/m^2/day days 1 to 10
[total dose/cycle = 400 mg/m^2]

◄ Bleomycin: I.V.: 15 mg day 14
  [total dose/cycle = 15 mg]
Doxorubicin: I.V.: 40 mg/m^2 day 1
  [total dose/cycle = 40 mg/m^2]
Procarbazine: Oral: 100 mg/m^2/day days 1 to 10
  [total dose/cycle = 1000 mg/m^2]

COPE

Use Brain tumors
Regimen
Cycle A:
  Vincristine: I.V.: 0.065 mg/kg/day (maximum 1.5 mg) days 1 and 8
    [total dose/cycle = 0.13 mg/kg]
  Cyclophosphamide: I.V.: 65 mg/kg day 1
    [total dose/cycle = 65 mg/kg]
Cycle B:
  Cisplatin: I.V.: 4 mg/kg day 1
    [total dose/cycle = 4 mg/kg]
  Etoposide: I.V.: 6.5 mg/kg/day days 3 and 4
    [total dose/cycle = 13 mg/kg]
Repeat cycle every 28 days in the following sequence: AABAAB

COPP

Use Lymphoma, non-Hodgkin
Regimen
Cyclophosphamide: I.V.: 450-650 mg/m^2/day days 1 and 8
  [total dose/cycle = 900-1300 mg/m^2]
Vincristine: I.V.: 1.4-2 mg/m^2/day (maximum 2 mg) days 1 and 8
  [total dose/cycle = 2.8-4 mg/m^2]
Procarbazine: Oral: 100 mg/m^2/day days 1 to 14
  [total dose/cycle = 1400 mg/m^2]
Prednisone: Oral: 40 mg/m^2/day days 1 to 14
  [total dose/cycle = 560 mg/m^2]
Repeat cycle every 3-4 weeks

CP (Leukemia)

Use Leukemia, chronic lymphocytic
Regimen
Chlorambucil: Oral: 30 mg/m^2 day 1
  [total dose/cycle = 30 mg/m^2]
Prednisone: Oral: 80 mg/day days 1 to 5
  [total dose/cycle = 400 mg]
Repeat cycle every 14 days

CP (Ovarian Cancer)

Use Ovarian cancer
Regimen
Cyclophosphamide: I.V.: 750 mg/m^2 day 1
  [total dose/cycle = 750 mg/m^2]
Cisplatin: I.V.: 75 mg/m^2 day 1
  [total dose/cycle = 75 mg/m^2]
Repeat cycle every 21 days

CT

Use Ovarian cancer
Regimen
Cisplatin: I.V.: 75 mg/m^2 day 2
  [total dose/cycle = 75 mg/m^2]
Paclitaxel: I.V.: 135 mg/m^2 continuous infusion day 1
  [total dose/cycle = 135 mg/m^2]
Repeat cycle every 21 days

CV

Use Retinoblastoma

Regimen
Cyclophosphamide: I.V.: 300 mg/m^2
  [total dose/cycle = 300 mg/m^2]
Vincristine: I.V.: 1.5 mg/m^2
  [total dose/cycle = 1.5 mg/m^2]
Repeat weekly for 6 weeks
followed by
Cyclophosphamide: I.V.: 200 mg/m^2
  [total dose/cycle = 200 mg/m^2]
Vincristine: I.V.: 1.5 mg/m^2
  [total dose/cycle = 1.5 mg/m^2]
Repeat weekly for 42 weeks

CVP (Leukemia)

Use Leukemia, chronic lymphocytic

Regimen NOTE: Multiple variations are listed below.
Variation 1:
  Cyclophosphamide: Oral: 400 or 300 mg/m^2/day days 1 to 5
    [total dose/cycle = 2000 or 1500 mg/m^2]
  Vincristine: I.V.: 1.4 mg/m^2 (maximum 2 mg) day 1
    [total dose/cycle = 1.4 mg/m^2]
  Prednisone: Oral: 100 mg/m^2/day days 1 to 5
    [total dose/cycle = 500 mg/m^2]
  Repeat cycle every 21 days
Variation 2:
  Cyclophosphamide: I.V.: 800 mg/m^2 day 1
    [total dose/cycle = 800 mg/m^2]
  Vincristine: I.V.: 1.4 mg/m^2 (maximum 2 mg) day 1
    [total dose/cycle = 1.4 mg/m^2]
  Prednisone: Oral: 100 mg/m^2/day days 1 to 5
    [total dose/cycle = 500 mg/m^2]
  Repeat cycle every 21 days

CVP (Lymphoma, non-Hodgkin)

Use Lymphoma, non-Hodgkin

Regimen NOTE: Multiple variations are listed below.
Variation 1:
  Cyclophosphamide: I.V.: 750 mg/m^2 day 1
    [total dose/cycle = 750 mg/m^2]
  Vincristine: I.V.: 1.2 mg/m^2 day 1
    [total dose/cycle = 1.2 mg/m^2]
  Prednisone: Oral: 40 mg/m^2/day days 1 to 5
    [total dose/cycle = 200 mg/m^2]
  Repeat cycle every 21 days for up to 10 cycles
Variation 2:
  Cyclophosphamide: I.V.: 750 mg/m^2 day 1
    [total dose/cycle = 750 mg/m^2]
  Vincristine: I.V.: 1.2 mg/m^2 day 1 (maximum 2 mg/dose)
    [total dose/cycle = 1.2 mg/m^2 (maximum 2 mg/dose)]
  Prednisone: Oral: 40 mg/m^2/day days 1 to 5
    [total dose/cycle = 200 mg/m^2]
  Repeat cycle every 28 days for up to 8 cycles
Variation 3:
  Cyclophosphamide: I.V.: 750 mg/m^2 day 1
    [total dose/cycle = 750 mg/m^2]
  Vincristine: I.V.: 1.4 mg/m^2 day 1 (maximum 2 mg/dose)
    [total dose/cycle = 1.4 mg/m^2 (maximum 2 mg/dose)]
  Prednisone: Oral: 40 mg/m^2/day days 1 to 5
    [total dose/cycle = 200 mg/m^2]
  Repeat cycle every 21 days for up to 8 cycles

◄ Variation 4:
   Cyclophosphamide: Oral: 400 mg/m^2/day days 1 to 5
   [total dose/cycle = 2000 mg/m^2]
   Vincristine: I.V.: 1.4 mg/m^2 day 1 (maximum 2 mg/dose)
   [total dose/cycle = 1.4 mg/m^2 (maximum 2 mg/dose)]
   Prednisone: Oral: 100 mg/m^2/day days 1 to 5
   [total dose/cycle = 500 mg/m^2]
   Repeat cycle every 21 days

Cyclophosphamide + Doxorubicin

Use Prostate cancer

Regimen
   Doxorubicin: I.V.: 40 mg/m^2 day 1
   [total dose/cycle = 40 mg/m^2]
   Cyclophosphamide: I.V.: 800-2000 mg/m^2 day 1
   [total dose/cycle = 800-2000 mg/m^2]
   Filgrastim: SubQ: 5 mcg/kg/day days 2 to 10 (or until ANC >10,000 cells/µL)
   [total dose/cycle = 45 mcg/kg or until ANC >10,000 cells/µL]
   Repeat cycle every 21 days

Cyclophosphamide + Estramustine

Use Prostate cancer

Regimen
   Cyclophosphamide: Oral: 2 mg/kg/day days 1 to 14
   [total dose/cycle = 28 mg/kg]
   Estramustine: Oral: 10 mg/kg/day days 1 to 14
   [total dose/cycle = 140 mg/kg]
   Repeat cycle every 28 days

Cyclophosphamide + Etoposide

Use Prostate cancer

Regimen
   Cyclophosphamide: Oral: 100 mg/day days 1 to 14
   [total dose/cycle = 1400 mg]
   Etoposide: Oral: 50 mg/day days 1 to 14
   [total dose/cycle = 700 mg]
   Repeat cycle every 28 days

Cyclophosphamide + Vincristine + Dexamethasone

Use Prostate cancer

Regimen
   Cyclophosphamide: Oral: 250 mg/day days 1 to 14
   [total dose/cycle = 3500 mg]
   Vincristine: I.V.: 1 mg/day days 1, 8, and 15
   [total dose/cycle = 3 mg]
   Dexamethasone: Oral: 0.75 mg twice daily days 1 to 14
   [total dose/cycle = 21 mg]
   Repeat cycle every 28 days

CYVADIC

Use Sarcoma

Regimen
   Cyclophosphamide: I.V.: 500 mg/m^2 day 1
   [total dose/cycle = 500 mg/m^2]
   Vincristine: I.V.: 1.4 mg/m^2/day days 1 and 5
   [total dose/cycle = 2.8 mg/m^2]
   Doxorubicin: I.V.: 50 mg/m^2 day 1
   [total dose/cycle = 50 mg/m^2]
   Dacarbazine: I.V.: 250 mg/m^2/day days 1 to 5
   [total dose/cycle = 1250 mg/m^2]
   Repeat cycle every 21 days

DA

Use Leukemia, acute myeloid (induction)

Regimen Induction:
  Daunorubicin: I.V.: 45 mg/m^2/day days 1, 2, and 3
    [total dose/cycle = 135 mg/m^2]
  Cytarabine: I.V.: 100 mg/m^2/day continuous infusion days 1 to 7
    [total dose/cycle = 700 mg/m^2]

Dacarbazine-Carboplatin-Aldesleukin-Interferon

Use Melanoma

Regimen
  Dacarbazine: I.V.: 750 mg/m^2/day days 1 and 22
    [total dose/cycle = 1500 mg/m^2]
  Carboplatin: I.V.: 400 mg/m^2/day days 1 and 22
    [total dose/cycle = 800 mg/m^2]
  Aldesleukin: SubQ: 4,800,000 units every 8 hours days 36 and 57
    [total dose/cycle = 28,800,000 units]
    then 4,800,000 units every 12 hours days 37 and 58
      [total dose/cycle = 19,200,000 units]
      then 4,800,000 units/day days 38 to 40, 43 to 47, 50 to 54, 59 to 61, 65 to 68, 71 to 75
        [total dose/cycle = 120,000,000 units]
  Interferon alpha-2a: SubQ: 6,000,000 units days 38, 40, 43, 45, 47, 50, 52, 54, 59, 61, 64, 66, 68, 71, 73, and 75
    [total dose/cycle = 96,000,000 units]
  Repeat cycle every 78 days for 3 cycles

Dartmouth Regimen

Use Melanoma

Regimen NOTE: Multiple variations are listed below.
  Variation 1:
    Cisplatin: I.V.: 25 mg/m^2/day days 1, 2, and 3
      [total dose/cycle = 75 mg/m^2]
    Dacarbazine: I.V.: 220 mg/m^2/day days 1, 2, and 3
      [total dose/cycle = 660 mg/m^2]
    Carmustine: I.V.: 150 mg/m^2 day 1 (every other cycle)
      [total dose/cycle = 150 mg/m^2; every other cycle]
    Tamoxifen: Oral: 10 mg twice daily (begin 1 week before chemotherapy)
      [total dose/cycle = 420 mg]
    Repeat cycle every 21 days
  Variation 2:
    Carmustine: I.V.: 150 mg/m^2 day 1
      [total dose/cycle = 150 mg/m^2]
    Cisplatin: I.V.: 25 mg/m^2/day days 1, 2, 3, 22, 23, and 24
      [total dose/cycle = 150 mg/m^2]
    Dacarbazine: I.V.: 220 mg/m^2/day days 1, 2, 3, 22, 23, and 24
      [total dose/cycle = 1320 mg/m^2]
    Tamoxifen: Oral: 10 mg twice daily days 1 to 42
      [total dose/cycle = 840 mg]
    Repeat cycle every 42 days
  Variation 3:
    Carmustine: I.V.: 150 mg/m^2 day 1
      [total dose/cycle = 150 mg/m^2]
    Cisplatin: I.V.: 25 mg/m^2/day days 1, 2, 3, 22, 23, and 24
      [total dose/cycle = 150 mg/m^2]
    Dacarbazine: I.V.: 220 mg/m^2/day days 1, 2, 3, 22, 23, and 24
      [total dose/cycle = 1320 mg/m^2]
    Tamoxifen: Oral: 160 mg/day days -6 to 0 (cycle 1 only)
      [total dose/cycle = 1120 mg]
      followed by Oral: 40 mg/day days 1 to 42
      [total dose/cycle = 1680 mg]
    Repeat cycle every 42 days

Variation 4:
  Carmustine: I.V.: 150 mg/m^2 day 1
    [total dose/cycle = 150 mg/m^2]
  Cisplatin: I.V.: 25 mg/m^2/day days 1, 2, 3, 29, 30, and 31
    [total dose/cycle = 150 mg/m^2]
  Dacarbazine: I.V.: 220 mg/m^2/day days 1, 2, 3, 29, 30, and 31
    [total dose/cycle = 1320 mg/m^2]
  Tamoxifen: Oral: 10-20 mg twice daily days 1 to 56
    [total dose/cycle = 1120-2240 mg]
  Repeat cycle every 56 days
Variation 5:
  Cisplatin: I.V.: 25 mg/m^2/day days 1, 2, and 3
    [total dose/cycle = 75 mg/m^2]
  Dacarbazine: I.V.: 220 mg/m^2/day days 1, 2, and 3
    [total dose/cycle = 660 mg/m^2]
  Carmustine: I.V.: 100 mg/m^2 day 1 (give in cycles 1, 3, and 6 **only**)
    [total dose/cycles 1, 3, and 6 = 100 mg/m^2]
  Tamoxifen: Oral: 160 mg loading dose immediately before cycle 1
    [total dose/loading dose + cycle 1 = 580 mg]
    followed by Oral: 20 mg daily days 1 to 21
      [total dose/subsequent cycles = 420 mg]
  Repeat cycle every 21 days
  Note: Tamoxifen is continued until 3 weeks after last cycle.

DAT

Use Leukemia, acute myeloid (induction)
Regimen Induction:
  Daunorubicin: I.V. bolus: 45 mg/m^2/day days 1, 2, and 3
    [total dose/cycle = 135 mg/m^2]
  Cytarabine: I.V. bolus: 200 mg/m^2
    [total dose/cycle = 200 mg/m^2]
  Thioguanine: Oral: 100 mg/m^2/day days 1 to 7
    [total dose/cycle = 700 mg/m^2]

DAV

Use Leukemia, acute myeloid
Regimen
  Daunorubicin: I.V.: 60 mg/m^2/day days 3, 4, and 5
    [total dose/cycle = 180 mg/m^2]
  Cytarabine I.V.: 100 mg/m^2/day continuous infusion days 1 and 2
    [total dose/cycle = 200 mg/m^2]
    followed by I.V.: 100 mg/m^2 over 30 minutes every 12 hours days 3 to 8 (12 doses)
      [total dose/cycle = 1200 mg/m^2]
  Etoposide: I.V.: 150 mg/m^2/day days 6, 7, and 8
    [total dose/cycle = 450 mg/m^2]
  Administer one cycle only

Decitabine (Low Dose Regimen)

Use Leukemia, chronic myelogenous; Myelodysplastic syndrome
Regimen
  Decitabine: I.V.: 20 mg/m^2/day days 1 to 5
    [total dose/cycle = 100 mg/m^2]
  Repeat cycle every 28 days for at least 3 cycles

DHAP

Use Lymphoma, non-Hodgkin
Regimen NOTE: Multiple variations are listed below.
  Variation 1:
    Dexamethasone: I.V. or Oral: 40 mg/day days 1 to 4
      [total dose/cycle = 160 mg]

Cisplatin: I.V.: 100 mg/m^2 day 1
  [total dose/cycle = 100 mg/m^2]
Cytarabine: I.V.: 2000 mg/m^2 every 12 hours for 2 doses day 2 (begins at the end of the cisplatin infusion)
  [total dose/cycle = 4000 mg/m^2]
Repeat cycle every 3-4 weeks for 6-10 cycles (salvage therapy) or 1-2 cycles (mobilization prior to high-dose therapy with peripheral hematopoietic progenitor cell support)
Variation 2:
Dexamethasone: I.V. or Oral: 40 mg/day days 1 to 4
  [total dose/cycle = 160 mg]
Oxaliplatin: I.V.: 130 mg/m^2 day 1
  [total dose/cycle = 130 mg/m^2]
Cytarabine: I.V.: 2000 mg/m^2 every 12 hours for 2 doses day 2
  [total dose/cycle = 4000 mg/m^2]
Repeat cycle every 3 weeks

Docetaxel-Bevacizumab

Use Breast cancer

Regimen NOTE: Multiple variations are listed below.
Variation 1:
Docetaxel: I.V.: 100 mg/m^2/day day 1
  [total dose/cycle = 100 mg/m^2]
Bevacizumab: I.V.: 7.5 mg/kg/day day 1
  [total dose/cycle = 7.5 mg/kg]
Repeat cycle every 21 days (administer docetaxel for up to 9 cycles, bevacizumab until disease progression or unacceptable toxicity)
Variation 2:
Docetaxel: I.V.: 100 mg/m^2/day day 1
  [total dose/cycle = 100 mg/m^2]
Bevacizumab: I.V.: 15 mg/kg/day day 1
  [total dose/cycle = 15 mg/kg]
Repeat cycle every 21 days (administer docetaxel for up to 9 cycles, bevacizumab until disease progression or unacceptable toxicity)

Docetaxel-Cisplatin

Use Lung cancer, nonsmall cell

Regimen
Docetaxel: I.V.: 75 mg/m^2 day 1
  [total dose/cycle = 75 mg/m^2]
Cisplatin: I.V.: 75 mg/m^2 day 1
  [total dose/cycle = 75 mg/m^2]
Repeat cycle every 21 days

Docetaxel-Cisplatin-Fluorouracil (Gastric Cancer)

Use Gastric cancer

Regimen
Docetaxel: I.V.: 75 mg/m^2 day 1
  [total dose/cycle = 75 mg/m^2]
Cisplatin: I.V.: 75 mg/m^2 day 1
  [total dose/cycle = 75 mg/m^2]
Fluorouracil: I.V.: 750 mg/m^2/day continuous infusion days 1 to 5
  [total dose/cycle = 3750 mg/m^2]
Repeat cycle every 21 days

Docetaxel-Cisplatin-Fluorouracil (Head and Neck Cancer)

Use Head and neck cancer

Regimen NOTE: Multiple variations are listed below.
Variation 1:
Docetaxel: I.V.: 75 mg/m^2 day 1
  [total dose/cycle = 75 mg/m^2]
Cisplatin: I.V.: 75 mg/m^2 day 1
  [total dose/cycle = 75 mg/m^2]
Fluorouracil: I.V.: 750 mg/m^2/day continuous infusion days 1 to 5
  [total dose/cycle = 3750 mg/m^2]
Repeat cycle every 21 days for 4 cycles

◄ Variation 2:
Docetaxel: I.V.: 75 mg/m^2 day 1
[total dose/cycle = 75 mg/m^2]
Cisplatin: I.V.: 75-100 mg/m^2 day 1
[total dose/cycle = 75-100 mg/m^2]
Fluorouracil: I.V.: 1000 mg/m^2/day continuous infusion days 1 to 4
[total dose/cycle = 4000 mg/m^2]
Repeat cycle every 21 days for total of 3 cycles

Docetaxel-Cyclophosphamide (TC)

Use Breast cancer

Regimen
Docetaxel: I.V.: 75 mg/m^2 day 1
[total dose/cycle = 75 mg/m^2]
Cyclophosphamide: I.V.: 600 mg/m^2 day 1
[total dose/cycle = 600 mg/m^2]
Repeat cycle every 21 days for 4 cycles

Docetaxel-FEC

Use Breast cancer

Regimen
Cycles 1, 2, and 3:
Docetaxel: I.V.: 80-100 mg/m^2 day 1
[total dose/cycle = 80-100 mg/m^2]
Repeat cycle every 21 days for 3 cycles
Cycles 4, 5, and 6 (FEC):
Fluorouracil: I.V.: 600 mg/m^2 day 1
[total dose/cycle = 600 mg/m^2]
Epirubicin: I.V.: 60 mg/m^2 day 1
[total dose/cycle = 60 mg/m^2]
Cyclophosphamide: I.V.: 600 mg/m^2 day 1
[total dose/cycle = 600 mg/m^2]
Repeat FEC cycle every 21 days for total of 3 cycles

Docetaxel-Prednisone

Use Prostate cancer

Regimen
Docetaxel: I.V.: 75 mg/m^2 day 1
[total dose/cycle = 75 mg/m^2]
Prednisone: Oral: 5 mg twice daily
[total dose/cycle = 210 mg]
Repeat cycle every 21 days for up to 10 cycles

Docetaxel-Thalidomide

Use Prostate cancer

Regimen
Docetaxel: I.V.: 30 mg/m^2/day days 1, 8, and 15
[total dose/cycle = 90 mg/m^2]
Thalidomide: Oral: 200 mg daily (at bedtime)
[total dose/cycle = 5600 mg]
Repeat cycle every 28 days

Docetaxel-Trastuzumab

Use Breast cancer

Regimen
Cycle 1:
Docetaxel: I.V.: 100 mg/m^2 day 1
[total dose/cycle 1 = 100 mg/m^2]
Trastuzumab: I.V.: 4 mg/kg (loading dose) day 1 cycle 1
followed by I.V.: 2 mg/kg/day days 8 and 15 cycle 1
[total dose/cycle 1 = 8 mg/kg]
Treatment cycle is 21 days

Subsequent cycles:
  Docetaxel: I.V.: 100 mg/m^2 day 1
    [total dose/cycle = 100 mg/m^2]
  Trastuzumab: I.V.: 2 mg/kg/day days 1, 8, and 15
    [total dose/cycle = 6 mg/kg]
  Repeat cycle every 21 days for a total of at least 6 cycles (continue weekly trastuzumab until disease progression)

Docetaxel-Trastuzumab-Carboplatin

Use Breast cancer

Regimen
Cycle 1:
  Trastuzumab: I.V.: 4 mg/kg (loading dose) day 1 cycle 1
  followed by I.V.: 2 mg/kg/day days 8 and 15 cycle 1
    [total dose/cycle 1 = 8 mg/kg]
  Docetaxel: I.V.: 75 mg/m^2 day 2
    [total dose/cycle 1 = 75 mg/m^2]
  Carboplatin: I.V.: AUC 6 day 2
    [total dose/cycle 1 = AUC = 6]
  Treatment cycle is 21 days
Subsequent cycles:
  Trastuzumab: I.V.: 2 mg/kg/day days 1, 8, and 15
    [total dose/cycle = 6 mg/kg]
  Docetaxel: I.V.: 75 mg/m^2 day 1
    [total dose/cycle = 75 mg/m^2]
  Carboplatin: I.V.: AUC 6 day 1
    [total dose/cycle = AUC = 6]
  Repeat cycle every 21 days for a total of ~6 cycles (continue weekly trastuzumab for 1 year after chemotherapy, or until disease progression or unacceptable toxicity)

Docetaxel-Trastuzumab-Cisplatin

Use Breast cancer

Regimen
Cycle 1:
  Trastuzumab: I.V.: 4 mg/kg (loading dose) day 1 cycle 1
  followed by I.V.: 2 mg/kg/day days 8 and 15 cycle 1
    [total dose/cycle 1 = 8 mg/kg]
  Docetaxel: I.V.: 75 mg/m^2 day 2
    [total dose/cycle 1 = 75 mg/m^2]
  Cisplatin: I.V.: 75 mg/m^2 day 2
    [total dose/cycle 1 = 75 mg/m^2]
  Treatment cycle is 21 days
Subsequent cycles:
  Trastuzumab: I.V.: 2 mg/kg/day days 1, 8, and 15
    [total dose/cycle = 6 mg/kg]
  Docetaxel: I.V.: 75 mg/m^2 day 1
    [total dose/cycle = 75 mg/m^2]
  Cisplatin: I.V.: 75 mg/m^2 day 1
    [total dose/cycle = 75 mg/m^2]
  Repeat cycle every 21 days for a total of ~6 cycles (continue weekly trastuzumab for 1 year after chemotherapy, or until disease progression or unacceptable toxicity)

Docetaxel-Trastuzumab-FEC

Use Breast cancer

Regimen
Cycle 1:
  Trastuzumab: I.V.: 4 mg/kg (loading dose) day 1 cycle 1
  followed by I.V.: 2 mg/kg/day days 8 and 15 cycle 1
    [total dose/cycle 1 = 8 mg/kg]

Docetaxel: I.V.: 80-100 mg/m^2 day 1
  [total dose/cycle 1 = 80-100 mg/m^2]
Treatment cycle is 21 days
Cycles 2 and 3:
  Trastuzumab: I.V.: 2 mg/kg/day days 1, 8, and 15
    [total dose/cycle = 6 mg/kg]
  Docetaxel: I.V.: 80-100 mg/m^2 day 1
    [total dose/cycle = 80-100 mg/m^2]
  Treatment cycle is 21 days
Cycles 4, 5, and 6 (FEC):
  Fluorouracil: I.V.: 600 mg/m^2 day 1
    [total dose/cycle = 600 mg/m^2]
  Epirubicin: I.V.: 60 mg/m^2 day 1
    [total dose/cycle = 60 mg/m^2]
  Cyclophosphamide: I.V.: 600 mg/m^2 day 1
    [total dose/cycle = 600 mg/m^2]
  Repeat FEC cycle every 21 days for total of 3 cycles

Docetaxel (Weekly Regimen)

Use Prostate cancer

Regimen
Docetaxel: I.V.: 40 mg/m^2 days 1, 8, and 15
  [total dose/cycle = 120 mg/m^2]
Repeat cycle every 4 weeks

Docetaxel (Weekly)-Trastuzumab

Use Breast cancer

Regimen
Cycle 1:
  Docetaxel: I.V.: 35 mg/m^2/day days 1, 8, and 15
    [total dose/cycle 1 = 105 mg/m^2]
  Trastuzumab: I.V.: 4 mg/kg (loading dose) day 0 cycle 1
  followed by I.V.: 2 mg/kg/day days 8 and 15 cycle 1
    [total dose/cycle 1 = 8 mg/kg]
  Treatment cycle is 28 days
Subsequent cycles:
  Docetaxel: I.V.: 35 mg/m^2/day days 1, 8, and 15
    [total dose/cycle = 105 mg/m^2]
  Trastuzumab: I.V.: 2 mg/kg/day days 1, 8, and 15
    [total dose/cycle = 6 mg/kg]
  Repeat cycle every 28 days

Dox-CMF (Sequential)

Use Breast cancer

Regimen
Doxorubicin: I.V.: 75 mg/m^2 day 1
  [total dose/cycle = 75 mg/m^2]
Repeat cycle every 21 days for 4 cycles
followed by (after completing Cycle 4)
Cyclophosphamide: I.V.: 600 mg/m^2 day 1
  [total dose/cycle = 600 mg/m^2]
Methotrexate: I.V.: 40 mg/m^2 day 1
  [total dose/cycle = 40 mg/m^2]
Fluorouracil: I.V.: 600 mg/m^2 day 1
  [total dose/cycle = 600 mg/m^2]
Repeat cycle every 21 days for 8 cycles

Doxorubicin + Ketoconazole

Use Prostate cancer

Regimen
Doxorubicin: I.V.: 20 mg/m^2 continuous infusion day 1
  [total dose/cycle = 20 mg/m^2]

Ketoconazole: Oral: 400 mg 3 times/day days 1 to 7
  [total dose/cycle = 8400 mg]
  Repeat cycle every 7 days

Doxorubicin + Ketoconazole/Estramustine + Vinblastine

Use Prostate cancer

Regimen
  Doxorubicin: I.V.: 20 mg/m^2/day days 1, 15, and 29
    [total dose/cycle = 60 mg/m^2]
  Ketoconazole: Oral: 400 mg 3 times/day days 1 to 7, 15 to 21, and 29 to 35
    [total dose/cycle = 25,200 mg]
  Estramustine: Oral: 140 mg 3 times/day days 8 to 14, 22 to 28, and 36 to 42
    [total dose/cycle = 8820 mg]
  Vinblastine: I.V.: 5 mg/m^2/day days 8, 22, and 36
    [total dose/cycle = 15 mg/m^2]
  Repeat cycle every 8 weeks

Doxorubicin (Liposomal)-Vincristine-Dexamethasone

Use Multiple myeloma

Regimen NOTE: Multiple variations are listed below.
  Variation 1:
  Doxorubicin, liposomal: I.V.: 40 mg/m^2 day 1
    [total dose/cycle = 40 mg/m^2]
  Vincristine: I.V.: 2 mg day 1
    [total dose/cycle = 2 mg]
  Dexamethasone: Oral or I.V.: 40 mg/day days 1 to 4
    [total dose/cycle = 160 mg]
  Repeat cycle every 4 weeks
  Variation 2:
  Doxorubicin, liposomal: I.V.: 40 mg/m^2 day 1
    [total dose/cycle = 40 mg/m^2]
  Vincristine: I.V.: 1.4 mg/m^2 (maximum 2 mg) day 1
    [total dose/cycle = 1.4 mg/m^2; maximum 2 mg]
  Dexamethasone: Oral: 40 mg/day days 1 to 4
    [total dose/cycle = 160 mg]
  Repeat cycle every 4 weeks

DTPACE

Use Multiple myeloma

Regimen
  Dexamethasone: Oral: 40 mg/day days 1 to 4
    [total dose/cycle = 160 mg]
  Thalidomide: Oral: 400 mg/day
    [total dose/cycle = 11,200 - 16,800 mg]
  Cisplatin: I.V.: 10 mg/m^2/day continuous infusion days 1 to 4
    [total dose/cycle = 40 mg/m^2]
  Doxorubicin: I.V.: 10 mg/m^2/day continuous infusion days 1 to 4
    [total dose/cycle = 40 mg/m^2]
  Cyclophosphamide: I.V.: 400 mg/m^2 continuous infusion days 1 to 4
    [total dose/cycle = 1600 mg/m^2]
  Etoposide: I.V.: 40 mg/m^2 continuous infusion days 1 to 4
    [total dose/cycle = 160 mg/m^2]
  Repeat cycle every 4-6 weeks

DVP

Use Leukemia, acute lymphocytic

Regimen Induction:
  Daunorubicin: I.V.: 25 mg/m^2/day days 1, 8, and 15
    [total dose/cycle = 75 mg/m^2]
  Vincristine: I.V.: 1.5 mg/m^2/day (maximum 2 mg) days 1, 8, 15, and 22
    [total dose/cycle = 6 mg/m^2]
  Prednisone: Oral: 60 mg/m^2/day days 1 to 28 then taper over next 14 days
    [total dose/cycle = 1680 mg/m^2 + taper over next 14 days]
  Administer single cycle; used in conjunction with intrathecal chemotherapy

EAP

Use Gastric cancer

Regimen
Etoposide: I.V.: 120 mg/m^2/day days 4, 5, and 6
  [total dose/cycle = 360 mg/m^2]
Doxorubicin: I.V.: 20 mg/m^2/day days 1 and 7
  [total dose/cycle = 40 mg/m^2]
Cisplatin: I.V.: 40 mg/m^2/day days 2 and 8
  [total dose/cycle = 80 mg/m^2]
Repeat cycle every 22-28 days

ECF

Use Gastric cancer

Regimen
Epirubicin: I.V.: 50 mg/m^2 day 1
  [total dose/cycle = 50 mg/m^2]
Cisplatin: I.V.: 60 mg/m^2 day 1
  [total dose/cycle = 60 mg/m^2]
Repeat cycle every 3 weeks
Fluorouracil: I.V.: 200 mg/m^2/day continuous infusion for up to 6 months
  [total dose/cycle = 36,000 mg/m^2]

EC (Nonsmall Cell Lung Cancer)

Use Lung cancer, nonsmall cell

Regimen
Etoposide: I.V.: 120 mg/m^2/day days 1, 2, and 3
  [total dose/cycle = 360 mg/m^2]
Carboplatin: I.V.: AUC 6 day 1
  [total dose/cycle = AUC = 6]
Repeat cycle every 21-28 days

EC (Small Cell Lung Cancer)

Use Lung cancer, small cell

Regimen NOTE: Multiple variations are listed below.
Variation 1:
  Etoposide: I.V.: 100-120 mg/m^2/day days 1, 2, and 3
    [total dose/cycle = 300-360 mg/m^2]
  Carboplatin: I.V.: 325-400 mg/m^2 day 1
    [total dose/cycle = 325-400 mg/m^2]
  Repeat cycle every 28 days
Variation 2:
  Etoposide: I.V.: 120 mg/m^2/day days 1, 2, and 3
    [total dose/cycle = 360 mg/m^2]
  Carboplatin: I.V.: AUC 6 day 1
    [total dose/cycle = AUC = 6]
  Repeat cycle every 21-28 days

EE

Use Wilms tumor

Regimen
Dactinomycin: I.V.: 15 mcg/kg/day days 1 to 5 of weeks 0, 5, 13, and 24
  [total dose/cycle = 300 mcg/kg]
Vincristine: I.V.: 1.5 mg/m^2 day 1 of weeks 1-10, 13, 14, 24, and 25
  [total dose/cycle = 21 mg/m^2]

EE-4A

Use Wilms tumor

Regimen
Dactinomycin: I.V.: 45 mcg/kg day 1 of weeks 0, 3, 6, 9, 12, 15, and 18
[total dose/cycle = 315 mcg/kg]
Vincristine: I.V.: 2 mg/m^2 day 1 of weeks 1-10, 12, 15, and 18
[total dose/cycle = 26 mg/m^2]

EFP

Use Gastric cancer

Regimen NOTE: Multiple variations are listed below.
Variation 1:
Etoposide: I.V.: 90 mg/m^2/day days 1, 3, and 5
[total dose/cycle = 270 mg/m^2]
Fluorouracil: I.V.: 900 mg/m^2/day (20-hour infusion) days 1 to 5
[total dose/cycle = 4500 mg/m^2]
Cisplatin: I.V.: 20 mg/m^2/day days 1 to 5
[total dose/cycle = 100 mg/m^2]
Repeat cycle every 24-28 days
Variation 2:
Etoposide: I.V.: 100 mg/m^2/day days 1, 3, and 5
[total dose/cycle = 300 mg/m^2]
Fluorouracil: I.V.: 800 mg/m^2/day (12-hour infusion) days 1 to 5
[total dose/cycle = 4000 mg/m^2]
Cisplatin: I.V.: 20 mg/m^2/day days 1 to 5
[total dose/cycle = 100 mg/m^2]
Repeat cycle every 3 weeks

ELF

Use Gastric cancer

Regimen
Leucovorin calcium: I.V.: 300 mg/m^2/day days 1, 2, and 3
[total dose/cycle = 900 mg/m^2]
followed by
Etoposide: I.V.: 120 mg/m^2/day days 1, 2, and 3
[total dose/cycle = 360 mg/m^2]
followed by
Fluorouracil: I.V.: 500 mg/m^2/day days 1, 2, and 3
[total dose/cycle = 1500 mg/m^2]
Repeat cycle every 21-28 days

EMA 86

Use Leukemia, acute myeloid

Regimen
Mitoxantrone: I.V.: 12 mg/m^2/day days 1, 2, and 3
[total dose/cycle = 36 mg/m^2]
Etoposide: I.V.: 200 mg/m^2/day continuous infusion days 8, 9, and 10
[total dose/cycle = 600 mg/m^2]
Cytarabine: I.V.: 500 mg/m^2/day continuous infusion days 1, 2, and 3 and days 8, 9, and 10
[total dose/cycle = 3000 mg/m^2]
Administer one cycle only

EMA/CO

Use Gestational trophoblastic tumor

Regimen NOTE: Multiple variations are listed below.
Variation 1:
Etoposide: I.V.: 100 mg/m^2/day days 1 and 2
[total dose/cycle = 200 mg/m^2]
Methotrexate: I.V.: 300 mg/m^2 continuous infusion over 12 hours day 1
[total dose/cycle = 300 mg/m^2]
Dactinomycin: I.V. push: 0.5 mg/day days 1 and 2
[total dose/cycle = 1 mg]

Leucovorin: Oral, I.M.: 15 mg twice daily for 2 days (start 24 hours after the start of methotrexate) days 2 and 3
[total dose/cycle = 60 mg]
Alternate weekly with:
Cyclophosphamide: I.V.: 600 mg/m^2 day 1
[total dose/cycle = 600 mg/m^2]
Vincristine: I.V. push: 0.8 mg/m^2 (maximum 2 mg) day 1
[total dose/cycle = 0.8 mg/m^2]
Repeat cycle every 2 weeks
Variation 2:
Dactinomycin: I.V.: 0.5 mg/day days 1 and 2
[total dose/cycle = 1 mg]
Etoposide: I.V.: 100 mg/m^2/day days 1 and 2
[total dose/cycle = 200 mg/m^2]
Methotrexate: I.V. bolus: 100 mg/m^2 then 200 mg/m^2 continuous infusion over 12 hours day 1
[total dose/cycle = 300 mg/m^2]
Leucovorin: Oral, I.M.: 15 mg every 12 hours for 4 doses (start 24 hours after methotrexate) days 2 and 3
[total dose/cycle = 60 mg]
Vincristine: I.V.: 1 mg/m^2 day 8
[total dose/cycle = 1 mg/m^2]
Cyclophosphamide: I.V.: 600 mg/m^2 day 8
[total dose/cycle = 600 mg/m^2]
Repeat cycle every 2 weeks
Variation 3:
Dactinomycin: I.V.: 0.5 mg/day days 1 and 2
[total dose/cycle = 1 mg]
Etoposide: I.V.: 100 mg/m^2/day days 1 and 2
[total dose/cycle = 200 mg/m^2]
Methotrexate: I.V.: 300 mg/m^2 continuous infusion over 12 hours day 1
[total dose/cycle = 300 mg/m^2]
Leucovorin: Oral, I.M.: 15 mg every 12 hours for 4 doses (start 24 hours after start of methotrexate) days 2 and 3
[total dose/cycle = 60 mg]
Vincristine: I.V.: 1 mg/m^2 day 8
[total dose/cycle = 1 mg/m^2]
Cyclophosphamide: I.V.: 600 mg/m^2 day 8
[total dose/cycle = 600 mg/m^2]
Repeat cycle every 2 weeks
Variation 4:
Dactinomycin: I.V.: 0.35 mg/m^2/day days 1 and 2
[total dose/cycle = 0.7 mg/m^2]
Etoposide: I.V.: 100 mg/m^2/day days 1 and 2
[total dose/cycle = 200 mg/m^2]
Methotrexate: I.V. bolus: 100 mg/m^2 then 200 mg/m^2 continuous infusion over 12 hours day 1
[total dose/cycle = 300 mg/m^2]
Leucovorin: Oral, I.M.: 15 mg every 12 hours for 4 doses (start 24 hours after start of methotrexate) days 2 and 3
[total dose/cycle = 60 mg]
Vincristine: I.V.: 1 mg/m^2 day 8
[total dose/cycle = 1 mg/m^2]
Cyclophosphamide: I.V.: 600 mg/m^2 day 8
[total dose/cycle = 600 mg/m^2]
Repeat cycle every 2 weeks
Variation 5 (patients with brain metastases):
Dactinomycin: I.V.: 0.5 mg/day days 1 and 2
[total dose/cycle = 1 mg]
Etoposide:I.V.: 100 mg/m^2/day days 1 and 2
[total dose/cycle = 200 mg/m^2]
Methotrexate: I.V.: 1 g/m^2 continuous infusion over 12 hours day 1
[total dose/cycle = 1 g/m^2]
Leucovorin: I.M.: 20 mg/m^2 every 6 hours for 12 doses (start 24 hours after start of methotrexate) days 2, 3, and 4
[total dose/cycle = 240 mg/m^2]

Vincristine: I.V.: 1 mg/m^2 day 8
[total dose/cycle = 1 mg/m^2]
Cyclophosphamide: I.V.: 600 mg/m^2 day 8
[total dose/cycle = 600 mg/m^2]
Repeat cycle every 2 weeks
Variation 6 (patients with brain metastases):
Dactinomycin: I.V.: 0.5 mg/day days 1 and 2
[total dose/cycle = 1 mg]
Etoposide: I.V.: 100 mg/m^2/day days 1 and 2
[total dose/cycle = 200 mg/m^2]
Methotrexate: I.V.: 1 g/m^2 continuous infusion over 12 hours day 1
[total dose/cycle = 1 g/m^2]
Leucovorin: Oral, I.M.: 30 mg/m^2 every 12 hours for 6 doses (start 32 hours after start of methotrexate)
days 2, 3, and 4
[total dose/cycle = 180 mg/m^2]
Vincristine: I.V.: 1 mg/m^2 day 8
[total dose/cycle = 1 mg/m^2]
Cyclophosphamide: I.V.: 600 mg/m^2 day 8
[total dose/cycle = 600 mg/m^2]
Repeat cycle every 2 weeks
Variation 7:
Dactinomycin: I.V.: 0.5 mg/day days 1 and 2
[total dose/cycle = 1 mg]
Etoposide: I.V.: 100 mg/m^2/day days 1 and 2
[total dose/cycle = 200 mg/m^2]
Methotrexate: I.V.: 1 g/m^2 continuous infusion over 24 hours day 1
[total dose/cycle = 1 g/m^2]
Leucovorin: Oral, I.M.: 15 mg every 8 hours for 9 doses (start 32 hours after start of methotrexate) days 2,
3, and 4
[total dose/cycle = 135 mg/m^2]
Vincristine: I.V.: 1 mg/m^2 day 8
[total dose/cycle = 1 mg/m^2]
Cyclophosphamide: I.V.: 600 mg/m^2 day 8
[total dose/cycle = 600 mg/m^2]
Repeat cycle every 2 weeks
Variation 8 (patients with lung metastases):
Dactinomycin: I.V.: 0.5 mg/day days 1 and 2
[total dose/cycle = 1 mg]
Etoposide: I.V.: 100 mg/m^2/day days 1 and 2
[total dose/cycle = 200 mg/m^2]
Methotrexate: I.V. bolus: 100 mg/m^2 then 200 mg/m^2 continuous infusion over 12 hours day 1
[total dose/cycle = 300 mg/m^2]
Leucovorin: Oral, I.M.: 15 mg every 12 hours for 4 doses (start 24 hours after start of methotrexate) days 2
and 3
[total dose/cycle = 60 mg]
Vincristine: I.V.: 1 mg/m^2 day 8
[total dose/cycle = 1 mg/m^2]
Cyclophosphamide: I.V.: 600 mg/m^2 day 8
[total dose/cycle = 600 mg/m^2]
Methotrexate: I.T.: 10 mg day 1 (every other cycle)
[total dose/cycle = 10 mg, every other cycle]
Repeat cycle every 2 weeks
Variation 9 (patients with lung metastases):
Dactinomycin: I.V.: 0.5 mg/day days 1 and 2
[total dose/cycle = 1 mg]
Etoposide: I.V.: 100 mg/m^2/day days 1 and 2
[total dose/cycle = 200 mg/m^2]
Methotrexate: I.V. bolus: 100 mg/m^2 then 200 mg/m^2 continuous infusion over 12 hours day 1
[total dose/cycle = 300 mg/m^2]
Leucovorin: Oral, I.M.: 15 mg every 12 hours for 4 doses (start 24 hours after start of methotrexate) days 2
and 3
[total dose/cycle = 60 mg]

Vincristine: I.V.: 1 mg/m^2 day 8
[total dose/cycle = 1 mg/m^2]
Cyclophosphamide: I.V.: 600 mg/m^2 day 8
[total dose/cycle = 600 mg/m^2]
Methotrexate: I.T.: 12.5 mg day 8
[total dose/cycle = 12.5 mg]
Repeat cycle every 2 weeks

EP (Adenocarcinoma)

Use Adenocarcinoma, unknown primary
Regimen
Cisplatin: I.V.: 60-100 mg/m^2 day 1
[total dose = 60-100 mg/m^2]
Etoposide: I.V.: 80-100 mg/m^2/day days 1, 2, and 3
[total dose = 240-300 mg/m^2]
Repeat cycle every 21 days

EP (Small Cell Lung Cancer)

Use Lung cancer, small cell
Regimen NOTE: Multiple variations are listed below.
Variation 1:
Etoposide: I.V.: 100 mg/m^2/day days 1, 2, and 3
[total dose/cycle = 300 mg/m^2]
Cisplatin: I.V.: 100 mg/m^2 day 1
[total dose/cycle = 100 mg/m^2]
Repeat cycle every 21 days
Variation 2:
Etoposide: I.V.: 80 mg/m^2/day days 1, 2, and 3
[total dose/cycle = 240 mg/m^2]
Cisplatin: I.V.: 80 mg/m^2 day 1
[total dose/cycle = 80 mg/m^2]
Repeat cycle every 21-28 days

EP/EMA

Use Gestational trophoblastic tumor
Regimen NOTE: Multiple variations are listed below.
Variation 1:
Etoposide: I.V.: 150 mg/m^2 day 1
[total dose/cycle = 150 mg/m^2]
Cisplatin: I.V.: 25 mg/m^2 infused over 4 hours for 3 consecutive doses, day 1
[total dose/cycle = 75 mg/m^2]
Alternate weekly with:
Etoposide: I.V.: 100 mg/m^2 day 1
[total dose/cycle = 100 mg/m^2]
Methotrexate: I.V.: 300 mg/m^2 infused over 12 hours day 1
[total dose/cycle = 300 mg/m^2]
Dactinomycin: I.V. push: 0.5 mg day 1
[total dose/cycle = 0.5 mg]
Leucovorin: Oral, I.M.: 15 mg twice daily for 2 days (start 24 hours after the start of methotrexate) days 2 and 3
[total dose/cycle = 60 mg]
Variation 2:
Dactinomycin: I.V.: 0.5 mg/day days 1 and 2
[total dose/cycle = 1 mg]
Etoposide: I.V.: 100 mg/m^2/day days 1 and 2
[total dose/cycle = 200 mg/m^2]
Methotrexate: I.V.: 300 mg/m^2 continuous infusion over 12 hours day 1
[total dose/cycle = 300 mg/m^2]
Leucovorin: Oral, I.M.: 15 mg every 12 hours for 4 doses (start 24 hours after start of methotrexate) days 2 and 3
[total dose/cycle = 60 mg]
Etoposide: I.V.: 150 mg/m^2 day 8
[total dose/cycle = 150 mg/m^2]

Cisplatin: I.V.: 75 mg/m^2 day 8
[total dose/cycle = 75 mg/m^2]
Repeat cycle every 2 weeks

Epirubicin-Oxaliplatin-Capecitabine

Use Esophageal cancer; Gastric cancer

Regimen
Epirubicin: I.V.: 50 mg/m^2 day 1
[total dose/cycle = 50 mg/m^2]
Oxaliplatin: I.V.: 130 mg/m^2 day 1
[total dose/cycle = 130 mg/m^2]
Capecitabine: Oral: 625 mg/m^2 twice daily days 1 to 21
[total dose/cycle = 26,250 mg/m^2]
Repeat cycle every 21 days for up to 8 cycles

EP (Nonsmall Cell Lung Cancer)

Use Lung cancer, nonsmall cell

Regimen
Etoposide: I.V.: 80-120 mg/m^2/day days 1, 2, and 3
[total dose/cycle = 240-360 mg/m^2]
Cisplatin: I.V.: 80-100 mg/m^2 day 1
[total dose/cycle = 80-100 mg/m^2]
Repeat cycle every 21-28 days

EPOCH

Use Lymphoma, non-Hodgkin

Regimen
Etoposide: I.V.: 50 mg/m^2/day continuous infusion days 1 to 4
[total dose/cycle = 200 mg/m^2]
Vincristine: I.V.: 0.4 mg/m^2/day continuous infusion days 1 to 4
[total dose/cycle = 1.6 mg/m^2]
Doxorubicin: I.V.: 10 mg/m^2/day continuous infusion days 1 to 4
[total dose/cycle = 40 mg/m^2]
Cyclophosphamide: I.V.: 750 mg/m^2 day 6
[total dose/cycle = 750 mg/m^2]
Prednisone: Oral: 60 mg/m^2/day days 1 to 6
[total dose/cycle = 360 mg/m^2]
Repeat cycle every 21 days

EP/PE

Use Lung cancer, nonsmall cell

Regimen
Etoposide: I.V.: 120 mg/m^2/day days 1, 2, and 3
[total dose/cycle = 360 mg/m^2]
Cisplatin: I.V.: 60-120 mg/m^2 day 1
[total dose/cycle = 60-120 mg/m^2]
Repeat cycle every 21-28 days

EP (Testicular Cancer)

Use Testicular cancer

Regimen NOTE: Multiple variations are listed below.
Variation 1:
Etoposide: I.V.: 100 mg/m^2/day days 1 to 5
[total dose/cycle = 500 mg/m^2]
Cisplatin: I.V.: 20 mg/m^2/day days 1 to 5
[total dose/cycle = 100 mg/m^2]
Repeat cycle every 21 days
Variation 2:
Etoposide: I.V.: 120 mg/m^2/day days 1, 2, and 3
[total dose/cycle = 360 mg/m^2]

◄ Cisplatin: I.V.: 20 mg/m^2/day days 1 to 5
   [total dose/cycle = 100 mg/m^2]
   Repeat cycle every 3 or 4 weeks
   Variation 3:
   Etoposide: I.V.: 120 mg/m^2/day days 1, 3, and 5
     [total dose/cycle = 360 mg/m^2]
   Cisplatin: I.V.: 20 mg/m^2/day days 1 to 5
     [total dose/cycle = 100 mg/m^2]
   Repeat cycle every 3 weeks

ESHAP

Use Lymphoma, non-Hodgkin

Regimen NOTE: Multiple variations are listed below.
   Variation 1:
   Etoposide: I.V.: 40 mg/m^2/day days 1 to 4
     [total dose/cycle = 160 mg/m^2]
   Methylprednisolone: I.V.: 250-500 mg/day days 1 to 5
     [total dose/cycle = 1250-2500 mg]
   Cytarabine: I.V.: 2000 mg/m^2 day 5
     [total dose/cycle = 2000 mg/m^2]
   Cisplatin: I.V.: 25 mg/m^2/day continuous infusion days 1 to 4
     [total dose/cycle = 100 mg/m^2]
   Repeat cycle every 21-28 days
   Variation 2:
   Etoposide: I.V.: 40 mg/m^2/day days 1 to 4
     [total dose/cycle = 160 mg/m^2]
   Methylprednisolone: I.V.: 500 mg/day days 1 to 5
     [total dose/cycle = 2500 mg]
   Cytarabine: I.V.: 2000 mg/m^2 day 5
     [total dose/cycle = 2000 mg/m^2]
   Cisplatin: I.V.: 25 mg/m^2/day continuous infusion days 1 to 4
     [total dose/cycle = 100 mg/m^2]
   Repeat cycle every 21-28 days
   Variation 3:
   Etoposide: I.V.: 60 mg/m^2/day days 1 to 4
     [total dose/cycle = 240 mg/m^2]
   Methylprednisolone: I.V.: 500 mg/day days 1 to 4
     [total dose/cycle = 2000 mg]
   Cytarabine: I.V.: 2000 mg/m^2 day 5
     [total dose/cycle = 2000 mg/m^2]
   Cisplatin: I.V.: 25 mg/m^2/day continuous infusion days 1 to 4
     [total dose/cycle = 100 mg/m^2]
   Repeat cycle every 21 days

Estramustine + Docetaxel

Use Prostate cancer

Regimen NOTE: Multiple variations are listed below.
   Variation 1:
   Docetaxel: I.V.: 20-80 mg/m^2 day 2
     [total dose/cycle = 20-80 mg/m^2]
   Estramustine: Oral: 280 mg 3 times/day days 1 to 5
     [total dose/cycle = 4200 mg]
   Repeat cycle every 21 days
   Variation 2:
   Docetaxel: I.V.: 20-80 mg/m^2 day 2
     [total dose/cycle = 20-80 mg/m^2]
   Estramustine: Oral: 14 mg/kg/day days 1 to 21
     [total dose/cycle = 294 mg/kg]
   Repeat cycle every 21 days
   Variation 3:
   Docetaxel: I.V.: 35 mg/m^2/day days 2 and 9
     [total dose/cycle = 70 mg/m^2]

Estramustine: Oral: 420 mg 3 times/day for 4 doses, then 280 mg 3 times/day for 5 doses days 1, 2, 3, 8, 9, and 10
[total dose/cycle = 6160 mg]
Repeat cycle every 21 days
Variation 4:
Docetaxel: I.V.: 60 mg/m^2 day 2 cycle 1
[total dose/cycle = 60 mg/m^2]
followed by I.V.: 60-70 mg/m^2 day 2 (subsequent cycles)
[total dose/cycle = 60-70 mg/m^2]
Estramustine: Oral: 280 mg 3 times/day days 1 to 5
[total dose/cycle = 4200 mg]
Repeat cycle every 21 days for up to 12 cycles

Estramustine + Docetaxel + Calcitriol

Use Prostate cancer

Regimen
Cycle 1:
Calcitriol: Oral: 60 mcg (in divided doses) day 1
[total dose/cycle = 60 mcg]
Estramustine: Oral: 280 mg 3 times/day days 1 to 5
[total dose/cycle = 4200 mg]
Docetaxel: I.V.: 60 mg/m^2 day 2
[total dose/cycle = 60 mg/m^2]
Treatment cycle is 21 days
Subsequent cycles:
Calcitriol: Oral: 60 mcg (in divided doses) day 1
[total dose/cycle = 60 mcg]
Estramustine: Oral: 280 mg 3 times/day days 1 to 5
[total dose/cycle = 4200 mg]
Docetaxel: I.V.: 70 mg/m^2 day 2
[total dose/cycle = 70 mg/m^2]
Repeat cycle every 21 days for up to 12 cycles

Estramustine + Docetaxel + Carboplatin

Use Prostate cancer

Regimen
Docetaxel: I.V.: 70 mg/m^2 day 2
[total dose/cycle = 70 mg/m^2]
Estramustine: Oral: 280 mg 3 times/day days 1 to 5
[total dose/cycle = 4200 mg]
Carboplatin: I.V.: Target AUC 5 day 2
[total dose/cycle = AUC = 5]
Repeat cycle every 3 weeks

Estramustine + Docetaxel + Hydrocortisone

Use Prostate cancer

Regimen
Docetaxel: I.V.: 70 mg/m^2 day 2
[total dose/cycle = 70 mg/m^2]
Estramustine: Oral: 10 mg/kg/day days 1 to 5
[total dose/cycle = 50 mg/kg]
Hydrocortisone: Oral: 40 mg daily
[total dose/cycle = 840 mg]
Repeat cycle every 3 weeks

Estramustine + Docetaxel + Prednisone

Use Prostate cancer

Regimen
Estramustine: Oral: 280 mg 3 times/day days 1 to 5 and days 7 to 11
[total dose/cycle = 8400 mg]
Docetaxel: I.V.: 70 mg/m^2 day 2
[total dose/cycle = 70 mg/m^2]

◄ Prednisone: Oral: 10 mg daily
  [total dose/cycle = 210 mg]
  Repeat cycle every 21 days for up to 6 cycles

Estramustine + Etoposide

Use Prostate cancer
Regimen NOTE: Multiple variations are listed below.
  Variation 1:
  Estramustine: Oral: 15 mg/kg/day days 1 to 21
    [total dose/cycle = 315 mg/kg]
  Etoposide: Oral: 50 mg/m^2/day days 1 to 21
    [total dose/cycle = 1050 mg/m^2]
  Repeat cycle every 4 weeks
  Variation 2:
  Estramustine: Oral: 10 mg/kg/day days 1 to 21
    [total dose/cycle = 210 mg/kg]
  Etoposide: Oral: 50 mg/m^2/day days 1 to 21
    [total dose/cycle = 1050 mg/m^2]
  Repeat cycle every 4 weeks
  Variation 3:
  Estramustine: Oral: 140 mg 3 times/day days 1 to 21
    [total dose/cycle = 8820 mg]
  Etoposide: Oral: 50 mg/m^2/day days 1 to 21
    [total dose/cycle = 1050 mg/m^2]
  Repeat cycle every 4 weeks

Estramustine + Vinorelbine

Use Prostate cancer
Regimen NOTE: Multiple variations are listed below.
  Variation 1:
  Estramustine: Oral: 140 mg 3 times/day days 1 to 14
    [total dose/cycle = 5880 mg]
  Vinorelbine: I.V.: 25 mg/m^2/day days 1 and 8
    [total dose/cycle = 50 mg/m^2]
  Repeat cycle every 21 days
  Variation 2:
  Estramustine: Oral: 280 mg 3 times/day days 1, 2, and 3
    [total dose/cycle = 2520 mg/m^2]
  Vinorelbine: I.V.: 15 or 20 mg/m^2 day 2
    [total dose/cycle = 15 or 20 mg/m^2]
  Repeat cycle weekly for 8 weeks, then every other week

EV

Use Prostate cancer
Regimen NOTE: Multiple variations are listed below.
  Variation 1:
  Estramustine: Oral: 10 mg/kg/day days 1 to 42
    [total dose/cycle = 420 mg/kg]
  Vinblastine: I.V.: 4 mg/m^2/day days 1, 8, 15, 22, 29, and 36
    [total dose/cycle = 24 mg/m^2]
  Repeat cycle every 8 weeks
  Variation 2:
  Estramustine: Oral: 600 mg/m^2/day days 1 to 42
    [total dose/cycle = 25,200 mg/m^2]
  Vinblastine: I.V.: 4 mg/m^2/day days 1, 8, 15, 22, 29, and 36
    [total dose/cycle = 24 mg/m^2]
  Repeat cycle every 8 weeks

EVA

Use Lymphoma, Hodgkin disease
Regimen
  Etoposide: I.V.: 100 mg/m^2/day days 1, 2, and 3
    [total dose/cycle = 300 mg/m^2]

Vinblastine: I.V.: 6 mg/m^2 day 1
  [total dose/cycle = 6 mg/m^2]
Doxorubicin: I.V.: 50 mg/m^2 day 1
  [total dose/cycle = 50 mg/m^2]
Repeat cycle every 28 days

FAC

Use Breast cancer
Regimen NOTE: Multiple variations are listed below.
  Variation 1:
    Fluorouracil: I.V.: 500 mg/m^2/day days 1 and 8
      [total dose/cycle = 1000 mg/m^2]
      or 500 mg/m^2 day 1
        [total dose/cycle = 500 mg/m^2]
    Doxorubicin: I.V.: 50 mg/m^2 day 1
      [total dose/cycle = 50 mg/m^2]
    Cyclophosphamide: I.V.: 500 mg/m^2 day 1
      [total dose/cycle = 500 mg/m^2]
    Repeat cycle every 21-28 days
  Variation 2:
    Fluorouracil: I.V.: 200 mg/m^2/day days 1, 2, and 3
      [total dose/cycle = 600 mg/m^2]
    Doxorubicin: I.V.: 40 mg/m^2 day 1
      [total dose/cycle = 40 mg/m^2]
    Cyclophosphamide: I.V.: 400 mg/m^2 day 1
      [total dose/cycle = 400 mg/m^2]
    Repeat cycle every 28 days
  Variation 3:
    Fluorouracil: I.V.: 400 mg/m^2/day days 1 and 8
      [total dose/cycle = 800 mg/m^2]
    Doxorubicin: I.V.: 40 mg/m^2 day 1
      [total dose/cycle = 40 mg/m^2]
    Cyclophosphamide: I.V.: 400 mg/m^2 day 1
      [total dose/cycle = 400 mg/m^2]
    Repeat cycle every 28 days
  Variation 4:
    Fluorouracil: I.V.: 600 mg/m^2/day days 1 and 8
      [total dose/cycle = 1200 mg/m^2]
    Doxorubicin: I.V.: 60 mg/m^2 day 1
      [total dose/cycle = 60 mg/m^2]
    Cyclophosphamide: I.V.: 600 mg/m^2 day 1
      [total dose/cycle = 600 mg/m^2]
    Repeat cycle every 28 days
  Variation 5:
    Fluorouracil: I.V.: 300 mg/m^2/day days 1 and 8
      [total dose/cycle = 600 mg/m^2]
    Doxorubicin: I.V.: 30 mg/m^2 day 1
      [total dose/cycle = 30 mg/m^2]
    Cyclophosphamide: I.V.: 300 mg/m^2 day 1
      [total dose/cycle = 300 mg/m^2]
    Repeat cycle every 28 days

FAM

Use Gastric cancer; Pancreatic cancer
Regimen NOTE: Multiple variations are listed below
  Variation 1:
    Fluorouracil: I.V.: 600 mg/m^2/day days 1, 8, 29, and 36
      [total dose/cycle = 2400 mg/m^2]
    Doxorubicin: I.V.: 30 mg/m^2/day days 1 and 29
      [total dose/cycle = 60 mg/m^2]
    Mitomycin: I.V.: 10 mg/m^2 day 1
      [total dose/cycle = 10 mg/m^2]
    Repeat cycle every 8 weeks

Variation 2:
  Fluorouracil: I.V.: 600 mg/m^2/day days 29 to 32
  [total dose/cycle = 2400 mg/m^2]
  Doxorubicin: I.V.: 50 mg/m^2 day 1
  [total dose/cycle = 50 mg/m^2]
  Mitomycin: I.V.: 10 mg/m^2 day 3
  [total dose/cycle = 10 mg/m^2]
  Repeat cycle every 8 weeks
Variation 3:
  Fluorouracil: I.V.: 500 mg/m^2/day days 1, 8, 21, and 28
  [total dose/cycle = 2000 mg/m^2]
  Doxorubicin: I.V.: 30 mg/m^2/day days 1 and 21
  [total dose/cycle = 60 mg/m^2]
  Mitomycin: I.V.: 10 mg/m^2 day 1
  [total dose/cycle = 10 mg/m^2]
  Repeat cycle every 6 weeks
Variation 4:
  Fluorouracil: I.V.: 275 mg/m^2/day days 1 to 5 and 36 to 40
  [total dose/cycle = 2750 mg/m^2]
  Doxorubicin: I.V.: 30 mg/m^2/day days 1 and 36
  [total dose/cycle = 60 mg/m^2]
  Mitomycin: I.V.: 10 mg/m^2 day 1
  [total dose/cycle = 10 mg/m^2]
  Repeat cycle every 10 weeks
Variation 5:
  Fluorouracil: I.V.: 600 mg/m^2/day days 1, 8, 22, and 29
  [total dose/cycle = 2400 mg/m^2]
  Doxorubicin: I.V.: 30 mg/m^2/day days 1 and 22
  [total dose/cycle = 60 mg/m^2]
  Mitomycin: I.V.: 10 mg/m^2 day 1
  [total dose/cycle = 10 mg/m^2]
  Repeat cycle every 6 weeks

FAMe

Use Gastric cancer

Regimen
  Fluorouracil: I.V.: 325 mg/m^2/day days 1 to 5 and days 36 to 40
  [total dose/cycle = 3250 mg/m^2]
  Doxorubicin: I.V.: 40 mg/m^2 day 1 and day 36
  [total dose/cycle = 80 mg/m^2]
  Lomustine: Oral: 110 mg/m^2 day 1
  [total dose/cycle = 110 mg/m^2]
  Repeat cycle every 10 weeks

FAMTX

Use Gastric cancer

Regimen NOTE: Multiple variations are listed below.
Variation 1:
  Methotrexate: I.V.: 1500 mg/m^2 day 1
  [total dose/cycle = 1500 mg/m^2]
  Fluorouracil: I.V.: 1500 mg/m^2 (1 hour after methotrexate) day 1
  [total dose/cycle = 1500 mg/m^2]
  Leucovorin: Oral: 15 mg/m^2 every 6 hours for 48 hours (start 24 hours after methotrexate) day 2
  [total dose/cycle = 120 mg/m^2]
  Doxorubicin: I.V.: 30 mg/m^2 day 15
  [total dose/cycle = 30 mg/m^2]
  Repeat cycle every 28 days
Variation 2:
  Methotrexate: I.V.: 1500 mg/m^2 day 1
  [total dose/cycle = 1500 mg/m^2]

Fluorouracil: I.V.: 1500 mg/m^2 (1 hour after methotrexate) day 1
  [total dose/cycle = 1500 mg/m^2]
Leucovorin: Oral: 30 mg/m^2 every 6 hours for 8 doses (start 24 hours after methotrexate)
  [total dose/cycle = 240 mg/m^2]
    followed by Oral: 30 mg/m^2 every 6 hours for 8 more doses if 24-hour methotrexate level ≥2.5 mol/L
      [total cumulative dose/cycle = 480 mg/m^2]
Doxorubicin: I.V.: 30 mg/m^2 day 15
  [total dose/cycle = 30 mg/m^2]
Repeat cycle every 28 days
Variation 3:
Methotrexate: I.V.: 1000 mg/m^2 day 1
  [total dose/cycle = 1000 mg/m^2]
Fluorouracil: I.V.: 1500 mg/m^2 (1 hour after methotrexate) day 1
  [total dose/cycle = 1500 mg/m^2]
Leucovorin: Oral: 15 mg every 6 hours for 8 doses (start 24 hours after methotrexate)
  [total dose/cycle = 120 mg/m^2]
Doxorubicin: I.V.: 30 mg/m^2 day 15
  [total dose/cycle = 30 mg/m^2]
Repeat cycle every 28 days

FAP

Use Gastric cancer
Regimen
Fluorouracil: I.V.: 300 mg/m^2/day days 1 to 5
  [total dose/cycle = 1500 mg/m^2]
Doxorubicin: I.V.: 40 mg/m^2 day 1
  [total dose/cycle = 40 mg/m^2]
Cisplatin: I.V.: 60 mg/m^2 day 1
  [total dose/cycle = 60 mg/m^2]
Repeat cycle every 5 weeks

FEC

Use Breast cancer
Regimen
Fluorouracil: I.V.: 500 mg/m^2 day 1
  [total dose/cycle = 500 mg/m^2]
Cyclophosphamide: I.V.: 500 mg/m^2 day 1
  [total dose/cycle = 500 mg/m^2]
Epirubicin: I.V.: 100 mg/m^2 day 1
  [total dose/cycle = 100 mg/m^2]
Repeat cycle every 21 days

FIS-HAM

Use Leukemia, acute lymphocytic; Leukemia, acute myeloid
Regimen
Fludarabine: I.V.: 15 mg/m^2/day every 12 hours days 1, 2, 8, and 9
  [total dose/cycle = 120 mg/m^2]
Cytarabine: I.V.: 750 mg/m^2/day every 3 hours days 1, 2, 8, and 9
  [total dose/cycle = 24,000 mg/m^2]
Mitoxantrone: I.V.: 10 mg/m^2/day days 3, 4, 10, and 11
  [total dose/cycle = 40 mg/m^2]

FL

Use Prostate cancer
Regimen NOTE: Multiple variations are listed below.
Variation 1:
Flutamide: Oral: 250 mg every 8 hours
  [total dose/cycle = 21,000 mg]
Leuprolide acetate: SubQ: 1 mg/day
  [total dose/cycle = 28 mg]
Repeat cycle every 28 days

Variation 2:
  Flutamide: Oral: 250 mg every 8 hours
    [total dose/cycle = 67,500 mg]
  Leuprolide acetate depot: I.M.: 22.5 mg day 1
    [total dose/cycle = 22.5 mg]
  Repeat cycle every 3 months

FLAG

Use Leukemia, acute myeloid
Regimen
  Fludarabine: I.V.: 30 mg/m^2/day days 1 to 5
    [total dose/cycle = 150 mg/m^2]
  Cytarabine: I.V.: 2 g/m^2/day days 1 to 5 (3.5 hours after end of fludarabine infusion)
    [total dose/cycle = 10 g/m^2]
  Filgrastim: SubQ: 5 mcg/kg day 1
    followed by SubQ: 300 mcg daily until ANC >500-1000 cells/mcL postnadir
    [total dose/cycle = 40-7800 mcg/kg]
  Repeat cycle every 3-4 weeks

FLAG-IDA

Use Leukemia, acute myeloid
Regimen
  Fludarabine: I.V.: 30 mg/m^2/day days 1 to 5
    [total dose/cycle = 150 mg/m^2]
  Cytarabine: I.V.: 2 g/m^2/day days 1 to 5
    [total dose/cycle = 10 g/m^2]
  Idarubicin: I.V.: 10 mg/m^2/day days 1, 2, and 3
    [total dose/cycle = 30 mg/m^2]
  Filgrastim: 5 mcg/kg from day 6 until neutrophil recovery
  Administer one cycle only

FLOX (Nordic FLOX)

Use Colorectal cancer
Regimen
  Oxaliplatin: I.V.: 85 mg/m^2 day 1
    [total dose/cycle = 85 mg/m^2]
  Fluorouracil: I.V.: 500 mg/m^2/day days 1 and 2
    [total dose/cycle = 1000 mg/m^2]
  Leucovorin: I.V.: 60 mg/m^2/day days 1 and 2
    [total dose/cycle = 120 mg/m^2]
  Repeat cycle every 2 weeks

Fludarabine-Cyclophosphamide (FC)

Use Leukemia, chronic lymphocytic
Regimen NOTE: Multiple variations are listed below.
  Variation 1:
    Fludarabine: I.V.: 25 mg/m^2/day days 1, 2, and 3
      [total dose/cycle = 75 mg/m^2]
    Cyclophosphamide: I.V.: 250 mg/m^2/day days 1, 2, and 3
      [total dose/cycle = 750 mg/m^2]
    Repeat cycle every 4 weeks for up to 6 cycles
  Variation 2:
    Fludarabine: I.V.: 30 mg/m^2/day days 1, 2, and 3
      [total dose/cycle = 90 mg/m^2]
    Cyclophosphamide: I.V.: 250 mg/m^2/day days 1, 2, and 3
      [total dose/cycle = 750 mg/m^2]
    Repeat cycle every 4 weeks for up to 6 cycles
  Variation 3:
    Cyclophosphamide: I.V.: 600 mg/m^2 day 1 only
      [total dose/cycle = 600 mg/m^2]
    Fludarabine: I.V.: 20 mg/m^2/day days 1 to 5
      [total dose/cycle = 100 mg/m^2]
    Repeat cycle every 4 weeks for up to 6 cycles

Variation 4:
  Fludarabine: I.V.: 30 mg/m^2/day days 1, 2, and 3
    [total dose/cycle = 90 mg/m^2]
  Cyclophosphamide: I.V.: 300 mg/m^2/day days 1, 2, and 3
    [total dose/cycle = 900 mg/m^2]
  Repeat cycle every 4 weeks for up to 6 cycles
Variation 5:
  Fludarabine: I.V.: 30 mg/m^2/day days 1, 2, and 3
    [total dose/cycle = 90 mg/m^2]
  Cyclophosphamide: I.V.: 300 mg/m^2/day days 1, 2, and 3
    [total dose/cycle = 900 mg/m^2]
  Repeat cycle every 4-6 weeks for up to 6 cycles

Fludarabine-Cyclophosphamide-Rituximab (CLL)

Use Leukemia, chronic lymphocytic

Regimen
  Cycle 1:
    Rituximab: I.V.: 375 mg/m^2 day 1
      [total dose/cycle = 375 mg/m^2]
    Fludarabine: I.V.: 25 mg/m^2/day days 2, 3, and 4
      [total dose/cycle = 75 mg/m^2]
    Cyclophosphamide: I.V.: 250 mg/m^2/day days 2, 3, and 4
      [total dose/cycle = 750 mg/m^2]
    Treatment cycle is 4 weeks
  Cycles 2-6:
    Rituximab: I.V.: 500 mg/m^2 day 1
      [total dose/cycle = 500 mg/m^2]
    Fludarabine: I.V.: 25 mg/m^2/day days 1, 2, and 3
      [total dose/cycle = 75 mg/m^2]
    Cyclophosphamide: I.V.: 250 mg/m^2/day days 1, 2, and 3
      [total dose/cycle = 750 mg/m^2]
    Repeat cycle every 4 weeks

Fludarabine-Cyclophosphamide-Rituximab (NHL)

Use Lymphoma, non-Hodgkin (Follicular lymphoma)

Regimen
  Cycle 1:
    Rituximab: I.V.: 375 mg/m^2 day 15
      [total dose/cycle = 375 mg/m^2]
    Fludarabine: I.V.: 25 mg/m^2/day days 1, 2, and 3
      [total dose/cycle = 75 mg/m^2]
    Cyclophosphamide: I.V.: 300 mg/m^2/day days 1, 2, and 3
      [total dose/cycle = 900 mg/m^2]
    Treatment cycle is 3 weeks
  Cycles 2-4:
    Rituximab: I.V.: 375 mg/m^2 day 1
      [total dose/cycle = 375 mg/m^2]
    Fludarabine: I.V.: 25 mg/m^2/day days 1, 2, and 3
      [total dose/cycle = 75 mg/m^2]
    Cyclophosphamide: I.V.: 300 mg/m^2/day days 1, 2, and 3
      [total dose/cycle = 900 mg/m^2]
    Each treatment cycle is 3 weeks

Fludarabine-Rituximab

Use Leukemia, chronic lymphocytic

Regimen
  Rituximab: I.V.: 375 mg/m^2/day days 1 and 4 (cycle 1); day 1 (cycles 2 to 6)
  Fludarabine: I.V.: 25 mg/m^2/day days 1 to 5
  Repeat cycle every 4 weeks

Fluorouracil + Carboplatin

Use Head and neck cancer

Regimen NOTE: Multiple variations are listed below.
  Variation 1:
    Fluorouracil: I.V.: 600 mg/m^2/day continuous infusion days 1 to 4
      [total dose/cycle = 2400 mg/m^2]
    Carboplatin: I.V.: 70 mg/m^2/day days 1 to 4
      [total dose/cycle = 280 mg/m^2]
    Repeat cycle every 3 weeks for 3 cycles
  Variation 2:
    Carboplatin: I.V.: 400 mg/m^2 day 1
      [total dose/cycle = 400 mg/m^2]
    Fluorouracil: I.V.: 1000 mg/m^2/day continuous infusion days 1 to 4
      [total dose/cycle = 4000 mg/m^2]
    Repeat cycle every 28 days

Fluorouracil-Leucovorin

Use Colorectal cancer

Regimen NOTE: Multiple variations are listed below.
  Variation 1 (Mayo Regimen):
    Fluorouracil: I.V.: 425 mg/m^2/day days 1 to 5
      [total dose/cycle = 2125 mg/m^2]
    Leucovorin: I.V.: 20 mg/m^2/day days 1 to 5
      [total dose/cycle = 100 mg/m^2]
    Repeat cycle every 28 days
  Variation 2:
    Fluorouracil: I.V.: 400 mg/m^2/day days 1 to 5
      [total dose/cycle = 2000 mg/m^2]
    Leucovorin: I.V.: 20 mg/m^2/day days 1 to 5
      [total dose/cycle = 100 mg/m^2]
    Repeat cycle every 28 days
  Variation 3:
    Fluorouracil: I.V.: 500 mg/m^2 day 1
      [total dose/cycle = 500 mg/m^2]
    Leucovorin: I.V.: 20 mg/m^2 (2-hour infusion) day 1
      [total dose/cycle = 20 mg/m^2]
      or 500 mg/m^2 (2-hour infusion) day 1
        [total dose/cycle = 500 mg/m^2]
    Repeat cycle weekly
  Variation 4:
    Fluorouracil: I.V.: 600 mg/m^2 weekly for 6 weeks
      [total dose/cycle = 3600 mg/m^2]
    Leucovorin: I.V.: 500 mg/m^2 (3-hour infusion) weekly for 6 weeks
      [total dose/cycle = 3000 mg/m^2]
    Repeat cycle every 8 weeks
  Variation 5:
    Fluorouracil: I.V.: 600 mg/m^2 weekly for 6 weeks
      [total dose/cycle = 3600 mg/m^2]
    Leucovorin: I.V.: 500 mg/m^2 weekly for 6 weeks
      [total dose/cycle = 3000 mg/m^2]
    Repeat cycle every 8 weeks
  Variation 6:
    Fluorouracil: I.V.: 600 mg/m^2 weekly
      [total dose/cycle = 600 mg/m^2]
    Leucovorin: I.V.: 500 mg/m^2 (2-hour infusion) weekly
      [total dose/cycle = 500 mg/m^2]
    Repeat cycle weekly
  Variation 7:
    Fluorouracil: I.V.: 2600 mg/m^2 continuous infusion day 1
      [total dose/cycle = 2600 mg/m^2]
    Leucovorin: I.V.: 500 mg/m^2 continuous infusion day 1
      [total dose/cycle = 500 mg/m^2]
    Repeat cycle weekly

Variation 8:
Fluorouracil: I.V.: 2600 mg/m^2 continuous infusion day 1
[total dose/cycle = 2600 mg/m^2]
Leucovorin: I.V.: 300 mg/m^2 (maximum 500 mg) continuous infusion day 1
[total dose/cycle = 300 mg/m^2; maximum 500 mg]
Repeat cycle weekly
Variation 9:
Fluorouracil: I.V.: 2600 mg/m^2 continuous infusion once weekly for 6 weeks
[total dose/cycle = 15,600 mg/m^2]
Leucovorin: I.V.: 500 mg/m^2 weekly for 6 weeks
[total dose/cycle = 3000 mg/m^2]
Repeat cycle every 8 weeks
Variation 10:
Fluorouracil: I.V.: 2300 mg/m^2 continuous infusion day 1
[total dose/cycle = 2300 mg/m^2]
Leucovorin: I.V.: 50 mg/m^2 continuous infusion day 1
[total dose/cycle = 50 mg/m^2]
Repeat cycle weekly
Variation 11:
Fluorouracil: I.V.: 200 mg/m^2/day continuous infusion days 1 to 14
[total dose/cycle = 2800 mg/m^2]
Leucovorin: I.V.: 5 mg/m^2/day continuous infusion days 1 to 14
[total dose/cycle = 70 mg/m^2]
Repeat cycle every 28 days
Variation 12:
Cycle 1:
Fluorouracil: I.V.: 200 mg/m^2/day continuous infusion for 4 weeks
[total dose/cycle = 5600 mg/m^2]
Leucovorin: I.V.: 20 mg/m^2/day days 1, 8, 15, 22
[total dose/cycle = 80 mg/m^2]
Treatment cycle is 6 weeks
Subsequent cycles (starting week 7):
Fluorouracil: 200 mg/m^2 continuous infusion days 1 to 21
[total dose/cycle = 4200 mg/m^2]
Leucovorin: I.V.: 20 mg/m^2/day days 1, 8, and 15
[total dose/cycle = 60 mg/m^2]
Repeat cycle every 4 weeks

Fluorouracil-Leucovorin-Irinotecan (Saltz Regimen)

Use Colorectal cancer

Regimen
Fluorouracil: I.V.: 500 mg/m^2/day days 1, 8, 15, and 22
[total dose/cycle = 2000 mg/m^2]
Leucovorin: I.V.: 20 mg/m^2/day days 1, 8, 15, and 22
[total dose/cycle = 80 mg/m^2]
Irinotecan: I.V.: 125 mg/m^2/day days 1, 8, 15, and 22
[total dose/cycle = 500 mg/m^2]
Repeat cycle every 42 days

FOIL

Use Colorectal cancer

Regimen
Irinotecan: I.V.: 175 mg/m^2 day 1
[total dose/cycle = 175 mg/m^2]
Oxaliplatin: I.V.: 100 mg/m^2 day 1
[total dose/cycle = 100 mg/m^2]
Leucovorin: I.V.: 200 mg/m^2 day 1
[total dose/cycle = 200 mg/m^2]
Fluorouracil: I.V.: 3800 mg/m^2/day continuous infusion days 1 and 2
[total dose/cycle = 7600 mg/m^2]
Repeat cycle every 14 days

FOLFOX 1

Use Colorectal cancer

Regimen
Oxaliplatin: I.V.: 130 mg/m^2 day 1 (every other cycle)
[total dose/cycle = 130 mg/m^2]
Leucovorin: I.V.: 500 mg/m^2/day days 1 and 2
[total dose/cycle = 1000 mg/m^2]
Fluorouracil: I.V.: 1.5-2 g/m^2/day continuous infusion days 1 and 2
[total dose/cycle = 3-4 g/m^2]
Repeat cycle every 14 days

FOLFOX 2

Use Colorectal cancer

Regimen
Oxaliplatin: I.V.: 100 mg/m^2 day 1
[total dose/cycle = 100 mg/m^2]
Leucovorin: I.V.: 500 mg/m^2/day days 1 and 2
[total dose/cycle = 1000 mg/m^2]
Fluorouracil: I.V.: 1.5-2 g/m^2/day continuous infusion days 1 and 2
[total dose/cycle = 3-4 g/m^2]
Repeat cycle every 14 days

FOLFOX 3

Use Colorectal cancer

Regimen
Oxaliplatin: I.V.: 85 mg/m^2 day 1
[total dose/cycle = 85 mg/m^2]
Leucovorin: I.V.: 500 mg/m^2/day days 1 and 2
[total dose/cycle = 1000 mg/m^2]
Fluorouracil: I.V.: 1.5-2 g/m^2/day continuous infusion days 1 and 2
[total dose/cycle = 3-4 g/m^2]
Repeat cycle every 14 days

FOLFOX 4

Use Colorectal cancer

Regimen
Oxaliplatin: I.V.: 85 mg/m^2 day 1
[total dose/cycle = 85 mg/m^2]
Leucovorin: I.V.: 200 mg/m^2/day days 1 and 2
[total dose/cycle = 400 mg/m^2]
Fluorouracil: I.V. bolus: 400 mg/m^2/day days 1 and 2
[total dose/cycle = 800 mg/m^2]
followed by I.V.: 600 mg/m^2 continuous infusion (over 22 hours) days 1 and 2
[total dose/cycle = 1200 mg/m^2]
Note: Bolus fluorouracil and continuous infusion are both given on each day.
Repeat cycle every 14 days

FOLFOX 6

Use Colorectal cancer

Regimen
Oxaliplatin: I.V.: 100 mg/m^2 day 1
[total dose/cycle = 100 mg/m^2]
Leucovorin: I.V.: 400 mg/m^2 day 1
[total dose/cycle = 400 mg/m^2]
Fluorouracil: I.V. bolus: 400 mg/m^2 day 1
[total dose/cycle = 400 mg/m^2]
followed by I.V.: 2.4-3 g/m^2 continuous infusion (46 hours) extending over days 1 and 2
[total dose/cycle = 2.4-3 g/m^2]
Repeat cycle every 14 days

FOLFOX 7

Use Colorectal cancer

Regimen
Oxaliplatin: I.V.: 130 mg/m^2 day 1
[total dose/cycle = 130 mg/m^2]
Leucovorin: I.V.: 400 mg/m^2 day 1
[total dose/cycle = 400 mg/m^2]
Fluorouracil: I.V. bolus: 400 mg/m^2 day 1
[total dose/cycle = 400 mg/m^2]
   followed by I.V.: 2.4 g/m^2 continuous infusion (46 hours) extending over days 1 and 2
   [total dose/cycle = 2.4 g/m^2]
Repeat cycle every 14 days

FU HURT

Use Head and neck cancer

Regimen
Hydroxyurea: Oral: 1000 mg every 12 hours for 11 doses days 0 to 5
Fluorouracil: I.V.: 800 mg/m^2/day continuous infusion (start AM after admission) days 1 to 5
Paclitaxel: I.V.: 5-25 mg/m^2/day continuous infusion days 1 to 5
Filgrastim: SubQ: 5 mcg/kg/day days 6 to 12 (start ≥12 hours after completion of fluorouracil infusion)
5-7 cycles may be administered

FU-LV-CPT-11

Use Colorectal cancer

Regimen NOTE: Multiple variations are listed below.
Variation 1:
  Irinotecan: I.V.: 350 mg/m^2 day 1
  [total dose/cycle = 350 mg/m^2]
  Leucovorin: I.V.: 20 mg/m^2/day days 22 to 26
  [total dose/cycle = 100 mg/m^2]
  Fluorouracil: I.V.: 425 mg/m^2/day days 22 to 26
  [total dose/cycle = 2125 mg/m^2]
  Repeat cycle every 6 weeks
Variation 2:
  Irinotecan: I.V.: 80 mg/m^2 day 1
  [total dose/cycle = 80 mg/m^2]
  Fluorouracil: I.V.: 2300 mg/m^2 continuous infusion day 1
  [total dose/cycle = 2300 mg/m^2]
  Leucovorin: I.V.: 500 mg/m^2 day 1
  [total dose/cycle = 500 mg/m^2]
  Repeat cycle weekly
  or
  Irinotecan: I.V.: 180 mg/m^2 day 1
  [total dose/cycle = 180 mg/m^2]
  Leucovorin: I.V.: 200 mg/m^2/day days 1 and 2
  [total dose/cycle = 400 mg/m^2]
  Fluorouracil: I.V.: 400 mg/m^2/day days 1 and 2
  [total dose/cycle = 800 mg/m^2]
    followed by I.V.: 600 mg/m^2/day continuous infusion days 1 and 2
    [total dose/cycle = 1200 mg/m^2]
  Repeat cycle every 2 weeks
Variation 3:
  Irinotecan: I.V.: 175 mg/m^2 day 1
  [total dose/cycle = 175 mg/m^2]
  Leucovorin: I.V.: 250 mg/m^2 day 2
  [total dose/cycle = 250 mg/m^2]
  Fluorouracil: I.V.: 950 mg/m^2 day 2
  [total dose/cycle = 950 mg/m^2]
  or
  Irinotecan: I.V.: 200 mg/m^2 day 1
  [total dose/cycle = 200 mg/m^2]

Leucovorin: I.V.: 250 mg/m^2 day 2
  [total dose/cycle = 250 mg/m^2]
Fluorouracil: I.V.: 850 mg/m^2 day 2
  [total dose/cycle = 850 mg/m^2]
Repeat cycle every other week

FUP

Use Gastric cancer

Regimen
Fluorouracil: I.V.: 1000 mg/m^2/day continuous infusion days 1 to 5
  [total dose/cycle = 5000 mg/m^2]
Cisplatin: I.V.: 100 mg/m^2 day 2
  [total dose/cycle = 100 mg/m^2]
Repeat cycle every 28 days

FZ

Use Prostate cancer

Regimen NOTE: Multiple variations are listed below.
Variation 1:
  Flutamide: Oral: 250 mg every 8 hours
    [total dose/cycle = 21,000 mg]
  Goserelin acetate: SubQ: 3.6 mg day 1
    [total dose/cycle = 3.6 mg]
  Repeat cycle every 28 days
Variation 2:
  Flutamide: Oral: 250 mg every 8 hours
    [total dose/cycle = 67,500 mg]
  Goserelin acetate: SubQ: 10.8 mg day 1
    [total dose/cycle = 10.8 mg]
  Repeat cycle every 3 months

GC

Use Lung cancer, nonsmall cell

Regimen
Gemcitabine: I.V.: 1000 mg/m^2/day days 1, 8, and 15
  [total dose/cycle = 3000 mg/m^2]
Cisplatin: I.V.: 100 mg/m^2 day 1 **or** 2 **or** 15
  [total dose/cycle = 100 mg/m^2]
Repeat cycle every 28 days for 2-6 cycles

Gemcitabine-Capecitabine

Use Biliary adenocarcinoma; Pancreatic cancer

Regimen
Gemcitabine: I.V.: 1000 mg/m^2/day days 1 and 8
  [total dose/cycle = 2000 mg/m^2]
Capecitabine: Oral: 650 mg/m^2 twice daily days 1 to 14
  [total dose/cycle = 18,200 mg/m^2]
Repeat cycle every 21 days

Gemcitabine-Carboplatin (Bladder Cancer)

Use Bladder cancer

Regimen
Gemcitabine: I.V.: 1000 mg/m^2/day days 1 and 8
  [total dose/cycle = 2000 mg/m^2]
Carboplatin: I.V.: AUC 5 day 1
  [total dose/cycle = AUC = 5]
Repeat cycle every 21 days for up to 6 cycles

Gemcitabine-Carboplatin (Nonsmall Cell Lung Cancer)

Use Lung cancer, nonsmall cell

Regimen NOTE: Multiple variations are listed below.
 Variation 1:
  Gemcitabine: I.V.: 1000 mg/m^2/dose days 1, 8, and 15
   [total dose/cycle = 3000 mg/m^2]
  Carboplatin: I.V.: AUC 5 day 1
   [total dose/cycle = AUC = 5]
  Repeat cycle every 28 days for up to 4 cycles
 Variation 2:
  Gemcitabine: I.V.: 1000 or 1100 mg/m^2/day days 1 and 8
   [total dose/cycle = 2000 or 2200 mg/m^2]
  Carboplatin: I.V.: AUC 5 day 8
   [total dose/cycle = AUC = 5]
  Repeat cycle every 28 days

Gemcitabine-Carboplatin (Ovarian Cancer)

Use Ovarian cancer

Regimen
 Gemcitabine: I.V.: 1000 mg/m^2/day days 1 and 8
  [total dose/cycle = 2000 mg/m^2]
 Carboplatin: I.V.: AUC 4 day 1
  [total dose/cycle = AUC = 4]
 Repeat cycle every 21 days for 6-10 cycles

Gemcitabine-Cisplatin (Bladder Cancer)

Use Bladder cancer

Regimen
 Gemcitabine: I.V.: 1000 mg/m^2/day days 1, 8, and 15
  [total dose/cycle = 3000 mg/m^2]
 Cisplatin: I.V.: 70 mg/m^2 day 2
  [total dose/cycle = 70 mg/m^2]
 Repeat cycle every 28 days for 6 cycles

Gemcitabine-Cisplatin (Lung Cancer)

Use Lung cancer, nonsmall cell

Regimen NOTE: Multiple variations are listed below.
 Variation 1:
  Gemcitabine: I.V.: 1000-1200 mg/m^2/day days 1, 8, and 15
   [total dose/cycle = 3000-3600 mg/m^2]
  Cisplatin: I.V.: 100 mg/m^2 day 2 **or** 15
   [total dose/cycle = 100 mg/m^2]
  Repeat cycle every 28 days
 Variation 2:
  Gemcitabine: I.V.: 1000-1200 mg/m^2/day days 1, 8, and 15
   [total dose/cycle = 3000-3600 mg/m^2]
  Cisplatin: I.V.: 100 mg/m^2 day 1 **or** 2 **or** 15
   [total dose/cycle = 100 mg/m^2]
  Repeat cycle every 28 days

Gemcitabine-Docetaxel (Bladder Cancer)

Use Bladder cancer

Regimen
 Docetaxel: I.V.: 40 mg/m^2/day days 1 and 8
  [total dose/cycle = 80 mg/m^2]
 Gemcitabine: 800 mg/m^2/day days 1 and 8
  [total dose/cycle = 1600 mg/m^2]
 Repeat cycle every 21 days for up to 6 cycles

Gemcitabine-Docetaxel (Sarcoma)

Use Osteosarcoma; Soft tissue sarcoma

Regimen
Gemcitabine: I.V.: 675 mg/m^2/day days 1 and 8
[total dose/cycle = 1350 mg/m^2]
Docetaxel: I.V.: 100 mg/m^2 day 8
[total dose/cycle = 100 mg/m^2]
Repeat cycle every 21 days

Gemcitabine-Erlotinib

Use Pancreatic cancer

Regimen
Cycle 1:
Gemcitabine: I.V.: 1000 mg/m^2/day days 1, 8, 15, 22, 29, 36, and 43 (cycle 1 only)
[total dose/cycle 1 = 7000 mg/m^2]
Erlotinib: Oral: 100 mg once daily days 1 to 56
[total dose/cycle 1 = 5600 mg]
Treatment cycle is 56 days
Subsequent cycles:
Gemcitabine: I.V.: 1000 mg/m^2/day days 1, 8, and 15
[total dose/cycle = 3000 mg/m^2]
Erlotinib: Oral: 100 mg once daily days 1 to 28
[total dose/cycle = 2800 mg]
Repeat cycle every 28 days

Gemcitabine-Irinotecan

Use Pancreatic cancer

Regimen
Gemcitabine: I.V.: 1000 mg/m^2/day days 1 and 8
[total dose/cycle = 2000 mg/m^2]
Irinotecan: I.V.: 100 mg/m^2/day days 1 and 8
[total dose/cycle = 200 mg/m^2]
Repeat cycle 21 days

Gemcitabine-Oxaliplatin

Use Pancreatic cancer

Regimen
Gemcitabine: I.V.: 1000 mg/m^2/day (infused at 10 mg/m^2/minute) day 1
[total dose/cycle = 1000 mg/m^2]
Oxaliplatin: I.V.: 100 mg/m^2/day (over 2 hours) day 2
[total dose/cycle = 100 mg/m^2]
Repeat cycle every 14 days

Gemcitabine-Paclitaxel

Use Ovarian cancer

Regimen
Paclitaxel: I.V.: 80 mg/m^2 infused over 60 minutes days 1, 8, and 15
[total dose/cycle = 240 mg/m^2]
Gemcitabine: I.V.: 1000 mg/m^2/day (start at end of paclitaxel infusion) days 1, 8, and 15
[total dose/cycle = 3000 mg/m^2]
Repeat cycle every 4 weeks

Gemcitabine-Vinorelbine

Use Lung cancer, nonsmall cell

Regimen NOTE: Multiple variations are listed below.
Variation 1:
Gemcitabine: I.V.: 1200 mg/m^2/day days 1 and 8
[total dose/cycle = 2400 mg/m^2]
Vinorelbine: I.V.: 30 mg/m^2/day days 1 and 8
[total dose/cycle = 60 mg/m^2]
Repeat cycle every 21 days for 6 cycles

Variation 2:
  Gemcitabine: I.V.: 1000 mg/m^2/day days 1, 8, and 15
    [total dose/cycle = 3000 mg/m^2]
  Vinorelbine: I.V.: 20 mg/m^2/day days 1, 8, and 15
    [total dose/cycle = 60 mg/m^2]
  Repeat cycle every 28 days for 6 cycles

GEMOX

Use Biliary adenocarcinoma

Regimen
  Gemcitabine: I.V.: 1000 mg/m^2 day 1
    [total dose/cycle = 1000 mg/m^2]
  Oxaliplatin: I.V.: 100 mg/m^2 day 2
    [total dose/cycle = 100 mg/m^2]
  Repeat cycle every 2 weeks

HDMTX

Use Osteosarcoma

Regimen
  Methotrexate: I.V.: 12 g/m^2/week for 2-12 weeks
    [total dose/cycle = 24-144 g/m^2]
  Leucovorin calcium rescue: Oral, I.V.: 15 mg/m^2 every 6 hours (beginning 30 hours after the beginning of
    the 4-hour methotrexate infusion) for 10 doses; **serum methotrexate levels must be monitored**
    [total dose/cycle = 150 mg/m^2]

HIPE-IVAD

Use Neuroblastoma

Regimen
  Cisplatin: I.V.: 40 mg/m^2/day days 1 to 5
    [total dose/cycle = 200 mg/m^2]
  Etoposide: I.V.: 100 mg/m^2/day days 1 to 5
    [total dose/cycle = 500 mg/m^2]
  Ifosfamide: I.V.: 3 g/m^2/day days 21 to 23
    [total dose/cycle = 9 g/m^2]
  Mesna: I.V.: 3 g/m^2/day continuous infusion days 21 to 23
    [total dose/cycle = 9 g/m^2]
  Vincristine: I.V.: 1.5 mg/m^2 day 21
    [total dose/cycle = 1.5 mg/m^2]
  Doxorubicin: I.V.: 60 mg/m^2 day 23
    [total dose/cycle = 60 mg/m^2]
  Repeat cycle every 28 days

Hyper-CVAD + Imatinib

Use Leukemia, acute lymphocytic

Regimen
  Cycle A: (Cycles 1, 3, 5, and 7)
    Imatinib: Oral: 400 mg/day days 1 to 14
      [total dose/cycle = 5600 mg]
    Cyclophosphamide: I.V.: 300 mg/m^2 every 12 hours, for 6 doses, days 1, 2, and 3
      [total dose/cycle = 1800 mg/m^2]
    Mesna: I.V. 600 mg/m^2/day continuous infusion days 1, 2, and 3
      [total dose/cycle = 1800 mg/m^2]
    Vincristine: I.V.: 2 mg/day days 4 and 11
      [total dose/cycle = 4 mg]
    Doxorubicin: I.V.: 50 mg/m^2/day continuous infusion day 4
      [total dose/cycle = 50 mg/m^2]
    Dexamethasone: Oral, I.V.: 40 mg/day days 1, 2, 3, 4, 11, 12, 13, and 14
      [total dose/cycle = 320 mg]
  Cycle B: (Cycles 2, 4, 6, and 8)
    Imatinib: Oral: 400 mg/day days 1 to 14
      [total dose/cycle = 5600 mg]

Methotrexate: I.V.: 1 g/m^2/day continuous infusion day 1
[total dose/cycle = 1 g/m^2]
Leucovorin: I.V.: 50 mg then 15 mg every 6 hours, for 8 doses (start 12 hours after the end of the methotrexate infusion)
[total dose/cycle = 170 mg]
Cytarabine: I.V.: 3 g/m^2 every 12 hours for 4 doses, days 2 and 3
[total dose/cycle = 12 g/m^2]
Repeat every 6 weeks in the following sequence: ABABABAB

CNS Prophylaxis
Methotrexate: I.T.: 12 mg/day day 2
[total dose/cycle = 12 mg/day]
or 6 mg into Ommaya day 2
[total dose/cycle = 6 mg/day]
Cytarabine: I.T.: 100 mg/day day 7 or 8
[total dose/cycle = 100 mg/day]
Repeat cycle every 3 weeks for 3 or 4 cycles

Maintenance (POMP)
Imatinib: Oral: 600 mg/day
[total dose/cycle = 18,000 mg]
Vincristine: I.V.: 2 mg/day day 1
[total dose/cycle = 2 mg]
Prednisone: Oral: 200 mg/day days 1 to 5
[total dose/cycle = 1000 mg/m^2]
Repeat cycle every month (except months 6 and 13) for 13 months

Intensification
Imatinib: Oral: 400 mg/day days 1 to 14
[total dose/cycle = 5600 mg]
Cyclophosphamide: I.V.: 300 mg/m^2 every 12 hours, for 6 doses, days 1, 2, and 3
[total dose/cycle = 1800 mg/m^2]
Mesna: I.V.: 600 mg/m^2/day continuous infusion days 1, 2, and 3
[total dose/cycle = 1800 mg/m^2]
Vincristine: I.V.: 2 mg/day days 4 and 11
[total dose/cycle = 4 mg]
Doxorubicin: 50 mg/m^2/day continuous infusion day 4
[total dose/cycle = 50 mg/m^2]
Dexamethasone: I.V. or Oral: 40 mg/day days 1, 2, 3, 4, 11, 12, 13, and 14
[total dose/cycle = 320 mg]
Cycle is given in months 6 and 13 during maintenance

Hyper-CVAD (Leukemia, Acute Lymphocytic)

Use Leukemia, acute lymphocytic

Regimen NOTE: Multiple variations are listed below.
Variation 1:
Cycle A: (Cycles 1, 3, 5, and 7)
Cyclophosphamide: I.V.: 300 mg/m^2 every 12 hours, for 6 doses, days 1, 2, and 3
[total dose/cycle = 1800 mg/m^2]
Mesna: I.V.: 1200 mg/m^2/day continuous infusion days 1, 2, and 3
[total dose/cycle = 3600 mg/m^2]
Vincristine: I.V.: 2 mg/day days 4 and 11
[total dose/cycle = 4 mg]
Doxorubicin: I.V.: 50 mg/m^2 day 4
[total dose/cycle = 50 mg/m^2]
Dexamethasone: (route not specified): 40 mg/day days 1, 2, 3, 4, 11, 12, 13, and 14
[total dose/cycle = 320 mg]
Cycle B: (Cycles 2, 4, 6, and 8)
Methotrexate: I.V.: 1 g/m^2 continuous infusion day 1
[total dose/cycle = 1g/m^2]
Leucovorin: (route not specified): 15 mg every 6 hours, for 8 doses (start 12 hours after end of methotrexate infusion)
[total dose/cycle = 120 mg]
Cytarabine: I.V.: 3 g/m^2 every 12 hours, for 4 doses, days 2 and 3
[total dose/cycle = 12 g/m^2]
Methylprednisolone: I.V.: 50 mg twice daily, for 6 doses, days 1, 2, and 3
[total dose/cycle = 300 mg/m^2]
Repeat every 6 weeks in the following sequence: ABABABAB

CNS Prophylaxis
Methotrexate: I.T.: 12 mg/day day 2
[total dose/cycle = 12 mg]
or 6 mg/day into Ommaya day 2
[total dose/cycle = 6 mg]
Cytarabine: I.T: 100 mg day 8
[total dose/cycle = 100 mg]
Repeat cycle every 3 weeks
Maintenance (POMP)
Mercaptopurine: Oral: 50 mg 3 times/day
[total dose/cycle = 4200-4650 mg]
Vincristine: I.V.: 2 mg day 1
[total dose/cycle = 2 mg]
Methotrexate: Oral: 20 mg/m^2/day days 1, 8, 15, and 22
[total dose/cycle = 80 mg/m^2]
Prednisone: Oral: 200 mg/day days 1 to 5
[total dose/cycle = 1000 mg/m^2]
or
Mercaptopurine: I.V.: 1 g/m^2/day days 1 to 5
[total dose/cycle = 5 g/m^2]
Vincristine: I.V.: 2 mg day 1
[total dose/cycle = 2 mg]
Methotrexate: I.V.: 10 mg/m^2/day days 1 to 5
[total dose/cycle = 50 mg/m^2]
Prednisone: Oral: 200 mg/day days 1 to 5
[total dose/cycle = 1000 mg/m^2]
Repeat cycles every month for 2 years
Variation 2:
Cycle A: (Cycles 1, 3, 5, and 7)
Cyclophosphamide: I.V.: 300 mg/m^2 every 12 hours, for 6 doses, days 1, 2, and 3
[total dose/cycle = 1800 mg/m^2]
Mesna: I.V.: 600 mg/m^2/day continuous infusion days 1, 2, and 3
[total dose/cycle = 1800 mg/m^2]
Vincristine: I.V.: 2 mg/day days 4 and 11
[total dose/cycle = 4 mg]
Doxorubicin: I.V.: 50 mg/m^2 day 4
[total dose/cycle = 50 mg/m^2]
Dexamethasone: Oral, I.V.: 40 mg/day days 1, 2, 3, 4, 11, 12, 13, and 14
[total dose/cycle = 320 mg]
Cycle B: (Cycles 2, 4, 6, and 8)
Methotrexate: I.V.: 1 g/m^2 continuous infusion day 1
[total dose/cycle = 1 g/m^2]
Leucovorin: I.V.: 50 mg (start 12 hours after end of methotrexate infusion)
followed by I.V.: 15 mg every 6 hours, for 8 doses
[total dose/cycle = 170 mg]
Cytarabine: I.V.: 3 g/m^2 every 12 hours, for 4 doses, days 2 and 3
[total dose/cycle = 12 g/m^2]
Repeat every 6 weeks in the following sequence: ABABABAB
CNS Prophylaxis
Methotrexate: I.T.: 12 mg day 2
[total dose/cycle = 12 mg]
or 6 mg into Ommaya day 2
[total dose/cycle = 6 mg]
Cytarabine: I.T.: 100 mg day 7
[total dose/cycle = 100 mg]
Repeat cycle every 3 weeks
Variation 3:
Cycle A: (Cycles 1, 3, 5, and 7)
Cyclophosphamide: I.V.: 300 mg/m^2 every 12 hours, for 6 doses, days 1, 2, and 3
[total dose/cycle = 1800 mg/m^2]
Mesna: I.V.: 600 mg/m^2/day continuous infusion days 1, 2, and 3
[total dose/cycle = 1800 mg/m^2]

Vincristine: I.V.: 2 mg/day days 4 and 11
[total dose/cycle = 4 mg]
Doxorubicin: I.V.: 50 mg/m^2 continuous infusion day 4
[total dose/cycle = 50 mg/m^2]
Dexamethasone: Oral, I.V.: 40 mg/day days 1, 2, 3, 4, 11, 12, 13, and 14
[total dose/cycle = 320 mg]
Cycle B: (Cycles 2, 4, 6, and 8)
Methotrexate: I.V.: 200 mg/m^2 day 1
followed by I.V.: 800 mg/m^2 continuous infusion day 1
[total dose/cycle = 1 g/m^2]
Leucovorin: I.V.: 50 mg (start 12 hours after end of methotrexate infusion)
followed by I.V.: 15 mg every 6 hours, for 8 doses
[total dose/cycle = 170 mg/m^2]
Cytarabine: I.V.: 3 g/m^2 every 12 hours, for 4 doses, days 2 and 3
[total dose/cycle = 12 g/m^2]
Repeat every 6 weeks in the following sequence: ABABABAB

CNS Prophylaxis
Methotrexate: I.T.: 12 mg day 2
[total dose/cycle = 12 mg]
or 6 mg into Ommaya day 2
[total dose/cycle = 6 mg]
Cytarabine: I.T.: 100 mg day 7 **or** 8
[total dose/cycle = 100 mg]
Repeat cycles every 3 weeks for 6 or 8 cycles

Maintenance (POMP)
Mercaptopurine: Oral: 50 mg 3 times/day
[total dose/cycle = 4200-4650 mg]
Vincristine: I.V.: 2 mg day 1
[total dose/cycle = 2 mg]
Methotrexate: Oral, I.V.: 20 mg/m^2/ day days 1, 8, 15, and 22
[total dose/cycle = 80 mg/m^2]
Prednisone: Oral: 200 mg/day days 1 to 5
[total dose/cycle = 1000 mg/m^2]
or
Mercaptopurine: I.V.: 1 g/m^2/day days 1 to 5
[total dose/cycle = 5 g/m^2]
Vincristine: I.V.: 2 mg day 1
[total dose/cycle = 2 mg]
Methotrexate: I.V.: 10 mg/m^2 /day days 1 to 5
[total dose/cycle = 50 mg/m^2]
Prednisone: Oral: 200 mg/day days 1 to 5
[total dose/cycle = 1000 mg]
Repeat cycles every month (except months 7 and 11 or 9 and 12) for 2 years

Intensification
Etoposide: I.V.: 100 mg/m^2/day days 1 to 5
[total dose/cycle = 500 mg/m^2]
Pegaspargase: I.V.: 2500 units/m^2 day 1
[total dose/cycle = 2500 units/m^2]
Given during months 9 and 12 of maintenance
or
Methotrexate: I.V.: 100 mg/m^2/day days 1, 8, 15, and 22
[total dose/cycle = 400 mg/m^2]
Asparaginase: I.V.: 20,000 units/day days 2, 9, 16, and 23
[total dose/cycle = 80,000 units]
Given during months 7 and 11 of maintenance
Variation 4:
Cycle A: (Cycles 1, 3, 5, and 7)
Cyclophosphamide: I.V.: 300 mg/m^2 every 12 hours, for 6 doses, days 1, 2, and 3
[total dose/cycle = 1800 mg/m^2]
Mesna: I.V.: 600 mg/m^2/day continuous infusion days 1, 2, and 3
[total dose/cycle = 1800 mg/m^2]
Vincristine: I.V.: 2 mg/day days 4 and 11
[total dose/cycle = 4 mg]

Doxorubicin: I.V.: 50 mg/m^{2}day 4
  [total dose/cycle = 50 mg/m^2]
Dexamethasone: (route not specified): 40 mg/day days 1, 2, 3, 4, 11, 12, 13, and 14
  [total dose/cycle = 320 mg]
Cycle B: (Cycles 2, 4, 6, and 8)
 Methotrexate: I.V.: 200 mg/m^2 day 1
  followed by I.V.: 800 mg/m^2 continuous infusion day 1
   [total dose/cycle = 1 g/m^2]
 Leucovorin: (route not specified): 15 mg every 6 hours, for 8 doses (start 24 hours after end of methotrexate infusion)
   [total dose/cycle = 120 mg]
 Cytarabine: I.V.: 3 g/m^2 every 12 hours, for 4 doses, days 2 and 3
   [total dose/cycle = 12 g/m^2]
 Repeat every 6 weeks in the following sequence: ABABABAB
CNS Prophylaxis
 Methotrexate: I.T.: 12 mg day 2
   [total dose/cycle = 12 mg]
 Cytarabine: I.T.: 100 mg day 8
   [total dose/cycle = 100 mg]
 Repeat cycle every 3 weeks for 4 or 8 cycles
Maintenance (POMP)
 Mercaptopurine: Oral: 50 mg 3 times/day
   [total dose/cycle = 4200-4650 mg]
 Vincristine: I.V.: 2 mg day 1
   [total dose/cycle = 2 mg]
 Methotrexate: Oral: 20 mg/m^2/day days 1, 8, 15, and 22
   [total dose/cycle = 80 mg/m^2]
 Prednisone: Oral: 200 mg/day days 1 to 5
   [total dose/cycle = 1000 mg/m^2]
 or
 Mercaptopurine: I.V.: 1 g/m^2/day days 1 to 5
   [total dose/cycle = 5 g/m^2]
 Vincristine: I.V.: 2 mg day 1
   [total dose/cycle = 2 mg]
 Methotrexate: I.V.: 10 mg/m^2/day days 1 to 5
   [total dose/cycle = 50 mg/m^2]
 Prednisone: Oral: 200 mg/day days 1 to 5
   [total dose/cycle = 1000 mg/m^2]
 or
 Interferon alfa: SubQ: 5 million units/m^2 daily
   [total dose/cycle = 140-155 million units/m^2]
 Cytarabine: SubQ: 10 mg daily
   [total dose/cycle = 280-310 mg]
 Repeat cycles every month for 2 years
Variation 5:
 Cycle A: (Cycles 1, 4, 6, and 8)
  Cyclophosphamide: I.V.: 300 mg/m^2 every 12 hours, for 6 doses, days 1, 2, and 3
   [total dose/cycle = 1800 mg/m^2]
  Mesna: I.V.: 600 mg/m^2/day continuous infusion days 1, 2, and 3
   [total dose/cycle = 1800 mg/m^2]
  Vincristine: I.V.: 2 mg/day days 4 and 11
   [total dose/cycle = 4 mg]
  Doxorubicin: I.V.: 50 mg/m^2 continuous infusion day 4
   [total dose/cycle = 50 mg/m^2]
  Dexamethasone: Oral, I.V.: 40 mg/day days 1, 2, 3, 4, 11, 12, 13, and 14
   [total dose/cycle = 320 mg]
 Cycle B: (Cycles 3, 5, 7, and 9)
  Methotrexate: I.V.: 200 mg/m^2 day 1
  followed by I.V.: 800 mg/m^2/day continuous infusion day 1
   [total dose/cycle = 1 g/m^2]
  Leucovorin: I.V.: 50 mg (start 12 hours after end of methotrexate infusion)
  followed by I.V.: 15 mg every 6 hours, for 8 doses
   [total dose/cycle = 170 mg]

Cytarabine: I.V.: 3 g/m^2 every 12 hours, for 4 doses, days 2 and 3
[total dose/cycle = 12 g/m^2]
Cycle C: Liposomal Daunorubicin/cytarabine (Cycle 2):
Daunorubicin, liposomal: I.V.: 150 mg/m^2/day days 1 and 2
[total dose/cycle = 300 mg/m^2]
Cytarabine: I.V.: 1.5 g/m^2/day continuous infusion days 1 and 2
[total dose/cycle = 3 g/m^2]
Prednisone: Oral: 200 mg/day days 1 to 5
[total dose/cycle = 1000 mg]
Administer in the following sequence: ACBABABA (Cycle C does not repeat)
CNS Prophylaxis
Methotrexate: I.T.: 12 mg day 2
[total dose/cycle = 12 mg]
or 6 mg into Ommaya day 2
[total dose/cycle = 6 mg]
Cytarabine: I.T.: 100 mg days 7 **or** 8
[total dose/cycle = 100 mg]
Repeat cycle every 3 weeks for 6 or 8 cycles
Maintenance (POMP)
Mercaptopurine: I.V.: 1 g/m^2/day days 1 to 5
[total dose/cycle = 5 g/m^2]
Vincristine: I.V.: 2 mg day 1
[total dose/cycle = 2 mg]
Methotrexate: I.V.: 10 mg/m^2/day days 1 to 5
[total dose/cycle = 50 mg/m^2]
Prednisone: Oral: 200 mg/day days 1 to 5
[total dose/cycle = 1000 mg]
Repeat cycles monthly, except months 6, 7, 18, and 19 for 3 years
Intensification
Methotrexate: I.V.: 100 mg/m^2/day days 1, 8, 15, and 22
[total dose/cycle = 400 mg/m^2]
Asparaginase: I.V.: 20,000 units/day days 2, 9, 16, and 23
[total dose/cycle = 80,000 units]
Given during months 6 and 18 of maintenance
Cyclophosphamide: I.V.: 300 mg/m^2 every 12 hours, for 6 doses, days 1, 2, and 3
[total dose/cycle = 1800 mg/m^2]
Mesna: I.V.: 600 mg/m^2/day continuous infusion days 1, 2, and 3
[total dose/cycle = 1800 mg/m^2]
Vincristine: I.V.: 2 mg/day days 4 and 11
[total dose/cycle = 4 mg]
Doxorubicin: I.V.: 50 mg/m^2/day continuous infusion day 4
[total dose/cycle = 50 mg/m^2]
Dexamethasone: Oral, I.V.: 40 mg/day days 1, 2, 3, 4, 11, 12, 13, and 14
[total dose/cycle = 320 mg]
Given during months 7 and 19 of maintenance

Hyper-CVAD (Lymphoma, non-Hodgkin)
Use Lymphoma, non-Hodgkin
Regimen
Cycle A: (Cycles 1, 3, 5, and 7)
Cyclophosphamide: I.V.: 300 mg/m^2 every 12 hours, for 6 doses, days 1, 2, and 3
[total dose/cycle = 1800 mg/m^2]
Vincristine: I.V.: 2 mg/day days 4 and 11
[total dose/cycle = 4 mg]
Doxorubicin: I.V.: 25 mg/m^2/day continuous infusion days 4 and 5
[total dose/cycle = 50 mg/m^2]
Dexamethasone: Oral, I.V.: 40 mg/day days 1, 2, 3, 4, 11, 12, 13, and 14
[total dose/cycle = 320 mg]
Cycle B: (Cycles 2, 4, 6, and 8)
Methotrexate: I.V.: 200 mg/m^2 day 1
followed by I.V.: 800 mg/m^2 continuous infusion day 1
[total dose/cycle = 1 g/m^2]

Leucovorin: Oral: 50 mg
  followed by Oral: 15 mg every 6 hours, for 8 doses (start 24 hours after end of methotrexate infusion)
    [total dose/cycle = 170 mg]
Cytarabine: I.V.: 3 g/m^2 every 12 hours, for 4 doses, days 2 and 3
  [total dose/cycle = 12 g/m^2]
Repeat every 6 weeks in the following sequence: ABABABAB

Hyper-CVAD (Multiple Myeloma)

Use Multiple myeloma
Regimen
Cyclophosphamide: I.V.: 300 mg/m^2 every 12 hours, for 6 doses, days 1, 2, and 3
  [total dose/cycle = 1800 mg/m^2]
Mesna: I.V.: 600 mg/m^2/day continuous infusion days 1, 2, and 3
  [total dose/cycle = 1800 mg/m^2]
Doxorubicin: I.V.: 25 mg/m^2/day continuous infusion days 4 and 5
  [total dose/cycle = 50 mg/m^2]
Vincristine: I.V.: 1 mg/day continuous infusion days 4 and 5
  followed by I.V.: 2 mg day 11
    [total dose/cycle = 4 mg]
Dexamethasone: Oral, I.V.: 20 mg/m^2/day days 1 to 5 and 11 to 14
  [total dose/cycle = 180 mg/m^2]
Repeat cycle once if ≥50% reduction in myeloma protein
Maintenance
Cyclophosphamide: Oral: 125 mg/m^2 every 12 hours, for 10 doses, days 1 to 5
  [total dose/cycle = 1250 mg/m^2]
Dexamethasone: Oral: 20 mg/m^2/day days 1 to 5
  [total dose/cycle = 100 mg/m^2]
Repeat maintenance cycle every 5 weeks

Hyper-CVAD + Rituximab

Use Lymphona, non-Hodgkin (Mantle cell)
Regimen
Cycle A: (Cycles 1, 3, 5 [and 7, if needed])
  Rituximab: I.V.: 375 mg/m^2 day 1
    [total dose/cycle = 375 mg/m^2]
  Cyclophosphamide: I.V.: 300 mg/m^2 every 12 hours, for 6 doses, days 2, 3, and 4
    [total dose/cycle = 1800 mg/m^2]
  Mesna: I.V.: 600 mg/m^2 continuous infusion days 2, 3, and 4
    [total dose/cycle = 1800 mg/m^2]
  Vincristine: I.V.: 1.4 mg/m^2 (maximum 2 mg) days 5 and 12
    [total dose/cycle = 2.8 mg/m^2; maximum 4 mg]
  Doxorubicin: I.V.: 16.7 mg/m^2 continuous infusion days 5, 6, and 7
    [total dose/cycle = 50.1 mg/m^2]
  Dexamethasone: Oral, I.V.: 40 mg/day days 2, 3, 4, 5, 12, 13, 14, and 15
    [total dose/cycle = 320 mg]
Cycle B: (Cycles 2, 4, 6 [and 8, if needed])
  Rituximab: I.V.: 375 mg/m^2 day 1
    [total dose/cycle = 375 mg/m^2]
  Methotrexate: I.V.: 200 mg/m^2 day 2
    followed by I.V.: 800 mg/m^{2}continuous infusion day 2
      [total dose/cycle = 1000 mg/m^2]
  Leucovorin: Oral: 50 mg (start 12 hours after the end of the methotrexate infusion)
    followed by Oral: 15 mg every 6 hours, for 8 doses
      [total dose/cycle = 170 mg]
  Cytarabine: I.V.: 3 g/m^2 every 12 hours, for 4 doses, day 3 and 4
    [total dose/cycle = 12 g/m^2]
Repeat every 6 weeks in the following sequence: ABABABAB

ICE (Lymphoma, non-Hodgkin)

Use Lymphoma, non-Hodgkin
Regimen
Etoposide: I.V.: 100 mg/m^2/day days 1, 2, and 3
  [total dose/cycle = 300 mg/m^2]

◀

Carboplatin: I.V.: AUC 5 (maximum 800 mg) day 2
  [total dose/cycle = AUC = 5]
Ifosfamide: I.V.: 5000 mg/m^2 continuous infusion day 2
  [total dose/cycle = 5000 mg/m^2]
Mesna: I.V.: 5000 mg/m^2 continuous infusion day 2
  [total dose/cycle = 5000 mg/m^2]
Filgrastim: SubQ: 5 mcg/kg/day days 5-12 (cycles 1 and 2 only)
  [total dose/cycle = 40 mcg/kg]
    followed by SubQ: 10 mcg/kg/day day 5 through completion of leukaphoresis (cycle 3 only)
Repeat cycle every 2 weeks for 3 cycles

ICE (Sarcoma)

Use Osteosarcoma; Soft tissue sarcoma
Regimen
Ifosfamide: I.V.: 1500 mg/m^2/day days 1, 2, and 3
  [total dose/cycle = 4500 mg/m^2]
Carboplatin: I.V.: 300-635 mg/m^2 day 3
  [total dose/cycle = 300-635 mg/m^2]
Etoposide: I.V.: 100 mg/m^2/day days 1, 2, and 3
  [total dose/cycle = 300 mg/m^2]
Mesna: I.V.: 500 mg/m^2 prior to each ifosfamide, and every 3 hours for 2 more doses/day days 1, 2, and 3
  [total dose/cycle = 4500 mg/m^2]
Repeat cycle every 21-28 days

ICE-T

Use Breast cancer; Soft tissue sarcoma
Regimen
Ifosfamide: I.V.: 1250 mg/m^2/day days 1, 2, and 3
  [total dose/cycle = 3750 mg/m^2]
Carboplatin: I.V.: 300 mg/m^2 day 1
  [total dose/cycle = 300 mg/m^2]
Etoposide: I.V.: 80 mg/m^2/day days 1, 2, and 3
  [total dose/cycle = 240 mg/m^2]
Paclitaxel: I.V.: 175 mg/m^2 day 4
  [total dose/cycle = 175 mg/m^2]
Mesna: I.V.: 250 mg prior to ifosfamide days 1, 2, and 3
  followed by: Oral: 500 mg at 4 and 8 hours after ifosfamide days 1, 2, and 3
    [total dose/cycle = I.V. 750 mg; Oral: 3000 mg]
  or
Mesna: I.V.: 1250 mg/m^2/day over 6 hours, days 1, 2, and 3
  [total dose/cycle = 3750 mg/m^2]
Repeat cycle every 28 days

Idarubicin, Cytarabine, Etoposide (ICE Protocol)

Use Leukemia, acute myeloid
Regimen
Idarubicin: I.V.: 6 mg/m^2/day days 1 to 5
  [total dose/cycle = 30 mg/m^2]
Cytarabine: I.V.: 600 mg/m^2/day days 1 to 5
  [total dose/cycle = 3000 mg/m^2]
Etoposide: I.V.: 150 mg/m^2/day days 1, 2, and 3
  [total dose/cycle = 450 mg/m^2]
Administer one cycle only

Idarubicin, Cytarabine, Etoposide (IDA-Based BF12)

Use Leukemia, acute myeloid
Regimen Induction:
Idarubicin: I.V.: 5 mg/m^2/day days 1 to 5
  [total dose/cycle = 25 mg/m^2]
Cytarabine: I.V.: 2000 mg/m^2 every 12 hours days 1 to 5 (10 doses)
  [total dose/cycle = 20,000 mg/m^2]

Etoposide: I.V.: 100 mg/m^2/day days 1 to 5
[total dose/cycle = 500 mg/m^2]
Second cycle may be given based on individual response; time between cycles not specified

IE

Use Soft tissue sarcoma

Regimen
Etoposide: I.V.: 100 mg/m^2/day days 1, 2, and 3
[total dose/cycle = 300 mg/m^2]
Ifosfamide: I.V.: 2500 mg/m^2/day days 1, 2, and 3
[total dose/cycle = 7500 mg/m^2]
Mesna: I.V.: 500 mg/m^2 prior to ifosfamide, after ifosfamide, and every 4 hours for 3 more doses (total of 5 doses/day) days 1, 2, and 3
[total dose/cycle = 7500 mg/m^2]
Repeat cycle every 28 days

IL-2 + IFN

Use Melanoma

Regimen
Cisplatin: I.V.: 20 mg/m^2/day days 1 to 4
[total dose/cycle = 80 mg/m^2]
Vinblastine: I.V.: 1.6 mg/m^2/day days 1 to 4
[total dose/cycle = 6.4 mg/m^2]
Dacarbazine: I.V.: 800 mg/m^2 day 1
[total dose/cycle = 800 mg/m^2]
Aldesleukin: I.V.: 9 million units/m^2/day continuous infusion days 1 to 4
[total dose/cycle = 36 million units/m^2]
Interferon alfa-2b: SubQ: 5 million units/m^2/day days 1 to 5, 7, 9, 11, and 13
[total dose/cycle = 45 million units/m^2]
Repeat cycle every 21 days

IMVP-16

Use Lymphoma, non-Hodgkin

Regimen
Ifosfamide: I.V.: 4 g/m^2 continuous infusion over 24 hours day 1
[total dose/cycle = 4 g/m^2]
Mesna: I.V.: 800 mg/m^2 bolus prior to ifosfamide, then 4 g/m^2 continuous infusion over 12 hours concurrent with ifosfamide, then 2.4 g/m^2 continuous infusion over 12 hours after ifosfamide infusion day 1
[total dose/cycle = 7.2 g/m^2]
Methotrexate: I.V.: 30 mg/m^2/day days 3 and 10
[total dose/cycle = 60 mg/m^2]
Etoposide: I.V.: 100 mg/m^2/day days 1, 2, and 3
[total dose/cycle = 300 mg/m^2]
Repeat cycle every 21-28 days

Interleukin 2-Interferon Alfa-2

Use Renal cell cancer

Regimen
Weeks 1 and 4:
Aldesleukin: SubQ: 20 million units/m^2 3 times weekly
[total dose/cycle = 120 million units/m^2]
Interferon Alfa-2: SubQ: 6 million units/m^2 once weekly
[total dose/cycle = 12 million units/m^2]
Weeks 2, 3, 5, and 6:
Aldesleukin: SubQ: 5 million units/m^2 3 times weekly
[total dose/cycle = 60 million units/m^2]
Interferon Alfa-2: SubQ: 6 million units/m^2 3 times weekly
[total dose/cycle = 72 million units/m^2]
Repeat cycle every 56 days

Interleukin 2-Interferon Alfa-2-Fluorouracil

Use Renal cell cancer

Regimen
Weeks 1 and 4:
  Aldesleukin: SubQ: 20 million units/m^2 3 times weekly
    [total dose/cycle = 120 million units/m^2]
  Interferon Alfa-2: SubQ: 6 million units/m^2 once weekly
    [total dose/cycle = 12 million units/m^2]
Weeks 2 and 3:
  Aldesleukin: SubQ: 5 million units/m^2 3 times weekly
    [total dose/cycle = 30 million units/m^2]
Weeks 5-8:
  Interferon Alfa-2: SubQ: 9 million units/m^2 3 times weekly
    [total dose/cycle = 108 million units/m^2]
  Fluorouracil: I.V.: 750 mg/m^2 once weekly
    [total dose/cycle = 3000 mg/m^2]
Repeat cycle every 56 days

IPA

Use Hepatoblastoma

Regimen
Ifosfamide: I.V.: 500 mg/m^2 day 1
  [total dose/cycle = 500 mg/m^2]
  followed by I.V.: 1000 mg/m^2/day continuous infusion days 1 to 3
    [total dose/cycle = 3000 mg/m^2]
Cisplatin: I.V.: 20 mg/m^2/day days 4 to 8
  [total dose/cycle = 100 mg/m^2]
Doxorubicin: I.V.: 30 mg/m^2/day continuous infusion days 9 and 10
  [total dose/cycle = 60 mg/m^2]
Repeat cycle every 21 days

Irinotecan-Cisplatin

Use Esophageal cancer

Regimen
Cisplatin: I.V.: 30 mg/m^2/day days 1, 8, 15, and 22
  [total dose/cycle = 120 mg/m^2]
Irinotecan: I.V.: 65 mg/m^2/day days 1, 8, 15, and 22
  [total dose/cycle = 260 mg/m^2]
Repeat cycle every 6 weeks

IVAC

Use Lymphoma, non-Hodgkin

Regimen
Ifosfamide: I.V.: 1500 mg/m^2/day days 1 to 5
  [total dose/cycle = 7500 mg/m^2]
Etoposide: I.V.: 60 mg/m^2/day days 1 to 5
  [total dose/cycle = 300 mg/m^2]
Cytarabine: I.V.: 2 g/m^2 every 12 hours days 1 and 2
  [total dose/cycle = 8 g/m^2]
Mesna: I.V.: 360 mg/m^2 every 3 hours days 1 to 5
  [total dose/cycle = 14,400 mg/m^2]
Methotrexate: I.T.: 12 mg day 5
Sargramostim: SubQ: 7.5 mcg/kg day 7 until ANC >1000 cells/mm^3
Repeat when ANC >1000 cells/mm^3

Ixabepilone-Capecitabine

Use Breast cancer

Regimen
Capecitabine: Oral: 1000 mg/m^2 twice daily days 1 to 14
  [total dose/cycle = 28,000 mg/m^2]
Ixabepilone: I.V.: 40 mg/m^2 day 1
  [total dose/cycle = 40 mg/m^2]
Repeat cycle every 3 weeks

Larson Regimen

Use Leukemia, acute lymphocytic

Regimen
  Cyclophosphamide: I.V.: 1200 mg/m^2 day 1
    [total dose/cycle = 1200 mg/m^2]
  Daunorubicin: I.V.: 45 mg/m^2/day days 1, 2, and 3
    [total dose/cycle = 135 mg/m^2]
  Vincristine: I.V.: 2 mg/day days 1, 8, 15, and 22
    [total dose/cycle = 8 mg]
  Prednisone: Oral or I.V.: 60 mg/m^2/day days 1 to 21
    [total dose/cycle = 1260 mg/m^2]
  Asparaginase: SubQ: 6000 units/m^2/day days 5, 8, 11, 15, 18, and 22
    [total dose/cycle = 36,000 units/m^2]
  Administer one cycle only

Lenalidomide-Dexamethasone

Use Multiple myeloma

Regimen
  Lenalidomide: Oral: 25 mg/day days 1 to 21
    [total dose/cycle = 525 mg]
  Dexamethasone: Oral: 40 mg/day days 1 to 4, 9 to 12, and 17 to 20 (cycles 1, 2, 3, and 4)
    [total dose/cycle = 480 mg]
  Dexamethasone: Oral 40 mg/day days 1 to 4 (cycle 5 and beyond)
    [total dose/cycle = 160 mg]
  Repeat cycle every 28 days

Lenalidomide-Dexamethasone (Low Dose)

Use Multiple myeloma

Regimen
  Lenalidomide: Oral: 25 mg/day days 1 to 21
    [total dose/cycle = 525 mg]
  Dexamethasone: Oral: 40 mg/day days 1, 8, 15, and 22
    [total dose/cycle = 160 mg]
  Repeat cycle every 28 days

Linker Protocol

Use Leukemia, acute lymphocytic

Regimen
Remission induction:
  Daunorubicin: I.V.: 50 mg/m^2/day days 1, 2, and 3
    [total dose/cycle = 150 mg/m^2]
  Vincristine: I.V.: 2 mg/day days 1, 8, 15, and 22
    [total dose/cycle = 8 mg]
  Prednisone: Oral: 60 mg/m^2/day days 1 to 28
    [total dose/cycle = 1680 mg/m^2]
  Asparaginase: I.M.: 6000 units/m^2/day days 17 to 28
    [total dose/cycle = 72,000 units/m^2]
If residual leukemia in bone marrow on day 14:
  Daunorubicin: I.V.: 50 mg/m^2 day 15
    [total dose/cycle = 50 mg/m^2]
If residual leukemia in bone marrow on day 28:
  Daunorubicin: I.V.: 50 mg/m^2/day days 29 and 30
    [total dose/cycle = 100 mg/m^2]
  Vincristine: I.V.: 2 mg/day days 29 and 36
    [total dose/cycle = 4 mg]
  Prednisone: Oral: 60 mg/m^2/day days 29 to 42
    [total dose/cycle = 840 mg/m^2]
  Asparaginase: I.M.: 6000 units/m^2/day days 29 to 35
    [total dose/cycle = 42,000 units/m^2]

◀ **Consolidation therapy:**
Treatment A (cycles 1, 3, 5, and 7)
Daunorubicin: I.V.: 50 mg/m²/day days 1 and 2
[total dose/cycle = 100 mg/m²]
Vincristine: I.V.: 2 mg/day days 1 and 8
[total dose/cycle = 4 mg]
Prednisone: Oral: 60 mg/m²/day days 1 to 14
[total dose/cycle = 840 mg/m²]
Asparaginase: I.M.: 12,000 units/m²/day days 2, 4, 7, 9, 11, and 14
[total dose/cycle = 72,000 units/m²]
Treatment B (cycles 2, 4, 6, and 8)
Teniposide: I.V.: 165 mg/m²/day days 1, 4, 8, and 11
[total dose/cycle = 660 mg/m²]
Cytarabine: I.V.: 300 mg/m²/day days 1, 4, 8, and 11
[total dose/cycle = 1200 mg/m²]
Treatment C (cycle 9)
Methotrexate: I.V.: 690 mg/m² continuous infusion day 1 (over 42 hours)
[total dose/cycle = 690 mg/m²]
Leucovorin: I.V.: 15 mg/m² every 6 hours for 12 doses (start at end of methotrexate infusion)
[total dose/cycle = 180 mg/m²]
Administer remission induction regimen for one cycle only. Repeat consolidation cycle every 28 days.

LOPP

Use Lymphoma, Hodgkin disease
Regimen
Chlorambucil: Oral: 10 mg/day days 1 to 10
[total dose/cycle = 100 mg/m²]
Vincristine: I.V.: 1.4 mg/m²/day (maximum 2 mg) days 1 and 8
[total dose/cycle = 2.8 mg/m²]
Procarbazine: Oral: 100 mg/m²/day days 1 to 10
[total dose/cycle = 1000 mg/m²]
Prednisone: Oral: 25 mg/m²/day (maximum 60 mg) days 1 to 14
[total dose/cycle = 350 mg/m²]
or
Prednisolone: Oral: 25 mg/m²/day (maximum 60 mg) days 1 to 14
[total dose/cycle = 350 mg/m²]
Repeat cycle every 28 days

M-2

Use Multiple myeloma
Regimen
Vincristine: I.V.: 0.03 mg/kg (maximum 2 mg) day 1
[total dose/cycle = 0.03 mg/kg]
Carmustine: I.V.: 0.5-1 mg/kg day 1
[total dose/cycle = 0.5-1 mg/kg]
Cyclophosphamide: I.V.: 10 mg/kg day 1
[total dose/cycle = 10 mg/kg]
Melphalan: Oral: 0.25 mg/kg/day days 1 to 4
[total dose/cycle = 1 mg/kg]
or 0.1 mg/kg/day days 1 to 7 or 1 to 10
[total dose/cycle = 0.7 or 1 mg/kg]
Prednisone: Oral: 1 mg/kg/day days 1 to 7
[total dose/cycle = 7 mg/kg]
Repeat cycle every 35-42 days

MACOP-B

Use Lymphoma, non-Hodgkin
Regimen
Methotrexate: I.V. bolus: 100 mg/m² weeks 2, 6, 10
followed by I.V.: 300 mg/m² over 4 hours weeks 2, 6, and 10
[total dose/cycle = 1200 mg/m²]
Doxorubicin: I.V.: 50 mg/m² weeks 1, 3, 5, 7, 9, and 11
[total dose/cycle = 300 mg/m²]

Cyclophosphamide: I.V.: 350 mg/m^2 weeks 1, 3, 5, 7, 9, and 11
  [total dose/cycle = 2100 mg/m^2]
Vincristine: I.V.: 1.4 mg/m^2 (maximum 2 mg) weeks 2, 4, 6, 8, 10, and 12
  [total dose/cycle = 8.4 mg/m^2; maximum 12 mg]
Bleomycin: I.V.: 10 units/m^2 weeks 4, 8, and 12
  [total dose/cycle = 30 units/m^2]
Prednisone: Oral: 75 mg/day for 12 weeks, then taper over 2 weeks
Leucovorin calcium: Oral: 15 mg/m^2 every 6 hours, for 6 doses (beginning 24 hours after methotrexate)
  weeks 2, 6, and 10
  [total dose/cycle = 270 mg/m^2]
Administer one cycle

MAID

Use Soft tissue sarcoma
Regimen
  Mesna: I.V.: 2500 mg/m^2/day continuous infusion days 1 to 4
    [total dose/cycle = 10,000 mg/m^2]
  Doxorubicin: I.V.: 20 mg/m^2/day continuous infusion days 1 to 3
    [total dose/cycle = 60 mg/m^2]
  Ifosfamide: I.V.: 2500 mg/m^2/day continuous infusion days 1 to 3
    [total dose/cycle = 7500 mg/m^2]
  Dacarbazine: I.V.: 300 mg/m^2/day continuous infusion days 1 to 3
    [total dose/cycle = 900 mg/m^2]
  Repeat cycle every 21-28 days

m-BACOD

Use Lymphoma, non-Hodgkin
Regimen
  Methotrexate: I.V.: 200 mg/m^2/day days 8 and 15
    [total dose/cycle = 400 mg/m^2]
  Leucovorin calcium: Oral: 10 mg/m^2 every 6 hours for 8 doses (beginning 24 hours after each methotrexate
    dose) days 9 and 16
    [total dose/cycle = 160 mg/m^2]
  Bleomycin: I.V.: 4 units/m^2 day 1
    [total dose/cycle = 4 units/m^2]
  Doxorubicin: I.V.: 45 mg/m^2 day 1
    [total dose/cycle = 45 mg/m^2]
  Cyclophosphamide: I.V.: 600 mg/m^2 day 1
    [total dose/cycle = 600 mg/m^2]
  Vincristine: I.V.: 1 mg/m^2 day 1
    [total dose/cycle = 1 mg/m^2]
  Dexamethasone: Oral: 6 mg/m^2/day days 1 to 5
    [total dose/cycle = 30 mg/m^2]
  Repeat cycle every 21 days

Melphalan-Prednisone-Thalidomide

Use Multiple myeloma
Regimen
  Melphalan: Oral: 4 mg/m^2/day days 1 to 7
    [total dose/cycle = 28 mg/m^2]
  Prednisone: Oral: 40 mg/m^2/day days 1 to 7
    [total dose/cycle = 280 mg/m^2]
  Thalidomide: Oral: 100 mg/day days 1 to 28
    [total dose/cycle = 2800 mg]
  Repeat cycle every 28 days for 6 cycles
  followed by
  Thalidomide: Oral: 100 mg daily (as maintenance)

MF

Use Breast cancer

Regimen

Methotrexate: I.V. 100 mg/m^2/day days 1 and 8
[total dose/cycle = 200 mg/m^2]
Fluorouracil: I.V.: 600 mg/m^2/day (start 1 hour after methotrexate) days 1 and 8
[total dose/cycle = 1200 mg/m^2]
Leucovorin: Oral, I.V.: 10 mg/m^2 every 6 hours for 6 doses (start 24 hours after methotrexate)
[total dose/cycle = 60 mg/m^2]
Repeat cycle every 28 days for 12 cycles

MINE

Use Lymphoma, non-Hodgkin

Regimen

Mesna: I.V.: 1.33 g/m^2/day concurrent with ifosfamide dose, then 500 mg orally (4 hours after each ifosfamide infusion) days 1, 2, and 3
[total dose/cycle = 3.99 g/m^2/1500 mg]
Ifosfamide: I.V.: 1.33 g/m^2/day days 1, 2, and 3
[total dose/cycle = 3.99 g/m^2]
Mitoxantrone: I.V.: 8 mg/m^2 day 1
[total dose/cycle = 8 mg/m^2]
Etoposide: I.V.: 65 mg/m^2/day days 1, 2, and 3
[total dose/cycle = 195 mg/m^2]
Repeat cycle every 28 days

MINE-ESHAP

Use Lymphoma, non-Hodgkin

Regimen

Mesna: I.V.: 1.33 g/m^2 concurrent with ifosfamide dose, then 500 mg orally (4 hours after ifosfamide) days 1, 2, and 3
[total dose/cycle = 4 g/m^2/1500 mg]
Ifosfamide: I.V.: 1.33 g/m^2/day days 1, 2, and 3
[total dose/cycle = 4 g/m^2]
Mitoxantrone: I.V.: 8 mg/m^2 day 1
[total dose/cycle = 8 mg/m^2]
Etoposide: I.V.: 65 mg/m^2/day days 1, 2, and 3
[total dose/cycle = 195 mg/m^2]
Repeat cycle every 21 days for 6 cycles, followed by 3-6 cycles of ESHAP

mini-BEAM

Use Lymphoma, Hodgkin disease

Regimen

Carmustine: I.V.: 60 mg/m^2 day 1
[total dose/cycle = 60 mg/m^2]
Etoposide: I.V.: 75 mg/m^2/day days 2 to 5
[total dose/cycle = 300 mg/m^2]
Cytarabine: I.V.: 100 mg/m^2 every 12 hours days 2 to 5 (8 doses)
[total dose/cycle = 800 mg/m^2]
Melphalan: I.V.: 30 mg/m^2 day 6
[total dose/cycle = 30 mg/m^2]
Repeat cycle every 4-6 weeks

Mitomycin-Vinblastine

Use Breast cancer

Regimen

Mitomycin: I.V.: 20 mg/m^2 day 1
[total dose/cycle = 20 mg/m^2]
Vinblastine: I.V.: 0.15 mg/kg/day days 1 and 21
[total dose/cycle = 0.3 mg/kg]
Repeat cycle every 6-8 weeks

Mitoxantrone + Hydrocortisone

Use Prostate cancer

Regimen
Mitoxantrone: I.V.: 14 mg/m^2 day 1
[total dose/cycle = 14 mg/m^2]
Hydrocortisone: Oral: 40 mg daily
[total dose/cycle = 840 mg]
Repeat cycle every 3 weeks

MOP

Use Brain tumors

Regimen
Mechlorethamine: I.V.: 6 mg/m^2/day days 1 and 8
[total dose/cycle = 12 mg/m^2]
Vincristine: I.V.: 1.5 mg/m^2/day (maximum 2 mg) days 1 and 8
[total dose/cycle = 3 mg/m^2]
Procarbazine: Oral: 100 mg/m^2/day days 1 to 14
[total dose/cycle = 1400 mg/m^2]
Repeat cycle every 28 days

MOPP/ABVD

Use Lymphoma, Hodgkin disease

Regimen NOTE: Multiple variations are listed below.
Variation 1:
Mechlorethamine: I.V.: 6 mg/m^2/day days 1 and 8
[total dose/cycle = 12 mg/m^2]
Vincristine: I.V.: 1.4 mg/m^2/day (maximum 2 mg) days 1 and 8
[total dose/cycle = 2.8 mg/m^2]
Procarbazine: I.V.: 100 mg/m^2/day days 1 to 14
[total dose/cycle = 1400 mg/m^2]
Prednisone: Oral: 40 mg/m^2/day days 1 to 14 (during cycles 1, 4, 7, and 10 only)
[total dose/cycle = 560 mg/m^2]
Doxorubicin: I.V.: 25 mg/m^2/day days 29 and 43
[total dose/cycle = 50 mg/m^2]
Bleomycin: I.V.: 10 units/m^2/day days 29 and 43
[total dose/cycle = 20 units/m^2]
Vinblastine: I.V.: 6 mg/m^2/day days 29 and 43
[total dose/cycle = 12 mg/m^2]
Dacarbazine: I.V.: 375 mg/m^2/day days 29 and 43
[total dose/cycle = 750 mg/m^2]
Repeat cycle every 56 days
Variation 2:
Mechlorethamine: I.V.: 6 mg/m^2/day days 1 and 8
[total dose/cycle = 12 mg/m^2]
Vincristine: I.V.: 1.4 mg/m^2/day (maximum 2 mg) days 1 and 8
[total dose/cycle = 2.8 mg/m^2]
Procarbazine: I.V.: 100 mg/m^2/day days 1 to 14
[total dose/cycle = 1400 mg/m^2]
Prednisone: Oral: 40 mg/m^2/day days 1 to 14 (during cycles 1 and 7 only)
[total dose/cycle = 560 mg/m^2]
Doxorubicin: I.V.: 25 mg/m^2/day days 29 and 43
[total dose/cycle = 50 mg/m^2]
Bleomycin: I.V.: 10 units/m^2/day days 29 and 43
[total dose/cycle = 20 units/m^2]
Vinblastine: I.V.: 6 mg/m^2/day days 29 and 43
[total dose/cycle = 12 mg/m^2]
Dacarbazine: I.V.: 375 mg/m^2/day days 29 and 43
[total dose/cycle = 750 mg/m^2]
Repeat cycle every 56 days

Variation 3:
  Mechlorethamine: I.V.: 6 mg/m^2/day days 1 and 8
   [total dose/cycle = 12 mg/m^2]
  Vincristine: I.V.: 1.4 mg/m^2/day (maximum 2 mg) days 1 and 8
   [total dose/cycle = 2.8 mg/m^2]
  Procarbazine: I.V.: 100 mg/m^2/day days 1 to 14
   [total dose/cycle = 1400 mg/m^2]
  Prednisone: Oral: 40 mg/m^2/day days 1 to 14 (every cycle)
   [total dose/cycle = 560 mg/m^2]
  Doxorubicin: I.V.: 25 mg/m^2/day days 29 and 43
   [total dose/cycle = 50 mg/m^2]
  Bleomycin: I.V.: 10 units/m^2/day days 29 and 43
   [total dose/cycle = 20 units/m^2]
  Vinblastine: I.V.: 6 mg/m^2/day days 29 and 43
   [total dose/cycle = 12 mg/m^2]
  Dacarbazine: I.V.: 375 mg/m^2/day days 29 and 43
   [total dose/cycle = 750 mg/m^2]
  Repeat cycle every 56 days
Variation 4:
  MOPP Regimen:
  Mechlorethamine: I.V.: 6 mg/m^2/day days 1 and 8
   [total dose/cycle = 12 mg/m^2]
  Vincristine: I.V.: 1.4 mg/m^2/day (maximum 2 mg) days 1 and 8
   [total dose/cycle = 2.8 mg/m^2]
  Procarbazine: I.V.: 100 mg/m^2/day days 1 to 14
   [total dose/cycle = 1400 mg/m^2]
  Prednisone: Oral: 25 mg/m^2/day days 1 to 14
   [total dose/cycle = 350 mg/m^2]
  ABVD Regimen:
  Doxorubicin: I.V.: 25 mg/m^2/day days 1 and 15
   [total dose/cycle = 50 mg/m^2]
  Bleomycin: I.V.: 6 units/m^2/day days 1 and 15
   [total dose/cycle = 12 units/m^2]
  Vinblastine: I.V.: 6 mg/m^2/day days 1 and 15
   [total dose/cycle = 12 mg/m^2]
  Dacarbazine: I.V.: 250 mg/m^2/day days 1 and 15
   [total dose/cycle = 500 mg/m^2]
  Each regimen cycle is 28 days. Administer regimens in alternating fashion as follows: 2 cycles of MOPP
   alternating with 2 cycles of ABVD for a total of 8 cycles
Variation 5 (pediatrics):
  Mechlorethamine: I.V.: 6 mg/m^2/day days 1 and 8
   [total dose/cycle = 12 mg/m^2]
  Vincristine: I.V.: 1.4 mg/m^2/day days 1 and 8
   [total dose/cycle = 2.8 mg/m^2]
  Procarbazine: Oral: 100 mg/m^2/day days 1 to 14
   [total dose/cycle = 1400 mg/m^2]
  Prednisone: Oral: 40 mg/m^2/day days 1 to 14
   [total dose/cycle = 560 mg/m^2]
  Doxorubicin: I.V.: 25 mg/m^2/day days 29 and 42
   [total dose/cycle = 50 mg/m^2]
  Bleomycin: I.V.: 10 units/m^2/day days 29 and 42
   [total dose/cycle = 20 units/m^2]
  Vinblastine: I.V.: 6 mg/m^2/day days 29 and 42
   [total dose/cycle = 12 mg/m^2]
  Dacarbazine: I.V.: 150 mg/m^2/day days 29 to 33
   [total dose/cycle = 750 mg/m^2]
  Repeat cycle every 56 days for 4 cycles
Variation 6 (pediatrics):
  Mechlorethamine: I.V.: 6 mg/m^2/day days 1 and 8
   [total dose/cycle = 12 mg/m^2]
  Vincristine: I.V.: 1.4 mg/m^2/day days 1 and 8
   [total dose/cycle = 2.8 mg/m^2]
  Procarbazine: Oral: 100 mg/m^2/day days 1 to 14
   [total dose/cycle = 1400 mg/m^2]

Prednisone: Oral: 40 mg/m^2/day days 1 to 14
  [total dose/cycle = 560 mg/m^2]
Doxorubicin: I.V.: 25 mg/m^2/day days 29 and 42
  [total dose/cycle = 50 mg/m^2]
Bleomycin: I.V.: 10 units/m^2/day days 29 and 42
  [total dose/cycle = 20 units/m^2]
Vinblastine: I.V.: 6 mg/m^2/day days 29 and 42
  [total dose/cycle = 12 mg/m^2]
Dacarbazine: I.V.: 375 mg/m^2/day days 29 and 43
  [total dose/cycle = 750 mg/m^2]
Repeat cycle every 56 days for 4 cycles

MOPP/ABV Hybrid

Use Lymphoma, Hodgkin disease

Regimen
Mechlorethamine: I.V.: 6 mg/m^2 day 1
  [total dose/cycle = 6 mg/m^2]
Vincristine: I.V.: 1.4 mg/m^2 (maximum 2 mg) day 1
  [total dose/cycle = 1.4 mg/m^2]
Procarbazine: Oral: 100 mg/m^2/day days 1 to 7
  [total dose/cycle = 700 mg/m^2]
Prednisone: Oral: 40 mg/m^2/day days 1 to 14
  [total dose/cycle = 560 mg/m^2]
Doxorubicin: I.V.: 35 mg/m^2 day 8
  [total dose/cycle = 35 mg/m^2]
Bleomycin: I.V.: 10 units/m^2 day 8
  [total dose/cycle = 10 units/m^2]
Vinblastine: I.V.: 6 mg/m^2 day 8
  [total dose/cycle = 6 mg/m^2]
Repeat cycle every 28 days

MOPP (Lymphoma, Hodgkin Disease)

Use Lymphoma, Hodgkin disease

Regimen NOTE: Multiple variations are listed below.
Variation 1:
Mechlorethamine: I.V.: 6 mg/m^2/day days 1 and 8
  [total dose/cycle = 12 mg/m^2]
Vincristine: I.V.: 1.4 mg/m^2/day days 1 and 8
  [total dose/cycle = 2.8 mg/m^2]
Procarbazine: Oral: 100 mg/m^2/day days 1 to 14
  [total dose/cycle = 1400 mg/m^2]
Prednisone: Oral: 40 mg/m^2/day days 1 to 14 (cycles 1 and 4)
  [total dose/cycle = 560 mg/m^2]
Repeat cycle every 28 days for 6-8 cycles
Variation 2:
Mechlorethamine: I.V.: 6 mg/m^2/day (maximum 15 mg) days 1 and 8
  [total dose/cycle = 12 mg/m^2]
Vincristine: I.V.: 1.4 mg/m^2/day (maximum 2 mg) days 1 and 8
  [total dose/cycle = 2.8 mg/m^2]
Procarbazine: Oral: 100 mg/m^2/day days 1 to 10
  [total dose/cycle = 1000 mg/m^2]
Prednisone: Oral: 25 mg/m^2/day (maximum 60 mg) days 1 to 14
  [total dose/cycle = 350 mg/m^2]
or
Prednisolone: Oral: 25 mg/m^2/day (maximum 60 mg) days 1 to 14
  [total dose/cycle = 350 mg/m^2]
Repeat cycle every 28 days
Variation 3:
Mechlorethamine: I.V.: 6 mg/m^2/day days 1 and 8
  [total dose/cycle = 12 mg/m^2]
Vincristine: I.V.: 1.4 mg/m^2/day days 1 and 8
  [total dose/cycle = 2.8 mg/m^2]
Procarbazine: Oral: 50 mg day 1, 100 mg day 2, 100 mg/m^2/day days 3 to 14
  [total dose/cycle = 150 mg / 1200 mg/m^2]

◄ Prednisone: Oral: 40 mg/m^2/day days 1 to 14
  [total dose/cycle = 560 mg/m^2]
Repeat cycle every 28 days
Variation 4:
  Mechlorethamine: I.V.: 6 mg/m^2/day days 1 and 8
    [total dose/cycle = 12 mg/m^2]
  Vincristine: I.V.: 1.4 mg/m^2/day days 1 and 8
    [total dose/cycle = 2.8 mg/m^2]
  Procarbazine: Oral: 50 mg day 1, 100 mg day 2, 100 mg/m^2/day days 3 to 10
    [total dose/cycle = 150 mg / 800 mg/m^2]
  Prednisone: Oral: 40 mg/m^2/day days 1 to 14
    [total dose/cycle = 560 mg/m^2]
  Repeat cycle every 28 days
Variation 5:
  Mechlorethamine: I.V.: 6 mg/m^2/day days 1 and 8
    [total dose/cycle = 12 mg/m^2]
  Vincristine: I.V.: 1.4 mg/m^2/day days 1 and 8
    [total dose/cycle = 2.8 mg/m^2]
  Procarbazine: Oral: 50 mg/m^2 day 1, then 100 mg/m^2/day days 2 to 14
    [total dose/cycle = 1350 mg/m^2]
  Prednisone: Oral: 40 mg/m^2/day days 1 to 14
    [total dose/cycle = 560 mg/m^2]
  Repeat cycle every 28 days

MOPP (Medulloblastoma)

Use Brain tumors
Regimen
Mechlorethamine: I.V.: 3 mg/m^2/day days 1 and 8
  [total dose/cycle = 6 mg/m^2]
Vincristine: I.V.: 1.4 mg/m^2/day (maximum 2 mg) days 1 and 8
  [total dose/cycle = 2.8 mg/m^2]
Prednisone: Oral: 40 mg/m^2/day days 1 to 10
  [total dose/cycle = 400 mg/m^2]
Procarbazine: Oral: 50 mg day 1
  [total dose/cycle = 50 mg]
    followed by Oral: 100 mg day 2
      [total dose/cycle = 100 mg]
      followed by Oral: 100 mg/m^2/day days 3 to 10
        [total dose/cycle = 800 mg/m^2]
Repeat cycle every 28 days

MP (Multiple Myeloma)

Use Multiple myeloma
Regimen
Melphalan: Oral: 8-10 mg/m^2/day days 1 to 4
  [total dose/cycle = 32-40 mg/m^2]
Prednisone: Oral: 40-60 mg/m^2/day days 1 to 4
  [total dose/cycle = 160-240 mg/m^2]
Repeat cycle every 28-42 days

MP (Prostate Cancer)

Use Prostate cancer
Regimen
Mitoxantrone: I.V.: 12 mg/m^2 day 1
  [total dose/cycle = 12 mg/m^2]
Prednisone: Oral: 5 mg twice daily
  [total dose/cycle = 210 mg]
Repeat cycle every 21 days

MTX/6-MP/VP (Maintenance)

Use Leukemia, acute lymphocytic

Regimen
Methotrexate: Oral: 20 mg/m^2 weekly
  [total dose/cycle = 80 mg/m^2]
Mercaptopurine: Oral: 75 mg/m^2/day
  [total dose/cycle = 2250 mg/m^2]
Vincristine: I.V.: 1.5 mg/m^2 day 1
  [total dose/cycle = 1.5 mg/m^2]
Prednisone: Oral: 40 mg/m^2/day days 1 to 5
  [total dose/cycle = 200 mg/m^2]
Repeat monthly for 2-3 years

MTX-CDDPAdr

Use Osteosarcoma

Regimen
Cisplatin: I.V.: 75 mg/m^2 day 1 of cycles 1-7, then 120 mg/m^2 for cycles 8, 9, and 10
Doxorubicin: I.V.: 25 mg/m^2/day days 1, 2, and 3 of cycles 1 to 7
Methotrexate: I.V.: 12 g/m^2/day days 21 and 28
Leucovorin calcium rescue: I.V.: 20 mg/m^2 every 3 hours (beginning 16 hours after completion of methotrexate) for 8 doses, then orally every 6 hours for 8 doses

MV

Use Leukemia, acute myeloid

Regimen Induction:
Mitoxantrone: I.V.: 10 mg/m^2/day days 1 to 5
  [total dose/cycle = 50 mg/m^2]
Etoposide: I.V.: 100 mg/m^2/day days 1 to 5
  [total dose/cycle = 500 mg/m^2]
Second cycle may be given based on individual response; time between cycles not specified

M-VAC (Bladder Cancer)

Use Bladder cancer

Regimen NOTE: Multiple variations are listed below.
Variation 1:
  Methotrexate: I.V.: 30 mg/m^2/day days 1, 15, and 22
    [total dose/cycle = 90 mg/m^2]
  Vinblastine: I.V.: 3 mg/m^2/day days 2, 15, and 22
    [total dose/cycle = 9 mg/m^2]
  Doxorubicin: I.V.: 30 mg/m^2 day 2
    [total dose/cycle = 30 mg/m^2]
  Cisplatin: I.V.: 70 mg/m^2 day 2
    [total dose/cycle = 70 mg/m^2]
  Repeat cycle every 4 weeks
Variation 2:
  Methotrexate: I.V.: 40 or 50 mg/m^2/day days 1, 15, and 22
    [total dose/cycle = 120 or 150 mg/m^2]
  Vinblastine: I.V.: 4 or 5 mg/m^2/day days 2, 15, and 22
    [total dose/cycle = 12 or 15 mg/m^2]
  Doxorubicin: I.V.: 40 or 50 mg/m^2 day 2
    [total dose/cycle = 40 or 50 mg/m^2]
  Cisplatin: I.V.: 100 mg/m^2 day 2
    [total dose/cycle = 100 mg/m^2]
  Repeat cycle every 4 weeks
Variation 3:
  Methotrexate: I.V.: 30 mg/m^2/day days 1, 15, and 22
    [total dose/cycle = 90 mg/m^2]
  Vinblastine: I.V.: 3 mg/m^2 day 2
    [total dose/cycle = 3 mg/m^2]
  Doxorubicin: I.V.: 30 mg/m^2 day 2
    [total dose/cycle = 30 mg/m^2]

Cisplatin: I.V.: 70 mg/m^2 day 2
  [total dose/cycle = 70 mg/m^2]
Repeat cycle every 4 weeks

Variation 4:
Methotrexate: I.V.: 60 mg/m^2 day 1
  [total dose/cycle = 60 mg/m^2]
  followed by I.V.: 30 mg/m^2 day 16
    [total dose/cycle = 30 mg/m^2]
Vinblastine: I.V.: 4 mg/m^2/day days 2 and 16
  [total dose/cycle = 8 mg/m^2]
Doxorubicin: I.V.: 60 mg/m^2 day 2
  [total dose/cycle = 60 mg/m^2]
Cisplatin: I.V.: 100 mg/m^2 day 2
  [total dose/cycle = 100 mg/m^2]
Repeat cycle every 23 days

Variation 5:
Methotrexate: I.V.: 30 mg/m^2/day days 1, 16, and 23
  [total dose/cycle = 90 mg/m^2]
Vinblastine: I.V.: 4 mg/m^2/day days 1, 16, and 23
  [total dose/cycle = 12 mg/m^2]
Doxorubicin: I.V.: 60 mg/m^2 day 2
  [total dose/cycle = 60 mg/m^2]
Cisplatin: I.V.: 100 mg/m^2 day 2
  [total dose/cycle = 100 mg/m^2]
Repeat cycle every 23 days

Variation 6:
Methotrexate: I.V.: 30 or 35 mg/m^2 day 1
  [total dose/cycle = 30 or 35 mg/m^2]
Vinblastine: I.V.: 3 or 3.5 mg/m^2 day 2
  [total dose/cycle = 3 or 3.5 mg/m^2]
Doxorubicin: I.V.: 30 or 35 mg/m^2 day 2
  [total dose/cycle = 30 or 35 mg/m^2]
Cisplatin: I.V.: 70 or 80 mg/m^2 day 2
  [total dose/cycle = 70 or 80 mg/m^2]
Repeat cycle every 2 weeks

Variation 7:
Methotrexate: I.V.: 30 mg/m^2 day 1
  [total dose/cycle = 30 mg/m^2]
Vinblastine: I.V.: 3 mg/m^2 day 2
  [total dose/cycle = 3 mg/m^2]
Doxorubicin: I.V.: 30 mg/m^2 day 2
  [total dose/cycle = 30 mg/m^2]
Cisplatin: I.V.: 70 mg/m^2 day 2
  [total dose/cycle = 70 mg/m^2]
Repeat cycle every 14 days

Variation 8:
Methotrexate: I.V.: 30 mg/m^2/day days 1, 15, and 22
  [total dose/cycle = 90 mg/m^2]
Vinblastine: I.V.: 3 mg/m^2/day days 1, 15, and 22
  [total dose/cycle = 9 mg/m^2]
Doxorubicin: I.V.: 45 mg/m^2 day 2
  [total dose/cycle = 45 mg/m^2]
Cisplatin: I.V.: 70 mg/m^2 day 2
  [total dose/cycle = 70 mg/m^2]
Repeat cycle every 4 weeks

Variation 9:
Methotrexate: I.V.: 40 mg/m^2/day days 1 and 15
  [total dose/cycle = 80 mg/m^2]
Vinblastine: I.V.: 4 mg/m^2/day days 1, 16, and 23
  [total dose/cycle = 12 mg/m^2]
Doxorubicin: I.V.: 60 mg/m^2 day 2
  [total dose/cycle = 60 mg/m^2]
Cisplatin: I.V.: 100 mg/m^2 day 2
  [total dose/cycle = 100 mg/m^2]
Repeat cycle every 23 days

Variation 10:
  Methotrexate: I.V.: 30 mg/m^2/day days 1, 15, and 22
    [total dose/cycle = 90 mg/m^2]
  Vinblastine: I.V.: 3 mg/m^2/day days 1, 16, and 22
    [total dose/cycle = 9 mg/m^2]
  Doxorubicin: I.V.: 30 mg/m^2 day 1
    [total dose/cycle = 30 mg/m^2]
  Cisplatin: I.V.: 70 mg/m^2 day 1
    [total dose/cycle = 70 mg/m^2]
  Repeat cycle every 4 weeks
Variation 11:
  Methotrexate: I.V.: 30 mg/m^2/day days 1, 15, and 22
    [total dose/cycle = 90 mg/m^2]
  Vinblastine: I.V.: 3 mg/m^2/day days 2, 15, and 22
    [total dose/cycle = 9 mg/m^2]
  Doxorubicin: I.V.: 30 mg/m^2 day 2
    [total dose/cycle = 30 mg/m^2]
  Cisplatin: I.V.: 70 mg/m^2 day 2
    [total dose/cycle = 70 mg/m^2]
  Leucovorin: Oral: 15 mg every 6 hours for 4 doses, days 2, 16, and 23
    [total dose/cycle = 180 mg]
  Repeat cycle every 4 weeks
Variation 12:
  Methotrexate: I.V.: 30 mg/m^2/day days 1 and 15
    [total dose/cycle = 60 mg/m^2]
  Vinblastine: I.V.: 3 mg/m^2/day days 2 and 15
    [total dose/cycle = 6 mg/m^2]
  Doxorubicin: I.V.: 30 or 40 mg/m^2 day 3
    [total dose/cycle = 30 or 40 mg/m^2]
  Cisplatin: I.V.: 70 mg/m^2 day 2
    [total dose/cycle = 70 mg/m^2]
  Repeat cycle every 4 weeks
Variation 13:
  Methotrexate: I.V.: 30 mg/m^2/day days 1 and 15
    [total dose/cycle = 60 mg/m^2]
  Vinblastine: I.V.: 3 mg/m^2/day days 2 and 15
    [total dose/cycle = 6 mg/m^2]
  Doxorubicin: I.V.: 30 or 40 mg/m^2 day 2
    [total dose/cycle = 30 or 40 mg/m^2]
  Cisplatin: I.V.: 70 mg/m^2 day 2
    [total dose/cycle = 70 mg/m^2]
  Repeat cycle every 4 weeks

M-VAC (Breast Cancer)

Use Breast cancer

Regimen
  Methotrexate: I.V.: 30 mg/m^2/day days 1, 15, and 22
    [total dose/cycle = 90 mg/m^2]
  Vinblastine: I.V.: 3 mg/m^2/day days 2, 15, and 22
    [total dose/cycle = 9 mg/m^2]
  Doxorubicin: I.V.: 30 mg/m^2 day 2
    [total dose/cycle = 30 mg/m^2]
  Cisplatin: I.V.: 70 mg/m^2 day 2
    [total dose/cycle = 70 mg/m^2]
  Leucovorin: Oral: 10 mg every 6 hours for 6 doses days 2, 16, and 23
    [total dose/cycle = 180 mg]
  Repeat cycle every 4 weeks

M-VAC (Cervical Cancer)

Use Cervical cancer

Regimen
Methotrexate: I.V.: 30 mg/m^2/day days 1, 15, and 22
[total dose/cycle = 90 mg/m^2]
Vinblastine: I.V.: 3 mg/m^2/day days 2, 15, and 22
[total dose/cycle = 9 mg/m^2]
Doxorubicin: I.V.: 30 mg/m^2 day 2
[total dose/cycle = 30 mg/m^2]
Cisplatin: I.V.: 70 mg/m^2 day 2
[total dose/cycle = 70 mg/m^2]
Repeat cycle every 4 weeks

M-VAC (Endometrial Cancer)

Use Endometrial cancer

Regimen
Methotrexate: I.V.: 30 mg/m^2/day days 1, 15, and 22
[total dose/cycle = 90 mg/m^2]
Vinblastine: I.V.: 3 mg/m^2/day days 2, 15, and 22
[total dose/cycle = 9 mg/m^2]
Doxorubicin: I.V.: 30 mg/m^2/day day 2
[total dose/cycle = 30 mg/m^2]
Cisplatin: I.V.: 70 mg/m^2/day day 2
[total dose/cycle = 70 mg/m^2]
Repeat cycle every 4 weeks

M-VAC (Head and Neck Cancer)

Use Head and neck cancer

Regimen
Methotrexate: I.V.: 30 mg/m^2/day days 1, 15, and 22
[total dose/cycle = 90 mg/m^2]
Vinblastine: I.V.: 3 mg/m^2/day days 2, 15, and 22
[total dose/cycle = 9 mg/m^2]
Doxorubicin: I.V.: 30 mg/m^2 day 2
[total dose/cycle = 30 mg/m^2]
Cisplatin: I.V.: 70 mg/m^2 day 2
[total dose/cycle = 70 mg/m^2]
Repeat cycle every 4 weeks

MVPP

Use Lymphoma, Hodgkin disease

Regimen
Mechlorethamine: I.V.: 6 mg/m^2/day days 1 and 8
[total dose/cycle = 12 mg/m^2]
Vinblastine: I.V.: 4 mg/m^2/day days 1 and 8
[total dose/cycle = 8 mg/m^2]
Procarbazine: Oral: 100 mg/m^2/day days 1 to 14
[total dose/cycle = 1400 mg/m^2]
Prednisone: Oral: 40 mg/m^2/day days 1 to 14
[total dose/cycle = 560 mg/m^2]
Repeat cycle every 4-6 weeks

N4SE Protocol

Use Neuroblastoma

Regimen
Vincristine: I.V.: 0.05 mg/kg/day days 1 and 2
[total dose/cycle = 0.1 mg/kg]
Doxorubicin: I.V.: 15 mg/m^2/day days 1 and 2
[total dose/cycle = 30 mg/m^2]
Cyclophosphamide: I.V.: 30 mg/kg/day days 1 and 2
[total dose/cycle = 60 mg/kg]

Fluorouracil: I.V.: 1 mg/kg/day days 3, 8, and 9
[total dose/cycle = 3 mg/kg]
Cytarabine: I.V.: 3 mg/kg/day days 3, 8, and 9
[total dose/cycle = 9 mg/kg]
Hydroxyurea: Oral: 40 mg/kg/day days 3, 8, and 9
[total dose/cycle = 120 mg/kg]
Repeat cycle every 21-28 days

N6 Protocol

Use Neuroblastoma

Regimen
Course 1, 2, 4, and 6:
Cyclophosphamide: I.V.: 70 mg/kg/day days 1 and 2
[total dose/cycle = 140 mg/kg]
Doxorubicin: I.V.: 25 mg/m^2/day continuous infusion days 1, 2, and 3
[total dose/cycle = 75 mg/m^2]
Vincristine: I.V.: 0.033 mg/kg/day continuous infusion days 1, 2, and 3
[total dose/cycle = 0.099 mg/kg]
Vincristine: I.V.: 1.5 mg/m^2 day 9
[total dose/cycle = 1.5 mg/m^2]
Course 3, 5, and 7:
Etoposide: I.V.: 200 mg/m^2/day days 1, 2, and 3
[total dose/cycle = 600 mg/m^2]
Cisplatin: I.V.: 50 mg/m^2/day days 1 to 4
[total dose/cycle = 200 mg/m^2]

NFL

Use Breast cancer

Regimen NOTE: Multiple variations are listed below.
Variation 1:
Mitoxantrone: I.V.: 12 mg/m^2 day 1
[total dose/cycle = 12 mg/m^2]
Fluorouracil: I.V.: 350 mg/m^2/day days 1, 2, and 3
[total dose/cycle = 1050 mg/m^2]
Leucovorin: I.V.: 300 mg/m^2/day days 1, 2, and 3
[total dose/cycle = 900 mg/m^2]
Repeat cycle every 21 days
Variation 2:
Mitoxantrone: I.V.: 10 mg/m^2 day 1
[total dose/cycle = 10 mg/m^2]
Fluorouracil: I.V.: 1000 mg/m^2/day continuous infusion days 1, 2, and 3
[total dose/cycle = 3000 mg/m^2]
Leucovorin: I.V.: 100 mg/m^2/day days 1, 2, and 3
[total dose/cycle = 300 mg/m^2]
Repeat cycle every 21 days

OPA

Use Lymphoma, Hodgkin disease

Regimen
Vincristine: I.V.: 1.5 mg/m^2/day (maximum 2 mg) days 1, 8, and 15
[total dose/cycle = 4.5 mg/m^2]
Prednisone: Oral: 60 mg/m^2/day days 1 to 15 in 3 divided doses
[total dose/cycle = 900 mg/m^2]
Doxorubicin: I.V.: 40 mg/m^2/day days 1 and 15
[total dose/cycle = 80 mg/m^2]
Second cycle may be given based on individual response; time between cycles not specified

OPEC

Use Neuroblastoma

Regimen
Vincristine: I.V.: 1.5 mg/m^2 day 1
[total dose/cycle = 1.5 mg/m^2]

◀ Cyclophosphamide: I.V.: 600 mg/m^2 day 1
   [total dose/cycle = 600 mg/m^2]
Cisplatin: I.V.: 100 mg/m^2 day 2
   [total dose/cycle = 100 mg/m^2]
Teniposide: I.V.: 150 mg/m^2 day 4
   [total dose/cycle = 150 mg/m^2]
Repeat cycle every 21 days

OPEC-D

Use Neuroblastoma
Regimen
Vincristine: I.V.: 1.5 mg/m^2 day 1
   [total dose/cycle = 1.5 mg/m^2]
Cyclophosphamide: I.V.: 600 mg/m^2 day 1
   [total dose/cycle = 600 mg/m^2]
Doxorubicin: I.V.: 40 mg/m^2 day 1
   [total dose/cycle = 40 mg/m^2]
Cisplatin: I.V.: 100 mg/m^2 day 2
   [total dose/cycle = 100 mg/m^2]
Teniposide: I.V.: 150 mg/m^2 day 4
   [total dose/cycle = 150 mg/m^2]
Repeat cycle every 21 days

OPPA

Use Lymphoma, Hodgkin disease
Regimen
Vincristine: I.V.: 1.5 mg/m^2/day (maximum 2 mg) days 1, 8, and 15
   [total dose/cycle = 4.5 mg/m^2]
Prednisone: Oral: 60 mg/m^2/day days 1 to 15 in 3 divided doses
   [total dose/cycle = 900 mg/m^2]
Doxorubicin: I.V.: 40 mg/m^2/day days 1 and 15
   [total dose/cycle = 80 mg/m^2]
Procarbazine: Oral: 100 mg/m^2/day days 1 to 15 in 2 or 3 divided doses
   [total dose/cycle = 1500 mg/m^2]
Second cycle may be given based on individual response; time between cycles not specified

PAC (CAP)

Use Ovarian cancer
Regimen
Cisplatin: I.V.: 50 mg/m^2 day 1
   [total dose/cycle = 50 mg/m^2]
Doxorubicin: I.V.: 50 mg/m^2 day 1
   [total dose/cycle = 50 mg/m^2]
Cyclophosphamide: I.V.: 1000 mg/m^2 day 1
   [total dose/cycle = 1000 mg/m^2]
Repeat cycle every 21 days for 8 cycles

PA-CI

Use Hepatoblastoma
Regimen NOTE: Multiple variations are listed below.
Variation 1:
Cisplatin: I.V.: 90 mg/m^2 day 1
   [total dose/cycle = 90 mg/m^2]
Doxorubicin: I.V.: 20 mg/m^2/day continuous infusion days 2 to 5
   [total dose/cycle = 80 mg/m^2]
Repeat cycle every 21 days
Variation 2:
Cisplatin: I.V.: 20 mg/m^2/day days 1 to 4
   [total dose/cycle = 80 mg/m^2]
Doxorubicin: I.V.: 100 mg/m^2 continuous infusion day 1
   [total dose/cycle = 100 mg/m^2]
Repeat cycle every 21-28 days

Paclitaxel-Bevacizumab

Use Breast cancer

Regimen
Paclitaxel: I.V.: 90 mg/m^2/day days 1, 8, and 15
[total dose/cycle = 270 mg/m^2]
Bevacizumab: I.V.: 10 mg/kg/day days 1 and 15
[total dose/cycle = 20 mg/kg]
Repeat cycle every 28 days

Paclitaxel-Carboplatin-Bevacizumab

Use Lung cancer, nonsquamous, nonsmall cell

Regimen
Paclitaxel: I.V.: 200 mg/m^2 infused over 3 hours day 1
[total dose/cycle = 200 mg/m^2]
followed by
Carboplatin: I.V.: Target AUC 6 day 1
[total dose/cycle = AUC = 6]
followed by
Bevacizumab: I.V.: 15 mg/kg day 1
[total dose/cycle = 15 mg/kg]
Repeat cycle every 21 days for 6 cycles

Paclitaxel-Carboplatin (Bladder Cancer)

Use Bladder cancer

Regimen
Paclitaxel: I.V.: 200 mg/m^2 or 225 mg/m^2 day 1
[total dose/cycle = 200 or 225 mg/m^2]
Carboplatin: I.V.: AUC 5-6 day 1
[total dose/cycle = AUC = 5-6]
Repeat cycle every 21 days

Paclitaxel-Carboplatin-Etoposide

Use Adenocarcinoma, unknown primary

Regimen
Paclitaxel: I.V.: 200 mg/m^2 infused over 1 hour day 1
[total dose/cycle = 200 mg/m^2]
followed by
Carboplatin: I.V.: Target AUC 6
[total dose = AUC = 6]
Etoposide: Oral: 50 mg/day days 1, 3, 5, 7, and 9
and Oral: 100 mg/day days 2, 4, 6, 8, and 10
[total dose/cycle = 750 mg]
Repeat cycle every 21 days

Paclitaxel-Carboplatin-Gemcitabine

Use Bladder cancer

Regimen
Paclitaxel: I.V.: 200 mg/m^2 day 1
[total dose/cycle = 200 mg/m^2]
Gemcitabine: I.V.: 1000 mg/m^2/day days 1 and 8
[total dose/cycle = 2000 mg/m^2]
Carboplatin: I.V.: AUC 5 day 1
[total dose/cycle = AUC = 5]
Repeat cycle every 21 days

Paclitaxel + Estramustine + Carboplatin

Use Prostate cancer

Regimen
Paclitaxel: I.V.: 100 mg/m^2 day 3 each week
[total dose/cycle = 400 mg/m^2]

Estramustine: Oral: 10 mg/kg/day days 1 to 5 each week
[total dose/cycle = 200 mg/kg]
Carboplatin: I.V.: Target AUC 6 day 3
[total dose/cycle = AUC = 6]
Repeat cycle every 28 days

Paclitaxel + Estramustine + Etoposide

Use Prostate cancer
Regimen
Paclitaxel: I.V.: 135 mg/m^2 day 2
[total dose/cycle = 135 mg/m^2]
Estramustine: Oral: 280 mg 3 times/day days 1 to 14
[total dose/cycle = 11,760 mg]
Etoposide: Oral: 100 mg/day days 1 to 14
[total dose/cycle = 1400 mg]
Repeat cycle every 21 days

Paclitaxel-Gemcitabine

Use Bladder cancer
Regimen
Paclitaxel: I.V.: 200 mg/m^2 day 1
[total dose/cycle = 200 mg/m^2]
Gemcitabine: I.V.: 1000 mg/m^2/day days 1, 8, and 15
[total dose/cycle = 3000 mg/m^2]
Repeat cycle every 21 days for a maximum of 6 cycles

Paclitaxel-Ifosfamide-Cisplatin

Use Testicular cancer
Regimen
Paclitaxel: I.V.: 250 mg/m^2 continuous infusion day 1
[total dose/cycle = 250 mg/m^2]
Ifosfamide: I.V.: 1500 mg/m^2/day days 2 to 5
[total dose/cycle = 6000 mg/m^2]
Cisplatin: I.V.: 25 mg/m^2/day days 2 to 5
[total dose/cycle = 100 mg/m^2]
Mesna: I.V.: 500 mg/m^2 prior to ifosfamide and every 4 hours for 2 doses, days 2 to 5
[total dose/cycle = 6000 mg/m^2]
Repeat cycle every 21 days for 4 cycles

Paclitaxel-Vinorelbine

Use Breast cancer
Regimen NOTE: Multiple variations are listed below.
Variation 1:
Paclitaxel: I.V.: 135 mg/m^2 day 1
[total dose/cycle = 135 mg/m^2]
Vinorelbine: I.V.: 30 mg/m^2 day 1
[total dose/cycle = 30 mg/m^2]
Repeat cycle every 21 days
Variation 2:
Paclitaxel: I.V.: 150 mg/m^2 day 1
[total dose/cycle = 150 mg/m^2]
Vinorelbine: I.V.: 25 mg/m^2 day 1
[total dose/cycle = 25 mg/m^2]
Repeat cycle every 21 days
Variation 3:
Paclitaxel: I.V.: 135 mg/m^2 day 1
[total dose/cycle = 135 mg/m^2]
Vinorelbine: I.V.: 30 mg/m^2/day days 1 and 8
[total dose/cycle = 60 mg/m^2]
Repeat cycle every 28 days

PCE

Use Adenocarcinoma, unknown primary

Regimen
Paclitaxel: I.V.: 200 mg/m^2 day 1
[total dose/cycle = 200 mg/m^2]
Carboplatin: I.V.: AUC = 6 day 1
[total dose/cycle = AUC = 6]
Etoposide: Oral: 50 mg/day days 1, 3, 5, 7, and 9
and Oral: 100 mg/day days 2, 4, 6, 8, and 10
[total dose/cycle = 750 mg]
Repeat cycle every 3 weeks

PC (Nonsmall Cell Lung Cancer)

Use Lung cancer, nonsmall cell

Regimen NOTE: Multiple variations are listed below.
Variation 1:
Paclitaxel: I.V.: 175-225 mg/m^2 day 1
[total dose/cycle = 175-225 mg/m^2]
Carboplatin: I.V.: Target AUC 5-7 day 1
[total dose/cycle = AUC = 5-7]
Repeat cycle every 21 days for 2-8 cycles
Variation 2:
Paclitaxel: I.V.: 175 mg/m^2 day 1
[total dose/cycle = 175 mg/m^2]
Cisplatin: I.V.: 80 mg/m^2 day 1
[total dose/cycle = 80 mg/m^2]
Repeat cycle every 21 days
Variation 3:
Paclitaxel: I.V.: 135 mg/m^2 continuous infusion day 1
[total dose/cycle = 135 mg/m^2]
Carboplatin: I.V.: AUC 7.5 day 2
[total dose/cycle = AUC = 7.5]
Repeat cycle every 21 days
Variation 4:
Paclitaxel: I.V.: 135 mg/m^2 continuous infusion day 1
[total dose/cycle = 135 mg/m^2]
Cisplatin: I.V.: 75 mg/m^2 day 2
[total dose/cycle = 75 mg/m^2]
Repeat cycle every 21 days

PCR

Use Leukemia, chronic lymphocytic

Regimen NOTE: Multiple variations are listed below.
Variation 1:
Cycle 1:
Cyclophosphamide: I.V.: 600 mg/m^2 day 1
[total dose/cycle = 600 mg/m^2]
Pentostatin: I.V.: 4 mg/m^2 day 1
[total dose/cycle = 4 mg/m^2]
Treatment cycle is 3 weeks
Cycles 2-6:
Cyclophosphamide: I.V.: 600 mg/m^2 day 1
[total dose/cycle = 600 mg/m^2]
Pentostatin: I.V.: 4 mg/m^2 day 1
[total dose/cycle = 4 mg/m^2]
Rituximab: I.V.: 375 mg/m^2 day 1
[total dose/cycle = 375 mg/m^2]
Repeat cycle every 3 weeks
Variation 2:
Cycle 1:
Pentostatin: I.V.: 2 mg/m^2 day 1
[total dose/cycle = 2 mg/m^2]

◄ Cyclophosphamide: I.V.: 600 mg/m² day 1
[total dose/cycle = 600 mg/m²]
Rituximab: I.V.: 100 mg/m² day 1 only
followed by I.V.: 375 mg/m²/day days 3 and 5 only
[total dose/cycle 1 = 850 mg/m²]
Treatment cycle is 3 weeks
Cycles 2-6:
Pentostatin: I.V.: 2 mg/m² day 1
[total dose/cycle = 2 mg/m²]
Cyclophosphamide: I.V.: 600 mg/m² day 1
[total dose/cycle = 600 mg/m²]
Rituximab: I.V.: 375 mg/m² day 1
[total dose/cycle = 375 mg/m²]
Repeat cycle every 3 weeks

PCV

Use Brain tumors
Regimen
Lomustine: Oral: 110 mg/m² day 1
[total dose/cycle = 110 mg/m²]
Procarbazine: Oral: 60 mg/m²/day days 8 to 21
[total dose/cycle = 840 mg/m²]
Vincristine: I.V.: 1.4 mg/m²/day (maximum 2 mg) days 8 and 29
[total dose/cycle = 2.8 mg/m²; maximum 4 mg]
Repeat cycle every 6-8 weeks

PE

Use Prostate cancer
Regimen NOTE: Multiple variations are listed below.
Variation 1:
Paclitaxel: I.V.: 30-35 mg/m²/day continuous infusion (given in 2-3 divided doses daily) either days 1 to 4
or days 2 to 5
[total dose/cycle = 120-140 mg/m²]
Estramustine: Oral: 600 mg/m²/day days 1 to 21
[total dose/cycle = 12,600 mg/m²]
Repeat cycle every 21 days
Variation 2:
Paclitaxel: I.V. 60-107 mg/m² infused over 3 hours weekly for 6 weeks
[total dose/cycle = 360-642 mg/m²]
Estramustine: Oral: 280 mg twice daily 3 days/week for 6 weeks
[total dose/cycle = 3360 mg]
Repeat cycle every 8 weeks
Variation 3:
Paclitaxel: I.V. 150 mg/m²/day days 2, 9, and 16
[total dose/cycle = 450 mg/m²]
Estramustine: Oral: 280 mg 3 times/day days 1, 2, 3, 8, 9, 10, 15, 16, and 17
[total dose/week = 7560 mg/m²]
Repeat cycle every 4 weeks
Variation 4:
Paclitaxel: I.V.: 100 mg/m²/day days 2, 9, and 16
[total dose/cycle = 300 mg/m²]
Estramustine: Oral: 280 mg 3 times/day days 1, 2, 3, 8, 9, 10, 15, 16, and 17
[total dose/cycle = 7560 mg]
Repeat cycle every 4 weeks

PE-CAdO

Use Neuroblastoma
Regimen
Cisplatin: I.V.: 100 mg/m² day 1
[total dose/cycle = 100 mg/m²]
Teniposide: I.V.: 160 mg/m² day 3
[total dose/cycle = 160 mg/m²]
alternating with
Cyclophosphamide: I.V.: 300 mg/m²/day days 1 to 5
[total dose/cycle = 1500 mg/m²]

Doxorubicin: I.V.: 60 mg/m^2 day 5
  [total dose/cycle = 60 mg/m^2]
Vincristine: I.V.: 1.5 mg/m^2/day days 1 and 5
  [total dose/cycle = 3 mg/m^2]
Repeat cycle every 21 days

Pemetrexed (Bladder Cancer Regimen)

Use Bladder cancer
Regimen
Pemetrexed: I.V.: 500 mg/m^2 infused over 10 minutes day 1
  [total dose/cycle = 500 mg/m^2]
Repeat cycle every 21 days

Pemetrexed-Carboplatin

Use Malignant pleural mesothelioma
Regimen
Pemetrexed: I.V.: 500 mg/m^2 infused over 10 minutes day 1
  [total dose/cycle = 500 mg/m^2]
Carboplatin: I.V.: AUC 5 infused over 30 minutes day 1 (start 30 minutes after pemetrexed)
  [total dose/cycle = AUC = 5]
Repeat cycle every 21 days

Pentostatin-Cyclophosphamide

Use Leukemia, chronic lymphocytic
Regimen
Cyclophosphamide: I.V.: 600 mg/m^2 day 1
  [total dose/cycle = 600 mg/m^2]
Pentostatin: I.V.: 4 mg/m^2 day 1
  [total dose/cycle = 4 mg/m^2]
Repeat cycle every 3 weeks for up to 6 cycles

PFL (Colorectal Cancer)

Use Colorectal cancer
Regimen
Cisplatin: I.V.: 25 mg/m^2/day continuous infusion days 1 to 5
  [total dose/cycle = 125 mg/m^2]
Fluorouracil: I.V.: 800 mg/m^2/day continuous infusion days 2 to 5
  [total dose/cycle = 3200 mg/m^2]
Leucovorin calcium: I.V.: 500 mg/m^2/day continuous infusion days 1 to 5
  [total dose/cycle = 2500 mg/m^2]
Repeat cycle every 28 days

PFL (Head and Neck Cancer)

Use Head and neck cancer
Regimen NOTE: Multiple variations are listed below.
Variation 1:
  Cisplatin: I.V.: 25 mg/m^2/day continuous infusion days 1 to 5
    [total dose/cycle = 125 mg/m^2]
  Fluorouracil: I.V.: 800 mg/m^2/day continuous infusion days 2 to 6
    [total dose/cycle = 4000 mg/m^2]
  Leucovorin: I.V.: 500 mg/m^2/day continuous infusion days 1 to 6
    [total dose/cycle = 3000 mg/m^2]
  Repeat cycle every 28 days
Variation 2:
  Cisplatin: I.V.: 100 mg/m^2 day 1
    [total dose/cycle = 100 mg/m^2]
  Fluorouracil: I.V.: 600-1000 mg/m^2/day continuous infusion days 1 to 5
    [total dose/cycle = 3000-5000 mg/m^2]

Leucovorin: Oral: 50 mg/m^2 every 4-6 hours days 1 to 6
[total dose/cycle = 1200-1800 mg/m^2]
Repeat cycle every 21 days

PFL + IFN

Use Head and neck cancer
Regimen
Cisplatin: I.V.: 100 mg/m^2 day 1
[total dose/cycle = 100 mg/m^2]
Fluorouracil: I.V.: 640 mg/m^2/day continuous infusion days 1 to 5
[total dose/cycle = 3200 mg/m^2]
Leucovorin calcium: Oral: 100 mg every 4 hours days 1 to 5
[total dose/cycle = 3000 mg/m^2]
Interferon alfa-2b: SubQ: 2 x 10^6 units/m^2 days 1 to 6
[total dose/cycle = 12 x 10^6 units/m^2]

POC

Use Brain tumors
Regimen
Prednisone: Oral: 40 mg/m^2/day days 1 to 14
[total dose/cycle = 560 mg/m^2]
Vincristine: I.V.: 1.5 mg/m^2/day (maximum 2 mg) days 1, 8, and 15
[total dose/cycle = 4.5 mg/m^2]
Lomustine: Oral: 100 mg/m^2 day 1
[total dose/cycle = 100 mg/m^2]
Repeat cycle every 6 weeks

POG-8651

Use Osteosarcoma
Regimen
(Surgery at week 10)
Methotrexate: I.V.: 12 g/m^2 weeks 0, 1, 5, 6, 13, 14, 18, 19, 23, 24, 37, and 38
[total dose/cycle = 144 g/m^2]
Leucovorin: (route not specified): 15 mg every 6 hours for 10 doses, weeks 0, 1, 5, 6, 13, 14, 18, 19, 23, 24, 37, and 38
[total dose/cycle = 1800 mg]
Doxorubicin: I.V.: 37.5 mg/m^2/day days 1 and weeks 2, 7, 25, and 28 and 30 mg/m^2 days 1, 2, and 3, week 20
[total dose/cycle = 390 mg/m^2]
Cisplatin: I.V.: 60 mg/m^2/day days 1 and 2, weeks 2, 7, 25, and 28
[total dose/cycle = 480 mg/m^2]
Cyclophosphamide: I.V.: 600 mg/m^2/day days 1, 2, and 3, weeks 15, 31, 34, 39, and 42
[total dose/cycle = 9000 mg/m^2]
Bleomycin: I.V.: 15 units/m^2/day days 1, 2, and 3, weeks 15, 31, 34, 39, and 42
[total dose/cycle = 225 units/m^2]
Dactinomycin: I.V.: 0.6 mg/m^2/day days 1, 2, and 3, weeks 15, 31, 34, 39, and 42
[total dose/cycle = 9 mg/m^2]
or
(Surgery at week 0)
Methotrexate: 12 g/m^2 weeks 3, 4, 8, 9, 13, 14, 18, 19, 23, 24, 37, and 38
[total dose/cycle = 144 g/m^2]
Leucovorin: (route not specified): 15 mg every 6 hours for 10 doses, weeks 3, 4, 8, 9, 13, 14, 18, 19, 23, 24, 37, and 38
[total dose/cycle = 1800 mg]
Doxorubicin: I.V.: 37.5 mg/m^2/day days 1 and 2, weeks 5, 10, 25, and 28 and 30 mg/m^2 days 1, 2, and 3, week 20
[total dose/cycle = 390 mg/m^2]
Cisplatin: I.V.: 60 mg/m^2/day days 1 and 2, weeks 5, 10, 25, and 28
[total dose/cycle = 480 mg/m^2]
Cyclophosphamide: I.V.: 600 mg/m^2/day days 1, 2, and 3, weeks 15, 31, 34, 39, and 42
[total dose/cycle = 9000 mg/m^2]

Bleomycin: I.V.: 15 units/m^2/day days 1, 2, and 3, weeks 15, 31, 34, 39, and 42
  [total dose/cycle = 225 units/m^2]
Dactinomycin: I.V.: 0.6 mg/m^2/day days 1, 2, and 3, weeks 15, 31, 34, 39, and 42
  [total dose/cycle = 9 mg/m^2]

POMP

Use Leukemia, acute lymphocytic
Regimen Maintenance:
  Mercaptopurine: Oral: 50 mg 3 times/day
    [total dose/cycle = 4200-4650 mg]
  Methotrexate: Oral: 20 mg/m^2 once weekly
    [total dose/cycle = 80 mg/m^2]
  Vincristine: I.V.: 2 mg day 1
    [total dose/cycle = 2 mg]
  Prednisone: Oral: 200 mg/day days 1 to 5
    [total dose/cycle = 1000 mg]
  Repeat cycle monthly for 2 years

Pro-MACE-CytaBOM

Use Lymphoma, non-Hodgkin
Regimen
  Prednisone: Oral: 60 mg/m^2/day days 1 to 14
    [total dose/cycle = 840 mg/m^2]
  Doxorubicin: I.V.: 25 mg/m^2 day 1
    [total dose/cycle = 25 mg/m^2]
  Cyclophosphamide: I.V.: 650 mg/m^2 day 1
    [total dose/cycle = 650 mg/m^2]
  Etoposide: I.V.: 120 mg/m^2 day 1
    [total dose/cycle = 120 mg/m^2]
  Cytarabine: I.V.: 300 mg/m^2 day 8
    [total dose/cycle = 300 mg/m^2]
  Bleomycin: I.V.: 5 units/m^2 day 8
    [total dose/cycle = 5 units/m^2]
  Vincristine: I.V.: 1.4 mg/m^2 (maximum 2 mg) day 8
    [total dose/cycle = 1.4 mg/m^2]
  Methotrexate: I.V.: 120 mg/m^2 day 8
    [total dose/cycle = 120 mg/m^2]
  Leucovorin: Oral: 25 mg/m^2 every 6 hours for 4 doses (start 24 hours after methotrexate dose) day 9
    [total dose/cycle = 100 mg/m^2]
  Repeat cycle every 21 days

PVA (POG 8602)

Use Leukemia, acute lymphocytic
Regimen
  Induction:
    Prednisone: Oral: 40 mg/m^2/day (maximum 60 mg) days 0 to 28 (given in 3 divided doses)
      [total dose/cycle = 1160 mg/m^2]
    Vincristine: I.V.: 1.5 mg/m^2/day (maximum 2 mg) days 0, 7, 14, and 21
      [total dose/cycle = 6 mg/m^2; maximum 8 mg]
    Asparaginase: I.M.: 6000 units/m^2 3 times per week for 2 weeks
      [total dose/cycle = 36,000 units/m^2]
    Intrathecal therapy (triple): Days 0 and 22
    Leucovorin: route and dose not specified: single dose 24 hours after every intrathecal treatment days 1 and 23
    Administer one cycle only
  CNS consolidation:
    Mercaptopurine: Oral: 75 mg/m^2/day days 29 to 43
      [total dose/cycle = 1125 mg/m^2]
    Intrathecal therapy (triple): Days 29 and 36
    Leucovorin: route and dose not specified: single dose 24 hours after every intrathecal treatment days 30 and 37
    Administer one cycle only

Intensification:
Regimen A:
Methotrexate: I.V.: 1000 mg/m^2 continuous infusion over 24 hours day 1
  [total dose/cycle = 1000 mg/m^2]
Cytarabine: I.V.: 1000 mg/m^2 continuous infusion over 24 hours day 1 (start 12 hours after start of methotrexate)
  [total dose/cycle = 1000 mg/m^2]
Leucovorin: I.M., I.V., or Oral: 30 mg/m^2 at 24 and 36 hours after the start of methotrexate
  [total dose/cycle = 60 mg/m^2]
    followed by I.M., I.V., or Oral: 3 mg/m^2 at 48, 60, and 72 hours after the start of methotrexate
      [total dose/cycle = 9 mg/m^2]
Repeat cycle every 3 weeks for 6 cycles (administered weeks 7, 10, 13, 16, 19, and 22)
Intrathecal therapy (triple): Weeks 9, 12, 15, and 18
Leucovorin: route and dose not specified: single dose 24 hours after every intrathecal treatment weeks 9, 12, 15, and 18
or
Regimen B:
Methotrexate: I.V.: 1000 mg/m^2 continuous infusion over 24 hours day 1
  [total dose/cycle = 1000 mg/m^2]
Cytarabine: I.V.: 1000 mg/m^2 continuous infusion over 24 hours day 1 (start 12 hours after methotrexate)
  [total dose/cycle = 1000 mg/m^2]
Leucovorin: I.M., I.V., or Oral: 30 mg/m^2 at 24 and 36 hours after the start of methotrexate
  [total dose/cycle = 60 mg/m^2]
    followed by I.M., I.V., or Oral: 3 mg/m^2 at 48, 60, and 72 hours after the start of methotrexate
      [total dose/cycle = 9 mg/m^2]
Repeat cycle every 12 weeks for 6 cycles (administer weeks 7, 19, 31, 43, 55, and 67)
Intrathecal therapy (triple): Weeks 9, 12, 15, and 18
Leucovorin: route and dose not specified: single dose 24 hours after every intrathecal treatment weeks 9, 12, 15, and 18

Maintenance:
Regimen A:
Methotrexate: I.M.: 20 mg/m^2 weekly, weeks 25 to 156
  [total dose/cycle = 2640 mg/m^2]
Mercaptopurine: Oral: 75 mg/m^2 daily, weeks 25 to 156
  [total dose/cycle = 69,300 mg/m^2]
Intrathecal therapy (triple): Every 8 weeks, weeks 26 through 105
Leucovorin: route and dose not specified: single dose 24 hours after every intrathecal treatment weeks 26 through 105
Prednisone: Oral: 40 mg/m^2/day (maximum 60 mg) days 1 to 7 (given in 3 divided doses), weeks 8, 17, 25, 41, 57, 73, 89, and 105
  [total dose/cycle = 2240 mg/m^2; maximum 3360 mg]
Vincristine: I.V.: 1.5 mg/m^2/day (maximum 2 mg) day 1, weeks 8, 9, 17, 18, 25, 26, 41, 42, 57, 58, 73, 74, 89, 90, 105, and 106
  [total dose/cycle = 24 mg/m^2; maximum 32 mg]
or
Regimen B:
Methotrexate: I.M.: 20 mg/m^2 weekly, weeks 22-28, 34-40, 46-52, and 58-64
  [total dose/cycle = 560 mg/m^2]
Mercaptopurine: Oral: 75 mg/m^2 daily for 7 weeks, weeks 22-28, 34-40, 46-52, and 58-64
  [total dose/cycle = 14700 mg/m^2]
followed by
Methotrexate: I.M.: 20 mg/m^2 weekly, weeks 70 to 156
  [total dose/cycle = 1720 mg/m^2]
Mercaptopurine: Oral: 75 mg/m^2 daily, weeks 70 to 156
  [total dose/cycle = 45,150 mg/m^2]
Intrathecal therapy (triple): Every 8 weeks, weeks 26 through 105
Leucovorin: route and dose not specified: single dose 24 hours after every intrathecal treatment weeks 26 through 105
Prednisone: Oral: 40 mg/m^2/day (maximum 60 mg) days 1 to 7 (given in 3 divided doses), weeks 8, 17, 25, 41, 57, 73, 89, and 105
  [total dose/cycle = 2240 mg/m^2]
Vincristine: I.V.: 1.5 mg/m^2/day (maximum 2 mg) day 1, weeks 8, 9, 17, 18, 25, 26, 41, 42, 57, 58, 73, 74, 89, 90, 105, and 106
  [total dose/cycle = 24 mg/m^2; maximum 32 mg]

PVB

Use Testicular cancer

Regimen NOTE: Multiple variations are listed below.
  Variation 1:
   Cisplatin: I.V.: 20 mg/m^2/day days 1 to 5
    [total dose/cycle = 100 mg/m^2]
   Vinblastine: I.V.: 0.2 mg/kg/day days 1 and 2
    [total dose/cycle = 0.4 mg/kg]
   Bleomycin: I.V.: 30 units/day days 2, 9, and 16
    [total dose/cycle = 90 units]
   Repeat cycle every 3 weeks
  Variation 2:
   Cisplatin: I.V.: 20 mg/m^2/day days 1 to 5
    [total dose/cycle = 100 mg/m^2]
   Vinblastine: I.V.: 0.15 mg/kg/day days 1 and 2
    [total dose/cycle = 0.3 mg/kg]
   Bleomycin: I.V.: 30 units/day days 2, 9, and 16
    [total dose/cycle = 90 units]
   Repeat cycle every 3 weeks
  Variation 3:
   Cisplatin: I.V.: 20 mg/m^2/day days 1 to 5
    [total dose/cycle = 100 mg/m^2]
   Vinblastine: I.V.: 6 mg/m^2/day days 1 and 2
    [total dose/cycle = 12 mg/m^2]
   Bleomycin: I.M.: 30 units/day days 2, 9, and 16
    [total dose/cycle = 90 units]
   Repeat cycle every 3 weeks

PVDA

Use Leukemia, acute lymphocytic

Regimen Induction:
  Prednisone: Oral: 60 mg/m^2/day days 1 to 28
   [total dose/cycle = 1680 mg/m^2]
  Vincristine: I.V.: 1.5 mg/m^2/day days 1, 8, 15, and 22
   [total dose/cycle = 6 mg/m^2]
  Daunorubicin: I.V.: 25 mg/m^2/day days 1, 8, 15, and 22
   [total dose/cycle = 100 mg/m^2]
  Asparaginase: I.M., SubQ, or I.V.: 5000 units/m^2/day days 1 to 14
   [total dose/cycle = 70,000 units/m^2]
  Administer one cycle only; used in conjunction with intrathecal chemotherapy

R-CVP

Use Lymphoma, non-Hodgkin

Regimen
  Rituximab: I.V.: 375 mg/m^2 day 1
   [total dose/cycle = 375 mg/m^2]
  Cyclophosphamide: I.V.: 750 mg/m^2 day 1
   [total dose/cycle = 750 mg/m^2]
  Vincristine: I.V.: 1.4 mg/m^2 day 1
   [total dose/cycle = 1.4 mg/m^2]
  Prednisone: Oral: 40 mg/m^2/day days 1 to 5
   [total dose/cycle = 200 mg/m^2]
  Repeat cycle every 21 days

Regimen A1

Use Neuroblastoma

Regimen
  Cyclophosphamide: I.V.: 1.2 g/m^2 day 1
   [total dose/cycle = 1.2 g/m^2]
  Vincristine: I.V.: 1.5 mg/m^2 day 1
   [total dose/cycle = 1.5 mg/m^2]

◀ Doxorubicin: I.V.: 40 mg/m^2 day 3
  [total dose/cycle = 40 mg/m^2]
  Cisplatin: I.V.: 90 mg/m^2 day 5
  [total dose/cycle = 90 mg/m^2]
  Repeat cycle every 28 days

Regimen A2

Use Neuroblastoma
Regimen
  Cyclophosphamide: I.V.: 1.2 g/m^2 day 1
  [total dose/cycle = 1.2 g/m^2]
  Etoposide: I.V.: 100 mg/m^2/day days 1 to 5
  [total dose/cycle = 500 mg/m^2]
  Doxorubicin: I.V.: 40 mg/m^2 day 3
  [total dose/cycle = 40 mg/m^2]
  Cisplatin: I.V.: 90 mg/m^2 day 5
  [total dose/cycle = 90 mg/m^2]
  Repeat cycle every 28 days

RICE

Use Lymphoma, non-Hodgkin
Regimen
  Rituximab: I.V.: 375 mg/m^2/day days -2 and 1 (cycle 1)
  [total dose/cycle = 750 mg/m^2]
  Rituximab: I.V.: 375 mg/m^2 day 1 (cycles 2 and 3)
  [total dose/cycle = 375 mg/m^2]
  Etoposide: I.V.: 100 mg/m^2/day days 3, 4, and 5
  [total dose/cycle = 300 mg/m^2]
  Carboplatin: I.V.: AUC = 5 (maximum 800 mg) day 4
  [total dose/cycle = AUC = 5]
  Ifosfamide: I.V.: 5000 mg/m^2 continuous infusion day 4
  [total dose/cycle = 5000 mg/m^2]
  Mesna: I.V.: 5000 mg/m^2 continuous infusion day 4
  [total dose/cycle = 5000 mg/m^2]
  Filgrastim: SubQ: 5 mcg/kg/day days 7 to 14 (cycles 1 and 2)
  [total dose/cycle = 40 mcg/kg]
  Filgrastim: SubQ: 10 mcg/kg/day days 7 to 14 (cycle 3)
  [total dose/cycle = 80 mcg/kg]
  Repeat cycle every 2 weeks

Rituximab-CHOP

Use Lymphoma, non-Hodgkin
Regimen
  Rituximab: I.V.: 375 mg/m^2 day 1
  [total dose/cycle = 375 mg/m^2]
  Cyclophosphamide: I.V.: 750 mg/m^2 day 1
  [total dose/cycle = 750 mg/m^2]
  Doxorubicin: I.V.: 50 mg/m^2 day 1
  [total dose/cycle = 50 mg/m^2]
  Vincristine: I.V.: 1.4 mg/m^2 (maximum 2 mg) day 1
  [total dose/cycle = 1.4 mg/m^2; maximum 2 mg]
  Prednisone: Oral: 40 mg/m^2/day days 1 to 5
  [total dose/cycle = 200 mg/m^2]
  Repeat cycle every 21 days

Stanford V

Use Lymphoma, Hodgkin disease
Regimen NOTE: Multiple variations are listed below.
  Variation 1:
  Mechlorethamine: I.V.: 6 mg/m^2 day 1
  [total dose/cycle = 6 mg/m^2]

Doxorubicin: I.V.: 25 mg/m^2/day days 1 and 15
  [total dose/cycle = 50 mg/m^2]
Vinblastine: I.V.: 6 mg/m^2/day days 1 and 15
  [total dose/cycle = 12 mg/m^2]
Vincristine: I.V.: 1.4 mg/m^2/day (maximum 2 mg) days 8 and 22
  [total dose/cycle = 2.8 mg/m^2; maximum 4 mg]
Bleomycin: I.V.: 5 units/m^2/day days 8 and 22
  [total dose/cycle = 10 units/m^2]
Etoposide: I.V.: 60 mg/m^2/day days 15 and 16
  [total dose/cycle = 120 mg/m^2]
Prednisone: Oral: 40 mg/m^2 every other day for 9 weeks
  followed by tapering of dose by 10 mg every other day, beginning at week 10
Repeat cycle every 28 days for 3 cycles; **Note:** In cycle 3, for patients ≥50 years of age, decrease
  vinblastine dose to 4 mg/m^2/dose and decrease vincristine dose to 1 mg/m^2/dose
Variation 2:
Mechlorethamine: I.V.: 6 mg/m^2/dose weeks 1, 5, and 9
  [total dose/cycle = 18 mg/m^2]
Doxorubicin: I.V.: 25 mg/m^2/dose weeks 1, 3, 5, 7, 9, and 11
  [total dose/cycle = 150 mg/m^2]
Vinblastine: I.V.: 6 mg/m^2/dose weeks 1, 3, 5, 7, 9, and 11
  [total dose/cycle = 36 mg/m^2]
Vincristine: I.V.: 1.4 mg/m^2/dose (maximum 2 mg) weeks 2, 4, 6, 8, 10, and 12
  [total dose/cycle = 8.4 mg/m^2; maximum 12 mg]
Bleomycin: I.V.: 5 units/m^2/dose weeks 2, 4, 6, 8, 10, and 12
  [total dose/cycle = 30 units/m^2]
Etoposide: I.V.: 60 mg/m^2/day for 2 consecutive days, weeks 3, 7, and 11
  [total dose/cycle = 360 mg/m^2]
Prednisone: Oral: 40 mg/m^2 every other day for 10 weeks
  [total dose prior to taper = 1400 mg/m^2]
  followed by tapering of prednisone dose during weeks 11 and 12
Treatment cycle is 12 weeks

TAC

Use Breast cancer

Regimen NOTE: Multiple variations are listed below.
Variation 1:
Docetaxel: I.V.: 75 mg/m^2 day 1
  [total dose/cycle = 75 mg/m^2]
Doxorubicin: I.V.: 50 mg/m^2 day 1
  [total dose/cycle = 50 mg/m^2]
Cyclophosphamide: I.V.: 500 mg/m^2 day 1
  [total dose/cycle = 500 mg/m^2]
Repeat cycle every 3 weeks
Variation 2:
Docetaxel: I.V.: 60 mg/m^2 day 1
  [total dose/cycle = 60 mg/m^2]
Doxorubicin: I.V.: 60 mg/m^2 day 1
  [total dose/cycle = 60 mg/m^2]
Cyclophosphamide: I.V.: 600 mg/m^2 day 1
  [total dose/cycle = 600 mg/m^2]
Repeat cycle every 3 weeks

TAD

Use Leukemia, acute myeloid

Regimen
Daunorubicin: I.V.: 60 mg/m^2/day days 3, 4, and 5
  [total dose/cycle = 180 mg/m^2]
Cytarabine: I.V.: 100 mg/m^2/day continuous infusion days 1 and 2
  [total dose/cycle = 200 mg/m^2]
  followed by I.V.: 100 mg/m^2/day over 30 minutes every 12 hours days 3 to 8
    [total dose/cycle = 1200 mg/m^2]
Thioguanine: Oral: 100 mg/m^2/day every 12 hours days 3 to 9
  [total dose/cycle = 1400 mg/m^2]
Administer one cycle only

Tamoxifen-Epirubicin

Use Breast cancer

Regimen
Tamoxifen: Oral: 20 mg daily
[total dose/cycle = 560 mg]
Epirubicin: I.V.: 50 mg/m^2/day days 1 and 8
[total dose/cycle = 100 mg/m^2]
Repeat epirubicin cycle every 28 days for 6 cycles; continue tamoxifen for 4 years

TCF

Use Esophageal cancer

Regimen
Paclitaxel: I.V.: 175 mg/m^2 day 1
[total dose/cycle = 175 mg/m^2]
Cisplatin: I.V.: 20 mg/m^2/day days 1 to 5 for Cycles 1, 2, and 3
[total dose/cycle = 100 mg/m^2]
   then 15 mg/m^2/day days 1 to 5
     [total dose/cycle = 75 mg/m^2]
Fluorouracil: I.V.: 750 mg/m^2/day continuous infusion days 1 to 5
[total dose/cycle = 3750 mg/m^2]
Repeat cycle every 28 days

TEX (Capecitabine + Docetaxel + Epirubicin)

Use Breast cancer

Regimen
Capecitabine: Oral: 1000 mg/m^2 twice daily days 1 to 14
[total dose/cycle = 28,000 mg/m^2]
Docetaxel: I.V.: 75 mg/m^2 day 1
[total dose/cycle = 75 mg/m^2]
Epirubicin: I.V.: 75 mg/m^2 day 1
[total dose/cycle = 75 mg/m^2]
Repeat cycle every 3 weeks

Thalidomide-Dexamethasone

Use Multiple myeloma

Regimen Note: Multiple variations are listed below.
Variation 1:
Thalidomide: Oral: 100 mg/day days 1 to 28
[total dose/cycle = 2800 mg]
Dexamethasone: Oral: 40 mg/day days 1 to 4
[total dose/cycle = 160 mg]
Repeat cycle every 28 days
Variation 2:
Thalidomide: Oral: 200 mg/day days 1 to 14 cycle 1
followed by Oral: 400 mg/day days 15 to 28 cycle 1
[total dose/cycle = 8400 mg]
Thalidomide: Oral: 400 mg/day days 1 to 28 (subsequent cycles)
[total dose/cycle = 11,200 mg]
Dexamethasone: Oral: 20 mg/m^2/day days 1 to 4, 9 to 12, and 17 to 20 cycle 1 (subsequent cycles)
[total dose/cycle = 240 mg/m^2]
Dexamethasone: Oral 20 mg/m^2/day days 1 to 4 (subsequent cycles)
[total dose/cycle = 80 mg/m^2]
Repeat cycle every 28 days
Variation 3:
Thalidomide: Oral: 100 mg/day days 1 to 7, 150 mg/day days 8 to 14, 200 mg/day days 15 to 21, 250 mg/day days 22 to 28, and 300 mg/day days 29 to 35 (cycle 1)
[total dose/cycle = 7000 mg]
Thalidomide: Oral: 300 mg/day days 1 to 35 (subsequent cycles)
[total dose/cycle = 10,500 mg]

Dexamethasone: Oral: 20 mg/m^2/day days 1 to 4, 9 to 12, and 17 to 20
  [total dose/cycle = 240 mg/m^2]
Repeat cycle every 35 days
Variation 4:
 Thalidomide: Oral: 200 mg/day days 1 to 28
  [total dose/cycle = 5600 mg]
 Dexamethasone: Oral: 40 mg/day days 1 to 4, 9 to 12, and 17 to 20 (odd cycles)
  [total dose/cycle = 480 mg]
 Dexamethasone: Oral: 40 mg/day days 1 to 4 (even cycles)
  [total dose/cycle = 160 mg]
 Repeat cycle every 28 days

TIP

Use Esophageal cancer; Head and neck cancer
Regimen
 Paclitaxel: I.V.: 175 mg/m^2 day 1
  [total dose/cycle = 175 mg/m^2]
 Ifosfamide: I.V.: 1000 mg/m^2/day days 1, 2, and 3
  [total dose/cycle = 3000 mg/m^2]
 Mesna: I.V.: 400 mg/m^2/day before ifosfamide days 1, 2, and 3
  plus I.V.: 200 mg/m^2 4 hours after ifosfamide days 1, 2, and 3
  [total dose/cycle = 1800 mg/m^2]
 Cisplatin: I.V.: 60 mg/m^2 day 1
  [total dose/cycle = 60 mg/m^2]
 Repeat cycle every 21-28 days

Topotecan-Cisplatin

Use Cervical cancer
Regimen Note: Body surface area capped at 2 m^2 maximum
 Topotecan: I.V.: 0.75 mg/m^2/day days 1, 2, and 3
  [total dose/cycle = 2.25 mg/m^2]
 Cisplatin: I.V.: 50 mg/m^2/day day 1 only
  [total dose/cycle = 50 mg/m^2]
 Repeat cycle every 21 days

Topotecan (Oral Regimen)

Use Lung cancer, nonsmall cell; Lung cancer, small cell; Ovarian cancer
Regimen
 Topotecan: Oral: 2.3 mg/m^2/day days 1 to 5
  [total dose/cycle = 11.5 mg/m^2]
 Repeat cycle every 21 days

Topotecan (Oral)-Cisplatin

Use Lung cancer, small cell
Regimen
 Topotecan: Oral: 1.7 mg/m^2/day days 1 to 5
  [total dose/cycle = 8.5 mg/m^2]
 Cisplatin: I.V.: 60 mg/m^2 day 5 only
  [total dose/cycle = 60 mg/m^2]
 Repeat cycle every 21 days for 4 cycles (or for 2 cycles beyond best response)

Topotecan (Weekly)

Use Lung cancer, small cell; Ovarian cancer
Regimen
 Topotecan: I.V.: 4 mg/m^2/day days 1, 8, and 15
  [total dose/cycle = 12 mg/m^2]
 Repeat cycle every 28 days

Trastuzumab-Paclitaxel

Use Breast cancer

Regimen NOTE: Multiple variations are listed below.
Variation 1:
Cycle 1:
Paclitaxel: I.V.: 175 mg/m^2 day 1
[total dose/cycle = 175 mg/m^2]
Trastuzumab: I.V.: 4 mg/kg (loading dose) day 1
followed by I.V.: 2 mg/kg/day days 8 and 15
[total dose/cycle 1 = 8 mg/kg]
Treatment cycle is 21 days
Subsequent cycles:
Paclitaxel: I.V.: 175 mg/m^2 day 1
[total dose/cycle = 175 mg/m^2]
Trastuzumab: I.V.: 2 mg/kg/day days 1, 8, and 15
[total dose/cycle = 6 mg/kg]
Repeat cycle every 21 days for a total of at least 6 cycles
Variation 2:
Cycle 1:
Trastuzumab: I.V.: 4 mg/kg (loading dose) day 1
followed by I.V.: 2 mg/kg/day days 8 and 15
[total dose/cycle 1 = 8 mg/kg]
Paclitaxel: I.V.: 175 mg/m^2 day 2
[total dose/cycle = 175 mg/m^2]
Treatment cycle is 21 days
Subsequent cycles:
Trastuzumab: I.V.: 2 mg/kg/day days 1, 8, and 15
[total dose/cycle = 6 mg/kg]
Paclitaxel: I.V.: 175 mg/m^2 day 2
[total dose/cycle = 175 mg/m^2]
Repeat cycle every 21 days for a total of at least 6 cycles (continue weekly trastuzumab after chemotherapy until disease progression or unacceptable toxicity)

Trastuzumab-Paclitaxel-Carboplatin

Use Breast cancer

Regimen
Cycle 1:
Trastuzumab: I.V.: 4 mg/kg (loading dose) day 1
followed by I.V.: 2 mg/kg/day days 8 and 15
[total dose/cycle 1 = 8 mg/kg]
Paclitaxel: I.V.: 175 mg/m^2 day 2
[total dose/cycle = 175 mg/m^2]
Carboplatin: I.V.: AUC 6 day 2
[total dose/cycle = AUC = 6]
Treatment cycle is 21 days
Subsequent cycles:
Trastuzumab: I.V.: 2 mg/kg/day days 1, 8, and 15
[total dose/cycle = 6 mg/kg]
Paclitaxel: I.V.: 175 mg/m^2 day 2
[total dose/cycle = 175 mg/m^2]
Carboplatin: I.V.: AUC 6 day 2
[total dose/cycle = AUC = 6]
Repeat cycle every 21 days for a total of at least 6 cycles (continue weekly trastuzumab after chemotherapy until disease progression or unacceptable toxicity)

Trastuzumab-Paclitaxel (Weekly)

Use Breast cancer

Regimen NOTE: Multiple variations are listed below.
Variation 1:
Week 1:
Trastuzumab: I.V.: 4 mg/kg (loading dose) day 1
[total dose/week 1 = 4 mg/kg]

Paclitaxel: I.V.: 90 mg/m^2 day 2
[total dose/week 1 = 90 mg/m^2]
Subsequent weeks:
Paclitaxel: I.V.: 90 mg/m^2 day 1
[total dose/week = 90 mg/m^2]
Trastuzumab: I.V.: 2 mg/kg day 1
[total dose/week = 2 mg/kg]
Repeat weekly
Variation 2:
Week 1:
Trastuzumab: I.V.: 4 mg/kg (loading dose) day 1
[total dose/week 1 = 4 mg/kg]
Paclitaxel: I.V.: 80 mg/m^2 day 1
[total dose/week 1 = 80 mg/m^2]
Subsequent weeks:
Trastuzumab: I.V.: 2 mg/kg day 1
[total dose/week = 2 mg/kg]
Paclitaxel: I.V.: 80 mg/m^2 day 1
[total dose/week = 80 mg/m^2]
Repeat weekly

Tretinoin-Idarubicin

Use Leukemia, acute promyelocytic

Regimen NOTE: Multiple variations are listed below.
Induction:
Variation 1:
Tretinoin: Oral: 45 mg/m^2/day day 1 up to 90 days
[total dose/cycle = up to 4050 mg/m^2]
≤20 years: 25 mg/m^2/day day 1 up to 90 days
[total dose/cycle = up to 2250 mg/m^2]
Idarubicin: I.V.: 12 mg/m^2/day days 2, 4, 6, and 8
[total dose/cycle = 48 mg/m^2]
Consolidation:
Course 1:
Idarubicin: I.V.: 5 mg/m^2/day days 1 to 4
[total dose/cycle = 20 mg/m^2]
or
Idarubicin: I.V.: 7 mg/m^2/day days 1 to 4
[total dose/cycle = 28 mg/m^2]
Tretinoin: Oral: 45 mg/m^2/day days 1 to 15
[total dose/cycle = 675 mg/m^2]
Course 2:
Mitoxantrone: I.V.: 10 mg/m^2/day days 1 to 5
[total dose/cycle = 50 mg/m^2]
or
Mitoxantrone: I.V.: 10 mg/m^2/day days 1 to 5
[total dose/cycle = 50 mg/m^2]
Tretinoin: Oral: 45 mg/m^2/day days 1 to 15
[total dose/cycle = 675 mg/m^2]
Course 3:
Idarubicin: I.V.: 12 mg/m^2 on day 1
[total dose/cycle = 12 mg/m^2]
or
Idarubicin: I.V.: 12 mg/m^2/day on days 1 and 2
[total dose/cycle = 24 mg/m^2]
Tretinoin: Oral: 45 mg/m^2/day days 1 to 15
[total dose/cycle = 675 mg/m^2]
Administer courses sequentially at 1-month intervals for 3 months
Maintenance:
Mercaptopurine: Oral: 50 mg/m^2 daily
[total dose/cycle = 4500 mg/m^2 (90 days)]
Methotrexate: I.M.: 15 mg/m^2 weekly
[total dose/cycle = 180 mg/m^2]

Tretinoin: Oral: 45 mg/m2/day days 1 to 15
   [total dose/cycle = 675 mg/m^2]
Repeat cycle every 3 months for 2 years
Variation 2:
Induction:
Tretinoin: Oral: 45 mg/m^2/day day 1 up to 90 days
   [total dose/cycle = up to 4050 mg/m^2]
<15 years: 25 mg/m^2/day day 1 up to 90 days
   [total dose/cycle = up to 2250 mg/m^2]
Idarubicin: I.V.: 12 mg/m^2/day days 2, 4, 6, and 8
   [total dose/cycle = 48 mg/m^2]
Consolidation:
Course 1:
Idarubicin: I.V.: 5 mg/m^2/day days 1 to 4
   [total dose/cycle = 20 mg/m^2]
Course 2:
Mitoxantrone: I.V.: 10 mg/m^2/day days 1 to 5
   [total dose/cycle = 50 mg/m^2]
Course 3:
Idarubicin: I.V.: 12 mg/m^2 day 1
   [total dose/cycle = 12 mg/m^2]
Administer courses sequentially at 1-month intervals for 3 months
Maintenance:
Mercaptopurine: Oral: 90 mg/m^2 daily
   [total dose/cycle = 8100 mg/m^2]
Methotrexate: I.M.: 15 mg/m^2 weekly
   [total dose/cycle = 180 mg/m^2]
Tretinoin: Oral: 45 mg/m^2/day days 1 to 15
   [total dose/cycle = 675 mg/m^2]
Repeat cycle every 3 months for 2 years

TVTG

Use Leukemia, acute lymphocytic; Leukemia, acute myeloid
Regimen
Topotecan: I.V.: 1 mg/m^2/day continuous infusion days 1 to 5
   [total dose/cycle = 5 mg/m^2]
Vinorelbine: I.V.: 20 mg/m^2/day days 0, 7, 14, and 21
   [total dose/cycle = 80 mg/m^2]
Thiotepa: I.V.: 15 mg/m^2 day 2
Gemcitabine: I.V.: 3600 mg/m^2 day 7
Dexamethasone: Oral or I.V.: 45 mg/m^2/day days 7 to 14 (given in 3 divided doses)
   [total dose/cycle = 315 mg/m^2]
Repeat cycle when ANC >500 cells/mm^3 and platelet count >75,000 cells/mm^3

VAC Alternating With IE (Ewing Sarcoma)

Use Ewing sarcoma
Regimen
Cycle A: (Odd numbered cycles)
Cyclophosphamide: I.V.: 1200 mg/m^2 day 1 (followed by mesna; dose not specified)
   [total dose/cycle = 1200 mg/m^2]
Vincristine: I.V.: 2 mg/m^2 (maximum: 2 mg) day 1
   [total dose/cycle = 2 mg/m^2; maximum 2 mg]
Doxorubicin: I.V.: 75 mg/m^2 day 1, for 5 cycles (maximum cumulative dose: 375 mg/m^2)
   [total dose/cycle = 75 mg/m^2; maximum cumulative dose: 375 mg/m^2]
Dactinomycin: I.V.: 1.25 mg/m^2 day 1, begin cycle 11 (after reaching maximum cumulative doxorubicin dose)
   [total dose/cycle = 1.25 mg/m^2]
Cycle B: (Even numbered cycles)
Ifosfamide: I.V.: 1800 mg/m^2/day days 1 to 5 (given with mesna)
   [total dose/cycle = 9000 mg/m^2]
Etoposide: I.V.: 100 mg/m^2/day days 1 to 5
   [total dose/cycle = 500 mg/m^2]
Alternate Cycles A and B, administering a cycle every 3 weeks (alternating in the following sequence: ABABAB) for 17 cycles

VAC Pulse

Use Rhabdomyosarcoma

Regimen
Vincristine: I.V.: 2 mg/m^2/dose (maximum 2 mg/dose) every 7 days, for 12 weeks
Dactinomycin: I.V.: 0.015 mg/kg/day (maximum 0.5 mg/day) days 1 to 5, every 3 months for 5 courses
Cyclophosphamide: Oral, I.V.: 10 mg/kg/day for 7 days, repeat every 6 weeks

VAC (Retinoblastoma)

Use Retinoblastoma

Regimen
Vincristine: I.V.: 1.5 mg/m^2 day 1
  [total dose/cycle = 1.5 mg/m^2]
Dactinomycin: I.V.: 0.015 mg/kg/day days 1 to 5
  [total dose/cycle = 0.075 mg/kg]
Cyclophosphamide: I.V.: 200 mg/m^2/day days 1 to 5
  [total dose/cycle = 1000 mg/m^2]

VAC (Rhabdomyosarcoma)

Use Rhabdomyosarcoma

Regimen
Induction (weeks 1 to 17):
  Vincristine: I.V. push: 1.5 mg/m^2 (maximum 2 mg) day 1 of weeks 1 to 13, then one dose at week 17
  Dactinomycin: I.V. push: 0.015 mg/kg/day (maximum 0.5 mg) days 1 to 5 of weeks 1, 4, 7, and 17
  Cyclophosphamide: I.V.: 2.2 g/m^2 day 1 of weeks 1, 4, 7, 10, 13, and 17
Continuation (weeks 21 to 44):
  Vincristine: I.V. push: 1.5 mg/m^2 (maximum 2 mg) day 1 of weeks 21 to 26, 30 to 35, and 39 to 44
  Dactinomycin: I.V. push: 0.015 mg/kg/day (maximum 0.5 mg) days 1 to 5 of weeks 21, 24, 30, 33, 39, and 42
  Cyclophosphamide: I.V.: 2.2 g/m^2 day 1 of weeks 21, 24, 30, 33, 39, and 42

VAD

Use Multiple myeloma

Regimen
Vincristine: I.V.: 0.4 mg/day continuous infusion days 1 to 4
  [total dose/cycle = 1.6 mg]
Doxorubicin: I.V.: 9 mg/m^2/day continuous infusion days 1 to 4
  [total dose/cycle = 36 mg/m^2]
Dexamethasone: Oral: 40 mg/day days 1 to 4, 9 to 12, and 17 to 20
  [total dose/cycle = 480 mg]
Repeat cycle every 28-35 days

VAD/CVAD

Use Leukemia, acute lymphocytic

Regimen Induction cycle:
Vincristine: I.V.: 0.4 mg/day continuous infusion days 1 to 4 and 24 to 27
  [total dose/cycle = 3.2 mg]
Doxorubicin: I.V.: 12 mg/m^2/day continuous infusion days 1 to 4 and 24 to 27
  [total dose/cycle = 96 mg/m^2]
Dexamethasone: Oral: 40 mg/day days 1 to 4, 9 to 12, 17 to 20, 24 to 27, 32 to 35, and 40 to 43
  [total dose/cycle = 960 mg]
Cyclophosphamide: I.V.: 1 g/m^2 day 24
  [total dose/cycle = 1 g/m^2]
Administer one cycle only

VATH

Use Breast cancer

Regimen
Vinblastine: I.V.: 4.5 mg/m^2 day 1
 [total dose/cycle = 4.5 mg/m^2]
Doxorubicin: I.V.: 45 mg/m^2 day 1
 [total dose/cycle = 45 mg/m^2]
Thiotepa: I.V.: 12 mg/m^2 day 1
 [total dose/cycle = 12 mg/m^2]
Fluoxymesterone: Oral: 10 mg 3 times/day days 1 to 21
 [total dose/cycle = 630 mg]
Repeat cycle every 21 days

VBAP

Use Multiple myeloma

Regimen
Vincristine: I.V.: 1 mg day 1
 [total dose/cycle = 1 mg]
Carmustine: I.V.: 30 mg/m^2 day 1
 [total dose/cycle = 30 mg/m^2]
Doxorubicin: I.V.: 30 mg/m^2 day 1
 [total dose/cycle = 30 mg/m^2]
Prednisone: Oral: 100 mg/day days 1 to 4
 [total dose/cycle = 400 mg]
Repeat cycle every 21 days

VBMCP

Use Multiple myeloma

Regimen
Vincristine: I.V.: 1.2 mg/m^2 (maximum 2 mg) day 1
 [total dose/cycle = 1.2 mg/m^2; maximum 2 mg]
Carmustine: I.V.: 20 mg/m^2 day 1
 [total dose/cycle = 20 mg/m^2]
Melphalan: Oral: 8 mg/m^2/day days 1 to 4
 [total dose/cycle = 32 mg/m^2]
Cyclophosphamide: I.V.: 400 mg/m^2 day 1
 [total dose/cycle = 400 mg/m^2]
Prednisone: Oral: 40 mg/m^2/day days 1 to 7 (all cycles)
 [total dose/cycle = 280 mg/m^2]
  followed by Oral: 20 mg/m^2/day days 8 to 14 (first 3 cycles only)
   [total dose/cycle = 140 mg/m^2]
Repeat cycle every 35 days

VBP

Use Testicular cancer

Regimen
Vinblastine: I.V.: 0.15 mg/kg/day days 1 and 2
 [total dose/cycle = 0.3 mg/kg]
Bleomycin: I.V.: 30 units/day days 2, 9, and 16
 [total dose/cycle = 90 units]
Cisplatin: I.V.: 20 mg/m^2/day days 1 to 5
 [total dose/cycle = 100 mg/m^2]
Repeat cycle every 21 days for 4 cycles

VCAP

Use Multiple myeloma

Regimen
Vincristine: I.V.: 1 mg/m^2 (maximum 1.5 mg) day 1
 [total dose/cycle = 1 mg/m^2]
Cyclophosphamide: Oral: 125 mg/m^2/day days 1 to 4
 [total dose/cycle = 500 mg/m^2]

Doxorubicin: I.V.: 30 mg/m^2 day 1
[total dose/cycle = 30 mg/m^2]
Prednisone: Oral: 60 mg/m^2/day days 1 to 4
[total dose/cycle = 240 mg/m^2]
Repeat cycle every 21 days for 6-12 months

VD

Use Breast cancer
Regimen
Vinorelbine: I.V.: 25 mg/m^2/day days 1 and 8
[total dose/cycle = 50 mg/m^2]
Doxorubicin: I.V.: 50 mg/m^2 day 1
[total dose/cycle = 50 mg/m^2]
Repeat cycle every 3 weeks

Vinorelbine-Cisplatin

Use Lung cancer, nonsmall cell
Regimen NOTE: Multiple variations are listed below.
Variation 1:
Cisplatin: I.V.: 50 mg/m^2/day days 1 and 8
[total dose/cycle = 100 mg/m^2]
Vinorelbine: I.V.: 25 mg/m^2/day days 1, 8, 15, and 22
[total dose/cycle = 100 mg/m^2]
Repeat cycle every 28 days for total of 4 cycles
Variation 2:
Vinorelbine: I.V.: 25 mg/m^2/day days 1, 8, 15, and 22
[total dose/cycle = 100 mg/m^2]
Cisplatin: I.V.: 100 mg/m^2 day 1
[total dose/cycle = 100 mg/m^2]
Repeat cycle every 28 days
Variation 3:
Vinorelbine: I.V.: 30 mg/m^2 weekly
Cisplatin: I.V.: 120 mg/m^2/day days 1 and 29, then once every 6 weeks
Variation 4:
Vinorelbine: I.V.: 30 mg/m^2/day days 1, 8, and 15
[total dose/cycle = 90 mg/m^2]
Cisplatin: I.V.: 80 mg/m^2 day 1
[total dose/cycle = 80 mg/m^2]
Repeat cycle every 21 days for total of 4 cycles
Note: Vinorelbine treatment is discontinued after day 1 of cycle 4
Variation 5:
Vinorelbine: I.V.: 30 mg/m^2/day days 1, 8, 15, and 22
[total dose/cycle = 120 mg/m^2]
Cisplatin: I.V.: 100 mg/m^2 day 1
[total dose/cycle = 100 mg/m^2]
Repeat cycle every 28 days for total of 3 or 4 cycles
Note: Vinorelbine treatment is discontinued after day 1 of last treatment cycle

Vinorelbine-FEC

Use Breast cancer
Regimen
Cycles 1 and 2:
Vinorelbine: I.V.: 25 mg/m^2/day days 1, 8, and 15
[total dose/cycle = 75 mg/m^2]
Treatment cycle is 21 days
Cycle 3:
Vinorelbine: I.V.: 25 mg/m^2/day days 1 and 8
[total dose/cycle 3 = 50 mg/m^2]
Treatment cycle is 21 days
Cycles 4, 5, and 6 (FEC):
Fluorouracil: I.V.: 600 mg/m^2 day 1
[total dose/cycle = 600 mg/m^2]

Epirubicin: I.V.: 60 mg/m^2 day 1
[total dose/cycle = 60 mg/m^2]
Cyclophosphamide: I.V.: 600 mg/m^2 day 1
[total dose/cycle = 600 mg/m^2]
Repeat FEC cycle every 21 days for total of 3 cycles

Vinorelbine-Gemcitabine

Use Lung cancer, nonsmall cell
Regimen
Vinorelbine: I.V.: 20 mg/m^2/day days 1, 8, and 15
[total dose/cycle = 60 mg/m^2]
Gemcitabine: I.V.: 800 mg/m^2/day days 1, 8, and 15
[total dose/cycle = 2400 mg/m^2]
Repeat cycle every 28 days

Vinorelbine-Trastuzumab

Use Breast cancer
Regimen
Week 1:
Trastuzumab: I.V.: 4 mg/kg (loading dose) day 1 week 1
[total dose/week 1 = 4 mg/kg]
Vinorelbine: I.V.: 25 mg/m^2 day 1
[total dose/week 1 = 25 mg/m^2]
Subsequent weeks:
Trastuzumab: I.V.: 2 mg/kg (loading dose) day 1
[total dose/week = 2 mg/kg]
Vinorelbine: I.V.: 25 mg/m^2 day 1
[total dose/week = 25 mg/m^2]
Repeat weekly

Vinorelbine-Trastuzumab-FEC

Use Breast cancer
Regimen
Cycle 1:
Trastuzumab: I.V.: 4 mg/kg (loading dose) day 1 cycle 1
followed by I.V.: 2 mg/kg/day days 8 and 15 cycle 1
[total dose/cycle 1 = 8 mg/kg]
Vinorelbine: I.V.: 25 mg/m^2/day days 1, 8, and 15
[total dose/cycle 1 = 75 mg/m^2]
Treatment cycle is 21 days
Cycle 2:
Trastuzumab: I.V.: 2 mg/kg/day days 1, 8, and 15
[total dose/cycle = 6 mg/kg]
Vinorelbine: I.V.: 25 mg/m^2/day days 1, 8, and 15
[total dose/cycle 2 = 75 mg/m^2]
Treatment cycle is 21 days
Cycle 3:
Trastuzumab: I.V.: 2 mg/kg/day days 1, 8, and 15
[total dose/cycle = 6 mg/kg]
Vinorelbine: I.V.: 25 mg/m^2/day days 1 and 8
[total dose/cycle 3 = 50 mg/m^2]
Treatment cycle is 21 days
Cycles 4, 5, and 6 (FEC):
Fluorouracil: I.V.: 600 mg/m^2 day 1
[total dose/cycle = 600 mg/m^2]
Epirubicin: I.V.: 60 mg/m^2 day 1
[total dose/cycle = 60 mg/m^2]
Cyclophosphamide: I.V.: 600 mg/m^2 day 1
[total dose/cycle = 600 mg/m^2]
Repeat FEC cycle every 21 days for total of 3 cycles

VIP (Etoposide) (Testicular Cancer)

Use Testicular cancer

Regimen NOTE: Multiple variations are listed below.

Variation 1:
  Etoposide: I.V.: 75 mg/m^2/day days 1 to 5
    [total dose/cycle = 375 mg/m^2]
  Ifosfamide: I.V.: 1200 mg/m^2/day days 1 to 5
    [total dose/cycle = 6000 mg/m^2]
  Cisplatin: I.V.: 20 mg/m^2/day days 1 to 5
    [total dose/cycle = 100 mg/m^2]
  Mesna: I.V.: 400 mg day 1 only
    followed by I.V.: 1200 mg/day continuous infusion days 1 to 5
    [total dose/cycle = 6400 mg]
  Repeat cycle every 21 days for 4 cycles

Variation 2:
  Etoposide: I.V.: 100 mg/m^2/day days 1 to 5
    [total dose/cycle = 500 mg/m^2]
  Ifosfamide: I.V.: 1200 mg/m^2/day days 1 to 5
    [total dose/cycle = 6000 mg/m^2]
  Cisplatin: I.V.: 20 mg/m^2/day days 1 to 5
    [total dose/cycle = 100 mg/m^2]
  Mesna: I.V.: 200 mg/m^2 every 4 hours, for 3 doses each day, days 1, 2, and 3
    [total dose/cycle = 1800 mg/m^2]
  Repeat cycle every 21 days

Variation 3:
  Ifosfamide: I.V.: 2500 mg/m^2/day days 1 and 2
    [total dose/cycle = 5000 mg/m^2]
  Mesna: I.V.: 2400 mg/m^2/day days 1 and 2
    [total dose/cycle = 4800 mg/m^2]
  Etoposide: I.V.: 100 mg/m^2/day days 3, 4, and 5
    [total dose/cycle = 300 mg/m^2]
  Cisplatin: I.V.: 40 mg/m^2/day days 3, 4, and 5
    [total dose/cycle = 120 mg/m^2]
  Repeat cycle every 21 days

Variation 4:
  Etoposide: I.V.: 75 mg/m^2/day days 1 to 5
    [total dose/cycle = 375 mg/m^2]
  Ifosfamide: I.V.: 1200 mg/m^2/day days 1 to 5
    [total dose/cycle = 6000 mg/m^2]
  Cisplatin: I.V.: 20 mg/m^2/day days 1 to 5
    [total dose/cycle = 100 mg/m^2]
  Mesna: I.V.: 120 mg/m^2 day 1 only
    followed by I.V.: 1200 mg/m^2/day continuous infusion days 1 to 5
    [total dose/cycle = 6120 mg/m^2]
  Repeat cycle every 21 days for 4 cycles

VIP (Small Cell Lung Cancer)

Use Lung cancer, small cell

Regimen
  Etoposide: I.V.: 75 mg/m^2/day days 1 to 4
    [total dose/cycle = 300 mg/m^2]
  Ifosfamide: I.V.: 1200 mg/m^2/day days 1 to 4
    [total dose/cycle = 4800 mg/m^2]
  Cisplatin: I.V.: 20 mg/m^2/day days 1 to 4
    [total dose/cycle = 80 mg/m^2]
  Mesna: I.V.: 300 mg/m^2 day 1 only
    followed by I.V.: 1200 mg/m^2/day continuous infusion days 1 to 4
    [total dose/cycle = 5100 mg/m^2]
  Repeat cycle every 21 days

VIP (Vinblastine) (Testicular Cancer)

Use Testicular cancer

Regimen NOTE: Multiple variations are listed below.
Variation 1:
Vinblastine: I.V.: 0.11 mg/kg/day days 1 and 2
[total dose/cycle = 0.22 mg/kg]
Ifosfamide: I.V.: 1200 mg/m^2/day days 1 to 5
[total dose/cycle = 6000 mg/m^2]
Cisplatin: I.V.: 20 mg/m^2/day days 1 to 5
[total dose/cycle = 100 mg/m^2]
Mesna: I.V.: 400 mg day 1
followed by I.V.: 1200 mg/day continuous infusion days 1 to 5
[total dose/cycle = 6400 mg]
Repeat cycle every 21 days for 4 cycles
Variation 2:
Vinblastine: I.V.: 6 mg/m^2/day days 1 and 2
[total dose/cycle = 12 mg/m^2]
Ifosfamide: I.V.: 1500 mg/m^2/day days 1 to 5
[total dose/cycle = 7500 mg/m^2]
Cisplatin: I.V.: 20 mg/m^2/day days 1 to 5
[total dose/cycle = 100 mg/m^2]
Mesna: I.V.: 300 mg/m^2 3 times/day days 1 to 5
[total dose/cycle = 4500 mg/m^2]
Repeat cycle every 21 days for 4 cycles

VM

Use Breast cancer

Regimen
Variation 1:
Mitomycin: I.V.: 10 mg/m^2 days 1 and 28, for 2 cycles
[total dose/cycle = 20 mg/m^2]
followed by I.V.: 10 mg/m^2 day 1 only for subsequent cycles
[total dose/cycle = 10 mg/m^2]
Vinblastine: I.V.: 5 mg/m^2/day days 1, 14, 28, and 42, for 2 cycles
[total dose/cycle = 20 mg/m^2]
followed by I.V.: 5 mg/m^2/day days 1 and 21
[total dose/cycle = 10 mg/m^2]
Repeat cycle every 6-8 weeks
Variation 2:
Mitomycin: I.V.: 10 mg/m^2/day days 1 and 28, for 2 cycles
[total dose/cycle = 20 mg/m^2]
followed by I.V.: 10 mg/m^2 day 1 only for subsequent cycles
[total dose/cycle = 10 mg/m^2]
Vindesine: I.V.: 2 mg/m^2/day days 1, 14, 28, and 42, for 2 cycles
[total dose/cycle = 8 mg/m^2]
followed by I.V.: 2 mg/m^2/ day days 1 and 21 for subsequent cycles
[total dose/cycle = 4 mg/m^2]
Repeat cycle every 6-8 weeks

VP (Small Cell Lung Cancer)

Use Lung cancer, small cell

Regimen
Etoposide: I.V.: 100 mg/m^2/day days 1 to 4
[total dose/cycle = 400 mg/m^2]
Cisplatin: I.V.: 20 mg/m^2/day days 1 to 4
[total dose/cycle = 80 mg/m^2]
Repeat cycle every 21 days

V-TAD

Use Leukemia, acute myeloid

Regimen Induction:
   Etoposide: I.V.: 50 mg/m^2/day days 1, 2, and 3
      [total dose/cycle = 150 mg/m^2]
   Thioguanine: Oral: 75 mg/m^2/day every 12 hours days 1 to 5
      [total dose/cycle = 750 mg/m^2]
   Daunorubicin: I.V.: 20 mg/m^2/day days 1 and 2
      [total dose/cycle = 40 mg/m^2]
   Cytarabine: I.V.: 75 mg/m^2/day continuous infusion days 1 to 5
      [total dose/cycle = 375 mg/m^2]
   Up to 3 cycles may be given based on individual response; time between cycles not specified

XelOx

Use Colorectal cancer

Regimen Note: Multiple variations are listed below.
   Variation 1:
      Oxaliplatin: I.V.: 130 mg/m^2 day 1
         [total dose/cycle = 130 mg/m^2]
      Capecitabine: Oral: 2500 mg/m^2/day days 1 to 14
         [total dose/cycle = 35,000 mg/m^2]
      Repeat cycle every 21 days
   Variation 2:
      Oxaliplatin: I.V.: 85 mg/m^2 day 1
         [total dose/cycle = 85 mg/m^2]
      Capecitabine: Oral: 3500 mg/m^2/day days 1 to 7
         [total dose/cycle = 24,500 mg/m^2]
      Repeat cycle every 14 days
   Variation 3:
      Oxaliplatin: I.V.: 50-80 mg/m^2/day days 1, 8, 22, and 29
         [total dose/cycle = 200-320 mg/m^2]
      Capecitabine: Oral: 1650 mg/m^2/day days 1 to 14 and 22 to 35
         [total dose/cycle = 46,200 mg/m^2]
   Variation 4:
      Oxaliplatin: I.V.: 70 mg/m^2/day days 1 and 8
         [total dose/cycle = 140 mg/m^2]
      Capecitabine: Oral: 2000 mg/m^2/day days 1 to 14
         [total dose/cycle = 28,000 mg/m^2]
      Repeat cycle every 21 days
   Variation 5:
      Oxaliplatin: I.V.: 120 mg/m^2 day 1
         [total dose/cycle = 120 mg/m^2]
      Capecitabine: Oral: 2500 mg/m^2/day days 1 to 14
         [total dose/cycle = 35,000 mg/m^2]
      Repeat cycle every 21 days
   Variation 6:
      Oxaliplatin: I.V.: 85 mg/m^2 day 1
         [total dose/cycle = 85 mg/m^2]
      Capecitabine: Oral: 2500 mg/m^2/day days 1 to 7
         [total dose/cycle = 17,500 mg/m^2]
      or Capecitabine: Oral: 3000 mg/m^2/day days 1 to 7 [total dose/cycle = 21,000 mg/m^2]
      or Capecitabine: Oral: 3500 mg/m^2/day days 1 to 7 [total dose/cycle = 24,500 mg/m^2]
      or Capecitabine: Oral: 4000 mg/m^2/day days 1 to 7
         [total dose/cycle = 28,000 mg/m^2]
      Repeat cycle every 14 days
   Variation 7:
      Oxaliplatin: I.V.: 130 mg/m^2 day 1
         [total dose/cycle = 130 mg/m^2]
      Capecitabine: Oral: 1000 mg/m^2 twice daily days 1 (beginning with evening dose) to 15 (ending with morning dose)
         [total dose/cycle = 28,000 mg/m^2]
      Repeat cycle every 21 days

CHEMOTHERAPY REGIMEN INDEX

Small Cell

LYMPHOID TISSUE (LYMPHOMA)
Lymphoma, Hodgkin Disease

Lymphoma, Non-Hodgkin

Lymphoma, Non-Hodgkin (Burkitt)

Lymphoma, Non-Hodgkin (Mantle cell)

MALIGNANT PLEURAL MESOTHELIOMA

MYELODYSPLASTIC SYNDROME

APPENDIX TABLE OF CONTENTS

Visit the Point http://thepoint.lww.com/QL2009 for exclusive access to:

Apothecary/Metric Conversions

Pounds/Kilograms Conversion

Temperature Conversion

Pharmaceutical Manufacturers and Distributors

Vitamin Products

Refer to the inside front cover of this book for your online access code.

ABBREVIATIONS & SYMBOLS COMMONLY USED IN MEDICAL ORDERS

Abbreviation	Meaning
$<$[1]	less than
$>$[1]	greater than
$\leq$	less than or equal to
$\geq$	greater than or equal to
5-HT	5-hydroxytryptamine
AACT	American Academy of Clinical Toxicology
AAP	American Academy of Pediatrics
ABG	arterial blood gases
ABW	adjusted body weight
ac	before meals or food
ACC	American College of Cardiology
ACE	angiotensin converting enzyme
ACLS	advanced cardiac life support
ACOG	American College of Obstetricians and Gynecologists
ACTH	adrenocorticotrophic hormone
ad	to, up to
ADH	alcohol dehydrogenase
ADHD	attention-deficit/hyperactivity disorder
ad lib	at pleasure
ADLS	activities of daily living
AED	antiepileptic drug
AHA	American Heart Association
AIDS	acquired immune deficiency syndrome
AIMS	Abnormal Involuntary Movement Scale
ALS	amyotrophic lateral sclerosis
ALT	alanine aminotransferase
AM	morning
ama	against medical advice
AMA	American Medical Association
amp	ampul
amt	amount
ANC	absolute neutrophil count
aq	water
aq. dest.	distilled water
ARB	angiotensin receptor blocker
ARDS	acute respiratory distress syndrome
AST	aspartate aminotransferase
ASAP	as soon as possible
a.u.[1]	each ear
AUC	area under the curve

Abbreviation	Meaning
BDI	Beck Depression Inventory
BEC	blood ethanol concentration
bid	twice daily
BLS	basic life support
bm	bowel movement
BMI	body mass index
BP	blood pressure
BPH	benign prostatic hyperplasia
BPRS	Brief Psychiatric Rating Scale
BSA	body surface area
BUN	blood urea nitrogen
C	Celsius, centigrade
CABG	coronary artery bypass graft
CAD	coronary artery disease
cal	calorie
CAN	Canadian
cap	capsule
CAPD	continuous ambulatory peritoneal dialysis
CAS	chemical abstract service
CBC	complete blood count
CBT	cognitive behavioral therapy
cc[1]	cubic centimeter
CDC	Centers for Disease Control and Prevention
CF	cystic fibrosis
CGI	Clinical Global Impression
CHD	coronary heart disease
CHF	congestive heart failure; chronic heart failure
Cl_{cr}	creatinine clearance
CIE	chemotherapy-induced emesis
C-II	schedule two controlled substance
C-III	schedule three controlled substance
C-IV	schedule four controlled substance
C-V	schedule five controlled substance
CIV	continuous I.V. infusion
C_{max}	maximum plasma concentration
C_{min}	minimum plasma concentration
cm	centimeter
CMV	cytomegalovirus
CNS	central nervous system or coagulase negative staphylococcus
COLD	chronic obstructive lung disease
comp	compound
cont	continue
COPD	chronic obstructive pulmonary disease
COX	cyclooxygenase
CPK	creatine phosphokinase

Abbreviation	Meaning
CRF	chronic renal failure
CRP	C-reactive protein
CRRT	continuous renal replacement therapy
CSF	cerebrospinal fluid
CT	computed tomography
CVVH	continuous venovenous hemofiltration
CVVHD	continuous venovenous hemodialysis
CVVHDF	continuous venovenous hemodiafiltration
CYP	cytochrome
d	day
D_5W	dextrose 5% in water
DBP	diastolic blood pressure
d/c[1]	discharge
DEHP	di(3-ethylhexyl)phthalate
DIC	disseminated intravascular coagulation
dil	dilute
disp	dispense
div	divide
DM	diabetes mellitus
DMARD	disease modifying antirheumatic drug
DSC	discontinued
DSM-IV	Diagnostic and Statistical Manual
dtd	give of such a dose
Dx	diagnosis
DVT	deep vein thrombosis
EBV	Epstein-Barr virus
ECG	electrocardiogram
ECMO	extracorporeal membrane oxygenation
ECT	electroconvulsive therapy
ED	emergency department
EEG	electroencephalogram
EF	ejection fraction
EG	ethylene glycol
EGA	estimated gestational age
EIA	enzyme immunoassay
ELISA	enzyme-linked immunosorbent assay
elix, el	elixir
emp	as directed
EPS	extrapyramidal side effects
ESR	erythrocyte sedimentation rate
ESRD	end stage renal disease
et	and
EtOH	alcohol
ex aq	in water
F	Fahrenheit

Abbreviation	Meaning
f, ft	make, let be made
FDA	Food and Drug Administration
FTT	failure to thrive
g	gram
GABA	gamma-aminobutyric acid
GAD	generalized anxiety disorder
GERD	gastroesophageal reflux disease
GFR	glomerular filtration rate
GGT	gamma-glutamyltransferase
GI	gastrointestinal
gr	grain
gtt	a drop
GU	genitourinary
GVHD	graft versus host disease
h	hour
HAM-A	Hamilton Anxiety Scale
HAM-D	Hamilton Depression Scale
HDL	high density lipoprotein
HF	heart failure
HFSA	Heart Failure Society of America
HIV	human immunodeficiency virus
HMG-CoA	3-hydroxy-3-methylglutaryl-coenzyme A
HOCM	hypertrophic obstructive cardiomyopathy
HPA	hypothalamic-pituitary-adrenal
hs[1]	at bedtime
HSV	herpes simplex virus
HTN	hypertension
HUS	hemolytic uremic syndrome
IBD	inflammatory bowel disease
IBS	irritable bowel syndrome
IBW	ideal body weight
ICD	implantable cardioverter defibrillator
ICH	intracranial hemorrhage
ICP	intracranial pressure
IDDM	insulin dependent diabetes mellitus
IDSA	Infectious Diseases Society of America
IHSS	idiopathic hypertrophic subaortic stenosis
I.M.	intramuscular
INR	international normalized ration
Int. unit	international unit
IOP	intraocular pressure
IUGR	intrauterine growth retardation
I.V.	intravenous
JIA	juvenile idiopathic arthritis
JNC	Joint National Committee

▶

Abbreviation	Meaning
kcal	kilocalorie
kg	kilogram
KIU	kallikrein inhibitor unit
L	liter
LAMM	L-α-acetyl methadol
LDH	lactate dehydrogenase
LDL	low density lipoprotein
LFT	liver function test
LGA	large for gestational age
liq	a liquor, solution
LR	lactated ringers
LVEF	left ventricular ejection fraction
LVH	left ventricular hypertrophy
M	Molar
MADRS	Montgomery Asbery Depression Rating Scale
MAOIs	monamine oxidase inhibitors
mcg	microgram
MDD	major depressive disorder
MDRD	modification of diet in renal disease
m. dict	as directed
mEq	milliequivalent
mg	milligram
MI	myocardial infarction
microL	microliter
mL	milliliter
mm	millimeter
mM	millimolar
mm Hg	millimeters of mercury
MMSE	mini mental status examination
M/P	milk to plasma ratio
MPS I	mucopolysaccharidosis I
MRHD	maximum recommended human dose
MRI	magnetic resonance imaging
MUGA	multiple gated acquisition scan
NAS	neonatal abstinence syndrome
NF	National Formulary
NFD	Nephrogenic fibrosing dermopathy
ng	nanogram
NIDDM	Noninsulin dependent diabetes mellitus
NKA	no known allergies
NKDA	no known drug allergies
NMDA	n-methyl-d-aspartic acid
NMS	neuroleptic malignant syndrome
NNRTI	non-nucleoside reverse transcriptase inhibitor
no.	number

Abbreviation	Meaning
noc	in the night
non rep	do not repeat, no refills
NPO	nothing by mouth
NRTI	nucleoside reverse transcriptase inhibitor
NS	normal saline
NSAID	nonsteroidal antiinflammatory drug
NSF	nephrogenic systemic fibrosis
NSTEMI	Non-ST-elevation myocardial infarction
NV	nausea and vomiting
O, Oct	a pint
OA	osteoarthritis
OCD	obsessive-compulsive disorder
o.d.[1]	right eye
OHSS	ovarian hyperstimulation syndrome
o.l.	left eye
o.s.[1]	left eye
OTC	over-the-counter
o.u.[1]	each eye
PAT	paroxysmal artrial tachycardia
pc, post cib	after meals
PD	Parkinson disease
PDA	patent ductus arteriosus
PDE-5	phosphodiesterase-5
PE	pulmonary embolus
PEG tube	percutaneous endoscopic gastrostomy tube
PHN	post-herpetic neuralgia
PID	pelvic inflammatory disease
PM	afternoon or evening
PMDD	premenstrual dysphoric disorder
P.O.	by mouth
PONV	postoperative nausea and vomiting
PPN	peripheral parenteral nutrition
P.R.	rectally
prn	as needed
PROM	premature rupture of membranes
PSVT	paroxysmal superventricular tachycardia
PT	prothrombin time
PTSD	post-traumatic stress disorder
PTT	partial thromboplastin time
PUD	peptic ulcer disease
pulv	a powder
PVD	peripheral vascular disease
q	every
qad	every other day
qd[1,2]	every day, daily

Abbreviation	Meaning
qh	every hour
qid	four times a day
qod[1,2]	every other day
qs	a sufficient quantity
qs ad	a sufficient quantity to make
QT_c	corrected QT interval
QT_c-F	corrected QT interval by Fredricia's formula
RA	rheumatoid arthritis
REM	rapid eye movement
RPLS	reversible posterior leukoencephalopathy syndrome
Rx	take, a recipe
SA	sinoatrial
SAD	seasonal affective disorder
SAH	subarachnoid hemorrhage
SBE	subacute bacterial endocarditis
SBP	systolic blood pressure
S_{cr}	serum creatinine
SERM	selective estrogen receptor modulator
SGA	small for gestational age
SGOT	serum glutamic oxaloacetic aminotransferase
SGPT	serum glutamic pyruvate transaminase
SI	International System of Units or Systeme international d'Unites
SIADH	syndrome of inappropriate antidiuretic hormone secretion
SL	sublingual
SLE	systemic lupus erythematosus
SNRI	serotonin norepinephrine reuptake inhibitor
SSKI	saturated solution of potassium iodide
SSRIs	selective serotonin reuptake inhibitors
stat	at once, immediately
STD	sexually transmitted disease
STEM I	ST-elevation myocardial infarction
SubQ	subcutaneous
supp	suppository
SVT	supraventricular tachycardia
SWFI	sterile water for injection
syr	syrup
$T_{1/2}$	half-life
tab	tablet
tal	such
TB	tuberculosis
TC	total cholesterol
TCA	tricyclic antidepressant
TD	tardive dyskinesia
TG	triglyceride
TIA	transient ischemic attack

Abbreviation	Meaning
tid	three times a day
TMA	thrombotic microangiopathy
T_{max}	time to maximum observed concentration, plasma
TNF	Tumor necrosis factor
TPN	total parenteral nutrition
tr, tinct	tincture
trit	triturate
tsp	teaspoonful
UC	ulcerative colitis
u.d., ut dict	as directed
ULN	upper limits of normal
ung	ointment
URI	upper respiratory infection
USAN	United States Adopted Names
USP	United States Pharmacopeia
UTI	urinary tract infection
UV	ultraviolet
V_d	volume of distribution
VEGF	vascular endothelial growth factor
VF	ventricular fibrillation
v.o.	verbal order
VT	ventricular tachycardia
VTE	venous thromboembolism
vWD	von Willebrand disease
VZV	varicella zoster virus
w.a.	while awake
x3	3 times
x4	4 times
YBOC	Yale Brown Obsessive-Compulsive Scale
YMRS	Young Mania Rating Scale

[1]ISMP error-prone abbreviation.
[2]JCAHO Do Not Use list.

NORMAL LABORATORY VALUES FOR ADULTS

Automated Chemistry (CHEMISTRY A)

Test	Values	Remarks
SERUM / PLASMA		
Acetone	Negative	
Albumin	3.2-5 g/dL	
Alcohol, ethyl	Negative	
Aldolase	1.2-7.6 IU/L	
Ammonia	20-70 mcg/dL	Specimen to be placed on ice as soon as collected.
Amylase	30-110 units/L	
Bilirubin, direct	0-0.3 mg/dL	
Bilirubin, total	0.1-1.2 mg/dL	
Calcium	8.6-10.3 mg/dL	
Calcium, ionized	2.24-2.46 mEq/L	
Chloride	95-108 mEq/L	
Cholesterol, total	≤200 mg/dL	Fasted blood required – normal value affected by dietary habits. This reference range is for a general adult population.
HDL cholesterol	40-60 mg/dL	Fasted blood required – normal value affected by dietary habits.
LDL cholesterol	<160 mg/dL	If triglyceride is >400 mg/dL, LDL cannot be calculated accurately (Friedewald equation). Target LDL-C depends on patient's risk factors.
CO_2	23-30 mEq/L	
Creatine kinase (CK) isoenzymes		
CK-BB	0%	
CK-MB (cardiac)	0%-3.9%	
CK-MM (muscle)	96%-100%	
CK-MB levels must be both ≥4% and 10 IU/L to meet diagnostic criteria for CK-MB positive result consistent with myocardial injury.		
Creatine phosphokinase (CPK)	8-150 IU/L	
Creatinine	0.5-1.4 mg/dL	
Ferritin	13-300 ng/mL	
Folate	3.6-20 ng/dL	
GGT (gamma-glutamyltranspeptidase)		
male	11-63 IU/L	
female	8-35 IU/L	
GLDH	To be determined	
Glucose (preprandial)	<115 mg/dL	Goals different for diabetics.
Glucose, fasting	60-110 mg/dL	Goals different for diabetics.
Glucose, nonfasting (2-h postprandial)	<120 mg/dL	Goals different for diabetics.
Hemoglobin A_{1c}	<8	
Hemoglobin, plasma free	<2.5 mg/100 mL	
Hemoglobin, total glycosolated (Hb A_1)	4%-8%	

Automated Chemistry (CHEMISTRY A) *continued*

Test	Values	Remarks
Iron	65-150 mcg/dL	
Iron binding capacity, total (TIBC)	250-420 mcg/dL	
Lactic acid	0.7-2.1 mEq/L	Specimen to be kept on ice and sent to lab as soon as possible.
Lactate dehydrogenase (LDH)	56-194 IU/L	
Lactate dehydrogenase (LDH) isoenzymes		
LD_1	20%-34%	
LD_2	29%-41%	
LD_3	15%-25%	
LD_4	1%-12%	
LD_5	1%-15%	

Flipped LD_1/LD_2 ratios (>1 may be consistent with myocardial injury) particularly when considered in combination with a recent CK-MB positive result.

Test	Values	Remarks
Lipase	23-208 units/L	
Magnesium	1.6-2.5 mg/dL	Increased by slight hemolysis.
Osmolality	289-308 mOsm/kg	
Phosphatase, alkaline		
adults 25-60 y	33-131 IU/L	
adults ≥61 y	51-153 IU/L	
infancy-adolescence	Values range up to 3-5 times higher than adults	
Phosphate, inorganic	2.8-4.2 mg/dL	
Potassium	3.5-5.2 mEq/L	Increased by slight hemolysis.
Prealbumin	>15 mg/dL	
Protein, total	6.5-7.9 g/dL	
SGOT (AST)	<35 IU/L (20-48)	
SGPT (ALT) (10-35)	<35 IU/L	
Sodium	134-149 mEq/L	
Thyroid stimulating hormone (TSH)		
adults ≤20 y	0.7-6.4 mIU/L	
21-54 y	0.4-4.2 mIU/L	
55-87 y	0.5-8.9 mIU/L	
Transferrin	>200 mg/dL	
Triglycerides	45-155 mg/dL	Fasted blood required.
Troponin I	<1.5 ng/mL	
Urea nitrogen (BUN)	7-20 mg/dL	
Uric acid		
male	2-8 mg/dL	
female	2-7.5 mg/dL	
CEREBROSPINAL FLUID		
Glucose	50-70 mg/dL	
Protein		
	15-45 mg/dL	CSF obtained by lumbar puncture.

Note: Bloody specimen gives erroneously high value due to contamination with blood proteins

Test	Values	Remarks
URINE		
(24-hour specimen is required for all these tests unless specified)		
Amylase	32-641 units/L	The value is in units/L and **not** calculated for total volume.
Amylase, fluid (random samples)		Interpretation of value left for physician, depends on the nature of fluid.
Calcium	Depends upon dietary intake	
Creatine		
male	150 mg/24 h	Higher value on children and during pregnancy.
female	250 mg/24 h	
Creatinine	1000-2000 mg/24 h	
Creatinine clearance (endogenous)		
male	85-125 mL/min	A blood sample must accompany urine specimen.
female	75-115 mL/min	
Glucose	1 g/24 h	
5-hydroxyindoleacetic acid	2-8 mg/24 h	
Iron	0.15 mg/24 h	Acid washed container required.
Magnesium	146-209 mg/24 h	
Osmolality	500-800 mOsm/kg	With normal fluid intake.
Oxalate	10-40 mg/24 h	
Phosphate	400-1300 mg/24 h	
Potassium	25-120 mEq/24 h	Varies with diet; the interpretation of urine electrolytes and osmolality should be left for the physician.
Sodium	40-220 mEq/24 h	
Porphobilinogen, qualitative	Negative	
Porphyrins, qualitative	Negative	
Proteins	0.05-0.1 g/24 h	
Salicylate	Negative	
Urea clearance	60-95 mL/min	A blood sample must accompany specimen.
Urea N	10-40 g/24 h	Dependent on protein intake.
Uric acid	250-750 mg/24 h	Dependent on diet and therapy.
Urobilinogen	0.5-3.5 mg/24 h	For qualitative determination on random urine, send sample to urinalysis section in Hematology Lab.
Xylose absorption test		
children	16%-33% of ingested xylose	
FECES		
Fat, 3-day collection	<5 g/d	Value depends on fat intake of 100 g/d for 3 days preceding and during collection.
GASTRIC ACIDITY		
Acidity, total, 12 h	10-60 mEq/L	Titrated at pH 7.

BLOOD GASES

	Arterial	Capillary	Venous
pH	7.35-7.45	7.35-7.45	7.32-7.42
pCO_2 (mm Hg)	35-45	35-45	38-52
pO_2 (mm Hg)	70-100	60-80	24-48
HCO_3 (mEq/L)	19-25	19-25	19-25
TCO_2 (mEq/L)	19-29	19-29	23-33
O_2 saturation (%)	90-95	90-95	40-70
Base excess (mEq/L)	-5 to +5	-5 to +5	-5 to +5

HEMATOLOGY Complete Blood Count

Age	Hgb (g/dL)	Hct (%)	RBC (mill/mm^3)	RDW
0-3 d	15.0-20.0	45-61	4.0-5.9	<18.0
1-2 wk	12.5-18.5	39-57	3.6-5.5	<17.0
1-6 mo	10.0-13.0	29-42	3.1-4.3	<16.5
7 mo to 2 y	10.5-13.0	33-38	3.7-4.9	<16.0
2-5 y	11.5-13.0	34-39	3.9-5.0	<15.0
5-8 y	11.5-14.5	35-42	4.0-4.9	<15.0
13-18 y	12.0-15.2	36-47	4.5-5.1	<14.5
Adult male	13.5-16.5	41-50	4.5-5.5	<14.5
Adult female	12.0-15.0	36-44	4.0-4.9	<14.5

Age	MCV (fL)	MCH (pg)	MCHC (%)	PLTS (x 10^3/mm^3)
0-3 d	95-115	31-37	29-37	250-450
1-2 wk	86-110	28-36	28-38	250-450
1-6 mo	74-96	25-35	30-36	300-700
7 mo to 2 y	70-84	23-30	31-37	250-600
2-5 y	75-87	24-30	31-37	250-550
5-8 y	77-95	25-33	31-37	250-550
13-18 y	78-96	25-35	31-37	150-450
Adult male	80-100	26-34	31-37	150-450
Adult female	80-100	26-34	31-37	150-450

WBC and Differential

Age	WBC (x 10^3/mm^3)	Segs	Bands	Lymphs	Monos
0-3 d	9.0-35.0	32-62	10-18	19-29	5-7
1-2 wk	5.0-20.0	14-34	6-14	36-45	6-10
1-6 mo	6.0-17.5	13-33	4-12	41-71	4-7
7 mo to 2 y	6.0-17.0	15-35	5-11	45-76	3-6
2-5 y	5.5-15.5	23-45	5-11	35-65	3-6
5-8 y	5.0-14.5	32-54	5-11	28-48	3-6
13-18 y	4.5-13.0	34-64	5-11	25-45	3-6
Adults	4.5-11.0	35-66	5-11	24-44	3-6

◀

Age	Eos	Basos	Atypical Lymphs	No. of NRBCs
0-3 d	0-2	0-1	0-8	0-2
1-2 wk	0-2	0-1	0-8	0
1-6 mo	0-3	0-1	0-8	0
7 mo to 2 y	0-3	0-1	0-8	0
2-5 y	0-3	0-1	0-8	0
5-8 y	0-3	0-1	0-8	0
13-18 y	0-3	0-1	0-8	0
Adults	0-3	0-1	0-8	0

Erythrocyte Sedimentation Rates and Reticulocyte Counts

Sedimentation rate, Westergren	Children	0-20 mm/hour
	Adult male	0-15 mm/hour
	Adult female	0-20 mm/hour
Sedimentation rate, Wintrobe	Children	0-13 mm/hour
	Adult male	0-10 mm/hour
	Adult female	0-15 mm/hour
Reticulocyte count	Newborns	2%-6%
	1-6 mo	0%-2.8%
	Adults	0.5%-1.5%

NORMAL LABORATORY VALUES FOR CHILDREN

<u>Normal Values</u>

CHEMISTRY

Albumin	0-1 y	2-4 g/dL
	1 y to adult	3.5-5.5 g/dL
Ammonia	Newborns	90-150 mcg/dL
	Children	40-120 mcg/dL
	Adults	18-54 mcg/dL
Amylase	Newborns	0-60 units/L
	Adults	30-110 units/L
Bilirubin, conjugated, direct	Newborns	<1.5 mg/dL
	1 mo to adult	0-0.5 mg/dL
Bilirubin, total	0-3 d	2-10 mg/dL
	1 mo to adult	0-1.5 mg/dL
Bilirubin, unconjugated, indirect		0.6-10.5 mg/dL
Calcium	Newborns	7-12 mg/dL
	0-2 y	8.8-11.2 mg/dL
	2 y to adult	9-11 mg/dL
Calcium, ionized, whole blood		4.4-5.4 mg/dL
Carbon dioxide, total		23-33 mEq/L
Chloride		95-105 mEq/L
Cholesterol	Newborns	45-170 mg/dL
	0-1 y	65-175 mg/dL
	1-20 y	120-230 mg/dL
Creatinine	0-1 y	≤0.6 mg/dL
	1 y to adult	0.5-1.5 mg/dL
Glucose	Newborns	30-90 mg/dL
	0-2 y	60-105 mg/dL
	Children to adults	70-110 mg/dL
Iron		
	Newborns	110-270 mcg/dL
	Infants	30-70 mcg/dL
	Children	55-120 mcg/dL
	Adults	70-180 mcg/dL
Iron binding	Newborns	59-175 mcg/dL
	Infants	100-400 mcg/dL
	Adults	250-400 mcg/dL
Lactic acid, lactate		2-20 mg/dL
Lead, whole blood		<10 mcg/dL
Lipase		
	Children	20-140 units/L
	Adults	0-190 units/L
Magnesium		1.5-2.5 mEq/L

NORMAL LABORATORY VALUES FOR CHILDREN

		Normal Values
Osmolality, serum		275-296 mOsm/kg
Osmolality, urine		50-1400 mOsm/kg
Phosphorus	Newborns	4.2-9 mg/dL
	6 wk to 19 mo	3.8-6.7 mg/dL
	19 mo to 3 y	2.9-5.9 mg/dL
	3-15 y	3.6-5.6 mg/dL
	>15 y	2.5-5 mg/dL
Potassium, plasma	Newborns	4.5-7.2 mEq/L
	2 d to 3 mo	4-6.2 mEq/L
	3 mo to 1 y	3.7-5.6 mEq/L
	1-16 y	3.5-5 mEq/L
Protein, total	0-2 y	4.2-7.4 g/dL
	>2 y	6-8 g/dL
Sodium		136-145 mEq/L
Triglycerides	Infants	0-171 mg/dL
	Children	20-130 mg/dL
	Adults	30-200 mg/dL
Urea nitrogen, blood	0-2 y	4-15 mg/dL
	2 y to Adult	5-20 mg/dL
Uric acid	Male	3-7 mg/dL
	Female	2-6 mg/dL

ENZYMES

Alanine aminotransferase (ALT)	0-2 mo	8-78 units/L
	>2 mo	8-36 units/L
Alkaline phosphatase (ALKP)	Newborns	60-130 units/L
	0-16 y	85-400 units/L
	>16 y	30-115 units/L
Aspartate aminotransferase (AST)	Infants	18-74 units/L
	Children	15-46 units/L
	Adults	5-35 units/L
Creatine kinase (CK)	Infants	20-200 units/L
	Children	10-90 units/L
	Adult male	0-206 units/L
	Adult female	0-175 units/L
Lactate dehydrogenase (LDH)	Newborns	290-501 units/L
	1 mo to 2 y	110-144 units/L
	>16 y	60-170 units/L

BLOOD GASES

	Arterial	Capillary	Venous
pH	7.35-7.45	7.35-7.45	7.32-7.42
pCO_2 (mm Hg)	35-45	35-45	38-52
pO_2 (mm Hg)	70-100	60-80	24-48
HCO_3 (mEq/L)	19-25	19-25	19-25
TCO_2 (mEq/L)	19-29	19-29	23-33
O_2 saturation (%)	90-95	90-95	40-70
Base excess (mEq/L)	-5 to +5	-5 to +5	-5 to +5

THYROID FUNCTION TESTS

T_4 (thyroxine)	1-7 d	10.1-20.9 mcg/dL
	8-14 d	9.8-16.6 mcg/dL
	1 mo to 1 y	5.5-16.0 mcg/dL
	>1 y	4.0-12.0 mcg/dL
FTI	1-3 d	9.3-26.6
	1-4 wk	7.6-20.8
	1-4 mo	7.4-17.9
	4-12 mo	5.1-14.5
	1-6 y	5.7-13.3
	>6 y	4.8-14.0
T_3 by RIA	Newborns	100-470 ng/dL
	1-5 y	100-260 ng/dL
	5-10 y	90-240 ng/dL
	10 y to adult	70-210 ng/dL
T_3 uptake		35%-45%
TSH	Cord	3-22 μIU/mL
	1-3 d	<40 μIU/mL
	3-7 d	<25 μIU/mL
	>7 d	0-10 μIU/mL

ACQUIRED IMMUNODEFICIENCY SYNDROME (AIDS) - LAB TESTS AND APPROVED DRUGS FOR HIV INFECTION AND AIDS-RELATED CONDITIONS

This list of tests is not intended in any way to suggest patterns of physician's orders, nor is it complete. These tests may support possible clinical diagnoses or rule out other diagnostic possibilities. Each laboratory test relevant to AIDS is listed and weighted. Two symbols (**) indicate that the test is diagnostic, that is, documents the diagnosis if the expected is found. A single symbol (*) indicates a test frequently used in the diagnosis or management of the disease. The other listed tests are useful on a selective basis with consideration of clinical factors and specific aspects of the case.

Acid-Fast Stain
Acid-Fast Stain, Modified, *Nocardia* Species
Antimicrobial Susceptibility Testing, Fungi
Antimicrobial Susceptibility Testing, Mycobacteria
Arthropod Identification
Babesiosis Serological Test
Bacteremia Detection, Buffy Coat Micromethod
Bacterial Culture, Blood
Bacterial Culture, Bronchoscopy Specimen
Bacterial Culture, Sputum
Bacterial Culture, Stool
Bacterial Culture, Throat
Bacterial Culture, Urine, Clean Catch
Beta$_2$-Microglobulin
Blood and Fluid Precautions, Specimen Collection
Bronchial Washings Cytology
Bronchoalveolar Lavage Cytology
Brushings Cytology
Candida Antigen
Candidiasis Serologic Test
Cat Scratch Disease Serology
CD4/CD8 Enumeration
Cerebrospinal Fluid Cytology
Cryptococcal Antigen Titer
Cryptosporidium Diagnostic Procedures
Cytomegalic Inclusion Disease Cytology
Cytomegalovirus Antibody
Cytomegalovirus Antigen Detection
Cytomegalovirus Culture
Cytomegalovirus DNA Detection
Darkfield Examination, Syphilis
Electron Microscopy
Folic Acid, Serum
Fungal Culture, Biopsy or Body Fluid
Fungal Culture, Blood
Fungal Culture, Cerebrospinal Fluid
Fungal Culture, Sputum
Fungal Culture, Stool
Fungal Culture, Urine
Hemoglobin A$_2$
Hepatitis B Surface Antigen
Herpes Cytology
Herpes Simplex Virus Antigen Detection
Herpes Simplex Virus Culture
Histopathology
Histoplasmosis Antibody
Histoplasmosis Antigen
**HIV-1/HIV-2 Serology
HTLV-I/II Antibody
*Human Immunodeficiency Virus Culture
*Human Immunodeficiency Virus DNA Amplification

India Ink Preparation
Inhibitor, Lupus, Phospholipid Type
KOH Preparation
Leishmaniasis Serological Test
Leukocyte Immunophenotyping
Lymphocyte Transformation Test
Microsporidia Diagnostic Procedures
Mycobacteria by DNA Probe
Mycobacterial Culture, Biopsy or Body Fluid
Mycobacterial Culture, Cerebrospinal Fluid
Mycobacterial Culture, Cutaneous and Subcutaneous Tissue
Mycobacterial Culture, Sputum
Mycobacterial Culture, Stool
Neisseria gonorrhoeae Culture and Smear
Nocardia Culture
Ova and Parasites, Stool
*p24 Antigen
Platelet Count
Pneumocystis carinii Preparation
Pneumocystis Immunofluorescence
Polymerase Chain Reaction
Red Blood Cell Indices
Risks of Transfusion
Skin Biopsy
Sputum Cytology
Toxoplasmosis Serology
VDRL, Serum
Viral Culture
Viral Culture, Blood
Viral Culture, Body Fluid
Viral Culture, Central Nervous System Symptoms
Viral Culture, Dermatological Symptoms
Viral Culture, Tissue
Virus, Direct Detection by Fluorescent Antibody
White Blood Count

FDA-APPROVED AND INVESTIGATIONAL ANTIRETROVIRAL DRUGS

Antiretroviral Drugs

Generic Name	Also Known As	Brand Name	FDA Status
NUCLEOSIDE/NUCLEOTIDE ANALOG REVERSE TRANSCRIPTASE INHIBITORS (NRTIs)			
abacavir	ABC	Ziagen®	Approved
apricitabine	AVX754	—	Investigational
didanosine	ddI	Videx®; Videx® EC	Approved
elvucitabine	ACH-126,443; Beta-L-Fd4C	—	Investigational
emtricitabine	FTC	Emtriva®	Approved
lamivudine	3TC	Epivir®	Approved
stavudine	d4T	Zerit®	Approved
tenofovir	TDF	Viread®	Approved
zidovudine	ZDV	Retrovir®	Approved
—	RCV	Racivir	Investigational
NONNUCLEOSIDE REVERSE TRANSCRIPTASE INHIBITORS (NNRTIs)			
delavirdine	DLV	Rescriptor®	Approved
efavirenz	EFV	Sustiva®	Approved
etravirine	TMC 125	Intelence™	Approved
nevirapine	NVP	Viramune®	Approved
rilpivirine	TMC 278	—	Investigational
PROTEASE INHIBITORS (PIs)			
atazanavir	ATV	Reyataz®	Approved
darunavir	DRV	Prezista™	Approved
fosamprenavir	FPV	Lexiva®	Approved
indinavir	IDV	Crixivan®	Approved
lopinavir and ritonavir	LPV/RTV	Kaletra®	Approved
nelfinavir	NFV	Viracept®	Approved
ritonavir	RTV	Norvir®	Approved
saquinavir	SQV	Invirase®	Approved
tipranavir	TPV	Aptivus®	Approved
FIXED-DOSE COMBINATION PRODUCTS			
abacavir and lamivudine	ABC/3TC	Epzicom®	Approved
abacavir, lamivudine, and zidovudine	ABC/3TC/ZDV	Trizivir®	Approved
efavirenz, emtricitabine and tenofovir	EFV/FTC/TDF	Atripla™	Approved
emtricitabine and tenofovir	FTC/TDF	Truvada®	Approved
zidovudine and lamivudine	ZDV/3TC	Combivir®	Approved
FUSION INHIBITORS			
enfuvirtide	ENF	Fuzeon®	Approved
—	TNX-355	—	Investigational
ENTRY INHIBITORS - CCR5 CO-RECEPTOR ANTAGONIST			
maraviroc	MVC	Selzentry™	Approved
vicriviroc	SCH-417690; SCH-D	—	Investigational

Antiretroviral Drugs *continued*

Generic Name	Also Known As	Brand Name	FDA Status
—	PRO 140	—	Investigational
—	INCB9741	—	Investigational
INTEGRASE INHIBITORS			
elvitegravir	GS-9137	—	Investigational
raltegravir	RAL	Isentress™	Approved
—	GSK364735	—	Investigational
MATURATION INHIBITORS			
bevirimat	PA-457	—	Investigational

DRUGS USED TO TREAT COMPLICATIONS OF HIV / AIDS

Brand Name	Generic Name (Synonym)	Use
Abelcet®, AmBisome®	amphotericin B, ABLC	Antifungal for aspergillosis
Bactrim™, Septra®	sulfamethoxazole and trimethoprim, SMZ/TMP	Antiprotozoal antibiotic used to treat and prevent *Pneumocystis carinii* pneumonia
Biaxin®	clarithromycin	Antibiotic used to treat and prevent *Mycobacterium avium*
Cytovene®	ganciclovir, DHPG	Antiviral used to treat CMV retinitis
DaunoXome®	daunorubicin citrate (liposomal)	Chemotherapy for Kaposi sarcoma
Diflucan®	fluconazole	Antifungal for candidiasis, cryptococcal meningitis
Doxil®	doxorubicin (liposomal)	Chemotherapy for Kaposi sarcoma
Eraxis™	anidulafungin	Antifungal (intravenous), used to treat *Candida* infections in the esophagus (candidiasis), blood stream (candidemia), and other forms of *Candida* infections, including abdominal abscesses and peritonitis (inflammation of the lining of the abdominal cavity)
Famvir®	famciclovir	Antiviral used to treat herpes
Foscavir®	foscarnet	Antiviral used to treat herpes and CMV retinitis
Gamimune® N	immune globulin, gamma globulin, IGIV	Immune booster used to prevent bacterial infections in children
Intron® A	interferon alfa-2b	Treat Kaposi sarcoma and hepatitis C
Marinol®	dronabinol	Treat loss of appetite
Megace®	megestrol acetate	Treat loss of appetite and weight
Mepron®	atovaquone	Antiprotozoal antibiotic used to treat and prevent *Pneumocystis carinii* pneumonia
Mycobutin®	rifabutin	Antimycobacterial used to prevent *Mycobacterium avium*
NebuPent®	pentamidine	Antiprotozoal antibiotic used to prevent *Pneumocystis carinii* pneumonia
Neutrexin®	trimetrexate glucuronate and leucovorin	Antiprotozoal antibiotic used to treat *Pneumocystis carinii* pneumonia
Panretin® Gel	alitretinoin gel 0.1%	AIDS-related Kaposi sarcoma
Procrit®, Epogen®	erythropoietin, EPO	Treat anemia related to AZT therapy
Roferon-A®	interferon alfa-2a	Treat Kaposi sarcoma and hepatitis C
Serostim®	somatropin rDNA	Treat weight loss
Sporanox®	itraconazole	Antifungal used to treat blastomycosis, histoplasmosis, aspergillosis, and candidiasis

DRUGS USED TO TREAT COMPLICATIONS OF HIV / AIDS *continued*

Brand Name	Generic Name (Synonym)	Use
Taxol®	paclitaxel	Kaposi sarcoma
Valcyte™	valganciclovir	Antiviral used to treat CMV retinitis
VFEND®	voriconazole	Antifungal for invasive aspergillosis and serious fungal infections due to *Fusarium sporotrichoides* and *Scedosporium apiospermum*, and Esophageal Candidiasis
Vistide®	cidofovir, HPMPC	Antiviral used to treat cytomegalovirus (CMV)
Vitrasert® Implant	ganciclovir insert	Antiviral used to treat CMV retinitis
Vitravene™ intravitreal injection	fomivirsen sodium injection	Antiviral used to treat CMV retinitis
Zithromax®	azithromycin	Antibiotic used to treat *Mycobacterium avium*

HERBS AND COMMON NATURAL AGENTS

The authors have chosen to include this list of natural products and their reported uses. Due to limited scientific evidence to support these uses, the information provided here is not intended as a cure for any disease, and should not be construed as curative or healing. In addition, the reader is strongly encouraged to seek other references that discuss this information in more detail, and that discuss important issues such as contraindications, warnings, precautions, adverse reactions, and interactions.

PROPOSED MEDICINAL CLAIMS

Herb	Reported Uses
Acetyl-L-carnitine (ALC)	Alzheimer disease; cerebral ischemia; coronary artery disease; depression; diabetic peripheral neuropathy; fibromyalgia; fragile X syndrome; infertility; mood disorder; neurologic function; neuropathy; Parkinson disease; Peyronie disease; sperm motility; tuberculosis
Adrenal extract	Depression; fatigue, stress; fibromyalgia
Aloe (*Aloe* spp)	Aphthous stomatitis; cancer (prevention); constipation; diabetes; dry skin; genital herpes; gingivitis; healing agent for wounds, minor burns, and other minor skin irritations; irritable bowel syndrome; psoriasis vulgaris; ulcerative colitis
Alpha-Lipoic acid	Alcohol-induced liver damage; cardiovascular outcomes (in end-state renal disease); cataract prevention; chemotherapy and radiation (adjunct); circulation; coronary artery disease; diabetes, diabetic peripheral neuropathy; drug-induced cardiotoxicity; glaucoma; hypertension; insulin resistance; liver protective effects; multiple sclerosis; neuralgias; neurologic disorders, including stroke
Andrographis (*Andrographis paniculata*)	Familial Mediterranean Fever (FMF); influenza; upper respiratory tract infection (treatment and prevention)
Aortic extract	Circulation structure, function, and integrity (arteries and veins); prevention of vascular disease including atherosclerosis, cerebral and peripheral arterial insufficiency, varicose veins, hemorrhoids, and vascular retinopathies such as macular degeneration
Arabinoxylan	Cancer; diabetes, type 2; HIV; immune support (antiviral and anticancer activity); leukopenia (chemotherapy-induced)
Arginine	Adrenoleukodystrophy (ALD); angina; burns; cancer; cardiovascular disease; chronic heart failure; circulation; critical illness; dental pain; erectile dysfunction; gastrointestinal cancer surgery; growth hormone reserve test/pituitary disorder diagnosis; heart protection during CABG; hypercholesterolemia; hypertension; immune support; inborn errors of urea synthesis; inflammatory bowel disease; increases lean body mass; male infertility; MELAS syndrome; migraine headache; myocardial infarction; peripheral vascular disease/claudication; pre-eclampsia; pressure ulcers; recovery after surgery; sexual vitality and enhancement; transplants; wound healing
Arnica (*Arnica montana*)	Bruising; coagulation; diabetic retinopathy; osteoarthritis; pain; swelling (postoperative); trauma
Artichoke (*Cynara scolymus*)	Bile flow; dyspepsia (nonulcer); eczema and other dermatologic problems; hepatic protection/stimulation; hypercholesterolemia; indigestion; irritable bowel syndrome (IBS)
Ashwagandha (*Withania somnifera*)	Adaptogen/tonic (promote wellness); chemotherapy and radiation (adjunct); diabetes (type 2); diuresis; hypercholesterolemia; longevity/anti-aging; osteoarthritis; Parkinson disease; stress, fatigue, nervous exhaustion
Astragalus (*Astragalus membranaceus*) [Milk Vetch]	Adaptogen/tonic (promote wellness); antiviral activity; athletic performance (enhancement); burns; chemotherapy and radiation (adjunct); coronary artery disease; diabetes; heart failure; immune support; liver protection; mental performance; multiple sclerosis; otitis media; renal failure; smoking cessation; tissue oxygenation; tuberculosis
Bacopa (*Bacopa monniera*)	Alzheimer disease/senility; anxiety; epilepsy; irritable bowel syndrome (IBS); memory enhancement and improvement of cognitive function
Barberry (*Berberis vulgaris*)	Bladder infection; bronchitis; sore throat; yeast infection

Herb	Reported Uses
Beta-Carotene	Age-related maculopathy; AIDS; asthma; breast cancer; carotenoid deficiency; cataract prevention; cervical dysplasia; chromosome damage (reduction); chronic obstructive pulmonary disease (COPD); coronary heart disease (risk reduction; in combination); cystic fibrosis; diabetes; diabetes, type 2; esophageal cancer; gastric cancer; immune support; laryngeal cancer; LDL oxidation (decrease in males); lung cancer (preventive); lung function; macular degeneration; night blindness; oral leukoplakia; osteoarthritis; photoprotection (erythropoietic protoporphyria); pregnancy-related complications
Betaine hydrochloride	Cardiovascular disease (in homocystinuric patients); cholesterol levels; digestive aid (hypochlorhydria and achlorhydria); hyperhomocysteinemia; hyperhomocysteinemia (in chronic renal failure patients); rosaceal; steatohepatitis (nonalcoholic); weight loss
Bifidobacterium bifidum (*bifidus*)	Atopic dermatitis; constipation; Crohn disease; diarrhea; gastrointestinal microflora recolonization (anaerobic); *Helicobacter pylori* infection; immune function; irritable bowel syndrome (IBS); pouchitis; ulcerative colitis
Bilberry (*Vaccinium myrtillus*)	Circulation, peripheral; diabetes; diarrhea; dysmenorrhea; fibrocystic breast disease (FBD); hemorrhoids; ophthalmologic disorders (antioxidant) including myopia, diminished acuity, glaucoma; dark adaptation, macular degeneration, night blindness, diabetic retinopathy, cataracts; peptic ulcer disease; scleroderma; vascular disorders including varicose veins, capillary permeability/stability, phlebitis
Biotin (Vitamin H)	Cardiovascular disease (risk reduction; in combination); diabetes; diabetic peripheral neuropathy; hypertriglyceridemia; nails, brittle; pregnancy supplementation; seborrheic dermatitis; total parenteral nutrition (TPN); uncombable hair syndrome
Bismuth	Diarrhea; ulcers
Bitter melon (*Momordica charantia*)	Antiviral; cancer; diabetes, including impaired glucose tolerance (IGT)
Black cohosh (*Cimicifuga racemosa*)	Arthritis; depression (mild); menopause symptoms (including vasomotor); premenstrual syndrome (PMS)
Bladderwrack (*Fucus vesiculosus*)	Anticoagulant; antioxidant; bacterial and fungal infections; cancer; diabetes; fibrocystic breast disease; hypothyroidism; nutrient (rich source of iodine, potassium, magnesium, calcium, and iron)
Borage (*Borago officinalis*)	Acute respiratory distress syndrome; alcohol hangover; atopic dermatitis (treatment and prophylaxis); atopic eczema; cystic fibrosis; diabetic neuropathy; fatty acids (preterm infants); growth and development (infants); hyperlipidemia; infantile seborrheic dermatitis; malnutrition-inflammation complex syndrome; periodontitis; rheumatoid arthritis; stress; weight regain
Boron	Cognitive function improvement; osteoarthritis; osteoporosis; rheumatoid arthritis; vaginitis
Boswellia (*Boswellia serrata*)	Antiinflammatory; arthritis; asthma; Crohn disease; ulcerative colitis
Branched-chain amino acids (BCAAs)	Amyotrophic lateral sclerosis; anorexia; cardiac atrophy; cirrhosis; diabetes; energy metabolism improvement (in cirrhosis patients); exercise performance; hepatic encephalopathy; muscle development and lean body mass (increase); muscle fatigue and soreness; protein metabolism (in COPD patients); tardive dyskinesia
Bromelain (*Anas comosus*)	Arthritis (antiinflammatory; proteolytic); burn debridement; cancer; cervical dysplasia; chronic obstructive pulmonary disease (COPD); digestive enzyme; osteoarthritis of the knee; sinusitis; steatorrhea; urinary tract infection (UTI)
Bupleurum (*Bupleurum falcatum*)	Brain damage (minimal, children); chronic inflammatory disease; fatigue; hepatic protection; hepatitis; systemic lupus erythematosus (SLE); thrombocytopenic purpura
Calcium	Antacid; black widow spider bite; blood pressure regulation; bone loss; bone stress injury prevention; cancer (prevention); colon cancer (distal); colorectal adenomas (recurrence); growth; hypercholesterolemia; hyperkalemia; hypermagnesemia; hyperparathyroidism; hyperphosphatemia; hypertension; kidney stones; lead toxicity; osteomalacia/rickets; poison ivy (topical; lactate form); premenstrual syndrome (PMS); pregnancy; pregnancy-induced hypertension; osteoporosis (prevention); weight loss

PROPOSED MEDICINAL CLAIMS *continued*

Herb	Reported Uses
Calendula (*Calendula officinalis*)	Antibacterial, antifungal, antiviral, antiprotozoal; radiation dermatitis; skin inflammation; wound healing
Caprylic acid	Antifungal/antiyeast; candidiasis; Crohn disease; dysbiosis; epilepsy (children)
Carnitine	Acute myocardial infarction (mortality); angina; athletic performance (enhancement); attention-deficit hyperactivity disorder (ADHD); chronic obstructive pulmonary disease (COPD); congestive heart failure (CHF); diabetes; fatigue; HIV/AIDS; hypercholesterolemia; hyperlipoproteinemia; hyperthyroidism; male infertility; myocardial infarction; neonatal growth and breathing; obesity; peripheral vascular disease; postexercise metabolic stress and muscle damage; quality of life (maintenance hemodialysis patients); renal failure/dialysis; sperm motility; weight loss
Cascara (*Rhamnus purshiana*)	Laxative
Cat's claw (*Uncaria tomentosa*)	Allergies; antiinflammatory; antimicrobial (antibacterial, antifungal, antiviral); antioxidant; arthritis; cancer; cervical dysplasia; Crohn disease; diverticulitis; endometriosis; fibromyalgia; immune support; multiple sclerosis; rosacea; systemic lupus erythematosus (SLE)
Cayenne (*Capsicum annuum, Capsicum frutescens*)	Antiinflammatory and analgesic (topical); cardiovascular circulatory support; cluster headache; digestive stimulant; fibromyalgia; postherpetic neuralgia; pruritus; rhinitis
Chamomile, German (*Matricaria chamomilla, Matricaria recutita*)	Anxiolytic; carminative, antispasmodic; colic; common cold; diaper rash; diarrhea (children); indigestion; insomnia (mild sedative); minor injury (topical antiinflammatory); nausea/vomiting; oral health (as mouth rinse/gargle); stress/anxiety; teething; uterine tonic; vaginitis
Chasteberry (*Vitex agnus-castus*)	Acne vulgaris; cervical dysplasia; corpus luteum insufficiency; hyperprolactinemia and insufficient lactation; cyclic mastalgia; menopause; menorrhagia; menstrual disorders including amenorrhea, endometriosis, premenstrual syndrome (PMS); rosacea
Chitosan	Antibacterial; dental plaque; hyperlipidemia; periodontitis; renal failure; weight loss; wound healing
Chlorophyll	Antiinflammatory, antioxidant, and wound healing properties; bacteriostatic; cancer; chemoprevention; herpes simplex, herpes zoster; odor absorbent/suppressant (breath freshener, toothpaste, mouthwash, and deodorant); pancreatitis; protectant; rheumatoid arthritis
Chondroitin sulfate	Coronary artery disease; interstitial cystitis; iron absorption enhancement; ophthalmologic uses; osteoarthritis; overactive bladder; psoriasis
Chromium	Atherosclerosis; cardiovascular disease (risk reduction; in combination); diabetes, type 1; diabetes, type 2; glaucoma; hypercholesterolemia; hypertriglyceridemia; hypothyroidism; immunosuppression; premenstrual syndrome (PMS); weight loss
Clove (*Syzygium aromaticum*)	Anal fissures; analgesic (toothache and teething); anesthetic; antiseptic; mosquito repellent
Coenzyme Q$_{10}$	Acute myocardial infarction; AIDS; Alzheimer disease; amyotrophic lateral sclerosis (ALS); angina; antioxidant; cancer (preventive); cardiomyopathy; cardioprotection during surgery; chemotherapy (adjunct); chronic fatigue syndrome; congestive heart failure (CHF); Down syndrome; exercise performance; fibromyalgia; gingivitis; HMG-CoA reductase inhibitors (may cause depletion of this nutraceutical); hypercholesterolemia; hypertension; migraine; mitochondrial disease and Kearns-Sayre syndrome; multiple sclerosis; muscle pain (associated with HMG-CoA reductase inhibitors); muscular dystrophy; myelodysplastic syndromes; Parkinson disease; periodontal disease; renal failure; tinnitus; weight loss
Coleus (*Coleus forskohlii*)	Antiinflammatory action after cardiopulmonary bypass; asthma and allergies; eczema; glaucoma; hypertension and congestive heart failure (CHF); lactagogue; psoriasis
Collagen (Type II)	Arthritis (rheumatoid and osteo); burns (first- and second-degree); soft tissue correction; ulcers (pressure, venous stasis, diabetic); wound healing (topical)
Colostrum	Antiviral (mild); athletic performance (enhancement); body composition; cryptosporidiosis; diarrhea; flu prevention; immune support; prevention of NSAID-induced GI injury; shigellosis; sore throat; upper respiratory tract infection

PROPOSED MEDICINAL CLAIMS *continued*

Herb	Reported Uses
Conjugated linoleic acid (CLA)	Cancer; muscle development and lean body mass (increase); obesity; oxidative stress and inflammatory disease in obese men; preeclampsia (in combination with calcium)
Copper	Age-related macular degeneration; anemia; atherosclerosis; copper deficiency; dental enamel demineralization (in combination with fluoride); growth promotion (children); marasmus; osteoporosis; plaque prevention; rheumatoid arthritis
Cordyceps (*Cordyceps sinensis*)	Adaptogen/tonic (promote wellness); antioxidant; chemotherapy and radiation (adjunct); endurance and stamina; fibromyalgia; hepatoprotection; hyperlipidemia; lung, liver, and kidney function (general support); sexual vitality (males and females); tissue oxygenation; fatigue; immunomodulator
Cranberry (*Vaccinium macrocarpon*)	Achlorhydria and B_{12} absorption; antioxidant; bacterial and fungal infections; cancer (prevention); *H. pylori* infection; nephrolithiasis (preventive); plaque; urinary tract infection, including prevention
Creatine	Congestive heart failure (CHF); enhancement of athletic performance (energy production and protein synthesis for muscle building); GAMT deficiency; Huntington disease; McArdle disease; muscle function and strength; mood; muscular dystrophy; Parkinson disease; resistance training in patients with Parkinson disease; schizophrenia; traumatic brain injury, prevention of complications (children)
Cyclo-hispro	Diabetes, type 2; hypoglycemia
Damiana (*Turnera diffusa*)	Female sexual dysfunction; weight loss/obesity
Dandelion (*Taraxacum officinale*)	Leaf used as a diuretic; root used for disorders of bile secretion (choleretic), appetite stimulation, dyspepsia
Dehydroepiandrosterone (DHEA)	Adrenal insufficiency; AIDS/HIV; antiaging; cardiovascular disease; cervical cancer; chronic fatigue syndrome; cocaine withdrawal; cognitive function; dementia; depression; diabetes, type 2; erectile dysfunction; extrapyramidal symptoms; fatigue; fibromyalgia; induction of labor; infertility; libido; lupus; muscle mass and strength; obesity; psoriasis; rheumatoid arthritis; schizophrenia; Sjögren syndrome
Devil's claw (*Harpagophytum procumbens*)	Antiinflammatory; back pain; osteoarthritis, gout, and other inflammatory conditions
Docosahexaenoic acid (DHA)	Alzheimer disease; angina pectoris; appetite; arrhythmias; asthma; attention-deficit disorder and attention-deficit hyperactivity disorder (ADD/ADHD); bipolar disorder; cancer (prevention); cardiovascular disease; colon cancer; coronary heart disease (risk reduction); Crohn disease; cystic fibrosis; depression; diabetes; diabetes, type 2; dysmenorrhea; eczema; hypercholesterolemia; hypertension; hypertriglyceridemia; IgA nephropathy; immune support; infant eye/brain development; lupus; nephrotic syndrome; preeclampsia; prevention of graft failure after heart bypass surgery; protection from cyclosporine toxicity in organ transplant patients; psoriasis; rheumatoid arthritis; schizophrenia; stroke (risk reduction); ulcerative colitis
Dong quai (*Angelica sinensis*)	Anemia; energy enhancement (particularly in females); hypertension; menopause, dysmenorrhea, premenstrual syndrome (PMS), and amenorrhea; menorrhagia; phytoestrogen; pulmonary hypertension
Echinacea (*Echinacea purpurea, Echinacea angustifolia*)	Antibacterial (topical; boils, abscesses, tonsillitis, poison ivy); antiviral; arthritis (*E. augustifolia*); genital herpes; immune support (cold and other upper respiratory infections); otitis media; radiation-associated leucopenia; upper respiratory infection; uveitis
Elder (*Sambucus nigra, Sambucus canadensis*)	Berry used as an antiviral, antioxidant, and for influenza; flower used as an antiinflammatory, for colds and influenza, diaphoretic, diuretic, fever, sinusitis, and sore throat
Ephedra (*Ephedra sinica*)	Allergies, sinusitis, hay fever; asthma; hypotension; sexual arousal; weight loss (monotherapy); weight loss (combination therapy)
Evening primrose (*Oenothera biennis*)	Amenorrhea; atopic dermatitis; attention-deficit disorder (ADD); depression; diabetes; diabetic peripheral neuropathy; eczema, dermatitis, and psoriasis; endometriosis; fatigue; fibrocystic breast disease (FBD); hypercholesterolemia; ichthyosis vulgaris; irritable bowel syndrome; mastalgia; menorrhagia; multiple sclerosis; obesity; omega-6 fatty acid supplementation; premenstrual syndrome (PMS) and menopause; pre-eclampsia; rheumatoid arthritis; Raynaud phenomenon; rosacea; scleroderma

PROPOSED MEDICINAL CLAIMS *continued*

Herb	Reported Uses
Eyebright (*Euphrasia officinalis*)	Conjunctivitis; eye fatigue; catarrh of the eyes; hepatoprotection
Fennel (*Foeniculum vulgare* Mill.)	ACE inhibitor-associated cough; colic, infantile; dysmenorrhea; ultraviolet skin protection
Fenugreek (*Trigonella foenum-graecum*)	Diabetes; hypercholesterolemia
Feverfew (*Tanacetum parthenium*)	Antiinflammatory, rheumatoid arthritis; migraine headache (preventive); muscle soreness
Fish oils	Acne vulgaris; angina pectoris; arrhythmias; asthma; bipolar disorder; body weight improvement; cancer (prevention); cardiac death (sudden; preventive); cardiac support (general; proposed benefits); cardiovascular disease; circulation; cognitive performance; colon cancer; coronary heart disease (preventive); Crohn disease; cystic fibrosis; depression; diabetes; diabetes, type 2; dysmenorrhea; eczema, psoriasis; fatigue; headache; heart disease and heart attack (risk reduction), including women; herpes simplex 2; hypercholesterolemia; hypertension; hypertriglyceridemia; IgA nephropathy; immune support; infant eye/brain development; lupus; memory enhancement; multiple sclerosis; nephrotic syndrome; preeclampsia; premenstrual syndrome (PMS); prevention of graft failure after heart bypass surgery; protection from cyclosporine toxicity in organ transplant patients; rheumatoid arthritis; rosacea; schizophrenia; scleroderma; stroke (risk reduction); ulcerative colitis
Flaxseed oil	Acne vulgaris; arthritis (rheumatoid); asthma; breast cancer; constipation; coronary heart disease (risk reduction); cyclic mastalgia; diabetes; hemorrhoids; HIV/AIDS; hyperlipidemia; hypertension; lupus nephritis; menopausal symptoms; multiple sclerosis; omega-3 essential fatty acid source (cell wall and cellular membrane structure; cholesterol transport and oxidation); premenstrual syndrome (PMS); prostaglandins production; psoriasis; stroke (risk reduction); systemic lupus erythematosus (SLE)
Folic acid	Alcoholism; anemia; atherosclerosis; beta-thalassemia; cancer (preventive; colon and breast); cardiovascular morbidity or mortality in patients with chronic renal failure; cervical dysplasia; cognitive function; coronary heart disease (risk reduction); coronary restenosis (rate reduction by decreasing plasma homocysteine levels); Crohn disease; dementia and Alzheimer disease (risk reduction); depression; endothelial dysfunction (in type 2 diabetes); gingivitis; hearing loss (slows progression); homocysteine; methotrexate toxicity; nitrate tolerance; osteoporosis; pregnancy (prevention of birth defects) and lactation; schizophrenia (risk reduction, by decreasing homocysteine levels); ulcer, aphthous; vitiligo
Gamma Linolenic Acid (GLA)	Acute respiratory distress syndrome; atopic dermatitis; attention-deficit hyperactivity disorder (ADHD); blood pressure control; cancer treatment (adjunct); diabetic neuropathy; immune enhancement; mastalgia; menopausal hot flashes; migraine; osteoporosis; preeclampsia; premenstrual syndrome (PMS); pruritus; rheumatoid arthritis; Sjögren syndrome; ulcerative colitis
Garcinia (*Garcinia cambogia*)	Exercise performance; halitosis; pancreatic function (supportive) and glucose regulation; weight loss
Garlic (*Allium sativum*)	Alopecia; antimicrobial (bacterial and fungal); antioxidant (practitioners should be aware that aged garlic extracts have been reported to improve this benefit); atherosclerosis; cancer (prevention); coagulation (mild inhibitor of platelet-activating factor); cryptococcal meningitis; hyperlipidemia; hypertension; immune support; peripheral vascular disease; tick repellant; upper respiratory tract infection
Ginger (*Zingiber officinale*)	Antiemetic, for nausea and vomiting in pregnancy; antiinflammatory (musculoskeletal); diverticulitis; indigestion/heartburn; motion sickness; osteoarthritis

◀ **PROPOSED MEDICINAL CLAIMS** *continued*

Herb	Reported Uses
Ginkgo (*Ginkgo biloba*)	Acute ischemic stroke; Alzheimer disease, dementia; anxiety; asthma; chemotherapy (adjunct); chronic cochleovestibular disorders; cognitive function; depression; epilepsy; functional measures (in patients with multiple sclerosis); gastric cancer; glaucoma; headache; intermittent claudication; macular degeneration; memory enhancement; mountain sickness; multiple sclerosis; ocular blood flow; Parkinson disease; peripheral blood flow (cerebral vascular disease, peripheral vascular insufficiency, impotence, tinnitus, and depression); premenstrual syndrome (PMS); quality of life; Raynaud phenomenon; retinopathy; seasonal affective disorder (SAD); seizures; sexual dysfunction (antidepressant-induced); tinnitus; vertigo; vitiligo
Ginseng, Panax (*Panax ginseng*)	Adrenal tonic; chemotherapy and radiation (adjunct); diabetes; immune support; physical and mental performance, energy enhancement
Ginseng, Siberian (*Eleutherococcus senticosus*)	Adaptogen/tonic (promote wellness); athletic performance (enhancement); stress (decreased fatigue); immune support
Glucosamine	Chronic venous insufficiency; inflammatory bowel disease; knee injury recovery; osteoarthritis and joint structure support; rheumatoid arthritis and other inflammatory conditions; temporomandibular joint (TMJ)
Glutamine	Alcoholism; athletic performance (enhancement); cancer (adjunct); catabolic wasting; chemotherapy (prevention of adverse effects); critical illness; fibromyalgia; HIV (adjunct); HIV wasting; immune support; muscular dystrophy; peptic ulcer disease; postsurgical healing; ulcerative colitis and other inflammatory bowel diseases
Glutathione	Antioxidant, chemoprotection; hepatoprotection (alcohol-induced liver damage); immune support; male infertility; peptic ulcer disease; peripheral artery disease
Golden seal (*Hydrastis canadensis*)	Antimicrobial (antibacterial/antifungal); bronchitis, cystitis, and infectious diarrhea; fever; gallbladder; gastritis; heart failure; immune stimulation; malaria (chloroquine resistant); mucous membrane tonifying (used in inflammation of mucosal membranes); narcotic concealment (urine analysis); sinusitis; sore throat; trachoma; urinary tract infection (UTI)
Gotu kola (*Centella asiatica*)	Anxiety; connective tissue (support); diabetic microangiopathy; hemorrhoids (topical); macular degeneration; memory enhancement; psoriasis; venous insufficiency; wound healing (topical)
Grapefruit seed (*Citrus paradisi*)	Antifungal, antibacterial, antiparasitic; diarrhea; diverticulitis; eczema; endometriosis; heart disease; irritable bowel syndrome (IBS); rosacea; sinusitis; sore throat; ulcerative colitis; urinary tract infection (UTI)
Grapeseed (*Vitis vinifera*)	Agitation (aromatherapy); allergies, antiinflammatory, asthma; antioxidant; cardiovascular health; chloasma; circulation, platelet aggregation inhibitor, capillary fragility, arterial/venous insufficiency (intermittent claudification, varicose veins); gingivitis; glaucoma; hyperlipidemia; macular degeneration; multiple sclerosis; Parkinson disease; scleroderma; sun protection
Green tea (*Camellia sinensis*)	Antioxidant; cancer and cardiovascular disease (preventive); chemotherapy and radiation (adjunct); diabetes; diarrhea; gingivitis; human T-cell lymphocytic virus; hypercholesterolemia; hypertension; hypertriglyceridemia; macular degeneration; photoprotection; platelet-aggregation inhibitor; weight loss
Guggul (*Commiphora mukul*)	Acne vulgaris; hypercholesterolemia; hypothyroidism; osteoarthritis; rheumatoid arthritis; weight loss
Gymnema (*Gymnema sylvestre*)	Diabetes, blood sugar regulation; hyperlipidemia
Hawthorn (*Crataegus oxyacantha*)	Angina; hypotension, hypertension, peripheral vascular disease, tachycardia; cardiotonic; congestive heart failure; heart failure
Hops (*Humulus lupulus*)	Sedative/hypnotic (mild)
Horse chestnut (*Aesculus hippocastanum*)	Scleroderma; venous insufficiency (varicose veins, hemorrhoids, deep venous thrombosis, lower extremity edema [oral and topical])
Horsetail (*Equisetum arvense*)	Bone and connective tissue strengthening, including osteoporosis; diuretic; high mineral content (including silicic acid)
HuperzineA (*Huperzia serrata*)	Myasthenia gravis; senile dementia and Alzheimer disease

PROPOSED MEDICINAL CLAIMS *continued*

Herb	Reported Uses
Hydroxymethyl butyrate (HMB)	AIDS wasting; athletic performance (enhancement); muscle damage
5-Hydroxytryptophan (5-HTP)	Anxiety; cerebellar ataxia; depression; fibromyalgia; headache; migraine; schizophrenia; sleep disorders, insomnia (stimulates the production of melatonin); weight loss/obesity
Hyssop (*Hyssopus officinalis*)	Kidney inflammation
Inositol hexaphosphate (IP-6)	Cancer (preventive); intermittent claudication
Iodine	Bacterial conjunctivitis; bladder irrigation; bowel irrigation; cancer; cognitive function; corpus vitreous degeneration; fibrocystic breast disease (FBD); filarial lymphoedema; goiter (preventive); Graves disease; hypothyroidism; molluscum; mucolytic; ophthalmia neonatorum (preventive); oral intubation; periodontitis/gingivitis; pneumonia; postcesarean endometriosis; renal pelvic instillation sclerotherapy; skin disinfectant (wound cleansing); thyrotoxicosis; water purification
Ipriflavone	Menopausal symptoms; prevention of osteoporosis (men and women)
Iron	ACE inhibitor-associated cough; anemia; athletic performance; attention-deficit hyperactivity disorder (ADHD); blood transfusions (reduction); cognitive performance; hyposalivation; menorrhagia; nutritional status (infants/children); pregnancy; restless legs syndrome
Isoflavones (soy)	Benign prostatic hyperplasia (BPH); bone mineral density (increase); cancer (preventive); cardiovascular effects; cervical dysplasia; chemotherapy (adjunct); cognitive function; diarrhea; endometriosis; hypercholesterolemia; immune function; menopausal symptoms; menstrual migraine; osteoarthritis; osteoporosis; premenstrual syndrome (PMS); weight loss
Kava kava (*Piper methysticum*)	Anxiety/stress, skeletal muscle relaxation, postischemic episodes; fibromyalgia; insomnia; muscle soreness
Kudzu (*Pueraria lobata*)	Alcoholism; cardiovascular disease/angina; deafness; diabetes; diabetic retinopathy; glaucoma; menopausal symptoms
Lactobacillus acidophilus	Allergies; bacterial vaginosis; colitis; constipation; diarrhea (infantile); eczema (preventive); gastrointestinal microflora recolonization; hepatic encephalopathy; hypercholesterolemia; immune support; irritable bowel syndrome (IBS); lactose intolerance; vaginal candidiasis
Lavender (*Lavendula officinalis*)	Anxiety; cancer; dementia; depression; hypnotic/sleep; perineal discomfort following childbirth; spasmolytic (oral); wound healing including minor burns (topical)
Lecithin	Acne vulgaris; dementia (ineffective); extrapyramidal disorders; hepatic steatosis; hypercholesterolemia
Lemon balm/Melissa (*Melissa officinalis*)	Agitation in dementia; antiviral (oral herpes virus); anxiety; attention-deficit hyperactivity disorder (ADHD); cognitive performance; colitis; dyspepsia; sedation (pediatrics); sleep quality; teething (topical)
Licorice (*Glycyrrhiza glabra*)	Adrenal insufficiency (licorice); aphthous ulcers/canker sores; atopic dermatitis; body fat mass reduction; Crohn disease; croup; expectorant and antitussive (licorice); familial Mediterranean fever (FMF); gastrointestinal ulceration (DGL chewable products); herpes simplex; hyperkalemia; viral hepatitis
Liver extract	Chronic fatigue syndrome; liver tonic; pernicious anemia
Lutein	Antioxidant; cataracts; colon cancer; macular degeneration; pre-eclampsia; visual acuity
Lycopene	Asthma (exercise induced); atherosclerosis; cancer (preventive; especially colon, lung, and prostate); macular degeneration; oral submucous fibrosis
Lysine	Angina pectoris; growth and development (children); herpes simplex; osteoporosis; ulcer, aphthous

PROPOSED MEDICINAL CLAIMS *continued*

Herb	Reported Uses
Magnesium	Acute tocolysis of preterm labor; arrhythmias/torsades de pointes; asthma; attention-deficit hyperactivity disorder (ADHD); cardiovascular disease; circulation; colic (magnesium salt); congestive heart failure (CHF); constipation; coronary artery disease; diabetes; dysmenorrhea; epilepsy; fatigue; fibromyalgia (magnesium salt); gallbladder (magnesium salt); hearing loss; heart disease; hypertension; hypoglycemia; insomnia; kidney stones; migraine headache; mitral valve prolapse (MVP); multiple sclerosis; muscle cramps; nervousness; neuropathic pain; osteoporosis; pre-eclampsia/eclampsia; premenstrual syndrome (PMS); stress/anxiety; tension headache
Maitake (*Grifola frondosa*)	Cancer
Malic acid	Aluminum toxicity; fibromyalgia
Manganese	Diabetes; epilepsy; menstrual symptoms; osteoporosis
Marshmallow (*Althaea officinalis*)	Cough; croup; mucilaginous, demulcent; peptic ulcer disease; skin inflammatory conditions; sore throat
Mastic (*Pistacia lentiscus*)	Dental plaque; *H. pylori* inhibitor; peptic ulcer disease
Melatonin	ADHD (sleep disorders); Alzheimer disease (sleep disorders); autism (sleep disorders); benzodiazepine tapering; bipolar disorder; cancer; cardioprotection; chemotherapy adverse effects; depression (sleep disturbances); dyspepsia; glaucoma; glycemic control; headache prevention; HIV/AIDS; hypertension; insomnia; irritable bowel syndrome; jet lag; nocturia; oxidative stress in dialysis patients (preventive); Parkinson disease; periodic limb movement disorder; preoperative sedation/anxiolysis; Rett syndrome; sarcoidosis, chronic; schizophrenia (sleep disorders); seasonal affective disorder (SAD); sedation (children); seizure disorders; skin damage; sleep disturbances; stroke; tardive dyskinesia; thrombocytopenia; tinnitus (sleep disorders)
Methionine	Acetaminophen toxicity; liver detoxification
Methyl sulfonyl methane (MSM)	Allergies; analgesic; arthritis (osteo and rheumatoid); interstitial cystitis; lupus; seasonal allergic rhinitis
Milk thistle (*Silybum marianum*)	*Amanita phalloides* mushroom toxicity; antidote for poisoning by Death Cup mushroom; antioxidant (specifically hepatic cells), acute/chronic hepatitis, jaundice, and stimulation of bile secretion/cholagogue; chemotherapy and radiation (adjunct); cirrhosis; constipation; diabetes; eczema; gallbladder; halitosis; hepatoprotective, including drug toxicities (ie, phenothiazines, butyrophenones, ethanol, and acetaminophen); hyperthyroidism; psoriasis; rosacea
Modified citrus pectin (MCP)	Anticarcinogenic; detoxification (toxic elements); diarrhea; hypercholesterolemia; prostate cancer
Muira puama (*Ptychopetalum olacoides*)	Athletic performance (enhancement); erectile dysfunction; sexual vitality (males)
N-Acetyl cysteine (NAC)	Acetaminophen toxicity; acute respiratory distress syndrome (ARDS); acute respiratory infection; angina; asthma (mucolytic, antioxidant); bronchitis; cancer; cardioprotection (during chemotherapy); cerebral adrenoleukodystrophy; chemotherapy adverse effects; chronic obstructive pulmonary disease (COPD); fatigue; glutathione production; heavy metal detoxification; HIV/AIDS; hyperthyroidism; hypothyroidism; influenza prevention; macular degeneration; multiple sclerosis; myocardial infarction; nephropathy (preventive); ovulation (induction in polycystic ovary syndrome); Parkinson disease; polycystic ovarian syndrome; renal impairment; scleroderma; sepsis; Sjögren syndrome; systemic lupus erythematosus (SLE)
Nicotinamide adenine dinucleotide (NADH)	Chronic fatigue syndrome; dementia; diabetes, type 1; hepatitis; Parkinson disease; stamina and energy
Octacosanol	Hypercholesterolemia; Parkinson disease
Olive leaf (*Olea europaea*)	Acne vulgaris; antibacterial; antifungal, antiviral; Crohn disease; diabetes; diarrhea; diverticulitis; eczema; endometriosis; hypertension; multiple sclerosis; scleroderma; ulcerative colitis; urinary tract infection (UTI)
Pancreatic extract	Antiinflammatory; cancer (adjunct); celiac disease; digestive disturbances; food allergies; immune complex diseases; malabsorption
Para-Aminobenzoic acid (PABA)	Peyronie disease; scleroderma; vitiligo

PROPOSED MEDICINAL CLAIMS *continued*

Herb	Reported Uses
Parsley (*Petroselinum crispum*)	Halitosis; antibacterial, antifungal
Passion flower (*Passiflora spp*)	Congestive heart failure (CHF); hyperthyroidism; insomnia (sedative)
Peppermint (*Mentha piperita*)	Brain injury (aromatherapy); carminative, spasmolytic; colic; cough; dyspepsia; gastrointestinal disorders, antispasmodic; indigestion; irritable bowel syndrome; motion sickness; nasal congestion; postherpetic neuralgia; postoperative nausea (inhalation); tension headache (topical)
Phenylalanine	Analgesic; depression; pain; Parkinson disease; reward deficiency syndrome in addiction; vitiligo
Phosphatidyl choline (PC)	Alcohol-induced liver damage; Alzheimer disease; gallstones; hepatitis; hypercholesterolemia; tardive dyskinesia
Phosphatidyl serine (PS)	Alzheimer disease; depression; memory enhancement
Phosphorus	Bowel cleansing; burns; diabetic ketoacidosis; hypercalcemia; hypercalciuria; hyperparathyroidism; hypophosphatemia; kidney stones; refeeding syndrome prevention; total parenteral nutrition (TPN); vitamin D resistant rickets
Policosanol	Coronary heart disease; hypercholesterolemia; intermittent claudication; platelet aggregation inhibition; reactivity/brain activity
Potassium	Bone loss; cardiac arrhythmias; congestive heart failure (CHF); hypercalciuria; hypertension; kidney stones; molluscum contagiosum; QT prolongation
Pregnenolone	Arthritis; hormone precursor (DHEA, cortisol, progesterone, estrogens, and testosterone); mental performance
Progesterone	Brain injury; breast cancer (preventive); dysmenorrhea; endometriosis; infertility; menopause; osteoporosis; premenstrual syndromes (PMS); preterm birth
Psyllium (*Plantago ovata, Plantago isphagula*)	Anal fissures; bulk-forming laxative (containing 10% to 30% mucilage); colon cancer; colonoscopy preparation; diarrhea; flatulence; halitosis; hemorrhoids; hypercholesterolemia; hyperglycemia; induction of labor; inflammatory bowel disease; irritable bowel syndrome (IBS); obesity
Pycnogenol (*Pinus pinaster*)	Asthma; attention-deficit hyperactivity disorder (ADHD); chronic venous insufficiency; climacteric syndrome; diabetes, type 2; diabetic microangiopathy; erectile dysfunction; gingival bleeding/plaque; hypertension; platelet aggregation (smokers); prevention of blood clots during long airplane flights; retinopathy; systemic lupus erythematosus (SLE); venous leg ulcers
Pygeum (*Pygeum africanum, Prunus africana*)	Benign prostatic hyperplasia (BPH)
Pyruvate	Athletic performance (enhancement); hyperlipidemia; photoaging; weight loss
Quercetin	Allergies; asthma; atherosclerosis; cardiovascular disease; cataracts; peptic ulcer disease; prostatitis; sinusitis
Red clover (*Trifolium pratense*)	Benign prostatic hyperplasia (BPH); endometriosis; hypercholesterolemia; liver and kidney detoxification (liquid extract); menopause symptoms (proprietary extract contains 4 phytoestrogens); menorrhagia; osteoporosis; prostate cancer
Red yeast rice (*Monascus purpureus*)	Hypercholesterolemia
Rehmannia (*Rehmannia glutinosa*)	Aplastic anemia (adjuvant); rheumatoid arthritis; Sheehan syndrome; systemic lupus erythematosus (SLE)
Reishi (*Ganoderma lucidum*)	Chemotherapy and radiation (adjunct); chronic hepatitis B; coronary heart disease; diabetes, type 2; fatigue; hypertension; immune support; poisoning; postherpetic neuralgia; proteinuria; seizure disorder
SAMe (S-adenosyl methionine)	Attention-deficit hyperactivity disorder (ADHD); cardiovascular disease; cholestasis; depression; fibromyalgia; headache; insomnia; liver disease; osteoarthritis; rheumatoid arthritis
Saw palmetto (*Serenoa repens*)	Androgenetic alopecia (topical); benign prostatic hyperplasia (BPH)

Herb	Reported Uses
Schisandra (*Schizandra chinensis*)	Adaptogen/tonic (to promote wellness); hepatic protection and detoxification; chemotherapy and radiation (adjunct); endurance, stamina, and work performance (enhancement); decreases fatigue
Selenium	Acne vulgaris (with vitamin E); AIDS/HIV; asthma; atherosclerosis; bronchial asthma; burns; cancer (preventive); cardiomyopathy; cardiovascular disease; cataracts; chemotherapy and radiation (adjunct); chromosome damage (reduction); circulation; cystic fibrosis; dandruff; diabetes; dialysis; eczema; epilepsy; esophageal cancer; gastric cancer; hemorrhoids; herpes simplex 1 and 2; hypothyroidism; infection; infertility; intracranial pressure symptoms; low birth weight; lymphedema; macular degeneration; myotonic dystrophy; pancreatitis; preeclampsia; prostate cancer (preventive); psoriasis; sepsis; thyroid conditions; tinea capitis; tinea versicolor; ulcerative colitis
Senna (*Cassia senna*)	Bowel preparation for colonoscopy; laxative
Shark cartilage	Analgesia; cancer therapy; macular degeneration; osteoarthritis, rheumatoid arthritis; psoriasis
Skullcap (*Scutellaria lateriflora*)	Anxiety; cancer (*in vitro*); inflammation (*in vitro*)
Slippery Elm (*Ulmus fulva, Ulmus rubra*)	Cancer; diarrhea; gastrointestinal disorders; sore throat
Spleen extract	Chemotherapy and radiation (adjunct); cold/influenza; fatigue; spleen function (supportive)
Stinging nettle (*Urtica dioica*)	Leaf used for allergic rhinitis, allergy, and hay fever symptoms, arthritis, joint pain, sinusitis, uric acid excretion; root used for benign prostatic hyperplasia (BPH)
St John's wort (*Hypericum perforatum*)	Antibacterial, antiinflammatory (topical: minor wounds, infections, bruises, muscle soreness, and sprains); antiviral; atopic dermatitis; climacteric symptoms (combination therapy); mild to moderate depression, depression (children), seasonal affective disorder (SAD), melancholia, stress and anxiety; obsessive compulsive disorder (OCD); perimenopausal symptoms; premenstrual syndrome (PMS); smoking cessation; social phobia; somatoform disorders
Taurine	Congestive heart failure (CHF); cystic fibrosis; diabetes; energy; gallbladder; hypercholesterolemia; hypertension; iron deficiency anemia; liver disease; myotonic dystrophy; nutritional supplement (infant formula); nutritional support (TPN); obesity; seizure disorders; surgery; vaccine adjunct; vision problems
Tea tree (*Melaleuca alternifolia*)	**Not for ingestion**; acne vulgaris; antifungal, antibacterial; mouthwash for dental and oral health; burns, cuts, scrapes, insect bites
Thyme (*Thymus vulgaris*)	Alopecia areata; antifungal; bronchitis with cough; cough (upper respiratory origin); croup; dental plaque; inflammatory skin disorders
Thymus extract	Fatigue; food allergies; immune support; otitis media; respiratory tract infection; sinusitis; systemic lupus erythematosus (SLE)
Thyroid extract	Fatigue; immune support; fibromyalgia; hypothyroidism
Tocotrienols	Atherosclerosis; cancer (preventive); heart disease; hypercholesterolemia; skin (supportive, protective)
Tribulus (*Tribulus terrestris*)	Athletic performance (enhancement); coronary artery disease; infertility; muscle strength; sexual vitality
Turmeric (*Curcuma longa*)	Antioxidant; antiinflammatory; antirheumatic; cancer; cholelithiasis prevention; hypercholesterolemia; dysmenorrhea; dyspepsia; HIV; muscle soreness; peptic ulcer disease; scabies; uveitis
Tylophora (*Tylophora asthmatica*)	Allergies; asthma
Tyrosine	Alzheimer disease; attention-deficit disorder and attention-deficit hyperactivity disorder (ADD/ADHD); cocaine cravings; depression; hypertension; hypothyroidism; narcolepsy; phenylketonuria (PKU); Rett syndrome; schizophrenia; stress; substance abuse
Uva Ursi (*Arctostaphylos uva-ursi*)	Hyperpigmentation; urinary tract infections and kidney stone prevention
Valerian (*Valeriana officinalis*)	Anxiety; hyperthyroidism; insomnia (sedative/hypnotic); premenstrual syndrome (PMS), menopause; restless motor syndromes and muscle spasms

PROPOSED MEDICINAL CLAIMS *continued*

Herb	Reported Uses
Vanadium	Diabetes, type 1; diabetes, type 2; hypercholesterolemia; hypoglycemia; pneumonia
Vinpocetine	Acute ischemic stroke; Alzheimer disease and senility; cognitive function; hearing impairment; joint disorders; urinary incontinence
Vitamin A (Retinol)	Acne vulgaris; AIDS; cancer (preventive); cervical dysplasia; circulation; cold/influenza; Crohn disease; diverticulitis; eczema; esophageal cancer; fibrocystic breast disease (FBD); gastric cancer; glaucoma; goiter; hemorrhoids; immune function; infant mortality; iron deficiency anemia; malaria; measles; menorrhagia; night blindness; norovirus; otitis media; photorefractive keratectomy; pneumonia; polp prevention; pregnancy related complications; premenstrual syndrome (PMS); psoriasis; respiratory infection; rosacea; skin aging, wrinkles; skin cancer preventive; sore throat; ulcerative colitis; urinary tract infection (UTI); weight loss; wound healing; xerophthalmia
Vitamin B_1 (Thiamine)	Alcoholism; Alzheimer disease; anemia (megaloblastic); cancer; cataract prevention; congestive heart failure (CHF); Crohn disease; diabetes; endothelial function; fibromyalgia; heart failure (cardiomyopathy); insomnia; metabolic disorders; neurological conditions (Bell palsy, trigeminal neuralgia, sciatica, sensory neuropathies); psychiatric illness; pyruvate dehydrogenase deficiency (PDH); total parenteral nutrition (TPN); Wolfram syndrome (DIDMOAD)
Vitamin B_2	Anemia; anorexia/bulimia; cataracts; depression; esophageal cancer; ethylmalonic encephalopathy; malaria; migraine; neonatal jaundice; pre-eclampsia
Vitamin B_3	Acne vulgaris (4% niacinamide topical gel); atherosclerosis; cataracts; coronary disease (preventive); diabetes, type 1; diabetes, type 2; hyperlipidemia (hypercholesterolemia, hypertriglyceridemia); impaired glucose tolerance; intermittent claudication; myocardial infarction (risk reduction); osteoarthritis; pellagra; Raynaud phenomenon; rheumatoid arthritis; schizophrenia
Vitamin B_5 (Pantothenic acid)	Adrenal support; allergies; arthritis; athletic performance (enhancement); attention-deficit hyperactivity disorder (ADHD); constipation; hyperlipidemia (pantethine, but not pantothenic acid, lowers cholesterol and triglycerides); osteoarthritis; rheumatoid arthritis; wound healing
Vitamin B_6 (Pyridoxine)	Akathisia; Alzheimer disease; angioplasty; arthritis; asthma; attention-deficit hyperactivity disorder (ADHD); autism; birth outcomes; cardiovascular disease; carpal tunnel syndrome; coronary heart disease (risk reduction); coronary restenosis (rate reduction by lowering plasma homocysteine levels); dementia (risk reduction); depression (associated with oral contraceptives); diabetic peripheral neuropathy; epilepsy, B_6 dependant; headache; hereditary sideroblastic anemia; homocysteine (reduction); hyperkinetic syndrome; immune function; insomnia; kidney stones; lactation suppression; monosodium glutamate (MSG) sensitivity; nausea and vomiting (in pregnancy); peptic ulcer disease; premenstrual syndrome (PMS); pyridoxine dependent seizures in newborns; tardive dyskinesia
Vitamin B_{12} (Cobalamin)	AIDS; angioplasty; asthma; atherosclerosis (due to homocysteine elevation); breast cancer; coronary heart disease; coronary restenosis (rate reduction by lowering plasma homocysteine levels); Crohn disease; dementia and Alzheimer disease (risk reduction); depression; diabetic peripheral neuropathy; fatigue; homocysteine (reduction); Imerslund-Grasbeck disease; male infertility; megaloblastic anemia; memory loss; multiple sclerosis; pernicious anemia; sickle cell disease; sulfite sensitivity
Vitamin B complex-25	See individual B vitamins

▶

Herb	Reported Uses
Vitamin C	AIDS; alkaptonuria; allergies; Alzheimer disease; asthma; atherosclerosis; cancer; cardiovascular disease (negative report); cataracts; cervical dysplasia; chromosome damage (reduction); circulation; cold; constipation; coronary heart disease (preventive, in patients taking lipid-lowering agents); Crohn disease; diabetes; diabetes, type 2; diverticulitis; eczema; endometriosis; fatigue; fever; fibrocystic breast disease (FBD); fibromyalgia; gallbladder disease (risk reduction); gingivitis; glaucoma; herpes simplex virus 1 and 2; *helicobacter pylori* (combination therapy); immune support; iron absorption enhancement; irritable bowel syndrome (IBS); LDL oxidation (decrease in males); macular degeneration; multiple sclerosis; myocardial infarction (risk reduction); nitrate tolerance (preventive); osteoporosis; otitis media; pain (complex regional pain syndrome with wrist fracture); Parkinson disease; peptic ulcer disease; plaque; pregnancy; psoriasis; reflex sympathetic dystrophy (preventive); sinusitis; sore throat; stress/anxiety; stroke (preventive); sunburn; ulcerative colitis; urinary tract infection (UTI); vaginitis; wound healing
Vitamin D	Cancer, congestive heart failure; Crohn disease; diabetes; epilepsy (during anticonvulsant therapy); fall prevention; familial hypophosphatemia; Fanconi syndrome; hearing loss; hepatic osteodystrophy; hyperparathyroidism; hypertension; hypocalcemia; immune response (prevents reactivation of latent tuberculosis infection); immune response to hepatitis B vaccine; multiple sclerosis; muscle weakness; Myelodysplastic syndrome; nutritional status (breast-feeding women and infants); osteogenesis imperfecta; osteomalacia; osteoporosis; physical performance; prostate cancer; proximal myopathy; psoriasis; renal osteodystrophy; rheumatoid arthritis; rickets; scleroderma; seasonal affective disorder (SAD); senile warts; tooth retention; weight loss (combination therapy)
Vitamin E	Acne vulgaris (with selenium); Alzheimer disease; anemia; angina; arterial elasticity; atherosclerosis; Benign prostatic hyperplasia (BPH); bladder cancer; breast cancer (preventive); cardiovascular disease; cataracts; cervical dysplasia; chromosome damage (reduction); circulation; colon cancer (preventive); congestive heart failure; diabetes; diabetes, type 2; dyslipidemias; dysmenorrhea; eczema; endometriosis; epilepsy; esophageal caner; fibrocystic breast disease (FBD); G6PD deficiency; gallbladder; gastric cancer; glomerulosclerosis (kidney disease); hemorrhoids; hyperlipidemia; immune support; intermittent claudication; LDL oxidation (decrease in males); macular degeneration; mucositis (chemotherapy-induced); multiple sclerosis; myocardial infarction (risk reduction); neurotoxicity; osteoarthritis; Parkinson disease; peptic ulcer disease; peripheral circulation; photorefractive keratectomy; platelet aggregation; premenstrual syndrome (PMS); prostate cancer; psoriasis; respiratory infection (preventive); rheumatoid arthritis; scleroderma; steatohepatitis; sunburn; systemic lupus erythematosus; tardive dyskinesia; ulcerative colitis; venous thromboembolism
Vitamin K	Hepatitis C (preventive effects); hepatocellular carcinoma; osteoporosis; synthesis of blood clotting factors; warfarin toxicity
White oak (*Quercus alba*)	Antiinflammatory (mild: throat and mouth as a soothing agent)
White willow (*Salix alba*)	Antipyretic; antiinflammatory; headache; low back pain; osteoarthritis
Wild yam (*Dioscorea villosa*)	Female vitality (conversion to progesterone in the body is poor); hyperlipidemia; menopause

PROPOSED MEDICINAL CLAIMS *continued*

Herb	Reported Uses
Yohimbe (*Pausinystalia yohimbe*)	Autonomic failure; male erectile dysfunction; platelet aggregation inhibition; sexual side effects of SSRIs; sexual vitality (men and women); xerostomia (psychotropic drug induced)
Zinc	Acne vulgaris; alopecia areata; aphthous ulcers; attention-deficit hyperactivity disorder (ADHD); benign prostatic hyperplasia (BPH); beta-thalassemia; cirrhosis; closed head injuries; cognitive deficits (children); common cold; Crohn disease; dandruff; diabetes; diabetic neuropathy; diaper rash; diarrhea; diverticulitis; Down syndrome; exercise performance; fungal infections; gastric ulcer healing; Gilbert syndrome; halitosis; hepatic encephalopathy; hepatitis C; herpes simplex; HIV/AIDS; hyperlipidemia; immune support; infection; infertility; kwashiorkor; leg ulcers; leprosy; lower respiratory tract infection (children); macular degeneration; malaria; mucositis; muscle cramps; osteoporosis; otitis media; parasite infection; plaque/gingivitis; pneumonia; poisoning (arsenic); pregnancy; prostatitis (chronic); rheumatoid arthritis; rosacea; sexual vitality (men); sickle cell anemia; skin conditions, eczema, psoriasis; sore throat; stomatitis; taste perception; tinnitus; trichomoniasis; ulcerative colitis; viral warts; Wilson disease; wound healing

NEW DRUGS ADDED SINCE LAST EDITION

Brand Name	Generic Name	Use
Alka-Seltzer Plus® Sinus Formula; Contac® Cold + Flu Maximum Strength Non-Drowsy; Mapap® Sinus Congestion and Pain Daytime; Sinutab® Sinus; Sudafed PE® Sinus Headache; Tylenol® Sinus Congestion & Pain Daytime	acetaminophen and phenylephrine	Temporary relief of sinus/nasal congestion and pressure, headache, and minor aches and pains
Arcalyst™	rilonacept	Treatment of cryopyrin-associated periodic syndromes (CAPS)
Azor™	amlodipine and olmesartan	Treatment of hypertension
Bystolic™	nebivolol	Treatment of hypertension
Cimzia®	certolizumab pegol	Treatment of Crohn disease
Cleviprex™	clevidipine	Management of hypertension
Deplin™	methylfolate	Medicinal food for management of patients with low plasma and/or low red blood cell folate
Doribax™	doripenem	Treatment of complicated intraabdominal infections and complicated urinary tract infections
Emend® for Injection	fosaprepitant	Prevention of nausea and vomiting associated with chemotherapy
Entereg®	alvimopan	Improve upper and lower GI recovery following resection surgery with primary anastomosis
Intelence™	etravirine	Treatment of HIV-1 infection
Isentress™	raltegravir	Treatment of HIV-1 infection
Ixempra™	ixabepilone	Treatment of metastatic or locally-advanced breast cancer
Kinrix™	diphtheria and tetanus toxoids, acellular pertussis, and poliovirus (inactivated) vaccine	Active immunization against diphtheria, tetanus, pertussis, and poliomyelitis
Kuvan™	sapropterin	Adjunct to dietary management in the treatment of tetrahydrobiopterin (BH4) responsive phenylketonuria (PKU)
—	LEVOleucovorin	Rescue agent after high-dose methotrexate therapy in osteosarcoma; antidote for impaired methotrexate elimination and for inadvertent overdosage of folic acid antagonists
Lexiscan™	regadenoson	Radionuclide myocardial perfusion imaging (MPI)
Lymphazurin™	isosulfan blue	Adjunct to lymphography
Nplate™	romiplostim	Thrombocytopenia
Normocarb HF™; PrismaSol	electrolyte solution, renal replacement	Used as a replacement solution
Pentacel®	diphtheria and tetanus toxoids, acellular pertussis, poliovirus (inactivated) and *Haemophilus* b conjugate vaccine	Active immunization against diphtheria, tetanus, pertussis, poliomyelitis, and invasive disease caused by *H. influenzae* type b
PrandiMet™	repaglinide and metformin	Management of type 2 diabetes mellitus
Pristiq™	desvenlafaxine	Treatment of major depressive disorder
Relistor™	methylnaltrexone	Treatment of opioid-induced constipation in patients receiving palliative care with inadequate response to conventional laxative regimens

Brand Name	Generic Name	Use
Sclerosol®; Sterile Talc Powder™	talc (sterile)	Prevention of recurrence of malignant pleural effusion in symptomatic patients
Simcor®	niacin and simvastatin	Treatment of primary hypercholesterolemia, mixed dyslipidemia, or hypertriglyceridemia
Tasigna®	nilotinib	Treatment of Philadelphia chromosome-positive chronic myelogenous leukemia
Tekturna HCT®	aliskiren and hydrochlorothiazide	Treatment of hypertension
Treanda®	bendamustine	Treatment of chronic lymphocytic leukemia
Treximet™	sumatriptan and naproxen	Treatment of migraine

PENDING DRUGS OR DRUGS IN CLINICAL TRIALS

Proposed Brand Name or Synonym	Generic Name	Use
Actemra®	tocilizumab	Rheumatoid arthritis
Akten®	AK 1015	Ocular anesthesia
AP23573	deforolimus	Cancer
Aquavan®	fospropofol	Sedation
Arcoxia®	etoricoxib	Osteoarthritis
Atryn®	antithrombin alfa	Antithrombin III deficiency
Bridion®	sugammadex	Reversal of nondepolarizing muscle relaxants
CNTO-1275	ustekinumab	Psoriasis
Fanapta®	iloperidone	Schizophrenia
Gemasense®	oblimersen	Chronic lymphocytic leukemia
Isovorin™	levofolinic acid	Osteogenic sarcoma, colorectal cancer
Kiacta™ (formerly Fibrillex™)	eprodisate	Amyloid A amyloidosis
MCC	mycobacterial cell wall-DNA complex	Bladder cancer
Mozobil®	plerixafor	Enhancement of mobilization of hematopoietic stem cells
Multag®	dronedarone	Atrial flutter or fibrillation
NBI-34060	indiplon	Insomnia
Onglyza®	saxagliptin	Diabetes mellitus type II
Orplanta®	satraplatin	Prostate cancer
OT-730	—	Glaucoma
Promacta®	eltrombopag	Chronic idiopathic thrombocytopenic purpura (ITP)
Provenge™	sipuleucel-T	Prostate cancer
Rezonic®	casopitant	Chemotherapy-induced nausea/vomiting
RSD1235	vernakalant	Atrial fibrillation
Spera™	satraplatin	Prostate cancer
Surfaxin™	lucinactant	Respiratory distress syndrome
Xiaflex®	clostridial collagenase	Dupuytren contracture
Vimpat®	lacosamide	Diabetic neuropathy, seizures
Xarelto®	rivaroxaban	Deep vein thrombosis
Zimulti® (formerly Acomplia™)	rimonabant	Weight loss agent

INDICATION / THERAPEUTIC CATEGORY INDEX

Amebicide

Antibiotic, Miscellaneous

Antibiotic, Topical

ALLERGIC DISORDERS (NASAL)

ALLERGIC DISORDERS (OPHTHALMIC)

ALOPECIA

ALPHA₁-ANTITRYPSIN DEFICIENCY (CONGENITAL)

ANESTHESIA (OPHTHALMIC)

Local Anesthetic

ANGINA PECTORIS

Beta-Adrenergic Blocker

Calcium Channel Blocker

Cardiovascular Agent, Miscellaneous

Vasodilator

ARTHRITIS (RHEUMATOID)

ASCARIASIS

ASCITES

Diuretic, Thiazide

ASPERGILLOSIS

ASTHMA

BITES (INSECT)

Anticholinergic Agent

Beta$_2$-Adrenergic Agonist Agent

Bronchodilator

Expectorant

Mast Cell Stabilizer

Theophylline Derivative

BRUCELLOSIS

Antibiotic, Aminoglycoside

Antitubercular Agent

Tetracycline Derivative

BULLOUS SKIN DISEASE

Antibacterial, Topical

Gold Compound

Immunosuppressant Agent

Vitamin D Analog

Vitamin, Fat Soluble

CISPLATIN TOXICITY

Antidote

CLAUDICATION

Blood Viscosity Reducer Agent

CMV RETINITIS

Antiviral Agent

COCCIDIOIDOMYCOSIS

Antifungal Agent

COLD SORE

Antiviral Agent

COLITIS (ULCERATIVE)

5-Aminosalicylic Acid Derivative

Antiinflammatory Agent

COLLAGEN DISORDERS

Adrenal Corticosteroid

COLONIC EVACUATION

Laxative

CONDYLOMA ACUMINATUM

Antiviral Agent

Biological Response Modulator

Immune Response Modifier

Keratolytic Agent

CONGENITAL SUCRASE-ISOMALTASE DEFICIENCY

Enzyme

CONGESTION (NASAL)

Adrenergic Agonist Agent

CONGESTIVE HEART FAILURE

CONJUNCTIVITIS (ALLERGIC)

CONSTIPATION

CONSTIPATION (CHRONIC IDIOPATHIC)

Gastrointestinal Agent, Miscellaneous

COPROPORPHYRIA

Beta-Adrenergic Blocker

CORNEAL EDEMA

Lubricant, Ocular

COUGH

Antihistamine/Antitussive

Antihistamine/Decongestant/Antitussive

DEPRESSION

DIABETES INSIPIDUS

Hormone, Posterior Pituitary

Vasopressin Analog, Synthetic

DIABETES MELLITUS, INSULIN-DEPENDENT (IDDM)

Antidiabetic Agent

Antidiabetic Agent, Insulin

DIABETES MELLITUS, NONINSULIN-DEPENDENT (NIDDM)

DIAGNOSTIC AGENT (CUSHING SYNDROME)

DIAPER RASH

DIARRHEA

DIARRHEA (BACTERIAL)

DIARRHEA (BILE ACIDS)

DYSTONIA

Neuromuscular Blocker Agent, Toxin

DYSURIA

Analgesic, Urinary

Antispasmodic Agent, Urinary

EAR WAX

Otic Agent, Ceruminolytic

EATON-LAMBERT SYNDROME

Cholinergic Agent

ECHOCARDIOGRAM AID

Diagnostic Agent

ECLAMPSIA

Barbiturate

Benzodiazepine

ECZEMA

Adrenal Corticosteroid

Antifungal/Corticosteroid

Corticosteroid, Topical

ECZEMA

EDEMA

Diuretic, Combination

Diuretic, Loop

ENCEPHALITIS (HERPES VIRUS)

ENDOCARDITIS TREATMENT

FEVER

Antipyretic

FIBROCYSTIC BREAST DISEASE

Androgen

GASTRITIS

GASTROESOPHAGEAL REFLUX DISEASE (GERD)

Uricosuric Agent

Xanthine Oxidase Inhibitor

GRAFT VS HOST DISEASE

Immunosuppressant Agent

GRAM-NEGATIVE INFECTION

Aminoglycoside (Antibiotic)

Antibiotic, Carbapenem

Antibiotic, Irrigation

Antibiotic, Lincosamide

GRAM-POSITIVE INFECTION

Antibiotic, Cyclic Lipopeptide

GRANULOMA (INGUINALE)

Antibiotic, Aminoglycoside

Antitubercular Agent

GRANULOMATOUS DISEASE, CHRONIC

Biological Response Modulator

GROWTH HORMONE DEFICIENCY

Growth Hormone

HEADACHE (TENSION)

HEART BLOCK

Adrenergic Agonist Agent

HEARTBURN

Antacid

Histamine H$_2$ Antagonist

Proton Pump Inhibitor

HEAT PROSTRATION

Electrolyte Supplement, Oral

HEAVY METAL POISONING

Antidote

HELICOBACTER PYLORI

Antibiotic, Miscellaneous

Macrolide (Antibiotic)

Penicillin

Tetracycline Derivative

HEMOLYTIC DISEASE OF THE NEWBORN

Immune Globulin

HEMOPHILIA

Vasopressin Analog, Synthetic

HOMOCYSTINURIA

Homocystinuria Agent

HOOKWORMS

Anthelmintic

HORMONAL IMBALANCE (FEMALE)

Progestin

HUMAN PAPILLOMAVIRUS (HPV) TYPES 6, 11, 16, 18

Vaccine

HUNTINGTON CHOREA

Monoamine Depleting Agent

HYDATIDIFORM MOLE (BENIGN)

Prostaglandin

HYPERACIDITY

Antacid

HYPERLIPIDEMIA

HYPERMAGNESEMIA

HYPERMENORRHEA (TREATMENT)

HYPERTRIGLYCERIDEMIA

HYPOKALEMIA

HYPOMAGNESEMIA

Electrolyte Supplement, Oral

Electrolyte Supplement, Parenteral

Magnesium Salt

HYPOMOBILITY

Anti-Parkinson Agent (Dopamine Agonist)

HYPONATREMIA

Alkalinizing Agent

Electrolyte Supplement, Oral

Vasopressin Antagonist

HYPOPARATHYROIDISM

Diagnostic Agent

Vitamin D Analog

HYPOPHOSPHATEMIA

Electrolyte Supplement, Oral

KERATITIS (EXPOSURE)

KERATITIS (FUNGAL)

Antifungal Agent

KERATITIS (HERPES SIMPLEX)

Antiviral Agent

KERATITIS (VERNAL)

Antiviral Agent

Mast Cell Stabilizer

KERATOCONJUNCTIVITIS (VERNAL)

Mast Cell Stabilizer

KERATOSIS (ACTINIC)

Porphyrin Agent, Topical

KIDNEY STONE

Alkalinizing Agent

Chelating Agent

Electrolyte Supplement, Oral

Irrigating Solution

Urinary Tract Product

Xanthine Oxidase Inhibitor

LABOR INDUCTION

Oxytocic Agent

Prostaglandin

LABOR (PREMATURE)

Adrenergic Agonist Agent

LACTATION (SUPPRESSION)

Ergot Alkaloid and Derivative

MRI ENHANCEMENT

Radiopaque Agents

MUCOPOLYSACCHARIDOSIS I (MPS I)

Enzyme

MUCOPOLYSACCHARIDOSIS II (MPS II, HUNTER SYNDROME)

Enzyme

MUCOSITIS

Keratinocyte Growth Factor

MULTIPLE SCLEROSIS

Antigout Agent

Biological, Miscellaneous

Biological Response Modulator

Monoclonal Antibody, Selective Adhesion-Molecule Inhibitor

Skeletal Muscle Relaxant

MUMPS

Vaccine, Live (Viral)

Vaccine, Live Virus

MUSCARINE POISONING

Anticholinergic Agent

MUSCLE SPASM

Skeletal Muscle Relaxant

MYASTHENIA GRAVIS

Cholinergic Agent

MYCOBACTERIUM AVIUM-INTRACELLULARE

Antibiotic, Aminoglycoside

Antibiotic, Miscellaneous

MYCOSIS (FUNGOIDES)

MYDRIASIS

MYELODYSPLASTIC SYNDROME (MDS)

MYELOMA

MYOCARDIAL INFARCTION

NEURITIS (OPTIC)

Adrenal Corticosteroid

NEUROBLASTOMA

Antineoplastic Agent

NEUROGENIC BLADDER

Antispasmodic Agent, Urinary

NEUROLOGIC DISEASE

Adrenal Corticosteroid

NEUTROPENIA

Colony-Stimulating Factor

Nonsteroidal Antiinflammatory Drug (NSAID), COX-2 Selective

OSTEODYSTROPHY

Vitamin D Analog

OSTEOMALACIA

Vitamin D Analog

Analgesic, Opioid

Skeletal Muscle Relaxant

PAIN (ANOGENITAL)

Anesthetic/Corticosteroid

Local Anesthetic

PAIN (BONE)

Radiopharmaceutical

PAIN (DIABETIC NEUROPATHY NEURALGIA)

Analgesic, Topical

PAIN (LUMBAR PUNCTURE)

Analgesic, Topical

PAIN (MUSCLE)

Analgesic, Topical

PAIN (NEUROPATHIC)

Analgesic, Miscellaneous

PAIN (SKIN GRAFT HARVESTING)

Analgesic, Topical

PAIN (VENIPUNCTURE)

Analgesic, Topical

PANCREATIC EXOCRINE INSUFFICIENCY

Enzyme

PLAGUE

Antibiotic, Aminoglycoside

Antitubercular Agent

PLANTAR WARTS

Topical Skin Product

PLATELET AGGREGATION (PROPHYLAXIS)

Antiplatelet Agent

PNEUMOCYSTIS CARINII

PNEUMONIA

PREMATURE LUTEINIZING HORMONE (LH) SURGES

PREMENSTRUAL DYSPHORIC DISORDER (PMDD)

PRURITUS

PSEUDOGOUT

PSEUDOHYPOPARATHYROIDISM

PSORIASIS

PSYCHOSES

SJÖGREN SYNDROME

Cholinergic Agent

SKELETAL MUSCLE RELAXANT (SURGICAL)

Skeletal Muscle Relaxant

SKIN INFECTION

Antibiotic, Glycylcycline

SKIN INFECTION (TOPICAL THERAPY)

Aminoglycoside (Antibiotic)

Antibacterial, Topical

Antibiotic/Corticosteroid, Topical

Antibiotic, Miscellaneous

SKIN PROTECTANT

Pharmaceutical Aid

SKIN ULCER

Enzyme

SLEEPING SICKNESS

Antiprotozoal

Topical Skin Product

SMALLPOX

Immune Globulin

Vaccine

TISSUE GRAFT

TOOTHACHE

TOPICAL ANESTHESIA

2009

QUICK LOOK DRUG BOOK

Top 200 Prescribed Tablets and Capsules with Images

The Quick Look Drug Book 2009 Top 200 Prescribed Drugs insert displays actual color photographs of the most commonly prescribed tablets and capsules.

Drugs are listed alphabetically by generic name, and, where applicable, the trade name is listed. Dosages appear under each individual image.

Use the white scale at the bottom of each image to determine the

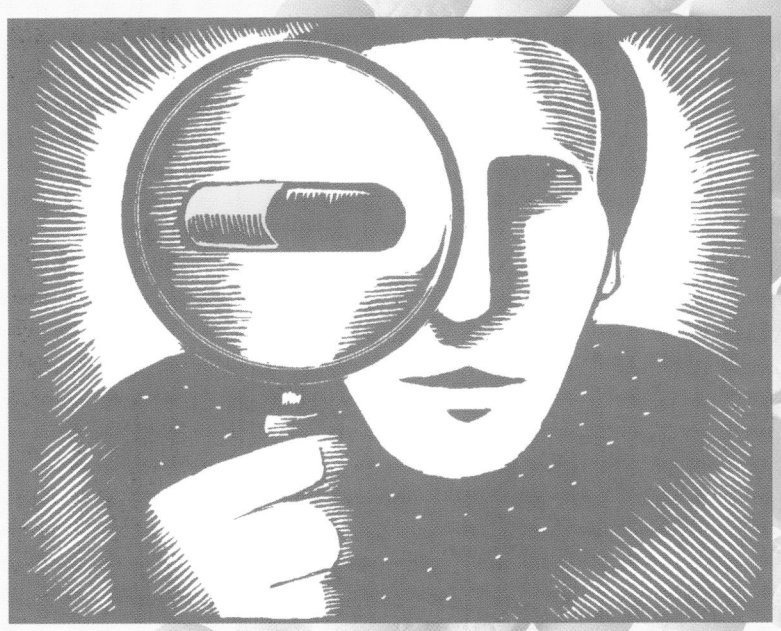

Acetaminophen and Codeine

(generic)

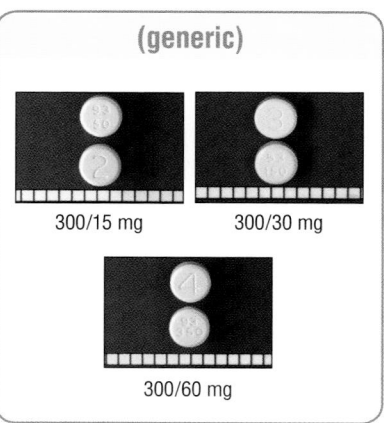

300/15 mg   300/30 mg

300/60 mg

Acyclovir

(generic)

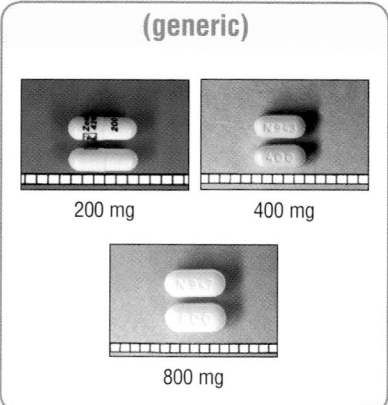

200 mg   400 mg

800 mg

Alendronate

Fosamax®

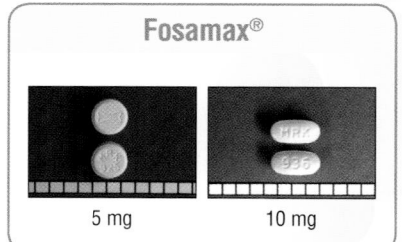

5 mg   10 mg

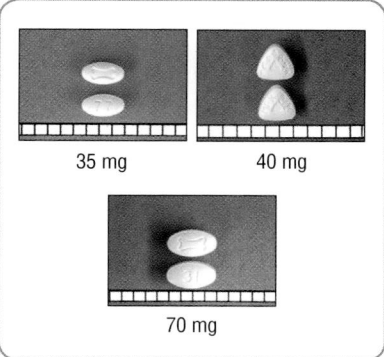

35 mg   40 mg

70 mg

Allopurinol

(generic)

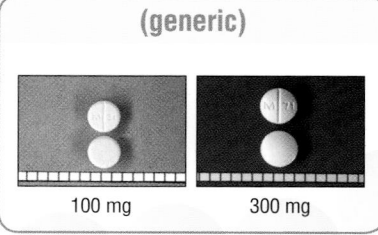

100 mg   300 mg

Alprazolam

(generic)

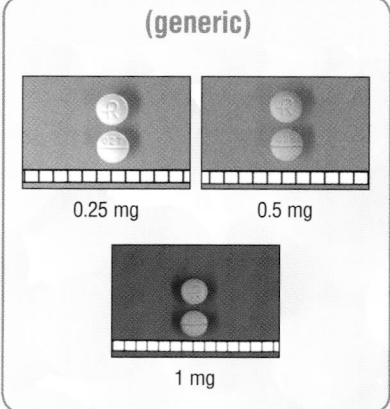

0.25 mg   0.5 mg

1 mg

Amitriptyline

(generic)

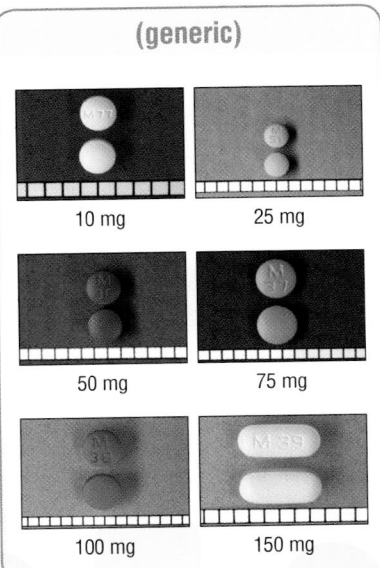

10 mg   25 mg

50 mg   75 mg

100 mg   150 mg

Amlodipine

(generic)

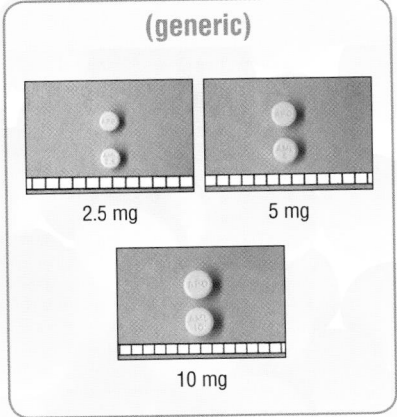

2.5 mg   5 mg

10 mg

Norvasc®

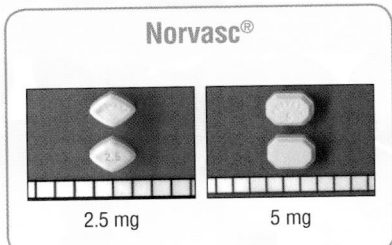

2.5 mg   5 mg

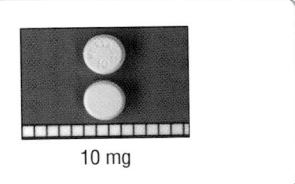

10 mg

Amlodipine and

Lotrel®

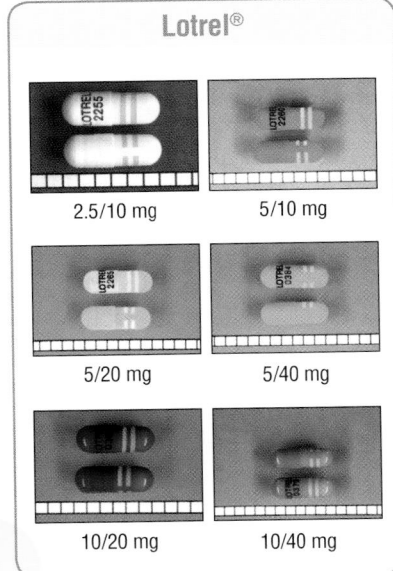

2.5/10 mg   5/10 mg

5/20 mg   5/40 mg

10/20 mg   10/40 mg

Amoxicillin

(generic)

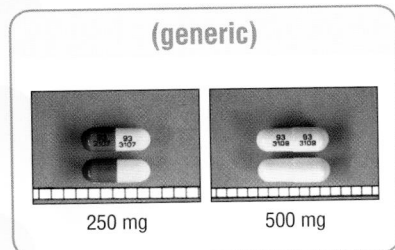

250 mg   500 mg

Amoxicillin and Clavulanate Potassium

(generic)

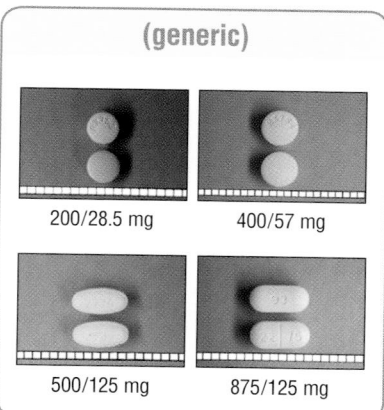

200/28.5 mg   400/57 mg

500/125 mg   875/125 mg

Aripiprazole

Abilify®

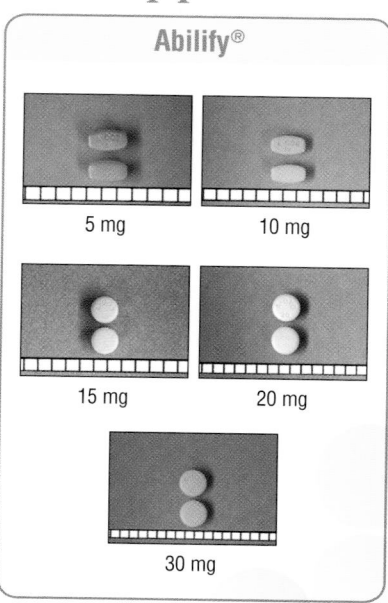

5 mg   10 mg

15 mg   20 mg

30 mg

Atenolol

(generic)

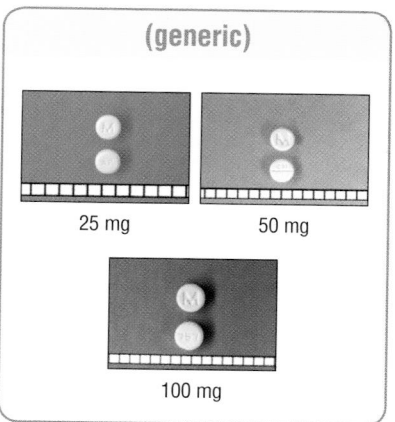

25 mg   50 mg

100 mg

Atorvastatin

Lipitor®

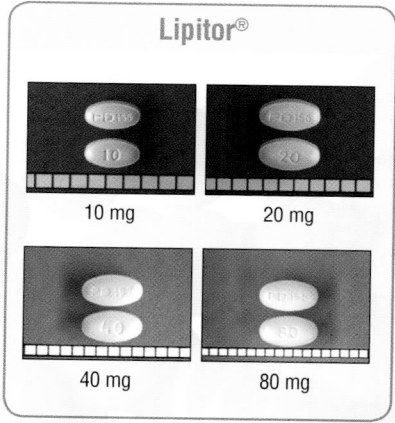

10 mg   20 mg

40 mg   80 mg

Azithromycin

(generic)

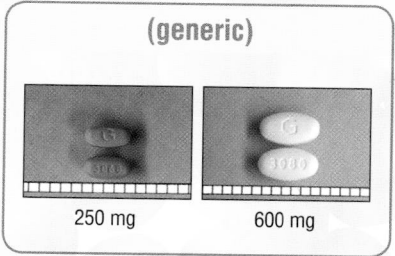

250 mg   600 mg

Benazepril

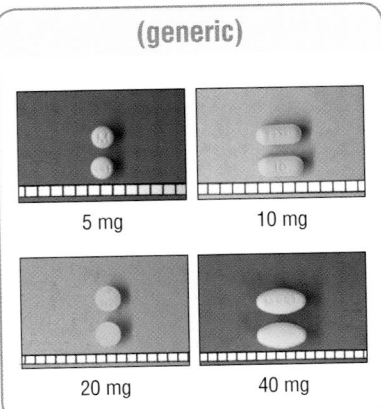

(generic)

5 mg · 10 mg · 20 mg · 40 mg

Bisoprolol and Hydrochlorothiazide

(generic)

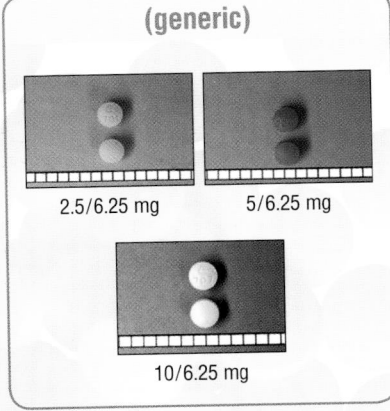

2.5/6.25 mg · 5/6.25 mg

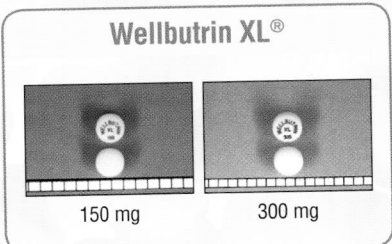

10/6.25 mg

Bupropion

Wellbutrin XL®

150 mg · 300 mg

(generic)

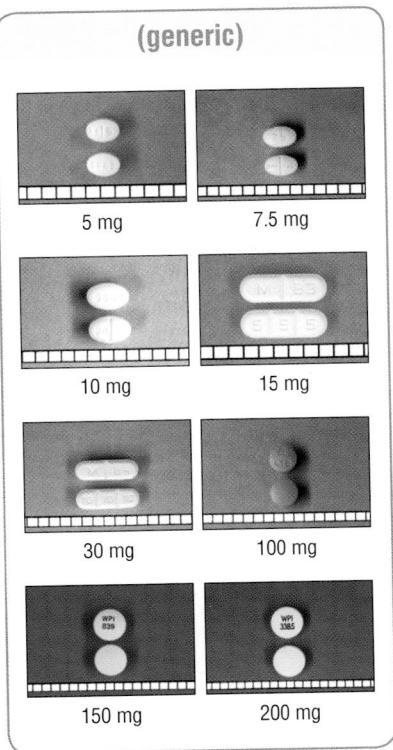

5 mg · 7.5 mg · 10 mg · 15 mg · 30 mg · 100 mg · 150 mg · 200 mg

Carisoprodol

(generic)

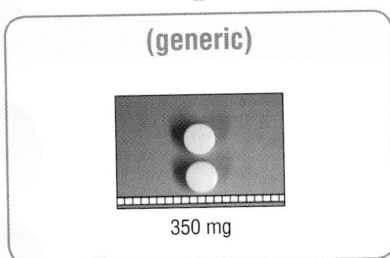

350 mg

Carvedilol

Coreg®

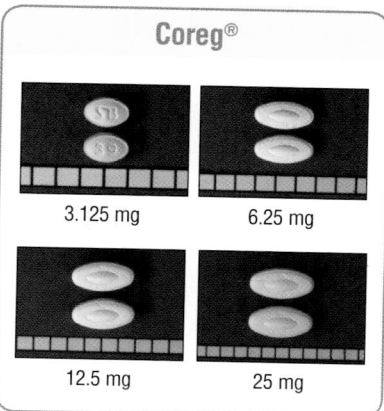

3.125 mg   6.25 mg

12.5 mg   25 mg

Celecoxib

Celebrex™

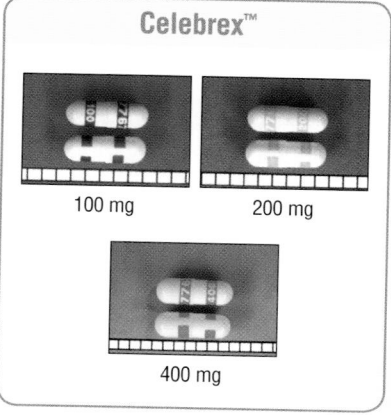

100 mg   200 mg

400 mg

Cephalexin

(generic)

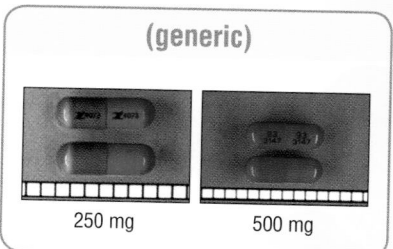

250 mg   500 mg

Cetirizine

Zyrtec®

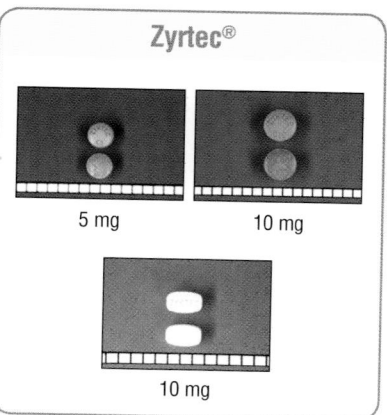

5 mg   10 mg

10 mg

Ciprofloxacin

(generic)

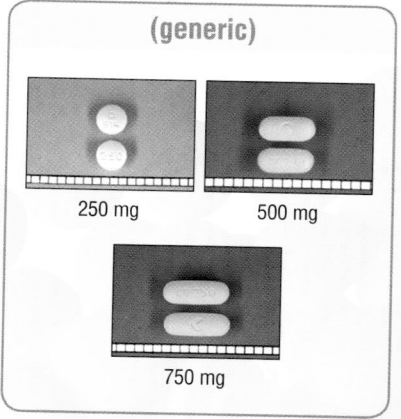

250 mg   500 mg

750 mg

Citalopram

(generic)

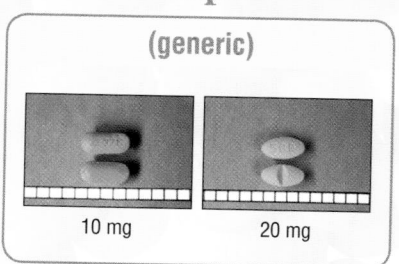

10 mg   20 mg

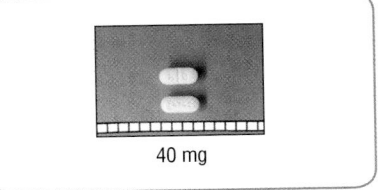

40 mg

Clindamycin

(generic)

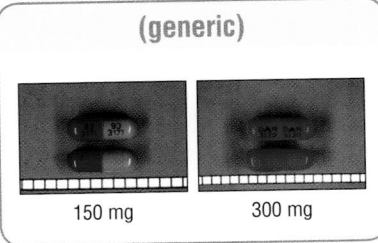

150 mg   300 mg

Clonazepam

(generic)

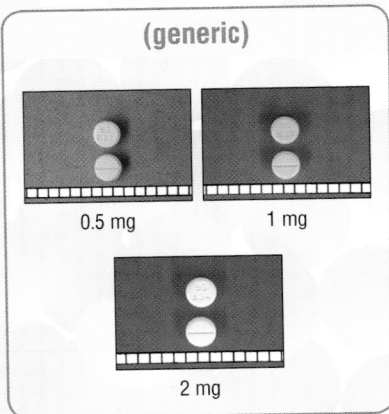

0.5 mg   1 mg

2 mg

Clonidine

(generic)

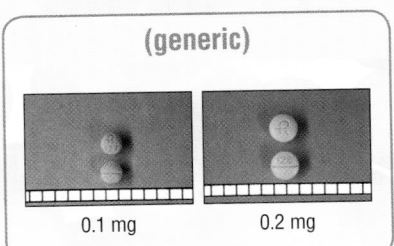

0.1 mg   0.2 mg

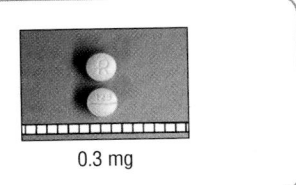

0.3 mg

Clopidogrel

Plavix®

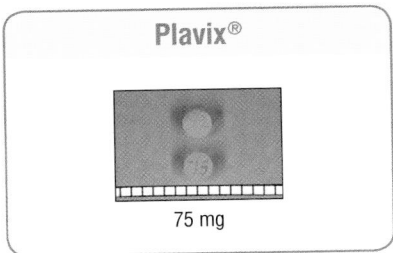

75 mg

Cyclobenzaprine

(generic)

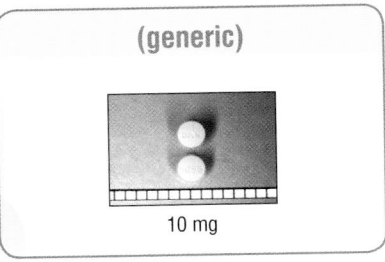

10 mg

Dextroamphetamine and Amphetamine

(generic)

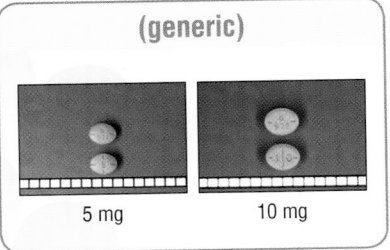

5 mg   10 mg

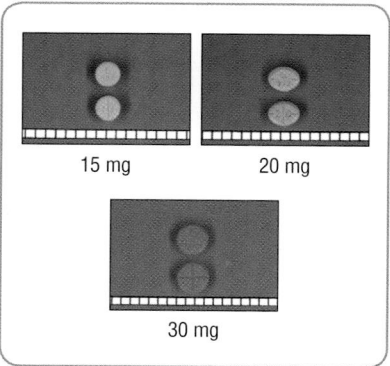

15 mg

20 mg

30 mg

Diazepam

(generic)

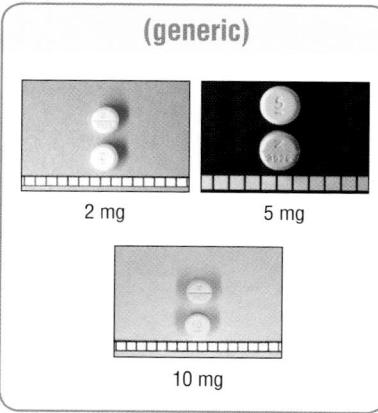

2 mg

5 mg

10 mg

Diclofenac

(generic)

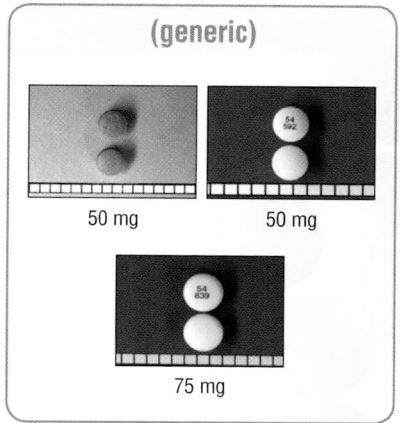

50 mg

50 mg

75 mg

Digoxin

Digitek®

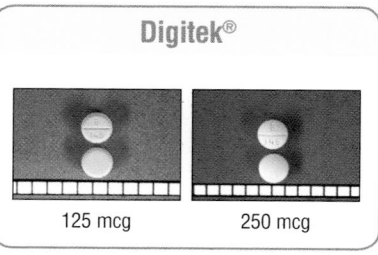

125 mcg

250 mcg

Diltiazem

(generic)

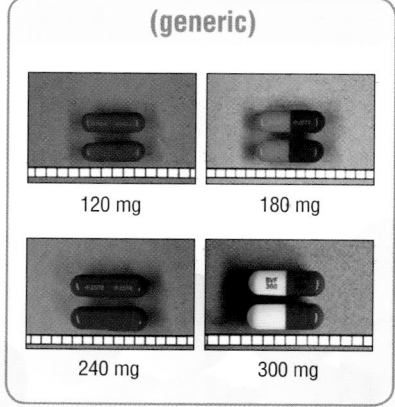

120 mg

180 mg

240 mg

300 mg

Donepezil

Aricept®

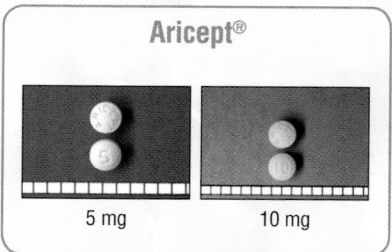

5 mg

10 mg

Doxazosin

(generic)

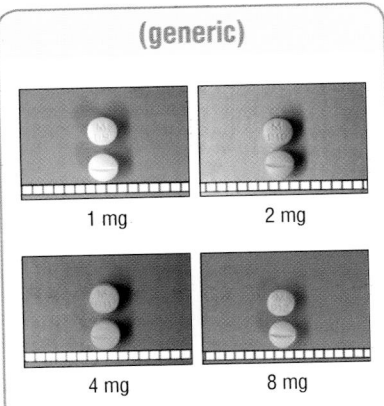

1 mg   2 mg

4 mg   8 mg

Doxycycline

(generic)

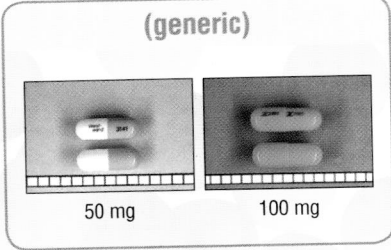

50 mg   100 mg

Duloxetine

Cymbalta®

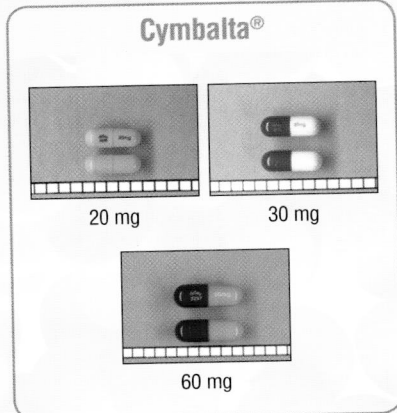

20 mg   30 mg

60 mg

Enalapril

(generic)

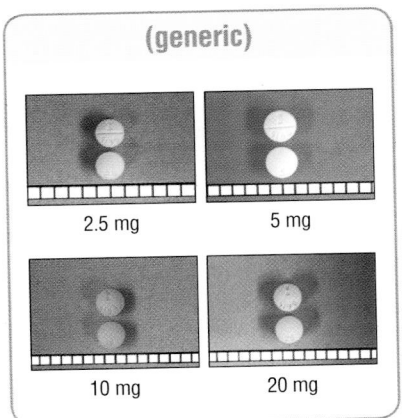

2.5 mg   5 mg

10 mg   20 mg

Escitalopram

Lexapro®

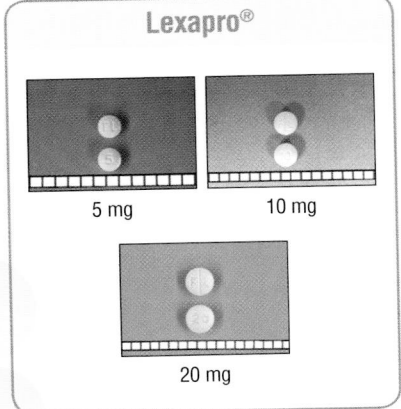

5 mg   10 mg

20 mg

Esomeprazole

Nexium®

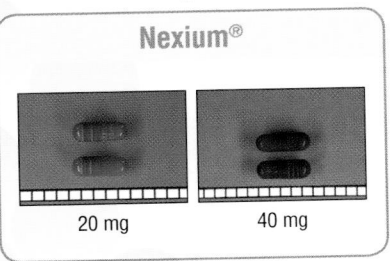

20 mg   40 mg

Estradiol

(generic)

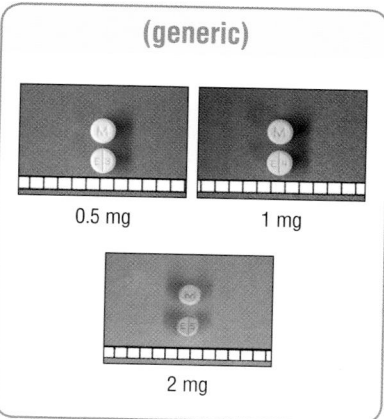

0.5 mg

1 mg

2 mg

Estrogens (Conjugated/Equine)

Premarin®

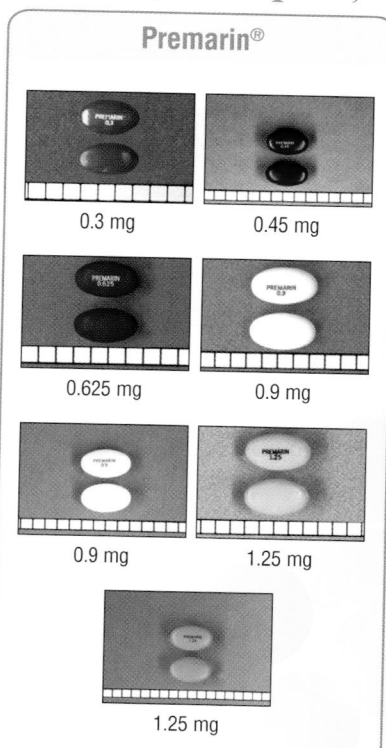

0.3 mg

0.45 mg

0.625 mg

0.9 mg

0.9 mg

1.25 mg

1.25 mg

Eszopiclone

Lunesta™

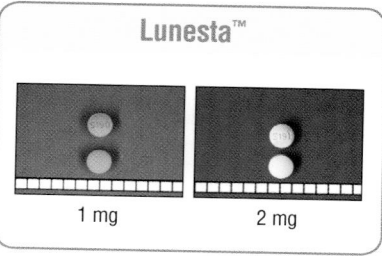

1 mg

2 mg

Ethinyl Estradiol and Drospirenone

Yasmin®

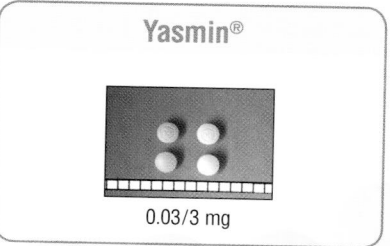

0.03/3 mg

Ezetimibe

Zetia™

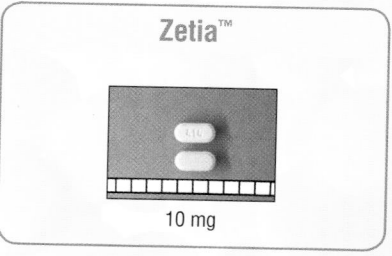

10 mg

Felodipine

(generic)

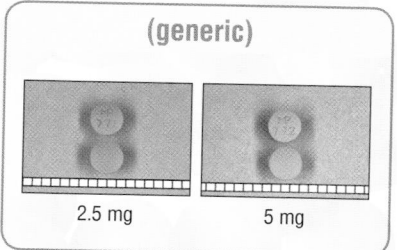

2.5 mg

5 mg

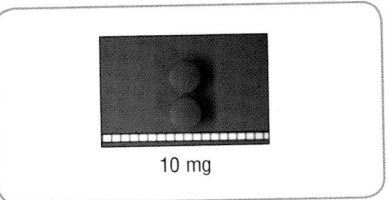

10 mg

Fenofibrate

TriCor®

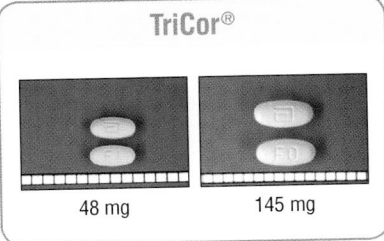

48 mg   145 mg

Ferrous Sulfate

(generic)

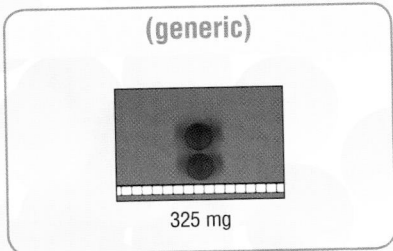

325 mg

Fluconazole

(generic)

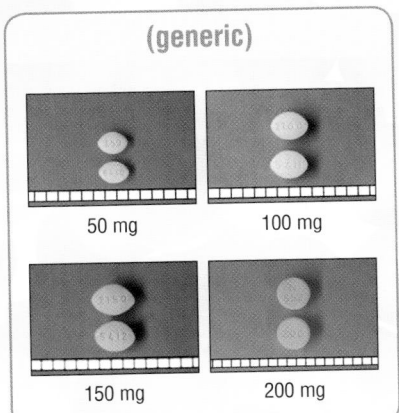

50 mg   100 mg

150 mg   200 mg

Fluoxetine

(generic)

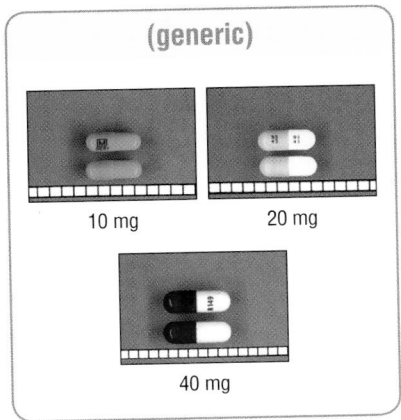

10 mg   20 mg

40 mg

Folic Acid

(generic)

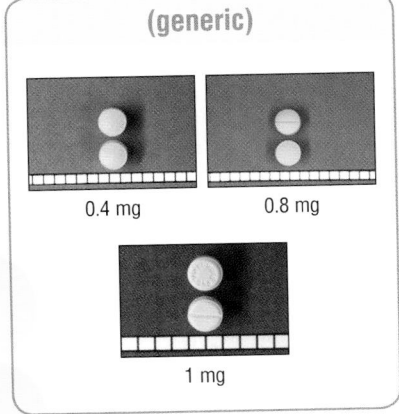

0.4 mg   0.8 mg

1 mg

Furosemide

(generic)

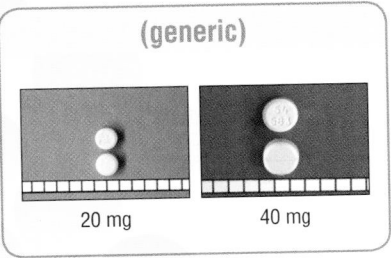

20 mg   40 mg

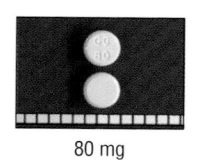

80 mg

Gabapentin

(generic)

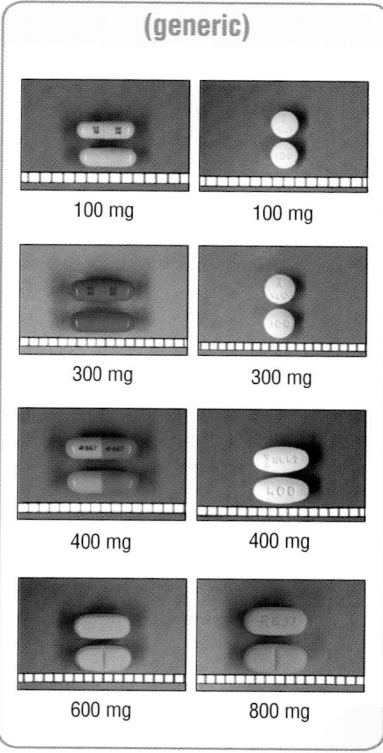

100 mg

100 mg

300 mg

300 mg

400 mg

400 mg

600 mg

800 mg

Gemfibrozil

(generic)

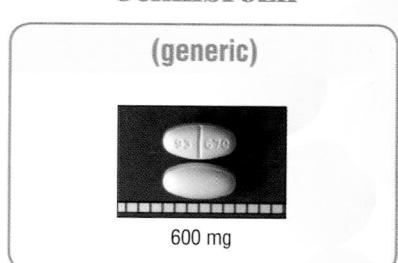

600 mg

Glimepiride

(generic)

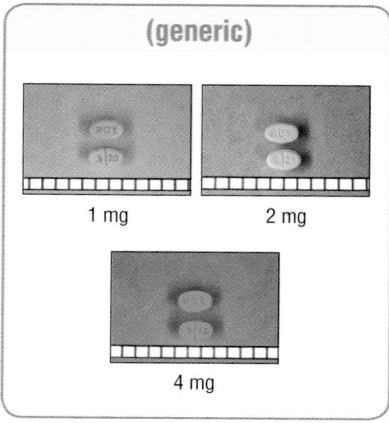

1 mg

2 mg

4 mg

Glipizide

(generic)

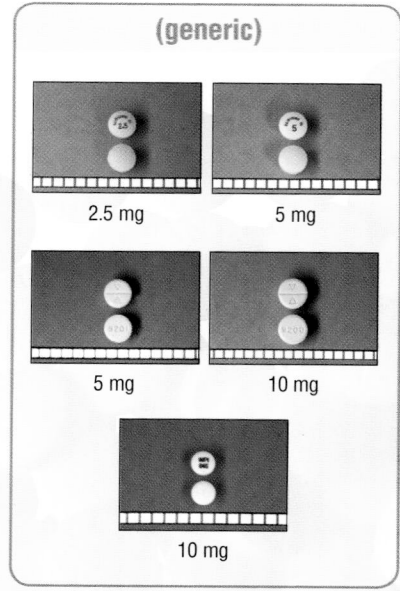

2.5 mg

5 mg

5 mg

10 mg

10 mg

Glyburide

(generic)

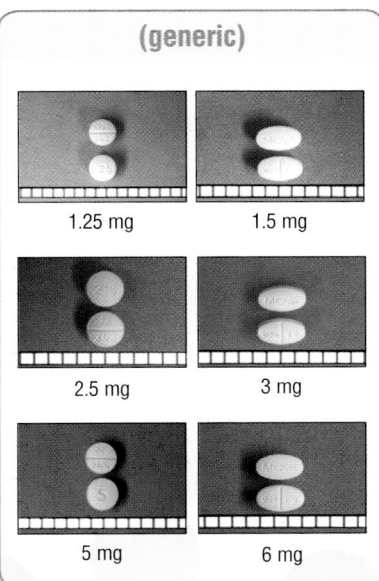

1.25 mg

1.5 mg

2.5 mg

3 mg

5 mg

6 mg

Glyburide Metformin

(generic)

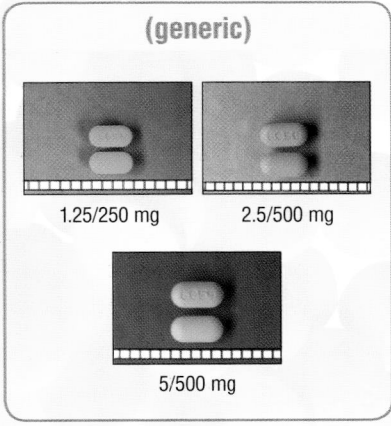

1.25/250 mg

2.5/500 mg

5/500 mg

Hydrochlorothiazide

(generic)

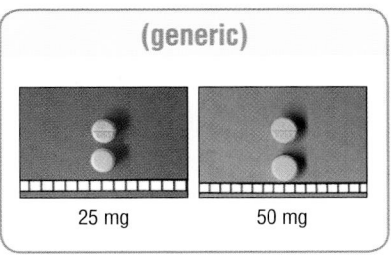

25 mg

50 mg

Hydrochlorothiazide and Triamterene

(generic)

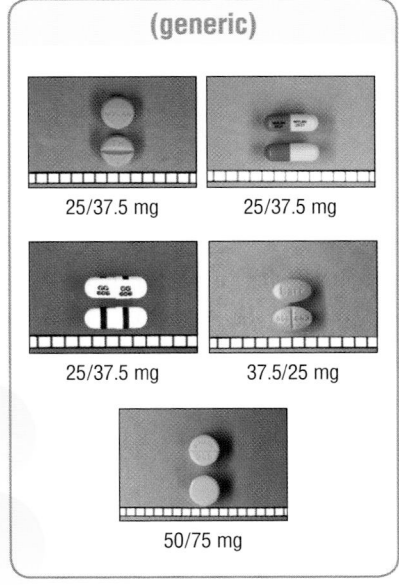

25/37.5 mg

25/37.5 mg

25/37.5 mg

37.5/25 mg

50/75 mg

Hydrocodone and Acetaminophen

(generic)

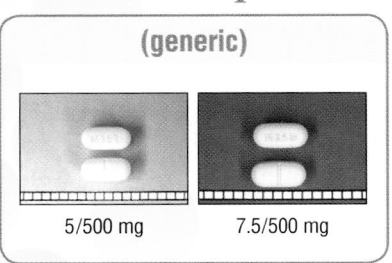

5/500 mg

7.5/500 mg

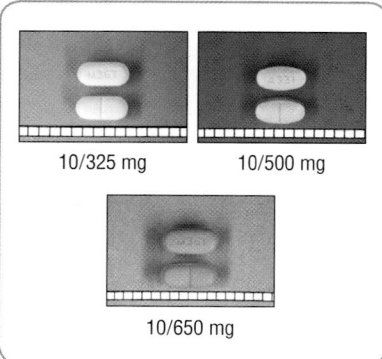

10/325 mg   10/500 mg

10/650 mg

Hydroxyzine

(generic)

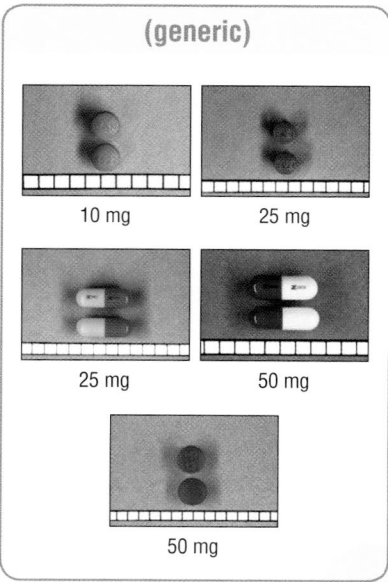

10 mg   25 mg

25 mg   50 mg

50 mg

Ibandronate

Boniva®

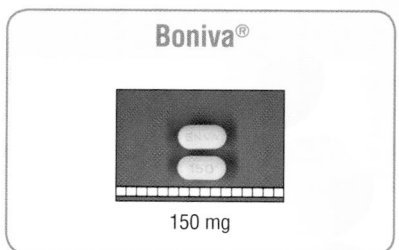

150 mg

Ibuprofen

(generic)

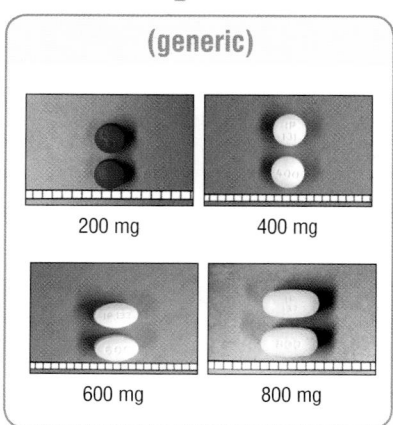

200 mg   400 mg

600 mg   800 mg

Irbesartan

Avapro®

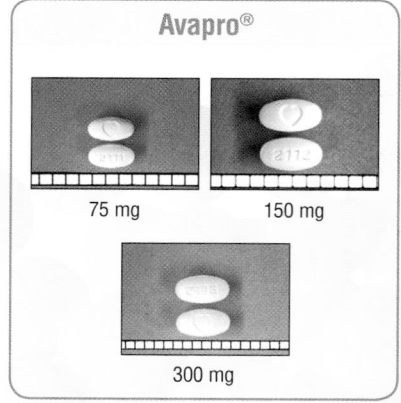

75 mg   150 mg

300 mg

Irbesartan and Hydrochlorothiazide

Avalide®

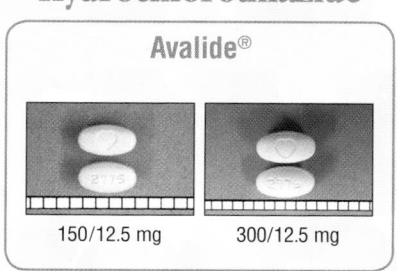

150/12.5 mg   300/12.5 mg

Isosorbide Mononitrate

(generic)

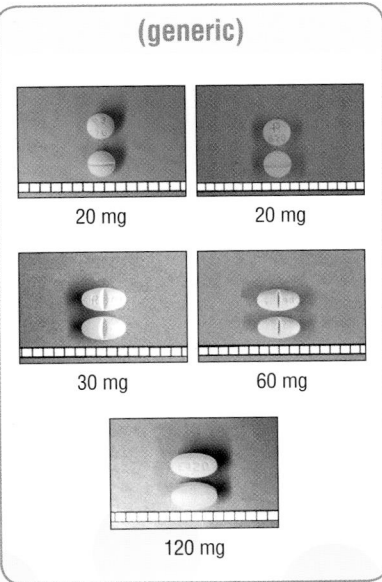

20 mg 20 mg

30 mg 60 mg

120 mg

Lamotrigine

Lamictal®

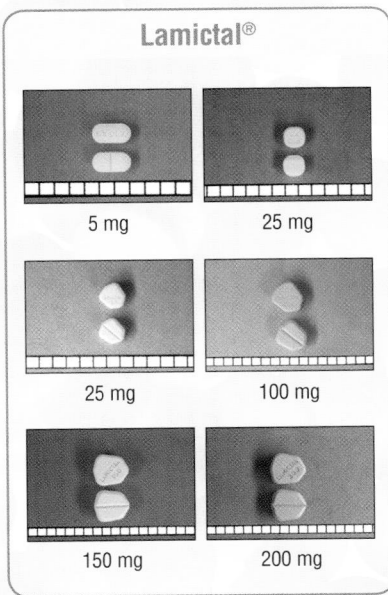

5 mg 25 mg

25 mg 100 mg

150 mg 200 mg

Lansoprazole

Prevacid®

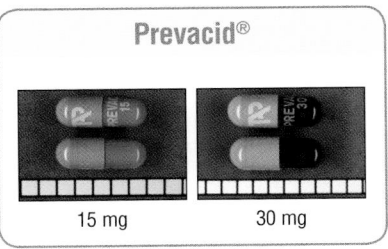

15 mg 30 mg

Levofloxacin

Levaquin®

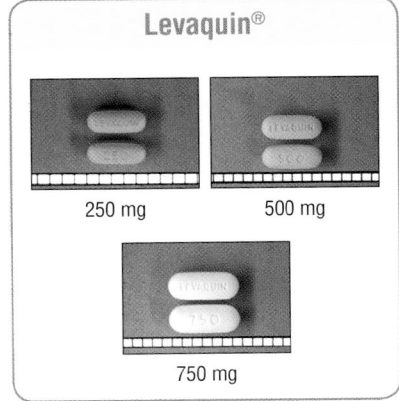

250 mg 500 mg

750 mg

Levothyroxine

(generic)

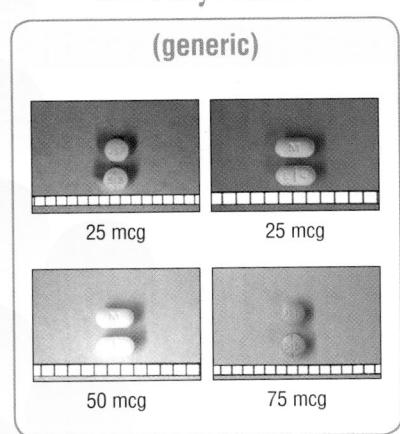

25 mcg 25 mcg

50 mcg 75 mcg

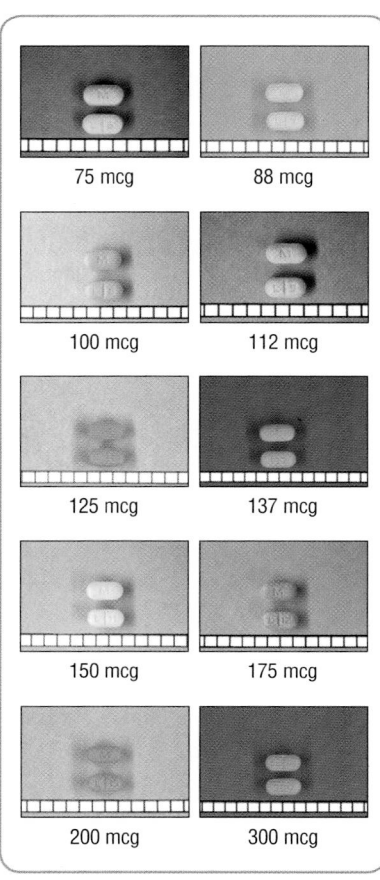

75 mcg

88 mcg

100 mcg

112 mcg

125 mcg

137 mcg

150 mcg

175 mcg

200 mcg

300 mcg

Levoxyl®

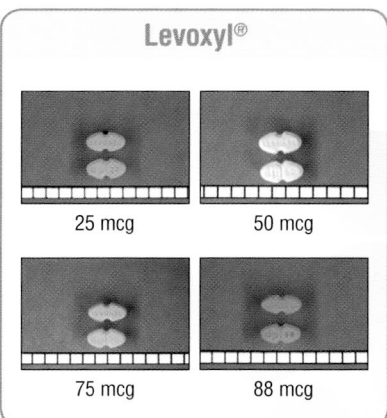

25 mcg

50 mcg

75 mcg

88 mcg

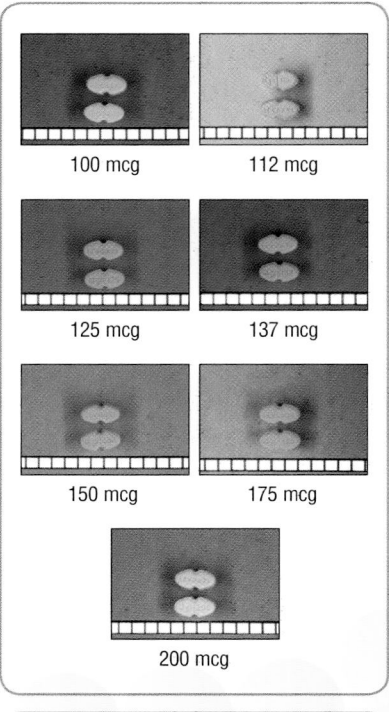

100 mcg

112 mcg

125 mcg

137 mcg

150 mcg

175 mcg

200 mcg

Synthroid®

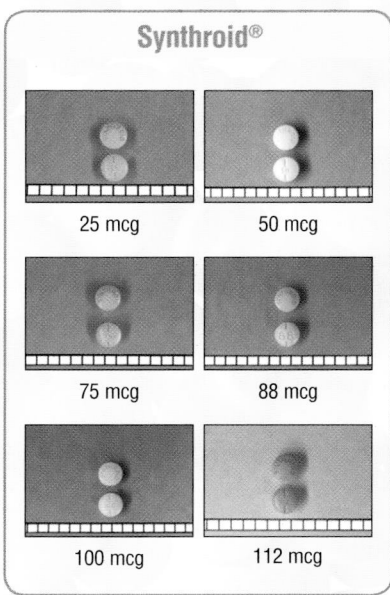

25 mcg

50 mcg

75 mcg

88 mcg

100 mcg

112 mcg

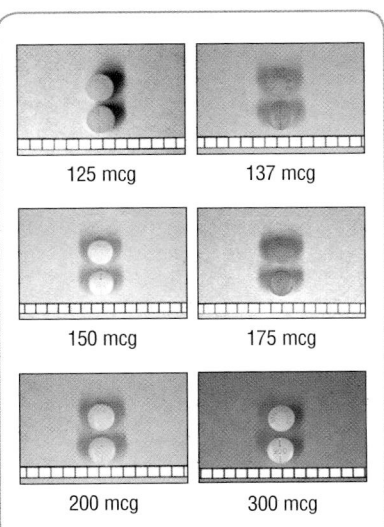

125 mcg   137 mcg

150 mcg   175 mcg

200 mcg   300 mcg

Lisinopril

(generic)

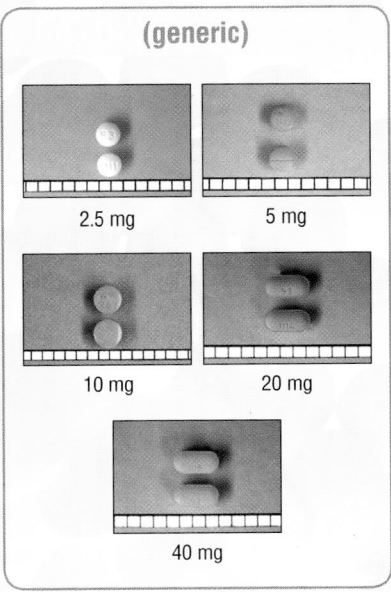

2.5 mg   5 mg

10 mg   20 mg

40 mg

Lisinopril and Hydrochlorothiazide

(generic)

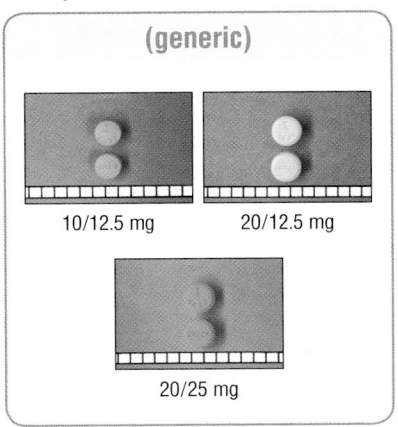

10/12.5 mg   20/12.5 mg

20/25 mg

Lorazepam

(generic)

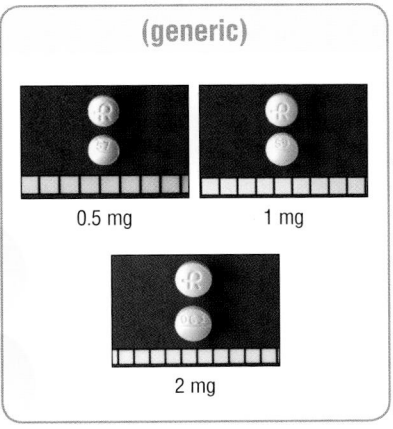

0.5 mg   1 mg

2 mg

Losartan

Cozaar®

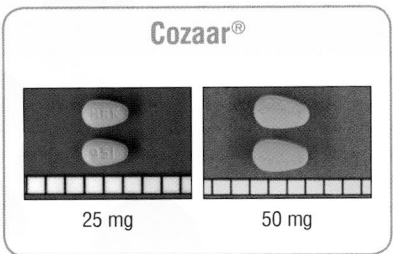

25 mg   50 mg

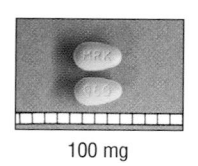
100 mg

Losartan and Hydrochlorothiazide

Hyzaar®

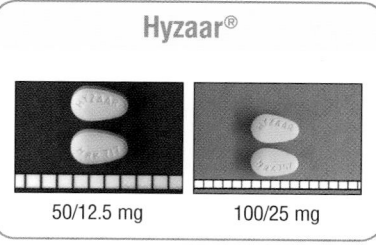

50/12.5 mg   100/25 mg

Lovastatin

(generic)

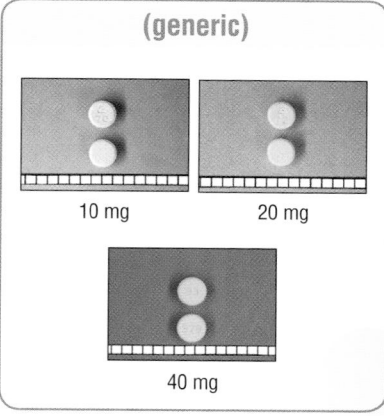

10 mg   20 mg

40 mg

Meclizine

(generic)

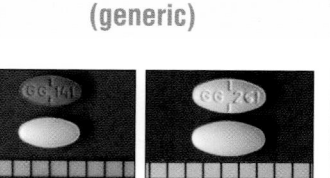

12.5 mg   25 mg

Meloxicam

(generic)

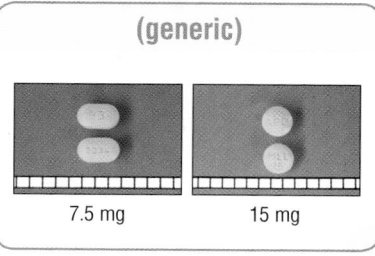

7.5 mg   15 mg

Metaxalone

Skelaxin®

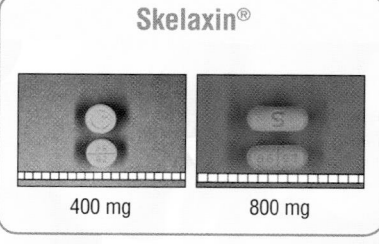

400 mg   800 mg

Metformin

(generic)

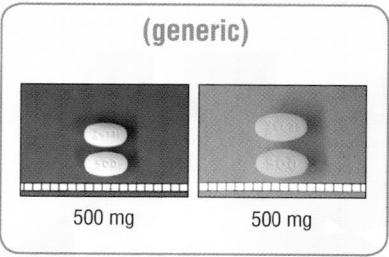

500 mg   500 mg

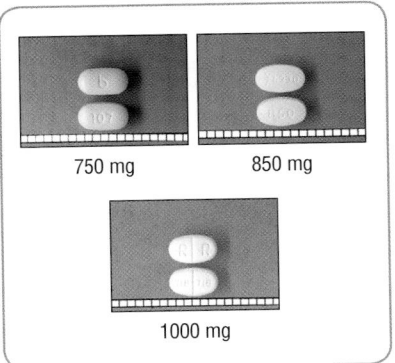

750 mg

850 mg

1000 mg

Methotrexate

(generic)

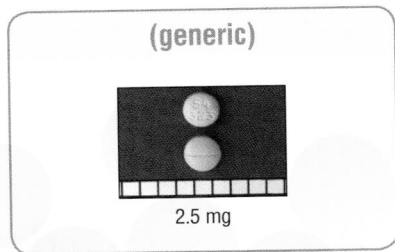

2.5 mg

Methylphenidate

Concerta®

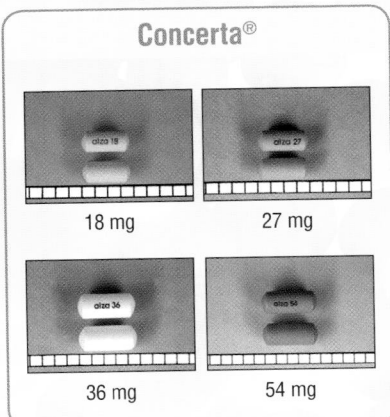

18 mg

27 mg

36 mg

54 mg

Methylprednisolone

(generic)

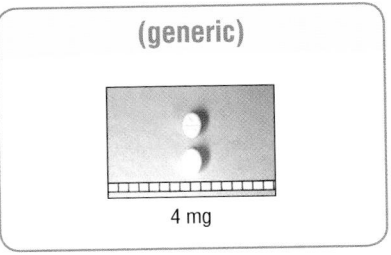

4 mg

Metoclopramide

(generic)

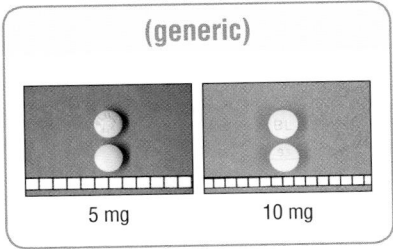

5 mg

10 mg

Metoprolol

(generic)

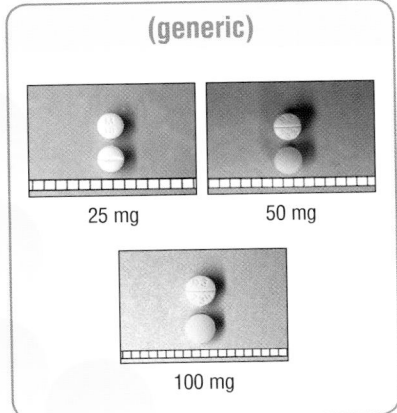

25 mg

50 mg

100 mg

Toprol-XL®

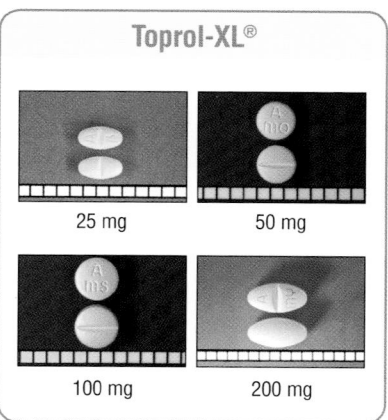

25 mg   50 mg

100 mg   200 mg

Metronidazole

(generic)

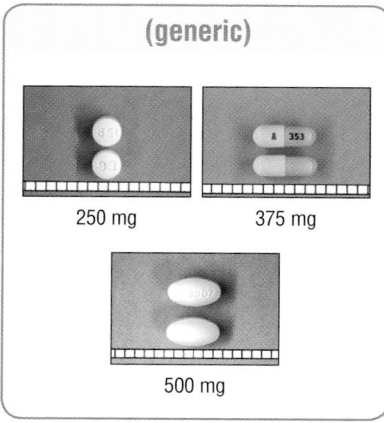

250 mg   375 mg

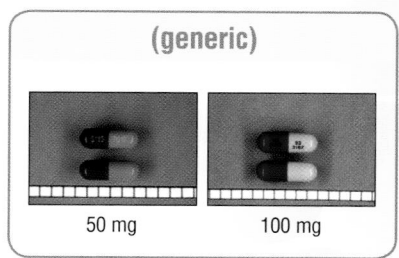

500 mg

Minocycline

(generic)

50 mg   100 mg

Mirtazapine

(generic)

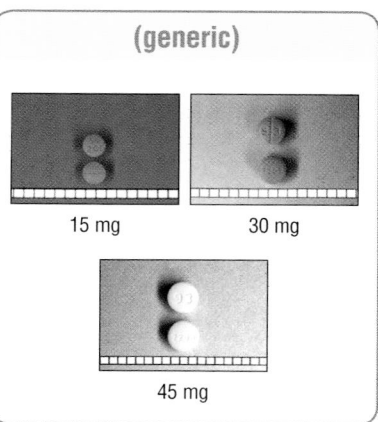

15 mg   30 mg

45 mg

Montelukast

Singulair®

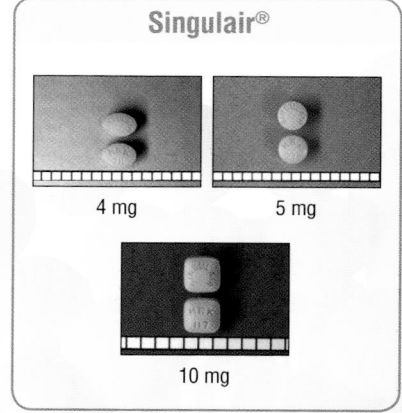

4 mg   5 mg

10 mg

Moxifloxacin

Avelox® ABC Pack

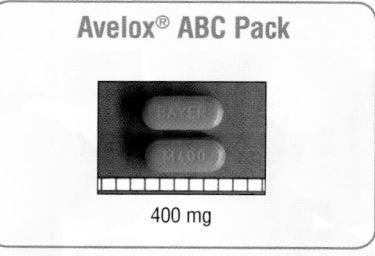

400 mg

Avelox®

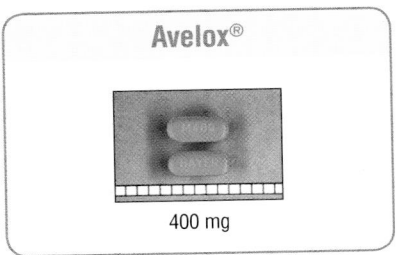

400 mg

Nabumetone

(generic)

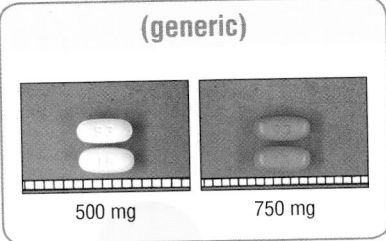

| 500 mg | 750 mg |

Naproxen

(generic)

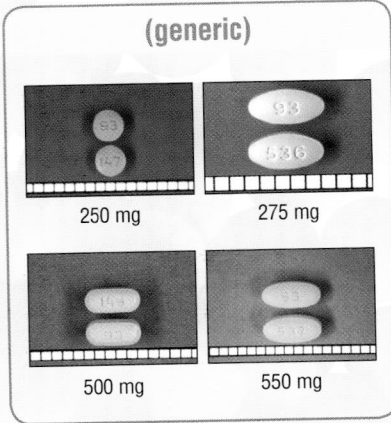

| 250 mg | 275 mg |
| 500 mg | 550 mg |

Niacin

Niaspan®

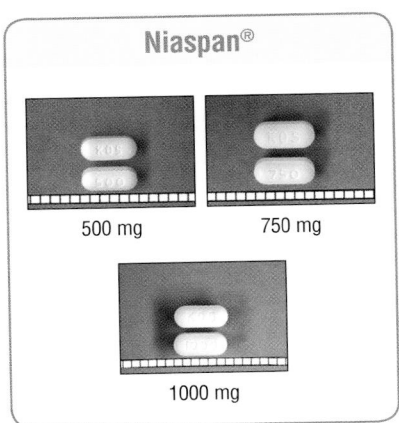

| 500 mg | 750 mg |
| 1000 mg | |

Nifedipine

(generic)

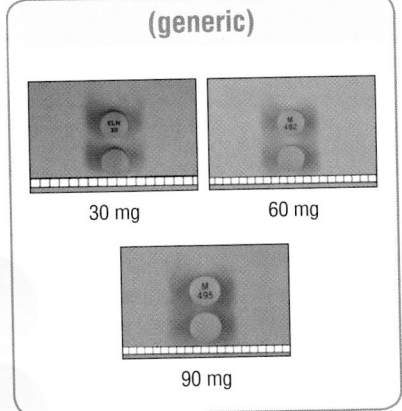

| 30 mg | 60 mg |
| 90 mg | |

Olanzapine

Zyprexa®

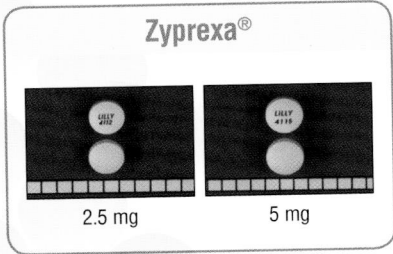

| 2.5 mg | 5 mg |

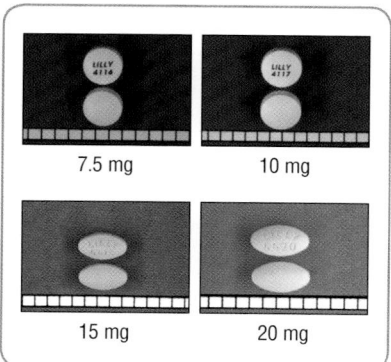

7.5 mg	10 mg
15 mg	20 mg

Olmesartan

Benicar®

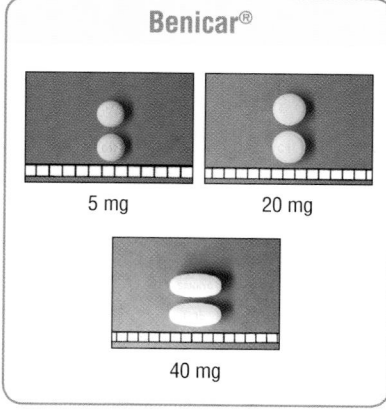

5 mg	20 mg
40 mg	

Olmesartan and Hydrochlorothiazide

Benicar HCT®

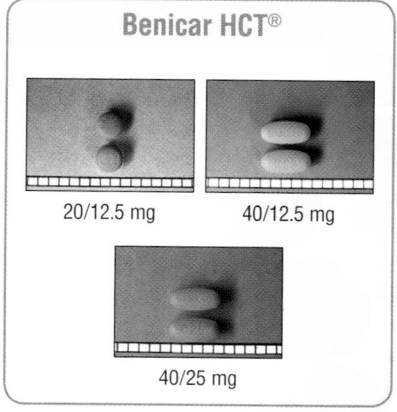

20/12.5 mg	40/12.5 mg
40/25 mg	

Omeprazole

(generic)

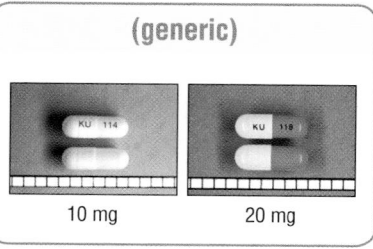

10 mg	20 mg

Oxycodone

(generic)

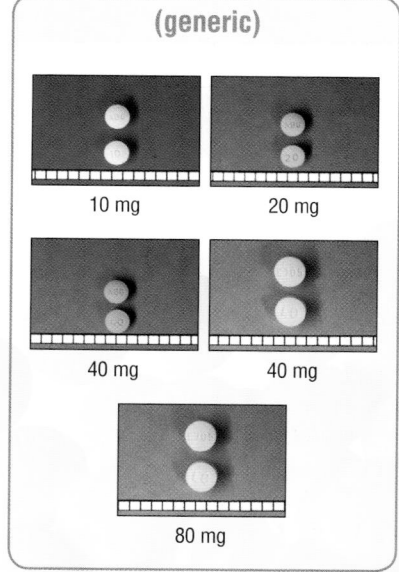

10 mg	20 mg
40 mg	40 mg
80 mg	

Oxycodone and Acetaminophen

(generic)

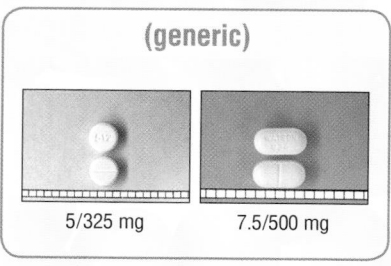

5/325 mg	7.5/500 mg

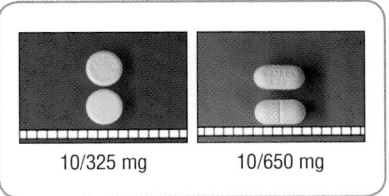

10/325 mg   10/650 mg

Pantoprazole

Protonix®

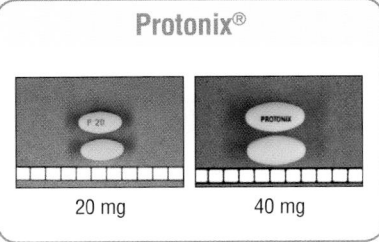

20 mg   40 mg

Paroxetine

(generic)

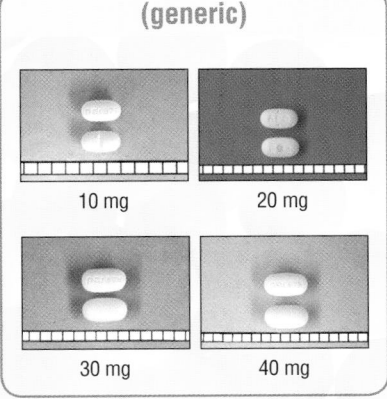

10 mg   20 mg

30 mg   40 mg

Penicillin V Potassium

(generic)

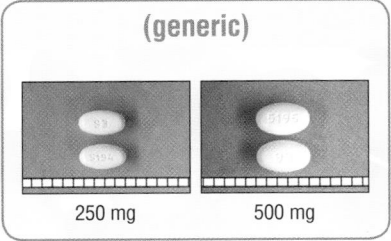

250 mg   500 mg

Phentermin

(generic)

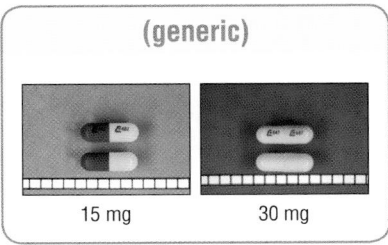

15 mg   30 mg

Pioglitazone

Actos™

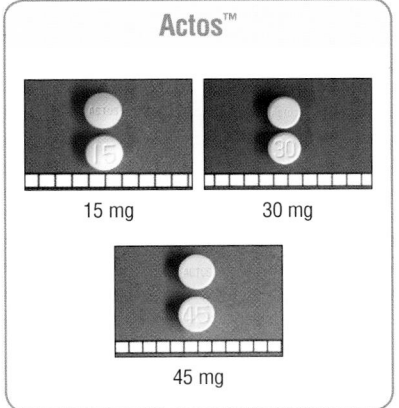

15 mg   30 mg

45 mg

Potassium Chloride

(generic)

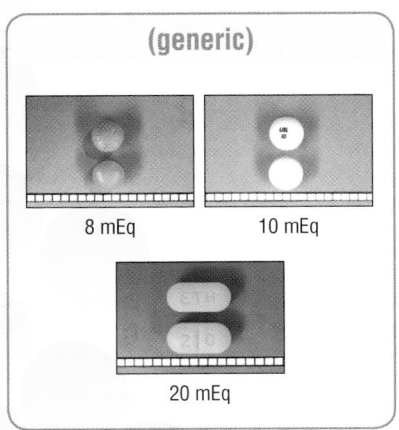

8 mEq   10 mEq

20 mEq

Klor-Con® 8

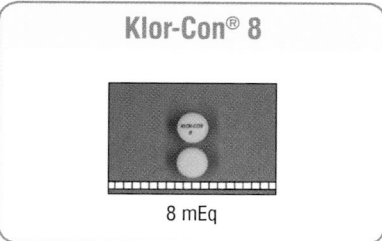

8 mEq

Klor-Con® 10

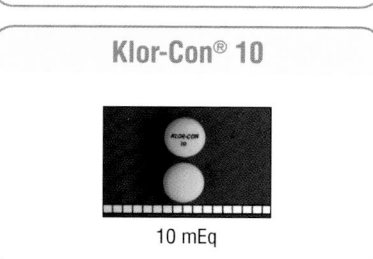

10 mEq

Pravastatin

(generic)

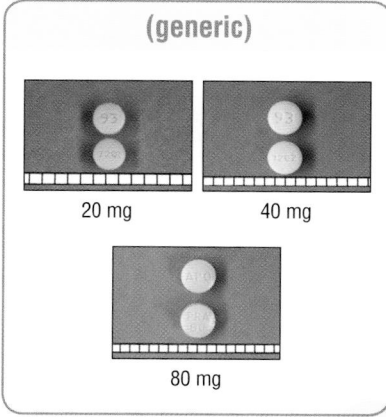

20 mg   40 mg

80 mg

Prednisone

(generic)

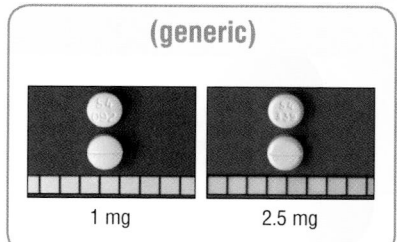

1 mg   2.5 mg

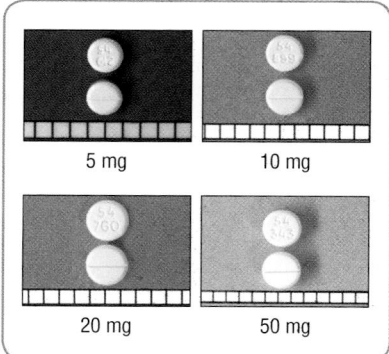

5 mg   10 mg

20 mg   50 mg

Pregabalin

Lyrica®

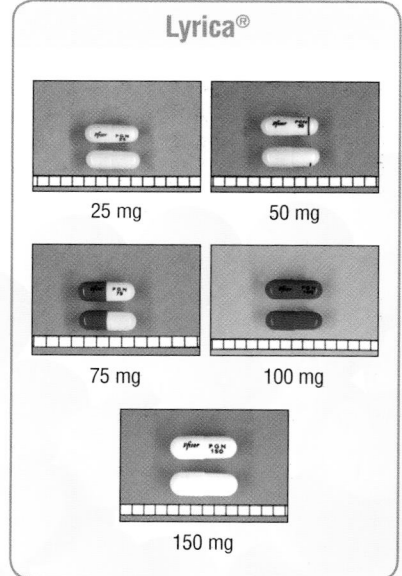

25 mg   50 mg

75 mg   100 mg

150 mg

Promethazine

(generic)

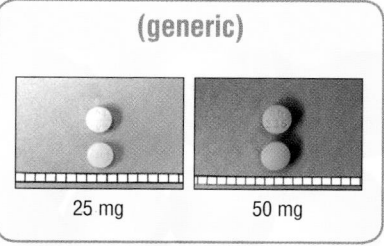

25 mg   50 mg

Propoxyphene and Acetaminophen

(generic)

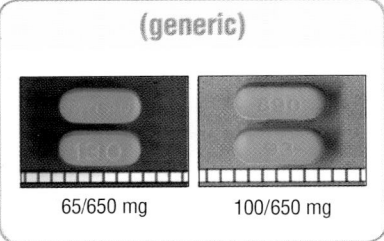

| 65/650 mg | 100/650 mg |

Propranolol

(generic)

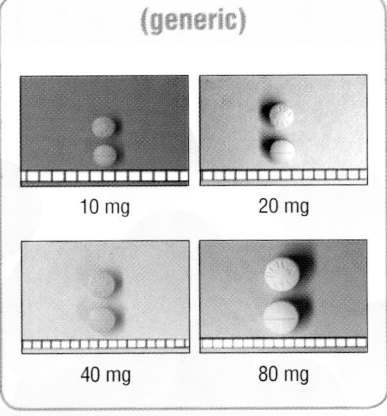

| 10 mg | 20 mg |
| 40 mg | 80 mg |

Quetiapine

Seroquel®

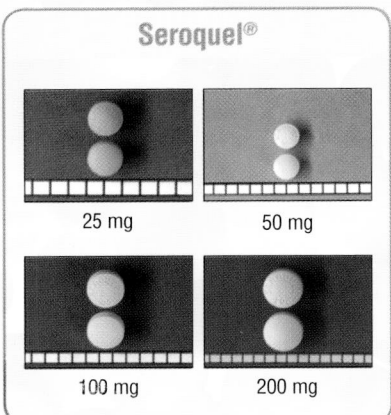

| 25 mg | 50 mg |
| 100 mg | 200 mg |

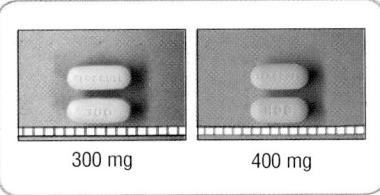

| 300 mg | 400 mg |

Quinapril

(generic)

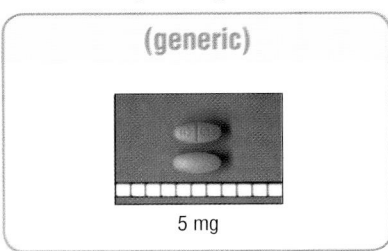

5 mg

Raloxifene

Evista®

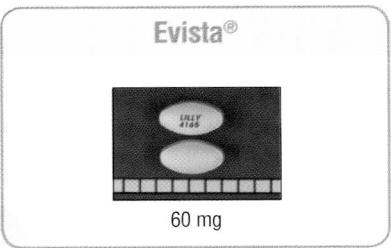

60 mg

Ramipril

Altace™

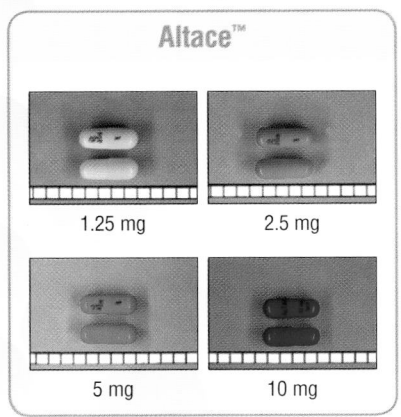

| 1.25 mg | 2.5 mg |
| 5 mg | 10 mg |

Ranitidine

(generic)

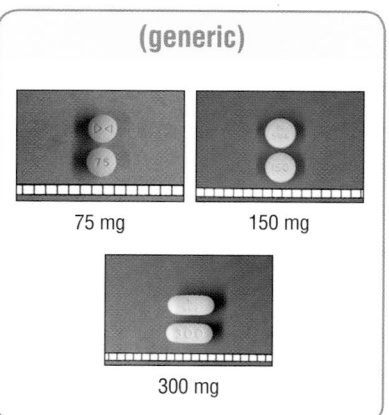

75 mg   150 mg

300 mg

Risedronate

Actonel®

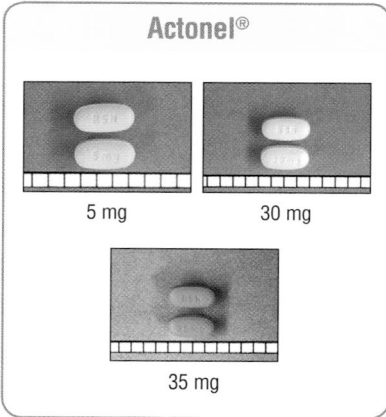

5 mg   30 mg

35 mg

Risperidone

Risperdal®

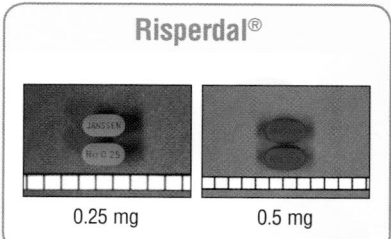

0.25 mg   0.5 mg

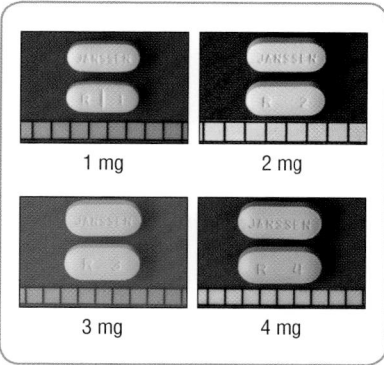

1 mg   2 mg

3 mg   4 mg

Ropinirole

Requip®

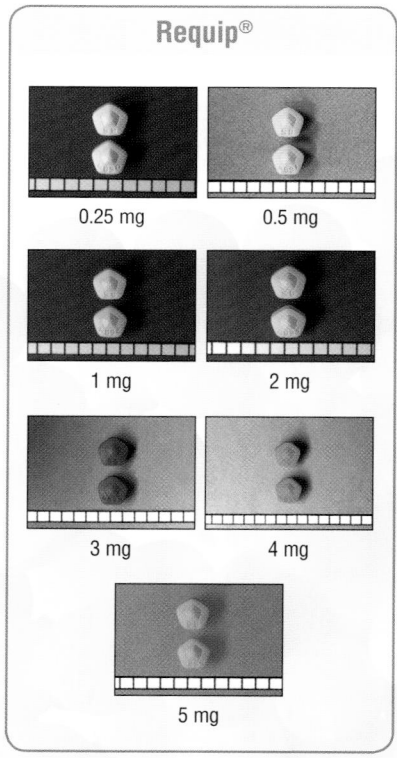

0.25 mg   0.5 mg

1 mg   2 mg

3 mg   4 mg

5 mg

Rosiglitazone

Avandia®

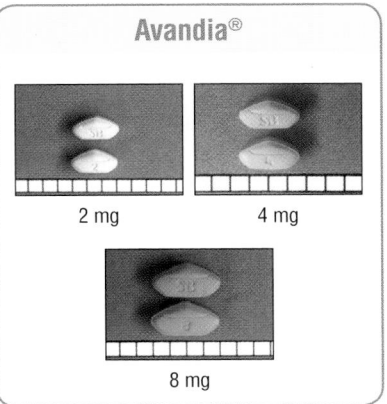

2 mg   4 mg

8 mg

Sertraline

(generic)

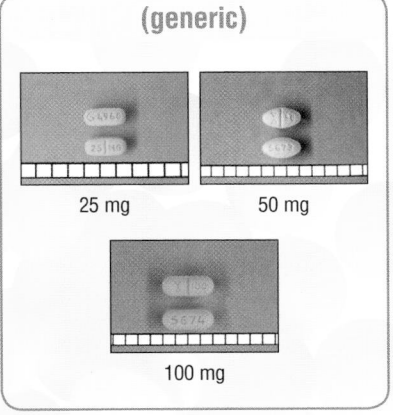

25 mg   50 mg

100 mg

Sildenafil

Viagra™

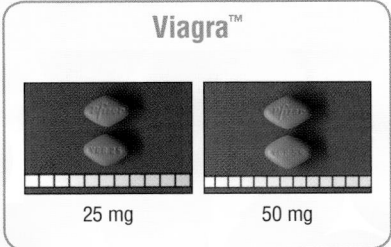

25 mg   50 mg

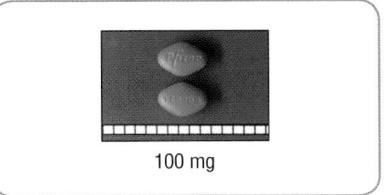

100 mg

Spironolactone

(generic)

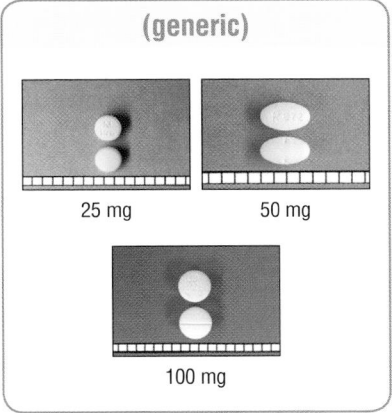

25 mg   50 mg

100 mg

Sulfamethoxazole and Trimethoprim

(generic)

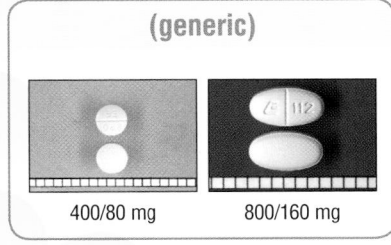

400/80 mg   800/160 mg

Tadalafil

Cialis®

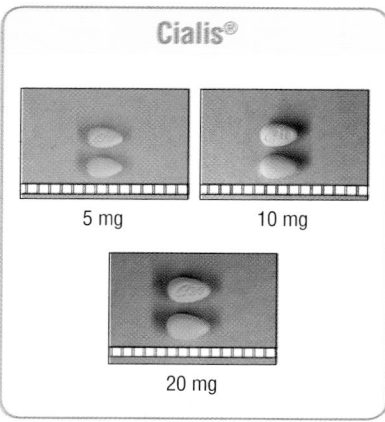

5 mg
10 mg
20 mg

Tamsulosin

Flomax®

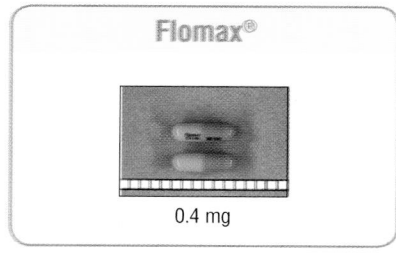

0.4 mg

Temazepam

(generic)

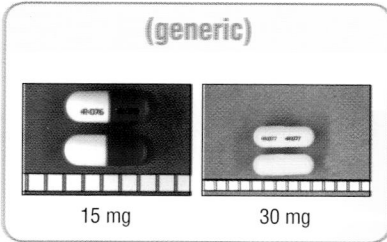

15 mg
30 mg

Terazosin

(generic)

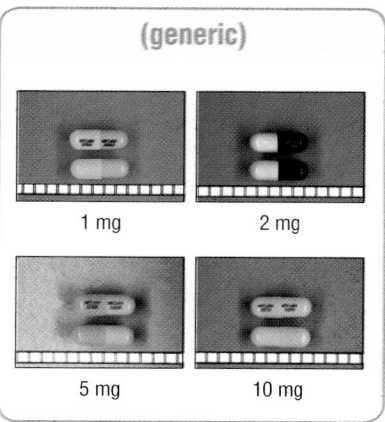

1 mg
2 mg
5 mg
10 mg

Tizanidine

(generic)

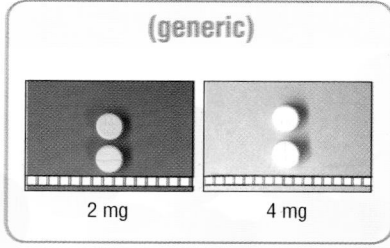

2 mg
4 mg

Tolterodine

Detrol® LA

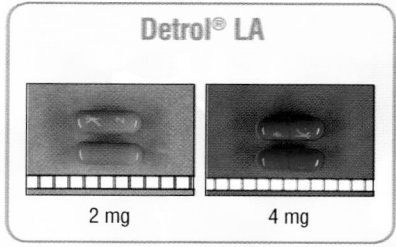

2 mg
4 mg

Topiramate

Topamax®

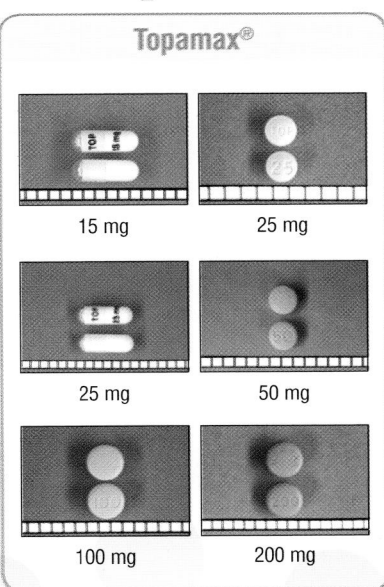

15 mg   25 mg

25 mg   50 mg

100 mg   200 mg

Tramadol

(generic)

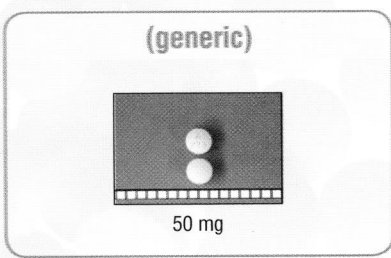

50 mg

Trazodone

(generic)

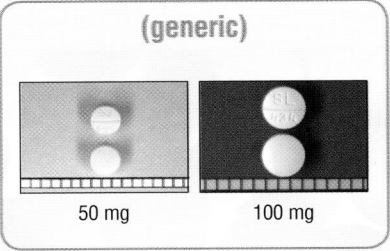

50 mg   100 mg

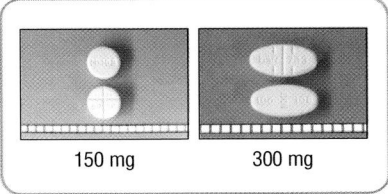

150 mg   300 mg

Valacyclovir

Valtrex®

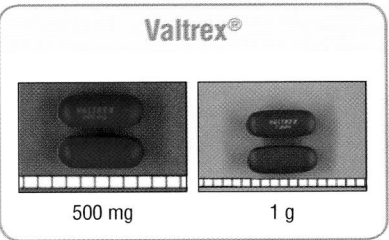

500 mg   1 g

Valproic Acid and Derivatives

Depakote® ER

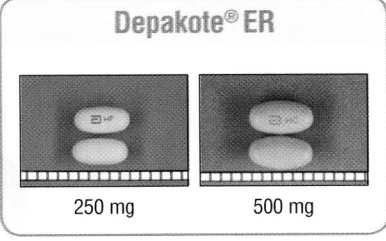

250 mg   500 mg

Valsartan

Diovan®

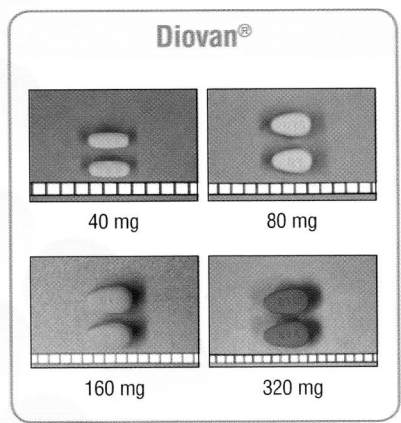

40 mg   80 mg

160 mg   320 mg

Valsartan and Hydrochlorothiazide

Diovan HCT®

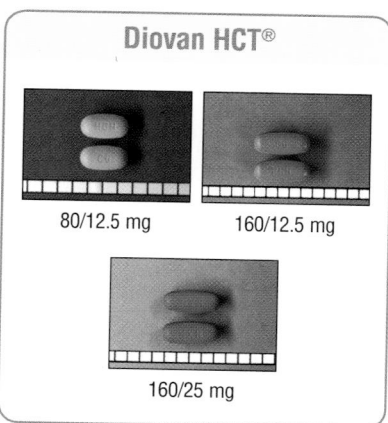

80/12.5 mg 160/12.5 mg

160/25 mg

Varenicline

Chantix®

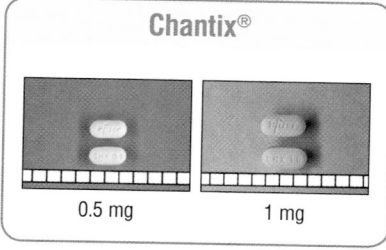

0.5 mg 1 mg

Venlafaxine

Effexor XR®

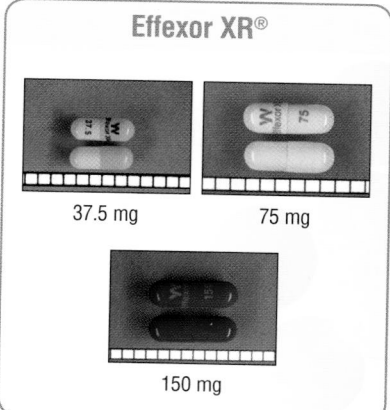

37.5 mg 75 mg

150 mg

Verapamil

(generic)

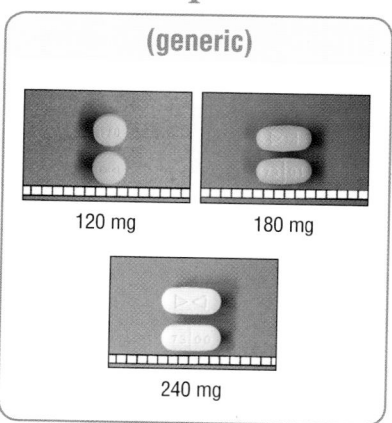

120 mg 180 mg

240 mg

Warfarin

(generic)

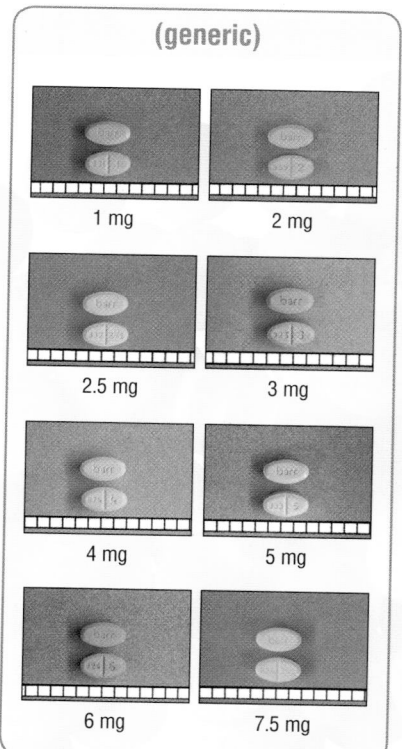

1 mg 2 mg

2.5 mg 3 mg

4 mg 5 mg

6 mg 7.5 mg

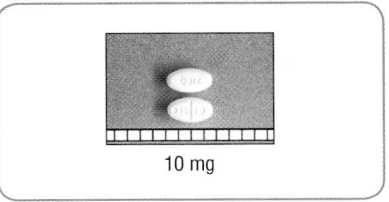

10 mg

Coumadin®

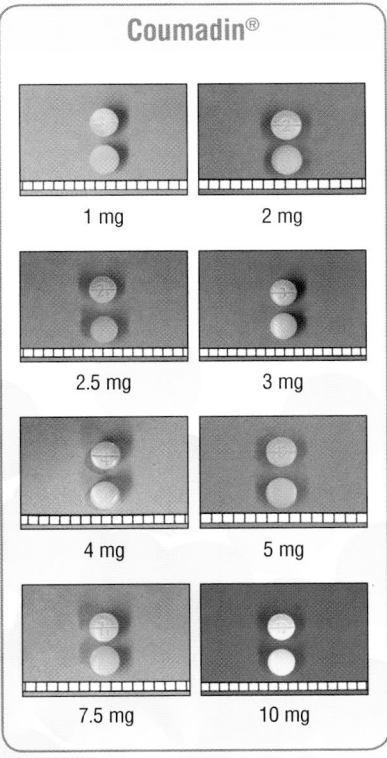

1 mg

2 mg

2.5 mg

3 mg

4 mg

5 mg

7.5 mg

10 mg

Zolpidem

(generic)

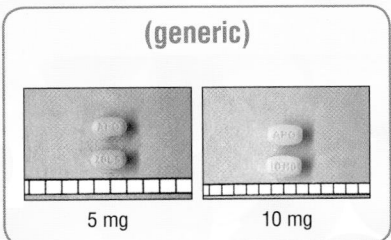

5 mg

10 mg

Ambien®

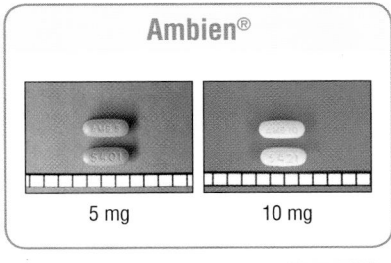

5 mg

10 mg

Ambien CR

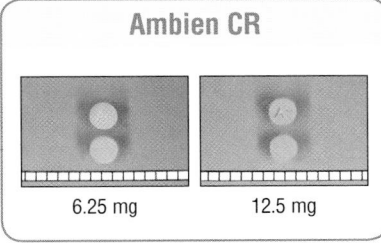

6.25 mg

12.5 mg